Expand research on specific topics of interest

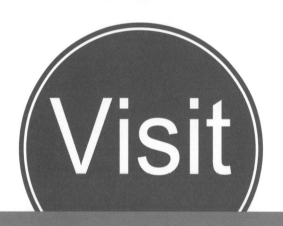

www.PathologyofDomesticAnimals.com

Further your understanding of pathology of domestic animals by accessing this book's companion website:

- Enhanced electronic image collection offers nearly 3,000 images from the print book, plus more than 325 bonus web-only images!

- A comprehensive references list, organized by volume and chapter, includes more than 11,500 references linked to original abstracts in PubMed.

ELSEVIER

Sixth Edition

Jubb, Kennedy, and Palmer's

Pathology of DOMESTIC ANIMALS

Volume 1

Sixth Edition

Jubb, Kennedy, and Palmer's
Pathology of DOMESTIC ANIMALS

Volume 1

EDITED BY:

M. GRANT MAXIE, DVM, PHD, DIPLOMATE ACVP
Co-Executive Director, Laboratory Service Division
Director, Animal Health Laboratory
University of Guelph
Guelph, Ontario
Canada

ELSEVIER

ELSEVIER

3251 Riverport Lane
St. Louis, Missouri 63043

JUBB, KENNEDY, AND PALMER'S PATHOLOGY OF DOMESTIC ANIMALS, SIXTH EDITION

ISBN: 978-0-7020-5322-1 (3 VOLUME SET)
978-0-7020-5317-7 (VOLUME 1)
978-0-7020-5318-4 (VOLUME 2)
978-0-7020-5319-1 (VOLUME 3)

Copyright © 2016 by Elsevier, Inc. All rights reserved.

No part of this publication may be reproduced or transmitted in any form or by any means, electronic or mechanical, including photocopying, recording, or any information storage and retrieval system, without permission in writing from the publisher. Details on how to seek permission, further information about the Publisher's permissions policies and our arrangements with organizations such as the Copyright Clearance Center and the Copyright Licensing Agency, can be found at our website: www.elsevier.com/permissions.

This book and the individual contributions contained in it are protected under copyright by the Publisher (other than as may be noted herein).

Notices

Knowledge and best practice in this field are constantly changing. As new research and experience broaden our understanding, changes in research methods, professional practices, or medical treatment may become necessary.

Practitioners and researchers must always rely on their own experience and knowledge in evaluating and using any information, methods, compounds, or experiments described herein. In using such information or methods they should be mindful of their own safety and the safety of others, including parties for whom they have a professional responsibility.

With respect to any drug or pharmaceutical products identified, readers are advised to check the most current information provided (i) on procedures featured or (ii) by the manufacturer of each product to be administered, to verify the recommended dose or formula, the method and duration of administration, and contraindications. It is the responsibility of practitioners, relying on their own experience and knowledge of their patients, to make diagnoses, to determine dosages and the best treatment for each individual patient, and to take all appropriate safety precautions.

To the fullest extent of the law, neither the Publisher nor the authors, contributors, or editors, assume any liability for any injury and/or damage to persons or property as a matter of products liability, negligence or otherwise, or from any use or operation of any methods, products, instructions, or ideas contained in the material herein.

Previous editions copyrighted 2007, 1993, 1985, 1970, 1963

Library of Congress Cataloging-in-Publication Data

Jubb, Kennedy, and Palmer's pathology of domestic animals / edited by M. Grant Maxie.—Sixth edition.
   p. ; cm.
   title: Pathology of domestic animals
   Includes bibliographical references and index.
   ISBN 978-0-7020-5322-1 (3 vol. set : alk. paper)—ISBN 978-0-7020-5317-7 (v. 1 : alk. paper)—ISBN 978-0-7020-5318-4 (v. 2 : alk. paper)—ISBN 978-0-7020-5319-1 (v. 3 : alk. paper)
   I. Maxie, M. Grant, editor. II. Title: Pathology of domestic animals.
   [DNLM: 1. Pathology, Veterinary. 2. Animals, Domestic. SF 769]
   SF769.P345 2016
   636.089'607—dc23

2015009121

Vice President and Publisher: Loren Wilson
Content Strategy Director: Penny Rudolph
Content Development Manager: Jolynn Gower
Content Development Specialist: Brandi Graham
Content Coordinator: Kayla Mugle

Publishing Services Managers: Anne Altepeter and Patricia Tannian
Senior Project Manager: Sharon Corell
Project Manager: Louise King
Designer: Brian Salisbury

Working together to grow libraries in developing countries

www.elsevier.com • www.bookaid.org

Printed in China

Last digit is the print number: 9 8 7 6 5 4 3 2 1

Contributors

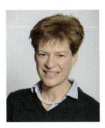

Dorothee Bienzle, DVM, PhD, Diplomate ACVP
Professor
Department of Pathobiology
Ontario Veterinary College
University of Guelph
Pathobiology
University of Guelph
Guelph, Ontario
Canada
Hematopoietic system

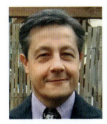

Carlo Cantile, DVM, PhD
Professor of Veterinary Pathology
Department of Veterinary Science
University of Pisa
Pisa, Italy
Nervous system

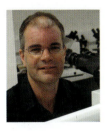

Jeff L. Caswell, DVM, DVSc, PhD, Diplomate ACVP
Professor
Department of Pathobiology
Ontario Veterinary College
University of Guelph
Guelph, Ontario
Canada
Respiratory system

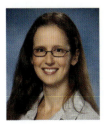

Rachel E. Cianciolo, VMD, PhD, Diplomate ACVP
Assistant Professor
Co-Director, International Veterinary Renal Pathology Service
Department of Veterinary Biosciences
College of Veterinary Medicine
The Ohio State University
Columbus, Ohio
USA
Urinary system

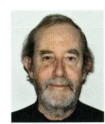

Barry J. Cooper, BVSc, PhD, Diplomate ACVP
Professor Emeritus of Pathology
Department of Biomedical Sciences
Cornell University
Ithaca, New York
USA
Muscle and tendon

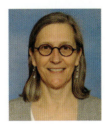

Linden E. Craig, DVM, PhD, Diplomate ACVP
Department of Biomedical and Diagnostic Sciences
University of Tennessee College of Veterinary Medicine
Knoxville, Tennessee
USA
Bones and joints

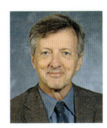

John M. Cullen, VMD, PhD, Diplomate ACVP
Professor
Department of Population Health and Pathobiology
College of Veterinary Medicine
North Carolina State University
Raleigh, North Carolina
USA
Liver and biliary system

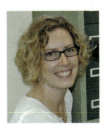

Keren E. Dittmer, BVSc, PhD, Diplomate ACVP
Institute of Veterinary, Animal, and Biomedical Sciences
Massey University
Palmerston North, Manawatu
New Zealand
Bones and joints

CONTRIBUTORS

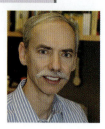

Robert A. Foster, BVSc, PhD, MACVSc, Diplomate ACVP
Professor
Department of Pathobiology
Ontario Veterinary College
University of Guelph
Guelph, Ontario
Canada
Female genital system
Male genital system

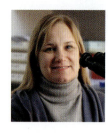

Elizabeth A. Mauldin, DVM, Diplomate ACVP, Diplomate ACVD
Associate Professor
Department of Pathobiology
School of Veterinary Medicine
University of Pennsylvania
Philadelphia, Pennsylvania
USA
Integumentary system

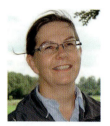

Andrea Gröne, DVM, PhD, Diplomate ACVP, Diplomate ECVP
Professor
Faculty of Veterinary Medicine
Department of Pathobiology
Utrecht University
Utrecht, The Netherlands
Endocrine glands

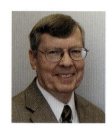

M. Grant Maxie, DVM, PhD, Diplomate ACVP
Co-Executive Director, Laboratory Service Division
Director, Animal Health Laboratory
University of Guelph
Guelph, Ontario
Canada
Introduction to the diagnostic process

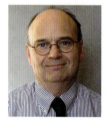

Jesse M. Hostetter, DVM, PhD, Diplomate ACVP
Associate Professor
Department of Veterinary Pathology
College of Veterinary Medicine
Iowa State University
Ames, Iowa
USA
Alimentary system

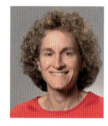

Margaret A. Miller, DVM, PhD, Diplomate ACVP
Professor
Department of Comparative Pathobiology
Purdue University
West Lafayette, Indiana
USA
Introduction to the diagnostic process

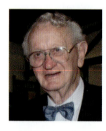

Kenneth V. F. Jubb†
Emeritus Professor
Faculty of Veterinary and Agricultural Sciences
University of Melbourne
Melbourne, Victoria, Australia
Pancreas

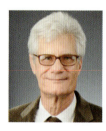

F. Charles Mohr, DVM, PhD, Diplomate ACVP
Professor of Clinical Anatomic Pathology
Department of Veterinary Pathology, Microbiology, and Immunology
School of Veterinary Medicine
University of California
Davis, California
USA
Urinary system

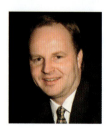

Matti Kiupel, Dr med vet habil, PhD, Diplomate ACVP
Professor
Department of Pathobiology and Diagnostic Investigation
College of Veterinary Medicine
Michigan State University
East Lansing, Michigan
USA
Hematopoietic system

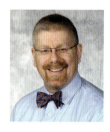

Bradley L. Njaa, DVM, MVSc, Diplomate ACVP
Anatomic Pathologist III
IDEXX Laboratories, Inc.
Professor (Adjunct)
Department of Veterinary Pathobiology
Oklahoma State University
Stillwater, Oklahoma
USA
Special senses

†Deceased.

CONTRIBUTORS

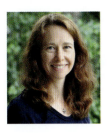

Jeanine Peters-Kennedy, DVM, Diplomate ACVP, Diplomate ACVD
Assistant Clinical Professor
Department of Biomedical Sciences
College of Veterinary Medicine
Cornell University
Ithaca, New York
USA
Integumentary system

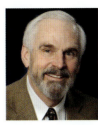

Donald H. Schlafer, DVM, PhD, Diplomate ACVP/ACVM/ACT
Emeritus Professor
Department of Biomedical Sciences
College of Veterinary Medicine
Cornell University
Ithaca, New York
USA
Female genital system

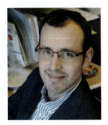

Brandon L. Plattner, DVM, PhD, Diplomate ACVP
Assistant Professor
Department of Pathobiology
Ontario Veterinary College
University of Guelph
Guelph, Ontario
Canada
Alimentary system

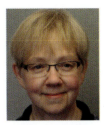

Margaret J. Stalker, DVM, PhD, Diplomate ACVP
Animal Health Laboratory
Laboratory Services Division
University of Guelph
Guelph, Ontario
Canada
Liver and biliary system

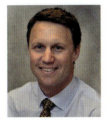

Nicholas A. Robinson, BVSc (Hons), PhD, MACVSc, Diplomate ACVP
Professor
College of Veterinary Medicine
University of Minnesota
St. Paul, Minnesota
USA
Cardiovascular system

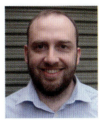

Andrew W. Stent, BVSc, MANZCVS, PhD
Faculty of Veterinary and Agricultural Sciences
University of Melbourne
Melbourne, Victoria
Australia
Pancreas

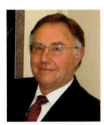

Wayne F. Robinson, BVSc, MVSc, PhD, MACVSc, Diplomate ACVP
Emeritus Professor
Federation University Australia
Victoria, Australia
Cardiovascular system

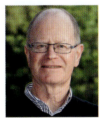

Keith G. Thompson, BVSc, PhD, Diplomate ACVP
Emeritus Professor
Pathobiology Section
Institute of Veterinary, Animal, and Biomedical Sciences
Massey University
Palmerston North, Manawatu
New Zealand
Bones and joints

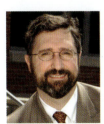

Thomas J. Rosol, DVM, PhD, Diplomate ACVP
Professor
Department of Veterinary Biosciences
Senior Advisor, Life Sciences, Technology Commercialization Office
College of Veterinary Medicine
The Ohio State University
Columbus, Ohio
USA
Endocrine glands

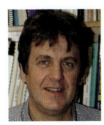

Francisco A. Uzal, DVM, FRVC, PhD, Diplomate ACVP
California Animal Health and Food Safety Laboratory
University of California
San Bernardino, California
USA
Alimentary system

CONTRIBUTORS

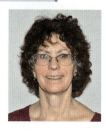

Beth A. Valentine, DVM, PhD, Diplomate ACVP
Professor
Department of Biomedical Sciences
College of Veterinary Medicine
Oregon State University
Corvallis, Oregon
USA
Muscle and tendon

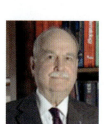

V.E.O. (Ted) Valli, DVM, PhD, Diplomate ACVP
Professor Emeritus
Department of Pathobiology
College of Veterinary Medicine
University of Illinois at Urbana-Champaign
Champaign, Illinois
USA
Hematopoietic system

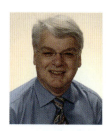

Brian P. Wilcock, DVM, PhD
Histovet Surgical Pathology
Guelph, Ontario
Canada
Special senses

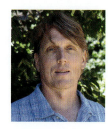

Kurt J. Williams, DVM, PhD, Diplomate ACVP
Department of Pathobiology and Diagnostic Investigation
College of Veterinary Medicine
Michigan State University
East Lansing, Michigan
USA
Respiratory system

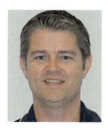

R. Darren Wood, DVM, DVSc, Diplomate ACVP
Associate Professor
Department of Pathobiology
Ontario Veterinary College
University of Guelph
Guelph, Ontario
Canada
Hematopoietic system

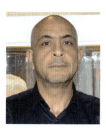

Sameh Youssef, BVSc, PhD, DVSc, Diplomate ACVP
Professor
Department of Pathology
Alexandria Veterinary College
Alexandria University
Alexandria, Egypt
Nervous system

Preface

In this sixth edition of *Pathology of Domestic Animals*, we continue the long tradition of surveying the literature and updating the information in this reference textbook in light of our own practical experience in the pathology of the major domestic mammals. True to the spirit of the first edition, this text is designed to explain the pathogenesis of common and not-so-common diseases, define the distinguishing features of these various conditions, and put them in a context relevant to both students and working pathologists. Knowledge has been generated incrementally since the publication of the fifth edition, particularly with respect to improved understanding of pathogenesis at the molecular level, as well as through the use of improved diagnostic tools, including the frontier of whole genome sequencing. My thanks to the contributors to this edition for their rigorous perusal of the literature in their areas of interest, for their addition of insightful information to their chapters, and for their inclusion of many new figures.

NEW TO THE SIXTH EDITION

The most noticeable, and I think very welcome, change in the sixth edition is the addition of full-color figures throughout the text. Nearly all of the images from prior editions have been replaced. These new images clearly depict the diagnostic features of hundreds of conditions.

We have also added a new chapter, "Introduction to the Diagnostic Process," to the usual lineup of chapters in these 3 volumes. The goal of this new chapter is to illustrate the whole-animal perspective and detail the approaches to systemic, multi-system, and polymicrobial disease.

The complete index is again printed in each volume as an aid to readers. "Further reading" lists have been pruned in the print book to save space. All references are available on any electronic version of the text as well as on the companion website that accompanies the purchase of any print book. These online references link to abstracts on PubMed.com.

COMPANION WEBSITE

In addition to updating the graphic design of these volumes, the print version of *Pathology of Domestic Animals* now has a companion website, accessible at:
PathologyofDomesticAnimals.com

Included on the companion website are:
- A complete image collection, including 325 bonus, electronic-only figures that have been called out in the text. These figures are identified in the printed version as "eFigs."
- An expanded list of useful references, each linked to the original abstract on PubMed.com.

I hope that we have captured significant changes and have synthesized this new knowledge to provide a balanced overview of all topics covered. Keeping pace with evolving agents and their changing impacts is a never-ending challenge. We have used current anatomical and microbial terminology, based on internationally accepted reference sources, such as the Universal Virus Database of the International Committee on Taxonomy of Viruses (http://www.ncbi.nlm.nih.gov/ICTVdb/index.htm). Microbial taxonomy is, of course, continually evolving, and classifications and names of organisms can be expected to be updated as newer phylogenetic analyses are reported. Debate continues, for example, over the taxonomy of *Chlamydophila/Chlamydia* spp. And change will continue.

We have attempted to contact all contributors of figures from previous editions and from various archives and apologize to any whom we were unable to contact or who were overlooked. If any individual recognizes an image as one of his/her own or as belonging to a colleague, we would be happy to correct the attribution in a future printing.

Acknowledgments

My thanks to Elsevier for their help and support throughout this project, beginning in the United Kingdom with Robert Edwards and Carole McMurray, and more recently in the United States, with Penny Rudolph, content strategy director; Brandi Graham, content development specialist; Sharon Corell, senior project manager; Louise King, project manager, and the entire behind-the-scenes production team.

Grant Maxie
Guelph, Ontario, 2015

These volumes are dedicated to Drs. Kenneth V.F. Jubb (1928-2013)[1], Peter C. Kennedy (1923-2006)[2], and Nigel C. Palmer, and to my family—Laura, Kevin, and Andrea.

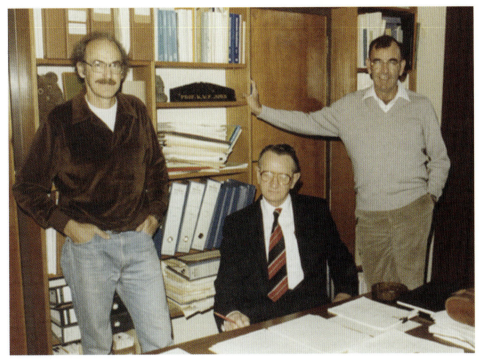

Drs. Palmer, Jubb, and Kennedy while working on the third edition in Melbourne, 1983. (Courtesy, University of Melbourne.)

---

[1] http://www.vet.unimelb.edu.au/news/2013/memorial.html
[2] http://senate.universityofcalifornia.edu/inmemoriam/peterckennedy.htm

Contents

VOLUME ONE

1 Introduction to the Diagnostic Process 1
   M. Grant Maxie, Margaret A. Miller

2 Bones and Joints 16
   Linden E. Craig, Keren E. Dittmer, Keith G. Thompson

3 Muscle and Tendon 164
   Barry J. Cooper, Beth A. Valentine

4 Nervous System 250
   Carlo Cantile, Sameh Youssef

5 Special Senses 407
   Brian P. Wilcock, Bradley L. Njaa

6 Integumentary System 509
   Elizabeth A. Mauldin, Jeanine Peters-Kennedy

VOLUME TWO

1 Alimentary System 1
   Francisco A. Uzal, Brandon L. Plattner, Jesse M. Hostetter

2 Liver and Biliary System 258
   John M. Cullen, Margaret J. Stalker

3 Pancreas 353
   Kenneth V.F. Jubb[†], Andrew W. Stent

4 Urinary System 376
   Rachel E. Cianciolo, F. Charles Mohr

5 Respiratory System 465
   Jeff L. Caswell, Kurt J. Williams

VOLUME THREE

1 Cardiovascular System 1
   Wayne F. Robinson, Nicholas A. Robinson

2 Hematopoietic System 102
   V.E.O. (Ted) Valli, Matti Kiupel, Dorothee Bienzle (with R. Darren Wood)

3 Endocrine Glands 269
   Thomas J. Rosol, Andrea Gröne

4 Female Genital System 358
   Donald H. Schlafer, Robert A. Foster

5 Male Genital System 465
   Robert A. Foster

[†]Deceased

CHAPTER 1

Introduction to the Diagnostic Process

M. Grant Maxie • Margaret A. Miller

INTRODUCTION	1
PURPOSE OF GROSS AND HISTOLOGIC EXAMINATIONS	2
Methodologies	2
Autopsy or biopsy formats	2
Types of investigations	2
Naturally occurring disease	2
Forensic (relating to the law)	2
Anesthetic deaths	2
Experimental disease, toxicopathology	3
Telepathology	3
Pattern recognition	3
Gross examination	4
Systematic	4
Problem-oriented	7
Aging changes and other incidental lesions	7
Postmortem changes	7
Sample selection and preservation, records	8
Trimming of fixed autopsy and biopsy specimens	8
Histologic examination	9
Hematoxylin and eosin	9
Special stains	9
Immunohistochemistry	9
Additional –ologies	10
Microbiology: bacteriology, mycoplasmology, mycology, virology	10
Parasitology	11
Immunology	11
Molecular biology	11
Clinical pathology, cytopathology	11
Toxicology	11
Imaging	11
Genetics	12
Photography	12
Case interpretations and client service	12
Decision analysis	12
Case coordination	12
Weighting of competing etiologies, cut-offs, explanations	12
Economic considerations	13
Final reports	14
Quality assurance of pathology services	14
Accreditation of laboratories: quality programs	14
Test validation	14
Occupational health and safety, biosafety/biocontainment	14
Initial and ongoing competence of pathologists	14
Certification of pathologists	14
Proficiency testing, peer review, requests for second opinions	14
Continuing education, documentation	14
CONCLUSION	15

INTRODUCTION

Diagnosis entails the integration of history, signalment, clinical signs, gross lesions, microscopic changes in tissues and cells, and any ancillary (microbiologic, immunologic, molecular, toxicologic/chemical) test results to arrive at a reliable conclusion with respect to the cause of disease or death. The ultimate outcome of establishing diagnoses of course includes aiding in the prevention and control of contagious diseases in herds and flocks, distinguishing the presence of new or emerging diseases, and in the case of pet animals, aiding grief counseling and case closure.

To be of more general and greater service to various animal industries, pathology investigations also contribute to *surveillance* efforts. Diagnoses must be accurate, terminology used should be standardized, and intelligence gathering networks must be harmonized. Rolled-up disease incident information can give useful insights into changes in the prevalence of endemic disease, the emergence of new diseases, and the reemergence of older diseases. Generation of disease surveillance data at the local, national, and international levels can contribute greatly to improved disease control policy and to the control, if not elimination, of individual diseases.

The diagnostic pathologist is both teacher and student at each step of the diagnostic process. It is essential to build on the knowledge base of general pathology, in which the cellular or tissue response to injury is studied, to comprehend the mechanisms of disease. With the basic principles of general pathology, the diagnostic pathologist learns to categorize a lesion by its gross or histologic features as *degenerative, inflammatory, a disturbance of growth,* or *a vascular insult.* In systemic pathology, the concepts of general pathology are applied at the organ system level, keeping in mind that the cellular response to, for example, a herpesvirus, tends to be stereotypical, whether in the respiratory tract, the liver, or another organ system. The student of systemic pathology must build on the knowledge of general pathology.

Although systemic pathology is usually categorized for teaching purposes into major organ systems, as in the chapters of this book, the diagnostician must constantly consider the interplay among organ systems and appreciate systemic pathology as the study of systemic disease, i.e., disease that affects the whole body. Few, if any, diseases are confined to one organ or tissue. A.B. Ackerman's assertion that general pathology and systemic pathology are "one" pathology is worth remembering. Finally, the concept of One Health is particularly appropriate in veterinary or comparative pathology, lest the pathologist be daunted by the variety of species encountered in practice. Thus, falling back on the example of herpesvirus infection, a horse is likely to respond to this or another particular type of injury as would a cow, dog, cat, pig, or even an avian species.

PURPOSE OF GROSS AND HISTOLOGIC EXAMINATIONS

- The gross and microscopic examinations of antemortem or postmortem specimens gather objective evidence regarding the pathogenesis and outcome of disease processes, and hence provide *quality control of medical practice*. These examinations add value to clinical examinations, such as hematology, serum biochemistry, diagnostic imaging, endoscopy, or exploratory surgery. The decline of autopsy rates is alarming in light of increased medical malpractice cases because pathology can be the single best way to confirm a clinical diagnosis, to determine the cause of death, and to evaluate the response to therapy. In cases of refused autopsies, postmortem computed tomography (PMCT) or magnetic resonance imaging (MRI) may be available as an alternative, and provide a *virtopsy* (virtual autopsy).
- In many cases of *unexpected death*, autopsy becomes the **initial** effort to establish a differential diagnosis on the way to determining the definitive morphologic and etiologic diagnoses.
- Antemortem microscopic examinations not only facilitate diagnosis, but allow prognostication and customization of *therapeutic plans*, primarily through phenotypic interpretations, and more recently, genotypic analyses.
- Through retrospective studies, pathologists *contribute to knowledge* of a particular disease or diseases of a specific organ system.
- Surveillance programs, such as autopsies mandated by horse racing commissions and screening programs for transmissible spongiform encephalopathies, and for endemic, emerging, or foreign animal diseases, are essential to document important causes of disease and death in different geographic regions or management situations so that *preventive measures* can be instituted to avoid injury or disease.
- As a *collaborator* in hypothesis-driven investigations, the pathologist interprets the cellular and tissue response in light of the other facets of the study.

Methodologies

Autopsy or biopsy formats

For *postmortem examination*, a thorough review of all information provided by the submitting veterinarian or obtained from interview of the animal owner is essential to formulate the diagnostic approach. This information directs microbiologic or toxicologic testing and sample collection/storage, indicates the need for photographic documentation, and can predict which organs or tissues require special attention. The objective is to determine the cause of disease and/or death, including infectious/contagious, toxic, or physical etiologies. Routine autopsies should follow a standard protocol. Most research investigations mandate a standardized autopsy protocol customized for the project.

Of course, some animals are submitted for autopsy with no history, either through careless omission or despite the submitter's best efforts. "Found dead" is an all too common history. In these situations, the pathologist must be especially thorough and systematic in the approach to postmortem examination.

With *surgical pathology*, or *autopsy-in-a-jar pathology*, in contrast to postmortem examination, the diagnostician may have the brief opportunity to evaluate a biopsy specimen(s) histologically without knowledge of the history, the submitting veterinarian's tentative diagnosis, tissue identification, or even the animal species. This, albeit momentary, opportunity to formulate an opinion, unbiased by the history, not only allows the pathologist to remain open-minded, but teaches and reinforces the integral components of the diagnostic process. How is the tissue or cellular response to injury recognized? How can this information be used to reach a diagnosis or at least a differential diagnosis? Of course, the pathologist who has had this brief unbiased glimpse at a biopsy specimen must then correlate the initial impression with all available history and the submitter's clinical observations. Arriving at a diagnosis and interpretation in these cases is truly a partnership between clinician and pathologist, and all possible facts must be shared to reach the most satisfactory conclusion.

In both autopsy and biopsy reports, the pathologist records objective evidence of his or her *findings* to recreate an accurate picture of the findings in the mind of the reader. In addition to these objective findings, the pathologist may add an *interpretation*, which is subjective and contains opinions based on personal experience or conventional wisdom.

Types of investigations

The diagnostic pathologist must remain versatile to deal effectively with a wide variety of specimens and the need for different protocols.

Naturally occurring disease

In the diagnostic laboratory, naturally occurring diseases comprise the majority of accessions. The pathologist should be familiar with the common diseases encountered in domestic animals in various settings and various stages of life, but must always remain open-minded and thorough so as not to overlook diagnostic clues in unusual situations. Not all juvenile pigs and ruminants die from pneumonia or diarrhea.

Forensic (relating to the law)

In cases of suspected animal abuse, cases may be submitted by law enforcement agencies for specialized documented investigations. Establishing a *chain-of-custody* is the first step in receipt of a specimen for autopsy in such investigations. The forensic autopsy requires photographic documentation of the identity of the animal as well as of any salient lesions. Whereas some forensic cases may be straightforward, others offer challenges, (e.g., age of skin wounds, age of bruises, diagnosis of drowning, estimating the time since death). Formalin-fixed and frozen (or otherwise preserved) specimens and other evidence must be securely stored for a length of time determined by the legal system. Many diagnostic laboratories also use a forensic or legal protocol for autopsy of insured animals.

Anesthetic deaths

Autopsy of animals that died during or shortly after anesthesia can be frustrating because, in many cases, lesions are not observed or are secondary to resuscitation attempts. The pathologist should keep in mind that anesthetic deaths could become a legal autopsy and therefore should document animal identity and any salient lesions. An underlying disease, such as a cardiac defect or cardiomyopathy, brachycephalic syndrome, or systemic infectious or noninfectious disease should be sought as an explanation for increased susceptibility to anesthesia. In many cases of anesthetic death, the end point of the autopsy is the *ruling out of underlying disease* that would explain why the animal succumbed during anesthesia.

Experimental disease, toxicopathology

The pathologist should always be involved in the experimental design for research investigations. Ideally, one pathologist should perform or supervise a team that performs all of the autopsies within a research study. In particular, the assigned pathologist develops the standardized protocol for postmortem examination of experimental subjects and collection of appropriate specimens for histologic examination and other assays. Good Laboratory Practice (GLP) mandates adherence to a set of guidelines to ensure the quality of data submitted to regulatory agencies. Although modifiers, such as mild, moderate, or severe, may be suitable in histologic reports in diagnostic practice, precise and reproducible *scoring of histologic lesions* is an integral part of toxicologic or other research investigations that allows comparison of lesions among treatment groups or comparison of treated animals with control animals.

Telepathology

Once limited mainly to research laboratories and the pharmaceutical industry, digital pathology has become more accessible, if not yet routine, in diagnostic laboratories and in teaching institutions. Transmission of still and/or video images from field autopsies is in use in various venues, and can be a very useful adjunct in sample selection and case resolution.

Although pathology residents are still trained mainly with glass slides viewed through microscopes, especially in their diagnostic practice, *virtual microscopy* is increasingly used in education, particularly that of professional students. Whereas the medical or veterinary student seeks to master concepts and theories to understand disease and interpret a pathology report, the pathologist-in-training must learn the actual thought processes involved in diagnosis. First and foremost, the trainee must learn to find the lesion, the area of interest, in a gross specimen or in a histologic section. Traditionally, histopathology was taught across a double-headed or multi-headed microscope. Today, ongoing innovations in slide scanners and software for viewing virtual slides have made this technology available to teaching institutions and diagnostic laboratories, so that even the eye movements of an experienced pathologist can be charted, and the pinpointing and categorization of a lesion can be taught to many students simultaneously or from a distance with virtual slides and digital images.

Even the most experienced pathologist requires continuing education and benefits from consultation with colleagues for both diagnostic and research cases. Telepathology, facilitated by the use of digital gross images and virtual histologic sections, makes consultation with experts around the world practical and rapid.

Pattern recognition

Often attributed to AB Ackerman and applied most extensively in dermatopathology, *pattern recognition is the key thought process in the making of a definitive diagnosis*, especially in histopathology. Equally applicable to organ systems other than the integument and to autopsy as well as surgical pathology, pattern recognition involves the mental sorting of the response to injury into categories to arrive at a specific etiologic diagnosis or at least to refine the differential diagnosis. Patterns of

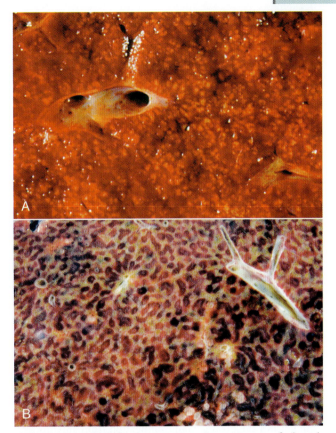

Figure 1-1 A. Multifocal necrotizing hepatitis in a foal with *Clostridium piliforme* infection (Tyzzer's disease). **B. Centrilobular hepatic degeneration and necrosis** in a horse with chronic passive congestion as a result of right heart failure.

the effects of hazards on the body, organs, and tissues can be recognized at the gross, subgross, and microscopic levels of examination, and these are detailed below.

The increasing availability of virtual histologic slides and the use of computer-assisted technology to link histologic pattern to a diagnostic algorithm have facilitated the automation of the process of pattern recognition, but the brain of the pathologist is still required in the "training" of the software program and in validation of the results. In certain situations, such as multifocal (random) hepatic necrosis versus a lobular or zonal pattern of hepatic degeneration or necrosis, pattern recognition is useful even at the macroscopic level to distinguish, in this example, between the effect of an infectious agent (Fig. 1-1A) and that of a metabolic, toxic, or ischemic insult, such as chronic passive hepatic congestion (Fig. 1-1B).

Recognition of the predominant pattern is not easy because of the frequent presence of more than one pattern. The diagnostic pathologist learns pattern recognition by practice, at low/scanning magnification, and, at least initially, when possible, without the benefit of knowledge of the case history or the submitter's presumptive diagnosis. Only after formulating an unbiased tentative diagnosis and differential diagnosis should the pathologist review the clinical data on the submission form.

Further reading

Ackerman AB. Histologic Diagnosis of Inflammatory Skin Diseases. A Method by Pattern Analysis. Philadelphia: Lea & Febiger; 1978.

Bille C, et al. Risk of anaesthetic mortality in dogs and cats: an observational cohort study of 3,546 cases. Vet Anaesth Analg 2012; 39:59-68.

Cooper JE, Cooper ME. Introduction to Veterinary and Comparative Forensic Medicine. Oxford: Blackwell Publishing; 2007.

Kuijpers CC, et al. The value of autopsies in the era of high-tech medicine: discrepant findings persist. J Clin Pathol 2014;67:512-519.

Lyle CH, et al. Sudden death in racing Thoroughbred horses: an international multicentre study of post mortem findings. Equine Vet J 2011;43:324-331.

Munro R, Munro HM. Some challenges in forensic veterinary pathology: a review. J Comp Pathol 2013;149:57-73.

Stover SM, Murray A. The California postmortem program: leading the way. Vet Clin North Am Equine Pract 2008;24:21-36.

Gross examination

Systematic

Traditionally, the word *autopsy*—literally, "to see for oneself"—was applied to postmortem examination of a human body; *necropsy*—"examine after death"—was the term for postmortem examination of a nonhuman body, but this is an artificial distinction. In step with the One Health approach to pathology, *autopsy has been proposed as the term for postmortem examination of any dead body, be it human or nonhuman*. One could argue that necropsy is the superior one-health term for postmortem examinations, because autopsy, etymologically, in no way implies that the subject viewed is dead, whereas necropsy distinguishes the postmortem examination from antemortem biopsy. To steer clear of the fray, in these volumes, autopsy is considered synonymous with postmortem examination, and the term necropsy is not used.

Colleges of veterinary medicine and pathology training programs adhere to a systematic approach to postmortem examination that is applicable to various animal species and varies somewhat among institutions. A systematic approach is important in the training of veterinary students and pathology residents. However, any approach should be adaptable when the need arises, for instance, when new pathologists join the program, when the caseload (number of cases, variation in species) changes, when safety issues demand it, or when postmortem laboratory facilities or equipment changes. New diagnostic laboratories should consult with existing laboratories and published references in designing a postmortem prosection protocol.

The systematic approach to postmortem examination remains important to even the most experienced pathologist when faced with a case of *"sudden death"* (in quotes because death is always sudden, but when it is also unexpected the term "sudden death" applies) with no historical facts or clinical signs for clues to the cause of death (Table 1-1). The systematic approach is also valuable to the busy pathologist, who, with little time for recording gross lesions during the postmortem examination, can more reliably remember details of multiple gross examinations at the end of the day if a systematic approach was followed for each case. Conduct of a *"routine"* or *"comprehensive"* autopsy is the usual response in the face of no or limited history; there is no such thing as a "complete" autopsy in which every muscle, nerve, joint, etc. is examined in detail.

The basic skills required in the autopsy process are prosection, description, and interpretation. The development of prosection skills requires a sharp knife plus a few other instruments, manual dexterity, a certain degree of strength, and knowledge

Table • 1-1

Major causes of unexpected death in domestic mammals

Species	Cause of death
Any species	Adverse drug reactions, anaphylaxis, anesthetic deaths, bacterial sepsis, drowning, electrocution, exsanguination, heat stroke, intestinal strangulation, physical trauma, toxicosis (e.g., Japanese yew)
Horses	Aortic rupture, colic (intestinal strangulation), exercise-induced pulmonary hemorrhage, ruptured uterine artery
Cattle	Anthrax, blackleg and other clostridial diseases, bloat, coliform mastitis, *Histophilus somni*, hypocalcemia, hypomagnesemia, lead poisoning, ruptured hepatic abscess, nutritional myopathy
Pigs	Bacterial infections (*Haemophilus parasuis, Actinobacillus suis, Actinobacillus pleuropneumoniae, Streptococcus suis, Salmonella* Choleraesuis), edema disease, gastric ulcer, manure pit gas poisoning, mulberry heart disease/hepatosis dietetica (vitamin E-selenium deficiency), porcine stress syndrome
Sheep/goats	Abomasal parasitism (*Haemonchus contortus*), bloat, clostridial enterotoxemia, copper poisoning, other bacterial infections (*Bibersteinia trehalosi*)
Dogs	Cardiac anomalies, dilated cardiomyopathy, gastric dilation/volvulus, hemorrhage from atrial or splenic hemangiosarcoma, hypoadrenocorticism (Addison's disease), parvoviral infection, pulmonary arterial thrombosis
Cats	Heartworm disease, hypertrophic cardiomyopathy, parvoviral infection

of anatomy (including interspecies variations). With practice, prosection skills are rapidly acquired. In contrast, description and interpretation of gross lesions is both science and art, and is fraught with the vagaries of individual variation, postmortem decomposition, secondary changes that obscure the primary lesion, and the co-existence of more than one disease or injury. In addition, interpretive abilities are based on extant knowledge of disease and disease mechanisms. Therefore the science and the art of gross examination evolve over a lifetime of learning.

Gross examination is followed by a written description of all salient lesions and at least an attempt at morphologic diagnosis. The best descriptions are factual, rather than interpretive, and employ lay (nonpathology) terminology to record size, shape, texture, color, odors, location, distribution (random or symmetric, focal, multifocal, coalescing, miliary, segmental, diffuse), and severity (mild, moderate, marked) of gross lesions, and weights of selected organs, such as heart, kidneys, and liver. The education required for writing a gross description includes knowledge of anatomy and of enough pathology to distinguish a lesion from a nonlesion or a change of no importance. Morphologic diagnosis, in contrast, places an interpretation on the described gross lesions. *Gross morphologic diagnosis* is not the be-all and end-all of the postmortem examination, but is a step along the way to definitive diagnosis. In its simplest form, it should imply the location of the lesion and the nature of the response to injury. In some instances, one word suffices. For example, a gross diagnosis of nephritis localizes the lesion to the kidneys and implies an inflammatory process. Appropriate modifiers can provide important additional information. In the example of nephritis, the addition of the word embolic or the prefix pyelo- tells the reader the likely route of infection. Likewise, the addition of descriptors of the inflammatory process, such as suppurative or granulomatous could, respectively, implicate different groups of infectious agents.

Morphologic diagnosis is the naming of a lesion and is made in two different ways. The first method is *pattern recognition*—a reflex, almost unthinking, response of the pathologist who recognizes the lesion, having seen it before, and names it accordingly. The second method of morphologic diagnosis—a *hypothetico-deductive strategy*—is applied to the lesion that is not immediately recognized, and entails contemplation of an unrecognized lesion and formulation of hypotheses in light of background knowledge in general and systemic pathology. In this situation, the pathologist realizes that a tissue change is a lesion, but does not recognize the lesion (either because it reflects a not previously encountered disease or because it is not a classic example of a well-known disease). A morphologic diagnosis can still be made accurately in many cases by categorizing a lesion according to the response to injury as degenerative/necrotic, inflammatory (acute, subacute, chronic, fibrinous, granulomatous), a vascular disturbance (hemorrhage, infarction, thrombosis, etc.), or a disturbance of growth (hypoplasia, atrophy, hypertrophy, hyperplasia, neoplasia, etc.). Principles of general and systemic pathology are invaluable in making a morphologic diagnosis for the lesion not implicitly recognized.

The ability to make a gross diagnosis at autopsy is arguably one of the more difficult and most important skills in pathology. Even in autopsy cases in which the organ system of interest is not indicated beforehand, the pathologist who has learned the gross characteristics of degenerative, inflammatory, vascular, and growth disturbances is well equipped to make a morphologic diagnosis.

- The cell swelling of *degeneration or necrosis* imparts pallor that is most easily appreciated in richly colored tissues, such as liver, renal cortex (Fig. 1-2), or muscle. Necrosis can be distinguished macroscopically from degeneration when it results in a change in structure; this is most visible when focal/segmental or multifocal, and well demarcated from adjacent viable tissue. In polioencephalomalacia of ruminants, necrosis imparts subtle swelling and yellow discoloration to the cerebral cortex (Fig. 1-3A); the laminar cerebrocortical necrosis is accentuated by autofluorescence under ultraviolet light (Fig. 1-3B).
- The gross diagnosis of *inflammation* is facilitated by the recognition of exudate, most obvious on serosal or mucosal surfaces (Fig. 1-4). However, even in the absence of pus, fibrin, or other gross exudate, inflammation may be intuited by reddening or swelling. Nodularity is a gross hallmark of granulomatous inflammation (Fig. 1-5).

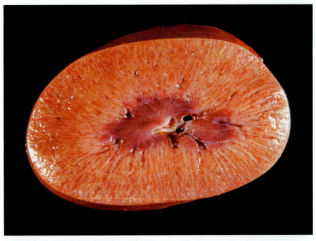

Figure 1-2 Renal tubular **degeneration** (fatty change/lipidosis) in an Ossabaw pig with metabolic syndrome.

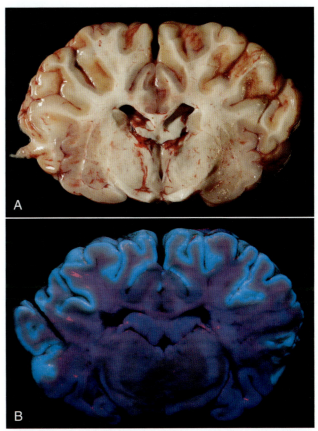

Figure 1-3 A. Cerebrocortical laminar necrosis in a calf with polioencephalomalacia. **B.** Necrotic cerebrocortical parenchyma is autofluorescent under ultraviolet light. (Courtesy K.G. Thompson.)

- Infarcts and thrombi (Fig. 1-6) are classic *vascular disturbances*. It is helpful to remember that vascular insults, such as thrombosis of renal artery and infarction of kidney, result in lesions in the organ or tissue supplied by the affected vessel, but reflect cardiac, systemic, or vascular disease at an upstream site.
- The category of *growth disturbances* can be divided into processes that make an organ or tissue too small

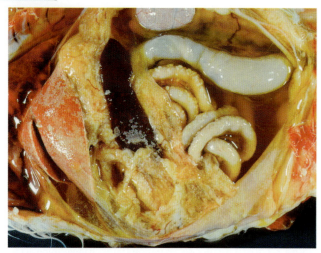

Figure 1-4 **Fibrinous exudate** on peritoneal surfaces and effusion in feline infectious peritonitis.

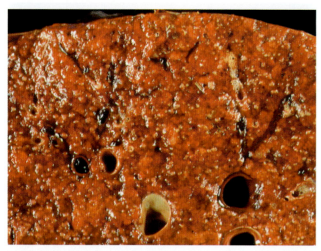

Figure 1-5 **Granulomatous** pneumonia in a horse with pulmonary aspergillosis.

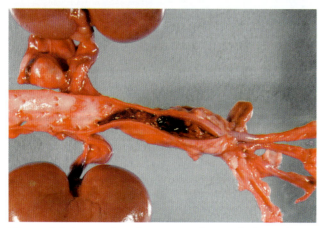

Figure 1-6 Aortic **thrombosis** in a dog with hyperadrenocorticism.

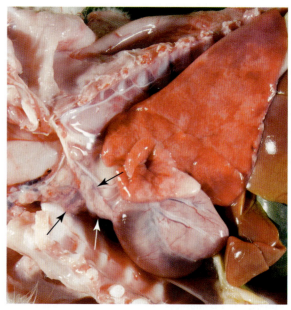

Figure 1-7 Thymic (arrows) **atrophy** in a puppy infected with canine parvovirus-2.

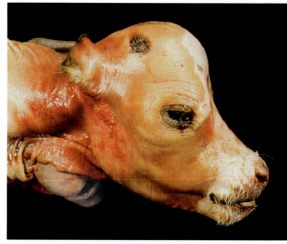

Figure 1-8 Diffuse thyroid **hyperplasia** (goiter) in a bovine fetus with maternal iodine deficiency. The lack of development of the hair coat in this near-term fetus is attributed to hypothyroidism.

(hypoplasia or atrophy) versus those that make it too large. Thymic atrophy (Fig. 1-7) can be easily overlooked because it is inconspicuous, but is a diagnostically useful lesion that, when severe, can implicate infection by certain viruses, such as canine or feline parvoviruses. Tissues or organs can be too large due to hyperplasia (enlargement caused mainly by an increased number of cells; Fig. 1-8), hypertrophy (enlargement the result of increased cellular size in postmitotic organs), or neoplasia. If the enlargement has a nodular or multinodular appearance, granulomatous inflammation is included in the differential diagnosis.

It takes practice to know how far to extend a morphologic diagnosis at the gross level (and when to hold the extra descriptors for the histologic diagnosis). Though a morphologic diagnosis is an interpretation, any autopsy record could become a legal document, so the limits of knowledge at that stage of the investigation should not be surpassed, especially if further testing is planned. That said, an **etiologic diagnosis** may be reached at autopsy for the occasional unique condition, such as *Actinobacillus pleuropneumoniae* pneumonia, osteochondrosis, or traumatic limb fracture.

Problem-oriented

A problem-oriented approach to postmortem examination can be useful in production (herd, flock, or kennel) situations in which, depending on the age of the affected animals and the environmental or management conditions, certain categories of disease, such as intestinal disease expressed as diarrhea or respiratory disease, predictably account for most of the loss from death or decreased production. Certainly, for any newly recognized clinical entity, the initial postmortem examinations should be thorough and systematic. However, once disease trends are established and the cause of disease can be predicted, and particularly if death or production loss is high, problem-oriented autopsy of animals, thoughtfully selected as those most likely to be in an early and untreated stage of the disease (and with minimal autolysis), can be performed. *The problem-oriented postmortem examination is focused on the tissues/organs of interest, which are examined early in the prosection and collected for histologic evaluation and microbiologic or other ancillary tests.*

In the diagnostic laboratory, it can be helpful to categorize *disease syndromes* (e.g., abortion, diarrhea, neurologic disease, respiratory disease, neoplasia, unexpected death, or suspected toxicosis). If, for example, the clinical problem is diarrhea, intestinal specimens should be collected as rapidly as possible to minimize autolysis and will preempt examination of other organs that might have preceded the intestine in the standardized autopsy protocol. Other tissues and organ systems may be neglected in the problem-oriented autopsy or may not be evaluated in each animal, when groups of animals with the same problem are examined. Nevertheless, the pathologist must keep an open mind and be keenly observant to avoid missing lesions indicative of a new or different disease entity ("more is missed by not looking than not knowing").

With sufficient history, the postmortem examination can be problem-oriented from the onset (upon receipt of the live animals, cadavers, or other specimens). However, in the situation of unexpected death (Table 1-1), postmortem examination should begin with an open-minded and thorough systematic gross evaluation; any focus on a particular problem or particular organ system should be based on available history, the signalment of the affected animals, and the environmental setting. Recognition of key gross lesions can narrow the differential diagnosis and guide the postmortem examination and selection of specimens for ancillary testing. In a research investigation, a standardized, but problem-oriented approach to postmortem examination is focused on those organs suspected or known to be targeted by the experimental treatment. The protocol should be based on background knowledge from previous studies and should be sufficiently systematic and thorough to avoid missing an important, but perhaps unexpected, lesion.

Aging changes and other incidental lesions

Lesions of little or no importance are commonly encountered in most species, especially in older animals. Although the presence of cholesterol granulomas in the choroid plexus of old horses may indicate previous hemorrhage, they are seldom associated with any clinical signs of brain disease. Even some neoplasms, such as the thyroid C-cell adenomas that are common in old horses, are unassociated with clinical disease. Siderotic plaques in the spleen of dogs are often attributed to hemorrhage, but are generally an incidental finding in old dogs,

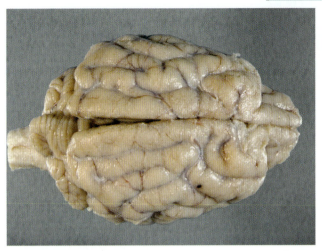

Figure 1-9 Cerebrocortical atrophy with leptomeningeal fibrosis in a geriatric dog.

along with nodular hyperplasia of splenic lymphoid tissue, hepatocytes, and pancreatic acinar cells. Prostatic hyperplasia is an expected lesion in older, sexually intact, male dogs; in contrast, the prostate gland of the castrated dog undergoes atrophy. Lipid vacuolation of renal tubular epithelial cells, especially prominent in intact male cats, imparts a fatty appearance to the feline renal cortex that would be considered lesion lipidosis in a nonfelid. Other lesions that are part of the debilitated state, but expected in geriatric animals, include osteopenia, degenerative joint disease, atrophy of skeletal muscle, and cerebrocortical atrophy (Fig. 1-9) along with meningeal fibrosis or even ossification.

Postmortem changes

The pathologist must distinguish postmortem changes from lesions. Depending on the postmortem interval before autopsy, the manner of death, body temperature and ambient conditions, and other factors, postmortem changes in tissues and organs can obscure lesions or be misinterpreted as lesions. Common postmortem changes, some of which are useful in estimating the time of death in a forensic autopsy, and some of which (or the lack thereof) can even be indicators of a particular disease, include onset of *rigor mortis* in skeletal and cardiac muscle, *clotting of blood* in vessels and heart, gravitational pooling of blood (*livor mortis*), and *autolysis*. Autolysis is especially severe in nonsterile tissues or in those exposed to pancreatic enzymes or bile. Postmortem bacterial overgrowth accelerates autolysis. Because many animals undergo euthanasia by an overdose of *barbiturate* before autopsy, the precipitation of barbiturate salts on tissues exposed to high concentration, especially the endocardium of the right ventricle in the case of intravenous injection, forms gray-tan gritty plaques (Fig. 1-10). Similar precipitates may be found on the pleural surfaces in the case of transthoracic or intrathoracic injections of barbiturate. In addition, inert ingredients, such as propylene glycol, in euthanasia solutions have caustic effects that result in a brown discoloration and friable texture to blood in the right ventricle (after intravenous injection) or, in the case of direct injection, discoloration and a coagulated appearance to perivascular tissues or in the cardiac ventricular wall.

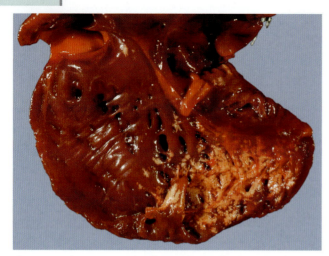

Figure 1-10 Precipitation of **pentobarbital salts** on right ventricular endocardium in a dog. (Courtesy K.M. Newkirk.)

Sample selection and preservation, records

The standard protocol for postmortem examination should include a list of tissues/organs to be fixed in formalin. The list will vary depending on the species, sex, and other factors (and may be shortened in the problem-oriented autopsy), but might include lymph node (a node draining tissues of interest is ideal; e.g., tracheobronchial lymph node in a case of pneumonia), thymus (especially in juvenile animals or in animals of any age with a thymic gross lesion or cranial mediastinal mass), spleen, bone marrow, liver, gallbladder, kidney, trachea, esophagus, lung, heart, ruminant forestomachs, stomach, duodenum, jejunum, ileum, colon, pancreas, adrenal glands, urinary bladder, gonads, uterus, thyroid/parathyroid glands, pituitary gland, eye, skin, mammary gland, diaphragm, tongue, other skeletal muscles, brain, spinal cord (a sample from the first cervical segment suffices in animals without a history of neurologic disease), and peripheral nerve. The list of tissues/organs to collect in formalin is especially important in the education of veterinary students and pathology residents, and in cases without gross lesions or an obvious cause of death at autopsy. Often, a question arises after the gross examination, or even after the preliminary histologic examination, that prompts examination of additional tissues. *It is always better to have representative samples of routine tissues and organs in the formalin container, even when there is no intent of histologic evaluation of every formalin-fixed tissue.* The list of tissues to collect in formalin should be reviewed during the description of gross findings to prevent omission of a lesion.

Phosphate-buffered 10% formalin is the standard fixative in diagnostic laboratories and is suitable for all tissues, including those for which immunohistochemistry is planned. Alternative fixatives should be used for selected tissues if electron microscopy is anticipated. Each laboratory should have a rotating schedule to store formalin-fixed tissues for a set period of time after the postmortem examination. Depending on available space and caseload, many laboratories keep formalin-fixed tissues in the original container for at least 30 days. The formalin container should be designed to resist evaporation, leakage, or damage from the fixative for the designated storage period. Subsequently, formalin-fixed tissues can be discarded or transferred to another type of container for long-term storage, if needed. Tissues that are kept too long in formalin are subject to cross-linking that masks antigens and interferes with immunohistochemistry. In contrast, paraffin-embedded tissue (that was not fixed too long in formalin) retains its antigenicity almost indefinitely. Few laboratories have sufficient space to store formalin containers from every autopsy and surgical biopsy for much longer than a month. However, many laboratories have space to store paraffin blocks for decades. All laboratories must store records and specimens from legal cases for a designated length of time in keeping with regulations.

Tissue specimens that are preserved for teaching gross pathology are generally thicker than those preserved for histologic examination, but can be stored for weeks to months in formalin. This may be preferable to freezing and thawing for certain pale tissues such as the brain. However, when preservation of color is important, *Klotz or Jores' solution* may be superior to formalin. *Plastination*, another method of long-term preservation of tissues for educational purposes, replaces liquids and fats in a formalin-fixed specimen with polymers, resulting in a museum specimen that emits negligible formalin fumes, has little odor, can be touched, and does not decay. In the diagnostic laboratory, unfixed tissue specimens can be refrigerated for a few days, pending the results of histologic examination. These refrigerated specimens can be submitted for microbiologic tests if deemed necessary after histologic evaluation. Perishable specimens that might be needed at a later date should be *frozen* at −70°C for long-term storage.

Photographs of lesions are paramount in legal cases, but photographic documentation also provides a record of routine diagnostic cases that can be used to write an accurate and descriptive autopsy report, explain the histologic findings, and teach pathology to veterinary students and residents. Each diagnostic laboratory should have a standard operating procedure for the labeling and storage of autopsy photographs. Likewise, the autopsy submission form, the gross report, histologic findings, and results from each laboratory section should be stored and accessible for the designated period of time after the autopsy. Similarly, radiographs can provide useful evidence of bony changes, fracture healing, tumor characteristics, and must also be indexed and archived.

Trimming of fixed autopsy and biopsy specimens

After thorough fixation, trimming of routine autopsy cases for preparation of histologic slides is often done by technicians. Complex cases (nervous system, cardiac conduction system), are usually trimmed by the case pathologist. Tissue sections are most useful if they include borders of normal and abnormal tissue, are ideally 1-2 mm thick, and fit easily in tissue cassettes.

Trimming of surgical biopsy specimens is perhaps best done by the pathologist who will interpret the histologic sections. The pathologist may be more capable than a nonveterinarian of understanding and interpreting the submission form and writing a gross description. In addition, a gross or differential diagnosis can often be construed from macroscopic examination of the formalin-fixed tissue. However, in a busy diagnostic laboratory, the histotechnologist can trim biopsy specimens more efficiently and, with training, quite well. Assigning the task of trimming biopsy specimens to a histotechnologist facilitates scheduling for maximum efficiency in the daily work flow of the laboratory. Gross descriptions of specimens can be recorded by the trimming technician, and can be supplemented by photographs. Second, and most important, the pathologist who did not read the submission form and trim the biopsy specimen has the brief opportunity to view the histologic sections with an unbiased eye.

The technician who trims biopsy specimens must know how to trim different types of specimens (different tissues, obtained with different biopsy instruments), how to trim painted surgical margins, and when to call the pathologist. The list of tissues that demand the attention of the assigned pathologist before trimming varies depending on the preferences of the pathologist, but may include whole organs (heart, brain, splenectomy specimens), amputation specimens, other large specimens, and tissues that may require photographic documentation or are designated as tissues of interest for teaching or research purposes.

Further reading

King JM, et al. The Necropsy Book. 5th ed. Gurnee, Ill: CL Davis Foundation; 2006.
Law M, et al. Necropsy or autopsy? It's all about communication! Vet Pathol 2012;49:271-272.
McGavin MD, Thompson SW. Specimen Dissection and Photography. Springfield, Ill: Charles C. Thomas; 1988.

Histologic examination

Examination of stained histology slides begins with subgross ("shirt-sleeve") examination of the slide—many tissues are easily identified, all tissues are located so as not to be missed when examining the slide on the microscope, and large, diffuse, or focal lesions can be seen and singled out for closer examination. The whole slide is scanned at low power before focusing on individual lesions and cells, and avoiding the possibility of missing lesions by jumping to conclusions. Histologic descriptions of common entities can be brief and focused. New entities bear further exposition. Clinically useful information should be reported. In the case of tumor biopsies, clinicians are of course intensely interested in the aggressiveness of the tumor—degree of anaplasia, evidence of invasion, completeness of removal, opportunity for recurrence, and hence prognosis. Malignant or potentially malignant neoplasms should be graded according to published criteria.

Hematoxylin and eosin

Hematoxylin and eosin (H&E) is the routine histologic stain and the basis for comparison with "special" histochemistry or immunohistochemistry procedures. H&E works so well in pathology because of the negatively charged affinity of acidic eosin for cytoplasmic proteins, and the positively charged affinity of basic hematoxylin for nuclear structures. Histologic evaluation typically begins with sections stained with H&E, so the pathologist must understand the mechanism of differential staining and know the factors that influence it to interpret lesions and troubleshoot problems with staining technique. In addition, *the periodicity of certain structures renders them birefringent in polarized light.* The pathologist uses this characteristic to accentuate structures such as collagen fibers, to distinguish between lamellar and woven bone, or to highlight crystals. Crystals, by their very nature, are birefringent, but only those resistant to dissolution in water or other solvents survive histologic processing. Birefringence may be accompanied by a color change for some compounds; therefore amyloid, especially with Congo red stain, has a characteristic apple-green birefringence.

Special stains

Histochemical techniques ("special stains") are used to label tissue components that cannot be distinguished or identified easily in the H&E-stained section. The pathologist must be familiar with histochemical techniques to identify connective tissues (e.g., fibrous collagen, elastin, reticulin fibers, muscle), carbohydrate moieties (e.g., glycogen, glycosaminoglycans, mucins), pigments (e.g., hemoglobin, bile, melanin, lipofuscin), mineral (e.g., iron, calcium, copper), amyloid, or microorganisms (bacteria, fungi, protozoa) in tissue sections. Metachromatic dyes, such as toluidine blue or Giemsa, are used to differentiate mucins, mast cell granules, and other proteoglycans that bind to blue dyes causing a color shift from blue to purple.

Immunohistochemistry

Immunohistochemistry (IHC, immunoperoxidase) has become a routine tool in the veterinary diagnostic laboratory with the increasing availability of antibodies that cross-react with antigens of veterinary species or were developed for use with veterinary species. Many of the technically difficult histochemistry techniques used in neuropathology have been replaced by IHC (Fig. 1-11). The use of IHC in oncology has broadened from diagnosis and classification of tumors (Fig. 1-12) to prognostic and therapeutic applications.

Immunohistochemistry is particularly useful in the diagnosis of infectious diseases because *the microbial antigens can be localized to the characteristic lesions*. Thus the presence of microbial proteins is evaluated in the context of the disease. Technically, IHC combines immune reactions (binding of antibody to microbial antigens or to intermediate filaments or some other cellular component) with chemical reactions that make the antigen-antibody complexes visible with light microscopy. Because IHC can be performed on formalin-fixed, paraffin-embedded tissue sections, the procedures for fixation and tissue processing are the routine procedures of the laboratory. That said, formalin-fixed tissue usually requires some form of antigen retrieval to unmask the tissue antigens and allow antibody binding.

With the sections for IHC just a few micrometers removed from the H&E-stained section, the H&E-stained section serves as a reference point for the evaluation of the IHC preparations. Important considerations in IHC include methodology, detection system, antibody type and source, tissue and reagent controls, equipment (autostainer), and quality control.

Further reading

Gibson-Corley KN, et al. Principles for valid histopathologic scoring in research. Vet Pathol 2013;50:1007-1015.
Kamstock DA, et al. Recommended guidelines for submission, trimming, margin evaluation, and reporting of tumor biopsy specimens in veterinary surgical pathology. Vet Pathol 2011;48:19-31.
McGavin MD. Factors affecting visibility of a target tissue in histologic sections. Vet Pathol 2014;51:9-27.
Ramos-Vara JA, Miller MA. When tissue antigens and antibodies get along: revisiting the technical aspects of immunohistochemistry. Vet Pathol 2014;51:42-87.

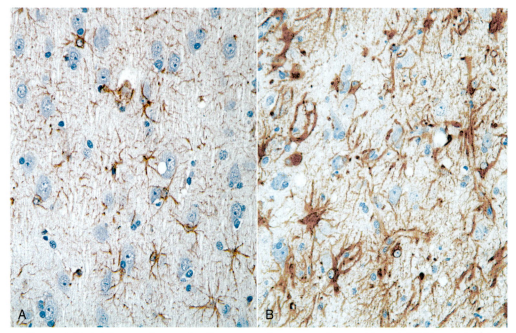

Figure 1-11 A. The cytoplasm and cell processes of astrocytes (not visible with H&E) are labeled with **immunohistochemistry for glial fibrillary acidic protein (GFAP)** in normal cerebral cortex of a dog. **B.** Hypertrophy of cerebrocortical astrocytes is demonstrated with **immunohistochemistry for GFAP** in a different cortical region of the same canine cerebrum.

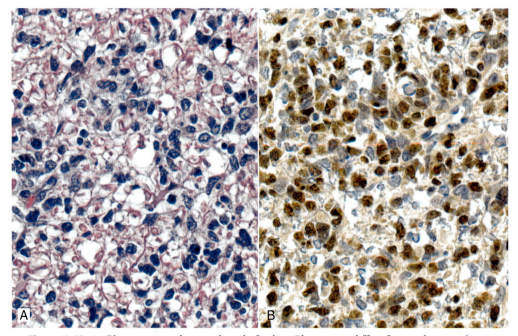

Figure 1-12 A. Gliomatosis in the spinal cord of a dog. Gliomatosis differs from a discrete glioma by the preservation of tissue architecture and lack of a mass effect. **B.** Nuclear labeling of the neoplastic cells with **immunohistochemistry for Olig-2** indicates their derivation from oligodendrocytes.

Additional –ologies

Ancillary testing may be required to reach definitive diagnoses. Tests available in each laboratory may advantageously be listed by disease syndrome and animal species. The common disease syndromes—respiratory disease, alimentary disease, abortion, unexpected death, suspected poisoning—may each have a template of available tests to ensure uniformity of investigations.

Microbiology: bacteriology, mycoplasmology, mycology, virology

The purpose of diagnostic microbiology is to confirm the suspicion of infectious disease and to identify the etiologic agent, often by bacterial or fungal culture or virus isolation. When the pathologist suspects infectious disease, microbiologic assays are selected based on the differential diagnosis established from the history, postmortem examination, or histologic evaluation, and on the availability of validated tests. Staying abreast of emerging diseases and rapidly developing diagnostic methods requires continuing education. The pathologist should consult the microbiologist (bacteriologist, mycologist, virologist, etc.) to learn the available (in-house) assays and preferred specimens to submit for the suspected disease.

Parasitology

The pathologist can diagnose many parasitisms by gross examination if the parasite is numerous enough to encounter and large enough to be seen with the naked eye (e.g., tapeworms, strongyles). Many of the clinical parasitology tests are also applicable in postmortem examination. Cytologic evaluation of scrapings is useful in the diagnosis of arthropod infestations of the skin. Fecal flotation examination is commonly used to detect parasite ova and is particularly useful in monitoring herd status or in the detection of those parasites that may not be evident on gross examination or in histologic sections. Cytology of a fecal smear augments the fecal examination and is used to detect organisms that may not float as well as parasitic eggs, such as coccidian oocysts, cryptosporidia, and other protozoa. The Baermann funnel technique is more cumbersome, and is used mainly in the diagnosis of lungworms. Finally, the pathologist may first encounter a parasitic organism in histologic sections. Knowledge of the appearance of protozoa, helminths, or arthropods in histologic sections helps to classify them to an extent, but molecular assays may be necessary for speciation for structurally similar organisms, such as the Apicomplexan protozoa.

Immunology

Immunologic assays augment microbiologic testing in screening for infectious disease and are used in the documentation of immunodeficiencies or immune-mediated/autoimmune diseases. Immunohistochemistry is one example of application of an immunologic assay to histologic evaluation. In frozen tissues, direct fluorescent antibody (FA) tests are used for rapid identification of bacterial or viral antigens. Conversely, indirect immunofluorescence employs a secondary antibody to detect host immunoglobulins, either antibodies to an infectious agent, or autoantibodies or immune complexes in immune-mediated diseases.

Serology usually refers to immunologic assays of serum or other fluids, including fetal fluids, for antibodies to infectious agents. These are typically quantitative assays in which the serum titer, especially a change in serum titer over a period of time, can indicate the state of the disease or distinguish between exposure and active infection. Immunoglobulin concentration can also be assayed in fetal fluids to indicate in utero exposure to infectious agents, or in serum to diagnose failure of passive transfer (of maternal antibodies) or other immunodeficiencies. Qualitative serology can document the presence of circulating autoantibodies.

Molecular biology

In diagnostic pathology, molecular biology technologies are used mainly for identification and characterization of infectious agents. Polymerase chain reaction (PCR) tests are based on amplification of a segment of nucleic acid, even down to the single molecule level; this makes PCR tests more sensitive than most other microbiologic assays. However, *the identification of nucleic acid of a microorganism does not equal diagnosis of a disease*. The pathologist must interpret the detection of an infectious agent, such as *Coxiella burnetii* in ovine or caprine fetal tissues, in context. The disadvantage of PCR tests on homogenized samples is that nucleic acid detection cannot be colocalized with a lesion or with a particular cellular location. When precise localization of the reaction is necessary, in situ tests must be used.

The PCR test can be used in *multiplex assays* for groups of bacterial, viral, protozoal, fungal, or tick-borne agents, or for groups of microorganisms that cause abortion, respiratory disease, or diarrhea in a particular species. If an unknown agent is isolated in pure culture, or if the biologic sample contains a single pathogen, universal PCR amplification of 16S or 18S rRNA followed by sequencing can allow speciation of the isolate or identification of the pathogen directly from the biologic sample. In addition, PCR can be used to validate another testing modality, for example, to document the presence of a cell marker when found by immunohistochemistry in an unusual site.

Detection of infectious agents by PCR may be augmented by, or even supplanted by, various *next generation gene sequencing* options, such as massively parallel sequencing to identify multiple organisms or microbiota, or whole genome sequencing. Other molecular diagnostic technologies, such as loop-mediated isothermal amplification and DNA microarrays, continue to be developed.

Clinical pathology, cytopathology

Clinical pathology, by definition, refers to the study of specimens from live animals; however, results from clinical pathology tests, such as serum biochemistries, often are the basis for biopsy and are used in establishing the differential diagnosis at postmortem examination. Many times, with biopsy or autopsy specimens, a preliminary diagnosis has been based on serum biochemistry or cytologic examination; the latter is particularly useful for mass lesions. Cytology is also used postmortem for rapid (within minutes) identification of parasites, preliminary diagnosis of masses, or evaluation of exudates. Cytology is the microscopic evaluation of cytoplasmic and nuclear detail that cannot be resolved in histologic sections of formalin-fixed, paraffin-embedded tissue. However, the structural relationships and patterns that are an integral part of histologic diagnosis are difficult or impossible to appreciate in cytologic preparations. Ideally, cytologic and histologic findings should be correlated and reconciled as the case is being closed.

Toxicology

Toxicosis should be suspected when illness or death is unexpected and not readily explained, when there has been an environmental change (new feed, new water source, change in premises), or when multiple animals in a group are affected simultaneously. Many toxic diseases do not have associated gross lesions. In these cases, tissue selection should be based on laboratory protocol, history, and consultation with the toxicologist. Tissues that are commonly frozen in suspected toxicosis cases with no specific lesions include brain, gastric content, aqueous humor, liver, kidney, urine, and adipose tissue. Suspected source material should be submitted and saved.

Imaging

Diagnostic imaging (radiology, computed tomography [CT], positron emission tomography [PET], ultrasound, magnetic resonance imaging [MRI]) is used to localize lesions, to determine their density and texture, and to recognize patterns antemortem. Radiology is the imaging modality that has been in use the longest. It is so applicable for bone pathology that many pathologists refuse to evaluate a bone biopsy without a radiograph. The different modalities are variably useful for evaluation of different tissues; for instance, a CT scan is better for bony tissue, whereas MRI is particularly useful in cross-sectional evaluation of the brain. Although certain lesions, such as edema, may be subtle or undetectable grossly at postmortem examination, they may be readily evident with brain MRI. In many cases, MRI cross-sections look strikingly like gross slices of brain.

Genetics

Diagnostic genetics has evolved from breeding studies used to classify Mendelian defects, through cytologic karyotyping of metaphase chromosome preparations, to molecular analysis of mutations with sequencing of amplified DNA. Genetic laboratories offer testing for animal diseases in which the mutated gene has been identified and the mutation is known. Typical requested specimens from live animals are EDTA-treated blood, pulled hairs (with the root), or cheek (buccal mucosa) swabs. The testing laboratory should be consulted for preferred specimens from cadavers. New genetic diseases are discovered when a new syndrome appears. Pathologists document the lesions in emerging genetic diseases and collaborate with geneticists to find the affected gene and characterize the mutation. When a similar disease is recognized in another species for which the mutated gene is known, genome sequencing data can direct the search for the mutated gene in the new species.

Photography

Macroscopic photography and photomicroscopy are integral parts of evaluation of lesions. Photographic documentation of animal identity and any pertinent lesions is paramount in the legal autopsy, but also useful in routine diagnostic pathology as a record to consult when writing reports and for teaching purposes. *Macroscopic photography* generally requires a lighting source (flash for handheld cameras to limit the exposure time). For close-up photography, the specimen and the camera must be immobile for sharp images. Other considerations for macrophotography include specimen base, such as nonglare glass over a black box; background color (to some degree, the pathologist's preference, but neutral [black or shades of gray] has been recommended); lighting source, position, and timing; and type of camera. Manual focus with a small aperture maximizes the depth of field for optimal focus of three-dimensional specimens; a larger aperture can be used to increase the lighting of flat surfaces.

For *photomicroscopy*, camera selection is, again, the major choice. Depending on the camera and software used, the photographer must adjust lighting, set the white balance, align the microscope for Köhler illumination to achieve optimal resolution and contrast, and focus. Most software programs include a focusing device, which is especially useful at low magnification. With virtual microscopic images, focusing is automatic.

Further reading

Chandler FW, et al. Color Atlas and Text of the Histopathology of Mycotic Disease. Chicago, Ill: Year Book Medical Publishers, Inc.; 1980.

Gardiner CH, et al. An Atlas of Protozoan Parasites in Animal Tissues. 2nd ed. Washington, DC: Armed Forces Institute of Pathology; 1998.

Gardiner CH, Poynton SL. An Atlas of Metazoan Parasites in Animal Tissues. Armed Forces Institute of Pathology. Gurnee, Ill: CL Davis DVM Foundation; 1999, revised 2006.

Case interpretations and client service
Decision analysis

Specimens generally are submitted either as whole bodies (live animals or cadavers) or as parts thereof (e.g., formalin-fixed or unfixed ["fresh"] surgical biopsy or postmortem specimens collected by a surgeon, internist, or other nonpathologist practitioner). Pathology specimens may be accompanied by other specimens for toxicology, bacteriology, virology, serology, molecular diagnostics, or other laboratory sections. Some specimens need only pathology examination, but in other cases, in which the submitting veterinarian has not specified the desired testing, *routing of specimens through the diagnostic laboratory may fall to the assigned pathologist*, who decides what additional testing beyond gross and histologic examination is needed to reach a diagnosis or case interpretation (Fig. 1-13).

Case coordination

In most diagnostic settings, *the final integration of results from various laboratory sections falls to the case pathologist* as the person most suited to interpret test results in light of the clinical and pathologic findings. A positive identification of an infectious agent or a toxic compound does not always equal disease diagnosis of an infection or poisoning.

Weighting of competing etiologies, cut-offs, explanations

In many cases, multiple and disparate lesions are encountered in the same cadaver at autopsy or even in the same surgical specimen. One or more of these lesions could account for, or contribute to, the reported clinical signs or death of the animal. Alternatively, an animal might have one disease condition of multifactorial cause. When more than one lesion or etiologic agent is encountered in a diagnostic case, the pathologist must summarize the findings, interpret results from laboratory tests, and explain the decision analysis to the submitting veterinarian.

Even when an accession is subjected only to histologic examination, the results can be complicated. Consider the following case: Multiple disparate lesions were found in a surgical biopsy specimen from a dog with sudden onset of "testicular" swelling. Histologically, an interstitial cell tumor was encountered in each testis. Ordinarily, in the surgical biopsy practice, a diagnosis of testicular interstitial cell tumor would be the end point. However, in this case, the dog also had arteriosclerosis of the testicular arteries bilaterally, which had resulted in atrophied (rather than swollen) testes. In addition, both interstitial cell tumors were so small that they could not have been palpated in the live animal and could not have accounted for the reported swelling. Fortunately, the scrotum was also submitted in formalin, and further examination detected pyogranulomatous dermatitis, which explained the swelling. Inflammation was severe and widespread in the ample scrotal samples, but yeasts were few and hard to find with H&E. Even with Gomori's methenamine

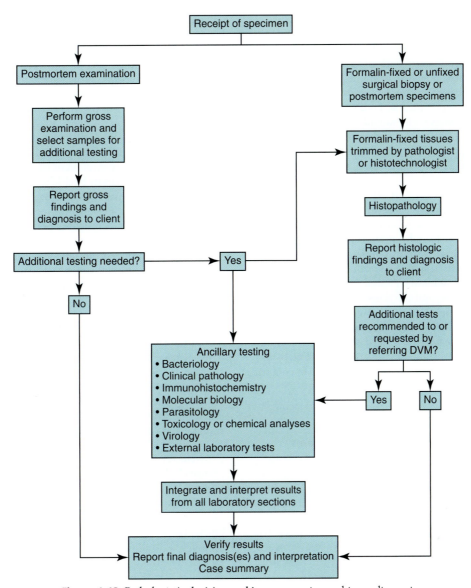

Figure 1-13 Pathologist's **decision-making process** in reaching a diagnosis.

silver histochemistry, few yeasts were encountered, but one yeast had a broad-based bud, allowing a presumptive diagnosis of blastomycosis. Inflammation did not involve the testes or vaginal tunics, but the submitting veterinarian should still be concerned about systemic blastomycosis. In summary, the dog had testicular lesions, including bilateral interstitial cell tumors, but these were all incidental findings and, in reality, the testes were smaller than normal rather than swollen. In a case such as this, a diagnosis of interstitial cell tumor is not useful to the client, and the pathologist must recall that scrotal swelling is often classified clinically as testicular swelling and must seek an explanation for the reported clinical problem.

The end point of a postmortem or surgical biopsy examination is the diagnosis that explains the reported clinical problem or the salient gross lesions, rather than a mere cataloguing of lesions.

Economic considerations

Economic considerations are a limiting factor in diagnostic testing. Realistically, diagnostic testing must be cost-efficient in herd, flock, kennel, and cattery settings, i.e., must be good for the group and can seldom be justified for an individual animal unless that animal has exceptional genetic potential. For companion animals, economic decisions are made, not for the good of the group, but for an individual animal; however, economic constraints of the pet owners, most of whom do not have medical insurance for their pets, still limit the extent of diagnostic testing, especially postmortem diagnostic testing. Agriculture departments may subsidize the cost of diagnostic testing for livestock. In diagnostic laboratories affiliated with teaching institutions, diagnostic testing and the development of new diagnostic tests is part of the educational process, so part of the expense may be borne by educational resources or grant monies. Retrospective and prospective studies by pathologists in conjunction with clinicians and other scientists are instrumental in the development of more effective and more efficient diagnostic assays. At autopsy, or in the surgical biopsy practice, it is usually the pathologist who decides which ancillary tests to use to reach the best diagnosis or case interpretation. The pathologist can cut expenses and shepherd resources by analyzing each case and requesting the most useful and efficient ancillary tests.

Final reports
In any case, the style of the final written report should suit the purpose of the report. Extensive descriptive detail may be important for board-style examinations and Good Laboratory Practice (GLP) reports; however, of more importance to the client in diagnostic laboratory reports are the final diagnoses and comments or interpretation of findings. Details that may contribute to case management should be included; exhaustive histologic descriptions may be of limited value. Findings must be communicated clearly, statements should be unambiguous, and all of the questions that led to the investigation should have been addressed.

Unfortunately, despite the best efforts of pathologists and ancillary services, a definitive cause of disease or death may not be obtained, and the final report may conclude "No diagnosis." The history may have been inadequate or misleading. The submission may have been incomplete (e.g., placenta not available or not submitted with an abortion case). Economics may have precluded additional confirmatory testing. The cause may have been beyond the scope of a pathology investigation (e.g., environmental, genetic, nutritional). *Although a definitive diagnosis cannot always be reached, several specific causes of disease should have been ruled out*, thereby avoiding unnecessary interventions. In some cases, the next step may be to request additional specimens in order to make or confirm a diagnosis.

Quality assurance of pathology services
Accreditation of laboratories: quality programs
Compliance with internationally recognized standards (e.g., ISO 9001:2008, ISO/IEC 17025), can be maintained to assure quality of laboratory testing, ensure the release of credible results, and to support continuous improvement. North American public veterinary diagnostic laboratories may be accredited periodically by the American Association of Veterinary Laboratory Diagnosticians (AAVLD) to ensure excellence in diagnostic service, conformity with regulatory requirements, quality of testing and equipment, and awareness of scientific advances. Accredited laboratories must implement and conform to a quality system that is monitored by a designated staff member and defines best practices for record maintenance, testing methods, physical facilities and equipment, specimen handling, personnel qualifications, and client satisfaction.

Test validation
Diagnostic tests, especially those for infectious diseases, are validated by documentation of internal or inter-laboratory performance using reference standards and relevant diagnostic specimens. This should be corroborated by the endorsement of diagnostic organizations, such as the World Organisation for Animal Health (WOAH/OIE), by publications in peer-reviewed scientific journals, or by direct comparison with an established method.

Occupational health and safety, biosafety/biocontainment
Biosafety and biocontainment are based on risk assessment to choose the most appropriate microbiologic practices, physical barriers, and personal protective equipment to prevent laboratory-acquired infections. Procedures must of course also be in place to prevent the spread of infectious agents from the laboratory, and to prevent cross-contamination of specimens under examination or testing.

In addition to protection from infectious agents, diagnostic laboratory staff must also be protected during postmortem examinations from physical injury by sharp instruments, power tools, heavy carcasses, noise, and slips and falls, and from chemical injury or hypersensitivity reactions to fixatives, disinfectants, cleaning solutions, animal-derived allergens, and toxins. Assessment of risk mandates handling of select agents at levels greater than Biosafety Level 2. Training in the use of safety equipment and enrollment of all at-risk laboratory personnel in an occupational health program ensures best practice protection against infectious agents and physical injury through vaccination, personal protective equipment, barriers, and other safeguards. Because the performance of postmortem examinations and long hours sitting at the microscope and computer can also result in fatigue and physical injury, ergonomic desks, chairs, and instruments, including microscopes, should be part of the occupational health program.

Initial and ongoing competence of pathologists
Certification of pathologists
The science and art of pathology are learned through advanced training and practice. Optimally, pathologists in an accredited diagnostic laboratory are certified by a college of veterinary pathology and have documented experience in the practice of diagnostic pathology. As a minimum, pathologists should have training and experience beyond the veterinary degree.

Proficiency testing, peer review, requests for second opinions
Perhaps because it is an art as well as a science, pathology may be the least-regulated discipline in the diagnostic laboratory. However, the pathologist in a diagnostic setting must work efficiently to keep up with the work flow. Furthermore, although a diagnosis is, to some extent, an opinion, the accuracy of diagnosis and the correlation of pathology reports with the clinical complaint should be subjected to proficiency testing and peer review. Proficiency tests are offered by various organizations, including the Veterinary Laboratory Association (VLA) and AAVLD (mainly for immunohistochemistry performance and interpretation).

More general peer review is usually an internal process in which staff pathologists review selected cases of other staff pathologists, and this review is documented. The clientele of a diagnostic laboratory should be invited to request second opinions (either from internal or external pathologists) if the pathology report is not in accord with the clinical impression or for any other reason. The second opinion should be rendered in the same manner as the first opinion, that is to say "blindly," at least initially and when possible, without knowledge of the signalment, history, clinical impression, or the first pathologist's opinion. Errors and opportunities for improvement are to be documented in the laboratory's corrective action/preventive action (CAPA) system within their quality program.

Continuing education, documentation
Documentation of continuing education and competence is as important as the initial specialty certification. The practicing pathologist must be aware of emerging diseases, changes in disease trends, and state of the art diagnostic testing.

Documentation of these activities contributes to the proof of continuous improvement of the laboratory's services, which is the intent of laboratory quality programs.

CONCLUSION

The purpose of this introductory chapter is to remind the reader that, although these volumes are organized into chapters based on particular organ systems, systemic pathology is a study of disease that affects the entire body. The pathologist is uniquely situated to extrapolate from the molecular level to the whole organism, and to study disease in individual animals or in herds, kennels, or other population settings. Because diagnostic specimens often arrive without antemortem evidence to incriminate a particular organ system or a particular category of injurious agents, or (worse) with misleading information, the pathologist must be well-educated (well-trained and continuously self-educated) and remain open-minded to:
- evaluate the body as a whole,
- correlate the structural with the biochemical/molecular changes of disease,
- interpret lesions and distinguish between primary and secondary lesions,
- coordinate pathologic changes with antemortem findings and ancillary postmortem test results, and
- render a final diagnosis (or, in some cases, the first diagnosis) that explains the events that led to disease or death, that addresses the identified problem, and that contributes to the health and productivity of livestock, companion animals, and research subjects.

Further reading

Munson L, et al. Elements of good training in anatomic pathology. Vet Pathol 2010;47:995-1002.

Obenson K, Wright CM. The value of 100% retrospective peer review in a forensic pathology practice. J Forensic Leg Med 2013; 20:1066-1068.

OECD Principles of Good Laboratory Practice (as revised in 1997), Environment Directorate, Organisation for Economic Co-operation and Development. Paris 1998. ENV/MC/CHEM(98)17 and OECD guidance on the GLP requirements for peer review of histopathology (draft, 2013).

Requirements for an accredited veterinary medical diagnostic laboratory. American Association of Veterinary Laboratory Diagnosticians, version 6.1, June, 2012.

World Organization for Animal Health (OIE). Principles and methods of validation of diagnostic assays for infectious diseases. In: OIE Manual of Diagnostic Tests and Vaccines for Terrestrial Animals. 7th ed. Paris: World Organization for Animal Health (OIE); 2012. p. 34-51.

 For more information, please visit the companion site: PathologyofDomesticAnimals.com

CHAPTER 2

Bones and Joints

Linden E. Craig • Keren E. Dittmer • Keith G. Thompson

DISEASES OF BONES	17
GENERAL CONSIDERATIONS	17
STRUCTURE AND FUNCTION OF BONE TISSUE	17
Cellular elements	17
Bone matrix	19
Matrix mineralization	20
Structural organization of bone tissue	20
Development and anatomy	21
Hormonal regulation of physeal growth	24
Modeling	24
Remodeling	26
Markers of remodeling	27
Blood supply	27
POSTMORTEM EXAMINATION OF THE SKELETON	28
Gross examination	28
Histologic techniques and stains	28
Preparation artifacts in histologic sections	29
Other laboratory techniques	29
RESPONSE TO MECHANICAL FORCES AND INJURY	30
Mechanical forces	30
Growth plate damage	30
Angular limb deformities	31
Periosteal damage	33
Fracture repair	33
Types of fractures	34
Process of fracture repair	34
Complications of fracture repair	35
Stress-related lesions in horses	36
GENETIC AND CONGENITAL DISEASES OF BONE	36
Generalized skeletal dysplasias	37
Chondrodysplasias	37
Chondrodysplasias of cattle	38
Chondrodysplasias of sheep	40
Chondrodysplasias of pigs	42
Chondrodysplasias of horses	42
Chondrodysplasias of dogs	43
Chondrodysplasias of cats	45
Osteogenesis imperfecta	46
Osteopetrosis	50
Congenital hyperostosis	53
Osteochondromatosis	54
Idiopathic multifocal osteopathy	54
Localized skeletal dysplasias	54
Limb dysplasias	54
Skull anomalies	56
Sternum and ribs	56
Pelvis	56
Vertebrae	57
Genetic diseases indirectly affecting the skeleton	57
Lysosomal storage diseases	57
Congenital erythropoietic porphyria	59
NUTRITIONAL AND HORMONAL BONE DISEASES	60
Nutritional imbalances affecting skeletal growth	60
Calcium, phosphorus, and vitamin D deficiency	61
Calcium and phosphorus homeostasis	61
Osteoporosis	63
Rickets and osteomalacia	68
Fibrous osteodystrophy	74
Other mineral imbalances	80
Other vitamin imbalances	82
TOXIC BONE DISEASES	84
Molybdenosis	84
Fluorosis	84
Lead toxicity	86
Vitamin A toxicity	86
Vitamin D toxicity	89
Plant toxicities	90
Other toxicities	91
HYPEROSTOTIC DISEASES	91
Craniomandibular osteopathy	91
Calvarial hyperostosis of Bullmastiffs	92
Hypertrophic osteopathy	92
Canine hepatozoonosis	94
OSTEONECROSIS	94
Morphology and fate of necrotic bone	95
Legg-Calvé-Perthes disease	97
INFLAMMATORY AND INFECTIOUS DISEASES OF BONES	97
Bacterial osteomyelitis	98
Fungal osteomyelitis	103
Viral infections of bones	104
Metaphyseal osteopathy	105
Canine panosteitis	106
TUMORS AND TUMOR-LIKE LESIONS OF BONES	107
Bone-forming tumors	109
Osteoma, ossifying fibroma, and fibrous dysplasia	109
Osteosarcoma	110
Cartilage-forming tumors	116
Chondroma	116
Osteochondroma	116
Multilobular tumor of bone	117
Chondrosarcoma	118
Fibrous tumors of bones	121
Vascular tumors of bones	122
Other primary bone tumors	122
Secondary tumors of bones	124
Tumor-like lesions of bones	125
DISEASES OF JOINTS	128
GENERAL CONSIDERATIONS	128
Fibrous joints	128
Cartilaginous joints	128
Synovial joints	129
Response of articular cartilage to injury	131
DEVELOPMENTAL DISEASES OF JOINTS	132
Osteochondrosis	132
Hip dysplasia	135
Cervical vertebral malformation-malarticulation	136
Luxations and subluxations	137
DEGENERATIVE DISEASES OF JOINTS	137
Synovial joints	137
Cartilaginous joints	143
Spondylosis	145
INFLAMMATORY DISEASES OF JOINTS	146
Fibrinous arthritis	146

Purulent (suppurative) arthritis	147	TUMORS AND TUMOR-LIKE LESIONS OF JOINTS	159
Infectious arthritis	148	Malignant tumors	159
Bacterial arthritis	148	Synovial cell sarcoma	159
Viral arthritis	154	Histiocytic sarcoma	159
Fungal arthritis	154	Other sarcomas	160
Protozoal arthritis	155	Benign tumors	160
Miscellaneous inflammatory lesions of joint structures	155	Synovial myxoma	160
Bursitis	155	Non-neoplastic lesions	162
Diskospondylitis	156	Synovial chondromatosis	162
Calcium crystal–associated arthropathy (pseudogout)	156	Synovial cysts	162
Immune-mediated polyarthritis	157	Synovial pad proliferation	163

ACKNOWLEDGMENTS

The update of the chapter is based on previous editions by Dr. Ken Jubb and Dr. Nigel Palmer. It is an honor to follow in their footsteps. We are grateful to the many pathologists who contributed illustrations to this chapter.

DISEASES OF BONES

GENERAL CONSIDERATIONS

Bone is a highly specialized connective tissue, its properties depending largely on the unique nature of its extracellular matrix. In addition to providing mechanical support and protecting key organ systems from traumatic injury, bone is intimately involved in the homeostasis of calcium, an essential cation in a wide range of bodily functions. Not only that, but new research suggests that bone is also involved in phosphorus metabolism and the regulation of glucose. In spite of their apparent inertia, *bones are dynamic organs, undergoing constant remodeling throughout life.* Even in mature individuals, bone tissue is continually undergoing localized resorption and replacement in response to the demands of mineral homeostasis and alterations in mechanical forces. The dynamic nature of bones is well illustrated by their impressive powers of repair following injury.

Because of the difficulties associated with processing mineralized tissue, the study of bones, both by researchers and diagnosticians, has lagged behind that of most other organ systems. The skeleton is seldom examined in detail during routine autopsy, and it is highly likely that many disorders go undiagnosed. Even in cases where a bone disease is suspected, many veterinary pathologists do not feel confident in their approach to making a diagnosis. *Familiarity with the gross and microscopic anatomy of bones, factors regulating bone formation and resorption, and an understanding of the responses of bone to injury are essential to an appreciation of the pathogenesis and pathology of bone diseases.* The initial sections of this chapter will therefore focus on these aspects and outline an approach to examining the skeleton at autopsy.

STRUCTURE AND FUNCTION OF BONE TISSUE

Cellular elements

Bone tissue consists of 4 cell types: *osteoblasts, osteocytes, lining cells,* and *osteoclasts.* The first 3 are derived from primitive osteoprogenitor cells of mesenchymal origin, which are present in bone as well as other tissues. Under the influence of the transcription factor Runx2 (runt-related transcription factor 2), mesenchymal cells differentiate to osteoprogenitor cells; subsequent differentiation depends on the balance of transcription factors. Chondrocytes are formed in the presence of SOX5, 6, and 9 (sex determining region Y—box 5, 6, 9); adipocytes are induced by PPARγ2 (peroxisome proliferator activator receptor); and osteoblasts develop when Runx2, osterix, and β-catenin signaling are high. Osteoclasts are derived from hematopoietic stem cells of the macrophage line.

Osteoblasts *are responsible for manufacturing osteoid,* the organic component of bone matrix. Active osteoblasts, which line surfaces where bone formation is occurring, have abundant rough endoplasmic reticulum and a prominent Golgi apparatus, reflecting their role in protein synthesis. Histologically, they appear as plump cuboidal cells with basophilic cytoplasm, their nuclei sometimes polarized away from the adjacent bone surface (Fig. 2-1). Not only do osteoblasts produce the osteoid of bone matrix, *they also play a role in initiating its mineralization,* although the mechanism is not fully understood. Osteoblasts are one of the central cells through

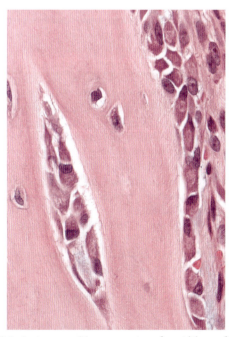

Figure 2-1 Active osteoblasts at a site of rapid bone formation in a newborn kitten. Note the eccentric nuclei, basophilic cytoplasm, and prominent Golgi zone in many of the cells. Some osteoblasts have surrounded themselves with osteoid to become osteocytes.

which bone resorption and formation are mediated. In addition to osteoid, they produce an array of regulatory factors that are deposited in bone matrix and that play a critical role in bone remodeling.

Inactive osteoblasts, or **bone-lining cells**, are flattened cells with few organelles that cover endosteal bone surfaces undergoing neither formation nor resorption. Although barely visible in histologic sections, these are the most abundant cells on the endosteal surface of the adult skeleton and link with each other to form a *functional barrier* between the extracellular fluid compartment of bone tissue and that of surrounding tissues; they also prevent association of osteoclast precursors with the bone surface. Bone-lining cells form the *bone-blood barrier* and control the movement of ions in and out of the extracellular fluid. When in areas of active remodeling, bone-lining cells express osteoblast markers such as RANKL (receptor activator of nuclear factor kappa B ligand), and may be the cell involved in direct cell-to-cell interaction with osteoclast precursors. In the bone remodeling unit, bone-lining cells are thought to *form a "roof" over the osteoclasts that are resorbing bone and osteoblasts that are resorbing bone*. In addition, under the action of intermittent parathyroid hormone (PTH), bone-lining cells *may revert to active osteoblasts*, thus allowing bone formation at sites of previous inactivity.

During active bone formation, ~10-20% of osteoblasts at regular intervals along a bone-forming surface surround themselves with osteoid and become **osteocytes** (see Fig. 2-1). *These are the most abundant cells of bone tissue, residing in small spaces (lacunae) within the mineralized matrix*. Newly formed osteocytes retain some morphologic and functional characteristics of osteoblasts, but as they mature and become embedded deeper in the mineralized matrix, the amount of rough endoplasmic reticulum in their cytoplasm is considerably reduced, and they develop features more typical of phagocytic cells. Osteocytes maintain contact with adjacent osteocytes, and with bone-lining cells or osteoblasts on the surface, by a network of branching cytoplasmic processes extending through *canaliculi*. In routinely stained histologic sections, the canaliculi are not visible and only the nuclei of osteocytes are usually apparent.

The direct effect of osteocytes on the formation and resorption of bone is controversial. The term *osteocytic osteolysis* was coined to describe the phenomenon whereby osteocytes could enlarge and fill in their lacunae, depending on PTH secretion and serum calcium concentrations; however, experimental evidence for this was lacking. Osteocytic osteolysis has been demonstrated in mice during lactation (resulting from increased parathyroid hormone–related protein, PTHrP), and may occur in hyperparathyroidism and under conditions that reduce mechanical loading.

Despite controversy surrounding the direct effects of osteocytes on bone formation and resorption, they are critical in the control of both processes. *Osteocytes produce the key bone regulatory factors* sclerostin, RANKL, and fibroblast growth factor 23 (FGF23), all likely under the control of PTH. Parathyroid hormone receptor activation (PTH/PTHrP receptor, PTH1R) results in decreased sclerostin, leading to increased Wnt signaling and subsequent activation of osteoblasts to form bone; at the same time, PTH leads to increased RANKL expression by osteocytes, resulting in increased osteoclastic bone resorption. *FGF23 produced by osteocytes is critical for phosphate homeostasis* and leads to phosphate excretion from the kidney.

Osteocytes form a *mechanosensation network* that assesses the mechanical loading of bone. The exact process by which this occurs is unclear; however, changes in fluid flow shear forces are detected by osteocyte processes, somehow activating them to produce nitric oxide, prostaglandins, bone morphogenetic proteins (BMPs), and Wnt proteins, which subsequently modify osteoblast and osteoclast activity. In humans, osteocytes can live for decades; however, osteocyte numbers do decrease with age, corresponding with a decrease in bone strength. Osteocyte apoptosis is an important part of the *response of bone to mechanical loading*. Both lack of mechanical stimulation and excessive mechanical loading resulting in fatigue damage lead to osteocyte apoptosis, which signals adjacent surviving osteocytes to express RANKL and stimulate osteoclastic resorption of the either unneeded or damaged bone. Mild to moderate mechanical loading inhibits osteocyte apoptosis and increases bone formation.

Osteoclasts *are primarily responsible for resorption of bone tissue*. They are derived through multiple fusions of cells from the monocyte/macrophage line. The key proteins involved in osteoclast formation are macrophage colony-stimulating factor (M-CSF) and receptor activator of nuclear factor kappa B (RANK). M-CSF production by the pre-monocyte allows differentiation to the osteoclast precursor, a cell that expresses RANK. This allows activation of osteoclast precursors by RANKL produced by osteoblasts and osteocytes, leading to fusion of osteoclast precursors and eventual formation of a mature osteoclast. Proinflammatory cytokines, particularly tissue necrosis factor-α (TNF-α), also stimulate production of RANK by osteoclast precursors.

Osteoclasts are rich in acid phosphatase and a range of other acid hydrolases that are packaged in primary lysosomes. The acid phosphatase isoenzyme present in osteoclasts is tartrate resistant (TRAP), unlike the tartrate-sensitive acid phosphatase found in monocytes and macrophages, and immunohistochemistry for TRAP may be used to identify osteoclasts in histologic sections. However, osteoclasts are usually easily recognizable histologically as *large, multinucleated cells* with eosinophilic cytoplasm, typically situated on bone surfaces and often within shallow pits called **Howship's lacunae** (Fig. 2-2). The presence of Howship's lacunae on a bone surface is convincing evidence of previous resorption at that site, even if no osteoclasts are present at the time of observation. Although not always apparent histologically, osteoclasts involved in active bone resorption have a highly specialized "ruffled" or brush border contiguous with the bone surface. A clear zone adjacent to the brush border is free of organelles but contains actin-like filaments, which may assist in anchoring the cell to the bone matrix. The attachment of active osteoclasts to the bone surface is an essential requirement for resorption to occur.

During **osteoclastic bone resorption**, an acid environment is created in the narrow space between the cell and the bone surface. Hydrogen and bicarbonate ions are generated from carbon dioxide and water by the action of carbonic anhydrase II. The protons are then pumped into the extracellular space by an H^+-ATPase, thereby creating the acidic environment required to dissolve bone mineral. To balance the charge and pH within the osteoclast, a chloride channel on the ruffled border allows movement of Cl^- into the extracellular space, and a HCO_3^-/Cl^- exchanger on the basolateral membrane removes bicarbonate from the cell. The activity of the acid hydrolases, released from osteoclasts when primary lysosomes

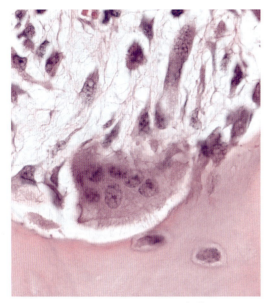

Figure 2-2 **Multinucleated osteoclast** in a shallow pit (Howship's lacuna) on a bone surface undergoing resorption. Note the ruffled border of the osteoclast adjacent to the bone.

fuse with the cell membrane of the brush border, is enhanced by the acidity of the local environment, and these enzymes break down the organic component of bone matrix. Fragments of degraded matrix are endocytosed by osteoclasts and further digested within secondary lysosomes.

The potential rate of removal of bone by osteoclasts is much greater than the rate of formation by osteoblasts. An individual osteoclast can erode ~400 µm^3 of bone, and travel 100 µm across a bone surface per hour. As a result, localized or generalized removal of bone during normal physiologic processes of modeling and remodeling, or in disease states, can occur very rapidly.

Once osteoclasts have completed their required phase of resorption, they undergo apoptosis and disappear from resorption sites. This is characterized by condensation of nuclear chromatin, loss of the ruffled border, and detachment from the bone surface. Inflammatory cytokines such as TNF-α and interleukin 1 (IL-1) enhance osteoclast survival, as does PTH. In cases of either nutritional or renal hyperparathyroidism, surviving osteoclasts are found in medullary spaces mixed with fibroblastic elements; this abnormal persistence of osteoclasts is an important aid to the diagnosis of these conditions.

Bone matrix

Bone matrix consists of *an organic component, called* **osteoid**, *and an inorganic component comprised predominantly of hydroxyapatite crystals*. The main constituent of osteoid (~90%) is **type I collagen**, which is also the predominant form of collagen in tendons, ligaments, dentine, and the ocular sclera. Each collagen molecule consists of 3 polypeptide chains assembled into a triple helix, a highly stable configuration resistant to proteolytic degradation, which forms the basic unit of all collagenous structures. The strength of bone and other collagenous structures is due in part to the manner in which individual collagen molecules are aggregated into fibrils, with each fibril overlapping its neighbor by about one quarter of its length. This creates a characteristic banding pattern, clearly evident on transmission electron microscopy. The tensile strength of collagenous structures is further enhanced by *intermolecular cross-links*, which form by the oxidative deamination of either lysyl or hydroxylysyl residues under the influence of the *copper-dependent enzyme lysyl oxidase*. The number of these cross-links in bone collagen is greater than that of the collagen types found in soft tissues. Interference with the formation of cross-links, as occurs in copper deficiency or certain toxicity diseases (see later), may significantly alter the mechanical properties of bone and other connective tissues.

Several *noncollagenous proteins* are produced by osteoblasts and consist of up to 10% of the organic matrix of bone. **Osteonectin** or **SPARC** (secreted protein, acidic, and rich in cysteine), a phosphoprotein that interacts with both type I collagen and hydroxyapatite, is found in the matrix immediately adjacent to osteoblasts and osteocytes. It may be important in the new intramembranous bone formation that occurs postfracture, and is thought to affect both osteoblast and osteoclast function.

Osteocalcin, also referred to as *bone-Gla protein* because of its γ-carboxyglutamic acid (Gla) residues, is abundant in bone, accounting for up to 10% of total noncollagenous proteins. Its synthesis by osteoblasts is *vitamin K dependent* and is increased 3-5 times by 1,25-dihydroxyvitamin D. Vitamin K is a cofactor of the carboxylase enzyme that adds 3 carboxyl-groups onto osteocalcin during post-translational modification. The carboxylated form of osteocalcin is deposited in osteoid before mineralization, and the presence of the carboxy- groups allows strong binding to calcium. Osteocalcin is thought to modify osteoblast and osteoclast activity, but its effects are controversial because osteocalcin has been shown to both increase and decrease bone formation by osteoblasts. It is also thought to increase the movement and activity of osteoclasts, and may be involved in the recruitment of osteoclasts to sites of bone resorption and remodeling. In vitro experiments suggest that osteocalcin inhibits matrix mineralization; however, osteocalcin-deficient mice have no change in bone mineral content or bone deposition rate, but the mice do have smaller less-perfect hydroxyapatite crystals. Osteocalcin's effects are not confined to bone. Recent research suggests that it is also involved in energy metabolism, where it enhances insulin sensitivity and pancreatic islet β-cell function. Other Gla-containing proteins, matrix-Gla protein and Gla-rich protein, are found in both cartilage and bone matrix, and because of this are thought to have roles in chondrogenesis and skeletal development, although their functions are not fully elucidated. Recently it has also been shown that matrix-Gla protein and Gla-rich protein are important inhibitors of vascular and soft tissue mineralization.

Other noncollagenous proteins found in bone matrix include the phosphorylated proteins **osteopontin** and **bone sialoprotein**. Bone sialoprotein is required for hydroxyapatite nucleation, whereas osteopontin physically blocks mineral formation. Both osteopontin and bone sialoprotein are involved in osteoclast differentiation and function. Many other glycoproteins and phosphoproteins are also found in bone, but their functions are either unknown or only just being clarified.

The **proteoglycans** (e.g., decorin, lumican, biglycan, epiphycan) of bone matrix are considerably smaller and less abundant than those found in cartilage matrix, possessing a relatively small protein core and only 1 or 2 glycosaminoglycan (chondroitin sulfate) side chains. The bone proteoglycans have important roles in all stages of bone formation, including matrix mineralization and cell proliferation. Proteoglycans are associated with various disease states; absence of proteoglycans is associated with a poorer prognosis in humans with osteosarcoma; proteoglycans are involved in soft tissue mineralization, and are also implicated in the pathogenesis of osteoporosis.

Bone matrix contains a *variety of growth factors* that are capable of inducing mitogenic responses in a range of cell types, including bone cells. These factors, which play important roles in bone development, modeling, and remodeling, especially at the local level, include bone morphogenetic proteins, fibroblast growth factors, platelet-derived growth factors, insulin-like growth factors, and transforming growth factor-β (TGF-β).

The **inorganic (mineral) component** of bone matrix is known to consist largely of **hydroxyapatite** [$Ca_{10}(PO_4)_6(OH)_2$], but its structure and properties are poorly understood. In addition to calcium and phosphate, bone mineral contains considerable quantities of *carbonate, magnesium, sodium,* and *zinc,* not all of which are available for exchange. *Fluoride* is also present in small amounts in bone matrix. Ultrastructurally, hydroxyapatite is present in bone matrix either as thin, needle-like crystals oriented in the same direction as collagen fibrils, or as an amorphous, granular phase, depending on the type of bone.

Matrix mineralization

The mineralization of skeletal tissues is a highly complex process, and is only partly understood. In organ systems throughout the body, extracellular tissue fluids in equilibrium with plasma are supersaturated with respect to hydroxyapatite. Many also contain type I collagen similar to that in bone, but mineralization does not normally occur. This is most likely due to the presence of potent inhibitors, which must be enzymatically degraded or activated before mineralization can be initiated. For example; although carboxylated matrix-Gla protein is a potent inhibitor of mineralization in soft tissues, either a lack of matrix-Gla protein or the presence of uncarboxylated matrix Gla-protein is associated with ectopic mineralization. In bone, the selective and localized degradation of such inhibitors, and the synthesis by osteoblasts of unique molecules that promote mineralization, could account for the orderly manner in which mineral deposition occurs in bone matrix. However, the presence of substrates that promote nucleation at humoral solute concentrations is also required.

Matrix vesicles, *tiny extracellular organelles originating as cytoplasmic blebs from osteoblasts, chondrocytes, and odontoblasts*, play an important role in initiating the mineralization process. These vesicles are rich in enzymes such as phospho1 (a phosphatase); ectonucleotide pyrophosphatase/phosphodiesterase 1 (ENPP1); metalloproteinases (MMPs) and tissue-nonspecific alkaline phosphatase (ALP); channels/transporters such as Pit 1 and 2 (Na^+/PO_4^{3-} symporter); phospholipids, particularly phosphatidylserine; and other components such as annexins and integrins. It is believed that the *key event in the initiation of mineralization is an alteration in the phosphate to inorganic pyrophosphate ratio*; inorganic pyrophosphate, together with osteopontin, inhibits mineralization. Two enzymes in the matrix vesicle are responsible for maintaining/altering the concentration of phosphate and inorganic pyrophosphate, ALP and ENPP1. Upregulation of ALP is the key event, and this leads to decreased pyrophosphate and increased phosphate, allowing mineralization to proceed. Two theories exist as to the mechanism involved in the initial nucleation of hydroxyapatite crystals: Either nucleation occurs within the matrix vesicle as a result of calcium and phosphate transportation into the vesicle by annexin (Ca^{2+}) and the Pit symporters (PO_4^{3-}), or direct nucleation of hydroxyapatite on collagen fibrils, perhaps using noncollagenous bone proteins.

Once the initial crystal has formed, the extracellular calcium and phosphate levels are generally adequate to allow continuous crystal propagation, with the preformed crystals acting as templates, until the entire aqueous space of the collagen fiber is filled with hydroxyapatite crystals. The mineralization of individual fibers occurs rapidly, as evidenced by the sharp division between highly and sparsely mineralized matrix at the junction between mineralized bone and osteoid seams. Osteoid does not become mineralized for 5-10 days after deposition. As a result, *a thin layer of unmineralized osteoid*, the **osteoid seam**, covers the surfaces where bone is being formed. Although not always apparent histologically in demineralized tissue sections, the osteoid seam is usually more eosinophilic than previously mineralized bone tissue and, in lamellar bone, separated from it by a *basophilic line*, the **mineralization front**. The osteoid seam may be 5-15 μm in depth, depending on the rate of bone formation. Once mineralization of osteoid begins, it occurs very rapidly, with >60% of the matrix becoming mineralized almost immediately. However, the remaining deposition of mineral is a slow cumulative process that can take weeks to complete.

Structural organization of bone tissue

Although the cellular elements of bone tissue, and the basic composition of the matrix, are relatively constant, there is variation in the organization of these components both at the macroscopic and microscopic level. The adult skeleton consists predominantly of mature **lamellar bone**, where the collagen fibers of the bone matrix are oriented in parallel layers. This pattern is clearly apparent in histologic sections viewed under polarized light. Osteocytes are in small slit-like lacunae between layers in a regular pattern, their distribution reflecting the orderly manner in which osteoblasts manufacture lamellar bone. In dense cortical bone, the lamellae are organized into **osteons** or **Haversian systems**, consisting of concentric lamellae surrounding a central vascular canal (Fig. 2-3). *Osteons run longitudinally through the cortex and are cemented together by interstitial lamellae.* The trabecular or cancellous bone of medullary cavities consists of variable numbers of lamellae arranged parallel to the surface rather than organized into osteons.

The alternating pattern of birefringent and nonbirefringent layers in lamellar bone has traditionally been interpreted as reflecting a 90° switch in orientation of collagen fibers between successive layers, creating a structure with physical strength similar to plywood. This model had remained unquestioned since the early 20th century, but has been challenged by recent studies using scanning electron microscopy. An alternative model proposes that lamellar bone consists of alternating layers of collagen organized into cylindrical rods and disordered collagen where loosely packed fibers are embedded in greater amounts of ground material run in multiple directions.

A variant of lamellar bone is often seen on the weight-bearing aspects of the long bones of rapidly growing animals, especially young ruminants. In these areas, the outer cortex is

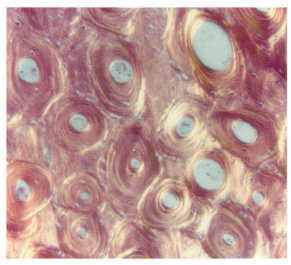

Figure 2-3 Transverse section of cortical bone viewed under polarized light to show the **osteons** or **Haversian systems,** which consist of concentric lamellae of bone surrounding a central vascular canal.

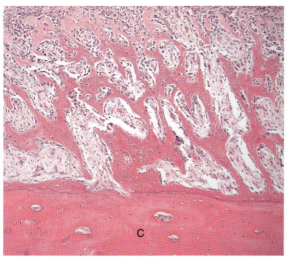

Figure 2-4 Trabeculae of **woven bone** emerging from the cortex (C) beneath an elevated periosteum. The osteocytes in the woven bone are more numerous than in the mature lamellar bone of the cortex and are irregularly distributed. The matrix of the woven bone is slightly more basophilic than that of the mature bone.

often arranged in laminar arrays rather than conventional Haversian systems, and is known as **laminar bone.**

In the developing fetus, and at sites of rapid bone formation during postnatal life, the *collagen fibers in bone matrix are arranged in a haphazard, interwoven fashion.* This immature form of bone tissue is referred to as **woven bone**, or coarse-bundle bone. Its matrix is more basophilic than that of lamellar bone, and the osteocytes are larger, more numerous, and are irregularly arranged (Fig. 2-4). During skeletal maturation and remodeling, woven bone is resorbed and replaced with lamellar bone, which has greater strength, but woven bone is seen in adults at sites where bone is produced rapidly in response to injury, inflammation or neoplasia. Fracture calluses invariably contain this form of bone tissue, as do bone-forming tumors.

A third type of bone, **chondroid bone**, arises directly from fibrocartilaginous origins and is found in ossifying tendon sheaths, bone derived from neural crest origins, and probably in some mixed tumors.

Further reading

Golub EE. Biomineralization and matrix vesicles in biology and pathology. Semin Immunopathol 2011;33:409-417.

Klein-Nulend J, et al. Mechanosensation and transduction in osteocytes. Bone 2013;54:182-190.

Neve A, et al. Osteocalcin: skeletal and extra-skeletal effects. J Cell Physiol 2013;228:1149-1153.

Reznikov N, et al. Three-dimensional structure of human lamellar bone: the presence of two different materials and new insights into the hierarchical organization. Bone 2014;59:93-104.

Zhou X, et al. Phosphate/pyrophosphate and MV-related proteins in mineralization: discoveries from mouse models. Int J Biol Sci 2012;8:778-790.

Development and anatomy

There are 2 distinct processes by which bone formation occurs in the developing fetus. *Most of the skull bones develop by intramembranous ossification.* The pathology of **the cranial bones** often differs from bones elsewhere in the body, and some of the cranial bones may be spared in disorders that affect other bones. This is probably because of the complex origins of the cranial bones. The bones of the skull can be divided into the *neurocranium* (cranial vault) of mesodermal origin, and the *viscerocranium* (facial skeleton) of neural crest origin. Most bones of the viscerocranium (with the exception of the ear bones and the ventral part of the mandible) are formed by intramembranous ossification. The neurocranium is further divided into the *dermatocranium*, which forms by intramembranous ossification, and the *chondrocranium* (the base of the skull plus the ethmoid bone), which forms by endochondral ossification. Some bones, such as the occipital bone, temporal bone, and sphenoid bone, have elements that form by both intramembranous and endochondral ossification before fusing to form a single bone.

Mesenchymal progenitor cells migrate from the cranial neural crest to form condensations at specific, highly vascular sites in the head region (and some other flat bones), where they differentiate directly into osteoblasts and produce anastomosing trabeculae of woven bone. Wnt signaling (canonical and noncanonical) is intimately involved in all stages of skeletal development, including craniofacial, limb, and joint development. A number of other transcription factors and genes also control craniofacial development, including homeobox-containing transcription factors, basic helix-loop-helix transcription factors, *Pax* genes, bone morphogenetic protein 4, and TGF-α. These centers of ossification expand by ongoing osteoblastic differentiation of mesenchymal cells at the periphery and apposition of new bone on the surface of trabeculae, to form a plate. A fibrous layer, the periosteum, separates the developing membrane bone from adjacent tissues and controls its shape. Individual bones of the developing skull are separated by connective tissue **sutures** that remain as active sites of intramembranous bone production, and are probably the site of origin for the distinctive tumor that arises in the skull, the multilobular tumor of bone. Growth factors involved in the regulation of suture formation include FGFR1,

2, 3; TGF-β1, 2, 3; ephrin-eph receptor signaling; BMPs; and MSX1 and 2 (msh homeobox-1, -2). It is thought that a gradient of growth factor signaling between the bones of a suture helps control and direct bone formation. Once growth stops, a bony union forms at the site of the sutures. With maturity, the woven bone is remodeled and replaced by lamellar bone. *Intramembranous bone formation also occurs at the periosteal surfaces of all bones during growth.*

Most bones of the skeleton, including those of the limbs, vertebral column, pelvis, and base of the skull, develop by **endochondral ossification**. In this process, cells from the lateral plate mesoderm, which form the appendicular skeleton, and cells from the paraxial mesoderm, which form the axial skeleton, arrange into condensations of primitive mesenchymal cells, which then differentiate into chondrocytes and produce crude cartilage models of the adult bone destined to form at that site. At this stage, chondrocytes are expressing type II, IX, and XI collagen, aggrecan, chondromodulin-1, and matrilin-3 under the control of the transcription factor SOX9. An avascular fibrous layer, the perichondrium, surrounds each cartilage model. As expansion of the model continues by interstitial growth, chondrocytes near the center become hypertrophic and start to express type X collagen. The matrix around mature hypertrophic chondrocytes undergoes mineralization, and the chondrocytes express osteopontin, metalloproteinases-9 and -13, and vascular endothelial growth factor. Meanwhile, the perichondrium becomes invaded with capillaries, converting it into a periosteum, and perichondrial chondrocytes differentiate into osteoblasts that form a narrow cuff of bone by intramembranous ossification around the midshaft region of the developing bone. Capillaries and chondroclasts (closely related to, or the same as, osteoclasts) invade the hypertrophic cartilage from the periosteum and establish a vascular network. Pre-osteoblasts also enter with the invading capillaries and differentiate into osteoblasts, which deposit osteoid on remnants of the mineralized cartilage, creating a **primary ossification center**. This process of endochondral ossification continues as the chondrocytes at either end of the developing bone continue to proliferate, and the model expands in length and width. Once the bone reaches a certain stage of development, **secondary ossification center**s appear at one or both ends (depending on the bone), and expand by endochondral ossification to form the **epiphyses** of long bones. As the epiphyses expand, they remain separated from the primary ossification center, now occupying the **diaphysis** and **metaphysis** of the developing bone, by the **physis** or **growth plate**. Limited growth in size of the epiphysis continues by endochondral ossification beneath the articular cartilage at the articular-epiphyseal cartilage complex. The epiphyseal side of the growth plate soon becomes capped by a layer of trabecular bone, preventing further growth from that side, but proliferation of chondrocytes in the growth plate and endochondral ossification on the metaphyseal side continues until maturity. The gross anatomy and terminology of a developing long bone, in this case the femur of a newborn calf, is illustrated in Figure 2-5.

During active bone growth, *the hyaline cartilage of the growth plate is organized into 3 easily recognizable zones* (Fig. 2-6). A **reserve, or resting zone**, with irregularly dispersed chondrocytes and pale staining matrix, is anchored to the trabecular bone of the epiphysis. The chondrocytes in this zone have the lowest concentration of intracellular ionized calcium, but the matrix has the highest concentration of type

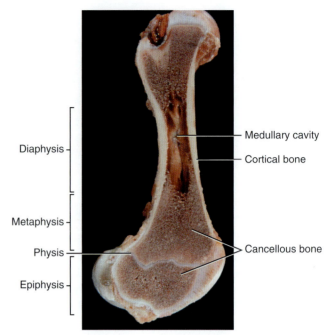

Figure 2-5 The femur from a newborn calf, illustrating the **gross anatomy and terminology** of the different regions.

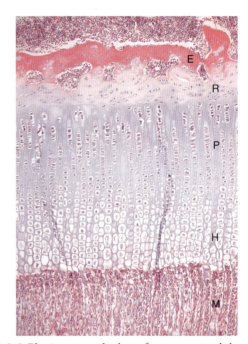

Figure 2-6 Physis or growth plate of a young animal showing the reserve (R), proliferative (P), and hypertrophic (H) zones. The reserve zone is anchored to trabecular bone of the epiphysis (E). Also note the abrupt transition from the hypertrophic zone of the physis to the metaphysis (M).

II collagen. In the **proliferative zone**, the chondrocytes are tightly packed into longitudinal columns, the cell at the top being the progenitor cell for longitudinal growth of each column. The chondrocytes in this zone are actively dividing, accumulating glycogen, and synthesizing matrix proteoglycans. The columns of chondrocytes are separated by deeply basophilic cartilage matrix rich in aggregated proteoglycans, which inhibit mineralization in spite of the presence of matrix vesicles. Within columns, only thin matrix septa separate individual chondrocytes. Indian hedgehog (Ihh) is a key regulator at this stage; via PTHrP, Ihh stimulates chondrocyte proliferation and inhibits chondrocyte hypertrophy, as well as regulating trabecular bone formation in the primary spongiosa. The transcription factor Runx2 has similar functions, and Wnt signaling is also important for chondrocyte survival, proliferation, and hypertrophy. Fibroblast growth factor receptor 3 (FGFR3) is a counterbalance to Ihh, and inhibits chondrocyte proliferation, whereas TGF-β inhibits chondrocyte maturation.

The chondrocytes of the **hypertrophic zone** become enlarged, but remain metabolically active and are responsible for preparing the matrix for mineralization. They rely on anaerobic glycolysis for energy production because of the distance from epiphyseal blood vessels, which terminate at the top of the proliferative zone, and the inability of oxygen to diffuse from the metaphysis through the mineralized matrix of the lower hypertrophic zone. The energy is used primarily in the accumulation, storage, and then release of calcium as part of the mineralization process. The lower region of the hypertrophic zone is commonly referred to as the zone of degeneration, because the chondrocytes appear to have separated from the pericellular matrix and become degenerate in sections prepared for histology and electron microscopy by routine methods. However, these chondrocytes are in fact highly differentiated cells capable of synthesizing type X collagen, chondrocalcin, and other macromolecules that, together with matrix vesicles, are likely to be involved in initiating matrix mineralization. *Mineralization of the cartilage matrix* occurs in the deepest layer of the hypertrophic zone and is an essential event in the process of endochondral ossification. This mineralized layer is not evident in histologic sections prepared after demineralization. *Hypertrophic chondrocytes in the lower mineralized zone undergo apoptosis so that the transition from growth plate to metaphysis is abrupt*, and is designated by the last intact layer of chondrocytes. This process of apoptosis is at least partially dependent on normal circulating concentrations of phosphate.

Around the perimeter of the growth plate there is a wedge-shaped groove of cells, termed the **ossification groove of Ranvier**. The cells in this groove proliferate and are responsible for increasing the diameter of the physis during growth. A dense layer of fibrous tissue, the **perichondrial ring of LaCroix**, surrounds the groove of Ranvier and is continuous with the fibrous layer of the periosteum. As such, it provides strong mechanical support at the bone-cartilage junction of the growth plate, an area that is prone to injury in fast-growing young animals. *Ext1* and *2* genes are important for perichondrial function, and mutations in these genes lead to decreased heparan sulfate, which results in increased cell responsiveness to bone morphogenetic proteins and subsequent excessive chondrogenesis, cartilage nodule formation, and hereditary multiple osteochondromas in humans.

From the metaphyseal side of the growth plate, chondroclasts attack the mineralized cartilage matrix and rapidly remove the delicate transverse septa between individual chondrocytes within columns, allowing vascular invasion. The thicker longitudinal septa of mineralized cartilage matrix between columns of chondrocytes are not resorbed at this stage. Instead, they provide a framework on which newly differentiated osteoblasts line up and deposit a layer of woven bone (Fig. 2-7). In the presence of Ihh, osteoblast progenitors differentiate and start to produce osteoblast markers, such as Runx2, alkaline phosphatase, osterix (Osx), and osteocalcin. Wnt signaling and the transcription factor Cfba1 are also key regulators of osteoblast differentiation and function. Runx2 and osterix are potent stimulators of extracellular matrix protein production by osteoblasts, including type I collagen, osteopontin, bone sialoprotein, and osteocalcin.

The lattice of trabeculae, with a basophilic core of mineralized cartilage covered by a thin, eosinophilic layer of bone, is termed the **primary spongiosa**. Trabeculae of the primary spongiosa extend at right angles to the direction of the growth plate, but deeper in the metaphysis, the trabeculae are remodeled by the coordinated action of osteoclasts and osteoblasts and are realigned in directions most suited to withstanding the mechanical forces acting on the bone. During this process, the cartilage cores and woven bone of the primary spongiosa are largely removed and replaced by thicker trabeculae of lamellar bone, which form the **secondary spongiosa**. While growth in length of a bone is continuing from the growth plate, osteoclastic resorption of trabeculae occurs at the metaphyseal-diaphyseal junction to create the medullary cavity.

The thickness of a growth plate is relatively constant across the width of the bone and is proportional to its rate of growth. So too is the distance to which trabeculae of the primary spongiosa extend into the metaphysis before they are remodeled. As growth slows, the different layers within the growth plate become narrow, and a transverse layer of trabecular bone forms on the metaphyseal side. The cartilage of the growth plate is then replaced with a bony scar, which is gradually remodeled into trabecular bone, blurring the margin between the epiphysis and metaphysis. The timing of growth plate closure varies both between and within bones and is

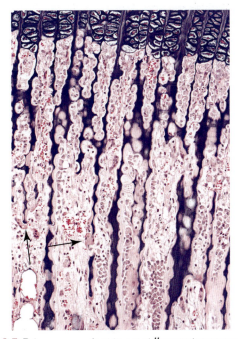

Figure 2-7 Primary spongiosa in a rapidly growing young animal. Basophilic spicules of mineralized cartilage matrix extend into the metaphysis at right angles to the growth plate and form a lattice on which osteoblasts are lining up and depositing osteoid. Osteoclasts (arrows) are resorbing some trabeculae from the medullary end.

controlled to a large degree by androgens and estrogens, but it is likely that nutritional factors can also play a role. At puberty a growth spurt occurs, likely caused by estrogen stimulation of the growth hormone–insulin-like growth factor I (GH-IGF-I) axis; this is followed by estrogen-induced senescence of growth plate chondrocytes, resulting in growth plate fusion. Androgen-induced stimulation of growth appears to be both a direct effect on the growth plate, as well as indirect GH-IGF-I. Growth hormone leads to increased proliferation of physeal chondrocytes, and increases IGF-I, which also increases chondrocyte proliferation and results in enlargement of hypertrophic chondrocytes.

In the radius, the distal growth plate remains open longer, and contributes significantly more to the length of the bone, than the proximal growth plate. In the humerus, femur, and tibia, the opposite is true. *The fastest growing growth plates are the ones that are most likely to suffer damage because of trauma or nutritional imbalances,* and are therefore worthwhile sites to examine at autopsy and to sample for histopathology. Compared to other species, the physes of the sheep and rat remain active for a longer time after sexual maturity. The dog, for example, reaches sexual maturity at 7-10 months of age, and growth plate closure (tibia and femur) occurs at 6-11 months of age. In the sheep, growth plate closure (metacarpal bone) does not occur until 17 months of age, even though sexual maturity is reached at 5.5 months of age. As a result, the bones of sheep remain susceptible to nutritional imbalances for a longer period than other species.

The growth in width of the diaphysis in young animals occurs by intramembranous ossification beneath the **periosteum**, *which covers the surface of bones except at their articular ends and at insertion points of muscles and tendons.* The periosteum has a tough outer fibrous layer and a more cellular inner layer, *the cambium,* which contributes preosteoblasts for new bone formation (Fig. 2-8). Where muscle fibers and tendons insert onto bones, dense collagen fibers, termed **Sharpey's fibers,** become embedded in the bone matrix. The periosteum has a rich supply of nerve endings and blood vessels. *The inner bone surface is lined by a thin layer of osteogenic lining cells called the* **endosteum.**

Hormonal regulation of physeal growth

In addition to the transcription and growth factors mentioned previously, many systemic hormones also influence growth plate function, in addition to regulating the formation and resorption of bone. Their effect may be on a particular zone of the growth plate, and may vary with the age of the animal. Table 2-1 summarizes the hormonal regulation of the growth plate.

Further reading

Baron R, Kneissel M. WNT signaling in bone homeostasis and disease: from human mutations to treatments. Nat Med 2013;19:179-192.
Burdan F, et al. Morphology and physiology of the epiphyseal growth plate. Folia Histochem Cytobiol 2009;47:5-16.
Del Fattore A, et al. Osteoclast receptors and signaling. Arch Biochem Biophys 2008;473:147-160.
Goltzman D. Studies on the mechanisms of the skeletal anabolic action of endogenous and exogenous parathyroid hormone. Arch Biochem Biophys 2008;473:218-224.
Hojo H, et al. Coordination of chondrogenesis and osteogenesis by hypertrophic chondrocytes in endochondral bone development. J Bone Miner Metab 2010;28:489-502.

Modeling

To establish the unique shape of a long bone, extensive architectural **modeling** *occurs throughout the growth phase.* As a bone increases in size, the diameter of its diaphysis increases by deposition of new bone beneath the periosteum and resorption from the endosteal surface. However, growth in length is more complex and involves the coordinated actions of osteoclasts and osteoblasts operating on different bone surfaces. The diameter of most long bones is greatest at the level of the growth plate, and then tapers through the metaphyseal region to its narrowest region in the diaphysis. This basic funnel shape is maintained during growth in length by continual osteoclastic resorption beneath the periosteum around the circumference of the metaphysis, thereby reducing its diameter. This is often referred to as the "cut-back" zone. Meanwhile, osteoblasts rapidly deposit new bone within tunnels between the peripheral trabeculae of the primary and secondary spongiosa, converting it into dense cortical bone (Fig. 2-9). During this process, spicules of mineralized cartilage originating from the growth plate become incorporated into the cortex and will remain there until they are removed by remodeling.

The peripheral metaphysis of a growing long bone is therefore an area of intense osteoclastic and osteoblastic activity. The cortex is relatively porous, consisting of trabecular bone undergoing compaction, and there is extensive peritrabecular fibrosis. This must be borne in mind when examining histologic sections from such areas in young animals with suspected metabolic bone diseases, particularly fibrous osteodystrophy.

The normal curvature present in some bones is produced during growth by a modeling process referred to as **osseous**

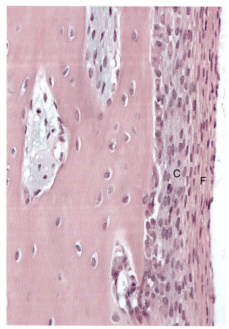

Figure 2-8 Periosteum in an actively growing young animal. Note the outer fibrous layer (F) and the cambium layer (C) containing primitive mesenchymal cells. A single layer of active osteoblasts lines the bone surface.

Table • 2-1

Systemic hormonal regulation of the physis, bone formation, and resorption

Hormone	Effect
1,25(OH)$_2$D$_3$	Maintain serum phosphorus concentrations required for chondrocyte apoptosis
	Nonessential role in growth plate chondrocytes → inhibits hypertrophic chondrocyte proliferation
	Stimulate and inhibit osteoblasts → response depends on stage of osteoblast differentiation
	↑ Runx2 and decreases PPARγ2 → ↑ osteoblast differentiation
	↑ RANKL expression by osteoblasts → ↑ bone resorption
Androgen	In bone, locally converted to estrogen compounds
	Indirect effects via GH-IGF-I
	Direct stimulation of chondrocyte proliferation
	Proapoptotic for osteoclasts
Calcitonin	Accelerates chondrocyte maturation and matrix mineralization
	Loss of ruffled border on osteoclasts, retraction from bone → ↓ osteoclastic resorption
	Inhibits the effects of RANKL
Estrogen	Indirect stimulation of growth via GH-IGF-I
	Senescence of growth plate chondrocytes
	Activates Runx2 and wnt/β-catenin signaling → ↑ osteoblast function and survival
	Induction of Fas ligand in osteoclasts → Proapoptotic
Glucocorticoids	Inhibit proliferation of chondrocytes
	Indirect effects via suppression of IGF-I and ↓ GH secretion
	Promote chondrocyte apoptosis
	Short term—↑ osteoclast resorption
	Long term—lead to inhibition of Wnt signaling → ↑ osteoblast apoptosis
	Long term—osteoclast cytoskeletal derangement → loss of bone formation/resorption coupling → ↓ bone mass
Growth hormone	Stimulates differentiation of resting chondrocytes into proliferating chondrocytes
	↑ IGF-I expression
	↑ Runx2 expression
IGF-I	Stimulates proliferation and hypertrophy of chondrocytes
	↑ Indian hedgehog expression
	Stimulates proliferation of osteoblast precursors and ↑ matrix synthesis
PTH	Indirect effects via ↑ IGF-I
	Low intermittent doses → anabolic effect → ↑ osteoblast proliferation, differentiation and ↓ osteoblast apoptosis
	Activates Runx2, inhibits Runx2 degradation → ↑ osteoblast function
	↑ Osterix expression and decreases PPARγ2
	↑ Osteoblast survival by promoting the β-catenin pathway
	High doses → ↑ RANKL expression by osteoblasts → ↑ bone resorption
	Stimulation of 1α-hydroxylase enzyme → ↑ 1,25(OH)$_2$D$_3$
Thyroid hormones	Essential for cartilage growth and maturation of chondrocytes
	Direct effects on growth via thyroid receptor α
	Stimulates differentiation to hypertrophic chondrocytes
	Indirect effects via GH-IGF-I
	Activates Wnt-β-catenin signaling

1,25(OH)$_2$D$_3$, 1,25-Dihydroxyvitamin D; GH-IGF-I, growth hormone–insulin-like growth factor I; PPARγ2, peroxisome proliferator activator receptor γ2; RANKL, receptor activator of nuclear factor kappa B ligand; Runx2, runt-related transcription factor 2.

drift, whereby the shaft of a bone moves on its long axis. This is accomplished by successive waves of osteoblastic and osteoclastic activity beneath appropriate periosteal and endosteal surfaces of the diaphyseal cortex, presumably under the influence of both genetic and mechanical forces, leading to the formation of laminar bone deposits. The same process is involved in efforts to correct shape abnormalities in long bones resulting from malunited fractures, or other acquired defects altering the mechanical forces acting on a bone.

Bones respond to increased usage during the growth phase by increasing bone mass, particularly in the density and thickness of the cortex. In adults, increased mechanical usage does not increase bone mass, but can decrease remodeling and conserve the amount of bone already present.

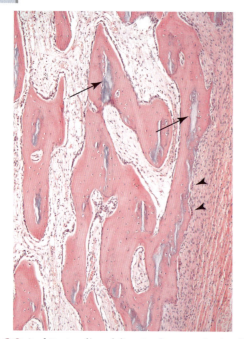

Figure 2-9 Architectural modeling in the metaphysis of a long bone during growth in length. To maintain the flare in the metaphyseal region, osteoclasts (arrowheads) resorb bone at the periosteal surface, whereas osteoblasts actively deposit bone along trabeculae of the primary and secondary spongiosa. Trabecular bone of endochondral origin is thus converted into dense cortical bone. The spicules of mineralized cartilage (arrows) derived from the growth plate persist until the cortex is remodeled.

Remodeling

In the cortex, activated osteoclasts form a "cutting cone," which bores longitudinally through the dense primary bone, creating a *resorption canal*. As the canal advances, it becomes lined by osteoblasts, which fill the space with concentric layers of new lamellar bone, creating a *secondary osteon or Haversian system*. This process provides a mechanism for ongoing internal replacement of cortical bone without altering its gross form or function. Remodeling of trabecular bone follows a similar sequence, but from the trabecular surface, without the formation of resorption canals.

Osteoclast precursors increase in number under the influence of M-CSF expression by osteoblasts, and *osteoclast formation is further regulated by osteoblasts through 3 other pathways*:

- RANK/RANKL—stimulate osteoclast formation
- Wnt-β-catenin—stimulate osteoclast formation
- Jagged 1/Notch 1—inhibit osteoclast formation

RANKL (receptor activator of NF-κB ligand) is a TNF-family molecule expressed by hypertrophic chondrocytes, osteoblasts, osteocytes, bone-lining cells, and activated T lymphocytes. Osteoclast precursor cells, mature osteoclasts, and dendritic cells express RANK, a TNF superfamily receptor. The third component of this pathway is osteoprotegerin (**OPG**), a decoy receptor expressed particularly by B lymphocytes in the bone marrow, in addition to osteoblasts and many other cells types. OPG binds and decreases the availability of RANKL. *Binding of RANKL to RANK* leads to the activation of a number of downstream signaling pathways, including RANK/TRAF-mediated protein kinase signaling, nuclear factor kappa B (NF-κB), AP-1, and nuclear factor of activated T cell 1 (NFATc1), *eventually resulting in the fusion of osteoclast progenitor cells to form the multinucleated osteoclasts. The ratio of RANKL to OPG, rather than the absolute quantity of each, is the important factor in the regulation of osteoclast formation;* either an increase in RANKL or a decrease in OPG leads to an increase in osteoclast number and activity. *Inflammatory conditions may lead to osteoclast formation* independent of the RANK system. TNF and IL-1 may directly activate NFATc1 signaling and therefore autonomous formation of osteoclasts. The increased rate of bone remodeling seen in a number of pathologic conditions, such as osteoporosis, hyperparathyroidism, and inflammation, is usually a result of increased expression of M-CSF and RANKL.

Bone is not a static organ and is continually being renewed. This is a tightly regulated process in which bone resorption is coupled to bone formation in the **basic multicellular unit (BMU)**, *which consists of osteoclasts, osteoblasts, osteocytes, bone-lining cells, and the capillary blood supply.* The bone resorption-formation cycle consists of 3 steps:

- *Initiation phase*: During this step, bone-lining cells, which normally prevent osteoclast precursors from interacting with the bone surface, retract from the surface and secrete collagenase. This digests the thin layer of nonmineralized bone, thus uncovering the mineralized matrix. Apoptosis of osteocytes, perhaps caused by mechanical stress, leads neighboring osteocytes to express RANKL. At the same time, production of sclerostin by osteocytes inhibits osteoblasts. M-CSF and RANKL produced by osteocytes and bone-lining cells recruit osteoclast precursors, which differentiate and start resorbing bone matrix. The bone-lining cells migrate and form a covering over the remodeling area.
- *Reversal or transition phase*: Osteoclasts undergo apoptosis, osteoblasts are recruited and differentiate. Pre-osteoblasts produce PTHrP, which stimulates osteoblast differentiation and inhibits osteoblast apoptosis.
- *Termination phase*: Wnt-β-catenin, BMPs (particularly BMP2), and TGF-β stimulate bone formation, followed by bone mineralization and later, movement into quiescence. This step accounts for three quarters of the time spent in the resorption-formation cycle. Osteomacs, resident tissue macrophages that are often associated with bone-lining cells, help regulate osteoblast mineralization.

Osteoclasts and osteoblasts together control the bone resorption-formation process. Resorption of bone releases factors, originally placed in the bone matrix by osteoblasts, such as osteocalcin and type I collagen, that attract osteoclasts to the site, and BMPs and IGF, which stimulate osteoblasts. There is direct cell-to-cell contact between osteoblasts and osteoclasts via RANKL and RANK, and also ephrinB2 (a ligand expressed by osteoclasts) and ephrinB4 (the corresponding receptor on osteoblasts). Binding of ephrinB2 to ephrinB4 promotes osteoblast differentiation and bone formation, while suppressing osteoclast differentiation. Both osteoclasts and osteoblasts also produce factors that regulate bone formation. Osteoclasts produce sphingosine-1-phosphate, which increases the migration and survival of osteoblasts and increases RANKL expression. Osteoblasts produce monocyte chemoattractant protein (MCP-1), which recruits osteoclast precursors. The capillary blood supply is also an important part of the process, supplying nutrients, oxygen, and hormones while removing calcium and waste products.

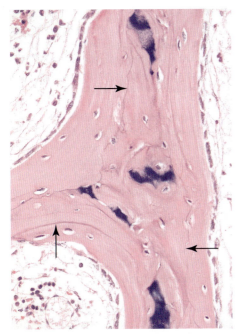

Figure 2-10 **Cementing lines** in a segment of trabecular bone. The smoothly contoured lines (vertical arrow) are referred to as **resting lines** and indicate sites at which bone formation had ceased for a period then restarted. The scalloped lines (horizontal arrows) are **reversal lines** and reflect previous resorption, followed by deposition of new bone.

A variety of systemic hormones influence the recruitment and action of differentiated osteoblasts and osteoclasts, as well as potentially stimulating the proliferation of their precursors. A list of the systemic factors involved in bone remodeling is presented in Table 2-1. Other local and systemic factors that can affect bone remodeling include leptin, nitric oxide synthase, neuropeptide Y, fibroblast growth factors, prostaglandins (particularly PGE_2), TGF-β, IL-1, IL-6, TNF-α, and BMPs.

In histologic sections, the separate units of secondary bone that form during remodeling can be distinguished from each other, and from adjacent primary bone, by the presence of deeply basophilic **cementing lines** (Fig. 2-10). These lines are created by the deposition of a thin layer of highly mineralized, collagen-free matrix at sites where bone resorption or formation ceases. Two types of cementing lines are recognized. Those with a scalloped appearance are termed **reversal lines**, and indicate a site where previous bone resorption had occurred, then new bone deposited in its place. Smoothly contoured cementing lines, or **resting lines**, mark sites where bone formation ceased for a period, then recommenced. The number and pattern of cementing lines may provide useful information on the recent history of an area of bone, particularly regarding the rate of turnover.

Markers of remodeling

Although not used routinely in veterinary medicine, various markers of bone remodeling or turnover can be measured in serum or urine and may add support to a clinical diagnosis, or be of value in research. *Serum alkaline phosphatase activity is a well-recognized indicator of osteoblastic activity*, increased levels occurring in diseases characterized by increased bone formation such as hyperparathyroidism. Its diagnostic value is limited, however, by the fact that high levels are also detected normally in rapidly growing young animals. Furthermore, other isoforms of alkaline phosphatase are commonly used as indicators of cholestatic liver disease in several species and hyperadrenocorticism in dogs; however, assays for bone-specific alkaline phosphatase overcome this limitation. Another potentially useful indicator of osteoblastic activity is serum osteocalcin. Three different forms of osteocalcin can be measured in plasma: intact osteocalcin, N-terminal osteocalcin, and unidentified fragments. *Plasma osteocalcin is thought to be a sensitive marker of bone formation.* Approximately 10-25% of the osteocalcin synthesized by osteoblasts escapes into the circulation, and serum concentrations are proportional to the rate of osteoid synthesis. However, some osteocalcin is released with bone resorption, and uncarboxylated osteocalcin may be a potential marker of bone turnover.

Bone resorption, associated with increased osteoclastic activity, is reflected by increased serum activity of *tartrate-resistant acid phosphatase isoform 5b*, an enzyme released by osteoclasts during the degradation of bone matrix. Other markers used to assess bone resorption include *serum carboxy-terminal telopeptide of type I collagen (ICTP), and urinary hydroxyproline, pyridinoline (PYD), and deoxypyrolidine (DPD)*, all breakdown products of type I collagen.

In dogs, horses, rats, and humans, considerable diurnal variation in the serum and urinary concentrations of bone markers has been demonstrated. This may reflect circadian rhythms in the rates of bone formation and resorption.

Blood supply

The blood supply to bones is derived from arteries entering the medullary cavity through foramina in the cortices of the diaphysis, metaphysis, and epiphysis, as well as periosteal arteries. In young growing animals, **nutrient arteries** supply the diaphyseal marrow and most of the central area of the metaphysis, whereas **metaphyseal arteries** supply the peripheral regions. Terminal branches from these vessels pass vertically toward the metaphyseal surface of the growth plate, where they end in fenestrated capillary loops immediately below the last intact transverse septum of the mineralized cartilage matrix. At this point, they turn back sharply into wide-bore venules characterized by low flow rate. Some terminal branches of the nutrient and metaphyseal arterial systems anastomose with each other, but they do not penetrate the growth plate.

Epiphyseal arteries supply the epiphyses or secondary centers of ossification, and small branches pass through narrow cartilage canals in the reserve zone of the growth plate to terminate at the start of the proliferative zone. This is the only source of oxygen and nutrients to the growth plate because no blood vessels terminate in the hypertrophic zone. Further branches of the epiphyseal artery pass to the under-surface of the overlying articular cartilage, where they form vascular loops similar to those on the metaphyseal side of growth plates, and participate in endochondral ossification.

Transphyseal blood vessels have been identified in newborn animals of several species, but their function remains obscure (Fig. 2-11). Most evidence suggests that the direction of arterial flow in these vessels is from the epiphysis to the metaphysis, but that venous flow occurs in the opposite direction. Whether the transphyseal vessels supply nutrients to the growth plate or just enhance blood supply to the metaphysis during the rapid growth phase is controversial. At sites where transphyseal vessels enter the metaphysis, they are surrounded

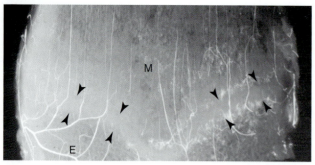

Figure 2-11 Transphyseal blood vessels. Cabinet radioangiogram of a 2-mm-thick slice of decalcified distal third metacarpal bone from a 13-day-old foal. The arterial blood supply to this area had been injected with radio-opaque dye immediately after death. Numerous transphyseal arteries cross from the epiphysis (E) to the metaphysis (M). The physis is between the pairs of arrowheads. (Courtesy E.C. Firth.)

by cartilage projections, which might be expected to strengthen the union between the epiphysis and metaphysis at a time when the growth plate is highly susceptible to shear forces. These vessels may also be involved in certain disease of bones, such as osteomyelitis, where they provide a possible route for spread of infection across the growth plate. The periphery of the growth plate is supplied by perichondrial arteries to the perichondrial ring of LaCroix, and by metaphyseal arteries.

The blood supply to the bone cortex in young animals is predominantly derived from the endosteal surface by way of nutrient arteries, and the flow of blood within the cortex is centrifugal. Arterial blood enters Haversian systems of the cortex through capillaries communicating with medullary sinusoids, but venous drainage occurs through the periosteal surface. With age, the cortex becomes increasing dependent on **periosteal arteries** for its blood supply.

Further reading

Boyce BF. Advances in the regulation of osteoclasts and osteoclast functions. J Dent Res 2013;92:860-867.

Kular J, et al. An overview of the regulation of bone remodelling at the cellular level. Clin Biochem 2012;45:863-873.

O'Brien CA, et al. Osteocyte control of osteoclastogenesis. Bone 2013;54:258-263.

POSTMORTEM EXAMINATION OF THE SKELETON

Of all organ systems, the skeleton is perhaps the most neglected during postmortem examination, even by experienced pathologists. Most organs are examined as part of the routine autopsy technique, but examination of the skeleton is more often confined to those occasions when the clinical history clearly indicates a skeletal problem. As a result, many skeletal disorders are likely to be missed. Furthermore, lack of familiarity with the normal appearance of skeletal structures commonly leads to misinterpretation in cases where a skeletal disease is suspected and a detailed examination of the skeleton is performed.

Gross examination

Complete examination of the skeleton is both impractical and unnecessary. A standard procedure for examining the skeleton should include an assessment of the shape, flexibility, and breaking strength of readily accessible bones, such as ribs, cranium, and key limb bones during routine autopsy. *No skeletal examination is complete without sectioning 1 or 2 representative long bones longitudinally* to reveal the growth plates, the thickness of the cortex, and the amount and density of trabecular bone in metaphyseal and epiphyseal regions. When the clinical history suggests the possibility of a skeletal disorder, a more detailed assessment is required. Antemortem radiographs are a valuable component of the gross examination in such cases and may highlight areas requiring special attention. The pathologist should insist on viewing them before commencing the autopsy. Radiographs of lesions identified during autopsy, either in the form of whole bones or sawn slabs, can also provide valuable information on the extent and severity of bone lysis or demineralization, but are an insensitive indicator of diffuse bone loss, as occurs in osteoporosis.

The manifestations of generalized skeletal diseases are likely to be most severe in certain bones. Even within bones, some regions may be affected more severely than others. For example, lesions associated with metabolic bone diseases, such as rickets and fibrous osteodystrophy, will be most marked at sites of rapid bone formation. The growth plates of the distal radius, proximal humerus, distal femur, and proximal tibia should therefore be targeted for gross and histologic examination. Costochondral junctions of the largest ribs are also useful sites to examine in such cases. In osteoporosis, the depletion of trabecular bone is more rapid than that of cortical bone, presumably because of the greater surface area available for resorption in trabecular bone tissue, and this may be more obvious in bones with a higher proportion of trabecular bone such as the vertebrae.

Histologic techniques and stains

Bone specimens for histologic processing should be *sawn at ~5-mm thickness*, immersed in neutral buffered formalin, and thoroughly fixed to preserve the osteoid matrix. Other than in a few specialist laboratories equipped to prepare undecalcified bone sections, the specimens must then be decalcified/demineralized before sectioning. In most laboratories, this involves the use of *commercial decalcifying agents*, usually consisting of strong acid solutions such as hydrochloric acid, which induce decalcification within 24-48 hours. In the interests of section quality and cellular detail, the specimen should not be left in the decalcifying fluid any longer than necessary. It is important that bone slabs are no thicker than 5 mm, to minimize the time they spend in the fluid. The end point for decalcification can be judged by probing the tissue with a needle, using a chemical test for calcium, or by radiography. The decalcified tissue should be immersed in flowing tap water for 2-4 hours to remove the acid, which would otherwise interfere with staining procedures. Although strong decalcifying solutions will allow the rapid preparation of sections for diagnostic purposes, they will also cause more tissue damage and may therefore impair interpretation. Hydrochloric acid–based solutions are unsuitable if the bone is to be used in downstream techniques, such as DNA/RNA extraction or in situ hybridization, and may be unsuitable for some immunohistochemical markers. Slower decalcification occurs with formic acid, but cell preservation is often superior to

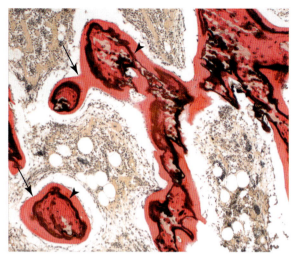

Figure 2-12 Section of femur from a sheep with inherited rickets stained with the method of **Tripp and MacKay** for demonstrating unmineralized **osteoid seams** in decalcified sections. The trabeculae consist of an inner core of mineralized bone stained black-brown (arrowheads), surrounded by seams of unmineralized osteoid stained pink-red (arrows).

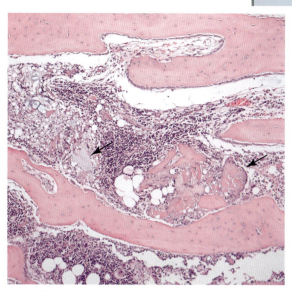

Figure 2-13 The multiple small fragments of bone and cartilage (arrows) embedded in the marrow spaces between trabeculae are **artifacts of sawing** ("sawdust") and should not be misinterpreted as lesions. Such artifacts are commonly present if sections are prepared close to a sawn surface.

hydrochloric acid, and a greater number of antibodies for immunohistochemistry have been used successfully. A chelating solution such as ethylenediaminetetraacetic acid (EDTA) will take ~7 days (for a small section), but enables preparation of higher-quality histologic sections, and can be used with techniques such as in situ hybridization.

The *preparation of undecalcified sections* requires the use of plastic embedding media, such as methyl methacrylate, and a heavy-duty sledge microtome. Several useful staining methods for undecalcified bone sections are available, including hematoxylin and eosin (H&E), von Kossa, toluidine blue, Villanueva's bone stain, and Masson trichrome method.

H&E is also a good general purpose stain for routine histologic examination of decalcified bone sections, allowing clear differentiation of bone and cartilage matrices and providing adequate cellular detail. However, it does not reliably allow assessment of the thickness of osteoid seams, which is of diagnostic significance in diseases such as rickets or osteomalacia. These seams generally appear pale orange/pink, in contrast to the slightly more basophilic bone that was previously mineralized, but the distinction is often too subtle or variable to allow confident interpretation. The Masson trichrome method is another useful general purpose stain for bone sections, but has similar limitations with regard to identifying osteoid seams. Staining methods that allow identification of unmineralized osteoid in demineralized sections have been published (see Ralis and Ralis, 1975; Tripp and MacKay, 1972 in Further reading) and, although not used routinely, can be easily performed in laboratories that are unable to cut undecalcified sections (Fig. 2-12). Toluidine blue is a useful stain for assessing the quality of cartilage matrix in decalcified sections, and may also be used to demonstrate mineralized osteoid in undecalcified sections.

Preparation artifacts in histologic sections

Because of the difficulty in preparing histologic sections from bones, artifactual changes are often present and could be misinterpreted as lesions. During the process of sawing bones before demineralization, multiple small, irregular-sized fragments of bone "*sawdust*" and soft tissue debris often become embedded in spaces between bone trabeculae (Fig. 2-13). Such fragments are commonly misinterpreted as necrotic bone. Rinsing the cut surface of the bone under running water, and gently brushing it before fixation, can minimize this artifact. Because the fragments will be most abundant near sawn surfaces, further trimming of the face to be sectioned, after demineralization, will further reduce them. In a section where "sawdust" is a problem, slicing deeper into the paraffin block is likely to yield cleaner sections for examination.

The heat generated by a bandsaw, or power drill in the case of bone biopsies, may create coagulative changes, resembling early ischemic necrosis, along the edges of the specimen. Overexposure to strong acid solutions during decalcification inhibits the staining of nucleic acids by hematoxylin and of collagen by eosin, resulting in poor cellular detail and difficulties in interpretation.

Another common histologic artifact is the presence of empty clefts between bone surfaces and the soft tissues of the marrow cavity. This reflects the much greater shrinkage of the soft tissues, when compared to bone, during fixation in formalin. Consequently, osteoblasts or osteoclasts lining the bone surface may become separated from their site of activity. However, where bone resorption has been occurring, the surface of the bone will have a characteristic scalloped appearance. Also, bone does not adhere to microscope slides as well as soft tissues of the marrow spaces and may become dislodged, leaving large spaces lined by osteoblasts. These could be misinterpreted as vascular spaces.

Other laboratory techniques

A variety of techniques may be used in the study of bones, but most are confined to the research laboratory. The periodic administration to growing animals of **fluorescent markers**, which are deposited at sites of active mineralization, allows objective measurement of the rate of bone formation in physiologic and disease states. The most commonly used marker is the antibiotic tetracycline, which fluoresces bright yellow when examined in undecalcified sections under blue or ultraviolet light. Other fluorochromes include alizarin red and calcein (green). Because the fluorochromes are only deposited at sites of active mineralization, a thin fluorescent line results from each dose. The distance is measured between lines representing sequential periods of exposure to the marker, and the rate of bone formation is estimated.

Microradiography of thick sections provides an indication of the pattern and degree of mineralization within the bone. Sections of bone, 60-100 μm thick, are placed in close contact with X-ray film and exposed. This creates an image of the bone section, which can be examined microscopically in association with histologic sections prepared from the same slab.

Bone ash measurements have historically been performed in animals with suspected metabolic bone diseases, but are of limited value for routine diagnosis because of the variability between individual bones and the lack of reliable reference ranges for animals of different age groups. More sophisticated and accurate methods for determining bone density, such as **dual energy X-ray absorptiometry (DEXA)** and **computed tomography (CT)**, have been developed for assessing bone mineral density in human patients, and CT scans, in particular, are becoming more accessible to veterinary clinicians and pathologists. An important consideration in interpreting bone mineral content (BMC) and bone mineral density (BMD) is the availability of age and sex-matched controls of the same species.

Technetium labeling to identify areas of metabolically active bone, detected by scintigraphy, can be used to detect bone abnormalities in the live animal. This technique greatly assists in locating multifocal lesions, such as the spread of metastatic disease within the skeleton, and although widely used in human medicine, has a relatively limited use for this purpose in animals.

DNA and RNA extraction from tissues is becoming more common in many research laboratories; however, extraction from a hard tissue such as bone presents a number of technical difficulties. Liquid nitrogen, tissue homogenizers, and even a mortar and pestle, allow the extraction of good-quality DNA and RNA from bone for subsequent use in both conventional and quantitative real-time polymerase chain reaction (qRT-PCR). Decalcification of bone with strong acids, such as hydrochloric or formic acid, significantly reduces the amount of DNA, and particularly RNA, that can be extracted; however, the use of EDTA as a decalcification agent may allow extraction of adequate amounts of RNA/DNA from decalcified bone sections.

Further reading

Chappard D, et al. New laboratory tools in the assessment of bone quality. Osteoporos Int 2011;22:2225-2240.

Dempster DW, et al. Standardized nomenclature, symbols, and units for bone histomorphometry: a 2012 update of the report of the ASBMR Histomorphometry Nomenclature Committee. J Bone Miner Res 2013;28:2-17.

Everts V, et al. Transmission electron microscopy of bone. In: Helfrich MH, Ralston SH, editors. Bone Research Protocols. New York: Humana Pr; 2012. p. 351-363.

RESPONSE TO MECHANICAL FORCES AND INJURY

The cells of bone tissue are capable of the same basic cellular responses as most other tissues, including *atrophy, hypertrophy, hyperplasia, metaplasia, neoplasia, degeneration,* and *necrosis*. Bones have an excellent capacity for repair or modification in response to a wide range of injurious stimuli or changes in mechanical demand. Depending on the stimulus, the response may be localized or generalized, but in general, the magnitude of skeletal response is greater in young growing animals than in adults. If the response is generalized, it is likely to be most prominent at sites of rapid bone growth or modeling.

Mechanical forces

Bone adapts or remodels in response to the mechanical demands placed upon it. According to **Wolff's law**, *it is deposited at sites where it is required and resorbed where it is not*. For example, trabeculae in the epiphyseal and metaphyseal regions of long bones are aligned in directions that best reflect the compressive forces associated with weight bearing, and the tension associated with mechanical insertions. In young individuals, increased mechanical stress on the skeleton increases the density of metaphyseal trabecular bone and the thickness of cortices. Increased mechanical usage in adults does not lead to an increase in bone mass, but reduces remodeling activity, conserving the amount of bone already present. Decreased activity accelerates bone loss by removing the inhibition of remodeling, and reduces formation, leading to a net reduction in bone mass. As discussed previously, osteocytes and osteoprogenitor cells are the key cells in this response to mechanical demand.

Reduced mechanical stress on bones because of partial or complete immobilization, as occurs during fracture repair, leads to increased resorption, resulting in decreased bone strength and stiffness. If an implant, such as a metal plate, remains attached to a bone after a fracture has repaired, it will share the mechanical load with the bone. The bone will then atrophy in proportion to the decreased load, and its strength will be greatly reduced. For this reason, *rigid implants should be removed soon after a fracture has healed*. Such implants may also trigger the development of an osteosarcoma at the site, particularly in dogs (see later), providing further reason for their removal.

Growth plate damage

In young growing animals, the growth plate is the weakest structure in the ends of long bones and is prone to traumatic injury resulting from shearing forces, compressive forces, or, in the case of traction epiphyses (e.g., lesser trochanter of the femur), excessive tension. In general, *the fastest growing growth plates are the most susceptible to injury, the distal radial physis being the most commonly affected*. Undulations in the growth plates of some bones increase their resistance to separation in response to shearing forces.

The consequences of growth plate injury depend on several factors, including the nature of the lesion, its location, the age of the animal, and the status of the blood supply. Growth plates subjected primarily to traction consist at least partly of fibrocartilage, which imparts increased resistance to tensile forces. Such growth plates are sometimes referred to as **apophyses**.

Complete separation through the growth plate, referred to as **slipped epiphysis** (or "epiphysiolysis"), is a relatively common sequel to severe trauma or horizontal shear forces acting in the region of the bone-physis interface. The Salter-Harris classification system is used to describe the 5 different types of physeal fracture that may occur. The separation almost invariably occurs through the hypertrophic zone, where the cell volume is greatest, and the matrix, which provides strength to the physis, is relatively sparse. Providing the epiphyseal vasculature has not been disrupted, the prognosis for this type of fracture is very good because the proliferative zone of the growth plate, and its blood supply, are likely to remain intact. However, separation of the capital femoral epiphysis, which may be associated with birth trauma in calves and occurs with some frequency in growing foals and puppies, may result in avascular necrosis of the femoral head. This reflects the greater risk of vascular damage as the nutrient vessels to the proximal femoral epiphysis travel along the neck of the femur and traverse the rim of the growth plate. The vessels supplying most other long bone epiphyses enter the bone some distance from the growth plate and are protected by the periosteum or the fibrous layer of the joint capsule.

Slipped capital femoral epiphysis occurs in pigs and deer as a manifestation of osteochondrosis, and in cats as a manifestation of physeal dysplasia, as a result of an underlying weakness in the growth plate. Slipped capital femoral epiphysis must be distinguished from Legg-Calvé-Perthes disease and fractures through the femoral neck.

The *most common type of physeal fracture* reported in dogs, cats, horses, and humans is characterized by extension of the fracture along the growth plate for a variable distance, then out through the metaphysis, leaving a triangular fragment of metaphyseal bone still attached to the growth plate. As with complete slipped epiphysis, the prognosis for further growth is very good. In contrast, fractures that cross the growth plate, with displacement of the fragments, will lead to the formation of a bony bridge between the metaphysis and epiphysis, precluding further growth in length at that site.

It is relatively common for epiphyseal separations, similar to those described previously, to be induced during postmortem examination of young animals when limb joints are disarticulated forcefully, particularly if the carcass is autolyzed. Such "fractures" are not accompanied by hemorrhage and are therefore easily distinguished from antemortem physeal fractures.

Growth plates of major limb bones, particularly the distal radius and ulna, are also susceptible to crushing injuries caused by compressive forces transmitted through the epiphysis. Such injuries, if severe enough, damage the epiphyseal blood supply as well as chondrocytes in the proliferating zone, leading to cessation of growth. *When the lesion is confined to one side of the growth plate, as it often is, continued growth on the other side leads to* **angular limb deformity**.

Detachment of the ischial tuberosity from the pelvis is a well-recognized entity in young breeding sows, resulting in acute lameness. The separation, which may be bilateral, usually occurs between 8 and 14 months of age, before the closure of the apophyseal growth plate between the tuber ischiadicum and the rest of the ischium. The tuber ischiadicum serves as the origin for the semitendinosus and semimembranosus muscles, and as an attachment for the sacrotuberous ligament. As such, it is subject to considerable traction force and any weakness in the growth plate, as may occur in osteochondrosis, predisposes it to fracture.

Angular limb deformities

Angular limb deformities ("bent-leg") are relatively common in young animals of several domestic species, particularly in fast-growing breeds. In many cases, the deformity can be traced to an asymmetrical lesion involving an active growth plate, such as the distal radius, but growth plate damage is not always the underlying cause, and even when it is, the cause is often not apparent. Abnormal development of carpal or tarsal bones is also reported as causing limb deformities, as is joint instability caused by laxity of supporting structures. Lateral deviation of the limb distal to the affected growth plate or joint is referred to as a **valgus deformity** and medial deviation as a **varus deformity**.

In **horses**, angular limb deformities occur primarily in young foals and are included with a group of disorders referred to as *developmental orthopedic diseases*. A variety of congenital and acquired lesions have been identified in foals with limb deformities, and in many cases, it is not possible to determine which changes are primary and which are secondary. *Developmental orthopedic diseases include juvenile osteochondral conditions related to immature joints or growth plates (osteochondrosis, subchondral cystic lesions, cuboidal bone disease, osteochondral fragmentation and avulsion fracture, physitis), flexural limb deformities (contractures and laxity), and wobbler disease.* Note that *"physitis" is a clinical term and should not be used by pathologists*, because it creates the misleading impression that the lesion is primarily inflammatory. Developmental orthopedic disease is fluid; deformities and lesions present at one time point may not be present at a later date. A radiographic survey found that of *juvenile osteochondral lesions* identified at 6 months of age, 46.6% had disappeared by 18 months of age, and 36.7% of the radiographic changes at 18 months of age were new lesions (see Osteochondrosis later).

Limb deformities are common in foals. A study found that 88.4% of foals had at least one limb deviation at 1 month of age, of which >50% were moderate to severe deviations. Of these limb deviations, 63.6% were angular limb deformities, most commonly carpal valgus and fetlock valgus deviations. Most carpal and fetlock valgus deviations were corrected by weaning, at which point flexural limb deformities were the predominant deviation (62.2%). Nonetheless, many angular and flexural limb deformities had disappeared by weaning, and some authors suggest that moderate limb deviations at birth may be "physiologic." As a foal grows, the chest becomes broader such that outward rotation of the limb is reduced, and periarticular supporting tissues are strengthened. In addition, any regions of the physis or developing joint surface that are subjected to extra strain or loading compensate by increasing the rate of endochondral ossification, and vice versa, until the load is balanced across the bone. If the deformity is severe, the compensatory mechanisms are exceeded and the deformity will persist without intervention.

Hypothyroidism (either congenital goiter or thyroid gland hyperplasia) has been associated with angular limb deformities in foals, caused by delayed ossification of carpal and tarsal bones and flexural deformities. Note that even in foals with no evidence of hypothyroidism, the bones of the carpus and tarsus can vary considerably in their degree of ossification at birth. *Septic infection* of bone in young foals may also involve physes, causing destruction of the growth cartilage (see

Osteomyelitis later). Foals that survive such infections may develop angular limb deformity.

In **dogs,** angular limb deformity is *most commonly associated with premature closure of the distal ulnar physis,* which is particularly susceptible to trauma, presumably because of its conical shape. Shearing forces acting on this growth plate result in crushing injury rather than physeal slippage or fracture, because of its conical shape, and are therefore more likely to result in retarded growth. If the growth plate of the adjacent radius escapes injury, the required synchrony between the 2 bones during development will be disturbed. Shortening of the limb will be accompanied by cranial bowing of the radius, valgus deformity, and outward rotation of the carpal and metacarpal bones. The syndrome occurs most often in large breeds, but is described as an autosomal recessive trait in the Skye Terrier.

Less frequently, angular limb deformity in young pups results from a lesion in either the proximal or distal physis of the radius, the latter being the most common. Such lesions may be caused by a fracture through the hypertrophic zone of the growth plate, or a crushing force transmitted through the epiphyseal bone. If the injury affects just one side of the growth plate and growth continues on the other side, angular deformity will result (Fig. 2-14). Premature closure of the distal tibial physis, resulting in curvature of the tibia/fibula, also occurs occasionally in pups.

Retarded endochondral ossification (retained endochondral cartilage core) *in giant-breed dogs* has been associated with angular limb deformities. The lesion is bilateral, and often clinically silent, healing uneventfully. However, large retained cores may interfere with longitudinal growth of the ulna and cause deviations. The lesion consists of a cone-shaped mass of unmineralized hypertrophic cartilage, with its base at the center of the ulnar growth plate and its apex projecting into the metaphysis (Fig. 2-15). The periphery of the growth plate is normal. The cause of the abnormality is unknown, but it could be a manifestation of osteochondrosis, or perhaps because of a temporary interruption or insufficiency in the metaphyseal blood supply. Radiolucent lesions caused by a cone-shaped wedge of retained cartilage may also be seen in the tibial tuberosity of dogs, particularly small breeds.

Angular limb deformities are described in young, rapidly growing **sheep** in different parts of the world and are *often referred to as "bent-leg" or "bowie."* It is relatively common in ram lambs in feedlots, but also occurs in pasture-fed lambs. Similar deformities also occur in young **goats,** especially fast-growing dairy breeds fed concentrate rations. The forelimbs are affected more frequently than the hindlimbs, and the deformity may be either unilateral or bilateral, and either valgus or varus (Fig. 2-16). The cause is not known, but there is a *strong association with high-energy rations and rapid growth.* Most reports of angular limb deformity in sheep and goats describe gross and microscopic lesions in the fast-growing *physis of the distal radius, and to a lesser extent in the distal metacarpals or metatarsals.* The lesions typically consist of *focal or segmental thickening of the physis,* caused by expansion of the hypertrophic zone, with extension into the proximal metaphysis. These lesions closely resemble the physeal manifestations of osteochondrosis in foals and pigs.

Varus and valgus deformities centered on the distal radial physis have been seen in yearling farmed male **red and wapiti-red crossbred (elk) deer** in New Zealand. Deer with heavy wide-beam antlers were particularly affected, and the deformities coincided with a period of rapid growth and hardening of velvet antler. Only the forelimbs were affected, and this was most commonly a carpal varus (bow-legged) deformity. Grossly, *segmental to multifocal thickening of the radial growth plate* was present, often with hemorrhage, necrosis, and destruction of thickened cartilage (Fig. 2-17). Lesions similar to physeal osteochondrosis were seen on microscopic

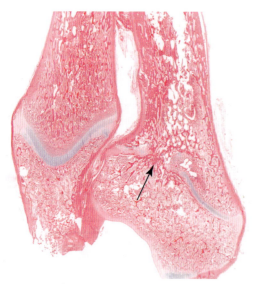

Figure 2-14 Distal radius and ulna from a pup with **angular limb deformity** secondary to traumatic damage to the radial physis. One side of the physis has been destroyed and is penetrated by thick bony trabeculae (arrow). Fusion of the epiphysis and metaphysis on this side has prevented further growth, whereas growth has continued from the undamaged segment of physis, resulting in angular deformity. (Courtesy D.H. Read.)

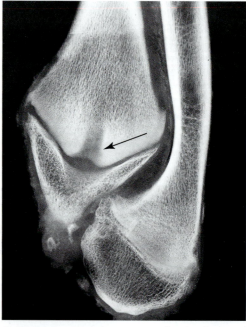

Figure 2-15 Retained cartilage core in the distal ulna of a dog. Slab radiograph showing retained cartilage core (arrow) in the distal ulna of a dog with angular limb deformity secondary to reduced growth from the affected ulnar physis.

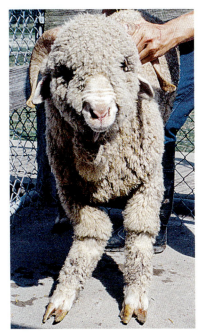

Figure 2-16 **Angular limb deformity** in a sheep. Valgus deformity of the right foreleg and varus deformity of the left in a young Rambouillet ram. There was focal duplication of the physeal cartilage in the right leg and focal thickening of the physis in the left leg. In both legs the physeal abnormalities are on the side that has grown more.

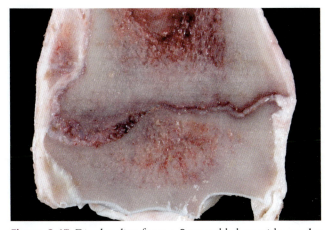

Figure 2-17 Distal radius from a 2-year-old deer with **angular limb deformity**. The left side of the physis is thickened, with areas of hemorrhage and gelatinous tissue indicating disruption of trabeculae and replacement with granulation tissue.

examination, with *hypertrophic chondrocytes extending into the metaphysis* and degenerate cartilage matrix, which in some areas was rarefied (Fig. 2-18). In severe cases, there was extensive disruption of both the physis and the primary spongiosa beneath the thickened cartilage, resulting from hemorrhage and microfractures. The pathogenesis of the disease is uncertain, but an association with copper deficiency has been postulated. In contrast, a high incidence of limb deformity centered on the metatarsus/metacarpus, and spontaneous fractures in fallow deer from a large deer park in the United Kingdom were considered to be caused by a metabolic bone disease, such as rickets.

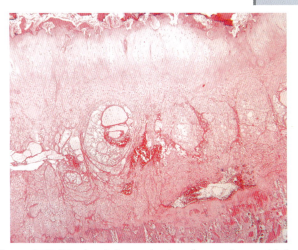

Figure 2-18 Distal radial growth plate from a 2-year-old deer with **angular limb deformity**. There are extensive horizontal clefts through the physis, with hemorrhage and rarefaction of cartilage matrix.

Further reading

Denoix JM, et al. A review of terminology for equine juvenile osteochondral conditions (JOCC) based on anatomical and functional considerations. Vet J 2013;197:29-35.

Jacquet S, et al. Evolution of radiological findings detected in the limbs of 321 young horses between the ages of 6 and 18 months. Vet J 2013;197:58-64.

Robert C, et al. Longitudinal development of equine forelimb conformation from birth to weaning in three different horse breeds. Vet J 2013;198(Suppl 1):e75-e80.1.

Periosteal damage

Periosteal damage caused by trauma stimulates rapid formation of new or **reactive bone** following activation and proliferation of osteoblast progenitors in the cambium layer. Trabeculae of woven bone extend from the underlying bone surface at acute angles, and can be readily distinguished histologically from the mature lamellar bone of the cortex (see Figure 2-4). *Separation of the periosteum from the bone surface* by hemorrhage, inflammatory exudate, or neoplasia, or following surgical intervention, is also followed by *subperiosteal new bone formation*. A pyramid-shaped region of new bone, referred to as **Codman's triangle**, may form beneath the periosteum in association with osteosarcoma, but can also occur in association with other bone lesions such as osteomyelitis. The mechanism of periosteal new bone formation is not clear, but it often precedes actual involvement of the periosteum by an underlying osteosarcoma or inflammatory process, suggesting that it may involve either local circulatory disturbances or the release of growth factors in response to bone resorption.

Localized outgrowths of new bone beneath the periosteum are referred to as **exostoses**. Depending on their size, and the inciting cause, they may either persist or gradually be removed by remodeling.

Fracture repair

Bone fractures are very common in animals and occur either when a bone is subjected to a mechanical force beyond that to which it is designed to withstand, or when there is an *underlying disease process that has reduced its normal breaking strength.* The latter is referred to as a **pathologic fracture** and, unless the predisposing disorder is corrected, the repair process is unlikely to be successful. The possibility of a localized bone disease (e.g., neoplasia or osteomyelitis) or a generalized disorder (e.g., fibrous osteodystrophy or osteoporosis) should always be considered if bone fracture has occurred without evidence of trauma.

Types of fractures

Fractures are classified as **simple**, if there is a clean break separating the bone into 2 parts, or **comminuted**, if several fragments of bone exist at the fracture site. When one segment of bone is driven into another, the fracture is referred to as an **impacted** fracture, and when there is a break in the overlying skin, usually because of penetration by a sharp fragment of bone, the fracture is referred to as **compound** or open. If there has been minimal separation between the fractured bone ends, and the periosteum remains intact, the lesion is classified as a **greenstick** fracture. An **avulsion** fracture occurs when there is excessive trauma at sites of ligamentous or tendinous insertions and a fragment of bone is torn away.

Microscopic fractures of individual trabeculae, or localized segments of cortical bone, also occur and are referred to as **microfractures**. Trabecular microfractures can sometimes be detected in histologic sections by the abnormal alignment of their cartilage cores, which are normally situated at right angles to the growth plate, and parallel to the cartilage cores of adjacent trabeculae (Fig. 2-19). Such microfractures, however, must, be differentiated from artifactual alterations in trabecular alignment that may occur when a bone is being sawn during processing. Once trabeculae have lost their cartilage core through remodeling, this does not apply, and because the direction of remodeled trabeculae is less predictable, detection of microfractures is more difficult. *Multiple microfractures involving several adjacent trabeculae without gross displacement of the bone ends are referred to as* **infractions**. These are sometimes seen in association with weight bearing on bones weakened by an underlying disease process, such as fibrous osteodystrophy (Fig. 2-20). Repeated bone trauma associated with strenuous exercise may lead to a **stress** fracture in the cortex of a limb bone. This represents the accumulation of several cortical microfractures, rather than a single traumatic event, and is typically seen in the dorsal or dorsomedial cortex of metacarpal III in young racehorses when they first enter training (see later).

Process of fracture repair

Unlike most other tissues, bone is capable of repair by regeneration rather than scar formation, and successful repair of a fracture can return the bone both to its original shape and strength. The process of fracture repair follows a consistent pattern, but can be modified by methods of stabilization and by interfering factors, such as infection or an underlying bone disease.

Fracture repair consists of 4 overlapping processes: inflammation, soft callus formation, hard callus formation, and remodeling. The initial event in uncomplicated fracture repair is the *formation of a hematoma* between the bone ends. With disruption of the blood supply, *ischemic necrosis* of bone and other tissues in the vicinity of the fracture is inevitable. An *acute inflammatory response* is triggered by mediators released from the hematoma and from necrotic tissues. Neutrophils and macrophages are the first cells to arrive at the fracture site, and secrete cytokines and growth factors, such as TGF-β, platelet-derived growth factor (PDGF), vascular endothelial growth factor (VEGF), and bone morphogenetic proteins (BMPs), among others, which attract multipotential mesenchymal stem cells to the site from the periosteum, bone marrow, and potentially other sites.

Fibroblasts producing fibrous connective tissue and chondrocytes producing cartilage are responsible for constructing the **soft callus**, which despite the name is semisolid and provides mechanical support. The early callus, consisting predominantly of hyaline cartilage, forms very rapidly and serves to anchor the fractured bone ends, allowing limited function while the repair process continues. Fibroblast and chondrocyte proliferation and differentiation are controlled by TGF-β,

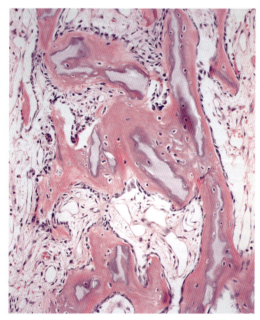

Figure 2-19 Trabecular microfractures in a calf with **osteogenesis imperfecta**. Note the abnormal alignment of cartilage cores in adjacent trabeculae that have been incorporated in a microcallus.

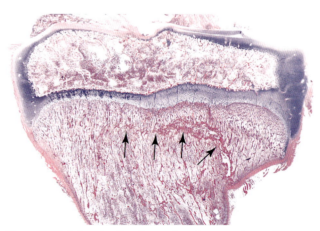

Figure 2-20 Infraction line (arrows) in the metaphysis of a young pig with fibrous osteodystrophy. The abnormal alignment of trabeculae across the center of the field represents a band of healed trabecular microfractures.

fibroblast growth factor 1 (FGF1), and BMPs. Vascular endothelial cells invade the callus under the influence of VEGF, BMPs, and FGF1; and angiopoietin I and II control vessel formation. Subperiosteal new bone formation commences on the bone surface adjacent to the bone ends, and osteoclasts appear and start to remove the dead bone.

New bone formation occurs in the **hard callus** *phase*, and BMPs are key regulators of osteoprogenitor cells and osteoblasts in this stage. The origin of the osteoprogenitor cells is unclear. They may arise from the periosteum or bone marrow, but could also originate from the circulation or blood vessels. Osteoblasts producing new bone have been identified ultrastructurally in the medullary callus as early as 24 hours after fracture. Improved oxygen tension in the area of the callus is required for cells to differentiate to the osteoblast form. As revascularization of the fracture site occurs, endochondral ossification within the callus leads to progressive replacement of the cartilage by trabeculae of woven bone. Although some bone in the callus may form from intramembranous ossification, most develops by endochondral ossification. The development of a bony callus further stabilizes the fracture and allows a return to normal function, although the repair process continues.

The *final phase* may take several months, or even years, and *involves the replacement of woven bone in the callus with mature lamellar bone*, and modeling of the callus to eventually restore the bone to its original shape. M-CSF, RANKL, TGF-β, BMPs, and TNF-α are involved in the regulation of this process. Once the remodeling process is completed, the strength of the bone will also be returned to its previous state. Modeling of the callus is more rapid in young animals than in adults and is more likely to result in complete resolution. In adults, residual changes such as persistence of medullary trabeculae and thickening of the periosteal bone surface are likely to persist at the fracture site.

The size of a fracture callus is proportional to the amount of movement between the fractured bone ends. Where there is considerable movement, callus formation will be exuberant, and may create diagnostic problems for the pathologist, especially in cases where the clinical history is incomplete and radiographs of the lesion are not available. In the early stages of callus formation, the abundance of pleomorphic spindle cells, sometimes exhibiting primitive osteoid formation, can easily be misinterpreted as an osteosarcoma in biopsy specimens (Fig. 2-21). As the callus matures, a more organized pattern develops, with osteoblasts lining up along trabeculae of woven bone and the cells between trabeculae appearing less primitive (Fig. 2-22). It must be remembered that an underlying osteosarcoma could have predisposed to fracture, and the 2 processes may in fact be present.

In fractures in which the separated ends have been perfectly aligned, and rigidly immobilized by metal plates or other methods of fixation, callus formation is minimal, or even non-existent. The repair process in this situation is more protracted as it relies on the process of Haversian system remodeling, whereby osteoclast cutting cones form resorption canals across the fracture line in the apposed cortices, followed by osteoblasts that form new osteons. This is referred to as **primary cortical healing** or primary fracture healing.

Complications of fracture repair

The repair process does not always proceed smoothly. In comminuted fractures, *fragments of necrotic bone that are too large*

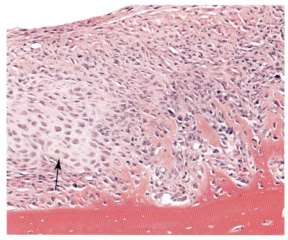

Figure 2-21 Periosteal reaction in a **repairing fracture**. In the early stages of callus formation, the abundance of pleomorphic spindle cells (arrow), sometimes exhibiting primitive osteoid formation, can easily be misinterpreted as an osteosarcoma in biopsy specimens.

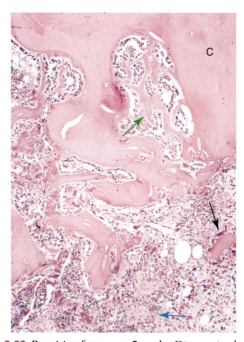

Figure 2-22 Repairing fracture at 2 weeks. Disorganized condensations of plump mesenchymal cells are producing osteoid (blue arrow) in a manner similar to that which occurs in some osteosarcomas. The pre-existing cortical bone (C) is still present and serves as an attachment site for some of the newly formed bone spicules (green arrow). Osteoclasts (black arrow) are resorbing fragments of necrotic bone.

for removal by osteoclastic resorption may persist at the site and interfere with the healing process. Such bone fragments are referred to as **sequestra**. The repair of compound fractures may be delayed by the development of bacterial osteomyelitis following contamination of the fracture site through the open skin wound. Failure to control the infection in the early stages will interfere with new bone formation and the resorption of dead bone. If the infection becomes chronic, new bone may form at the margin of healthy and diseased tissue in an attempt to wall off the infected area. The result may be the development of a large callus containing pockets of infection or fistulae surrounded by granulation tissue and trabecular bone. Any large fragments of bone engulfed by the inflammatory process are likely to persist as sequestra, causing irritation, delayed healing, or nonhealing.

Excessive movement between bone ends during the repair process may inhibit the formation of a bony callus by continually disrupting attempts at revascularization. This favors the formation of cartilage and fibrous tissue and may lead to the development of a false joint or **pseudoarthrosis** at the fracture site. A pseudoarthrosis may also develop if soft tissues separate the fractured bone ends or if persistent infection inhibits callus formation.

Stress-related lesions in horses

A spectrum of stress-related lesions, including **bucked shins** and **incomplete cortical fractures**, *commonly affect the dorsal cortex of the third metacarpal bone in young sport horses*, particularly Thoroughbreds and Quarter horses, undergoing intensive training for their first season of racing. Estimations of prevalence for bucked shins vary from 30-90% of all young horses in training. Incomplete cortical fractures (so-called *saucer fractures*) may occur several months after the initial signs of bucked shins. Both lesions affect the left metacarpal bone more often than the right, but may be bilateral.

Bucked shins is characterized by the formation of smoothly contoured foci of periosteal new bone on the dorsal aspect of the metacarpal bone, accompanied by pain and swelling. The pathogenesis of bucked shins is controversial. For many years, it was considered to be the result of fatigue injuries leading to microfractures in the dorsal cortex of the metacarpal bone, with subsequent callus formation. However, the extent of new bone formation is in excess of what would be expected as a response to such microfractures, with negligible bone displacement and instability. An alternative hypothesis based on Wolff's law suggests that the repeated high-strain fatigue during training or racing decreases bone stiffness, thus inducing formation of reactive bone on the periosteal surface in an effort to increase the inertial properties of the bone and increase its resistance to bending.

Incomplete cortical fractures (stress or saucer fractures) seldom occur in horses that have not previously had bucked shins, suggesting that the conditions are related, but only about 12% of horses with bucked shins develop such fractures. They usually occur 6-12 months after the onset of bucked shins and involve the periosteal new bone that forms on the dorsal or dorsolateral aspect of the third metacarpal. Until this bone is remodeled and strengthened, it is susceptible to fatigue injury during the high-strain cyclic loading associated with training or racing. Failure of the bone may be in the form of many small saucer-shaped stress fractures, extending part way into the cortex before returning to the surface.

Stress-related lesions are often found incidentally in the *distal condyles of the third metacarpal and metatarsal bones* of Thoroughbred racehorses. Linear defects in the articular cartilage adjacent to the sagittal ridge on either side are closely related to microcracks, increased density of the subchondral bone with increased numbers of atypical osteocytes, and intense focal remodeling of the bone. These changes are presumably a response to the increased strain associated with training and may predispose to **condylar fractures**. Similar **parasagittal fractures** that start in the sagittal groove may also occur in the *proximal phalanx*.

Further reading

Ai-Aql ZS, et al. Molecular mechanisms controlling bone formation during fracture healing and distraction osteogenesis. J Dent Res 2008;87:107-118.

Muir P, et al. Exercise-induced metacarpophalangeal joint adaptation in the Thoroughbred racehorse. J Anat 2008;213:706-717.

Schindeler A, et al. Bone remodeling during fracture repair: the cellular picture. Semin Cell Dev Biol 2008;19:459-466.

GENETIC AND CONGENITAL DISEASES OF BONE

A variety of genetic abnormalities primarily affecting bone formation or remodeling have been reported in humans and domestic animals. These are collectively known as skeletal dysplasias and are *usually associated with short stature, abnormally shaped bones, and/or increased bone fragility*. Not surprisingly, human skeletal dysplasias have been subjected to much greater scientific scrutiny than those in animals, leading to the development of detailed and sometimes confusing systems of classification, based on their radiographic appearance, the bones involved, age of onset, or pathogenesis. A comprehensive international classification system for skeletal dysplasias, proposed in 1991 and revised in 2010, includes >100 entities. Advances in molecular biology have allowed the development of a more precise classification system based on the actual genetic defect, and some disorders previously thought to be separate entities are merely examples of variable expression of the same genetic defect. Skeletal dysplasias of animals are seldom investigated in as much detail as their human counterparts and classification is often imprecise, but it is clear that a similar range of conditions exist, creating opportunities for the development of potentially useful animal models. Studies in animals, particularly laboratory mice, are already proving valuable in helping to identify the molecular basis of inherited disorders of the skeleton and other body systems. Such studies also generate new information on the role of specific proteins in bone function and physiology.

The diversity of skeletal dysplasias reflects the complexity of the processes involved in bone formation and remodeling, and the large number of genes required for normal development. In some dysplasias, the entire skeleton is involved, whereas in others the defect is confined to individual bones or regions within bones. The terminology generally reflects either the distribution of lesions or the nature of the defect. Some examples of commonly used terms are listed in Table 2-2.

Most skeletal dysplasias in animals are lethal or semilethal, but the gene frequency of some disorders in some breeds has reached surprisingly high levels. This most likely reflects either inbreeding or excessive use of a sire carrying a defective gene. The latter has clearly been responsible for the very high prevalence reached by certain genetic diseases in cattle, where artificial breeding is widely practiced.

Not all skeletal abnormalities are caused by genetic defects. Exposure of developing fetuses to toxins, mineral deficiencies,

Table • 2-2

Terminology of some congenital abnormalities in skeletal development

Term	Nature of the defect
Generalized	
Achondroplasia	Absence of cartilage development
Chondrodysplasia	Disordered cartilage development
Osteogenesis imperfecta	Genetic defect in type I collagen formation characterized by osteopenia and excessive bone fragility
Osteopetrosis	Persistence of primary and/or secondary spongiosa caused by defect in osteoclastic bone resorption
Skeletal dysplasia	Disordered skeletal development
Head	
Brachycephalic	Shortening of the head
Brachygnathia	Abnormally short jaw (inferior or superior)
Campylognathia	Harelip
Palatoschisis	Cleft palate
Prognathia	Abnormal projection of the jaw
Spine	
Kyphosis	Abnormal dorsal curvature of the spinal column
Lordosis	Abnormal ventral curvature of the spinal column
Scoliosis	Lateral deviation of the spinal column
Limbs	
Amelia	Absence of one or more limbs
Hemimelia	Absence of the distal part of a limb
Micromelia	Presence of abnormally small limbs
Notomelia	Accessory limb attached to the back
Peromelia	Congenital deformity of the limbs
Phocomelia	Absence of the proximal portion of one or more limbs
Digits	
Adactyly	Absence of a digit
Dactylomegaly	Abnormally large digits
Ectrodactyly	Partial or complete absence of a digit
Polydactyly	Presence of supernumerary digits
Polypodia	Presence of supernumerary feet
Syndactyly	Fusion of digits

or infectious agents at appropriate stages of gestation can create skeletal lesions indistinguishable from those with a genetic cause. For the veterinary pathologist, it is as important to determine the cause of the problem as it is to characterize the lesions. Otherwise valuable stud animals may be slaughtered unnecessarily, or teratogenic agents may go undetected. In this section, discussion will focus on those skeletal dysplasias of domestic animals that are known, or strongly believed, to be genetic in origin. Acquired skeletal abnormalities will be discussed in the nutritional and hormonal bone diseases, and toxic bone disease sections.

Further reading

Warman ML, et al. Nosology and classification of genetic skeletal disorders: 2010 revision. Am J Med Gen A 2011;155:943-968.

Generalized skeletal dysplasias

Several important generalized disorders of bones are recognized in animals, all of them having analogous human counterparts. The underlying defect may lie in the formation of cartilage, thus affecting all bones that form by endochondral ossification. Such disorders are referred to as **chondrodysplasias** and affected individuals, no matter what the species, usually *show various degrees of dwarfism*. The term **achondroplasia** is often used in place of chondrodysplasia to describe diseases characterized by *disproportionate dwarfism*, especially in human medicine, and although it is less accurate, the term is entrenched in the literature. In animals, **chondrodystrophy** is used interchangeably with chondrodysplasia. Alternatively, the defect may involve the synthesis of a specific component of bone matrix (e.g., type I collagen), as occurs in **osteogenesis imperfecta**. A defect in bone remodeling is the mechanism involved in another group of skeletal dysplasias, the **osteopetroses**. Only those disorders reported in domestic animals are included in this section, but from time to time, the veterinary pathologist will be confronted with bone deformities that do not resemble any of the syndromes currently recognized in animals. In such cases, reference to the substantial human literature on skeletal dysplasias may be useful.

Chondrodysplasias

The dwarfism of the chondrodysplasias is disproportionate, in contrast to the proportionate or primordial dwarfism associated with somatotropin deficiency or defects in the insulin-like growth factor pathway. The chondrodystrophic dog breeds (e.g., Dachshund, Pekingese, and Basset Hound) are actually variant forms of disproportionate dwarfism. The short-legged trait in chondrodystrophic dog breeds is associated with a fibroblast growth factor 4 (Fgf4) retrogene inserted in chromosome 18, and expressed in the cartilage of the long bones. Similarly, the brachycephalic skull shape, at least in part, is associated with a single nucleotide polymorphism (SNP) in bone morphogenetic protein 3 (BMP3).

The underlying molecular defects of a number of animal chondrodysplasias have now been determined. The human skeletal dysplasia classification system groups disorders based on radiographic, biochemical, and molecular criteria, and 22 out of the 40 groups are associated with chondrodysplasia. Once more of the molecular defects associated with chondrodysplasias in animals have been determined, a similar classification system for animals could be developed.

Cartilage grows by both interstitial proliferation and surface apposition. Longitudinal growth of the cartilage model in the fetus, and at growth plates in young animals, relies on interstitial proliferation of chondrocytes, whereas transverse growth occurs by both interstitial and appositional growth. In some chondrodysplasias, appositional growth is normal but interstitial growth of cartilage is defective, resulting in premature closure of growth plates and reduced length of long bones. The intersphenoid, spheno-occipital, and interoccipital synchondroses at the base of the skull also develop by interstitial proliferation of chondrocytes and close prematurely in such disorders. In some chondrodysplastic calves, bony ridges project into the cranial cavity, possibly resulting from early fusion of the spheno-occipital synchondrosis and altered growth in this region of the skull. Although there is hypoplasia of basocranial bones and impaired development of the ethmoids and turbinates, the mandible, which enlarges by appositional growth, develops normally, leading to prognathia inferior. As the brain continues to grow, the cranium becomes domed and hydrocephalus may develop. The spinal column is shorter than normal because of reduced length of individual vertebrae, as are the ribs, but costochondral junctions may be enlarged because the cartilage expands by appositional growth.

Chondrodysplasias of cattle

Several forms of inherited chondrodysplasia occur in different breeds of cattle and are broadly classified on the basis of their morphologic characteristics into *"bulldog," Telemark, "snorter" (brachycephalic), and long-headed (dolichocephalic) types*.

The *most severe form of bovine chondrodysplasia is the lethal* **bulldog type**, which occurs in the Dexter and a number of other miniature cattle, including miniature Jersey, miniature Scottish Highland, and miniature Belted Galloway. Some short-legged Dexters are heterozygous for an *incompletely dominant gene*, which, when homozygous, gives rise to a bulldog calf. It is likely that Dexter cattle heterozygous for the bulldog mutation were used in the development of the other miniature cattle breeds in which bulldog calves have been seen.

Bulldog calves may be carried to full term but are usually aborted before the seventh month of gestation. Aborted calves may or may not have hair and are much smaller than normal for the stage of pregnancy; in fact, they may be so small they are not noticed by the owner. In all cases, they possess severe, relatively consistent, skeletal abnormalities. Bulldog calves have *extremely short limbs, which are usually rotated; a short, domed head with protruding mandible; a short vertebral column; cleft palate; and a large ventral abdominal hernia* (Fig. 2-23). The tongue is normal size but, because of the shortened skull bones, protrudes markedly. The shortened limb bones consist of mushroom-shaped, cartilaginous epiphyses, which make up 50-70% of bone length and are separated by a short central segment of diaphyseal bone.

Histologically, the long bones lack distinct growth plates. Instead, the physeal cartilage consists of densely packed chondrocytes showing no orderly arrangement into columns, and a fibrillar eosinophilic intercellular matrix surrounding large, vascular, cartilage canals. Because of failure of endochondral ossification at the growth plates, there is no distinct primary or secondary spongiosa and little growth in length of long bones (Fig. 2-24). However, intramembranous ossification beneath the periosteum proceeds normally, and contributes disproportionately to the bone volume.

Dexter chondrodysplasia is associated with 2 different mutations in the *aggrecan (ACAN) gene*, and a test for carriers of these mutations is commercially available. Aggrecan is the main matrix proteoglycan expressed by chondrocytes during cartilage formation in the mesenchymal primordial limb buds. The specific roles of cartilage matrix proteoglycans are for the most part unknown.

Bulldog calves have also been described in the Holstein breed, where the calves are similar to those of the Dexter breed; however, *in Holsteins the defect has autosomal recessive inheritance* and, as such, the heterozygous parents are phenotypically normal. Other features described in Holstein bulldog calves include pulmonary hypoplasia resulting from reduced ribs and tapering of the thorax, and a stenotic trachea at the cranial thoracic inlet.

The **Telemark lethal** form of bovine chondrodysplasia is also inherited as an *autosomal recessive trait*. Affected calves are born alive but cannot stand, and die of suffocation shortly after birth. The head and facial abnormalities are similar to those of bulldog calves, and the limbs, although not quite as short as in bulldog calves, are much shorter than normal and rotated to various degrees. A similar disorder, characterized by

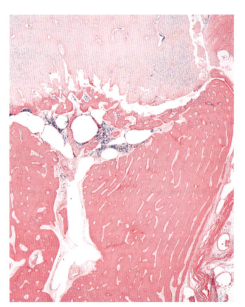

Figure 2-24 Physeal and metaphyseal regions of a long bone from a Dexter bulldog calf with **bovine chondrodysplasia**. There is no arrangement of chondrocytes into a recognizable growth plate. The metaphysis is markedly abbreviated and consists of thick bony trabeculae incorporating only occasional cartilage spicules. The intramembranous bone of periosteal origin greatly exceeds the volume of bone derived from endochondral ossification at the growth plates. (Microscope slide courtesy R.W. Cook.)

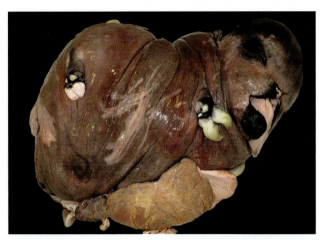

Figure 2-23 **Bovine chondrodysplasia.** Aborted Scottish Highland bulldog calf with extremely short, rotated limbs; a short domed head with protruding mandible; short spine; and large umbilical hernia.

autosomal recessive inheritance, occurs in Jersey cattle, but shows much greater phenotypic variability. The lesions in Jerseys may include a short, broad head, deformed mandible, cleft palate, and short, spiraled limbs, but many calves have mild lesions and are viable.

Brachycephalic ("snorter") type dwarfism was common in the *Hereford breed* in North America, during the late 1940s through to the 1960s, but was also seen in other countries because of importation of North American bulls. Snorter dwarfism has also been reported in other beef breeds, especially the Angus. The disease is inherited as an *autosomal recessive trait*, but appears to be partially expressed in heterozygotes, some of which are slightly smaller and more compact than normal. However, clinical detection and elimination of carriers based on size, and other tests, were found to be unreliable because of the large overlap between carriers and normal animals. With the introduction of programs to eliminate the defective gene and a change in breeding emphasis to larger-frame beef cattle, *snorter dwarfism is now rare*.

Snorter dwarfism is a much milder form of chondrodysplasia than the bulldog types. Affected animals have noisy labored respiration, which gives rise to the snorter name, and chronic ruminal tympany. Affected calves have *a short, broad head with bulging forehead and a slightly protruding mandible* (Fig. 2-25). The eyes are prominent and laterally displaced. The vertebral column is short, and radiographically, the ventral borders of the vertebral bodies and the ends of the transverse processes have characteristic exostoses; these changes are most obvious in the lumbar region, and radiography of this area can be used to diagnose snorter dwarfism in affected animals. Bony projections into the cranium are the result of premature closure of the basocranial synchondroses. The distal limb bones are proportionately shorter than proximal bones, with the metacarpi showing the greatest degree of shortening. Long bones have a short diaphyseal length but normal epiphyseal length. *The ratio of total metacarpal length to diaphyseal diameter is a useful diagnostic indicator for snorter dwarfism.* In snorter dwarfs the ratio is usually ≤4.0, whereas in normal animals it is >4.5. Histologic changes in the growth plates of snorter dwarfs are relatively mild and are not of diagnostic value. The microscopic organization of growth plates into their different zones is normal, but the columns of palisading chondrocytes are shorter, less hypertrophied, and more irregular.

Long-headed or **dolichocephalic dwarfs** are slightly larger than snorter dwarfs, but the main difference is that *the head is proportionately much longer and tapers to a narrow muzzle*.

The defect has been reported in a number of beef cattle including Angus, Holstein, and Simmental. Affected animals may have crooked limbs, and a slow growth rate. In Angus cattle, a nonsense mutation in cGMP-dependent type II protein kinase (PRKG2) was shown to be the cause of an outbreak of long-headed dwarfs in the United States. PRKG2 regulates phosphorylation of SOX9, a transcription factor required for translocation and regulation of collagen type II (Col2) and X (Col10) in the growth plate, and is therefore critical for growth plate development. PRKG2 is found on bovine chromosome 6, adjacent to quantitative trait loci for production traits, such as growth rate and milk yield, and therefore was likely under considerable selection pressure.

Another form of chondrodysplasia, caused by mutations in the **Ellis van Creveld syndrome 2** *(EVC2)* gene (previously called the *LIMBIN* gene), has been described in *Japanese Brown cattle and Tyrolean Grey cattle*. The dwarfism has autosomal recessive inheritance, and affected cattle have short rotated long bones (Fig. 2-26) with enlarged distal and proximal ends (Fig. 2-27). Histologically, there is disorganization of the growth plate with decreased thickness of the proliferative and hypertrophic chondrocyte zones; in a number of animals, the physes close prematurely. Some chondrocytes contain cytoplasmic vacuoles. The EVC2 protein forms part of the primary cilia and is thought to be involved in regulating sonic hedgehog signaling. In mice, EVC2 was found to be expressed in proliferating chondrocytes; however, the function of the gene is unknown.

Further reading

Agerholm JS, et al. Familial chondrodysplasia in Holstein calves. J Vet Diagn Invest 2004;16:293-298.

Koltes JE, et al. A nonsense mutation in cGMP-dependent type II protein kinase (PRKG2) causes dwarfism in American Angus cattle. Proc Natl Acad Sci U S A 2009;106:19250-19255.

Rimbault M, Ostrander EA. So many doggone traits: mapping genetics of multiple phenotypes in the domestic dog. Hum Mol Genet 2012;21:R52-R57.

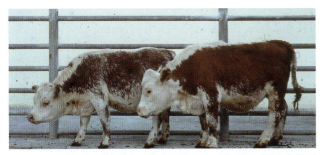

Figure 2-25 Two brachycephalic ("snorter") dwarf Hereford calves with **bovine chondrodysplasia** showing the characteristic short stature, short broad head with bulging forehead, and distended abdomen. (Courtesy R.D. Jolly.)

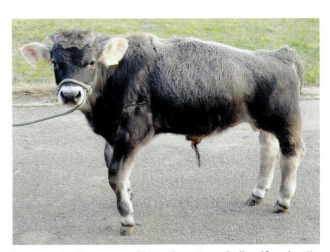

Figure 2-26 Six-month-old Tyrolean Grey bull calf with **Ellis van Creveld syndrome 2**. The calf has disproportionately shortened limbs, enlarged epiphyses, and carpal flexion. (Courtesy A. Gentile.)

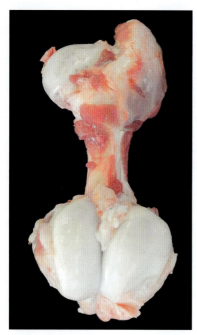

Figure 2-27 Femur from a Tyrolean Grey calf with **chondrodysplasia** showing the shortened diaphyses and enlargement of the epiphyses. (Courtesy C. Benazzi.)

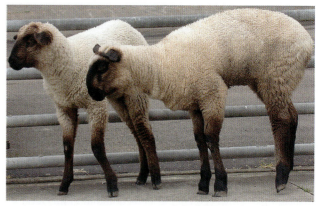

Figure 2-28 Lambs with **spider lamb syndrome** showing the long legs, straight hocks, and lumbar kyphosis. One has a pronounced Roman nose. Both lambs had severe valgus deformity of the hind limbs giving a "cow-hocked" appearance not evident in this image.

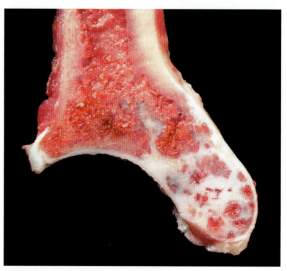

Figure 2-29 **Spider lamb syndrome.** Distal scapula showing persistent islands and bands of cartilage surrounding multiple, small ossification centers in the supraglenoid tubercle.

Chondrodysplasias of sheep

The most common, and potentially important, form of hereditary chondrodysplasia in sheep is **spider lamb syndrome**, *a semilethal condition of Suffolk and Hampshire sheep*. Spider lambs were first recognized in North America in the late 1970s, and the defect was subsequently introduced to other countries with imported Suffolk genetic material. The trait is characterized by *autosomal recessive inheritance with complete penetrance*, but with variation in expressivity between individuals, perhaps depending on genetic background. The prevalence of spider lamb syndrome in North America reached a much higher level than would normally be expected for a semilethal genetic disorder, because of selection for growth and long-legged animals heterozygous for the "spider" gene. The mutant allele results in enhancement of long bone growth.

Lambs with spider syndrome may be aborted or stillborn, but most are born alive, showing skeletal deformities of variable severity. Some appear clinically normal at birth but develop typical signs of the disease by 4-6 weeks of age, including *disproportionately long limbs and neck, shallow body, scoliosis and/or kyphosis of the thoracic spine, concave sternum and other sternal deformities, and valgus deformity of the forelimbs below the carpus, creating a knock-kneed appearance* (Fig. 2-28). Hindlimb deformities may also be present, but are less severe than those involving the forelimbs. Facial deformities, including Roman nose, and deviation and shortening of the maxilla, are common, but not consistent. The deformities of the limbs and spinal column become progressively more severe with age.

Diagnosis is best confirmed by demonstrating characteristic radiographic changes in the elbow, sternum, and shoulder. Multiple, irregular islands of ossification are present in the anconeal area, olecranon, and distal humerus, and there is malalignment of cuboidal-shaped sternebrae, with wedge-shaped vertebral bodies. In addition, there is *elongation of occipital condyles in a craniocaudal direction*. There may be dorsal deviation of the sternum between the second and sixth sternebrae, and the caudal sternebrae often fail to fuse across the midline. Cervical and thoracic vertebral bodies are often abnormal in shape and contain excessive quantities of cartilage that form tongues and islands extending into the middle of the vertebrae. The olecranon and distal scapula also contain an *excess of cartilage surrounding the multiple, irregular-shaped islands of ossification* (Fig. 2-29). Severe degenerative arthropathy, particularly involving the atlanto-occipital, elbow, and carpal joints, is present in lambs >3 months of age (Fig. 2-30).

Histologically, the changes reflect abnormal development of ossification centers in bones that develop by endochondral ossification. Multiple small ossification centers develop in nodules of hypertrophic cartilage but fail to coalesce and expand in the normal fashion toward articular surfaces (Fig. 2-31). The thick articular cartilage and lack of subchondral bone predispose to flap formation, erosion, and degenerative arthropathy.

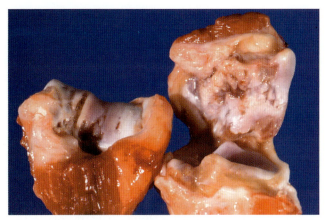

Figure 2-30 Severe degeneration of the elbow joint in a lamb with **spider lamb syndrome**. The olecranon is thickened, and there is loss of articular cartilage with irregular pitting of the subchondral bone in the trochlear notch. The humeral condyle is devoid of articular cartilage and the subchondral bone is pitted.

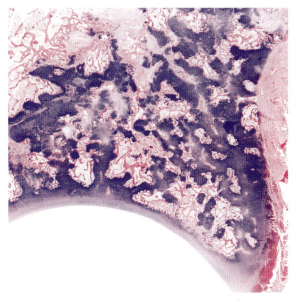

Figure 2-31 Subgross preparation of the scapula from a **spider lamb** showing multiple ossification centers separated by irregular bands of cartilage.

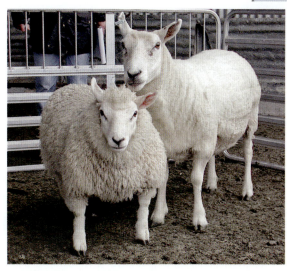

Figure 2-32 Phenotypically normal heterozygous Texel ewe with lamb affected by **Texel chondrodysplasia**. Note the short limbs and characteristic wide-based stance.

The proliferative and hypertrophic zones of vertebral and long bone growth plates are disorganized and irregularly thickened, with tongues and islands of cartilage extending into the metaphysis or epiphysis.

An interesting feature of the disease is that the ossification centers most severely affected are those that develop around the time of birth. Those growth plates (proximal metatarsal and metacarpal) that complete their development before birth, and are not subjected to the mechanical forces of weight bearing and locomotion, appear normal. The lesions associated with spider lamb syndrome therefore may reflect the influence of mechanical stress on a defective cartilage model, and could help to explain some of the variable expressivity that is a feature of the disease.

A *point mutation* (T→A at position 1719) in ovine fibroblast growth factor receptor 3 (FGFR3) has been identified as the underlying defect in spider lamb syndrome. FGFR3 is strongly expressed in resting and proliferating chondrocytes, wherein it limits the number of chondrocytes that enter the hypertrophic phase, thereby limiting growth. A test for detecting heterozygous animals is available.

Chondrodysplastic syndromes characterized by **disproportionate dwarfism** are uncommon in sheep. The best known of these is the *Ancon mutant*, which historically gained popularity as a breed for its inability to jump walls. Although the Ancon breed is now extinct, the mesomelic, short-limbed dwarfism has reappeared in different breeds, presumably because of new mutations.

A *chondrodysplasia characterized by dwarfism and varus deformity of the forelimbs has been described in* **Texel sheep** in New Zealand. The syndrome is inherited as an *autosomal recessive trait*, but with variable expression. Affected lambs appear normal at birth, but by 2-4 weeks of age show reduced growth rate, *shortened neck and legs, varus forelimb deformities, and a wide-based stance* (Fig. 2-32). Severely affected lambs show progressive reluctance to walk and often die within the first 4 months of life. In such cases, the articular cartilage on major weight-bearing surfaces of the hip and shoulder joints may be completely eroded, exposing the subchondral bone. The trachea is flaccid, sometimes kinked, and tracheal rings are partially flattened. Histologically, there is *disorganization of chondrocytes in both articular and physeal cartilage, and multiple foci of chondrolysis, which sometimes coalesce to form large clefts and cystic spaces* crossed by basophilic strands or clumps of granular material. Chondrocytes are enlarged and surrounded by *concentric rings of basophilic fibrillar and granular matrix* (Fig. 2-33). Chondrocyte columns in the physis are disorganized, and broad tongues of hypertrophic cartilage extend into the metaphysis close to healing trabecular microfractures. Similar microscopic changes are also present in tracheal cartilage. Chondroitin-4-sulfate levels in articular cartilage are decreased, and a 1-bp deletion, resulting in a premature stop codon, has been found in SLC13A1, a sodium-sulfate transporter.

Disproportionate dwarfism is a feature of **brachygnathia, cardiomegaly, and renal hypoplasia syndrome** in Merino

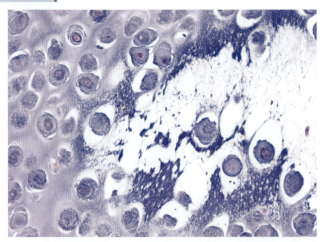

Figure 2-33 Articular cartilage from a 3-week-old Texel lamb with **chondrodysplasia** showing a focus of chondrolysis and the characteristic concentric rings around chondrocytes.

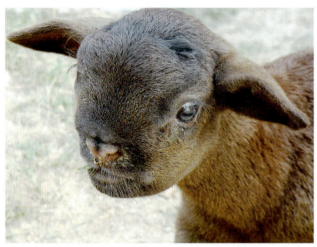

Figure 2-34 Skeletal dysplasia in a Cabugi lamb with domed head, exophthalmos, short maxilla, and protruding mandible. (Courtesy F. Riet.)

sheep in Australia. The syndrome has *autosomal recessive* inheritance, and lambs are born dead at full term. The abnormalities include disproportionate dwarfism; inferior brachygnathia; a short, broad cranium; small thoracic cavity with increased heart size and right-sided ventricular hypertrophy; abdominal distension; and hepatomegaly. Histologically, renal hypoplasia and liver congestion are present, but bone lesions are not reported.

A skeletal dysplasia with craniofacial abnormalities and dwarfism has been reported in *hair sheep of the* **Cabugi breed** in Brazil. Dwarf lambs die at 2-6 months of age, have short straight limbs, *a domed head with widely separated eyes and prominent exophthalmos, a short muzzle, and mandibular prognathia* (Fig. 2-34). In addition, there is aplasia of sternebrae 1 and 7. The limb bones (except the scapula and humerus) are shorter than normal with the metacarpal and metatarsal bones most decreased in length. Of the skull bones, *the nasal bone is most reduced in size*. Microscopically, no lesions are reported in any organs or bones. The disease may have dominant inheritance with incomplete penetrance, as the shortened face is a feature of the Cabugi breed and may represent heterozygous animals.

Chondrodysplasias of pigs

Disproportionate dwarfism was reported in 3 litters of **Danish Landrace pigs** sired by the same boar. The abnormalities were confined to the long bones of the limbs, and were most severe in the forelimbs. The first signs of limb shortening were noticed by 3 weeks of age, and became more obvious with time. Affected pigs had an abnormal gait caused by loose attachment of the limbs to the body and excessive mobility of joints. Animals developed a degenerative arthropathy that worsened with age. Few animals reached breeding age, and those that did had low fertility. Histologically, the physes had decreased thickness of the proliferative zone and an irregular hypertrophic zone, but the chondrocytes within each zone appeared normal. Breeding trials indicated autosomal recessive inheritance.

Dwarfism analogous to Schmid metaphyseal chondrodysplasia of humans has been described in the progeny of an apparently normal **Yorkshire** sow. Animals were normal at birth, but developed shorter, wider long bones with age. Long bones and the costochondral junctions had excessive physeal cartilage that extended into the metaphysis; articular cartilage was normal. Microscopically, the zone of hypertrophy was expanded, with disorganized chondrocyte columns and variably sized chondrocytes. Areas of hemorrhage and necrosis were present near tongues of cartilage that extended into the metaphysis. Breeding indicated autosomal dominant inheritance, and a missense mutation was found in the α1 chain of type X collagen (COL10A1) that led to impaired ability of the type X collagen chains to interact and undergo trimerization. Type X collagen is specifically expressed by hypertrophic chondrocytes during endochondral ossification.

Chondrodysplasias of horses

Disproportionate dwarfism is recognized in the **Friesian** breed of horse, with affected horses having a proportionately larger head, broad chest and long back, with short limbs and hyperextension of the fetlock joints. Histologically, there is disorganization of the proliferative and hypertrophic chondrocyte zones of the growth plate. The defect has been linked to a 2-MB region in chromosome 14.

Four distinct types of dwarfism have been described in miniature horses, associated with 4 different *mutations in the ACAN gene*. One form closely resembles the "bulldog" dwarfism of Dexter cattle (Fig. 2-35).

Further reading

Dantas FP, et al. Skeletal dysplasia with craniofacial deformity and disproportionate dwarfism in hair sheep of Northeastern Brazil. J Comp Pathol 2014;150:245-252.

Eberth JE. Chondrodysplasia-like Dwarfism in the Miniature Horse. Thesis. University of Kentucky; 2013. Available at: <http://uknowledge.uky.edu/gluck_etds/11>.

Shariflou MR, et al. Lethal genetic disorder in Poll Merino/Merino sheep in Australia. Aust Vet J 2011;89:254-259.

Smith LB, et al. Fibroblast growth factor receptor 3 effects on proliferation and telomerase activity in sheep growth plate chondrocytes. J Anim Sci Biotechnol 2012;3:39.

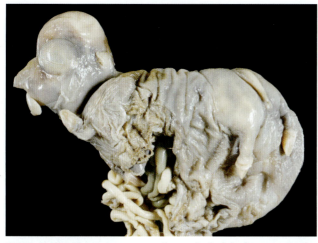

Figure 2-35 Aborted miniature horse foal with features similar to bulldog **chondrodysplasia**; extremely short, rotated limbs; protruding tongue; and umbilical hernia.

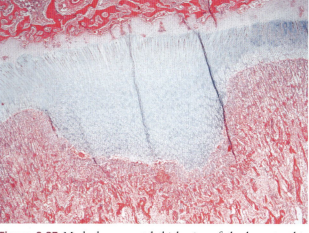

Figure 2-37 Marked, segmental thickening of the hypertrophic zone in the physis of an **Alaskan Malamute puppy with chondrodysplasia**.

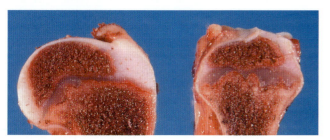

Figure 2-36 Irregular thickening of the proximal humeral (left) and distal radial physes of an **Alaskan Malamute puppy with chondrodysplasia**.

Chondrodysplasias of dogs

A variety of forms of inherited chondrodysplasia are recognized in dogs of different breeds. Some breeds, such as Dachshund, Corgi, and Basset Hound, are in fact defined by their chondrodysplasia.

Chondrodysplasia in the Alaskan Malamute is characterized by *disproportionate, short-legged dwarfism and autosomal recessive inheritance* with complete penetrance and variable expression. At birth, the growth plates of affected puppies appear normal radiographically and microscopically. Radiographic changes become apparent as early as 7-10 days of age, but are more pronounced after 3 weeks. During growth, the changes become marked, including bowing of radius and ulna, lateral deviation and enlargement of the carpus, wide irregular growth plates, and sclerotic mushroomed metaphyses (Fig. 2-36). This suggests that mechanical force is required to create the clinical and pathologic changes. Abnormal endochondral ossification occurs throughout the body, but the most striking lesions occur in the distal ulna and radius, likely reflecting the proportionately greater weight-bearing responsibility of the forelimbs compared to the hindlimbs, and the greater susceptibility to injury. Irregular thickening of the growth plates in the limb bones is a feature of the disease, and microscopically, broad tongues of hypertrophic cartilage extend into the metaphysis in close proximity to healing trabecular microfractures (Figs. 2-37, 2-38). Disruption of the metaphyseal blood supply, leading to impaired vascular invasion of the developing growth plate, is considered responsible for the

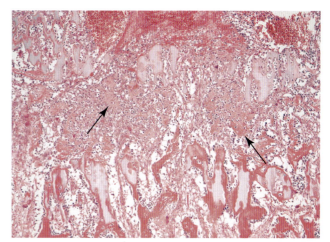

Figure 2-38 Primary spongiosa immediately beneath a thickened segment of physis in the same **Alaskan Malamute puppy with chondrodysplasia**. Note the disruption of the normal trabecular architecture and replacement by proliferating osteoblasts producing disorganized spicules of osteoid (arrows). An area of hemorrhage is present closer to the physis.

physeal thickenings. *The growth plate lesions bear a remarkable resemblance to rickets*, both grossly and in demineralized bone sections, but appositional bone formation rates and mineralization of cartilage are normal. Hemolytic anemia, characterized by stomatocytosis, macrocytosis, reticulocytosis, increased osmotic fragility, and decreased life-span of erythrocytes, accompanies the chondrodysplasia in this breed. Animals have low hemoglobin concentrations and red cell numbers but normal packed cell volumes. Heterozygotes have intermediate hemoglobin concentrations, suggesting that this manifestation of the syndrome is inherited as an incompletely dominant trait.

Chondrodysplasia in the Norwegian Elkhound and Karelian Bear dog *is also a disproportionate, short-legged dwarfism*. Affected animals have bowing of the radius and ulna, and shortened vertebral bodies. The proliferative zone of the growth plate is markedly reduced. *A highly distinctive feature is the presence of one or more large, intracytoplasmic inclusions* *in the chondrocytes of all* zones. The inclusions stain deep blue with the alcian blue–periodic acid–Schiff method at pH 1.0 and 2.6, and on electron microscopy consist of homogeneous finely granular material bound by a smooth discontinuous membrane. Inclusions that escape from degenerate chondrocytes persist free in lacunae. The chondrocyte columns in the zone of hypertrophy and degeneration are generally disorganized and separated by wide matrix bars. Trabeculae in the primary spongiosa are coarse and short, with many horizontal bridges and thick osteoid seams. No inclusions are present in osteoblasts or osteocytes. A nonsense mutation with autosomal recessive inheritance in the integrin-α10 *(ITGA10)* gene that results in a premature stop codon and loss of nearly half the protein has been associated with this form of chondrodysplasia in the Norwegian Elkhound and Karelian Bear dog. The *ITGA10* gene is expressed by growth plate chondrocytes, and binds type II, IV, and VI collagens. Its function is unknown, but is thought to be associated with matrix fibril assembly and chondrocyte proliferation.

Chondrodysplasia in the English Pointer has been reported in the United Kingdom and Australia. Inheritance appears to be autosomal recessive. Affected puppies are smaller than their littermates, have lateral deviation of the forelimbs, and develop locomotory abnormalities, including a bunny-hopping gait. Some also have inferior prognathism, dorsoventral flattening of the thorax and enlarged costochondral junctions. Growth plates are irregularly thickened, resulting from increased width of the hypertrophic zone, but the lesion varies in severity between different bones. Increased mineralization of laryngeal and tracheal cartilage occurs in some affected animals. At around 10 weeks of age, articular cartilages appear normal, but by 16-18 weeks, there are abnormalities in the cartilage of all major limb joints, including wrinkles, projections, and sometimes fibrillation. In the epiphyseal cartilage beneath these lesions, initially there is decreased staining density of the matrix, followed by irregular cystic spaces containing degenerate chondrocytes and strands of collagen. Severe degenerative arthropathy develops in some joints.

Chondrodysplasia in the Great Pyrenees also appears to be inherited as an autosomal recessive trait. Affected pups are normal at birth but by 2 weeks are shorter and lighter than their littermates, and by 12 weeks of age develop angular limb deformities. Mature dwarfs are less than half of normal size. Radiographic abnormalities are restricted to the metaphyses of long bones and vertebrae and are characterized by *delayed ossification*. Histologically, chondrocyte columns in growth plates are disorganized, and many chondrocytes contain cytoplasmic vacuoles that consist of dilated cisternae of rough endoplasmic reticulum. Metaphyseal trabeculae are thicker than normal and are often joined by lateral bridges.

Pseudoachondroplastic dysplasia occurs in **Miniature Poodles,** and inheritance of the trait is *autosomal recessive*. The disease is not apparent at birth, but by 2-3 weeks of age affected pups are noticeably smaller than their littermates and have difficulty standing and walking. The skull is usually normal, but mild inferior prognathism may be present. Vertebral bodies are short and show delayed ossification, costal cartilages are longer than normal, and costochondral junctions are enlarged. Severely affected pups have dorsoventral flattening of the rib cage, presumably caused by persistent recumbency. The limb bones are also short and bowed, particularly those of the forelimbs, and possess enlarged epiphyses that are sometimes flared over the metaphyses. Histologically, the cartilage matrix is sparse and lacks basophilia. *Chondrocytes vary in size, may be surrounded by haloes,* and are sometimes clumped together in enlarged lacunae. Chondrocyte columns in growth plates are irregular, and the proliferative zone is abnormal. Ossification centers develop later than normal and are multifocal, creating a stippled appearance of epiphyses radiographically (Fig. 2-39). The articular surface is irregular, and degenerative arthropathy and spondylosis may develop in pups <1 year of age. A 130-kb deletion leads to loss of most of exon 1 of the *SLC13A1* (the sodium-sulfate cotransporter) gene and results in decreased sulfation of glycosaminoglycans. *The underlying defect in cartilage matrix formation not only causes defective endochondral ossification but also results in abnormal formation of the trachea and nasal septum.*

Multiple epiphyseal dysplasia is a rare condition of **Beagle dogs**, probably inherited as an autosomal recessive trait. Affected puppies walk with a swaying gait, but in adults, lameness is only apparent after exercise. The earliest radiographic signs are not visible until 3 weeks of age and consist of *stippled epiphyseal mineralization* (Fig. 2-40), particularly in the tarsal bones. The carpal bones; femoral, humeral, metacarpal, and metatarsal epiphyses; and the bodies of the sixth and seventh lumbar vertebrae may also be affected. By 4-6 months, the stippling is no longer apparent, having been incorporated into the normal ossification centers. The abnormal foci of epiphyseal mineralization develop in a specific subarticular zone of the epiphyses. The initial lesion is a floccular accumulation of chondroitin sulfate and glycoprotein in chondrocyte lacunae. As adjacent lacunae coalesce and liquefy, their contents mineralize.

Osteochondrodysplasia in the Scottish Deerhound becomes apparent at around 4-5 weeks of age, with affected puppies showing exercise intolerance and retarded growth. These pups develop a bunny-hopping gait, kyphosis, marked bowing of the limbs, and joint laxity. Mature dogs have

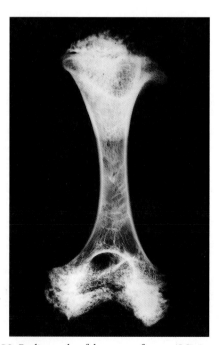

Figure 2-39 Radiograph of humerus from a **Miniature Poodle with pseudoachondroplastic dysplasia** showing irregular, multifocal development of ossification centers creating a stippled appearance.

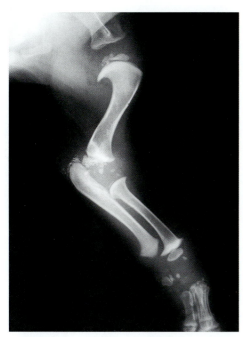

Figure 2-40 **Multiple epiphyseal dysplasia** in a Beagle dog showing stippled epiphyses in shoulder, elbow, and carpal regions. (Courtesy G.P. Rasmussen.)

shortened, porotic long bones, shortened vertebrae, distorted carpal and tarsal bones, incongruences of hip and elbow joints, and enlargement of muscle attachment sites. Growth plates are irregular in width, and physeal-metaphyseal junctions are uneven. The subchondral bone of the humeral head and distal femoral condyles may be flattened. Histologically, there are islands of enlarged basophilic, vacuolated chondrocytes in epiphyses, but physeal and metaphyseal lesions are intermittent. Physes contain some areas that are normal, in addition to areas that are narrow and hypocellular, or lack proliferative or hypertrophic zones. A characteristic feature is the *presence of periodic acid–Schiff-positive, diastase-resistant cytoplasmic inclusions in proliferative and hypertrophic chondrocytes*. The metaphyses may consist of normal primary and secondary spongiosa in some areas, whereas elsewhere the trabeculae are thin, sparse, and largely replaced by fibrovascular connective tissue. The irregularity of the physeal and metaphyseal lesions may reflect localized trauma. The condition is probably inherited as an autosomal recessive trait.

A syndrome with **combined ocular and skeletal dysplasia** occurs in the **Labrador Retriever and Samoyed** breeds. The bone lesions are confined to the appendicular skeleton and include *shortening of the limb bones, abducted elbows, valgus deformity of the carpi, and abnormally shaped radii and ulnas*. Affected dogs have a characteristic "downhill" conformation because of more severe involvement of the forelimbs. In some dogs, the coronoid processes are ununited, and there is hypoplasia of both the coronoid and anconeal processes, but these changes may be incidental because they occur as separate defects in these breeds. Retained cartilage cores may be present in the distal ulna. Although clinical evidence of dwarfism may not be evident until about 8 weeks of age, a radiographic image classification system allows identification of affected puppies at birth. Histologically, the growth plate contains disorganized chondrocyte columns, with cells forming nests and wide bands of unevenly stained matrix. Tongues of cartilage may extend down into the metaphysis. The ocular lesions in both breeds consist of *cataracts and retinal detachment*. The ocular and skeletal lesions appear to be inherited together, but the *defective gene has recessive effects on the skeleton and incomplete dominance in the eye*. Heterozygotes may have mild eye lesions but a clinically normal skeleton. Two different mutations, both of which affect the COL3 domain of collagen IX, have been found to cause oculoskeletal dysplasia: drd1 dwarfism with retinal dysplasia type 1 in Labrador Retrievers caused by a 1-bp insertion in *COL9A3* (collagen IX, α3 chain) and drd2 dwarfism with retinal dysplasia type 2 in Samoyeds caused by a large deletion at the 5′ end of *COL9A2* (collagen IX, α2 chain).

Two other types of **disproportionate dwarfism** without ocular lesions have been described in **Labrador Retrievers**. Mild dwarfism, termed *skeletal dysplasia 2*, has been described in Europe. Affected animals have shortened legs with a normal body length and width; however, considerable overlap in size occurs with normal dogs. The disease has *autosomal recessive inheritance with incomplete penetrance* and is caused by a point mutation in a highly conserved area of *COL11A2* (collagen XI, α2 chain). The mutation has not been determined for the other, *more severe form*, also described in Labrador Retrievers in Europe. The disease is suggested to have autosomal recessive inheritance, and affected dogs have short front legs with deviation of the radius. Histologically, there is disorganization of chondrocyte columns and irregularities in endochondral ossification.

Chondrodysplasia of cats

There are *few reports of chondrodysplasias in cats*. One report describes a severe form in a stillborn kitten with homozygous Pelger-Huët anomaly, after test-mating of a brother and sister with heterozygous Pelger-Huët anomaly. The kitten was small and had a dome-shaped skull, flat face, and protruding tongue. Vertebrae were short, as were ribs and long bones of the limbs. The limbs were thick and had broad, mushroom-shaped epiphyses. Growth plates were incompletely formed, with partial or irregular ossification at the center of the physis and more normal peripheral regions. Cartilage matrix was mottled with areas of cystic degeneration. The skeletal lesions in the stillborn kitten were very similar to those seen in rabbits with homozygous Pelger-Huët anomaly. Skeletal defects were also present in a littermate with normal leukocytes, suggesting that the skeletal abnormalities may have been the result of inbreeding rather than associated with Pelger-Huët anomaly.

A *possible metaphyseal chondrodysplasia* was diagnosed in 2 unrelated kittens with short limbs, bowed forelimbs, marked widening of the physes, and flaring of the metaphyses. The most severe physeal lesions were present in the distal radius and proximal humerus. The radiographic changes initially led to a diagnosis of rickets, but neither kitten responded to treatment, and there was no evidence of defective mineralization. One kitten had 2 siblings with similar limb deformities, and its probable sire was also known to have short, deformed forelimbs, suggesting a genetic cause.

An **osteochondrodysplasia** characterized by short, misshapen distal limbs is reported in **Scottish Fold cats**. Affected animals may be lame, reluctant to jump, and have a stiff gait. Some animals may have a short, inflexible tail. Abnormal bone growth results in irregularity in the size and shape of tarsal, carpal, metatarsal, and metacarpal bones; phalanges; and caudal vertebrae. Secondary degenerative arthropathy may

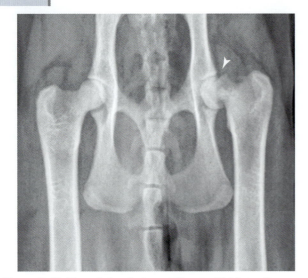

Figure 2-41 Physeal dysplasia in a 2-year-old Maine Coon cat. Radiograph showing unilateral slipped capital femoral epiphysis (white arrowhead). The physis on the opposite femoral head is still open, despite the age of the cat.

lead to narrowing of joint spaces and progressive new bone formation and exostoses, which in severe cases is responsible for swelling of plantar tarsometatarsal regions. Histologically, there is evidence of defective endochondral ossification in physes and beneath articular cartilage. Cartilage columns in physes are disorganized, with irregular thickening of physeal cartilage. Islands of cartilage may extend from articular cartilage into epiphyses; the articular cartilage may have necrotic foci and a discontinuous tide mark. Enthesophytes may also occur at ligamentous insertions. Lesions can be detected in kittens as young as 7 weeks of age, but the bony changes are slowly progressive and may not be detected for several years. The condition appears to have autosomal dominant inheritance with incomplete penetrance. Affected cats homozygous for the *fd* (fold-eared) gene are severely affected, whereas heterozygous animals tend to develop milder lesions, but because all possess some degree of osteochondrodysplasia of the distal limbs, the breed is not recognized in the United Kingdom.

A syndrome characterized by **physeal dysplasia** and atraumatic slipped capital femoral epiphysis occurs in cats (Fig. 2-41), most of which are *male and overweight*. Affected females often have affected male littermates. The Siamese and Maine Coon breeds are over-represented, but the lesion is common in domestic shorthair cats. Affected cats are typically young (2-4 years), but older than the age of expected physeal closure (7-9 months). The lesion is *persistence of dysplastic growth plates characterized by disorganized clusters of chondrocytes* surrounded by abundant matrix (Fig. 2-42A, B). These changes are also present in other physes but only the proximal femoral physis fractures, presumably because of the shear forces at that site. A similar syndrome in humans is recognized in adolescent, overweight boys.

Further reading

Goldstein O, et al. COL9A2 and COL9A3 mutations in canine autosomal recessive oculoskeletal dysplasia. Mamm Genome 2010;21:398-408.

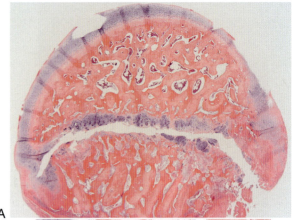
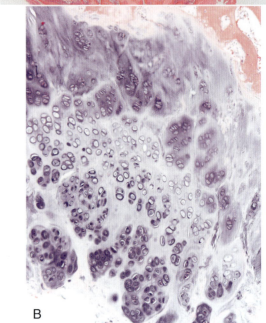

Figure 2-42 A. Femoral head and neck from a cat with **physeal dysplasia.** Note the fracture through the persistent dysplastic physis. The articular cartilage loss is artifactual. **B.** Higher magnification of physis showing clusters of abnormal hypertrophic chondrocytes.

Kyöstilä K, et al. Canine chondrodysplasia caused by a truncating mutation in collagen-binding integrin alpha subunit 10. PLoS One. 2013;8:e75621.

Neff MW, et al. Partial deletion of the sulfate transporter SLC13A1 is associated with an osteochondrodysplasia in the Miniature Poodle breed. PLoS One 2012;7:e51917.

Takanosu M, et al. Incomplete dominant osteochondrodysplasia in heterozygous Scottish Fold cats. J Small Anim Pract 2008;49: 197-199.

Osteogenesis imperfecta

Osteogenesis imperfecta is one of the most frequently observed inherited connective tissue disorders of humans, but *occurs rarely in domestic animals*. The disease is characterized by *excessive bone fragility*, which in severe cases may result in multiple intrauterine fractures, skeletal deformities, and either stillbirth or perinatal death. Milder forms may be inapparent at birth but lead to increased incidence of postnatal fractures, bowing of the limbs, and reduced growth. Other abnormalities include fragile, opalescent teeth (dentinogenesis imperfecta), joint laxity, and blue sclerae. *At least 4 distinct forms of osteogenesis imperfecta are recognized in human patients*, and up to 9 forms have been described. Osteogenesis imperfecta types 1 to 4 are inherited as autosomal dominant traits because of mutations in either the *COL1A1* or *COL1A2* genes that code for the α1 and α2 collagen chains, respectively. Type I collagen is the predominant collagen type in bone, dentin, ligaments, tendons, and in the ocular sclera, thus accounting for the characteristic distribution of lesions. The other types account for only 2-5% of osteogenesis imperfecta cases and have autosomal recessive inheritance. These forms are associated with defects in proteins associated with the production, folding, maintenance of structure, and secretion of type I collagen.

Most reports of osteogenesis imperfecta in animals are in calves and lambs and appear analogous to the most severe form of the disease in humans (type II). *Typically "outbreaks" of disease occur in these species resulting from new dominant mutations in germ cell lines of a sire.* As such, the disease is not necessarily breed-related and can occur in crossbred animals. In **cattle**, the disease has occurred in Australia, the United States, and Denmark in the offspring of 3 clinically normal, unrelated **Holstein-Friesian** bulls, and also in **Charolais** calves in Denmark and **Angus** calves in Brazil. A single crossbred **Hereford** calf with osteogenesis imperfecta has been identified in New Zealand. There is convincing evidence to support an autosomal dominant mode of inheritance in Holstein-Friesian cattle, although the percentage of calves affected from the 3 Holstein-Friesian bulls varied from 9-44%. This presumably reflects different degrees of gonadal mosaicism following mutations in the germ cell lines of each bull. The manifestations of the disease in each report have been similar, but with minor variations, such as different changes in bone noncollagenous proteins, suggesting that different mutations may be involved. The mode of inheritance in Charolais cattle was not determined.

Affected calves are usually born alive and are of normal size, but most are unable to stand because of marked hypermobility of the joints, and in some cases, the presence of limb fractures. Some affected Holstein-Friesian calves are able to stand and can walk with difficulty, but have a characteristic crouched stance with pasterns almost touching the ground (Fig. 2-43). Some calves have dentinogenesis imperfecta, characterized by small, translucent pink-gray teeth, which are barely erupted at birth, and in one of the reports, may fracture in calves that survive for a few weeks (Fig. 2-44). The sclerae are typically dark blue, but this is more evident during postmortem examination following enucleation of the eye (Fig. 2-45). Skin fragility is not a feature of the disease in calves.

The main findings during postmortem examination relate to the skeleton. *Although the bones are essentially normal in shape, they are extremely brittle* and can usually be broken with little effort. Acute fractures are common in the mandibles and major limb bones. Severely affected calves may have multiple, well-developed calluses on their ribs, indicating intrauterine fractures (Fig. 2-46). In young Holstein-Friesian calves, cones of bone may project well into the medullary cavity, whereas in older calves, the bones are severely osteopenic. In both Charolais calves and in an affected Holstein-Friesian calf that had survived long enough to stand and support weight, multiple transverse lines were present grossly and radiographically in the metaphyses and epiphyses of long bones. These represented bands of healing trabecular microfractures (infraction lines), presumably resulting from trauma during weight-bearing. Tendons are thinner than normal and discolored pink.

Histologically, osteoblast numbers and activity vary from appearing normal in younger calves to trabeculae being lined by atrophic flat osteoblasts in older calves. Calcified cartilage spicules in the primary spongiosa are lined by only a thin layer of basophilic bone matrix, and there is little osteoclastic resorption or realignment of trabeculae. Deeper in the secondary spongiosa trabeculae may be lined by woven bone. Infractions and trabecular microfractures are common. Bone cortices are porous because of incomplete compaction of osteons and

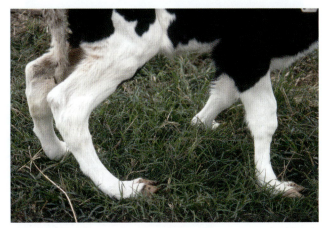

Figure 2-43 **Bovine osteogenesis imperfecta** in a 2-week-old Holstein calf. Because of excessive joint laxity, the calf has a crouched stance, and its pasterns almost touch the ground.

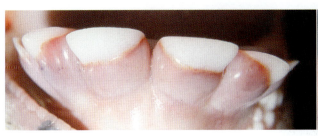

Normal

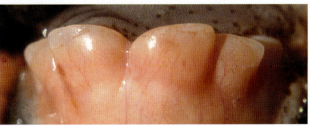

Affected

Figure 2-44 Dentinal dysplasia, with small pink-gray barely erupted teeth in a 2-week-old Holstein calf with **osteogenesis imperfecta** (right). The left image shows the incisor teeth of an age-matched control calf.

consist predominantly of deeply basophilic woven bone with few lamellae, interspersed by loose mesenchymal tissue (Fig. 2-47). The dentin in affected calves is basophilic, coarsely laminated and approximately one-fifth as thick as in control calves. Dentinal tubules are irregularly oriented, irregularly mineralized, reduced in number, and have an undulating margin with the pulp cavity (Fig. 2-48). The sclera is approximately one-fifth normal thickness. The tendons are hypercellular and contain large fibroblasts with a vacuolated cytoplasm. Ultrastructurally, collagen fibrils in the tendons, dentin, sclera, and skin of affected calves are significantly narrower than normal.

Skin fragility is not reported in calves with osteogenesis imperfecta, but **Belgian blue calves with dermatosparaxis** do have skeletal lesions. These calves have a mutation in the procollagen I N-proteinase gene, an enzyme that removes the N-propeptide from type I and II procollagen and is involved in the conversion of procollagen to collagen. Although the bones are grossly normal and *not prone to spontaneous fractures*, they are *abnormally brittle when processed*. Histologically, cortical bone of periosteal origin is disorganized and hypermineralized with radially oriented lamellae. Bone derived from compaction of the chondro-osseous complex is normal.

Arachnomelia, a lethal defect of Italian Brown, Simmental, German Fleckvieh, and Brown Swiss cattle is also *accompanied by increased bone fragility*. Features of the disease include facial deformities, such as *brachygnathia inferior and turning up of the nose, abnormally thin diaphyses of the long bones, angular limb*

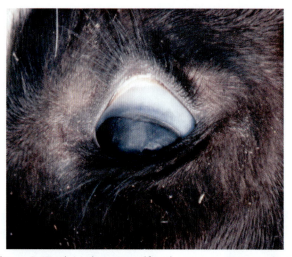

Figure 2-45 Blue sclera in a calf with **osteogenesis imperfecta**.

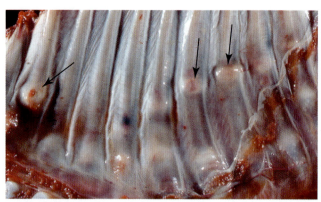

Figure 2-46 Several mature calluses (arrows) on the ribs of a newborn calf with **osteogenesis imperfecta**, indicating intrauterine fractures due to extreme bone fragility.

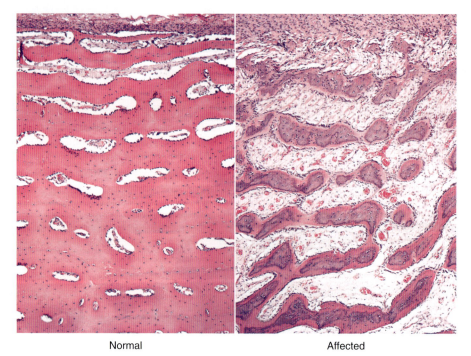

Normal   Affected

Figure 2-47 Periosteum and developing cortical bone in a **normal newborn calf** on the left. Similar view of the developing cortex in a calf with **osteogenesis imperfecta** on the right, showing basophilic spicules of woven bone and minimal compaction by the addition of lamellar bone.

Diseases of Bones

Genetic and Congenital Diseases of Bone

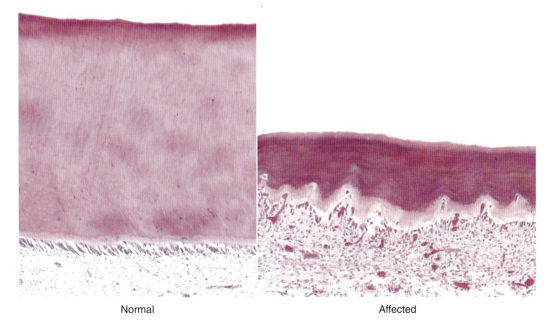

Normal   Affected

Figure 2-48 Tooth dentin in a normal newborn calf on the left. Similar view of the dentin in a calf with **osteogenesis imperfecta** on the right, showing the basophilic thin layer of dentin, and the undulating margin with the pulp cavity.

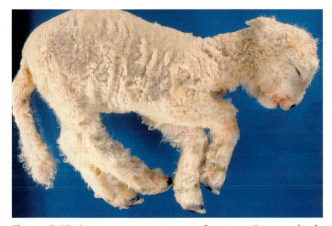

Figure 2-49 Ovine osteogenesis imperfecta in a Romney lamb. Note the domed forehead and brachygnathia inferior.

deformities with massive hyperextension of the fetlocks, and spinal deformities (kyphosis and scoliosis). The cortex of the long bones is of normal thickness; however, the overall diameter is reduced, resulting in fractures of the metacarpal and metatarsal bones, particularly in association with assisted births. The disease has autosomal recessive inheritance, and mutations have been found in 2 different genes. In Simmental and German Fleckvieh breeds, a 2-bp deletion has been found in the molybdenum cofactor synthesis step 1 *(MOCS)* gene, whereas in Brown Swiss, a 1-bp insertion occurs in the sulfite oxidase *(SUOX)* gene. Both mutations likely result in increased sulfite levels, possibly leading to the abnormal bone development.

In **sheep**, severe forms of osteogenesis imperfecta have been reported in 2 flocks in New Zealand and one in the United Kingdom, but many "outbreaks" likely remain unreported. In both New Zealand reports, one of which involved the **Romney** breed, affected lambs died either during parturition or soon after. The Romney lambs had a domed head with brachygnathia inferior, dark blue sclerae, fragile pink teeth, and marked joint laxity (Fig. 2-49). A feature of the disease in Romneys, which involved about 50 lambs, was the presence of *marked skin fragility*. This has not been described in any of the other reports of osteogenesis imperfecta in humans or animals but was a feature of unreported cases diagnosed in crossbred lambs in New Zealand. Test-matings of the Romney ram and unrelated ewes confirmed dominant inheritance. In affected lambs, the bones could be easily bent or cut with a knife, and were often abnormally shaped with thick diaphyseal regions (Fig. 2-50). Most lambs had recent fractures surrounded by hemorrhage and older (in utero) fractures with poorly formed calluses, especially involving the ribs. Microscopic changes were similar to those described in calves with osteogenesis imperfecta, but more severe. Persistent trabeculae of calcified cartilage, lined by a thin layer of basophilic bone, extended deep into the diaphyses of long bones, filling the marrow cavities (Fig. 2-51). Osteoclastic resorption of the primary spongiosa was impaired, with no formation of a recognizable secondary spongiosa. The cortices were extremely porous, but thicker than normal, and consisted of narrow, basophilic trabeculae separated by loose connective tissue. There was no evidence of compaction into normal cortical bone.

Similar gross and microscopic bone lesions, tooth abnormalities, and skin fragility occurred in lambs from the other New Zealand flock, the breed of which was not disclosed. The United Kingdom outbreak occurred in lambs of the **Clun Forest** breed. These lambs often survived parturition and were bright and alert, but usually could not stand. Multiple recent and intrauterine fractures were present in most lambs, and in lambs <3 weeks of age, there was persistence of the primary spongiosa filling most of the marrow cavity, similar to the New Zealand outbreaks. Blue sclerae were reported, but there was

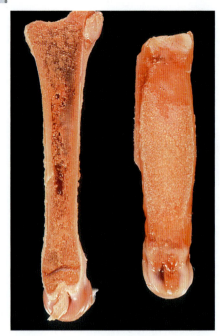

Figure 2-50 Ovine osteogenesis imperfecta in a Romney lamb. Metatarsal bones from a **normal newborn lamb** (left) and a **lamb with osteogenesis imperfecta**. The bone from the affected lamb is shorter, has a thick diaphysis and no medullary cavity.

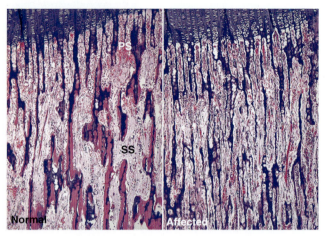

Figure 2-51 Metaphysis from a long bone of a **normal newborn lamb** (left) showing primary spongiosa (PS) and secondary spongiosa (SS). Similar microscopic field from a **newborn lamb with osteogenesis imperfecta** on the right. The primary spongiosa persists deep into the metaphysis and consists of delicate trabeculae lined by a thin layer of basophilic bone.

no mention of tooth abnormalities. The histologic lesions in bone closely resembled those in the New Zealand lambs.

A milder form of osteogenesis imperfecta is described in **Barbados Blackbelly** sheep. Although fractures occur in utero, affected lambs are born alive and can stand, in spite of joint laxity. The teeth of these lambs are normal. Autosomal recessive inheritance is suspected in this breed.

Osteogenesis imperfecta has been described in **puppies and kittens**, although it is likely that early reports of the disease in these species were misdiagnoses of fibrous osteodystrophy caused by nutritional secondary hyperparathyroidism. More recently, convincing cases have been recognized in both species. The disease has been reported in **Dachshunds** throughout Europe. Affected animals show signs of pain when handled, have brittle, translucent teeth that fracture easily, and hyperlaxity of the joints, particularly the tibiotarsal joint. Microscopically, although the primary spongiosa appears normal, long bones lack a secondary spongiosa, and trabeculae that are present consist of woven bone lined by a layer of small osteoblasts that often contain a single cytoplasmic vacuole. No Haversian systems are present in the cortices, which consist of thin trabeculae of woven bone separated by loose fibrovascular tissue. The dentin of the teeth is one-quarter normal thickness. The disease in Dachshunds has *autosomal recessive inheritance* and is caused by a missense mutation in the *SERPINH1* gene, which codes for an essential collagen chaperone, HSP47. This protein is involved in the correct folding of collagen and stabilizes the collagen triple helix. Other cases of osteogenesis imperfecta have occurred in **Golden Retriever, Beagle,** and **Standard Poodle** pups. Histologically, the Golden Retriever and Beagle had only thin trabeculae in the secondary spongiosa lined by atrophic osteoblasts. The Beagle had a heterozygous deletion-insertion mutation in the *COL1A2* gene, and the Golden Retriever a heterozygous missense mutation in the *COL1A1* gene. The disease has also been diagnosed in a 12-week-old domestic longhair kitten and a 4.5-month-old domestic shorthair kitten. Both cases had similar lesions, including fractures of both bones and teeth, thin trabeculae in the metaphysis, and a marked reduction in the quantity of cortical bone.

Further reading

Evason MD, et al. Suspect osteogenesis imperfecta in a male kitten. Can Vet J. 2007;48:296-298.

Kamoun-Goldrat AS, Le Merrer MF. Animal models of osteogenesis imperfecta and related syndromes. J Bone Miner Metab 2007; 25(4):211-218.

Seeliger F, et al. Osteogenesis imperfecta in two litters of Dachshunds. Vet Pathol 2003;40:530-539.

Testoni S, Gentile A. Arachnomelia in four Italian brown calves. Vet Rec 2004;155:372.

Widmer C, et al. Molecular basis for the action of the collagen-specific chaperone Hsp47/SERPINH1 and its structure-specific client recognition. Proc Natl Acad Sci U S A 2012;109:13243-13247.

Osteopetrosis

Osteopetrosis, or *"marble bone disease,"* is a group of rare disorders characterized by *defective osteoclastic bone resorption and accumulation of primary spongiosa in marrow cavities*. Two main forms are recognized in humans: a severe, recessively inherited, lethal (malignant) form with lesions present at birth, and a dominant (benign) form, which has variable penetrance and becomes manifest in adolescence or adults. In animals, most descriptions of osteopetrosis appear analogous to the malignant form, and *autosomal recessive inheritance is suspected in most cases*. Because of the complexity of osteoclast differentiation and function, there are many points at which bone resorption can be interrupted, thus accounting for the clinical and morphologic variability associated with the osteopetroses. Osteoclasts may be present in abundance but

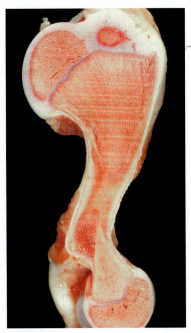

Figure 2-52 **Bovine osteopetrosis.** Humerus with unresorbed cones of primary spongiosa extending from the proximal and distal growth plates into the diaphysis. No medullary cavity is evident. (Courtesy R.A. Fairley.)

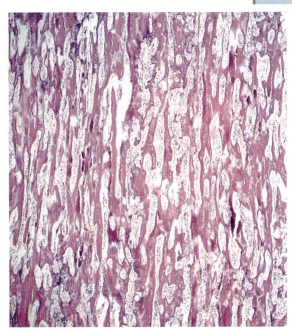

Figure 2-53 **Bovine osteopetrosis.** Metaphysis showing a dense lattice of delicate interconnected trabeculae consisting of cartilage matrix covered by a thin layer of bone.

incapable of resorbing bone because of proton pump (ATP6i) or chloride channel (ClCN7) mutations that interfere with the acidification ability of osteoclasts. In other forms, such as mutations in the *RANKL* gene (which promotes osteoclast differentiation), osteoclasts are either absent or markedly reduced in number.

In **cattle**, osteopetrosis is best studied in the **Angus** breed. Affected calves are small, premature (250-275 days of gestation), and usually stillborn. Clinically, they show brachygnathia inferior, impacted molar teeth, and a protruding tongue. The long bones are shorter than normal and easily fractured. The bone fragility is much less marked than in osteogenesis imperfecta. Research in mice has shown that the increased bone fragility seen in osteopetrosis may be associated with structural or geometric changes in the bone. Radiographically, the medullary cavities are dense, without clear differentiation between the cortex and medulla. Vertebrae are short and bones of the skull are thick. On a cut surface, the *metaphyses and diaphyses of long bones are filled with dense, unresorbed cones of primary spongiosa extending from the metaphysis to the center of the diaphysis* (Fig. 2-52). Nutrient foramina and cranial nerve foramina in the skull are either absent or hypoplastic. As a result of the skull abnormalities, the cerebral hemispheres are rectangular and flattened dorsoventrally, the cerebellum is partially herniated through the foramen magnum, and optic nerves are hypoplastic. The liver may be enlarged because of increased extramedullary hematopoiesis.

Histologically, growth plates are essentially normal, but metaphyses are relatively avascular. Dense chondro-osseous tissue, consisting of cartilage matrix lined by a thin layer of woven bone fills the medulla (Fig. 2-53). In the long bones, osteoclasts are rare and, when present, have scant cytoplasm that may be vacuolated. However, osteoclasts in the skull may be numerous. Osteoblasts lining trabeculae are widely separated and also have minimal cytoplasm. Cortical bone is apparently normal. In the teeth, dentin, enamel, cementum, and bone are interwoven, likely contributing to tooth impaction. In the brain, there is mineralization of blood vessel walls and neurons in the thalamus, cerebellum, meninges, choroid plexus, and around the aqueduct of Sylvius. There is chromatolysis of cranial nerve nuclei, periventricular corpora amylacea, and in the eye, loss of retinal ganglion cells and atrophy of the optic nerve.

In Red Angus cattle, osteopetrosis has been associated with a large 2.8-kb deletion in the anion exchange gene, *SLC4A2*. This protein exports bicarbonate ions in exchange for chloride ions, thus preventing the toxic buildup of bicarbonate ions inside the osteoclast during the acidification process. The same mutation was not found in a sample of Black Angus cattle. Interestingly, some Red Angus calves with osteopetrosis were found to be heterozygous for the mutation. These calves survived up to a week postparturition, in contrast to homozygous mutant animals that were stillborn. This suggests that the *inheritance maybe more complicated than simple autosomal recessive.*

Osteopetrosis of **Hereford** and **Simmental** breeds resembles that of Angus calves in most respects, but in affected Herefords the frontal bones are markedly thickened and filled with cystic spaces. The domed forehead of these calves could be misinterpreted as hydrocephalus unless the skull is sectioned. Similar cystic spaces may also be present in the metaphyseal areas of long bones.

Osteopetrosis, in combination with abnormal skull formation and mandibular gingival hamartomas, has been described in **Belgian Blue cattle** in Europe. Affected calves were usually premature (210-260 days of gestation), stillborn, and small. Those born alive were blind. All calves had brachygnathia inferior, and most had gingival hamartomas (up to 15 cm) on the cranial mandible, possibly associated with defective tooth eruption. The epiphyses and metaphyses of the long bones were dense, and the medullary cavity was absent. There was increased bone fragility and fractures of the long bones. Pedigree analysis suggested autosomal recessive inheritance, and a missense mutation was found in the chloride/proton exchanger lysosomal anion transporter (*CLCN7*). ClC-7 and its obligate subunit, osteopetrosis-associated transmembrane protein (Ostm1), are found in the lysosomes of all cells but also on the ruffled border of osteoclasts, where it is involved in acidification of resorption lacunae. Osteopetrosis was not considered as a diagnosis in these calves until genetic analysis suggested a *CLCN7* mutation; the bones were subsequently sectioned revealing the osteopetrosis. This highlights the importance of sectioning a selection of bones during postmortem examination.

Brachygnathia inferior and osteopetrosis has been described in a small inbred flock of **Polypay sheep** in Oregon. Six out of 40 lambs died during the first week of life. A particular feature of this disease was the presence of multiple limb fractures, suggesting a diagnosis of osteogenesis imperfecta. However, the absence of skin fragility, blue sclera, and pink teeth, combined with persistence of the primary spongiosa, suggested that osteopetrosis was the more likely diagnosis. Histologically, the medullary cavity was filled with chondro-osseous tissue and *large numbers of osteoclasts that lacked a ruffled border* and were not in intimate contact with bony trabeculae (Fig. 2-54).

Osteopetrosis in **horses**, with clinical, radiographic, and pathologic features similar to the severe lethal form in Angus calves, has been reported in **Peruvian Paso** foals and one **Appaloosa**. Affected foals are of normal size at birth and are born alive but unable to stand. Brachygnathia inferior is a consistent finding, and there is malpositioning and impaction of the teeth, reflecting the requirement of osteoclastic activity for normal tooth eruption. Long bones and vertebrae contain cones of primary spongiosa extending from the physis to the center of the diaphysis, filling the medullary cavity (Fig. 2-55). The fragility of the bones is illustrated by the presence of multiple rib fractures, some of which probably occur in utero. Histologic changes are similar to those described for Angus calves, except for the presence of normal to increased numbers of osteoclasts in affected foals. The osteoclasts appear larger than normal, with increased numbers of nuclei. No ruffled border and only a few lysosomes are present ultrastructurally, *suggesting a functional defect in osteoclasts* as the basis of the disease in foals. Although the total number of cases is small, it is likely that the disease in Peruvian Paso horses is inherited as an autosomal recessive trait.

Osteopetrosis has also been reported in an inbred captive herd of **white-tailed deer**. In addition to marked brachygnathia inferior, impacted teeth and protruding tongue, affected fawns had characteristic radiodense bones, and calluses on several ribs, indicating in utero fractures.

In **dogs**, osteopetrosis was reported in 3 neonatal Dachshund puppies from the same litter. Their bones were of normal size and shape (for that breed) but had increased fragility. Osteoclasts were present histologically. Isolated cases of osteopetrosis in an Australian Shepherd and a Pekingese were diagnosed at 12 and 30 months, respectively. Both dogs developed severe myelophthisic anemia.

Acquired osteopetrosis occurs with a number of viral infections, such as bovine viral diarrhea, feline leukemia virus, and canine distemper virus (see later). A sclerosing dysplasia of the radial and ulnar metaphyses has been described in Newfoundland dogs (see later). Diffuse osteosclerosis may also occur in cats secondary to lymphoma, myeloproliferative disease, or systemic lupus erythematosus.

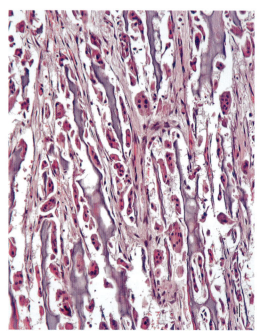

Figure 2-54 Ovine osteopetrosis in a Polypay sheep. The metaphysis consists of thin cartilage spicules lined by numerous osteoclasts that are not in intimate contact with the bone. (Courtesy R. Bildfell.)

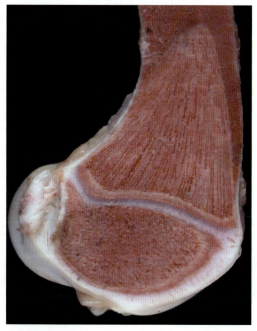

Figure 2-55 Equine osteopetrosis distal femur of a foal. Note the cone of unresorbed primary spongiosa extending into the metaphysis from the physis. (Courtesy M.W. Leach.)

Genetic and Congenital Diseases of Bone

Further reading

Ihde LL, et al. Sclerosing bone dysplasias: review and differentiation from other causes of osteosclerosis. Radiographics 2011;31:1865-1882.

Meyers SN, et al. A deletion mutation in bovine SLC4A2 is associated with osteopetrosis in Red Angus cattle. BMC Genomics 2010;11:337.

O'Toole D, et al. Neuropathology and craniofacial lesions of osteopetrotic Red Angus calves. Vet Pathol 2012;49:746-754.

Sartelet A, et al. A missense mutation accelerating the gating of the lysosomal Cl-/H+-exchanger ClC-7/Ostm1 causes osteopetrosis with gingival hamartomas in cattle. Dis Model Mech 2014;7: 119-128.

Congenital hyperostosis

Congenital hyperostosis (cortical hyperostosis, diaphyseal dysplasia) is a rare disease of newborn **pigs**. Affected piglets are either stillborn or die within the first few days of life, and show various degrees of thickening of one or both forelimbs (Fig. 2-56), and sometimes the hindlimbs as well. The thickened limbs are hard and may be up to twice their normal size. The radius and ulna are the most severely affected, and in some cases are the only bones involved. Grossly, a thick layer of periosteal bone extends along the diaphyses (Fig. 2-57). Marked edema of the surrounding soft tissues contributes to the thickness of the limb. Histologically, radiating trabeculae of woven bone extend from the surface of apparently normal cortical bone beneath a thickened periosteum containing multiple layers of active osteoblasts (Fig. 2-58). The periosteum merges with edematous, poorly vascular connective tissue containing scattered, stellate fibroblasts, which infiltrate adjacent muscle bundles and the overlying dermis. No lesions are found in bones of the axial skeleton.

The pathogenesis of congenital hyperostosis is unknown. Initial suggestions that the disease is inherited as an autosomal recessive trait have not been supported by subsequent observations. Another possibility is that local impairment of blood flow to the forelimbs, because of abnormal intrauterine positioning of the fetus, results in prolonged edema and a bony periosteal reaction. In support of this hypothesis, arteriosclerotic vascular lesions, consistent with acute hypertension, have been found in small arteries and arterioles supplying the radioulnar region of affected piglets.

Infantile cortical hyperostosis, or Caffey's disease, in children resembles some aspects of congenital hyperostosis of pigs. The human disease may be either familial and congenital with autosomal dominant inheritance of mutations in the *COL1A1* gene, or sporadic and environmentally induced (possibly viral). It is characterized by extensive periosteal new bone formation at multiple sites, most commonly the mandible, clavicle, and long bones, including those of the forearm, with or without histologic evidence of inflammation. However, the human syndrome is self-limiting and regresses over several years. A hyperostotic disease similar to infantile cortical hyperostosis was reported in an 18-month-old West Highland White terrier dog that had periosteal new bone formation involving the pelvis, scapulae, humeri, ulnae, femora, and to a lesser extent the radii and tibiae. The dog had a leukocytosis and histologically the lesions were consistent with a polyostotic periostitis.

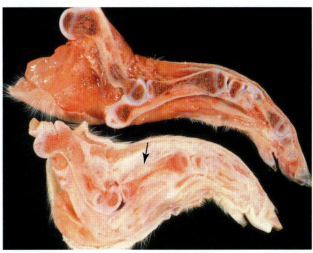

Figure 2-57 Porcine congenital hyperostosis. Comparison of forelegs from a normal piglet (top) and an affected piglet (bottom). The radius of the affected limb is thickened due to increased periosteal bone (arrow). There is extensive edema and swelling of soft tissues throughout the entire limb. (Courtesy R.A. Fairley.)

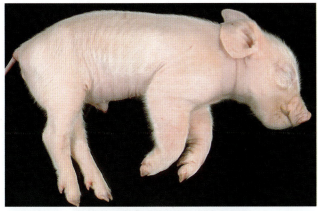

Figure 2-56 Porcine congenital hyperostosis with marked swelling of both forelegs and less severe involvement of the hind legs. (Courtesy R.A. Fairley.)

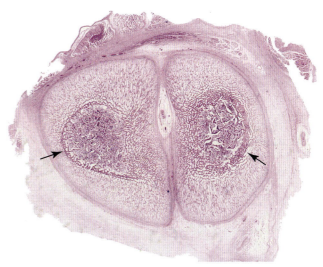

Figure 2-58 Porcine congenital hyperostosis. Transverse sections showing radiating trabeculae of woven bone extending out from the cortex (black arrows) beneath a thickened periosteum.

Osteochondromatosis

Osteochondromatosis, also known as *multiple cartilaginous exostosis*, is a skeletal dysplasia characterized by the formation of single or multiple tumor-like exostoses. In humans, dogs, and horses, the disease is inherited as an autosomal dominant trait. In dogs, the lesions usually are not present at birth but arise in young animals on the surface of endochondral bones adjacent to physes or subarticular growth cartilages, and continue to enlarge until the skeleton matures. In affected horses, the lesions are often present at birth and tend to be bilaterally symmetrical. Because of their tumor-like appearance, these lesions are discussed in more detail in the section on cartilage-forming tumors (see Tumors and tumor-like lesions of bones).

Idiopathic multifocal osteopathy

This syndrome, characterized by multifocal absence of bone in the skull, cervical vertebrae, and proximal regions of the radius, ulna, and femur has been reported in 4 Scottish Terrier dogs. Three of the 4 dogs were related, suggesting a genetic cause. It was not clear whether the disorder was acquired or congenital, because the abnormalities were not detected until the dogs were young adults, by which time the lesions were well developed. The localized areas of absent bone were replaced with fibrous tissue and an acellular mineralized matrix with scalloped areas of bone and osteoclasts at the edge of the lesion, suggesting lysis of bone and replacement fibrosis. A similar condition characterized by multicentric bone lysis and replacement fibrosis occurs in humans, in whom it is referred to as *Winchester syndrome or "vanishing bone disease"*; although the bone lysis usually starts in the bones of the hand. It has autosomal recessive inheritance and has been associated with mutations in metalloproteinase-2 (MMP2) and other proteins in the MMP2 activation pathway.

Further reading

Cerruti-Mainardi P, et al. Infantile cortical hyperostosis and COL1A1 mutation in four generations. Eur J Pediatr 2011;170:1385-1390.

Evans BR, et al. Mutation of membrane type-1 metalloproteinase, MT1-MMP, causes the multicentric osteolysis and arthritis disease Winchester syndrome. Am J Hum Genet 2012;91:572-576.

Localized skeletal dysplasias

Skeletal dysplasias characterized by localized anomalies of the appendicular or axial skeleton are included in this section. The vertebral abnormalities associated with wobbler disease in dogs, and horses are discussed in the Joints section of this chapter.

Limb dysplasias

The most frequent malformations of the limbs are the localized chondrodysplasias seen in chondrodystrophic breeds of dog and cat. The defect is usually confined to the appendicular bones, producing the sort of dwarfism seen in such breeds as the Basset Hound, Dachshund, and Munchkin cat. The short-limbed chondrodystrophic trait in dogs has been linked to the expression of a retrogene lacking some of the regulatory sequences in fibroblast growth factor 4 (FGF4), possibly resulting in premature growth plate closure. In some breeds, such as the Boston Terrier and Boxer, only the cranium is affected, and single nucleotide polymorphisms in bone morphogenetic protein 3 (BMP3) have been linked with brachycephalic skull types.

A wide range of defects of the limbs and/or digits has been reported in domestic animals, often as isolated cases of unknown cause. Rather than attempt to present a comprehensive list, discussion in this section will focus on those conditions known or suspected to be genetic in origin.

Syndactyly, a defect characterized by *partial or complete fusion of functional digits*, occurs in several breeds of cattle, including Holstein-Friesian, Angus, Chianina, Hereford, Simmental, German Red Pied, Indian Hariana, and Japanese native cattle. Inheritance in cattle is *autosomal recessive with incomplete penetrance and variable expression*. The disorder became very common in the Holstein-Friesian breed following extensive use of a heterozygous bull for artificial breeding, but is rare in other breeds. In Holstein-Friesians, the disorder seldom affects all 4 digits. The right forelimb is most frequently affected, followed by the left forelimb, then the right hindlimb. In contrast, the defect in Angus cattle usually affects all 4 digits. *The lesions of syndactyly may vary from complete horizontal fusion of all paired phalangeal bones to fusion of only one of the phalangeal pairs, or fusion of only the interdigital soft tissues not the bones.* Vertical fusion of phalanges is reported in some affected Angus cattle. In the Holstein-Friesian breed, syndactyly is linked to increased susceptibility to hyperthermia, and affected cattle often die of heat stress. In Angus, Holstein-Friesian, and Simmental breeds, the defect has been linked to a number of different causal mutations in lipoprotein receptor–related protein-4/multiple epidermal growth factor-7 (LRP4/Mefg7). LRP4 can regulate canonical Wnt signaling and likely acts as a cofactor or modulator to control BMP, fibroblast growth factor, and Sonic hedgehog signaling in limb development.

Syndactyly has been reported in Shorthorn cattle in association with **dactylomegaly**, a form of club foot (talipes). The condition was characterized by various degrees of dew claw enlargement. *Syndactyly is also reported in pigs* (Fig. 2-59), in

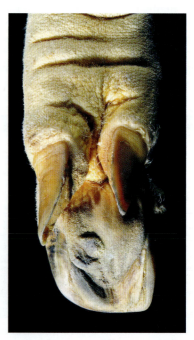

Figure 2-59 **Syndactyly** in a pig. There is complete fusion of the normally paired third and fourth digits.

which the right forelimb is also thought to be the most commonly affected limb; it is presumed to have simple dominant inheritance. Syndactyly has been observed occasionally in a number of different species, including sheep, dogs, and cats.

Polydactyly is an *increase in the number of digits*. The anomaly is observed in all species but is perhaps best known in cats, dogs, horses, and cattle. Polydactyly is an inherited trait in various bovine breeds, but the inheritance pattern is poorly understood. A polygenic mode of inheritance requiring a dominant gene at 1 locus and 2 recessive genes at another is postulated in Simmental cattle, whereas in other breeds, autosomal dominant inheritance with incomplete penetrance is hypothesized. In most cases, it is the medial digit that is duplicated, and although all 4 feet may be affected, the anomaly is more frequently confined to the forelimbs. In horses, 3 forms of polydactyly are described; however, there is frequently overlap between categories. The common atavistic type features an extra medial digit, usually involving a forelimb, which articulates with a second metacarpal. It is thought to have come down through the generations from ancient horses, which had more than one toe. The rare, teratogenic form is characterized by duplication of bones distal to the fetlock joint, producing a cloven hoof. The third category is a hereditary form in which the polydactyly is bilaterally symmetrical. In goats a Shami buck with 2 extra digits on both hindlegs sired a doe kid with a similar defect, suggesting a genetic cause. Polydactyly has been reported in Yorkshire pigs from a closed breeding farm in the United States. The inheritance of the anomaly was determined to be most likely recessive, but with incomplete penetrance and possibly lethal expression. *Polydactyly is most common in cats* (Fig. 2-60), *in which it has simple dominant inheritance with variable* expression. An inherited syndrome of multiple skeletal defects, including polydactyly and syndactyly together with cleft palate, shortened tibia, brachygnathism, and scoliosis, occurred in a family of Australian Shepherd dogs. An X-linked lethal gene was suspected.

Hindlimb preaxial polydactyly is a feature of some breeds of dog, such as *Great Pyrenees and Saint Bernard*. This has been linked to single nucleotide polymorphisms in the ZPA (sonic hedgehog) regulatory sequence in intron 5 of the Limb region 1 protein *(LMBR1)* gene. In humans and mice, mutations in this region are associated with ectopic expression of sonic hedgehog in the anterior limb bud; however, this was not seen in the dog.

Polymelia is an increase in the number of limbs (Fig. 2-61). One form of polymelia, called *developmental duplication*, occurs as an *autosomal recessive defect in Angus cattle*. The number of affected calves is small, however, because of increased embryonic mortality of homozygous animals. The disease usually involves *duplication of a forelimb*, which arises from the neck or shoulder region. Mortality is associated with difficult calving; once born, and the limb surgically removed, the calves grow well. A test is available to detect carriers of the disease, but the mutation has not been published.

Incomplete fusion of the paw resulting in a cleft foot or limb is reported in dogs and cats and referred to as **ectrodactyly**. In cats, *a dominant gene with variable expressivity* is responsible, and the defect is bilateral. In dogs, there does not appear to be any breed, sex, or limb predilection; the inheritance pattern is unknown, but a dominant mode is postulated. *The cleft in the paw extends to the level of the metacarpals*, occasionally the carpus. Various other limb defects may accompany the ectrodactyly, including aplasia or hypoplasia of carpal and metacarpal bones, duplication of digits, fusion of metacarpals, and particularly elbow joint luxation. Syndromes characterized by total or partial absence of phalanges have been reported as ectrodactyly in calves and lambs. These defects differ from the disease in cats and dogs and may be better termed **adactyly**, a condition characterized by the *absence of phalanges* and reported as a possible inherited defect in Southdown lambs, in which the hindlimbs 3 cm distal to the tarsal joint failed to develop.

Hemimelia refers to the *partial absence of part of the distal limb*, for example, tibial hemimelia, absence of the tibia. Such a defect with autosomal recessive inheritance occurs in Galloway calves, which have bilateral agenesis or shortening of the tibial bones. Other bones of the hindlimbs are apparently normal, highlighting the localized nature of the defect. Affected animals also have a ventral abdominal hernia,

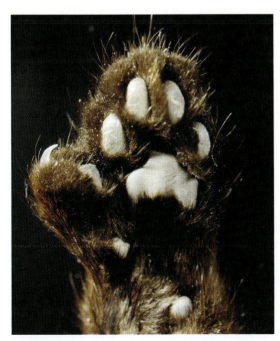

Figure 2-60 Polydactyly in a cat. The forelimb has 6 digits instead of the usual 5.

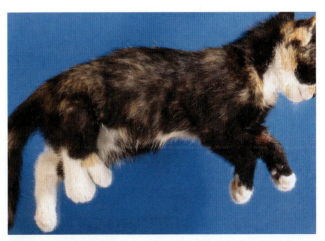

Figure 2-61 A kitten with **polymelia**. All right hindlimb bones are duplicated.

nonfusion of the pelvic symphyses and Müllerian ducts, bilateral cryptorchidism, and meningocele. A similar syndrome, also believed to be transmitted as an autosomal recessive trait, occurs in Shorthorn cattle. A recessively inherited form of hemimelia involving the distal forelimbs is reported in Chihuahua dogs. The abnormality may be either *transverse*, in which case the entire forearm is absent, or *paraxial*, where there is aplasia of only some metacarpals and digits. Paraxial hemimelia with bilateral agenesis of radial bones is reported in goat kids.

Peromelia, *a severe congenital malformation of a limb or absence of the extremity of a limb*, is a term sometimes used synonymously with hemimelia. It has been used to describe a syndrome characterized by agenesis of distal parts of the limbs of Angora goats. Affected kids lacked phalanges and parts of the metacarpus or metatarsus on one or more limbs. Autosomal recessive inheritance was suspected. In isolated cases in which the distal limb is absent, it is important to exclude the possibility that the missing component was accidentally ingested by the dam when she was eating the placenta. This is most likely to occur in goats. Congenital absence of one or more limbs, **amelia**, has been reported in a foal and calves.

A focal bone dysplasia has been described in the *metaphyses of the distal radial and ulnar bones* of **Newfoundland dogs**. On sagittal sections of bone, linear striations, parallel to the long axis of the bone, of pale firm homogeneous material are visible. Histologically, these consist of poorly cellular fibrous tissue that infiltrates between and merges with thin delicate bony trabeculae. It is suggested that the disease may be a form of *sclerosing bone dysplasia*.

Skull anomalies

Brachygnathia inferior, *shortening of the mandibles* (Fig. 2-62), and **brachygnathia superior**, *shortening of the maxillae*, may occur alone or in combination with other skeletal defects. Brachygnathia inferior is commonly encountered in otherwise normal domestic animals and, although generally not life threatening, is considered an undesirable characteristic. In brachycephalic dogs, brachygnathia superior is often a breed standard. Genetic and teratogenic causes have been suggested, and both are likely to occur. In cattle, some breeding trials have been able to reproduce brachygnathia inferior in offspring with numbers suggestive of autosomal recessive inheritance, whereas others have not. In East Friesian milking sheep, breeding trials suggested brachygnathia inferior had oligogenic inheritance with possibly a dominant and recessive locus involved. Brachygnathia inferior is a part of the inherited disorder of *Polled Merino/Merino sheep* called *brachygnathia, cardiomegaly, and renal hypoplasia syndrome*. Brachygnathia superior occurs in association with degenerative joint disease in Angus calves. In addition to brachygnathia superior, affected calves have a dome-shaped head and degenerative changes are present in articular cartilage throughout the body. The nature of the underlying defect is not known, but histologically there is degeneration of cartilage matrix and necrosis of chondrocytes in articular cartilage.

Sternum and ribs

Lateral curvature of the sternum occurs in association with vertebral scoliosis, especially when the latter shows simultaneous torsion. *Pectus excavatum* is a deformity of the thoracic wall that is uncommon but seen most frequently in cats and dogs. Abnormal growth of the sternum and ribs results in a concave appearance to the ventral thorax. It may be congenital or the result of "swimmer pup" syndrome in dogs. There may be a familial tendency to thoracic wall deformities (pectus excavatum, unilateral thoracic wall concavity) in Bengal kittens, and chondrodystrophic Munchkin cats may also have an increased incidence of pectus excavatum and spinal lordosis. This retraction of the caudal sternebrae and xiphoid is also seen in lambs and calves, and is apparently caused by shortness of the tendinous portions of the diaphragm. C*lefts of the sternum* may occur as isolated defects but are usually accompanied by ectopia cordis or form part of the defect known as *schistosomus reflexus*. In this syndrome, there is lordosis, dorsal reflection of the ribs with more or less total eventration, nonunion of the pelvic symphysis, and dorsal reflection of the pelvic bones. Sternal deformity also occurs in "spider lamb" chondrodysplasia. Costal abnormalities are usually secondary to malformation of the vertebral column or sternum. Absent or fused ribs correspond to absent or fused vertebrae and may accompany severe scoliosis.

Pelvis

Lesions of the lumbosacral region, arising from abnormalities of the notochord failing to give rise to appropriate dermatomes, occur in humans and lead to various abnormalities often collectively termed **caudal regression syndrome**. Abnormalities of this derivation result in lumbosacral agenesis, as seen in English bulldogs, and are often accompanied by anorectal abnormalities, urogenital anomalies, various anomalies of the spinal cord, and in humans the development of a variety of tumors and cysts. The sacrum may be absent, or it may be hypoplastic or deviated in association with absence of the coccygeal vertebrae. Hypoplastic chondrodysplasia of the coccygeal vertebrae is a characteristic of French bulldogs and occurs occasionally, with kinking of the remnants, in cattle and cats. Malformations of the sacrum accompany other severe spinal defects. The pubic bones are separated and may be absent, in association with ectropion of the bladder.

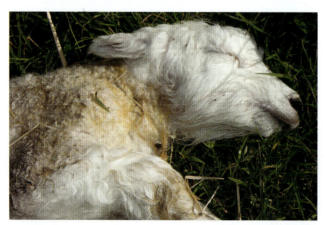

Figure 2-62 Brachygnathia inferior in a newborn lamb.

Further reading

Charlesworth TM, Sturgess CP. Increased incidence of thoracic wall deformities in related Bengal kittens. J Feline Med Surg 2012;14:365-368.

Gorbach D, et al. Polydactyl inheritance in the pig. J Hered 2010; 101:469-475.

Madgwick R, et al. Syndactyly in pigs: a review of previous research and the presentation of eight archaeological specimens. Int J Osteoarchaeol 2013;23:395-409.

Park K, et al. Canine polydactyl mutations with heterogeneous origin in the conserved intronic sequence of LMBR1. Genetics 2008; 179:2163-2172.

Vertebrae

The development of the vertebrae and intervertebral disks is a complex process involving interactions between ectodermal and mesodermal elements. Defects can arise from errors at many stages of development and, because of the proximity of the spinal cord, the consequences are often serious. **Spina bifida** results from *defective closure of dorsal vertebral laminae in a segment of the vertebral column*. It has been reported in several different breeds of cattle, and there is some evidence to support autosomal recessive inheritance. Teratogenic agents acting early in pregnancy can no doubt produce similar lesions. The lesions vary markedly in severity and are often accompanied by defects in the overlying skin, meningocele, and sometimes myelodysplasia. The defect may occur at any level of the vertebral column but appears to favor the lumbar and sacral regions. Various nonskeletal defects have been described in association with spina bifida, including arthrogryposis caused by spinal damage and defective innervation of some muscle groups, fusion of the kidneys, unilateral aplasia of one uterine horn, atresia ani, and kyphoscoliosis.

Perosomus elumbus, a rare congenital defect characterized by *partial to complete agenesis of the lumbosacral spinal cord and vertebrae*, is reported in cattle, sheep, pigs, horses, and dogs. It may be accompanied by other skeletal defects, cryptorchidism, renal agenesis, cerebellar hypoplasia, atresia ani, and arthrogryposis, among other defects. It has been suggested, but not proved, that perosomus elumbus in Holstein cattle is inherited.

Block vertebra results from *improper segmentation of the somites in the embryo, resulting in complete or partial fusion of adjacent vertebrae*. The fused structure may be equal to or shorter than the pair of vertebrae it replaces. There are usually no clinical signs. **Butterfly vertebrae** are so called because of the appearance of the indented vertebral end plates on ventrodorsal radiographs. The cause is persistence of notochord, or a sagittal cleft of notochord, which leads to a dorsoventral sagittal cleft in the vertebral body. The halves may spread laterally, but the condition is usually an incidental radiographic finding in screw-tailed dogs such as Bulldogs, Pugs, and Boston Terriers. **Hemivertebrae** may arise as a result of displacement and inappropriate fusion of somites. In this case, one member of a pair of somites fuse diagonally with a somite cranial or caudal to it, forming a vertebra but leaving the other members of the pairs to persist as hemivertebrae. *Lumbosacral transitional vertebrae complex* occurs in a number of dog breeds, in which the most common abnormality is separation of the first spinous process from the median crest of the sacrum. These abnormalities predispose dogs to degeneration at the lumbosacral junction and cauda equina syndrome. Subluxations, fusions, and other anomalies of cervical vertebrae are described in developmental disturbances of joints.

Complex vertebral malformation (CVM) is a *lethal congenital defect of Holstein calves characterized by shortening of the cervical and thoracic vertebral column resulting from multiple hemivertebrae, fused and misshapen vertebrae, and scoliosis*. Affected calves are smaller than normal, sometimes aborted or born premature, and consistently show arthrogryposis of the forelimbs. The hindlimbs may also show mild arthrogryposis. Approximately 50% have heart malformations, particularly interventricular septal defects and dextraposition of the aorta. Other abnormalities that may be seen include rib deformities, and head malformations, including cleft palate. The defect has *autosomal recessive inheritance;* however, a decreased number of affected animals are obtained in breeding trials because of *intrauterine mortality of homozygous mutant calves*. CVM is caused by a missense mutation in *SLC35A3* (UDP-N-acetylglucosamine transporter), a nucleotide sugar transporter that may result in abnormal Notch (a family of receptors important for fetal development) function. The mutation was traced to a single bull used for artificial insemination, and at the peak, carrier rates in some countries reached 30% as a result of the widespread use of this sire.

Brachyspina, *shortening of the spine, is another hereditary defect of Holstein Friesian cattle*. Affected animals have decreased birth weights, growth retardation, heart, kidney, and ovarian malformations. *The shortening of the vertebral column occurs as a result of incomplete development of intervertebral disks and fusion of the epiphyses of adjacent vertebrae.* Affected animals also have long, slender limbs. Histologically, there are irregularly ossified areas separated by cartilage, with incomplete formation, and sometimes absence, of epiphyses, allowing the merging of the diaphyses of adjoining vertebrae. Brachyspina has *autosomal recessive inheritance* and is associated with a 3.3-kb deletion in the *FANCI* (Fanconi anemia, complementation group I) gene. *FANCI* is required for DNA cross-link repair. Approximately 2% of human Fanconi anemia cases have a mutation in this gene and similar clinical signs to those in affected Holstein calves. There is a low incidence of clinical cases of brachyspina in calves as at least half the homozygous mutant fetuses die during pregnancy.

Further reading

Agerholm JS, et al. Morphological variation of "complex vertebral malformation" in Holstein calves. J Vet Diagn Invest 2004;16: 548-553.

Charlier C, et al. A deletion in the bovine FANCI gene compromises fertility by causing fetal death and brachyspina. PLoS One 2012;7:e43085.

Lappalainen AK, et al. Alternative classification and screening protocol for transitional lumbosacral vertebra in German shepherd dogs. Acta Vet Scand 2012;54:27.

Thomsen B, et al. A missense mutation in the bovine SLC35A3 gene, encoding a UDP-N-acetylglucosamine transporter, causes complex vertebral malformation. Genome Res 2006;16:97-105.

Genetic diseases indirectly affecting the skeleton

Lysosomal storage diseases

The lysosomal storage diseases are a large group of inherited or acquired deficiencies in the activity of specific lysosomal enzymes, culminating in the accumulation of otherwise digestible substrates in the lysosomal systems of various cell types. Although many such diseases have been reported in domestic animals, only the mucopolysaccharidoses, mucolipidoses, and gangliosidoses affect the skeleton. In all groups of diseases, there are lesions of significance in other organ systems, particularly the central nervous system (CNS) (see Vol. 1, Nervous system).

The **mucopolysaccharidoses** (MPS) are characterized by the *accumulation of partially catabolized glycosaminoglycans in lysosomes* and are classified on the basis of the specific enzyme defect and clinical phenotype as MPS I through MPS VII (with several subgroups). The clinical phenotype depends on the type of product stored. Storage of dermatan and keratan sulfate (IV A, VI) results in severe skeletal disease, whereas storage of heparan sulfate (MPS III) leads to neurologic disease. As would be expected, storage of both dermatan and heparan sulfate (MPS I, II) produces both skeletal and CNS defects. MPS I, VI, and VII, in particular, are associated with moderate to severe skeletal defects.

MPS I: Hurler's syndrome, caused by a deficiency of *α-L-iduronidase*, is reported in *domestic shorthaired cats* and most likely has autosomal recessive inheritance. Affected animals have facial dysmorphia, corneal opacity, bilateral coxofemoral subluxation, pectus excavatum, and fusion of cervical vertebrae, but no dwarfism. Nor are there metachromatic granules in circulating neutrophils. Although the number of cases is small, cats with MPS I appear to have a high incidence of meningiomas. MPS I also occurs in *Plott Hounds* as an autosomal recessive trait. Affected dogs are stunted, with facial dysmorphia, and develop progressive lameness in addition to diffuse, bilateral corneal opacity. A feature of the canine disease is the development of osteopenia and severe degenerative joint disease with extensive periarticular bone proliferation. This degenerative process extends to the spine, in which vertebral dysplasia and an increased rate of intervertebral disk degeneration result in kyphoscoliosis and spinal cord compression (Fig. 2-63). Fibroblasts and fixed macrophages in most tissues contain storage product, as do hepatocytes and chondrocytes. As with cats with MPS I, no metachromatic granules are in neutrophils, but occasional vacuoles may be present in lymphocytes. MPS I has also been described in a Rottweiler, an Afghan Hound, and a Boston Terrier.

MPS II: Hunter syndrome, defect in *iduronate-2-sulphatase* activity, has been described in a *Labrador retriever*. The skeletal lesions were mild but included coarse facial features, enlarged digits, and generalized osteopenia.

MPS VI: Maroteaux-Lamy syndrome, *arylsulfatase-B deficiency*, *occurs in Siamese cats*, and it is inherited as an autosomal recessive trait. By 2 months of age, the typical features of the syndrome, including broad flattened face, small ears, diffuse corneal clouding, large forepaws, and pectus excavatum, are evident. Affected kittens can be recognized at 1 week of age by excessive concentrations of urinary dermatan sulfate and metachromatic granules in the cytoplasm of circulating neutrophils. Radiographic lesions are present in the axial and distal skeleton by 6 months of age and are progressive. Most affected cats have symmetrical epiphyseal dysplasia, short stature, and develop degenerative joint disease. The early onset of degenerative joint disease is thought to relate to increased numbers of inflammatory cytokines as a result of increased mechanical stress, leading to increased apoptosis of articular chondrocytes and depletion of proteoglycans and collagen in the cartilage matrix. Thoracic vertebral bodies are short, and there are fusions of cervical and lumbar vertebrae, absence or dysplasia of cervical and thoracic vertebral spinous processes, and increased width of intervertebral spaces. The ribs broaden at the costochondral junctions. In older animals, the epiphyses and metaphyses of long bones are distorted by bony proliferation, and articular surfaces are irregular. Some animals develop posterior ataxia and paresis at <1 year of age because of compression of the spinal cord by osteophytes. *Microscopic abnormalities in the skeleton are centered on articular and physeal cartilage*. Growth plates are poorly organized, with lack of column formation and an uneven chondro-osseous junction. Chondrocytes are swollen with abundant, finely vacuolated cytoplasm. Membrane-bound cytoplasmic inclusions are also present in hepatocytes, bone marrow granulocytes, transitional epithelium, skeletal and cardiac muscle, vascular smooth muscle cells, and fibroblasts of the skin, heart valves, and cornea. Two different mutations in the arylsulfatase gene have been found in Siamese cats. One mutation, L476P, results in serious disease, whereas the other, D520N, results only in very mild disease. The D520N mutation is present in 11.4% of Siamese cats, and a subset of these carries both mutations. These cats have a higher incidence of degenerative joint disease than the general population. In dogs, MPS VI has been reported in miniature Doberman Pinschers, Miniature Schnauzers, Miniature Poodles, Chesapeake Bay Retrievers, and Welsh Corgis.

MPS VII: Sly syndrome, *β-glucuronidase deficiency*, has been described in *Brazilian Terriers*, a German Shepherd, and a mixed-breed dog. The Brazilian Terriers had brachycephalic skull morphology, dwarfism, and delayed ossification of the epiphyses, with cartilaginous carpal and tarsal bones. The German Shepherd and mixed-breed dog were older at presentation but had similar bone lesions, with epiphyseal dysplasia, vertebral dysplasia, joint hyperlaxity, corneal opacity, and thickened atrioventricular valves. Neutrophils contained metachromatic granules. Isolated cases of MPS VII have also been reported in domestic shorthaired cats, with similar skeletal lesions to those described for MPS VI.

Mucolipidosis II: I-cell disease, caused by deficient activity in the *N-acetylglucosamine-1-phosphotransferase*, has been reported in *domestic shorthaired cats*, with similar skeletal lesions to MPS I, VI, and VII, including facial dysmorphism, growth retardation, angular limb deformities, epiphyseal dysplasia, and fusion of cervical and lumbar vertebral bodies, but no corneal opacity.

GM$_1$ gangliosidosis *occurs in cats, calves, sheep, and dogs* and is caused by a *deficiency of β-galactosidase*. In sheep, there is a concomitant deficiency of α-neuraminidase. In dogs, GM$_1$ gangliosidosis has been described in the Shiba Inu, Portuguese Water dog, Alaskan Husky, Beagle cross, and English Springer Spaniel. Proportional dwarfism was seen in the Alaskan Husky

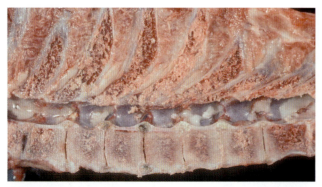

Figure 2-63 Mucopolysaccharidosis I in a 23-month-old Plott hound with premature intervertebral disk degeneration and collapse of the thoracic disk spaces.

and the English Springer Spaniel. The English Springer Spaniel also had coarse facial features, including frontal bossing and widely spaced eyes. Widely spaced irregular intervertebral spaces are seen in affected Alaskan Huskies, Portuguese water dogs, and English Springer Spaniels. Although retarded endochondral ossification of vertebrae has been described in the Alaskan Husky, it has been hypothesized that this is caused by malnutrition rather than a direct effect of the storage disease. The English Springer Spaniel may also have abnormally shaped femoral heads and degenerative changes in the femoral and tibial articular cartilages. In the Beagle and other species with GM_1 gangliosidosis, only neurovisceral changes are present.

Further reading

Crawley AC, et al. Prevalence of mucopolysaccharidosis type VI mutations in Siamese cats. J Vet Intern Med 2003;17:495-498.

Hordeaux J, et al. Histopathologic changes of the ear in canine models of mucopolysaccharidosis types I and VII. Vet Pathol 2011;48:616-626.

Hytonen MK, et al. A novel GUSB mutation in Brazilian terriers with severe skeletal abnormalities defines the disease as mucopolysaccharidosis VII. PLoS One 2012;7:e40281.

Simonaro CM, et al. Mechanism of glycosaminoglycan-mediated bone and joint disease: implications for the mucopolysaccharidoses and other connective tissue diseases. Am J Pathol 2008;172:112-122.

Congenital erythropoietic porphyria

Red-brown discoloration of the teeth and bones, caused by a recessively inherited defect in porphyrin metabolism, is reported in several breeds of cattle, including Hereford, Holstein, Ayrshire, Shorthorn, and Jamaica Red and Black. A deficiency of uroporphyrin III cosynthetase (UROS) leads to the accumulation of uroporphyrin I and coproporphyrin I in blood, bone, and a variety of other tissues. The urine may be red-brown or turn red on exposure to sunlight. The action of sunlight on porphyrins accumulated in the skin results in photodynamic dermatitis, and accumulation of porphyrins in erythrocytes leads to hemolytic anemia. The teeth, bones, and urine of affected animals show bright red-pink fluorescence (Fig. 2-64A) on exposure to ultraviolet light in a dark room. Congenital erythropoietic protoporphyria in Limousin cattle, caused by a deficiency of the mitochondrial enzyme ferrochelatase, is associated with photosensitivity but no discoloration of the bones or teeth.

Inherited forms of porphyria associated with discoloration of the bones and teeth have been reported in *cats and Duroc pigs*. There are *2 forms of inherited porphyria in cats* that result in red-brown discoloration of the teeth and bones. The first, **congenital erythrocytic porphyria**, has clinical features similar to that described in cattle and is caused by homozygous mutations in UROS. The other, **acute intermittent porphyria,** has autosomal dominant inheritance, normal UROS activity, and no photosensitization, but increased urinary 5-aminolevulinic acid and porphobilinogen (porphyrin precursors). This form of porphyria is caused by mutations in the hydroxymethylbilane synthase (HMBS) gene, which results in induction of hepatic δ-aminolevulinate synthase 1, leading to increased heme synthesis and subsequent porphyrin accumulation.

Acquired porphyria with pink discoloration of bones was recognized at slaughter in ~300 of 390 crossbred lambs in

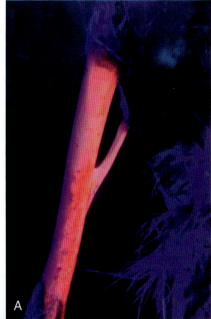

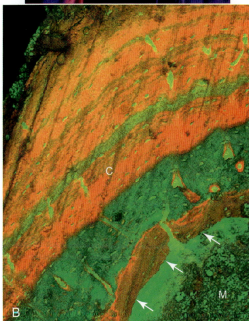

Figure 2-64 A. Porphyria in a wild rat. Fluorescent pink tibia under ultraviolet light. **B.** Confocal microscopy of the same rat. Porphyrins (orange) have been deposited at sites of active ossification in layers in the cortex (**C**). The arrows indicate the endosteal surface, and the medullary cavity is marked by (M).

Australia. Similar "outbreaks" have also occurred occasionally in lambs and young deer in New Zealand. In the New Zealand cases, the discoloration was relatively subtle but was most prominent in the cortices of long bones and fluoresced on exposure to ultraviolet light, but teeth were not affected. On cut surfaces of long bones in a sample of affected lambs and deer, the pink discoloration was confined to areas of bone that had formed in the weeks before death, in particular the outer cortex. This reflects the fact that *porphyrins are only deposited at sites of active mineralization* (Fig. 2-64B). In congenital porphyria, the constant availability of porphyrins during dental and skeletal mineralization results in diffuse discoloration of all mineralized tissues. The extraction of coproporphyrin and protoporphyrin from the bones of lambs in the Australian outbreak suggested an enzyme block toward the end of the heme synthetic pathway, most likely induced by a toxin. Although lead toxicity can induce porphyrin accumulation, no lead was detected in affected lambs. Toxicity caused by some chlorinated hydrocarbons can also result in impaired heme synthesis, and the detection of 1,2,4-trichlorobenzene in fat samples supported this possibility in the lambs. This compound is a *major metabolite of lindane*, an organochlorine insecticide that was widely used in parts of Australia and New Zealand before being banned. The occurrence of acquired porphyria in grazing animal may therefore reflect environmental contamination caused by leakage from chemical dumpsites.

Further reading

Agerholm JS, et al. A molecular study of congenital erythropoietic porphyria in cattle. Anim Genet 2012;43:210-215.

Clavero S, et al. Feline acute intermittent porphyria: a phenocopy masquerading as an erythropoietic porphyria due to dominant and recessive hydroxymethylbilane synthase mutations. Hum Mol Genet 2010;19:584-596.

NUTRITIONAL AND HORMONAL BONE DISEASES

Bone growth and maturation is a complex process, requiring an interaction between genetic factors, local and systemic hormones, dietary nutrients, and mechanical forces. Anything that interferes with the synthesis of proteoglycans or collagen by chondroblasts or osteoblasts, the differentiation of precursor cells, or the resorption of bone by osteoclasts can result in a skeletal abnormality. The expression of an abnormality depends on many factors, including the phase of skeletal development that is altered, the severity of the defect, the age of the animal at the time of the insult, and how long it persists. As a result, the range of possible skeletal defects is huge, and a single cause may vary considerably in its manifestations.

An accurate diagnosis is not always possible in an animal with a skeletal defect, particularly because the inciting cause is often no longer present at the time of examination. In many cases, the pathologist is presented with lesions reflecting an insult that occurred several weeks or months earlier and can only speculate as to its cause. It may not even be possible to determine with confidence whether a defect is genetic or acquired. Such decisions should not be taken lightly because they can greatly influence the actions of the owner, sometimes leading to unnecessary culling of related animals, resulting in considerable wastage of valuable breeding stock. *Many teratogenic agents have been shown to mimic genetic diseases of the skeleton and other organ systems*, and unless there is clear evidence that the problem is inherited, or it resembles an established genetic disorder, any temptation to attribute a genetic cause should be resisted.

Nutritional imbalances affecting skeletal growth

Bone development by endochondral ossification is sensitive to quantitative and qualitative alterations in nutrition, both in fetal and postnatal life. **Malnutrition or starvation**, if severe enough, will retard longitudinal bone growth, resulting in narrow growth plates that may become sealed by a horizontal plate of bone on the metaphyseal side. If the nutritional abnormality is corrected, physeal growth will resume and the plate of bone will be displaced into the metaphysis, persisting for some time as a radiographically and grossly visible **growth arrest line**, parallel to the growth plate (Fig. 2-65). The presence of several parallel lines of transverse trabeculae indicates recurrent episodes of retarded growth. Growth arrest lines are often accompanied by osteoporosis caused by reduced bone formation and increased resorption in response to starvation, and the contents of the marrow cavity may be gelatinous because of *serous atrophy of medullary adipose tissue*. Growth arrest lines may be detected in fetuses, in which case they imply either defective maternal nutrition or retarded fetal development resulting from some other cause, such as intrauterine infection. Similar, but less well-defined, lines in the metaphysis also occur in fetuses and in postnatal animals in association with certain infectious (growth retardation lattices with bovine viral diarrhea virus infection) or toxic agents (such as lead) that interfere with osteoclastic resorption of the primary or secondary spongiosa and must be differentiated from growth arrest lines. These are discussed in the sections Toxic bone diseases of bones, and Inflammatory and infectious diseases of bones.

Deficiencies or excesses of specific nutrients, including minerals and vitamins, can have a major impact on the developing skeleton. So too can a variety of toxic principles, primarily of plant origin, that an animal is exposed to during skeletal development. These will be discussed in some detail in the Toxic diseases of bones section. The so-called metabolic bone diseases—rickets, osteomalacia, fibrous osteodystrophy, and osteoporosis—caused by deficiencies or imbalances of vitamin D, calcium, or phosphorus are discussed in detail later. Other

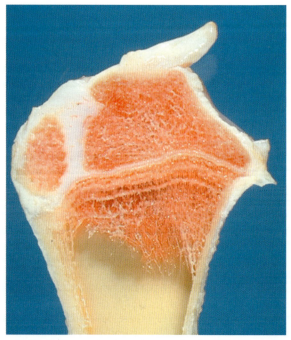

Figure 2-65 Proximal tibia from a lamb with **osteoporosis** showing several **growth arrest lines** parallel to the physis.

nutrient deficiencies that affect bone will also be reviewed in this section.

Calcium, phosphorus, and vitamin D deficiency

Deficiencies in calcium, phosphorus, or vitamin D lead to disturbed bone growth, modeling, or remodeling, resulting in the group of diseases known as osteodystrophies or metabolic bone disease. Because of the complexity of the processes involved in bone development, errors may occur at many stages, the consequences varying with the nature and severity of the imbalance. Genetic defects involving specific enzymes or receptors critical to the activity of hormones or cells participating in bone formation are also reported as causing metabolic bone disease in humans and animals, but these are rare. The manifestations of metabolic bone diseases are generally most severe in young animals, where the skeleton is undergoing rapid turnover, but lesions also occur in adults because of an effect on the quality or quantity of bone formed during remodeling. In addition to variations with age, there are variations between species in the manifestations of dietary mineral imbalances.

Metabolic bone diseases are traditionally classified as **rickets, osteomalacia, fibrous osteodystrophy, or osteoporosis**. Although these are distinct morphologic entities with characteristic pathogenesis and lesions, *they can occur in combination in the same individual.* This may create confusion diagnostically. Furthermore, *their cause can vary between species.* For example, calcium deficiency in sheep is likely to result in osteoporosis, but in a rapidly growing pig, fibrous osteodystrophy is a more likely result. Also, each of these disorders can be caused by more than one dietary or endocrine imbalance. In reality, metabolic bone diseases seldom result from a deficiency of a single dietary nutrient. *More often, there is either a deficiency of several nutrients or a dietary imbalance in the ratio of calcium to phosphorus.* The distinguishing features of each entity, together with their cause, pathogenesis, and occurrence in different species are discussed in detail later.

The term **osteopenia** is often used to describe syndromes associated with increased radiolucency of bone, but makes no inference as to its quality. As such, it includes osteoporosis, wherein only the quantity of bone is abnormal, as well as osteomalacia, fibrous osteodystrophy, and osteogenesis imperfecta, wherein the bone is not only reduced but is abnormal in quality.

Metabolic disease can usually be treated successfully, providing the problem is recognized early and there are no lasting effects caused by pathologic fractures or disruption of growth plates in young growing animals. However, in cases where severe generalized osteoporosis has developed, insufficient bone surfaces may remain to allow appositional bone deposition to proceed, and affected animals remain susceptible to hypocalcemic crises and the deleterious effects of chronically weakened bones. In production animals, an early and accurate diagnosis is important if significant economic loss is to be avoided. This requires a good history, recognition of species differences, and an ability to accurately interpret radiographic and/or pathologic alterations. Whenever possible, more than one affected animal should be examined because lesions may vary in severity between animals, even if they are being fed the same ration. *It is important to examine and sample bones from several sites, particularly those that are showing obvious abnormalities and those from sites of rapid growth or movement.* *This includes the physes of the distal radius, proximal humerus, proximal tibia, distal femur, and the costochondral junctions of the largest ribs.*

Because bone matrix is composed largely of calcium and phosphate ions in the form of hydroxyapatite crystals, any dietary or physiologic factors affecting the metabolism of calcium and/or phosphorus can interfere with the formation of bone tissue and cause an osteodystrophy. Because of the importance of these 2 elements in bone formation, and hence in the cause of metabolic bone diseases, a brief review of their homeostasis is presented later. Vitamin D and parathyroid hormone are integral components of homeostatic control mechanisms for calcium and phosphorus, and their role is also discussed.

Calcium and phosphorus homeostasis

Calcium and phosphorus are required for a variety of essential bodily functions in addition to those involving skeletal development. *Approximately 99% of the calcium in the body is in the skeleton as hydroxyapatite; the remaining 1% is in extracellular fluids and soft tissues.* The concentration of calcium in extracellular fluids and in the cytosol must be kept within narrow limits to maintain critical functions such as muscle contraction, neuromuscular irritability, blood coagulation, and mineralization of bone matrix. A small fraction of the calcium in bone (about 1%) is freely exchangeable with the extracellular fluid compartment. The skeleton is therefore an important storage site for calcium, providing a readily available source should dietary levels become temporarily deficient. Phosphorus is also a component of hydroxyapatite in bone matrix and, like calcium, has other essential functions, in particular, the generation and transfer of cellular energy. *Approximately 85% of the phosphorus in the body is in the skeleton.*

There are *3 distinct fractions of calcium* in extracellular fluids (including plasma); an ionized fraction (about 50%), a protein-bound fraction mostly bound to albumin (about 40%), and calcium complexed to other ions such as citrate and phosphate (about 10%). The *ionized fraction of calcium (Ca^{2+}) is the physiologically active form and is tightly controlled* by the actions of parathyroid hormone (PTH), 1,25-dihydroxyvitamin D ($1,25(OH)_2D_3$), and calcitonin in the intestine, skeleton, and kidney.

Inorganic phosphate also exists in ionized, protein-bound, and complexed forms in plasma. The protein-bound fraction is relatively small (about 10%), and 35% of plasma phosphate is complexed to sodium, calcium, and magnesium; the remaining 55% is ionized. The predominant form of ionized phosphate in plasma is the divalent anion HPO_4^{2-}. Plasma phosphorus concentration is controlled by the action of PTH, $1,25(OH)_2D_3$, and the phosphatonin system, particularly fibroblast growth factor 23 (FGF23). An inverse relationship exists between plasma ionized phosphate and plasma ionized calcium concentrations, an *increase in phosphate resulting in a reduction in ionized calcium.*

Parathyroid hormone is secreted by the parathyroid gland when calcium-sensing receptors on chief cells detect low serum ionized calcium concentrations. *The net effect of PTH is to increase plasma ionized calcium and reduce plasma phosphate concentrations.* In the renal tubules, PTH binds to the PTH receptor 1 (PTHR1), leading to activation of adenylate cyclase and phospholipase C signaling. Ultimately, the actions of PTH in the kidney result in opening of the TRPV5 (transient receptor potential vanilloid 5) calcium channel, allowing increased resorption of calcium from the renal filtrate; and increased breakdown of NPT2 (Na-P$_i$ ATPase pump 2) phosphate channels, leading to decreased resorption of phosphorus from the renal filtrate.

In bone, depending on the dose, the actions of PTH may be antagonistic. As discussed previously, high doses of PTH result in upregulation of RANKL expression on osteoblasts and subsequent recruitment and activation of osteoclasts, leading to increased osteoclastic resorption of bone and release of calcium and phosphorus into blood. PTH also decreases expression of the decoy receptor osteoprotegerin (OPG). Intermittent low-dose treatment of humans with osteoporosis with PTH results in increased bone formation because of increased differentiation of osteoblasts. This functional linkage between osteoblasts and osteoclasts may account for the concurrent increase in osteoblastic and osteoclastic activity in the bones of animals with hyperparathyroidism.

PTH in combination with low serum ionized calcium stimulates the renal 1α-hydroxylase enzyme, leading to increased synthesis of 1,25-dihydroxyvitamin D (1,25(OH)$_2$D$_3$, calcitriol) from 25-hydroxyvitamin D. **Vitamin D** is biologically inert, but undergoes 2 successive hydroxylations in the liver and kidney to form the *active form, 1,25-dihydroxyvitamin D. Vitamin D exists in 2 forms: vitamin D$_2$* (ergocalciferol), obtained from yeasts and plants, and *vitamin D$_3$* (cholecalciferol), obtained from radiation of skin with ultraviolet light or from the diet (fatty fish, cod liver oil). Ultraviolet B radiation of skin leads to the photochemical conversion of 7-dehydrocholesterol in keratinocytes and the dermis to pre-vitamin D$_3$, which then undergoes thermal isomerization to vitamin D$_3$. Latitude, time of day, season, and amount of skin pigmentation can all affect vitamin D$_3$ production in the skin. At lower angles, the sun does not have the intensity required to form vitamin D in the skin. Furthermore, high levels of melanin in the skin absorb ultraviolet photons, making them unavailable for vitamin D formation. A dense hair/wool coat also reduces cutaneous vitamin D$_3$ synthesis. Dogs and cats are unusual in mammalian species because they do not appear to make vitamin D in the skin, owing to the presence of a 7-dehydrocholesterol-Δ^7-reductase enzyme, which breaks down 7-dehydrocholesterol, making it unavailable for conversion to vitamin D. Cats and dogs are therefore reliant on their diet for vitamin D.

Vitamin D$_2$ from the diet and vitamin D$_3$ from the skin/diet are transported in the circulation bound to a vitamin D–binding protein. In the liver, vitamin D undergoes a 25-hydroxylation to form 25-hydroxyvitamin D (25OHD), the major form of vitamin D in circulation. A number of hepatic enzymes are capable of performing the 25-hydroxylation reaction, and this step is not closely regulated; the serum 25OHD concentration therefore reflects the level of cutaneous vitamin D$_3$ formation and/or dietary levels of vitamin D. Measurement of serum 25OHD is used to determine whether an individual has adequate or deficient vitamin D status. The most active form of vitamin D is 1,25-dihydroxyvitamin D, which is formed in the mitochondria of renal proximal tubular epithelial cells by the 25-hydroxyvitamin D-1α-hydroxylase enzyme. This step is closely regulated, and *1,25(OH)$_2$D$_3$ formation is stimulated directly by high PTH and low phosphorus, and indirectly by low ionized calcium*, which acts through PTH. When plasma phosphorus and ionized calcium concentrations are adequate, and PTH levels are low, 25OHD is converted to either 24,25-dihydroxyvitamin D or 1,24,25-trihydroxyvitamin D, biologically inert metabolites that represent the initial step in the degradation pathways.

Active vitamin D binds to the vitamin D receptor-retinoid X receptor complex in the nucleus of renal tubular and intestinal epithelial cells, resulting in increased expression of vitamin D–responsive genes, such as *TRPV5* and *6*, *NPT2a, 2b, 2c* (Na$^+$-P$_i$ ATPase pump 2a, b, c), *calbindin-D$_{9k}$* and *D$_{28k}$*, and *NCX1* (Na$^+$/Ca^{2+} exchanger). The increased production of these calcium and phosphorus channels and pumps, and calcium-binding proteins, results in

- Increased absorption of calcium and phosphorus from the kidneys and intestine. In the intestine, 1,25(OH)$_2$D$_3$ increases the efficiency of calcium absorption from about 10-70%.
- Inhibition of PTH production in the parathyroid gland by increasing the sensitivity of calcium-sensing receptors to calcium
- Negative feedback on the 1α-hydroxylase enzyme to decrease its own production

As with PTH, vitamin D may have antagonistic effects in bone. Decreasing serum ionized calcium concentrations lead 1,25(OH)$_2$D$_3$ to stimulate bone resorption by upregulating RANKL expression and inhibiting OPG expression, likely in association with PTH. Local production of 1,25(OH)$_2$D$_3$ by chondrocytes, osteoblasts, osteocytes, and osteoclasts in bone can lead to increased bone formation and mineralization depending on the stage of bone development, and chondrocyte and osteoblast differentiation. Although vitamin D is required for normal mineralization of bone matrix, there is controversy as to whether vitamin D has a direct effect or whether its effects are mediated through maintenance of adequate extracellular concentrations of calcium and phosphorus.

Historically, the sole role of vitamin D has been in the maintenance of calcium and phosphorus. However, it has been shown that *many cells in the body express the vitamin D receptor*, and increasingly vitamin D is being associated with a number of diseases in humans, including neoplasia, autoimmune disease, psychiatric disease, cardiovascular disease, hypertension, and diabetes mellitus. Many of the studies linking vitamin D and human disease have been epidemiologically based, and therefore more research is required to clarify the associations and attempt to remove the many confounding factors. However, research has showed that vitamin D is intimately involved in both the innate and adaptive immune system. Macrophages contain the 1α-hydroxylase enzyme and are capable of producing 1,25(OH)$_2$D$_3$. Active vitamin D may increase the production of the bactericidal peptide cathelicidin as part of the innate immune response, while increasing the numbers of Th2 and Treg lymphocytes, and decreasing the numbers of Th1 and B lymphocytes in the adaptive immune response. Research is lacking in animals, but it seems reasonable that vitamin D has a similar role in the immune system in domestic animal species.

Calcitonin *is the counterbalance to vitamin D and PTH, and acts to decrease serum ionized calcium concentrations*. As discussed previously, calcitonin is secreted by thyroidal C-cells in response to increased concentrations of serum ionized calcium. It inhibits osteoclast action and leads to decreased osteoclastic bone resorption, subsequently resulting in decreased release of calcium and phosphorus into the blood, allowing serum ionized calcium to return to normal.

Traditionally, it has been thought that the control of serum phosphorus concentration was indirect, as a result of the tighter control of calcium. However, a number of proteins, termed **phosphatonins**, have recently been found to be involved in phosphorus metabolism. The most important of these is *fibroblast growth factor 23* (FGF23). FGF23 is produced by osteocytes in bone, and *its production is increased by either hyperphosphatemia or increased $1,25(OH)_2D_3$*. The kidney is the main target organ for FGF23, and together with its cofactor, klotho, they downregulate the NPT2a and 2c phosphorus channels in the kidney, resulting in decreased resorption of phosphorus from the renal tubules. FGF23 also decreases the production of $1,25(OH)_2D_3$ by inhibiting the 1α-hydroxylase enzyme and activating the 24-hydroxylase enzyme that catabolizes $1,25(OH)_2D_3$. In the parathyroid gland, FGF23 decreases secretion of PTH. *The result of FGF23 activity is to decrease plasma phosphorus concentration.* Other phosphatonins include PHEX and the SIBLING proteins (MEPE, DMP1, and ASARM peptides), also produced by bone osteocytes. Decreases in PHEX and DMP1 lead to increased FGF23. ASARM peptides are cleaved from MEPE and DMP1; these small peptides inhibit mineralization and inhibit phosphorus uptake in the kidney. Phosphatonin research is relatively new and has received little attention in the veterinary literature; it remains to be seen if the functions and metabolism of these proteins are similar in the wide array of veterinary species.

Further reading

Caudarella R, et al. Role of calcium-sensing receptor in bone biology. J Endocrinol Invest 2011;34:13-17.

Penido MG, Alon US. Phosphate homeostasis and its role in bone health. Pediatr Nephrol 2012;27:2039-2048.

Rowe PS. Regulation of bone-renal mineral and energy metabolism: the PHEX, FGF23, DMP1, MEPE ASARM pathway. Crit Rev Eukaryot Gene Expr 2012;22:61-86.

Silva BC, et al. Catabolic and anabolic actions of parathyroid hormone on the skeleton. J Endocrinol Invest 2011;34:801-810.

Osteoporosis

Osteoporosis is easily the most common of the metabolic bone diseases, both in humans and animals. Rather than being a specific disease, osteoporosis is a lesion characterized by a reduction in the quantity of bone, the quality of which is normal. In effect, osteoporosis represents an imbalance between bone formation and resorption in favor of the latter, resulting in bone that is structurally normal but with reduced breaking strength.

The development of a negative balance between bone formation and resorption is recognized as a *normal part of the aging process* in humans and animals. Osteoporosis could therefore be considered a natural phenomenon, but there are several physiologic situations and disease states that either accelerate bone loss or increase bone resorption, leading to premature depletion of the skeleton. Those of most importance in animals are discussed in detail later.

Many mild cases of osteoporosis in animals remain undetected, even at postmortem examination, because the shape of individual bones is not altered, and unless there have been pathologic fractures, lameness is not likely to have been observed clinically. The *occurrence of a bone fracture without evidence of excessive trauma may be the first indication that an animal, or human, is suffering from osteoporosis*. In farmed livestock, there may be an unusually high incidence of fractures in the herd or flock, suggesting increased bone fragility.

Confirmation of osteoporosis can be difficult, especially when the degree of bone depletion is relatively mild. Routine radiographic procedures are insensitive in the early stages of osteoporosis because ~30-50% of skeletal calcium must be lost before the change can be reliably detected by this method. For this reason, dual-energy X-ray absorptiometry (DEXA), computed tomography (CT), and quantitative ultrasound are used for early diagnosis of osteoporosis in human patients, and to allow quantitation of bone mineral content and density (BMC and BMD). *Subjective assessment of the cut surface of bones at autopsy will allow diagnosis of advanced cases of osteoporosis*, but knowledge of what is normal for an animal of the age and species in question is essential, especially when the changes are equivocal. Radiography of isolated bones can detect much smaller alterations in bone density than whole-body radiographs, but comparison with age, breed, and sex-matched controls may still be necessary before osteoporosis can be diagnosed with confidence; the same applies for more precise imaging techniques such as DEXA and CT.

Objective measurement of histologic parameters such as bone volume, trabecular thickness, osteoid volume, osteoblastic and osteoclastic activity, and bone mineral apposition rate is commonly used by medical pathologists, but *histomorphometry* remains largely a research tool in veterinary pathology. *Bone ash measurements* have been traditionally used for the diagnosis of osteoporosis in animals, and although they may provide information on the matrix-mineral relationship, reliable reference ranges are seldom available and interpretation of results is difficult. Because the ratio of calcium to phosphorus is fixed in deposits of hydroxyapatite within bone, bone ash samples do not identify low calcium or low phosphorus as causes for osteopenic bone disease, merely that the matrix to mineral ratio is abnormal.

Osteoporosis in human patients is defined as bone mass 2.5 standard deviations below the young adult mean. In animals, such precise data are not available, and the cutoff point between a normal and osteoporotic skeleton is somewhat arbitrary. For this reason, the diagnosis tends to be restricted to cases in which there is an obvious reduction in bone mass.

Gross lesions of osteoporosis are generally most marked in bones, and areas of bones, which *consist predominantly of cancellous bone*, presumably because trabecular bone has a greater surface area to volume ratio than cortical bone and is resorbed more rapidly. Vertebral bodies, in particular, are affected early in humans and animals with osteoporosis and may contain pathologic fractures. Flat bones of the skull, scapula, ilium, and ribs may also be severely affected, and the breaking strength of the ribs, as assessed during autopsy, may be noticeably reduced. Cancellous bone in the metaphysis and epiphyses of long bones may be reduced in amount and more porous than normal (Fig. 2-66). Trabeculae that are most concerned with transmission of weight-bearing stress are relatively spared and may become more prominent. Thickened trabeculae extending partially or completely across the medullary cavity may be present in the metaphysis or diaphysis of humans and animals with chronic osteoporosis (Fig. 2-67). The pathogenesis of these so-called *reinforcement lines or bone bars* is

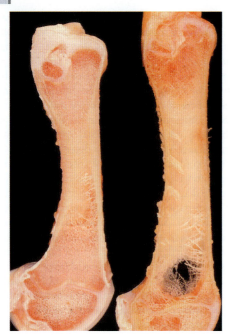

Figure 2-66 Femur from a pig with **severe osteoporosis** (right) compared to that of a normal pig. Note the marked depletion of cancellous bone in the metaphyses and epiphyses and the very thin cortices in the affected pig. (Courtesy R.A. Fairley.)

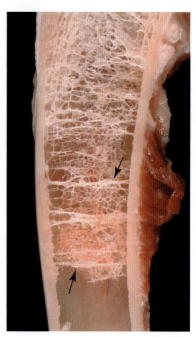

Figure 2-67 Narrow cortices, depletion of cancellous bone, and formation of transverse reinforcement trabeculae (arrows) in a dog with chronic **osteoporosis**. (Courtesy R.A. Fairley.)

uncertain, but they may represent an attempt to reinforce weakened bones at locations of biomechanical stress. In most forms of osteoporosis, an exception being disuse osteoporosis (see later), cortical bone is resorbed most rapidly from the endosteal surface and long vascular channels. In advanced stages, the medullary cavities of affected bones are enlarged and the cortices thin. Osteoporotic bones are usually light and fragile, but an accompanying reduction in soft tissue mass and muscular power in many cases tends to preserve the skeleton against stress fractures.

Histologic examination of severely osteoporotic bones will not necessarily yield diagnostic information, because the depletion of bone tissue is likely to have been established on the basis of radiography or gross examination. However, it may allow assessment of bone quality, thus allowing differentiation from other metabolic bone diseases and other forms of osteopenia. Furthermore, *although it is not likely to determine the cause, histology may provide an indication of the pathogenesis of bone loss*. For example, there is evidence that osteoporosis caused by increased resorption is characterized by a decline in trabecular numbers, whereas osteoporosis caused by decreased formation is characterized by normal numbers of thin trabeculae. Quantitative histomorphometry may be of value in the diagnosis of osteoporosis in equivocal cases, but this is essentially a research tool rather than one used for routine diagnosis.

In severely osteoporotic young animals, the hypertrophic zone of the growth cartilages may be narrowed or absent, and when growth ceases, the physis is sealed by a plate of bone (Fig. 2-68). The chondrocytes in the growth plate are small, with a relative increase in the amount of cartilage matrix. In immature metaphyses, the primary spongiosa may be removed completely, so that there is no framework remaining for the production of secondary spongiosa. In cases resulting from starvation or malnutrition, characteristic transverse trabeculae may be evident grossly and microscopically in the metaphysis. These **growth arrest lines**, which differ from the reinforcement lines referred to previously, result from intermittent cessation and reactivation of physeal growth and represent a succession of sealing layers from the physis. Microscopically, trabeculae are reduced in number and/or size and often are fractured. Depending on the cause of the osteoporosis, evidence of abnormal activity of osteoblasts and/or osteoclasts may be present. Intracortical resorption in long bones occurs along vascular channels and is produced by teams of osteoclasts working parallel to the long axis of the bone, the so-called *cutting cones*. Intracortical resorption is functionally important because a small loss of compact bone has a greater effect on bone stiffness than a comparable loss of cancellous bone.

Postmenopausal osteoporosis is the most important form of osteoporosis in human patients and, although the cause is multifactorial, estrogen deficiency around the time of menopause plays a significant role. An equivalent form of osteoporosis is not recognized in animals, but there are several other causes, many of which are discussed later. Nevertheless, sheep are commonly used as a model for studying postmenopausal osteoporosis in humans.

Senile osteoporosis is common in humans and occurs in other animals, but *seldom appears as a clinical problem in veterinary medicine*. This may reflect the considerably shorter life-span of most domestic animals when compared to humans, although in reality, it is often difficult for the veterinary pathologist to distinguish between the effects of age and other factors that might contribute to reduced skeletal mass in old animals. Beagle dogs aged 7-8 years have ~8% less bone tissue in their forelimbs than do young adults, but this reduction is not clinically significant.

Most cases of osteoporosis in animals, especially farm animals, are **nutritional** in origin and may be caused by a

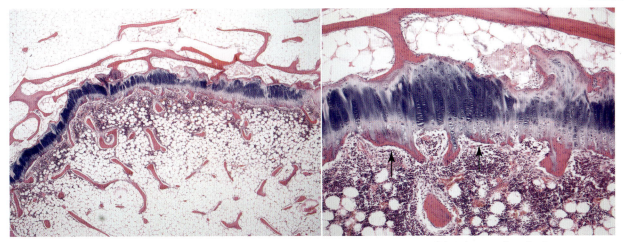

Figure 2-68 Osteoporosis and physeal closure in a young pig. Narrowing of the physis and marked deficiency of trabecular bone in the epiphysis and metaphysis of a young pig with severe osteoporosis (left). On the right is a closer view of the physis in the same animal, showing almost complete absence of hypertrophic chondrocytes and sealing of the metaphyseal side of the physis with narrow plates of bone (arrows). Occasional trabeculae extend for a short distance into the metaphysis.

deficiency of a specific nutrient, such as calcium, phosphorus, or copper, or by **starvation**, whereby there is restricted intake of an otherwise balanced ration. Starvation is relatively common in grazing animals in areas prone to drought or because of overstocking in seasons when pasture growth is below expectations. Poor-quality milk replacers fed to young calves or other young animals may also result in starvation because of inadequate digestibility and absorption of nutrients. In starved animals, the mechanism of osteoporosis is complex, but studies indicate that *bone formation is decreased*, as evidenced by inactive osteoblasts seen histologically and sparse or absent sites of bone formation after tetracycline administration in dogs with malabsorption. The reasons for the lack of bone formation are not entirely clear, but a lack of dietary protein and energy likely contribute. In addition, starvation leads to decreased IGF-1 and estrogen, and increased PPARγ (peroxisome proliferator activator receptor), which diverts osteoprogenitor cells to becoming adipocytes rather than osteoblasts, as shown by the initial increase in bone marrow fat seen in the early stages of starvation in humans. With increasing time of starvation, the bone marrow fat is mobilized and replaced with fluid rich in hyaluronic acid, and this serous atrophy of medullary adipose tissue is a common feature of starvation-induced osteoporosis in animals (Fig. 2-69). Studies in mice and humans suggest that bone resorption is increased in starvation, perhaps either because of concurrent hypocalcemia and PTH-induced osteoclastic resorption or mechanical factors such as weight loss–induced decline in the weight-bearing functions of the skeleton. The effects of starvation on the skeleton are greater in young growing animals than adults, and growth of the skeleton is retarded. Animals affected with osteoporosis at a young age may not fully recover on a return to balanced nutrition. Long-term studies in human survivors of post–World War II starvation show that affected individuals had a premature onset of senile osteoporosis, in addition to other metabolic disturbances.

Severe under-nutrition also has a profound effect on tooth development. Delayed formation and eruption of the whole dentition, with a relatively greater delay in the growth of the

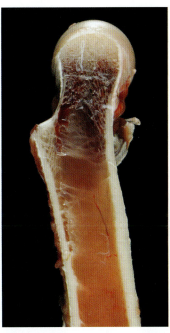

Figure 2-69 Starvation-induced osteoporosis in an alpaca. Marked depletion of metaphyseal cancellous bone, thin cortices, and serous atrophy of medullary adipose tissue.

jaws, leads to overcrowding of the teeth, especially the permanent molars. This causes malocclusion and malalignment of teeth, and there is partial or complete elimination of the diastemata between incisors and canines, and between canines and deciduous molars. Nutritional rehabilitation allows rapid growth of jaws and teeth, but malocclusion of permanent dentition persists, and often there is abnormal development of parts of some teeth.

Uncomplicated **calcium deficiency**, in the presence of optimum dietary levels of phosphorus and vitamin D, causes osteoporosis experimentally in mature and immature animals, but rarely if ever occurs as a natural disease. In gilts, **lactational osteoporosis** occurs when rations marginally deficient in calcium, and with normal or excess phosphorus, are fed over extended periods during gestation and/or lactation. Generalized osteoporosis, and a tendency to fracture vertebrae, femurs, and phalanges, characterizes the condition. The condition may be complicated by disuse osteoporosis caused by confinement in farrowing crates, or by other deficiencies, and affected animals may have microscopic evidence of concurrent fibrous osteodystrophy.

The *osteoporosis induced by calcium deficiency is caused by excess bone resorption* as a result of increased activity of parathyroid hormone following a reduction in serum ionized calcium concentration. *Rickets/osteomalacia are not features of uncomplicated calcium deficiency* because calcium resorption from bone ensures that this mineral is not a limiting factor at sites of mineralization. Parathyroid glands are slightly enlarged because of hyperplasia, and fibrous osteodystrophy sometimes develops but is less florid than the osteodystrophy of calcium deficiency induced by phosphorus excess or vitamin D deficiency.

Prolonged calcium deficiency causes dental abnormalities in sheep, including delayed eruption and increased susceptibility to wear resulting from mild enamel hypoplasia. When adequate calcium becomes available, superior brachygnathia develops because of inadequate repair of the upper skull compared to the mandible.

A form of lactational osteoporosis has been seen in dairy cows, particularly first-calving heifers, in New Zealand. Animals are affected in the first month after calving, with spiral fractures of the mid-diaphysis of the humerus and no history of trauma. The humeri have decreased metaphyseal trabeculae with porous cortices (Fig. 2-70), and histologically, there is evidence of increased osteoclastic bone resorption. The pathogenesis of the osteoporosis is uncertain but is thought to be caused by poor nutrition during growth, resulting in reduced bone mineral density and increased susceptibility to bone loss and fracture during the demands of late pregnancy and/or early lactation, when there is extensive mobilization of calcium from bone.

Classically, **phosphorus deficiency** *produces osteomalacia in adults and rickets in growing animals, both under natural and experimental conditions. However, under some circumstances, it causes osteoporosis.* The reasons for this are not clear, but it may be related to the anorexia that often accompanies phosphorus deficiency, the age and growth rate of the animals, and the severity and duration of phosphorus deficiency. It is not clear whether osteoporosis and osteomalacia are interconvertible or whether osteoporosis is a stage in the development of osteomalacia.

Osteoporosis is recognized as a feature of naturally occurring and experimental **copper deficiency** in lambs, calves, foals, pigs, and dogs. As a component of the enzyme lysyl oxidase, *copper is required for the cross-linkage of collagen and elastin*, and this most likely accounts for the increased bone fragility in copper-deficient animals when compared to animals with osteoporosis of other causes. The bone lesions associated with copper deficiency are discussed in the section Other mineral imbalances. It should be mentioned, however, that the *gross lesions and microscopic bone lesions of copper deficiency may also resemble the lesions of rickets and of osteochondrosis*.

Osteoporosis is often present in animals with **severe gastrointestinal parasitism**, most likely *secondary to malabsorption*. However, there is convincing evidence that subclinical parasitism may also cause osteoporosis, probably by a different mechanism. In one study, continuous dosing of lambs with *Trichostrongylus colubriformis* between 4 and 7 months of age led to osteoporosis and concurrent rickets. The lambs had low plasma phosphorus concentrations and normal plasma calcium, suggesting that the bone lesions were caused by induced phosphorus deficiency. Trichostrongyle infections have been shown to lower the concentration of phosphorus carrier proteins in the intestinal mucosa, leading to phosphorus malabsorption in parasitized animals. Subclinical infection of lambs with *Teladorsagia circumcincta* has also been shown to produce osteoporosis, in this case because of decreased availability of protein and energy for matrix deposition. *The importance of parasite-induced osteoporosis in grazing animals is unknown*, but it is undoubtedly more common than is recognized and may be responsible for some of the unexplained cases of spontaneous fractures in cattle and sheep (Fig. 2-71).

Osteoporosis is a complication of **inflammatory bowel disease (IBD)** in humans and has been described in dogs with **malabsorption syndrome** and IBD, the mechanism for which is still being determined. It is thought that the generation of proinflammatory cytokines such as TNF, IL-1 and, IL-6, of which IL-6 is the most important, plays a role in the osteoporosis associated with IBD of humans, and may also be important in various parasitic and other enteric diseases of animals. B lymphocytes, T lymphocytes, and macrophages in chronic inflammation can activate osteoclasts via RANKL expression and cytokine production. TNF, IL-1, and IL-6 have effects on both osteoblasts and osteoclasts. Inhibition of osteoblasts is mediated by cytokine inhibition of Runx2, increased Dickkopf-related protein 1 (Dkk1), and sclerostin, which inhibit the Wnt-frizzled pathway and antagonize BMPs. The result is increased expression of RANKL and sclerostin by osteoblasts, but decreased expression of Runx2, osteocalcin,

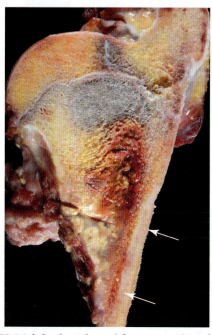

Figure 2-70 Mid-diaphyseal spiral fracture resulting from **osteoporosis** in the humerus of a 2-year-old dairy cow. Note the porous metaphyseal bone and linear red streaks (arrows) in the cortex consistent with cortical resorption cavities.

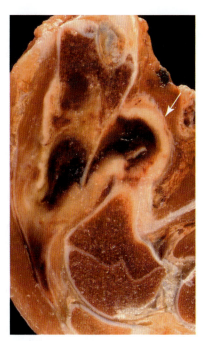

Figure 2-71 Spontaneous femoral fracture (~1-week duration) in a heavily parasitized young sheep with **severe osteoporosis.** Note the thin cortices and porous cancellous bone. There is hemorrhage and early callus formation (arrow) between the misaligned bone ends.

PTHR1, osterix, and osteoprotegerin, thus decreasing osteoblast formation and function. TNF, IL-6, and IL-1 also upregulate osteoclast formation and activity by activating the NF-κB, MAPK, and JAK-STAT pathways, resulting in increased TRAP; cathepsin K; MMP9 and 13; carbonic anhydrase; and TNF, IL-1, and IL-6 expression by osteoclasts. The presence of immune complexes or inflammatory cytokines may activate osteoclasts independent of RANKL. Th17 cells produce IL-17, which is also a potent stimulator of RANKL. In addition, it is likely that reduced dietary intake and/or absorption of vitamin D and calcium may have a role, as may chronic corticosteroid therapy used to treat IBD. A postmortem study of Portuguese Water dogs found that 54% of dogs with IBD had osteoporosis, whereas 32% of dogs without IBD had osteoporosis. In the dogs without IBD, osteoporosis was significantly correlated with age.

Corticosteroid-induced osteoporosis is common in humans, and its occurrence in animals may be under-estimated. In humans on long-term corticosteroid treatment, 30-50% of patients develop fractures and 9-40% osteonecrosis. In the first year on glucocorticoids, bone mineral density declines 3-12%, and then 0.5-3% every year after, as long as the patient is on corticosteroids. Glucocorticoids increase the expression of Dickkopf-related protein 1, which inhibits Wnt-β-catenin signaling and BMPs. Corticosteroids may also inhibit Wnt-β-catenin signaling directly. At the same time, PPARγ expression is increased and Runx2 expression is decreased. The result is diversion of osteoprogenitor cells to the adipocyte line and decreased formation of mature osteoblasts. Corticosteroids also increase caspase-3 expression, which increases osteoblast and osteocyte apoptosis. This apoptosis of osteocytes is thought to lead to the loss of bone strength seen before the loss of bone mineral density, and is thought to be caused by disruption of mechanosensory function. Although corticosteroids decrease osteoclast production, they also prolong their life-span. In vitro, corticosteroids have been shown to increase RANKL expression and decrease OPG expression. Indirect effects of corticosteroids on the skeleton are mediated through reduced calcium absorption in the intestine and reduced calcium reabsorption in renal tubules, both of which would be expected to enhance bone resorption through secondary hyperparathyroidism.

The clinical importance of osteoporosis in dogs and other animal species with *spontaneous and iatrogenic hyperadrenocorticism* is not clear because few studies have been reported, but hyperadrenocorticism is considered one of the most common causes of generalized osteopenia detected radiographically in dogs. In one study, a 25% reduction in mean trabecular bone volume was detected in Beagle dogs with clinical hyperadrenocorticism, resulting from reduced bone formation rather than increased osteoclastic activity. However, another study in dogs found that 92% of dogs with hyperadrenocorticism had serum PTH concentrations greater than the reference range.

Other causes of *generalized osteoporosis* in humans and domestic animals include **vitamin A toxicity, hyperthyroidism, chronic metabolic acidosis,** and possibly chronic exposure to **cadmium.** The **immunosuppressive agent** cyclosporin and certain **anticonvulsant drugs** (e.g., phenobarbital, diphenylhydantoin, carbamazepine) have also been associated with osteoporosis in human patients.

Disuse osteoporosis is loss of bone mass resulting from muscular inactivity and reduced weight bearing. It may be localized, following paralysis or fracture of a limb, or more generalized, in association with prolonged recumbency or inactivity. Measurable loss of mineral occurs in horses that have a limb cast for prolonged periods and in experimental disuse of the forelimb in young adult Beagle dogs. Rapid bone loss occurs in the first 6 weeks in the Beagle dog model, followed by slower bone loss between 8 and 32 weeks, with a total reduction in bone mass of 30-50% of normal. *Bones that normally carry the greatest loads suffer the greatest proportional loss in mass from disuse.* Equivalent muscle atrophy occurs at the same time as bone loss. Although the mechanism behind disuse osteoporosis is unclear, it is the result of both increased bone resorption and decreased bone formation. Disuse is thought to result in microdamage to bone, which leads to osteocyte apoptosis and release of prostaglandin-E_2, RANKL, and nitric oxide, all of which stimulate bone resorption. At the same time, osteocytes increase synthesis of sclerostin, which decreases Wnt signaling, resulting in decreased osteoblast formation and function. Patients on bed rest tend to have increased fat reserves that lead to increased serum leptin concentrations. Leptin, via the hypothalamus and sympathetic nervous system, inhibits osteoblast activity and increases bone resorption.

The effects of remobilization on disuse osteoporosis are not clearly defined. Recovery from relatively short periods of immobilization does occur, but the age of the patient influences the response. The effect of weightlessness associated with prolonged space travel is well documented, and the loss of bone strength remains for a prolonged period after returning to normal gravity.

Further reading

Alexandre C, Vico L. Pathophysiology of bone loss in disuse osteoporosis. Joint Bone Spine 2011;78:572-576.

Braun T, Schett G. Pathways for bone loss in inflammatory disease. Curr Osteoporos Rep 2012;10:101-108.
Gow AG, et al. Hypovitaminosis D in dogs with inflammatory bowel disease and hypoalbuminaemia. J Small Anim Pract 2011;52:411-418.
Oheim R, et al. Large animal model for osteoporosis in humans: the ewe. Eur Cell Mater 2012;24:372-385.
Weinstein RS. Glucocorticoid-induced osteoporosis and osteonecrosis. Endocrinol Metab Clin North Am 2012;41:595-611.

Rickets and osteomalacia

It is convenient to consider these 2 diseases together because they have *a similar cause and pathogenesis, differing only in the age at which they occur*. **Rickets** is a disease of the developing skeleton in young animals and is accompanied by *abnormal endochondral ossification at growth plates, in addition to defective bone formation*. Its expression is greatly influenced by the level of physical activity undertaken; sedentary animals are less likely to suffer from fractures, infractions, and joint collapse. **Osteomalacia** occurs only in adults, and although there are no lesions associated with growth cartilages, *the bone changes are the same as those that occur in rickets*. Both diseases occur in all domestic animal species and wildlife, but there are differences between species in the circumstances under which they occur, and in the most likely cause.

The pathogenesis of both rickets and osteomalacia involves **defective mineralization**. In young animals with rickets this includes cartilage matrix at sites of endochondral ossification, as well as newly formed osteoid. In adults, in whom skeletal growth by endochondral ossification is no longer occurring, the defective mineralization affects only the osteoid formed during skeletal remodeling. The nature of the lesions varies, depending on the cause, the age and growth rate of the animal, and the duration of the disease process. Furthermore, the dietary abnormality may involve a deficiency of more than one nutrient. As a result, the macroscopic and microscopic changes are not always classic, and the lesions may overlap with those of other metabolic bone diseases. Diagnosis on the basis of morphology alone may therefore be difficult.

Anything that interferes with the mineralization of cartilage or bone matrix may cause rickets or osteomalacia, but most cases in animals result from dietary deficiencies of either vitamin D or phosphorus.

Vitamin D deficiency may occur in grazing animals where the combination of relatively high latitudes and temperate climates allows them to graze pasture for much of the year. Such conditions occur in parts of the United Kingdom, South America, New Zealand, and southern Australia. Ultraviolet light–induced activation is a more important source of vitamin D than diet in grazing animals, but may be inadequate during the winter months in some regions. When the winter sun is at an angle of <30° to the horizontal, the short-wavelength ultraviolet rays required for the activation of 7-dehydrocholesterol are reflected by the atmosphere, and cutaneous synthesis of previtamin D_3 is impaired. Mature grass and sun-cured hay are relatively good alternative sources of vitamin D_2, but the levels present in immature pasture are likely to be inadequate. This may be further compounded by the anti–vitamin D activity of carotenes present in lush pasture and green cereal crops. The extra demands of pregnancy and lactation during winter and early spring may also contribute significantly to the development of clinical osteomalacia. *It is likely that many grazing animals are vitamin D deficient for a period during the late winter and early spring*, but clinical rickets or osteomalacia are only likely to develop if the deficiency is marked or persists for longer than usual. Problems may also occur if vitamin D deficiency is combined with deficiencies of other essential nutrients, such as phosphorus or copper.

Sheep appear to be more susceptible to vitamin D deficiency than cattle, possibly because dense fleece covers much of their skin. Not surprisingly, the concentration of vitamin D in blood increases following shearing. *Alpacas and llamas may be even more susceptible to vitamin D deficiency than sheep*. Rickets has been diagnosed in young camelids in New Zealand, South Australia, and northern regions of North America. The disease occurs during winter months and is accompanied by low blood concentrations of both 25-hydroxyvitamin D (25OHD) and phosphorus. In the New Zealand report, lambs grazing the same pasture had normal serum phosphorus concentrations, and the phosphorus content of the pasture was normal. Vitamin D deficiency was considered the most likely cause; the low serum phosphorus concentrations were likely secondary to reduced absorption of phosphorus from the intestine. The natural environment for alpacas and llamas is at high altitude near the equator, where solar irradiation is intense. Their dense fiber and pigmented skin may have evolved as a protective mechanism to prevent excessive solar irradiation reaching the skin. This could be a disadvantage in animals moved to lower altitudes, especially at latitudes with limited solar irradiation during winter.

Dietary deficiency of vitamin D also occurs in housed animals, particularly piglets and calves (at higher latitudes), because of lack of sunlight and errors in the formulation of rations. Piglets grow rapidly and are weaned early. If exposed to rachitogenic diets while the cartilages are still growing rapidly, the lesions tend to be florid. Affected piglets may also develop tetany and muscle fasciculations caused by severe hypocalcemia. *Vitamin D deficiency rickets occurs only rarely in puppies and kittens*, even though neither species seems capable of manufacturing vitamin D in their skin. The widespread availability of balanced commercial diets has reduced the likelihood of deficient rations being fed to dogs and cats, and the most common inappropriate diet fed to puppies and kittens is meat and offal, which contain adequate vitamin D and high levels of phosphorus. However, inadequate rations are occasionally incriminated in the cause of osteodystrophies in puppies; a diet of milk and meat was thought to be the cause in 2 reports of rickets in a Greyhound litter and a Collie puppy, presumably the diet met calcium and phosphorus requirements but not vitamin D. The vitamin D concentration of milk is low, but deficiency in neonatal puppies is unlikely, providing sufficient vitamin D has been stored in the liver of puppies during pregnancy.

Phosphorus deficiency *is well-established as a cause of rickets and osteomalacia*, although the exact mechanism is uncertain. Presumably, the delayed mineralization in phosphorus-deficient animals reflects inadequate extracellular concentrations of the phosphate ions required for formation of hydroxyapatite. Segmental growth plate thickening is a feature of rickets and is likely a direct effect of phosphorus deficiency because normal serum phosphorus concentrations are required for apoptosis of hypertrophic chondrocytes. *Rickets and osteomalacia caused by phosphorus deficiency are uncommon but do occur in animals grazing pastures low in* *phosphorus*. There are many areas of the world, including South America, South Africa, northern Australia, and New Zealand, where soil phosphorus levels are very low, and successful livestock production requires application of phosphorus either to the soil or the animals. Supplementation of individual animals is often not practical, but the problem can be prevented by regular application of phosphorus-containing fertilizers. Reduced fertilizer use in an effort to cut production costs has led to an increased incidence of rickets, osteomalacia, and other diseases associated with phosphorus deficiency in some countries. *Cattle appear to be more susceptible than sheep to phosphorus deficiency, whereas horses seem remarkably resistant.* Rickets has also been diagnosed in farmed red deer grazing phosphorus-deficient pastures in New Zealand. *Phosphorus deficiency rickets is not recognized in piglets*, but hypophosphatemia may be a complication of vitamin D deficiency.

Signs of phosphorus deficiency develop slowly, especially in the mature skeleton, and many animals with subclinical osteomalacia no doubt remain undiagnosed. Clinical disease is most likely to occur in cows where the deficiency is exacerbated by the extra demands of pregnancy or lactation. Such animals lose condition, develop transient, shifting lameness, and show an increased susceptibility to fractures. They may crave phosphorus-rich materials, and *osteophagia and pica are characteristic signs of the deficiency*. Fertility can be severely reduced, and estrus may be irregular, inapparent, or absent. Newborn calves are of normal size and development, but while suckling, their growth is subnormal, and this is accentuated after weaning. Maturity is delayed and deficient animals appear long and lean, and have a rough hair coat. Hypophosphatemia develops early, but blood phosphorus concentrations return to normal rapidly if the animals are supplemented. Serum calcium concentrations are usually normal or increased. The presence of normal serum phosphorus concentration in an animal with osteodystrophy does not therefore exclude phosphorus deficiency as the cause. The poorly mineralized bone is removed slowly and will persist until well after the underlying dietary deficiency has been corrected.

Dietary phosphorus deficiency is virtually impossible in carnivores because of the high levels of phosphorus normally present in their rations. In fact, the opposite, excess dietary phosphorus resulting in nutritional secondary hyperparathyroidism and fibrous osteodystrophy is relatively common in puppies and kittens. However, rickets has been reported in a 10-week-old Shetland sheep dog on a commercial renal failure diet, designed to be low in phosphorus and protein, thus providing inadequate phosphorus for a growing animal, leading to phosphorus deficiency and rickets. Similarly, osteomalacia was reported in an adult dog with food allergies fed an unbalanced elimination ration.

Calcium *is also required for mineralization, but there is doubt that uncomplicated calcium deficiency is capable of inducing rickets.* Calcium deficiency rickets has been diagnosed in children in Africa; however, other complicating factors are usually involved, such as phosphorus deficiency, renal compromise, and iron deficiency. Because any decrease in extracellular concentrations of ionized calcium is rapidly corrected by the actions of PTH and $1,25(OH)_2D_3$ on bone and the small intestine, calcium is unlikely to be a limiting factor at sites of mineralization. *Persistent dietary deficiency or unavailability of calcium is more likely to lead to fibrous osteodystrophy or osteoporosis* (depending on age and species) resulting from hyperparathyroidism and excessive bone resorption. Hypocalcemia does not occur until the advanced stages of calcium deficiency, by which time skeletal growth will be retarded and any effect on growth plates reduced. It is important to recognize however, that vitamin D deficiency will be accompanied by hypocalcemia resulting from impaired resorption of calcium from bone and absorption from the small intestine. The skeletal lesions of vitamin D deficiency in young animals would therefore be expected to include changes characteristic of both rickets and fibrous osteodystrophy. In contrast, lesions attributable to hyperparathyroidism should not complicate phosphorus deficiency rickets or osteomalacia. More likely, chronic phosphorus deficiency will be accompanied by anorexia, and the skeletal changes may therefore reflect a combination of osteomalacia and osteoporosis.

Rickets and osteomalacia are recognized in human patients with **gastrointestinal malabsorption** resulting from chronic disorders of the small intestine, hepatobiliary system, or pancreas. Because vitamin D is fat soluble, any interference with the digestion or absorption of fat can reduce dietary vitamin D absorption and predispose to deficiency. Reduced absorption of calcium may also occur. A recent study of dogs with inflammatory bowel disease and hypoalbuminemia found that low plasma ionized calcium, low 25OHD, and high PTH was common. However, this form of rickets is reported rarely in animals, likely because of less complete radiographic and pathologic evaluation of the skeleton in animals with such diseases, or the fact that affected animals do not live long enough for the skeletal lesions to become manifest clinically. Nonetheless, rickets has been described in a 17-month-old Border Collie with extrahepatic biliary atresia.

Rickets has been reproduced experimentally in rats by the addition of iron to a normal, nonrachitogenic diet. *Iron interferes with the absorption of phosphorus* and high dietary levels may induce phosphorus deficiency. High dietary levels of other phosphorus antagonists, such as *calcium and aluminum*, might also be expected to induce phosphorus-deficiency rickets. Aluminum toxicity caused by chronic antacid administration or long-term total parenteral nutrition has caused rickets and osteomalacia in humans. Lesions resembling osteomalacia have been observed in cattle ingesting high concentrations of fluoride, which interferes with mineralization when incorporated into bone matrix.

Hereditary forms of rickets *resulting from inborn errors in metabolism have been only rarely recognized in animals*. Some cases of inherited rickets reported in the literature are more consistent with a diagnosis of nutritional fibrous osteodystrophy; the diagnosis of inherited rickets should be confirmed with genetic testing. There are 3 main groups of inherited rickets: vitamin D–dependent rickets type I, hereditary vitamin D–resistant rickets (also called vitamin D–dependent rickets type II), and hypophosphatemic rickets.

Vitamin D–dependent rickets type I is caused by a defect in the renal 1α-hydroxylase enzyme (CYP27B1), which converts 25OHD to $1,25(OH)_2D_3$. The disease is inherited as an autosomal recessive trait in people and the Hannover strain of pigs; sporadic, often unconfirmed, cases have been reported in a Saint Bernard dog and in cats. The disease is characterized by high levels of serum PTH and 25OHD but low or undetectable serum $1,25(OH)_2D_3$ concentrations. Affected pigs are clinically normal until 4-6 weeks of age, but then plasma calcium and phosphorus concentrations fall and alkaline phosphatase activity increases. Florid rickets develops over the next

3-5 weeks, and the pigs die unless treated. Two different deletions in the *CYP27B1* gene have been found in pigs with vitamin D–dependent rickets type I. Causative mutations in the *CYP27B1* gene have also been found in 2 cats.

Hereditary vitamin D–resistant rickets is caused by a defect in the vitamin D receptor-effector system in the cells of target organs. The common marmoset *(Callithrix jacchus)* has relative end-organ resistance to $1,25(OH)_2D_3$, with concentrations 4-10 times higher than Rhesus monkeys, without hypercalcemia. Despite the high $1,25(OH)_2D_3$ concentrations, some marmosets develop rickets. The vitamin D receptor is normal in marmosets; however, they have overexpression of a vitamin D–response element binding protein, which interferes with vitamin D–regulated gene expression. Hereditary vitamin D–resistant rickets has been confirmed in a Pomeranian dog and a cat. Animals have autosomal recessive mutations in the vitamin D receptor with severe rickets, hypocalcemia, hypophosphatemia, and serum $1,25(OH)_2D_3$ concentrations 5-20 times greater than normal. Approximately 70-80% of affected humans also have partial to total alopecia, but this has not been described in animals to date.

Hypophosphatemic rickets may have X-linked, autosomal dominant, or autosomal recessive inheritance in humans, depending on the mutant gene. This form of rickets is characterized by hypophosphatemia, normocalcemia, and low to low-normal serum $1,25(OH)_2D_3$. In humans, mutations have been found in the *PHEX* (phosphate regulating gene with homologies to endopeptidases on the X-chromosome), *FGF23*, *DMP1* (dentin matrix protein 1), and *ENPP1* (ecto-nucleotide pyrophosphate/phosphodiesterase 1) genes. Regardless of the mutated gene, the end result is an increase in serum FGF23 concentration, resulting in phosphaturia and inhibition of the renal 1α-hydroxylase. Autosomal recessive hypophosphatemic rickets type 1, caused by a nonsense mutation in dentin matrix protein-1, has been described in Corriedale sheep in New Zealand. The sheep are affected from birth; a fetus and newborn lambs had growth plate lesions, rib fractures, and infraction lines (Fig. 2-72). Those that survive the birth process have the classic lesions of rickets, decreased growth rate, angular limb deformities (Fig. 2-73), and collapse of the subchondral bone of the humeral head. An unusual feature of the hypophosphatemic rickets in humans and sheep is the formation of large exostoses at the sites of tendon and ligament insertions.

Animals with rickets are generally stiff or lame and in severe cases reluctant to stand. The limbs, especially the forelimbs, may be bowed or knock-kneed, reflecting asymmetrical involvement of growth plates. Swelling of the carpal and other joints, caused by enlarged ends of long bones, may lead to an initial suspicion of arthritis. Affected pigs may stand with a hunched back, walk on the tips of their toes, or adopt a dog-sitting position. Knuckling of the carpus is also described in pigs with rickets. In many animals, however, the clinical signs are mild and nonspecific.

Macroscopic lesions of rickets *are most prominent at sites of rapid growth, including metaphyseal and epiphyseal regions of long bones and costochondral junctions of the large middle ribs*. Enlargement of costochondral junctions is a classic feature of the human disease and is referred to as the "*rachitic rosary.*" Costochondral junctions are normally prominent in fast-growing young animals, and any enlargement must be interpreted with caution. In rickets, the metaphysis of the rib is often wider than the cartilaginous portion, and on sagittal section, the chondro-osseous junction is irregular, with tongues of unresorbed cartilage extending into the metaphysis (Fig. 2-74A, B). Segmental thickening of the physis is a feature of the disease (Fig. 2-75), often with replacement of the normal architecture of the metaphysis by a mixture of disorganized trabeculae, irregular tongues and islands of cartilage, fibrous tissue, and sometimes hemorrhage. Loss of the normal trabecular arrangement in the metaphysis is best appreciated radiographically, at least in severe cases (Fig. 2-76). Similar changes may be evident in sagittal sections of long bones, especially at sites of rapid growth, such as distal radius, proximal humerus, distal femur (Fig. 2-77), and proximal tibia. Metacarpal and metatarsal physes are also likely to show gross changes. The severity of lesions between different physes may vary considerably, even within the same animal, and although

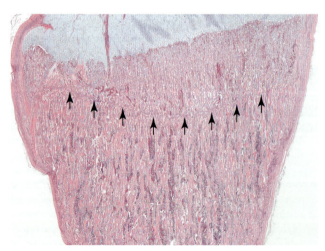

Figure 2-72 Rib from a 5-day-old lamb with **inherited rickets**. The arrows indicate an infraction line extending across the metaphysis.

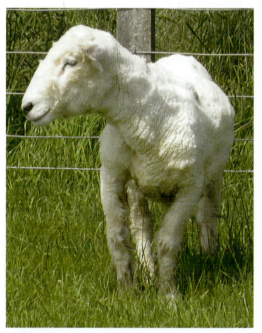

Figure 2-73 Angular limb deformity in a 1-year-old sheep with **inherited rickets**. Valgus deformity of the left forelimb and varus deformity of the right forelimb.

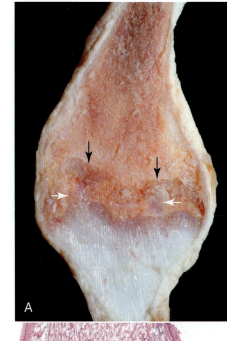

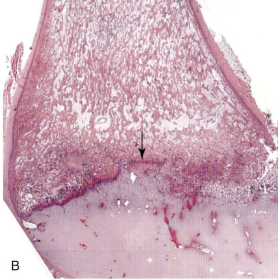

Figure 2-74 Phosphorus deficiency **rickets** in a 1-year-old steer. **A.** Swelling of metaphysis at the costochondral junction and disruption of normal architecture of the primary spongiosa. Broad tongues of cartilage extend into the metaphysis from the physeal cartilage (red arrows). The stage at which defective bone formation began is indicated by the black arrows. **B.** Subgross preparation showing irregular tongues of cartilage in the metaphysis (arrow) and disorganization of metaphyseal bone.

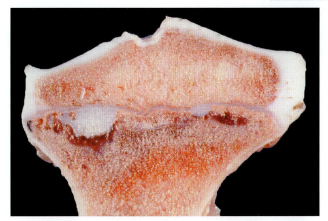

Figure 2-75 Focal thickening of the physis in the proximal tibia of a pig with **rickets**. The dark red gelatinous areas indicate trabecular disruption and replacement with vascular fibrous connective tissue.

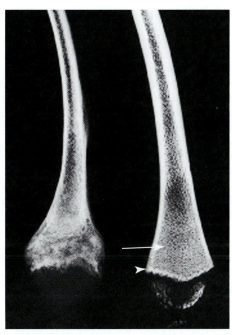

Figure 2-76 Rickets in a calf. A normal rib is on the right in this radiograph. There is metaphyseal swelling and disorganization of trabecular bone in the rachitic bone. Note the regular trabecular pattern in the primary (arrowhead) and secondary spongiosa (arrow) in the normal rib.

the disease is systemic, the physeal lesions are often multifocal rather than diffuse. This emphasizes the importance of examining sagittal sections of several bones during postmortem examination.

Focal thickening of physeal cartilage, similar to that observed in rickets, is also described in osteochondrosis in various species and in the inherited dwarfism of Alaskan Malamute dogs. In rickets, however, the physeal lesions are generally accompanied by evidence of bone fragility, including trabecular disruption, hemorrhage, and infractions. Pathologic fractures may be present in the limbs, ribs, or vertebrae in severe cases. When the deficiency is relatively recent but severe, a distinct zone where abnormal bone formation began may be present in the metaphysis. This reflects a change from adequate to inadequate dietary phosphorus or vitamin D and may be of value in relating the disease to a particular change in diet or environment.

Endochondral ossification occurring beneath articular cartilage is also abnormal in animals with rickets, but because the rate of epiphyseal bone formation is slower than that of the metaphysis, the lesions are milder. The articular cartilage may be irregularly thickened, and in severe cases, there may be

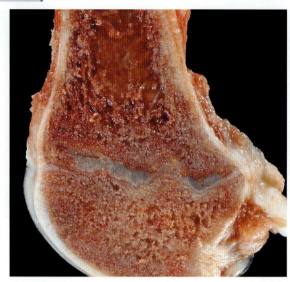

Figure 2-77 The physis of the distal femur is segmentally thickened in an alpaca with **rickets**.

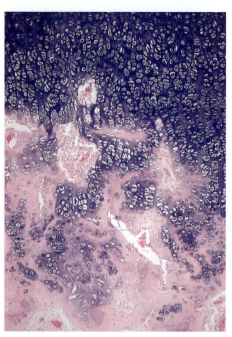

Figure 2-78 Thickening and disorganization of the hypertrophic zone in the physis of a pig with **rickets**. The metaphysis consists of persistent tongues and islands of hypertrophic chondrocytes surrounded by a thick layer of osteoid.

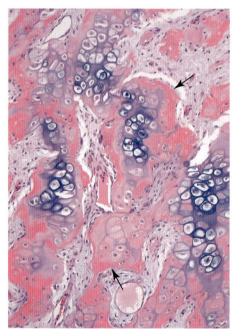

Figure 2-79 The metaphysis of a pig with **rickets** showing clusters of hypertrophic chondrocytes, some of which are degenerate, surrounded by unmineralized osteoid (arrows).

infolding and irregularity of the articular surface caused by collapse of weakened subchondral bone. These articular lesions of rickets occur most often in pigs, but also occur in association with fibrous osteodystrophy, and tend to involve large, weight-bearing joints such as the shoulder and hip. Similar macroscopic lesions occur in the articular cartilage of pigs with osteochondrosis, but because this disease is not associated with defective bone formation, the subchondral bone does not collapse.

In mild rickets, the lesions may not be apparent grossly or radiographically. Furthermore, reduced growth rate in animals with phosphorus-deficiency rickets may reduce the severity of lesions. In such cases, histology is essential for confirmation.

The **microscopic lesions of rickets** *reflect the failure of mineralization of cartilage at sites of endochondral ossification, and of osteoid deposited during bone growth and remodeling. Persistence of hypertrophic chondrocytes at sites of endochondral ossification, both at physes and beneath articular cartilage, is the hallmark of rickets in histologic preparations* (Fig. 2-78). The lesions are often irregular and are usually accompanied by disruption of the underlying trabecular bone. As the cartilage continues to accumulate, its growth rate slows, possibly because of inadequate diffusible nutrients, and the hypertrophic cells form irregular clumps instead of characteristic columns. Some of these clumps are bypassed by the irregular ingrowth of vascular and osteogenic tissue and are left behind in the metaphysis as unmineralized, often degenerate, clusters of hypertrophic chondrocytes surrounded by osteoid (Fig. 2-79). Occasionally, the persistent tongues of cartilage are replaced by connective tissue in which metaplastic osteoid forms. If the dietary deficiency is corrected, plates of rachitic cartilage may become undermined by invading vessels and stranded in the metaphysis, forming a grossly visible translucent band parallel to the growth plate.

Metaphyseal trabeculae are thicker than normal, irregular in shape, and may be partly covered by seams of unmineralized osteoid. Trabecular microfractures are common (Fig. 2-80). Infractions (incomplete fractures) in various stages of repair are also relatively common and reflect the fragility of the trabeculae. *In vitamin D deficiency, the histologic lesions may have features of fibrous osteodystrophy in addition to rickets, caused by hypocalcemia and secondary hyperparathyroidism.* In such cases, osteoblastic and osteoclastic activity is prominent, and trabeculae are separated by loose fibrous connective tissue, even in areas distant from repairing infractions.

A combination of rickets and fibrous osteodystrophy can, at least in theory, also occur in association with chronic renal disease resulting from renal secondary hyperparathyroidism and impaired renal synthesis of $1,25(OH)_2D_3$. However, in animals with renal disease, the lesions of fibrous osteodystrophy generally predominate.

Cortical bone is also affected in rickets, but the lesions are generally overshadowed by those involving growth plates. Grossly, the diaphyses of long bones may appear shorter and thicker than normal with a narrow medullary cavity. In spite of their increased thickness, the cortices are more susceptible to weight-bearing trauma and in severe cases may be soft, bent, or contain pathologic fractures. Histologically, a layer of poorly mineralized osteoid may accumulate within partly filled Haversian systems and on the periosteal surface.

Osteoid seams are best illustrated in undecalcified sections, but can be appreciated in decalcified sections stained with H&E as pale, eosinophilic matrix against the darker staining mineralized bone (Fig. 2-81). Special stains for demonstrating unmineralized osteoid in demineralized sections can be of value (Fig. 2-82) but are not used routinely, and sections may be difficult to interpret in the absence of controls. *It is important to recognize that osteoid seams are not pathognomonic for rickets and osteomalacia*, nor are they invariably present. They also may occur in other syndromes at sites of rapid bone formation rather than caused by delayed mineralization.

The **lesions of osteomalacia** *are similar to those of rickets but because they occur in adult animals, growth plates are not involved*. Osteomalacic bones have reduced resistance to pressure and tension, and increased susceptibility to the stress and strain of ordinary activity. As a result, there is *excessive deposition of matrix where mechanical stimuli are strongest*, such as at insertions of tendons and fascia, places of angulation and curvature, and on stress-oriented epiphyseal trabeculae. When the disease is advanced, the bones fracture readily; the marrow cavity is expanded and may extend into the epiphysis; and the cortex is thin, spongy, and soft. In affected cattle, fractures are most common in the ribs, pelvis, and long bones, whereas in pigs they occur most often in the vertebral column. Deformities are often present, including kyphosis or lordosis, medial displacement of the acetabula with compression of pubic bones, twisting of the ilia, and narrowing of the pelvis. The ribs and transverse processes of the lumbar vertebrae droop so that the thorax is narrowed and flattened and the sternum prominent. Collapse of articular surfaces and degeneration of cartilages is sometimes observed, and tendons may separate from their attachments. In long-standing cases of osteomalacia, cachexia and anemia are often present.

The histologic changes of osteomalacia reflect the inadequate mineralization of osteoid formed during remodeling; the lesions resemble those in the cortex of animals with rickets. In many cases, particularly those caused by phosphorus deficiency, osteoporosis associated with concurrent deficiency of protein and other nutrients is superimposed. The lesions develop

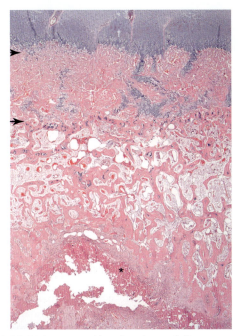

Figure 2-80 **Rickets** caused by phosphorus deficiency in a farmed red deer. Costochondral junction showing an irregular line of recent trabecular fractures deep in the metaphysis (asterisk). Note the disruption of trabecular architecture and persistent islands of cartilage in the primary and secondary spongiosa (between arrows).

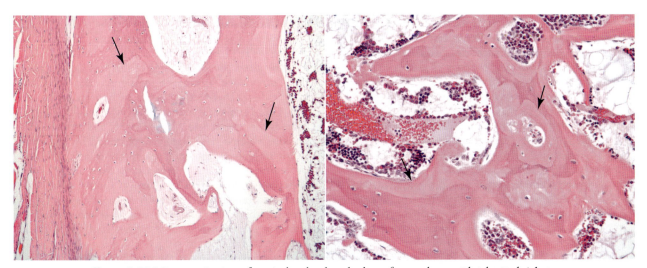

Figure 2-81 Microscopic view of cortical and trabecular bone from a sheep with inherited **rickets**. In the cortex (left), Haversian systems are filled with pale pink, unmineralized osteoid (arrows), whereas pale pink seams of unmineralized osteoid cover trabeculae on the right (arrows).

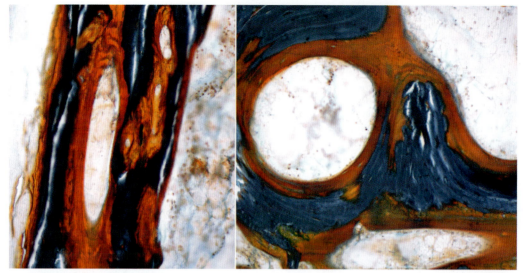

Figure 2-82 Undecalcified sections of a rib from a sheep with inherited **rickets** stained with Goldner's trichrome method. Unmineralized osteoid seams filling cortical Haversian systems (left) and lining trabeculae (right) are orange-gold, whereas mineralized bone stains blue-green.

slowly, but in advanced cases, trabeculae are reduced in size and number, and the cortices are thin and porous. Osteoid covers the trabeculae and lines the expanded Haversian canals. Localized accumulations of osteoid occur at sites of mechanical stress.

Further reading

Dittmer KE, Thompson KG. Vitamin D metabolism and rickets in domestic animals: a review. Vet Pathol 2011;48:389-407.

Dittmer KE, et al. Pathology of inherited rickets in Corriedale sheep. J Comp Pathol 2009;141:147-155.

Madson DM, et al. Rickets: case series and diagnostic review of hypovitaminosis D in swine. J Vet Diagn Invest 2012;24:1137-1144.

Fibrous osteodystrophy

Fibrous osteodystrophy (osteodystrophia fibrosa, osteitis fibrosa cystica) is a relatively common metabolic bone disease characterized by extensive bone resorption, accompanied by proliferation of fibrous tissue and poorly mineralized, immature bone. The pathogenesis involves *persistent elevation of plasma PTH*, and the lesion can be considered to represent the skeletal manifestation of primary or secondary hyperparathyroidism. Different animal species vary in their susceptibility to fibrous osteodystrophy and, to some degree, in the distribution of lesions. Horses, pigs, dogs, cats, ferrets, and goats are often affected, as are reptiles and New World nonhuman primates, but the disease is rare in sheep and goats.

Primary hyperparathyroidism *is usually the result of a functional parathyroid gland adenoma* (see Vol. 3, Endocrine glands). This occurs rarely in adult dogs, and there are isolated reports in horses and cattle. Hereditary primary hyperparathyroidism associated with diffuse parathyroid hyperplasia has been reported in a litter of German Shepherd puppies with fibrous osteodystrophy. Familial primary hyperparathyroidism also occurs in Keeshond dogs, but no mutations have thus far been found in dogs in genes that are associated with primary hyperparathyroidism in humans. *In primary hyperparathyroidism autonomous secretion of PTH results in persistent hypercalcemia and hypophosphatemia*, the latter reflecting increased urinary clearance of phosphate. This differs from secondary hyperparathyroidism, in which plasma total calcium concentrations are usually either normal or slightly decreased, and depending on the cause, plasma phosphorus concentrations are either normal or increased. The persistent hypercalcemia in primary hyperparathyroidism is generally accompanied by polydipsia/polyuria, muscular weakness, and widespread mineralization of soft tissues. Affected animals may succumb to the effects of *nephrocalcinosis* before the skeletal changes are severe enough to become clinically apparent. The skeletal changes in the German Shepherd puppies with primary hyperparathyroidism are more severe than those described in adult dogs with functional parathyroid adenomas. This probably reflects the more rapid turnover of bone in young animals. Generalized bone resorption also occurs in **pseudohyperparathyroidism** or **hypercalcemia of malignancy** caused by the production of calcitropic hormones, most commonly parathyroid hormone–related peptide (PTHrP), by tumors such as malignant lymphoma and apocrine gland adenocarcinoma of the anal sac. Occasionally, other carcinomas, malignant melanoma, and other tumors may produce other factors that cause hypercalcemia, such as $1,25(OH)_2D_3$, prostaglandins, and cytokines (TGF-β, IL-1β). Although increased osteoblastic activity and reduced trabecular bone volume have been demonstrated by histomorphometric techniques, the bone lesions are usually mild and are not apparent clinically or even radiographically.

Secondary hyperparathyroidism is a much more common cause of fibrous osteodystrophy in animals than primary hyperparathyroidism and *may stem from either chronic renal disease or dietary imbalance of calcium and phosphorus*. PTH secretion is stimulated by reduction in plasma ionized calcium, whatever the cause, and if the stimulus persists, then generalized bone resorption results.

Renal secondary hyperparathyroidism occurs most often in dogs, and occasionally in cats, as a complication of chronic renal failure. Impaired glomerular filtration in animals with renal failure leads to progressive hyperphosphatemia caused by reduced renal clearance of phosphate. Hypocalcemia develops as a result of the inverse relationship between plasma ionized phosphate and calcium concentrations, and stimulates the release of PTH. The hyperphosphatemia also triggers the production of FGF23 by osteocytes. FGF23 acts to increase renal excretion of phosphate, but also suppresses renal 1α-hydroxylase, leading to decreased production of $1,25(OH)_2D_3$, and stimulates 24-hydroxylase, thus increasing the breakdown of 25OHD and $1,25(OH)_2D_3$ and exacerbating the hypocalcemia. It is now thought that the action of FGF23 leads to reduced serum $1,25(OH)_2D_3$ concentration before any decreased production as a result of renal tissue loss. In humans, serum FGF23 concentration is a sensitive marker of early renal failure and increases progressively as renal function declines. Similar results have been reported in cats with renal failure, wherein FGF23 concentrations have been found to precede the development of azotemia in old cats, and FGF23 increases with increased stage of chronic renal disease. The increase in PTH results in increased osteoclastic bone resorption and increased bone turnover. Increased bone formation also occurs because of PTH inhibition of sclerostin, but the mineralization of newly formed bone is defective, possibly because of defects in the regulatory proteins DMP1 and ENPP1, and the decrease in $1,25(OH)_2D_3$. This gives rise to a bone disease with features of both fibrous osteodystrophy and osteomalacia, and for this reason, the disorder is often referred to by the more general term **renal osteodystrophy** in animals and has been renamed "*chronic renal failure–mineral and bone disorder*" (CKD-MBD) in human medicine. In addition, increased FGF23 in human patients with chronic renal disease is associated with cardiovascular changes, including left ventricular hypertrophy and cardiovascular mineralization.

Nutritional secondary hyperparathyroidism *may be caused by a simple dietary deficiency of calcium, excess dietary phosphorus, or in association with vitamin D deficiency*. As discussed previously in this chapter, vitamin D deficiency alone is a cause of rickets or osteomalacia, but reduced calcium absorption from the intestine in animals with vitamin D deficiency often results in concurrent fibrous osteodystrophy. Excess dietary phosphorus may cause fibrous osteodystrophy even in animals receiving adequate dietary calcium. Increased plasma phosphate concentration, resulting from increased intestinal absorption of phosphorus, depresses plasma ionized calcium and indirectly stimulates the release of PTH.

In practice, *nutritional secondary hyperparathyroidism is most often caused by diets containing low calcium and a relatively high concentration of phosphorus* and, with the exception of horses, affects young, rapidly growing animals. Horses seem to be remarkably sensitive to the effects of high phosphorus diets and relatively resistant to the effects of rations low in phosphorus. In all species, there are several factors that influence the development and severity of lesions in secondary hyperparathyroidism. These include the degree to which dietary calcium is deficient and, perhaps more important, the degree to which dietary phosphorus is in excess. Although the efficiency of calcium absorption decreases markedly at high intakes, that of phosphorus seems to be unchanged. Furthermore, over a wide range of intakes, plasma calcium concentration is more sensitive to dietary phosphorus than to dietary calcium.

Differences between species in the susceptibility, likely cause, and distribution of lesions in fibrous osteodystrophy are discussed later in some detail.

In the **horse**, the disease occurs at any time after weaning, but the prevalence, and possibly the susceptibility, declines after about the seventh year. Horses require a calcium:phosphorus ratio of ~1:1. Diets in which the calcium:phosphorus ratio is 1:3 or wider can result in fibrous osteodystrophy, depending to some extent on individual and familial susceptibility, and on additional sources of calcium, such as drinking water. The condition usually occurs after maintenance for some months on diets consisting largely of grain, corn, and grain byproducts such as bran, hence the term *bran disease*. Fibrous osteodystrophy also occurs in horses grazing tropical grasses high in oxalate, even though the dietary calcium and phosphorus are normal. Lush pastures are most hazardous, some containing as much as 7.8% oxalate on a dry weight basis. Those with total oxalate >0.5% and calcium:oxalate ratios <0.5 are potentially dangerous because oxalate binds calcium and makes it unavailable for absorption. Several grasses, including *Setaria sphacelata*, *Cenchrus ciliaris* (buffel grass), *Brachiaria mutica* (para grass), *Digitaria decumbens* (pangola grass), *Pennisetum clandestinum* (kikuyu grass), and *Panicum* spp. contain sufficient oxalate to produce clinical disease. Renal secondary hyperparathyroidism is not reported in horses because renal failure in this species typically results in hypercalcemia rather than hypocalcemia.

The *clinical signs and gross lesions* of fibrous osteodystrophy generally develop more rapidly in young, growing horses because of their increased rate of bone formation and remodeling. Early signs consist of minor changes in gait, stiffness, transient and shifting lameness, and lassitude. Loss of appetite with progressive cachexia and anemia develop later. The anemia may be caused by PTH-induced depression of erythropoiesis by an unknown mechanism. *The most characteristic feature is bilateral enlargement of the bones of the skull*, affecting both the maxillae and mandibles, hence the term *big-head* (Fig. 2-83A). The bony enlargement begins along the alveolar margins of the mandibles, producing cylindrical thickenings and reducing the intermandibular space. The molar margins of the maxillae then begin to enlarge, and the enlargement spreads to involve the palate, the remainder of the maxillae, and the lacrimal and zygomatic bones. In severe cases, the nasal and frontal bones are also enlarged (Fig. 2-83B). Initially, the enlargements are soft, but later they harden. Involvement of the palate reduces the nasal passages and may cause dyspnea. Palatine and mandibular thickening causes reduction of the buccal cavity and mastication is impaired. The teeth loosen and are partially buried or may exfoliate, and the softened bone yields to pressure, further impairing prehension and mastication. The face may be continually wet from occlusion of the lacrimal canals. In advanced cases, the enlargement of the head may be extreme, and although it is invariably bilateral, it is not always symmetrical.

Gross lesions in the remainder of the skeleton indicate advanced disease. In such cases, the scapulae may be thickened and curved so that the shoulder joint is displaced forward and the trunk droops in the pectoral girdle, giving undue prominence to the sternum. The vertebral column curves downward, sometimes upward, and the arch of the ribs is reduced. There is increased susceptibility to fractures, and to avulsion of ligaments, particularly in the lower limbs. Some animals escape the fractures and ligamentous detachments and pass

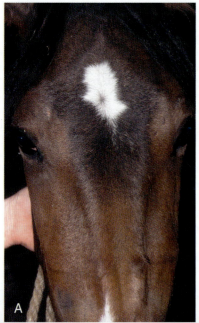

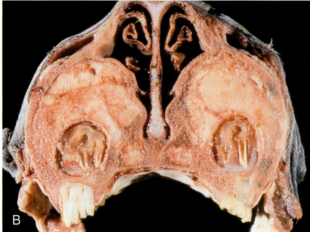

Figure 2-83 **Fibrous osteodystrophy** in a horse. **A.** Bilateral enlargement of the maxillary bones. **B.** Marked, bilateral enlargement of maxillary bones with obliteration of the maxillary sinuses and attenuation of the nasal passages. (Courtesy P.C. Stromberg.)

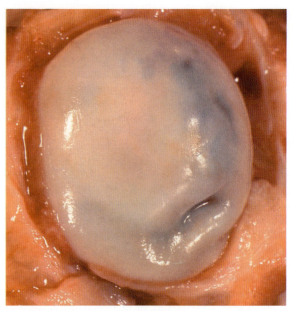

Figure 2-84 **Fibrous osteodystrophy** in a pig. The articular surface of the humerus is irregular because of collapse of subchondral bone. (Courtesy R.A. Fairley.)

into cachectic recumbency, but multiple fractures may occur if such animals are forced to rise. Radiography of affected bones may show generalized osteopenia but not until the relatively advanced stages of the disease. Macerated bones from severely affected animals are finely cancellous or pumice-like and may be brittle and crumbly. The weight of the macerated bones may be <50% of normal.

Severe cases of fibrous osteodystrophy in horses are now rare, and animals with facial swelling resulting from nutritional secondary hyperparathyroidism are seldom seen. However, milder forms of the disease may still be a cause of poorly defined lameness and could perhaps predispose to spontaneous fractures of sesamoid bones or phalanges in racehorses in training, which are fed rations high in grain.

Serum concentrations of calcium and phosphorus are of limited value in the diagnosis of nutritional secondary hyperparathyroidism in horses, although a slight increase in serum phosphorus is reported as a common finding in affected horses. Serum concentrations of PTH are likely to be of more diagnostic value, and the test has been validated in horses. Increased urinary fractional clearance of phosphorus is also considered a sensitive indicator of secondary hyperparathyroidism. In one survey, abnormally high phosphorus clearance ratios were detected in 87.5% of racehorses in Hong Kong, suggesting that subclinical hyperparathyroidism is relatively common.

In **swine**, *fibrous osteodystrophy usually occurs in young growing animals fed unsupplemented grain rations*. The disease also accompanies rickets in association with vitamin D deficiency. Clinical signs include stiffness, reluctance to rise and, in severe cases, lameness. Some affected animals may develop enlargement of the skull similar to that seen in horses. The mandibles may be affected first, and sometimes are the only site of gross lesions, but in other cases, the basocranium is also enlarged. The teeth are mobile and often deeply and obliquely embedded in the fibro-osseous connective tissue. Radiographically, there is a generalized reduction in bone density.

At postmortem examination, the ribs may bend or snap with little effort. Recent or healing pathologic fractures are often present. Articular surfaces of major joints may be irregular and focally depressed because of collapse of subchondral bone (Fig. 2-84). Growth plates are of normal thickness, except in cases caused by vitamin D deficiency in which rickets and fibrous osteodystrophy occur concurrently.

Severe fibrous osteodystrophy is relatively common in **goats** fed rations high in concentrates, but there are no convincing reports of the disease in either **sheep** or **cattle**, suggesting species variation in susceptibility. In goats, fibro-osseous enlargement of the mandibles and maxillae is a characteristic clinical feature (Fig. 2-85). Respiratory distress may be present because of encroachment by enlarged maxillary bones on the nasal cavity. The relative severity of lesions in bones of the skull in goats and certain other species may be related to the mechanical stimulus associated with chewing. The bones of the limbs are also affected in goats with fibrous osteodystrophy, and the limbs may be markedly bowed.

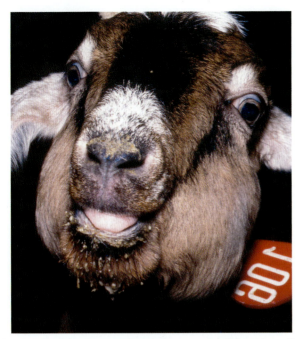

Figure 2-85 **Fibrous osteodystrophy** in a goat. Bilateral swelling of maxillae and mandibles.

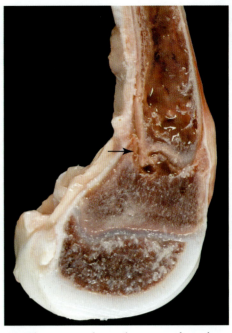

Figure 2-86 **Fibrous osteodystrophy** in a greyhound puppy. Fracture (arrow) in the distal femur with attempts to form a fibrous callus.

In **dogs** and **cats**, nutritional secondary hyperparathyroidism is usually caused by *diets consisting largely or entirely of meat or offal*. The calcium content of such diets is low, and the calcium:phosphorus ratio very wide. For example, the calcium content of cardiac and skeletal muscle is ~10 mg/100 g, and the ratio of calcium to phosphorus ~1:20. The calcium:phosphorus ratio of liver is ~1:50. The ideal ratio is about 1:1, and skeletal abnormalities develop when ratios are 1:2 or greater. Supplementation of all-meat diets with appropriate levels of calcium corrects the imbalance and prevents fibrous osteodystrophy.

Clinical signs of nutritional secondary hyperparathyroidism usually begin a few weeks after weaning. Kittens fed exclusively on beef heart develop signs of fibrous osteodystrophy within 4 weeks. In both kittens and puppies, signs of the disease are progressive and include reluctance to move, hindlimb lameness, and incoordination. Enlargement of facial bones is uncommon. Affected animals become depressed and may develop sudden lameness caused by infractions or fractures of long bones (Fig. 2-86) or vertebrae, the latter resulting in paralysis. Callus formation at fracture sites does occur but consists primarily of fibrous tissue with little evidence of mineralization. Radiographically, there is generalized, often marked, osteopenia (Fig. 2-87). Fibrous osteodystrophy in cats has been inappropriately referred to as *osteogenesis imperfecta* in the early veterinary literature because of the osteopenia and bone fragility. Osteogenesis imperfecta has, however, been diagnosed in the cat and remains a differential for fibrous osteodystrophy.

Renal secondary hyperparathyroidism *may occur in adult dogs with renal failure*, but the skeletal lesions are usually of secondary importance to the manifestations of uremia. Resorption of alveolar socket bone occurs early in the disease and may be evident radiographically. As the disease progresses, there is accelerated resorption of cancellous bones of the maxilla and mandibles, occasionally resulting in soft, pliable

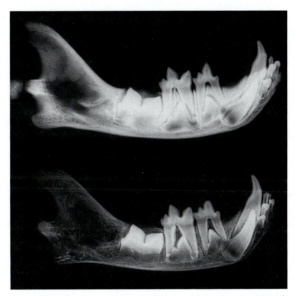

Figure 2-87 **Fibrous osteodystrophy** in a kitten. Mandible from a normal kitten (top) and a kitten with fibrous osteodystrophy. Note the marked, diffuse rarefaction and loss of alveolar bone in the affected mandible.

mandibles (so-called "rubber jaw"). Skull bones may have a moth eaten appearance resulting from localized areas of accentuated resorption. Facial enlargement is a feature of some dogs with renal secondary hyperparathyroidism, but usually occurs in dogs with familial renal disease that develop slowly progressive renal failure from a young age (Fig. 2-88). In such dogs, there is symmetrical enlargement of the head caused by marked enlargement of the maxillae and mandibles. The bones are firm rather than hard and can usually be cut with a knife. Focal red-brown areas of recent or old

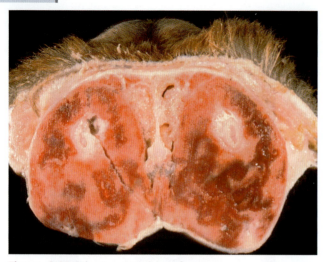

Figure 2-88 **Fibrous osteodystrophy** in a puppy. Transverse section through the maxillae of a Chow puppy with renal secondary hyperparathyroidism. Note the massive enlargement of the bone. In older dogs with renal secondary hyperparathyroidism, the bones are less enlarged, but softer.

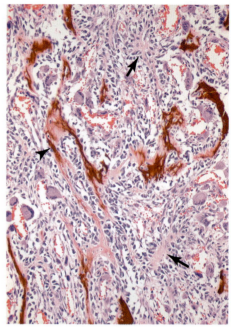

Figure 2-89 **Fibrous osteodystrophy** in a ferret. Undecalcified section stained by the von Kossa method and counterstained with H&E. Active osteoblasts are forming delicate spicules of poorly mineralized osteoid (arrowhead) or unmineralized osteoid (arrows). Many large osteoclasts are also present.

hemorrhage may be evident on cut surface. Young dogs with renal osteodystrophy may also have enlarged costochondral junctions and irregularly thickened physes, reflecting concurrent rickets caused by impaired formation of $1,25(OH)_2D_3$.

The microscopic features of fibrous osteodystrophy are similar in all domestic animal species and are characterized by increased osteoclastic bone resorption, marked fibroplasia, and increased osteoblastic activity with formation of immature woven bone. These are also features of normal bone during development, and can be found in other diseases. For example, longitudinal growth of long bones in rapidly growing young animals is accompanied by prominent osteoclastic and osteoblastic activity and intertrabecular fibrosis in the peripheral metaphyses as part of the normal modeling process. Such areas must be avoided when examining bone for histologic evidence of fibrous osteodystrophy. Healing fractures at certain stages of maturity, and diseases associated with hyperostosis (discussed elsewhere in this chapter), may also be confused with fibrous osteodystrophy if histologic sections are examined without an awareness of their exact location and adequate clinical and/or radiographic knowledge of the case.

The lesions of fibrous osteodystrophy vary between different bones, depending on their rate of turnover, and with stage of the disease process. It is important therefore to examine several sections from different parts of the skeleton, particularly those areas that are growing most rapidly. In early lesions, the increase in bone resorption is reflected by increased numbers of plump, active osteoclasts, often within Howship's lacunae along the surface of trabeculae. Osteoblastic activity is also prominent (Fig. 2-89), and it is not unusual to find bone trabeculae being resorbed on one side while new bone is being added on the other. Wide osteoid seams may be present at sites of rapid bone formation, especially in renal osteodystrophy, wherein there may be concurrent rickets or osteomalacia. Resorption cavities lined by osteoclasts may be present in cortical bone (Fig. 2-90), and even within trabeculae (Fig. 2-91), providing convincing evidence for exaggerated bone resorption. Fibrillar connective tissue initially surrounds

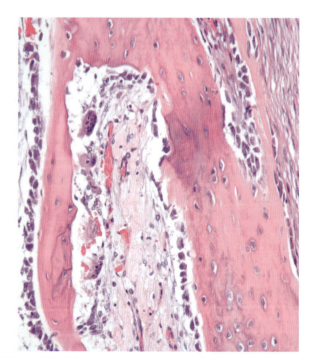

Figure 2-90 **Fibrous osteodystrophy** in a kitten. Large resorption cavities in the cortex with osteoclasts and Howship's lacunae indicating active resorption.

trabeculae undergoing resorption (Fig. 2-92), but later progresses to fill the intertrabecular spaces. As the disease progresses, *mature trabecular and cortical bone are extensively replaced by a combination of loose fibrous connective tissue and irregular trabeculae of poorly mineralized or unmineralized*

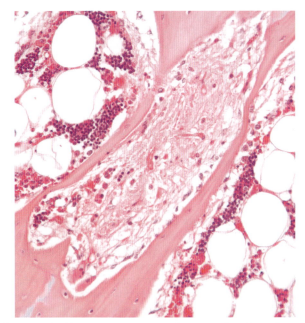

Figure 2-91 Resorption cavity within a trabecula indicating severe hypocalcemia and **fibrous osteodystrophy**.

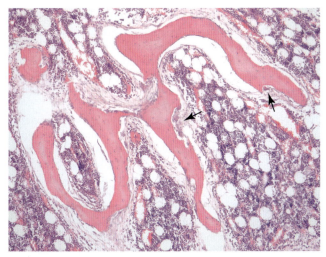

Figure 2-92 Early lesion of **fibrous osteodystrophy** in a pig with peritrabecular fibrosis and osteoclastic resorption (arrows).

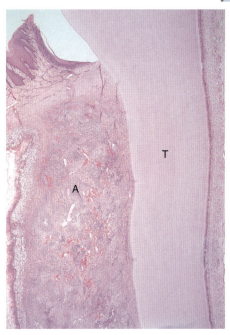

Figure 2-93 Fibrous osteodystrophy in a dog. Section of tooth (T) and alveolar bone (A) from a young dog with renal secondary hyperparathyroidism. The normally dense alveolar bone has been completely replaced by disorganized trabecular bone and fibrous connective tissue.

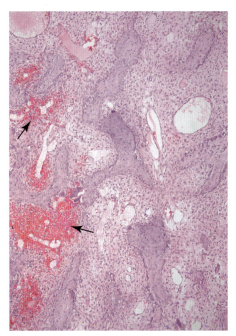

Figure 2-94 Fibrous osteodystrophy in a dog. Alveolar bone showing the irregular trabeculae of woven bone surrounded by highly cellular fibrous connective tissue. The trabeculae are surrounded by active osteoblasts and occasional osteoclasts. Foci of hemorrhage (arrows) are also present.

woven bone, which may encroach on the medullary cavity and expand peripherally to elevate the periosteum. The compact bone of the cortex is resorbed from endosteal and periosteal surfaces, and from within. In advanced lesions, only porous remnants of the original cortex may remain. The soft, enlarged mandibles and maxillae consist of highly cellular fibrous connective tissue surrounding delicate trabeculae of poorly mineralized woven bone (Figs. 2-93, 2-94). Osteoclastic activity may be largely absent in such advanced lesions, or remain in isolated pockets where remnants of the original bone are still being resorbed. In the absence of an adequate history or gross description, such lesions could be confused with benign or malignant bone tumors, or perhaps a fracture callus. Cyst-like cavities are sometimes present, possibly secondary to localized hemorrhage, and there may be sufficient hemosiderin in some areas to cause brown discoloration grossly.

Growth plates are histologically normal in fibrous osteodystrophy unless there is concurrent rickets or interference with vascular invasion resulting from trabecular fractures in the adjacent metaphysis. *Premature resorption of the primary spongiosa* is a feature of fibrous osteodystrophy in young,

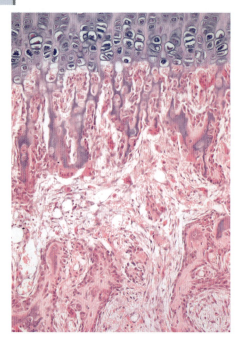

Figure 2-95 Fibrous osteodystrophy in a kitten. The physis is normal, but there is premature osteoclastic resorption of trabeculae in the primary spongiosa and replacement with disorganized spicules of woven bone.

growing animals. In fibrous osteodystrophy, the newly formed trabeculae, usually extending into the metaphysis at right angles to the growth plate, are resorbed almost as rapidly as they form and are replaced by disorganized spicules of woven bone lacking the cartilage core (Fig. 2-95). The spicules are often lined by osteoclasts and/or active osteoblasts, 2-3 cells deep, and separated by a moderate amount of fibrous connective tissue.

In severe cases, the articular cartilage of weight-bearing joints may herniate into the epiphysis, causing an irregular articular surface. This is the result of osteoclastic resorption of the calcified zone of articular cartilage, as well as resorption and collapse of subchondral epiphyseal bone.

In humans with renal failure, histologic lesions of osteomalacia are a prominent feature, but in dogs with renal secondary hyperparathyroidism, fibrous osteodystrophy predominates. Even in relatively young puppies, histologic evidence of rickets is unlikely because the characteristic physeal lesions of rickets require relatively rapid growth and puppies with renal failure grow poorly. *The lesions of renal osteodystrophy in dogs are usually most severe in the bones of the skull.* Histologic evidence of bone resorption by numerous large osteoclasts is prominent, particularly around the teeth where alveolar bone may be removed completely. Although facial enlargement occurs in some cases, osteopenia is more common in dogs with renal failure.

Further reading

Christov M, et al. Bone biopsy in renal osteodystrophy: continued insights into a complex disease. Curr Opin Nephrol Hypertens 2013;22:210-215.

Geddes RF, et al. Fibroblast growth factor 23 in feline chronic kidney disease. J Vet Intern Med 2013;27:234-241.

Koizumi M, et al. Parathyroid function in chronic kidney disease: role of FGF23-Klotho axis. Contrib Nephrol 2013;180:110-123.

Stillion JR, Ritt MG. Renal secondary hyperparathyroidism in dogs. Compend Contin Educ Vet 2009;31:E8.

Other mineral imbalances

Manganese is an essential trace element in animals, being required for the activation of glycosyltransferases involved in the biosynthetic pathway of sulfated glycosaminoglycans. *A deficiency of manganese causes decreased production and increased degradation of cartilage glycosaminoglycans* and therefore potentially affects all bones that develop by endochondral ossification.

Manganese deficiency has been incriminated as the cause of skeletal deformities in newborn calves and other farmed livestock in several countries. The deficiency does not appear to affect adult animals, but calves born to cows fed manganese-deficient rations during pregnancy may show various degrees of **skeletal deformity**. A number of different names have been given to the collection of defects associated with manganese deficiency, including congenital joint laxity and dwarfism, congenital spinal stenosis, crooked calf disease, and congenital chondrodystrophy of unknown origin.

In one study, pregnant cows fed 183 mg of manganese per day produced normal calves, whereas those fed 115-123 mg manganese per day produced calves with deformities of the limbs, including reduced length and breaking strength of humeri, enlarged joints, and twisted legs. Similar skeletal defects occur in lambs and kids. The reduced breaking strength of bones in this syndrome may reflect the fact that manganese is necessary for the glycosylation of collagen as well as the synthesis of cartilage glycosaminoglycans.

In New Zealand, manganese deficiency was incriminated in a naturally occurring "outbreak" of **chondrodystrophy** involving 32 purebred Charolais calves to various degrees. Because of severe drought, the pregnant cows had been fed a diet of apple pulp and corn silage, both of which are low in manganese. The calves had short limbs with enlarged joints and collapsed tracheas with thick cartilage rings. The limb bones were short and had large mushroom-shaped epiphyses. Microscopic lesions included irregular alignment and degeneration of physeal chondrocytes, absence of hypertrophic cells and degeneration of matrix with unmasking of collagen fibers. Calves with mild lesions that were able to walk gradually recovered, but their legs remained bent and shortened for several months. Similar outbreaks have occurred in other breeds of cattle in New Zealand (Fig. 2-96), usually associated with periods of drought. The number of animals affected, and the variability of clinical signs, often helps differentiate it from a hereditary chondrodysplasia.

In Australia, outbreaks of **congenital chondrodystrophy of unknown origin** (CCUO) are often associated with periods of drought, low pasture availability, and supplemental feeding. Affected calves have disproportionate dwarfism, axial rotation of the limbs, and growth arrest lines. Histologically, there is premature closure of physes with reduced numbers of hypertrophic chondrocytes, disorganized chondrocyte columns, and cartilage matrix degeneration. The disease has been associated with manganese deficiency, although this has not been confirmed in all cases. Zinc deficiency has also been postulated as a potential cause for CCUO, but evidence is currently lacking for this as a definitive cause of CCUO.

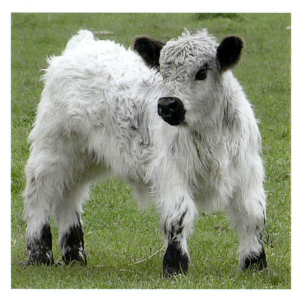

Figure 2-96 Chondrodystrophy due to **manganese deficiency** in a Galloway calf born after a drought to a dam fed grape marc during pregnancy. Note shortened rotated limbs and enlarged epiphyses. (Courtesy S.A. Atkinson.)

Manganese deficiency was suggested as a possible cause of unusual skeletal deformities in calves from several properties in western Canada. **Congenital spinal stenosis** and myelomalacia, together with premature closure of growth plates, malformations of the cranial base and shortening of long bones characterize the syndrome. The spinal stenosis appears to be the result of flaring of the ends of vertebral bodies and protrusion of vertebral articular processes. Focal closure of growth plates is found in the offspring of manganese-deficient rats.

Similar congenital skeletal malformations, particularly disproportionate dwarfism, have been reported in a number of different outbreaks around the world. Feeding manganese-deficient silage during the winter has been associated with congenital joint laxity and dwarfism in the Northern Hemisphere. Soils high in iron, copper, zinc, and sulfur may interfere with manganese bioavailability; during drought conditions, animals likely ingest more soil, perhaps contributing to manganese deficiency. Liver manganese concentrations are thought to be the most reliable indicator of manganese status; however, the deficiency in manganese during pregnancy may have been temporary, and liver manganese concentrations in suckling calves return to normal within a few days of birth. Although manganese deficiency is often suspected as the cause of these outbreaks, the evidence to support this is often lacking, highlighting the difficulty in establishing a definitive cause in a disease that is not discovered until several months after the initial damage has occurred.

There is no doubt that **copper deficiency** influences skeletal development, but full appreciation of the range of manifestations and the mechanisms involved is lacking. The role of copper deficiency in **osteoporosis** and its association with **osteochondrosis** is some species are discussed further elsewhere in this chapter. *As a component of the enzyme lysyl oxidase, copper is required for cross-linkage of collagen molecules.* This is an important step in strengthening the matrix elements of bone tissue, cartilage, and other connective tissues that rely on collagen for support. It is not surprising therefore that increased fragility of bone, and possibly cartilage, is a feature of copper deficiency. Studies in dogs and swine have demonstrated reduced osteoblastic activity in animals with copper deficiency, leading to narrow cortices of long bones and reduced deposition of bone on persistent spicules of mineralized cartilage in the primary spongiosa. These metaphyseal changes resemble those of vitamin C deficiency, which is not surprising because both deficiencies interfere with collagen synthesis and cross-linkage.

In calves, foals, pigs, deer, and dogs, copper deficiency has been associated with grossly visible thickenings in rapidly growing growth plates. These foci consist of *retention of hypertrophic zone chondrocytes*, which protrude into the metaphysis, but the mechanism for this lesion in copper deficiency is not clear. It is possible that the stress of weight bearing causes microfractures of fragile trabeculae in the primary spongiosa, with local disruption of the metaphyseal blood supply and impaired invasion of the mineralized cartilage. A similar mechanism has been proposed for the focal thickening of growth plates in chondrodysplastic Alaskan Malamutes and for the physeal thickening seen in some cases of osteochondrosis. In support of this hypothesis, trabecular microfractures, adjacent to foci of physeal thickening, are described in copper-deficient swine, calves, and foals, but it is seldom possible to accurately assign cause and effect in natural cases as the lesions are frequently too advanced to provide clues to their origin. Whatever the mechanism, these *growth plates bear a strong resemblance, grossly and histologically, to those of rickets and osteochondrosis*. Differentiation from rickets may be further complicated by the possibility of spontaneous long bone fractures in copper-deficient animals resulting from osteoporosis and increased bone fragility.

Physeal changes are not a feature of copper deficiency in lambs. In one report, lambs with experimentally induced copper deficiency developed osteoporosis, but no lesions were detected in growth plates. Nor are there any descriptions of growth plate thickening in sheep with natural copper deficiency, suggesting either a species difference, or the fact that lambs, because of their lower body weight, are less likely to develop trabecular microfractures than foals, calves, or pigs.

Copper deficiency may be either *primary*, caused by inadequate dietary copper, or *secondary* to increased dietary levels of copper antagonists, but the mechanisms vary between species. Absorption of copper is reduced by the presence of divalent cations, such as zinc, iron, and cadmium, that compete with copper for a common transport mechanism. Zinc may also induce the formation of metallothionein, a protein that binds copper in the intestine, liver, and kidney and reduces its availability. Phytates in carbohydrate diets may form insoluble ligands with copper and prevent its absorption. Skeletal lesions consistent with osteochondrosis are described in pigs and foals fed experimental diets high in zinc, and in foals grazing pastures contaminated with zinc close to industrial plants. The possibility of a direct toxic effect of zinc on developing bone or cartilage must be considered, but a secondary effect through induction of copper deficiency is favored.

Calves and lambs grazing pastures containing high levels of **molybdenum** have developed skeletal lesions consistent with copper deficiency. This is believed to be due to the formation of thiomolybdates in the sulfide-rich environment of the rumen and induction of secondary copper deficiency. Thiomolybdates do not form in the digestive tract of nonruminants, providing a possible explanation for the higher tolerance of monogastric species to dietary molybdenum. However, although dietary molybdenum has little effect on copper uptake in horses, skeletal lesions resembling those of copper deficiency have been reproduced in rats and rabbits fed rations with high levels of molybdenum (see also Toxic bone diseases).

Further reading

Hansen SL, et al. Feeding a low manganese diet to heifers during gestation impairs fetal growth and development. J Dairy Sci 2006;89:4305-4311.

Palacios C. The role of nutrients in bone health, from A to Z. Crit Rev Food Sci Nutr 2006;46:621-628.

White PJ, Windsor PA. Congenital chondrodystrophy of unknown origin in beef herds. Vet J 2012;193:336-343.

Other vitamin imbalances

Deficiencies and excesses of vitamins A and D can significantly influence skeletal development and remodeling, as can deficiency of vitamin C. The skeletal manifestations of imbalances in these enzymes will be discussed here, except for vitamin D deficiency, which has been included previously with calcium and phosphorus deficiency because of its role in the causation of rickets and osteomalacia.

Vitamin A may be obtained from either preformed vitamin A in animal-based products or provitamin A carotenoids in plant-based products. The preformed vitamin A, in the form of retinyl esters, is hydrolyzed in the gut by intestinal and pancreatic enzymes to retinol, which is absorbed by intestinal epithelial cells and bound to cellular retinol-binding protein. Approximately 50% of the provitamin A carotenoids are oxidized to retinal, followed by reduction to retinol, whereas the remaining 50% is absorbed intact by intestinal epithelial cells. All forms are incorporated into chylomicrons and released into circulation, from which remnants of the chylomicrons are taken up by hepatocytes. If retinol is not required, it is re-esterified and stored in liver stellate cells. Retinol to be used is bound to retinol-binding protein (RBP) and released into circulation, where it combines with transthyretin. Most of the vitamin A taken up by cells in the body is the retinol-RBP-transthyretin form, whereas a small amount may be chylomicron remnants or all-*trans*-retinoic acid bound to albumin. On uptake into cells, the retinol is oxidized to all-*trans*retinal, then all-*trans*-retinoic acid (ATRA), the main biologically active form. ATRA binds to the retinoic acid receptor, which then forms a heterodimer with the retinoid X receptor; this complex binds to retinoic acid response elements in the promoter of target genes and modulates gene transcription.

The functions of vitamin A, other than that of retinal in relation to vision (see Vol. 1, Eye and ear), are incompletely understood. ATRA has been shown to have conflicting effects on osteoclasts. Whereas ATRA treatment of osteoclast progenitor cells inhibits RANKL-induced differentiation of the progenitor cells, in mouse calvarial bone culture, ATRA increases RANKL expression and decreases OPG expression, thus *stimulating periosteal bone resorption*. Mature osteoclasts express the retinoic acid receptor, and treatment with ATRA increases bone resorption. The effects of vitamin A on bone formation are less well studied than those on bone resorption; however, retinoids have been shown to inhibit adipocyte differentiation in favor of stimulating osteoblast differentiation. By themselves, retinoids induce osteoblast differentiation but not bone formation, but with bone morphogenetic proteins, they stimulate both osteoblast differentiation and bone formation. Vitamin A deficiency has been shown to decrease *BMP2*, *collagen α1 type 1*, and *osteocalcin* expression in bone. Other skeletal genes that are known to be directly altered by vitamin A include *collagen X* and *metalloproteinase-13* (see Toxic bone diseases for vitamin A toxicity).

Vitamin A deficiency *occurs in cattle and pigs fed unsupplemented rations of grain and/or old hay*. Yellow corn, new hay, and fresh silage are adequate sources of carotene, but potency decreases with storage. Animals grazing green pasture or crops are unlikely to suffer from vitamin A deficiency, but dry summer pastures may be deficient. Although deficiency of vitamin A affects many tissues, the emphasis here is on the skeletal manifestations and their sequelae. *The underlying skeletal abnormality in vitamin A deficiency involves defective remodeling of membranous bone, presumably because of the stimulatory effect of vitamin A on osteoclastic activity.* Consequently, there is asynchrony between the developing central nervous system (CNS) and the bones of the skull and spinal column. Failure of the cranial cavity and spinal canal to enlarge sufficiently to accommodate the brain, cranial nerves, and spinal cord results in secondary changes in the CNS and a variety of neurologic signs. Membrane bones in other locations, including the periosteal surface of long bones, are also affected and may develop a coarse profile, but these changes are not significant clinically.

In the cranium, the defect is particularly severe in the bones of the caudal fossa, and the *cerebellum may herniate into the foramen magnum*. In puppies with vitamin A deficiency, deafness is a prominent sign because of changes in the internal auditory meatus, whereas affected *calves and pigs develop blindness caused by the narrow optic foramina and compression of optic nerves*. The basis for these variations between species is not clear, but lesions are modified according to the severity of the deficiency and the stage of skeletal growth. Spinal nerve roots, especially those in the cervical cord, may herniate into the intervertebral foramina, although the lesions are not always bilaterally symmetrical.

The pathogenesis of the asynchrony in development between the nervous system and skeleton is complex and is related to altered patterns of drift in bones that are growing during the period of deficiency. Normally, osteoclasts are responsive to vitamin A, and in the cranium of deficient animals, there is inadequate resorption of endosteal bone. Often, bone is produced at sites where resorption should be occurring, thus exacerbating the retarded expansion of the cranial cavity and the various foramina. Endochondral bone does not appear to be directly influenced by vitamin A deficiency.

The effect of vitamin A deficiency on dental development is well studied in the continuously growing incisors of rats and guinea pigs, but not in the teeth of other species. Inadequate differentiation and spatial organization of odontoblasts leads to irregular formation of poor quality dentin. Ameloblastic differentiation is also suboptimal and results in enamel hypoplasia. In addition, undifferentiated ameloblasts invade the dental pulp, where they induce the odontoblasts to form concretions.

Vitamin A deficiency, like excess, is **teratogenic**, and swine and large felids appear to be very susceptible. Abortions, stillbirths, and a variety of lesions, including subcutaneous edema, microphthalmia, retinal dysplasia, hypotrichosis, supernumerary ears, polydactyly, arthrogryposis, cleft palate, pulmonary hypoplasia, diaphragmatic hernia, hepatic cysts, and cardiac, renal, and gonadal malformations, may occur in the offspring of vitamin A–deficient swine. Hydrocephalus, and protrusions of spinal cord through intervertebral foramina, may also occur. The frontal and parietal bones may be thin and the basioccipital bone thicker than normal. The latter bone is also thickened in neonatal calves from vitamin A–deficiency dams, as are the squamous, occipital, basisphenoid, and presphenoid bones. Lesions in calves include stillbirths, congenital blindness, incoordination, thickened carpal joints, hydrocephalus, herniation of cerebellar vermis through the foramen magnum, constriction and degeneration of optic nerves, and retinal dysplasia.

Vitamin C (ascorbic acid) is a cofactor for the prolyl and lysyl hydroxylases, which are required for the hydroxylation of proline and lysine during procollagen synthesis, and it is also an important antioxidant. In **vitamin C deficiency**, there is *reduction or failure of the secretion and deposition of collagen.* Furthermore, the deficiency of hydroxylysine and hydroxyproline results in *impaired formation of intermolecular cross-links,* and any collagen that is produced is of reduced strength. Vitamin C is required for carnitine hydroxylation, and deficiency in carnitine may explain the early clinical sign of fatigue in humans with vitamin C deficiency. Proteoglycan synthesis, particularly on cell membranes involved in receptor-ligand interactions, requires vitamin C. Vitamin C is also required for hypoxia-inducible transcription factor-1α (HIF-1α) activity, and although usually associated with antioxidant activity, vitamin C may also act as a pro-oxidant.

Most mammals synthesize ascorbic acid from glucose via glucuronic acid. The last step in vitamin C synthesis involves oxidation of L-gulonolactone to L-ascorbic acid by the action of L-gulonolactone oxidase. Vitamin C is also present in large quantities in food of plant origin, but it may be broken down by heat, ultraviolet radiation, and oxygen. It is absorbed in the ileum via active transport, and there is no storage in the body. Some species, including humans, primates, guinea pigs, and bats, lack the hepatic microsomal enzyme L-gulonolactone oxidase and, in the absence of a dietary source of ascorbic acid, develop **scurvy**. Humans and guinea pigs have the *L-gulonolactone* gene; however, it is highly mutated with missing exons and base substitutions, making it nonfunctional. *A spontaneous mutation involving L-gulonolactone oxidase is recorded in pigs.* The defect in pigs is inherited as an autosomal recessive trait, and homozygous recessive piglets develop classic scorbutic lesions shortly after weaning. Maternal milk is a rich source of vitamin C and prevents signs of deficiency before weaning. A similar defect is recognized in the Shionogi rat, a mutant rat of the Wistar strain.

The **lesions of scurvy** in guinea pigs with dietary vitamin C deficiency and in pigs with an inherited deficiency of L-gulonolactone oxidase are similar, although the lesions described in pigs are more severe. This probably reflects the complete absence of vitamin C in affected pigs, and the effect of greater body mass on weakened connective tissues. In guinea pigs, a dietary deficiency of vitamin C may be partial rather than absolute, or may be sporadic, and the bone lesions therefore vary in severity. Pigs with inherited L-gulonolactone oxidase deficiency are normal at birth but lose condition, become reluctant to stand or move, and develop swellings around their joints. Gross lesions are dominated by *subperiosteal accumulations of clotted blood* around the shafts of the long bones, the scapulae, the bones of the head, and on the ribs. The metaphyses are fragile, discolored by hemorrhage and separate easily from the adjacent physes. Similar hemorrhages occur around major joints, along costochondral junctions, and on mandibles of affected guinea pigs; there may also be petechiae and bruising visible on the skin. The bones are osteopenic and fragile. Subclinical scurvy in guinea pigs is accompanied by such nonspecific signs as diarrhea, weight loss, and dehydration, and may be more common than is generally appreciated because the early bone lesions may not be detected clinically or at autopsy. In humans, there may also be hypertrophy and bleeding of the gums, abnormal dentine production, and loss of teeth.

The most characteristic microscopic lesion of scurvy is in the metaphysis; naked spicules of mineralized cartilage, derived from the zone of provisional mineralization in the growth plate, persist as a "scorbutic lattice" (Figs 2-97, 2-98). The layer of bone that is normally deposited on this cartilage framework by active osteoblasts is absent or deficient, because osteoblasts are unable to produce osteoid. Osteoblasts are sparse and appear to have lost their polarity. The marrow cavity may be filled with a population of poorly differentiated mesenchymal cells showing little if any collagen formation. In some cases, apparently normal bone trabeculae are present in the secondary spongiosa, representing bone formed during a period when dietary vitamin C was adequate. The cartilage spicules of the scorbutic lattice do not have the strength of normal trabeculae. Microfractures or infractions associated with hemorrhage and fibrin, but with little evidence of normal repair, are often present. Mechanical forces no doubt influence the development of such lesions. The cartilage spicules of the scorbutic lattice have a high mineral content and may be visible radiographically as a radiodense band in the metaphysis.

Physes are generally thin and contain a reduced number of chondrocytes, poorly organized into columns. Cortices of long bones are thin and the periosteum may be elevated by hemorrhage or thin, irregular spicules of basophilic, woven bone separated by loose connective tissue.

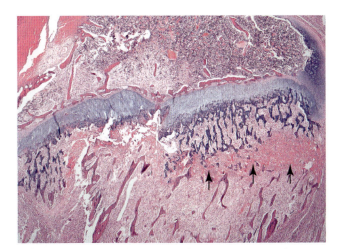

Figure 2-97 Physis and metaphysis from a guinea pig with **scurvy**. Note the basophilic spicules of cartilage matrix without osteoid deposition in the primary spongiosa. This is referred to as a *scorbutic lattice*. Trabeculae in the secondary spongiosa do possess an osteoid layer, indicating that the deficiency of vitamin C is relatively recent. An infraction line (arrows) between the primary and secondary spongiosa reflects the trabecular fragility.

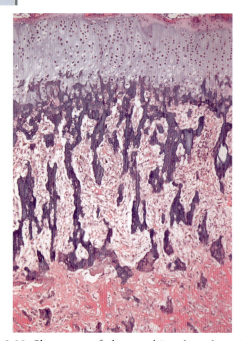

Figure 2-98 Closer view of physis and "scorbutic lattice" in the same guinea pig with **scurvy**. The mineralized cartilage spicules are devoid of an osteoid layer, and no osteoblasts are apparent. The spaces between trabeculae are filled with poorly differentiated mesenchymal cells. Trabecular fragments surrounded by fibrin at the bottom of the image are part of the infraction shown in **Figure 2-97**. There is no evidence of repair.

Further reading

Conaway HH, et al. Vitamin A metabolism, action, and role in skeletal homeostasis. Endocr Rev 2013;34:766-797.

Fain O. Musculoskeletal manifestations of scurvy. Joint Bone Spine 2005;72:124-128.

Hill B, et al. Clinical and pathological findings associated with congenital hypovitaminosis A inextensively grazed beef cattle. Aust Vet J 2009;87:94-98.

Mandl J, et al. Vitamin C: update on physiology and pharmacology. Br J Pharmacol. 2009;157:1097-1110.

TOXIC BONE DISEASES
Molybdenosis

In sheep **molybdenosis** is associated with *epiphysiolysis of the greater trochanter and subperiosteal hemorrhages of long bones*, leading to formation of bony excrescences. Subperiosteal new bone formation at sites of muscle and tendon insertion has also been described in rats fed a low-copper diet supplemented with tetrathiomolybdate. In feedlot cattle, molybdenum poisoning caused weight loss, and animals died over many months despite a short exposure to toxic levels; fatal cases showed both severe nephrosis and hepatotoxicity. Although it has been suggested that bone lesions, at least in lambs, may be caused by molybdenum toxicity rather than copper deficiency, the latter seems to be a better option. In ruminants, molybdenum may also interfere with the metabolism of sulfur and affect ruminal microflora. Weakening of connective tissues with tearing of insertion sites, resulting from reduced strength of tendons and ligaments, would not be surprising in copper-deficient animals with reduced cross-linkage of collagen. The formation of reactive bone would be an expected response to periosteal elevation induced by hemorrhage at such sites. In affected animals, the other commonly associated lesions of copper deficiency are absent, so the exact pathogenesis of bone lesions in molybdenosis remains uncertain.

Fluorosis

Fluorine is an essential trace element that is capable of inducing *characteristic dental and/or bony changes* when ingested in chronic excess. **Fluorosis** *is the term used to denote chronic fluoride toxicity*. All species are susceptible, but because of the manner in which chronic poisoning occurs, *fluorosis is most common in herbivorous animals*. Discussion here is based on fluorosis in cattle, which are more susceptible than sheep and horses and for which the abnormalities are better described.

Toxic levels may be obtained from subsurface waters, especially where *rock phosphate* is plentiful. Rock phosphates vary considerably in their fluoride content, and chronic poisoning has occurred in cattle and sheep given rock phosphates as "licks." Contamination of pastures adjacent to *mineral ore refineries* may also cause toxicity, either directly or by uptake of fluorine by plants, because fluorine is volatile at high temperatures and is part of the gaseous and particulate effluent of many industrial processes. *Dust from volcanic eruptions* also contains abundant fluorides. Because of the widespread distribution of fluorine in nature, many animals obtain small nontoxic doses, partly from drinking water and partly from windblown dust that settles on pastures.

Fluoride is removed rapidly from the blood by renal excretion and deposition in bones and teeth. A small amount is deposited in soft tissues. Some fluorine crosses the placental barrier, and although plasma levels are lower in fetal than maternal circulation, under certain circumstances, fetal fluorosis may develop. Evidence regarding fluorine levels in milk is conflicting. The deposition of fluoride in bone may be functionally comparable to that of other elements, such as lead and strontium, and may represent a detoxification mechanism. Unless the intake of fluoride is very low, there is a steady accumulation of fluorine because it is deposited as calcium fluoride or fluorapatite, both of which have low solubility. Many normal cattle have 600-900 μg/g in their bones, but fetal lesions apparently occur at concentrations as low as 100-200 μg/g. Fluorosis does not develop in older cattle until the concentration reaches 2,500-3,000 μg/g. A level of 40-60 mg/kg (dry matter) in feed will produce such concentrations in the bone of cattle after 2-3 years. In general, the toxicity of fluorine depends on the aqueous solubility of the compound fed; sodium compounds are more soluble and more toxic than calcium compounds.

Fluoride toxicity is enhanced by poor nutrition and alleviated somewhat by high dietary intakes of calcium and aluminum. While ingesting toxic levels of fluorine, urine of cattle usually contains 10 μg/g fluorine or more; high urinary concentrations may persist for some time after excess fluorine is removed from the diet. Plasma fluorine is also elevated during periods of exposure but declines a few days after fluorine is removed from the diet.

The characteristic changes of severe fluorosis occur in teeth and bones and are accompanied by shifting lameness, loss of production, and a variety of nonspecific signs of debility. **Dental lesions** develop only if intoxication occurs while teeth are in the developmental stages and enamel is forming. Ameloblasts and odontoblasts are extremely sensitive to fluorine, which causes them to produce a matrix that mineralizes abnormally and is reduced in quality and quantity. In particular, *the outer layer of enamel is hypomineralized.* The incremental lines in the enamel are disrupted, and the normal subsurface pigment band of bovine incisors is distorted.

The mildest macroscopic evidence of dental fluorosis is the *presence of small foci of dry, chalky enamel.* These mottled areas are readily visible as opacities when the tooth is transilluminated. In more severe cases, *all the enamel in affected teeth may be chalky, opaque, and show various degrees of yellow, dark brown, or black discoloration* (Fig. 2-99), *which is virtually pathognomonic for fluorosis.* Affected teeth show accelerated wear and may develop chip fractures. In chronic cases, they may be worn to the gum line. The pigment is present in the enamel layer and possibly in the dentin, and may reflect oxidation of the organic matrices of the teeth. Unlike the pigment of food stains and tartar, it is not limited to the surface and cannot be removed by scraping. Hypoplasia of enamel may occur in severe fluorosis and is evident as punctate pits or horizontal grooves, usually most prominent on the lateral aspect of the tooth. The horizontal disposition of the grooves and pits is attributable to periodic interference with mineralization of enamel during odontogenesis.

Although the fetus does not accumulate high levels of fluorine, under some circumstances, lesions may develop in the deciduous teeth of calves exposed during gestation. Microscopically, the odontoblasts are disorganized and have vacuolated cytoplasm. There is excessive predentin and formation of globular dentin. Fibrosis of the pulp cavity with ectopic bone formation is also seen. Lesions in permanent teeth, especially those that are last to erupt, are much more common, with those that erupt first showing little or no damage. In cattle, the permanent teeth are sensitive to fluorosis from about 6-36 months of age. The most severe effects occur when exposure coincides with initiation of crown formation. In areas of endemic fluorosis, where ingestion of the element is more or less continuous, the lateral incisors of cattle show the most obvious lesions and, together with the second premolars and second and third molars, the most severe lesions. Lesions of similar severity are typically present in teeth that develop simultaneously. These associations include the first incisor with the second molar, second incisor with the third molar, and the third incisor with the second premolar. Lesions in the second incisor must be severe before lesions are prominent in the third molar, and in general, incisor abrasion develops before molar abrasion. Lesions may develop in the fourth incisor in the absence of changes in other teeth.

The bone lesions of fluorine toxicity, **osteofluorosis**, are generalized but not uniform and, in severe cases, are characterized grossly by the formation of *periosteal hyperostoses*, which give the macerated bones a chalky rough appearance (Fig. 2-100). Lesions occur first on the medial surface of the proximal third of the metatarsal and later on the mandible, metacarpals, and ribs. The pelvis, vertebrae, and other bones of the distal limbs are also affected. In chronically affected cattle, fracture of the digital bones in the medial claw is common, leading to lameness and a preference for affected animals to stand cross-legged. A similar pattern of development occurs in horses. Although exostoses often develop at sites of tendinous or fascial insertions, this is not the rule, and the reasons for their occurrence and distribution are unknown. Endostoses seldom occur in farm animals. Articular surfaces are normal, and lameness is due to involvement of the periosteum, encroachment of osteophytes on tendons and ligaments and, in some cases, to mineralization and even ossification of the latter structures. Fluorine is incorporated into bone matrix during mineralization and will therefore be most abundant in young animals at sites of active formation but is also deposited in older animals during remodeling. *Exposure of cattle >3 years of age may therefore produce osteofluorosis but not dental fluorosis.*

Depending on the level of exposure to fluoride and its concentration in bone, the bones may appear grossly and radiographically normal. A characteristic microscopic feature that may be detected in ground bone sections in such cases is brown discoloration of osteons, similar to that in enamel. The discoloration is apparently due to the effect of fluoride on osteoblasts, and its extent depends on the rates of bone growth or remodeling. Both endosteal and periosteal osteoblasts are affected and produce an abnormal matrix, which mineralizes abnormally. Sections of cortex may have a mottled appearance, with some lamellae in some osteons showing discoloration and others appearing normal, depending on whether they were exposed to toxic levels of fluorine during formation. In fetuses, brown mottling of lamellar bone occurs at much lower concentrations of fluorine than in older cattle.

At *highly toxic levels*, the gross lesions of osteofluorosis occur rapidly. Not only is any new bone abnormal, preformed bone is apparently altered in its mechanical properties and has a reduced life-span. The rate of remodeling is correspondingly increased both for fluoridated normal bone and for bone formed under the influence of fluoride. The medullary cavity is enlarged, and resorption spreads progressively outward through the cortex and may involve the laminar periosteal bone. Resorption cavities may be excavated much more rapidly than they can be refilled, and the cortex becomes porotic. The impaired mechanical properties induce periosteal reinforcement with laminar bone or, if the need is greater and

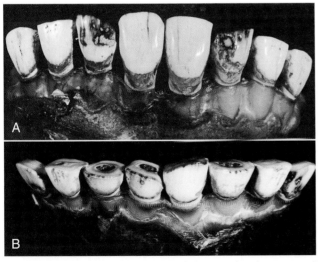

Figure 2-99 Fluorosis, cow. A. Dark brown discoloration and hypoplasia of enamel in the incisors of a cow. The variable involvement of the teeth reflects variation in levels of the toxin during enamel formation. **B.** Accelerated wear of incisor teeth in a cow with fluorosis. (Courtesy J.L. Shupe.)

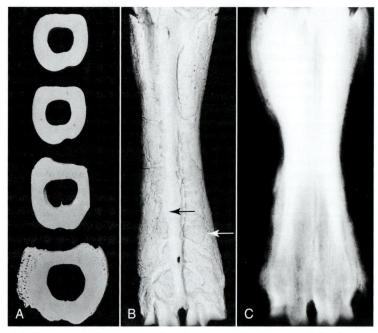

Figure 2-100 **Chronic osteofluorosis** in a bovid. **A.** Transverse sections of the diaphysis of metatarsals from an ox with increasing severity of osteofluorosis (top to bottom). Note the increased thickness of the cortex resulting from periosteal new bone formation. **B. Extensive periosteal new bone formation** (arrows) on the metatarsal bone. **C.** Radiograph of a metatarsal from an affected animal illustrating the extent of the periosteal hyperostosis. (Courtesy J.L. Shupe.)

the deposition of new bone more rapid, by coarse woven cancellous bone. When fluoride levels are very high, the new matrices produced are abnormal and remain unmineralized, as in osteomalacia.

In young, growing dogs and pigs, and presumably in other species, *fluorine intoxication produces lesions, which, in many respects, resemble rickets.* This is presumably caused by inhibition of mineralization when fluorine is present in high doses. The ends of long bones and the costochondral junctions are enlarged, whereas physes are usually increased in depth, softer than normal, and yield to the pressure of weight bearing. The change at osteochondral junctions appears to be caused by continued proliferation of chondrocytes, which fail to mature and align themselves. Associated with immaturity, there is a reduced amount of cartilaginous matrix, and although this appears to mineralize normally, albeit intermittently, the mineralized spicules are thin and fragile. The wide seams of osteoid that are deposited are poorly and irregularly mineralized.

Lead toxicity

Lead toxicity is better recognized for its effects on the nervous system but also causes bone lesions. *The characteristic lesion is a band of sclerosis, referred to as a* **"lead line,"** *visible radiographically and grossly in the metaphysis of developing bones.* This is a relatively early morphologic lesion in children with lead poisoning and also occurs in animals (Fig. 2-101A). The sclerosis is caused by persistence of mineralized cartilage trabeculae in the metaphysis (Fig. 2-101B) because of impaired osteoclastic resorption. Microscopically, many osteoclasts are present, but they may be separated from the surface of bone trabeculae (Fig. 2-101C) and appear poorly able to degrade mineralized matrix. Some osteoclasts may contain *acid-fast intranuclear inclusions*. Ultrastructurally, a large amount of mineralized cartilage matrix is in the cytoplasm of osteoclasts, suggesting a defect in intracellular processing of the matrix. The metaphyseal sclerosis associated with lead toxicity radiographically and grossly resembles that seen in association with some cases of canine distemper viral infection and intrauterine bovine viral diarrhea virus infection, both of which may interfere with osteoclast function or number.

Vitamin A toxicity

Vitamin A toxicity is well recognized as a cause of skeletal disease in humans and animals. Natural cases of toxicity usually follow an accidental overdose with vitamin A concentrate or excessive feeding of diets containing high concentrations of the vitamin, such as liver. Depending on the age and species of animal, and the duration and level of exposure to excess vitamin A, *the manifestations of toxicity may include physeal damage, osteoporosis, or the development of exostoses (osteophytes).* High concentrations of carotenes in green feed oats may predispose to rickets in lambs through inhibition of vitamin D activity.

The **physeal lesions** of vitamin A toxicity are characterized by reduced chondrocyte proliferation and reduced size of hypertrophic chondrocytes, resulting in narrowing of growth plates. Loss of proteoglycans and unmasking of collagen fibers occur, and with high doses, there is sometimes complete destruction of segments of growth plates. Rapidly growing physes, especially those subjected to the greatest compressive forces, are most likely to show changes resulting in reduced length of certain long bones. In organ culture, vitamin A

Diseases of Bones

Toxic Bone Diseases

87

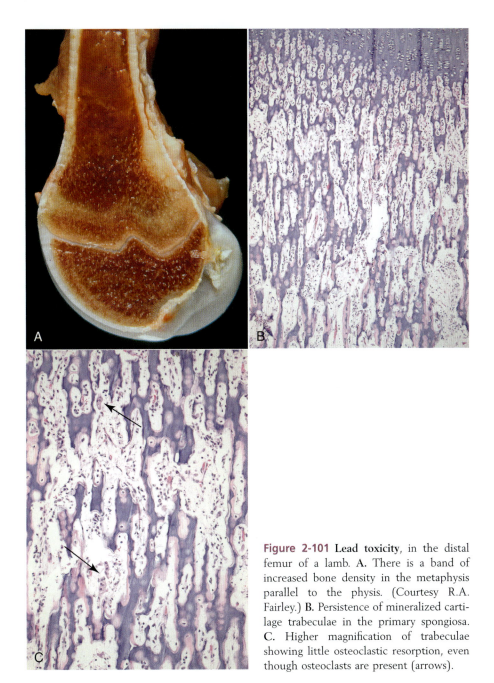

Figure 2-101 **Lead toxicity**, in the distal femur of a lamb. **A.** There is a band of increased bone density in the metaphysis parallel to the physis. (Courtesy R.A. Fairley.) **B.** Persistence of mineralized cartilage trabeculae in the primary spongiosa. **C.** Higher magnification of trabeculae showing little osteoclastic resorption, even though osteoclasts are present (arrows).

inhibits chondrocyte proliferation and reduces RNA and protein synthesis. Lysis of matrix may be the result of destabilization of lysosomal membranes, with the release of acid proteases that attack matrix proteins.

The **osteoporosis** of vitamin A toxicity is associated with decreased numbers of osteoblasts and fewer, thinner osteoid seams than normal; it is most severe in cortical bone and some of the membranous bones of the skull. Periosteal bone formation is more severely affected than endosteal and intracortical formation. In long bones, this results in thin cortices, reduced diaphyseal diameter, and an exaggerated metaphyseal flare. Metaphyseal trabeculae tend to be reduced in number but thicker than normal. Hypervitaminosis A interferes with cell differentiation in the embryonic skeleton and may have similar effects on osteoblasts in postnatal bone. The decrease in osteoid production also suggests a direct toxic effect on osteoblasts. The osteoporosis may be exacerbated by continued bone resorption, osteoclasts apparently being less sensitive than osteoblasts to the effects of increased vitamin A. Fractures are not a feature of vitamin A toxicity in farm animals and pets as they are in some laboratory species. Osteoporosis is reversible in animals removed from diets high in vitamin A, but the physeal damage is permanent and the consequences emphasized with time.

The *formation of exostoses* in association with vitamin A toxicity is often extensive. The pathogenesis of this lesion is not clear but may be associated with fragility of periosteal attachments, and provoked by tensions and minor trauma.

Toxicity associated with *single, large doses of vitamin A* has been recognized in pigs and calves. In baby **pigs** given excess vitamin A orally as part of disease prevention programs, a characteristic syndrome develops. Grossly, there is shortening of long bones and prolongation of the traction epiphyses of the tibial tuberosity, the greater trochanter of the femur, and the humeral tuberosity. Rotation of epiphyses, particularly those of the distal femur and proximal and distal humerus, is also described, and tarsal and carpal bones may be distorted. The medial and lateral metatarsal bones, and to a lesser extent the metacarpal bones, may be of different lengths. Pigs treated shortly after birth show an abnormal gait and possess noticeably short legs by 6-8 weeks of age. The condition occurs with as little as twice the recommended dose of vitamin A. *The basis for the gross lesions is destruction and focal closure of growth plates.* Continued growth of the intact parts of the physis and superimposed adaptational deformities account for the characteristic appearance of the bones.

Similar lesions occur in **kittens** given daily oral doses of 40-100 µg/g body weight of vitamin A for 4-5 weeks, followed by a 6-15 week recovery period. The metacarpal lesions tend to be more severe than in piglets; the tibial lesions are similar, whereas those in the distal femur and other sites are less severe.

In 7-week-old **pigs** given about 20 µg/g vitamin A for 5 weeks then killed, osteoporosis is prominent. Lesions are especially severe in the squamous occipital bone, which may be so thin that the cerebellum can be crushed by manual pressure to the overlying skin. The long bones are short and fragile with thin cortices, flared metaphyses, and typical physeal lesions, but the latter are less severe than at higher dose rates, and gross deformities do not occur. Exostoses may be present, especially near the insertion of the brachialis muscle on the proximal radius.

Vitamin A toxicity has been incriminated as the cause of "**hyena disease**" in **calves**. This unusual form of dwarfism is characterized by *relative under-development of the caudal body structures* resulting from premature closure of growth plates, particularly in the pelvic limbs, and has been associated with the injection of newborn calves with vitamins A and D. Affected calves have a characteristic "bunny-hopping" gait and a sloped back with small hindquarters, resembling a hyena. Although the lesions are most severe in the bones of the pelvic limbs and lumbosacral vertebrae, the pectoral limbs are also affected. Physes are narrow, but many focal triangular projections of physeal cartilage may protrude into the metaphysis. Administration of excess vitamin A to calves has been shown to induce premature mineralization of physeal cartilage, leading to early closure of growth plates and impaired longitudinal bone growth, supporting vitamin A toxicity as the cause of hyena disease. An autoimmune mechanism associated with bovine viral diarrhea virus has also been suggested but is not supported by convincing evidence.

Osteophyte formation is the hallmark of prolonged exposure to excess vitamin A in many species and is the outstanding feature of *chronic vitamin A poisoning in* **cats,** producing the syndrome referred to as **deforming cervical spondylosis**. The syndrome in adult cats results from prolonged feeding of bovine livers, which ordinarily contain large amounts of vitamin A when derived from grazing animals. The disease was common in Australia and Uruguay, where beef livers are plentiful and relatively cheap, but also occurs sporadically in other countries when domestic cats are given unconventional diets.

In young growing cats, this same diet would be expected to result in fibrous osteodystrophy because of the imbalance in calcium and phosphorus.

Deforming cervical spondylosis is typically *seen in cats >2 years of age* and is characterized by postural changes, cervical ankylosis, and forelimb lameness, sometimes accompanied by cutaneous hyperesthesia or anesthesia. The vertebral lesions are similar to those of mucopolysaccharidosis VI, but the age of the cat should prevent confusion. *Extensive confluent exostoses develop, especially on the dorsal and lateral aspects of the cervical vertebrae and sometimes on the occipital bone.* In general, the exostoses do not encroach on the neural canal and only occasionally involve ventral aspects of the vertebrae (Fig. 2-102A, B). The intervertebral foramina are considerably altered in shape and reduced in size, causing compression and degeneration of nerves, leading to denervation atrophy of muscles. Exostoses occasionally occur on the cranial thoracic vertebrae and may be accompanied by similar outgrowths on the sternum and fixation of the ribs. Periarticular osteophytes also occur about the proximal joints of one or both forelimbs and, if extensive, may cause fixation of the shoulder and elbow joints, usually in the flexed position. Lumbar vertebrae and pelvic limbs are seldom affected. The osteophytes consist initially of either osteocartilaginous tissue that overgrows joints and causes ankylosis, or of woven bone that develops at the site of muscle insertions and extends into the perimysium. Later, the woven bone and cartilage are replaced by lamellar bone. The stress on cervical intervertebral joints associated with regular grooming probably accounts for the concentration of exostoses in the cervical region of cats. In animals with chronic lesions, patches of ungroomed fur may develop in inaccessible sites. Interestingly, cats fed bovine liver tend to have higher and more persistently elevated plasma vitamin A concentration than cats supplemented with the vitamin, even at a higher equivalent dosage.

Oral and dental lesions, including hypermobility and loss of incisor teeth, may also occur in older cats in association with vitamin A toxicity and cervical spondylosis, but it is

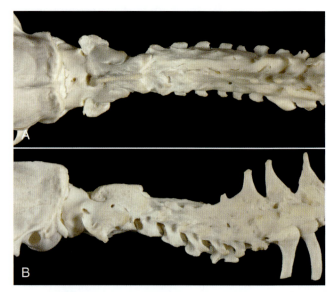

Figure 2-102 Vitamin A toxicity in a cat. **A, B.** Dorsal and lateral views of cervical vertebrae showing extensive exostoses leading to ankylosis.

difficult to determine whether the changes are primary or secondary. Liver has a low calcium content, which could lead to resorption of alveolar bone, but excess vitamin A causes dental lesions even when dietary calcium is normal.

Several *other lesions* are associated with vitamin A toxicity. In some species, including humans, rats, rabbits, and dogs, it causes *ectopic mineralization* in internal organs. In cattle, pigs, and dogs, there is decreased cerebrospinal fluid pressure and, in calves at least, this is associated with *thinning of the fibrous cap of arachnoid granulations*. Vitamin A is stored in the liver in *Ito cells*, which increase in size with dietary excess. Peliosis-like changes in the liver, in addition to hemorrhages around joints and hair loss, are reported in people with hypervitaminosis A. *Alopecia and dermatitis* are features of toxicity in **horses**.

Like vitamin A deficiency, *excess vitamin A is* **teratogenic**, the effects depending to some extent on dose, stage of gestation, and the compound administered. Teratogenicity is increased by protein or protein-energy malnutrition. Vitamin A is used extensively to treat skin disease in people and to a lesser extent in dogs. The half-life of some retinoids is many months, and anomalies in children exposed in utero are well recognized, but are not reported in puppies. *Experimental hypervitaminosis A during pregnancy produces defects in many systems in a variety of animals.* Vitamin A toxicity was incriminated as the cause of continued high prevalence of cleft palate and lip, pulmonary hypoplasia, and abortions near term in a swine herd. The problem in this herd ceased following reduction of vitamin A supplementation to normal levels. The mechanism of teratogenesis is unknown, but excess vitamin A in the embryo inhibits chondrogenesis and osteogenesis, possibly by modifying the differentiation of mesenchyme.

Vitamin D toxicity

Vitamin D is essential for normal bone development, in particular mineralization of cartilage during endochondral ossification and of newly formed osteoid, but in excess, it is highly toxic. Vitamin D toxicity may result from accidental oversupplementation of young animals, ingestion of plants that contain the active form of the vitamin, or accidental ingestion of rodenticide containing cholecalciferol (vitamin D_3). The potency of the latter toxin is illustrated by the fact that cats and dogs may be poisoned by ingesting the carcasses of poisoned rats. Cats appear to be more sensitive to vitamin D toxicity than dogs. When administered as 1 or 2 massive doses shortly before parturition, vitamin D appears to prevent postparturient hypocalcemia ("milk fever") in cows, but mineralization of soft tissues may result, particularly in pregnant Jersey cows, and in this breed, its use is contraindicated. Vitamin D is stored in muscle and fat, and meat from vitamin D–treated "downer cows" is a potential hazard to dogs and cats. Significant amounts of vitamin D may be secreted in milk, and soft tissue mineralization in suckling puppies has been attributed to high dietary levels in the bitch.

Several plants, including *Solanum malacoxylon* (syn *glaucum, glaucophyllum*), *Cestrum diurnum*, and *Trisetum flavescens* cause diseases similar to hypervitaminosis D in grazing animals in various parts of the world (see Enteque seco and Manchester wasting disease, in Vol. 3, Endocrine glands). Traditionally, vitamin D_2 (ergocalciferol) is regarded as the plant form of vitamin D, but *the toxic principle in these plants is 1,25-dihydroxycholecalciferol-glycoside.* Lesions in poisoned animals are indistinguishable from those produced by excess vitamin D. Other calcinogenic plants in which the active principle is less well defined include *Solanum torvum, S. verbascifolium*, possibly *S. esuriale*, and *Dactylis glomerata*. Alfalfa *(Medicago sativa)* contains vitamin D_3 in addition to vitamin D_2.

The *mechanism of vitamin D toxicity* is related primarily to its effect on increasing calcium absorption from the intestine, mobilizing it from bone, and reducing its excretion by the kidney. The end result is *hypercalcemia* together with *hyperphosphatemia*, which, if persistent, will lead to widespread mineralization of soft tissues, in particular the kidneys, gastric mucosa, lungs, endocardium, and arterial walls. Death from renal failure is likely to occur before noticeable changes develop in the skeleton. In fact, there are few reports of the skeletal lesions of vitamin D toxicity in animals.

The skeletal changes in hypervitaminosis D may be characterized by either sclerosis or rarefaction, depending on the level of dietary calcium and the pattern of exposure. An early response in bone is widespread, intense osteoclastic activity, which may remove most of the primary spongiosa and cause active resorption in other sites. With continued administration, the matrix produced by osteoblasts accumulates, sometimes in large amounts and in a distinctive pattern. It often has a tangled fibrillary arrangement and appears somewhat mucoid, floccular, and intensely basophilic. Osteoblasts are abundant. Mineralization of this basophilic matrix is delayed, but it is gradually converted to a relatively homogeneous eosinophilic substance resembling osteoid. Initially, the maturation of the matrix is local, irregular in distribution, and is unrelated to normal patterns of osteogenesis. If toxicity is prolonged, the abnormal matrices continue to accumulate and virtually obliterate the marrow spaces. This produces a mosaic of basophilic and acidophilic matrix, and newly formed woven bone. *The presence of abundant basophilic matrix is virtually pathognomonic for vitamin D toxicity* and is valuable diagnostically when plasma levels of the vitamin are not known.

Skeletal lesions of vitamin D toxicity are usually associated with intermittent toxic doses of the vitamin. This results in surges of osteoblastic activity during periods of withdrawal and rapid production of large amounts of abnormal matrix. This matrix may slowly mature and mineralize, but the process is hastened by further administration of the vitamin. With continued intermittent administration of vitamin D, there are further cycles of matrix deposition, maturation, and mineralization. *Broad, basophilic, resting lines separate the layers of bone produced in each cycle.* Necrosis of osteocytes occurs with high doses of vitamin D, and groups of empty lacunae are often present in cortical bone and in the center of trabeculae.

Virtually all bones are affected to some extent in vitamin D toxicity, but *the outstanding changes occur in long bones, especially in the ends where growth is most rapid*. The epiphyses are usually normal and appear to escape even the resorptive changes. The growth plates are also normal. The lesions involve the metaphyseal spongiosa and extend well into the diaphysis to fill the medullary cavity. Little active bone marrow remains and is gradually replaced by dilated veins and loose fibrous tissue, which is sparsely populated with hematopoietic cells. Areas of sclerosis may alternate with transverse bands of resorption, indicating intermittent toxicity. Active resorption of primary spongiosa may be accompanied by an intense neutrophilic reaction. Both the periosteum and endosteum are involved, and new periosteal bone contributes to the thickness of the metaphysis. Usually, the perichondrium is not affected, but sometimes it produces new cartilage and bone. In addition, there is rapid metaplastic bone formation in the thickened fibrous layer of the periosteum, producing a collar of new bone around the metaphysis.

Plant toxicities

Many plant species are known or suspected to cause skeletal abnormalities, either by inducing a teratogenic effect on the developing fetus or influencing skeletal remodeling in young growing animals. Those with a teratogenic action typically exert their influence early in pregnancy and require ingestion by the dam during a specific stage of fetal development. The classic example is **Veratrum californicum** (false hellebore, wild corn, or skunk cabbage), which causes cyclopia in the progeny of **ewes** that consume the plant on day 14 of gestation. *V. californicum* contains several steroidal alkaloids, the most active being cyclopamine, cycloposine, and jervine. *Cyclopamine is most abundant in the plant and is responsible for the craniofacial defects*, but the cause of the other anomalies is unknown. Ingestion of *V. californicum* by pregnant ewes near day 29 produces *marked shortening* of the metacarpals, metatarsals, and tibiae, and sometimes the radii, whereas tracheal and laryngeal stenosis occurs in the offspring of ewes ingesting the plant on or about day 31 of gestation. There is variation in the degree of susceptibility, but lesions are usually bilaterally symmetrical, and twins tend to be affected equally. Fusion of metacarpals may result in postnatal bowing of the legs, and fusion or deformities of joints may cause arthrogryposis. Obviously, not all ewes will graze the plant at precisely the same time of gestation, and in a natural outbreak, the changes detected in affected lambs include a range of abnormalities. Prolonged gestation is also a feature of malformed fetal lambs, and embryonic losses may be substantial. Death of about 17% of embryos occurs with maternal ingestion of *V. californicum* on days 19-21 of gestation, and up to 75% of embryos when the plant is ingested on day 14.

Ingestion of *V. californicum* by *pregnant cows* between days 12 and 30 of gestation may induce a range of anomalies, including cleft palate, harelip, brachygnathia, hypermobility of hock joints, syndactyly, and reduced number of coccygeal vertebrae. The length and diameter of all limb bones may be reduced, or the changes may be restricted to the metacarpals and metatarsals. Between days 30 and 36 of gestation the teratogens selectively inhibit growth in length of the metacarpal and metatarsal bones.

A syndrome referred to as **crooked-calf disease** occurs when pregnant cows ingest certain **wild lupins**, including *Lupinus caudatus*, *L. sericeus*, and *L. formosus*, especially between days 40 and 80 of gestation. Malformation of the limbs, notably the forelimbs, is the most common alteration, but the axial skeleton may also be involved. The limb abnormalities consist of flexion contracture and arthrogryposis, in addition to shortening and variable rotation of the bones. Torticollis, and either scoliosis or kyphosis are common, involvement of the thoracic spine being associated with costal deformities. There are various subtle and often asymmetrical changes in the skull, in which the most definable malformations are cleft palate or brachygnathia superior. Affected calves are usually born alive and may survive, depending on the nature and severity of their malformations, but growth is retarded, and the malformations persist, often becoming more severe with age. Neuromuscular structure and function are regarded as normal, or at least not primarily responsible for the skeletal deformity. No remarkable or consistent histologic changes are reported in crooked calves.

Lupins contain several alkaloids, some of which are teratogenic. The quinolizidine alkaloid *anagyrine* is present in *L. caudatus* and *L. sericeus*, and is almost certainly a teratogen. In *L. formosus*, the piperidine alkaloid *ammodendrine* may be responsible. Inhibition of fetal movement caused by a sedative or anesthetic effect of the alkaloids may be the basis for the skeletal deformities. Alternatively, secondary effects of direct toxicity to the dam may be involved; sustained uterine contractions producing deformities in the fetus have been suggested. *L. caudatus* (tailcup lupine) does not produce lesions in fetal lambs or kids, suggesting differences between cattle and other species in the metabolism of anagyrine.

Lupins cause 2 other distinct diseases in animals: a nervous disorder associated with the alkaloids in bitter lupins (see Vol. 1, Nervous system) and a mycotoxicosis caused by *Phomopsis leptostromiformis* (see Vol. 2, Liver and biliary system).

Conium maculatum (poison hemlock, European hemlock, spotted hemlock) is toxic to various species and causes a syndrome characterized by excitation and subsequent depression. There are 5 piperidine alkaloids in *C. maculatum*, the major ones being *coniine* and *γ-coniceine*. Both are thought to be toxic and the latter teratogenic. Cattle are most susceptible, and there is decreasing susceptibility through sheep, horses, and pigs. *C. maculatum* is also teratogenic, especially for cattle, with pigs being less susceptible and sheep relatively resistant. The plant causes *arthrogryposis and spinal deformities* in the offspring of sows and cows when fed between days 43-53 and 55-75 of gestation, respectively. *Cleft palate* occurs in the offspring of pigs exposed to the plant between days 30 and 45 and goats exposed between days 30 and 60 of gestation. *Carpal flexure* occurred in lambs and kids when *Conium* was fed to pregnant ewes and goats from days 30-60 of gestation, but resolved spontaneously as they grew.

Nicotiana tabacum (burley tobacco) causes arthrogryposis and sometimes brachygnathia and kyphosis in piglets exposed to the plant in utero. **Nicotiana glauca** (wild tree tobacco) causes similar lesions and also produces arthrogryposis and spinal deformities in calves exposed between days 45 and 75 of gestation. The teratogen is an α-substituted piperidine alkaloid, anabasine, which is present also in *N. tabacum*. It produces the lesions when given between days 43 and 53 of gestation and causes cleft palate when administered between days 30 and 37.

Jimsonweed (*Datura stramonium*) and **wild black cherry** (*Prunus serotina*) are suspected teratogens in sows, both being linked to *arthrogryposis*.

Various etiologies, including plant toxicities, have been incriminated in a limb deformity syndrome of lambs referred to as *bent leg*. In Australia, the syndrome has been associated with ingestion of *Trachymene ochracea* (white parsnip), *T. cyanantha*, and *T. glaucifolia* (wild parsnip) by ewes, which preferentially graze the flowers of *Trachymene* spp. The toxic principle is unknown, but the deformity may either be congenital because of exposure of lambs in utero, or may develop during postnatal growth, probably following exposure of lambs through the milk. Gross deformities are usually most prominent in the forelimbs and include outward bowing, flexion, and lateral rotation of the carpal joints, and medial or lateral rotation of the fetlocks. Similar syndromes are described in New Zealand (where it is called **"bowie"**) and South Africa, but plant toxicities are not suspected. Further discussion of these syndromes is included with angular limb deformities.

Outbreaks of congenital limb deformity and abortion have been reported in cattle, sheep, and horses in association with ingestion of **locoweed** (species of *Astragalus* and *Oxytropis*) by pregnant animals. The abnormalities include brachygnathia, contracture or overextension of joints, limb rotations, osteoporosis, and bone fragility. The toxic agent responsible for the skeletal defects is not known but is most likely unrelated to that responsible for the neurologic manifestations of locoweed toxicity, which inhibits the lysosomal enzyme α-mannosidase, inducing a lysosomal storage disease.

The leguminous plant **Lathyrus odoratus** (sweet pea) contains the amino acid β-aminopropionitrile, which inhibits lysyl oxidase and interferes with the formation of intermolecular cross-links in collagen and elastin. Skeletal deformities have been produced experimentally when the plant was fed to young rats, but natural disease associated with ingestion by grazing animals is unlikely.

Fetal ankylosis and abortion are recorded in foals whose dams graze **hybrid sorghum and Sudan grass** *(Sorghum sudanense)* during days 20-50 of gestation, and a similar association has been made in cattle. The lesions in foals involve many joints but are not well described. It is not clear whether the foals have ankylosis or arthrogryposis.

Other toxicities

An **equine bone fragility syndrome** characterized by diffuse or patchy osteoporosis has been associated with *pulmonary silicosis* in horses in California. The horses have chronic lameness or stiffness with skeletal deformities, including lateral bowing of the scapulae and ribs, lordosis, and decreased cervical vertebral range of motion. The axial skeleton and proximal appendicular skeleton are most severely affected. Pathologic fractures most commonly affect the ribs and pelvis. Grossly, the scapulae and ribs are thickened, rough, and more curved than normal (Fig. 2-103). Rib cortices are either thick or indistinguishable from the medulla. Microscopically, there is an increase in the size and number of resorption cavities, beginning along the trabecular surfaces and eventually affecting the cortex.

Overdosing of ewes with the anthelmintic **parbendazole** between days 12 and 24 of gestation may produce skeletal abnormalities in a high proportion of lambs. Neurologic lesions may also be present (see Vol. 1, Nervous system). The skeletal malformations include compression and/or fusion of vertebral bodies, fusion of proximal ribs, curvature of long bones, hypoplasia of articular surfaces, and absence of various bones such as ulna, humerus, and metacarpals. Lesions are reliably reproduced by a double dose of the drug and may even occur with less than twice the recommended dose.

A range of fetal abnormalities, including twisted limbs, brachygnathia inferior, and arthrogryposis, is reported in several sheep flocks in New Zealand where ewes had been affected by **nitrate toxicity** during early pregnancy. The ewes had been fed during the winter on crops containing high levels of nitrate, and although the evidence to incriminate nitrate toxicity as the cause of fetal abnormalities was circumstantial, agents such as pestivirus and Akabane virus were excluded. The problem occurred on 7 properties, and the incidence of abnormal lambs varied from 1-11%.

Further reading

Arens AM, et al. Osteoporosis associated with pulmonary silicosis in an equine bone fragility syndrome. Vet Pathol 2011;48:593-615.

Schultheiss WA, et al. Chronic fluorosis in cattle due to the ingestion of a commercial lick. 1995;66:83-84.

Welch KD, et al. Cyclopamine-induced synophthalmia in sheep: defining a critical window and toxicokinetic evaluation. J Appl Toxicol. 2009;29:414-421.

HYPEROSTOTIC DISEASES

Excessive bone formation, or hyperostosis, occurs as a nonspecific response to various forms of bone injury, including trauma, infection, metabolic disturbances, mineral and vitamin imbalances, subperiosteal hemorrhage, and neoplasia. Many of these are discussed elsewhere in this chapter. This section includes a group of poorly understood diseases characterized by marked hyperostosis in the absence of a direct cause.

Craniomandibular osteopathy

Craniomandibular osteopathy, also known as *"lion jaw," is a proliferative disorder usually confined to the bones of the skull, in particular the mandibles, and occipital and temporal bones.* The tympanic bullae are often severely affected. Lesions are bilateral but irregular and may also involve the parietal, frontal, and maxillary bones. Occasionally, there is subperiosteal and extraperiosteal proliferation of new bone associated with long bones. The disease is most common in West Highland White Terriers, but is also described in several other breeds, including Scottish Terriers, Labrador Retrievers, Great Danes, Doberman Pinschers, Cairn Terriers, German Wirehaired Pointers, Pyrenean Mountain Dogs, and in a Boxer, a Boston Terrier, and an English Bulldog.

The disease is usually recognized at ~4-7 months of age because of either discomfort while chewing or inability to open the mouth to eat. Proliferative changes may be palpable

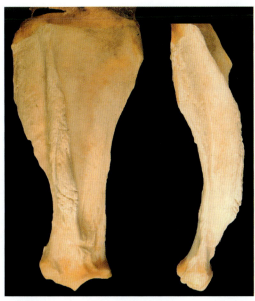

Figure 2-103 Equine pulmonary silicosis in the scapula of a horse. The scapular spine is thickened and roughened by new bone proliferation. There is also increased convex curvature to the scapula. (Courtesy S.M. Stover.)

or grossly visible, and pain is elicited when attempting to open the mouth. Radiographic findings are characterized by more or less symmetrical enlargement of the mandibles and tympanic bullae, although the lesions may occur independently. Ossification of soft tissues, especially near the angular processes of the mandibles, may result in fusion of the processes to the bullae and ankylosis. The disease has an intermittent, progressive course lasting several weeks to a few months. It is often self-limiting and nonfatal, although some dogs are euthanized because they cannot eat. During clinical exacerbations, which tend to recur every 2-3 weeks, fever is present but laboratory data are normal.

At the height of the disease, atrophy of the muscles of mastication and increased fibrous and osseous tissue of the head are obvious. The full extent of the bone changes is best demonstrated in radiographs and macerated specimens (Fig. 2-104A, B). In the mandible, new bone deposition is usually most prominent in the region of the angle, involving medial, ventral, and lateral aspects but tending to avoid the alveolar bone. The tympanic bullae are often enlarged 2-3 times and filled with new bone.

Histologic changes in the mandible involve the endosteum, periosteum, and trabecular bone and present a complex pattern of intermittent and concurrent bone formation and resorption.

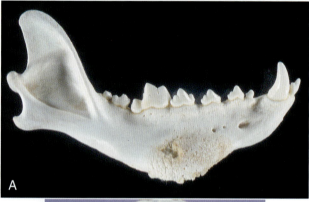

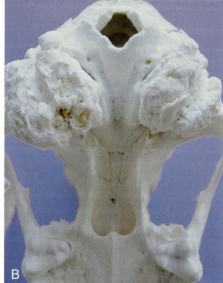

Figure 2-104 Craniomandibular osteopathy in dogs. Macerated specimens from 2 different dogs showing new bone formation along the mandible (**A**) and tympanic bullae (**B**).

The mosaic of reversal and resting lines resulting from this cellular activity bears some resemblance to the changes seen in Paget's disease of humans, but further comparison is unjustified. The significance of this mosaic pattern is easily overemphasized because the mandible of growing dogs is a site of intense bone modeling as teeth mature, erupt, and drift during normal development. Bone resorption in craniomandibular osteopathy is random and disoriented, involving both preexisting lamellar trabeculae and newly formed woven bone. Similarly, bone formation occurs simultaneously in many areas, evolving from fibrous tissue, which frequently fills the marrow spaces and thickens the periosteum. Lymphocytes, plasma cells, and neutrophils are sometimes present in areas of active osteogenesis.

As the disease subsides, formation of woven bone may be superseded by lamellar bone production, and existing woven trabeculae are replaced by lamellar bone, which is then gradually resorbed. In some cases, especially where fusion of mandibles to tympanic bullae is present, resorption is insufficient to allow restitution of normal function.

The cause of craniomandibular osteopathy is not known. The presence of inflammatory infiltrates raises the possibility of an infectious agent, but none has been demonstrated. In West Highland White and Scottish Terriers, there is evidence of a genetic etiology with autosomal recessive inheritance. However, the occurrence of the syndrome in diverse breeds suggests that there may be more than one cause of the condition. Alternatively, there may be an inherited predisposition in several breeds, but the presence of an additional factor, perhaps an infectious agent, is required for the disease to be expressed. The etiology and pathogenesis of a similar condition in children, infantile cortical hyperostosis, are also unknown.

Calvarial hyperostosis of Bullmastiffs

Calvarial hyperostosis is an idiopathic condition occurring in young Bullmastiff dogs. It differs from craniomandibular osteopathy in the breed affected, the distribution, and the inflammatory nature of the lesion. Although the condition was originally described in males, both male and female Bullmastiffs are affected. The dogs are typically presented for pain and swelling of the skull at 5-10 months of age. Fever and lymphadenopathy may also be present. The lesions consist of asymmetrical hyperostosis of the skull *without involvement of the mandibles*. There is occasional limb involvement. Microscopically, the lesion consists of *subperiosteal woven bone proliferation with foci of neutrophils and necrosis*. The disease is typically self-limiting.

Hypertrophic osteopathy

This syndrome, which is also known as hypertrophic pulmonary osteopathy, is *characterized by diffuse, periosteal new bone formation along the diaphyses and metaphyses of certain limb bones in association with a chronic inflammatory or neoplastic lesion, usually in the thoracic cavity.* It occurs in a wide variety of species but is most often reported in dogs. Occasionally, hypertrophic osteopathy occurs in association with nonthoracic lesions, such as botryoid rhabdomyosarcoma of the urinary bladder in dogs and ovarian tumors in horses. Rarely, the disease occurs in animals with no detectable visceral lesions.

The thoracic lesions associated with hypertrophic osteopathy are diverse. In dogs, it occurs most often with primary or secondary pulmonary neoplasms, but also with granulomatous pleuritis, granulomatous lymphadenitis of bronchial or mediastinal nodes, chronic bronchitis, bacterial endocarditis, *Dirofilaria immitis* infection, esophageal granulomas, tumors provoked by *Spirocerca lupi*, and with neoplastic disease of the thoracic wall. In horses, hypertrophic osteopathy is more often associated with granulomatous inflammatory diseases involving the thoracic cavity. Hypertrophic osteopathy is present only in a minority of animals with thoracic lesions, but the incidence is much higher in some types than in others. For example, dogs with pulmonary metastases from osteosarcoma are much more likely to develop the syndrome than are dogs with metastatic carcinoma. It is also possible that many mild cases of hypertrophic osteopathy are missed both clinically and postmortem.

The *periosteal new bone formation in hypertrophic osteopathy is usually confined to the limbs*, and in the dog involves particularly the radius, ulna, tibia, metacarpals, and metatarsals, with relative sparing of the bones of the proximal limbs and phalanges (Fig. 2-105). The more distal limb bones are generally affected first, the lesions then extending proximally. The extent of the hyperostosis is best demonstrated in radiographs and macerated specimens where, in florid cases, they appear as wart or cauliflower-like accretions extending along the whole length of the bone (Fig. 2-106). Cross-sections of bone demonstrate the asymmetrical development of these accretions (Fig. 2-107), which tend to occur initially and most severely where the periosteum is free of tendinous insertions or adjacent bones. Articular surfaces are not involved. Occasionally, hyperostosis occurs on the vertebrae and skull, and minor endosteal lesions occur infrequently. Although the lesions of hypertrophic osteopathy are progressive, they regress if the primary thoracic lesion is removed.

Histologically, the earliest changes are hyperemia and edema, with proliferation of highly vascular connective tissue in the periosteum, in some cases leading to extensive hemorrhage. These changes are associated with a rapid increase in peripheral blood flow in the distal half of the limbs and may be accompanied by a light infiltrate of lymphocytes and plasma cells. Shortly thereafter, osteoblasts deposit osteoid on the existing cortical bone, and then, if the disturbance persists, begin to lay down new trabeculae perpendicular to the original cortex. The new bone may be deposited with extraordinary rapidity, and the width of the cortex may be doubled in a few weeks. In the early and active stages of the disease, the new bone is clearly distinguishable from the original cortex because the former is trabecular and the latter compact. Later, the difference may be less distinct because the original cortex is converted to trabecular bone by resorption from the endosteal surface within cortical vascular canals. The periosteal new bone is surrounded by dense collagen, which infiltrates and thickens the adjacent soft tissues of the limbs.

The pathogenesis of hypertrophic osteopathy is obscure, but *increased blood flow* to the limbs is a consistent early change. Several hypotheses have been proposed, including hypoxia, arteriovenous shunting, and neurogenic and humoral mechanisms, but none consistently fits the clinical and experimental observations. According to the *neurogenic theory*, impulses originating in the thoracic lesion travel via the vagus nerve to the brainstem and initiate reflex vasodilation in the limbs, either by humoral or neural means. Limited support for this theory is provided by the regression of bone lesions in

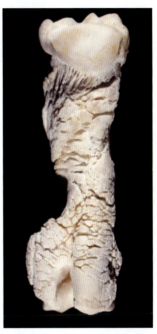

Figure 2-106 Hypertrophic osteopathy in a horse. Florid periosteal reaction along the shaft of the humerus.

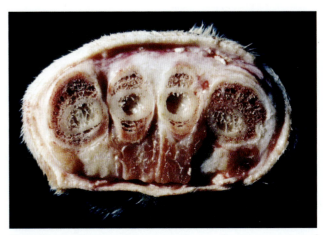

Figure 2-107 Hypertrophic osteopathy in a dog. Cross-section of metacarpal bones showing eccentric periosteal bone proliferation that avoids adjacent bones.

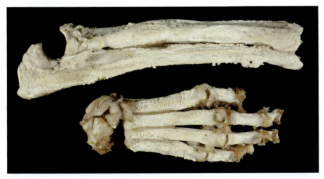

Figure 2-105 Hypertrophic osteopathy in a dog. Periosteal new bone involving the radius, ulna, and metacarpal bones, with relative sparing of the phalanges.

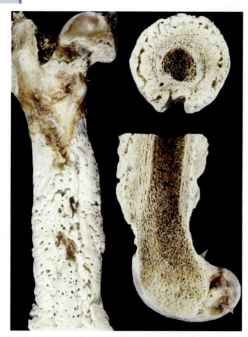

Figure 2-108 Canine hepatozoonosis in a dog. Femur with periosteal new bone along the diaphysis. The cross-section shows concentric layers of new bone surrounding the porous original cortex. Endosteal proliferation is not present. (Courtesy R.J. Panciera.)

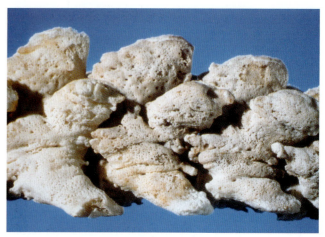

Figure 2-109 Canine hepatozoonosis. Vertebrae markedly affected by periosteal new bone. (Courtesy of Texas A&M University.)

some, but not all, cases treated by vagotomy. The *humoral hypothesis* proposes either that the primary thoracic lesion produces a hormone or hormone-like substance or that arteriovenous anastomoses in the primary lesion prevent catabolism of such a substance in the lung. Support for this hypothesis is derived from the production of typical skeletal lesions following experimental venoarterial shunts in dogs, but there is no evidence of such shunts in most spontaneous cases. Another theory is that vascular endothelial growth factor and platelet-derived growth factor released from platelets within abnormal limb circulation contribute to the development of the bone lesions. In a very limited number of cases, the disease has been restricted to one limb, and vascular abnormalities are generally found in those cases.

Canine hepatozoonosis

Periosteal new bone formation, similar to that occurring in hypertrophic osteopathy, is a feature of canine hepatozoonosis caused by *Hepatozoon americanum* infection of dogs in the United States. Transmission is by ingestion of an infected tick by the canid host, which may occur during self-grooming or by ingestion of a prey species infested with ticks. The osseous lesions also consistently develop in experimentally infected dogs and coyotes.

The periosteal reaction occurs primarily on the diaphyseal regions of the more proximal limb bones (Fig. 2-108), but also may involve bones of the axial skeleton, including the ilium and vertebrae (Fig. 2-109); the distribution of lesions differs therefore from that of hypertrophic osteopathy. Microscopically, the lesions are similar to those of hypertrophic osteopathy, with periosteal woven bone forming trabeculae perpendicular to the diaphyseal cortex. The parasite is not present within the bone, and the periosteal new bone formation is not related to *H. americanum* cysts in adjacent muscle fibers. The widespread, often symmetrical, distribution of lesions suggests that humoral rather than local factors are involved in the pathogenesis of the bony lesions.

Clinical signs of canine hepatozoonosis include pyrexia, depression, weakness, muscle atrophy, and gait abnormalities ranging from stiffness to recumbency. Leukocytosis resulting from mature neutrophilia, and sometimes a left shift, is a consistent laboratory finding. Different stages of this protozoon agent are present in skeletal muscles throughout the body, often inducing a pyogranulomatous inflammatory response. The disease can lead to debilitation and death.

Hepatozoon canis, a species once only found in the Old World, has been increasingly detected in dogs in the United States, alone and in combination with *H. americanum*. It is unclear whether *H. canis* is capable of causing the same bone lesions as *H. americanum*.

Further reading

Allen KE, et al. *Hepatozoon* spp infections in the United States. Vet Clin Sm Anim 2011;41:1221-1238.

McConnell JF, et al. Calvarial hyperostosis syndrome in two bullmastiffs. Vet Rad Ultrasound 2006;47:72-77.

Panciera RJ, et al. Skeletal lesions of canine hepatozoonosis caused by *Hepatozoon americanum*. Vet Pathol 2000;37:225-230.

Withers SS, et al. Paraneoplastic hypertrophic osteopathy in 30 dogs. Vet Comp Oncol 2013 March 14; doi: 10.1111/vco.12026. [Epub ahead of print.]

OSTEONECROSIS

Like any living tissue, *bone will die when deprived of its blood supply*. This is referred to as **osteonecrosis**, or the synonymous term **osteosis**. In animals, bone ischemia is most often associated with trauma, particularly fractures, wherein vascular disruption to part of the fractured bone is inevitable. Osteonecrosis also occurs in many acute inflammatory diseases of bones, where the periosteal or myeloid vascular supplies may be disrupted by exudate accumulating either beneath the periosteum or between trabecular bone in marrow spaces. In such cases, the presence of *a large fragment of necrotic bone*, or

sequestrum, often proves to be a major hindrance to successful repair. This is discussed in more detail in the following section: Inflammatory and infectious bone diseases. Other causes of ischemic necrosis of bone, or **bone infarction**, include infiltrating neoplasms, thromboembolism and peripheral vasoconstriction in association with ergotism, fescue foot, or chronic anemia. Animals in cold climates may also develop peripheral vasoconstriction and necrosis of bone, together with ischemic necrosis of other tissues in peripheral regions (frostbite); the necrosis is more severe if the animal is dehydrated or at high altitude.

In humans, bone infarction occurs in association with steroid therapy, bisphosphonate treatment, alcoholism, hyperviscosity, hemoglobinopathies, and in divers or tunnel workers who work in dysbaric conditions. **Steroid-induced bone necrosis** is most often found in the femoral head, distal femur, and proximal humerus. Increased adipogenesis and adipocyte hypertrophy is thought to compress venous blood flow in the bone, resulting in increased intraosseous pressure such that arterial blood flow is prevented. In animals, corticosteroid-induced bone necrosis has been induced experimentally in rabbits and horses, but its prevalence in association with routine steroid therapy is unknown. Similar changes in adipogenesis are also thought to be behind alcohol-induced osteonecrosis. Other causes of impaired lipid metabolism in animals, such as hyperlipidemia in miniature Schnauzers, may predispose to bone infarction. Idiopathic ischemic necrosis of the radial carpal bone has been described in a Staffordshire Bull Terrier, and of the accessory carpal bone in a mixed-breed dog. As a rule, regions of bone that are served by end-arteries and have poor collateral circulation, such as the femoral head and part of the carpal bones, are most prone to nonseptic osteonecrosis.

Necrosis of bone and bone marrow is described in calves with the juvenile form of sporadic lymphosarcoma. Infarcts of various sizes are found both in vertebral bodies and long bones (Fig. 2-110). The pathogenesis of the lesion is not known but may involve vascular obstruction caused by increased intraosseous pressure associated with neoplastic infiltration of the bone marrow.

A possible sequel to bone infarction is the *development of osteosarcoma*. Multiple bone infarcts have been associated with the formation of osteosarcoma in breeds of dogs not usually susceptible to this tumor (e.g., Miniature Schnauzer). The reparative process triggered by the infarcts may be responsible for initiating the malignancy, similar to the proposed mechanism of tumor induction at sites of fracture repair and osteomyelitis in dogs and cats (see later).

Morphology and fate of necrotic bone

In the early stages, necrotic bone is often impossible to recognize on gross examination. Furthermore, its mineral composition will be unaltered, and its radiographic appearance will therefore resemble that of normal healthy bone. The *earliest recognizable alteration is usually a change in the periosteum to a dull, dry, parchment-like sheath, which can be detached easily.* This contrasts with the normal periosteum and cortical surface, which is smooth, white, glistening, and firmly adherent, except where muscles and fascia are inserted. The sharp contrast in color between a pale tan area of ischemia and the adjacent areas of normal marrow is an early indication of necrosis during gross examination, especially in young animals where the marrow is red due to active hematopoiesis (Fig. 2-111). Necrotic bone is slowly but progressively resorbed by osteoclasts, but these cells can only gain access to areas where the blood supply is intact and oxygen tension is maintained. Within a few weeks, evidence of the resorptive process will be apparent grossly as a margin of fibrous connective tissue separating the necrotic bone from adjacent viable bone. The necrotic bone will remain chalky white or become light brown. Gas gangrene occasionally develops in necrotic bone of livestock, but is rare in companion animals.

Microscopically, zones of empty lacunae caused by loss of osteocytes characterize necrotic bone (Fig. 2-112), but pyknotic

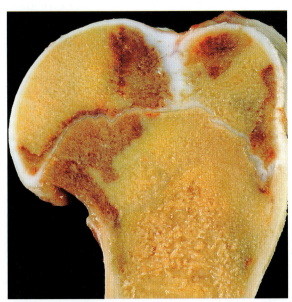

Figure 2-110 Infarcts in malignant lymphoma in a 6-month-old calf. Multiple irregular yellow foci representing medullary infarcts throughout the epiphysis and metaphysis of the proximal humerus. Similar lesions were present in most other long bones.

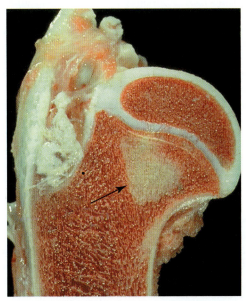

Figure 2-111 Necrosis of bone in the metaphysis of a young foal with **acute osteomyelitis**. The necrotic bone (arrow) is pale tan compared to the surrounding hematopoietic bone marrow.

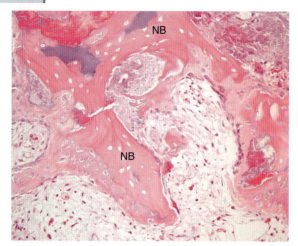

Figure 2-112 **Necrotic bone** surrounded by new, woven bone at the site of collapse of the femoral head in a dog with **Legg-Calvé-Perthes disease**. Note the empty lacunae in the necrotic bone (NB) and the more basophilic matrix of the new woven bone. The necrotic bone has a scalloped margin, reflecting a period of osteoclastic resorption before the new bone was deposited on its surface.

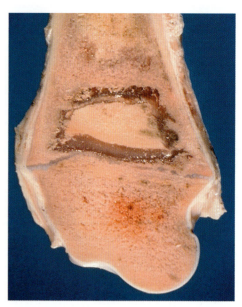

Figure 2-113 **Large sequestrum** surrounded by an **involucrum** of granulation tissue in the distal radius of a foal with salmonellosis.

nuclei from dead osteocytes may take anywhere from 2 days to 4 weeks to disappear. Hematopoietic tissue in the marrow cavity will show evidence of necrosis within 2-3 days after ischemia and can therefore provide an early indication, but adipose tissue is more resistant to ischemia and will not show evidence of necrosis for about 5 days. If an ischemic event is only transient, then there may be death of hematopoietic cells and perhaps osteocytes, but not adipocytes. The discovery of scattered empty lacunae in a section of bone does not justify a diagnosis of osteonecrosis as this may reflect normal turnover or even be an artifact of preparation. Prolonged immersion in acidic demineralizing solutions can mimic osteocyte death. In osteonecrosis, all the lacunae in an area of bone should be empty, and the contents of the marrow cavity should be necrotic. Sometimes dystrophic calcification occurs in the necrotic medullary fat.

The fate of necrotic bone depends on several factors, the most important being its volume, whether it is accompanied by sepsis, and whether it is in contact with viable tissue. In pyogenic infections of bone, sequestration is a common problem and usually has serious implications. The prognosis is more favorable if the necrotic bone is at a site that is both sterile and has good collateral circulation, and the volume of necrotic bone is small. In such cases, a zone of granulation tissue develops at the interface between the necrotic and viable tissue. This encroaches on the dead tissue and over a period of several weeks, the necrotic fat is replaced by collagenous connective tissue. *Osteoblasts derived from local progenitor cells begin to deposit seams of new woven bone on the remnants of necrotic bone* (see Fig. 2-112). This new bone is sharply demarcated from the necrotic bone, which will usually be lamellar, and can be easily distinguished by its increased basophilia and the presence of viable osteocytes. Meanwhile, osteoclasts are recruited to the site and commence removal of the necrotic bone that is being used as a framework for deposition of new bone. This repair process, sometimes referred to as *"creeping substitution,"* therefore involves the gradual resorption of dead bone at the same time as it is being replaced by new bone. Eventually, the new woven bone will be replaced with lamellar bone, but until such remodeling is complete, the combination of woven bone and partly resorbed dead bone may not be strong enough to withstand the forces of weight bearing and may collapse.

When the volume of necrotic bone is small, and is not in an area predisposed to further damage during the repair process, resolution is likely to be uncomplicated and complete. In fact, many such events probably occur throughout life but do not become clinically apparent. Repetitive injury at the same site may lead to an exaggerated response with the formation of local exostoses.

The healing process is more complex when the necrotic bone is separated from viable connective tissue, as occurs frequently with necrosis or detachment of the periosteum. In such lesions, resorption of necrotic bone may still be complete if its volume is small, but if a relatively large volume of cortical bone is involved, sequestration may occur. Even when infection is not present, the sequestrum may interfere with the healing process by acting as a foreign body. *Attempts to wall off the sequestrum will lead to the formation of a layer of granulation tissue and reactive bone; this layer is referred to as an* **involucrum** (Fig. 2-113).

The efficacy of the collateral circulation is another important factor in the likely outcome of osteonecrosis. When the nutrient artery is occluded, large areas of the bone marrow become necrotic, along with the adjacent cancellous and compact bone. If the damage is restricted to the diaphyseal extremities, the prognosis is more favorable because this region has a dual blood supply of osseous origin, from the nutrient vessels on the diaphyseal side and from the vessels of the joint capsule and ligaments on the epiphyseal side, as well as that from adjacent soft tissues.

As a rule, *the collateral circulation in cortical bone is inefficient* because, in spite of abundant anastomoses, the vessels are small and, because they are confined within narrow canals, are incapable of effective compensatory dilation. The resting and proliferative cartilage of the major growth plates depends on the epiphyseal circulation, whereas the sinusoidal circulation of the primary spongiosa is derived from metaphyseal vessels and is vulnerable to trauma. In contrast, the articular cartilages are relatively insensitive to regional ischemia because their nutrient supply is obtained by diffusion from the synovial fluid.

Osseous sequestration is a relatively common sequel to distal limb wounds in horses and cattle, the most common sites being the third metatarsal and metacarpal bones. Although the initial event may be traumatic, it is likely that the introduction of infection to the site predisposes to sequestration, rather than reduced peripheral cortical circulation alone. Sequestra may be detected at about 14 days after injury, when there is some separation from adjacent viable bone and early formation of an involucrum. In a study of sequestra in llama and alpacas, only 19% of cases were associated with trauma, and hematogenous spread of bacteria to bone was considered to be the most common cause of the sequestra.

Legg-Calvé-Perthes disease

This disease, characterized by *avascular necrosis of the femoral head*, is a well-recognized entity in children but also occurs with some frequency in dogs, especially smaller breeds. Miniature Poodles, West Highland White Terriers, and Yorkshire Terriers are particularly susceptible, and there is evidence to suggest that the disease is inherited as an *autosomal recessive trait*. Avascular necrosis of the femoral head may also occur in other breeds of dog, and in other species, as a result of fractures of the femoral head, but such cases should not be confused with Legg-Calvé-Perthes disease, which has a different pathogenesis. Clinically, the disease has an insidious onset, usually between 4 and 8 months of age, and is bilateral in ~15% of cases. There is no obvious sex or leg preference in dogs, unlike children, among whom boys are affected 5 times more frequently than girls.

Anatomic and experimental evidence supports the theory that the *osteonecrosis in Legg-Calvé-Perthes disease is initiated by one or more episodes of ischemia*. As skeletal maturation takes place, the developing blood vessels supplying the femoral head are progressively incorporated into fibro-osseous canals, which offer protection as they travel along the femoral neck. In highly susceptible Miniature Poodles, the incorporation of vessels into these canals is delayed, or is incomplete, in contrast to mongrels, for which the vessels run mainly intraosseously. In experimental studies, even a relatively slight degree of intracapsular tamponade produces lesions similar to those in the naturally occurring disease, probably by occluding veins that drain the femoral head. A transient increase in intra-articular pressure caused by an effusion associated with synovitis or trauma would therefore be expected to interfere with venous drainage from the femoral head and produce the natural disease.

In the early stages of the disease, the shape of the femoral head, and the outlines of the articular cartilage and physis, appear grossly and radiographically normal, even though the subchondral bone may be necrotic. If the area of necrosis is small, and the vascular supply is quickly re-established, healing may occur uneventfully. When the subchondral infarct is more extensive, *continued weight bearing leads to fracture and collapse of the necrotic trabecular bone and flattening of the femoral head* (Fig. 2-114), predisposing to degenerative arthropathy. The physis of the femoral head is also disrupted, and may close prematurely, because of interruption of the epiphyseal blood

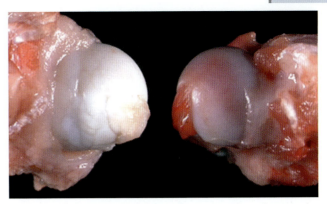

Figure 2-114 **Legg-Calvé-Perthes** disease in a dog. The articular surface of the femoral head on the left is irregular because of collapse of necrotic subchondral bone. The unaffected femoral head from the same dog is included for comparison. (Courtesy M.W. Leach.)

supply to the resting and proliferative zones at the time of the initial insult.

The repair process involves initial revascularization, thought to be stimulated by increased hypoxia-inducible factor 1α and vascular endothelial growth factor expression, and proliferation of mesenchymal cells from the margin of the necrotic area. This is followed by increased bone morphogenetic protein 2 expression, deposition of woven bone on the remnants of necrotic trabeculae, and formation of new thin trabeculae of woven bone between existing trabeculae. Gradually, the dead bone is removed by osteoclasts, and eventually the woven bone is replaced by lamellar bone.

Further reading

Fan M, et al. Experimental animal models of osteonecrosis. Rheumatol Int 2011;31:983-994.

Kamiya N, et al. Acute BMP2 upregulation following induction of ischemic osteonecrosis in immature femoral head. Bone 2013;53:239-247.

Kim HK, et al. Effects of non-weight-bearing on the immature femoral head following ischemic osteonecrosis: an experimental investigation in immature pigs. J Bone Joint Surg Am 2012;94:2228-2237.

Rousseau M, et al. Osseous sequestration in alpacas and llamas: 36 cases (1999-2010). J Am Vet Med Assoc 2013;243:430-436.

Valentino LW, et al. Osseous sequestration in cattle: 110 cases (1987-1997). J Am Vet Med Assoc 2000;217:376-383.

INFLAMMATORY AND INFECTIOUS DISEASES OF BONES

Inflammation of bones originates in vascular areas of the medullary cavity or periosteum and is referred to as either **osteomyelitis** or **periostitis**, respectively. **Osteitis** is a more general term for inflammation of bones but is used less frequently. Most inflammatory diseases of bones are caused by bacterial infections, although other agents can also infect bones.

Noninfectious osteitis also occurs, usually in response to local periosteal injury, and typically results in the formation of **exostoses**. The exostoses may be due to a single insult, if there is damage to the periosteum, or to repeated minor trauma. For example, tearing of ligamentous insertions will often induce local periostitis and the development of exostoses or osteophytes. Small exostoses may be completely resorbed if the stimulus is removed, but larger ones may be converted from woven to lamellar bone and persist indefinitely. Exostoses often remain clinically inapparent but may interfere with the function of adjacent structures, such as tendons or ligaments, as occurs in some cases of "splints" on the second and fourth metacarpal bones of horses. There is evidence to suggest that traumatic injury to the periosteum may predispose to bacterial periostitis at the site, even if the overlying skin is intact. The mechanism is uncertain, but damage to adjacent tissues may increase their susceptibility to infection.

Hepatozoon americanum causes a disseminated and symmetrical periosteal proliferation that is neither inflammatory nor associated with the location of the organism. The bony lesion of canine hepatozoonosis is discussed with other hyperostotic diseases. Rare causes of osteomyelitis, such as *Halicephalobus gingivalis* in horses and *Leishmania* spp. in dogs, are not included in this chapter.

Bacterial osteomyelitis

Bacteria infect bone by 3 routes: *hematogenous, local extension, and implantation*. Hematogenous osteomyelitis is very common in animals, especially young horses and ruminants. There is little doubt that bacterial osteomyelitis is more common than is diagnosed, because affected animals often die of septicemia before the bone lesions become evident, and the skeleton is generally not closely examined at postmortem examination unless clinical signs suggest a skeletal disorder.

During bacteremia or septicemia, there is a predilection for bacteria to localize to sites of active endochondral ossification within the metaphyses and epiphyses of long bones and vertebral bodies. This reflects the unique nature of the vascular architecture at the physis and at the equivalent site in expanding epiphyses. Capillaries invading the mineralized cartilage make sharp loops before opening into wider sinusoidal vessels that communicate with the medullary veins. The capillaries are fenestrated, thus permitting ready escape of bacteria into the bone marrow. Furthermore, sluggish circulation in the sinusoidal system, and the relative inefficiency of the phagocytic cells lining it, also tend to favor the development and persistence of infection. Experiments in rabbits suggest that trauma, or some other factor that alters the metaphyseal environment, enhances the establishment of bone infection in animals with bacteremia. Thus a combination of *injury and concurrent bacteremia* may be involved in the pathogenesis of hematogenous osteomyelitis. As the skeleton matures, the vascular morphology at chondro-osseous junctions becomes less suitable for bacterial localization. In fact, there is probably only a narrow window during which bacteria are able to establish in bones, whether the bacteria are derived from umbilical infections in colostrum-deprived animals or from infections in the respiratory or alimentary tracts. The clinical manifestations of osteomyelitis may not develop until several months later when the bone lesion becomes extensive enough to cause pain, disfigurement, or pathologic fracture.

Some bacteria have a predilection for bone. *Staphylococcus aureus*, for example, can invade osteoblasts. This intracellular location may favor persistence of the infection by protecting the organisms from host defense mechanisms and antibiotics. Other bacteria that commonly establish in bones (e.g., *Salmonella* spp.) may possess similar mechanisms of survival. At sites of bacterial infection, cytokines such as tumor necrosis factor α (TNF-α), interleukin-1 (IL-1), and IL-6 produced by inflammatory cells and osteoblasts stimulate osteoclast proliferation, differentiation, and bone resorption.

There are several possible sequelae to hematogenous bacterial infection of bone. The initial response is characterized by *edema and acute purulent inflammation*. Many infections are probably eliminated spontaneously by host defenses at this early stage, perhaps assisted by prompt and vigorous treatment with specific antibacterial agents. If the infection is not eliminated, it may become segregated by fibrous inflammatory tissue and woven bone, with development of a *metaphyseal or epiphyseal abscess (Brodie's abscess)* (Fig. 2-115). Alternatively, the exudate may percolate through the adjacent marrow cavity, causing necrosis of soft tissues and trabecular bone. These early lesions appear grossly as discrete areas of pallor, sharply demarcated from normal red bone marrow (see Fig. 2-112). *Resorption of necrotic trabecular bone* from the edge of the lesion, and *proliferation of granulation tissue*, results in separation of the necrotic, infected bone from adjacent viable tissues (see Fig. 2-113). It is not unusual to find several foci of osteomyelitis in different bones within the same animal (Fig. 2-116A), or even within the same bone. Osteoclasts or inflammatory cells may resorb small foci of necrotic bone, but larger foci persist as **sequestra**, harboring bacteria and interfering with the repair process. *The granulation tissue or reactive bone that forms a layer around the sequestrum* is referred to as an **involucrum** (Fig. 2-116B; see also Fig. 2-113).

The physis usually prevents the spread of infection from the metaphysis to the epiphysis, but transphyseal blood vessels in very young animals may transmit infection from one side to the other. In such cases, the physis is usually involved in the septic inflammatory process and is destroyed locally (Fig. 2-117). The cortex is relatively porous in young animals and offers little resistance to the spread of infection when it penetrates through vascular canals to the periosteum. If cortical penetration occurs within the attachment of a joint capsule, then *septic arthritis* may result, but more commonly, a *subperiosteal abscess* develops. Disruption or thrombosis of the blood supply from the metaphysis to the inner portion of the cortex, together with periosteal elevation and interference with periosteal blood vessels, causes segmental cortical necrosis and formation of sequestra. In severe cases of bacterial

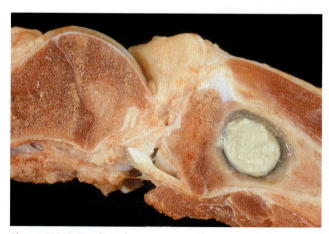

Figure 2-115 **Brodie's abscess** in a pig. There is a well-demarcated abscess in the proximal tibia.

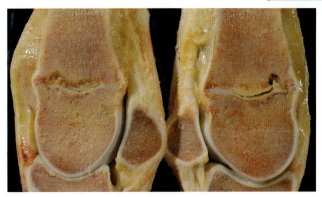

Figure 2-117 Osteomyelitis with physeal destruction in a foal. The metaphyseal bone is soft, yellow, and separated from the physis.

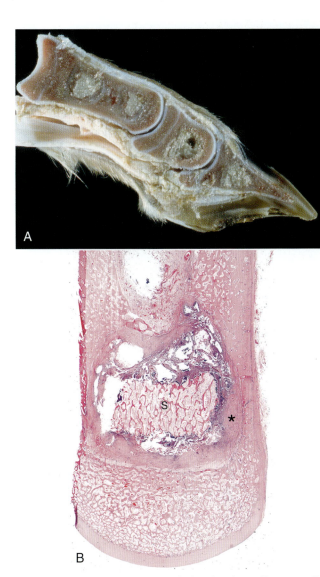

Figure 2-116 Osteomyelitis in a foal with salmonellosis. **A.** All 3 phalangeal bones contain sequestra. **B.** Sequestrum in the distal metaphysis of P1 from the same foal. Note the thick involucrum of granulation tissue (asterisk) surrounding the sequestrum of necrotic cancellous bone (S).

osteomyelitis, there may be locally extensive necrosis and sequestration of metaphyseal and cortical bone, with an exuberant involucrum formed beneath an elevated periosteum, resulting in swelling and disfigurement of the bone (Fig. 2-118A-C).

The *predilection sites* for hematogenous osteomyelitis vary between species. There is also variation in the bacteria involved and the age of affected animals. In **foals,** osteomyelitis seldom occurs after 4 months of age, and the lesions occur more often in the secondary ossification centers of the epiphyses than in the metaphysis. *Most infections establish immediately beneath the thickest part of the articular cartilage,* particularly in the caudal aspect of the lateral and medial femoral condyles, dorsal to the weight-bearing articular surface. Other common sites for epiphyseal osteomyelitis in foals include the distal intermediate ridge of the tibia, medial styloid process of the radius, and the proximal humerus, but many other sites may be involved. The vascular arrangement at sites of thickened cartilage is characterized by an increased arterial supply and greater sinusoidal filling than in areas where the articular cartilage is thinner. If the infection becomes established, there may be extensive destruction of subchondral bone with collapse of the articular cartilage and communication with the joint space (Fig. 2-119A, B). Metaphyseal lesions in foals are most common at sites where the physis deviates greatest from a horizontal plane. Approximately 70% of foals with bacterial osteomyelitis, including virtually all of those with epiphyseal lesions, also have septic arthritis. This may reflect either concurrent establishment of infection in the synovium during bacteremia, or direct spread from bone. The bacteria most commonly involved in foals with osteomyelitis are *Escherichia coli, Streptococcus* spp., *Salmonella* spp., *Klebsiella* spp., and *Rhodococcus equi.* Hematogenous osteomyelitis of the tarsal bones, usually in association with infectious arthritis, is reported as an entity in young foals <1 month of age.

In **cattle,** hematogenous osteomyelitis is not confined to young animals, as it is in foals. In one study, the age range in cattle was 2 weeks to 5 years. *Metaphyseal osteomyelitis* in this study occurred at many sites in long bones, but particularly the distal metacarpus, metatarsus, radius, and tibia. *Epiphyseal osteomyelitis* occurred most often in the distal femoral condyle, distal radius, and the patella, and was usually associated with infection by *Salmonella* spp. In contrast, metaphyseal infections were most often caused by *Trueperella (Arcanobacterium) pyogenes.* The *Salmonella* spp. infections were almost invariably in calves <3 months of age, whereas *T. pyogenes* usually affected cattle >6 months of age. As in foals, septic osteomyelitis generally accompanies bacterial arthritis in calves. Hematogenous osteomyelitis and arthritis also frequently occur together in young **lambs, goats,** and **deer,** and are associated with a range of organisms.

Hematogenous bacterial osteomyelitis is rare in dogs but may occur in puppies that survive canine parvovirus infection, or other conditions associated with neutropenia or neutrophil adhesion defects (such as canine leukocyte adhesion deficiency). *Bartonella vinsonii* has been reported to cause hematogenous osteomyelitis in a cat. More often, bacterial osteomyelitis in dogs and cats is via the local extension or implantation routes. *Local extension* of severe bacterial periodontitis into the maxilla and mandible is common in older **dogs** and cats (Fig. 2-120). In **cats,** if the maxillary canine teeth become loose and infected, the surrounding alveolar bone forms a smooth nodular proliferation (Fig. 2-121) called

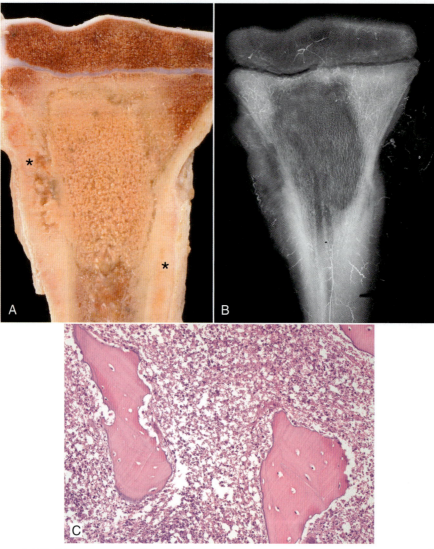

Figure 2-118 Chronic osteomyelitis, foal. *Rhodococcus equi* infection. **A.** Large sequestrum filling most of the metaphysis in the proximal radius. New bone formation along the periosteum (asterisks) has caused enlargement of the bone. **B.** Radioangiogram of the same specimen showing the periosteal reaction and lack of blood supply to the sequestrum. (Courtesy E.C. Firth.) **C.** Ragged trabeculae of necrotic bone surrounded by necrotic inflammatory debris. The scalloped margins of trabeculae indicate previous osteoclastic resorption.

feline buccal bone expansion or alveolar osteitis, which will persist even after loss or removal of the affected canine tooth.

In small animals, osteomyelitis is commonly the result of *implantation* of bacteria in open fractures, contamination during surgical fracture repair, bite wounds, or gunshot injury. Staphylococci, especially *Staphylococcus pseudintermedius*, and streptococci are the most common organisms involved, although mixed infections including gram-negative bacteria and anaerobic bacteria also occur. Because of the association with fractures, osteomyelitis in dogs is most common in long bones of the appendicular skeleton. Foreign material implanted traumatically beneath the skin, or surgical implants, may act as a nidus for infection. The mucopolysaccharide glycocalyx layer (biofilm) produced on the surface of implants by staphylococci and other bacteria protects the bacteria from phagocytosis, antibodies, and some antibiotics. Even after apparent resolution, bacterial infections of bone may recur as a result of proliferation of bacteria that have survived within the biofilm or in necrotic bone.

Histologic changes in bacterial osteomyelitis are predictable but depend on the causative agent and the stage of infection. *Acute osteomyelitis* in young animals may be *distinguished from active myelopoiesis* by the presence of fibrin and a dense population of neutrophils and necrotic cells in the primary spongiosa, where hematopoietic tissue is usually absent. Excessive osteoclastic resorption of bone trabeculae is another characteristic feature, and there may be necrosis of physeal or articular cartilage. In the epiphysis, inflammatory foci typically start immediately beneath the articular cartilage, resulting in local destruction of subchondral trabecular bone (Fig. 2-122A, B). Degeneration or necrosis of the overlying articular cartilage is common in young animals with hematogenous bacterial osteomyelitis resulting from septic embolism or thrombosis of blood vessels in cartilage canals. In *chronic osteomyelitis*,

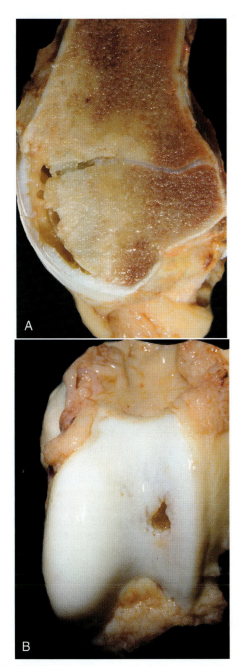

Figure 2-119 Osteomyelitis in a foal, the result of *Salmonella enterica* serovar Typhimurium infection. **A.** Extensive destruction of subchondral bone in the distal femur. The infection has spread to involve much of the epiphysis, as well as the physis and part of the metaphysis. **B.** Same lesion before sectioning, showing communication with the stifle joint through a defect in the trochlear groove.

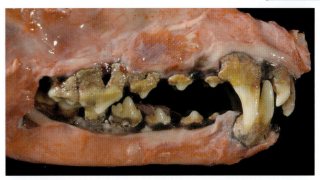

Figure 2-120 Periodontal osteomyelitis in a Greyhound. Severe dental calculus with gingival recession and alveolar bone osteomyelitis of the maxilla and mandible.

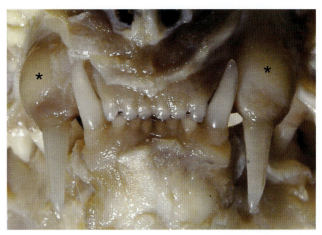

Figure 2-121 Periodontal bone expansion in a cat. The alveolar bone surrounding maxillary canine teeth of cats forms smooth proliferations (asterisks) as a response to chronic periodontal osteomyelitis.

marrow spaces between necrotic, partly resorbed bone trabeculae may be filled with necrotic debris, fibrous connective tissue, or a mixed population of inflammatory cells. A thick layer of granulation tissue infiltrated with neutrophils may surround larger areas of necrotic bone, with prominent osteoclastic activity at the margins. Proliferation of connective tissue and woven bone in chronic lesions may make it difficult to distinguish the reaction from neoplasia, especially in biopsy specimens where the sample is small. *The presence of neutrophils and plasma cells within the reactive bone and connective tissue supports a diagnosis of chronic osteomyelitis.* Osteomyelitis secondary to an open fracture may present a considerable diagnostic challenge, because the inflammatory changes will be superimposed on the proliferative components of fracture repair. In such cases, patient history and radiographic changes are indispensable.

Vertebral osteomyelitis is a relatively common manifestation of bacterial osteomyelitis in horses and farmed livestock. Most cases probably result from hematogenous spread of infection to the bones during the neonatal period in animals with inadequate passive immunity. Bacteria may enter via the umbilicus, respiratory tract, digestive tract, or perhaps via the placenta immediately before parturition. In piglets and lambs, tail biting and tail docking, respectively, are believed to provide a portal of entry for bacteria in some cases of vertebral osteomyelitis. Following localization to the epiphysis or metaphysis of a vertebral body, or adjacent to a growth plate in a developing vertebral arch, the infection causes progressive destruction and weakening of the affected vertebral bone. As in long bones, sequestration and abscessation may occur. The *most common sequela is pathologic fracture and collapse of affected vertebrae* with dorsal displacement of pus and necrotic bone fragments into the spinal canal (Fig. 2-123). Such an event is

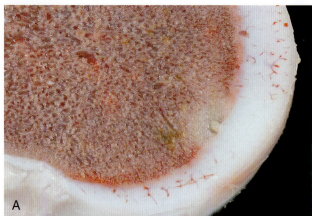

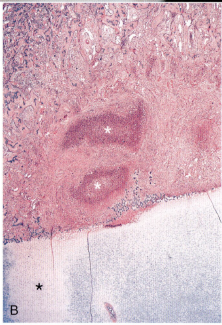

Figure 2-122 Suppurative osteomyelitis in the epiphysis of a calf. **A.** Focus of suppuration and trabecular destruction immediately beneath the articular surface. **B.** Intense, suppurative inflammation and effacement of epiphyseal trabecular bone (white asterisks) adjacent to the articular cartilage. There is also a pale pink focus of necrotic cartilage (black asterisk).

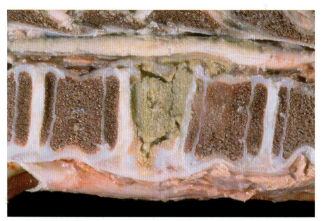

Figure 2-123 Vertebral osteomyelitis in a calf, the result of *Escherichia coli* infection. The vertebral body is completely necrotic and collapsed. Fragments have been forced into the spinal canal, compressing the cord. (Courtesy P.C. Stromberg.)

accompanied by the sudden onset of neurologic signs caused by compression of the spinal cord. In cases where vertebral fracture does not occur, the suppurative process may permeate the cortex in any direction, spreading to involve the pleura, peritoneum, or spinal muscles, or protrude as an encapsulated abscess into the spinal canal and cause partial compression of the cord. If the infection is contained or does not result in cord compression, it may go undetected or be found incidentally at slaughter.

Trueperella (Arcanobacterium) pyogenes is the most common causative organism in vertebral osteomyelitis in large animals, but a range of other bacteria may be involved. These include: *Escherichia coli*, *Salmonella enterica* serovar Typhimurium, staphylococci, streptococci, and *Rhodococcus equi* in foals; *Fusobacterium necrophorum* in calves; *Mannheimia haemolytica*, *F. necrophorum*, and staphylococci in sheep; and *Erysipelothrix rhusiopathiae*, staphylococci, and streptococci in pigs. In dogs, vertebral osteomyelitis has been linked to migration of plant material. In cats, bite wounds are the most likely route of infection. Diskospondylitis is discussed with other joint infections.

Localized bacterial periostitis is often associated with primary inflammatory conditions in adjacent tissues. Examples include infections of the feet of cattle with *F. necrophorum* ("footrot"), necrotic stomatitis of cattle caused by the same organism, infections of the paranasal sinuses as an extension from perforating injuries, bite wounds that produce cellulitis or abscesses, chronic paronychia, and pressure sores over bony prominences. Penetrating wounds of the hoof in cattle or horses may also spread to involve the adjacent third phalanx.

Atrophic rhinitis of pigs is mediated by bacterial toxins produced by *Pasteurella multocida* and *Bordetella bronchiseptica*. These toxins inhibit osteoblast differentiation and stimulate osteoclast activity, resulting in bone loss. The disease is discussed in more detail in Vol. 2, Respiratory system. A similar lytic condition may affect the turbinates of dogs.

Mandibular osteomyelitis caused by *Actinomyces bovis* is most common in **cattle** but occasionally occurs in horses, pigs, deer, sheep, and dogs. In cattle, the disease is known as actinomycosis or **"lumpy jaw,"** and the classic lesion is confined to the mandible. The maxilla is rarely involved, and the organism rarely spreads even to regional lymph nodes, which, although large and indurated, are not infected. *A. bovis* is probably an obligate parasite of the oropharyngeal mucosa in a number of animal species, and most infections involve the buccal tissues. Most, if not all, cases follow a penetrating injury to the oral mucosa. *A. bovis* may invade bone directly though the periosteum, but *osteomyelitis usually develops from periodontitis*, presumably via lymphatics, which drain into the mandibular bone. Once in the bone, *A. bovis* causes a chronic, pyogranulomatous inflammatory reaction. Suppurative tracts permeate the medullary spaces, leading to multiple foci of bone resorption and proliferation. Large sequestra do not develop, even when the cortex is invaded, probably because of the slow, progressive nature of the disease. Fistulae often discharge through the skin or mucous membranes. Periosteal proliferation is excessive, and the bone may become enormously enlarged, with destruction of the normal architecture of the mandible. The teeth in the affected portion of the jaw become loose, lost, or buried in granulation tissue. On cut surface, the affected mandible has a "honeycomb" appearance with reactive bone surrounding pockets of inflammatory tissue (Fig. 2-124A). Fragments of necrotic trabecular bone

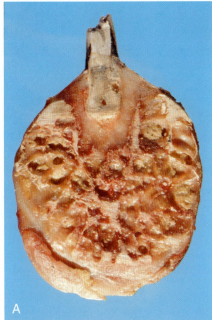

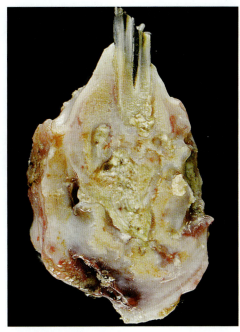

Figure 2-125 **Mandibular osteomyelitis** in a sheep. Bony expansion and suppurative inflammation of the mandible surrounding the affected tooth root.

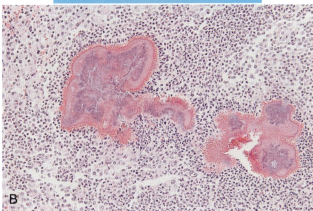

Figure 2-124 **Mandibular osteomyelitis** in a cow, resulting from *Actinomyces bovis* infection. **A.** Section through mandible showing "honeycomb" appearance caused by pockets of inflammatory tissue surrounded by reactive bone. **B. Colonies of *A. bovis*** surrounded by characteristic brightly eosinophilic clubs of Splendore-Hoeppli material and suspended in a dense neutrophilic exudate.

accumulate in purulent exudate as "bone sand." The pus is also likely to contain many 1-2 mm diameter, soft, light yellow granules referred to as *"sulfur granules."* These consist of an internal mass of tangled, gram-positive filaments mixed with some bacillary and coccoid forms, and a periphery consisting of closely packed, club-shaped, eosinophilic bodies (Splendore-Hoeppli material) (Fig. 2-124B). A similar tissue reaction, accompanied by club-colonies, occurs in association with some other bacteria, in particular *Actinobacillus lignieresi*, but the colonies are smaller and the clubs larger. Furthermore, actinobacillosis is a disease of soft tissues rather than bone. *Fusobacterium necrophorum* and a variety of nonspecific bacteria may cause osteomyelitis by direct spread from periodontitis, but the lesions are usually more destructive and less proliferative than with *A. bovis*. Similar lesions may be produced by *Trueperella pyogenes*.

Mandibular osteomyelitis associated with loosening or loss of molar teeth (Fig. 2-125) is sometimes detected in ill-thrifty **sheep** in the absence of other likely causes of weight loss, and may be a more important problem than is currently recognized in commercial sheep flocks. Grass awns or other plant matter may be wedged into pockets between teeth and the alveolar bone, providing a route of entry for opportunistic bacteria into the mandible.

Further reading

Lewis JR, et al. Significant association between tooth extrusion and tooth resorption in domestic cats. J Vet Dent 2008;25:86-95.
Sutton A, et al. Spinal osteomyelitis and epidural empyema in a dog due to migrating conifer material. Vet Rec 2010;166:693-694.
Wright JA, Nair SP. Interaction of staphylococci with bone. Int J Med Microbiol 2010;300:193-204.

Fungal osteomyelitis

Mycotic infections of bone are less common than those caused by bacteria, but certain pathogenic fungi, in particular *Coccidioides immitis*, *Blastomyces dermatitidis*, and *Cryptococcus neoformans*, may cause osteomyelitis. Most are dimorphic, having a filamentous form in the environment and a yeast form in tissues.

Coccidioides spp. are dimorphic fungi geographically restricted to the southwestern United States, Mexico, and a few areas in Central and South America. Infection is typically subclinical, and bone involvement can manifest months to years after exposure. *Coccidioides* can infect a wide variety of domestic animals. Horses, llamas, cats, and dogs are most likely to get the disseminated form, which can include osteomyelitis. Bone is the most common site of dissemination in **dogs**, and the appendicular skeleton is more commonly affected than the axial. Clinical signs include fever, weight loss, and bone pain. Bone lesions most often occur in the distal diaphysis of

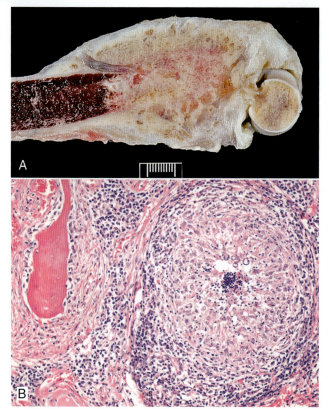

Figure 2-126 **Coccidioides osteomyelitis** in the distal humerus of a dog. **A.** There is periosteal and endosteal new bone proliferation with loss of the cortical bone within the affected area. (Courtesy B. Murphy.) **B.** A pyogranuloma centered on spherules and endospores adjacent to a scalloped trabecula of bone surrounded by fibrosis.

long bones; a single bone lesion is the most common presentation (Fig. 2-126A). Lung lesions have often resolved by the time osteomyelitis manifests. Radiographic and gross findings are similar to neoplasia, with a mix of lysis and proliferation. Microscopically, the inflammation is pyogranulomatous; the spherules are poorly chemotactic, and the endospores attract large numbers of neutrophils (Fig. 2-126B). However, the organisms can often be difficult to find within the lesion, even with silver staining. Culture of the organism results in mycelial growth that is highly infectious; therefore the laboratory should be contacted before sending in suspected *Coccidioides* spp. samples.

Blastomyces dermatitidis primarily occurs in North America, but has also been diagnosed in Central America, Europe, Africa, and India. Male sporting dogs 1-5 years of age are most commonly affected, but the disease is also seen in females and older dogs. Dogs may act as a sentinel species for humans, because they are 10 times more likely to become infected. Inhalation of spores is the most common route of infection, and pneumonia is the most common presentation. Dissemination to skin, eyes, and bone are common; 30% of infected dogs have bone involvement. These dogs are lame, with soft tissue swelling. The bone lesion is typically osteolytic, solitary, and distal to the elbow or stifle. The pneumonia may have resolved by the time the bone lesion manifests. Like the other fungal osteomyelitides, the lesion is pyogranulomatous with rare intralesional organisms.

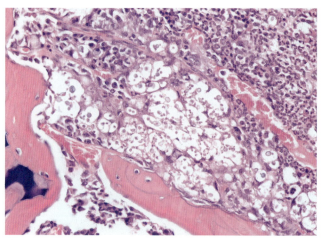

Figure 2-127 **Cryptococcus osteomyelitis** in the rib of a dog. Numerous clusters of organisms with characteristic thick capsule in the marrow space. The adjacent bone is scalloped.

Cryptococcus spp. have a worldwide distribution and can affect a wide variety of domestic animals. It is one of the few systemic mycoses in which **cats** are more commonly affected than dogs. The route of infection is thought to be inhalation, with the lungs and nasal cavity most commonly affected. In cats, bone lesions are typically in the maxilla (nasal turbinates, sinuses, and cribriform plate), and there is often soft tissue swelling of the bridge of the nose. Histologically, the lesion is remarkable for the large numbers of organisms relative to the scant amount of inflammation (Fig. 2-127). Most affected cats are not immunosuppressed, and feline immunodeficiency virus infection does not worsen the prognosis.

Histoplasma capsulatum rarely involves bone, even in disseminated infections. When it does cause osteomyelitis, the lesion is typically in the metaphysis of long bones, especially around the carpal and tarsal joints of cats. *Aspergillus* and *Candida* occasionally cause osteomyelitis in dogs, less so in other species. Other organisms, such as *Pythium insidiosum*, localize sporadically to bone and cause osteomyelitis.

Viral infections of bones

Bovine viral diarrhea virus (BVDV) has been associated with **growth retardation lattices** (zones of metaphyseal sclerosis parallel to the growth plate) in aborted calves following maternal infection (Fig. 2-128). These lattices consist of zones of persistent primary spongiosa with increased mineralized cartilage and trabecular bone density, presumably reflecting viral destruction of osteoclasts and the time required for new osteoclasts to differentiate from precursors. Similar zones of persistent primary spongiosa have been linked to BVDV infection in older calves, up to 4 months of age. Although these have been called *"transient osteopetrosis,"* the term *osteopetrosis* is more appropriately used for genetic, diffuse increased bone density. Similarly, the term *growth arrest lines* should be reserved for bands of increased bone volume resulting from transient decreases in longitudinal bone growth.

Classical swine fever virus and border disease virus, which are closely related to BVDV, cause similar lesions in pigs and lambs, respectively.

Growth retardation lattices also occur in dogs with natural and experimental infection with **canine distemper virus**. In experimental infections in puppies, impaired osteoclastic resorption of the primary spongiosa was supported by the detection of necrotic osteoclasts. The lesions were transient and resolved once viral antigen disappeared.

Canine adenovirus type I infection in pups may be accompanied by grossly visible metaphyseal hemorrhages at costochondral junctions, caused by virus-induced injury to endothelial cells, some of which contain characteristic intranuclear inclusion bodies. Necrosis of all cellular elements in the metaphysis also occurs, possibly caused by ischemia, but there are no reports of residual lesions.

Feline herpesvirus causes necrosis of the turbinate bones of germ-free cats following intranasal inoculation, and produces necrosis in the metaphyses and periosteum of growing bones when administered intravenously. Sites of active osteogenesis are most susceptible. The virus infects osteoprogenitor cells, osteoblasts, osteoclasts, and endothelial cells, all of which may contain intranuclear inclusions.

Medullary sclerosis may occur in cats infected with **feline leukemia virus** and is associated with nonregenerative anemia (see Vol. 3, Hematopoietic system). It is not clear whether the osteosclerosis is a direct result of the viral infection or is secondary to chronic anemia or hypoxia. Myelofibrosis may also be a feature of this infection.

Metaphyseal osteopathy

Although commonly referred to as *hypertrophic osteodystrophy* (HOD), in many cases of metaphyseal osteopathy, there is no periosteal proliferation, whereas metaphyseal necrosis and inflammation are consistent findings.

Metaphyseal osteopathy is a *disease of young growing dogs*, mainly those of large and giant breeds, especially Great Danes, Boxers, German Shepherds, Irish Setters, and Weimaraners. In Weimaraners, entire litters may be affected, and puppies with an affected littermate are more likely to relapse. Affected dogs are usually 3-4 months of age, but puppies 7 weeks to 8 months can be affected. Clinical signs include fever, anorexia, malaise, and lameness associated with swelling and pain of the metaphyseal regions of long bones. The *distal radius and ulna* are most often affected, but the femurs, humeri, scapulae, vertebrae, ribs, mandible, and optic foramina may also be involved. Bones distal to the tarsus and carpus are usually spared. Radiographs taken early in the disease show alternating radiodense and radiolucent zones in the metaphysis parallel to the physis, and there is often lipping of the metaphyseal margins. Acute cases are characterized grossly by a narrow band of pallor in the primary spongiosa adjacent to rapidly growing physes. Infractions (antemortem or postmortem) may be present through the primary spongiosa of some bones (Fig. 2-129), reflecting the fragility of the trabeculae in these areas of acute inflammation. In most cases, the lesion does not progress, but in others, periosteal and extraperiosteal ossification develops, and the ends of the long bones become swollen and hard. Occasionally, these swellings are extensive and involve almost two thirds of the length of the bone, excluding only the mid-diaphysis and epiphyses (Fig. 2-130). The lesions

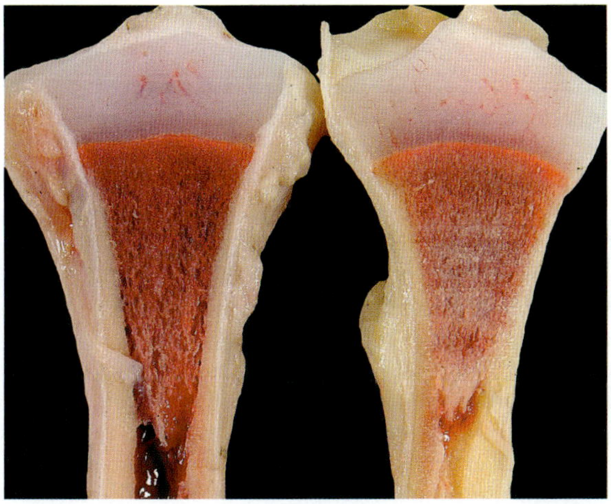

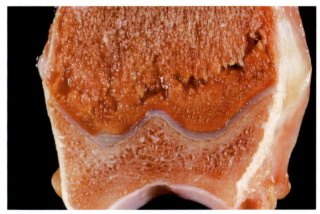

Figure 2-129 Metaphyseal osteopathy in a dog. Acute lesion showing an infraction line through weakened trabeculae in the primary spongiosa of the distal radius. Note the lack of periosteal bone proliferation.

Figure 2-128 Bovine viral diarrhea virus growth retardation lattices in a calf tibia. The affected tibia (right) has multiple lines of increased bone density in the metaphysis parallel to the articular-epiphyseal growth complex. The tibia on the left is normal for comparison. (Courtesy B.T. Webb.)

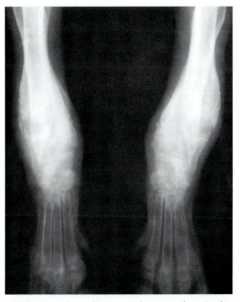

Figure 2-130 Metaphyseal osteopathy in a dog. Radiograph of chronic lesions with extensive periosteal reaction involving the radii and ulnae.

are *usually bilaterally symmetrical*. Relapses may occur over a period of weeks to months, but most animals recover, and the excess metaphyseal bone is gradually removed.

The *histologic lesions* in acute cases are characteristic. The growth plates are structurally normal, but there is *persistence of the mineralized cartilage lattice of the primary spongiosa and intense intertrabecular suppurative inflammation with necrosis and disappearance of osteoblasts* (Fig. 2-131A, B). Deposition of osteoid on the mineralized cartilage spicules of the primary spongiosa is absent, and the delicate trabeculae frequently fracture. Osteoclastic activity is prominent in some areas. The suppurative inflammation and necrosis of marrow contents may extend throughout much of the metaphysis, and fibrin thrombi may be present in small blood vessels. Aggregates of neutrophils are often in the periosteum, associated with hemorrhages, as well as in cartilage canals of the epiphyses and in bones such as vertebrae, mandibles, and turbinates. Enamel hypoplasia associated with inflammation of the dental crypt may also occur.

If the disease progresses, periosteal and extraperiosteal woven bone may develop in areas of previous hemorrhage and inflammation, eventually forming a collar of bone around metaphyses. There is also proliferation of mesenchymal tissue in the marrow spaces, replacing the suppurative exudate and providing precursor cells for the reconstruction of the damaged tissues. In those animals that have recurrences of the disease, acute inflammatory changes are superimposed on the osteogenic fibrous tissue in marrow spaces.

Although there have been numerous proposed causes for metaphyseal osteopathy, none has been proved. A possible link has been suggested between metaphyseal osteopathy and canine distemper vaccination, but the link may only be temporal, because metaphyseal osteopathy and vaccinations both occur in young dogs. A study of 53 cases in Weimaraners showed that the disease responds better to corticosteroids than nonsteroidal anti-inflammatory drugs, suggesting that the disease is sterile and immune-mediated. This condition may represent an inappropriate inflammatory response by an immature immune system.

Canine panosteitis

Canine panosteitis (panostosis, juvenile osteomyelitis, enostosis, eosinophilic panosteitis) is a disease of unknown cause that, like metaphyseal osteopathy, usually affects dogs of the large and giant breeds between 5 and 12 months of age. Basset Hounds, Chinese Shar Pei, Giant Schnauzers, German Shepherds, and Mastiffs are over-represented. The name is a misnomer, because inflammation is rarely a feature. Males are affected more often than females.

Clinical signs vary from *mild to severe lameness*, which may shift from one bone to another. The disease is prone to remission and exacerbation, and is *usually self-limiting* after 1 to several months. The lameness is associated with abnormalities in the diaphysis of a long bone, usually in the foreleg. Multiple bone involvement occurs in about 50% of cases, and rarely, other bones such as ilium and metatarsals are affected.

Because the disease is self-limiting and is well recognized by radiologists, pathologic studies are few, and the lesions are defined in terms of their radiographic appearance. When clinical signs begin, no lesions may be visible. About 10 days later, initial involvement of the long bone is seen as an increased density or densities of the medulla in the region of the nutrient foramen. The density may increase in size, sometimes filling the entire medullary cavity, or may remain localized (Fig. 2-132). If the reaction extends to the cortex, marked cortical thickening may result because of periosteal proliferation. When the animal recovers, the increased density disappears over a period of weeks to months.

The initial increased radiodensity is due to expanding areas of fibrovascular tissue in the bone marrow, which are rapidly replaced by woven bone. This bone is subject to consecutive episodes of formation and resorption, thus reversal and resting

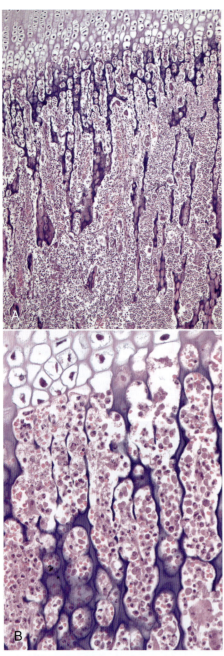

Figure 2-131 **Metaphyseal osteopathy** in a dog. **A.** Acute disease showing normal physis and intense inflammatory reaction between trabeculae of the primary spongiosa. Trabeculae are delicate and consist of calcified cartilage with little, if any, osteoid. **B.** Higher magnification image from the same animal showing mineralized cartilage spicules devoid of osteoid separated by neutrophils and necrotic cellular debris. No osteoblasts are apparent.

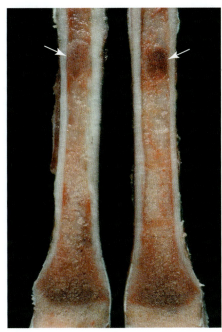

Figure 2-132 **Panosteitis** in a German Shepherd dog. Patchy foci of increased bone density within the medullary cavity (arrows).

lines are often present in the same trabeculae, and osteoclasts and osteoblasts are active in the same microscopic field. Cartilage is sometimes formed in the fibrovascular tissue. Periosteal woven bone formation may be stimulated, and this, like the medullary bone, is replaced by lamellar bone before being replaced over the ensuing months. The older, more mature bone in the center of the medullary lesions is removed first.

In most dogs, there is no inflammation in the lesions, but sometimes plasma cells and histiocytes are present. Eosinophilia is an inconstant feature, and serum chemistry is unremarkable. Abnormalities in clotting times are inconstant findings. *The cause of canine panosteitis is not known.* Genetic, allergic, and dietary factors, hyperestrogenism, filterable agents, and various bacteria have been proposed, but the evidence is inconclusive.

Further reading

Safra N, et al. Clinical manifestations, response to treatment, and clinical outcome for Weimaraners with hypertrophic osteodystrophy: 53 cases. J Am Vet Med Assoc 2013;242:1260-1266.

Trivedi SR, et al. Variation in clinical presentation and epidemiology of cryptococcosis in cats and dogs from California. J Am Vet Med Assoc 2011;239:357-369.

Webb BT, et al. Bovine viral diarrhea virus cyclically impairs long bone trabecular modeling in experimental persistently infected fetuses. Vet Pathol 2012;49:930-940.

TUMORS AND TUMOR-LIKE LESIONS OF BONES

Primary tumors of bones are common in dogs and to a lesser extent in cats, but occur infrequently or rarely in other domestic animals. They may arise from any of the mesenchymal tissues present in bones, including precursors of bone, cartilage, fibrous tissue, adipose tissue, and vascular tissue, *but tumors of bone and cartilage-forming cell lines are the most common*. In humans, most primary tumors of bones are benign, but this does not apply to all animal species. In dogs, most tumors of bones are malignant. Benign and malignant tumors of bone occur with approximately equal frequency in cats, but in horses, cattle, and other domestic animals, benign tumors of bones are much more common than malignant ones. Secondary tumors of bones, in particular metastatic carcinomas, are very common in humans but are seldom diagnosed in animals. The prevalence of secondary bone tumors in animals is no doubt under-estimated because the skeleton is seldom examined in detail either radiographically or postmortem, but it is almost certainly much lower than in humans. Several comprehensive surveys and reviews of bone tumors have been published and are included in Further reading.

The classification of primary tumors and tumor-like lesions of bones in domestic animals is generally similar to that developed for humans, but there are too many differences in morphology and prognosis to allow direct extrapolation. The system used in this chapter is based on a modification of the World Health Organization (WHO) fascicle on *Histological Classification of Bone and Joint Tumors of Domestic Animals* (Box 2-1). Rather than discuss benign and malignant tumors separately, as in the WHO system, *the most important of these tumors will be grouped according to the nature of the predominant matrix that they produce*. This reflects the manner in which a pathologist is likely to approach the diagnosis of a bone tumor.

It is often difficult to classify a bone tumor into one category or another with confidence, because the predominant matrix may vary throughout the tumor, and poorly differentiated sarcomas may reveal little evidence of their lineage. Because the prognosis of different bone tumors varies markedly, accurate classification by the pathologist will greatly assist the clinician or surgeon and should be attempted, but only in cases where sufficient tissue and information is provided. The pathologist must not feel pressured into making a definitive diagnosis in cases where either the specimen or history is inadequate. There are many benign lesions of bones that may resemble malignant tumors, and the consequences of an incorrect diagnosis can be substantial.

The clinical history and radiographic appearance are often crucial to an accurate diagnosis of a bone lesion, and the pathologist should not rely on microscopic features alone, particularly with small biopsy specimens. For example, a biopsy specimen of predominantly chondroid matrix and cells with features of malignancy may be a chondrosarcoma; however, it may also be an area of chondroid matrix production in an osteosarcoma, in which neoplastic osteoblasts are producing osteoid elsewhere. If tumor cells are obviously producing osteoid, then the diagnosis should be osteosarcoma because this is the most malignant component. The potential treatment and prognosis differ substantially between the different diagnoses, and if there is any doubt, the pathologist should request more/deeper biopsy specimens from the lesion. In addition to knowledge of the species, breed, and age of the animal, it is important to be aware of the location of the lesion and its duration. Certain bone tumors of humans and animals occur with increased frequency at specific sites, hence the value of knowing the exact location of the lesion. It is also important to know if there has been a previous fracture or infection at the site, whether the animal is on immunosuppressive therapy, or whether the animal has recently suffered from a systemic

BOX • 2-1

Histologic classification of tumors and tumor-like lesions of bones

Benign tumors
- Chondroma
- Feline osteochondromatosis
- Hemangioma
- Myxoma of the jaw
- Ossifying fibroma
- Osteoma
- Osteochondroma

Malignant tumors
- Chondrosarcoma
  - Central
  - Periosteal
  - Extraskeletal
- Fibrosarcoma
  - Central
  - Periosteal
  - Maxillary and mandibular (dogs)
- Hemangiosarcoma
- Giant cell tumor of bone
- Liposarcoma
- Multilobular tumor of bone
- Osteosarcoma
  - Central
    - Chondroblastic
    - Fibroblastic
    - Giant cell type
    - Osteoblastic
      - Nonproductive
      - Productive
    - Poorly differentiated
    - Telangiectatic
  - Peripheral
    - Periosteal
    - Parosteal
  - Extraskeletal
- Tumors of bone marrow
  - Malignant lymphoma of bone
  - Multiple myeloma

Secondary tumors
- Metastatic
- Invasive

Tumor-like lesions
- Cysts
  - Aneurysmal bone cyst
  - Benign (unicameral) bone cyst
  - Intraosseous epidermoid cyst
  - Subchondral cystic lesions
- Exuberant fracture callus
- Fibrodysplasia ossificans progressiva
- Fibrous dysplasia

Based on World Health Organization International Histological Classification of Tumors of Domestic Animals, with modifications.

disease or soft tissue tumor, which may have spread to the bone.

Radiographs provide valuable additional information on the extent, nature, and behavior of a bone tumor. Surgeons or clinicians should be encouraged to send digital radiographs with cytologic and biopsy samples of bone. Radiographs can also be of considerable value to the surgeon or pathologist in establishing a list of likely differential diagnoses, and selecting sites for histologic or cytologic examination. Postmortem radiographs of a bone lesion will often provide more information of diagnostic relevance than gross examination of the affected bone, but the radiographic appearance can seldom allow reliable differentiation of primary tumors, secondary tumors, and inflammatory conditions of bones. However, it is often more useful at demonstrating the presence of aggressive behavior than gross or histologic examination.

Proliferation of new, woven bone is a common response to various forms of bone injury and should not be misinterpreted as osteosarcoma. This reactive bone may be deposited beneath an elevated periosteum and form the so-called *Codman's triangle*, which often occurs in osteosarcoma but also in other lesions in which the periosteum is separated from the underlying bone. When the periosteum is breached, the radiating spicules of reactive bone expanding out from the original lesion may create a "sunburst" effect in radiographs. Reactive bone is not just confined to the periosteal surface. Many primary and secondary tumors growing within the bone marrow cavity stimulate endosteal new bone formation, as do many inflammatory lesions. In the early stages of formation, reactive bone consists of rapidly proliferating, immature mesenchymal cells producing spicules of unmineralized osteoid. These spicules usually merge with broader trabeculae of woven bone lined by a single layer of plump osteoblasts (Fig. 2-133), unlike

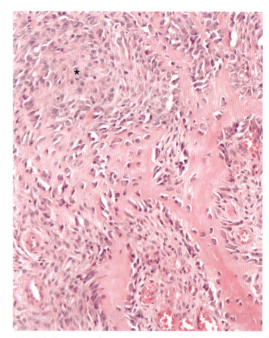

Figure 2-133 Section of a recent fracture showing trabeculae of **reactive, woven bone** covered by a single layer of plump osteoblasts. If the pathologist receives only a biopsy of the tissue marked by the asterisk (*), the lesion may be misinterpreted as an osteosarcoma.

osteosarcoma, where the spaces between spicules or islands of tumor bone are generally filled with malignant osteoblasts. However, in small biopsy samples, differentiation of early reactive bone from osteosarcoma may be extremely difficult, if not impossible.

In addition to new bone formation, *osteolysis is also a feature of many bone tumors*, and osteoclasts can often be seen resorbing mature bone as the advancing tumor permeates the marrow cavity or invades the cortex. The gross and radiographic appearance of a bone tumor reflect the balance between bone resorption and new bone formation. *Biopsy samples or samples collected for histology or cytology from a suspected bone tumor postmortem should always include areas of lysis, because these areas are most likely to contain cells of diagnostic significance.* Too often, samples submitted to the pathologist consist entirely of reactive bone, and no diagnosis is possible. In such cases, it is important that the pathologist does not exclude the possibility of an underlying tumor, and if the history and radiographic appearance suggest neoplasia, examination of further biopsies, including areas of lysis, is recommended.

Further reading

Dernell WS, et al. Tumors of the skeletal system. In: Withrow SJ, Vail DM, editors. Withrow & MacEwens Small Animal Clinical Oncology. 4th ed. St. Louis: Saunders Elsevier; 2006. p. 540-582.

Egenvall A, et al. Bone tumors in a population of 400 000 insured Swedish dogs up to 10 y of age: incidence and survival. Can J Vet Res 2007;71:292-299.

Slayter MV, et al. Histological Classification of Bone and Joint Tumors of Domestic Animals. Washington, DC: World Health Organization/Armed Forces Institute of Pathology, American Registry of Pathology; 1994.

Thompson KG, Dittmer KE. Tumors of bones. In: Meuten DJ, editor. Tumors in Domestic Animals. 6th ed. Forthcoming.

Bone-forming tumors

Osteoma, ossifying fibroma, and fibrous dysplasia

These benign tumors are uncommon in domestic animals, and there is considerable confusion over their classification and diagnosis. Some reports of osteoma in the literature are likely ossifying fibromas and vice versa, and it is possible the two represent different stages of the same tumor. All 3 arise most commonly from the bones of the skull, particularly those bones that develop by intramembranous ossification. Fibrous dysplasia is not a true neoplasm of bones but is included in this group because of the need to differentiate it from osteoma and ossifying fibroma.

An **osteoma** is a *dense, smoothly contoured, protruding, slowly progressive mass of well-differentiated bone* that most commonly arises from a sessile or pedunculated base on the periosteum. They are rare but are found most often in the mandible, maxilla, nasal sinuses, and craniofacial bones in horses and cattle, but also occur in other species. Osteomas occasionally arise from the bones of the pelvis, or tubular bones of the limbs, and *must be differentiated from osteochondromas*. In osteochondroma, the bone forms by endochondral ossification beneath a cap of hyaline cartilage, and there is continuity between the intertrabecular spaces of the tumor and the marrow cavity of the bone.

The tumors can become very large and are often extremely hard and must be cut with a saw. Clinical signs, other than disfigurement, may be non-existent or may relate to compression of adjacent structures.

Histologically, osteomas consist of trabecular bone formed by osteoblasts, remodeled by osteoclasts, and ultimately converted almost entirely to *lamellar bone*. The trabeculae are gradually thickened by appositional growth so that ultimately the spaces between them are relatively inconspicuous, and the density of the tumor mass approaches that of mature cortex. Actively expanding tumors have a zonal configuration, with an outer layer of connective tissue resembling periosteum; beneath this are slender trabeculae of woven bone arranged approximately perpendicular to the surface, whereas in deeper regions, trabeculae are broader and consist largely or completely of lamellar bone. The spaces between trabeculae are filled with sparse numbers of spindle cells and possibly adipose and hematopoietic tissue. Some tumors are virtually indistinguishable from exostoses; location and clinical history should be considered in differentiating the 2.

Ossifying fibroma *is a rare fibro-osseous tumor of the head*, occurring most frequently in young horses <1 year of age, and primarily involving the rostral mandible. There are occasional reports of the tumor in cats, dogs, and sheep, and occasionally involving the long bones. Typically, ossifying fibroma is a firm to hard, sharply demarcated, expansile, intraosseous mass, which distorts the normal contours of the affected bone (Fig. 2-134). The tumor consists of a *dense fibrovascular stroma of spindle-shaped fibroblasts within which are irregularly shaped, usually interconnected, trabeculae of woven bone* lined by plump osteoblasts. *The stroma is denser than that in an osteoma*, and the cells show no signs of malignancy. Lamellar bone is rare in ossifying fibroma, but may be formed where woven bone trabeculae are resorbed and replaced; if so, then a maturing ossifying fibroma may eventually resemble an osteoma. Ossifying fibromas exhibit slow progressive enlargement, but there are no reports of malignant transformation.

Fibrous dysplasia *is a rare, fibro-osseous lesion of bone* that, in humans, is associated with a somatic activating mutation of the Gsα subunit of G-protein, which results in increased cyclic adenosine monophosphate (cAMP), leading to abnormalities in osteoblast differentiation. Although well documented in humans, there are few reliable reports of fibrous dysplasia in animals, but there seems little doubt that the condition does occur in several animal species, including horses, dogs, and domestic cats. As in humans, young animals

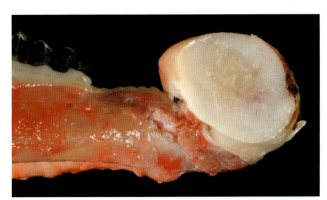

Figure 2-134 **Ossifying fibroma** in the rostral mandible of a sheep.

are most commonly affected. Fibrous dysplasia is not a neoplasm and may be monostotic or polyostotic, but the craniofacial bones are most commonly affected. The expansile lesion consists of *proliferating mesenchymal cells that form poorly organized, disoriented trabeculae of woven bone*, without any obvious transition of cells to osteoblasts. The lesion is surrounded by a thin shell of dense bone produced by the periosteum. There is no cure for fibrous dysplasia, and in humans, it often recurs postsurgery. Malignant transformation has been reported in humans, but not in animals.

There are several lesions that must be distinguished from each other, including osteoma, ossifying fibroma, fibrous dysplasia, osteosarcoma, and perhaps even fibrous osteodystrophy, especially in horses. In osteomas, the spaces between trabeculae may contain marrow rather than fibrous connective tissue, and the trabeculae are larger and denser with a much greater proportion of lamellar bone. The spicules of fibrous dysplasia are usually more uniform and are not rimmed by osteoblasts. The connective tissue cells of ossifying fibroma lack the pleomorphism and high mitotic index of osteosarcoma, and the bone is formed in a more regular and uniform manner. Confusion with fibrous osteodystrophy is unlikely as long as an adequate history accompanies a small bone biopsy. The lesions of fibrous osteodystrophy are bilaterally symmetrical, and large osteoclasts are often present among the loose fibrous connective tissue surrounding trabeculae of woven bone.

Osteosarcoma

This malignant tumor is the most common primary neoplasm of the appendicular skeleton in dogs and cats. In general, it is a rapidly progressive tumor with early metastasis to the lungs leading to early mortality. Most osteosarcomas arise from within bones, particularly in the metaphyseal regions of long bones, and are referred to as **central osteosarcomas**. Less commonly, osteosarcomas arise in the periosteum or even in extraskeletal tissues. Two types of peripheral osteosarcoma may arise in the periosteum. One is referred to as **periosteal osteosarcoma** and may show similar biologic behavior to central osteosarcoma; the other is **parosteal osteosarcoma**, which shows greater differentiation, slower growth, and a much better prognosis than central osteosarcoma.

Osteosarcoma accounts for up to 85% of malignant bone tumors in dogs and 70% in cats. It occurs in middle-aged to older dogs, with a median age of ~7 years, but the range is broad, and a small peak in incidence occurs at 18-24 months of age. The tumor occurs predominantly in large and giant breeds, and has been variously associated with increasing height and weight. Osteosarcomas of the appendicular skeleton are reported to be slightly more common in male dogs compared to females. Cats tend to develop the tumor at an older average age; again there is a broad age range, but for appendicular osteosarcomas, the mean age of occurrence is 8 years and for axial osteosarcomas 10.4 years. There is no reported sex predilection in cats.

The tumor has a strong site preference in **dogs**, and is 3-4 times more likely to occur in the appendicular skeleton, and 1.6-1.8 times more likely to occur in the forelimbs compared to the hindlimbs. Most osteosarcomas of the forelimbs involve *the metaphyses of either the distal radius or proximal humerus. The distal femur and distal tibia, followed closely by the proximal femur and proximal tibia, are favored sites in the hindlimb* (Fig. 2-135A). Approximately 50% of osteosarcomas of the axial skeleton occur in bones of the head, and 50% in the ribs,

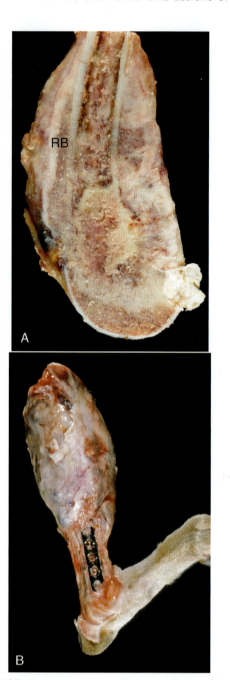

Figure 2-135 Osteosarcoma. **A.** The metaphysis of the distal femur is a common site. Note the extensive periosteal reactive bone (RB) along the cortex. **B.** An **implant-associated osteosarcoma** in the proximal tibia of a dog that occurred 7 years after the fracture and plating.

vertebrae, and pelvis. Most rib tumors occur near the costochondral junctions. In **cats**, like dogs, osteosarcomas are more common in the appendicular than axial skeleton, and there is an apparent predilection for the hindlimbs. Digital osteosarcomas are more common in cats than dogs. In addition to the sites mentioned previously, osteosarcomas occasionally occur at sites of chronic irritation and repair, such as those associated with osteomyelitis, bone infarcts, or the presence of a fixation device (Fig. 2-135B). In such cases, the tumor may originate from the diaphyseal region of long bones, or other locations not normally considered predilection sites for osteosarcoma.

Osteosarcomas are rare in domestic animals other than dogs and cats, but are reported occasionally in horses, cattle and sheep. In these species, the tumor generally involves bones of the head, particularly the mandible. Some reports in horses are more consistent with ossifying fibroma rather than osteosarcoma.

The *gross and radiographic appearance* of central osteosarcoma varies markedly, depending on the behavior of the tumor cells and the matrix they produce. Some subtypes are predominantly lytic, some are productive, whereas others comprise a mixture of both destructive and proliferative elements. Assessment of the gross features is greatly enhanced by radiographs of dissected and bisected specimens. Radiolucent or osteolytic tumors are usually hemorrhagic and soft, consisting of fleshy tumor tissue, and often contain light yellow areas of necrosis. Pathologic fractures may accompany erosion of cortical bone, and osteolytic tumors tend to invade the adjacent soft tissues early in their course. Radiodense tumors are various shades of gray on gross examination, and areas of tumor bone and tumor cartilage give a stippled appearance to radiographs and a gritty texture when cut. In compound osteosarcomas, a tumor that produces multiple types of matrix, tumor cartilage is sometimes recognizable by its texture and color, and tends to be located at the periphery of the neoplasm. The amount of periosteal reaction is usually not proportional to the degree of cortical destruction. Osteosarcomas of long bones commonly, perhaps invariably, erode cortical bone, but although they tend to invade the epiphysis rather than the diaphysis, they rarely penetrate the adjacent articular cartilage. Telangiectatic osteosarcomas are soft and dark red, indistinguishable grossly from hemangiosarcomas (Fig. 2-136).

Although cytology is usually less reliable than histology in the diagnosis of mesenchymal tumors, *central osteosarcomas can often be diagnosed with confidence on examination of fine-needle aspirates* or imprints prepared from tissue biopsy samples. Cytologic preparations from osteosarcomas are usually more cellular than aspirates or imprints from soft tissue sarcomas, and the cells may have characteristic features of malignant osteoblasts. In many cases, the cytologic characteristics, together with clinical history and radiography, will be sufficient to allow a definitive diagnosis of osteosarcoma, but malignancy cannot be excluded on the basis of cytology, as the sample may not be sufficiently representative of the lesion. Because most osteosarcomas originate from within the medullary cavity, shallow aspirates may be largely acellular or, at best, just contain a small number of reactive osteoblasts. Furthermore, some productive subtypes of osteosarcoma with extensive tumor bone formation may not yield significant numbers of tumor cells to cytologic preparations, and aspirates from telangiectatic osteosarcomas may be too heavily contaminated with blood to be of value. Even in cases where a cytologic diagnosis of osteosarcoma can be made, classification of the tumor into one of the subtypes listed later is not possible.

Malignant osteoblasts may be present individually or in clusters in cytologic preparations and are sometimes associated with *brightly eosinophilic strands or islands of matrix, consistent with osteoid* (Fig. 2-137). They vary from *round or oval to plump, fusiform cells, often with an eccentric nucleus* and deeply basophilic cytoplasm. The cytoplasm may have a pale Golgi zone adjacent to the nucleus, and in some cases, there are variable numbers of small, clear, intracytoplasmic vacuoles and/or fine pink granules. Similar pink granules may also be present in tumor cells from chondrosarcomas, or occasionally fibrosarcomas. In anaplastic osteosarcomas, there may be marked anisokaryosis, multiple large, irregularly shaped nucleoli, and a variable nuclear-to-cytoplasmic ratio. Mitotic figures are common and may be abnormal. In contrast, well-differentiated osteosarcomas may consist largely of relatively uniform-sized cells with many features of reactive osteoblasts. A similar population of reactive osteoblasts associated with strands of matrix may be harvested from an early fracture

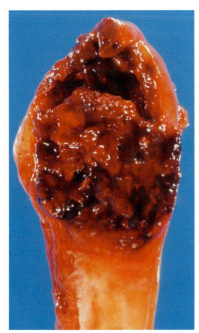

Figure 2-136 **Telangiectatic osteosarcoma** in the proximal tibia of a cat showing multiple, blood-filled spaces resembling hemangiosarcoma.

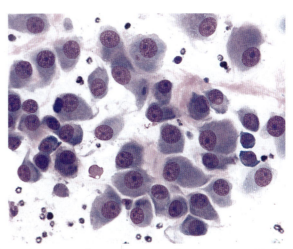

Figure 2-137 Cytologic appearance of **osteosarcoma.** Moderate numbers of oval to pyriform-shaped cells with eccentric nuclei, basophilic cytoplasm, and pale perinuclear Golgi zone in some cells. There is moderate variation in nuclear size and nucleus:cytoplasm ratio. Cells are producing pink strands of matrix.

callus, highlighting the importance of clinical history and knowledge of the radiographic appearance of the lesion. *Unless the characteristics of malignancy are unequivocal, histologic examination is recommended*. In cases where the determination of cell type is difficult, the application of a stain, ideally to an unstained smear, for *alkaline phosphatase* is helpful. If membrane-bound alkaline phosphatase is present on cells, the application of BCIP/NBT (5-bromo, 4-chloro, 3-indoylphosphate/nitroblue tetrazolium) leads to brown-black granular staining of the cytoplasm (Fig. 2-138). Expression of alkaline phosphatase is a feature of osteoblasts, and one study suggested the technique had 89% specificity and 100% sensitivity for diagnosing osteosarcoma. Care must be taken in assessing the cells for features of malignancy, because reactive osteoblasts will also stain positive for alkaline phosphatase.

The *histologic appearance of osteosarcomas varies markedly*, but the production of osteoid and/or tumor bone by malignant osteoblasts is a common factor. The tumor matrix may also contain variable quantities of cartilage and collagen, but *if tumor osteoid is present, then the tumor is classified as an osteosarcoma*. This reflects the greater malignant potential of malignant osteoblasts than either chondroblasts or fibroblasts. Bone formation also occurs in some chondrosarcomas, but indirectly through endochondral ossification of tumor cartilage, and should not be misinterpreted as tumor bone. Similarly, osseous metaplasia of multipotential mesenchymal cells in tumors of non-osseous origin, such as mammary carcinomas, may create confusion.

Low-power examination may allow identification of cortical destruction and permeation between pre-existing bone trabeculae of tumor cells. *Malignant osteoblasts* may be spindle-shaped cells resembling fibroblasts, or plump, oval or round cells with basophilic cytoplasm and eccentric, hyperchromatic nuclei, more closely resembling non-neoplastic osteoblasts. Mitotic figures are often very common, and may be atypical. The nature and amount of osteoid is highly variable. In some cases, it consists of hyaline, eosinophilic material arranged in thin strands or narrow ribbons between the malignant cells, producing a lace-like pattern. In others, the osteoid is present as irregular islands or spicules separated by malignant osteoblasts. Thin strands of osteoid may closely resemble collagenous fibrous tissue, and distinguishing between the 2 forms of matrix may be impossible. Both are birefringent, reflecting their collagen content, and reliable differentiation is not possible using histochemical stains. Fibrin in areas of hemorrhage may also be mistaken for osteoid, but is not birefringent. In general, osteoid is less fibrillar than collagen, more amorphous, and often partly or completely surrounds the tumor cells, entrapping them in lacunar spaces. If the matrix is mineralized, it is probably osteoid.

Formation of endosteal and periosteal new bone is a feature of a variety of inflammatory and neoplastic bone lesions, not just osteosarcoma, and must be differentiated from tumor bone. This may be difficult in small biopsy samples. In reactive bone, trabeculae are interconnected and lined by a *single layer* of osteoblasts, with the spaces in between trabeculae filled with non-neoplastic connective tissue. In tumor bone, the spicules are disorganized, are not interconnected, and the spaces between trabeculae are filled with malignant osteoblasts. Distinguishing between osteosarcoma and an early fracture callus presents an even greater challenge. Rapidly proliferating, plump mesenchymal cells surrounding themselves with osteoid are a feature of fracture repair, especially during the first few days, and may easily be confused with osteosarcoma. Evidence of maturation within the callus is a useful differentiating feature, with progression of undifferentiated mesenchymal cells producing osteoid to formation of bone trabeculae with increasing width. The cell population in a fracture callus would be expected to show less atypia than most osteosarcomas. Not surprisingly, the histologic appearance may be extremely difficult to interpret in cases where pathologic fracture has occurred in association with an osteosarcoma. *Knowledge of the clinical history and radiographic findings are particularly important adjuncts to histology in such cases*.

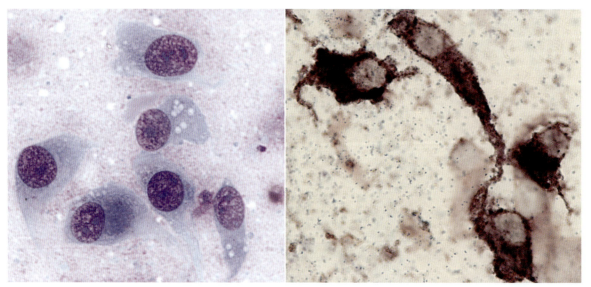

Figure 2-138 Scraping from an **osteosarcoma** in the distal humerus. The unusual location and fibroblastic appearance of the cells (left) made a definitive diagnosis on cytology challenging. The same cells when stained for alkaline phosphatase using BCIP/NBT substrate (right), however, showed dark brown staining of the cytoplasm supporting a diagnosis of osteosarcoma.

Multinucleated giant cells with features of osteoclasts are often scattered throughout osteosarcomas because of RANKL expression by the neoplastic osteoblasts. In rapidly growing osteosarcomas, large areas of coagulative necrosis and hemorrhage are often present, probably resulting from ischemia.

As shown in Box 2-1, osteosarcomas may be subclassified according to the predominant histologic pattern. This scheme is an adaptation of a system developed for use in human medicine and is now well accepted by veterinary pathologists. *Subclassification of osteosarcomas can be justified in that it may lead to the identification of correlations of osteosarcoma subtype with prognosis and susceptibility to therapy.* For example, fibroblastic osteosarcomas in dogs may have a relatively favorable prognosis, whereas the prognosis for the telangiectatic form is very poor. However, the exercise is not always straightforward because of the inherent variability present within many osteosarcomas, and the fact that a subdominant pattern may appear to be the most malignant. *Classification into one of the 6 categories is determined by the predominant pattern in representative sections from the tumor*, but if no single pattern is dominant, the tumor is best characterized as a *combined-type osteosarcoma*. In cases where only small fragments of tissue are received for examination, the main aim should be to determine whether the tumor is an osteosarcoma, rather than what subtype it belongs to.

- In **poorly differentiated osteosarcoma**, the tumor cells vary from small cells resembling those of bone marrow stroma, to large pleomorphic cells of an undifferentiated sarcoma (Fig. 2-139). The only clue that the tumor is an osteosarcoma is the presence of small quantities of *unequivocal tumor osteoid*. These tumors are generally highly aggressive, forming lytic bone lesions, and often are associated with pathologic fractures
- **Osteoblastic osteosarcomas** are recognizable by the presence of *cells with features of anaplastic osteoblasts* throughout much of the tumor. The tumor cells have hyperchromatic, often eccentric nuclei and variable quantities of basophilic cytoplasm. The cell borders are often angular, and there may be a pale Golgi zone adjacent to the nucleus. Osteoblastic osteosarcomas may be further *subclassified into nonproductive and productive osteosarcomas*, depending on the quantity of tumor bone produced. Osteoid may vary from hard to find, to lacy strands (Fig. 2-140) and irregular islands, to extensive accumulations (Fig. 2-141). Moderately productive osteoblastic osteosarcoma is the *most common subtype* of osteosarcoma in dogs. Radiographically, there is a mixed pattern of destruction and production. In some cases, with abundant tumor bone formation, differentiation of tumor bone from reactive bone may be difficult or impossible.
- In **chondroblastic osteosarcomas**, *the malignant mesenchymal cells directly produce both osteoid and chondroid matrices*. Although the 2 components are usually intermixed, they remain separate in some tumors, and small

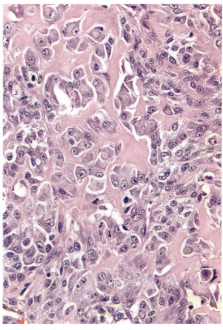

Figure 2-140 Histologic patterns of osteosarcoma. Lacy strands of osteoid between malignant osteoblasts in a **moderately productive osteoblastic osteosarcoma.**

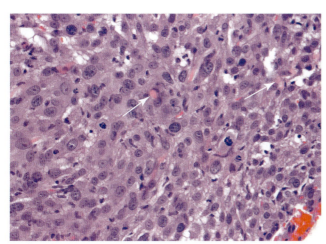

Figure 2-139 Histologic patterns of osteosarcoma. Sheets of anaplastic mesenchymal cells with features of osteoblasts in a **poorly productive osteoblastic osteosarcoma.** Mitotic figures are common. Only small quantities of osteoid are in this field (arrows).

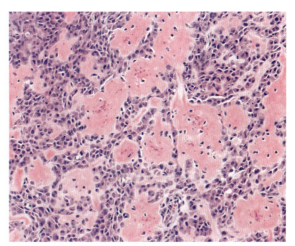

Figure 2-141 Histologic patterns of osteosarcoma. Broad lakes of osteoid separated by malignant osteoblasts in a **productive osteoblastic osteosarcoma.** Some tumor cells are trapped in the osteoid as pairs or clusters.

biopsy specimens may lead to an incorrect diagnosis of chondrosarcoma.

- **Fibroblastic osteosarcomas** consist of a population of *spindle cells* similar to those of fibrosarcoma (Fig. 2-142), within which there is *evidence of osteoid or bone formation by tumor cells*. The spicules of bone may be sparse, especially in early lesions, and it is not uncommon for such tumors to initially be diagnosed as fibrosarcomas then later reclassified as osteosarcoma following examination of further biopsies. In one study, the prognosis for dogs with fibroblastic osteosarcoma was more favorable than for other subtypes. Care must be taken to differentiate collagenous matrix from osteoid (see previously).
- **Telangiectatic osteosarcoma** is an *aggressive, osteolytic tumor* consisting of a mixture of solid areas and blood-filled spaces, grossly and radiographically resembling hemangiosarcoma and aneurysmal bone cyst (see Fig. 2-136). Histologically, telangiectatic osteosarcoma can *be differentiated from hemangiosarcoma by the presence of occasional spicules of osteoid among pleomorphic, malignant mesenchymal cells* (Fig. 2-143), although a careful search is often required to detect osteoid. Furthermore, the blood-filled spaces present throughout the tumor are lined by tumor cells negative for factor VIII on immunohistochemistry, and therefore not endothelium. The nuclear pleomorphism and high mitotic rate help differentiate osteosarcoma from aneurysmal bone cysts. Metastases of telangiectatic osteosarcomas generally resemble the primary tumor, containing many cystic spaces filled with blood. In dogs, *this subtype is associated with the least favorable prognosis of all forms of osteosarcoma.*
- **Giant cell–rich osteosarcomas** resemble nonproductive osteoblastic osteosarcoma histologically, but possess areas in which *tumor giant cells predominate* and must be differentiated from giant cell tumor of bone. The differentiation is important, because giant cell tumor of bone is often benign and has a better prognosis than osteosarcoma. Mononuclear cells with nuclear atypia, a high mitotic rate, and other features of malignancy are consistent with osteosarcoma.

Central osteosarcoma is perhaps the most malignant group of tumors of animals, at least in dogs. *The prognosis for all subtypes is very poor. Hematogenous metastasis to the lungs* commonly occurs early in the disease, and vascular invasion can sometimes be detected at the tumor margins (Fig. 2-144). Pulmonary metastases are detected radiographically in ~10% of canine appendicular and axial osteosarcomas at the time of initial diagnosis, and it is likely that most dogs with osteosarcoma will eventually develop metastases if their lives are prolonged by surgery or other forms of treatment. In one study, dogs with telangiectatic osteosarcoma had a 100%

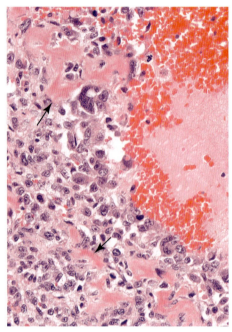

Figure 2-143 **Telangiectatic osteosarcoma** in a dog. Malignant mesenchymal cells are forming spicules of osteoid (arrows) and blood-filled spaces.

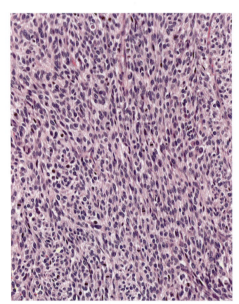

Figure 2-142 Histologic patterns of osteosarcoma. Sheets of elongate spindle-shaped mesenchymal cells with features of malignancy that could be a fibrosarcoma. Although no osteoid is apparent in this field small quantities were present elsewhere in the tumor, consistent with a **fibroblastic osteosarcoma.**

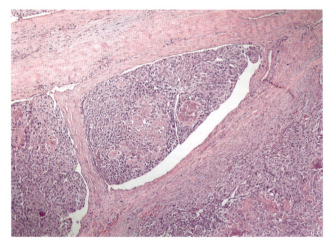

Figure 2-144 Tumor tissue containing osteoid within large veins at the margin of an **osteosarcoma.**

metastatic rate. Hematogenous metastasis to other organs, including the lymph nodes, brain, and skeleton, can also occur. When metastasis to regional lymph nodes, although rare, is present, it is associated with a poorer prognosis. The median survival time for dogs with appendicular skeletal osteosarcomas in one study was only 14-19 weeks. Survival time is only marginally better (22 weeks) in dogs with osteosarcomas of the axial skeleton, although osteosarcomas of the mandible and maxilla generally have a better prognosis.

Grading systems for osteosarcoma have been developed based on scoring of different attributes, such as nuclear and cellular pleomorphism, mitotic index, amount of tumor necrosis, amount of tumor matrix, tumor cell density, number of multinucleated cells, and vascular invasion. Tumors with a high grade were associated with reduced survival times and increased risk of metastasis. However, no histologic grading system for osteosarcomas has gained widespread acceptance by veterinary pathologists, especially because the histologic appearance can vary widely within different regions of the same tumor.

Serum total and bone-specific alkaline phosphatase (ALP) may be useful as a prognostic factor. Increased ALP before surgery has been associated with a shorter survival time post-surgery in dogs with appendicular osteosarcomas. The failure of ALP to decline post surgery is also associated with a short survival time.

The incidence of metastasis in cats with central osteosarcoma is considerably less than in dogs, and the prognosis is therefore more favorable. A median survival time of 49.2 months has been reported in cats with appendicular osteosarcoma following treatment by amputation, but the number of animals in most studies of feline osteosarcoma has been small.

Two types of peripheral osteosarcoma arising from the periosteal surface of bones have been recognized in dogs. The first, also called a **periosteal osteosarcoma**, has similar histologic features and biologic behavior as central osteosarcoma. It arises from the *undifferentiated mesenchymal cells of the periosteal cambium layer*. The tumor initially spreads into the adjacent soft tissue but may also invade the underlying cortex. Histologically, a periosteal osteosarcoma is most commonly the chondroblastic osteosarcoma subtype. Too few cases of periosteal osteosarcomas have been reported in dogs and other domestic animals to provide reliable data on the age, sex, and site incidence.

Parosteal osteosarcoma also arises from the surface of bones, but in this case, *from the outer fibrous layer of the periosteum*. Published reports of these tumors are rare and the tumor is poorly defined, but they have been reported in dogs, cats (Fig. 2-145), horses, a pig, and a cow. Most cases are presented as a firm, slowly enlarging mass on the surface of a bone, and they tend to follow a longer clinical course than central osteosarcomas. Radiographically, the tumor has an evenly contoured margin, and the *underlying cortex is generally intact*. This is in contrast to osteochondroma, wherein the marrow cavity of the tumor is continuous with that of the adjacent bone. The histologic appearance in animals is not well characterized, and cases reported as parosteal osteosarcomas have varied markedly. In animals, as in humans, parosteal osteosarcoma consists of *broad trabeculae of well-differentiated bone separated by moderately cellular fibrous connective tissue showing some pleomorphism, but no convincing evidence of malignancy*. Mitotic figures are uncommon. Some tumors may have a cartilaginous cap, similar to that of

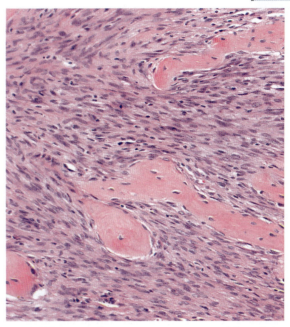

Figure 2-145 **Parosteal osteosarcoma** in a cat with broad, disoriented, bony trabeculae separated by uniformly cellular tissue resembling immature fibrous tissue.

osteochondroma. Differentiation from reactive bone may also present a challenge. Metastasis of parosteal osteosarcoma to the lungs occurs late, if at all, and may be associated with differentiation of the tumor to a more aggressive form.

Osteosarcomas occasionally arise in soft tissues of dogs and cats, in the absence of a primary bone lesion. These **extraskeletal osteosarcomas** occur most often in the mammary gland, but may also arise in the gastrointestinal tract, subcutaneous tissues, spleen, urinary tract, liver, skin, muscle, eye, and thyroid gland. They also arise in the esophagus in association with *Spirocerca lupi* infestation. In general, extraskeletal osteosarcomas are more likely to occur in older dogs (mean age 10.6-11.5 years) than are skeletal osteosarcomas, and show no apparent predilection for large breeds. Although distant metastases are common, the lungs are involved less often than in skeletal osteosarcomas, and death is usually caused by either local recurrence or euthanasia at the time of diagnosis. The mean survival time is reported to be lower than for skeletal osteosarcomas, in part because of the later detection of intra-abdominal tumors and limited surgical options for tumors at some sites. Osteosarcoma of the mammary gland in bitches should not be confused with *the more common, non-neoplastic, osseous metaplasia* that occurs in association with mixed mammary tumors. Osseous metaplasia also occurs in some malignant peripheral nerve sheath tumors and malignant melanomas. However, malignant transformation of metaplastic bone may occur in mammary, thyroid, and salivary carcinomas.

Although extraskeletal osteosarcoma appear to be less common in cats than in dogs, a recent study found that of 145 feline osteosarcomas, 38% were extraskeletal. The most frequent location was subcutaneous tissues, particularly those associated with vaccination sites. Similarly, intraocular osteosarcomas in cats may occur following trauma to the eye. Other reported sites include the liver and mammary gland.

Further reading

Barger A, et al. Use of alkaline phosphatase staining to differentiate canine osteosarcoma from other vimentin-positive tumors. Vet Pathol 2005;42:161-165.

Boerman I, et al. Prognostic factors in canine appendicular osteosarcoma—a meta-analysis. BMC Vet Res 2012;8:56.

Dimopoulou M, et al. Histologic prognosticators in feline osteosarcoma: a comparison with phenotypically similar canine osteosarcoma. Vet Surg 2008;37:466-471.

Selvarajah GT, Kirpensteijn J. Prognostic and predictive biomarkers of canine osteosarcoma. Vet J 2010;185:28-35.

Cartilage-forming tumors

Tumors consisting entirely or predominantly of cartilage are *uncommon* in the skeleton of domestic animals. They are diagnosed most frequently in dogs, where ~10% of skeletal tumors are cartilaginous, and in sheep, where chondromas comprise a relatively high proportion of skeletal tumors. Cartilaginous tumors often contain areas of bone formed by endochondral ossification of tumor cartilage. This should not be mistaken for the tumor bone formed directly from neoplastic mesenchymal cells in osteosarcoma. Repairing fractures also contain cartilage and bone in various proportions at different stages of maturity and could be confused with cartilage- or bone-forming tumors.

Extraskeletal tumors containing cartilage also occur, particularly those arising as a component of lipomatous soft tissue masses (chondrolipomas). Cartilaginous tissue is also present and may become dominant in mixed tumors of mammary and salivary gland origin.

Chondroma

A chondroma is a benign neoplasm of cartilage, but in veterinary medicine, the term has often been used loosely to include benign proliferations of cartilage in several extraskeletal tissues. Primary chondromas of bone can be separated into *enchondromas,* which originate within the medullary cavity of a bone, and *ecchondromas,* which arise from cartilage elsewhere in the skeleton. Both forms are rare in animals. Enchondromas are sometimes polyostotic, in which case the syndrome is referred to as *enchondromatosis.* It is likely that many tumors diagnosed as chondromas in animals are in fact osteochondromas or low-grade chondrosarcomas, especially in cases where the pathologist is not provided with an adequate history or access to radiographs of the lesion.

Chondromas occur rarely in dogs, cats, and cattle, and although considered to be more common than other skeletal tumors in sheep, they are infrequently diagnosed in this species. The tumors are typically firm to hard, smooth or nodular, roughly spherical masses with a fibrous capsule. They involve flat bones and ribs more commonly than long bones. On cut surfaces, a lobular pattern may be evident because of dissection of the blue-white cartilage by fibrous septa. Areas of mineralization or ossification appear as chalky white stippling. Myxomatous tissue, which occurs in some chondromas, has a gelatinous texture grossly and is prone to hemorrhage and necrosis.

Histologically, these benign tumors consist of irregular lobules of hyaline cartilage with cells that are, by definition, quite regular in size and appearance and typically chondrocytic. This is especially true of enchondromas. The matrix is usually more fibrous than that of normal hyaline cartilage. Foci of endochondral ossification and mineralization may be present, and lobules of myxomatous tissue sometimes develop. Differentiation between chondroma and low-grade chondrosarcoma is difficult on the basis of histopathology and may require the assessment of biologic behavior in sequential radiographs. Chondromas are normally discrete lesions and do not permeate through the marrow cavity and trabeculae of bone.

Chondromas expand slowly, and a rapid change in size may indicate malignant transformation. Expanding tumors within the medullary cavity cause bone deformation and may predispose to fracture, but with complete excision, the prognosis for chondromas is good.

Osteochondroma

An osteochondroma is a benign, cartilage-capped tumor-like exostosis arising from the surface of an endochondral bone adjacent to a physis or subarticular growth cartilage. The tumor may be monostotic or polyostotic, in which case the terms **multiple cartilaginous exostosis, hereditary multiple exostoses,** or **osteochondromatosis** are often used. In humans, dogs, and horses, the polyostotic form is inherited as an autosomal dominant trait and would be more appropriately classified as a *skeletal dysplasia* than a neoplasm, but is included here for convenience. A similar polyostotic form has also been diagnosed in a pig. In humans, mutations in the *EXT1* and *2 genes* are associated with hereditary multiple exostoses. These mutations lead to decreased heparan sulfate, which results in increased responsiveness to bone morphogenetic proteins and subsequent *excessive chondrogenesis at the perichondrial ring.*

In horses, the lesions are often present at birth, and in both dogs and horses, the lesions tend to be bilaterally symmetrical. The lesions increase in size corresponding with the period of active bone growth in young animals. Osteochondromas may develop on any bone that forms by endochondral ossification, and common sites in dogs and horses are the metaphyses of long bones, the pelvis, ribs, scapulae, and vertebrae. Although many cases are merely of esthetic rather than clinical significance, lesions in some locations interfere with the action of ligaments or tendons, and exostoses derived from vertebrae sometimes protrude into the spinal canal, resulting in spinal cord compression. The caudal distal radius is the most common site for monostotic osteochondromas in Thoroughbred horses, and this often causes damage to the deep digital flexor tendon. In dogs, osteochondromas have also occasionally been reported in the trachea.

During the phase of expansion, the outgrowths consist of a thin outer cap of hyaline cartilage resembling a poorly organized growth plate, adjacent to trabeculae of bone that have formed by endochondral ossification from the deep surface of the cartilage (Fig. 2-146). It is important that biopsies of osteochondromas are properly oriented to show the architecture of the lesion. *Trabecular bone and bone marrow within the mass are continuous with the marrow cavity of the parent bone. This is a useful diagnostic feature in the differentiation of osteochondromas from some hyperplastic or neoplastic bone masses.* Once bone growth ceases, the cartilage columns in the cap become discontinuous and are replaced by bone. The trabecular bone in osteochondromas is not remodeled, and the mineralized cartilage cores persist.

Once growth of the animal ceases, growth of the osteochondroma also comes to an end. Even though the lesions are benign, the prognosis in dogs is poor because of progression

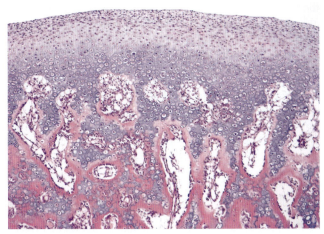

Figure 2-146 Osteochondroma in a dog. The outer layer of proliferating chondrocytes is differentiating into disorganized hyaline cartilage with randomly distributed hypertrophic chondrocytes. Endochondral ossification is occurring at the deep surface of the cartilage cap.

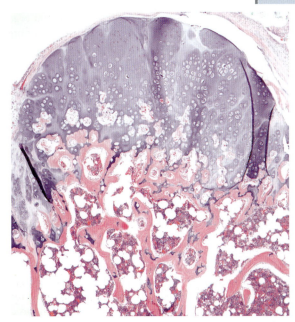

Figure 2-147 Osteochondroma in a cat showing a cap of disorganized hyaline cartilage with multiple nodules of proliferating chondrocytes. At the deep surface of the cartilage cap, endochondral ossification is occurring, and the marrow cavity contains hematopoietic and adipose tissue.

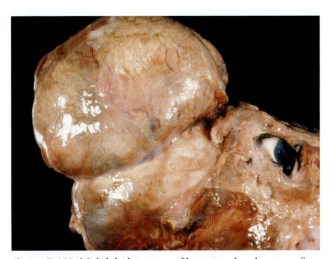

Figure 2-148 Multilobular tumor of bone in a dog showing a firm immovable mass protruding from the skull. (Courtesy D.J. Meuten.)

of clinical signs and *malignant transformation of lesions*. Continued growth of an osteochondroma in an adult animal suggests that malignant transformation into a chondrosarcoma or osteosarcoma has occurred. From 5-25% of human patients with the syndrome eventually develop chondrosarcoma, and similar cases have occurred in dogs. There are no reports of malignant transformation of osteochondromas in horses.

Despite the similar name, **osteochondromatosis in cats** differs from the condition in dogs and horses. Osteochondromatosis in cats occurs in mature animals and tends to involve flat bones, including bones derived from intramembranous ossification. Long bones are seldom affected, and when they are, the distribution is random and shows no inclination toward the metaphysis. It appears to be less common in cats compared to dogs, and although reported cases have a wide age distribution, most affected cats are aged between 2 and 4 years. The lesions in cats are dense bony masses and appear to arise as *multifocal areas of osteocartilaginous hyperplasia in the periosteum that undergo progressive enlargement* (Fig. 2-147). Their behavior is therefore more consistent with that of a true tumor, unlike osteochondromas in dogs and horses. Furthermore, *the lesions in cats are not continuous with the marrow cavity of the adjacent bone*; the underlying cortex often remains intact. The cause of the disease in cats is uncertain, but virus particles that resemble feline leukemia virus and transmissible feline sarcoma have been found in the cartilage of lesions, although their significance is uncertain. Malignant transformation of feline osteochondroma is also reported. A syndrome of cranial osteochondromas has been reported in white-tailed **deer** in the United States.

Multilobular tumor of bone

Multilobular tumor of bone is a slow-growing but locally aggressive and potentially malignant tumor, occurring most often in the skull of dogs, and rarely in the cat and horse. Many alternative terms have been proposed for the tumor, including chondroma rodens, cartilage analogue of fibromatosis, calcifying aponeurotic fibroma, multilobular chondroma or osteoma, and multilobular osteochondrosarcoma. The term multilobular tumor of bone is now preferred, because the aforementioned syndromes in animals differ from the equivalent forms in humans, and it recognizes that the tumors may be malignant or benign.

In dogs, multilobular tumor of bone is primarily a disease of middle-aged to older animals, occurring most often, but not exclusively, in medium or large breeds. In one study of 39 cases, the median age was 8 years (range 4-17 years), and the median weight was 29 kg. Three cases have been recorded in cats, varying in age from 9 months to 8 years, and there is one report in a 12-year-old Thoroughbred mare.

The tumor is usually a *firm, immovable mass involving skull bones* (Fig. 2-148), and clinical signs are related to compression and disturbance of function in adjacent structures. The swelling visible on the skull surface may provide little indication of the degree to which the tumor impinges on adjacent organs, such as the brain. The tumor is surrounded by a tough fibrous membrane, and on cut surface, multiple gritty foci are intersected by bands of fibrous tissue, consistent with the stippled appearance often present in radiographs of the tumor.

Histologically, the multilobular tumor of bone has a characteristic pattern consisting of multiple circular, oval or irregularly-shaped nodules of cartilaginous, osseous, or osteocartilaginous tissue separated by narrow fibrous septa (Fig. 2-149). In certain areas of some tumors, broad, ill-defined zones of mesenchymal tissue merge with the nodules. The cartilaginous nodules usually are surrounded by spindle-shaped septal cells, contiguous with the plump oval nuclei of the neoplastic chondrocytes in the center of each lobule. Resorption of mineralized cartilage and endochondral bone formation sometimes occurs, and osteoclastic remodeling of bone develops occasionally. In these nodules, the matrix-producing cells are unequivocally chondrocytic in appearance. In some tumors, the bone is produced by angular osteoblasts with abundant basophilic cytoplasm, but in others, oval cells of indeterminate type produce a tissue reminiscent of chondroid bone. The mineralization process tends to progress centrifugally to involve the entire nodule, and the septal tissue then consists of dense collagen. In these areas, the tumor is extremely hard. Osseous and cartilaginous tissue may be present in the same nodule, and some tumors contain separate osseous and cartilaginous nodules. Although the nodular pattern predominates, resorption of the hard tissues does occur, and nodules may be replaced by dense connective tissue containing areas of cartilaginous metaplasia.

Surgical removal is difficult because of the location of these tumors, and local recurrence occurs in 47-58% of cases, with a median time to recurrence of 420-797 days, depending on the study. Malignant transformation often occurs in tumors that are long-standing or recurrent. Indicators of malignancy include mitotic activity, loss of the orderly lobular architecture, necrosis, hemorrhage, and overgrowth of one of the mesenchymal elements. *A grading system*, based on these indicators has been proposed and provides useful prognostic information. Grade III tumors have shorter median times to local recurrence, metastasis, and survival. The lungs are the most common site for metastasis of multilobular tumor of bone, and the characteristic appearance of multilobular tumors is retained in the metastases. Approximately 20-58% of dogs develop metastases despite treatment; however, dogs can survive for several months with pulmonary metastases because of the slow growth of the tumor.

Chondrosarcoma

Chondrosarcomas are malignant mesenchymal tumors in which the neoplastic cells produce variable quantities of cartilaginous or fibrillar matrix, but not osteoid. Although bone may be present in chondrosarcomas, it forms by endochondral ossification of tumor cartilage, rather than being produced directly by malignant mesenchymal cells.

Primary chondrosarcomas are those that arise either from within a bone (central or medullary chondrosarcoma) or from the periosteal surface (peripheral chondrosarcoma), the former being the most common in animals. The term *secondary chondrosarcoma* refers to those that develop by malignant transformation of cartilage in an osteochondroma.

Chondrosarcoma is *reported most frequently in the dog*, where it accounts for ~10% of primary tumors of bones and is second only to osteosarcoma in incidence. In most other domestic species, chondrosarcoma is a relatively rare tumor, and too few cases are reported to provide reliable information on its clinicopathologic features. In sheep, chondrosarcoma is considered to occur more frequently than osteosarcoma, but it remains a rare tumor in this species.

In dogs, chondrosarcoma occurs most often in medium to large breeds (weighing 20-40 kg), particularly Boxers, German Shepherds, Golden Retrievers, and various mixed breeds, but is rare in small and giant breeds. Although a broad age range is reported, the tumor is *most common in middle-aged to older dogs*, the mean age of affected animals varying from 5.9-8.7 years. Conflicting results have been found with regard to sex predilection, although one study found a higher incidence in females than males. There is less information on the age incidence in cats, but one retrospective study found a mean age of 9.6 years and a higher incidence in male cats than females.

In all species, *chondrosarcomas involve the flat bones more often than long bones*. The ribs, turbinates, and pelvis are common sites in dogs, although nasal chondrosarcomas are rare in Boxers. Chondrosarcomas may also occur in the appendicular skeleton of dogs including, but not restricted to, sites of predilection for osteosarcomas. In cats, chondrosarcomas are reported in both flat bones and long bones, particularly the scapula and digits. In sheep, the cartilages of the sternocostal complex were the most common site for chondrosarcoma in one survey, followed by the scapulae and tuber coxae. In cattle and horses, chondrosarcomas are found most often on flat bones, but long bones are occasionally affected.

Grossly, central chondrosarcomas are firm or hard and may consist of either several large lobules resembling hyaline cartilage or multiple small, contiguous nodules of translucent, blue-white or pink tissue (Fig. 2-150). In some tumors, there are soft mucoid areas; in others, cavitation with myxoid change may be present, as may chalky white foci of mineralization or

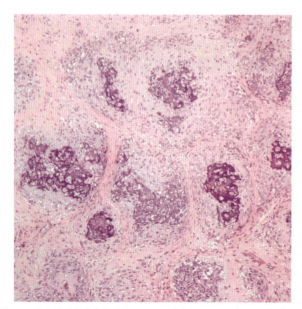

Figure 2-149 **Multilobular tumor of bone** in a dog. Lobules of cartilage and mineralized osteocartilaginous tissue separated by narrow bands of fibrous stroma.

Diseases of Bones
Tumors and Tumor-Like Lesions of Bones

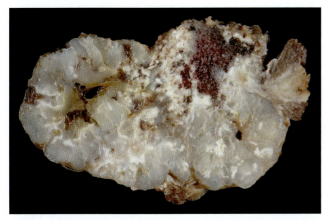

Figure 2-150 **Chondrosarcoma** from the rib of a dog. Note the firm translucent blue-white nodules of cartilage, interspersed by chalky white foci of mineralization. (Courtesy B. Murphy.)

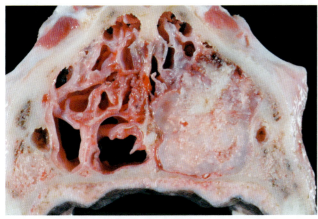

Figure 2-151 **Nasal chondrosarcoma** in a dog. Nodules of tumor tissue resembling hyaline cartilage unilaterally fill the nasal cavity and replace nasal turbinates.

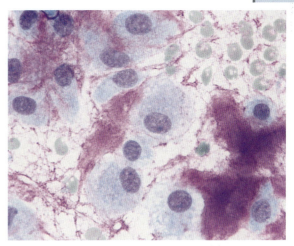

Figure 2-152 Cytologic preparation from a **chondrosarcoma** in a dog. Several oval to fusiform cells, often with eccentric nuclei, prominent nucleoli, and basophilic cytoplasm, are closely associated with a background of brightly magenta matrix.

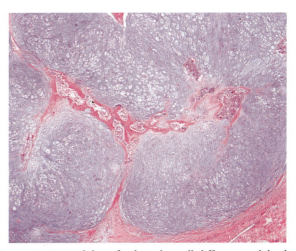

Figure 2-153 Nodules of relatively well-differentiated hyaline cartilage from a **chondrosarcoma**. Note areas where cartilage has undergone endochondral ossification, forming trabeculae of bone.

ossification. Chondrosarcomas tend to grow expansively and can reach a large size; they have a smooth surface and a capsule that merges with surrounding fibrous tissue. The more highly malignant tumors may contain areas of necrosis and hemorrhage. Nasal chondrosarcomas tend to destroy turbinates (Fig. 2-151), fill the nasal cavity, and may either spread into adjacent sinuses or penetrate overlying bone and infiltrate adjacent soft tissues. When in long bones, chondrosarcomas may produce lytic lesions similar to osteosarcomas. Chondrosarcomas may extend through the cortex into soft tissues, may permeate through the diaphysis of long bones, and unlike osteosarcomas may invade and cross joint spaces. Periosteal chondrosarcomas are less common in animals than central chondrosarcomas and usually occur as slow growing, nodular masses on the surface of flat bones in older dogs and cats.

Fine-needle aspirates from chondrosarcomas usually contain fewer cells than osteosarcomas but, on low-power examination, *lakes of bright pink-purple chondroid matrix* may be evident (Fig. 2-152). The tumor cells are similar to those from osteosarcomas, varying from round to fusiform, possessing large, hyperchromatic nuclei and basophilic cytoplasm, which sometimes contains fine pink granules. Anisokaryosis is generally a prominent feature, and there may be multinucleated tumor cells. Although a presumptive diagnosis of chondrosarcoma may be possible in cytologic specimens, confirmation requires histopathology. *Malignant chondroblasts and osteoblasts have too many features in common to allow reliable differentiation cytologically*, and some osteosarcomas have extensive chondroid matrix.

Histologically, well-differentiated chondrosarcomas show few indications of malignancy and closely resemble benign tumors of cartilage. Differentiation of chondrosarcomas from chondromas can be difficult. Endochondral ossification of tumor cartilage may be present and should not be mistaken for the formation of tumor bone (Fig. 2-153). *Knowledge of the clinical and radiographic features is often essential for accurate classification of cartilaginous tumors*. Fortunately for the veterinary pathologist, most chondrosarcomas in animals are well advanced before the owner seeks veterinary advice and biopsy samples are collected. In fact, the challenge may be to decide whether a malignant mesenchymal tumor involving bone is a chondrosarcoma, osteosarcoma, or some other sarcoma of bone. Such a decision is important, given the differences in prognosis. In some chondrosarcomas, the matrix becomes fibrillar and hyalinized, resembling osteoid, and differentiation from osteosarcoma may be very difficult, especially in small biopsy samples. Chondrosarcomas in the sinonasal region of dogs are often characterized by nodules of variously differentiated chondroid tissue forming within poorly differentiated mesenchymal elements (Fig. 2-154).

Chondrosarcomas generally consist of *lobules of mesenchymal cells producing variable quantities of disorganized hyaline cartilage*. Endochondral ossification and coagulative necrosis are common. Microscopic features of malignancy in central chondrosarcomas include the presence of many tumor cells with plump nuclei and prominent nucleoli, binucleate tumor cells, and large chondrocytes with single or multiple nuclei (Fig. 2-155). Mitotic figures are seldom present in well-differentiated chondrosarcomas, and *even a single mitotic figure strongly supports a diagnosis of malignancy in this tumor*. In poorly differentiated, more malignant chondrosarcomas, mitotic figures may be relatively common (Fig. 2-156). Neoplastic chondrocytes invading the medullary cavity of bone (Fig. 2-157), penetrating the cortex, or invading adjacent soft tissues also suggest malignancy. Grading of chondrosarcomas is not common in dogs, but grading classification systems based variably on matrix production, architecture, cellularity, pleomorphism, cellular atypia, necrosis, and mitotic rate have been proposed.

Chondrosarcomas tend to grow more slowly and metastasize later than osteosarcomas, and typically follow a longer clinical course. Local invasion is common, as is recurrence following surgical removal, but the chance of successful removal from accessible sites is much greater than for osteosarcoma. Metastasis is usually to the lungs, but other visceral organs such as the kidney, liver, heart, and skeleton are sometimes involved. Sinonasal chondrosarcomas tend to metastasize less frequently than other chondrosarcomas.

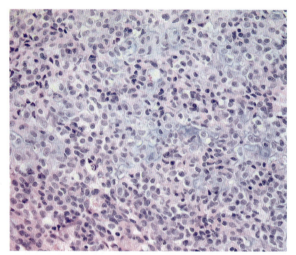

Figure 2-154 Anaplastic mesenchymal cells with chondroid differentiation in some areas, consistent with a **poorly differentiated chondrosarcoma**.

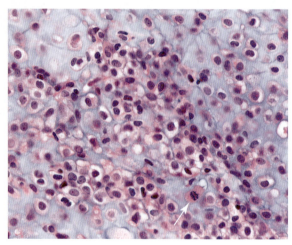

Figure 2-156 **Nasal chondrosarcoma** from a dog. Areas of chondroid matrix surround poorly differentiated neoplastic cells. Note the mitotic figure (arrow).

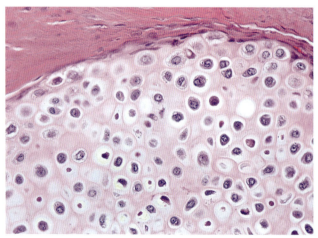

Figure 2-155 **Chondrosarcoma** from the distal radius of a dog. Plump neoplastic chondrocytes are compressing a ligament. Most of the tumor cells have large, variably sized nuclei and prominent nucleoli; some lacunae contain more than one cell.

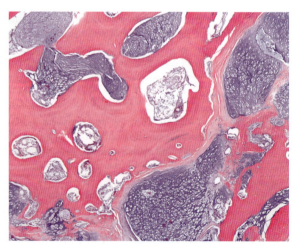

Figure 2-157 Malignant transformation of synovial chondromatosis to a **chondrosarcoma** in a dog. Note invasion of the chondrosarcoma between cortical and trabecular bone.

Further reading

Durham AC, et al. Feline chondrosarcoma: a retrospective study of 67 cats (1987-2005). J Am Anim Hosp Assoc 2008;44:124-130.

Farese JP, et al. Biologic behavior and clinical outcome of 25 dogs with canine appendicular chondrosarcoma treated by amputation: a Veterinary Society of Surgical Oncology retrospective study. Vet Surg 2009;38:914-919.

Waltman SS, et al. Clinical outcome of nonnasal chondrosarcoma in dogs: thirty-one cases (1986-2003). Vet Surg 2007;36:266-271.

Wright IM, Minshall GJ. Clinical, radiological and ultrasonographic features, treatment and outcome in 22 horses with caudal distal radial osteochondromata. Equine Vet J 2012;44:319-324.

Fibrous tumors of bones

Fibrous tumors of bones are less common in domestic animals than tumors forming bone or cartilage. Ossifying fibroma and fibrous dysplasia are discussed previously with osteoma, because of the similarities among these 3 benign tumors. Skeletal fibromas are extremely rare in animals, unlike humans, in whom non-ossifying fibromas are relatively common.

Skeletal **fibrosarcomas** arise from connective tissue stroma in either the medullary cavity or periosteum. Their histologic and gross appearances are essentially the same as that of fibrosarcomas elsewhere, although their innocuous microscopic appearance often belies their invasive tendencies. Central (medullary) fibrosarcomas (Fig. 2-158) are less common than those originating from the periosteum. Fibrosarcomas comprise ~5-9% *of bone tumors in dogs* and occur predominantly in mature male dogs of large and medium breeds, but are rarely reported in the bone of other species. Fibrosarcomas are also occasionally reported in dogs post radiation therapy for oral lesions.

In dogs, **central fibrosarcomas** *arise most often in metaphyses of long bones*, particularly the proximal femur, proximal tibia, distal radius, and proximal ulna, and cause lytic lesions that must be differentiated from fibroblastic osteosarcomas. They are also reported in the mandible, maxilla, pelvis, vertebra, and ribs of dogs. It is likely, however, that the prevalence of skeletal fibrosarcoma is overestimated. In one study, 6 of 11 tumors originally diagnosed as skeletal fibrosarcomas were reclassified as osteosarcoma following re-examination and identification of areas of osteoid production by tumor cells. Because of the poorer prognosis of osteosarcoma, an accurate diagnosis carries considerable clinical relevance. The pathologist should not be tempted to diagnose skeletal fibrosarcoma if the quantity of tissue available for examination is inadequate. Sequential radiographs of the lesion may be of diagnostic value because *fibrosarcomas of bone, although they are primarily destructive, usually progress more slowly than osteosarcomas or other highly malignant bone tumors*. Immunohistochemistry for osteocalcin or alkaline phosphatase staining of cytology smears may help distinguish between osteoblasts and fibroblasts.

Periosteal fibrosarcomas occur in most species and *tend to involve flat bones*, especially those of the head, but also occur on the scapula and occasionally on long bones. They enlarge slowly, causing disfigurement of the bone involved. They are intimately attached to the bone surface, and erosion of the adjacent bone cortex may eventually predispose to pathologic fracture.

Maxillary or mandibular fibrosarcoma of the dog is technically a periosteal fibrosarcoma, but it is classified separately from other tumors of this type because of its more frequent occurrence and *deceptively benign histologic appearance*. Maxillary or mandibular fibrosarcomas occur primarily in middle-aged dogs, usually around 8-9 years of age. They appear to be most common in the Golden Retriever and Golden Retriever mixed-breed dogs, followed by the Doberman Pinscher, German Shepherd, and other large-breed dogs. Typically, the mass is broadly adherent to the periosteal surface of the bone, with invasion into other adjacent structures, such as the nasal cavity, hard palate, and orbit.

Classification of maxillary and mandibular fibrosarcomas as malignant is based more on their invasive behavior than their histologic appearance, and they can present a challenge to the pathologist, particularly with small biopsy specimens. They are nonencapsulated, typically less cellular than fibrosarcomas from other locations, lack the characteristic pattern of interwoven bundles, have minimal pleomorphism, and produce an abundant collagenous matrix (Fig. 2-159). The

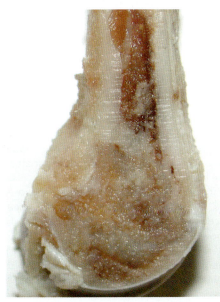

Figure 2-158 Central fibrosarcoma in the distal femur of a cat showing replacement of metaphyseal and cortical bone with tumor tissue.

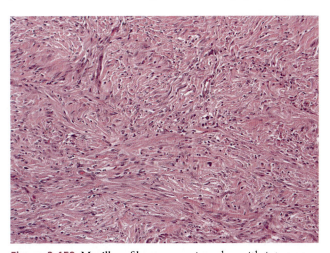

Figure 2-159 Maxillary fibrosarcoma in a dog with interwoven bundles of well-differentiated fibrous tissue showing little microscopic evidence of malignancy.

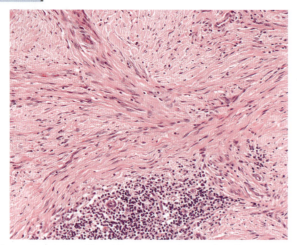

Figure 2-160 Maxillary fibrosarcoma from a dog showing superficial tumor tissue with a lymphocytic infiltrate.

grading systems described for soft tissue sarcomas do not predict prognosis for maxillary and mandibular fibrosarcomas. Superficial tumor tissue may have multifocal lymphocytic infiltrates (Fig. 2-160), and there may be fibrous organization of edematous soft tissue. On biopsy, these tumors are often misdiagnosed as nodular fasciitis, chronic inflammatory nodules, or granulation tissue, especially if the pathologist is unaware of the clinical history or radiographic findings. Evidence of invasion of surrounding tissues, such as muscle or bone, assists in diagnosis. *Local recurrence after surgical removal is common*, even with clean margins, and reported metastasis rates vary from 10-24%.

Vascular tumors of bones

Although tumors of vascular tissue are described with the circulatory system, they can occur as primary bone tumors and will therefore be mentioned briefly here. Intraosseous **hemangioma** is extremely rare in domestic animals. **Hemangiosarcoma** occurs occasionally as a primary bone tumor, especially in dogs, and is considered slightly less common than primary fibrosarcoma of bone, with a reported incidence of 2-3%. Skeletal hemangiosarcomas have also been described in cats, horses, and cattle. The tumor is found mainly in large and medium-sized breeds of dog, with Boxers, German Shepherds, and Great Danes over-represented. The *proximal and distal ends of long bones* are most often affected, but tumors are also reported in the scapula, pelvic bones, sternum, ribs, maxilla, and vertebrae.

Skeletal hemangiosarcoma is an aggressive tumor causing bone destruction and often predisposing to pathologic fracture. The tumor tends to remain within the medullary cavity rather than invade adjacent soft tissues, but erodes and weakens the cortex. Grossly, the tumor resembles hemangiosarcomas of other organs, consisting of spongy, dark red tissue, and *cannot be reliably differentiated from telangiectatic osteosarcoma and aneurysmal bone cysts*. Diagnosis is based on the demonstration in microscopic sections of malignant endothelial cells forming vascular channels, at least in some areas of the tumor. The supporting stroma may become impregnated with blood proteins, forming a hyaline material resembling osteoid, and leading to an incorrect diagnosis of telangiectatic osteosarcoma. *In telangiectatic osteosarcoma, malignant osteoblasts, rather than endothelial cells, line the blood-filled spaces*, but the distinction is often difficult, especially in small biopsy samples or at sites of pathologic fracture. Immunohistochemistry for factor VIII or osteocalcin may assist in distinguishing between the 2 entities. Hemangiosarcomas occasionally metastasize to bones from other tissues, and thorough postmortem examination of an affected animal is required before the tumor can be considered to be of bone origin.

Other primary bone tumors

Giant cell tumor of bone is a recognized entity in humans but is rare in domestic animals, with only isolated reports in dogs, cats, and horses. Some reported cases in animals are not convincing and may represent other tumors in which osteoclasts are prominent. Giant cell tumors of humans and animals *typically cause expansile osteolytic masses in the ends of long bones*, often involving much of the subchondral epiphyseal bone. Involvement of metacarpal bones and of the axial skeleton is also recorded in dogs and cats. As the mass expands, it destroys cortex but tends to remain at least partly circumscribed by a thin shell of bone. The osteolytic nature of the tumor combined with its bony shell creates a characteristic "soap-bubble" appearance in radiographs.

In cytologic preparations, the presence of a *large percentage of multinucleated giant cells* among many plump, spindle-shaped, or ovoid mesenchymal cells suggests the possibility of giant cell tumor. Giant cells may also be present in aspirates from other bone lesions, particularly osteosarcoma, but the percentage in giant cell tumors is likely to be much higher. In one report of this tumor in a dog, 25% of all cells obtained by fine-needle aspirates were multinucleated giant cells. However, definitive diagnosis still requires histologic examination of sections from representative areas of the mass.

The tumor is characterized *histologically by the presence of large numbers of multinucleated giant cells closely associated with neoplastic mononuclear cells*. The mononuclear cells consist of 2 types: a round cell with nuclear features similar to osteoclasts, and a spindle-shaped cell of likely osteoblastic lineage. The osteoblast-like cells are thought to produce RANKL, TGF-β, TNF-α and M-CSF, which promote fusion of mononuclear cells into osteoclast-like giant cells. The giant cells, which resemble osteoclasts, are often very large, and may contain >50 nuclei, which resemble the nuclei of the mononuclear cells. The giant cells are scattered uniformly throughout the tumor. In some tumors, there may be areas of collagen and/or osteoid formation, but this is not a prominent feature, and the matrix may be produced by reactive fibroblasts and/or osteoblasts, respectively, rather than by the tumor cells. The tumor is highly vascular and may contain cavernous spaces and areas of hemorrhage, leading to possible confusion with aneurysmal bone cyst, which also contains variable numbers of multinucleated cells. Osteosarcomas may also contain osteoclasts in some areas and be mistakenly diagnosed as giant cell tumors, but osteosarcomas contain more tumor osteoid than giant cell tumor of bone, and the tumor cells of an osteosarcoma show greater pleomorphism.

Because there are so few documented cases of giant cell tumor in animals, there is inadequate information to provide an indication of their biologic behavior. Benign and malignant forms are reported in animals, benign being most common. In humans, most giant cell tumors are benign, but they commonly recur following surgery, and ~5-10% are malignant, metastasizing predominantly to the lungs.

Because of the marked differences in prognosis between giant cell tumor and osteosarcoma, both of which may contain many multinucleated giant cells, *a diagnosis of giant cell tumor should never be made from small biopsy samples that are not representative of the lesion.*

Liposarcoma is a rare primary bone tumor in animals, resembling its soft tissue counterpart but forming osteolytic bone lesions. The tumor cells typically contain variable numbers of intracytoplasmic vesicles, often with an eccentrically positioned nucleus but, in some areas, may consist of less well-differentiated spindle cells. **Osteoliposarcoma**, a form of malignant mesenchymoma, is a malignant neoplasm containing liposarcomatous and osteosarcomatous tissue and is recorded in the dog.

Plasma cell myeloma or multiple myeloma, a malignant tumor of plasma cells within the bone marrow, typically produces discrete, multicentric, lytic lesions in bones, especially those involved in active hematopoiesis. Although plasma cell myeloma is thought to occur most often in **dogs**, it is also reported in **cats** and occasionally **horses**. In fact, a recent study found that multiple myeloma was just <1% of all feline malignancies at their institution, whereas it was only 0.3% of canine malignancies. The mean age of affected dogs is ~9.2 years, and one study found that male dogs were more likely to be affected, whereas another found no sex predilection. In cats, there is a higher incidence in males, but no sex predilection is recognized in the small number of cases reported in horses.

A feature of plasma cell myeloma in all species is the *production of a homogeneous immunoglobulin or immunoglobulin fragment* (paraprotein or M-component), which appears as a monoclonal, occasionally biclonal, spike on serum protein electrophoresis. The disease may also be accompanied by Bence-Jones proteinuria, hyperviscosity syndrome, and hypercalcemia. Involvement of vertebral bodies may result in paraplegia caused by protrusion of tumor masses into the spinal canal, or secondary to pathologic fractures of vertebral bodies. Discrete, "punched-out" foci of osteolysis, of various sizes, and often involving multiple bones, are present in ~50% of dogs and cats with plasma cell myeloma, but appear to be less common in affected horses. In dogs, the principal sites of bone involvement are vertebrae, especially in the thoracolumbar region, femur, pelvis, humerus, and ribs. Bones of the distal limb are seldom involved in dogs, unlike cats, where they appear to be involved as often as proximal bones of the limb.

Grossly, the lytic foci consist of soft, fleshy or gelatinous, dark red nodules, replacing trabecular bone (Fig. 2-161). The lesions are often multiple and may be associated with a pathologic fracture. Histologic or cytologic examination reveals a relatively pure, dense population of plasma cells, which may be well differentiated or large, anaplastic round cells with a high mitotic index (Figs. 2-162, 2-163).

Malignant lymphoma may also occur as a primary tumor of bone in humans and animals, but more frequently, bone involvement occurs in association with multicentric lymphoma. There are few reported cases of primary skeletal lymphoma in **dogs**; most have occurred in animals <1 year of age, with Boxers and German Shepherds over-represented. The lesions in dogs are typically lytic and multiple, and cannot be distinguished radiographically or grossly from plasma cell myeloma. Pathologic fractures and hypercalcemia are reported, but hypercalcemia is not a consistent feature of the disease, even when the bone lesions are extensive. Microscopically,

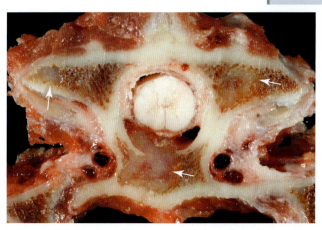

Figure 2-161 **Plasma cell myeloma** in the vertebra of a dog. Note the foci of soft gray-tan tissue (arrows) replacing trabecular bone, and extending into the spinal canal.

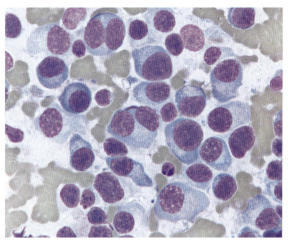

Figure 2-162 Cytologic preparation from a **plasma cell myeloma** in a dog, consisting of a population of round cells with eccentric nuclei, basophilic cytoplasm and pale Golgi area adjacent to nucleus. There are binucleate cells and moderate anisocytosis and anisokaryosis. Plasma cells have many features in common with osteoblasts, but the smaller size of the plasma cells assists in differentiation between the two. (Compare to **Figure 2-137**.)

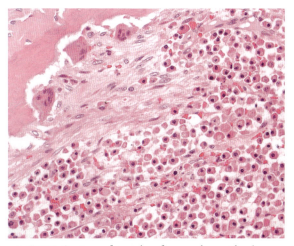

Figure 2-163 Section of vertebra from a dog with **plasma cell myeloma**. The medullary cavity is filled with a monomorphic population of plasma cells. Osteoclasts on the edge of the tumor are resorbing bone.

sheets of monomorphic lymphocytes replace bone trabeculae and the contents of the marrow cavity in areas of lysis.

Infiltration of bone marrow, together with multifocal to locally extensive bone infarction, is reported in **calves** with the juvenile, sporadic form of malignant lymphoma. Affected calves also have generalized lymph node enlargement and variable involvement of other organs, including liver, kidney, and spleen. The bone infarcts are readily visible grossly as discrete, pale tan areas, but are not detected unless the bones are sectioned during postmortem examination (see Figure 2-110). The mechanism of the tumor-associated bone marrow necrosis is not clear, but ischemia secondary to infiltration of the marrow with malignant cells is the most likely explanation. Histologically, the infarcted areas may include either neoplastic or non-neoplastic tissue and are often bordered by a zone of edematous connective tissue.

Further reading

Frazier SA, et al. Outcome in dogs with surgically resected oral fibrosarcoma (1997-2008). Vet Comp Oncol 2012;10:33-43.
Patel RT, et al. Multiple myeloma in 16 cats: a retrospective study. Vet Clin Pathol 2005;34:341-352.
Thompson KG, Dittmer KE. Tumors of bones. In: Meuten DJ, editor. Tumors in Domestic Animals. 6th ed. Forthcoming.

Secondary tumors of bones

Malignant neoplasms originating in soft tissues or in the skeleton may involve bone secondarily either by hematogenous metastasis or direct extension. **Metastatic bone disease** is very common in humans but is *generally considered rare in domestic animals*. Several explanations for this discrepancy have been proposed. The life-span of most farm animals is abbreviated by slaughter, and that of many pets by euthanasia, thus limiting the time for tumors to develop, metastasize, and, perhaps most important, produce signs of metastatic disease.

Although there appears to be a genuine difference between the frequency of skeletal metastases in humans and domestic animals, *metastatic bone disease in animals is likely to be much more common than is realized*. The skeleton of animals with malignancies at other sites is seldom examined in detail, either radiographically or at postmortem examination, and skeletal metastases could easily be missed. In one survey, skeletal metastases were identified in 5.8% of dogs with metastatic carcinoma, but because <20% of the dogs underwent bone scan, skeletal radiography, or postmortem examination, the true prevalence was probably much greater. In another study, 98 dogs with a variety of carcinomas were subjected to thorough examination of the skeleton at autopsy. The spine, pelvis, and long bones were sectioned longitudinally and the ribs inspected visually. Macroscopic metastases were detected in 21.4% of the dogs. The prevalence of metastases would almost certainly have been higher had the bones been scanned or radiographed, or if the skeleton had been subjected to detailed microscopic examination.

Carcinomas metastasize to the skeleton of dogs much more commonly than sarcomas. The most common tissues of origin are the mammary gland, thyroid, prostate, ovary, lung, and malignant pilomatricoma of the skin (Fig. 2-164). The ribs, vertebrae, and proximal long bones are the favored locations for skeletal metastases in dogs.

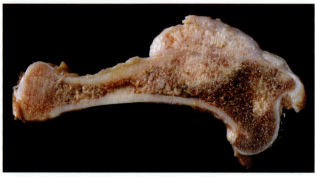

Figure 2-164 **Metastatic carcinoma** (malignant pilomatricoma) in the proximal humerus of a dog.

Information on the prevalence of skeletal metastases in cats is scarce, but there are occasional reports of pulmonary and mammary carcinomas metastasizing to the bones in this species. Interestingly, metastatic carcinomas in the skeleton of cats more frequently involve bones of the distal limb, unlike humans and dogs, wherein skeletal metastases are uncommon in bones distal to the elbow or stifle.

Skeletal bone tumors generally produce osteolytic lesions that are difficult, if not impossible, to distinguish radiographically from primary bone tumors. This may contribute to the under-diagnosis of secondary bone tumors in cases where the radiographic diagnosis is not confirmed by cytologic or histologic examination of biopsy specimens. A secondary bone tumor should at least be considered as a differential diagnosis when an osteolytic lesion is seen radiographically at a site that is uncommon for a primary bone tumor.

The molecular mechanisms behind metastatic bone disease are an important area of research in human medicine, particularly with regard to breast cancer. From this research, the concept of the "vicious cycle" has been developed. Metastatic tumors in bone produce factors, notably PTHrP, that lead to recruitment and fusion of osteoclasts and subsequent osteoclastic resorption of bone. Bone resorption results in the release of growth factors from the bone matrix, particularly TGF-β, which stimulate further growth of tumor cells, thus allowing expression of more bone resorbing factors by tumor cells—hence the "vicious cycle." TGF-β promotes PTHrP expression by tumor cells but may also increase osteoclast formation independent of RANKL and M-CSF. At the same time, TGF-β inhibits osteoblast maturation and matrix mineralization, consequently inhibiting bone formation. Some tumors may also inhibit bone formation by secreting Wnt signal inhibitors such as dickkopf1. Some breast tumor cells have been found to express bone matrix proteins, such as bone sialoprotein, that allow binding of the tumor cells to bone matrix assisting with the establishment of tumor growth in bone.

In general, dogs with skeletal metastases are older than dogs with primary tumors of bones (median age 8.5-10 years), and there is no obvious breed predilection. However, in one study, metastatic skeletal carcinomas were found most commonly in dogs weighing <25 kg, and ~30% of such tumors were found in small dogs weighing <15 kg.

A definitive diagnosis of metastatic bone tumor is based on either cytologic or histologic examination of fine-needle aspirates or tissue biopsies, respectively, but in most cases, the

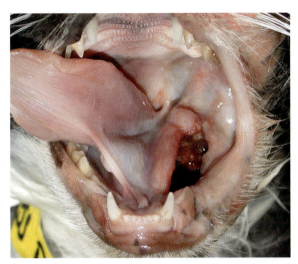

Figure 2-165 Squamous cell carcinoma in the oral cavity and left mandible of a cat. Note the ulceration of the gingiva and enlargement of the mandible.

tumor cells provide few indications as to the tissue of origin. Even after thorough postmortem examination, the primary site of a metastatic skeletal carcinoma may not be apparent, although malignant epithelial cells within skeletal lesions can only be derived from an extraskeletal carcinoma (except in birds). In one report, all carcinomas that metastasized to bone also metastasized to soft tissues. Osteosarcomas sometimes metastasize from the bone of origin to other skeletal sites, in which case the secondary lesions may be in atypical locations and may appear to have been present for different lengths of time. Reactive bone is common in association with secondary bone tumors and should not be misinterpreted as tumor bone produced by neoplastic osteoblasts. For some sarcomas, such as hemangiosarcoma, which may originate in bone or other tissues, it may be impossible to determine whether skeletal involvement is primary or secondary, but if the tumor is present in several skeletal sites, then metastasis is more likely.

Malignant tumors in soft tissues adjacent to a bone may penetrate the bone by direct extension and can be referred to as **invasive tumors of bones**. This is a feature of some types of tumor, in particular, *squamous cell carcinoma of the digits and oral cavity in dogs and cats* (Fig. 2-165). These aggressive tumors frequently invade the periosteum of the underlying bone, erode the cortex, and penetrate the medullary cavity. In dogs, bone invasion is reported to occur in 77% of oral squamous cell carcinomas. Microscopically, cords of anaplastic epithelial cells with squamous differentiation permeate the osseous and non-osseous tissues (Fig. 2-166A, B), and are accompanied by either an osteoblastic reaction or a prominent fibroblastic response with osteoclastic resorption of adjacent bone. Squamous cell carcinomas of the canine digit not only invade bone but can also metastasize to local lymph nodes, and eventually to the lungs.

Other tumors that appear to have an affinity for bone invasion *are malignant melanomas of the oral cavity in dogs and fibrosarcomas of the canine skull and long bones*. Tumors of dental origin may also extend into the maxilla or mandible of dogs and cats. Synovial histiocytic sarcomas and myxomas often invade bones and may create lytic lesions on both sides of the affected joint (see Tumors of joints).

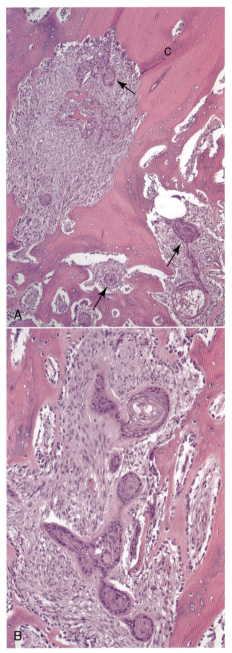

Figure 2-166 Squamous cell carcinoma in the mandible of a cat. **A.** Cords of epithelial cells (arrows) surrounded by a marked fibroblastic response are invading the dense cortical bone (C) and adjacent reactive bone. **B.** Closer view of tumor cells showing squamous differentiation.

Further reading

Carroll EE, et al. Malignant pilomatricoma in 3 dogs. Vet Pathol 2010;47:937-943.

Gottfried S, et al. Metastatic digital carcinoma in the cat: a retrospective study of 36 cats (1992-1998). J Am Anim Hosp Assoc 2000; 36:501-509.

Tumor-like lesions of bones

Several non-neoplastic lesions of bones occur in humans and domestic animals and must be differentiated from primary and secondary bone tumors. Included among these are various forms of bone cysts, most of which are not true cysts as defined by pathologists, but appear cystic radiographically. Other diseases that must be differentiated include exuberant fracture callus, synovial chondromatosis, ectopic ossification, and fibrodysplasia ossificans progressiva.

Benign or unicameral (also called *solitary* or *simple*) **bone cysts** are reported in long bones of children, *young, particularly male, large-breed dogs*, and there is one report in a cat. The cysts are most common in the distal radius and distal ulna; they start in the metaphysis, but with growth of the animal, move into the diaphysis. The lesions may be monostotic or polyostotic and are generally lytic and expansile, with erosion of the cortex and little or no periosteal new bone formation. Pathologic fracture may occur because of local bone destruction. The cyst is considered unicameral; however, it may appear multiloculated radiographically and grossly because of incomplete bony ridges projecting into the lumen. The cyst cavity is cone shaped, filled with clear or serosanguineous fluid, and lined by a fibrous connective tissue membrane of variable thickness, with scattered multinucleated giant cells, hemosiderin-laden macrophages, cholesterol crystals, and dilated blood vessels. There appears to be a breed predisposition in Doberman Pinschers. The cysts in this breed usually affect the distal radius and ulna, and are generally polyostotic. The pathogenesis of benign bone cysts is unknown, but the most widely accepted hypothesis is that obstruction of venous outflow from the bone leads to increased intraosseous pressure, and production of cytokines such as prostaglandins, IL-1β, and metalloproteinases, resulting in localized bone resorption and subsequent cyst formation. Others, however, consider them to be due to disturbance of growth at the physis, because in humans, the cysts reach their maximum size before cessation of growth. Recurrence following curettage, steroid injections, or bone grafts is uncommon.

Aneurysmal bone cysts have been reported rarely in dogs, cats, horses, and cattle. Radiographically, they appear as expansile, osteolytic lesions contained by a thin, "ballooned" periosteum with an internal "soap-bubble" appearance caused by internal septa; the cysts must be differentiated from osteosarcoma, hemangiosarcoma, fibrosarcoma, and plasma cell myeloma. Too few cases are reported in animals to establish age or site prevalence, although lesions are described in bones of both the axial and appendicular skeleton. The gross appearance of aneurysmal bone cysts closely resembles that of benign bone cysts, telangiectatic osteosarcoma, and hemangiosarcoma. Aneurysmal bone cysts typically exude blood from the cut surface, and may contain solid areas in addition to multiple blood-filled cysts. In contrast to benign bone cysts, which are unicameral, aneurysmal bone cysts are multiloculated. Pathologic fracture may be present.

Fine-needle aspirates are unlikely to be useful in the diagnosis of either aneurysmal or benign bone cysts as the preparations are likely to be heavily contaminated with blood. Confirmation of the diagnosis requires histologic examination of biopsy specimens. An aneurysmal bone cyst consists of cavernous blood-filled spaces, usually located eccentrically in the bone, separated by septa of loosely arranged spindle cells with scattered multinucleated giant cells and hemosiderin-containing macrophages (Fig. 2-167), similar to the lining of benign bone cysts. It is unusual for the spaces to be lined by endothelial cells. Osteoid or spicules of reactive bone may be present in the surrounding connective tissue and should not

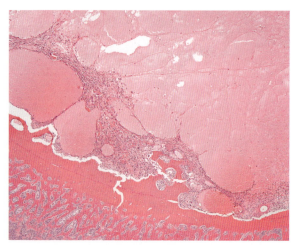

Figure 2-167 **Aneurysmal bone cyst** from a cat. Large blood-filled spaces are surrounded by loose connective tissue, cortical bone, and an extensive periosteal reaction.

be mistaken for tumor bone. *There may be more solid areas of spindle cell proliferation* with increased mitotic figures, and solid areas may predominate in some aneurysmal bone cysts. The pathogenesis of the lesions is not known, but a local alteration in blood flow has been thought to play a role. Increased venous pressure may occur secondary to trauma or a tumor, resulting in dilation of the vascular bed and subsequent erosion of bone. Two cases of aneurysmal bone cysts in dogs were reported to occur after a history of trauma, 6 weeks and 8 years previously. However, in humans, ~70% of aneurysmal bone cysts are primary, and associated with consistent chromosomal abnormalities, a TRE17/USP6 translocation, suggesting *these cysts may be neoplastic rather than reactive lesions*. The translocation results in TRE17 upregulation and activation of matrix metalloproteinases. Recurrence, postcomplete surgical excision of the lesion, has not been reported in animals. Malignant transformation of an aneurysmal bone cyst to a chondrosarcoma has been reported in a dog.

Subchondral (juxtacortical) bone cysts occur in young horses, pigs, and occasionally in other species, as a manifestation of osteochondrosis (see Osteochondrosis).

Intraosseous epidermoid cysts *are reported rarely in dogs and horses as a cause of lytic lesions in the distal phalanx*. At this site in dogs, they must be differentiated from nail bed squamous cell carcinomas, malignant melanomas, and osteomyelitis. In horses, they must be differentiated from keratomas. Two cases in dogs have been reported in vertebral bodies. Radiographically, there may be a sclerotic reaction around one or more lytic foci and extensive periosteal new bone formation. Grossly, the lesion consists of multilocular cysts containing pale cream-colored, crumbly material. Microscopically, *the cysts are lined by well-differentiated, stratified squamous, keratinizing epithelium and filled with layers of keratinized squames*. The squamous epithelium may show marked epithelial hyperplasia and could be mistaken for squamous cell carcinoma if a biopsy sample is inadequate. The cysts are generally supported by a dense fibrous stroma and surrounded by thickened bone trabeculae. The pathogenesis of intraosseous epidermoid cysts is uncertain, but the digital lesions are believed to be *secondary to a penetrating wound*, with traumatic implantation of epidermal fragments into the underlying bone. Cysts involving the skull of humans, and vertebral body of the dog, may represent *rests of heterotopic ectoderm* that have become sequestered along lines of closure during embryonic development.

An **exuberant fracture callus** containing extensive areas of disorganized and primitive bone, cartilage, and fibrous tissue may also resemble a primary bone tumor. Even in cytologic and histologic preparations, differentiation of an early callus from osteosarcoma and chondrosarcoma can present a significant challenge, especially in cases where the clinical and radiographic history is inadequate.

Tumoral calcinosis in *horses* has an unknown pathogenesis. It usually occurs in animals about 2-4 years of age, and 90% of lesions develop on the *lateral aspect of the stifle* (Fig. 2-168). The lesions may be single or multiple and are sometimes attached to the joint capsule, but not to the overlying skin. They usually appear as *hard, well-circumscribed, nonpainful, subcutaneous swellings* ranging in size from 3-12 cm in diameter. Individual lesions consist of a tough, outer, fibrous capsule with collagenous trabeculae dividing the interior into numerous variable-sized locules consisting of finely granular, chalky white accumulations of calcium salts, surrounded by a rim of granulomatous inflammatory cells. The lesions usually do not cause lameness and do not recur after surgical removal. Tumoral calcinosis in humans is an inherited disease, with affected individuals developing calcified masses in the skin. Two forms of the disease occur: one form associated with hyperphosphatemia and caused by mutations in genes involved in phosphorus metabolism *(FGF23, klotho, GALNT3)*, the other with normophosphatemia and mutations in *SAMD9*, a gene of unknown function. In the few cases described in horses, increased serum phosphorus concentrations have not been reported, and a hereditary basis to the disease has not been determined.

Ectopic ossification refers to the *formation of non-neoplastic trabecular bone in non-osseous sites*, presumably following the induction of pluripotential stem cells by appropriate growth factors. In most cases, ectopic bone is detected as an incidental finding at autopsy without an obvious predisposing cause. Typical sites include the pulmonary connective tissue of dogs and cattle, and the cervical and lumbosacral dura mater of aged dogs ("ossifying pachymeningitis"). Ectopic ossification also occurs in the supporting connective tissue of certain tumors, particularly mammary, thyroid, and salivary carcinomas in dogs and intestinal carcinomas in cats. Ectopic bone may form in lesions that have been mineralized for an extended period, such as calcinosis circumscripta, possibly because of metaplasia of cells involved in the initial process of mineralization or resulting from local production of growth factors (TGF-β, FGFs, BMPs).

Where ectopic bone forms in close association with, or becomes attached to, a bone, differentiation of the lesion from a fracture callus or a parosteal osteosarcoma may prove difficult. Depending on its stage of maturation, a fracture callus is likely to contain remnants of cartilage or chondro-osseous bone, whereas ectopic bone is composed exclusively of trabecular bone. In parosteal osteosarcoma, the spaces between trabeculae will be populated with mesenchymal cells showing features of malignancy, rather than a single layer of osteoblasts lined up along the surface of bone trabeculae.

A syndrome resembling human **fibrodysplasia ossificans progressiva** (FOP) has been described in several cats, and occasionally in the dog, although some of these cases more closely resemble myositis ossificans. In cats, the disease is characterized by *progressive, symmetrical hyperplasia and ossification of connective tissue* in the subcutis, epimysium, and joint capsules of the neck, dorsum, and limbs (Fig. 2-169A). Affected cats have ranged in age from 16 weeks to 6 years. A feature of the disease in humans, and in some reported cases in animals, is the formation of *nodules of disorganized hyaline cartilage that undergo multifocal endochondral ossification* (Fig. 2-169B), which in some areas may have microscopic features suggestive of chondrosarcoma. The progressive nature of the disease around multiple joints allows diagnosis of FOP. As in humans, a heterozygous mutation has been found in the *ACVR1* gene (ACVR1/ALK2 activin receptor–like kinase 2, a BMP type 1 receptor) of a 16-week-old and a 20-week-old cat with FOP. The mutation leads to constitutive activity of the BMP type I receptor, resulting in osteoblast differentiation and bone formation. *Myositis ossificans* differs from fibrodysplasia ossificans in being localized and asymmetrical. The lesions characteristically possess a peripheral zone of orderly maturation from fibrous tissue to mineralized osteoid, which is gradually replaced by lamellar bone (see Vol. 1, Muscle and tendon).

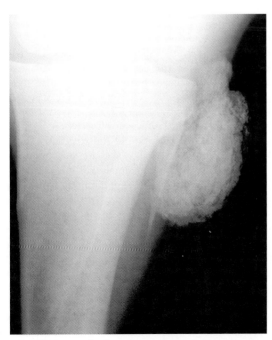

Figure 2-168 Tumoral calcinosis in a horse. A large, discrete mass lateral to the femorotibial joint contains multiple radiodense deposits.

Further reading

Berkowitz A, et al. Detailed analyses of feline fibrodysplasia ossificans progressiva. Vet Pathol 2010;47:52S.

Lipitz L, et al. Intramedullary epidermoid cyst in the thoracic spine of a dog. J Am Anim Hosp Assoc 2011;47:e145-149.

Ye Y, et al. TRE17/USP6 oncogene translocated in aneurysmal bone cyst induces matrix metalloproteinase production via activation of NF-kappaB. Oncogene 2010;29:3619-3629.

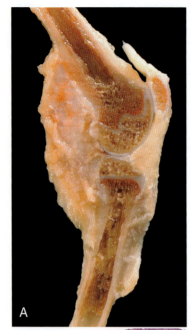

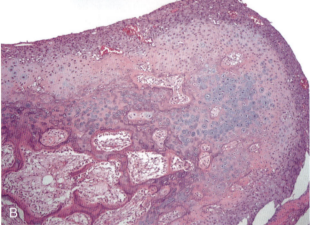

Figure 2-169 **Fibrodysplasia ossificans progressiva** in the left stifle from a 5-month-old kitten. **A.** Massive thickening of the joint capsule on the caudal aspect with tissue resembling cartilage. Similar lesions involved the right stifle and several other limb joints. **B.** Disorganized hyaline cartilage containing many plump chondrocytes and undergoing multifocal endochondral ossification.

DISEASES OF JOINTS

GENERAL CONSIDERATIONS

Three main types of joints or articulations unite adjacent bones and/or cartilaginous structures throughout the skeleton. These are classified on the basis of their morphology and tissue composition as *fibrous, cartilaginous,* or *synovial joints*. This method of classification has limitations; some joints contain a mixture of the different tissue types, whereas others change their composition during maturation. Furthermore, even within each category, there is considerable variation in the amount of movement between adjacent skeletal structures. In spite of these limitations, the system is widely accepted in the medical and veterinary literature and is used throughout this chapter.

Fibrous joints

In these joints, the *bones are united by fibrous tissue*, which allows little movement between them. Fibrous joints are *subdivided into sutures, syndesmoses, and gomphoses*.

- **Sutures** are limited to the *skull*, where they allow continued growth of cranial bones by intramembranous ossification as the brain matures. Osteogenic cells form a cambial layer adjacent to the bone-forming surfaces and are separated by intervening layers of fibrous tissue, which vary in thickness depending on their location. Broader sheets of fibrous tissue often occur at the junctions of 3 adjacent skull bones and are referred to as **fontanelles**. A bony union or **synostosis** replaces the fibrous tissue of many sutures once growth ceases.
- **Syndesmoses** are fibrous joints in which *adjacent bones are united by an interosseous ligament or membrane*, such as occurs in some species between the shafts of the tibia and fibula and between the radius and ulna. Syndesmoses contain fibrous and elastic connective tissue in variable proportions. Consequently, minor movement may occur between the bones because of stretching of the ligament or membrane.
- **Gomphoses** are specialized fibrous *joints between the teeth and either the mandible or maxilla*. The membrane between tooth and bone is termed the **periodontal ligament**, and although it contains no elastic fibers, it allows slight movement of the tooth.

Cartilaginous joints

These are joints in which the *union consists of either hyaline or fibrocartilage*, or a combination of the 2. There are 2 types of cartilaginous joints: *synchondroses and symphyses*.

Synchondroses are *temporary joints* that exist only while the skeleton is growing and are replaced by bone once the skeleton matures. *Physeal growth plates*, which unite the separate centers of ossification in long bones, are synchondroses consisting of well-organized hyaline cartilage. Synchondroses also exist between bones forming by endochondral ossification in the basicranium.

Symphyses are located in the *midsagittal plane of the body and are permanent joints*, unlike synchondroses. The adjacent bones are capped by a thin layer of hyaline cartilage, which blends with fibrocartilage, forming a joint that has great strength while still allowing a limited amount of movement. Examples are the *pubic symphysis* and *intervertebral disks*. Intervertebral disks unite each pair of vertebrae in the vertebral column, with the exception of the atlas and axis.

Diseases of **intervertebral disks** are very common in humans and certain domestic animals. For this reason, a brief discussion of the unique structure and function of these joints is appropriate. Each disk contains *a central core*, the **nucleus pulposus**, which is a remnant of the notochord. In young animals, the nucleus pulposus is gelatinous and translucent. The matrix consists of glycosaminoglycans, particularly chondroitin-6-sulfate, keratan sulfate, and hyaluronan (hyaluronic acid), collagen (mainly type II), and a large amount of water. The cellular concentration is relatively sparse and consists predominantly of *chondrocytes*, which are often arranged in small clusters, and fibrocytes. The nucleus pulposus of immature animals may also contain clusters of notochordal or physaliferous cells, which have abundant, finely vacuolated cytoplasm filled with glycogen. With aging, the glycosaminoglycan and water concentration of intervertebral disks declines, and the number of fibrocytes increases. *The nucleus pulposus is surrounded by the* **annulus fibrosus,** which is broader ventrally than dorsally and consists of concentric layers of fibrocartilage. The direction of the collagen fibers alternates between each layer. The matrix of the annulus fibrosus consists predominantly of type I collagen. Fine nerve endings are present in the outer third of the annulus fibrosus. *The cranial and caudal boundaries of intervertebral disks are occupied by* **cartilaginous end plates,** which consist of hyaline cartilage and are in direct apposition to the vertebral bodies on either side of the joint. Collagen fibers from the annulus fibrosus merge with those of the cartilaginous end plates and become embedded in the bony trabeculae of the vertebral body, forming a strong, stable union.

Dorsally and ventrally the intervertebral disks merge with the **dorsal and ventral longitudinal ligaments,** which run the length of the spinal column. The dorsal longitudinal ligament lies in the floor of the vertebral canal, merging with each disk as it passes, except between the second and tenth thoracic vertebrae. In this region, *conjugal ligaments* connecting the heads of the corresponding ribs cross the floor of the canal between the dorsal longitudinal ligament and the dorsal portion of the annulus fibrosus. The extra support provided by the conjugal ligaments contributes to the low incidence of disk protrusions between the second and tenth thoracic vertebrae in dogs.

Intervertebral disks are designed to allow limited movement between adjacent vertebral bodies when the vertebral column is subjected to a wide variety of different loading conditions, including compression, tension, bending, shear forces, and torsion. Degenerative changes occurring in the nucleus pulposus (as part of chondrodysplasia) or annulus fibrosus (as part of the aging process) can markedly alter the ability of intervertebral disks to withstand such forces.

Synovial joints

Synovial or **diarthrodial** joints are found predominantly in the appendicular skeleton and allow considerable movement between adjacent bones. The bone ends in these specialized joints are covered by *hyaline articular cartilage,* and an *articular capsule* surrounds a central cavity filled with *synovial fluid.* Some synovial joints are supported by ligaments, whereas others, such as the femorotibial joint, contain fibrocartilaginous menisci. Because of the importance of these joints, and the frequency with which they are involved in disease processes, the individual components of synovial joints will be discussed in more detail.

Articular cartilage is the key component of synovial joints, being required to withstand the compressive forces associated with weight bearing in addition to the shear forces that occur during motion. Grossly, it is smooth, pale blue-white, and turgid in young animals, but with advancing age, it becomes yellow, opaque, and less elastic. The thickness of articular cartilage varies between and within joints, tending to be thickest at points of maximum weight bearing.

Microscopically, articular cartilage is divided into 4 layers. In the *superficial or gliding layer,* which makes up only 10-20% of the total cartilage thickness, the chondrocytes are relatively small and flat, with their long axis parallel to the articular surface. Beneath this layer is an *intermediate (transitional) layer* in which the chondrocytes are round or ovoid, then a *radial layer,* in which large, round chondrocytes line up vertically in short columns reminiscent of those in the physis. The fourth layer is *calcified cartilage,* which is separated from the subchondral bone by an irregular basophilic line, referred to as the *tidemark.* Within the tidemark, the chondrocyte-derived type II collagen fibers are structurally cemented to the osteoblast-derived type I collagen. In immature animals, endochondral ossification beneath the articular cartilage contributes to the growth of the epiphysis.

Articular cartilage is devoid of blood vessels and nerves. Chondrocytes are the only cell type in articular cartilage and make up only 5% of the tissue. The remaining 95% is matrix secreted by the chondrocytes. This matrix is composed of proteoglycans, collagen, and water. The *proteoglycans* consist predominantly of aggrecan, a highly glycosylated protein that contains the glycosaminoglycans chondroitin sulfate and keratan sulfate. Aggrecan molecules bind to hyaluronic acid to form a large aggregate with a negative charge. The glycosaminoglycan molecules in these aggregates are negatively charged because of the presence of many carboxyl and sulfate groups and therefore remain separated when attached to the core protein. Water molecules are trapped by the negative charges and result in a matrix that is 70-80% water.

Collagen fibers are responsible for the tensile strength of articular cartilage. Type II collagen is predominant in articular cartilage, but types V, VI, IX, X, and XI are also present. Although not apparent in routine histologic preparations, type II collagen fibrils are arranged in loops with either end firmly embedded in the calcified zone. Therefore the fibrils located in the superficial layer are oriented parallel to the articular surface, whereas those in the radial layer are more vertical. This arrangement presumably enhances the ability of articular cartilage to withstand shear and compressive forces. Water moves slowly within this proteoglycan and collagen meshwork, thus allowing articular cartilage to maintain its turgidity when subjected to a compressive load. This flow of water during movement is important in promoting the transport of nutrients and growth factors to chondrocytes within the articular cartilage.

The metachromasia of the cartilage matrix with stains such as toluidine blue is due to its glycosaminoglycan content. When proteoglycans are lost, metachromasia is reduced, the intercellular substance stains positively by the periodic acid–Schiff method, and collagen fibers are more prominent. Chondrocytes in articular cartilage must continually synthesize new matrix components to replace those that are degraded and lost. As chondrocytes age, they secrete less matrix with smaller aggrecan complexes. Collagen cross-linking also increases with age, resulting in loss of tensile strength and resiliency of the articular cartilage. Because of the absence of nerve endings, damage to articular cartilage does not cause pain unless there is concomitant injury to the subchondral bone and/or joint capsule, both of which are well supplied with nerves.

The thin plate of **subchondral bone,** to which the articular cartilage is attached, is ~10 times more deformable than cortical bone. This is important in allowing more even distribution of the load between the articular cartilage and the bone at times of peak loading. In chronic degenerative joint diseases, the subchondral bone may become denser. In such cases, the articular cartilage is required to bear an increased proportion of the burden, and the degenerative process is accelerated. There is some debate as to whether thickening of the subchondral bone precedes degeneration of the articular cartilage in degenerative joint diseases, or if it occurs as a sequel, but it is likely that the 2 processes occur concurrently.

In some joints of ruminants, horses, and pigs, nonarticulating depressions known as **synovial fossae** (Fig. 2-170) are present near the midline of the joints. These normal structures are bilaterally symmetrical (Fig. 2-171) and are acquired during the first months of postnatal life as a consequence of joint modeling. Synovial fossae appear as central depressions having distinct borders and a smooth, blue to pink surface, reflecting the proximity of the subchondral capillary bed. A study in swine found that synovial fossae were not present at birth, but were present after 4-5 months of age on the articular surfaces of the scapula, distal humerus, proximal radius, distal radius, and distal surface of the intermediate carpal bone. *It is important that synovial fossae are not mistaken for lesions in the articular cartilage or as indicators of collapsed subchondral bone.* In general, they are of no significance, although in horses they may be structural points where infection can be passed between the joint cavity and the subchondral bone. In diseased joints, synovial fossae may become more prominent because of hyperemia of the synovium or the underlying epiphyseal bone.

An **articular capsule** surrounds each synovial joint and consists of an outer fibrous capsule and an inner synovial membrane. The **fibrous capsule** consists of parallel bundles of dense, fibrous connective tissue and merges with the periosteum of the bones on either side of the joint. This strong capsule restricts the range of movement possible between articulating bone ends and is supported in some areas by focal thickenings or **ligaments**. Intra-articular ligaments, such as the cruciate ligaments of the stifle, add further support. **Tendons** may also attach to the articular capsule, adding strength to areas that require it. Collagen fibers from ligaments and tendons may be attached to the fibrous capsule or may attach to bone at sites referred to as **entheses**. At these sites, collagen fibers from the tendon merge with zones of unmineralized then mineralized fibrocartilage, before becoming incorporated into bone as **Sharpey's fibers**. Entheses are well served by blood vessels and nerves. Excessive tension on ligaments may lead to rupture of the ligament, or to an avulsion fracture, where a fragment of bone is detached with the enthesis intact. The latter is not uncommon in animals with rickets or fibrous osteodystrophy. The fibrous capsule is well supplied with blood vessels, lymphatics, proprioceptive nerves, and pain receptors. Thickening of the fibrous capsule in animals with chronic joint diseases leads to reduced motion or stiff joints.

In the *femorotibial joints* of domestic animals, *semilunar fibrocartilaginous disks*, or **menisci**, provide additional stability. These structures are firmly attached to ligaments, or to the fibrous layer of the joint capsule, and extend into the joint space between the articulating bone surfaces. Menisci are not lined by a synovial membrane but are innervated and have a blood supply. Similar, but more circular or oval structures, referred to as **articular disks**, *are in the temporomandibular joint*. Articular disks may possess a central perforation. Meniscal mineralization and ossification in the stifle joint occurs uncommonly in humans and has been reported in cats. Such lesions must be differentiated from intra-articular avulsion fractures or loose bodies in radiographs.

The **synovial membrane** is a smooth, glistening, highly vascular layer that lines the inner surface of the joint. It also covers any intra-articular ligaments or tendons and is reflected on intra-articular bone, where it merges with the periosteum or the perichondrium. In the transition zone, it merges with the articular margins and spreads for a short distance over the non–weight-bearing articular cartilage. In some areas, particularly in recesses of the joint, the synovial membrane has many small, villus projections. These synovial villi are not easily discerned macroscopically in normal joints but may become enlarged, hyperemic, and more numerous in some chronic inflammatory or degenerative diseases of joints. In addition, thickened folds of synovial membrane, often containing adipose tissue, extend into the joint cavity. These *fat pads* generally occupy triangular intra-articular spaces formed by the round bone ends within the joint capsule. Synovial membranes lining tendon sheaths and bursae are similar to those lining diarthrodial joints.

The *synovial membrane generally consists of 2 layers*, a thin, cellular **intima** on the inner surface and a **subintima**, which

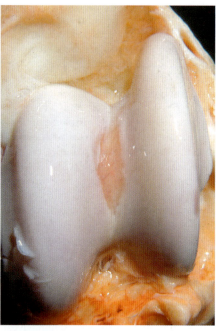

Figure 2-170 Synovial fossa in a horse talus. This island of synovium in the groove between articular condyles should not be confused with cartilage erosion.

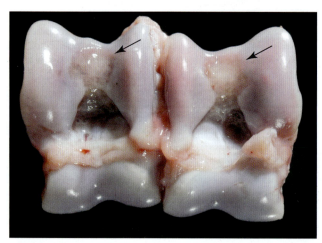

Figure 2-171 Synovial fossae in goat tali. The bilateral symmetry of these normal hourglass-shaped islands of synovium (arrows) is typical.

contains variable quantities of areolar, adipose, and fibrous tissue. The loose fibrous connective tissue of the subintima merges with the dense fibrous capsule. The subintima is richly vascular, and contains lymphatics and nerves, together with a small number of antigen-presenting dendritic cells. In areas where the synovial membrane lines intra-articular ligaments or tendons, the subintimal layer is usually attenuated or inapparent.

The synovial intima consists of **synoviocytes** forming an ill-defined layer, 1-3 cells deep. The cells vary in shape from fusiform to polygonal. No basement membrane exists between the synovial intima and subintima, and the *synoviocytes are of mesenchymal rather than epithelial origin*. Two types of synoviocytes, referred to as type A (macrophage-like) and type B (fibroblast-like) cells, are recognized on the basis of their morphology, function, and immunochemical staining. *Type A synoviocytes originate from bone marrow and have phagocytic and antigen-processing functions*. Ultrastructurally, they resemble tissue macrophages, possessing a dense, heterochromatin-rich nucleus, many cytoplasmic vacuoles, and poorly developed rough endoplasmic reticulum. They are primarily responsible for removing and degrading particulate matter from the joint cavity and possess antigen-processing properties. Immunohistochemically, they stain with CD18. *Type B synoviocytes are probably of fibroblastic origin*. They have a well-developed Golgi apparatus, prominent rough endoplasmic reticulum, and are responsible for the synthesis of hyaluronan in addition to matrix components, including collagen. They are also equipped with various enzymes capable of degrading cartilage and bone. Both cell types produce cytokines and other mediators. Immunohistochemically, both types of synoviocytes are vimentin positive and cytokeratin negative.

The synovial membrane is freely permeable in either direction to molecules of small dimension, which may be removed by the capillaries and lymphatics. Larger particles are phagocytized by type A synoviocytes. The removal of particulate matter from the joint and its deposition in the subintimal layer is a continuous process. Because of the long life-span of type A synoviocytes, estimated to be from 3-6 months, phagocytosed particulate matter may persist in the synovium for long periods. When the volume is large, as may occur in diseased joints, its presence in the synovial membrane stimulates fibrosis of the capsule, contributing to the swelling and fixation of diseased joints. *The synovial membrane proliferates markedly in certain disease states* and has considerable powers of regeneration following injury or synovectomy. In chronic synovitis, lymphocytes and plasma cells infiltrate the synovial membrane and may accumulate in hypertrophic synovial villi. The lymphocytes are often perivascular and sometimes arranged in follicles.

Synovial fluid is a viscous, clear, colorless or slightly yellow fluid and is the main source of nutrients for articular cartilage. Essentially, *it is a dialysate of plasma, modified by the addition of hyaluronan, glycoprotein, and various other macromolecules by type B synoviocytes*. Electrolytes and small molecules such as glucose, lactate, and some small plasma proteins are able to move freely into and out of the synovial fluid through the synovial membrane, but large proteins such as fibrinogen are excluded. The viscous nature of synovial fluid reflects its high concentration of hyaluronan and varies between joints, as does the volume of fluid.

Hyaluronan is believed to function as a lubricant for the synovial membrane and periarticular tissues, but it probably plays little, if any part, in lubricating the motion between cartilage surfaces. Lubrication of synovial joints relies on the presence of the glycoprotein **lubricin**, which provides boundary lubrication and promotes survival of chondrocytes.

Normal diarthrodial joints contain only a very small volume of synovial fluid, but the volume generally increases greatly in response to injury or inflammation. This is most likely caused, in part, by increased vascular permeability in the synovial membrane following the release of inflammatory mediators such as prostaglandins and cytokines. The resulting increase in protein concentration of synovial fluid alters the normal oncotic balance and therefore fluid volume. In damaged joints, increased lymphatic drainage accelerates the clearance of proteins and cartilage breakdown products from synovial fluid.

Synovial fluid normally contains a small number of mononuclear cells and occasional free synoviocytes. Neutrophils and erythrocytes are uncommon unless the joint has been damaged, the synovial membrane is inflamed, or the sample has been contaminated with blood during collection. *The number of neutrophils increases markedly in both septic and sterile inflammatory diseases of the joint*. The synovial fluid may become turbid and less viscous depending on the number of neutrophils present.

Response of articular cartilage to injury

Because of its avascular nature and the absence of undifferentiated cells with the ability to respond to injury, *articular cartilage has only limited powers of regeneration*. The chondrocytes of mature articular cartilage show little, if any, sign of mitotic activity and have limited capacity for increasing matrix synthesis. Furthermore, their encasement in lacunae restricts their capacity to migrate to areas of damage. The regenerative potential of articular cartilage decreases even further with advancing age as the number of chondrocytes declines and the size of matrix proteoglycans decreases.

The response of articular cartilage to injury varies with the nature of the insult and with the depth of the lesion. *Superficial lacerations that do not penetrate the tidemark, and therefore fail to cause hemorrhage or inflammation, do not heal*. Chondrocytes adjacent to the lesion may proliferate, forming small clusters (*chondrones*), and may produce new matrix, but they do not migrate into the lesion. Within a few weeks of injury, the chondrocyte response subsides; the lesion persists for long periods but without progressing to chondromalacia or degenerative joint disease.

The repair of injuries that involve the full depth of the articular cartilage and penetrate subchondral bone differs markedly from the repair of superficial lesions. Hemorrhage occurs from blood vessels in the subchondral bone, and the lesion becomes filled with a hematoma. Inflammatory cells and primitive mesenchymal cells invade the hematoma, probably under the influence of local growth factors, such as PDGF and TGF-β, derived from platelets and from the damaged bone. Within ~2 weeks of injury, some of the mesenchymal cells in the lesion have features of chondrocytes and begin to produce a matrix rich in proteoglycans, which also contains type II collagen. By 6-8 weeks, the defect is filled with fibrocartilage, which is firmly bonded to the adjacent hyaline articular cartilage. New bone formation occurs at the base of the lesion, restoring the subchondral bone plate, but the new bone does not extend into the area previously occupied by articular cartilage; instead, it remains well below the articulating surface. Fibrocartilage repair tissue is analogous to the fibrous scar that repairs most other tissues, and although it is an adequate replacement for articular cartilage at sites of deep injury, it does not perform as well when subjected to mechanical loading. In general, *most large defects in articular cartilage will eventually progress to degeneration after being filled with fibrocartilaginous repair tissue*. Early signs of degeneration may be present within a year of injury, although in some situations, the repair tissue appears to function satisfactorily for a prolonged period and may become remodeled to more closely resemble normal articular cartilage. Interestingly, continuous passive motion of articular surfaces subjected to full-thickness injury has been shown to stimulate more rapid and successful healing of the articular cartilage than either complete immobilization or intermittent active motion.

Further reading

Waller KA, et al. Role of lubricin and boundary lubrication in the prevention of chondrocyte apoptosis. Proc Natl Acad Sci USA 2013;110:5852-5857.

DEVELOPMENTAL DISEASES OF JOINTS
Osteochondrosis

Osteochondrosis is characterized by a focal failure of endochondral ossification that occurs in both the physeal growth plate and the articular-epiphyseal cartilage of *growing animals*. The disease occurs in pigs, horses, large breed dogs, cattle, and sheep. The term osteochondrosis is ambiguous but entrenched. This umbrella term includes 3 forms of osteochondrosis affecting the *articular-epiphyseal cartilage*:

- **Osteochondrosis latens**—focal ischemic cartilage necrosis that involves the growth cartilage, but not the articular cartilage, of the articular-epiphyseal cartilage complex (subclinical, may resolve without progression).
- **Osteochondrosis manifesta**—retention of the necrotic cartilage resulting in failure of endochondral ossification and a grossly or radiographically visible focus of necrotic cartilage within the subchondral bone (may or may not show clinical signs, can resolve by gradual removal of the necrotic cartilage focus).
- **Osteochondrosis dissecans**—focal cartilage necrosis that dissects through the articular cartilage to form a cleft, often resulting in a flap of articular cartilage (clinically relevant lesion that is not reversible). The previously used term *osteochondritis dissecans* should not be used, because the lesion is not inflammatory.

Osteochondrosis is multifactorial, and numerous risk factors have been studied, especially in pigs and horses.
- **Genetics** influences conformation, which contributes to development of lesions. For example, pigs genetically predisposed to have joint conformation that overloads the medial condyle of the distal femur are more likely to develop lesions than those with normal joints. Osteochondrosis is common in commercial pigs but not miniature pigs or wild pigs, indicating an inadvertent selection by producers for genetically predisposed animals.
- **Trauma** contributes to the progression of osteochondrosis latens to more advanced lesions. Many young pigs have latens lesions, but most of those lesions resolve. In commercial pigs that get more exercise, those lesions are more likely to progress to manifesta or dissecans. The fact that predilection sites are those bearing the highest load also supports a role for trauma in development of lesions. The role of trauma is thought to be limited to normal weight bearing, rather than major traumatic incidents, which is supported by the bilateral distribution of the lesions.
- **Nutrition** was once thought to play a role, but experiments have shown no difference in the development of lesions in animals raised on restricted feed, even when it leads to slower growth. Although imbalances in calcium, phosphorus, vitamin D, copper, and other minerals have been suspected to contribute to osteochondrosis, there is no evidence to support such an association.
- **Growth rate** does not affect the development of osteochondrosis latens lesions or the development of more advanced lesions in animals that are not exercised. The combination of exercise and rapid growth rate increases the development of lesions.

The primary lesion of osteochondrosis is a *focal failure of blood supply to the growing cartilage*. During growth, the epiphyseal growth cartilage is supplied by vessels within cartilage canals, whereas the overlying articular cartilage is avascular. As growth slows, the epiphyseal growth cartilage becomes thinner, the vessels regress, and the canals fill with cartilage (chondrification). In growing animals, the vessels in the epiphyseal growth cartilage enter from the perichondrium, and then anastomose with vessels entering from the advancing ossification front. It is these vessels that cross the ossification front that are prone to failure. Although the vessels are necrotic, thrombi are rarely, if ever, detected. The necrotic vessels are surrounded by areas of ischemic necrosis of the epiphyseal growth cartilage (**osteochondrosis latens**) (Fig. 2-172). If this necrotic cartilage persists as the ossification front reaches it, then it results in an area of delayed endochondral ossification (**osteochondrosis manifesta**) (Fig. 2-173). If a cleft forms within the necrotic area of epiphyseal growth cartilage and

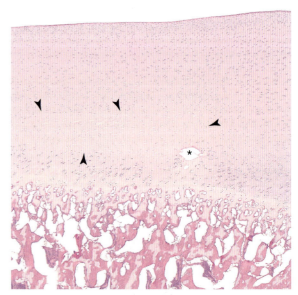

Figure 2-172 Osteochondrosis latens in a 12-week-old pig. The earliest lesion of osteochondrosis is a necrotic cartilage canal (asterisk) surrounded by necrotic epiphyseal growth cartilage (bounded by arrowheads). Notice that the overlying articular cartilage is unaffected. (Courtesy C.S. Carlson.)

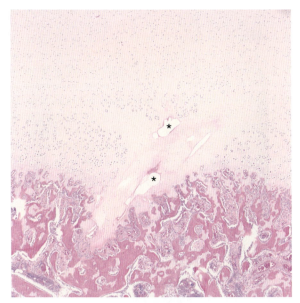

Figure 2-173 Osteochondrosis manifesta in a 12-week-old pig. Persistent focus of necrotic cartilage (with necrotic cartilage canals, asterisks) being incorporated into the epiphysis by the ossification front. (Courtesy C.S. Carlson.)

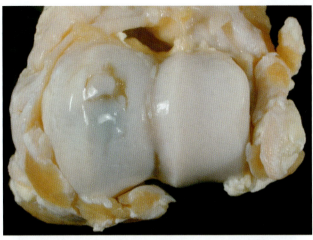

Figure 2-175 Osteochondrosis dissecans in the distal humerus of a 6-month-old pig. Flaps of articular cartilage separated by fissures and clefts from the surrounding intact cartilage of the medial humeral condyle. (Courtesy C.S. Carlson.)

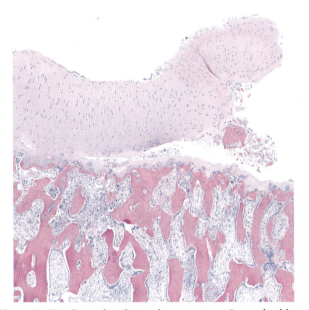

Figure 2-174 Osteochondrosis dissecans in a 6-month-old pig. A flap of cartilage formed by a dissecting band of necrosis and separation extending along the deep growth cartilage and communicating with the articular surface. (Courtesy C.S. Carlson.)

extends to the articular surface, this lesion is referred to as **osteochondrosis dissecans** (Fig. 2-174). If the cleft extends parallel to the articular surface, a flap of articular cartilage forms. This flap can become detached, survive, and even enlarge within the joint space, deriving nutrients from the synovial fluid. The remaining epiphyseal cartilage within some of these flaps may undergo endochondral ossification. Some eventually become attached to or embedded within the synovial membrane.

The physeal lesions of osteochondrosis differ morphologically from those involving the articular-epiphyseal cartilage complex, suggesting a different pathogenesis. *Early lesions in the growth plate consist of cone-shaped foci of retained cartilage extending into the metaphysis*, but rather than containing necrotic cartilage, these foci of metaphyseal dysplasia consist of viable hypertrophic chondrocytes. This does not exclude the possibility of an ischemic origin, because experimental vascular disruption has been shown to induce similar changes in the growth plate of young pigs and lesions identical to tibial dyschondroplasia in chickens. It has also been suggested that these retained wedges of hypertrophic cartilage are secondary to trabecular microfractures in the primary spongiosa that interfere with vascular invasion of the mineralized cartilage during endochondral ossification, leading to persistence of hypertrophic zone chondrocytes.

In some studies of **swine**, up to 100% of commercial piglets have osteochondrosis latens lesions. Many of these lesions resolve completely. Predilection sites in pigs are the joint surfaces of the medial femoral condyle, humeral condyles (Fig. 2-175), humeral head, and dorsal acetabulum. The articular lesions of osteochondrosis are often bilateral and may be symmetrical. It is important to distinguish them from synovial fossae, which are normal in some joints (see Figs. 2-170, 2-171). Early articular lesions appear as *thickened, white foci of articular cartilage*, which are sharply demarcated from adjacent normal areas of cartilage. In some cases, the articular cartilage that is not directly affected by osteochondrosis will be *depressed or wrinkled* because of collapse of necrotic cartilage in the underlying epiphyseal cartilage. In more advanced lesions, the affected cartilage usually shows evidence of separation and flap formation (osteochondrosis dissecans). In other cases, segments of articular cartilage may be detached completely, leaving a deep ulcer with exposure of subchondral bone. The defect in the articular surface is initially filled with vascular connective tissue, which eventually is converted to fibrocartilage. Even if a dissecting lesion does not result, necrotic cartilage may persist in the subchondral bone, resulting in a focal radiolucent area; these lesions are sometimes called *"bone cysts,"* although they contain no epithelial lining.

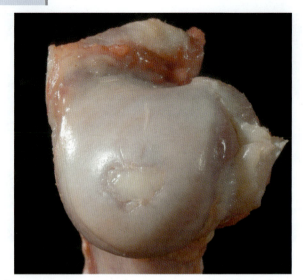

Figure 2-176 **Osteochondrosis dissecans** in a dog. A focus of articular cartilage is encircled by fissures forming a partially attached flap.

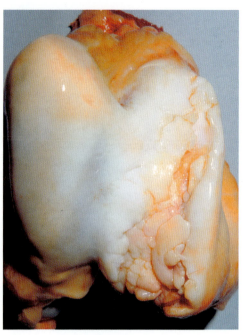

Figure 2-177 **Osteochondrosis dissecans** in a 6-month-old foal. Extensive under-running and displacement of articular cartilage on the lateral trochlear ridge. The many small cartilage nodules represent attempts at repair.

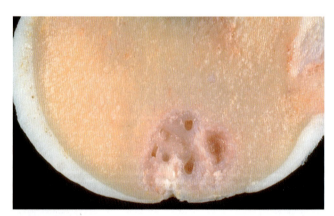

Figure 2-178 **Osteochondrosis** in a horse. Subchondral cystic lesion in the medial femoral condyle. (Courtesy D. Meuten, North Carolina State College of Veterinary Medicine.)

Degenerative joint disease may be a long-term sequela if the pig lives long enough.

The physeal cartilage can also be affected in swine. The predilection sites for physeal osteochondrosis in swine are distal ulna and femur, costochondral junction, femoral head, humeral head, and ischial tuberosity. When the physis of the femoral head is affected, the resulting abnormal physis is prone to fracture, resulting in a *slipped capital femoral epiphysis*. This condition was termed epiphysiolysis in the past, but the lesion is not epiphyseal.

Osteochondrosis in **dogs** usually occurs in young males of large and giant breeds. Osteochondrosis dissecans of the humeral head is the classic presentation of the disease (Fig. 2-176), but should *be diagnosed only in growing dogs*. A grossly similar lesion commonly develops in middle-aged and older dogs as a result of cartilage erosion without pre-existing osteochondrosis. Elbow dysplasia was once thought to be caused by osteochondrosis, but is now thought to be due to heritable joint incongruities.

Although microscopic evidence of articular osteochondrosis is present in 50% of **horses** 2-18 months of age, only a small percentage of these will be clinically, radiographically, or grossly apparent. Many small lesions heal spontaneously, and some previously described small lesions are now thought to be normal anatomic variations. Predilection sites include the lateral trochlear ridge (Fig. 2-177) and medial condyle of the femur, patella, distal tibia, and various sites in the tarsal and fetlock joints. Ossification of attached cartilage flaps seems to be more common in the horse than in other species. Lesions of osteochondrosis may also involve articular facets of cervical vertebrae, which may contribute to cervical vertebral malformation. However, primary and secondary lesions of the articular facets can be difficult to distinguish.

Osteochondrosis manifesta lesions in horses are sometimes called *subchondral bone cysts*, which are most common on the distal aspect of the medial femoral condyle (Fig. 2-178), distal aspect of the metacarpus, and the carpus, elbow, and phalanges. Such lesions have also been reproduced experimentally in young horses following traumatic damage to the articular cartilage and its supporting subchondral bone, suggesting that not all subchondral cysts are related to osteochondrosis. Histologically, the cysts usually consist of variable quantities of fibrous tissue and fibrocartilage, and are surrounded by sclerotic bone trabeculae.

Foals with congenital and neonatal angular limb deformities sometimes have concomitant hypoplasia of carpal bones and osteochondrosis dissecans. These may be manifestations of defective growth and maturation of cartilage.

There are only occasional reports of osteochondrosis in **cattle**, but the disease may be more common in this species than is currently recognized. Because of financial constraints and difficulties in detailed radiologic examination, many lame cattle are sent for slaughter without definitive diagnosis. In bulls, degenerative joint disease and osteochondrosis have a predilection for the lateral trochlear ridge, suggesting that at least some cases of degenerative joint disease are secondary to osteochondrosis. Other predilection sites for osteochondrosis in cattle are the humeral head, distal radius, elbow joint, and the tibial tarsal and occipital condyles.

Osteochondrosis appears to be rare in **sheep** but has been reported as a cause of lameness in young, rapidly growing Suffolk ram lambs. Microscopic lesions are common in growth plates of fast-growing lambs, but few of these progress to gross lesions.

Further reading

Olstad K, et al. Early lesions of articular osteochondrosis in the distal femur of foals. Vet Pathol 2011;48:1165-1175.

Ytrehus B, et al. Etiology and pathogenesis of osteochondrosis. Vet Pathol 2007;44:429-448.

Hip dysplasia

Hip dysplasia is the most common skeletal disease of large- and giant-breed dogs, but may occur in all dog breeds and is occasionally reported in cats, cattle, and horses. *The disease is characterized by a lack of conformity between the femoral head and acetabulum, resulting in excessive joint laxity and degenerative joint disease.* A polygenic mode of inheritance is postulated in dogs. Comparing affected (Labrador Retriever) and unaffected (Greyhound) breeds has identified dozens of potential contributing genes. Environmental effects are believed to play a role in the severity of lesions. In particular, ad libitum food consumption and rapid growth rate contribute to the incidence and severity of the disease.

Increased joint laxity is a common feature in **dogs** with hip dysplasia and appears to have a hereditary basis. Radiographic evidence of hip dysplasia in affected pups may be apparent as early as 7 weeks of age. Another factor that may contribute to subluxation is excessive joint fluid; however, it is difficult to discern whether the larger volume of joint fluid within dysplastic joints is a cause or effect of the subluxation.

The *gross lesions* of canine hip dysplasia vary with the stage of the disease. In the early stages, acetabula appear shallow, there is subluxation of the femoral head, and the articular cartilage may be dull or rough. *The lesions are most prominent in weight-bearing areas of the femoral head and the dorsal rim of the acetabulum.* As the disease progresses, the articular cartilage becomes yellow or gray, and erosion leads to fibrillation and eburnation, with sclerosis of the subchondral bone. Osteophytes may develop at joint margins. The shape of the femoral head may be altered because of the abnormal forces associated with subluxation, and the femoral neck may become thickened and encircled by a solid ring of osteophytes. The joint capsule may be thickened by fibrous connective tissue and villus proliferation of the synovium (Fig. 2-179). In advanced stages, evidence of hip dysplasia may be masked by the manifestations of severe, degenerative joint disease. In some cases, the formation of osteophytes around the acetabular rim may disguise its original shallowness. In dogs with severely dysplastic joints, advanced changes of degenerative joint disease may be present by 1 year of age.

Microscopic changes in hip dysplasia are those of degenerative joint disease (see later) and contribute nothing specific to the diagnosis. Early lesions include edema of the ligament of the head of the femur, and hypertrophy and hyperplasia of synoviocytes in the synovial membrane. Later in the disease,

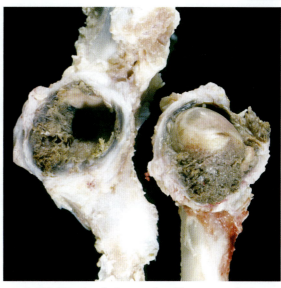

Figure 2-179 Hip dysplasia in a dog. There is marked synovial proliferation and hemosiderosis within the acetabulum and surrounding the flattened and eburnated femoral head.

synovial villi may be infiltrated by mononuclear cells, the joint capsule will thicken with fibrous tissue, and the eroded articular cartilage will contain clusters of proliferating chondrocytes.

Hip dysplasia is much less common in **cats** than in dogs, but its frequency in the general cat population is probably under-estimated. Many cats with radiographic evidence of hip dysplasia are asymptomatic, and *the diagnosis is often incidental*. In a survey of 648 cats representing 12 breeds, the overall frequency of hip dysplasia was about 6.6%. Persians and Himalayans had a higher prevalence rate (15.8% and 25.0%, respectively). Other studies have indicated a high prevalence of hip dysplasia in the Maine Coon breed, which, like the Persian and Himalayan breeds, has a larger body size and a relatively small gene pool. As in dogs, no sex predilection is apparent in cats.

The role of joint laxity in the pathogenesis of feline hip dysplasia is uncertain and requires further investigation. A consistent observation in cats with hip dysplasia is an *abnormally shallow acetabulum*, rather than subluxation of the joint, which is a feature of the disease in dogs. The shallow acetabulum predisposes to degenerative joint disease, but the distribution of lesions in cats differs from that in dogs. The most extensive remodeling and proliferative changes in affected cats involve the craniodorsal acetabular margin, whereas in dogs, the dorsal rim of the acetabulum is most severely affected. A further difference is the lack of remodeling of the femoral neck in cats with hip dysplasia.

Hip dysplasia in **cattle** is best known in *Herefords* but also occurs in the Aberdeen Angus, Galloway, and Charolais breeds. An inherited component is suspected, but too few cases are reported to allow confirmation or characterization of the mode of inheritance. The disease is *largely confined to males*. Although some calves may be affected at birth, clinical lameness usually commences from 3 months to 2 years of age. Because lame bulls are more often sent for slaughter than subjected to postmortem examination, the true prevalence of hip dysplasia in cattle may be much higher than is realized. The lesions are generally bilateral and are characterized by

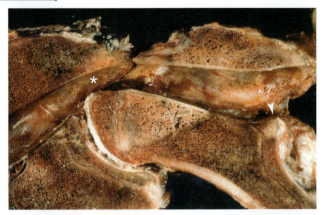

Figure 2-180 Cervical vertebral malformation-malarticulation in a horse. Flexion of the cervical vertebrae results in stenosis of the spinal canal (asterisk). There is also flaring of the caudal epiphysis (arrowhead), which can also contribute to spinal cord compression.

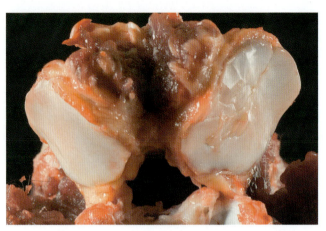

Figure 2-181 Cervical vertebral malformation-malarticulation in a horse. Osteochondrosis of the articular facet joints can contribute to the intervertebral joint instability.

shallow acetabula and degenerative arthropathy involving both the femoral head and acetabulum.

Cervical vertebral malformation-malarticulation

Cervical vertebral malformation-malarticulation (also known as cervical stenotic myelopathy and **wobbler syndrome**) is a common cause of spinal cord compression in horses and dogs. In both species, the lesion is thought to be at least partially hereditary, with males more often affected than females.

Horses have 2 forms of spinal cord compression: dynamic and static. **Dynamic compression** occurs when the neck is flexed and is most commonly seen at C3-C4 and C4-C5 in horses 8-18 months of age. **Static compression** is present regardless of the neck position and is most commonly seen at C5-C6 and C6-C7 in horses 1-4 years of age and older. Thoroughbreds, Warmbloods, and Tennessee Walking Horses are most often affected. Postmortem disarticulation of vertebrae allows detailed examination of each vertebra, including the articular facets. Another method involves sectioning the cervical spine along a parasagittal plane within the spinal canal, but outside the spinal cord to allow removal of the cord intact, and flexion to look for dynamic compression (Fig. 2-180). *Gross findings* contributing to static compression include thickening of the ligamentum flavum, thickened dorsal lamina, and osteophytes that surround the articular facets and encroach on the spinal canal. Osteochondrosis of the articular facets is also present in some cases (Fig. 2-181). Imaging findings are only moderately correlated with postmortem findings, so all cervical vertebrae should be examined, regardless of radiographic localization. Vertebrae are complex bones with multiple structures that can lead to narrowing of the canal. If changes are not apparent after parasagittal sectioning, opening the articular facet joints is warranted; however, changes in these joints may be secondary in chronic cases.

Microscopic findings within the ligamentum flavum and dorsal lamina include excess disorganized fibrocartilage, bone proliferation, and siderophages. Gross examination of the spinal cord at sites of suspected compression may reveal areas of flattening; microscopic findings are typical of compression (see Vol. 1 Nervous system).

Dogs can be affected by static cervical canal stenosis, intervertebral disk herniation, and osseous encroachment on the

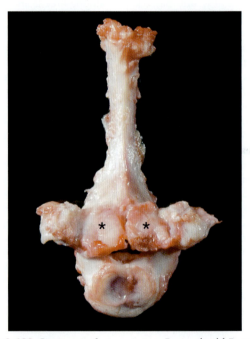

Figure 2-182 Static spinal stenosis in a 5-month-old Rottweiler. The cranial articular processes (asterisks) of the first thoracic vertebra are displaced medially and ventrally, resulting in dorsoventral narrowing of the spinal canal. This lesion more commonly affects the cervical vertebrae.

spinal canal (Fig. 2-182). Instability leading to dynamic compression is not thought to play a role in canine cervical vertebral malformation-malarticulation. *Doberman Pinschers* can have congenitally stenotic vertebrae, particularly affecting the caudal cervical vertebrae. Intervertebral disk herniation affects older Dobermans, but the presence of disk degeneration and protrusion in clinically normal Dobermans calls into question the significance of this finding. *Great Danes* are most often affected by osseous encroachment of the articular processes on the spinal canal. Although large head size was thought to contribute to development of spinal cord compression in both Dobermans and Great Danes, no correlation has been found between conformation and this condition.

Luxations and subluxations

Congenital luxations are rare in animals, but **atlantoaxial subluxations** are reported in dogs, goats, cattle, and horses. In dogs, miniature and toy breeds are usually affected. *The underlying lesion appears to be failure of fusion of the odontoid process to the body of the axis.* Clinical signs vary from neck pain to tetraplegia, with age of onset varying from a few months to several years. Absence or hypoplasia of the odontoid process occurs in calves, often in conjunction with atlanto-occipital fusion. Tetraplegia may be present at birth or develop at several months of age. In both dogs and calves, fusion of the odontoid process with the axis normally occurs in the early months of life, and it is possible that in some cases postnatal influences are responsible for the condition.

Atlantoaxial subluxations occur in some *Arabian foals* with a familial, probably inherited, syndrome. Affected foals may be dead or tetraparetic at birth, or develop progressive ataxia within a few months. Congenital atlanto-occipital fusion and cervical scoliosis also occurs in horses as a sporadic defect unrelated to the Arabian condition.

Patellar luxations and subluxations are common in dogs, less so in horses, and rare in other species. In **dogs**, most are associated with anatomic defects and are probably inherited as polygenic traits. The condition may be unilateral or bilateral, and luxations of variable severity may occur either medially or laterally. Occasionally, they occur in both directions. Medial luxations are most common in both small- and large-breed dogs. Lateral luxations are less common but tend to occur in larger dogs, including some giant breeds. Under normal circumstances, the presence of the patella within the trochlear groove during growth creates a groove of adequate depth. Developmental anomalies affecting the angle of the stifle joint and the direction of tension on the patellar ligament result in patellar luxation or subluxation; the result is a shallow trochlear groove, continued or worsening luxation, and degenerative joint disease (Fig. 2-183).

Patellar luxation in **horses** is uncommon and typically congenital. The luxations may be lateral, medial, distal, and unilateral, or bilateral. Lateral luxation is most common and is associated with hypoplasia of the lateral ridge of the femoral trochlea. The condition is inherited in miniature horses and ponies. Patellar luxation is uncommon in cats and may be an incidental finding. Medial luxation is most common in **cats**, and the condition is often bilateral.

The consequences of luxations and subluxations vary with the species of animal and the joint involved. In general, subluxations, whether they are genetic or traumatic in origin, predispose to degenerative joint disease because of instability of the joint.

Abnormal positioning of joints in terms of overextension or overflexion occurs in animals with **arthrogryposis**, but only in the most severe cases are the articular surfaces deformed. The primary lesion is in the central nervous system, resulting in lack of movement in utero and fixation of the joints in the flexed position.

Further reading

Da Costa RC. Cervical spondylomyelopathy (wobbler syndrome) in dogs. Vet Clin N Am Small Anim Pract 2010;40:881-913.

Smith GK, et al. Pathogenesis, diagnosis, and control of canine hip dysplasia. In: Tobias KM, Johnston SA, editors. Veterinary Surgery: Small Animal, vol. 1. St. Louis: Elsevier Saunders; 2012. p. 824-848.

DEGENERATIVE DISEASES OF JOINTS
Synovial joints

Degenerative diseases involving the major weight-bearing joints of the limbs are very common in humans and domestic animals. In human medicine, the term "osteoarthritis" is preferred for this group of diseases, although it incorrectly implies an inflammatory origin. **Degenerative joint disease** is a more appropriate term, based on the putative pathogenesis, and will be used in this chapter. Other commonly used *synonyms include osteoarthrosis and degenerative arthropathy.*

Degenerative joint disease is not a specific entity but a common sequel to various forms of joint injury. It involves an interaction between biologic and mechanical factors on the articular cartilage, subchondral bone, and synovium and can be either *monoarticular* or *polyarticular*. It may be classified as either *primary* or *secondary*. **Primary** *degenerative joint disease refers to those cases where there is no apparent predisposing cause, and it generally occurs in older animals.* Such cases may reflect an acceleration of the normal aging changes that occur in joints. Mild degenerative changes in weight-bearing articular surfaces, including yellowing and fibrillation of cartilage, are common incidental findings in adult dogs at postmortem examination. In the absence of clinical signs of lameness, it is difficult to justify a diagnosis of degenerative joint disease in such cases, but it is likely that these represent the early manifestations of the disease.

Secondary *degenerative joint disease is associated with an underlying abnormality in the joint or supporting structures, predisposing to premature degeneration of the cartilage. Any condition that causes direct damage to the articular cartilage, creates instability, or results in abnormal directional forces can predispose to degenerative joint disease.* For example, secondary degenerative joint disease is an inevitable consequence of the joint laxity in dogs with hip dysplasia or ruptured cranial cruciate ligament, because of the effect of abnormal mechanical forces

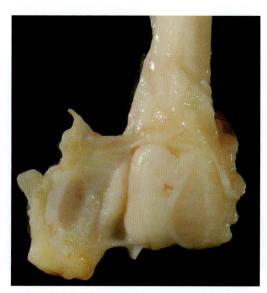

Figure 2-183 **Patellar luxation** in a dog. The trochlear groove is shallow and there is eburnation of the patella and medial trochlear ridge.

on articular cartilage. Incongruity of opposing articular surfaces, as occurs in animals with osteochondrosis, can also cause degenerative joint disease. Other disorders that may predispose to secondary degenerative joint disease include misaligned limb fractures, angular limb deformities, aseptic necrosis, metabolic bone diseases with collapse of subchondral bone, inherited defects in cartilage or collagen formation, and septic arthritis.

The *gross lesions* of degenerative joint disease are similar whether the disease is primary or secondary, although the lesions of secondary degenerative joint disease are generally more severe by the time an affected animal is examined postmortem. *The earliest gross lesion is roughening of the articular cartilage in areas of weight bearing* (Fig. 2-184A) resulting from loss of proteoglycans from the matrix and unmasking of the collagen fibrils. This is referred to as **fibrillation**. Initially, only the superficial layers are involved (Fig. 2-184B), but with continued abrasion of the degenerate cartilage, vertical fissures develop in deeper layers in the direction of collagen fibril alignment and may extend to the subchondral bone. In hinge-type joints, such as the hock, fetlock, and elbow, *linear grooves (wear lines)* may be present in the cartilage in the direction of joint movement. These are relatively common in the joints of adult horses. Progressive erosion of fibrillated cartilage is accompanied by sclerosis of the subchondral bone. In advanced lesions, *the articular cartilage may be completely absent and the exposed bone polished to a smooth surface by rubbing against the opposing bone, a process referred to as* **eburnation**, which means to become ivory-like (Fig. 2-185). This is the most painful stage of degenerative joint disease. Increased stiffness of the sclerotic subchondral bone may accelerate the loss of the overlying cartilage because of reduced flexibility during weight bearing. In fact, some investigators have proposed that sclerosis of subchondral bone may be the initial lesion in degenerative joint disease. More likely, this is just one of a combination of factors involved in progression of the disease. Cystic lesions are often present beneath eburnated surfaces in human patients with degenerative joint disease but are seldom seen in domestic animals. *Another consistent gross feature of degenerative joint disease is the formation of* **osteophytes** *at the margin of articular cartilage and bone* (Fig. 2-186). These small, nodular, outgrowths of bone, covered by a thin layer of hyaline cartilage may surround the articular surface and either distort its shape or obscure the boundary between the articular surface and the supporting bone. Osteophytes develop rapidly following joint injury and can be detected as early as 7 days after a joint has been experimentally destabilized. Changes also occur in the synovium and joint capsule of animals with degenerative joint disease. The joint capsule is thickened with fibrous connective tissue, and there may be hypertrophy of synovial villi.

A variety of *histologic changes* have been reported in the articular cartilage of animals and humans with degenerative joint disease. *Reduction in metachromatic staining of the superficial cartilage matrix*, presumably associated with the loss of proteoglycans, is a common early change and may be accompanied by necrosis of chondrocytes in the tangential layer (Fig. 2-187). Clusters of proliferative chondrocytes (isogenous groups or chondrones) may be present, especially adjacent to fissures in areas of fibrillation. Elsewhere, the density of

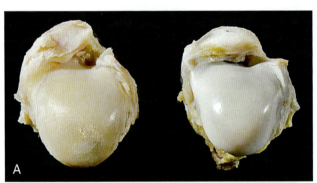

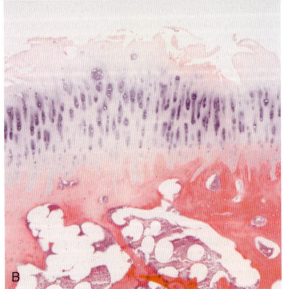

Figure 2-184 Degenerative joint disease in dogs. **A.** Humeral heads from 2 different dogs. The left is from an 11-year-old dog. The articular cartilage is diffusely yellow and slightly roughened. There is a focus of **fibrillation** of the caudal humeral head. The right is from a 7-month-old dog. Note the smooth, shiny white articular cartilage. **B.** Microscopic appearance of fibrillation. The superficial cartilage is necrotic and ragged. There are isogenous groups of chondrocytes (chondrones) within the remaining articular cartilage.

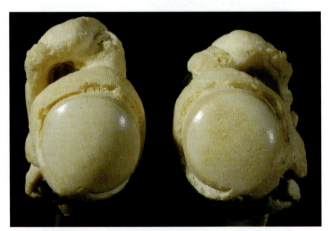

Figure 2-185 Degenerative joint disease in a dog. Both femoral heads are flattened and the subchondral bone is **eburnated**. There are also complete smooth rings of osteophytes around the femoral necks.

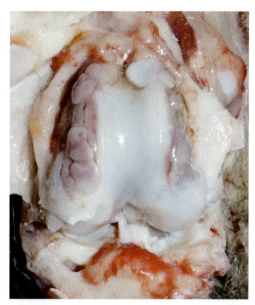

Figure 2-186 **Degenerative joint disease** in a dog. **Osteophytes** along the margins of the articular cartilage of the distal end of the femur.

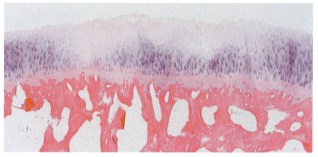

Figure 2-188 **Degenerative joint disease** in a dog. The articular cartilage is thinned, necrotic, and contains deep fissures.

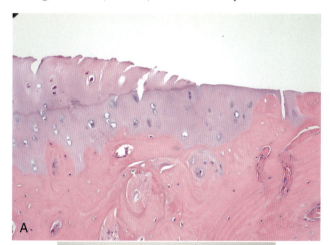

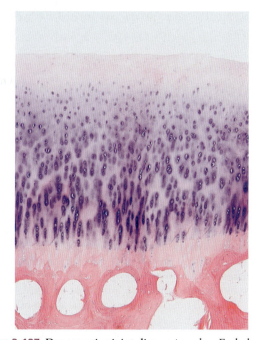

Figure 2-187 **Degenerative joint disease** in a dog. Early lesion of degenerative joint disease characterized by loss of staining in the superficial articular cartilage stroma.

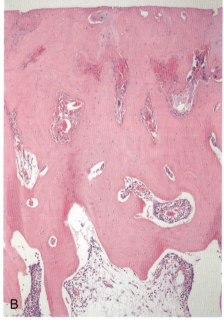

Figure 2-189 **Degenerative joint disease** in a dog. **A.** Junction between areas of fibrillation and **eburnation**. **B.** Densely sclerotic **eburnated subchondral bone**.

chondrocytes is often reduced, but remnants of degenerate cells may still be apparent. In advanced lesions, *the overall thickness of the degenerate cartilage may be markedly reduced*, the surface irregular, and deep clefts present (Fig. 2-188). Collagen fibrils within the matrix appear more prominent. The tidemark is often duplicated or disrupted and may be penetrated by blood vessels. *Fibrillated cartilage merges with areas of eburnation* (Fig. 2-189A), where the articular cartilage is absent and the trabeculae of subchondral bone show variable degrees of thickening and/or remodeling (Fig. 2-189B). In chronic degenerative joint disease, *synovial villi are hypertrophic*, sometimes branching, and are lined by hyperplastic synoviocytes (Fig. 2-190A). Small to moderate numbers of *inflammatory cells*, predominantly lymphocytes and plasma cells, in addition to hemosiderin-containing macrophages, are often present (Fig. 2-190B). *Fragments of degenerate cartilage,*

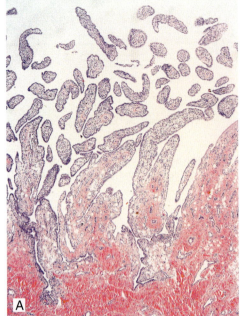

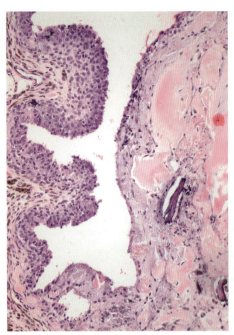

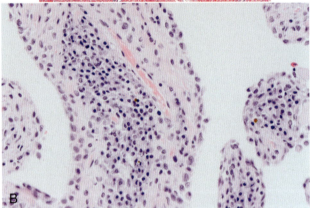

Figure 2-190 Chronic degenerative joint disease. **A.** Hypertrophic synovial villi with rare inflammatory cells (atlanto-occipital joint of a horse). **B.** Mild predominantly plasmacytic synovitis with occasional siderophages from the shoulder joint of a dog.

Figure 2-191 Chronic degenerative joint disease. Fragments of degenerate cartilage and occasional spicules of bone, most likely derived from the eroded articular surface, embedded in the synovium. The adjacent villi are covered by hyperplastic synoviocytes.

presumably derived from the eroded articular surface, may be embedded in the synovium or attached to its surface (Fig. 2-191). Such fragments may enlarge through proliferation of surviving chondrocytes and may be an early stage of secondary osteochondromatosis.

The *pathogenesis of degenerative joint disease is complex* and continues to be debated in human medicine, even after many decades of research and observation. Although there are differing hypotheses on the exact sequence of events, most investigators conform to the view that the disease is *primarily degenerative in nature and that the accompanying inflammatory changes are secondary*. It must be recognized, however, that lesions of degenerative joint disease will also develop as a sequel to chronic inflammation in primary inflammatory conditions of humans and domestic animals. There is convincing evidence that the *chondrocytes* of articular cartilage play an important role in the early stages of disease development. These postmitotic cells normally survive throughout the life of the individual and maintain a balance between degradation and repair of the cartilage matrix under the influence of cytokines, growth factors, and direct physical stimuli. Disruption of this balance in favor of matrix catabolism occurs in the early stages of degenerative joint disease and is reflected by depletion of the proteoglycan aggregates of aggrecan, which are a major component of the cartilage matrix. Continued reduction in the proteoglycan content of the matrix, together with damage to collagen fibrils, interferes with the viscoelastic properties of articular cartilage. As a result, progressive loss of cartilage occurs under the influence of normal biomechanical forces.

The early loss of matrix components in degenerative joint disease is mediated by degradative enzymes, including metalloproteinases, serine proteinases, cysteine proteinases, and aggrecanase. Many of these enzymes are derived from chondrocytes, but synoviocytes and inflammatory cells may also produce them. Natural inhibitors of these enzymes are normally present in articular cartilage but are deficient in degenerative joint disease. Several zinc-dependent metalloproteinases are recognized, but the collagenases, stromelysins, and gelatinases appear to be the most important in cartilage degradation. Collagenase and stromelysin are synthesized as latent enzymes in cartilage and can be activated by plasmin and plasminogen activator or inhibited by plasminogen activator inhibitor-1. Collagenase breaks down the scaffolding of type II collagen, whereas stromelysin cleaves aggrecan in addition to some types of collagen. Degradation products of aggrecan and type II collagen may remain in the cartilage matrix or diffuse into the synovial fluid, where they can be detected. Proteoglycan fragments in synovial fluid may be either phagocytosed by synovial cells or enter lymphatics in the synovium.

Various cytokines and growth factors are also believed to be involved in the pathogenesis of degenerative joint disease, particularly in the generation of the inflammatory response. Most attention has focused on the role of the cytokines interleukin-1 (IL-1), interleukin-6 (IL-6), and tumor necrosis factor-α (TNF-α). IL-1 and TNF-α have been shown to increase the synthesis of metalloproteinases and plasminogen activators, and to induce the resorption of cartilage both in vitro and in vivo. IL-1 also stimulates fibroblasts to synthesize collagen type I and type II, and may therefore contribute to fibrous thickening of the joint capsule in degenerative joint disease. The role of IL-6 is less clear, but it is released in vitro by chondrocytes from normal and degenerate cartilage and may be involved in autocrine stimulation of chondrocyte proliferation. It has also been detected in the synovial fluid of human patients with various arthropathies and may be an important intermediate signal for the activities of IL-1 and TNF-α. Growth factors, such as insulin-like growth factor-1 and transforming growth factor-β, have an anabolic effect on connective tissues and have been shown to stimulate proteoglycan and collagen synthesis. They can also inhibit or reverse some of the catabolic effects of IL-1. Similarly, the cytokine interferon-γ inhibits the action of IL-1 on metalloproteinase production and proteoglycan depletion from cartilage. These observations support the concept of a complex interaction between cytokines and growth factors in the pathogenesis of degenerative joint disease.

Inflammatory changes in the synovium of humans and animals with degenerative joint disease are most likely secondary to the stimulation of IL-1 and TNF-α by synoviocytes following the release of degraded collagen and proteoglycan fragments from degenerate cartilage. The neuropeptide substance P may also be involved. This peptide has been detected in the synovial membrane and fluid of human patients with degenerative joint disease and has been shown to activate both inflammatory cells and synoviocytes, in addition to stimulating the secretion and action of IL-1.

Primary and secondary degenerative joint diseases are common in most domestic animal species, but in dogs, horses, and cattle, certain types are either sufficiently common or important to warrant discussion as separate entities.

Although **degenerative joint diseases of horses** may affect a wide range of synovial joints, those involving the *interphalangeal, metacarpophalangeal, and hock joints* are of particular importance. *These joints are subjected to considerable biomechanical loading during motion*, especially in performance horses, and are therefore predisposed to traumatic injury to the articular cartilage, subchondral bone, or supporting structures. In joints subjected to considerable motion, such as the metacarpophalangeal (fetlock) joints, the changes of degenerative joint disease are usually characterized by *gradual erosion of articular cartilage, sclerosis of subchondral bone, chronic synovitis, and gradual stiffening of the joint resulting from fibrous thickening of the joint capsule*. In low-motion joints, such as the proximal and distal interphalangeal, distal intertarsal, and tarsometatarsal joints, maximum loading during motion is focused on a restricted area. In these joints, the lesion typically is characterized by full-thickness necrosis of the articular cartilage with limited wearing, focal damage to subchondral bone, and bony ankylosis. Degenerative changes involving the navicular bone and the adjacent deep digital flexor tendon, referred to as *navicular syndrome*, probably have a similar pathogenesis as other degenerative joint diseases and will be discussed here.

Traumatic and degenerative diseases of the **metacarpophalangeal (fetlock) joint** of the foreleg are *more common than similar lesions affecting any of the other limb joints*. This susceptibility to injury presumably reflects the relatively small surface area of this joint in comparison to most others and the considerable range of motion expressed by the joint. Furthermore, during racing, the entire weight of the animal is transmitted to the ground through this joint during one phase of the stride. *Poor conformation and excessive training of horses at a young age no doubt contribute to the development of lesions in this and other joints.* **Traumatic synovitis** of the dorsal joint capsule often results from repeated overextension of the fetlock joint in the racehorse. At the point of maximum extension, the *proximodorsal margin of the proximal phalanx traumatizes the synovial pad* covering the dorsal surface of the distal end of the cannon bone. In response to constant trauma, the fibrous pad becomes enlarged because of hyperemia, edema, and fibroplasia, and extends across the adjacent dorsal articular margin of the cannon bone. Degeneration of the underlying articular cartilage occurs as a result of impaired access to synovial fluid and release of inflammatory mediators from the inflamed synovium. In cases where the inflammation resolves and the synovial pad retracts, the degenerate, pitted articular surface remains as evidence. The histologic features of these lesions vary with their duration. In the subacute stages, they include a mixture of hemosiderin-containing macrophages and well-ordered granulation tissue. Chronic lesions consist of dense, poorly vascularized fibrous tissue infiltrated by mononuclear inflammatory cells and covered by a layer of synoviocytes.

Another common change involving the metacarpophalangeal joint in performance horses is the *formation of a periarticular lip along the dorsal articular margin of the proximal phalanx*. With repeated trauma, microscopic or macroscopic chip fractures may develop in the bony support of the lip. The repair of such fractures is often compromised by the continued trauma of racing or training, and loosened chip fractures, attached to the adjacent bone by granulation tissue, may cause synovitis and acute clinical signs.

In racehorses, foci of subchondral bone lysis and collapse occur on the palmar articular surface of the condyle of the cannon bone (Fig. 2-192). This lesion was once called traumatic osteochondrosis, but it is thought to be an acquired lesion caused

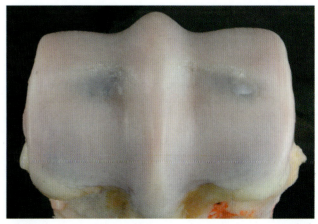

Figure 2-192 Subchondral bone lysis in an equine distal cannon bone. There are 2 blue-gray depressed foci of bone lysis and collapse of the articular surface. These lesions are caused by repetitive overload trauma rather than osteochondrosis. (Courtesy C.M. Riggs.)

by repetitive overload trauma, rather than a developmental lesion. There is also an association between development of this lesion and other lesions of degenerative joint disease, such as linear wear lines and cartilage erosion.

Transverse ridge arthrosis *is a degenerative lesion involving the transverse ridge of the condyle of the cannon bone, particularly in the foreleg.* The lesions vary from mild fibrillation to the development of deep ulcers extending into the underlying bone. The transverse ridge develops between the dorsal articular surface of the condyle, which articulates with the proximal phalanx, and the palmar surface of the condyle, which articulates with the proximal sesamoid bones. If the fetlock joint is overextended during racing, the base of the proximal sesamoid bone over-rides the transverse ridge, exposing it to shearing forces and eventually leading to degeneration.

Degenerative diseases of **interphalangeal joints** are commonly referred to as **ringbone**. *High* or *low* ringbone refers to involvement of the *proximal (pastern)* or *distal (coffin) interphalangeal joints*, respectively. The condition is most common in the forelimbs of older horses and is related to joint instability secondary to traumatic injuries, repeated episodes of minor trauma from athletic activity, or mechanical stresses associated with faulty conformation. The condition may also be caused by fractures or osteochondrosis, which more commonly affect the hindlimbs.

The severity of the articular and periarticular lesions of high ringbone varies markedly between individuals. In the *early stages of the disease*, affected joints may be partly immobilized by fibrous thickening of the dorsal joint capsule, and there may be early cartilage degeneration of one or both condyles of the distal first phalanx and the apposed glenoid cavity of the proximal second phalanx. The periarticular response, which includes fibrous thickening of the dorsal joint capsule and bone formation beginning in the joint capsule insertion line, is much more prominent than the cartilaginous changes. *The periarticular bony response on the dorsal surface of the joint gives the lesion its name.* In *advanced lesions*, full-thickness necrosis of the articular cartilage, followed by erosions in the subchondral bony plate, may lead to *ankylosis*. In cases where there is residual joint motion, there is eburnation of the articular surfaces, thickening of the subchondral bony plates, and inhibition of ankylosis.

Degenerative disease of the distal interphalangeal (coffin) joint or low ringbone has a similar pathogenesis as high ringbone. The periarticular osteophytes result in a ring of bone just above the coronary band. The most severe cases are due to fracture of the extensor process of the distal phalanx.

Spavin is a term for degenerative joint disease of the **tarsal joint** of horses. Early lesions involving only soft tissues are termed *bog spavin* (excess synovial fluid), *blind spavin*, or *jack spavin*. Once bony lesions are radiographically or grossly visible, the condition is *true* or *bone spavin*. The *major lesions develop on the medial side of the tarsus*, primarily involving the distal intertarsal joint and, less commonly, the tarsometatarsal and proximal intertarsal joints. Early lesions show full-thickness necrosis of the apposed cartilage surfaces and intense bone remodeling within the thickened subchondral bony plate. Intermediate lesions show penetration of the necrotic cartilage by granulation tissue from the areas of intense subchondral bone remodeling. As the lesion progresses, granulation tissue extends across the joint space through areas of necrotic cartilage and establishes a *fibrous ankylosis*, which later gives way to a more stable *bony ankylosis*.

Navicular syndrome is a common and controversial degenerative disorder of the distal sesamoid or navicular bone. There is a navicular bursa between the navicular bone and the deep digital flexor tendon that is normally lined with synoviocytes; this bursa forms a synovial joint-like space between the 2 structures. The lesions of the navicular bone are similar to those in diarthrodial joints, that is, loss of cartilage and subchondral bone along with periarticular osteophytes. The lesions in the deep digital flexor tendon can progress to granulation tissue and fibrosis, which results in adhesions to and lysis of the subchondral bone (Fig. 2-193). The resorptive process follows the pathway of the nutrient arteries into the medullary cavity of the distal border of the navicular bone, creating deep synovial invaginations that are recognized on radiographs as enlarged vascular channels. The forelimbs are most often affected, and the lesions are typically bilateral. The pathogenesis of the disease is not completely understood, but both the shape of the navicular bone and the angle of the hoof contribute, and both are heritable.

Primary and secondary **degenerative joint diseases of dogs** are relatively common, particularly medium and large breeds, and usually involving the major weight-bearing joints. Secondary degenerative joint disease in dogs most often occurs as a sequel to joint instability or incongruity owing to chondrodystrophy, dysplastic diseases of the hip and elbow, or to the various manifestations of osteochondrosis.

Primary degenerative joint disease is sufficiently common in aged dogs to be regarded by many as an *inevitable consequence of aging.* Gross lesions are often found incidentally at postmortem examination in animals that had shown no clinical evidence of lameness. In one study, 31 (21%) of 150 randomly selected dogs had degenerative lesions in the stifle joint at autopsy. In 23 of these dogs, the lesions were bilateral. Degenerative joint disease of the shoulder and hip joints are

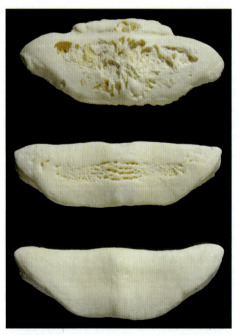

Figure 2-193 Navicular bones from 3 different horses. The bottom navicular bone is normal. The center bone has moderate osteolysis of the flexor surface. The top navicular bone has severe osteolysis of the flexor surface.

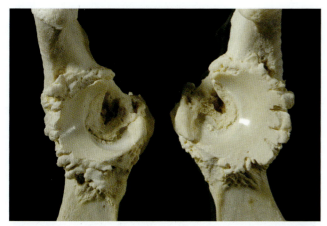

Figure 2-194 **Degenerative joint disease** in the acetabula of a dog. Osteophytes encircle the articular surface, which is shiny and polished by eburnation.

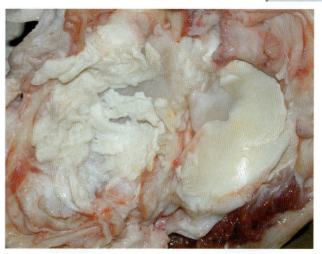

Figure 2-195 **Degenerative joint disease** in an ox. Proximal tibia with shredding of medial meniscus.

also common in middle-aged and old dogs. The lesions are usually bilateral and develop slowly, starting at around 5-6 years of age, as areas of softening and yellow discoloration on regions of articular cartilage subjected to maximum weight-bearing stress; the lesions then progress to fibrillation (see Fig. 2-184) and sometimes eburnation. Osteophytes frequently line the chondro-osseous junction and may encircle the articular surface (Fig. 2-194). In severe cases, the joint capsule is thickened and synovial villi are hypertrophic.

Degenerative joint disease of the *shoulder joint* is common (see Fig. 2-184) and may be related to joint laxity. In one study, 74% of adult dogs had gross cartilage lesions of the humeral head at postmortem examination. Shoulder lesions of primary degenerative joint disease may be difficult to distinguish from osteochondrosis, especially in the advanced stages. Both typically affect the caudal aspect of the humeral head, and both are generally bilateral. However, as described earlier in this chapter, osteochondrosis develops at a much earlier age, and although healed lesions of osteochondrosis may be found incidentally in older dogs, the majority of caudal humeral head lesions in adult dogs are due to degenerative joint disease and not osteochondrosis.

Degenerative joint disease of cats is much less common than in dogs. The shoulder, elbows, hips, and tarsal joints are most commonly affected. In radiographic surveys, 61% of cats >5 years of age have degenerative joint disease, and 90% of those >11 years of age do. Siamese cats with worse than expected degenerative joint disease of the shoulders and stifles should be screened for mucopolysaccharidosis VI; >10% of Siamese cats carry the D520N mutation that causes only mild disease, but which can lead to a high incidence of degenerative joint disease.

Degenerative joint disease of cattle is likely more common than is realized. Degenerative joint disease of the *stifle joint* occurs in mature dairy cows and is reported as a *possible inherited trait in Holsteins and Jerseys*. Clinical signs include lameness and muscle atrophy. The lesions are bilateral and appear to develop in the conventional manner. Cartilage degeneration, erosion, eburnation, and osteophyte formation occur on the distal femur and are most severe on the medial aspect. Complementary lesions are present in the proximal tibia, and shredding of the medial meniscus is common (Fig. 2-195). *Stifle arthropathy also occurs in stud dairy and beef bulls* and may be secondary to poor conformation, ligament damage, a ruptured meniscus, or as a consequence of osteochondrosis. The latter may be an important cause of wastage of well-grown beef bulls that have been fed for optimal growth before sale or showing.

Further reading

Barr ED, et al. Postmortem evaluation of palmar osteochondral disease (traumatic osteochondrosis) of the metacarpo/metatarsophalangeal joint in Thoroughbred horses. Eq Vet J 2009;41:366-371.

Craig LE, Reed A. Age-associated cartilage degeneration of the canine humeral head. Vet Pathol 2013;50:264-268.

Crawley AC, et al. Prevalence of mucopolysaccharidosis type VI mutations in Siamese cats. J Vet Intern Med 2003;17:495-498.

Slingerland LI, et al. Cross-sectional study of the prevalence and clinical features of osteoarthritis in 100 cats. Vet J 2011;187:304-309.

Cartilaginous joints

The most important degenerative diseases of cartilaginous joints are those affecting *intervertebral disks*. Such diseases are of particular importance in humans and dogs but are rare in other species. **Degeneration of intervertebral disks** occurs in all dog breeds as part of the aging process, but there are significant differences between chondrodystrophic and nonchondrodystrophic breeds in the nature of the degeneration and the age at which it occurs.

Chondrodystrophic breeds, such as the Dachshund, Pekingese, Corgi, and Basset Hound are defined by an expressed fibroblast growth factor 4 *(fgf4)* retrogene that affects the length and curvature of their legs, as well as the composition of their nucleus pulposus. In affected breeds, the nucleus pulposus contains up to 12 times more collagen than proteoglycan. The collagen composition increases rapidly with maturity and by 11 months of age averages 25%. In nonchondrodystrophic breeds, the collagen content of intervertebral disks remains <5% for most of the animal's life (Fig. 2-196A). At all ages, the proteoglycan content of the intervertebral disk in chondrodystrophic breeds is significantly less than that of nonchondrodystrophic breeds. In chondrodystrophic breeds, the nucleus pulposus starts to degenerate early in life, and by

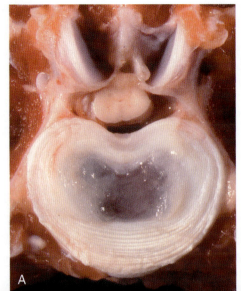

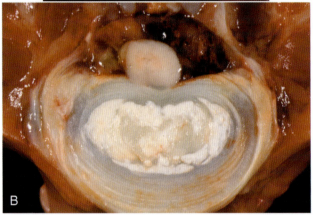

Figure 2-196 **Intervertebral disks** from dogs. **A. Normal** translucent gelatinous nucleus pulposus surrounded by annulus fibrosus. **B.** Degeneration and chalky white mineralization of the nucleus pulposus of a chondrodystrophic dog. (A and B, Courtesy R.A. Fairley.)

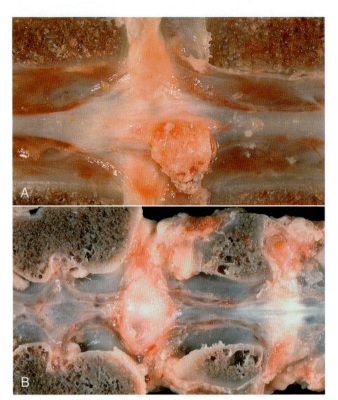

Figure 2-197 Intervertebral disk herniation. **A.** Hansen type I herniation of a crumbly mass of degenerate disk material into the spinal canal through a tear in the dorsal longitudinal ligament. **B.** Hansen type II herniation causing the dorsal longitudinal ligament to bulge into the spinal canal.

1 year of age, it has become largely replaced by dry, gray/white or yellow, cartilaginous material. The initial microscopic change is thickening of the delicate fibrocartilaginous septa between cellular clusters, dividing the nucleus pulposus into lobules. Chondrocyte proliferation within the nucleus leads to *replacement of the original structure with chondroid tissue* within the first year of life. No lesions are apparent in the annulus fibrosus at this stage. The change in the nucleus pulposus in chondrodystrophic dogs *occurs in all disks* throughout the length of the vertebral column and is accompanied by a decline in the glycosaminoglycan and water content, and an increase in the collagen content of the matrix. Beginning at the periphery, *the chondroid tissue in the nucleus pulposus degenerates and mineralizes*, eventually becoming a friable mass (Fig. 2-196B). At this stage, there is *degeneration of the inner lamellae of the annulus fibrosus*, probably because of the altered viscoelastic properties of the degenerate nucleus pulposus. Individual lamellae may tear and allow degenerate nuclear material to escape into the annulus. Meanwhile, degeneration of the annulus fibrosus continues until the outer lamellae are also involved.

These mineralized, friable intervertebral disks in chondrodystrophic breeds are predisposed to Hansen **type I intervertebral disk herniations,** *which are characterized by a massive extrusion of degenerate nuclear material through the annulus fibrosus and dorsal longitudinal ligament into the spinal canal* (Fig. 2-197A). The sudden compression of the spinal cord and/or peripheral nerve roots typically causes *acute pain, paresis,* or *paralysis,* depending on the volume of extruded material and its location. Extradural hemorrhage may accompany laceration of longitudinal venous sinuses in the spinal canal. In some cases, severe damage to the spinal cord or its vascular supply results in *extensive hemorrhagic myelomalacia and ascending syndrome.* More commonly, the myelomalacia remains localized to a few cord segments. *The irritant nuclear material induces an inflammatory reaction* within the spinal canal and may become adhered to the dura. Type I herniations of intervertebral disks are largely confined to chondrodystrophic dogs, particularly Dachshunds, and generally occur between 3 and 7 years of age. Increased chance of disk herniation in Dachshunds is associated with shorter leg and spine length, which are indicators of the severity of their chondrodystrophy. The appearance of a long back in chondrodystrophic breeds is an optical illusion created by their relatively short legs; it does not contribute to the pathogenesis of intervertebral disk extrusion.

In **nonchondrodystrophic dogs,** *the normal mucoid nature of the nucleus pulposus persists, at least until middle age,* and although it may become dry and more fibrous with advancing age, it seldom mineralizes. Occasionally, fibrous metaplasia of the nucleus pulposus occurs in relatively young dogs of nonchondrodystrophic breeds, but such changes are believed to be secondary to *focal disruption of lamellae in the annulus fibrosus,* presumably as a result of trauma. In support of this belief is the observation that these lesions are *generally confined to a single disk,* unlike the generalized changes that occur in the nucleus pulposus of chondrodystrophic dogs. Traumatic damage to the annulus fibrosus would be expected to alter the biomechanical properties of the entire disk, leading to adaptive, and eventually degenerative, changes in the nucleus pulposus.

Nonchondrodystrophic breeds are more likely to have Hansen **type II herniations,** which generally develop slowly and are characterized by *partial herniation of the nucleus pulposus through ruptured annular fibers,* eventually resulting in bulging of outer lamellae and the intact dorsal longitudinal ligament into the spinal canal (Fig. 2-197B). Damage to the cord or peripheral nerve roots is less than in type I herniations, and clinical signs may be milder. Type II herniations are usually seen in nonchondrodystrophic dogs between 6 and 8 years of age but can occur in any breed, as well as in humans, cats, and occasionally other species. Type I herniations can also occur in nonchondrodystrophic dogs.

Because of the eccentric location of the nucleus pulposus within the annulus fibrosus, most herniations occur through the narrower dorsal or dorsolateral regions of the annulus. In fact, dorsal herniation of disk material into the spinal canal is considered the most common cause of paresis or paralysis in dogs. Ventral herniation also occurs and may predispose to spondylosis (see later); on rare occasions, nuclear material may herniate through the cranial or caudal cartilaginous end plate into a vertebral body, forming a so-called *"Schmorl's node."*

Disk protrusions occur most frequently at sites of greatest vertebral mobility. In dogs, 70% of clinical cases of intervertebral disk herniations occur between the 12th thoracic and 2nd lumbar vertebrae. Approximately 15% of cases occur in the cervical region. Neurologic signs associated with cervical disk protrusions are usually less severe than those involving the thoracolumbar region because the cervical cord occupies comparatively less space in the spinal canal, allowing more room for displacement before compressive damage occurs.

In **horses,** the nucleus pulposus is more fibrous than that of dogs, and its demarcation from the annulus fibrosus is less distinct. Although the nucleus pulposus of horses becomes less cellular with age, no chondroid or fibrous metaplasia occurs. Herniations of intervertebral disks are *rare in horses* but occasionally are reported in the *cervical region.* Furthermore, in one study of cervical intervertebral disks in 17 clinically normal horses, partial extrusion of nuclear material through the annulus fibrosus, similar to type II lesions in dogs, was detected histologically in 5 horses. No intervertebral disk herniations have been reported in the thoracolumbar region of horses, probably because of the relative inflexibility of the equine spine in comparison to dogs and humans, and the strong longitudinal ligaments supporting the spine in this species. The mechanism of the cervical herniations in horses is not clear, but traumatic damage to the disk or adjacent vertebrae is a likely possibility, at least in some cases. In *cats,* macroscopic signs of intervertebral disk degeneration are not apparent until old age, if then. Degenerative changes similar to those occurring in nonchondrodystrophic dogs are described in *adult sows and boars,* but dorsal herniation of the nucleus pulposus into the spinal canal has not been reported in swine.

Spondylosis

Spondylosis (spondylosis deformans, ankylosing spondylosis, ventral bridging spondylosis) is a common degenerative disease of the vertebral column; it is characterized by the formation of osteophytes at the ventral and lateral margins of vertebral bodies adjacent to intervertebral spaces. The osteophytes may appear as spurs growing toward the adjacent vertebral body or as complete bony bridges with fusion of vertebrae (Fig. 2-198). Osteophytes may also be found dorsolaterally, projecting into the vertebral canal, but these are small and uncommon. In some cases, spondylosis is accompanied by degeneration of the synovial joints of the articular facets, and the reactive osteophytes may produce concurrent ankylosis of these articulations.

The *pathogenesis* of spondylosis is believed to involve a *degenerative change in the ventral annulus fibrosus.* Separation or tearing of the collagenous attachment of the annulus fibrosus from the adjacent vertebral body predisposes to mild ventral displacement of the annulus fibrosus and stretching of the ventral longitudinal ligament. This induces formation of bony outgrowths or spurs at the ventral margin of the intervertebral disk. As the disease progresses, further displacement of the annulus fibrosus and stretching of the ventral longitudinal ligament leads to more extensive osteophyte formation and eventually to bony bridging of the intervertebral space.

Spondylosis occurs most frequently in bulls, rams, pigs, and dogs. It is important in **bulls** kept in artificial breeding centers, where it is presumably related to repeated traumatic damage to intervertebral disks during semen collection; *lesions are found in almost any bull past middle age.* Osteophytes develop mainly on the caudal end of thoracic vertebrae and the cranial end of lumbar vertebrae, and their incidence and size tend to decrease in either direction from the thoracolumbar junction. The greatest number and size of osteophytes is therefore in the area of greatest spinal curvature, where maximum pressure on the disks during the thrust of service would be expected. The sequence of osteophyte development begins with degeneration of the annulus fibrosus, which may be present in bulls as young as 2 years of age. The osteophytes develop first in the outer annulus fibrosus and at its insertion to the rim of the vertebra. Growth is also caused in part by periosteal apposition and osseous metaplasia of ligaments. The trabecular bone of the osteophytes becomes continuous with that of the vertebral body and eventually is densely sclerotic. A thick layer of bone may be deposited along the ventral and

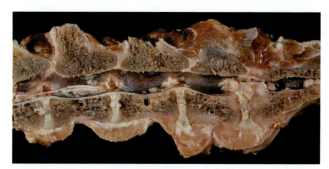

Figure 2-198 Ankylosing spondylosis of the lumbar vertebrae in a dog. Fusion of adjacent vertebral bodies by bridging osteophytes formed ventral to the intervertebral disks.

ventrolateral aspects of the vertebral bodies. In late stages, the heads of many ribs and the articular processes of the vertebrae bear large irregular osteophytes, which frequently cause ankylosis of the corresponding joint.

Although spondylosis is a *common incidental finding in breeding bulls and rams, the disease is sometimes associated with clinical signs.* Affected bulls may show caudal weakness and ataxia, or even paralysis, after dismounting from service. They may continue to be mildly ataxic or recover, only to be affected again later. The onset of signs is usually associated with fracture of the vertebral bodies and of the ankylosing new bone, which is dense, but brittle. The line of fracture tends to follow a large penetrating vessel to the intervertebral disk, which is frequently separated, and then to diverge across the dorsal corner of one or other vertebra. There is little displacement of the fractured ends in most cases, which accounts for the incomplete spinal syndrome. Trauma to the spinal cord is usually mild, and paralysis is usually secondary to either hemorrhage or repeated trauma.

Spondylosis is common in cull **rams,** where it affects the thoracic vertebrae more than the lumbar. Lesions are most common between T10 and T11. Degeneration and necrosis in the ventral annulus fibrosus are the most common microscopic findings.

In **dogs**, the incidence of spondylosis increases with age after about the fifth year, and *vertebral osteophytes are a common incidental finding during radiography or at postmortem examination.* As in bulls, the primary morphologic change in dogs and cats with spondylosis is in the *annulus fibrosus.* In dogs, most lesions occur in the region of the first and second lumbar vertebrae, an area of relatively high mobility. The lumbosacral articulation is also often involved. Clinical signs are often absent but can include stiffness and back pain. A similar but more severe condition termed *diffuse idiopathic skeletal hyperostosis (DISH)* has also been described in dogs. This condition differs from spondylosis in that the ventral bridging ossification occurs without disk degeneration or herniation. There is "flowing" ossification along the ventral longitudinal ligament involving at least 4 contiguous vertebrae. In humans, the condition also involves the appendicular skeleton (tendons, ligaments, and joint capsules), but this aspect has not been described in dogs.

Ankylosing spondylosis is a relatively common incidental finding in adult **pigs**. Although no specific predisposing factors have been identified, degenerate intervertebral disks or narrow disk spaces are often associated with the lesions. The osteophytes most commonly involve *lumbar vertebrae*, especially those in the lumbosacral region. Ankylosis, if present, may be confined to the ventral aspect of the vertebral bodies, but in some cases, there is extensive new bone formation in the vertebral arches, thus fusing the articular processes and encroaching on the spinal canal.

Spondylosis in *horses* is comparable to that in other species, but the evolution of the osteophytes has not been studied in detail. Vertebral ankylosis in *cats* with chronic vitamin A toxicity is discussed elsewhere.

Further reading

Kranenburg HC, et al. Diffuse idiopathic skeletal hyperostosis (DISH) and spondylosis deformans in purebred dogs: a retrospective study. Vet J 2011;190:84-90.

Levine JM, et al. Association between various physical factors and acute thoracolumbar intervertebral disk extrusion or protrusion in Dachshunds. J Am Vet Med Assoc 2006;229:370-375.

Orbell GMB, et al. Severity and distribution of ventral thoracolumbar spondylosis and histological assessment of associated intervertebral disc degeneration in cull rams. N Z Vet J 2007;55:297-301.

Parker HG, et al. An expressed fgf4 retrogene is associated with breed-defining chondrodysplasia in domestic dogs. Science 2009;325:995-998.

INFLAMMATORY DISEASES OF JOINTS

Inflammatory diseases of joints are generally referred to as either **arthritis** or **synovitis**. Although these terms are sometimes used interchangeably, they have slightly different meanings. Synovitis refers to inflammation of the synovial membrane, whereas arthritis implies inflammation of other joint components in addition to the synovial membrane. Inflammation of tendon sheaths often accompanies inflammation of an adjacent synovial joint and is referred to as **tenosynovitis**. Secondary inflammation occasionally follows chronic degenerative joint diseases, hence the commonly used term osteoarthritis, but in this section discussion will be confined to joint diseases that are primarily inflammatory in origin.

Arthritis may be either *infectious or noninfectious. Infectious arthritis occurs most frequently in farmed livestock and horses*, especially in young animals, in which it commonly affects the carpal and tarsal joints as a sequel to neonatal bacteremia. Most cases of noninfectious arthritis occur in dogs and cats and are immune mediated.

Fibrinous arthritis

Fibrinous arthritis is typical of many *acute inflammatory diseases* of synovial joints, particularly those caused by *bacterial infections*. The presence of fibrin within synovial fluid indicates increased permeability of blood vessels in the synovial membrane, as fibrinogen and other large molecules are normally excluded. *Fibrin clots* may be floating free within the joint fluid, attached to the synovial membrane, or lodged within recesses of the joint (Fig. 2-199). In some cases, sheets of yellow fibrin partially or completely cover the synovial membrane, which is often edematous and hyperemic or may be studded with petechiae. *Synovial villi*, which are barely noticeable in normal joints, may become prominent macroscopically because of edema and hyperemia. The synovial fluid is increased in volume and is usually slightly turbid. When the inflammatory reaction is severe, there may be gross edema of the periarticular tissues. At this early stage, microscopic changes in the synovial membrane consist of edema and vascular engorgement, with few inflammatory cells. Serous fluid or serofibrinous exudate often infiltrate the fibrous layer of the articular capsule and the adjacent periarticular tissue.

In arthritis of longer duration, edema of synovial tissues is less apparent, but the joint capsule and synovial membrane are thickened because of proliferation of stromal cells and synoviocytes, the latter often becoming several layers thick. Sheets of fibrin containing variable numbers of neutrophils and fibroblasts may be attached to the surface. Villi continue to enlarge as a result of cellular proliferation and may become extensively branched, with increasing numbers of

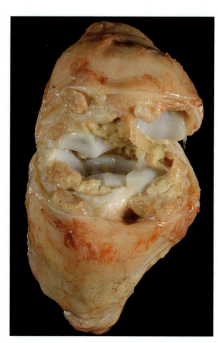

Figure 2-199 **Fibrinous arthritis** in the carpus of a calf. Abundant yellow fibrin fills the recesses of the joint. The articular cartilage is smooth and unaffected.

lymphocytes and plasma cells, but few neutrophils. Extravasated neutrophils pass quickly into the synovial fluid but seldom in sufficient numbers to give the fluid a purulent character. *Hypertrophy of villi* is greatest in the transition zone, and the proliferating fibrous stroma is joined by proliferating perichondrium to produce a fringe of granulation tissue, which can spread across the articular cartilage as a pannus and cause degeneration of the underlying cartilage.

Early resolution of infection with fibrinous arthritis is common, especially in smaller joints. However, the extensive deposits of fibrin in severe cases cannot be effectively removed by fibrinolytic mechanisms. Instead, the fibrin, which is deposited on the synovial membrane and within the layers of the articular capsule and periarticular tissue, is progressively invaded by fibrous tissue, leading to enlargement and restricted movement of affected joints. The synovial lining is repaired by proliferation of synoviocytes. *Articular cartilage generally remains intact* in fibrinous arthritis, except in areas where it is covered by pannus. Pannus formation in joints with restricted movement may result in adhesions between apposed articular surfaces, leading to ankylosis.

Low-grade inflammation, with intense lymphocytosis, may persist in the synovial membrane, even in cases where the infection has apparently resolved. This may be due to either the persistence of an infectious agent that cannot be cultured or ineffective removal of the peptidoglycan components of microbial cell walls by macrophages. For example, the cell wall of group A streptococci is relatively resistant to degradation by mammalian lysosomal enzymes, and is capable of provoking *persistent inflammation* in synovial tissues. Cell-wall peptidoglycans from various other organisms, including *Erysipelothrix rhusiopathiae*, also have this ability. All bacterial cell walls contain peptidoglycans, but there is considerable structural heterogeneity among bacterial species, and the types of side chains on the molecules probably determine their arthritogenic potential.

Purulent (suppurative) arthritis

This type of arthritis is characterized by the presence of *significant numbers of neutrophils in the synovial fluid, synovial membrane, and sometimes in adjacent structures*. When caused by bacterial infection, the neutrophils are usually abundant and may show *degenerative changes* in cytologic preparations of joint fluid. This is often referred to as **septic arthritis**. Neutrophilic inflammation is a feature of arthritis caused by *Mycoplasma* spp., *Borrelia burgdorferi*, and certain viruses, but in these infections, the neutrophils in synovial fluid are *nondegenerate*. Noninfectious, *immune-mediated arthritis* is also characterized by the presence of viable neutrophils in synovial fluid, and differentiation from infectious arthritis is often difficult. *Bacteria are seldom detected in synovial fluid of animals with septic arthritis, and false negatives on bacterial culture are common.*

Septic arthritis is often monoarticular and is *potentially a much more destructive process than fibrinous arthritis*. The synovial fluid is initially thin and cloudy but may resemble frank pus after a few days. *Destruction of articular cartilage* is much more likely to occur in septic arthritis than in fibrinous arthritis. *Lysosomal enzymes*, particularly collagenase, released from neutrophils probably play an important role in cartilage destruction. Cytokines of macrophage origin, such as interleukin-1 and tumor necrosis factor-α, have also been shown to induce the resorption of cartilage both in vitro and in vivo and are most likely involved in chondrocyte-mediated cartilage degradation by stimulating the synthesis of metalloproteinases and plasminogen activators.

Complete resolution of septic arthritis is possible if the infection is eliminated spontaneously or by antibiotic therapy before erosion of cartilage occurs, but if the inflammatory process persists, the joint and adjacent structures will be severely altered. Cartilage degeneration occurs mainly at sites of weight bearing or at the articular margins, the latter in association with pannus formation. *Erosion of the degenerate cartilage may allow infection to enter the subchondral bone, resulting in purulent osteomyelitis* with extensive separation of the articular cartilage. In such cases, it may be difficult to determine whether the arthritis preceded the osteomyelitis or vice versa, or whether the infectious agent gained access to both sites independently. Granulation tissue originating in the subchondral bone may grow over the degenerate articular surface and predispose to ankylosis.

The suppurative process may extend to involve adjacent tendon sheaths and outward from the synovial membrane of the articular capsule to produce cellulitis in periarticular tissues (Fig. 2-200). The joint region is then greatly enlarged, and the proliferation of fibrous tissue in response to inflammation, or during the healing process, results in permanent joint stiffness. In some cases, localization of cellulitis into a periarticular abscess may be followed by fistulation to the skin. Fistulation to the skin surface may also result directly from empyema of the joint. Adhesions between tendons and tendon sheaths frequently occur in cases where tenosynovitis has developed in association with septic arthritis.

Although it is convenient to classify inflammatory diseases of joints as fibrinous or purulent, in reality, many are **fibrinopurulent arthritis** because the exudate consists of both fibrin and neutrophils. In the chronic stages of many infectious and noninfectious forms of arthritis, lymphocytes and/or plasma cells are the major cell types infiltrating the synovial membrane. In such cases, **lymphocytic/plasmacytic synovitis**

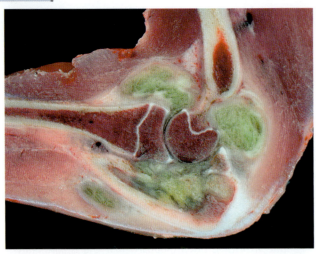

Figure 2-200 Suppurative arthritis in a lamb. Suppurative exudate fills the elbow joint and extends into the surrounding tendon sheaths and soft tissue. There is suppurative osteomyelitis of the proximal ulna.

is a more appropriate morphologic diagnosis. The term **proliferative arthritis** is often used to describe *chronic inflammatory diseases of joints where hypertrophy and hyperplasia of synovial villi are prominent features.*

An accurate etiologic diagnosis in animals with inflammatory diseases of joints may be crucial to a successful clinical outcome. In particular, failure to differentiate infectious and noninfectious causes of purulent arthritis can lead to inappropriate treatment and significantly alter the prognosis. *It is also important for septic arthritis to be recognized early and treated appropriately to prevent degeneration of articular cartilage.* In addition to clinical history, analysis of synovial fluid often provides useful information but seldom allows a definitive diagnosis. Many infectious and noninfectious forms of arthritis are characterized by increased numbers of neutrophils in synovial fluid. The neutrophils may show degenerative changes in bacterial infections, but this is often difficult to appreciate in synovial fluid where the high concentration of hyaluronan prevents the cells from flattening on the slide. Furthermore, not all bacteria induce such changes in neutrophils. Culture of bacteria or other agents from an inflamed joint allows a definitive diagnosis, but false negatives are common. Use of blood culture medium enrichment may improve the sensitivity of synovial culture. Broad-range 16S rRNA gene PCR is also useful for detecting microorganisms within synovial fluid or tissues. Microscopic examination of synovial membrane biopsies provides information on the nature of the inflammatory response and may be useful in differentiating chronic inflammatory and degenerative diseases of joints.

Infectious arthritis

This section is limited to inflammatory lesions of the joint(s) in which a live organism is present. A variety of infectious agents, including *bacteria, viruses, and fungi,* are capable of infecting diarthrodial joints in humans and domestic animals. *In many, if not most situations, the arthritis is but one manifestation of a systemic infection,* with inflammatory lesions involving several tissues. In other cases, the infection may appear to be confined to one or more joints, suggesting either an affinity for synovial membranes or persistence of the infection in joints after being cleared from other sites.

A list of microorganisms that are commonly associated with infectious arthritis in domestic animals is presented in Box 2-2. Many agents other than those included in the list are capable of causing arthritis but usually in isolated cases. Cats are not included in the list because infectious arthritis in this species is rare.

Some generalizations may be made about the prevalence of these infections relative to age. In *sheep,* with the exception of infection by *Mycoplasma* spp., infectious arthritis is primarily a disease of lambs. In *cattle,* streptococcal and coliform polyarthritis are neonatal, whereas infections caused by *Trueperella pyogenes* and *Salmonella* spp. may occur at any age. Streptococcal polyarthritis in *swine* is often a neonatal disease, but the other infections usually occur in weaned pigs. In *horses,* the organisms listed, other than *Salmonella* spp., generally cause intrauterine or neonatal infections.

Bacterial arthritis

Bacterial arthritis is common in horses and food animals, usually as a sequel to neonatal bacteremia following omphalophlebitis ("navel ill"), or infections of the gastrointestinal tract or lungs. In many cases, the origin of the infection is not apparent either clinically or at postmortem examination, but inadequate transfer of colostral immunoglobulins is a common predisposing factor. The richly vascular synovial membrane appears to be a favored site for localization of blood-borne bacteria. Experimental studies have shown that viable bacteria injected intravenously lodge in the synovial membrane and gain access to synovial fluid more readily than to spinal fluid, aqueous humor, or urine.

Hematogenous bacterial infections in neonatal animals typically cause *polyarthritis.* Infected joints are generally hot, painful, and swollen because of the hyperemia and edema of the synovial membrane and joint capsule, and the increased quantity of synovial fluid. Although the infection may resolve in some joints, it often persists in others, particularly the large joints of the limbs, causing severe septic arthritis with destruction of articular cartilage. *Many, if not most young animals with septic arthritis of hematogenous origin also have osteomyelitis in the adjacent bones.* This may be due to concurrent localization of the organism in the bone and synovial membrane, or it may reflect the close vascular relationship between the epiphyseal bone and synovial membrane in young animals, with spread of infection from one site to the other. Foci of osteomyelitis originating at sites of endochondral ossification in the epiphysis, immediately beneath the articular cartilage, may under-run and penetrate the cartilage, spreading the infection directly into the synovial fluid. In joints where the capsule attaches beyond the physis, inflammatory foci in the metaphysis may contaminate the synovial fluid by penetrating the cortex near the physeal margin. This region is relatively porous in young animals because of the intense structural modeling that occurs in the metaphyseal cortex during rapid growth. The prevalence of concurrent bone involvement should always be considered in animals with bacterial arthritis, because even if the arthritis can be successfully treated, the animal may eventually succumb to the effects of chronic osteomyelitis.

The reason certain organisms are more likely to localize in the synovial membrane than others during bacteremia is not clear, but experimental evidence suggests that it is not purely

> **BOX • 2-2**
>
> ### Common causes of infectious arthritis in domestic animals
>
> **Sheep**
> - Chlamydophila pecorum
> - Erysipelothrix rhusiopathiae
> - Escherichia coli
> - Histophilus somni
> - Mycoplasma spp.
> - Staphylococcus aureus
> - Streptococcus spp.
>
> **Goats**
> - Mycoplasma spp.
> - Caprine arthritis-encephalitis virus
>
> **Swine**
> - Actinobacillus suis
> - Brucella suis
> - Erysipelothrix rhusiopathiae
> - Escherichia coli
> - Haemophilus parasuis
> - Mycoplasma spp.
> - Salmonella spp.
> - Staphylococcus aureus
> - Staphylococcus hyicus subsp. hyicus
> - Streptococcus spp.
> - Streptococcus suis
> - Trueperella pyogenes
>
> **Cattle**
> - Chlamydophila pecorum
> - Escherichia coli
> - Histophilus somni
> - Mycoplasma bovis
> - Salmonella spp.
> - Streptococcus spp.
> - Trueperella pyogenes
>
> **Horses**
> - Actinobacillus equuli
> - Escherichia coli
> - Klebsiella spp.
> - Rhodococcus equi
> - Salmonella spp.
> - Streptococcus spp.
>
> **Dogs**
> - Blastomyces dermatitidis
> - Borrelia burgdorferi
> - Ehrlichia ewingii
> - Escherichia coli
> - Staphylococcus spp.
> - Streptococcus spp.

Spread of infection to joints from adjacent soft tissues is uncommon because the dense, fibrous layer of the joint capsule provides an effective barrier, but spread may occur in necrotizing disorders such as necrobacillosis and footrot in cattle.

Direct implantation of bacteria into a synovial joint may occur as a sequel to a *penetrating wound* from the skin surface. This is the most common cause of bacterial arthritis in *dogs and cats*, where the disease occurs more often in adolescent and adult animals than in neonates. The arthritis is *monoarticular*, and a mixed population of opportunistic bacteria is likely to be involved, often resulting in a highly destructive inflammatory response. Surgery or collection of synovial fluid may also introduce bacteria to a joint.

Although many different bacteria have been associated with arthritis in domestic animals, some specific types of bacterial arthritis are sufficiently important to warrant discussion in more detail.

Erysipelas. *Erysipelothrix rhusiopathiae*, the cause of porcine erysipelas and erysipeloid in humans, is a gram-positive bacillus with a wide geographic distribution and host range. It causes outbreaks of disease in pigs, lambs, and birds, and sporadic disease in the other domestic species. The organism is widespread in nature and is capable of survival, and perhaps growth, in decaying material of animal origin. It may be present in the soil of pig pens and in pit slurry, and survives for 2-3 weeks on pasture spread with slurry. It is resistant to many disinfectants and is capable of infecting many species, some of them in epidemic proportions. In spite of these epidemiologic features, *pigs are probably the principal source of infection for other pigs*. E. rhusiopathiae can persist for many months in the lesions of diseased pigs, and it is often carried in the tonsils, intestine, bone marrow, and gall bladder of healthy swine.

Porcine erysipelas occurs in pigs of all ages, but the most susceptible are pregnant sows and pigs 2-12 months of age. The disease can be produced by ingestion of the organism, contamination of cutaneous wounds, or as a result of bites of infected flies. The manifestations of erysipelas in pigs vary from an *acute septicemic form*, which is usually fatal, to *mild and chronic forms* characterized by necrosis of the skin, endocarditis, and polyarthritis. *In epidemics, the septicemic form predominates, whereas in endemic areas, the disease tends to be sporadic, with cases of septicemia, polyarthritis, or endocarditis occurring in varying proportions.*

The articular lesions of acute erysipelas are typically those of *fibrinous polyarthritis*. The volume of synovial fluid is increased, and the synovial membrane is hyperemic. In some cases, the synovial arterioles show necrotizing inflammation and extensive plugging by cellular thrombi.

Arthritis is a common expression of **chronic erysipelas** in pigs and may be unassociated with earlier acute or subacute signs of infection. It can be reproduced experimentally by injections of the organism and also occurs in vaccinated swine. *Although vaccination seems useful in preventing the acute syndrome and mortality, it appears to enhance susceptibility to polyarthritis.* In pigs with acute arthritis, organisms may be isolated from grossly normal as well as inflamed joints, but isolation from affected joints may be difficult in the chronic disease. Persistence of the inflammation in such cases may be due to the presence of bacterial antigens, rather than intact organisms, in synovial tissues. Antigens persist for up to 18 months in arthritic joints, and specific antibodies found in synovial

due to chance. Studies in mice have indicated that adherence of *Staphylococcus aureus* to collagen is likely to be involved in the pathogenesis of septic arthritis and osteomyelitis. Other organisms causing arthritis have also been shown to possess *collagen-binding components*.

fluid may be produced by plasma cells in the synovial membrane. Culture of the sediment from centrifuged synovial fluid, however, usually yields few organisms, even in very chronic erysipelas.

The *lesions in chronic erysipelas arthritis* vary in severity. In mild cases, there is excess synovial fluid and villus hypertrophy, but the articular capsule may appear normal. In severe cases, there is extensive villus hyperplasia and hypertrophy over much of the synovial membrane (Fig. 2-201A), together with pannus formation and cartilage degeneration. The hypertrophic villi are hyperemic and infiltrated with mononuclear cells, including plasma cells (Fig. 2-201B). *Diskospondylitis* is also a feature of chronic erysipelas.

Acute and chronic arthritis, similar to that caused by *E. rhusiopathiae* infection, also occur in pigs in association with certain other bacterial and mycoplasmal infections, and *in many cases, the cause is undetermined*. Molecular biologic techniques capable of demonstrating the presence of small quantities of persistent antigen may improve diagnostic success with such cases.

Erysipelas in **sheep** is usually the result of *percutaneous infection*, entry being gained through *the umbilicus, docking and castration wounds, shearing wounds, and cuts or abrasions acquired during dipping*. The lesion in sheep may be confined to the skin and subcutis at the point of entry, or there may be bacteremia with localization in joints. Rarely, death may occur from septicemia.

Fibrinopurulent polyarthritis and osteomyelitis make up the usual form of erysipelas in young lambs after docking or castration, and sometimes following umbilical infections. The arthritis is subacute or chronic, and associated morbidity may be as high as 50%. Mortality is low and is a consequence of severe lameness rather than a direct result of the infection. The main limb joints are involved. In the early stages, there is synovitis with an increased volume of turbid synovial fluid. Later, the fibrinous exudate may coagulate into firm pads. Articular cartilage is initially unaffected, but foci of osteomyelitis in the subchondral epiphyseal bone may lead to collapse of the overlying articular surface and formation of irregular pits or ulcers with a base of granulation tissue. In the chronic stages, the joints are stiffened and deformed by periarticular fibrosis and by periosteal and perichondral osteophytes. *Histologically*, there are lymphocytes and plasma cells within the synovium and neutrophils within the synovial fluid.

Cutaneous infections following dipping are associated with contamination of nonbactericidal dips with *E. rhusiopathiae*. Lesions occur most often about the *fetlocks*, but invasion may occur wherever the skin is injured and contaminated. Postdipping infections, which mimic cutaneous erysipelas, are occasionally caused by both *Trueperella pyogenes* and *Corynebacterium pseudotuberculosis*. Cutaneous erysipelas may also occur when sheep are confined in wet, contaminated pens. *Lameness is severe* and out of proportion to the gross changes in affected feet. The disease is febrile in some animals and associated with rapid wasting, but recovery occurs in 2-3 weeks. The affected pasterns are hot and painful, and there is regional lymphadenitis. The coronary band may be swollen, and the swelling, which is always slight, may extend to the metacarpal or metatarsal regions. The affected areas are progressively depilated. Incision reveals moderate erythema and slight edema of the subcutis. *Histologically*, there are superficial pustules in the epidermis. In the outer layers of the dermis, there is perivascular edema, accumulation of neutrophils, and cellular thrombi within vessels. The reaction is more severe in the deeper layers of the dermis and is characterized by suppurative hydradenitis, necrotizing vasculitis, and vascular thrombosis. Similar changes occur in the *sensory laminae of the foot* and are responsible for the severe lameness.

Streptococcal arthritis. Streptococci cause a variety of infections in domestic animals, including *septicemia, meningitis, polyarthritis, bronchopneumonia, and endocarditis*. In **swine**, there are well-defined syndromes of streptococcal septicemia, with localization in synovial structures, meninges, and elsewhere, caused by **Streptococcus suis**. There are at least 35 serotypes of *S. suis* based on capsular antigens, but serotype 2 is the most commonly isolated from pigs and is also a common cause of meningitis in humans, especially in Asia. The organism is carried in the palatine tonsils of pigs, and infection is probably by the respiratory route. In infected herds, it

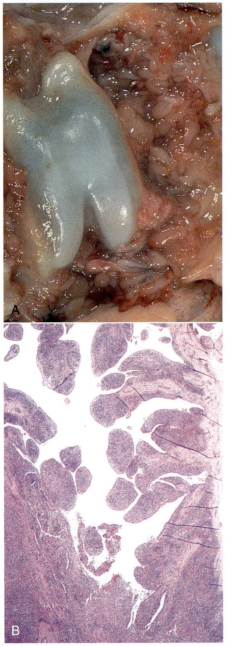

Figure 2-201 *Erysipelothrix arthritis* in a pig. **A.** Marked synovial hyperplasia in the stifle joint. (Courtesy R.A. Fairley.) **B.** Hyperplastic villi with dense lymphoplasmacytic infiltrates.

is isolated from up to 80% of clinically normal pigs and is commonly found in nasal turbinates and pneumonic lungs, where it is probably a secondary invader. Limited outbreaks occur, but *sporadic, isolated disease is more common*. The incubation period varies from 1-14 days and the clinical course from 4-48 hours. Affected pigs are usually ~10-14 weeks of age, and the most significant lesion is *purulent meningitis*, which, along with *polyserositis*, is visible grossly in ~50% of pigs. The bacteria probably enter the cerebrospinal fluid within monocytes via the choroid plexuses. *Purulent arthritis* occurs in a few animals (Fig. 2-202), usually those at the lower end of the age range. *Fibrinopurulent pericarditis, endocarditis, or hemorrhagic, necrotizing myocarditis* occurs in some pigs.

Streptococcus dysgalactiae subsp. **equisimilis** was the most common isolate in one study of piglets with arthritis attributed to abrasions from rough flooring.

Streptococci also cause *polyarthritis and meningitis* in **calves**. Embolic iridocyclitis occurs in many bacterial infections in which polyarthritis occurs, but in none is it so consistent or prominent as in the *streptococcal disease of neonatal calves*. The disease is probably secondary to *umbilical infection* in most cases, but because ocular lesions may be visible grossly by 24 hours of life, there is a possibility that some infections are intrauterine. The clinical signs are *hypopyon, corneal opacity, and meningitis*, and because of the strong affinity of the organisms for the meninges and eyes, the disease is without a chronic phase. The arthritis is acute, and there is no obvious joint swelling.

In **lambs**, *Streptococcus* spp. are probably second only to *Erysipelothrix rhusiopathiae* as a cause of polyarthritis, although in the United Kingdom, *S. dysgalactiae* is the most common isolate from the joints of arthritic lambs. The *umbilicus* is accepted as the likely route of entry in most cases, and this is supported by the high prevalence of the disease in sucklings. Localization of *Streptococcus* spp. in the joints and other organs of lambs is a sequel to bacteremia. Some lambs die acutely of septicemia and show few gross lesions. Infection of various tissues occurs in the course of 1-2 days and may involve any one or a combination of sites, including *the uvea, cerebrospinal meninges, valvular endocardium, myocardium, kidneys, and joints*. Meningeal localization seldom occurs in the absence of polyarthritis, but the latter may not be clinically evident in cases with a short clinical course. Polyarthritis may, however, occur alone. The infection may subside in many joints, persisting only in the larger limb joints and causing chronic lesions of purulent arthritis. In ~20% of lambs with subacute or chronic polyarthritis, there is coincident valvular endocarditis.

Coliform arthritis. *Escherichia coli often localizes in the joints or meninges (or both) in farm animals and is a rare cause of arthritis in dogs*. In septicemic colibacillosis of neonatal **calves**, polyarthritis and tenosynovitis are common but easily overlooked or overshadowed by other manifestations of acute septicemia, including meningitis and polyserositis. The organism may enter the blood from the gut, oropharynx, or umbilicus. The lesions in calves are similar to those of streptococcal infection, although iridocyclitis, with grossly visible hypopyon, occurs less frequently with coliform polyarthritis. In some cases, the polyarthritis is chronic, with lesions restricted to one or 2 of the larger limb joints and tending to be symmetrical. Chronic coliform arthritis in calves is often coincident with interstitial nephritis (white-spotted kidney), which may develop into descending pyelonephritis. Polyarthritis caused by *E. coli* also occurs commonly in horses and pigs, but does not appear to be a common isolate from the joints of lambs with polyarthritis.

Staphylococcal arthritis. *Staphylococcus aureus is a relatively common cause of polyarthritis in farm animals and monoarticular arthritis in dogs*. In lambs, *S. aureus* may occur as a sporadic infection or as a complication of tick pyemia. In the United Kingdom, the latter syndrome occurs in lambs born onto tick-infested ground, particularly during spring when tick activity is at a peak. The agent gains entry to the blood through bites of the blood-sucking nymphal stage of the tick *Ixodes ricinus*, then localizes in the synovial membrane and various internal organs. Vertebral osteomyelitis is a frequent complication of *S. aureus* septicemia in affected lambs, often leading to ataxia or paralysis following collapse of necrotic bone into the spinal canal.

Staphylococcus hyicus subsp. *hyicus* is an important cause of fibrinopurulent arthritis in **pigs**. Lesions are most common in the *elbow and tarsal joints*. The palatine tonsil is an important site of entry for this organism in pigs. *Staphylococcus* spp. were the most common bacteria isolated from the synovial fluid in a study of 19 cases of *septic arthritis* in **dogs**. Interestingly, although all dogs in the study had increased numbers of neutrophils in their synovial fluid, the *neutrophils were nondegenerate* in all but one case. This reinforces the point that detection of toxic neutrophils in synovial fluid is not a reliable means of differentiating septic arthritis from noninfectious, immune-mediated arthritis in dogs.

***Haemophilus* and *Histophilus* septicemia and arthritis.** Glasser's disease *is a fibrinous meningitis, polyserositis, and/or polyarthritis of* **pigs** *caused by* **Haemophilus parasuis**. Glasser's disease is peracute, with high fever, lameness, and neurologic disturbances, including paresis, stupor, and hyperesthesia. As in other septicemic diseases of pigs, the skin may show purple discoloration. The course is 1-2 days, and without treatment, the mortality rate is very high. Usually, *serofibrinous meningitis, pericarditis, pleuritis, peritonitis*, and *synovitis of many joints* characterize the morbid picture. In individual cases, all these tissues, or any combination of them, may be inflamed. Occasionally, the lesions occur in only one site, and in some pigs or some outbreaks, gross lesions are absent. *Predilection sites* for lesions of Glasser's disease are *meninges, joints, peritoneum, pleura*, and *pericardium, in descending order*. Meningitis, which is more severe in the cranial than the spinal

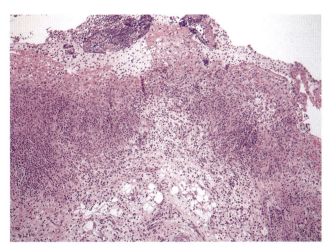

Figure 2-202 Streptococcal arthritis in a pig. The synovium is ulcerated, infiltrated by neutrophils, and covered with fibrin.

meninges, occurs in >80% of affected pigs. *Polyarthritis is most severe in the atlanto-occipital and large-limb joints.* The synovial fluid is increased in volume and turbid because of increased numbers of neutrophils. The *synovitis* is characterized by gray-yellow fibrin, which covers the membrane or accumulates as a meniscus-like pad between articular surfaces. The *gastric fundic mucosa* is often intensely red because of venous infarction, a change that accompanies septicemia of several causes in pigs.

The *microscopic lesions* of *H. parasuis* infection in pigs are those of septicemia and fibrinous inflammation. Thrombosis of vessels in the skin, meninges, and renal glomeruli is often prominent. The organism can best be cultured from visceral pleura, providing the interval from death to postmortem examination is relatively short. It is seldom isolated from other sites. Glasser's disease is defined on an etiologic basis because there are other organisms, such as *Streptococcus suis*, that produce similar lesions and similar diseases. *Mycoplasma* spp. also produce serositis and arthritis in swine, but the diseases are more chronic, and meningitis is either absent or lymphocytic, depending on the species of mycoplasma involved.

Histophilus somni, previously known as *Haemophilus agni*, *Histophilus ovis*, or *Haemophilus somnus*, produces an acute, fulminating, septicemic disease in **lambs** and a more chronic disease in older sheep. Lambs with *H. somni* septicemia are usually *found dead*, the course of the disease being <12 hours. Animals that survive for >24 hours develop *fibrinopurulent arthritis, choroiditis, and basilar meningitis*. The disease tends to remain enzootic in a flock, and losses may continue for several months. *The most constant postmortem findings are multiple hemorrhages throughout the carcass.* The hemorrhages vary in severity but are usually most obvious in lambs dying acutely. The intermuscular connective tissue is wet and slightly stained with blood. The large blotchy hemorrhages of the serosa lack specificity, but *tiny streaks of hemorrhage that are quite diagnostic can usually be seen in the muscles.* They are best appreciated by viewing the intact muscle through the perimysium, and are usually most common near the tendinous attachments. In all cases except the most acute, small foci of necrosis, surrounded by a red halo, are present in the liver. The *absence of pulmonary lesions* usually allows differentiation of this infection from *Mannheimia haemolytica* septicemia, which produces similar hepatic lesions. In *mature animals*, a more extended course is usual, and lesions include myocarditis, embolic nephritis, and meningoencephalitis, similar to the lesions of *H. somni* infection in cattle.

Histologically, there is evidence of *overwhelming intravascular bacterial multiplication*. Blood vessels in many tissues are plugged with bacteria, and some of the emboli give rise to *acute vasculitis and secondary infarctions.* All tissues share in this reaction to some extent, but there is preferential involvement of liver and muscle. In these organs, there is often severe inflammation in the parenchyma adjacent to the damaged vessels.

Acute serofibrinous arthritis involving 1 or 2 joints, usually including the atlanto-occipital joint, occurs regularly in **cattle** with meningoencephalitis caused by **H. somni**. These animals die suddenly and usually have hemorrhagic necrosis in the brain.

Borreliosis. *Borrelia burgdorferi* is the cause of a multisystemic disease *(Lyme disease, Lyme borreliosis)* in humans and domestic animals, including *dogs, horses, cattle, and cats*. In all species, *infection is far more common than disease*, but the host-bacterium interactions responsible are not well defined. *Arthritis is a common feature of disease in animals and human patients with borreliosis.* Other lesions include *myocarditis and nephritis in dogs, ocular disease and probably encephalitis in horses, and abortion in cattle.*

In the northeastern United States, the disease is endemic and transmitted by hard ticks, *Ixodes scapularis and I. pacificus*. The most common clinical signs in **dogs** with borreliosis are anorexia, lethargy, and lameness in association with fever and lymphadenopathy. Severe depression occurs in some cases and may be due to meningitis. The *arthritis is typically intermittent and involves one or more joints*. The affected joint may be related to the tick attachment site. In endemic areas, most dogs are seropositive and asymptomatic. Experimental infection of Beagle puppies results in lameness and joint effusion in only a minority. However, microscopic synovitis was present in all experimentally infected puppies. *Microscopic lesions are nonspecific* and consist of lymphocytes and plasma cells in the synovial subintima. Fibrin exudation and Mott cells are rare. Definitive diagnosis in naturally infected dogs is difficult, but *B. burgdorferi* DNA can be detected by PCR using fresh and formalin-fixed, paraffin-embedded tissue from experimentally infected animals. Immunohistochemistry on formalin-fixed, paraffin-embedded tissue can be used in both experimental and natural infections.

In *horses* and *cattle*, a wide array of clinical signs, including arthritis and lameness, has been attributed to *B. burgdorferi*, but confirmed reports of infection causing disease are lacking.

Chlamydial arthritis. The genera **Chlamydia** and **Chlamydophila** contain several species of obligate intracellular, gram-negative bacteria characterized by the absence of cell-wall peptidoglycans. Only **Chlamydophila pecorum** is a cause of arthritis in domestic animals. *Sporadic or epidemic C. pecorum polyarthritis occurs in calves and lambs*, and occasionally in other animals. The natural habitat of chlamydiae is the intestinal tract, where the organism multiplies in the mucosal epithelium before entering the lamina propria. Nonvirulent strains rarely progress beyond the mesenteric nodes. Following oral exposure of calves to virulent strains, the chlamydiae spread to the liver and mesenteric nodes via blood vessels and lymphatics of the lower small intestine. Multiplication in these sites is followed by a primary, low-level chlamydemia with localization and multiplication in the spleen, liver, lungs, and kidneys. The joints are infected during a secondary chlamydemia, and arthritogenic strains produce their most severe effects in synovial membranes, with clinical arthritis developing about 10 days after oral inoculation. Severe watery or bloody diarrhea often occurs a few days before the development of arthritis.

The disease in calves is severe, causing a high mortality rate both naturally and experimentally. Affected calves may be weak at birth, suggesting intrauterine infection. In these animals, fever, anorexia, reluctance to stand or move, and swelling of joints develop in 2-3 days, and death occurs 2 days to 2 weeks after the onset of signs. *All or many joints are affected*, those of the limbs most severely. The subcutaneous and adjacent periarticular tissues are edematous with clear fluid, which also extends around tendon sheaths. Surrounding muscles are hyperemic and edematous with petechiae in the fascia. Joint cavities are distended with turbid yellow-gray fluid, and strands or wads of fibrin adhere to the synovium. Viscera may show changes attributable to systemic infection.

The ovine syndrome is less severe, being characterized by high morbidity but negligible mortality, even though the infection is systemic. Affected lambs show conjunctivitis, depression, anorexia, reluctance to move, joint stiffness that disappears with exercise, and weight loss. Most lambs recover, but a few are permanently lame. Articular lesions in lambs are similar to those in calves, although the milder reaction and longer course allows fibrotic thickening of tendon sheaths and articular capsules and hyperplasia of synovial villi. In soft tissues, including the central nervous system, histologic traces of inflammation are present.

Chlamydophila felis causes upper respiratory disease, conjunctivitis, and rarely, arthritis in cats.

Further reading

Fittipaldi N, et al. Virulence factors involved in the pathogenesis of the infection caused by the swine pathogen and zoonotic agent *Streptococcus suis*. Future Microbiol 2012;7:259-279.

Oliveira S, Pijoan C. *Haemophilus parasuis*: new trends on diagnosis, epidemiology, and control. Vet Microbiol 2004;99:1-12.

Susta L, et al. Synovial lesions in experimental canine Lyme borreliosis. Vet Pathol 2012;49:453-461.

Zoric M, et al. Incidence of lameness and abrasions in piglets in identical farrowing pens with four different types of floor. Acta Vet Scand 2009;51:23.

Mycoplasmal arthritis. *Mycoplasmas are ubiquitous organisms that are difficult to isolate, propagate, and identify*, in addition to often being difficult to associate with specific diseases. Polyserositis and polyarthritis produced by these organisms are problems of considerable magnitude in farm animals and often complicate mycoplasma ("enzootic") pneumonia or other disease syndromes. The diseases are seldom fatal but produce a lingering debility from which animals never completely recover. Mycoplasmas can be difficult to culture, but PCR and immunohistochemistry can detect the organisms within affected tissue. Continued inflammation in the absence of viable organisms may be due to an immune response to persistent mycoplasma antigen.

Three *Mycoplasma* spp. are pathogenic for **swine:** *Mycoplasma hyopneumoniae* causes enzootic pneumonia; *M. hyorhinis* causes polyserositis and *polyarthritis*, usually in animals about 3-10 weeks of age; *M. hyosynoviae* also causes *polyarthritis* (usually in pigs >10 weeks of age) but not polyserositis. Other mycoplasmas are sometimes associated with various diseases of swine, but they are not primary pathogens.

M. hyorhinis has a predilection for collagen-containing structures, including serous and synovial membranes and cartilage, but meningitis is either absent or mild. Although the effects of polyserositis predominate early in the disease, signs of *polyarthritis* become evident once villus hypertrophy, synovial thickening, and organization of fibrinous exudate replace the initial synovial edema and hyperemia. In the chronic disease, thickening and brown discoloration of joint capsules, erosion and discoloration of articular cartilages, and pannus formation are observed. Discoloration of joint structures is probably a sequel to synovial hemorrhage. Early microscopic changes consist of hyperemia, diffuse lymphocyte and macrophage infiltration, and mild villus hypertrophy, followed by ulceration of synovial membranes. *Fibrinopurulent exudate is consistently present in virtually all joints* and is most abundant in the recesses, where the synovial membrane is reflected from the articular cartilage. Later, perivascular lymphoplasmacytic accumulations and more pronounced villus hypertrophy become evident, and fibrinous exudate is less prominent. Erosions, developing first at the periphery of the articular cartilages, later occur centrally, and *erosion of cartilage and subchondral bone by pannus* is not unusual in advanced cases. Joint contractures are associated with the chronic arthritis and thickened joint capsules.

M. hyosynoviae infection in pigs <6 weeks of age is uncommon, and separation of piglets from their dams by 5 weeks of age usually prevents transmission. Clinical disease often develops following management stress and is more frequent, and more severe, in pigs with poor conformation and gait. Lesions are not fully described but are likely to be similar to those of *M. hyorhinis*.

Mycoplasma spp. cause several important disease syndromes in small ruminants, including contagious caprine pleuropneumonia in goats *(Mycoplasma capricolum* subsp. *capripneumoniae)* and contagious agalactia in **sheep and goats**. The agents causing contagious agalactia occur *worldwide*. Contagious agalactia is caused by *M. agalactiae* in sheep and goats, but in goats, many other *Mycoplasma* spp. can also cause the same syndrome, including *M. mycoides* subsp. *capri, M. capricolum* subsp. *capricolum*, and *M. putrefaciens*. Goats are more susceptible than sheep, especially pregnant or lactating females and young kids. Specific disease features vary with the *Mycoplasma* spp. involved. Mastitis, agalactia, polyarthritis (carpi and tarsi), and conjunctivitis/keratitis are most common. The articular lesion is a *hyperplastic synovitis with severe fibrinopurulent inflammation* (Fig. 2-203), which may result in ankylosis.

Mycoplasma bovis sporadically causes polyarthritis in **cattle** of any age, often concurrently with pneumonia or mastitis. Calves can be affected by drinking milk from cows with mastitis. Approximately half of feedlot cattle with *Mycoplasma* pneumonia will also have arthritis. *Gross lesions* are extremely variable. The shoulder, elbow, carpus, hip, stifle, and hock are most often affected, but severe lesions usually affect only one limb. In acute disease, the joints are distended by turbid fluid with fibrin; extension into tendon sheaths and periarticular soft tissues is common. Severely affected animals can have erosion of the articular cartilage, thickened joint

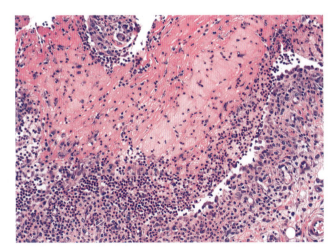

Figure 2-203 *Mycoplasma mycoides* **arthritis** in a goat kid. The synovium is inflamed and hyperplastic with a thick fibrinosuppurative exudate attached to the surface.

capsule, and foci of caseous necrosis in the periarticular tissues. *Microscopically*, fibrin and neutrophils adhere to the synovium, which has areas of ulceration and hyperplasia. The subintima is edematous with neutrophils, macrophages, lymphocytes, and plasma cells. There can also be lymphoid follicle formation and fibroblast hyperplasia. The organism can be detected by culture, PCR, and/or immunohistochemistry within affected joints.

Most affected animals recover in 1-2 months, but a few develop chronic arthritis characterized by proliferative and erosive arthritis with well-vascularized pannus extending from the thickened synovial membrane across the articular cartilage. Spread of inflammation to the subchondral bone with development of osteomyelitis occurs in some animals. The predominant cells in the chronic synovial lesions are lymphocytes and plasma cells, with fewer neutrophils and macrophages. Isolation of mycoplasma is often difficult in chronic stages.

Mycoplasma mycoides subsp. *mycoides* small colony type (*M. m. mycoides* SC), the agent of contagious bovine pleuropneumonia, is endemic in Africa and East Asia, with occasional cases reported in Europe. *M. m. mycoides* SC rarely causes *polyarthritis and endocarditis* in calves in which it is used as a vaccine. *Mycoplasma alkalescens, M. californicum,* and *M. canadense* have also been associated with arthritis and mastitis in cattle.

Another member of the family *Mycoplasmataceae,* **Ureaplasma diversum**, has been associated with severe polyarthritis in bovine fetuses aborted during the last trimester. The coxofemoral joint, elbow, stifle, and carpus can be affected. The lesions are severe, with erosion and deformation of the articular surfaces and thickening of the periarticular soft tissues. Histologically the synovial membrane is replaced by granulation tissue, which also extends across and into the articular cartilage. These findings emphasize the importance of examining multiple joints in aborted fetuses.

Occasionally, mycoplasma arthritis occurs in **cats and dogs.** *Mycoplasma gateae* and *Mycoplasma felis* have been associated with feline polyarthritis. *Mycoplasma spumans* and *Mycoplasma edwardii* have been associated with canine arthritis. Immunosuppression is a predisposing factor in some cases.

Viral arthritis

The best-characterized example of viral arthritis in animals is **caprine arthritis-encephalitis virus (CAEV)**. This syndrome in **goats** is caused by persistent infection with the CAE *lentivirus*. The neurologic, mammary, respiratory and systemic features are described in Vol. 1, Nervous system. *In many herds, arthritis is the major or only clinical manifestation of infection*, with signs of lameness often associated with carpal hygromas, weight loss, and reduced milk production. The prevalence of infection in a herd may reach 100%, but expression of disease is variable and rarely exceeds 25-30%.

A high prevalence of unilateral or bilateral **carpal hygromas** is a characteristic clinical feature of caprine arthritis-encephalitis. The hygromas are chronic lesions that appear as flattened, fluctuant, subcutaneous distensions over the cranial carpus, and are filled with yellow or bloody fluid, often containing fibrinous or gelatinous masses. *Usually, there is no communication with the carpal joint or tendon sheaths.* The tendon sheaths and joint capsule are thickened by fibrous tissue, in which collagen degeneration and mineralization may occur. In many cases, the major joints, especially carpus and stifle, are distended with clear yellow fluid. Other gross changes, which are also seen most often in the carpus and stifle, include hypertrophy of synovial villi, fibrillation and erosion of cartilage, and destruction of joint structures by pannus. Lymphocytic/plasmacytic arthritis is present microscopically in many joints.

CAEV is readily transmitted to kids in colostrum and milk, and horizontal transmission probably occurs. Although the colostrum may contain antibody, this does not influence viral transmission. In blood, the virus is present in monocytes and is activated when they mature into macrophages. Following infection there is vascular injury to synovial structures, with exudation of plasma proteins into synovial fluid. Synovial villi become hypertrophic and edematous, and accumulate infiltrates of plasma cells, lymphocytes (Fig. 2-204), and scattered macrophages, which are sometimes multinucleated. Some villi may be fibrotic, and there is hyperplasia of synoviocytes on their surfaces. Hyalinized masses of fibrin also form villus structures in inflamed joints, and layers of fibrin may cover the synovial membrane in some areas.

A related lentivirus, the **visna/maedi virus**, causes chronic arthritis in **sheep**. Arthritis is less common in lentivirus-infected sheep than in goats. The lesion is a lymphoplasmacytic synovitis that also may contain macrophages and lymphoid follicles. Genetic analysis of lentiviruses in mixed flocks of sheep and goats suggests that there is transmission between these species.

Lameness caused by acute arthritis is reported in **cats** in association with feline **calicivirus** infection, or 5-7 days after live-virus vaccination. Feline **foamy (syncytium-forming) virus** has been associated with chronic polyarthritis in cats. Young male cats are most often affected, and coinfection with feline leukemia virus may play a role.

Fungal arthritis

Arthritis involving one or more joints rarely occurs in dogs with systemic fungal infections. In some cases, the arthritis may be immune mediated, following the deposition of immune complexes in the synovial membrane, but hematogenous localization of fungal agents in joints, or direct spread from osteomyelitis in adjacent bones also occurs. Fungi identified in arthritic joints of dogs include *Blastomyces, Histoplasma,*

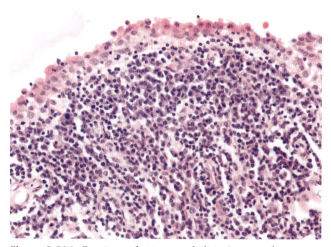

Figure 2-204 Caprine arthritis-encephalitis. Intense plasmacytic infiltration of the synovium and hypertrophy of synoviocytes on the surface.

Coccidioides, *Cryptococcus*, and *Sporothrix* spp. Radiography may reveal a destructive process in a bone or bones adjacent to the joint and erosive changes in articular cartilage. The causative agent is sometimes evident on cytologic examination of synovial fluid obtained by arthrocentesis. Histologically, the synovial inflammation is usually *pyogranulomatous*.

Protozoal arthritis

Proliferative synovitis in **dogs** may be associated with *visceral leishmaniasis* caused by the protozoal agent *Leishmania donovani* or *Leishmania infantum*. Synovial villi in affected joints are hypertrophic and infiltrated with plasma cells and macrophages, some of which may contain the organism. The agent is occasionally demonstrated in macrophages collected from synovial fluid.

Further reading

Blacklaws BA. Small ruminant lentiviruses: immunopathogenesis of visna-maedi and caprine arthritis encephalitis virus. 2012;35:259-269

Gagea MI, et al. Naturally occurring *Mycoplasma bovis*-associated pneumonia and polyarthritis in feedlot beef calves. J Vet Diagn Invest 2006;18:29-40.

Maunsell FP, et al. *Mycoplasma bovis* infection in cattle. J Vet Intern Med 2011;25:772-783.

Nicolet J. Mycoplasmas and mycoplasmoses. In: Lefèvre P-C, et al, editors. Infectious and Parasitic Diseases of Livestock, vol 2. Oxfordshire, UK: CABI; 2010. p. 785-789.

Miscellaneous inflammatory lesions of joint structures

Bursitis

Bursae are periarticular pockets of synovial fluid that may be part of the normal anatomy (synovial bursae) or acquired lesions (adventitious bursae). In horses, there are 3 **synovial bursae** associated with the nuchal ligament and the underlying vertebrae: the cranial nuchal bursa (between the atlas and the nuchal ligament), the caudal nuchal bursa (between the axis and the nuchal ligament), and the supraspinous bursa (between the spinous process of the second thoracic vertebra and the nuchal ligament). When bursitis affects the cranial and/or caudal nuchal bursa, the condition is known as **poll evil**. Inflammation of the supraspinous bursa is known as **fistulous withers**. In either location, the condition may be sterile or bacterial. Bacterial bursitis is more likely to fistulate. In brucellosis-endemic areas *Brucella abortus* is often isolated, and vaccination is considered a useful method of treatment. *Actinomyces bovis*, a common component of the normal bovine oral flora, sometimes can be cultured from closed lesions in horses, and exposure to cattle is considered a predisposing factor. In North America and other locations where brucellosis and the exposure of horses to cattle are declining, *Streptococcus* and *Staphylococcus* spp. are the most common isolates, but several other bacteria have also been implicated. The infections are probably *hematogenous*, but it is not clear whether a predisposing bursal lesion is required. A penetrating wound is rarely found. The microscopic findings are typical of a bacterial infection; there is synovial proliferation along with fibrin, neutrophils, and macrophages. Over time, the wall of the bursa thickens with dense collagen. Sterile bursitis, which is thought to be caused by acute or chronic trauma, is characterized by nonsuppurative inflammation, fibroplasia, and fibrosis.

Adventitious bursae occur outside the joint capsule over bony prominences subjected to trauma (similar to a sterile seroma). **Capped elbow** (over the olecranon) and **capped hock** (over the tuber calcaneus) in **horses** occur with kicks, falls, and prolonged recumbency. Carpal bursitis, also known as **hygroma**, is not uncommon in cattle, sheep, and goats. The distended bursae are sometimes filled with fibrin concretions (Fig. 2-205). Carpal hygromas are common in adult goats infected with *caprine arthritis encephalitis virus*. Adventitious bursae over the olecranon in dogs are termed **elbow hygroma**. These lesions are not lined by a true synovial membrane, but by mesenchymal cells that have taken on a synoviocyte-like morphology (Fig. 2-206). The wall becomes increasingly fibrous with chronicity. Although inflammation may be present, these are not primarily inflammatory lesions.

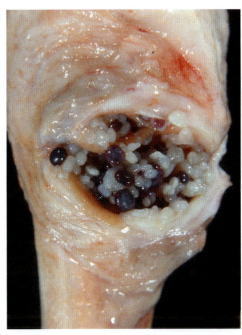

Figure 2-205 Chronic carpal bursitis in a sheep. Thickened fibrous wall surrounding numerous fibrin concretions.

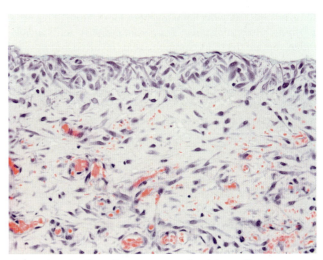

Figure 2-206 Elbow **hygroma** in a dog. The wall is composed of granulation tissue in which the lining cells resemble synoviocytes.

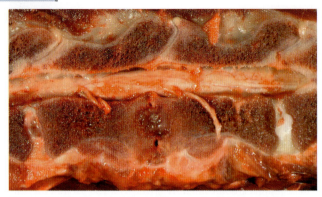

Figure 2-207 Fungal (*Aspergillus* spp.) diskospondylitis in a German Shepherd dog. The intervertebral disk is replaced by a gray liquefied focus surrounded by sclerotic bone. (Courtesy K.M. Newkirk.)

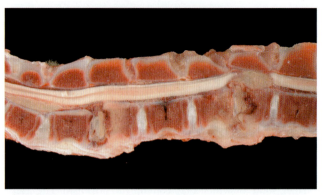

Figure 2-208 Bacterial diskospondylitis in a 3-week-old lamb. Two sites of diskospondylitis with destruction of disks and extension of inflammation into the spinal canal and adjacent vertebrae.

Capped hocks (over the tuber calcaneus) and adventitious bursitis (over the distal lateral hock) are common in finishing **pigs**. The prevalence is 20-60%, and increased prevalence is associated with increasing age and hard slippery floors/falling. The walls of both lesions frequently have evidence of previous hemorrhage, further supporting the role of trauma rather than inflammation in these lesions.

Diskospondylitis

Diskospondylitis is inflammation of an intervertebral disk and the contiguous vertebrae. It occurs occasionally in dogs and pigs, and less often in cats, horses, cattle, and sheep. Most cases are caused by bacteria, usually as a result of primary bacteremia, but also secondary to a chronic infection elsewhere in the body.

In **dogs**, diskospondylitis occurs most often in large males and usually involves the lumbosacral spine, causing hyperesthesia, stilted gait, and/or pelvic limb lameness. *Staphylococcus pseudintermedius* is the most common cause, although streptococci, *Brucella canis*, and *E. coli* are also causative. Often, the primary source of the hematogenous bacteria is not identified, but when present is most often a urogenital infection, skin infection, or valvular endocarditis. Intervertebral disks can also be involved in systemic *Aspergillus terreus* in dogs (Fig. 2-207).

In **pigs**, most lesions occur in the upper thoracic and upper lumbar spine following hematogenous localization of bacteria. *Erysipelothrix rhusiopathiae*, *Trueperella pyogenes*, and *Staphylococcus* spp. are the most common agents involved, but in some geographic areas, *Brucella suis* may be an important cause of the disease. Diskospondylitis in **horses** most often involves the cervical vertebrae, inducing signs of neck pain. In some cases, there is a history of a penetrating wound to the neck. The pathogenesis of hematogenous infection of the intervertebral disk is unknown because the disk is avascular in adults. Organisms may localize initially in the vascular outer part of the annulus fibrosus. Alternatively, localization in the vertebral body or end plate with extension to the disk may occur. However, early changes are centered on the intervertebral disk, suggesting that the infection originates there.

Gross lesions are soft, gray, or yellow areas of discoloration and disruption in the disk, often extending into the spinal canal and adjacent vertebrae (Fig. 2-208). Complete destruction of disks, with fibrous replacement and formation of vertebral osteophytes, occurs late in the disease (Fig. 2-209); such lesions are easily confused with ventral bridging spondylosis.

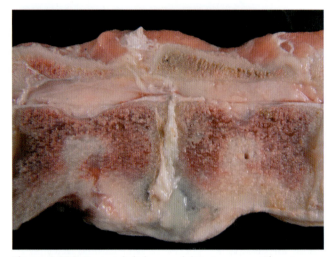

Figure 2-209 Bacterial diskospondylitis in a ram. Chronic suppurative inflammation of the intervertebral disk with ventral bony bridging.

The inflammatory reaction may extend dorsally into the spinal canal, causing meningomyelitis, or laterally, causing paravertebral abscessation. *Microscopic lesions* of diskospondylitis vary with the stage of the disease and the nature of the causative organism. Early bacterial infections are characterized by suppurative inflammation, hemorrhage, and necrosis of intervertebral structures and adjacent bones. In chronic lesions, vascular connective tissue, infiltrated with mononuclear or mixed inflammatory cells, predominates.

Calcium crystal–associated arthropathy (pseudogout)

A syndrome characterized by the deposition of *calcium pyrophosphate dihydrate* ($Ca_2P_2O_7 \cdot 2H_2O$) *crystals* in articular and para-articular tissues is well recognized in humans and is reported occasionally in *aged dogs*, where it occurs as single, tumor-like, periarticular masses developing over a period of several months or even years. Grossly, the lesions consist of *multiple, hard, chalky white nodules separated by fibrous septa.* Although the masses are adherent to the joint capsule, they do not involve joint cavities or articular surfaces. Microscopically, the chalky nodules consist of variably sized deposits of pale brown crystalline material separated by fibrous or cartilaginous connective tissue. A *granulomatous inflammatory reaction*, including many large, multinucleated giant cells, is closely associated with the crystalline deposits. The crystals are weakly birefringent, rhomboidal or rectangular, and stain positively with alizarin red and von Kossa stains.

A more severe and polyarthritic form of the disease occurs in young Great Danes, where it is thought to be caused by an autosomal dominant defect in calcium metabolism. The crystals are deposited within and around the joints, resulting in granulomatous inflammation, fibrosis, and cartilaginous metaplasia. Cytologic examination of synovial fluid may reveal weakly birefringent rectangular and rhomboid crystals within neutrophils, monocytes, and synovial lining cells.

The pathogenesis of this syndrome, now referred to as *calcium pyrophosphate dihydrate crystal deposition disease*, is unknown. *True gout*, which is associated with the deposition of urate crystals within joint structures, occurs commonly in humans, birds, and reptiles, but does not occur in mammalian species possessing the enzyme uricase. There are no convincing reports of gout in dogs; even Dalmatian dogs, with their high serum uric acid concentrations, do not develop the disease.

Further reading

Burkert BA, et al. Signalment and clinical features of diskospondylitis in dogs: 513 cases (1980-2001). J Am Vet Med Assoc 2005;227:268-275.

García-López JM, et al. Diagnosis and management of cranial and caudal nuchal bursitis in four horses 2010; 237:823-829.

KilBride AL, et al. A cross-sectional study of the prevalence and associated risk factors for capped hock and the associations with bursitis in weaner, grower and finisher pigs from 93 commercial farms in England. Vet Prev Med 2008;83:272-284.

Immune-mediated polyarthritis

The term **immune-mediated polyarthritis** is used to classify a group of *inflammatory but noninfectious diseases of joints*. These occur most often in **dogs** and **cats**. The *lesions may resemble those of infectious arthritis*, which is not surprising, as the mediators produced during the inflammatory process are quantitatively and qualitatively similar. Furthermore, *synovial fluid from both forms of arthritis is characterized by the presence of increased numbers of* **neutrophils**. *Demonstration of toxic change in the neutrophils is often mentioned as a means of differentiating infectious from immune-mediated arthritis, but this is unreliable.* First, not all bacteria induce significant toxic change in synovial neutrophils. Second, unless the viscosity of the synovial fluid is reduced by the lytic action of lysosomal enzymes on hyaluronan, the neutrophils may not "flatten" sufficiently in direct smears for signs of degeneration to be apparent. The hocks, carpi, and stifles are most often affected by immune-mediated polyarthritis, whereas the larger more proximal joints are more likely to be affected by infectious arthritis. Immune-mediated polyarthritis is divided into *erosive and non-erosive forms*, based on the presence or absence of articular cartilage destruction.

Erosive polyarthritis. Erosive polyarthritis is very rare, representing only about 1% of all canine polyarthritis. The pathogenesis involves antibodies against immunoglobulins (rheumatoid factors), heat shock proteins, type II collagen, and other self-antigens within the joint. Immune complex deposition within the synovium results in complement fixation, inflammatory cell recruitment, and cytokine production, leading to activation of fibroblasts, macrophages, and T lymphocytes that produce matrix-degrading enzymes, such as metalloproteinases. These enzymes are partially responsible for the cartilage erosion that characterizes the disease.

- **Rheumatoid arthritis** is very rare in animals. In dogs, it typically affects the stifle, carpus, and digits of small-breed, middle-aged dogs. Antibodies to immunoglobulins (**rheumatoid factors**) are often present in the blood and synovial fluid, but these can occur in a variety of infectious diseases as well. Antibodies to canine distemper virus, heat shock proteins, and type II collagen have also been implicated. The lesions are typically symmetrical and severe. There is synovial villus hypertrophy, synoviocyte proliferation, fibrin deposition, synovial necrosis, lymphoplasmacytic synovitis, and destruction of cartilage and subchondral bone. Degeneration of articular cartilage begins at the margins, where *granulation tissue from the inflamed synovium either spreads across the articular cartilage as a pannus or invades the epiphysis, destroying subchondral bone and undermining the articular cartilage*. Erosion of central regions of articular cartilage (Fig. 2-210) occurs later in the disease process.
- **Felty's syndrome** is a triad of rheumatoid arthritis, leukopenia, and splenomegaly. This syndrome has been diagnosed in a small proportion of dogs with erosive polyarthritis.
- **Erosive polyarthritis of greyhounds** has been reported most often in England and Australia. The disease begins insidiously between 3 and 30 months of age. Clinically, there is lameness and joint swelling involving limb joints distal to, and including, elbows and stifles. Superficial lymph nodes are enlarged. Despite considerable effort, no infectious agent has yet been identified, and the syndrome does not appear to be related to athletic activity. *Gross findings* in affected joints include an excess of turbid synovial fluid, with fibrin clots in severe cases; yellow/brown discoloration, and thickening of synovial membranes, sometimes with adherent fibrin plaques; ecchymotic hemorrhages in the synovial membrane; and erosions of articular cartilage. *Lesions are common in the first and second phalangeal joints, and in carpal, tarsal, elbow, and stifle joints.* Occasionally, shoulder, hip, and atlanto-occipital joints are

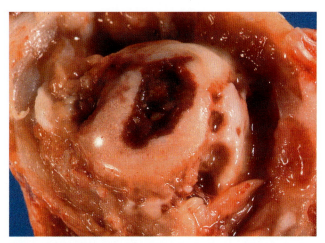

Figure 2-210 Rheumatoid arthritis in the humeral head of a dog. Severe erosion of the articular cartilage and subchondral bone.

involved. *Microscopic lesions* include *necrosis of articular cartilage and proliferative synovitis*. The articular cartilage shows either full-thickness necrosis or necrosis of deep layers with relative sparing of superficial zones. Typical changes in the synovium include villus hypertrophy, proliferation of synoviocytes, and infiltration by lymphocytes, plasma cells, and neutrophils. In some areas, the lymphocytic infiltrates are intense and may form follicles. There is no evidence of vasculitis. Pannus formation is often present, but never extensive, and changes in subchondral bone are usually minimal.

- **Feline chronic progressive polyarthritis** of **older cats** has an *insidious onset*, *chronic progression*, and clinical signs restricted to symmetrical deformities of the *carpus, tarsus, and digits* caused by loss of joint margins, subluxation, collapse of joint space, and ankylosis. The synovial fluid contains low to moderate numbers of neutrophils and lymphocytes. Synovial membranes are heavily infiltrated with lymphocytes and plasma cells, and enlarged synovial villi often contain prominent lymphoid follicles with germinal centers. *Rheumatoid factor is absent*. Infection with feline leukemia virus is present in about 50% of affected cats.
- **Feline chronic progressive polyarthritis** of **young cats** has been associated with feline foamy (syncytium-forming) virus but may represent an immune-mediated disease, as the same virus can be found in unaffected cats. The disease is characterized by *sudden onset* of high fever, severe pain in joints and tendon sheaths, and lymphadenomegaly associated with affected joints. Synovitis is initially characterized by *fibrinopurulent synovitis, but later, plasma cells and lymphocytes predominate*. Rheumatoid factor is absent. Enlarged lymph nodes may have exuberant lymphoid hyperplasia, including marked extracapsular extension, mimicking lymphosarcoma. The skeletal lesions are bilateral and *most frequently involve the tarsometatarsal and carpometacarpal joints*, but the elbow and stifle joints, and the articular facets of the thoracic and lumbar spine, may also be affected. The periosteal new bone consists of trabeculae of woven bone, and the intertrabecular spaces often are infiltrated with lymphocytes and plasma cells. Pannus formation usually occurs late in the disease and leads to erosions of joint margins, collapse of joint spaces, and fibrous ankylosis, but subluxation is not a feature.

Non-erosive polyarthritis. The pathogenesis of non-erosive polyarthritis involves circulating antigen-antibody complexes deposited in multiple joints, leading to lymphoplasmacytic synovitis and neutrophils within the synovial fluid, but no cartilage erosion. *Synovial fluid cytology* is useful in confirming the disease as inflammatory, but is not specific and often does not allow differentiation from infectious arthritis or from erosive polyarthritis. The characteristic feature is a mild to moderate increase in cellularity, and most of the cells are nondegenerate neutrophils.

- **Idiopathic polyarthritis** is the *most common* form and occurs most often in young adult sporting and large-breed dogs. Labrador Retrievers, Golden Retrievers, German Shepherds, Cocker Spaniels, and American Eskimos dogs are over-represented. Most studies do not show a sex predisposition. Idiopathic polyarthritis is divided into 4 subtypes:
  - Type I, or uncomplicated polyarthritis, is the *most common* subtype, representing 50-65% of all idiopathic polyarthritis cases in dogs. No underlying disease is present, and the source of the antigen-antibody complexes is unknown.
  - Type II, or reactive polyarthritis, is associated with infectious or inflammatory conditions distant from the joints, such as pancreatitis, urinary tract infections, otitis, heartworm disease, pyometra, and pneumonia.
  - Type III, or enteropathic polyarthritis, is associated with gastrointestinal or hepatic disease.
  - Type IV polyarthritis is associated with neoplasia, including carcinomas from a variety of sites, leiomyosarcoma, and lymphoma.
- **Vaccine-induced polyarthritis** occurs within 30 days of an initial or booster vaccine. The disease is typically transient, but in some breeds, such as the Akita, prolonged disease occurs, and the prognosis can be guarded.
- **Drug-induced polyarthritis** occurs most commonly following *sulfonamide* administration, especially in *Doberman Pinschers*. Other drugs such as phenobarbital, erythropoietin, penicillin, lincomycin, erythromycin, and cephalosporins have also been implicated. Clinical signs typically resolve within 5 days of discontinuing the drug.
- **Polyarthritis-polymyositis syndrome** is most common in Spaniels. The condition begins with fever, muscle and joint pain, and elevated creatine kinase. The myositis leads to fibrosis and contracture, limiting joint mobility.
- **Steroid-responsive meningitis-arteritis,** formerly known as *Beagle pain syndrome*, affects young medium- and large-breed dogs. A small proportion of dogs with immune-mediated polyarthritis will also have meningitis, reflecting an overlap between these 2 conditions.
- **Juvenile-onset polyarthritis** of **Akitas** affects puppies 9 weeks to 8 months of age. Cyclic fever, polyarthritis, and meningitis can occur. Puppies may also have nonregenerative anemia, neutrophilic leukocytosis, hypoalbuminemia, and hyperglobulinemia. A temporal relationship to vaccines is thought to be coincidental. The disease is inherited.
- **Familial Chinese Shar Pei fever** is an inherited autoimmune disease that occurs in 23% of Shar Pei dogs. Shar Pei dogs have an unstable duplication upstream of the gene hyaluronic acid synthetase 2 *(HAS2)*, leading to increased production of hyaluronic acid by dermal fibroblasts. This excess hyaluronic acid is responsible for the breed-defining skin folds, but degradation of this material is thought to trigger the immune system, leading to cyclic fever and pain. One component of the disease is hock swelling, which is caused by periarticular cellulitis with or without intra-articular inflammation.
- **Systemic lupus erythematosus (SLE)** is thought to account for <20% of immune-mediated polyarthritis in dogs. Onset is typically between 2 and 4 years of age. Polyarthritis may be accompanied by evidence of disease in other organs, such as the skin, kidney, bone marrow, or neuromuscular system. Predisposed breeds include German Shepherds, Shetland Sheepdogs, Beagles, Afghan Hounds, Irish Setters, Old English Sheepdogs, Cocker Spaniels, Collies, and Poodles. Neutrophils containing phagocytosed, partially degraded nuclear material, referred to as *lupus erythematosus cells (LE cells)*, are rarely detected in the synovial fluid of animals with systemic lupus erythematosus. The phagocytosed nuclear material in LE cells is dense, diffusely pink or purple, and displaces the nucleus to the periphery of

the cell. Leukophagocytic macrophages and neutrophils containing more granular nuclear remnants are common in the synovial fluid of acutely inflamed joints and should not be misinterpreted as LE cells. Interestingly, dogs owned by humans with SLE are more likely to develop the disease, suggesting a common environmental or infectious agent.
- **Plasmacytic/lymphocytic synovitis** is an insidious, non-erosive arthritis involving primarily the *stifle joint of small- and medium-sized breeds of dog*. The syndrome may be accompanied by joint laxity and partial or complete rupture of the cranial cruciate ligament, but it is seldom possible to determine which lesion came first. It is possible that the synovitis in these animals reflects an exaggerated immune response to mediators or antigens released following ligament damage, surgery, or degenerative joint disease. Radiographic evidence of degenerative joint disease may be present in some cases. The synovial membrane is thickened, edematous, and red/yellow on gross examination. Microscopic examination reveals a *marked diffuse and/or nodular plasmacytic/lymphocytic infiltration of the synovium and hypertrophy of synovial cells*. Villus hypertrophy may also be a feature. Unlike other forms of immune-mediated arthritis, the increase in cellularity of the synovial fluid is due predominantly to small mononuclear cells rather than neutrophils, the latter composing only 10-40% of the cell population.

Further reading

Johnson KC, Mackin AM. Canine immune-mediated polyarthritis part I: pathophysiology. J Am Anim Hosp Assoc 2012;48:12-17.

Olsson M, et al. A novel unstable duplication upstream of HAS2 predisposes to a breed-defining skin phenotype and a periodic fever syndrome in Chinese Shar-Pei dogs. PLoS Genet 2011;7:e1001332.

TUMORS AND TUMOR-LIKE LESIONS OF JOINTS

Malignant tumors

Historically, synovial cell sarcoma has been reported to be the most common or only malignant tumor of joints. However, more recent studies using immunohistochemistry have shown that multiple types of mesenchymal tumors with very different behaviors occur within and around joints.

Synovial cell sarcoma

In humans, there is a sarcoma that often occurs on the limbs but *outside* the joint capsule. It was originally named *synovial cell sarcoma* based on its microscopic appearance, which mimics the embryonic synovium. It is now known that the cell of origin is not synovial, but a pluripotential mesenchymal stem cell that occurs throughout the body. The tumor in humans (now called *synovial sarcoma*) has monophasic (spindle cells only) and biphasic (spindle and epithelial cells) forms. Although the epithelial component is cytokeratin-positive, immunohistochemistry is not used to identify the tumor in humans because a molecular test for a genetic translocation is more sensitive and specific. Therefore in humans, a synovial sarcoma is defined as a soft tissue sarcoma that is sometimes biphasic and has a specific genetic translocation. *In canine sarcomas, the identification of cytokeratin-positive cells does not indicate synovial origin*. Normal synoviocytes are not cytokeratin positive, and the tumor in humans called synovial sarcoma is known to *not* be of synoviocyte origin. *There is no tumor of synovial origin recognized in humans*. Additionally, veterinary pathologists have no marker to identify tumors of synoviocyte origin, except those of histiocytic (type A) origin, in which CD18 can be used. If a tumor of type B synoviocytes exists, we have no way of recognizing it, that is, no specific marker of type B synoviocyte origin. The intra-articular tumors previously diagnosed as synovial cell sarcoma likely represent a variety of soft tissue sarcomas, some of which may have arisen from type B synoviocytes, but more likely represent typical soft tissue sarcomas, including perivascular wall tumors, nerve sheath tumors, and fibrosarcomas. Although the type B synoviocytes are sometimes called fibroblastic, they produce the viscous glycosaminoglycan component of synovial fluid, not collagen. Therefore tumors arising from type B synoviocytes would be expected to produce viscous fluid. One candidate for this type of tumor is the synovial myxoma; however, it has not been proven to be of synoviocyte origin and is benign. Therefore *the term synovial cell sarcoma should not be used* for this or any other tumor until a way of identifying them is found.

Histiocytic sarcoma

Histiocytic sarcoma is a malignancy of dendritic cell origin that may be localized or disseminated. In veterinary medicine, this neoplasm is best characterized in dogs. The disseminated form involves multiple sites and may represent a later stage of the localized form. The neoplastic cells express leukocyte surface markers characteristic of dendritic cells, such as CD1, CD11c, and MHC II. Because most leukocyte surface markers are detectable only in frozen tissue, CD18, a formalin-resistant marker of hematopoietic origin, is used to help diagnose histiocytic sarcoma in formalin-fixed tissue. Although it is not specific for histiocytic sarcoma, *CD18 membrane staining of cells with the appropriate morphology is considered diagnostic*. These tumors may arise from type A or histiocytic synoviocytes, but they may also arise from the dendritic cells within the subintima. Because their appearance and behavior is similar to histiocytic sarcomas arising in other tissues, histiocytic sarcoma is the appropriate diagnosis, rather than histiocytic synovial cell sarcoma. *Histiocytic sarcoma is the most commonly occurring tumor within the joints of dogs*. Bernese Mountain Dogs, Rottweilers, Bullmastiffs, Golden Retrievers, Labrador Retrievers, and Flat-Coated Retrievers are predisposed, especially if they have a pre-existing joint problem, such as ruptured cranial cruciate ligament. This is hypothesized to be due to malignant transformation of dendritic cells within a chronically inflamed synovium. Histiocytic sarcoma also occurs in the joints of cats, but much less frequently. Histiocytic sarcoma is a *grossly* multilobulated, infiltrative tumor that often fills the joint and extends into the surrounding bones and soft tissues (Fig. 2-211). The stifle is the joint most commonly affected, followed by the elbow, shoulder, coxofemoral, carpal, and tarsal joints. *Cytologically*, the cells have abundant, often vacuolated cytoplasm (Fig. 2-212). Microscopically, the neoplastic cells are round, polygonal, to spindle shaped with abundant eosinophilic cytoplasm and distinct cell borders (Fig. 2-213A). The cytoplasm sometimes contains vacuoles to such a degree that, before the use of immunohistochemistry, some of these tumors were diagnosed as liposarcomas. By immunohistochemistry, there is

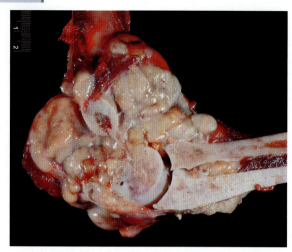

Figure 2-211 Histiocytic sarcoma in the elbow of a dog. Multiple soft lobules fill the joint and extend into the surrounding tissues. (Courtesy B.K. Harrington.)

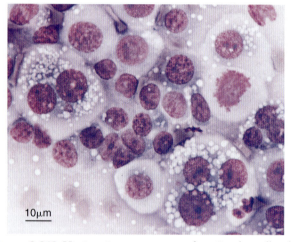

Figure 2-212 Histiocytic sarcoma in a dog. Cytologically, the neoplastic cells have abundant finely vacuolated cytoplasm and occasional multinucleation.

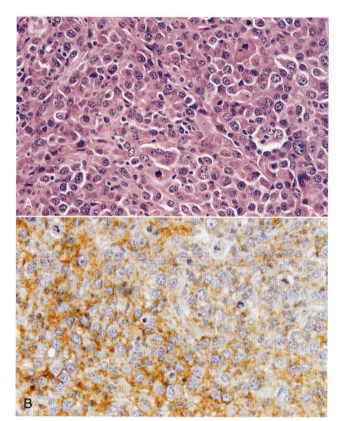

Figure 2-213 Histiocytic sarcoma in a dog. **A.** The neoplastic cells are pleomorphic with abundant eosinophilic cytoplasm, frequent mitoses, and occasional multinucleation. There are non-neoplastic lymphocytes and neutrophils intermingled with the neoplastic cells. **B.** Immunohistochemistry for CD18 is variably intense within the cytoplasm and along the cell membranes.

membrane staining for CD18 (Fig. 2-213B). The cells are also positive for CD1 and CD11c, but these markers require frozen tissue. Although the tumor cells are negative for CD3 and CD79a, there are often numerous non-neoplastic lymphocytes, as well as other inflammatory cells, such as eosinophils, neutrophils, and plasma cells, throughout the tumor. Nuclear features such as size, shape, chromatin distribution, and nucleoli are highly variable, but pleomorphic nuclei and coarse chromatin are common. Mitoses are usually frequent and sometimes bizarre. Multinucleated cells are often, but not always, present. *Compared to histiocytic sarcoma at other sites, the joint location has a more favorable outcome.* Common metastatic sites include lymph nodes, lung, liver, and spleen.

Other sarcomas

Fibrosarcoma, myxosarcoma, hemangiosarcoma, hemangiopericytoma, liposarcoma, peripheral nerve sheath tumors, and other soft tissue sarcomas can also arise within joints and should be diagnosed using the same morphologic and immunohistochemical techniques used for soft tissue sarcomas in other sites. Rhabdomyosarcoma and osteosarcoma can also involve joints by extension from adjacent muscles and bones, respectively. Multicentric lymphosarcoma can affect the synovium, with lameness as the presenting clinical sign; this has been reported in dogs, cats, sheep, and cattle. Chondrosarcomas of the joint are thought to arise from nodules of synovial chondroid metaplasia or chondrocytes within the periarticular fibrocartilage, rather than the articular cartilage chondrocytes, which are mitotically inactive. There are 2 reports of chondrosarcoma arising from malignant transformation of primary synovial chondromatosis in dogs. Chondrosarcomas arising in bone can also extend into adjacent joints.

Benign tumors
Synovial myxoma

This is the second most common neoplasm occurring in the joints of dogs. Cats can also be affected. Large-breed, middle-aged dogs, especially Doberman Pinschers and Labrador Retrievers, are most commonly affected. This neoplasm occurs in a single joint; the stifle and digit are most commonly affected, followed by the tarsus, elbow, carpus, and vertebral facets. The abundant viscous fluid produced by these tumors suggests they are of type B synoviocyte origin; however, this has not been proved, as there are no reliable markers of type B synoviocytes. In the past these were often diagnosed as myxosarcoma or nodular synovial hyperplasia. Synovial

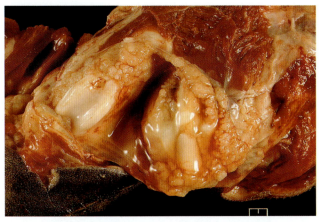

Figure 2-214 Synovial myxoma in the stifle of a dog. Numerous soft translucent nodules line the synovium and fill the joint. (Courtesy A.J. Cooley.)

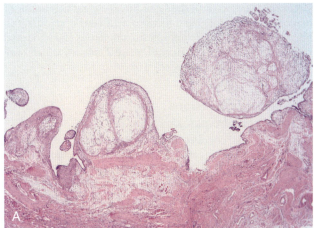

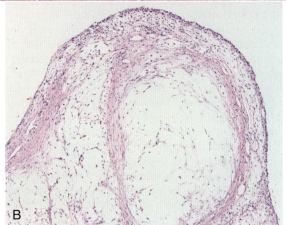

Figure 2-215 Synovial myxoma in a dog. **A.** Round myxoid nodules expand the synovium. **B.** The nodules are composed of stellate to spindle cells within an abundant clear myxoid matrix.

myxomas are slow-growing tumors that often have a long (months to years) history of clinical signs before diagnosis. Although synovial myxoma is a benign tumor, it can cause bony lysis on both sides of the affected joint. Therefore this benign tumor cannot always be distinguished radiographically from malignant joint tumors, such as histiocytic sarcoma. *Grossly*, synovial myxomas consist of soft, white translucent nodules and pockets of viscous fluid. The nodules often line the entire inner surface of the joint capsule (Fig. 2-214) and exude abundant clear viscous fluid on cut section. These nodules are softer than synovial chondromatosis and more distinctly nodular than histiocytic sarcoma. The translucent nodules and pockets of viscous fluid can extend outside the joint capsule and into adjacent bones and muscle. *Microscopically*, these tumors have a characteristic appearance consisting of variably sized, sparsely cellular round *nodules* (Fig. 2-215A) composed of stellate to spindle cells with long cell processes suspended in an abundant hypovascular myxoid matrix (Fig. 2-215B). Mitotic figures are rare, and nuclei are small and hyperchromatic. Foamy non-neoplastic macrophages are frequently scattered throughout. The intra-articular portions of the tumor are covered with synovium, which is often hyperplastic and inflamed. There are occasional cystic spaces filled with fluid and lined by synovium or compressed mesenchymal cells. In some cases, the myxomatous nodules extend into bone, causing lysis, as well as infiltrating beyond the joint capsule along fascial planes, sometimes to the surgical margins of amputation sites. Despite this, *the prognosis is good, and metastases have not been reported.*

Periarticular fibroma is an uncommon tumor that most often occurs in dogs as a solitary mass in the tissues surrounding the carpal joint. The tarsal joint can also be affected, as can the more distal joints of the limbs. More proximal joints are rarely affected. Periarticular fibromas are slow-growing tumors that are often asymptomatic. There are no radiographic changes except for the periarticular soft tissue mass. The *gross appearance* is of a discrete, firm nodular white mass attached to the lateral or medial joint capsule or tendon sheath. Because some cases include a history of trauma, these masses may represent focal fibrous scar tissue; however, they are typically discrete from the overlying skin and more spherical than expected for a fibrous scar. *Microscopically*, they are similar to fibromas occurring elsewhere, consisting of dense collagen and sparse fibroblasts; some periarticular fibromas will have dissecting bands of myxomatous stroma. The mass is distinct from the surrounding subcutaneous collagen, but is often continuous with the joint capsule or tendon sheath, making complete excision difficult. However, the prognosis is good, even with incomplete excision. The lameness does not always resolve with removal, indicating that these masses are not always the cause of the lameness.

Giant cell tumor of tendon sheath is a rare tumor occurring in the distal limbs of cats. In humans, this is the most common primary tumor of the hand; the cell of origin is unknown. Middle-aged cats are most commonly affected. *Grossly*, this tumor forms a fusiform mass on the distal limb with intimate involvement of flexor or extensor tendons. *Microscopically*, these are multilobular masses composed of polygonal to spindle-shaped cells mixed with multinucleated giant cells. Multinucleated giant cells vary in number but are often more frequent at the periphery. Mitoses are rare in both populations. The stroma varies from dense and collagenous to loose and myxomatous. The prognosis is good with complete excision (which often requires amputation). These tumors will recur following incomplete excision. Metastasis has not been reported. In cats, *an important differential diagnosis for any spindle cell tumor with giant cells is vaccine-associated sarcoma*. Some feline vaccine protocols have recommended vaccinating distal to the elbow and stifle; therefore vaccine-associated sarcomas could occur in the same site as a giant cell tumor of tendon sheath. Malignant features within the spindle cell populations (nuclear pleomorphism, numerous and abnormal mitoses, etc.) will help distinguish these 2 entities, which have very different prognoses.

Non-neoplastic lesions
Synovial chondromatosis

Primary synovial chondromatosis is rare and occurs spontaneously rather than in response to degenerative joint disease. Most reports are in dogs, but cats, horses, and pigs are also rarely affected. The term synovial *osteo*chondromatosis is also used, reflecting that many of the nodules undergo endochondral ossification. Affected dogs are mostly large- and giant-breed males. The shoulder is most often affected, followed by the digits, stifle, elbow, and hock. *Grossly*, there are numerous masses in a single joint without significant pre-existing degenerative joint disease. The joint is lined and filled with hard, pearly nodules ranging from 1 mm to 1 cm in diameter. The number of nodules can be in the thousands. Most of the nodules are attached to the synovium, but many become detached "loose bodies." There may be grooves and erosions in the articular cartilage caused by the nodules, but the degree of cartilage erosion is mild compared to the nodular proliferation. In rare cases, there can be malignant transformation into chondrosarcoma (see Fig. 2-157).

Secondary synovial chondromatosis *occurs in association with degenerative joint disease.* The nodules are less numerous (5-10) and often mixed with other forms of synovial proliferation and metaplasia. The erosive changes in the articular cartilage are more marked than is the degree of synovial proliferation (Fig. 2-216). There are 2 possible mechanisms of

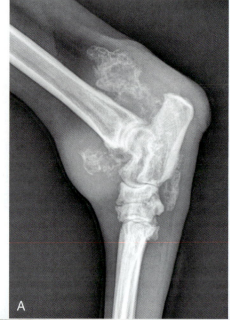

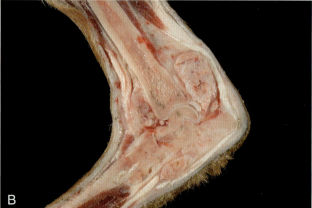

Figure 2-217 Synovial chondromatosis in the tarsal joint of a 6-year-old German Shepherd dog. **A.** Radiograph showing the partially ossified cartilaginous nodules within the joint, which has relatively mild degenerative joint disease. **B.** Longitudinal section of the same joint with multiple, variably sized nodules filling the joint. Note the intact articular cartilage.

formation: Either pieces of articular cartilage break free and lodge in the synovium or, more likely, there is metaplasia of the hyperplastic synovium into cartilage, which undergoes ossification to form bony nodules. These lesions can detach and become free floating within the synovial fluid. In some cases, it is difficult to distinguish whether the lesion is primary or secondary (Fig. 2-217A, B).

Synovial cysts

Synovial cysts are rare periarticular synovium-lined structures filled with synovial fluid. They typically communicate with the adjacent joint, which is often affected by degenerative joint disease. The pathogenesis is thought to be joint capsule herniation caused by increased intra-articular pressure. They can also form adjacent to tendon sheaths. *Grossly*, synovial cysts typically affect a single joint and are most common as fluctuant swellings in and around the elbow of geriatric **cats**.

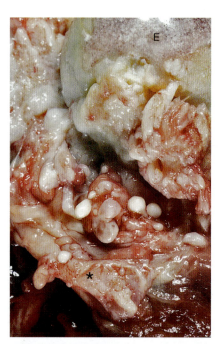

Figure 2-216 Synovial chondromatosis in the coxofemoral joint of a dog. There are variably sized, smooth white and gray cartilaginous nodules within the hyperplastic synovium. Also note the marked thickening of the joint capsule (asterisk) and eburnation of the femoral head (E). (Courtesy R.A. Fairley.)

They have also been reported in feline digits. The cysts can be numerous and extensive, extending distally and proximally to the carpus and shoulder, respectively. Radiographs usually reveal degenerative joint disease with osteophytes of both elbows, even though the synovial cysts affect only one joint. Rarely, the cysts contain 1-2 mm calculi. Affected joints also have cartilage erosion and osteophytes. In **dogs**, clinically relevant cysts are most often intraspinal and extradural, arising from the articular facet joints and compressing the spinal cord. Extradural cysts within the spinal canal have also been reported in **horses**, but the more common site in horses is adjacent to the digital flexor tendon sheath. *Microscopically*, the synovial cysts of cats are lined by synoviocytes, which are in turn surrounded by a thin collagenous wall, or adipose, muscle, or granulation tissue. Low numbers of siderophages, lymphocytes, and plasma cells may be present in the surrounding tissue. **Ganglion cysts** contain viscous fluid but do not have a synovial lining. These may form by loss of the synovial lining from a true synovial cyst, escape of synovial fluid without herniation of the synovial membrane, or by mucinous degeneration of periarticular connective tissue. Ganglion cysts may be similar to adventitious bursae described previously with miscellaneous inflammatory conditions of joints.

Synovial pad proliferation

This is a soft tissue mass that occurs in the *fetlock joint of horses, typically racing horses*. It was formerly termed chronic proliferative or villonodular synovitis. The *metacarpophalangeal joint is most commonly affected*; involvement of the hindlimb (metatarsophalangeal joint) is rare. The synovial pad of the fetlock joint is a fold (plica) of fibrous connective tissue in the dorsal recess of the joint capsule at its attachment to the cannon bone. The lesion is formed by enlargement of this plica secondary to injury. Causes include osteochondral fractures of the dorsal proximal phalanx, degenerative joint disease, and hyperextension of the joint causing impact trauma to the normal synovial plica. *Grossly*, these occur as a visible or palpable mass at the proximal dorsal aspect of the affected fetlock. Most masses are 7-10 mm in diameter. The medial portion of the mass is usually thicker than the lateral portion. The mass is often rubbery and pedunculated. The color varies from tan to red-brown, depending on the age of the lesion and amount of hemorrhage. *Microscopically*, acute lesions may contain blood, hemosiderin, and granulation tissue. As the lesion ages, granulation tissue is replaced by dense collagen.

Further reading

Aeffner F, et al. Synovial osteochondromatosis with malignant transformation to chondrosarcoma in a dog Vet Pathol 2012;49:1036-1039.

Affolter VK, et al. Localized and disseminated histiocytic sarcoma of dendritic cell origin in dogs. Vet Pathol 2002;39:74-83.

Craig LE, et al. The diagnosis and prognosis of synovial tumors in dogs: 35 cases. Vet Pathol 2002;39:66-73.

Craig LE, et al. Canine synovial myxoma: 39 cases. Vet Pathol 2010;47:931-936.

Klahn SL, et al. Evaluation and comparison of outcomes in dogs with periarticular and nonperiarticular histiocytic sarcoma. J Am Vet Med Assoc 2011;239:90-96.

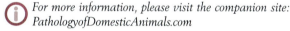

For more information, please visit the companion site: PathologyofDomesticAnimals.com

CHAPTER 3

Muscle and Tendon

Barry J. Cooper • Beth A. Valentine

MUSCLE	**165**
STRUCTURE AND DEVELOPMENT	**165**
Motor units	165
Muscle structure	165
Microscopic structure	165
Ultrastructure	167
Myogenesis and muscle development	167
Histochemical fiber types	169
Specialized structures	170
Techniques for the study of muscle	171
BASIC REACTIONS OF MUSCLE	**173**
Atrophy	173
Denervation atrophy	173
Disuse atrophy	175
Atrophy resulting from malnutrition or cachexia	177
Atrophy of endocrine disease	178
Myopathic atrophy and myopathic change	178
Hypertrophy	178
Muscle injury and necrosis	180
Muscle regeneration	182
Muscle fibrosis	184
Other myofiber alterations	185
Postmortem changes	186
CONGENITAL AND INHERITED DISEASES	**186**
Primary central nervous system conditions	187
Arthrogryposis and dysraphism	187
Congenital flexures	189
Muscular defects	189
Forelimb-girdle muscular anomaly of Japanese black cattle	189
"Splayleg" (myofibrillar hypoplasia) in piglets	189
Myostatin defects leading to muscular hyperplasia	190
Muscular steatosis	191
Congenital clefts of the diaphragm	191
Muscular dystrophy	192
Canine X-linked muscular dystrophy	192
Feline X-linked muscular dystrophy	194
Other muscular dystrophies in cats	196
Ovine muscular dystrophy	196
Inherited and congenital myopathies	197
Breed-associated myopathies in the dog	197
Inherited and congenital myopathies of cats	198
Inherited and congenital myopathies of cattle	199
Inherited and congenital myopathies of sheep	200
Inherited and congenital myopathies of horses	200
Myotonic and spastic syndromes	200
Myotonia in the dog	201
Myotonia in the cat	201
Myotonia in the goat	201
Periodic paralyses	202
Myotonic dystrophy-like disorders in dogs and horses	202
Spastic syndromes	203
Metabolic myopathies	204
Metabolic myopathies of the dog	204
Metabolic myopathy of the cat	205
Metabolic myopathies of the horse	205
Metabolic myopathies of cattle and sheep	207
Other metabolic myopathies	208
Congenital myasthenia gravis	209
Canine congenital myasthenia	209
Feline congenital myasthenia	209
Malignant hyperthermia	209
Malignant hyperthermia in pigs (porcine stress syndrome)	209
Malignant hyperthermia in dogs	210
Malignant hyperthermia in horses	210
CIRCULATORY DISTURBANCES OF MUSCLE	**210**
Compartment syndrome	211
Downer syndrome	212
Muscle crush syndrome	212
Vascular occlusive syndrome	212
Postanesthetic myopathy in horses	213
PHYSICAL INJURIES OF MUSCLE	**213**
Ossifying fibrodysplasia	213
Strains/tears/ruptures/fibrotic myopathies/contractures	213
NUTRITIONAL MYOPATHY	**214**
Etiology and pathogenesis	214
Nutritional myopathy of cattle	215
Nutritional myopathy of sheep and goats	216
Nutritional myopathy of pigs	217
Nutritional myopathy of horses	218
Nutritional myopathy of other species	218
TOXIC MYOPATHIES	**218**
Ionophore toxicosis	219
Toxic plants and plant-origin toxins	219
DEGENERATIVE (NECROTIZING) MYOPATHIES INCLUDING RHABDOMYOLYSIS	**221**
Exertional myopathies	221
Exertional rhabdomyolysis in the horse	221
Canine exertional rhabdomyolysis	223
Exertional myopathy in other species ("capture myopathy")	223
Equine systemic calcinosis	223
Other degenerative myopathies	224
MYOPATHIES ASSOCIATED WITH ENDOCRINE DISORDERS	**224**
Hypothyroidism	224
Hyperthyroidism	224
Hyperadrenocorticism	224
Other endocrinopathies	225
MYOPATHIES ASSOCIATED WITH SERUM ELECTROLYTE ABNORMALITIES	**225**
Hypokalemia in cats	225
Hypokalemia in cattle	225
Hypernatremia in cats	225
Hypophosphatemia in dogs	225
IMMUNE-MEDIATED CONDITIONS	**225**
Masticatory myositis of dogs	226
Polymyositis of dogs	227
Other immune-mediated myositides of dogs	228
Polymyositis of cats	228
Immune-mediated myositis of horses	229
Acquired myasthenia gravis	229
MYOSITIS RESULTING FROM INFECTION	**230**
Suppurative myositis	230

Clostridial myositis	230	**NEOPLASTIC DISEASES OF MUSCLE**	240
Malignant edema and gas gangrene	232	Rhabdomyoma	241
Blackleg	232	Rhabdomyosarcoma	241
Pseudo-blackleg	233	Nonmuscle primary tumors of muscle	244
Specific infectious diseases with muscle alterations	233	Secondary tumors of skeletal muscle	245
Granulomatous lesions	233	Muscle pseudotumors	246
Staphylococcal granuloma	233		
Roeckl's granuloma of cattle	234	**TENDONS AND APONEUROSES**	246
Changes in muscle secondary to systemic infections	234	**GENERAL CONSIDERATIONS**	246
PARASITIC DISEASES	234	**TENDON AGING AND INJURY**	247
Sarcocystosis	234	**PARASITIC DISEASES OF TENDONS AND APONEUROSES**	247
Eosinophilic myositis of cattle, sheep, and camelids	236	**FIBROMATOUS DISORDERS OF TENDONS AND APONEUROSES**	248
Toxoplasma and *Neospora* myositis	237	Musculoaponeurotic fibromatosis (desmoid tumor) of the horse	248
Trichinellosis	237	Fibrodysplasia ossificans progressive	248
Cysticercosis	239		
Hepatozoonosis	240		
Leishmaniasis	240		

ACKNOWLEDGMENTS

Dr. Thomas J. Hulland (University of Guelph), author of this chapter in the 2nd, 3rd, and 4th editions, is fully acknowledged for his contributions to the original text and illustrations. Dr. M. Donald McGavin (University of Tennessee) generously gave his time and energy to assist with photomicrographs. We acknowledge the contributions of the late Dr. John van Vleet to the previous edition. Some of the material provided by these authors in previous editions has been retained.

MUSCLE

This chapter is concerned with skeletal muscle, *the most abundant tissue in the mammalian body*. Skeletal muscle is also sometimes referred to as *striated muscle* (although, of course, cardiac muscle is also striated) or voluntary muscle. We use the term *skeletal muscle* throughout this chapter.

It is unfortunate that, in veterinary medicine, skeletal muscle is often overlooked in routine pathology studies, especially in autopsy cases. Muscle expresses a wide variety of lesions, some of them secondary but many reflecting primary muscle disease. Indeed, whole textbooks have been devoted to muscle disease and muscle pathology of humans. Without routine sampling of muscle, lesions can be missed. For example, one autopsy study involving a large number of horses found muscle lesions (excluding polysaccharide inclusions) in 65% of animals. In this chapter, we attempt to document the variety of diseases and lesions that are currently recognized in animals.

STRUCTURE AND DEVELOPMENT
Motor units

In veterinary medicine, skeletal muscle is often included as part of the "musculoskeletal system" in which the pathology of muscle is grouped with that of bone. However, it is more appropriate to *consider muscle as part of the neuromuscular system* because of the interactions of the nervous system and muscle both in health and disease. Fundamental to that idea is the concept of the motor unit.

A motor unit consists of a motor neuron, located in the spinal cord, and all the muscle fibers that it innervates. Functionally, when the motor neuron fires, all of the muscle fibers that it innervates are stimulated. Graded muscle contraction is accomplished by recruitment of additional motor units. The number of muscle fibers in a motor unit varies, both within and between muscles, ranging from the low 10s to thousands depending on the "fineness" of control needed. The muscle fibers in a particular motor unit overlap and are admixed with those in adjacent motor units. Many of the properties of the muscle fibers in a motor unit are determined by the neuron that innervates it. This is of particular importance, from the point of view of pathology, to the determination of fiber type and the changes that occur in denervating diseases, which are discussed more fully later.

Muscle structure

Muscles are made up of muscle fibers, also called *myofibers*, which are variable in both diameter and length. Fiber diameter varies within and between muscles and depending on age, exercise, nutritional status, and species, although the fibers of such disparately sized species as mouse and horse are not much different. Muscle fibers in the extrinsic muscles of the eye are consistently small (10-30 μm in diameter) and round; those of the major limb muscles vary, with an average least diameter of 40-65 μm and appear polygonal in cross-sections that lack shrinkage artifact, such as in frozen sections. The size of fibers increases with age until puberty, at which time males have slightly larger fibers than females. In old age, the fiber diameter slowly decreases. In those domestic animals that have been studied, the size distribution of muscle fibers conforms more or less to a normal unimodal distribution curve. A distinctly bimodal curve develops in a muscle when disease, pregnancy, or nutritional status prompts either atrophy or hypertrophy of fibers.

Microscopic structure

Myofibers are long tubular cells up to ~10 cm in length (Fig. 3-1). The longer length of many whole muscles is accomplished by either a pinnate arrangement or by overlapping of fibers. Physiologically, the limited length of individual muscle fibers makes sense so as to limit the amount of time required for the action potential to be conducted along the full length of the fiber to produce synchronous contraction. Individual muscle fibers are delimited by a plasma membrane, the *sarcolemma*, surrounding which is the *basal lamina*. (It should be noted that in the older literature the term *sarcolemma* was applied to the plasma membrane, the basal lamina, and the endomysial connective tissue as a collective supporting structure. However, modern usage is to apply the term to the plasma membrane.) Muscle fibers contain a large number of nuclei, which characteristically are situated immediately below the sarcolemma (Fig. 3-2A; see also Fig. 3-1). In normal muscle, <3% of the nuclei of the multinucleated myofiber are displaced internally, although the number tends to be higher adjacent to the myotendinous junction where muscle and tendon interdigitate. An increased number of internal nuclei may occur in diseased muscle. Myonuclei are slender, oval, and have evenly distributed chromatin and 1 or 2 small nucleoli. Most of the volume of the fiber is occupied by myofibrils, which, in quality longitudinal sections, can be seen to have cross-striations. Muscle fibers contain numerous

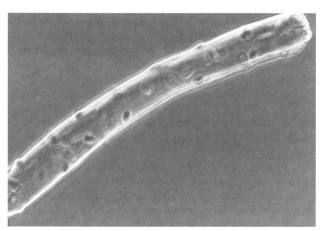

Figure 3-1 A small **isolated muscle fiber** from a mouse showing cross-striations and numerous subsarcolemmal nuclei. Phase contrast microscopy. (From Zachary JF, McGavin MD. Pathologic Basis of Veterinary Disease. 5th ed. St. Louis: Mosby/Elsevier; 2012.)

mitochondria, most clearly visible in frozen sections; their number depends on the type of fiber (see later). Other organelles are present and are discussed under Ultrastructure.

Supporting the muscle fibers and their satellite cells is a connective tissue framework. Intimately applied to the basal lamina of each muscle fiber is the scant *endomysium*, which carries the capillary network with its longitudinal orientation. Around each primary bundle, or fascicle, of 40-150 fibers is the more abundant *perimysium*, in which run larger vessels, nerve trunks, and sensory neuromuscular spindles. Finally, surrounding the whole muscle lies the *epimysium*, which carries tendon organ sensory endings and, sometimes, prominent tendinous bands.

Closely associated with the muscle fibers is a second population of cells, the **satellite cells**. These occupy a position between the basal lamina and the sarcolemma (Fig. 3-2B). These cells are resting myoblasts that play an important role in early muscle fiber growth and muscle regeneration. In the resting state they contain a nucleus and a minimal amount of cytoplasm with a few mitochondria and tubules and cannot be distinguished in routine light microscopic sections from the subsarcolemmal myonuclei. Satellite cell numbers progressively decrease from the neonatal period to old age.

Unlike mature muscle fibers, satellite cells are capable of mitotic division. When these cells divide in a developing muscle they give rise to daughter cells, some of which become postmitotic and fuse with the enlarging multinucleated myofiber. Other daughter cells remain as part of the satellite cell pool outside the myofiber and retain mitotic capability. It is clear that this mechanism makes the satellite cells a progressively smaller proportion of the total nuclear population within the basal lamina.

Satellite cells unquestionably play an *essential role in muscle repair*. However, the old view that muscle repair is the exclusive domain of these cells is changing. Recent studies have demonstrated that stem cells, either mesenchymal stem cells or those derived from bone marrow, can become myoblasts

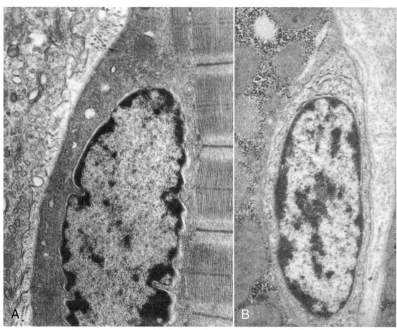

Figure 3-2 A. Myofiber nucleus and adjacent myofibril. **B. Satellite cell** lying between the sarcolemma and the basal lamina. Transmission electron micrograph. (Courtesy T.J. Hulland.)

and potentially can participate in regeneration of skeletal muscle. However, the contribution of these myogenic stem cells in the overall process of muscle cell regeneration is still unclear. What is clear is that experimental depletion of satellite cells prevents muscle regeneration so they are essential for repair of injured muscle. Both satellite cells, themselves *true stem cells* (because of their ability to replicate the resting pool), and *other tissue stem cells with myogenic potential* may play a role in the development of muscle neoplasms, a concept discussed later in this chapter.

The ability of myoblasts, whether derived from stem cells or satellite cells, to participate in the repair of muscle in diseases such as muscular dystrophy, has aroused interest in delivering these cells to diseased muscle, either hematogenously or via direct injection into the affected muscle. To date success has been limited, but studies continue.

Ultrastructure

The most distinctive ultrastructural characteristic of skeletal muscle cells is the presence of *striated myofibrils*, approximately 0.5-1.0 μm in diameter, consisting, in cross-section, of thousands of regularly sized and regularly oriented *myofilaments* (Fig. 3-3A, B). In longitudinal section, contractile units or *sarcomeres*, about 20 μm long, extend from one Z band to the next, and consist of bands and lines created by the interdigitation of thick and thin filaments. The *thin filaments*, 6 nm wide, consist of *actin*, associated with which are the proteins *tropomyosin* and *troponin*. They are attached to the electron-dense Z band containing noncontractile proteins, including α-actinin, and incompletely overlap the 16-nm wide myosin *thick filaments*. The zone of no overlap adjacent to the Z band is referred to as the I band. The central zone between the ends of the thin filaments in which only thick filaments are visible is the H band, which is divided by the M line. The A band is the wide central zone that extends from one end of the thick filaments to the other and alternates with the I band. In muscle contraction, the actin filaments and myosin filaments slide over one another, causing the Z bands to move closer together and reducing the widths of the I and H band. In cross-section at a central point where thick and thin filaments are present, one myosin filament is surrounded at regular intervals by 6 thin filaments, or 12 when the sarcomere is in strong contraction.

Myofibrils are surrounded by *sarcoplasm* (the muscle cell cytoplasm), which makes up 30-40% of the fiber volume, and in it are elements of the T-tubular system, the sarcoplasmic reticulum, mitochondria, lysosomes, glycogen granules and, often, fat droplets. The sarcoplasmic reticulum in the muscle fibers of all mammals forms a labyrinth that surrounds myofibrils and abuts at the triads with the T tubule, located between 2 terminal cisternae of sarcoplasmic reticulum (see Fig. 3-3A, B). The T tubule is an invagination of the sarcolemma, allowing action potentials to be conducted deep into the cell, and the close association with the sarcoplasmic reticulum is important in excitation-contraction coupling. In mammals, these triads can be found at each end of each sarcomere. Sarcoplasm between the myofibrils and the outer cell membrane is often rich in mitochondria and glycogen granules.

Muscle cells contain a complex cytoskeleton that functions to maintain the organization and structural integrity of the fiber. It is beyond the scope of this chapter to discuss all the cytoskeletal proteins in detail but some deserve mention because of their usefulness in studying muscle disease. The *intermediate filament desmin* is important as an immunohistochemical marker for muscle differentiation, particularly in tumors. Closely associated with the sarcolemma is the important protein *dystrophin*, which is linked to *laminin* in the basal lamina via a complex of membrane proteins. Mutations in different members of this complex are responsible for various forms of muscular dystrophy.

Quite apart from their ability to shorten in active contraction, myofibrils are capable of length adjustment accomplished by shedding or adding sarcomeres. This can be important when muscles are immobilized in either a shortened or lengthened state, as in a cast. This, along with accompanying changes in interstitial connective tissue, can result in reduction in range of motion after removal of the cast. During hypertrophy or atrophy, the breadth of myofibers can also be increased or decreased by building or discarding myofilaments and myofibrils.

Muscle has a high requirement for arginine, glucogenic amino acids, and energy, the last reflected in part by the content of glycogen or the numerous mitochondria observable in different muscle fiber types.

Myogenesis and muscle development

Development of skeletal muscle is a complex process that is still under intense study. The advent of sophisticated molecular techniques has led to an explosion of understanding of the genes and signaling mechanisms involved in the process, a topic that is too complex to discuss in detail here. However, a brief outline is relevant to our understanding of some disease processes in muscle.

The majority of skeletal muscle precursor cells, including those that will become the limb and axial muscles, arise in the embryo from *mesodermal somites*, which give rise to *myotomes*. Some muscles, such as muscles of the head and neck, arise from sites outside the somites. Within each myotome, which corresponds roughly to a vertebral body segment with its spinal nerve, the individual muscles develop by a process of aggregation and migration of presumptive myogenic cells.

The first clear sign of differentiation is the migration of myogenic cells, destined to become myocytes, into the regions where future muscles will appear. This occurs before any neural influence is exerted. The direct connection of the nerve to the myotome determines the subsequent route of innervation, but because migration occurs, the mature muscle may receive nerve fibers derived from more than one myotome.

During development, these precursor cells undergo determination to become *committed myoblasts* and in turn become *mononuclear myocytes*, which subsequently fuse to form the multinucleated *myofibers*, the early immature fibers being referred to as *myotubes*. Multiple gene products are involved in the determination and commitment of the precursor cells to the myogenic lineage. Among these are the transcription factors Pax3 and Pax7, and an array of 4 myogenic regulatory factors (MRFs), specifically Myf5, MyoD, Mrf4 (also known as Myf6), and myogenin. As discussed later, Pax3 and Pax7 can be involved in the development of muscle tumors (rhabdomyosarcomas), whereas MyoD and myogenin are sensitive markers of muscle cell lineage in tumors.

Myogenesis is similar in a number of species in which it has been studied, including rodents, pigs, and sheep. It is considered to occur in 4 somewhat overlapping phases, namely

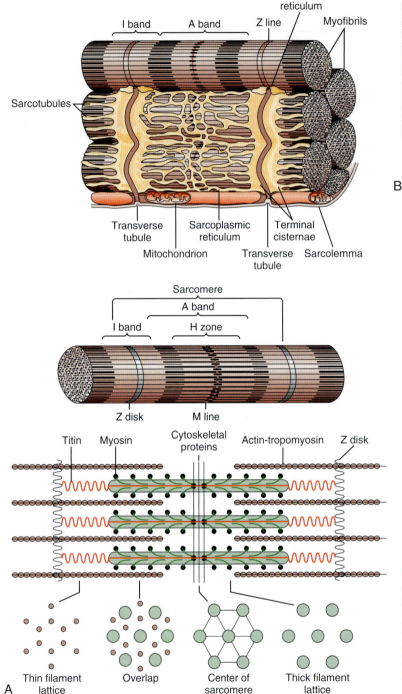
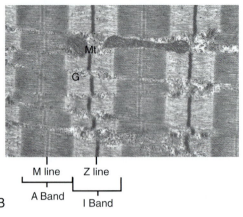

Figure 3-3 A. Schematic diagram showing muscle structure, including sarcomeric arrangement and orientation of the T-tubules and sarcoplasmic reticulum. (From Copstead-Kirkhorn LE, et al. Pathophysiology: Biological and Behavioral Perspective. 4th ed. St. Louis: Saunders; 2010.) B. Ultrastructure of skeletal muscle showing Z line, A and I bands, and the M line. Mitochondria (Mt) and glycogen granules (G) are also shown.

embryonic, fetal, neonatal, and *adult,* each involving the MRFs, the proliferation of myogenic precursors, the commitment to become postmitotic myoblasts and myocytes, and fusion to form multinucleated myofibers. During the embryonic phase, myoblasts fuse to form primary myofibers, whereas in the fetal phase myoblasts fuse both with the primary fibers, and with other myoblasts to form a series of generations of secondary myofibers, aligned along previous generations, which in a sense act as templates. During the fetal and neonatal phases, myoblasts continue to fuse with existing myofibers, thus increasing their number of nuclei. In the adult, incorporation of myoblasts into the growing myofibers can still occur, but much of the enlargement of fibers involves hypertrophy without fusion. Embryonic, fetal, and adult myoblasts are not identical, in that they demonstrate distinct differences in their requirements for various MRFs as well as in other characteristics. Similarly, primary, secondary, and adult myofibers differ, including in the type of *myosin heavy chains (myHC)* and other proteins of the contractile apparatus that they express. Importantly, many of the events involved in muscle development are recapitulated in regeneration of muscle after injury.

Further development of the immature myotube, allowing it to become a mature muscle fiber, consists of construction of actin and myosin filaments, incorporation of multiple other essential proteins, formation of the Z band into which the thin actin filaments insert, and evolution of the tubular systems. The last of these involves the invagination of the T tubular system from caveolae or other small, regular recesses on the sarcoplasmic membrane. As the myofiber matures, myonuclei move to the subsarcolemmal position.

Initial development of muscle, until about the end of the first trimester, is independent of innervation, but subsequent development is dependent on a functional neural connection. During initial formation of myofibers, fast myHC isoforms are expressed. As fibers become innervated, other myHC isoforms, including type I, are expressed. Differentiation of skeletal muscle, including the determination of fiber type (see later), is therefore largely determined by the characteristics of the innervating neuron, although locally acting myogenic factors also contribute.

Histochemical fiber types

Skeletal *muscle fibers are heterogeneous* and show differences in a variety of biochemical and physiologic characteristics. Classically, fiber types have been divided into *red slow oxidative* and *white fast glycolytic*, referring to the gross color of muscles, and to contractile properties, fatigue resistance and major source of energy supply. Based on enzyme histochemical stains, the former are referred to as **type 1** and the latter as **type 2**. The most useful of these stains for fiber typing is the stain for *myosin ATPase*, which uses variations in acid and alkali lability to identify the fiber types (Fig. 3-4A). Additional stains are used to demonstrate other properties, in particular stains for mitochondrial oxidative activity. The latter include the NADH-tetrazolium reductase (NADH-TR) and the succinate dehydrogenase (SDH) stains. In many species, type 2 fibers can be further divided based on myosin ATPase staining at particular pH and on mitochondrial stains. These subtypes have been classically referred to as *type 2A*, which are *fast twitch oxidative, fatigue resistant*, and *type 2B*, which are *fast twitch glycolytic, fatigable*. However, recent work characterizing myHC isoforms in muscle have shown that this scheme is an oversimplification.

Based on expression of myHC isoforms, *4 basic fiber types are now recognized*. These are **type 1, type 2A, type 2B,** and **type 2X**. *Type 2X* fibers have moderately high staining for mitochondrial stains and resistance to fatigue intermediate between type 2A and type 2B. To complicate matters, it is now well recognized that *hybrid fibers exist*, expressing a mix of myHC isoforms. In addition, specific myHC isoforms are expressed in the embryo and fetus and *unique isoforms are* expressed in some head muscles, extraocular muscles, and laryngeal muscles. In the muscles of mastication, an isoform termed *myHC-M*, is expressed in several species, including carnivores, primates (except for humans), and a few others, such as some marsupials and some bats. This isoform is of particular interest in the dog, where it is thought to be involved in the pathogenesis of myositis of masticatory muscles.

Fiber type proportions vary among regions of muscles, among muscles, among individuals, between males and females, and among species. This variation largely reflects the functional demands made on particular muscles. Muscles involved in posture, for example, are typically rich in type 1 fibers, whereas those involved in short-term bursts of activity contain more type 2 fibers. Knowledge of the fiber type characteristics of particular muscles and species is important in investigating and understanding pathologic states. Some diseases affect one fiber type more than others and this can determine what muscles should be sampled. For example, in the horse, one should sample a muscle rich in type 1 fibers when investigating a suspected case of equine motor neuron disease versus a

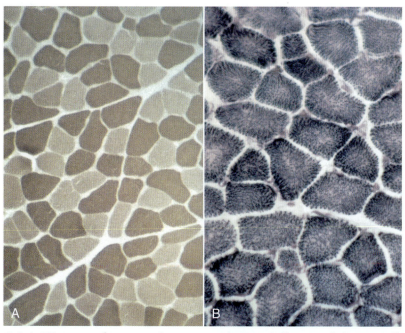

Figure 3-4 **A. Fiber types** from normal canine muscle. Type 2 fibers are dark, type 1 fibers are light. ATPase stain, alkaline preincubation. **B.** Normal canine muscle showing relatively uniform staining for mitochondria in this species. NADH-TR stain.

muscle rich in type 2 fibers when equine polysaccharide myopathy is suspected.

Knowledge of the differences in fiber type distribution between species is of obvious importance in veterinary medicine. For example, in rodents such as the rat and the mouse, type 2B fibers, expressing myHC-2B are abundant, yet they are not present in most large animals, except for certain specialized muscles. In the dog, for example, limb muscles express type 2A and 2X but not 2B. Accordingly, staining for oxidative enzymes is relatively high in all muscle fibers in the dog (Fig. 3-4B). Similarly, fibers expressing myHC-2B are essentially absent in the limb muscles of horses and cattle. However, in contrast in the pig, muscle fibers do express myHC-2B.

Although detailed knowledge of fiber types and fiber type and subtype distribution can be important in the investigation of muscle diseases, particularly at the research level, in diagnostic practice the pathologist is looking for alterations in fiber type distribution, and the demonstration of the pattern formed in sections stained for type 1 and type 2 is often sufficient. Examples illustrating this will be discussed later in this chapter. For now, it is important to recognize several aspects of fiber type development and distribution. First, muscle fibers in the same motor unit have essentially the same fiber type characteristics. Second, fiber type in the embryo is initially determined by intrinsic mechanisms, later modulated by the influence of neural activity and hormonal influences. Third, functional demands correlate with fiber type characteristics, not only in the expression of myHC isoforms and the level of oxidative and glycolytic activity but in many other biochemical properties of the fibers. Fourth, muscle fiber types are matched to the neuron innervating a motor unit. In short, *muscle fiber types are determined by the activity of the innervating motor neuron.* Finally, under some conditions, including some disease states, fiber types can switch.

An obvious limitation that pathologists face when working with formalin-fixed tissues is that enzyme histochemical fiber typing will not be possible. One possible solution to this may be to use immunohistochemical stains for specific myHC. Such antibodies are often used on frozen sections, but not all of them work on fixed tissue. Nevertheless, some antibodies do work on fixed tissue and, although not optimal, their use may give some indication of fiber type distribution (Fig. 3-5).

Specialized structures

The **neuromuscular junction** (Fig. 3-6A, B) is the site of synaptic transmission of an impulse from motor nerve terminals to muscle fibers so as to initiate a propagated action potential and contraction. This is accomplished by the release of acetylcholine from the nerve terminal, which diffuses across the synaptic cleft to act on acetylcholine receptors on the muscle membrane. The interface takes the form of a complex, "pretzel-shaped" neural termination, which is pressed into a shallow but convoluted, synaptic gutter of matching shape on the myofiber surface. Close to the neuromuscular junction, the nerve fiber loses its myelin sheath, the bare axon being covered by Schwann cell processes. Within the nerve terminal there are hundreds of synaptic vesicles, which contain acetylcholine, as well as numerous mitochondria. On the complexly folded postsynaptic membrane (that is, the muscle membrane) there are acetylcholine receptors, which function as ion channels that open when acetylcholine is bound. When sufficient receptors are activated, a muscle action potential is generated. Acetylcholinesterase is also associated with the

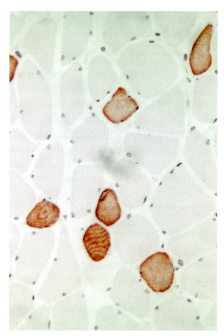

Figure 3-5 **Immunostain for type 1 myHC** showing type 1 fibers in a cat. Immunohistochemistry for slow myHC.

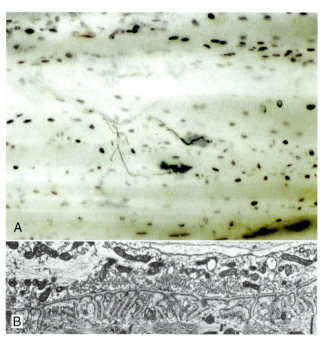

Figure 3-6 A. **Neuromuscular junction** (blue patches) with terminal nerve fibers (black). Combined silver/cholinesterase stain. B. Transmission electron micrograph of a **neuromuscular junction** from a mouse. Postsynaptic folds are apparent in the muscle membrane of the muscle fiber and numerous synaptic vesicles and mitochondria are present in the nerve terminal.

postsynaptic muscle membrane, its function being to destroy acetylcholine after the impulse has occurred.

Each muscle fiber bears one neuromuscular junction. However, as previously discussed, a single motor neuron can innervate anywhere from a few to hundreds, even thousands, of muscle fibers, forming the motor units. Muscles requiring fine motor control have motor units made up of relatively small numbers of muscle fibers, whereas large postural muscles have motor units containing many muscle fibers.

Abnormalities of the neuromuscular junction can be seen in certain disease states. The classic example is myasthenia gravis, in which loss of acetylcholine receptors occurs, associated with simplification of the postsynaptic membrane (that is, reduction in the complexity of the postsynaptic folds).

Sensory **muscle spindles** are found in all skeletal muscles in and anchored to the perimysial connective tissue, associated with a small nerve radicle. They are more numerous in some muscles than others, and are generally difficult to find in the larger muscles of mature animals. Spindles are about 0.5-3.0 mm long and 200-500 µm wide (Fig. 3-7A, B). They contain several *intrafusal fibers* enclosed within a fibrous capsule. Muscle spindles act as *mechanoreceptors* that monitor muscle stretch and contribute to proprioception. Intrafusal fibers are histochemically different from the *extrafusal skeletal muscle fibers* and express some unique myHC isoforms. The intrafusal fibers are referred to as nuclear bag fibers or nuclear chain fibers, based on their distribution of nuclei. Abundant sensory axons entering the spindle have "flower-spray," "grape-cluster," or spiral endings on the intrafusal fibers. Intrafusal fibers generally do not participate in the pathologic processes affecting extrafusal fibers and are also resistant to atrophy. For the pathologist, the main point in being able to recognize muscle spindles in muscle sections is to be aware that they do not represent an abnormality.

Techniques for the study of muscle

The choice of muscles to sample depends on several factors, including which muscles are clinically involved, the distribution of lesions and whether the samples are from biopsy or autopsy. It is obvious that in autopsy cases many muscles can potentially be sampled whereas for biopsy more limited sites must be selected, based on clinical involvement. As has already been stated, in the case of some suspected diseases it is advisable to select muscle with predominantly one fiber type or the other, which requires knowledge of the disease in question as well as the distribution of fiber types in particular muscles of a particular species.

Muscle lesions can be studied histologically using either fixed tissue for light and/or electron microscopy, or frozen sections for light microscopy. In many dedicated muscle pathology laboratories, conventional paraffin-embedded sections for light microscopy are rarely used. The use of frozen sections avoids contraction and shrinkage artifacts that can occur in fixed samples and has the advantage of allowing enzyme histochemistry for fiber typing and the investigation of certain specific diseases. Frozen sections can also be used for immunohistochemistry, utilizing many useful antibodies that cannot be used on fixed tissue (e.g., the immunostain for resident histiocytes shown later in this chapter). Finally, frozen sections are advantageous for visualization of cell outlines and of certain cellular structures such as mitochondria (see Fig. 3-7A).

Unfortunately, many laboratories are not equipped to prepare and study frozen sections of muscle, necessitating that examination be done using routine sections. Furthermore, longitudinal sections are very difficult to prepare from frozen

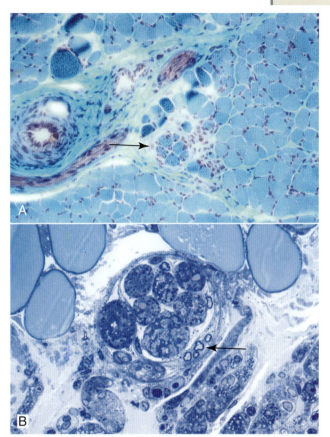

Figure 3-7 Muscle spindles. A. In dystrophic canine muscle (arrow). The fine granules present in extrafusal skeletal muscle fibers are mitochondria, which are shown well with this stain. Gomori trichrome stain. **B.** A 1-µm plastic section from a cat with nemaline myopathy showing intrafusal fibers and small myelinated nerve fibers (arrow). Toluidine blue stain.

tissue and, in the opinion of the authors, recognition of some histologic features, particularly infiltrating cells, is easier using fixed sections, including longitudinal sections. Thus in this chapter we discuss and illustrate both methods.

Whether for fixation or frozen sections, it is necessary to select samples in which the orientation of muscle fibers is known. Typically, strips of muscle are collected in which muscle fibers run along the length of the sample. This requires knowledge of the orientation of fibers within a particular muscle, but allows for the preparation of precisely oriented transverse or longitudinal sections.

One of the most important considerations relating to fixation of muscle tissue for light or electron microscopy is the avoidance of contraction artifacts. For this purpose, *muscle should be fixed in a slightly stretched condition*, ideally using some sort of muscle clamp or by pinning the slightly stretched sample to a piece of tongue depressor (Fig. 3-8A, B). At postmortem, the latter method has the advantage of allowing samples to be labeled with the identity of the muscles sampled. Either method helps to avoid contraction artifact, such as contraction bands (Fig. 3-9A-C). After fixation, the muscle sample can be removed from the clamp, discarding the damaged ends. Even when muscle samples are clamped, the pathologist must recognize that artifacts can still occur, in particular hypercontracted fibers, which in cross-section can

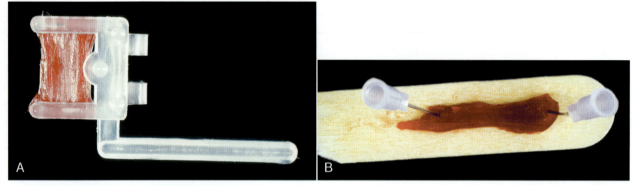

Figure 3-8 **Sampling of muscle. A.** Muscle sample in a muscle clamp. **B.** Muscle sample pinned on a tongue depressor.

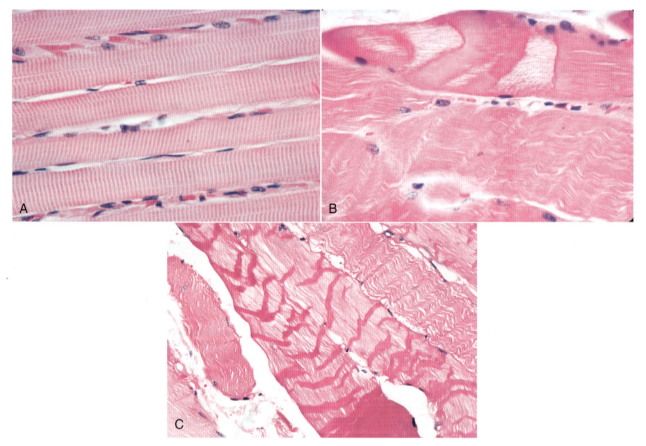

Figure 3-9 Effect of clamping is apparent in these sections. **A.** Normal canine skeletal muscle fixed in a muscle clamp. **B, C.** Examples of muscle fixed without clamping. Severe artifact is apparent, including contraction bands in (**C**). Artifactual contraction bands can be difficult to differentiate from hyperacute injury. H&E stain.

appear as "dark fibers" resembling those seen in acute necrosis (see section on Muscular dystrophies).

When collecting samples for the preparation of frozen sections, it is not necessary to clamp the muscle. However, the same requirements to ensure the proper orientation of fibers apply. Again, narrow strips of muscle are collected, preferably with the muscle fibers running along the length of the sample (Fig. 3-10). If there is any question of the orientation of fibers

within a sample, it is advisable to use a dissecting microscope while trimming to ensure precise transverse sections.

The procedure for preparation of frozen sections has been described in numerous textbooks, some of which are in the recommended reading list, and will not be repeated here. The most important consideration, however, is to *ensure rapid freezing to avoid the formation of ice crystals*, which result in artifactual vacuolation in the sections. For this reason,

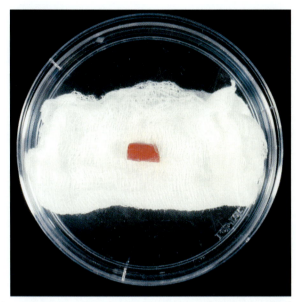

Figure 3-10 Sampling for frozen sections. The muscle sample is unclamped and is kept in a humid environment until segments are frozen.

samples should be snap frozen in isopentane cooled in liquid nitrogen.

In the case of paraffin-embedded sections, **routine stains** are used. For frozen sections an array of stains are used, including H&E, Gomori trichrome, ATPase at acid and alkaline pH, mitochondrial stains such as NADH-TR and SDH, PAS and, where appropriate, various immunostains. Stains for other enzymes are used for investigation of specific diseases, such as mitochondrial myopathies.

Further reading

Acevedo LM, Rivero J-LL. New insights into skeletal muscle fibre types in the dog with particular focus towards hybrid myosin phenotypes. Cell Tissue Res 2006;323:283-303.

Bentzinger DF, et al. Building muscle; molecular regulation of myogenesis. Cold Spring Harb Perspect Biol 2012;4:a008342.

Dubowitz V, et al. Muscle Biopsy: A Practical Approach. 4th ed. St. Louis: Saunders Elsevier; 2013.

Floeter MK. Structure and function of muscle fibers and motor units. In: Karpati G, et al., editors. Disorders of Voluntary Muscle. 8th ed. New York: Cambridge University Press; 2010. p. 1-19.

Grounds MD, Relaix F. Myogenic precursor cells. In: Karpati G, et al., editors. Disorders of Voluntary Muscle. 8th ed. New York: Cambridge University Press; 2010. p. 20-36.

Montarras D, et al. Lying low but ready for action: the quiescent muscle satellite cell. FEBS J 2013;280:4036-4050.

Murphy M, Kardon G. Origin of vertebrate limb muscle: the role of progenitor and myoblast populations. Curr Topics Dev Biol 2011;96:1-32.

Schiaffino S, Reggiani C. Fiber types in mammalian skeletal muscles. Physiol Rev 2011;91:1447-1531.

Toniolo L, et al. Fiber types in canine muscles: myosin isoform expression and functional characterization. Am J Physiol Cell Physiol 2007;292:C1915-C1926.

BASIC REACTIONS OF MUSCLE

Atrophy

At the gross or clinical level, the term *muscle atrophy* refers to a reduction in muscle volume or mass, which may be generalized or limited to certain muscles. At the cellular level, muscle atrophy most often reflects decreased myofiber diameter rather than loss of fibers. Fiber atrophy can be generalized or can involve only some fibers, sometimes selectively involving particular muscle fiber types. Histochemical evaluation of fiber types is often necessary to determine the likely cause of the atrophy. For example, in some circumstances, type 2 fibers are more sensitive to atrophy than are type 1 fibers. Morphometric analysis of overall fiber diameter may be necessary to confirm grossly apparent atrophy resulting from mild overall reduction of myofiber diameter. In other words, widespread but modest atrophy of individual fibers can result in obvious reduction in muscle mass at the gross level.

There are a number of possible **causes** of muscle atrophy. These include denervation, disuse, malnutrition, endocrine disorders, and cachexia associated with neoplasia or other chronic diseases. Muscle fiber *atrophy occurs when cellular catabolism exceeds synthesis* of cellular components. The relative importance of each of these processes varies according to the nature of the insult causing atrophy. In some circumstances, catabolism is increased while synthesis is decreased. In others, synthesis may actually be increased but catabolism is enhanced such that it still exceeds synthesis. Essentially, muscle fibers undergoing atrophy suffer a net loss of cytoplasmic components, including myofibrils, mitochondria, glycogen, and other organelles. Two major pathways have been shown to be involved in muscle atrophy, namely, the *ubiquitin-proteasome system* and the *autophagy-lysosome system*.

Simple myofiber atrophy does not involve sarcolemmal damage and therefore should not be expected to result in increased serum activity of CK or AST. Having said that, if atrophy is severe, stress on remaining functional fibers can cause injury and thus modest increases in these enzymes. Provided that the time interval is relatively short, if the influences inducing atrophy are removed and the muscle environment is returned to normal, the sequence can be reversed and fibers can be restored to normal size.

Denervation atrophy

Myofibers that have lost connection with peripheral nerves because of neuropathy or neuronopathy undergo rapid and severe atrophy caused by denervation. Denervation atrophy is usually characterized histologically by *fiber atrophy involving both type 1 and type 2 fibers* (Fig. 3-11A, B), although there are exceptions to this. It is important to recognize that when a motor neuron is lost or its axon is injured all muscle fibers within that motor unit undergo atrophy. However, it is also important to remember that muscle fibers belonging to any one motor unit are intermixed with those of neighboring motor units. Thus the histologic pattern seen depends on the number of neurons lost or the extent of peripheral nerve injury. Mild denervation, where limited numbers of motor units are involved, results in scattered single or small contiguous groups of atrophic fibers. These become compressed by adjacent normal innervated fibers into angular shapes, the lesion being referred to as *angular atrophy* (see Fig. 3-11A, B). More extensive denervation will result in large groups of small fibers, which remain rounded in transverse section, as there

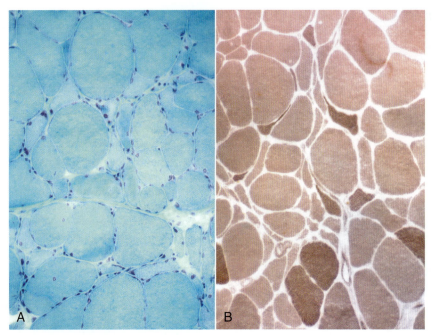

Figure 3-11 Small group atrophy. Angular atrophic fibers are present individually and in small clusters. Both type 1 and type 2 fibers are atrophic. **A.** Gomori trichrome stain. **B.** ATPase stain, alkaline preincubation. This lesion is strongly suggestive of denervation.

are no neighboring innervated fibers to cause them to adopt the angular shape. When there are small groups of atrophic fibers the lesion is referred to as *small group atrophy*, whereas larger groups of atrophic fibers are, logically enough, referred to as *large group atrophy* (Fig. 3-12A, B). Even in the absence of histochemical preparations, muscle containing extensive small group and large group atrophy is most likely to be denervated, and a careful examination of intramuscular nerves (Fig. 3-13A, B) and, where applicable, peripheral nerve trunks, ventral nerve roots, and motor neurons is indicated.

Denervation atrophy is relatively common in animals, and is always accompanied by some degree of muscle weakness. Clinical signs may be mild if only small numbers of motor units are involved. Some of the best-known examples of denervation atrophy in animals are laryngeal hemiplegia in horses caused by axonal degeneration of the left recurrent laryngeal nerve, injury to the supraspinatus nerve by trauma or the pressure of a poorly fitting collar in a work horse ("sweeney"), equine motor neuron disease (causing symmetrical atrophy), or equine protozoal myeloencephalitis (causing asymmetrical atrophy) in the horse, and radial or brachial paralysis in dogs and horses owing to trauma. Other common causes of denervation atrophy are lesions involving the ventral gray matter of the spinal cord or the ventral roots emerging from the spinal canal, and inherited or acquired peripheral neuropathies, including polyneuritis.

Denervation atrophy is typically rapid and severe. It is accompanied by abnormal spontaneous activity (fibrillations, positive sharp waves, and sometimes pseudomyotonic bursts) detectable with concentric needle electromyography. Reduction in mass may be readily observed or may require careful palpation of muscle mass for detection. Given the variable muscling of different breeds of dogs and horses, a diagnosis of mild symmetric muscle atrophy can be difficult.

As stated previously, the hallmark of denervation atrophy is involvement of both type 1 and type 2 fibers. Type 2 fibers, however, can be affected preferentially, especially early in the denervation process. The denervation of equine motor neuron disease is somewhat unique, in that there is often preferential atrophy of type 1 fibers, presumably because of oxidative injury to type 1 motor neurons as a result of vitamin E deficiency (Fig. 3-14).

As discussed previously, the type of muscle fibers in a motor unit is determined by the electrical activity of the nerve supplying that motor unit. Denervated motor units can become reinnervated. This is accomplished by sprouting from adjacent intact axons, the sprouting occurring at the last node of Ranvier. In such a case, muscle fiber size can be restored to normal but the reinnervated muscle fibers adopt the fiber type of the reinnervating neuron, which can result in the normal mosaic pattern being replaced by clusters of fibers all of the same fiber type. This lesion, which is referred to as *fiber type grouping*, can only be demonstrated using histochemical preparations and is diagnostic of denervation followed by reinnervation (Fig. 3-15A-C). If the reinnervating neuron or its axon is subsequently lost, the cluster of muscle fibers will undergo atrophy, resulting in groups of atrophic fibers of the same fiber type. This lesion is called *type-specific group atrophy* and is indicative of ongoing denervating disease (Fig. 3-16).

In denervated muscle, any remaining innervated fibers often undergo hypertrophy. Although both type 1 and type 2 fibers can undergo hypertrophy, the hypertrophic fibers often appear to be predominantly type 1 (Fig. 3-17A, B). There are a couple of possible explanations for this. Type 1 fibers might not undergo atrophy to the same extent as type 2 fibers, or type 1 neurons (and hence type 1 motor units) might be relatively spared in the disease process. However, it is likely, when denervation is fairly extensive, that the relatively small number of remaining intact fibers, even if originally both type 1 and

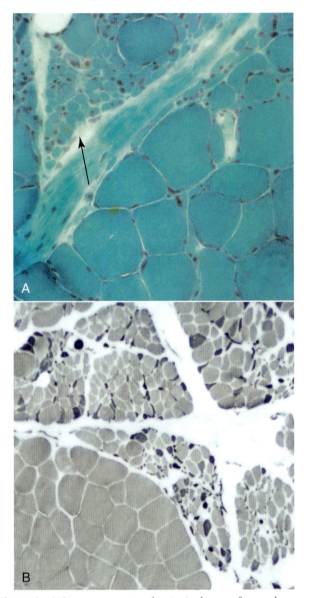

Figure 3-12 **Large group atrophy. A.** A cluster of severely atrophic fibers (arrow) with endomysial fibrosis resulting from chronic denervation in the medial head of the triceps of a horse with chronic equine motor neuron disease. There is marked compensatory hypertrophy of other fibers. Frozen section, Gomori trichrome. **B.** Extensive large group atrophy in a dog with denervating disease. Both type 1 and type 2 fibers are affected. ATPase stain, alkaline preincubation.

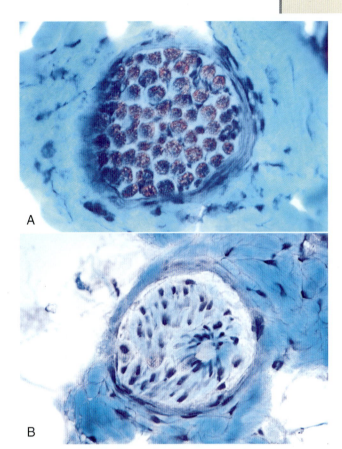

Figure 3-13 **Degeneration of intramuscular nerve. A.** A normal intramuscular nerve contains numerous myelinated fibers. **B.** A similar sized intramuscular nerve from a horse with motor neuron disease has severe loss of myelinated fibers, with proliferation of Schwann cells. Frozen sections, Gomori trichrome.

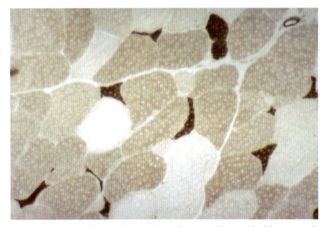

Figure 3-14 **Preferential atrophy of type 1 fibers** (darkly stained) in a horse with equine motor neuron disease. ATPase, acid preincubation.

type 2, are forced to do more work, mimicking the activity of type 1 motor units and thus converting to that fiber type. Even without histochemical preparations to determine fiber types, *a pattern of modest numbers of large-diameter fibers among severely atrophic fibers is very suggestive of severe chronic denervation.* In very severe cases, there can be eventual loss of denervated myofibers, with replacement of muscle by fibrous connective tissue and often by adipose tissue (Fig. 3-18). Determining the cause of the severe atrophy in such "end-stage muscles" can be very difficult because both severe chronic neuropathic processes and severe chronic myopathic processes can result in a similar appearance.

Disuse atrophy

Disuse atrophy occurs because of decreased contractile activity of innervated muscle. Decreased muscular activity caused by painful lameness (Fig. 3-19A), bone fracture or disease, or limb immobilization are most common. Disuse atrophy in humans and experimental animals classically involves type 2

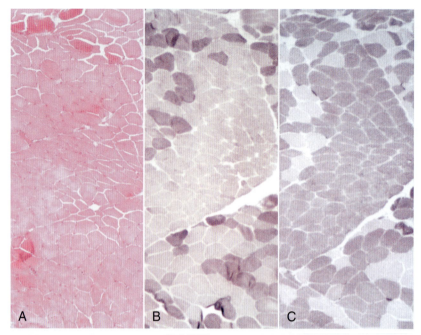

Figure 3-15 Fiber type grouping in muscle from a dog. Serial sections stained with (**A**) H&E (**B**) ATPase, alkaline preincubation (**C**) ATPase, acid preincubation. **B** and **C** show grouping of type 1 fibers indicating denervation and reinnervation. This diagnosis could not be made on the H&E stain alone.

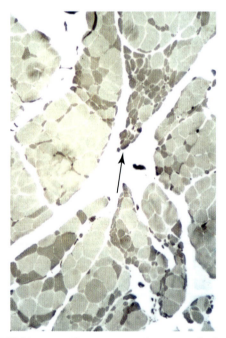

Figure 3-16 Type-specific group atrophy in muscle from a dog. In addition to grouping of type 1 fibers, there is a cluster of severely atrophic type 2 fibers (arrow), indicating denervation of previously reinnervated fibers. A single type 1 fiber is present among the atrophic type 2 fibers. ATPase, alkaline preincubation.

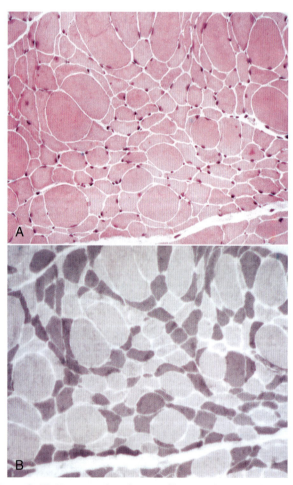

Figure 3-17 Hypertrophy of type 1 fibers in denervated muscle, from a horse with protozoal myelitis. There is extensive denervation atrophy of both type 1 and type 2 fibers. Intact fibers are hypertrophic, all staining as type 1. **A.** H&E stain. **B.** ATPase, alkaline preincubation.

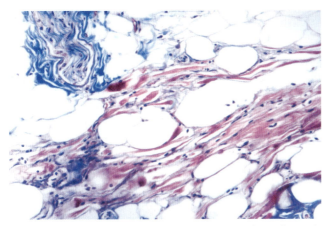

Figure 3-18 Chronic denervation atrophy, with loss of muscle fibers and replacement by fibrous and adipose tissue. Masson trichrome stain.

fibers preferentially, although this pattern is not seen in all muscles in people with disuse atrophy. Although type 2 preferential atrophy is seen in some cases of disuse atrophy in domestic animals (Fig. 3-19B), in many cases there is overall atrophy of all fiber types with no clear preferential pattern. Because no workload is imposed on muscle fibers undergoing disuse atrophy, there is no compensatory hypertrophy of other fibers.

Atrophy resulting from malnutrition or cachexia

Atrophy resulting from malnutrition occurs when an animal is unable to supply enough dietary nutrients to maintain muscle mass. Muscle proteins are continuously turned over and can be mobilized as a source of nutrients for the rest of the body. The large bulk of body muscle represents a very large pool of protein that can be used in this way. Net loss of muscle protein probably starts hours after negative nitrogen balance has been reached. The muscle atrophy of cachexia associated with chronic illness and neoplasia is mediated by circulating cytokines such as tumor necrosis factor (TNF, "cachectin"), which act systemically to increase catabolism, including catabolism of myofibers. The atrophy of cachexia is gradual, and the process may take place over a prolonged period.

In the dog, atrophy of temporal muscles is often prominent and can occur fairly rapidly in animals that are ill for any reason. The back and thigh muscles are also susceptible to severe atrophy resulting from cachexia. Histochemically, type 2 fibers are affected preferentially in cachexia (Fig. 3-20). Similar to the case in denervation atrophy and some cases of disuse atrophy, type 1 muscle fibers are relatively resistant to atrophy caused by cachexia. In most cases the degree of atrophy achieved through cachexia is not as severe as that seen in denervation atrophy, and the history provides clinical information and a time frame for the atrophy that should enable differentiation of cachexia from disuse and denervation atrophy.

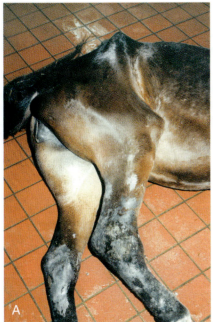

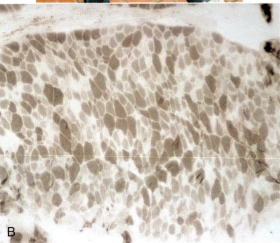

Figure 3-19 Disuse atrophy (A) in the right hind limb of a horse with septic arthritis of the tarsus (B). There is overall diffuse atrophy but type 2 fibers (light) are more severely affected. ATPase, acid preincubation.

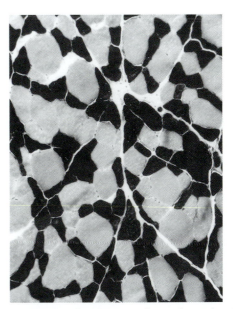

Figure 3-20 Atrophy of cachexia. Preferential atrophy of type 2 (dark-staining) fibers in an emaciated sheep; frozen section, ATPase, alkaline preincubation. (Courtesy T.J. Hulland.)

Atrophy of endocrine disease

Neuromuscular weakness and muscle atrophy can accompany hypothyroidism and hyperadrenocorticism in the dog. Selective atrophy of type 2 fibers is seen in both disorders (Fig. 3-21). No compensatory type 1 hypertrophy occurs. The finding of individual or small groups of mildly angular atrophic fibers, as can be seen in routine sections, can suggest denervation atrophy, and histochemical preparations to reveal the selective type 2 involvement may be necessary. In general, the atrophy of type 2 fibers in endocrine myopathy is not as severe as in the atrophy of denervation.

In summary, preferential atrophy of type 2 fibers can suggest endocrine disease, disuse, malnutrition, or cachexia. These possibilities must be differentiated based on clinical information and additional diagnostic testing.

Myopathic atrophy and myopathic change

Atrophy of fibers commonly occurs in myopathic conditions, that is, in primary muscle disease, and the atrophy contributes to the nonspecific myopathic change of increased fiber size variation. Selective type 1 fiber atrophy is seen in many congenital myopathies in humans and also has been seen in cats with nemaline myopathy (Fig. 3-22). In such cases, the use of histochemical procedures is essential to distinguish the selective type 1 atrophy that is suggestive of primary myopathy. Severe and/or chronic *myopathic change* can result in a wide variation of fiber size, including both atrophic and hypertrophic fibers, as well as increased central nuclei and various cytoarchitectural changes (Fig. 3-23). Hypertrophic fibers are prone to *fiber splitting*, and some of the small-diameter fibers interpreted as atrophic in chronic myopathic conditions may represent fiber splitting.

Hypertrophy

As with atrophy, *hypertrophy can refer to the gross appearance of muscle or to increased diameter of individual myofibers*. Increase in muscle fiber size can be due to incorporation of proliferating myoblasts into existing myofibers and/or to increase in fiber size resulting from synthesis of new myofibrils and other cellular components. The former process is important in muscle growth during early development but in adults is less often involved. Although there are exceptions, such as some forms of muscle injury, most muscle fiber hypertrophy in adults does not involve incorporation of additional satellite cells. Muscle hypertrophy can occur under physiologic conditions or as a consequence of pathologic processes.

Two main pathways mediating muscle fiber hypertrophy have been recognized, namely, that initiated by IGF1 and that involving myostatin, a member of the transforming growth factor β (TGF-β) family. The role of myostatin is to negatively regulate muscle growth. It inhibits myoblast differentiation and is able to cause decreased protein synthesis in muscle fibers. Its absence consequently results in increased muscle mass due to increased fiber numbers and fiber hypertrophy, as seen in animals with so-called *double muscling* caused by a mutation in the gene for myostatin. The extent to which increased muscle mass is due to hypertrophy versus hyperplasia varies among species (see Congenital and inherited defects).

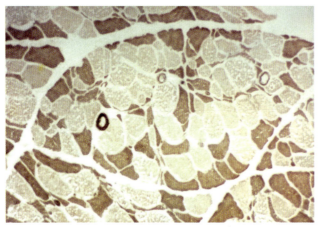

Figure 3-21 Preferential atrophy of type 2 (dark staining) fibers in a dog with hypothyroid myopathy. ATPase, alkaline preincubation.

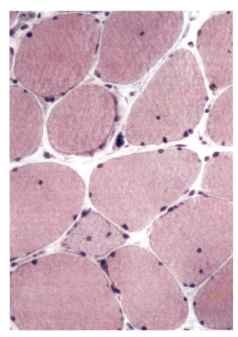

Figure 3-23 Chronic myopathic change in a horse. There is excessive fiber size variation, with both atrophic and hypertrophic fibers, as well as numerous central nuclei. Frozen section, H&E stain.

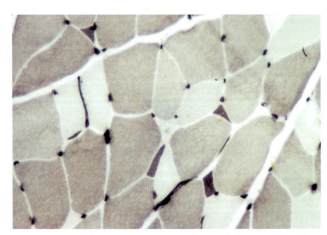

Figure 3-22 Selective atrophy of type 1 (dark staining) fibers in a cat with congenital nemaline myopathy. ATPase, acid preincubation.

Physiologic hypertrophy is typically associated with muscles undergoing increased workload. It is a desirable process in athletes and a well-recognized form in humans is the increase in muscle mass that occurs in weightlifters. There are upper limits for this type of hypertrophy, and for animals it lies somewhere between 80 and 100 µm in fiber diameter. There are also breed differences in the degree of muscle development, an obvious example being in greyhound dogs.

Pathologic hypertrophy occurs in a variety of disease situations. In some cases as a compensatory mechanism, hypertrophy of remaining functional fibers can occur in muscles affected by neuropathic (see Fig. 3-17A, B) or myopathic processes. In a sense this is a type of workload-induced hypertrophy caused by increased workload imposed on fibers less severely affected or unaffected by the myopathic or neuropathic condition. Hypertrophic fibers in myopathic and neuropathic conditions are often abnormal, may contain one or more internal nuclei, and *may undergo fiber splitting*. Fiber splitting presumably allows more efficient diffusion of nutrients to nourish the fiber. When division is more or less complete, 2 or often more fibers can take the place of one large one (Fig. 3-24A-C) and, on histochemical preparations, appear as a cluster of the same fiber type that should not be mistaken for fiber type grouping. Other possible changes include *bizarre cytoarchitectural changes* such as the formation of ring fibers and whorled fibers (see later).

Fiber hypertrophy occurs in a variety of other disease states, including myotonia, where it is presumably caused by abnormally increased muscle contractile activity, and in the already mentioned "double muscling." In some species, including the cat and the mouse, but to a lesser degree in dogs, muscular dystrophy of the Duchenne type can result in marked muscle hypertrophy. In Quarter Horses, hyperkalemic periodic paralysis can result in heavy muscling. In some of these diseases, selection for what was thought to be a desirable characteristic has led to selection for a disease state.

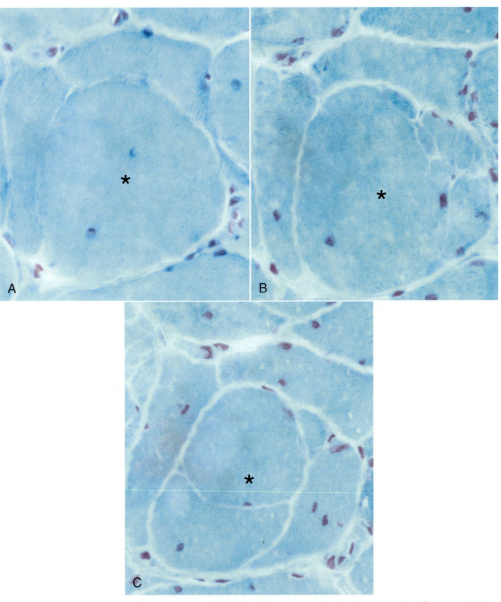

Figure 3-24 A-C. **Fiber splitting** in a cat with nemaline myopathy. The hypertrophic fiber marked with * is intact in (**A**), shows some splitting in (**B**), and is split into 4 fibers in (**C**). Serial skip frozen sections. Frozen section, Gomori trichrome stain.

Finally, muscle may appear enlarged because of *pseudohypertrophy*, as in chronically damaged muscles in which muscle tissue has been replaced by masses of fibrous tissue and/or adipose tissue, or because of fascial thickening, as seen in cats with fibrodysplasia ossificans progressiva (see Tendons and aponeuroses).

Muscle injury and necrosis

Skeletal muscle is subject to a variety of degenerative lesions ranging from focal interruptions of the sarcolemma to outright necrosis. Small sarcolemmal disruptions, such as may be caused by eccentric contraction, can be repaired by resealing, mediated by fusion of subsarcolemmal membrane vesicles. This process requires the protein *dysferlin*, defects in which cause a form of limb girdle muscular dystrophy in humans and a myopathy in mice. However, dysferlinopathies have not yet been identified in domestic animals. Other subtle forms of injury include myofibrillar alterations and Z band streaming. Such subtle injuries are not usually obvious on routine histologic examination, although they may be apparent ultrastructurally. Some of these subtle forms of injury do not elicit an inflammatory reaction, although there is evidence that infiltration by macrophages is important in repairing injury resulting from eccentric contraction.

Necrosis, which can range in severity from single necrotic fibers to extensive involvement of muscles, can result from many different causes, including ischemia, trauma, inherited diseases such as the muscular dystrophies, inflammatory myopathies, and extreme exertion (such as in so-called capture myopathy) (Fig. 3-25A, B). A unique feature of necrosis in skeletal muscle fibers is that *it can be segmental*, affecting only part of a fiber, which is a consequence of the multinucleated nature of these cells (Fig. 3-26). In the necrotic segments, myofibrils and other cytoplasmic components and the sarcolemma are degraded, but the basal lamina and the endomysium often remain intact. Satellite cells also remain intact in most forms of injury and are required for successful regeneration.

Histologic evidence of segmental or extensive necrosis of muscle fibers, often together with evidence of regeneration, is a common expression of many muscle diseases in animals. A classification scheme previously was developed for the description of necrotic lesions of muscle based on spatial distribution and temporal patterns, which is often useful to identify broad etiologic categories of muscle disease. The 4 categories of muscle necrosis are as follows:

- *Focal monophasic reactions* result from an isolated single mechanical injury, such as external trauma or needle insertion.
- *Multifocal monophasic reactions* result from a single insult, such as exposure to myotoxic drugs or chemicals, or metabolic disorders, which may initiate widespread muscle lesions, but all the alterations are synchronous (that is, in the same phase of injury and repair).
- *Focal polyphasic reactions* result from repeated injury to the same site.
- *Multifocal polyphasic reactions* are common in muscle diseases of animals and result from ongoing insults occurring over a prolonged period, such as from nutritional deficiencies, inflammatory myopathies, or genetic disorders (as in the muscular dystrophies). The lesions are widespread in the musculature and are at various stages of necrosis, leukocytic infiltration, and regeneration.

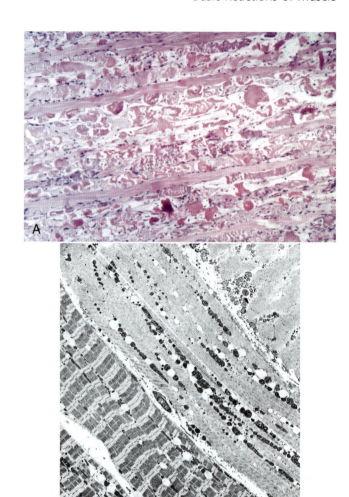

Figure 3-25 A. Massive (*multifocal monophasic*) **coagulative necrosis** in a wallaby, presumed to be due to overexertion ("capture myopathy"). H&E stain. **B.** Myofibrillar lysis in a foal. Transmission electron micrograph. (Courtesy T.J. Hulland.)

Because muscle necrosis involves damage to and eventually destruction of the sarcolemma, normal ionic gradients cannot be maintained. Sodium ions diffuse from the extracellular fluid into the damaged fiber and potassium ions diffuse out. More important, calcium ions, which are normally maintained at a much lower concentration in the cytosol than in the extracellular fluid, diffuse into the cell. They are important in the process of necrosis, as discussed later. Furthermore, larger molecules can leak from the cell into the extracellular fluid and eventually into the blood. These include muscle proteins and enzymes such as myoglobin, *creatine kinase (CK) and aspartate aminotransferase (AST)*. The latter 2 are of great diagnostic value in detecting muscle injury. *Serum CK is the most sensitive and the most specific indicator of muscle injury.* Aspartate aminotransferase is also found within hepatocytes. Alanine aminotransferase, an enzyme most often associated with hepatocellular injury, can also increase slightly in dogs with severe muscle injury. The degree to which activities of CK and AST are increased in serum depends on the extent and duration of muscle injury. Mild injury may not increase these serum enzyme activities above the normal range or may do so only modestly. It is important to be aware of the kinetics of these processes. Following muscle necrosis, CK rises quickly,

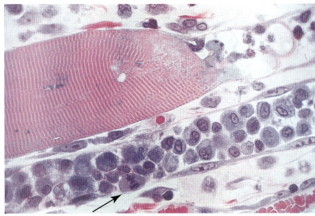

Figure 3-26 Segmental necrosis. A muscle fiber (top) is intact on the left but has undergone lysis on the right, leaving an empty tube formed by the basal lamina. Some macrophages are present in the tube. There is myofibrillar disarray in the junctional area between intact and lysed segments. Below there is another tube densely infiltrated by macrophages and lined by plump activated satellite cells. One satellite cell is in mitosis (arrow). (Courtesy A. Kelly, University of Pennsylvania. From Zachary JF, McGavin MD. Pathologic Basis of Veterinary Disease. 5th ed. St. Louis: Mosby/Elsevier; 2012.)

peaking at ~4-6 hours after muscle injury in the animal species studied (horse and dog). It is assumed that kinetics in other species are similar. Serum activity of AST rises more slowly, with a peak at ~24 hours. However, CK has a short half-life of only 6-12 hours, and it disappears fairly quickly in the case of a monophasic injury. AST has a longer half-life of ~48 hours, so increases persist for a longer period after such an injury. Thus both enzymes are useful in determining the degree and duration of muscle necrosis. In a monophasic injury, CK may be increased only slightly or even within normal range, but AST may still be increased if samples are taken more than ~24 hours after injury. In ongoing muscle disease (i.e., polyphasic injury), as occurs in the muscular dystrophies, for example, both CK and AST are persistently elevated.

As mentioned previously, damage to the sarcolemma in muscle necrosis results in the influx of calcium ions into injured muscle fibers (Fig. 3-27A). This can cause contraction of myofibrils, producing contraction bands similar to those shown in Figure 3-9C. Contraction bands caused by hyperacute muscle injury can be very difficult to differentiate from artifactual contraction bands. If there is evidence of infiltration of neutrophils and macrophages, the pathologist can be confident that the lesion is real. Clamping of samples reduces the incidence of artifactual contraction bands.

Entry of calcium ions leads to activation of calcium-dependent proteases, such as the calpains, which then degrade myofibrils and other cellular components. As in other tissues, *there appears to be a final common destructive pathway of mitochondrial calcium overload, which begins with many different causes of membrane or energy failure and ends with hypercontraction, coagulation, and dissolution of contractile proteins.* Many animal myopathies seem to fit well into this sequence of events, particularly the nutritional myopathies. Histologically apparent mineralization (Fig. 3-27B) occurs within hours after the onset of protein coagulation during which striations are lost. It is most likely that this mineralization involves

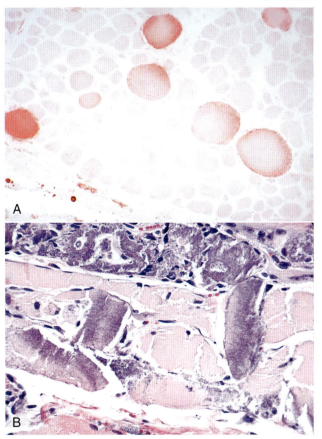

Figure 3-27 Calcium entry into necrotic fibers. A. Acutely injured fibers in canine muscular dystrophy, showing increased intracellular levels of calcium. Frozen section, Alizarin red S stain. B. Mineralization of necrotic fibers in a case of bovine nutritional myopathy, H&E stain.

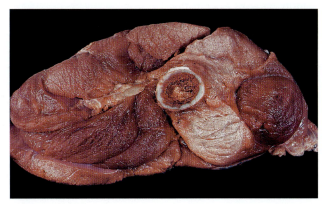

Figure 3-28 Necrotic muscle in the thigh of a foal with nutritional myopathy. Grossly necrotic muscle typically is pale and often nearly white in color.

calcium ions taken up from the blood. Its sequestration in mitochondria can maintain a gradient for calcium entry and it is most likely to be seen in those conditions in which the blood supply to the injured muscle is intact. Marked mineralization may contribute to the white appearance of necrotic muscle in the nutritional myopathies, but it is fair to say that any extensive areas of muscle necrosis will appear pale or "white" (Fig. 3-28; see also feline ischemic myopathy, under Circulatory disturbances of muscle). Thus, although the nutritional myopathies are sometimes referred to as *white muscle*

Figure 3-29 **Resident histiocytes** (dendritic macrophages) in normal canine muscle. Frozen section immunostained for CD1c, no counterstain.

disease, we prefer not to use that term because of its nonspecificity. Muscle necrosis is sometimes referred to as *rhabdomyolysis* or *myodegeneration*, although the latter could also refer to changes that do not lead to outright necrosis. It should also be mentioned that, in the older veterinary literature, muscle necrosis is sometimes referred to as *hyaline degeneration* or *Zenker's degeneration*. Less severe forms of muscle necrosis, in which a minority of fibers are affected, may be difficult to identify on gross examination.

Necrosis of muscle fibers is quickly followed by an inflammatory response, with an initial transient influx of neutrophils, followed by a more prolonged infiltration by macrophages, which are derived from circulating monocytes (see Fig. 3-26). It should be mentioned that *resident histiocytes* are present in normal muscle, in the perimysium and epimysium, and, rarely, in the endomysium (Fig. 3-29). These do not appear to contribute to the cellular infiltrate, but secrete chemokines that attract infiltrating neutrophils and monocytes. Macrophages have long been recognized to be involved in the phagocytosis of necrotic muscle cell debris but apparently play a more complicated role than that. Initial infiltrating macrophages are proinflammatory (so-called *M1 macrophages*), releasing cytokines such as TNF and interleukin 1 and do function to phagocytose debris. Soon after, there is a switch, such that the macrophages become anti-inflammatory (*M2 macrophages*), expressing different cell surface markers and secreting cytokines such as interleukin 10. This sequence appears to be a mechanism for controlling and terminating the inflammatory response to muscle injury. Macrophages also have been shown to play an important role in promoting satellite cell activation and proliferation and are thus important in muscle regeneration.

Muscle regeneration

Skeletal muscle has a remarkable ability to regenerate. *Along with the influx of macrophages, there is activation of satellite cells* (see Fig. 3-26), which reside in a resting state between the sarcolemma and the basal lamina. These cells are capable of proliferation, generating daughter cells that both renew the satellite cell population and differentiate to form muscle fibers. Thus they are true stem cells.

Regeneration of skeletal muscle is often said to recapitulate embryonic myogenesis, which at the morphologic level at least is a reasonable concept. However, the 2 processes, particularly at the molecular level, are not identical. Nevertheless, in response to muscle fiber injury, satellite cells proliferate, the process occurring within a couple of days. Those cells that are destined to form new myofibers subsequently express the MRFs myoD, myf5, mrf4, and myogenin. They quickly begin to fuse to form myotubes and to express muscle proteins such as myosin heavy chain (myHC), initially as the embryonic and fetal forms.

Several factors are important in the successful regeneration of skeletal muscle. Among these is the persistence of the basal lamina after the removal of necrotic material. *Given the existence of the basal lamina scaffold, muscle fibers can regenerate very rapidly* and, in time, become mature muscle fibers that are almost indistinguishable from normal (Fig. 3-30A-C). In the later stages of regeneration the basal lamina of the original fiber is phagocytosed. If the basal lamina scaffold is disrupted, such as in trauma, especially in the presence of hemorrhage, scar tissue is likely to form, possibly admixed with disorganized muscle regeneration (Fig. 3-31).

The presence of macrophages is also essential for muscle regeneration. The initial infiltrating macrophages are of the proinflammatory M1 phenotype, later switching to the anti-inflammatory M2 type. Both types are thought to be derived from the initial infiltrate of monocytes (Fig. 3-32A, B). With respect to regeneration, current evidence is that M1 macrophages stimulate proliferation of muscle precursor cells, whereas M2 macrophages promote differentiation to form myotubes.

Another factor important in muscle regeneration is neural activity. The initial stages of regeneration, including the expression of developmental forms of myHC, are independent of innervation. However, if regenerating fibers are not reinnervated, they remain small. Formation of new neuromuscular junctions may be from existing nerve terminals. However, if a regenerated fiber segment is separated from the parent fiber in some way, nerve sprouting is required to accomplish this. Furthermore, regenerating muscle fibers can switch from developmental forms of myHC to fast adult type without neural influence, but the further switch to type 1 myHC requires neural activity.

In the case of *segmental necrosis*, the end of the intact segment is sealed by fusion of the sarcolemma, with subsequent fusion of regenerating myoblasts. Under some circumstances, regenerating myoblasts may fail to fuse, possibly because of residual debris preventing successful contact. Under these circumstances, more than one small muscle fiber may be formed, connected to a pre-existing intact portion of the parent fiber. In transverse section, these fibers are small and resemble split fibers. However, they have not actually split, but have failed to fuse laterally. The term *forked fibers* has been used by some authors to describe this process. In addition, the presence of debris or scar tissue may prevent regenerating fibers from fusing end to end. Under those circumstances, new myotendinous junctions can be formed, resulting in 2 new fibers connected in series.

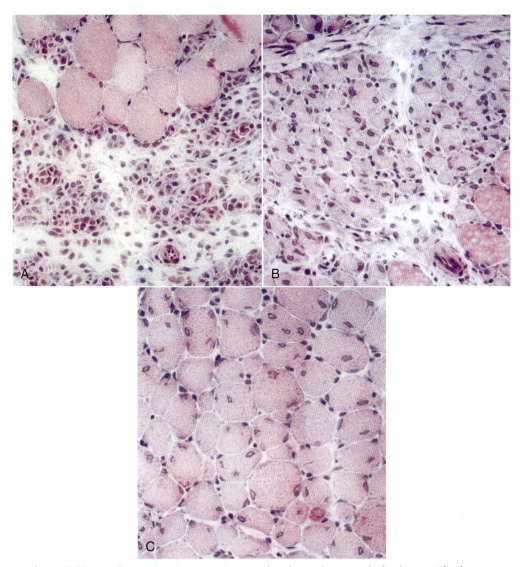

Figure 3-30 **Muscle regeneration** in canine muscle subjected to a single focal injury (*focal monophasic necrosis*) induced by local injection of the myotoxin notexin. **A.** 3 days after injury, there are clusters of macrophages and activated satellite cells within pre-existing basal lamina tubes. **B.** 5 days after injury, small myotubes have formed. **C.** 7 days after injury, the regenerating fibers have enlarged almost to normal size. All micrographs are at the same magnification. Frozen sections, H&E stain.

Early in the process, regenerating muscle fibers can be recognized by their relative basophilia and the presence of central nuclei (Fig. 3-32C). In most species, the nuclei are quickly relocated to their normal subsarcolemmal position. However, in rodents, central nuclei persist and can be a useful marker for past regeneration (Fig. 3-33). If longitudinal sections are examined, young regenerate fibers, or myotubes, can be recognized by having chains of closely spaced nuclei (see Fig. 3-32C). Regenerating muscle fibers also can be identified using immunohistochemistry for embryonic or neonatal myHC isoforms (Fig. 3-34A, B), or enzyme histochemical fiber typing. In the latter case, the regenerating fibers stain dark at both acid and alkaline pH and are referred to as *type 2c fibers*.

Finally, regenerate muscle fibers undergo an increase in fiber diameter, associated with the production of new myofibrils and other organelles. This is associated with a loss of basophilia. In the case of simple injury without disruption of the basal lamina and supporting connective tissue, mature regenerate fibers may be indistinguishable from normal muscle. Where there is disruption of the tissue, regenerate muscle may be disorganized and, in severe cases, may form so-called *muscle giant cells* (see Fig. 3-31), a sign of abortive muscle regeneration.

In aged animals or in long-term myopathic processes, such as the muscular dystrophies, regeneration may be relatively inefficient compared with young animals. The reasons for this are not completely agreed upon. In some cases long-term repetitive necrosis may result in loss of satellite cells or in loss of their regenerative capacity, perhaps as a result of proliferative exhaustion. However, the situation is more complicated than that because there is evidence that the muscle environment also may be altered such that regeneration is less effective. For example, there is experimental evidence that some uncharacterized serum factors from young animals can enhance muscle regeneration in aged animals.

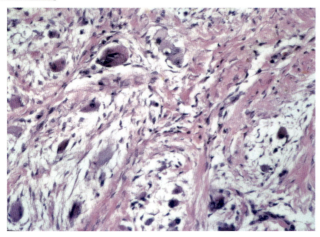

Figure 3-31 Abortive regeneration in muscle adjacent to a carcinoma. The tissue is composed chiefly of collagenous fibrous and adipose tissue, embedded in which are several misshapen regenerative myocytes ("muscle giant cells"). H&E stain.

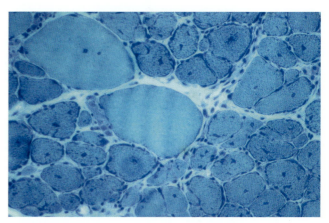

Figure 3-33 Muscle regeneration in muscle from an *mdx* mouse, a model of Duchenne muscular dystrophy. Many fibers have central nuclei, which persist in regenerated murine muscle. Frozen section, trichrome stain.

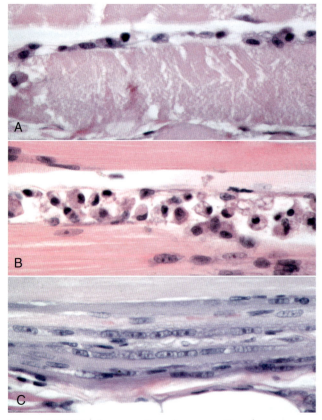

Figure 3-32 Muscle necrosis and regeneration showing areas from the muscle of a cat with ischemic myopathy, showing (**A**) an acutely necrotic fiber (coagulative necrosis) (**B**) another fiber infiltrated by macrophages and (**C**) basophilic regenerating fibers with chains of central nuclei. H&E stain.

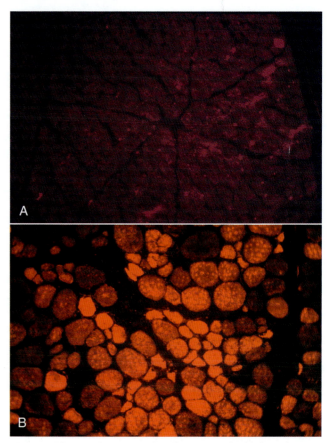

Figure 3-34 Muscle regeneration from 8-week-old dogs, showing the expression of fetal myHC. **A.** In normal muscle at this age there is no expression of fetal myHC. **B.** In muscle from a dystrophic pup there are numerous regenerating fibers staining for fetal myHC. Immunofluorescence staining.

Muscle fibrosis

Some proliferation of the interstitial connective tissues always accompanies necrosis and regeneration of muscle. Indeed, it has been shown that *fibroblasts are essential for both muscle development and muscle regeneration*. The temporary proliferation of connective tissue elements can serve as additional support for muscle fibers, nerves, and blood vessels. Furthermore, chemotactic factors secreted by fibroblasts appear to be important in promoting migration of activated satellite cells, which may serve to increase their numbers at sites of injury and regeneration.

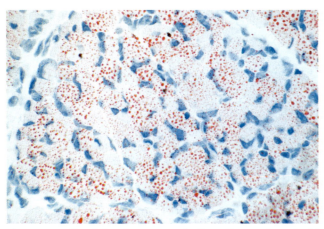

Figure 3-35 Lipid droplets in muscle fibers from a 4-week-old dog. This is a normal finding. Oil Red O stain.

Under normal circumstances, this additional connective tissue is removed after the muscle is repaired. However, in the presence of ongoing injury, such as occurs in the muscular dystrophies, there is persistence of inflammation, dominated by infiltrating macrophages. These cells, as well as others, secrete a wide array of cytokines. There is also ongoing deposition of fibrin, which over time can become organized and replaced by fibrous tissue. Finally, there is evidence that in chronic muscle injury myogenic cells can switch to a fibroblastic or adipocytic phenotype. The end result is that *in chronic degenerative muscle disease there is loss of muscle tissue with replacement by collagenous fibrous tissue and adipose tissue* (see discussion of muscular dystrophy in Congenital and inherited defects). Of course, in the event of severe tissue disruption and hemorrhage, the hematoma and damaged tissue may become organized as fibrous tissue.

Another situation in which muscle fibrosis and fat infiltration may be seen is *chronic denervation*. In such situations there can be loss of muscle fibers with replacement by fibrous tissue and adipose tissue. This is the case, for example, in fibrotic myopathy in horses, which can be due to chronic denervation (see Fig. 3-18).

Other myofiber alterations

Vacuolar degeneration is an infrequent alteration in muscle fibers (see figure in the discussion of myotonic dystrophy-like disease in the horse in Myotonic and spastic syndromes) sometimes associated with electrolyte abnormalities. It can also occur in myotonia because of dilation of the sarcoplasmic reticulum (see the discussion of Feline myotonia). The presence of lipid is also commonly observed (Fig. 3-35) and appears as vacuolation. The presence of **lipid vacuoles** can be normal. For example, we have observed numerous lipid droplets in the muscle of young puppies. However, large numbers in older animals may indicate a pathologic condition, raising the possibility of a lipid storage myopathy or mitochondrial myopathy.

A variety of inclusion-like structures or focally abundant or altered structural components, termed **cytoarchitectural changes**, occur in myopathies of animals. These include *whorled fibers* and *ringbinden* (Fig. 3-36A, B). Such alterations in the muscles of humans sometimes are associated with specific diseases. *Nemaline rods* have been found in nemaline myopathy of cats and, as a nonspecific change, in occasional

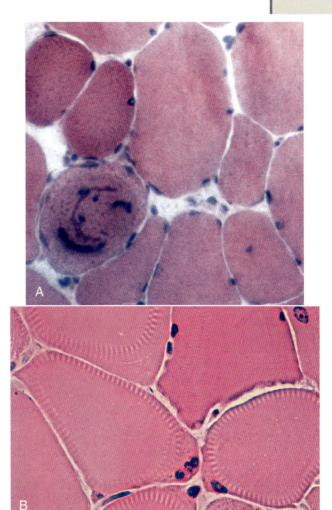

Figure 3-36 A. A whorled fiber from a cat with muscular dystrophy (Duchenne type). H&E stain. **B.** Ringbinden. Plastic thin section.

cases in dogs, with or without hypothyroidism. The rods represent accumulations of Z band material as confirmed by electron microscopy (see feline nemaline myopathy in Congenital and inherited diseases). *Targetoid fibers* (with central zones of myofibrillar disruption) and *ragged red fibers* (containing increased numbers of mitochondria, which are sometimes enlarged, mostly at the periphery of the fiber) are sometimes seen. In people ragged red fibers are the hallmark of mitochondrial myopathies. It can be difficult to assess the presence of ragged red fibers in dogs because all of their muscle fibers contain numerous mitochondria and therefore stain strongly for SDH and NADH-TR. Peripheral and central sarcoplasmic masses have been reported in the muscles of sheep and cattle in diseases designated as muscular dystrophy. Abnormal glycogen accumulation may develop in the muscles of dogs, sheep, cattle, cats, and horses (see also Congenital and inherited defects). In all species, these are generally non–membrane-bound collections. The deposits are PAS positive and digested by amylase (diastase) and are usually just under the sarcolemma. More complex *polysaccharide inclusions* occur in polysaccharide storage myopathy of horses (see later) or as a nonspecific finding in a number of other species.

Ringbinden (ring fibers) (see Fig. 3-36B) are one of the unusual findings that may occur experimentally when denervation or tenotomy is combined with atrophy and regeneration or occasionally in naturally occurring lesions. Ringbinden are seen in transverse sections and involve a circumferentially arranged band of myofibrils at the periphery of the fiber. Circular myofibrils accompanied by a mass of disrupted subsarcolemmal contractile elements presumably represent a true pathologic change of myofibers. Ring fibers most often occur naturally in animals as a nonspecific myopathic change.

The *role of apoptosis* in skeletal muscle disease is still unclear. Although apoptosis represents an important activity in myoblasts during normal differentiation and development, its role in postmitotic mature myofibers is uncertain, although it is thought to occur. Activated satellite cells may also undergo apoptosis. In several models of muscle disease (X-linked muscular dystrophy in mouse, bupivacaine injury of immature rat muscle), apoptosis precedes the development of necrosis. Apoptosis is also thought to be involved in the sarcopenia of aging. Further studies are needed to establish the role and the importance of apoptosis in muscle diseases of animals and human beings.

Postmortem changes

Veterinary pathologists are often faced with the challenge of interpreting changes in tissues that have undergone significant postmortem autolysis. Postmortem changes in muscle are common but variable, making interpretation of the gross appearance of muscle difficult. Postmortem changes may include pallor or the muscles may become unusually dark after death. A wide range of differences in color and consistency of muscle normally exists among various muscles and among species. Pallor of muscles is also present in animals that are anemic and is often seen normally in neonatal animals. Given the difficulty in interpretation of gross changes, it behooves the pathologist to take multiple muscle samples for histologic evaluation.

Rigor mortis *refers to contracture of skeletal muscles that develops after death.* Rigor mortis is characterized by stiffening of the muscles and immobilization of the joints. It proceeds in orderly fashion from the muscles of the jaw to those of the trunk and then to those of the extremities, and it passes off in the same order. The time of onset, in average circumstances, is 2-4 hours after death and maximum rigor is achieved in 24-48 hours, after which it disappears. The intensity of rigor varies considerably as does the time of onset. *The factors influencing the time of onset and degree of rigor are glycogen reserves, the pH of the muscles at the time of death, and the environmental temperature.* Rigor is slight or absent in cachectic or chronically debilitated animals. Rigor occurs with extraordinary rapidity in animals that die during or shortly after intense muscular activity, when muscle pH and glycogen stores are low. Onset of rigor can be delayed in well-rested, well-fed animals. It is hastened in onset and disappearance in a warm environment and retarded in a cold environment. Rigor occurs as a result of adenosine triphosphate (ATP) depletion and develops because muscle fibers deprived of energy are unable to maintain calcium in sequestered stores. The resulting diffusion of calcium ions results in activation of the contractile mechanism. *As a result of ATP depletion, cross-bridging of myosin and actin cannot be released, resulting in a prolonged state of contraction.* The eventual disappearance of rigor is due to autolytic processes, in which contractile proteins are broken down.

Skeletal muscle is also prone to various artifactual changes that interfere with accurate histologic evaluation. Muscle collected from *freshly dead animals*, especially horses, is often still capable of vigorous contraction when myofiber ends are cut, allowing calcium-rich extracellular fluid to enter the myofiber and trigger the contractile apparatus. *Exposure to formalin* can also trigger contraction in fresh muscle samples (see Fig. 3-9B, C). Various procedures have been advocated for elimination of the resultant contraction band artifact in muscle. It has been suggested that delayed sampling, or allowing relaxation of the sample after collection, will result in better histologic preparations. Although the myofilamentous elements of myofibers are somewhat resistant to autolysis, and overall architecture of muscle is better preserved postmortem than that of tissues such as nervous tissue or gastrointestinal mucosa, this type of processing must still be considered less than ideal. Rapid postmortem loss of glycogen may result in inability to diagnose a glycogen storage myopathy, and postmortem alterations in mitochondria and other organelles certainly interfere with ultrastructural evaluation. Histochemical procedures also may be affected by postmortem autolysis, with resultant loss of fiber typing ability.

As discussed previously, *samples taken at postmortem should be clamped in some way to avoid contraction artifacts*. Strips of muscle a few centimeters long and no more than 1 cm in thickness should be collected. Certainly the pathologist should avoid simply throwing a chunk of fresh muscle into formalin, which will result in severe artifacts.

Further reading

Ciciliot S, Schiaffino S. Regeneration of mammalian skeletal muscle; Basic mechanisms and clinical implications. Curr Pharmaceut Des 2010;16:906-914.

Grounds MD. Towards understanding skeletal muscle regeneration. Pathol Res Pract 1991;187:1-22.

McGavin MD, Valentine BA. Muscle. In: McGavin MD, et al., editors. Thomson's Special Veterinary Pathology. 3rd ed. St. Louis: Mosby; 2001. p. 461-473.

Saclier M, et al. Monocyte/macrophage interactions with myogenic precursor cells during skeletal muscle regeneration. FEBS J 2013;280:4118-4130.

Schiaffino S, et al. Mechanisms regulating skeletal muscle growth and atrophy. FEBS J 2013;296:4294-4314.

Serrano AL, et al. Cellular and molecular mechanisms regulating fibrosis in skeletal muscle repair and disease. Curr Topics Dev Biol 2011;96:167200.

Shelton DG. Routine and specialized laboratory testing for the diagnosis of neuromuscular diseases in dogs and cats. Vet Clin Pathol 2010;39:278-295.

Yusuf F, Brand-Saberi B. Myogenesis and muscle regeneration. Histochem Cell Biol 2012;138:187-199.

CONGENITAL AND INHERITED DISEASES

Numerous conditions affect skeletal muscle development, integrity, and function in animals. Congenital myopathic and neuropathic conditions are apparent at birth or soon thereafter, usually within the first year of life, and may or may not be inherited. *Pedigree analysis and breeding studies often help to distinguish those congenital disorders that are also inherited.* Inherited disorders affecting skeletal muscle in animals in

Table • 3-1

Animal myopathies in which the gene defect is known

Disorder	Gene affected	Type of disease	Species/breed affected
Phosphofructokinase (PFK) deficiency	PFK, muscle isozyme	Carbohydrate metabolic defect	English Springer Spaniels, American Cocker Spaniels
Myophosphorylase deficiency	Myophosphorylase	Carbohydrate metabolic defect	Charolais cattle
Polysaccharide storage myopathy	Glycogen synthase 1 (GYS1)	Carbohydrate metabolic defect	Horses—especially draft and Quarter Horse-related breeds
Glycogen branching enzyme defect	Glycogen branching enzyme (GBE1)	Carbohydrate metabolic defect	Quarter Horses, Norwegian Forest Cats
Centronuclear myopathy	PTPLA	Centronuclear myopathy	Labrador Retriever
X-linked myotubular myopathy	Myotubularin *MTM1*	Centronuclear myopathy	Labrador Retriever
Hyperkalemic periodic paralysis (HYPP)	Skeletal muscle sodium channel	Channelopathy leading to myotonia and paralysis	Impressive line of Quarter Horses
Canine myotonia	Skeletal muscle chloride channel—ClC-1	Channelopathy leading to myotonia	Miniature Schnauzer
Exercise-induced collapse	Dynamin 1	Episodic collapse associated with exercise	Labrador Retriever
X-linked muscular dystrophy	Dystrophin	Muscular dystrophy	Various dog breeds, DSH cats
Double muscling	Myostatin	Muscular hyperplasia	Various beef breeds, Whippets
Callipyge phenotype	CLPG1	Muscular hyperplasia	Sheep
Porcine stress syndrome	Ryanodine receptor	Malignant hyperthermia	Various pig breeds
Malignant hyperthermia	Ryanodine receptor 1	Malignant hyperthermia	Quarter Horses, dogs

which the gene defect is known are listed in Table 3-1. Gene mutations leading to skeletal muscle dysfunction are most often *point mutations*, such as hyperkalemic periodic paralysis (HYPP) in horses, phosphofructokinase (PFK) deficiency in dogs, and myophosphorylase deficiency in cattle. Some disorders, such as canine X-linked muscular dystrophy, can occur because of either point mutations or deletions, and the genetically characterized cases of feline X-linked muscular dystrophy have been due to a gene deletion.

Following tradition, congenital and inherited defects of skeletal muscle are discussed separately from the congenital and inherited myopathies, although it is recognized that the distinction between these 2 groups is not always clear. Numerous disorders are difficult to classify using traditional classification schemes, and diseases or syndromes can change their status as a result of investigation and new information.

Abnormal development of neuroectoderm that involves the lower motor neuron portion of the nervous system will also affect skeletal muscle. Although the primary defect is in the nervous system, the profound effect these disorders can have on skeletal muscle development and function warrant a brief discussion here.

Primary central nervous system conditions

Neuroectodermal defects affecting the innervation of individual myotomes and the muscles that form from them can result in abnormal muscle development. Given the complex interaction of myogenic and neurogenic cells during development, it is often difficult to define the exact nature of the defect. Neuroectodermal defects can result in abnormal muscle development or structure owing to lack of innervation, loss of innervation, or abnormal motor neuron activity.

For proper in utero development, muscles require normal innervation. Without it they atrophy or fail to develop normally (hypotrophy) and are more or less replaced by fibrous tissue and fat (Fig. 3-37A, B). Associated with each embryonic spinal cord segment is a myotome, a collection of cells with myoblastic potential, which migrate as the fetus develops and that ultimately form muscle. Committed myoblastic cells from one myotome may contribute to several muscles. Later, nerves from the same spinal segment follow the route of the myoblastic cells and innervate the same muscles. Most developing muscles are formed from myoblastic cells and nerves from 2 to 6 cord segments, but a few small muscles of the distal limbs receive contributions from only one. This explains why some muscles innervated from only one segment are vulnerable to denervation or lack of innervation resulting from a cord lesion involving a single segment, whereas a cord lesion of similar extent contributing innervation to muscles receiving cells and nerves from multiple segments can be associated with apparently normal muscle and nerve development. In the latter case, collateral innervation from nerves arising in normal cord segments can develop.

Developing skeletal muscle motor units are innervated by more than one nerve and, in some species, such as the dog, this polyinnervation is still present at birth. With maturation of the neuromuscular unit, the innervation pattern is simplified to one nerve fiber per motor unit. This pattern of polyinnervation can further complicate the pathologic findings in muscle from animals with neuroectodermal defects.

Arthrogryposis and dysraphism

Arthrogryposis literally means *crooked joint*. The terms *congenital articular rigidity* and *arthrogryposis multiplex congenita*

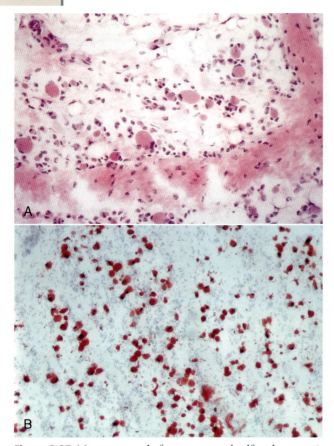

Figure 3-37 Masseter muscle from a neonatal calf with **congenital trigeminal nerve hypoplasia**. There is severe **lack of myofibers with replacement by adipocytes**. Remaining myofibers exhibit marked variation in diameter with many hypotrophied fibers. Frozen sections. **A.** H&E. **B.** Oil red O.

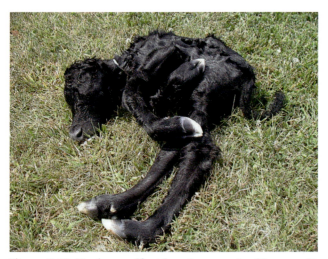

Figure 3-38 Newborn calf with **arthrogryposis**. (Courtesy D. Steffen.)

are also used to describe this syndrome. Arthrogryposis can involve one or more limbs, depending on the underlying neuroectodermal defect. Severely affected animals may also have scoliosis, kyphosis, and torticollis, and the limbs or parts of limbs may be rotated, abducted, or curled backward or forward in grotesque positions (Fig. 3-38). Newborn animals afflicted with arthrogryposis are sometimes stillborn and may show autolysis indicative of in utero death 2-4 days earlier.

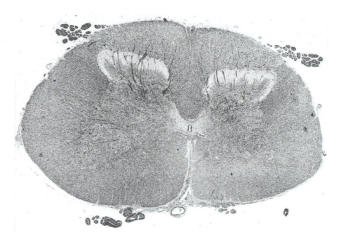

Figure 3-39 Failure of development of the right ventral horn in a calf with **myelodysplasia**. (Courtesy T.J. Hulland.)

Hydramnios is disproportionately associated with these, as is dystocia. Many, perhaps most, are of normal skeletal size, although some are considerably smaller than normal or smaller than littermates. In the rare cases in which limb involvement is unilateral, the animal is likely to be born alive.

The causes of arthrogryposis are often not clear, although one common underlying cause is decreased limb movement in utero. Both myogenic and neurogenic disorders can result in decreased limb movement and arthrogryposis, but *denervation is by far the most common cause*. Arthrogryotic fixation of the joints of lambs, calves, piglets, and foals, and less frequently of kittens and puppies, occurs with some regularity, and sometimes in epidemics. In cases of epidemic incidence, viral infections or toxins affecting the nervous system are most likely (see later). In black Angus cattle, an autosomal recessive genetic defect causing arthrogryposis has been identified.

Unequivocal links exist between arthrogryposis and *the recognizable lesions caused by arrest or delay of neural tube closure* (**dysraphism**). These include, in the extreme, spina bifida and cord agenesis, but also anomalies of the dorsal septum, anomalies of the central canal such as hydromyelia and syringomyelia, anomalies of the dorsal, central, or ventral gray matter (Fig. 3-39), and anomalies of the ventral median fissure (see Vol. 1, Nervous system). Dysraphism does not always lead to arthrogryposis; segmental lesions are sometimes found in clinically normal animals.

Obvious spinal cord and/or peripheral nerve abnormalities are present in a proportion, perhaps a majority, of arthrogryotic domestic animals. In the rest, although an absence of primary myogenic or osteogenic lesions seems to point to a neurologic cause, the identity of the failed neural component is not obvious on routine investigation. Several careful studies of unilateral arthrogryposis in animals and children have indicated that the neural changes can be subtle and varied. The number of motor neurons in an apparently normal cord may be segmentally reduced, particularly in the caudal portion of the thoracic and lumbar eminences; or the number of motor neurons may be increased, or the neurons may be disoriented. Beyond this, conjecturally, there could be failure of neural direction, or connection, or of end plate development.

Affected animals may have obvious reduction in mass of affected muscle because of atrophy or hypotrophy. Muscle mass can, however, appear superficially normal if there is replacement of the lost muscle mass by fat (see Fig. 3-37).

Dissection of major nerve trunks and muscle often is very difficult. Nerve trunks often appear to be normal on gross examination. Where comparisons are possible, peripheral nerve trunks in affected limbs may be demonstrably smaller and lacking some fascicles, although individual axons are normal.

Histologically, marked fiber size variation resulting from irregularity of muscle development may be evident. Normal diameter muscle fibers can occur admixed with, or adjacent to, groups of small round muscle fibers (see Fig. 3-37). Rarely, a typical denervation pattern of clusters of large and clusters of small fibers can be seen. Abnormalities resulting in denervation and reinnervation result in fiber type grouping. Other alterations in the fiber type pattern, such as type 1 fiber predominance, are more difficult to explain but may reflect abnormal innervation or neural activity.

As noted previously, it is often impossible to relate lesions to a specific cause. The critical event must occur early in pregnancy. *Genetic causes* are postulated or confirmed in calves, and postulated in sheep and pigs, but the establishment of such a relationship does not require a different pathogenetic mechanism since the gene effect apparently would be directed at the neural component. Syndromes in the Charolais, Friesian, Swedish, and Red Danish breeds of cattle, sometimes associated with cleft palate, are consistent with that of a simple recessive or modified recessive characteristic. *Environmental toxins or viruses* may result in a similar disease pattern. Akabane virus, Cache Valley virus, bluetongue virus, border disease virus, and Schmallenberg virus cause outbreaks of arthrogryposis in cattle and/or sheep. *Lupinus laxiflorus* (wild lupine), and other plant toxins, also cause deformities in fetuses when they are ingested by the dam during early pregnancy (see Vol. 1, Bones and joints).

Congenital flexures

Pastern contracture and immobility by itself can sometimes be part of arthrogryposis. If the flexure is combined with some degree of distal limb rotation, the pathogenesis is likely to be associated with neural and muscle changes as a minor expression of arthrogryposis. Many lambs, foals, and calves are born with an apparent inability to straighten the fetlock and sometimes other distal joints, yet deformities are minimal and muscle loss is not apparent. The problem in these cases seems to relate to the holding of the affected joint or joints in flexion without relief during a period of time in late gestation. The affected muscles appear to have reacted as they would after tenotomy by losing sarcomeres from the ends of myofibrils. This makes the joint initially incapable of extension, but under more or less constant tension the lost sarcomeres are quickly returned in hours or days. Such an explanation seems applicable because many affected foals and lambs recover completely within a few days to weeks. The original joint-fixing event can only be guessed at, but it would be easy to understand how it might happen in species in which the fetal size and limb length are high in relation to dam size.

Further reading

Banker BQ. Arthrogryposis multiplex congenita: spectrum of pathologic changes. Human Pathol 1986;17:656-672.

van den Brom R, et al. Epizootic of ovine congenital malformations associated with Schmallenberg virus infection. Tijdschr Diergeneeskd 2012;137:106-111.

Windsor P, et al. Neurological diseases of ruminant livestock in Australia. V: congenital neurogenetic disorders of cattle. Aust Vet J 2011;89:394-401.

Muscular defects

This section describes developmental defects affecting muscle that are not associated with lesions in nervous tissue.

Forelimb-girdle muscular anomaly of Japanese black cattle

An autosomal recessive disorder in Japanese black cattle leads to hypoplasia of forelimb-girdle musculature with reduced myofiber diameter in affected muscles. Affected cattle develop tremors, abnormal forelimb gait, and abnormal shape of the shoulder area. The gene has been mapped to bovine chromosome 26.

"Splayleg" (myofibrillar hypoplasia) in piglets

Splayleg, also called spraddle-leg, is a disease of neonatal piglets. It occurs in all countries with a well-developed pig-rearing industry. The incidence of the disease fluctuates inexplicably but frequently appears as a farm or regional outbreak. The disease incidence within litters is variable and a sow may produce consecutive litters with the disease. Genetic predisposition and infectious or nutritional causes are postulated but not proved.

Piglets with splayleg assume a posture with the hindlegs or all 4 legs laterally extended (Fig. 3-40). They are apparently unable to adduct them or retrieve them from a forward or backward position. Mobility is reduced and affected pigs are susceptible to accidents or may starve because of an inability to compete to suckle. *The locomotor defect is transient and within a week, or at most 2, survivors appear normal.*

The clinical signs of splayleg reflect muscle weakness. Not all piglets suffering from splayleg have primary muscle disease; other conditions cause similar signs, but much less frequently.

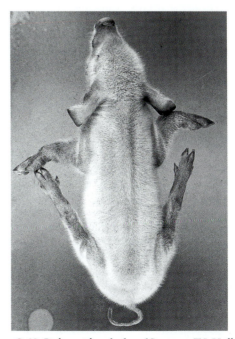

Figure 3-40 Piglet with **splayleg**. (Courtesy T.J. Hulland.)

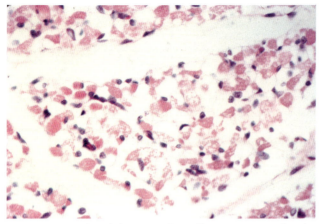

Figure 3-41 Reduced diameter of myofibers in a neonatal piglet with **splayleg**. H&E stain.

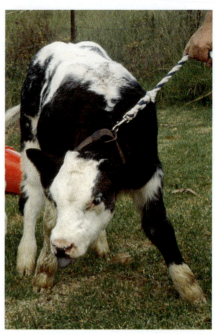

Figure 3-42 Congenital muscular hyperplasia ("double muscling") caused by defective myostatin in a calf. There is increase in muscle bulk and an enlarged protruding tongue. (Courtesy P. Windsor.)

Developmental abnormalities of spinal closure may be responsible (see Arthrogryposis and dysraphism) and myopathy induced by the injection of saccharated iron may produce a similar syndrome in one or more litters. The splayleg syndrome described here is unrelated to either of the preceding causes. The most common finding in skeletal muscle of affected pigs is *reduced diameter of myofibers with an abnormally small mass of myofibrils within individual muscle fibers* (Fig. 3-41), and increased cytoplasmic glycogen filling the large extramyofibrillar spaces. It is also possible, however, to find a similar histologic picture of apparent myofiber immaturity in clinically normal neonatal piglets. It may be that subtle differences in the degree of myofiber immaturity explain the variable clinical expression.

In pigs, the early postnatal period seems to mark the end of vigorous new muscle fiber production, although some increase may continue in some circumstances. In the critical period just before and just after birth, splayleg pigs show an irregularity or retardation in the transition of type 2 fibers to type 1 fibers in the developing muscle. *These findings in pigs with splayleg suggest delayed maturation of muscle in utero.* Examination of muscle from recovered piglets indicates that postnatal maturation continues, and eventually the muscles from such pigs are indistinguishable from control piglets.

The characteristic lesions of myofibrillar hypoplasia are only partly revealed by light microscopy. Affected muscles, chiefly the longissimus, semitendinosus, and triceps, are incompletely or irregularly involved, and *the most obvious change is lightness of staining with eosin caused by the low volume of myofibrils within outer cell membranes of normal volume.* The remainder of the fiber sheath appears to be empty but sometimes contains a nucleus or thin pink proteinaceous fluid. In longitudinal section, myofibrils appear to be diluted by watery fluid or clear strips of space. Periodic acid-Schiff staining reveals *marked accumulation of cytoplasmic glycogen.*

Electron microscopic examination of muscle from pigs with splayleg reveals segmental Z-line distortion with dispersal of the electron-dense material (Z-line streaming), loss of register and alignment of sarcomeres, reduced volume of myofilaments, and myofilament splitting and disarray. Glycogen granules are abundant, and there are increased numbers of ribosomes. Although degenerative changes, including increased phagolysosomes and lysis of myofilaments, have been described, this is not a consistent finding.

Myofibrillar hypoplasia has been reported as an isolated case in a 6-week-old **calf**. Lesions very similar to those in splayleg pigs were seen. A clinical syndrome similar to splayleg occurs in **puppies**, and affected pups are known as *swimmer pups*. Affected pups may have underlying myopathy or neuropathy, but more often this syndrome is seen in rapidly growing, overnourished pups. Dorsoventral flattening of the sternum often occurs. Affected pups often recover completely if measures such as use of a type of harness to help keep legs under the body and assisted exercise are employed.

Myostatin defects leading to muscular hyperplasia

Economic pressure to produce beef cattle with increased muscling has undoubtedly led to perpetuation of multiple genetic defects involving muscle development. The best characterized of these is the defect known as **double muscling**. This disorder occurs within several beef breeds, including Charolais, Santa Gertrudis, South Devon, Angus, Belgian Blue, Belgian White, and Piedmontese cattle. It is characterized primarily by an *increase in the number of fibers in affected muscles. The individual fibers are of normal size and structure.* This is in contrast to findings in other cattle with increased muscle bulk that are not double-muscled, in which a normal number of hypertrophied muscle fibers is found. In double-muscled homozygotes showing the full effect of the hyperplasia, the increase in gross muscle size is substantial, although not twice normal as the common name "double muscle" might suggest (Fig. 3-42). In fact, the contours of the large muscles are regular and normal except for rather prominent topographic clefts between muscles that are associated with large individual muscle size, reduced body fat proportion and thin skin. Bones may be lighter than normal and are often marginally shorter. Probably all striated muscles of the body are affected to some degree but *the muscles showing the most obvious change are those of the thighs, rump, loin, and shoulder*, giving the calf a very athletic

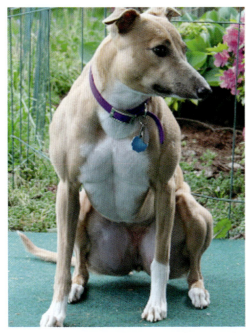

Figure 3-43 Whippet dog with muscular hypertrophy ("bully whippet") caused by defective myostatin. (From Mosher DS, et al. A mutation in the myostatin gene increases muscle mass and enhances racing performance in heterozygote dogs. PLoS Genet 2007;3:e79.)

appearance and predisposing to dystocia, and *hypertrophy of the tongue*. Some fiber increase is manifested by heterozygotes, but the level of heritability seems to be low and subject to capricious variability of penetrance or expression. A higher proportion of type 2 glycolytic fibers and a decreased capillary density are found in muscle from doubled-muscled cattle.

This disorder has been found to be due to *genetic defects in the myostatin gene*, which normally functions to limit skeletal muscle growth. Other genes are likely to be involved in the development of double muscling, as the degree of double muscling in Belgian Blue cattle is significantly greater than in double-muscled Piedmontese cattle, despite the fact that both breeds have genetic defects that apparently result in inactivation of myostatin.

A unique 2-nucleotide deletion in the myostatin gene leads to double muscling in Whippet **dogs** ("bully whippets"). Affected dogs display remarkable gross muscle hypertrophy and have episodic muscle cramping and stiffness (Fig. 3-43). Heterozygote dogs are more muscular than wild-type dogs and race faster, suggesting the possibility of selection pressure for this mutation within racing whippet lines.

Muscular hyperplasia most pronounced in hindquarter musculature occurs in the *callipyge phenotype* in **sheep**. This disorder has an unusual pattern of inheritance known as *polar dominance*, in which only heterozygotes having received the mutation from the sire are affected. Parental imprinting may play a role. The callipyge phenotype is due to a point mutation in the *CLPG1* gene on chromosome 18, but the manner in which this defect results in muscular hypertrophy is complex. The genetic defect results in upregulated activity of several genes involved in determination of skeletal muscle myotube size and myosin expression. Affected genes include *DLK1*, *RTL1*, and *PARK7*. Affected lambs are normal at birth and develop muscular hypertrophy by 1 month of age. Meat quality may be reduced in affected sheep.

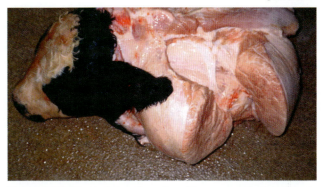

Figure 3-44 Cervical muscle replaced by a mass of adipocytes in a newborn calf with **steatosis** (muscular pseudohypertrophy). (Courtesy I.M. Langohr.)

Muscle steatosis

Muscle steatosis *is a disease characterized by too much fat deposited within muscles*. It carries an inference that the fat is where muscle once was or ought to have been; effectively, fat *replacement of muscle fibers, often forming an area of enlargement (muscular pseudohypertrophy*; Fig. 3-44). Fat infiltration of muscle is a common nonspecific finding in chronic myopathic and neuropathic disorders that affect muscle. The adipocytes that infiltrate muscle are derived from intramuscular mesenchymal cells. Fat infiltration may be accompanied by variable degrees of fibrosis. Steatosis of muscle is *best considered a reaction of chronically damaged or denervated muscle*, rather than a true developmental muscular defect.

The syndrome in livestock, often known as muscular steatosis, is not typically associated with fibrosis. *It appears in clinically healthy animals, and it is usually a problem only in meat inspection*. Although previous damage resulting from neural lesions, nutritional myopathy, exertional myopathy, ischemia, or trauma are possible underlying causes, in most cases an exact cause is not determined. Studies on steatosis in normal market pig carcasses indicate that about 1-5% of pigs have small steatotic lesions and that a smaller proportion of pigs have extensive lesions of the cranial thigh or loin muscles.

Sometimes the steatosis affects several muscles of one limb, but more often it affects only one or several muscles in one region. It may be bilaterally symmetrical or asymmetrical. Rarely does it affect all of one muscle, and the dividing line between normal and fatty muscle is not sharp. Surviving muscle fibers in the marginal areas may be normal or smaller than normal but are often angular in fixed tissue as a result of adjacent pressure from turgid lipocytes.

Congenital clefts of the diaphragm

The embryologic development of the diaphragm is complex, with contributions from several different tissues. The septum transversum forms the central tendon, the dorsal aspect of the caudal mediastinum (the dorsal mesoesophagus) forms the diaphragm surrounding the esophagus and aorta, and the right and left pleuroperitoneal membranes fuse to close the pleuroperitoneal canals and form the final complete diaphragm.

Congenital diaphragmatic clefts affect all species either alone or as part of a more generalized malformation. *The most common defect involves the left dorsolateral and central portions of the diaphragm, indicative of failure of closure of the left pleuroperitoneal* canal. The clefts may permit the herniation of tissues ranging in size from a small button of liver to extensive displacement of viscera. In very large congenital clefts, the diaphragm may be represented by only a narrow rim of muscle that does little more than mark the diaphragmatic origin. Congenital clefts must be differentiated from acquired but healed lacerations of the diaphragm. The occurrence of congenital diaphragmatic hernia is best documented in the *dog* and *rabbit*. In the dog, incomplete closure of the left pleuroperitoneal canal is most common. In the rabbit both defective closure of the left pleuroperitoneal membrane and absence of the major portion of the left diaphragm have been reported. Autosomal recessive inheritance has been proposed in both dogs and rabbits. The occurrence of congenital diaphragmatic hernias in 5 of 27 puppies from 3 father-daughter matings would support this form of inheritance; however, further inbreeding of this particular colony of dogs failed to produce any subsequent pups with diaphragmatic hernias, suggesting that the genetic defect is likely to involve multiple genes.

Further reading

Ducatelle R, et al. Spontaneous and experimental myofibrillar hypoplasia and its relation to splayleg in newborn pigs. J Comp Pathol 1986;96:433-445.

Langohr IM, et al. Muscular pseudohypertrophy (steatosis) in a bovine fetus. J Vet Diagn Invest 2007;19:198-201.

Mosher DS, et al. A mutation in the myostatin gene increases muscle mass and enhances racing performance in heterozygote dogs. PLoS Genet 2007;3:e79.

Rodgers BD, Garikipati DK. Clinical, agricultural, and evolutionary biology of myostatin; a comparative review. Endocrine Rev 2008; 29:513-534.

Yu H, et al. Park7 expression influences myotube size and myosin expression in muscle. PLoS ONE 2014;9:e92030.

Muscular dystrophy

The muscular dystrophies of humans are defined as inherited progressive myopathies characterized histologically by ongoing muscle fiber necrosis and regeneration. Peripheral nerves and neuromuscular junctions are normal. The advent of molecular genetics has begun to further characterize these disorders according to their genetic basis and has aided in validating several animal disorders as true animal models of human disease. Given the high conservation of genes on the mammalian X chromosome, it was suspected that progressive degenerative myopathies inherited as an X-linked recessive trait in animals were likely to be homologs of the X-linked Duchenne and Becker muscular dystrophies of humans. Molecular genetic analysis has proved this to be the case. **True muscular dystrophy**, *homologous to Duchenne and Becker muscular dystrophy of humans, occurs in the dog, cat, and mouse.* Duchenne and Becker muscular dystrophy are X-linked recessive disorders of humans caused by defects in the gene coding for *dystrophin*, a sarcolemmal-associated cytoskeletal protein. Immunostaining of frozen sections of muscle and Western blot analysis for dystrophin in snap-frozen muscle samples are typically necessary for confirmation of dystrophin-deficient muscular dystrophy. A few dystrophin antibodies react with formalin-fixed, routinely processed tissue. It is interesting that dystrophin deficiency results in progressive gross muscle atrophy in most breeds of dogs, but causes marked muscular hypertrophy in the mouse, cat, and Rat Terrier dog. Muscle fiber hypertrophy occurs, especially in early stages of the disorder, but extensive fiber necrosis leads to overall muscle atrophy in most cases. At this time there is no explanation for this phenomenon, although it would appear that muscle hypertrophy is more apparent in animals of small stature. Dystrophin has been found to be linked to several other proteins that function as a transmembrane complex, and other defects in this dystrophin complex, such as *α-dystroglycan deficiency*, can produce similar diseases inherited as autosomal recessive traits.

In animals, a number of muscle disorders have been erroneously designated as "muscular dystrophy," most notably those degenerative myopathies occurring secondary to nutritional deficiency. An inherited progressive myopathy in sheep has been described as a muscular dystrophy and is included in this section, although this disorder might be better classified as a congenital progressive myopathy because cytoarchitectural alterations are the hallmarks of this disorder, and ongoing fiber degeneration and regeneration are not typical features. Other inherited myopathies in dogs and cattle, many of which have been described as muscular dystrophies, are considered to be less likely candidates for true muscular dystrophy and are described in the Congenital myopathy section.

Canine X-linked muscular dystrophy

Sporadic reports from around the world of a severe progressive degenerative myopathy affecting young male dogs led to the establishment of a breeding colony of affected Golden Retriever dogs. Although a similar disorder has now been identified in many breeds, including Irish Terrier, Samoyed, Rottweiler, Dalmatian, Shetland Sheepdog, Labrador Retriever, German Shorthaired Pointer, Brittany Spaniel, Rat Terrier, Belgian Groenendael Shepherd, and Schnauzer, *the disease is best characterized in the Golden Retriever.* Being X-linked, this disorder can also occur in crossbred dogs.

Affected pups may be normal or slightly small at birth. Some affected pups may show severe progressive weakness leading to death within the first few weeks of life. This may be particularly true of affected pups in large litters that include normal and carrier pups, and may in part be due to an inability to compete for food. Other pups show no signs of disease until ~8 weeks of age, when reduced jaw mobility, exercise intolerance, and a stiff-legged gait become apparent. Serum activities of creatine kinase (CK) and aspartate aminotransferase (AST) are, however, markedly increased, indicative of severe myonecrosis, even in neonates with inapparent disease, and levels of CK and AST continue to rise until peaking at ~6 months of age. Serum CK and AST levels in older dogs are always high, but tend to be decreased as compared with younger dystrophic dogs. Serum activities of CK and AST are highest if blood is drawn 4-6 hours after exercise. *Clinical signs of neuromuscular weakness are progressive until approximately 8-12 months of age, when the disease tends to stabilize.* The severity of the disorder is variable, with some dogs developing severe muscle atrophy and contractures by 6 months of age (Fig. 3-45) and others remaining stiff, muscle wasted, and exercise intolerant but without severe impairment of joint mobility. Dystrophic dogs have a characteristic stiff-legged shuffling gait and a thickening of the muscles of the base of the tongue and under the jaw, tend to drool excessively, and develop abdominal breathing and often deformation of the ribcage caused by diaphragmatic contracture. Esophageal dysfunction is common, and dystrophic dogs may develop aspiration pneumonia caused by regurgitation. The severity of the disease

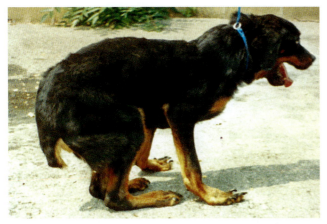

Figure 3-45 One-year-old male Rottweiler dog with severe **X-linked muscular dystrophy**.

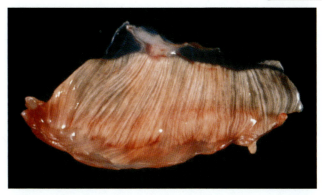

Figure 3-46 Pale streaking of diaphragm muscle caused by **massive necrosis** in a neonatal pup with fulminant X-linked muscular dystrophy. (From Zachary JF, McGavin MD. Pathologic Basis of Veterinary Disease. 5th ed. St. Louis: Mosby/Elsevier; 2012.)

varies among breeds. Although muscle atrophy is more obvious than hypertrophy in the Golden Retriever and Rottweiler, in other breeds such as the Rat Terrier there is progressive development of muscular hypertrophy resulting in obvious increased bulk, particularly involving muscles of the thigh, neck, and shoulder girdle. Breed size may have some role in the type and severity of changes, with larger breeds being most severely affected. A study of histologic lesions in golden retrievers with muscular dystrophy compared with Golden Retriever × yellow Labrador Retriever dog with muscular dystrophy found reduced severity in the cross-breds. As these breeds are approximately the same size, findings suggest that breed size is not the only factor related to phenotype in dystrophic dogs. Female carriers are clinically normal, although higher than normal levels of serum CK and AST are apparent, particularly in carriers <6 months of age.

Concentric needle electromyography reveals marked spontaneous activity in the muscles of dystrophic dogs. Although the complex repetitive activity generated by canine dystrophic muscle was initially interpreted as myotonia, resulting in characterization of this disorder as a myotonic myopathy, careful analysis of the electrical activity indicates that these bursts do not wax and wane, but rather start and stop abruptly and are *characteristic of pseudomyotonia*. Although the exact cause of this electrical activity is not known, membrane instability associated with clusters of degenerating and regenerating fibers is suspected.

Pups dying with fulminant neonatal disease have characteristic gross pathologic findings of severe degeneration of the diaphragm and strap muscles, including the trapezius and sartorius muscles of the limbs, characterized by pale white streaks within affected muscles (Fig. 3-46). Histologic evaluation reveals massive acute muscle fiber necrosis and mineralization, and similar findings are present in tongue muscle. This selective involvement of muscles in neonatal pups may reflect exercise-induced injury in muscles used for breathing, crawling, and suckling and may also involve the susceptibility to injury of more mature, larger-diameter fibers.

Postmortem examination of affected dogs that survive the neonatal period typically reveals pale musculature that may be slightly firm, which is especially true of the sartorius muscles of the hindlimbs. The diaphragm often exhibits the most striking changes, with thickening, contracture, and fibrosis evident (Fig. 3-47). On histologic examination, muscle

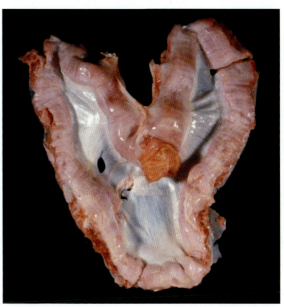

Figure 3-47 Severe diaphragmatic **muscle fibrosis and contraction** in a young adult dog with X-linked muscular dystrophy.

samples exhibit the characteristic findings of muscular dystrophy. *Numerous swollen and dark staining fibers (so-called* **large dark fibers***) are seen throughout the sections and are considered to be the earliest stage of muscle fiber degeneration*. Small clusters of overtly *necrotic fibers*, either in a coagulative state or macrophage-infiltrated, and of *regenerate fibers* are seen (multifocal, polyphasic necrosis; Fig. 3-48). Scattered *mineralized fibers* are common. The basal lamina of necrotic fiber segments is preserved, resulting in the presence of "empty sarcolemmal tubes" and the ability to fully regenerate affected fiber segments. Muscle spindles are unaffected. With increasing age, the degree of overt fiber necrosis and regeneration decreases. In *older dystrophic dogs*, marked fiber size variation, with internal nuclei, cytoarchitectural changes including nemaline rods, and a type 1 fiber predominance may be seen. Endomysial fibrosis and fat infiltration, the hallmark of advanced Duchenne dystrophy in boys, occurs in some muscles (Fig. 3-49), but is variable and typically less apparent in the dog.

In addition to evidence of fiber necrosis and regeneration, ultrastructural studies of muscle from dystrophic dogs have

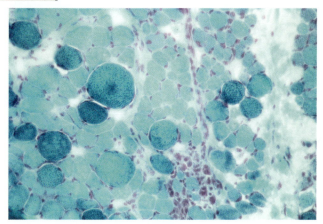

Figure 3-48 Characteristic **multifocal polyphasic necrosis** in muscle from a dog with X-linked muscular dystrophy. There are characteristic large dark fibers as well as clusters of overtly necrotic fibers with macrophage infiltration. Frozen section, Gomori trichrome.

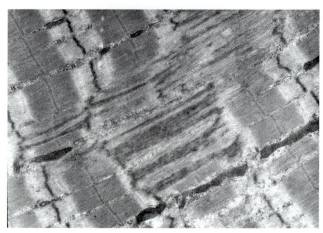

Figure 3-50 **Streaming of Z bands** in a pup with X-linked muscular dystrophy. Transmission electron micrograph.

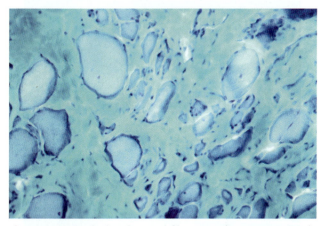

Figure 3-49 **Marked endomysial fibrosis** in the sartorius muscle of a dog with X-linked muscular dystrophy. Remaining fibers have variable diameter and frequently contain internal nuclei. Frozen section, Gomori trichrome.

found small areas of apparent sarcolemmal defects in otherwise normal-appearing fibers. *Nonspecific cytoarchitectural changes,* including increased mitochondrial content and Z-line streaming are also seen (Fig. 3-50). Alizarin red staining of frozen sections has confirmed that influx of calcium, probably through defects in the sarcolemma, is an early event leading to muscle fiber necrosis in dystrophic muscle (see Fig. 3-27A). Although considered to be an essential cytoskeletal protein and known to be part of a membrane-associated complex, *the exact function of dystrophin and the cause of muscle fiber necrosis in dystrophin-deficient muscle is still not clear.* The dystrophin complex links the cytoskeleton to the extracellular matrix and basal lamina, and therefore may serve to "strengthen" the sarcolemma.

Cardiac muscle of dystrophic dogs 6 months or older exhibits myofiber necrosis, mineralization, and fibrosis in a *subepicardial pattern.* The left ventricular wall and right side of the interventricular septum are most severely affected. The development of *progressive degenerative cardiomyopathy* is a hallmark of Duchenne and Becker muscular dystrophy in humans, and often eventually results in congestive heart failure in older dystrophic dogs.

Immunostaining of frozen sections for dystrophin typically reveals complete absence of this sarcolemmal-associated protein (Fig. 3-51A, B), although partial expression may be present in Becker-type mutations or in so-called revertant fibers, which are fibers that have undergone secondary somatic mutation allowing for dystrophin expression. Cardiac muscle in dystrophic dogs completely lacks dystrophin. Although dystrophin expression has been absent or nearly absent in the dystrophic dogs studied to date, it is possible that animals expressing an abnormal truncated or elongated dystrophin will be found.

Muscle from young female carriers often contains numerous large dark fibers and scattered necrotic and regenerating fibers. This reflects the mosaic pattern of dystrophin expression in muscle of young carrier dogs. The degree of overt necrosis and regeneration appears to be less than the proportion of large dark fibers, suggesting that membrane repair in some large dark fibers is possible. By about 6 months of age, evidence of necrosis or regeneration is rare because of loss of skeletal muscle mosaicism, and histologic findings in muscle from carriers 6 months of age or older are of essentially normal muscle. This loss of dystrophin mosaicism is thought to reflect up-regulation or translocation of dystrophin throughout the mosaic muscle fibers. Cardiac muscle, composed of uninucleate cells incapable of regeneration, maintains a striking mosaicism for dystrophin for the life of the animal, and carrier females also develop cardiac muscle necrosis and progressive fibrosis in a pattern similar to that seen in dystrophic males. Curiously, although the fibrosis of cardiac muscle in older female carriers is quite striking, overt cardiac failure does not occur.

Feline X-linked muscular dystrophy

As in studies of canine muscular dystrophy, the recognition of a severe progressive degenerative myopathy in young male cats led to breeding studies of affected cats. To date, this disorder has only been reported in cats of mixed breeding. Its occurrence in Europe as well as North America suggests that, as in humans and dogs, the feline dystrophin gene is prone to spontaneous mutation.

Affected cats develop marked muscle hypertrophy, stiff gait, "bunny-hopping" in the rear limbs, reduced activity, and difficulty jumping up onto furniture and other objects. Clinical signs may be recognized as early as 5 months or as late as 2 years of age.

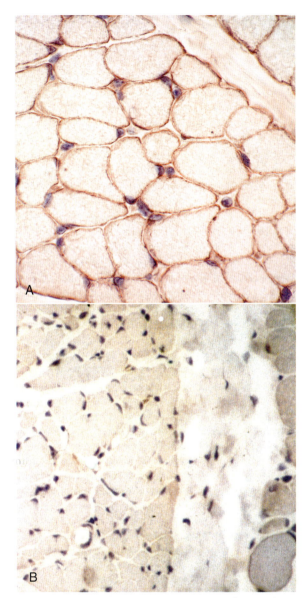

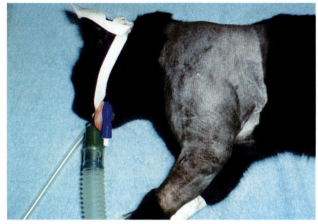

Figure 3-52 Marked hypertrophy of cervical and proximal forelimb muscles in a **cat with X-linked muscular dystrophy**.

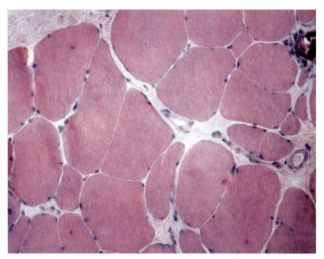

Figure 3-53 Excessive fiber size variation with both atrophy and hypertrophy, internal nuclei, and with scattered mineralized fibers, in a **cat with X-linked muscular dystrophy**. Frozen section H&E.

Figure 3-51 A. Dystrophin immunostaining of **normal** canine muscle, showing uniform sarcolemmal staining. Fiber size variation is normal in this 8-week-old dog. Frozen section, immunoperoxidase. **B. Dystrophin is completely absent** in muscle from an 8-week-old dog with X-linked muscular dystrophy. Frozen section, immunoperoxidase.

Thickening of tongue muscle may result in difficulties prehending food and in drooling. Regurgitation resulting from esophageal dysfunction also may be evident. Given the fairly subtle signs, it is likely that affected cats may not be recognized by owners as being abnormal. Muscular hypertrophy is most evident in the muscles of the neck and proximal limbs (Fig. 3-52). Dystrophic cats are prone to development of a *malignant hyperthermia-like syndrome* associated with restraint or general anesthesia. Serum activities of CK and AST are typically very high, and increases can be detected in kittens as young as 3 weeks of age. Electromyographic studies of affected cats reveal bizarre complex repetitive activity similar to that seen in the dystrophic dog.

At autopsy, affected cats have thickening of the muscular wall of the esophagus as well as marked thickening and contraction of the diaphragm. Skeletal muscle is often diffusely pale as well as displaying various degrees of hypertrophy. Pale streaks are often visible in the left ventricular wall and interventricular septum.

Histologic evaluation reveals *marked fiber size variation with numerous hypertrophied fibers often containing multiple internal nuclei*. Scattered clusters of necrotic and regenerating fibers with scattered mineralized myofibers are seen, and fibers with bizarre cytoarchitecture can occur. The degree of myofiber degeneration and regeneration is often less than that seen in dystrophic dogs (Fig. 3-53). Endomysial fibrosis occurs, but is minimal.

Foci of necrosis and mineralization of cardiac myofibers, followed by progressive fibrosis, can be seen in the left ventricular wall and interventricular septum of affected cats in a pattern similar to that seen in dystrophic dogs and in Duchenne and Becker muscular dystrophy. Cardiac lesions are not, however, a consistent finding in dystrophic cats, and clinical signs of cardiac insufficiency have not been reported, although experimental studies using inbred cats demonstrated left ventricular hypertrophy in all affected animals.

Other muscular dystrophies in cats

A muscular dystrophy associated with α-dystroglycan deficiency occurs in Sphynx and Devon Rex cats. This disorder is inherited as an autosomal recessive trait with variable clinical severity. Affected cats exhibit neuromuscular dysfunction from an early age, typically from 3 to 23 weeks of age. Ventroflexion of the neck, exercise intolerance, megaesophagus, a hypermetric forelimb gait, muscle tremors, and collapse with exercise are characteristic. Serum activities of CK and AST are generally within the normal range. Sudden death resulting from laryngospasm is common. Histopathologic findings are consistent with a primary myopathy and are characterized by excessive fiber size variation caused by rounded and angular atrophy and marked hypertrophy, internal nuclei, fiber splitting, and scattered necrotic and regenerate fibers. Endomysial fibrosis occurs in older affected cats.

Muscular dystrophy associated with laminin deficiency also has been described in cats. Affected cats developed progressive muscle weakness and atrophy, and also had peripheral neuropathies. In cases that survive for extended periods, fibrous replacement of atrophic muscle is severe. An autosomal recessive inheritance is suspected. This disorder is analogous to laminin-deficient congenital muscular dystrophies in humans.

Ovine muscular dystrophy

Muscular dystrophy of Merino sheep is an autosomal recessive disorder that occurs in widely separated flocks in Australia. This disorder affects about 1-2% of the progeny each year. The sexes are equally affected and *skeletal muscle of affected sheep expresses dystrophin in a normal manner, consistent with the non–X-linked nature of this disorder.* Although similarities to myotonic dystrophy of humans have been proposed, there is no compelling evidence that this is the case.

Initial signs are *lack of normal growth and reduced flexion of the hindlimbs* that lead to aberrations of gait or, in mild cases, just stiffness. Subtle clinical signs may be detected in lambs at 3-4 weeks of age. The rate of progression of this disorder is extremely variable but the majority of cases have clear-cut signs of hindlimb gait abnormalities by 6-12 months of age and are severely affected by 2-3 years of age. Under field conditions, the animals often die of inanition at 6-18 months of age. With care, some animals can be maintained for up to 5 years, during which time the clinical disease is slowly progressive. Serum activity of CK is increased at rest in animals with unequivocal clinical signs of muscle dysfunction and is increased further after exercise. No electromyographic abnormalities are found.

On postmortem examination, apart from emaciation, the prominent changes are in the vastus intermedius, soleus, anconeus, and medial head of the triceps, where normal muscle may be replaced by mature adipose tissue. The muscles in advanced cases appear gray, and are hard and atonic. Involvement of other muscles, most often the extensors of the hip, stifle, and hock joints and flexors of the shoulder, carpus, and digits, is limited to microscopic changes only, although these muscles may exhibit some degree of pallor. Affected muscles have a high proportion of type 1 fibers, and it appears that this accounts for the distribution of lesions, as this disorder affects only type 1 fibers.

The initial stages of the dystrophic lesion are heralded by a general hypertrophy of type 1 fibers followed by loss of myofibrils and formation of *characteristic sarcoplasmic masses* at the periphery or in the central portion of the cell (Fig.

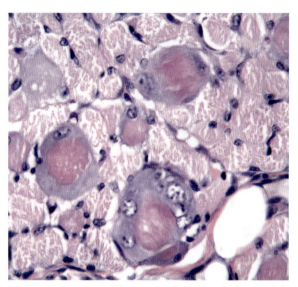

Figure 3-54 Variation in fiber size with enlarged fibers with large vesicular nuclei and pale amphophilic sarcoplasmic masses in muscle from a **sheep with muscular dystrophy**. H&E stain.

3-54). This is followed by an irregular atrophy of fibers. Fiber proportions remain normal. Compensatory hypertrophy of fibers is often accompanied by fiber splitting, resulting in fiber nesting ("orange section" clusters). A few fibers develop peripheral annular fibrils ("ring fibers" or "ringbinden"). Many fibers acquire internally located nuclei. Hypercontracted fiber segments are observed only sporadically, and regenerative fibers are rare or nonexistent. Muscles undergo progressive loss of fibers that may reach 80-100% in animals >2 years of age, and undergo progressive fat infiltration and/or endomysial fibrosis. In advanced muscle lesions, aggregates of lymphoid and histiocytic cells occur but these seem to be unimportant in the genesis of lesions.

Ultrastructural findings include *focal myofibril degeneration and Z-line abnormalities, including nemaline rods.* The distinctive sarcoplasmic masses are found to contain a mixture of normal organelles and tubular and fibrillar structures, including abnormal Z-line material. Immunocytochemical studies indicate profound alterations in cytoskeletal elements, including *loss of alpha actinin and proliferation of desmin.* Desmin forms the major constituent of the sarcoplasmic masses. Similar abnormal expression of desmin has been demonstrated in a growing number of myopathies affecting people and animals, and the term *myofibrillar myopathy* has been proposed for such disorders.

Further reading

Baroncelli AB, et al. Muscular dystrophy in a dog resembling human becker muscular dystrophy. J Comp Pathol 2014;150:429-433.

Blunden AS, Gower S. Hypertrophic feline muscular dystrophy: diagnostic overview and a novel immunohistochemical diagnostic method using formalin-fixed tissue. Vet Rec 2011;168:510.

Cozzi F, et al. Development of muscle pathology in canine X-linked muscular dystrophy. II. Quantitative characterization of histopathologic progression during postnatal skeletal muscle development. Acta Neuropathol 2001;101:469-478.

Gaschen F, Burgunder JM. Changes in skeletal muscle in young dystrophin-deficient cats: a morphological and morphometric study. Acta Neuropathol 2001;101:591-600.

Kane AM, et al. Cardiac structure and function in female carriers of a canine model of Duchenne muscular dystrophy. Res Vet Sci 2013;94:610-617.

Martin PT, et al. Muscular dystrophy associated with α-dystroglycan deficiency in Sphynx and Devon Rex cats. Neuromusc Dis 2008;18:942-952.

O'Brien DP, et al. Laminin alpha 2 (merosin)–deficient muscular dystrophy and demyelinating neuropathy in two cats. J Neurol Sci 2001;189:37-43.

Richards RB, et al. Skeletal muscle pathology in ovine congenital progressive muscular dystrophy. Part I. Histopathology and histochemistry. Acta Neuropathol 1988;77:95-99, 161-167.

Shelton GD, Engvall E. Canine and feline models of human inherited muscle diseases. Neuromusc Dis 2005;15:127-138.

Inherited and congenital myopathies

Many animal disorders have been compared with similar disorders in humans, but such comparisons are rarely validated. Several disorders are included in this section that have previously been designated as muscular dystrophies; the myopathy of sheep included in the muscular dystrophy section might be better classified as an inherited progressive myopathy. Inherited metabolic disorders are described in the Metabolic myopathies section. *The classification of myopathies in animals, similar to those in people, is subject to modification based on findings of ongoing genetic and pathogenetic studies as well as on changes in disease definitions.*

Breed-associated myopathies in the dog

Several myopathic disorders are recognized in dogs that are breed-specific and it is likely that many more will be identified in the future. An inherited basis is suspected, if not confirmed, in most cases of breed-associated myopathies.

Centronuclear myopathy of Labrador Retrievers. An inherited myopathy in Labrador Retrievers has been reported from Europe, North America, and Australia. The disorder occurs in working dog lines and not in show lines and is inherited as an *autosomal recessive disorder*. Both yellow and black Labrador Retrievers are affected. Various names attributed to this disorder include type 2 fiber deficiency, Labrador myopathy, and muscular dystrophy. Extensive genetic studies have identified a short interspersed repeat element (SINE) exonic insertion in the protein tyrosine phosphatase-like A (*PTPLA*) gene, which leads to *PTPLA* splicing defects. Although the function of the *PTPLA* gene in dogs is still unknown, it is thought that impaired *PTPLA* signaling is the cause of centronuclear myopathy in Labrador Retriever dogs. This syndrome is considered to be similar to centronuclear myopathy in people.

Clinical severity is quite variable. Evidence of *stunting, reduced exercise tolerance, and a stiff "bunny hopping" gait* may be apparent soon after birth or may not occur until ~6 months of age. Affected dogs may always have a slightly stiff gait and low head carriage, or may be apparently normal at rest. Exercise in affected dogs leads to increasing signs of weakness and collapse. Clinical signs are exacerbated by cold ambient temperature. Muscle atrophy may or may not be apparent. *The temporalis muscles appear to be particularly prone to atrophy.* Decreased or absent patellar reflexes is a consistent finding in affected dogs. Megaesophagus leading to regurgitation may occur, but is uncommon. This disorder may progress, but often stabilizes by 6 months to 1 year of age, and affected

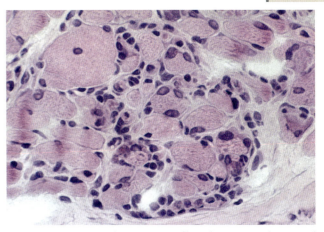

Figure 3-55 Increased variation in fiber diameter with internal nuclei in a Labrador Retriever with **congenital centronuclear myopathy**. Frozen section, H&E.

dogs may show some degree of improvement with age. Electromyography reveals bizarre spontaneous, high-frequency activity. Serum activities of CK and AST are normal or only slightly increased.

Postmortem examination may indicate normal or slightly reduced muscling. On histologic examination, *affected muscles exhibit a marked increase in fiber size variation that is most severe in older dogs.* Although initial reports indicated a type 2 fiber deficiency, subsequent studies indicate that, although alterations in fiber type are typical, atrophy or deficiency of type 2 fibers is variable. Scattered angular atrophied fibers may be seen. Fiber type grouping and small and large group atrophy are common. Alterations in mitochondrial distribution are often striking, with peripheral mitochondrial aggregates and cytoplasmic zones devoid of mitochondria. Fibers with internal nuclei are a common finding (Fig. 3-55) and whorled and split fibers can be seen. There are scattered necrotic and regenerate fiber segments. Endomysial fibrosis is minimal. Despite the angular atrophy and fiber type grouping suggestive of denervation, motor nerve conduction velocities are normal and no abnormalities have been found in the peripheral or central nervous systems.

Genetic testing for the abnormal *PTPLA* gene is available to identify carrier dogs as well as affected dogs. This testing will likely greatly reduce the incidence and prevalence of this disorder.

X-linked myotubular myopathy in Labrador Retrievers. A mutation in the myotubularin gene *MTM1* causes an X-linked myotubular myopathy in Labrador Retriever dogs and humans. Affected dogs are presented at an early age (<6 months) with generalized muscle weakness and atrophy that progress to recumbency. Affected dogs develop dysphagia, a hoarse bark, and masticatory muscle weakness. Histopathologic findings are excessive fiber size variation with type 1 fiber predominance and many central nuclei within small diameter fibers. Ultrastructural changes are reduction in number of triads, disorganization of remaining triads, myofibrillary disarray, and membranous whorls. The molecular defect results in sequestration of mutant myotubularin protein within proteasomes, and abnormal folding leading to premature degradation has been proposed.

Inherited myopathy of Great Dane dogs. A myopathy with scattered degenerate and regenerate fibers and intramyofiber core-like structures occurs in young adult Great Dane dogs. Affected dogs have exercise intolerance, an exercise-induced tremor, and progressive muscle weakness and atrophy. Increase in serum concentration of CK and abnormal spontaneous activity with electromyography are common. Clinical signs are apparent before 1 year of age, both males and females are affected, and affected dogs are typically fawn or brindle colored. Autosomal recessive inheritance is suspected. Ultrastructural features of the cores are disarray of myofilaments and thickened Z-lines. Genetic studies indicate that the cause is a mutation in the *BIN1* muscle specific exon, a gene that codes for amphiphysin 2, an important factor in membrane function in multiple cell types. The Great Dane myopathy may be a model for human BIN1-related centronuclear myopathy.

Myopathy of Bouvier des Flandres dogs. A *degenerative polymyopathy* occurs in the Bouvier des Flandres dog. Although the inheritance is not known, both sexes are affected. *Esophageal muscle and muscles of deglutition appear to be preferentially involved*, although generalized weakness occurs and histopathologic changes are seen in multiple muscles.

Affected dogs may not be recognized until 1-2 years of age when regurgitation caused by megaesophagus becomes apparent. Clinical severity is variable, however, and affected pups may be slightly stunted and display locomotor and swallowing difficulties as early as 7 weeks of age. Generalized muscle atrophy, weakness, and a peculiar paddling gait are characteristic. Serum activities of CK and AST are typically moderately increased. Bizarre high-frequency activity is seen with concentric needle electromyography.

Postmortem findings are *generalized muscle atrophy and pallor and megaesophagus*. Histopathologic changes include moderate to severe increase in fiber size variation with rounded atrophy and hypertrophy of both fiber types. Severe cytoarchitectural changes are seen, including whorled fibers, split fibers, and fibers with internal nuclei. Multifocal myofiber necrosis and regeneration occurs, but is generally not striking. Endomysial and perimysial fibrosis occurs, but is relatively mild. Cardiac myofiber degeneration and fibrosis also may be present.

Canine dermatomyositis. A syndrome of crusting and alopecic skin lesions and associated myositis has been described in Shetland Sheepdogs, Collies, and in a Pembroke Welsh Corgi dog. Canine dermatomyositis is thought to be inherited as an *autosomal dominant disorder* based on genetic studies in the Collie dog. This disorder has been likened to human dermatomyositis, which is thought to involve autoimmune mechanisms. In people, characteristic findings are a skin rash of the face, upper chest, and skin overlying joints, and muscle weakness with perifascicular atrophy and immune complex deposition and damage in skeletal muscle capillaries. Dogs with dermatomyositis develop distinctive skin lesions with basal cell degeneration and subepidermal cleft formation, but muscle lesions are not consistently found. Serum activities of CK and AST are normal. Nonsuppurative inflammation and atrophy of temporal and masseter muscles have been seen in affected dogs. However, *electrodiagnostic and histologic studies of a group of affected Shetland Sheepdogs did not reveal convincing evidence of a primary myositis*. Muscle inflammation, when present, appeared to represent extension of inflammation from overlying ulcerated and inflamed skin lesions. Therefore the relationship of this canine disorder to the human disorder remains questionable.

Other canine myopathies. A *juvenile-onset distal myopathy occurs in Rottweiler dogs*. Both males and females are affected, and clinical signs of muscle weakness and plantigrade and palmigrade stance are evident at ~2 months of age. The disorder is progressive, and is characterized histologically by *marked myofiber atrophy and fat infiltration with mild myonecrosis and endomysial fibrosis*. Serum activities of CK and AST are normal or only slightly increased. Electromyographic studies reveal rare fibrillations and positive sharp waves. The finding of decreased serum and muscle carnitine levels and improvement following carnitine supplementation suggest that *this may be a form of metabolic myopathy involving lipid metabolism*.

A *polymyopathy* with involvement of esophageal musculature occurs in association with dyserythropoiesis and cardiomegaly in *English Springer Spaniel dogs*. Findings in affected skeletal muscle include marked increase in fiber size variation with both rounded atrophy and hypertrophy and many fibers with internal nuclei. Central linear or irregular granular inclusions within myofibers that are visible on hematoxylin and eosin (H&E) and Gomori trichrome–stained frozen sections are characteristic. Inclusions are often associated with fiber splitting.

Nemaline rods within myofibers (see Nemaline myopathy of cats) occur as a nonspecific change in various canine myopathic conditions, and have been described in dogs with *X-linked muscular dystrophy*, hypothyroidism, and Cushing's syndrome. *Nemaline rods are formed by expanded Z-lines and are visible only in frozen sections stained with Gomori trichrome stain or on ultrastructural evaluation*. Ultrastructurally, nemaline rods are electron-dense structures with periodicity similar to the Z-band material from which these structures arise. Congenital nemaline myopathy has been described in a 10-month-old Border Collie dog and adult-onset nemaline myopathy occurred in an 11-year-old Schipperke dog. Affected dogs displayed exercise intolerance and muscle weakness.

Exercise-induced collapse occurs in *Labrador Retrievers with a mutation in the canine dynamin 1 (DNM1) gene*. Dynamin 1 is involved in neurotransmission and it is likely that this disorder reflects failure of neuromuscular transmission during strenuous exercise. As such no muscle lesions are expected and none have been reported.

Centronuclear myopathy has also been reported in a Border Collie.

Inherited and congenital myopathies of cats

Primary congenital myopathies are less commonly described in cats than in dogs. Some are better characterized than others. It is possible that, given the relatively sedentary life of most house cats, a subtle neuromuscular dysfunction could be overlooked.

Nemaline myopathy of cats. An *apparently inherited congenital myopathy characterized by intramyofiber nemaline rods occurs in mixed-breed cats*. Both males and females are affected. This congenital myopathy is similar to congenital nemaline rod myopathy of humans.

Affected cats exhibit signs of *progressive neuromuscular dysfunction* characterized by reluctance to move, a crouched "jerky" and hypermetric gait, muscle twitching, muscle atrophy, and hyporeflexia. Serum activities of CK and lactic dehydrogenase are mildly increased. No abnormalities are detected on electromyographic studies.

Muscle atrophy, most severe in the proximal limb muscles and muscles of mastication, is seen on gross examination. Characteristic histopathologic findings are seen with frozen section histochemistry, and include *atrophy of type 1 and type 2A fibers and presence of nemaline rods*. Nemaline rods are only visible with Gomori trichrome stain (Fig. 3-56) and occur primarily within atrophied type 1 and 2A fibers and only rarely in type 2B fibers. Nemaline rods are also seen in toluidine blue–stained Epon-Araldite embedded sections and in sections examined by electron microscopy (Fig. 3-57). Fiber size variation and marked fiber splitting also are seen. Fiber typing is often indistinct in areas in which myofibers exhibit extensive fiber splitting. Fiber necrosis and regeneration are uncommon but may be seen, especially in younger cats.

Other feline myopathies. A syndrome of *feline hyperesthesia* has been recognized for many years. Detailed studies of frozen section muscle biopsies of epaxial muscle from affected cats have found numerous rimmed vacuoles. The contents of these vacuoles stain with monoclonal antibodies to paired helical filaments and beta amyloid, and this disorder has been likened to *human inclusion-body myositis*. Myopathy with tubulin-reactive inclusions has been described in 2 unrelated cats with a slowly progressive muscular weakness.

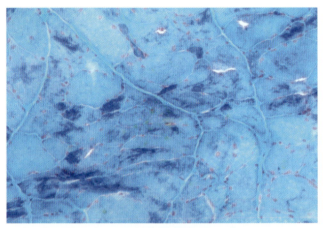

Figure 3-56 Numerous aggregates of dark staining nemaline rods in muscle from a cat with **congenital nemaline myopathy**. Frozen section, Gomori trichrome.

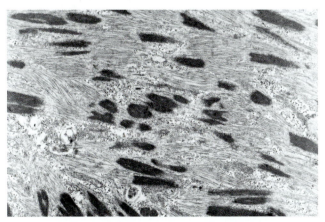

Figure 3-57 Dense staining elongate bodies composed of Z-disk material with associated myofilaments characteristic of nemaline rods in a cat with **congenital nemaline myopathy**. Transmission electron micrograph.

Inherited and congenital myopathies of cattle

Congenital and inherited myopathies have been described in beef and dairy breeds. Double muscling in beef breeds, a genetic defect in the myostatin gene, is discussed under the heading Congenital and inherited defects. Myopathy caused by glycogen storage disease is described in the Metabolic myopathy section.

Myopathy of the diaphragmatic muscle (diaphragmatic dystrophy). An inherited myopathy affecting primarily diaphragmatic and intercostal muscles has been described in *Meuse-Rhine-Yssel cattle in the Netherlands and in Holstein-Friesian cattle in Japan*. The disorder in these 2 breeds appears to be identical. The disorder affects males and females, and is suspected to be transmitted as an autosomal recessive trait.

Clinical signs in affected cattle occur in adults from 2 to 10 years of age and include *loss of appetite and condition, decreased rumen activity, and recurrent bloat*. Serum activities of CK, AST, and LDH are normal. Abnormal spontaneous activity was not seen in an electromyographic study of the diaphragm of affected Meuse-Rhine-Yssel cattle, although subtle changes in motor unit potentials were found.

The most severe gross pathologic changes are found in the *diaphragm, which is swollen, pale, and inflexible*. Similar changes are seen in intercostal muscles. Microscopic changes of myopathy occur in many other muscles and become more obvious as the disease progresses. Affected fibers exhibit marked cytoarchitectural alterations, including vacuolar change, sarcoplasmic masses, atrophy and hypertrophy of fibers, numerous internal nuclei, marked fiber splitting, and central core-like lesions. *These core-like lesions are the most distinctive finding in this disorder*. Frozen section histochemistry studies demonstrate lack of mitochondrial enzyme staining within the cores, but strong staining at the periphery, similar to the cores and rimmed vacuoles described in several human myopathies. Scattered necrotic fiber segments are seen, often with macrophage infiltration. Endomysial fibrosis occurs and appears to be progressive. *Myocardial fibers contain distinctive centrally located inclusions* that are intensely acidophilic on H&E stain and dark green with Gomori trichrome stain. On ultrastructural examination, the core-like lesions in skeletal muscle and the inclusions within cardiac myocytes consist of *disordered myofilaments with streaming of Z-line material*. Immunohistochemical studies of affected Holstein-Friesian cattle demonstrate that the core-like lesions in skeletal muscle contain actin and ubiquitin, but lack α actinin, desmin, and vimentin. Similar studies of myocardial fibers found variable ubiquitin reactivity of cardiac inclusions, and increased desmin reactivity on the periphery of the inclusions. It is proposed that this bovine disorder *may be a form of myofibrillar myopathy*.

Other bovine myopathies. Congenital myopathy occurs in *Braunvieh × Brown Swiss calves*. Both males and females are affected. These calves are abnormal at or soon after birth, with rapidly progressive muscle weakness and recumbency developing within 2 weeks of birth. Histologic findings are marked fiber size variation resulting from fiber atrophy and hypertrophy, fiber splitting of hypertrophied fibers, disorganization of myofibrils, nemaline rods, internal nuclei, and peripheral eosinophilic inclusions. Fiber necrosis, regeneration, and endomysial fibrosis are not seen. Ultrastructural evaluation reveals that peripheral inclusions consist of tightly packed filamentous structures. Myofibrillar and mitochondrial disarray are also seen.

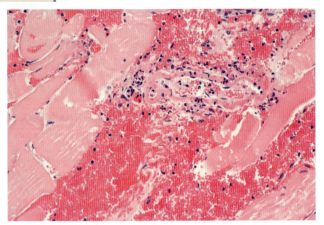

Figure 3-58 Necrotizing vasculitis and hemorrhagic necrosis of muscle in a Gelbvieh steer.

A congenital myopathy has been reported in a single Friesian calf that showed progressive weakness from birth. Muscle fibers were poorly developed and often exhibited lack of adequate myofibrils similar to myofibrillar hypoplasia of piglets. The most striking abnormality was the absence of Z-lines and presence of intracytoplasmic electron dense inclusions.

A degenerative myopathy characterized by necrotizing vasculopathy within skeletal muscle occurs in *young Gelbvieh cattle* (Fig. 3-58). The cause of this disorder is not known, although both immune-mediated and vitamin E deficiency–associated vasculopathy have been proposed.

Inherited and congenital myopathies of sheep

The progressive inherited myopathy of *Merino sheep* in Australia has been described in the Muscular dystrophy section. A suspected autosomal recessive congenital myopathy has been described in *Border Leicester sheep*. At birth, affected lambs have clinical signs similar to lambs with cerebellar cortical atrophy ("daft lambs"), but central nervous system lesions are absent. Clinical signs consist of difficulty or inability to rise and a peculiar arching of the neck with the head pressed back in an opisthotonos-like position. Pathologic findings in muscle are primarily within the cervical muscle and consist of abnormal fiber size variation resulting from fiber atrophy and hypertrophy. It has been proposed that small-diameter fibers represent delayed myofiber differentiation and maturation rather than atrophy. Ultrastructural abnormalities, including electron-dense bodies within axons of intramuscular nerves, suggest that myofiber lesions may reflect functional deficits of peripheral nerves rather than a primary myopathic process.

Inherited and congenital myopathies of horses

The majority of inherited and congenital muscle disorders of horses are described under the headings of Metabolic muscle disease and Myotonia and spastic disorders. Myopathy with central cores has been described in a 10-month-old pony.

Further reading

Beggs AH, et al. *MTM1* mutation associated with X-linked myotubular myopathy in Labrador Retrievers. PNAS 2010;107:14697-14702.

Böhm J, et al. Altered splicing of the BIN1 muscle-specific exon in humans and dogs with highly progressive centronuclear myopathy. PLoS Genet 2013;9:e1003430.

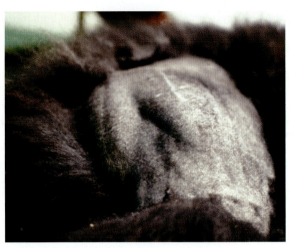

Figure 3-59 Dimpling following percussion in a Chow Chow dog with **congenital myotonia**. (Courtesy L. Fuhrer.)

Braund KG, et al. Investigating a degenerative polymyopathy in four related Bouvier des Flandres dogs. Vet Med Small Anim Clinician 1990;85:558-570.

Chang KC, et al. Molecular and cellular insights into a distinct myopathy of Great Dane dogs. Vet J 2010;183:322-327.

Cooper BJ, et al. Nemaline myopathy of cats. Muscle Nerve 1986;9:618-625.

Maurer M, et al. Centronuclear myopathy in Labrador retrievers; a recent founder mutation in the PTPLA gene has rapidly disseminated worldwide. PLoS ONE 2012;7:e46408.

Nakamura N. Dystrophy of the diaphragmatic muscles in Holstein-Friesian steers. J Vet Med Sci 1996;58:79-80.

Patterson EE, et al. A canine *DNM1* mutation is highly associated with the syndrome of exercise-induced collapse. Nat Genet 2008;40:1235-1239.

Myotonic and spastic syndromes

Myotonia is defined clinically as a temporary inability of skeletal muscle fibers to relax, resulting in transient uncontrollable muscle tension as a result of voluntary muscle contraction, and is manifested clinically as muscle stiffness. Electromyographically, myotonia is characterized by waxing and waning spontaneous electrical activity ("dive bomber" sounds) evident following needle insertion or muscle percussion during concentric needle electromyography. In many, but not all, myotonic syndromes, prolonged focal muscle contraction may be elicited by muscle percussion, a phenomenon known as "dimpling" (Fig. 3-59). Myotonia may be inherited or acquired. Myotonia is most obvious on initiation of muscle contraction and often improves with continued exercise. Affected individuals may be normal between episodes or have persistent muscle stiffness resulting in a stiff gait. Myotonic syndromes reflect muscle membrane electrical abnormalities, most often associated with ion channel defects. Ion channel disorders are a diverse group of disorders, collectively termed the **channelopathies**, and many involve the abnormal regulation of chloride and sodium ions.

In animals, confirmed or suspected inherited myotonias are most common. Drug- or toxin-induced myotonia occurs in humans, and a report of transient myotonia in a dog following ingestion of a phenoxy herbicide indicates that such induced forms of myotonia are possible in animals. Hypercortisolism owing to endogenous or exogenous corticosteroids can induce a myotonia-like syndrome in dogs, although this disorder is best classified as a *pseudomyotonia*. Pseudomyotonic electrical discharges are also a feature of X-linked Duchenne-type muscular dystrophy in the dog and cat, and the canine disorder has been erroneously described as a myotonic myopathy.

Several syndromes involving *episodic spasticity of limb movements* are recognized in animals. The cause of these spastic syndromes is poorly understood, although an inherited basis is often suspected. Although primary myopathy is suspected in some cases, it is also possible for abnormal peripheral or central nervous system activity to result in episodic spasticity.

Myotonia in the dog

A *congenital myotonic syndrome* has been described in several breeds of dog, including Chow Chow, Staffordshire Terrier, and Miniature Schnauzer dogs. A suspected *adult-onset myotonic syndrome* has been described in the Rhodesian Ridgeback and Boxer dog. Clinical signs in myotonic dogs are often misinterpreted as a shifting leg lameness. Myotonia has been best characterized in the Chow Chow and Miniature Schnauzer dog.

Myotonia in the Chow Chow. This disorder occurs in Chow Chow dogs worldwide, including North America, Europe, Australia, and New Zealand. It may be that breeding for heavy muscling has concentrated the trait in this breed. Myotonia in Chow Chows affects both sexes, and is likely to be an *autosomal recessive trait*. Mildly affected animals, however, may go undetected. The specific muscle defect leading to myotonia in the Chow Chow is still not known.

Clinical signs of stiff gait and muscular spasm on initiation of movement may be apparent as early as 6 weeks of age. Electromyographic evidence of myotonia precedes obvious clinical signs and persists for the life of the animal. Laryngospasm is common, causing episodic collapse or cyanosis, and affected dogs often have a weak or hoarse bark. Muscular contraction occurring when affected dogs attempt to rise often results in transient splaying of the forelimbs followed by sufficient relaxation to allow the dog to stand and ambulate, although affected Chow Chows often have a persistent stiffness of gait. Affected dogs may have a stiff "bunny hopping" gait in the pelvic limbs, and muscular hypertrophy is evident in early stages. Percussion of limb or tongue musculature results in dimpling (see Fig. 3-59). Serum activity of creatine kinase may be mildly increased.

In young myotonic dogs, the muscles may appear hypertrophied. In older affected dogs, muscle atrophy may be more obvious, and muscles may appear slightly pale. Histopathologic findings in affected muscle are minimal in early stages of the disorder. Only rare necrotic fibers are seen. With time *progressive myopathic changes*, including excessive fiber size variation, resulting from both hypertrophy and atrophy, internal nuclei, and mild endomysial fibrosis may be apparent. *Chronic myopathic changes, in particular numerous fibers with one or more internal nuclei, are the most consistent finding in muscle from older myotonic Chow Chows.*

Myotonia in the Miniature Schnauzer. Myotonia congenita in the Miniature Schnauzer, also reported as "myotonic myopathy," is an autosomal recessive disease that is clinically and histopathologically similar to myotonia in the Chow Chow. Abnormal muscle membrane chloride conductance in the Miniature Schnauzer is due to mutations in a skeletal muscle voltage–dependent chloride channel, CIC-1. Testing for the DNA defect by PCR is available and should help to reduce the prevalence and incidence of this disease.

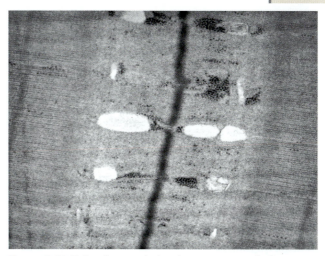

Figure 3-60 Dilated sarcotubular elements in muscle from a cat with **congenital myotonia**. Transmission electron micrograph. (Courtesy J.F. Cummings.)

Myotonia in the cat

A suspected inherited congenital myotonia occurs in mixed-breed cats. Clinical signs include a *crouched and stiff hindlimb gait and marked hypertrophy of proximal appendicular muscle evident at ~4 months of age*. These clinical signs of myotonia resemble those of male cats with muscular dystrophy; however, serum activities of CK and AST in myotonic cats are normal. Vocalization is weak, facial muscle spasms may be seen, and transient laryngospasm may occur. Electromyography reveals characteristic waxing and waning myotonic activity. Muscle percussion induces "dimpling." *Increased variation in fiber size resulting from prominent fiber hypertrophy is the primary histopathologic finding*. Fibers with multiple tiny clear cytoplasmic vacuoles may be seen, especially in plastic-embedded sections. Ultrastructural evaluation reveals mild dilation of T-tubules and terminal cisternae of the sarcoplasmic reticulum (Fig. 3-60). Clinical signs are apparently not progressive. Both males and females are affected, and the underlying defect is as yet unknown.

Myotonia in the goat

Congenital myotonia in the goat has been recognized for many years. *The myotonic goat is said to be the oldest recognized animal model of an inherited human skeletal muscle disease*. In fact, these so-called *"fainting goats"* are prized by certain breeders. If nothing else, the advantages of keeping such goats include the difficulty myotonic goats have in jumping fences because of muscle spasms associated with initiation of muscle contraction.

Myotonia in goats is inherited as *an autosomal dominant trait, with probable incomplete penetrance*. This disorder has been shown to be due to mutation in a skeletal muscle voltage-dependent chloride channel, CIC-1, which causes decreased skeletal muscle chloride channel conductance. This condition is very similar to congenital myotonia (Thomsen's disease) in humans.

Affected goats show clinical signs of myotonia within 2 weeks of birth. Attacks are most often initiated by startling an affected goat. Affected goats assume a "sawhorse" stance and often fall over. Myotonic episodes are transient and affected goats are normal in between episodes. Percussion induces a prolonged muscle "dimpling," and concentric needle electromyography reveals characteristic waxing and waning myotonic potentials. Serum activities of CK and AST are normal.

There are no gross abnormalities in myotonic goats, and affected goats do not appear to be heavily muscled. Histopathologic changes in muscle examined by light microscopy are minimal, with only mild increase in fiber size variation owing primarily to fiber hypertrophy and, in some cases, increased internal nuclei. On ultrastructural examination, dilated and proliferated sarcoplasmic reticulum and T-tubules are evident.

Periodic paralyses

The periodic paralyses are a group of inherited muscle disorders. In humans, hypokalemic, normokalemic, and hyperkalemic periodic paralyses are recognized. Although electrical myotonia and pseudomyotonia is a feature of many of the periodic paralyses, the transient attacks of paralysis are associated with muscle hypotonia rather than hypertonicity. These disorders are sometimes referred to as *paramyotonias* rather than true myotonic syndromes. The periodic paralyses are *due to ion channel defects that affect muscle sodium channel activity* and alter the muscle membrane potential. To date, only hyperkalemic periodic paralysis has been recognized in animals. The most common and the best-characterized syndrome occurs in horses. A similar disorder has been seen in a young American Pit Bull dog.

Hyperkalemic periodic paralysis in horses. *Hyperkalemic periodic paralysis (HYPP) occurs in horses related to the Quarter Horse stallion "Impressive" and is inherited as an autosomal dominant trait.* Homozygotes exhibit more severe signs of muscle dysfunction than do heterozygotes. The diagnosis of HYPP in horses can be confirmed by DNA testing.

Foals homozygous for HYPP often exhibit a peculiar respiratory noise caused by *laryngospasm*, and may develop dysphagia and emaciation during the first 2 years of life. Laryngospasm and pharyngeal collapse associated with exercise is common. Such horses must be considered nonviable as performance animals. Heterozygotes may appear to be clinically normal, but are prone to transient attacks of paralysis. Initial signs include muscle fasciculations, flashing of the third eyelid, muscle spasm, and inspiratory stridor. In severe attacks these signs will be followed by collapse to sternal or lateral recumbency associated with limb hypotonia. Attacks typically last from a few minutes to a few hours. Electromyography performed when animals are apparently normal reveals myotonic discharges and complex repetitive activity (pseudomyotonia).

Serum chemistry analysis often reveals higher than normal potassium levels in affected horses, particularly during attacks of weakness, but this finding is variable. Serum activities of CK and AST are normal or only very slightly increased. Clinical signs of weakness can be induced in HYPP horses with an oral potassium challenge test, high potassium feeds such as alfalfa or molasses-containing feeds, stress, or cold weather. *Sudden death* may occur in HYPP horses, perhaps caused by effects of increased blood potassium on cardiac function. Attacks also may be precipitated by inhalant anesthetic agents, and may resemble malignant hyperthermia.

The underlying defect in HYPP in horses, as in humans, is a mutation in the muscle sodium channel leading to increased open time. The increased influx of sodium through defective channels results in compensatory loss of muscle potassium, hence the hyperkalemia. Increased concentration of potassium ions outside the cell may further activate the abnormal sodium channels. The alteration in resting muscle membrane potential can lead to increased muscle action potentials and muscle fasciculations and spasms as well as to complete depolarization with inactivation of sodium channel activity and collapse.

There are no gross findings in horses with HYPP, other than frequent heavy and well-defined muscling. Although a vacuolar myopathy similar to humans with hyperkalemic periodic paralysis has been reported, in most cases of equine HYPP, *abnormalities are not found on light microscopy.* Ultrastructural findings of dilated sarcotubular elements are characteristic of HYPP, and are similar to those seen in myotonia in the cat and goat. DNA testing is now available on cells obtained from mane hairs rather than on blood, which is a boon for the pathologist who can now obtain the appropriate sample for testing in cases of otherwise unexplained death in Quarter-Horse–related breeds.

Myotonic dystrophy–like disorders in dogs and horses

Myotonic dystrophy is the most common inherited myotonic disorder in humans, affecting ~5 per 100,000 people, and is inherited as an autosomal dominant condition. Onset of obvious clinical signs is most often in late childhood, although this is quite variable, and a congenital form is also recognized. Myotonic dystrophy is a multisystem disorder associated with a constellation of signs, including cataracts and testicular atrophy. Muscle dysfunction is progressive, although the clinical signs of muscle dysfunction remain relatively mild. Findings in muscle biopsies include selective atrophy of type 1 fibers, hypertrophy of type 2 fibers, internal nuclei, ring fibers, and sarcoplasmic masses. However, these histopathologic findings are not specific for myotonic dystrophy. Attempts have been made to classify a group of animal disorders as animal models of myotonic dystrophy based on some similarities in clinical and pathologic findings, but the evidence for this is unconvincing. In particular, the involvement of other organ systems is generally lacking. The genetic defect in human myotonic dystrophy has been shown to be an abnormal expansion of a trinucleotide (CTG) repeat in a gene coding for a serine-threonine protein kinase. Similar molecular studies are lacking in animals. Myotonic dystrophy–like disease has been reported in a Rhodesian Ridgeback dog and in a Boxer dog. The best characterized of the myotonic dystrophy–like disorders occurs in the horse.

Myotonic dystrophy–like disease in the horse. A progressive early-onset myopathy associated with clinical and electrical myotonia and profound cytoarchitectural alterations in muscle occurs sporadically in horses. Breeds affected include Quarter Horse, Thoroughbred, and Standardbred, and both males and females appear to be equally represented. Although the early onset of clinical signs suggests that this disorder is congenital, to date there is no proof that it is inherited, and affected foals appear to occur only sporadically.

Affected foals may have difficulty standing at birth or, more commonly, develop a *progressive stiff gait with marked prominence of proximal limb muscles*, especially the gluteal muscle, evident at ~1 month of age. Percussion of muscle induces prolonged muscle dimpling. Affected foals become progressively weaker and have difficulty rising, with later development of muscle atrophy. Serum activities of CK and AST may be mildly increased. Concentric needle electromyography reveals characteristic myotonic and pseudomyotonic discharges.

At autopsy, affected muscles are often hypertrophied and may contain fibrous tissue and linear streaks caused by fat infiltration. Severe lesions are pale and yellow-white. Atrophy of affected muscles also may be seen. There is selective involvement of muscle, with *the most severe lesions found in the longissimus, iliopsoas, medial gluteal, biceps femoris, semitendinosus, semimembranosus, and sartorius muscles*. The triceps brachii and rectus femoris are less severely affected.

Histopathologic findings are a marked increase in fiber size variation with fiber hypertrophy as well as rounded atrophy and severe cytoarchitectural changes including pale-staining peripheral sarcoplasmic masses, internal nuclei, and small clear vacuoles (Fig. 3-61). Ring fibers and fiber splitting also can be seen. Only scattered necrotic and regenerate fibers are seen. Alterations in fiber type distribution in affected muscles include type 1 fiber predominance and fiber type grouping. Peripheral and intramuscular nerves, however, are histologically normal. Endomysial and perimysial fibrosis occurs, but is variable.

On ultrastructural examination, sarcoplasmic masses are composed of ribosomes, mitochondria, and disarrayed myofibrils.

Other myotonic-like disorders in the horse. A syndrome resembling *stiff-man syndrome* occurs in the horse. *Affected horses exhibit periodic muscle stiffness and spasms*. Muscle spasms are initiated by voluntary movement. Muscle hypertrophy may be evident. Electromyography reveals persistent motor unit activity, but no abnormal primary spontaneous activity of muscle is seen. Muscle biopsy samples are reported to be normal. A disorder involving *autoantibodies to glutamic acid decarboxylase*, resulting in a neuromyotonic syndrome similar to that occurring in humans, is proposed.

A syndrome of episodic painful muscle spasms associated with prolapse of the third eyelid has been described in horses with ear tick (Otobius megnini) infestation. Percussion of affected muscle groups results in muscle dimpling. Serum activities of CK and AST are often moderately to markedly increased. Electromyographic studies are normal unless muscle contracture occurs secondary to needle placement. No abnormalities have been reported in muscle biopsy samples. Clinical signs resolve following removal or insecticidal treatment of the ear ticks.

Spastic syndromes

"Scotty cramp" is an episodic motor disease, primarily of Scottish Terrier dogs. This disorder most often begins at 2-6 months of age, but adult onset is also possible. It is characterized by *hindlimb and pelvic muscle hypertonicity* along with upward arching of the back for periods of 1-30 minutes, and is precipitated by exercise or excitement. No consistent gross or histologic abnormalities are found in the central nervous system, peripheral nerves, or skeletal muscles.

Muscle hypertonicity precipitated by exercise or excitement has been described in several *Cavalier King Charles Spaniels*. Vacuolation of scattered muscle fibers and several minor ultrastructural changes occur, but there is no clear indication of the cause.

"Dancing Doberman" disease has been described as a spastic disease of one or both hocks in Doberman Pinschers of any age. The animals are reluctant to bear weight continuously and exhibit a peculiar shifting hindleg action resembling dancing. This appears to be a nonspecific sign because some of these dogs apparently have a localized myopathy and others have evidence of a neuropathy.

Spastic paresis of cattle affecting one or both hindlegs is usually seen in calves 3-7 months of age, although onset of signs can occur in adults. The disease appears first as an exaggerated straightness of the hock that increases to the point of *inability to flex the hock*. In the later stages, in animals with unilateral involvement, the affected limb may swing stiffly like a pendulum or be held out in an abnormal cranial or caudal position. The disease, also called *contraction of the Achilles tendon, straight hock*, or *Elso heel* (the latter derived from the name of the Friesian bull, some of whose progeny had the disease), is worldwide in distribution. It primarily affects Holstein-Friesian cattle but has been found in several other dairy and beef breeds, and has a distinct familial pattern. Deafferentation (cutting of the sensory nerve root) of the gastrocnemius muscle relieves the effect, suggesting that the defect is an *unmodulated or uncontrollable sensory-motor reflex loop*.

A related syndrome, referred to as *spastic syndrome, crampy spasticity*, or *stretches* affects mature animals, usually *bulls*, and causes periodic and sudden extension and stiffening of both hindlegs. During episodes, the back is arched and the neck is extended. Episodes last for a period of seconds to minutes. The disease is progressive and it is reportedly associated with straight hocks and a variety of other abnormalities of bone, joints, or spinal column.

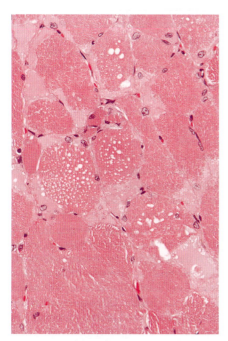

Figure 3-61 Excessive fiber size variation, pale peripheral sarcoplasmic masses, and fine cytoplasmic vacuoles, in muscle from a **foal with myotonic dystrophy-like disease**. H&E stain.

Further reading

Broeckx BJ, et al. The prevalence of nine genetic disorders in a dog population from Belgium, the Netherlands and Germany. PLoS ONE 2013;8:e74811.

Finnigan DF, et al. A novel mutation of the CLCN1 gene associated with myotonia hereditaria in an Australian cattle dog. J Vet Intern Med 2007;21:458-463.

Lehmann-Horn F, et al. Periodic paralysis: understanding channelopathies. Curr Neurol Neurosci Rep 2002;2:61-69.

Lobetti RG. Myotonia congenita in a Jack Russell terrier. J S Afr Vet Assoc 2009;80:106-107.

Ludvikova E, et al. Histopathological features in subsequent muscle biopsies in a warmblood mare with myotonic dystrophy. Vet Q 2012;32:187-192.

Nollet H, Deprez P. Hereditary skeletal muscle diseases in the horse. A review. Vet Q 2005;27:65-75.

Shelton GD. Muscle pain, cramps and hypertonicity. Vet Clin North Am Small Anim Pract 2004;34:1483-1496.

Toll J, et al. Congenital myotonia in 2 domestic cats. J Vet Int Med 1998;12:116-119.

Vite CH. Myotonia and disorders of altered muscle cell membrane excitability. Vet Clin N Am Small Anim Pract 2002;32:169-187.

Metabolic myopathies

Abnormal skeletal muscle metabolism leading to neuromuscular dysfunction most often is due to inborn errors of metabolism, but can result from acquired metabolic defects. In some disorders, a metabolic defect is suspected based on clinical and pathologic findings but an exact cause remains elusive. Metabolic defects can affect multiple organ systems, with metabolically active organs such as skeletal muscle, cardiac muscle, nervous tissue, and liver being most severely compromised. Muscle dysfunction, however, can be the primary or the only clinical sign. In some such cases, the occurrence of tissue-specific isozymes of enzymes involved in metabolism can explain selective organ dysfunction, and in other cases the cause is not clear.

In *humans* metabolic myopathies are broadly classified into 4 groups according to the type of metabolism affected:
- Carbohydrate metabolic disorders
- Disorders of lipid metabolism
- Disorders of mitochondrial metabolism (mitochondrial myopathies)
- Disorders of adenine nucleotide metabolism (myoadenylate deaminase deficiency)

Clinical signs of progressive muscle weakness, or exercise-induced muscle cramping, contracture, and rhabdomyolysis are most common. Skeletal muscle dysfunction may occur because of inadequate energy production, disruption of myofibrillar structure resulting from storage of carbohydrate or lipid, or a combination of these factors. To date, the confirmed or suspected metabolic myopathies in animals that have been identified include disorders of carbohydrate metabolism, mitochondrial function, and lipid metabolism.

Note that the terminology is confusing regarding *periodic acid-Schiff (PAS) positive, amylase-resistant inclusions* that occur within myofibers in some metabolic disorders. The terms *amylopectin, amylopectin-like, polyglucosan bodies, Lafora bodies,* and *complex polysaccharide* have all been applied to this material. Until detailed biochemical analysis of this type of stored material is available, it is safe to say that *all these terms describe a similar type of material*.

Metabolic myopathies of the dog

Glycogen storage disease type II in Lapland dogs. A canine model of Pompe's disease caused by acid maltase (acid α-glucosidase) deficiency has been recognized in the Lapland dog. Massive glycogen storage occurs in multiple organs, but skeletal, myocardial, and smooth muscle are most severely involved. The disorder is inherited as an autosomal recessive trait.

Clinical signs of progressive weakness and regurgitation owing to megaesophagus are present from ~6 months of age. Myocardial dysfunction is also a feature. Affected dogs typically die at 10-18 months of age.

Overall muscle atrophy and megaesophagus are found on postmortem examination. Histologic examination reveals massive glycogen storage in multiple organs. Stored material is visible in routine preparations as clear vacuoles. This material stains positively with PAS stain and is digested by amylase (diastase), consistent with glycogen. Ultrastructural studies indicate that *the stored glycogen is membrane-bound within lysosomes*.

Phosphofructokinase deficiency (glycogenosis type VII) in English Springer Spaniels and American Cocker Spaniels. Phosphofructokinase (PFK) is a rate-controlling glycolytic enzyme. Quantitative and qualitative alterations in PFK activity can significantly alter energy metabolism in cells such as erythrocytes and skeletal muscle cells that rely heavily on glucose metabolism for energy. PFK is a tetramer composed of liver, muscle, and platelet type subunits in tissue-specific patterns. *The genetic mutation is a point mutation in the muscle isozyme of PFK, and a PCR-based test can detect affected and carrier animals.*

In English Springer Spaniels and American Cocker Spaniels, deficiency of the muscle isozyme of PFK results in *recurrent hemolytic episodes due to defective erythrocyte carbohydrate metabolism*. Variable hematocrit and persistent high reticulocyte counts are typical findings. Episodes are most often initiated by exercise or excitement, as PFK-deficient erythrocytes are particularly sensitive to lysis associated with a mildly increased pH of blood (alkalemia) resulting from hyperventilation. Skeletal muscle cells are apparently protected by up-regulation of the liver isozyme of PFK. Exercise intolerance, exercise-induced muscle cramps, and progressive muscular atrophy and weakness can occur, however, particularly in older PFK-deficient dogs. Erythrocyte PFK activity is markedly reduced in affected dogs, and moderately decreased in heterozygotes.

In humans with PFK deficiency, clinical signs are entirely caused by muscular dysfunction, with exercise-induced cramps and myoglobinuria being most common. Late-onset progressive muscle weakness may also occur. The differences in clinical signs in affected dogs reflect the sensitivity of canine erythrocytes to alkalosis-induced lysis and possibly also to the high reliance of canine muscle on oxidative metabolism and less reliance on anaerobic glycolysis.

Studies of skeletal muscle from older PFK-deficient dogs have revealed *chronic myopathic changes, including excessive fiber size variation and intramyofiber vacuoles and inclusions of material* that is stained lightly by hematoxylin in H&E-stained sections. This material is *intensely PAS-positive* and resists digestion by amylase (diastase), consistent with an amylopectin-like complex polysaccharide. Ultrastructural studies indicate that this material is composed of non–membrane-bound granular filamentous and amorphous material. These complex polysaccharide inclusions are not a consistent finding and, given that these types of inclusions can occur in dogs for other reasons (see Other metabolic myopathies); it is possible that those reported were not related to the PFK deficiency. Other histopathologic findings at autopsy of PFK-deficient dogs include marked extramedullary hematopoiesis and hemosiderosis resulting from recurrent hemolysis.

Other canine metabolic myopathies
- *Mitochondrial myopathy* causing episodic weakness and exercise-induced lactic acidosis has been described in a litter of Old English Sheepdogs.
- *Familial myoclonic epilepsy* with polyglucosan bodies in skeletal muscle occurs in miniature wire-haired Dachshunds.
- Neuromuscular weakness associated with *increased lipid accumulation and decreased carnitine activity* within skeletal muscle has been described as an acquired disorder in a variety of dog breeds.
- *Lipid storage myopathy* is thought to reflect abnormal lipid metabolism. It should be noted that increased intramyofiber lipid is normal in pups up to ~2 months of age and should not be interpreted as a lipid storage myopathy (see Fig. 3-35)

Metabolic myopathy of the cat

A glycogen storage disease type IV resulting from deficiency of glycogen branching enzyme occurs as an autosomal recessive trait in **Norwegian Forest cats**. Although glycogen storage occurs in multiple organ systems in the cat, it is dysfunction of skeletal muscle, cardiac muscle, and nervous tissue that characterizes the feline disorder. In contrast, glycogen storage type IV of humans typically results in early-onset and progressive hepatic cirrhosis and liver failure. The molecular basis for this difference between cats and humans is as yet unknown.

Two clinical syndromes have been identified. The most common is the birth of fully developed kittens that are either stillborn or that die within a few hours of birth. Affected kittens that survive the neonatal period develop *progressive neuromuscular weakness, muscle atrophy, and cardiac dysfunction* beginning at ~5-7 months of age. Affected cats are often mildly febrile, exhibit generalized muscle tremors and a "bunny hopping" pelvic limb gait. *Progression to tetraplegia is rapid*, occurring within ~2 months following onset of clinical signs. Electromyography reveals abnormal spontaneous activity in multiple muscles. Cardiologic abnormalities include concentric left ventricular hypertrophy, left atrial dilation, decreased relaxation of the left ventricular wall during diastole, and focal hyperechoic areas in the subendocardial region of the left ventricular wall. Serum activities of CK and ALT are often increased. Glycogen branching enzyme activity in muscle, liver, and leukocytes is markedly reduced in affected cats, and moderately to severely reduced in clinically normal parents of affected cats.

Gross pathologic findings are absent in stillborn kittens or kittens dying soon after birth. In older affected animals, *severe generalized skeletal muscle atrophy* is evident. Fibrous replacement of muscle may be seen. *Left ventricular hypertrophy and left atrial dilation* are typical, and foci of fibrosis may be evident within the left ventricular myocardium.

Characteristic histopathologic findings are non–membrane-bound inclusions of *pale pink to amphophilic material within cells of many organs* (Fig. 3-62). This material is PAS-positive and amylase-resistant. Skeletal muscle, cardiac muscle, and central and peripheral nervous tissue are most severely affected and accumulation of stored material in these organs is accompanied by severe degenerative changes.

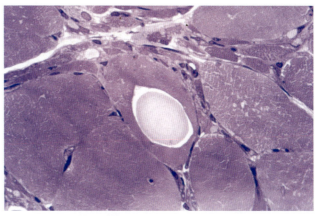

Figure 3-62 A pale hyaline ovoid inclusion of complex polysaccharide in muscle from a Norwegian Forest cat with **glycogen branching enzyme deficiency** (glycogenosis type IV). Thin section. (Courtesy T.J. Van Winkle.)

Metabolic myopathies of the horse

Equine polysaccharide storage myopathy. A glycogen storage myopathy occurs in many breeds of horses worldwide. This disorder has been recognized sporadically for many years. Only recently have studies begun to reveal the variety of clinical disorders associated with polysaccharide storage myopathy in horses as well as the wide range of breeds affected.

Equine polysaccharide storage myopathy is most common in draft, warm-blood, and Quarter-Horse–related breeds. In draft-related breeds, a prevalence of >50% has been reported. This disorder has also been recognized in virtually all other breeds, including ponies and miniature horses. Clinical signs range from recurrent exertional rhabdomyolysis, to progressive weakness that may or may not be accompanied by overt muscle atrophy, to mechanical lameness of the pelvic limbs. Subclinical cases are common. Serum activities of CK and AST may or may not be increased in affected horses. This disorder is inherited as an autosomal dominant trait with variable clinical expression.

Gross pathologic findings vary from no significant findings to obvious pale streaks within affected muscle. Muscle atrophy may or may not be evident. Red staining of muscle because of myoglobin release may be seen at postmortem examination of horses dying as a result of rhabdomyolysis. Careful evaluation of the diaphragm is indicated in animals dying with respiratory failure following clinical rhabdomyolysis because *severe diaphragmatic necrosis can occur*.

Histopathologic findings are variable. In the most severe cases, numerous round to irregularly shaped *pale pink to blue-gray inclusions are seen within skeletal muscle fibers* on H&E-stained sections (Fig. 3-63). *Inclusions may be single or multiple and are segmental, replacing up to 90% or more of the cross-sectional area of affected fiber segments* (Fig. 3-64). These inclusions are PAS-positive and amylase-resistant, consistent with a form of *complex polysaccharide* (Fig. 3-65). *Inclusions occur only in type 2X glycolytic* (traditionally reported as type 2B) *and 2A oxidative-glycolytic fibers*. Muscles that are strongly type 2 in composition, including semimembranosus, semitendinosus, gluteal, longissimus, and pectoral muscles, are most severely affected. In all cases in which inclusions of complex polysaccharide are seen, other fibers contain subsarcolemmal rounded vacuoles that are either clear or that contain pale pink hyaline material on H&E-stained sections. This material

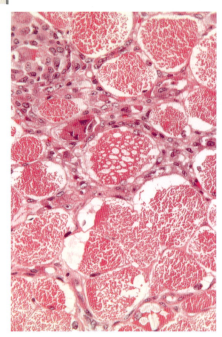

Figure 3-63 Marked fiber size variation with numerous fibers containing multiple subsarcolemmal to intracytoplasmic vacuoles containing pale pink glycogen and complex polysaccharide in a draft horse with **polysaccharide storage myopathy**. A focus of macrophages indicates previous segmental necrosis. H&E stain.

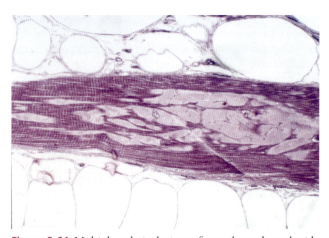

Figure 3-64 Multiple pale inclusions of complex polysaccharide replace large portions of fiber segments in a horse with **polysaccharide storage myopathy**. Thin section. (Courtesy J.F. Cummings.)

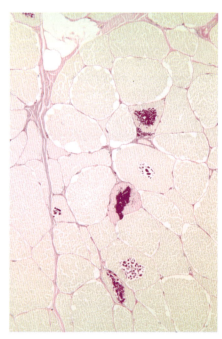

Figure 3-65 Amylase resistant inclusions of complex polysaccharide in muscle from a horse with **polysaccharide storage myopathy**. Periodic acid-Schiff with amylase digestion.

is PAS-positive and amylase-sensitive, consistent with *glycogen*. Fibers with complex polysaccharide or glycogen inclusions often occur in clusters, particularly at the periphery of fascicles. A more subtle pathologic change, involving only subsarcolemmal inclusions of glycogen, is seen in horses believed to have a form of the same disorder (Fig. 3-66A, B). Numerous clear vacuoles within the fiber interior as well as in a subsarcolemmal location may also be seen. Aggregates of glycogen and of amylase-resistant material often contain ubiquitin. *Chronic myopathic changes* are often found, especially in older affected horses, and include excessive fiber size variation due to fiber atrophy and/or hypertrophy and increase in internal nuclei within myofibers. Scattered myofiber necrosis or regeneration may or may not be seen. Macrophages within necrotic fiber segments or found as small clusters within the interstitium often contain PAS-positive, amylase-resistant complex polysaccharide. In very severe cases, to date only documented in draft-related horses with apparent sudden onset of inability to rise, massive replacement of skeletal muscle by infiltrating adipose tissue can be seen. Other organs, with the exception of rare cases with inclusions of complex polysaccharide within cardiac myofibers, are unaffected.

Ultrastructural examination of affected muscle indicates that *glycogen storage is not intralysosomal but rather is dispersed within the cytoplasm*. Loss or attenuation of myofibrils occurs (Fig. 3-67). Organized inclusions of PAS-positive, amylase-resistant material are composed of tangled fibrillar material studded with glycogen particles. Immunohistochemical studies have found that abnormal glycogen within the skeletal muscle fibers becomes bound to ubiquitin (Fig. 3-68), which may play a role in the development of amylase resistance.

Despite the clinical and pathologic similarities to myopathies caused by carbohydrate metabolic defects in people, dogs, and cats, extensive studies have failed to document a defect in either glycolytic or glycogenolytic pathways in muscle from affected horses. However, diets designed to minimize starch and sugar intake and maximize fat intake have proved to be extremely successful in controlling clinical signs of skeletal muscle dysfunction. Curiously, studies of a small number of horses indicate that pathologic findings are not obviously altered by dietary therapy.

Genetic studies have linked a single nucleotide polymorphism in the skeletal muscle glycogen synthase 1 gene (*GYS1*) to one form of equine polysaccharide storage myopathy. This mutation is most common in breeds prone to develop the most severe accumulation of abnormal and especially of amylase-resistant complex polysaccharide. The defect may lead to increase in glycogen synthase activity resulting in excess glycogen production and storage. Interestingly, horses

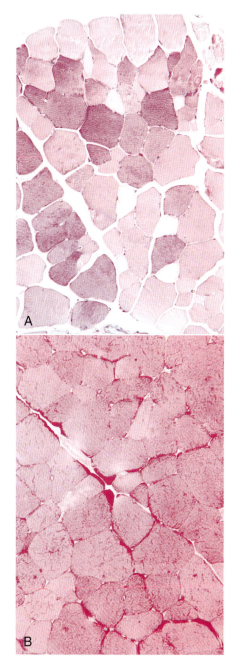

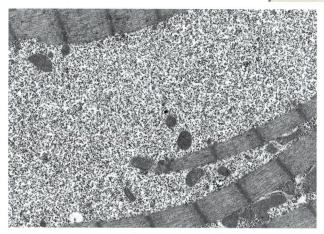

Figure 3-67 Aggregates of granular glycogen with attenuation of myofibrils in a horse with **polysaccharide storage myopathy**. Transmission electron micrograph. (Courtesy J.F. Cummings.)

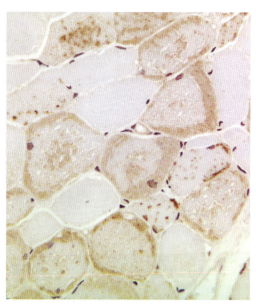

Figure 3-68 Inclusions of glycogen and complex polysaccharide in a horse with **polysaccharide storage myopathy** are positive for **ubiquitin**. Immunohistochemistry for ubiquitin.

Figure 3-66 A. Normal glycogen staining pattern of horse muscle. **B.** Multiple myofibers with peripheral aggregates of densely stained glycogen in an Arabian horse with **polysaccharide storage myopathy**. Fibers in this horse also contain increased coarse granular glycogen. Periodic acid-Schiff.

with the *GYS1* mutation that also have a ryanodine receptor 1 (*RYR1*) mutation have more severe clinical disease. Genetic testing has greatly aided the diagnosis of this form of equine polysaccharide storage myopathy. Histopathology of muscle samples is still necessary to diagnose *GYS1* mutation-negative cases.

Glycogen brancher enzyme deficiency in horses. *Glycogen brancher enzyme deficiency (glycogenosis type IV)* occurs in Quarter Horse and Paint foals. Affected foals may be aborted or stillborn, or develop weakness and die of cardiac failure in the first few months of life. Characteristic spherical or ovoid inclusions of PAS-positive amylase-resistant amylopectin are seen within skeletal myofibers (Fig. 3-69) and myocardiocytes, particularly Purkinje fibers. Similar material is seen to a lesser degree in many other organs. This disorder is inherited as an autosomal recessive trait and the defect is in the *GBE1* gene. Genetic testing to identify carriers and affected foals is available and should reduce the incidence and prevalence of this disorder.

Other metabolic myopathies of horses. A *mitochondrial myopathy* caused by deficiency of complex 1 respiratory chain enzyme has been described in an Arabian. Profound exercise intolerance and exercise-induced lactic acidosis without evidence of exercise-induced muscle necrosis were seen.

Metabolic myopathies of cattle and sheep

Biochemical abnormalities leading to abnormal glycogen storage within skeletal muscle occur in sheep and cattle. In some cases, the disorder is generalized and in others it is

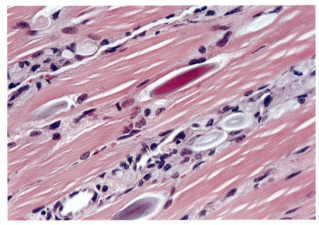

Figure 3-69 Spherical-to-ovoid bodies of complex polysaccharide within skeletal muscle myofibers in a Quarter Horse foal with **glycogen branching enzyme deficiency**. (Courtesy M.D. McGavin.)

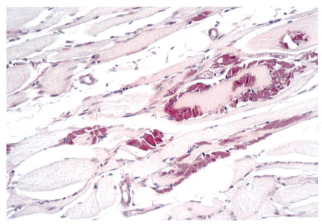

Figure 3-70 Inclusions of complex polysaccharide that are PAS positive and amylase resistant in skeletal **muscle adjacent to a synovial sarcoma** in a dog. Periodic acid-Schiff with amylase digestion.

confined to skeletal muscle. *Clinical signs of neuromuscular weakness in young sheep and cattle resulting from metabolic myopathy must be distinguished from the more common nutritional myopathies.*

Bovine metabolic myopathy caused by myophosphorylase deficiency. Glycogen phosphorylase is an essential glycolytic enzyme. Tissue-specific isoforms exist, and the skeletal muscle isoform is known as myophosphorylase. *An autosomal recessive defect in the myophosphorylase gene similar to McArdle's disease in people occurs in Charolais cattle, and results in metabolic dysfunction confined to skeletal muscle.* Clinical signs of exercise intolerance and exercise-induced collapse can be seen in affected cattle as young as 7 weeks of age. Increased serum activities of CK and AST are characteristic. Subsarcolemmal vacuoles due to glycogen storage within myofibers are characteristic, and biochemical and histochemical studies reveal a *complete lack of myophosphorylase activity*. Testing of DNA from peripheral white blood cells will detect homozygotes and heterozygotes.

Glycogenosis type II (Pompe's disease) in cattle. Glycogen storage disease caused by acid maltase (acid α-glucosidase) deficiency occurs as an autosomal recessive trait in Shorthorn and Brahman cattle. Two clinical syndromes are reported in Shorthorn cattle. An early-onset form results in intralysosomal glycogen storage within skeletal, cardiac, and smooth muscle, and in neurons of the central and autonomic nervous systems. Clinical signs of cardiac dysfunction predominate, leading to death resulting from cardiac failure. A late-onset form develops clinical signs predominantly of muscle weakness. Serum activity of CK is often increased, sometimes markedly. In Brahman cattle glycogenosis type II results in early-onset signs of poor growth and neurologic dysfunction.

Glycogen storage diseases of sheep. A *generalized form* of glycogen storage disease occurs in sheep. Glycogen storage confined to skeletal muscle resulting from *myophosphorylase deficiency* also occurs, and is similar to the disease in cattle.

Other metabolic myopathies

Acid maltase deficiency (glycogenosis type II) resulting in generalized glycogen storage occurs in *Japanese quail*. These birds have been studied as an animal model of acid maltase deficiency of people. Clinical signs of muscle dysfunction predominate, and include inability to right themselves following placement in dorsal or lateral recumbency, and poor wing movements. Weakness is progressive. Abnormal accumulation of membrane-bound glycogen particles occurs as early as day 16 of embryonal development. Progressive glycogen storage resulting in *vacuolar myopathy*, with formation of autophagic vacuoles followed by fiber loss and fatty replacement, are characteristic. Abnormal glycogen storage also occurs in cardiac and smooth muscle as well as in neurons in the brain and spinal cord.

It should be noted that inclusions of PAS-positive, amylase resistant complex polysaccharide (amylopectin; proteoglycans) can occur within skeletal muscle of a variety of species under a variety of circumstances that are not related to inborn errors of metabolism. In particular polysaccharide inclusions occur in dog muscle associated with adjacent malignant neoplasia (Fig. 3-70) and in some dogs with hypothyroidism. In many cases the cause is unknown. This is particularly true of amylase-resistant inclusions in hedgehog muscle.

Further reading

Aleman M. A review of equine muscle disorders. Neuromusc Dis 2008;18:277-287.

Bilstrom JA, et al. Genetic test for myophosphorylase deficiency in Charolais cattle. Am J Vet Res 1998;59:267-270.

Finno CJ, et al. Equine diseases caused by known genetic mutations. Vet J 2009;179:336-347.

Inal Gultekin G, et al. Missense mutation in PFKM associated with muscle-type phosphofructokinase deficiency in the Wachtelhund dog. Mol Cell Probes 2012;26:243-247.

McCue ME, et al. Glycogen synthase (GYS1) mutation causes a novel skeletal muscle glycogenosis. Genomics 2008;9:458-466.

McCue ME, et al. Polysaccharide storage myopathy phenotype in quarter horse-related breeds is modified by the presence of an RYR1 mutation. Neuromus Dis 2009;19:37-43.

Valberg SJ, et al. Glycogen branching enzyme deficiency in quarter horse foals. J Vet Intern Med 2001;15:572-580.

Valentine BA, Cooper BJ. Incidence of polysaccharide storage myopathy: necropsy study of 225 horses. Vet Pathol 2005;42:823-827.

Valentine BA, et al. Ubiquitin expression in muscle from horses with polysaccharide storage myopathy. Vet Pathol 2006;43:270-275.

Ward TL, et al. Glycogen branching enzyme (GBE1) mutation causing equine glycogen storage disease IV. Mamm Genome 2004;15: 570-577.

Congenital myasthenia gravis

Two clearly defined types of myasthenia gravis occur in humans and animals; both congenital and acquired myasthenia gravis have been described in dogs and cats.
- The *congenital disease* is due to an inherent defect in acetylcholine end plate receptors.
- The more common *acquired disease* is an immune-mediated disorder caused by circulating anticholinesterase receptor antibodies and is discussed in the section on Immune-mediated conditions.

Canine congenital myasthenia

In the dog, congenital myasthenia gravis has been described in Jack Russell Terriers, Springer Spaniels, Smooth Fox Terriers, the Gammel Dansk Hønsehund, and smooth-haired miniature Dachshund dogs. The disorder is inherited as an *autosomal recessive trait*. Affected dogs are clinically normal at birth but develop clinical signs of *exercise-induced weakness and collapse* at an early age. Clinical signs are apparent at ~5-8 weeks of age in affected Springer Spaniels and Jack Russell Terriers, and at ~12-16 weeks of age in the Gammel Dansk Hønsehund. Clinical signs are progressive in growing Jack Russell Terriers and Springer Spaniels, often leading to recumbency. The disorder is not progressive in the Gammel Dansk Hønsehund, and clinical signs resolved by 6 month of age in affected Smooth-haired Miniature Dachshunds. Esophageal dysfunction leading to megaesophagus may occur in the Springer Spaniel and Smooth Fox Terrier. A decremental response occurs with repetitive nerve stimulation studies. Circulating antibodies to acetylcholine receptors are not found, but affected dogs improve with anticholinesterase therapy.

No abnormalities are seen in the motor end plate by light microscopy. Ultrastructural evaluation reveals *decreased density of postsynaptic acetylcholine receptors and shallow secondary clefts in the end plate synaptic gutters*. Studies in the Jack Russell Terrier have shown a decreased rate of insertion of acetylcholine receptors into the postsynaptic membrane. Young animals are apparently able to function normally, but with growth this reduced acetylcholine receptor density results in neuromuscular weakness.

Feline congenital myasthenia

Myasthenia gravis is less commonly described in cats. This disorder has been described in Siamese and in domestic short-haired cats. Mode of inheritance is not known. Clinical signs of *episodic weakness* are first noted at about 4-5 months of age. Affected cats may have a weak voice and the disorder may progress to tetraplegia. Megaesophagus has not been reported. A decremental response is seen with repetitive nerve stimulation, and circulating antibodies to acetylcholine receptors are not found. Clinical improvement can be seen with oral or intravenous anticholinesterase therapy. Acetylcholine receptor density was found to be 66% of normal in one cat studied.

Further reading

Dickinson PJ, et al. Congenital myasthenia gravis in smooth-haired miniature dachsund dogs. J Vet Intern Med 2005;19:920-923.

Shelton GD. Myasthenia gravis and disorders of neuromuscular transmission. Vet Clin North Am Small Anim Pract 2002;32:189-206.

Shelton GD. Routine and specialized laboratory testing for the diagnosis of neuromuscular diseases in dogs and cats. Vet Clin Pathol 2010;39:278-295.

Malignant hyperthermia

Malignant hyperthermia (MH) is a condition that results in a sudden increase in myoplasmic calcium concentration leading to prolonged myofiber contraction and muscle rigidity, hypermetabolism, tachycardia, dyspnea, metabolic acidosis, and life-threatening hyperthermia. Severe acute rhabdomyolysis is the primary histopathologic finding. Episodes are triggered by a variety of circumstances, including stress and pharmacologic agents such as halothane anesthesia. Malignant hyperthermia is an inherited disorder in humans, pigs, horses, and some dogs. The defect is in the ryanodine receptor, a calcium-release channel of the sarcoplasmic reticulum that serves a critical role in triggering release of calcium from the sarcoplasmic reticulum during excitation-contraction coupling. Malignant hyperthermia in humans is associated with >100 mutations within the ryanodine receptor gene *RYR1*. Other myopathic disorders leading to susceptibility to MH occur, and therefore MH is best regarded as a syndrome rather than a single entity. Susceptible individuals may have mildly increased serum CK activities and increased erythrocyte fragility. Testing for MH susceptibility classically involved in vitro exposure of muscle biopsy samples to various concentrations of caffeine and halothane. Muscle from MH-susceptible individuals exhibits contraction at relatively low concentrations of these pharmacologic agents as opposed to normal individuals. Genetic testing for specific ryanodine receptor defects is now available for pigs, dogs, horses, and people.

Malignant hyperthermia-like episodes may also occur in people or animals with other underlying myopathies. This is certainly the case in cats with X-linked muscular dystrophy, in which anesthesia or the stress of restraint can trigger episodes of fatal hyperthermia. Underlying HYPP has been associated with malignant hyperthermia-like episodes associated with anesthesia in horses, and it is possible that other myopathic conditions may predispose horses to this disorder.

Malignant hyperthermia in pigs (porcine stress syndrome)

Malignant hyperthermia in pigs renders them susceptible to episodes associated with stresses such as handling, transportation, or fighting, and *may result in sudden death*. The muscle of affected pigs is usually *pale, soft, and exudative (PSE pork)*. Porcine stress syndrome has been recognized in Europe and North America for a long time as *herztod* or *back muscle necrosis* of pigs, and occurs in all pork-producing countries of the world. *Susceptible pigs exhibit intense, immobilizing limb and torso muscle rigidity, respiratory difficulty, tachycardia, acidosis and, often, rapid death*. Heavy-muscled pigs seem to be most susceptible to the clinical disease. Before identification of the ryanodine receptor gene defect, a large body of literature accumulated regarding various biochemical abnormalities detected in affected muscle and in affected animals. *A single point mutation in the skeletal muscle ryanodine receptor (RYR1) at locus HAL-1843 leading to increased channel open time has been shown to be the cause of MH* in domestic pigs, including Pietrain, Yorkshire, Poland China, Duroc, and Landrace breeds.

DNA testing of peripheral blood for the *HAL-1843* gene defect is available commercially. Genetic studies point to a single affected founder pig followed by widespread dissemination of the gene, and it has been suggested that these pigs have been selected based on their heavy muscling and decreased body fat. It has been estimated that 2-30% of purebred breeding pigs are susceptible to malignant hyperthermia. A similar syndrome of MH appears to occur in *Vietnamese pot-bellied pigs*. In one case of a pot-bellied pig dying because of anesthesia-induced hyperthermia, a gene defect at *HAL-1843* was detected. Testing of parents of another pot-bellied pig with suspect malignant hyperthermia, however, did not reveal *HAL-1843* defects, suggesting that in pigs, as in humans, *more than one gene defect may lead to MH*.

Postmortem examination of the muscles of susceptible pigs that have not endured an episode of hyperthermia recently reveals normal muscles. *Pigs dying of hyperthermia have pale muscles that are wet and apparently swollen. Rigor mortis develops unusually rapidly.* In addition to lesions of skeletal muscle, *lesions of acute heart failure*, such as pulmonary edema and congestion, hydropericardium, hydrothorax, and hepatic congestion, often are present. The muscles most likely to be affected are those of the *back, loin, thigh,* and *shoulder*. Although both type 1 and type 2 myofibers undergo necrosis, muscles with a high proportion of type 2 fibers such as longissimus, psoas, and semitendinosus are most extensively and most frequently affected, and these should be examined histologically. Hemorrhages sometimes are present in muscles, and in the warm carcass a marked lowering of muscle pH to 5.8 or lower can be detected. On cooling, the pH rises rapidly toward neutrality. Myocardial pallor involving the ventricular muscles sometimes occurs, but the clinical signs of tachycardia are probably related to acidosis.

Microscopic examination of malignant hyperthermia susceptible animals not recently affected by hyperthermic episodes reveals normal muscle fibers, or there may be a few degenerate fibers. *There is nothing distinctive about the appearance of the degenerate fibers.* In pigs dying acutely of malignant hyperthermia, *muscle fibers are separated by edema fluid*. This is evident in rapidly fixed specimens only and may be lost in processing. Changes in muscle fibers are widespread and are typically characterized as *multifocal monophasic injury*. It is possible, however, to find polyphasic injury in pigs with recent nonfatal episodes of MH, and underlying chronic myopathic changes also may be observed. Degenerative changes vary from segmental hypercontraction to overt coagulative necrosis. *Hypercontraction* is the most common lesion in skeletal muscle. Myocardial lesions include multifocal granular degeneration of myocytes, contraction band necrosis, and myocytolysis.

Malignant hyperthermia in dogs

There are sporadic reports of MH like episodes in various breeds of dogs. *Exercise-induced hyperthermia* has been seen in English Springer Spaniels and in Labrador Retrievers. *Ingestion of hops* can trigger a MH-like episode in susceptible dogs, and this condition has been most commonly seen in Greyhounds. Studies of a breeding colony of mixed-breed dogs susceptible to anesthesia-induced MH determined that the disorder was inherited as a dominant trait with variable severity. The genetic defect in autosomal dominant canine MH is a mutation in the skeletal muscle calcium release channel (*RYR1*). Chronic myopathic changes including internal nuclei, increased fiber size variation, and fiber hypertrophy may be seen in muscle from MH-susceptible dogs. Histologic lesions in dogs dying because of hyperthermia are similar to those seen in other MH-susceptible species.

Malignant hyperthermia in horses

Severe acute rhabdomyolysis caused by malignant hyperthermia occurs in horses and can be triggered by inhalant anesthetic agents or by injection of succinylcholine. An inherited defect in the ryanodine receptor 1 has been documented in Quarter Horses, and MH episodes in Quarter Horses can also be triggered by exercise, breeding, illness, concurrent myopathy, illness, or other stress. Interestingly, horses with the GYS1 mutation-positive form of polysaccharide storage myopathy as well as the MH defect are much more difficult to treat.

Further reading

Adami C, et al. Unusual perianesthetic malignant hyperthermia in a dog. J Am Vet Med Assoc 2012;240:450-453.

Aleman M, et al. Malignant hyperthermia associated with ryanodine receptor 1 (C7360G) mutation in Quarter Horses. J Vet Intern Med 2009;23:329-334.

O'Brien PJ, et al. Use of a DNA-based test for the mutation associated with porcine stress syndrome (malignant hyperthermia) in 10,000 breeding swine. J Am Vet Med Assoc 1993;203:842-851.

Roberts MC, et al. Autosomal dominant canine malignant hyperthermia is caused by a mutation in the gene encoding the skeletal muscle calcium release channel (RYR1). Anesthesiology 2001;95: 716-725.

Rosenberg H, et al. Malignant hyperthermia. Orphanet J Rare Dis 2007;2:21.

CIRCULATORY DISTURBANCES OF MUSCLE

Skeletal muscle is a highly vascular tissue with an abundant capillary bed that forms an extensive system of anastomoses. It is generally not possible to induce muscle fiber necrosis by ligation of, or damage to, intermuscular arteries, because most muscles receive small collateral arterioles from tendons, fascial sheaths, and major nerve trunks. Naturally occurring examples of ischemic muscle necrosis most often are due to vascular occlusion secondary to pressure. Occlusion of major arteries such as aortic-iliac thrombosis ("saddle thrombi") can also cause ischemic muscle necrosis, as can widespread vascular injury (vasculitis, necrotizing vasculopathy) involving intramuscular vasculature.

Each muscle fiber is served, at any given level, by 3-12 capillaries that run mainly longitudinally in the endomysium. Type 1 fibers are served by slightly more capillaries than are type 2 fibers of comparable size. *Maximum myofiber diameter is limited to some extent by the distance from the capillary to the center of the fiber(s) supplied.* When the distance becomes abnormally great, the fiber is likely to form a cleft (*fiber splitting*) allowing the entry of a capillary, effectively serving the fiber interior (see Fig. 3-24). Myofiber splitting appears to be a mechanism primarily initiated to improve the capillary-to-fiber ratio. This hypothesis is supported by the finding that most myofibers exhibiting fiber splitting are hypertrophied fibers.

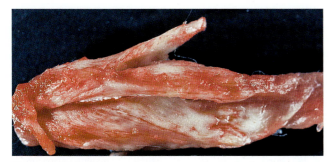

Figure 3-71 **Infarct** in a lumbar epaxial muscle from a cat presumed to have been run over by a car. There is a locally extensive zone of pallor and slight swelling. (Courtesy A. de Lahunta.)

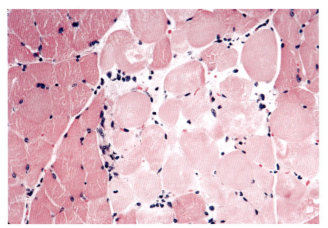

Figure 3-72 Focal muscle **infarct** characterized by myofiber pallor, loss of cytoplasmic detail, and fragmentation in a dog. There is little cellular reaction. H&E stain. (Courtesy M.D. McGavin.)

Ischemic damage to muscle fibers, and the capacity to repair, depends on the completeness and duration of oxygen and nutrient deprivation. Severe ischemia causes infarcts, which may be visible grossly as areas of muscle pallor similar to other necrotizing lesions. Areas of infarcted muscle are often slightly swollen (Fig. 3-71). Histologically, muscle infarcts consist of discrete zones of coagulative necrosis similar to infarcts in any other tissue (Fig. 3-72). Inflammation is lacking in the infarcted zone but may be present at margins. If the margin with intact muscle is not included in histologic sections, it will be difficult to recognize infarcted muscle.

Ischemic injury also can be exacerbated by reperfusion injury, especially in cases of crush injury or muscle necrosis secondary to recumbency in a large animal, such as downer cow syndrome. Use of devices such as hip clamps and slings to aid in treatment of recumbent animals can also result in ischemic muscle injury.

Provided that satellite cells are still viable, regeneration following ischemic injury is possible (see Fig. 3-32). As with regeneration in any other circumstance, effective regenerative repair is most likely in lesions with intact basal laminae. Crush injury is particularly likely to result in damage to the muscle basal lamina.

Regardless of the duration and extent of the ischemic change, *the muscle fiber plasma membrane becomes permeable to enzymes and myoglobin*. Serum creatine kinase activity is markedly increased but, because of the short half-life of CK in serum (6-12 hours in most species), often returns to near normal in 4-5 days after monophasic necrosis, even when destruction of muscle is extensive. Myoglobin is released from damaged muscle and the amount released will vary directly with the severity and extent of damage. When a large mass of muscle is physically injured or when ischemic degenerative changes are extensive, large amounts of myoglobin are released into the bloodstream. Much of this is excreted by the kidneys. Myoglobin has a direct toxic effect on convoluted tubules leading to nephrosis. Renal ischemia and hypoxic injury caused by shock and circulatory collapse contribute to the potential for severe renal damage and renal shutdown. Hyperkalemia caused by massive muscle fiber breakdown can result in acute heart failure.

Syndromes of ischemic muscle necrosis recognized in humans and animals are compartment syndrome, downer syndrome, muscle crush syndrome, and vascular occlusive syndrome. The distinctions among these syndromes are not always clear. In veterinary medicine, *hypotensive myopathy in anesthetized horses constitutes another syndrome*. In compartment syndrome, downer syndrome, and muscle crush syndrome, ischemia is caused by increased intramuscular pressure. The vascular occlusive syndrome results from physical obstruction of the blood supply to muscle, and hypotension leading to poor muscle perfusion is thought to be the cause of hypotensive myopathy in horses.

Compartment syndrome

Muscles that are surrounded by either a heavy aponeurotic sheath or by bone and sheath are vulnerable to ischemia when muscle fibers are subjected to moderately vigorous but not exhaustive contraction. This syndrome occurs in well-conditioned athletes, but nowhere is the syndrome more clearly primary and specific than in the infarction that occurs in the supracoracoid muscles of some breeds of broiler chickens and in some breeds of turkeys. In these birds, a brief, vigorous flapping of the wings increases intramuscular pressure of the supracoracoid muscle within the inelastic breastbone and the outer muscle sheath. Muscle in full contraction increases in diameter up to 20% and this causes partial or transient collapse of the venous outflow. At the same time, muscle activity increases arterial blood flow to the muscle. Subsequent muscle contractions tend to build internal pressure until the intramuscular pressure exceeds first venous and then arterial blood pressure. Metabolites of the muscle fibers exerting an increased osmotic tension coupled with increased arteriolar blood pressure cause accumulation of interstitial water early in the process and this further increases intramuscular pressure. Once blood flow has stopped, ischemic changes of both muscle and vessels begin, and further water escapes via damaged endothelial cells. Pressure builds for 1-4 hours after muscle exercise and the extent and severity of damage to muscle increases with time. In both humans and birds, early fasciotomy releases intramuscular pressure and restores the potential for complete regenerative repair.

The so-called *spontaneous rupture of the gastrocnemius muscle of Channel Island breeds of cattle* may represent an example of compartment syndrome leading to ischemia and subsequent rupture. Similarly, the swelling of muscle that can occur in dogs and horses with *masticatory myopathy*, and in horses with *exertional rhabdomyolysis*, may occur at least partly because of compartment syndrome, with initial muscle damage leading to increased pressure against thick overlying fascia.

Downer syndrome

Humans and most of the domestic species share a muscle ischemia syndrome that is initiated by external pressure of objects or by pressure created by the weight of body, torso, or head on a limb tucked under the body for prolonged periods. This condition in humans is usually related to drug overdose, whereas in animals it is induced by prolonged anesthesia, muscle, joint, or bone damage causing prostration, or metabolic or neurologic disease causing paresis. Absolute size and body weight have some influence on the incidence of the disease. Animals in good condition are particularly susceptible, and thin animals seldom suffer from ischemic muscle necrosis. Rams and heavy ewes, boars, and sows, and even large dogs are occasionally susceptible, but this disorder does not occur in cats. Cows are the species most frequently affected, partly because of their weight and their muscle bulk and partly because they are subject to diseases in which paresis is common.

The pathogenesis of the downer syndrome depends upon the fact that the weight of the body can cause pressure within muscles to rise to levels considerably higher than both venous and arterial pressure. Muscles of limbs in a flexed or tucked position are particularly susceptible. The intramuscular pressure soon serves to collapse veins of the fascial sheaths and skin, causing congestion, and then collapses arteries. In cows and horses, extensive ischemic lesions are sometimes created by a period of inertia as short as 6 hours, whereas some cows seem to be able to tolerate 12 or even more hours of immobility with minimal residual lesions. As time passes and as the pressure is removed, the affected limb continues to swell as edema fluid increases under returned arterial flow. Reperfusion injury is likely to contribute to ischemic damage in the downer syndrome. The extent of lesions within a muscle mass is quite variable but seldom involves more than half of the mass. The degree of damage will reflect the extent, duration, and severity of the ischemic episode as well as the extent and rapidity of reflow.

The clinical presentation of downer syndrome can be complicated by *pressure-induced peripheral nerve injury*. Even 6 hours of anesthesia or comparable inactivity in horses and cows can cause sciatic or other nerve damage leading to *peroneal nerve paralysis* and a flexed rear fetlock, or a dropped shoulder and elbow because of *radial paralysis*. This peripheral nerve dysfunction is, however, more often caused by nerve conduction block than to structural nerve damage, allowing for the possibility of a relatively rapid recovery. If there is actual structural damage to nerves, effective recovery and mobilization may be delayed until nerves to muscles are regenerated, and complete recovery is not always possible.

Muscle crush syndrome

This form of muscle ischemia has characteristics in common with downer syndrome. *It is usually initiated by acute accidental trauma, often including bone fracture.* It occurs less frequently in animals than in humans, but has been seen in the dog and perhaps the cow. Initial events center on the *traumatic laceration of muscle*, which leads to a combination of high osmotic tension and hyperemia that result in accumulation of abundant edema fluid in the area. Edema causing increased pressure can exacerbate the muscle damage. If the damaged muscle and bone are still confined within a relatively firm sheath, conditions resembling those of compartment syndrome are set up. The limb swells and extends, and becomes turgid. Ischemia of variable extent ensues but, because of the great amount of myoglobin released, *renal dysfunction* may dominate the syndrome.

Vascular occlusive syndrome

When a *major vessel to a limb is occluded*, the limb becomes cool, the arterial pulse is lost, skin over the limb loses its ability to sweat, and some limitation of movement may be apparent. When this occurs as a result of *aortic-iliac arterial thrombosis in the horse*, the effects are usually transient, apparently because of effective collateral circulation. Some muscle degeneration probably occurs but is repaired rapidly and completely. In the *cat with aortic-iliac thrombosis* associated with underlying cardiomyopathy more of the aorta is likely to be occluded than is the case in the horse, and collateral circulation may be less effective at restoring circulation to hindlimb muscles. Muscle lesions vary from mild to severe (Fig. 3-73). The *anatomic pattern of degeneration* varies from one case to another and more distal muscles are not necessarily more vulnerable. Hindlimb muscle from cats with aortic-iliac thrombosis can also exhibit chronic myopathic changes indicative of previous bouts of subclinical ischemic myopathy.

An ischemic lesion of muscle seen in *sheep in advanced pregnancy* appears also to be caused by arterial occlusion. Ewes carrying twins or triplets sometimes suffer from ischemic necrosis of the internal abdominal oblique muscle without evidence of congestion or hemorrhage. This muscle does not have a confining sheath, thus the necrosis is not part of a compartment syndrome. The arterial supply to the abdominal oblique is via a tortuous branch of the internal iliac artery that turns back on itself inside the iliac tuberosity, and it may be vulnerable to stretch and/or trauma. Ischemia of the muscle is followed by rupture, and subsequently the other abdominal muscles also rupture. In spite of this, the ewes sometimes lamb at term without difficulty.

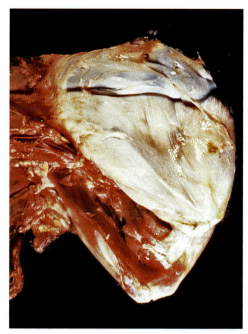

Figure 3-73 Pale thigh muscle caused by infarction in a cat with **ischemic myopathy** resulting from aortic-iliac thrombosis. This is the same case as shown in Figure 3-32A-C.

Postanesthetic myopathy in horses

Postoperative weakness as a result of neuromuscular dysfunction occurs with some regularity in horses. *Various etiologies are possible.* Heavily muscled horses anesthetized and laid on poorly padded surfaces can develop *pressure-induced ischemic damage* to muscle similar to downer syndrome. *Compartment syndrome* affecting selected muscles can also occur. Cases of compartment syndrome in which a hemorrhagic infiltrate is prominent suggest predominantly venous occlusion. Pressure-induced neuropathy is a frequent complication. Horses with underlying myopathy, such as hyperkalemic periodic paralysis (HYPP) (see Myotonic and spastic syndromes) and polysaccharide storage myopathy (see Metabolic myopathies) are particularly prone to postanesthetic myopathy. A hyperthermia-like condition is also possible.

A syndrome of ischemic myopathy associated with hypotension and decreased muscle perfusion occurs in horses, most often associated with *halothane anesthesia*. This syndrome can be reproduced experimentally. Marked increases in serum CK and AST activities and lactate concentration occur. Swelling is most common in downside muscles, with increased intracompartmental pressure indicative of associated compartment syndrome.

Further reading

Genthon A, Wilcox SR. Crush syndrome: a case report and review of the literature. J Emerg Med 2014;46:313-319.

Lindsay WA, et al. Induction of equine postanesthetic myositis after halothane induced hypotension. Am J Vet Res 1989;50:404-410.

Mabvuure NT, et al. Acute compartment syndrome of the limbs; current concepts and management. Open Orthop J 2012;6:535-543.

Maxie MG, Physick-Sheard PW. Aortic-iliac thrombosis in horses. Vet Pathol 1985;22:238-249.

PHYSICAL INJURIES OF MUSCLE

Traumatic injuries of muscle (*laceration, contusion, tearing, penetrating wounds*) are common and may be the result of external trauma, or they may be a result of a muscle rupture or tear of the fascia as occurs occasionally in violent contraction, rarely in overextension. The effects of external trauma are very variable and depend on the qualities of the applied force, the presence or absence of concomitant fracture of the adjacent bones, and especially on the degree of hemorrhage, injury to blood vessels, and injury to motor nerves. The principles governing the outcome of these types of lesions have been discussed earlier in this chapter.

Violent contraction of muscle may result in either hernia or rupture with hemorrhage. A hernia occurs when the belly of the muscle protrudes through a rent in the overlying fascia and epimysium. The hernia can be reduced by pressure when the muscle is relaxed and it hardens and bulges further when the muscle contracts, providing thereby a point of useful distinction between hernia and tumor of soft tissue.

Actual rupture of muscle tissue may also occur during violent exercise and is probably more common than rupture of the tendon. The muscle bulges at the end opposite to that which is torn. Such ruptures are not necessarily complete from the outset, but may become so later from additional strain or degeneration caused by infiltrating hemorrhage with pressure and ischemia. Regeneration in large defects is ineffective and the gap is filled in by scar tissue. The muscle most frequently ruptured in animals is the diaphragm. Trauma, with acute abdominal compression, is the usual cause in the dog. In cattle, it tends to follow diaphragmatic myositis secondary to traumatic reticulitis. In horses, it is a consequence (in foals) of abdominal compression at parturition, and diaphragmatic rupture occurs occasionally with acute gastric dilation. Acquired ruptures must be differentiated from congenital and postmortem ruptures by attention to the edges of the cleft. Hemorrhage is indicative of antemortem trauma. Rounded edges are indicative of chronicity, as seen in congenital diaphragmatic hernia.

The histologic appearance of traumatic injury depends on the age of the lesions. Initially it includes sarcolemmal rupture with myofiber necrosis that can be accompanied by edema, hemorrhage, and neutrophilic infiltration. Bleeding into muscle, whether caused by trauma or spontaneous hemorrhage, as in some hemorrhagic diatheses, is often sufficient in volume to result in hematoma, the fate of which will depend largely on its volume. Metaplastic bone may form in the capsule of the hematoma. Severe trauma-induced swelling in muscle results in secondary ischemic injury, which causes muscle necrosis. Healing includes fibrosis, and regeneration attempts often are disordered because of damage to the basal lamina.

Ossifying fibrodysplasia

Also termed *myositis ossificans* or *fibrodysplasia ossificans*, this infrequent condition of the dog, cat, pig, and horse represents heterotopic ossification within the connective tissues of skeletal muscle. It occurs as either a localized or a generalized form. The generalized form is described under Fibromatous disorders of tendons and aponeuroses.

The *localized form* of myositis ossificans occurs in the dog and horse. In the dog, the lesion often, but not always, occurs secondary to trauma and results in firm swollen areas in the affected muscles, generally in the caudal hip, shoulder, quadriceps, or neck. Microscopically, the lesion typically has 3 zones—a central area of actively proliferating undifferentiated connective tissue, a middle zone with osteoid and immature bone, and an outer zone of mature trabecular bone.

Strains/tears/ruptures/fibrotic myopathies/contractures

Strains are the result of *overstretching of muscles* that have disrupted muscle fibers, most commonly at the muscle-tendon junction. The severity of damage varies from mild localized disruption to complete rupture of muscle fibers. Hemorrhage and edema accompany the muscle damage, and healing is by fibrosis.

Fibrotic myopathy of the semitendinosus, semimembranosus, and gracilis muscles occurs most often in Quarter Horses performing sliding halts. Physical tearing and hemorrhage from these abrupt maneuvers initiates the damage with fibrous replacement as an outcome. Additionally, some cases are the result of denervation injury.

Several syndromes of limb muscle dysfunction, possibly associated with trauma, are described in dogs. A variety of names have been applied, including infraspinatus contracture, quadriceps contracture, gracilis contracture, fibrotic myopathy of semitendinosus, and gracilis-semitendinosus myopathy. The contractures are the result of functional shortening of affected muscles following injury and healing by fibrosis.

Fibrotic myopathy of the gracilis and semitendinosus fibrotic myopathy occur most often in German Shepherds, especially males. The affected muscle may contain a thin fibrous band.

A myopathy of the tail muscles occurs in dogs, especially hunting dogs, and is known as *limber tail* or *frozen tail*. This myopathy appears to be associated with overexertion. Environmental factors such as overly cold or warm temperature of water the dog is swimming in also may play a role.

Further reading

Braund KG. Idiopathic and exogenous causes of myopathies in dogs and cats. Vet Med 1997;92:629-634.

Dabareiner RM, et al. Gracilis muscle injury as a cause of lameness in two horses. J Am Vet Med Assoc 2004;224:1630-1633.

Lewis DD, et al. Gracilis or semitendinosus myopathy in 18 dogs. J Am An Hosp Assoc 1997;33:177-188.

Tambella AM, et al. Myositis ossificans circumscripta of the triceps muscle in a Rottweiler dog. Vet Comp Orthop Traumatol 2013;26:154-159.

NUTRITIONAL MYOPATHY

Historically, myopathy resulting from nutritional deficiency (also called nutritional myodegeneration, white muscle disease, stiff-lamb disease and, inappropriately, nutritional muscular dystrophy) formed a large portion of the veterinary literature related to muscle disease in animals. These disorders are still important today, particularly in livestock and zoo animals.

Nutritional myopathies are *principally diseases of calves, lambs, swine, and foals.* They infrequently affect carnivores. *The most common nutritional deficiency leading to nutritional myopathy in most species is* **deficiency of selenium**. Nutritional myopathy resulting from vitamin E deficiency in the absence of selenium deficiency is uncommon in mammals, but may be more common in birds and reptiles. It is possible that vitamin E deficiency in association with marginal selenium status can lead to nutritional myopathy in a variety of species. Selenium was established as an essential nutrient and implicated in nutritional myopathy in the late 1950s. Muscle fiber necrosis, as seen in nutritional myopathy, was discussed earlier (see Muscle injury and necrosis); *it is a selective, segmental multifocal and polyphasic necrosis of myofibers* that leaves the ensheathing basal lamina and satellite cells intact, which therefore enables rapid and efficient regenerative repair. Myoglobinuria is usually absent in the enzootic disease of young animals but may occur in the sporadic cases in young adult animals, as those have a higher concentration of myoglobin in skeletal muscle. Frequently, skeletal muscle damage is concurrent with myocardial lesions.

Etiology and pathogenesis

Nutritional myopathy is a problem around the world but it occurs most often in those countries with intensive livestock-rearing operations. Selenium moves through a soil-plant-animal cycle. Sedimentary rocks provide most of the selenium that becomes incorporated into soils. Alkaline and well-aerated soils provide much higher amounts of selenium available to growing plants than acid, poorly aerated soils. This difference in availability from soils is related to the chemical form of selenium and not to the selenium concentration in the soil. *Soluble selenates* predominate in alkaline soils, and sparingly soluble *selenites* complexed with iron salts are in acid soils. As selenium moves from soils into growing plants, it is largely incorporated into organic compounds, mainly in those selenoproteins with abundant selenomethionine. The selenium content in the lush forage of heavily fertilized and watered soils is low because of dilution by the abundant plant tissue. Surveys of plants grown in soils throughout the United States and other countries have provided data and have been used to map areas of selenium deficiency and excess. Deficient areas include the southeastern, northeastern, midwestern, and far northwestern portions of the United States. The prevalence of nutritional myopathy in animals throughout the United States correlates closely with the areas having low (<0.05 ppm dry weight) plant selenium concentrations. Animals are able to use selenium from inorganic salts (selenites and selenates) as well as from the organic forms in plants. In most of the studies that compared the efficacy of various chemical forms of selenium to prevent deficiency disease in animals, *organic selenium was found to have greater protection than inorganic selenium (selenite)*. However, because selenite is readily available and inexpensive, this form is commonly used as a dietary selenium supplement.

Selenium is distributed widely in animal tissues, and the concentration is directly related to dietary intake. Highest concentrations are found in kidney and liver, intermediate amounts are found in heart and skeletal muscle, and low content is found in blood and fat. Animals fed rations in which small amounts (0.1-0.2 ppm) of selenium are added to meet their nutritional requirements do not develop large increases in tissue selenium content; therefore human consumption of the tissues of animals so fed offers no risk of causing selenium toxicosis. Tissue or whole blood *glutathione peroxidase activity* is a reliable indicator of selenium availability. Glutathione peroxidases are labile enzymes and enzyme analysis is more challenging than tissue or whole blood selenium analysis. Liver or whole blood selenium analysis is preferred under most circumstances and results correlate well with glutathione peroxidase activity.

Vitamin E content of compounded animal feeds is generally low because many of the feedstuffs used are poor sources of that vitamin. Vitamin E degradation because of prolonged storage of feedstuffs can also occur. Rich sources of vitamin E include wheat bran, many vegetable oils, green pasture grass, and legumes such as alfalfa. The biological activity of vitamin E is concentrated in the α-tocopherol fraction, and thus determinations of total tocopherol content of feeds may be of limited value for determining their vitamin E potency and ability to prevent deficiency disease. Diets that contain large amounts of polyunsaturated fats (e.g., those in fish oils) require greater amounts of vitamin E, which limits oxidation and the development of rancidity. Also, if diets with low selenium content are fed, vitamin E supplements may need to be increased to prevent deficiency disease.

Of the domestic mammals, *cattle, sheep, and pigs are most susceptible to nutritional myopathy*. Horses and goats are moderately susceptible, and occasional cases have been reported in dogs and cats. Most zoo ungulates should be regarded as susceptible to the disease. Historically, nutritional myopathy has been thought of as a disease of young animals, particularly the very young. *Rapid postnatal growth seems to predispose*, a problem perhaps of outgrowing a scarce resource or of biochemical transition as fiber types develop into the adult patterns. Although nutritional muscle degeneration occasionally does occur in mature animals, it is rare in most species and most areas. Horses are an exception, and nutritional myopathy with strong predilection for masticatory muscle necrosis ("equine masticatory myopathy/myositis") occurs in adult horses of all ages. This syndrome is particularly common in the Pacific Northwest, where soil and plant selenium concentrations are very low, and the ready access to grass pasture and alfalfa products may lead to lack of trace mineral supplementation and severe selenium deficiency. Cases have also been reported from the northeastern United States. Nutritional myopathy in adult horses varies from relatively mild disease responsive to selenium supplementation to severe disease nonresponsive to selenium and aggressive supportive therapy. It is possible that ischemic injury secondary to compartment syndrome (see Circulatory disturbances of muscle) in involved masticatory muscle may result in fibrosis rather than regeneration.

In cattle, spontaneous nutritional myopathy can occur in utero in 7-month-old fetuses, and muscle lesions are seen in lambs and calves at birth. However, lesions do not necessarily occur in calves or lambs born of cows or ewes, which themselves have extensive lesions of nutritional myopathy before, or at the time of, parturition. It is equally true that dams of calves or lambs with extensive lesions seldom show clinical disease or even clinicopathologic evidence of muscle fiber breakdown.

Nutritional myopathy occurs in all of the susceptible domestic species on widely variable planes of nutrition. Neonatal disease usually affects the thrifty, well-grown suckling animal and the sporadic disease in yearlings and adults usually occurs in animals in good physical condition. The disease in adult ruminants affects animals fed marginal-quality rations, such as turnips or poor-quality hay, and can appear as clinical or subclinical disease in animals in very poor condition because of neglect or chronic disease.

One of the most perplexing aspects of these myopathies is the irregularity and unpredictability of their occurrence. Natural disease is seldom a serious problem in consecutive years, yet sometimes it will occur in most years in any given region. A good deal of correlative and circumstantial evidence indicates that climate-related conditions, such as the length and the amount of sunshine of the growing season, and the length of the housing season, may be very important. Because the disease often occurs while animals are consuming stored feeds, the condition and duration of storage of the fodder can be relevant. Detailed investigation sometimes reveals comparable concentrations of vitamin E and selenium in forage from one year to the next, yet the incidence of nutritional myopathy in animals consuming it may be quite different. Grazing of dry pastures may be associated with an increase in the incidence of disease and also may have an influence later through the stored hay or grain harvested from them. On the other hand, ingestion of lush pasture also may cause problems. *In most parts of the world, nutritional myopathy occurs in late winter or early spring,* but in sheep it may occur more often in the fall, in both pastured and feedlot animals that are immature.

The patterns of nutritional myopathy seem, in a general way, to obey the rules of straightforward deficiency of 1 or 2 essential nutrients. The metabolism of vitamin E and selenium is incompletely understood. Understanding of factors involved in membrane integrity and membrane alterations in disease has elucidated the role of the subcellular changes, which seem to be a basic result of deficiency of these substances.

In many cells, *vitamin E- and selenium-containing enzymes are required as physiologic antagonists to a group of chemically varied substances known as free radicals.* **Free radicals** are molecules with an odd number of electrons; they can be either organic or inorganic. Some free radicals are products of normal cell function, and several participate in, or are products of, oxidative metabolism. They may also be produced outside the cell as products of tissue radiation, drug reactions, and inflammation. One of the major sources of free radicals is the cell detoxification process, which renders materials less harmful by converting them to epoxides. Many intracellular and extracellular free radicals contain oxygen, and are involved in electron transfer reactions. They are highly reactive and this is responsible for their rapid alteration (instability), which occurs in oxidation-reduction reactions within a wide range of cellular structures and enzyme systems.

Free radicals may initiate cellular injury by causing peroxidation of membrane lipids and by causing physicochemical damage to protein molecules, including those of mitochondria, endoplasmic reticulum, and cytosol. Protection against the effects of free radicals is provided partly by the constant presence of *small scavenger molecules* such as tocopherols, ascorbate, and beta-carotene. These "quench" free radicals, but both free radicals and scavengers are consumed in the process. Protection is also provided in part by selenium-containing enzymes of the *glutathione peroxidase/glutathione reductase* system. This system is capable, under normal circumstances, of more or less constant renewal by a complex sequence that makes use of several enzymes, although some consumption of the selenium-containing component does occur.

From the preceding, certain conclusions seem to emerge. *Although vitamin E- and the selenium-containing glutathione system perform many similar functions at the cellular level in quenching destructive metabolites and by-products, they likely function independently.* The development of vitamin E deficiency-related neurodegenerative diseases rather than myopathy in horses, that is, equine degenerative myeloencephalopathy and equine motor neuron disease, support this theory. The circumstantial clinical evidence that one can relieve the need for the other in the prevention of muscle disease is also reasonably explained. The need for some of both at all times within the cell, and vitamin E outside the cell, perhaps is explained by the fact that the 2 mechanisms quench a different array of free radicals and that tocopherol operates both outside and inside the cell while the glutathione system operates only inside the cell. The practical interpretation of deficiency of vitamin E or selenium should relate to the consumption of these elements during a steady intracellular production of free radicals, rather than an interpretation of these nutrients as structural cellular components that may be deficient.

In the absence of sufficient protection by selenium and/or vitamin E, cellular membranes are modified by free radicals, and the ability of those membranes to maintain essential differential ionic gradients is diminished or lost. This initiates the sequence of events discussed earlier (see Muscle injury and necrosis) in which calcium entry results in hypercontraction of myofibrils and necrosis of myofibers.

Nutritional myopathy of cattle

Clinicopathologic descriptions of the disease in calves appeared in the 1890s and the disease was well known at that time in Germany, France, Switzerland, and Scandinavia. *Nutritional* myopathy occurs, sometimes in endemic proportions, in calves 4-6 weeks of age, mostly of beef type. It is also common in animals up to 6 months of age and occurs sporadically in older cattle. In calves there is often a typical history indicating that the dam has been housed at least 3-4 months and had been fed poor-quality hay or not enough hay. Similar problems occur in calves in the United States, Australia, and New Zealand when legume hay alone or irrigated legume pasture is fed. Sulfur fertilizers applied to the pasture, and copper deficiency in the dam, may be contributing factors. *The precipitating event in many cases is unaccustomed physical activity that converts subclinical to clinical disease.* The feeding of cod liver oil that has become rancid destroys vitamin E in the ration and has been blamed for producing the disease. The presenting sign in calves is often stiffness or dyspnea, but a shuffling gait, a dropping of the chest between the shoulders, and outward rotation of the forelimbs have also been noted. Some calves become recumbent and die rapidly with signs of respiratory failure. Calves >3-4 months of age may show myoglobinuria.

Postmortem lesions in calves are usually dominated by marked mineralization of necrotic skeletal and/or cardiac muscle. When the heart is extensively affected, intercostal muscles and the diaphragm are usually also affected, but other skeletal muscle lesions may not be widespread. *Heart lesions in calves usually involve the left ventricle more than the right.* Small lesions just under the epicardium or endocardium may appear as scattered white "brush" strokes. The mineralized lesions are creamy white and opaque. Small streaks of hemorrhage also may be seen. Lungs are often filled with pink frothy fluid and an excess of fluid may be present in the thorax indicating heart failure. *In those cases in which skeletal muscle lesions predominate, the most extensive lesions can be found in the large weight-bearing muscles of the thigh and shoulder* (Fig. 3-74), but many others are affected and the lesions are bilaterally symmetrical.

Suckling animals often have extensive lesions in the *highly active tongue and neck muscles*, and occasionally in the voluntary muscles of rectum, urethra, and esophagus. Affected muscles are pale, irregularly opaque and yellow to creamy white. Minimal myocardial lesions are sometimes present, but not accompanied by evidence of cardiac failure.

In older calves and young adult cattle, the patterns of disease vary considerably and are unrelated to age. Dairy and beef calves 6-12 months of age show stiffness and lethargy just after winter housing, or sometimes while they are housed.

The disease is often related to poor-quality feed. In similar circumstances, extensive myopathy occurs in pregnant heifers and they may suffer a high incidence of abortion, stillbirth, placental retention, and parturient recumbency. Feedlot steers fed high-moisture corn, which has been treated with propionic acid to control fungal growth and stored for 6-8 months, show initial signs of diarrhea and unthriftiness, and become recumbent. Many have lesions in muscles at slaughter. Most mature animals with extensive skeletal muscle lesions have myoglobinuria.

Young adult cattle with bilateral dorsal scapular displacement ("flying scapula") have rupture of the serratus ventralis muscle; this may be of sufficient duration to have extensive fibrosis and multifocal osseous and cartilaginous metaplasia underlying the displaced scapulae. Presumably, nutritional myopathy of the subscapular muscles has preceded rupture and displacement.

Histologic lesions of nutritional myopathy in cattle are multifocal polyphasic necrosis with or without mineralization (Fig. 3-75), followed by macrophage infiltration and myofiber regeneration. By electron microscopy the earliest detectable change is *degeneration of mitochondria*, and this is followed by loss of some parts of the sarcomere and then disintegration of the tubular systems. By histochemical examination, it can be determined that *type 1 fibers degenerate preferentially but not exclusively*. Apart from this preference, the pattern of degeneration appears to be random. This random pattern is helpful in distinguishing this from other muscle diseases such as ischemic degeneration.

Changes in *myocardium* are very similar to those seen in skeletal muscle. Mineralization of necrotic fibers is often pronounced and the coagulated, mineralized myofibrils appear to be rapidly removed by macrophages. Necrotic myocardial fibers are not regenerated; they are replaced by condensed fibrous stroma.

Nutritional myopathy of sheep and goats

Nutritional myopathy in **sheep** *is probably more prevalent in more areas of the world than the disease in cattle.* The disease was first described in Germany in 1925. The names *white muscle disease, rigid lamb disease*, and *stiff lamb disease* were coined to describe the most frequently encountered clinical patterns in 2-4 week-old lambs, which very often are *spring*

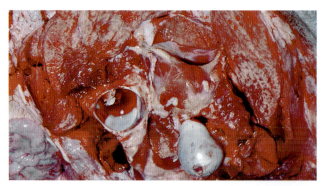

Figure 3-74 Pale areas of necrosis in cross-section of caudal thigh muscles from a calf with **nutritional myopathy**. (Courtesy M.D. McGavin.)

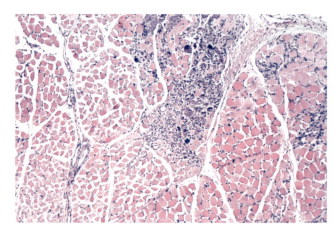

Figure 3-75 Extensive zones of myofiber necrosis and mineralization in laryngeal muscle from a calf with **nutritional myopathy**. H&E stain.

lambs, recently turned out onto the first green pasture. Congenital nutritional myopathy does occur in lambs, but not often. The typical disease may occur as an outbreak among lambs from 1 day to 2 months of age or beyond. Mortality at this stage may be very low or may reach 50%. The next peak of incidence occurs at 4-8 months of age as weaned lambs are put onto lush pastures following mowing or into feedlots. Mortality is not usually very high, but the incidence of minimal clinical disease may be moderately high and that of subclinical disease may be higher still. Beyond these age groups, nutritional myopathy in more mature sheep is clinically apparent sporadically, but subclinical disease may involve from 5-30% of a group. Under special circumstances, the incidence of clinical disease and mortality may rise dramatically. Thus, in various parts of the world, the disease has been precipitated by stress from bad weather, prolonged winter feeding, subsistence on root crops, or forced activity, as well as feeding on stubble, legume pastures, dry pastures, and pastures with too much copper. Outbreaks in lambs and yearlings have also occurred on pastures on which copper had been made unavailable by top-dressing with molybdenum.

Lesions and their corresponding clinical signs are as varied as the circumstances under which myopathy occurs. The lesions may be detectable in lamb fetuses at least 2 weeks before parturition. In the congenital disease, *tongue and neck muscles* used in suckling movements often contain the most severe lesions. When the lesions occur in lambs a few days older, they are likely to be much more extensive and involve primarily the *major muscles of the shoulder and thigh but also back, neck, and respiratory (diaphragm and intercostal) muscles.* The gross appearance of affected muscles is similar to that described for calves, although *the likelihood of muscle mineralization is probably greater.* Lambs normally have pale muscles; consequently, the recognition of the mineralized flecking is almost essential if diagnosis is to be made grossly with any confidence. It is necessary to confirm the gross diagnosis by histologic examination.

In older sheep, lesions are more varied in distribution, location, and extent, but some similarity to the distribution in young animals may exist. For example, bilaterally symmetrical lesions of the thigh muscles may occur but they may predominate in or be confined to the intermediate head of the triceps, or the tensor fascia latae. Lesions in pregnant ewes may be more or less confined to the abdominal muscles subjected to increased work load from supporting the pregnant uterus and may rupture, allowing viscera to herniate.

Microscopically, the changes seen in affected muscle are *multifocal polyphasic necrosis* as seen in nutritional myopathy in other species.

Reports of nutritional myopathy in **goats** are relatively few, but this may be due to the fact that the goat is less often reared under intensive animal agriculture practices. Caprine nutritional myopathy has been observed in Europe, the Middle East, New Zealand, Australia, and North America. In most instances it appears in goats on pasture, and clinical and pathologic changes are similar to those seen in sheep.

Nutritional myopathy of pigs

Nutritional myopathy in swine has been reported as a spontaneous disease wherever intensive pig rearing is practiced, but particularly in northern, central, and eastern continental Europe, the United Kingdom, the United States, and Canada. Classical lesions involving only skeletal muscles are less common than some of the other expressions of porcine vitamin E/selenium deficiency such as hepatosis dietetica and mulberry heart disease, but *systematic microscopic study of muscles has revealed a much higher incidence of muscle lesions than was thought to exist.* Because the pig is an easily managed experimental animal, much more is known about experimental vitamin E/selenium deficiency in this species than in others.

Naturally occurring nutritional myopathy is not known to be congenital in pigs, but piglets as young as 1 day of age may have extensive lesions, which cause paresis or extreme weakness. Growing pigs of all sizes up to 65 kg may be affected in outbreaks, but *most commonly affected are weaned pigs 6-20 weeks of age.* A special circumstance is that caused in pigs a few days old by the *injection of iron dextran products*, which precipitates acute widespread degenerative and usually fatal myopathy. It is believed that iron acts as a catalyst for lipid peroxidation of cell membranes. Older pigs, and particularly sows that have recently farrowed, are occasionally susceptible to widespread nutritional myopathy of sufficient severity to cause prostration, although more often clinical signs, if present at all, consist of lethargy and slowness of movement.

Apart from deficiencies in diet, the factors that trigger the disease in pigs seem to be relatively few. Unaccustomed exercise does not seem to play a part, but *feeding rancid or oxidized fish liver oils, which destroy vitamin E, may do so.* Newly harvested grain sometimes seems to contain a myopathy-inducing factor, and pigs fed quantities of peas (*Pisum sativum*) may be particularly prone to the disease. Metals occurring as contaminants in ground mineral mixes can induce an increased requirement for vitamin E and/or selenium. Silver, copper, cadmium, cobalt, vanadium, tellurium, and zinc, and possibly other metals, in some way bind selenium or prevent its participation in free radical protective activities. This leads to a 2-fold or greater demand for selenium to prevent lesions that can be only partly alleviated by vitamin E supplementation.

Mineralization of degenerate fibers is often not abundant and even when it is present and visible, it is difficult to detect grossly in the naturally pale muscles of the pig. This, and the fact that lesions in heart and liver are much more dramatic, may explain why there are relatively few reports of skeletal muscle lesions in natural outbreaks of vitamin E/selenium deficiency disease. In the experimental disease in pigs, gross lesions may be seen in muscle, but many skeletal muscle lesions are microscopic, whereas the liver and heart lesions are grossly visible.

Microscopic muscle lesions are similar to the multifocal polyphasic necrosis seen in lambs and calves. Type 1 fibers are principally affected and, in view of the orderly central arrangement of type 1 fibers within muscle fascicles in the pig, this leads to a *distinct central degeneration within fascicles.* Regeneration is often rapid and complete in surviving piglets, but the mortality rate may be as high as 80% of a litter, and usually 100% when secondary to iron injection. The survival rate for older pigs is higher except in those instances in which the cardiac lesions are prominent. Relatively few pigs survive mulberry heart disease.

Myocardial degeneration (mulberry heart disease) is the most common manifestation of vitamin E/selenium deficiency in growing weaned pigs 6-20 weeks of age. It is described in Vol. 3, Cardiovascular system. The liver lesions associated with vitamin E/selenium deficiency are referred to as *nutritional hepatic necrosis or hepatosis dietetica* and are described in Vol. 2, Liver and biliary system.

Nutritional myopathy of horses

Nutritional myopathy in *foals* has been recognized for many years. *The usual age range is 1 day to 12 weeks and it may be present at birth.* Cases have been reported from North America, Europe, and Australia in most breeds of light horses and in pony, zebra, and donkey foals. Serum creatine kinase concentrations may be very high; over 2 million IU/L in nonsurviving cases, and as high as 200,000 IU/L in surviving animals. Nutritional myopathy occurs in horses of all ages in areas in which severe selenium deficiency is common. *The clinical signs of nutritional myopathy may be nonspecific* and may be mistaken for evidence of colic, cardiac failure, general depression, or botulism. In foals and young adult horses *the most common features are stiffness and muscular weakness. In adults, trismus and inability to prehend and masticate feed are most common, although stiff gait and sudden onset of recumbency are also possible.* The most convincing indications of nutritional myopathy are the myocardial lesions that are similar to those seen in other species. The presence of myocardial necrosis separates the syndrome from the exertional, metabolic, and ischemic myopathies, but does not rule out toxic myopathy.

It is important to realize that there are other causes of myodegeneration in foals (as well as adult horses) that are not related to nutritional deficiency. This may at least help to explain perplexing findings of normal selenium and vitamin E in foals with degenerative myopathy. When such cases occur, careful evaluation and genetic testing for polysaccharide storage myopathy and for glycogen branching enzyme defect are needed.

Postmortem lesions of nutritional myopathy in foals are similar in many respects to those in calves and lambs— *multifocal polyphasic necrosis.* Foals dying acutely may have myocardial lesions. In the *subacute syndrome, shoulder, neck,* and *thigh muscles* may be bilaterally and extensively involved and this usually accounts for an inability to rise or to assume certain postures such as the one for suckling. Involvement of the lingual, pharyngeal, and masticatory muscles results in dysphagia. Involvement of digital flexors and extensors may be more frequent than in calves. Affected muscle may be pale tan (see Fig. 3-28). Areas of necrotic muscle with *chalky opaque flecking of muscle* also can be seen, especially within temporal and masseter muscle of adult horses with nutritional myopathy. Myoglobinuria may be present and reflects the severity of muscle damage. In adult horses (and also donkeys and mules), there is severe involvement of the masticatory and tongue muscles.

Histologic lesions in both foals and older horses with selenium-deficiency myopathy are similar to those seen in calves or pigs—*multifocal polyphasic necrosis.* The repair process in foals is rapid and usually complete in 2 weeks if the foal survives, but some lasting retardation of growth may result. Older animals may have the same capability for regeneration, especially in subclinical disease, but it is expected that in older animals the repair process may be less effective, and healing will be by scarring in severely affected muscles. Scarring may be responsible for limitations of gait or deviation of the neck. Severe cases of masticatory muscle necrosis in adult horses with nutritional myopathy may not be capable of adequate regeneration, as evidenced by inability to successfully treat some severely affected horses despite aggressive medical, dietary, and supportive therapy. It is possible that compartment syndrome contributes to severe injury and impaired regenerative capacity in these cases.

Steatitis is apparently not seen in older horses with nutritional myopathy but it is common in foals and may, in the healing stage, lead to lumpiness in subcutaneous adipose tissue, especially along the nuchal crest and over the gluteal muscles and the abdominal wall. The affected fat is firm and yellow-brown. Microscopically, neutrophilic infiltration and necrosis and mineralization of fat cells are present.

Nutritional myopathy of other species

Nutritional myopathy is unusual in carnivores and primates. Clinical, morphologic, and therapeutic evidence suggests that it does occur. There are several reports in dogs fed prolonged diets unusually low in vitamin E and selenium, and dogs with chronic biliary fistulas developing nutritional myopathy and myocardial damage. *Cats fed vitamin E–deficient diets develop steatitis (yellow fat disease).*

Nutritional myopathy and steatitis in *ranch mink* has largely disappeared following addition of vitamin E to commercial mink feed. A number of *zoo animals* appear to be susceptible to nutritional myopathy, but details are scarce and evidence largely circumstantial. Outbreaks within species of interest such as brown pelicans and geckoes have precluded additional testing that would require sacrifice of remaining animals, and diagnosis in these cases has relied on characteristic clinical and pathologic findings and response to diet therapy, often supplementation with vitamin E. A small nocturnal wallaby, the Rottnest quokka *(Setonix brachyurus)*, and the nyala *(Tragelaphus angasi)* seem to be exquisitely susceptible. Problems of diagnosis arise in such populations in which capture myopathy is a complication (see Exertional myopathies), but cases that circumstantially appear to be due to nutritional myopathy are reported in several species of gazelle and antelope in Africa, roe deer in Scotland, and white-tailed deer and Rocky Mountain bighorn sheep in North America. Nutritional myopathy also occurs, but is apparently uncommon, in camelids.

Further reading

Brigelius-Flohe R, Traber MG. Vitamin E: function and metabolism. FASEB 1999;13:1145-1155.

Da Costa LA, et al. Nutrigenetics and modulation of oxidative stress. Ann Nutr Metab 2012;60(Suppl. 3):27-36.

Pearson EG, et al. Masseter myodegeneration as a cause of trismus or dysphagia in adult horses. Vet Rec 2005;156:642-646.

Streeter RM, et al. Selenium deficiency associations with gender, breed, serum vitamin E and creatine kinase, clinical signs and diagnoses in horses of different age groups: a retrospective examination 1996-2011. Equine Vet J Suppl 2012;43:31-35.

Van Vleet JF, Ferrans VJ. Etiologic factors and pathologic alterations in selenium-vitamin E deficiency and excess in animals and humans. Biol Trace Elem Res 1992;33:1-21.

TOXIC MYOPATHIES

A large group of chemical and biological agents are recognized as producing skeletal muscle degeneration and necrosis, either experimentally in laboratory animals or as sporadic clinical occurrences in human patients treated with various therapeutic agents. However, in veterinary medicine, naturally occurring toxicities are largely limited to disease syndromes associated with ingestion of *ionophores, toxic plants,* and *plant-origin toxins.*

Skeletal muscle is a metabolically active tissue that is susceptible to various toxic injuries. Skeletal muscle toxic injury most often a result of membrane damage, altered protein synthesis, increased intracellular calcium concentration, or mitochondrial damage. Some agents, such as oxytetracycline, cause direct local injury at injection sites.

Clinical expression of myotoxicities is highly variable. Possible clinical presentations include lack of overt clinical signs but elevated serum concentrations of skeletal muscle cytoplasmic enzymes; stiffness and muscle pain with or without myoglobinuria; and severe muscle weakness accompanied by recumbency usually with myoglobinuria. Mortality rates may be high in severely affected animals; death is often caused by concurrent myocardial damage by the same toxin, although necrosis of respiratory muscle can also result in death.

Ionophore toxicosis

Ionophores *used in agriculture are monensin, lasalocid, salinomycin, narasin,* and *maduramicin.* Ionophores are compounds that alter membrane permeability to electrolytes by influencing transmembrane transport. In excess, all of these agents damage skeletal and cardiac muscle but *horses are uniquely susceptible.* Most reports of toxicosis involve monensin, an ionophore used widely for years.

Monensin, an antibiotic produced by the fermentation of *Streptomyces cinnamonensis,* has a growth-promoting effect in ruminants and is an efficient coccidiostat in birds and other animals. Monensin is produced commercially in very large quantities in North America and Europe, where it is added, as a concentrated premix, to pelleted or bulk feeds fed to cattle, sheep, and other ruminants. Toxicity develops when monensin is fed to monogastric animals, which have a much reduced tolerance for the drug, or when human or mechanical error leads to concentrations of monensin in the ration that are abnormally high for the species being fed. Toxic effects have been recorded in horses, donkeys, mules, zebras, cattle, sheep, dogs, wallabies, camels, blesbok, Stone sheep, turkeys, and chickens. Many episodes of monensin poisoning have been caused by mixing errors in packaged, pelleted, commercial animal feeds, either concentrates or final mix, which has put hundreds or thousands of animals at risk, sometimes over wide geographic areas. In North America alone, such mixing errors have been reported in horse, cattle, dog, and zoo feeds. Some indication of susceptibility of different species is provided by the *estimated LD_{50} for different animals.* Horses and other equids that are sensitive have an LD_{50} of 2-3 mg of monensin/kg body weight. LD_{50} values for other species are: dogs, 5-8 mg/kg; sheep and goats, 12-24 mg/kg; cattle, 50-80 mg/kg; and various types of poultry 90-200 mg/kg. Pigs, which may be given the drug for its coccidiostatic properties or be exposed by mistake, have an LD_{50} of 16-50 mg/kg body weight. The toxic effects of monensin or salinomycin are potentiated by the addition of tiamulin, triacetyloleandomycin, or sulfonamides to the ration, usually for therapeutic purposes.

Ingestion of **maduramicin**, an ionophore antibiotic used as a coccidiostat in poultry, has caused *cardiotoxicity in cattle and sheep.* Cases occurred in South Africa and Israel, where dried poultry litter was used as a source of protein for ruminants. The clinical and pathologic features of this toxicosis are similar to those of monensin cardiotoxicity.

When a single large toxic dose of an ionophore is fed to an animal, clinical signs of *lethargy, stiffness, muscular weakness,* and *recumbency* occur within 24 hours. Horses and other equids are likely, in the early stages, to show marked signs of colic, apprehension, shifting or fidgeting, sweating, myoglobinuria, and muscle tremors. Dogs show apprehension and progressive weakness. If sublethal doses are fed, the toxic effect will be cumulative, and the clinical onset may be delayed for 2-3 days to weeks depending on the total amount and the period over which it is fed, but the debility is likely to be more pronounced. Animals on low-level toxicity experiments often have delayed progression of the toxic signs because consumption of these feeds is reduced. These animals frequently scour and lose weight. At dose levels capable of inducing clinical signs of toxicity in a few days, many animals show evidence of *progressive cardiac failure caused by a high incidence of myocardial lesions.* Animals recovering from the acute disease may subsequently develop, within several months, signs of progressive cardiac insufficiency from myocardial fibrosis. Sometimes renal failure, in addition to poor growth or poor weight gain, occurs, although the signs referable to skeletal muscle injury may disappear.

Postmortem lesions of ionophore toxicity may be difficult to detect in acute cases dying within 24 hours. *In horses, myocardial damage predominates, in sheep and swine the skeletal muscles are the main site of damage and myoglobinuria is generally present, and in cattle skeletal and cardiac muscle are about equally affected.* Skeletal muscle may lack normal rigor, and ill-defined pale streaks may be visible in both myocardium and skeletal muscle. Later, the white streaking of affected skeletal muscles becomes more prominent. Hindlimb muscles may be the sites of major degenerative changes. Cases with terminal cardiac damage will have features of congestive heart failure including fluid accumulations in body cavities, pulmonary congestion and edema, and hepatic congestion.

Microscopic lesions of ionophore toxicity typically are *multifocal monophasic necrosis* by 48 hours after exposure and thus differ from the polyphasic lesions of nutritional myopathy. One of the earliest electron-microscopically visible lesions in muscle fibers is *marked swelling and disintegration of mitochondria.* Monensin is an ionophore that distorts membrane transport of sodium and potassium. This apparently leads to abnormalities of the electrolyte-modulated calcium gating mechanism and then mitochondrial failure, energy exhaustion, failure of calcium ion removal from the cytosol, and eventually myofibrillar hypercontraction and segmental degeneration. *Both type 1 and type 2 fibers are involved with necrosis and macrophage infiltration.* Satellite cell nuclei as well as endomysial cells apparently survive acute toxicity, and the early stages of regeneration are initiated during the first few days after exposure.

Myocardial lesions in monensin toxicity are not reparable and, particularly in a growing animal, the probability of lasting cardiac insufficiency is high.

Toxic plants and plant-origin toxins

In the southern United States, mature cattle and goats on pasture may ingest the beans of the **senna or coffee senna plant** (*Cassia occidentalis* or *C. obtusifolia*) or **coyotillo** (*Karwinskia humboldtiana*) late in the year, after a killing frost has made the plant more palatable than normal. Horses and pigs also may be affected. After eating the plant for a few days, animals develop diarrhea, show evidence of weakness, and

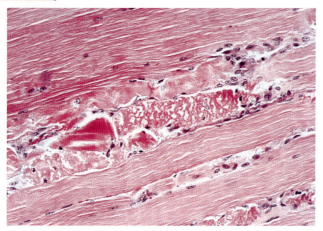

Figure 3-76 Segmental myodegeneration caused by ***Cassia occidentalis*** poisoning of a heifer. H&E stain. (Courtesy M.D. McGavin.)

display a swaying, stumbling gait that is related to the developing muscle lesions. The disease progresses rapidly and most of the animals affected become recumbent and develop myoglobinuria and high concentrations of muscle-origin enzymes in serum. Recumbent animals may live for several days, but usually do not recover. The morbidity rate may reach 60%.

Postmortem lesions in recumbent animals consist of *ill-defined pallor of much of the muscle mass*. Histologic changes are typically *multifocal monophasic necrosis*. The destruction of muscle fibers is segmental (Fig. 3-76). Myocardium is not extensively involved but animals dying acutely show some myocardial lesions. The specific toxins have not been identified.

In swine, natural outbreaks of *Cassia* spp. toxicity on several pig farms occurred when animals were fed grain contaminated with *C. occidentalis* seeds. Several pigs died after a short period of reduced weight gain and a progressively wobbly, unsteady gait. Experimentally, the clinical disease was reproduced after 40 days with diets with as little as 1% of ground seeds. Postmortem examination revealed no gross lesions, but microscopic degeneration of the myocardium and diaphragm were characterized by *vacuolation and segmental hypercontraction of fibers*. The lesions were unexpectedly limited in the skeletal musculature, considering the marked locomotor clinical signs.

Gossypol *is a yellow, pigmented, polyphenolic substance present in cottonseeds* (*Gossypium* spp.). It is toxic to swine, and toxicosis occurs when swine are fed cottonseed cake or meal at a concentration of 10% or more of rations to which it is added as a protein supplement. Lesions occur after feeding such rations for a month or more, which suggests that the toxic effects are cumulative. Gossypol is toxic to experimental lambs and calves at concentrations of <450 ppm in the feed (the level of free gossypol permitted in human and some animal foods). Dogs also may be affected. Lesions are present in several organs, including the heart, skeletal muscles, liver, and lungs, and *death is due to cardiac failure*, which causes fluid accumulation in body cavities. Histologically, *segmental necrosis of skeletal muscle and myocardial necrosis* is present, the liver has centrilobular necrosis and the lungs are congested and edematous. Affected animals are pot-bellied and poorly grown, and most die acutely. Natural outbreaks of disease in calves and lambs circumstantially linked to cottonseed meal ingestion have similar patterns of poor growth and sudden death. Serum enzyme concentrations are generally not significantly increased, which seems to confirm that the heart is the only striated muscle generally affected. Other circumstantial evidence suggests, however, that in calves, skeletal muscle lesions can be locally extensive but unpredictable in distribution. *Both type 1 and 2 muscle fibers undergo segmental necrosis* that is indistinguishable from the lesions of other toxic myopathies.

Degenerative myopathy is also reported in sheep with lupinosis (*Diaporthe toxica*), in sheep with water hemlock (*Cicuta douglasii*) toxicosis, in calves with false lupine (*Thermopsis montana*) toxicosis, in horses and ruminants with white snakeroot (*Ageratina*, formerly *Eupatorium* spp.) and rayless goldenrod (*Isocoma pluriflora*) toxicosis, and in pigs, cattle, sheep, and other species with selenium toxicosis.

A myoglobinuric disease of pastured horses has been described as *seasonal pasture myopathy* and *atypical myopathy* in Great Britain and in the United States. Extensive myolysis is triggered by ingestion of **hypoglycin A** within seeds of the box elder tree (*Acer negundo*, North America; *Acer pseudoplatanus*, Europe), which leads to acquired multiple acyl-CoA dehydrogenase deficiency (MADD). Affected horses have characteristic changes in serum acylcarnitines and in urinary organic acids as well as reduced muscle tissue concentrations of short- and medium-chain acyl-CoA dehydrogenase and isovaleryl-CoA dehydrogenase. Risk factors in affected horses are young age (mean ~3 years), poor to normal body condition, longer time on pasture, and less supplemental feeding. Other risk factors are season (fall), poor pasture drainage, and pasture vegetation of low nutritional value.

Autopsy findings are typical of rhabdomyolysis, with areas of pale musculature in multiple muscles. Histopathologic findings are of severe, acute, locally extensive and generally monophasic myonecrosis. Affected fibers are predominantly type 1, and there is an accompanying increase in intramyofiber lipid. Muscles most likely to be severely affected are neck, proximal limb, intercostal, and diaphragm. Myocardial necrosis can also occur.

Further reading

Bautista AC, et al. Diagnostic value of tissue monensin concentrations in horses following toxicosis. J Vet Diagn Invest 2014;26: 423-427.

East NE, et al. Apparent gossypol-induced toxicosis in adult dairy goats. J Am Vet Med Assoc 1994;204:642-643.

Panter KE, et al. Water hemlock (*Cicuta douglasii*) toxicosis in sheep: pathologic description and prevention of lesions and death. J Vet Diag Invest 1996;8:474-480.

Scimeca JM, Oehme FW. Postmortem guide to common poisonous plants of livestock. Vet Hum Toxicol 1985;27:189-199.

Unger L, et al. Hypoglycin a concentrations in seeds of *Acer pseudoplatanus* trees growing on atypical myopathy-affected and control pastures. J Vet Intern Med 2014;28:1289-1293.

Vashishtha VM, et al. Clinical and pathological features of acute toxicity due to *Cassia occidentalis* in vertebrates. Indian J Med Res 2009;130:23-30.

Westermann CM, et al. Acquired multiple Acyl-CoA dehydrogenase deficiency in 10 horses with atypical myopathy. Neuromus Dis 2008;355:355-364.

DEGENERATIVE (NECROTIZING) MYOPATHIES INCLUDING RHABDOMYOLYSIS

It is worth a brief introduction to *terminology related to rhabdomyolytic diseases*. Although the term *degeneration* is not synonymous with necrosis, *degenerative myopathy by definition is a muscle disease characterized by myofiber necrosis*. As such, various muscle disorders that have been previously discussed in this chapter, most prominently the muscular dystrophies, malignant hyperthermia, equine polysaccharide storage myopathy, nutritional myopathies, and toxic myopathies, which are characterized by ongoing or episodic myonecrosis, are also classified as degenerative myopathies. To add to the potential confusion, in clinical medicine the term *rhabdomyolysis*, which simply means lysis of myofibers, often has been applied to cases of severe acute myonecrosis. Often this is associated with exercise, hence the term *exertional rhabdomyolysis*. Technically the term *rhabdomyolysis* could be employed in any situation in which sufficient muscle necrosis to result in obvious clinical signs and clear-cut increase in serum CK and AST concentrations occurs.

This section focuses on muscle disorders characterized by myofiber necrosis that are not congenital and are not due to nutritional deficiency or toxins. There is some overlap of inherited disorders with equine recurrent rhabdomyolysis, which is traditionally described under the heading of *exertional myopathy*, but which has now been shown to be an inherited muscle disorder.

Exertional myopathies

*The term **exertional myopathy** should be reserved for myofiber damage occurring as a result of exercise stress as the primary cause.* In cases of apparent exertional myopathy, a thorough search for underlying conditions is warranted. For example, acute myofiber injury is precipitated by exercise in X-linked muscular dystrophy, nutritional myopathy, metabolic myopathies, malignant hyperthermia, and myopathy resulting from hypokalemia. In such cases, the initiation of abnormal excitation-contraction coupling, inadequate energy metabolism, ionic imbalance, or simply the mechanical stresses occurring during contraction are thought to lead to myofiber damage of predisposed muscle.

Historically, the syndrome of passage of *myoglobin-pigmented urine (myoglobinuria)* was recognized long before it was determined that massive *skeletal muscle necrosis (rhabdomyolysis)* was the cause. Small wonder that so many names exist for the various manifestations of exertional myopathy. In a broad sense, *exertional myopathy has included the group of diseases in which acute muscle fiber necrosis is initiated by muscle activity of the major muscle groups but in which the underlying cause is unknown or poorly understood.* Such activity may be intensive or exhaustive, but in susceptible individuals exertional myopathy may occur with only minimal exercise. Continued research into causes of exertional rhabdomyolysis is clearly warranted and, as is true of equine exertional rhabdomyolysis (see later), may lead to better understanding of causes and preventive measures.

Exertional rhabdomyolysis in the horse

Various manifestations of exertional myopathy have been recognized in horses for many, many years. There are numerous names for the disorder, including *azoturia* (presumably named for nitrogen-containing compounds in the urine, and possibly related to the resemblance of myoglobin to the red-purple azo dyes), *black water*, *paralytic myoglobinuria*, *Monday-morning disease*, *set fast*, and *tying up*. Various classifications have distinguished the disorder in heavy horse breeds that are prone to severe and often life-threatening muscle injury, particularly when worked after a day of rest and full grain ration (hence the term *Monday-morning disease*), from the often less severe disorder in light horse breeds. Muscle injury severe enough to result in myoglobinuria, profound weakness, and recumbency is common in heavy horse breeds, hence the terms *azoturia*, *black water*, and *paralytic myoglobinuria*. Exertional myopathy in light horse breeds is typically less severe, resulting in episodic muscle pain, sometimes associated with swelling, and reluctance to move, hence the names *set fast* and *tying up*. Given the recent recognition of a metabolic myopathy leading to exertional rhabdomyolysis in both heavy and light breeds (see later), it becomes clear that *the same underlying disorder can result in a spectrum of clinical signs*.

It has long been suspected that the clinical disorder represents a syndrome with multiple possible etiologies. It has been proposed that exertional myopathy in the horse be classified as either sporadic exertional rhabdomyolysis or recurrent exertional rhabdomyolysis, with sporadic exertional rhabdomyolysis possibly resulting from muscle exhaustion or electrolyte depletion in any horse, and recurrent exertional rhabdomyolysis occurring in horses somehow predisposed to this disorder. Studies of serum activities of CK and AST after exercise have shown, however, that *subclinical exertional myopathy is common in horses*. As exertional myopathy can occur without obvious clinical signs other than, perhaps, poor performance, it is possible that so-called sporadic cases really represent recurrent disease, and therefore this classification is difficult to justify based on current knowledge of equine muscle disease.

Previously, *etiologies* proposed for equine exertional rhabdomyolysis have included muscle lactic acidosis, hypothyroidism, electrolyte imbalance, and vitamin E and/or selenium deficiency. Of these, *only electrolyte imbalance, in particular hypokalemia, is still considered possible*. Extensive studies have shown that lactic acid levels in the muscle of exercising horses prone to exertional rhabdomyolysis are no different than those of control horses. Removal of thyroid glands results in poor cardiac output and performance without evidence of muscle damage, and vitamin E and selenium status varies widely in affected horses. More recently, a *metabolic myopathy* thought to involve abnormal starch and sugar metabolism (equine polysaccharide storage myopathy, see Metabolic myopathies) has been shown to be the most common cause of exertional rhabdomyolysis in many breeds of horses, including Quarter Horse, Warmblood, draft, Arabian, Standardbred, Tennessee Walker, Morgan, and Welsh pony–related breeds. It is possible that a similar metabolic disorder is the cause of recurrent exertional rhabdomyolysis in Thoroughbreds, although this is controversial, with one group reporting evidence for abnormal calcium handling in muscle fibers of affected Thoroughbreds. Defective ryanodine receptor function similar to malignant hyperthermia has not, however, been found in affected Thoroughbreds. Whether the abnormal muscle contracture testing reported in in vitro studies of muscle from Thoroughbreds with recurrent exertional rhabdomyolysis is a primary or secondary abnormality is still unknown. *There is strong evidence that there is an autosomal* dominantly inherited basis for the predisposition to exertional rhabdomyolysis in horses with polysaccharide storage myopathy and in Thoroughbreds with recurrent exertional rhabdomyolysis. Although further studies are needed, *it is now accepted that exertional rhabdomyolysis in horses most often is due to underlying metabolic abnormalities of muscle rather than simply poor management of diet and exercise conditioning.*

Although diets high in starches and sugars (grains) are associated with increased severity of exertional rhabdomyolysis, clinical signs can still occur in horses fed only forage. Despite differing opinions regarding cause, *almost all horses with recurrent exertional rhabdomyolysis respond positively after a diet change to one that is high in fat, high in fiber, and low in starches and sugars.* Stall rest appears to exacerbate the signs of equine exertional rhabdomyolysis but the mechanism by which daily exercise benefits such horses is still unknown.

Weakness and/or pain in the hindlimbs occurs suddenly, and the animal soon becomes unable or very reluctant to move. This may be accompanied by sweating and generalized tremors. The affected muscles, which are typically those of the *gluteal, femoral, and lumbar groups*, may be swollen and board-like in their rigidity. *Myoglobinuria* can appear early in the disease, causing dark red-brown discoloration of the urine. Severely affected horses become recumbent, a sign that is often a prelude to death from myoglobinuric nephrosis or problems associated with being down and attempting to rise. Considerable variation occurs between cases as to the nature and duration of the initiating exercise and severity of clinical signs. Recovery from mild attacks in quiet animals may occur in a few hours. Recovery from severe episodes may take days. But, if an animal continues to struggle and is unable to rise, death or euthanasia is the most likely outcome. *Atrophy of the gluteal muscles* may be a feature of recovery in moderate to severe cases. Exertional rhabdomyolysis occurs in both males and females, although *females appear to be predisposed*. The activity of the ovarian hormones estrogen and progesterone does not, however, appear to be directly related to onset of exertional rhabdomyolysis in females, and ovariectomy is not an effective therapy.

The apparent pain and muscle swelling associated with many cases of equine exertional rhabdomyolysis is curious, as muscle necrosis per se is neither painful nor does it cause muscle swelling. It is suspected that *increased intramuscular pressure, perhaps exacerbated by oxidative membrane injury, may cause painful muscle injury in this disorder.* This may explain the often-reported improvement obtained following vitamin E and selenium supplementation in affected horses.

Exertional rhabdomyolysis typically leads to marked increase in serum CK and AST. The degree of CK and AST increase does not, however, correlate with severity of clinical signs. It is possible that muscle cramping or stiffness in the absence of overt necrosis may occur in some horses. If increased serum CK activity is not reduced by at least 50% every 24 hours in a horse with rhabdomyolysis resulting from exercise, this is evidence of continued muscle injury, and the possibility of an underlying myopathy should be considered.

Grossly visible changes in muscle may be inapparent. In severe cases, they are most obvious in the gluteal, lumbar, and caudal thigh regions but lesions often are widespread. *Muscles may be moist, swollen, and dark, and streaks of pallor may be visible in the more extensively involved muscles* (Fig. 3-77). If ischemic complications occur, the muscles also may show blotchy or linear hemorrhage. In animals that have survived

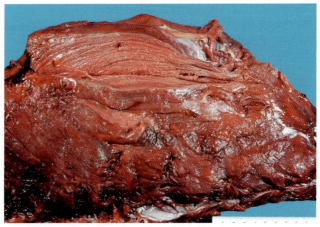

Figure 3-77 Equine exertional rhabdomyolysis. Affected muscle has pale areas as well as red-tinged zones. These gross findings do not aid in diagnosis of possible underlying causes. (Courtesy M.D. McGavin.)

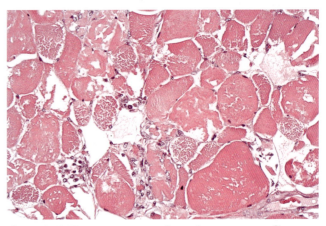

Figure 3-78 Transverse section of acutely necrotic myofibers in a horse with **rhabdomyolysis.** H&E stain.

for 2-3 days, muscles may become paler and, although edema may surround larger muscle divisions, the locally damaged areas appear dry compared with normal muscle.

Necrosis affects primarily the strongly glycolytic fibers (type 2X—traditionally referred to as type 2B—glycolytic, and type 2A oxidative-glycolytic fibers) in contrast to the primary involvement of type 1 oxidative fibers in the nutritional myopathies. *Damaged fiber segments generally undergo hypercontraction followed by coagulative necrosis* (Fig. 3-78). Mineralization is not typically seen. There is also potential for perpetuation of myofiber injury due to release of free radicals and subsequent oxidative membrane injury. Oxidative injury to muscle capillary endothelium can result in interstitial edema and increase in intramuscular pressure that can predispose to ischemia (*compartment syndrome*) (see Circulatory disturbances of muscle). Lesions are multifocal and often monophasic, but can be polyphasic in horses with repeated bouts of necrosis or ongoing injury. Cardiac involvement is not expected.

In horses with *polysaccharide storage myopathy*, abnormal inclusions of pale pink glycogen and, in severe cases, blue-gray complex polysaccharide may be seen within scattered myofibers on H&E stain (see section in Metabolic myopathies; see also Fig. 3-63). Given the high incidence of underlying equine polysaccharide storage myopathy in horses with histories of exertional rhabdomyolysis or postanesthetic myopathy (see later), *PAS staining and careful evaluation of muscle from all such cases for evidence of chronic myopathy and abnormal glycogen and complex polysaccharide storage are warranted.*

Canine exertional rhabdomyolysis

Rhabdomyolysis is recognized as a syndrome affecting racing Greyhounds and racing sled dogs. Given the vast difference in type of exercise (i.e., sprint vs. endurance racing) in these 2 breeds of dog, there are likely to be differing underlying etiologies.

In **racing Greyhounds**, the disorder primarily affects longissimus, quadriceps, and biceps femoris muscles. Affected dogs may display distress and generalized muscle pain associated with a stiff gait. Myoglobinuria can lead to death caused by renal failure. In less severe cases, myoglobinuria is not evident, and muscle pain may only be mild to moderate. Similar to exertional rhabdomyolysis in horses, affected muscles may be swollen as well as painful, indicative of mechanisms besides simple muscle necrosis as a cause of pain and swelling. Predisposing factors that have been proposed include an *excitable nature, lack of physical fitness, hot and humid conditions,* and *overexertion of physically fit dogs.* Gross lesions are not often seen in affected muscles, although histopathologic evidence of acute degenerative changes is found in susceptible muscles.

Racing sled dogs may undergo massive rhabdomyolysis during racing that can lead to *sudden death.* There is often selective involvement of certain muscle groups; in one case studied there were moderate to severe multifocal monophasic necrotizing lesions involving quadriceps, psoas, deep digital flexor, and gastrocnemius muscles, with sparing of triceps brachii, epaxial, and cranial tibial muscles. Gross lesions are not typically seen, and sampling of multiple muscle groups may be necessary to determine the extent of injury. It has been suggested that prolonged endurance-type exercise leads to increased lipid peroxidation and reduced plasma antioxidant concentrations; however, vitamin E supplementation does not appear to ameliorate exercise-induced muscle injury in racing sled dogs, and pre-race plasma vitamin E levels do not appear to correlate with risk of exertional rhabdomyolysis. As in horses, dietary management is likely to play a role in canine exertional rhabdomyolysis; a high-fat and low-carbohydrate diet has been reported to reduce exercise-induced muscle injury in these dogs.

Exertional myopathy in other species ("capture myopathy")

Massive muscle injury caused by overexertion or associated with transport can occur in sheep and cattle. Underlying nutritional myopathy (see the section on Nutritional myopathy) or metabolic myopathy (see the section on Metabolic myopathies) predisposing to exercise-induced muscle injury is also possible. *Of special interest is exertional myopathy occurring in wild animals after capture and/or immobilization, an entity known as* **capture myopathy**. First described in wild ungulates, this disorder has been seen in multiple species, including wild ruminants, captured otters, cetaceans, mustelids, canids, marsupials, and wild birds. Clinically affected animals can exhibit *dyspnea, weakness, muscle tremors or muscle rigidity, hyperthermia, collapse, and often death.* Thigh muscle rupture may occur. Those that do not die acutely show myoglobinuria and increased levels of muscle enzymes in the blood and may

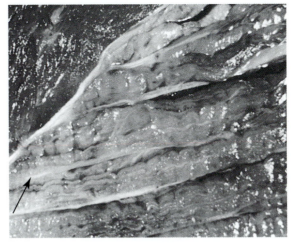

Figure 3-79 Marked pallor of affected muscle (arrow) in **bovine transport myopathy**. (Courtesy T.J. Hulland.)

subsequently die of renal failure. When the animal is down, secondary ischemic complications may occur (see Circulatory disturbances of muscle). If the animal survives the muscle lesions are capable of more or less complete repair over a few weeks unless infarction has intervened.

Capture myopathy is associated with stress to the affected animal, and *increased circulating catecholamines may play a role*, particularly in the cardiac damage that can be seen. Hyperthermia and metabolic acidosis also have been associated with capture myopathy. Extreme overexertion likely also contributes. In some cases marginal selenium status or an electrolyte abnormality such as hypokalemia or hyperkalemia may be predisposing factors.

Gross and histologic lesions are often similar to those occurring as a result of other causes of severe exertional myopathy. They may also resemble those of hyperthermia in pigs, with *prominent muscle edema* in animals dying acutely. Muscles may contain *indistinct pale streaks* (Fig. 3-79), and *hemorrhagic streaking* is not uncommon. Degenerative lesions in skeletal muscle are typically *multifocal and monophasic* (see Fig. 3-25A). In most cases death occurs during the degenerative phase and therefore acute myodegeneration, often with macrophage invasion of affected segments, is seen affecting various muscles. Cardiac lesions, when present, are most often acute, although animals that survive capture myopathy may die acutely at a later date as a result of myocardial fibrosis. Myoglobinuric nephrosis may be seen.

Equine systemic calcinosis

A mineralizing degenerative myopathy associated with vascular wall and other soft tissue mineralization occurs in horses. Affected horses are typically young to young adult Quarter Horse and Paint horse breeds, although horses up to 9 years of age have been reported. Common clinical signs are fever and malaise, with marked increase in serum CK and AST activities. Atrophy of paraspinal and gluteal muscle is common. Histopathologic findings are multifocal and polyphasic degenerative myopathy with prominent mineralization in multiple muscle groups (Fig. 3-80). Kidneys, lung, and heart also show degenerative change with mineralization, and mineralization within arterial walls can be striking (Fig. 3-81). Lesions resemble hypervitaminosis D but no exposure to

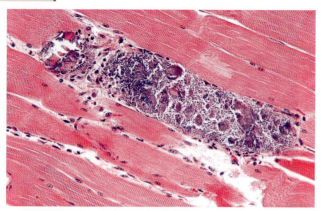

Figure 3-80 Muscle from a horse with **systemic calcinosis**. There is segmental necrosis with prominent mineralization. H&E stain.

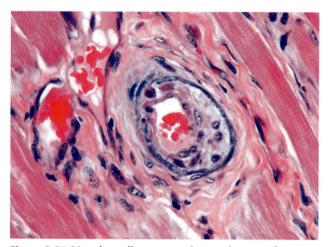

Figure 3-81 Vascular wall necrosis and mineralization of an intramuscular blood vessel in a horse with **systemic calcinosis**. H&E stain.

calcinosis-calinogenic plants (e.g., *Solanum malacoxylon*) or to excess vitamin dietary vitamin D has been found. The cause is not known, but evaluation of history indicates coexisting inflammatory conditions such as exposure to or infection with *Streptococcus zooepidemicus* subsp. *equi*, other nondiagnosed respiratory conditions, and injection of an immunostimulant suggest that this may be an unusual response to a systemic inflammatory condition. This is supported by a consistent finding of hyperfibrinogenemia, a finding not associated with most other equine rhabdomyolytic disorders.

Other degenerative myopathies

Equine postanesthetic degenerative myopathy has been discussed (see Circulatory disturbances of muscle). A form of malignant hyperthermia also has been proposed as a cause of anesthetic-related myopathy in horses. This may be appropriate for those cases in which hyperthermia occurs during inhalant anesthesia, but most affected horses develop myopathy during recovery rather than during anesthesia. Although such horses may develop dangerously high body temperatures during recovery, this condition is best considered to be a hypermetabolic state rather than malignant hyperthermia. Underlying myopathy of any type may be a predisposing factor in horses that develop life-threatening hyperthermia either during or after general anesthesia.

Paraneoplastic necrotizing myopathy is recognized in people, and one author (BAV) has seen a case of suspect paraneoplastic necrotizing myopathy in a dog with colonic adenocarcinoma.

Further reading

Barrey E, et al. Muscular microRNA expressions in healthy and myopathic horses suffering from polysaccharide storage myopathy or recurrent exertional rhabdomyolysis. Equine Vet J Suppl 2010;38:303-310.

Hinchcliff KW, et al. Oxidant stress in sled dogs subjected to repetitive endurance exercise. Am J Vet Res 2000;61:512-517.

Shelton GD. Rhabdomyolysis, myoglobinuria, and necrotizing myopathies. Vet Clin North Am Small Anim Pract 2004;34:1469-1482.

Tan J-Y, et al. Suspected systemic calcinosis and calciphylaxis in 5 horses. Can Vet J 2010;51:993-999.

Wilberger MS, et al. Prevalence of exertional rhabdomyolysis in endurance horses in the Pacific Northwestern United States. Equine Vet J 2014;doi:10.1111/evj.12255.

Williams ES, Thorne ET. Exertional myopathy (Capture Myopathy). In: Fairbrother A, et al., editors. Noninfectious Diseases of Wildlife. Ames, IA: The Iowa State Press; 1996. p. 181-193.

MYOPATHIES ASSOCIATED WITH ENDOCRINE DISORDERS

Hypothyroidism

Some dogs with hypothyroidism may develop clinical signs of weakness, stiffness, reluctance to move, decreased exercise tolerance, and *muscle wasting* in addition to the usual signs of alopecia and obesity. The likelihood of development of myopathy is increased if concomitant endocrinopathies are present such as diabetes mellitus and hyperadrenocorticism.

Muscle biopsies reveal *atrophy of type 2 fibers* (see Fig. 3-21). The atrophic fibers appear oval or angular in outline and are present throughout all muscle fascicles. Nemaline rods may be found, especially in type 1 fibers. No evidence of muscle fiber degradation or inflammatory cell infiltration is present. Initiation of thyroid hormone replacement therapy leads to resolution of the lesions. Selective involvement of type 2 fibers has been attributed to alterations in carbohydrate metabolism with subsequent loss of energy from glycolysis and glycogenolysis. Peripheral neuropathy with axonal degeneration can also occur due to hypothyroidism (and hyperadrenocorticism) with subsequent denervation atrophy of type 1 and type 2 fibers.

Hyperthyroidism

Affected cats may exhibit muscular tremors, ventroflexion of the neck, disturbances in gait, generalized weakness, and collapse. Microscopic alterations usually are absent, but *nonspecific myofiber damage may be present*.

Hyperadrenocorticism

Cushing's disease caused by pituitary-dependent hyperadrenocorticism, adrenal-dependent hyperadrenocorticism, and iatrogenic hyperadrenocorticism may result in muscular weakness, stiff stilted gait, *muscle atrophy*, and inability to walk in dogs. The pelvic limbs are mainly affected.

In muscle biopsies, there is *selective atrophy of type 2 fibers, fiber splitting, and focal necrosis*. Medical or surgical treatment of Cushing's disease may lead to resolution of the muscle lesions unless severe atrophy or contracture is present in the pelvic limb musculature. The muscle fiber alterations are attributed to *increased catabolism and inhibited synthesis of muscle proteins.*

Other endocrinopathies

Hypoadrenocorticism (Addison's disease) in dogs and cats often results in muscle weakness presumed to be related to accompanying *hyperkalemia*. Muscle alterations have not been characterized.

Primary hyperaldosteronism in cats leads to hypokalemia, hypertension, and muscular weakness.

Beagle dogs given *exogenous porcine growth hormone* had hypertrophy of types 1 and 2 fibers. However, skeletal muscle alterations have not been described in dogs or cats with acromegaly.

Further reading

Braund KG. Endogenous causes of myopathies in dogs and cats. Vet Med 1997;92:618-628.

Djajadiningrat-Laanen S, et al. Primary hyperaldosteronism: expanding the diagnostic net. J Feline Med Surg 2011;13:641-650.

Platt SR. Neuromuscular complications in endocrine and metabolic diseases. Vet Clin North Am Small Anim Pract 2002;32:125-146.

MYOPATHIES ASSOCIATED WITH SERUM ELECTROLYTE ABNORMALITIES

Hypokalemia in cats

In 1984, a *polymyopathy* was identified in cats and in more than half of the affected animals, there was a coexisting hypokalemia. Subsequently, a distinct syndrome of **hypokalemic myopathy** was characterized, and the disorder was also termed *feline kaliopenic polymyopathy/nephropathy syndrome* and *sporadic feline hypokalemic polymyopathy.*

Clinically, affected cats have generalized weakness, ventroflexion of the neck, a stiff stilted gait, exercise intolerance, reluctance to walk, and muscle pain. Serum activity of skeletal muscle enzymes (CK, AST) are elevated and serum potassium levels are low (<3 mEq/L). Hypokalemia is attributed to low dietary intake or to excessive renal loss. Low intake has occurred in cats fed potassium-depleted regular diets or high-protein vegetarian diets. Excessive renal loss of potassium can be present in cats with chronic renal disease and in those fed acidic diets to prevent urolithiasis. The periodic hypokalemic polymyopathy syndrome in Burmese kittens 2-6 months of age is a *WNK4*-associated autosomal recessive trait that may result in potassium-losing nephropathy.

In general, *the skeletal muscle lesions are either mild or absent*. Lesions are *polyphasic necrosis*. However, muscle biopsy samples and even many autopsy muscle samples can be normal. In a case studied at autopsy by one of the authors (BAV), myofiber necrosis and regeneration were only found in diaphragm and intercostal muscles. It is possible that these muscles are preferentially involved, and inclusion of samples of respiratory muscles in autopsy samples from suspect cases is advised. The skeletal muscle damage has been attributed to influx of sodium with a decrease in resting membrane potential and hypopolarization, altered glycogen metabolism in skeletal muscle fibers, and ischemic injury from hypokalemia-induced vasoconstriction. Treatment with potassium supplementation is generally successful but the syndrome may recur unless supplementation is maintained.

Hypokalemia in cattle

A hypokalemic syndrome with *muscle weakness and myopathy* occurs in postparturient dairy cattle treated for ketosis with *isoflupredone*, a glucocorticoid with high mineralocorticoid activity leading to severe hypokalemia. Affected cattle are weak, recumbent, and unable to elevate their heads off the ground and instead hold them against their flanks. They are severely hypokalemic (1.4-2.3 mEq/L; normal 3.9-5.8). Vacuolar change and multifocal acute necrosis occur in both weight-bearing and non–weight-bearing muscle. In addition, weight-bearing musculature often develops ischemic necrosis.

Hypernatremia in cats

Muscle weakness evident as ventroflexion of the neck has been observed with hypernatremia and hypodipsia in the cat.

Hypophosphatemia in dogs

Muscle weakness occurs in dogs with hypophosphatemia. Necrosis of skeletal muscle with myoglobinuria was present in severe acute phosphorus depletion.

Further reading

Gandolfi B, et al. First WNK4-hypokalemia animal model identified by genome-wide association in Burmese cats. PLoS ONE 2012;7:e53173.

Sattler N, Fecteau G. Hypokalemia syndrome in cattle. Vet Clin North Am Food Anim Pract 2014;30:351-357.

Taylor SM. Selected disorders of muscle and the neuromuscular junction. Vet Clin North Am Small Anim Pract 2000;30:59-75.

IMMUNE-MEDIATED CONDITIONS

Immune-mediated disorders are those in which abnormal activation of the immune system results in tissue damage. *Immune-mediated muscle damage can involve circulating antibodies directed against muscle cell components, cytotoxic T lymphocytes that infiltrate and attack muscle cells, or immune-complex deposition that subsequently exposes muscles to inflammatory mediators and ischemia.*

It is important to distinguish primary immune-mediated myositis from florid degenerative myopathy in which cellular infiltrates, primarily composed of macrophages, can mimic those of true inflammatory disease. It may be necessary to employ special procedures to identify the type of infiltrating cells or detect specific antibody binding to muscle components. *Immune-mediated disease of muscle is characterized by interstitial and perivascular infiltration of lymphocytes and/or plasma cells* (Fig. 3-82). These cells may be mixed with macrophages and with eosinophils and neutrophils, particularly in cases accompanied by severe myofiber necrosis. *The diagnosis is dependent on determining that cellular infiltrates actually cause the myofiber necrosis and are not secondary to the muscle damage.* The finding of mononuclear leukocytic invasion of otherwise intact myofibers is the hallmark of primary myositis. Infiltrating cells may be seen surrounding intact myofibers, or may be seen centrally, causing a characteristic "coring out" of myofibers with otherwise intact peripheral myofibrils (Fig. 3-83).

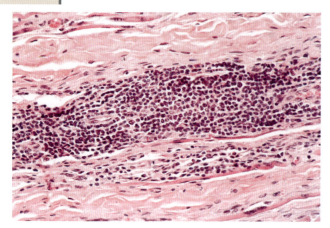

Figure 3-82 Interstitial and perivascular infiltration of mononuclear inflammatory cells characteristic of **immune-mediated myositis** in muscle from a dog. H&E stain.

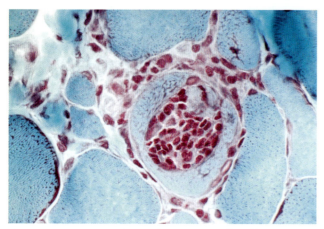

Figure 3-83 Mononuclear inflammatory cell infiltrate at the periphery and "coring out" the interior of an otherwise intact myofiber characteristic of **immune-mediated myositis** in a dog. Frozen section, Gomori trichrome.

Lymphocytic myositis must be distinguished from infiltration of skeletal muscle by malignant lymphoma (see Neoplastic Diseases of Muscle).

Masticatory myositis of dogs

An immune-mediated myositis localized to the masticatory muscles occurs in dogs. The masseter, temporal, and pterygoid muscles are selectively affected. Although previously designated as 2 separate disorders—eosinophilic myositis and atrophic myositis—these are now recognized to be 2 ends of the spectrum of a single disease known as **masticatory myositis**. Given the thick fascia of the masticatory muscles in dogs, the swelling that can occur in masticatory myositis may be due, at least in part, to ischemic damage resulting from compartment syndrome initiated by increased pressure within inflamed muscle. *Atrophic myositis is the result of prominent atrophy of temporal and masseter muscles.* The masticatory muscles of dogs have a unique myosin isoform, known as *type 2M myosin. Dogs with masticatory myositis have antibodies directed against this unique myosin isoform*, and diagnostic testing for type 2M antibodies in canine serum is available. It has been proposed that various bacterial infections may result in antibodies that cross-react between bacterial antigens and type 2M myosin. In addition,

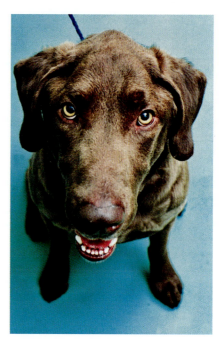

Figure 3-84 Chronic **masticatory myositis** in a dog; severe atrophy of masticatory muscles. (Courtesy W. Hornbuckle.)

antibodies to myositigen, a masticatory muscle protein in the myosin binding protein C family, have been identified in dogs with masticatory myositis.

Affected dogs are unable to fully open the mouth (*trismus*). Muscle swelling or atrophy is most obvious in the temporal and masseter muscles and is bilateral (Fig. 3-84). Pain upon opening the jaw is common, and jaw immobility persists during general anesthesia. Swelling of muscle may result in a degree of exophthalmos. Attacks, if untreated, last up to 2-3 weeks and the periods between attacks may be a few weeks, months, or 2-3 years. If left unchecked, *this inflammatory myopathy leads to progressive destruction of the muscles of mastication and permanent inability to fully open the jaw*. Muscle atrophy gradually becomes very obvious and the head appears to have a fine fox-like contour with unusual prominence of the zygomatic arches.

This disorder occurs in many breeds, although the *German Shepherd* breed appears to be predisposed. Serum activities of CK and AST may be normal, or may be mildly to moderately increased. Masticatory myositis with a strong eosinophilic inflammatory component may be accompanied by peripheral blood eosinophilia, but this is not a consistent finding. Clinical response to immunosuppressive doses of corticosteroids may be rapid, but cases may relapse once corticosteroid therapy is discontinued. *Masticatory myositis is progressive*, but now that this disorder is often recognized and treated in early stages, fewer chronic cases are presented for postmortem examination. Affected dogs may, however, develop aspiration pneumonia or complications of corticosteroid therapy leading to death or euthanasia.

Grossly visible changes in the muscle vary with the stage of disease. The acutely affected muscles are swollen, dark red, doughy or hard, and the cut surface reveals hemorrhagic streaks and irregular yellow-white patches. In the late stages, there is advanced atrophy and fibrosis.

Histologically, this disorder most often has *multifocal polyphasic necrosis. Inflammatory infiltrates are interstitial and often perivascular.* Previous corticosteroid therapy can reduce and alter the inflammatory component present. Eosinophils may or may not be the predominant cell type seen in affected muscle, but, if present, *eosinophils will always be admixed with lymphocytes.* Eosinophils can be seen in muscle damaged by a variety of insults. The primary inflammatory cells causing destruction of myofibers in masticatory muscle myositis of dogs are lymphocytes, presumably recruited following binding of antibody. Lymphocytes may be admixed with plasma cells, and plasma cells may predominate in some cases. Immunophenotyping of lymphocytic infiltrates in masticatory myositis reveals a *mixture of T cells and B cells, with more CD4+ T cells than CD8+ T cells*. These findings help to distinguish masticatory myositis from polymyositis involving masticatory muscles, in which infiltrating lymphocytes are T cells, with more CD8+ T cells than CD4+ T cells (see Polymyositis section). Macrophages are also prominent in cases with marked myofiber necrosis. Sarcolemmal expression of major histocompatibility complex (MHC) class I and class II antigens in canine masticatory myositis and inflammatory cell infiltration have been found to be independent events, suggesting that MHC expression may play a role in this condition. Fiber atrophy is common, and atrophic fibers can be seen associated with inflammation (Fig. 3-85) or with dense fibrosis.

Histologic examination of muscle from suspect masticatory myositis dogs often can be frustrating. The inflammatory lesions are patchy in some cases, and biopsy may reveal only generalized fiber atrophy. *Any evidence of fiber degeneration or regeneration, even in the absence of obvious inflammation, should be considered suspicious if the clinical history is consistent with masticatory myositis.* Examination for evidence of endomysial and perimysial fibrosis is important, as severe fibrosis will negatively impact on the prognosis for return of full jaw mobility and muscle mass. Those cases with numerous inflammatory cells and minimal fibrosis are more likely to recover with corticosteroid therapy than cases in which inflammatory infiltrates are minimal and fibrosis is the predominant finding. An apparent increase in connective tissue may also occur because of loss of damaged myofibers and condensation of existing fibrous stroma.

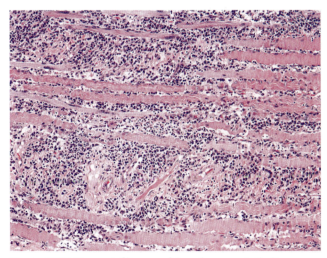

Figure 3-85 Dense infiltrates of lymphocytes, including many plasma cells, separating myofibers in temporal muscle from a dog with **masticatory myositis**. This is a particularly florid lesion. H&E stain.

The masticatory muscles of dogs, especially the temporal muscles, appear to be particularly prone to a variety of generalized myopathic and systemic disorders. Dogs with X-linked muscular dystrophy have prominent atrophy of the temporal muscle and are unable to fully open their mouths, although this condition is not painful. Labrador Retrievers with inherited myopathy also have prominent temporal muscle atrophy. Polymyositis (see later) may appear primarily as a problem with muscles of mastication, although careful evaluation will reveal abnormalities in other muscles. Dogs with any generalized illness often develop rapid atrophy of the temporal muscles that resolves with treatment for the primary problem. Persistent bilaterally symmetric atrophy of masticatory muscles not associated with pain, immobility of the jaw, or generalized disease also occurs in dogs. These latter cases of masticatory muscle atrophy appear to be idiopathic and are not associated with inflammation. If atrophy of temporal and/or masseter muscle occurs unilaterally, denervation atrophy is most likely.

Polymyositis of dogs

Immune-mediated polymyositis occurs most commonly in dogs. Dogs with polymyositis may be presented with primary signs of masticatory muscle involvement, and both masticatory myositis and polymyositis should be considered in the differential diagnosis of such dogs. Testing for serum antibodies to type 2M myosin may be useful, as *most dogs with polymyositis do not have serum antibodies to 2M myosin*. It is possible, however, for nonspecific myosin antibodies to be found in the serum of dogs with polymyositis or other myopathies associated with myofiber necrosis. *Muscle fiber damage in polymyositis is mediated by T lymphocytes.*

Polymyositis occurs mostly commonly in *adult dogs of various breeds*, although large breeds are overrepresented and German Shepherds may be predisposed. *A breed-associated polymyositis has been recognized in Newfoundlands* in which signs of muscle weakness may be apparent in dogs as young as 6 months of age. *Clinical signs of polymyositis are variable*, and include exercise intolerance, overall muscle weakness, stiff gait, and muscle atrophy. Muscle pain, elicited by deep muscle palpation, may be evident. Esophageal muscle involvement leads to regurgitation. Fever may also occur. Increase in serum activities of CK and AST is quite variable, and values may be within normal limits. Polymyositis may occur as part of the spectrum of disease in dogs with *systemic lupus erythematosus*, which is often accompanied by a positive antinuclear antibody (ANA) titer. Dogs with polymyositis can also have concurrent myocarditis, inflammatory bowel disease, and thyroiditis. Polymyositis may also be associated with neoplasia in dogs. In particular, a link to round cell tumors such as lymphoma, plasmacytoma, and anaplastic round cell tumor has been postulated. Polymyositis can occur as a paraneoplastic disease in dogs with thymoma. Treatment with immunosuppressive doses of corticosteroids often results in resolution of signs, although if esophageal muscle fibrosis has occurred there will be persistent esophageal dysfunction. The ability to successfully treat canine polymyositis in chronic phases in which there is extensive fiber loss and fibrosis is much reduced as compared with treatment in early stages of the disease.

Gross pathologic findings include mild to severe generalized muscle atrophy. In cases with esophageal involvement, *dilation of the esophagus may be evident*. Examination of multiple samples from different sites on the head and limbs may be necessary to detect inflammatory lesions. The disorder is *multifocal and polyphasic. The most common finding is of interstitial and perivascular lymphocytic infiltration in affected muscle* (see Fig. 3-82). *Invasion of otherwise intact skeletal muscle fibers by lymphocytes is characteristic* (see Fig. 3-83). Regenerating fibers as well as degenerating fibers are common, and eosinophils also can be seen (Fig. 3-86), and severe chronic disease may result in some degree of endomysial/perimysial fibrosis. Fibrosis may be most apparent in masticatory muscles and in the esophageal wall. Immunophenotypic studies have confirmed that, similar to polymyositis in humans, *invading lymphocytes in canine polymyositis are primarily cytotoxic (CD8+) T cells* (Fig. 3-87A, B). Infiltrates of B lymphocytes, as seen in masticatory myositis (see Masticatory myositis of dogs), are not found in polymyositis. An admixture of eosinophils and neutrophils, however, can be seen in particularly florid lesions.

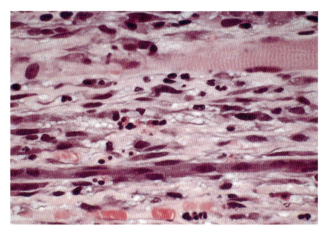

Figure 3-86 **Polymyositis** in a dog. There is a regenerating myotube as well as active inflammation consisting of eosinophils and lymphocytes.

Other immune-mediated myositides of dogs

*A bilateral extraocular muscle myositis involving only the **extraocular rectus and oblique muscles** has been described in dogs.* The retractor bulbi and all other skeletal muscles are normal. Golden Retriever dogs appear to be predisposed. This disorder affects young to young-adult dogs, with age range of onset from about 6 to 18 months. *Clinical signs are of sudden onset of bilateral nonpainful exophthalmos.* Gross lesions of swelling and pallor can be seen within extraocular muscles. *Interstitial lymphocytic inflammatory cell infiltrates are associated with myofiber necrosis and regeneration in a multifocal polyphasic pattern.* Given the localization within extraocular muscles, an immune-mediated disorder directed at a unique epitope within these muscles is suspected. Corticosteroid therapy is usually curative, which supports an immune-mediated basis for this disorder.

An inflammatory myopathy leading to severe tongue atrophy has been described in *Pembroke Welsh Corgi dogs in Japan*. Affected dogs have tongue and facial muscle atrophy. Histopathologic findings are myofiber atrophy with intramuscular fibrosis and fat infiltration, with moderate to severe infiltrates of predominantly B lymphocytes and macrophages. No antibodies to type 2M fibers have been detected, but an autoantibody that binds a 42-kDa molecule in skeletal muscle has been identified by western blot analysis.

An inflammatory myopathy with histopathologic features similar to polymyositis, including infiltration by T lymphocytes, has been described in 2 *adult Boxer dogs*. Severe progressive dysphagia was the presenting sign. Inflammation was predominantly found within thyropharyngeal, tongue, and masseter muscles. One dog had been treated with corticosteroids with no apparent clinical response.

Polymyositis of cats

Most reported cases of polymyositis in cats have instead proved to be degenerative polymyopathy resulting from hypokalemia. A

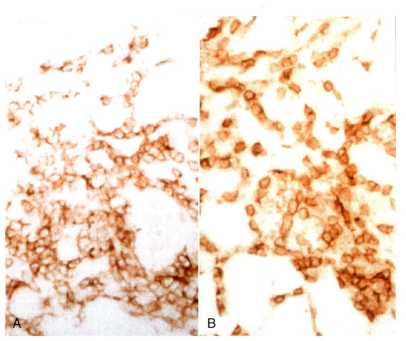

Figure 3-87 Immunophenotyping of cellular infiltrates in muscle from a dog with **polymyositis**. **A.** Infiltrating cells are **CD3+** T lymphocytes. **B.** Infiltrating T lymphocytes are further characterized to be **CD8β+** cytotoxic T cells. Immunohistochemistry.

lymphocytic polymyositis associated with retroviral disease has been identified in adult cats experimentally infected with feline immunodeficiency virus (FIV). Clinical signs of neuromuscular dysfunction are not apparent, but serum activity of CK is moderately increased. Inflammation has the typical interstitial and perivascular pattern of immune-mediated myositis. Infiltration of muscle and myofiber necrosis of multiple muscles is mediated by cytotoxic CD8+ T lymphocytes. Other lymphocyte subsets are not found. Pelvic limb musculature is more commonly affected than thoracic limb muscles. This disorder in cats is similar to HIV-associated polymyositis in people and SIV-associated polymyositis in monkeys. A severe chronic polymyositis associated with progressive weakness and muscle atrophy has been reported in a captive Bengal tiger. Histopathologic evidence of a multifocal and polyphasic myositis characterized by interstitial infiltrates of lymphocytes and invasion of intact myofibers by mononuclear cells typical of polymyositis were seen. Because this case occurred before the recognition of FIV infection in cats, it is tempting to speculate that this may also have been viral associated.

Immune-mediated myositis of horses

Although exertional and postanesthetic myopathies in horses are often called "myositis," this term is not appropriate for these conditions. These disorders are degenerative myopathies and are not primary inflammatory conditions.

An interstitial lymphocytic myositis suspected to be immune-mediated occurs in horses but is uncommon. Infiltrating cells are predominantly T cells.

Hemorrhagic necrosis of muscle resulting from vascular injury occurs in horses with immune-complex disease caused by *Streptococcus equi*–associated *purpura hemorrhagica*. In some cases, the involvement of skeletal muscle is severe enough for neuromuscular dysfunction to be the primary presenting sign. Affected horses typically have markedly increased serum activities of CK and AST associated with muscle weakness and pain. Dependent edema also can be seen. *Hemorrhagic infarcts can be found within affected muscles, and fibrinoid necrosis of vascular walls and vasculitis are seen in tissue sections* (Fig. 3-88). Inflammatory infiltrates are not seen except at the periphery of necrotic zones. Infarcts in other organs, such as lung and intestine, are common. *Streptococcus equi* often can be isolated from lymph nodes or guttural pouches. Immune complexes in purpura hemorrhagica are composed of IgA and streptococcal M protein.

Another syndrome of degenerative myopathy and rapid muscle atrophy occurs in young to young-adult Quarter Horses after exposure to *Streptococcus equi*. Skeletal muscle appears to be the only tissue affected in these horses. The cause is not yet known, although cross-reacting antibodies to streptococci affecting skeletal muscle myosin have been proposed.

Acquired myasthenia gravis

Two clearly defined types of myasthenia gravis occur in dogs and cats. The *congenital disease* is due to abnormal neuromuscular junction formation and is discussed in the section on Congenital myasthenia gravis. The *acquired disease* occurs when circulating antibodies to motor end plate acetylcholine receptors bind and form immune complexes at the neuromuscular junction. The cross-linking of bound antibodies leads to increased endocytosis of acetylcholine receptors and therefore reduction in receptor density.

As in people, a link between thymic abnormalities and development of acquired myasthenia gravis occurs in dogs and cats. *Thymic follicular hyperplasia or thymoma is associated with development of myasthenia gravis in people, and thymoma can cause myasthenia gravis in dogs and cats.* The normal thymus contains myoid cells that express muscle proteins and acetylcholine receptors. The presence of these cells is thought to be important for induction of self-recognition of these proteins. Myoid cells are readily seen by light microscopy in the thymus of neonatal or late-term aborted ruminants. Myoid cells occur in the thymic medulla and consist of large round cells with central euchromatic nuclei and abundant eosinophilic cytoplasm. These cells are scattered amongst the epithelial cells of Hassall's corpuscles, and express muscle actin and myoglobin with immunohistochemical procedures. It is thought that abnormal immune regulation occurs because of thymoma. Removal of the thymic mass often results in resolution of signs of thymoma-induced myasthenia gravis.

Acquired myasthenia gravis in dogs also has been *associated with concurrent hypothyroidism*, and sporadic cases have occurred apparently *associated with malignant neoplasia*. In most cases, myasthenia gravis occurs unassociated with an underlying neoplastic or systemic disease process. Three clinical forms of acquired myasthenia gravis are recognized in dogs.

- The classic form is the *generalized form* in which episodic weakness, primarily of appendicular muscles, leads to exercise-induced collapse. Signs of weakness are alleviated by rest. Generalized myasthenia may also appear as selective and persistent weakness primarily of pelvic limbs. Megaesophagus is common in generalized myasthenia gravis in dogs.
- A *localized form* with selective involvement of esophageal, facial, and pharyngeal muscle leads to megaesophagus and regurgitation without generalized weakness.
- The third form is *a fulminating form* in which rapid development of sustained generalized weakness occurs.

Breeds at risk for development of acquired myasthenia gravis include German Shepherds, Golden Retrievers, Akitas, terrier breeds, German Shorthaired Pointers, and Chihuahuas. An inherited predisposition to myasthenia gravis has been described in Newfoundland dogs and the occurrence of

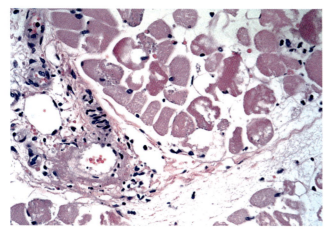

Figure 3-88 *Streptococcus equi*–associated **purpura hemorrhagica** involving skeletal muscle. Acute myofiber necrosis is associated with fibrinoid necrosis of the wall of an interstitial blood vessel. H&E stain. (From Zachary JF, McGavin MD. Pathologic Basis of Veterinary Disease. 5th ed. St. Louis: Mosby/Elsevier; 2012.)

adult-onset myasthenia gravis in 3 Great Dane littermate dogs supports the possibility of a genetic predisposition to development of this immune-mediated disease. But most cases appear to be sporadic.

A bimodal age distribution occurs in dogs, with peak incidences of acquired myasthenia gravis occurring at ~3 years of age and at ~10 years of age. There does not appear to be a sex predisposition in dogs. Only the generalized form of myasthenia gravis has been reported in cats, and Abyssinian cats may be predisposed.

Diagnosis of myasthenia gravis can be made in many cases with *electrodiagnostic testing*, using repetitive nerve stimulation, in which a decremental response in the amplitude of the compound motor action potential is demonstrated. A positive response to anticholinesterase therapy (edrophonium) is also considered diagnostic. *Detection of circulating antiacetylcholine receptor antibodies is considered the most definitive test.*

Abnormalities are not seen in muscle or peripheral nerves by light microscopy, but immune complexes can be detected at neuromuscular junctions using immunohistochemical procedures. Reduction in acetylcholine receptor density resulting from increased internalization of receptors can be demonstrated with specialized techniques such as bungarotoxin binding assay. Simplification of synaptic clefts is seen on ultrastructural examination. Dogs with associated megaesophagus often have concurrent aspiration pneumonia.

To date, thymic follicular hyperplasia has not been described as a cause of myasthenia gravis in animals. Thymoma can be associated with either the generalized form or the fulminant form of myasthenia gravis in dogs, and with generalized myasthenia gravis in cats.

Further reading

Evans J, et al. Canine inflammatory myopathies: a clinicopathologic review of 200 cases. J Vet Intern Med 2004;18:679-691.

Kaese HJ, et al. Infarctive purpura hemorrhagica in five horses. J Am Vet Med Assoc 2005;226:1893-1898.

Paciello O, et al. Expression of major histocompatibility complex class I and class II antigens in canine masticatory muscle myositis. Neuromusc Dis 2007;17:313-320.

Pumarola M, et al. Canine inflammatory myopathy: analysis of cellular infiltrates. Muscle Nerve 2004;29:782-789.

Shelton GD. Myasthenia gravis and disorders of neuromuscular transmission. Vet Clin North Am Small Anim Pract 2002;32:189-206.

Shelton GD. From dog to man: The broad spectrum of inflammatory myopathies. Neuromusc Dis 2007;17:663-670.

Sponseller BT, et al. Severe acute rhabdomyolysis associated with *Streptococcus equi* infection in four horses. J Am Vet Med Assoc 2005;227:1800-1807.

MYOSITIS RESULTING FROM INFECTION

Depending on the nature of the causative agent, *myositis resulting from infection can be suppurative, granulomatous, or necrotizing, hemorrhagic, and edematous.* Pyogenic organisms can cause cellulitis as well as myositis or can organize to form muscle abscesses.

Suppurative myositis

Abscesses in muscle can be due to hematogenous bacterial infection, but more often they result from *inoculation*

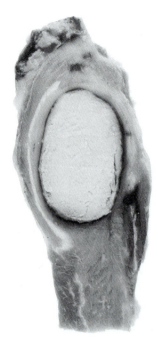

Figure 3-89 Abscess in the gluteal muscles of a goat. (Courtesy W. Hadlow.)

(penetrating wound, contaminated injection, contamination of surgical site or laceration), or by *extension from a suppurative focus* in adjacent structures, such as joints, tendon sheaths, or lymph nodes. The most common causes of abscesses in muscle are *Trueperella pyogenes* in cattle and swine; *Corynebacterium pseudotuberculosis* in sheep, goats, and horses; *Streptococcus equi* in horses; and *Pasteurella multocida* in cats. Acute cellulitis and myositis may occur in *Haemophilus parasuis* infection (Glasser's disease) in swine.

The development of an intramuscular abscess is comparable to abscess development elsewhere. The early stage consists of *local, ill-defined, cellulitis*. Healing may take place after this with a minimum of scarring, or it may proceed to the formation of a *typical abscess with a liquefied center, a pyogenic membrane, and an outer fibrous sheath* (Fig. 3-89). The lesion may slowly organize if it is effectively sterilized, expand if it is not or, alternatively, fistulate to the surface, collapse, and heal.

In horses, *Corynebacterium pseudotuberculosis* abscesses within muscle are most common in the axillary and triceps region. Swelling of infected pectoral muscle has led to the name *pigeon fever*. Another common name is *dryland distemper*, although cases occurring in horses in the Willamette Valley of Oregon indicate that infection can also occur in moist climates. Cases are most common in the fall. Lameness is a common clinical sign that can occur without obvious muscle swelling. Infection by *Corynebacterium pseudotuberculosis* can also lead to purpura hemorrhagica.

Clostridial myositis

Clostridial infection of muscle is common and is an important disease in livestock. Several clostridial organisms can cause myositis, most commonly *Clostridium septicum*, *C. chauvoei*, *C. perfringens*, *C. novyi*, and *C. sordellii*. Mixed infection is also possible. Muscle necrosis is the characteristic lesion, with various degrees of edema, hemorrhage, and gas production (Figs. 3-90, 3-91A, B, 3-92). Necrosis of interstitial tissue as

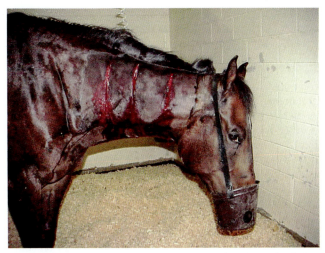

Figure 3-90 Subcutaneous swelling over neck as a result of **clostridial myositis** in a horse. The incisions in the skin have been made to relieve pressure and to expose the lesion to oxygen. (Courtesy D.J. Meuten.)

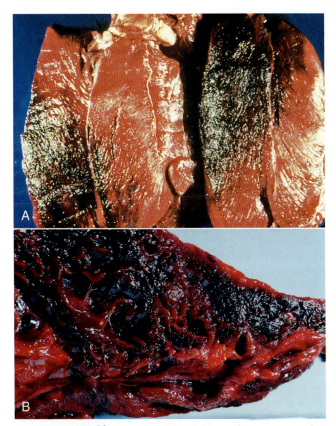

Figure 3-91 **Blackleg** in a cow. **A.** Dark hemorrhagic zones within affected muscle. (Courtesy College of Veterinary Medicine, Cornell University. In: Zachary JF, McGavin MD. Pathologic basis of veterinary diseases, 5th edition. St. Louis, 2012, Mosby/Elsevier.) **B.** Muscle bundles separated by hemorrhage and gas bubbles. (Courtesy Dr. M.D. McGavin, College of Veterinary Medicine, University of Tennessee. In: Zachary JF, McGavin MD. Pathologic basis of veterinary diseases, 5th edition. St. Louis, 2012, Mosby/Elsevier.)

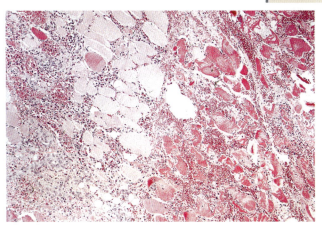

Figure 3-92 Separation of necrotic myofibers by edema and hemorrhage in muscle from a cow with **clostridial myositis (blackleg)**. There is little inflammatory response. H&E stain.

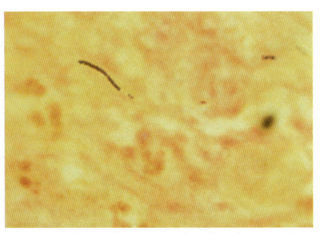

Figure 3-93 Clostridial organisms within affected tissue are **large gram-positive bacilli**. Gram stain.

well as muscle is typical. Tissue damage and systemic illness are due to production of bacterial exotoxins, and *clostridial myositis is often fatal*. Clinically recognized syndromes of clostridial myositis are *malignant edema, gas gangrene, blackleg and pseudo-blackleg*. These clinical syndromes have been linked to specific clostridial organisms, but considerable overlap exists. For example, malignant edema can be caused by *C. novyi, C. septicum, C. chauvoei*, and *C. sordellii*. Gas gangrene can be caused by *C. novyi, C. perfringens*, and *C. septicum*. The only organism-specific disease is blackleg caused by *C. chauvoei*. In many cases it might be best to use a general term of *clostridial myositis*. Clinical and postmortem findings do not reliably distinguish the different syndromes. Diagnosis must rely on laboratory identification of the organism involved, such as by anaerobic culture or fluorescent antibody testing. Bacteria within the lesion can be sparse or abundant, and can sometimes be demonstrated in histologic or cytologic preparations (Fig. 3-93). Care must be taken to distinguish pathogenic organisms from clostridia invading tissue because of postmortem overgrowth.

Clostridia are gram-positive, anaerobic, spore-forming bacilli that occur within soil and feces. Clostridial infection occurs within damaged muscle with reduced oxygen tension, which allows for vegetative growth from spores and production of exotoxins. Once the bacteria are established and producing toxins, they cause additional necrosis allowing spread of infection. Traumatic injury that can lead to clostridial myositis can be bruising or perforation (including injection of nonantibiotic substances). Dormant clostridial spores within muscle are thought to be the cause of infection associated with muscle bruising, and wound contamination is suspected in infections at sites of perforating wounds. Clostridial myositis is most common in ruminants, horses, and swine.

Malignant edema and gas gangrene

Malignant edema often is due to *C. septicum*, and gas gangrene often is due to *C. perfringens*. Both malignant edema and gas gangrene are associated with muscular hemorrhage and edema as well as necrosis (see Fig. 3-90). When gas is produced within the lesion the term gas gangrene is appropriate. In the absence of gas, malignant edema is the usual term. *These infections are due to wound infection, but activation of dormant spores within muscle is also possible.* Horses with injection site infections are also often horses that have been treated for colic, and it has been proposed that clostridia that have entered the bloodstream through compromised gastrointestinal mucosa can "seed" muscle damaged by the injection. Deep wounds are the most likely to develop clostridial infection. In addition to injection sites, common causes of such wounds in animals are castration, shearing, penetrating stake wounds, and injuries to female genitalia during parturition.

In malignant edema and gas gangrene, there is extensive necrosis of muscle with serosanguineous exudate. When lysis of exuded red cells occurs, the tissues become stained darkly by free hemoglobin as well as hemorrhage (see Fig. 3-91A, B). The tissues have a rancid odor in the beginning and an exceedingly foul odor in the end.

Histologically, *edema fluid*, poor in protein, often accompanied by hemorrhage, separates necrotic muscle fibers from each other and the endomysium. *Neutrophils are not numerous*; a few are loosely scattered at the advancing margin of the lesion, but they are rapidly and effectively destroyed by the toxins (see Fig. 3-92). Deeper within the lesions, muscle fibers are fragmented. *Bacteria are seldom numerous in the lesions.*

It is not uncommon for animals to die within 24 hours of the onset of local signs of **gas gangrene**. Invasion, sometimes massive, of the bloodstream occurs shortly before death, or shortly after, and the offending organisms can then be obtained from most tissues. As well as the local lesion, at postmortem there is *severe pulmonary congestion* and evidence of *profound postmortem degradation of internal organs*. Within a few hours of death there is extensive gas formation in all organs, which then crepitate. The liver, especially, may be honey-combed with bubbles, and cut blood vessels may continuously release gas bubbles.

In rams, wound infection by *C. novyi* causes a condition known as **"swelled head."** The wounds are acquired on the top of the head during fighting. This is a rapidly fatal condition, death usually occurring within 48 hours. There is extensive infiltration of clear, gelatinous fluid in the tissues of the head, throat, neck, and cranial thorax and sometimes also in the pleural and pericardial sacs. There is no discoloration of muscle and no, or scant, extravasation of erythrocytes. The bacilli are very few in number and can only be cultured from the primary focus of infection. *Clostridium novyi* may also predominate in wound infections of horses and, when it does, these lesions are also a nonhemorrhagic variety of malignant edema.

Blackleg

Blackleg, also known as black quarter and emphysematous gangrene, is a gangrenous myositis of ruminants caused by C. chauvoei and characterized by the activation of latent spores in muscle. This definition of blackleg separates it from gas gangrene in which, if *C. chauvoei* is involved, it is as a wound contaminant.

Blackleg occurs most often in cattle and sheep and rarely in other domestic animals. Blackleg in **cattle** primarily affects animals 9 months to 2 years of age with a reduced incidence at 6-9 months and 2-3 years, and an even lower incidence in animals >3 years of age. It affects animals in good condition, and often selectively causes death in the best-grown or best-fattened animals in a group. *Blackleg is chiefly a disease of pastured animals with a tendency to be seasonal in summer.* It is often associated with moist pastures and rapid growth of both forage and cattle, but it is also a problem on some arid ranges. Because the source of *C. chauvoei* organisms appears to be persistent on certain fields, it has been assumed that the organism is soil-borne, but it is unlikely that it grows in soil. Growth does take place readily in the intestinal tract of cattle, and it is now thought that soil contamination persists by a process of constant replenishment by fecal contamination.

The detailed pathogenesis of blackleg is still somewhat uncertain, but many of the critical points in the following proposed sequence of events have been confirmed in the natural disease and in experimental infections in cattle. *The infection is acquired by the ingestion of spores,* and either these spores, or spores produced following one or more germinative cycles in the gut, are taken across the intestinal mucosa in some way. *Spores are distributed to tissues, including muscle, where they may survive for long periods. The latent spores in muscle are stimulated to germinate when a local event creates muscle damage or low oxygen tension.* It appears that all that is required to establish a medium for the organisms to multiply is a small intramuscular hemorrhage or a hypoxic degenerative focus initiated by traumatic damage to muscle. Additional tissue damage is due to various bacterial exotoxins, including neuraminidase.

The clinical manifestations of blackleg are often not observed and because of the rapid clinical course, *animals are often found dead*. When animals are seen ill, signs consist of lameness, swelling, and crepitation of the skin over a thigh or shoulder if the lesion is superficial, and fever. It is typical for swellings to increase rapidly in size and to be hot initially and cold later. Affected animals subsequently show depression and circulatory collapse. *Death rapidly ensues and seldom does an animal survive >24-36 hours after the onset of any signs of lameness.* If the muscle lesions are deep within a muscle mass or in the diaphragm, no localizing signs may be evident and no palpable changes detectable. Similarly, lesions in the tongue, heart, or sublumbar muscles may escape clinical detection.

An animal that has died of blackleg swells and bloats rapidly, but on incision it is often not as putrid as its external appearance suggests. Blood-stained froth flows from the nose but not usually from other orifices. Blotchy hemorrhages may be present on the conjunctivae. A poorly circumscribed swelling may be visible on superficial inspection and crepitation detectable on palpation. The skin overlying crepitant swellings is taut and resonant, but normal or dark in color and of normal strength. The subcutaneous tissues and fascia around the lesion are thick with yellow gelatinous fluid that is copiously blood-stained close to the lesion. Gas bubbles may be apparent in the fluid. Muscle affected by blackleg often smells sweet and butyric, like rancid butter.

The lesions of blackleg are usually found in the large muscles of the pectoral and pelvic girdles, but they may be found in any striated muscle including the myocardium. Lesions in the crura of the diaphragm and in the tongue are quite common, and if lesions are present in 2 or 3 sites simultaneously, they may be lethal before any of them is very large. This makes their clinical detection more difficult, and their detection at postmortem dependent on detailed examination of many muscles. Even with small widely separated lesions, however, the rancid butter odor may be pervasive.

In addition to the specific muscle lesions of blackleg, changes are present in the rest of the carcass. *There is severe and rapid postmortem degeneration of internal organs.* There is often *fibrinohemorrhagic pleuritis.* The parietal pleura is hemorrhagic, and large or delicate blood-stained clots of fibrin overlie the ventral mediastinum and epicardium. Pneumonia is not part of the intrathoracic lesion, but the lungs are congested, and they may be quite edematous. The myocardium may be pale and friable, or dark red; some of the latter areas contain foci of *emphysematous myocarditis and necrosis.* It is these areas that give rise to fibrinohemorrhagic pericarditis. Endocardial lesions sometimes occur, particularly in young animals. The endocardium is hemorrhagic and may be ulcerated or contain thrombi. If there is atrioventricular valve involvement, it is usually on the right side. Organisms often can be recovered from many organs and from the blood shortly after death. Because *C. chauvoei* is not a postmortem contaminant, identification of *C. chauvoei* is diagnostic.

Blackleg in **sheep** closely resembles the disease in cattle and the causative organism is the same. *The disease in sheep, however, is much less common than in cattle,* and although there is some overlap in enzootic distribution, *the disease in sheep usually occurs in locales quite apart from those where it occurs in cattle.* The clinical signs are similar to those in cattle except that crepitation may not be palpable during life, and there is usually dark discoloration of the overlying skin. The lesions resemble those in cattle, but there are usually fewer gas bubbles, and the muscle remains moister.

Pseudo-blackleg

Pseudo-blackleg is due to *C. septicum* infection and closely mimics blackleg. This disease of cattle produces lesions that are deep within muscle, like those of blackleg. A diagnosis of pseudo-blackleg is made when there is no detectable wound, the lesion is deeply located, and *C. septicum* is demonstrated in the lesions of a carcass examined immediately after death. This latter precaution is necessary to avoid, as far as possible, misdiagnosis based on the postmortem invasion of *C. septicum* and other organisms from the alimentary tract.

The lesions of pseudo-blackleg differ quantitatively and somewhat qualitatively, from those of blackleg. They tend to be multiple in widely separated muscles. There is very extensive blood-stained gelatinous exudate in the connective tissues, and this exudate contains only occasional small gas bubbles. The lesions may become confluent as very large patches throughout the connective tissues. *The muscle lesions, although always present, are less extensive than in blackleg.* The muscles are dark red and moist, and only after examination by multiple incisions is the lack of a distinct primary focus evident. When

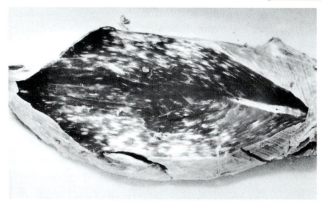

Figure 3-94 Disseminated pale areas of myonecrosis in **foot-and-mouth disease** in a calf. (Courtesy W. Hadlow.)

bubbles of gas are present in necrotic muscle, they are smaller and not as numerous as they are in blackleg.

Pseudo-blackleg is reported in *pigs* in which the muscle lesions are part of a generalized body invasion by *C. septicum* organisms following entry via a primary gastric focus.

Specific infectious diseases with muscle alterations

Muscle lesions can occur in *foot-and-mouth disease* of calves (see Vol. 2, Alimentary system), *bluetongue* of sheep (see Vol. 2, Alimentary system), *Teschen disease* of swine, and leptospirosis (*Leptospira icterohaemorrhagiae*) of dogs. In 5-10% of calves affected with foot-and-mouth disease, pale areas with or without white streaks of mineralization are present (Fig. 3-94) and represent areas of necrosis histologically. Myocarditis also may be found in calves. Sheep with bluetongue may have scattered small hemorrhagic lesions in skeletal muscle. Microscopic findings are myofiber necrosis, vasculitis, and hemorrhage.

Granulomatous lesions

Various diseases discussed elsewhere may produce granulomatous lesions in skeletal muscle. *Actinobacillosis* ("wooden tongue" in cattle) (see Vol. 2, Alimentary system), *actinomycosis* ("lumpy jaw in cattle") (see Vol. 1, Bones and joints), and *tuberculosis* are examples.

Beef cattle given injections of oil-adjuvant bacterins into paravertebral muscles may develop pyogranulomatous myositis with extension into the vertebral canal. Affected cattle showed lameness and paraparesis.

Other diseases with granulomatous lesions in skeletal muscle are *botryomycosis* and *Roeckl's granuloma* described in detail later.

Staphylococcal granuloma

Chronic granulomas of muscle or connective tissue caused by staphylococci, and referred to as **botryomycosis** in early literature, are much less common than they once were, but they still occur, particularly in the *horse and pig.* They represent a persistent, low-grade infection by *Staphylococcus aureus*, but it is not clear why the same organism at other times produces a conventional abscess or a gangrenous phlegmon. In horses, lesions are most frequent on the neck and pectoral region ("breast boils"), whereas in the pig, castration wounds and the mammary glands are the most common sites.

The lesion begins as a microabscess around a small colony of organisms and progresses rapidly, sometimes to a very large size. The *fully formed granuloma* is a hard, nodular, gray-white mass of dense, fibrous tissue, irregularly cavitated by small abscesses. The abscesses may be joined by tracts or they may fistulate to the surface. They contain a small quantity of thick, orange-yellow pus, which in turn contains minute granules. The granules consist of a central colony of the organisms, whereas the bulk of the granule mass is made up of "clubs" of reactive protein material; hence the *typical club colony of botryomycosis*. Histologically, the organisms are readily visible in tissues because they stain with hematoxylin and are relatively large. Variable numbers of neutrophils, lymphocytes, and plasma cells are present in the loose fibrous tissue outside of the club colony. Muscle is involved at the periphery of the expanding granulomatous lesion where fibrous septa surround fibers causing atrophy and segmental degeneration.

Roeckl's granuloma of cattle

This nodular lesion of skeletal muscle is apparently specific for cattle, and it may be associated with similar lesions in liver, lungs, lymph nodes, and testes. The lesion is sometimes referred to as *nodular necrosis*, and it is well known in Europe but rare elsewhere. Included in the list of suggested causes are tuberculosis, pseudotuberculosis, sarcocystosis, blastomycosis, and larvae of *Hypoderma bovis*, but none has been regularly found in typical lesions. Acid-fast organisms are usually not present, and although *Trueperella pyogenes* is sometimes recovered, it is not considered to be the cause of the multiple granulomas.

The lesions occur in cattle of all ages. In any single animal, nodules are all of the same size but the size varies from one animal to the next, from 0.5 to 5 cm in diameter, in or under the skin. *Sites of predilection are the skin around the base of the tail, the limbs, the withers, and the abdominal wall*, but lesions are seldom seen deep in muscle masses.

When nodules are cut, surfaces tend to bulge and consist of 3 zones. The *central zone* is dry, dull, necrotic-looking, and often distinctly yellow. The *reactive zone* is gray-pink, semi-translucent, and elastic. The *outer layer* is thin, white fibrous tissue that radiates out along trabecular divisions in adjacent muscle. Larger nodules may be laminated, indicating periodic growth, and small nodules may be reduced to a hard scar with or without mineralization.

Histologically, the early stages of Roeckl's granuloma are small abscesses surrounded by granulation tissue that may contain abundant eosinophils. In other animals, the predominant inflammatory cell may be the lymphocyte. Epithelioid cells and a few giant cells may be present in the reactive zone. The capsule is made up of mature collagen. *These lesions seem to be the modified or exaggerated response of a sensitized animal to a persistent or repetitively introduced antigen.*

Changes in muscle secondary to systemic infections

Lesions in muscle caused by the specific presence of an infectious agent are described elsewhere. More common than these lesions of muscle are the degenerative changes of muscle fibers that occur in acute systemic infections such as pneumonic pasteurellosis of cattle ("shipping fever"); these may be the result of endotoxemia. The lesions, although widespread, cannot be appreciated grossly and consist of scattered segmental necrosis of single myofibers or small groups of myofibers (Fig. 3-95).

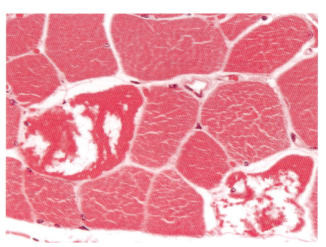

Figure 3-95 Scattered necrotic fiber segments as a result of **endotoxic muscle injury** in a horse.

Further reading

Hauptmann S, et al. Skeletal muscle oedema and muscle fibre necrosis during septic shock. Observations with a porcine septic shock model. Virchows Archiv 1994;424:653-659.

Nogradi N, et al. Musculoskeletal *Corynebacterium pseudotuberculosis* infection in horses; 35 cases (1999-2009). J Am Vet Med Assoc 2012;241:771-777.

Peek SJ, et al. Clostridial myonecrosis in horses (37 cases 1985-2000). Equine Vet J 2003;35:86-92.

Useh NM, et al. Pathogenesis and pathology of blackleg in ruminants; the role of toxins and neuraminidase. A short review. Vet Q 2003;25:155-159.

Valentine BA, Löhr CV. Myonecrosis in three horses with colic: evidence for endotoxic injury. Vet Rec 2007;161:786-789.

PARASITIC DISEASES

Sarcocystosis

Sarcocystis spp. *are protozoal parasites of animal muscle that in many respects resemble coccidia, the main difference being their obligatory development in 2 hosts.* The sexual stages develop in a predator host, whereas the asexual phases develop in the prey animal. Some animals, such as the opossum and humans, are vehicles for both parts of the *Sarcocystis* spp. cycle but not for the same species, there being considerable specificity on the part of both the intermediate and definitive hosts. There is, however, some latitude. For example, several individual parasites develop in dogs, or coyotes, or foxes, or wolves as a definitive host, and a number of intermediate host species of the same general type may be "accidentally" infected at low level. More than 90 *Sarcocystis* species are recognized in mammals, birds, and reptiles, and 14 of these are regularly found in muscles of domestic animals as part of the intermediate host infection. The prevalence of infection in cattle, sheep, and horses can approach 100%, but there is great geographic variation. For example, studies of horses within the United States reveal a prevalence of 0.5-21%, whereas in Mongolia a prevalence of 97.5% has been reported. In llamas in South America, prevalence varies by year studied, up to ~50% of animals studied at slaughter. Where it was once thought that the muscle phase of infection was asymptomatic and safe for the intermediate host, it is now known that particularly the schizogonous phase may cause severe clinical disease and death under both natural and experimental conditions. The production of enteric disease by the sexual phase in the predator host is considered elsewhere (see Vol. 2, Alimentary system). Fetal infection with abortion and neonatal mortality is described in Vol. 3, Female genital system.

Consideration here is primarily given to those *Sarcocystis* spp. infections affecting the muscles of domestic animals as intermediate hosts. *Sporocysts* are ingested when herbage contaminated by carnivore or human fecal material is consumed. *Sporozoites* are released and these invade many tissues. One or 2 generations of *schizogony* take place within endothelial cells, the first in small arterioles, the second (if there is one) in capillaries. The second or third generation of *schizonts* develops within striated muscle fibers as thin-walled cysts initially containing round *metrocytes*, which repeatedly divide to produce numerous banana-shaped *bradyzoites*. The much-enlarged mature cyst persists in muscle for long periods and the cycle is completed when muscle is consumed by the predator host and the *sexual cycle* of the parasite is developed in the intestinal epithelial cells. Large cysts can be seen as discrete pale nodules within affected muscle (Fig. 3-96).

In almost all cases *Sarcocystis* cysts within muscle are found as an incidental finding with no evidence of inflammation or clinical disease (Fig. 3-97). When *clinical disease* occurs in an intermediate host, it may occur at either of 2 stages of the developmental cycle. It may take the form of fever, petechiation of mucous membranes, edema, icterus, and macrocytic hypochromic anemia 3-5 weeks after initial infection and lasting for 6-8 weeks during the *schizogonous (parasitemic)* stage. These signs seem to be related to many small episodes of intravascular coagulation, although endothelial schizonts are not the site of thrombus formation. The parasites are also present in perivascular macrophages. In food and fiber animal species, this acute syndrome has also been called Dalmeny disease. The second stage, in which clinical signs and death may occur, comes as the *schizonts enter muscle at ~40 days after infection*, sometimes with extensive fiber degeneration and marked enzyme release, which attracts macrophages and plasma cells. Another wave of muscle disease may be associated with enlargement of the cysts in a massive infestation and this can cause lameness. Maturation of cysts may take 60-100 days, by which time any tissue reaction has subsided.

Sarcocystis species that have been recognized in the muscles of the **horse** are *S. bertrami* (*S. equicanis*) and *S. fayeri*. Both species complete their cycle in the dog. Cysts in horse muscle are microscopic in size and rarely numerous, but occasionally there is massive involvement of skeletal muscles. The tongue is a common site. Similar to other species, most equine sarcocystosis is an incidental finding. But equine sarcocystosis of the tongue is seen as a localized eosinophilic glossitis with myonecrosis (Fig. 3-98).

Sarcocystis species in **cattle** are presently considered to be: *S. cruzi* with a cycle completed in domestic and wild canids; *S. hirsuta* with a cycle completed in the domestic cat; and *S. hominis* with a cycle completed in humans. Two additional species are found in the water buffalo; *S. fusiformis* with a cat-buffalo cycle, and *S. levinei* with a dog-buffalo cycle. Only *S. cruzi* seems to be capable of causing significant clinical disease in cattle. Clinical signs exhibited during the schizogonous stage may include evidence of hemolysis as described earlier as well as progressive debility, abortion, drooling, lymphadenitis, sloughing of the tip of the tail and, in some outbreaks, death in a high proportion of affected animals. See also Eosinophilic myositis of cattle, sheep, and camelids.

Four species of *Sarcocystis* regularly affect **sheep,** namely *S. tenella* (*S. ovicanis*) and *S. arieticanis*, which have a

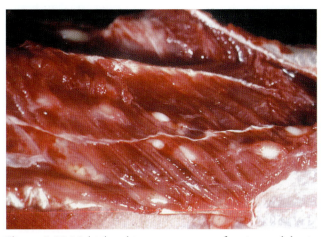

Figure 3-96 Multiple white-tan **sarcocysts** forming nodules in alpaca muscle. (Courtesy College of Veterinary Medicine, Cornell University. From Zachary JF, McGavin MD. Pathologic Basis of Veterinary Disease. 5th ed. St. Louis: Mosby/Elsevier; 2012.)

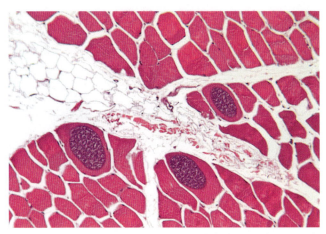

Figure 3-97 **Sarcocysts** as an incidental finding within muscle from a cougar. H&E stain.

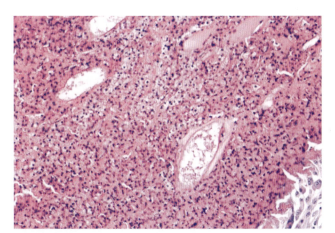

Figure 3-98 Degenerate sarcocysts associated with intense granulomatous inflammation in tongue muscle from a horse with **Sarcocystis glossitis**. H&E stain.

sheep-dog cycle, and *S. gigantea* and *S. medusiformis*, which have a sheep-cat cycle. *Sarcocystis tenella* is quite virulent in lambs if infective doses are large, and naturally occurring encephalomyelitis in mature sheep with neurologic disease has been blamed on this organism. Chronically debilitated sheep often have an enormous number of cysts in their muscles. This ought to have some effect on muscle performance, but lameness is not apparent. *Sarcocystis gigantea* cysts are very large (1-3 mm) and distend segments of esophageal striated muscle fibers well above the adventitial surface of the esophagus. Two species (*S. capricanis* and *S. hericanis*) have a goat-dog cycle, and another (*S. moulei*) has a goat-cat cycle. None appears to be pathogenic for **goats** as natural infections but, experimentally, even moderate levels of infectious sporocysts led to death of some animals.

Three species of *Sarcocystis* are found in **swine**; *S. miescheriana* with a pig-dog and pig-wild Canidae cycle, *S. porcifelis* with a pig-cat cycle, and *S. suihominis*, which completes its cycle in humans. Of the 3, only *S. miescheriana* is known to produce clinical signs of diarrhea, myositis, and lameness.

Sarcocystis organisms have been observed in the muscles of **dogs** and **cats** from time to time. It was thought that these represented host parasites traveling to an abnormal site, but it now appears that such cysts are morphologically unlike the species that originate in the cat or dog and that these species in dogs and cats complete their cycle in the sheep, horse, or cow. Severe myositis caused by *Sarcocystis* infection has been reported in dogs. Sarcocystosis occurs in many wild species; for example, deer have at least 5 distinct species all of which complete their cycle in the dog or in wild canids.

Histologically, *Sarcocystis* organisms are rarely accompanied by an acute inflammatory reaction, and *schizonts in endothelial cells cause little or no evidence of endothelial cell destruction*. As the organisms enter muscle, a wide range of change may be encountered. Usually there is no muscle fiber degeneration but there may be thin, linear collections of lymphocytes between fibers in the region. Sometimes the muscle fiber undergoes segmental hyaline change in the region of the invading parasite and rarely, extensive floccular degeneration of muscle fibers occurs. The extent of muscle change bears little relationship to the numbers of developing cysts, but generally, very low numbers of *Sarcocystis* produce no reaction (see Fig. 3-97).

As cysts mature, and the contained bradyzoites become more distinct, the cyst capsule within the enlarged muscle fiber becomes thicker and more clearly differentiated from the muscle sarcoplasm. Muscle sarcoplasm and muscle nuclei surround the parasite in the early stages. In some parasitic species, the outer capsular zone develops distinct radial striations, which, on electron microscopy, prove to be complex convolutions of the cyst wall. Small pores allow communication between cyst contents and muscle cell content, but apart from the obvious nutritional dependence of the parasite on the muscle fiber, little is known of the biochemical interplay which must take place.

Microscopic inspection of *Sarcocystis*-infected muscle often reveals occasional degenerate parasitic cysts surrounded by variable numbers of inflammatory cells (very few of which are eosinophils), or, at a later state, macrophages and granulation tissue. It is not known whether these represent "over-age" cysts or simply random changes in an easily modified host-parasite relationship. Such reactions in muscle increase with host age.

Eosinophilic myositis of cattle, sheep, and camelids

Eosinophilic myositis *is a relatively rare condition in cattle, sheep, and camelids of all ages* that has some significance for meat inspection because the lesions are usually discovered in skeletal muscle and myocardium of animals slaughtered for human consumption. *Sudden deaths in cattle and sheep have been ascribed to the myocarditis.* The disease is included here because *there is good evidence that eosinophilic myositis in cattle, sheep, and camelids may be caused by degeneration of Sarcocystis* spp. *Sarcocystis* spp. remnants are often found in the center of the lesions, and IgE specific for the parasite is associated with degranulated eosinophils. Animals with parasites but not myositis have serum levels of IgE comparable to those in animals with lesions, suggesting that the inflammatory reaction in eosinophilic myositis is stimulated by parasite cyst rupture. A heat-stable, eosinophil-chemotactic substance has been isolated from affected bovine muscle in which eosinophilic myositis lesions were present. The substance has a molecular size less than bovine albumin, and its activity seems to correlate with lesion size and severity.

The gross lesions of eosinophilic myositis in ruminants are characteristic, being well-demarcated, green, focal stripes or patches that fade to off-white when exposed to air (Fig. 3-99). Some lesions have a brown-green or gray-green color. Single muscles or groups of muscles may be involved or the lesions may be widespread through all muscles, including the heart. Individual lesions may be 2-3 mm to 5-6 cm in diameter in both heart and skeletal muscle, and no part of the muscle mass seems to be exempt.

Histologically, both acute and more chronic fibrotic reactions may exist side by side. The reaction is characterized by large numbers of eosinophils, and it is these that impart the green color to the gross lesion. Dense masses of mature eosinophils separate adjacent endomysial sheaths and perimysial trabeculae (Fig. 3-100). Muscle fiber degeneration is not an obvious feature of the disease, but occasional segments of fibers do undergo hypercontraction and degeneration. These may be later evident only as endomysial sheaths stuffed with

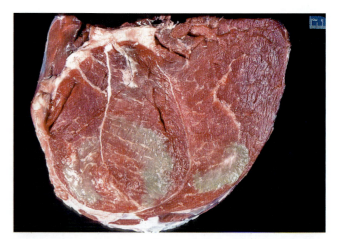

Figure 3-99 Zones of green-bronze discoloration resulting from *Sarcocystis*-associated **eosinophilic myositis** in bovine muscle. (Courtesy Dr. M.D. McGavin, College of Veterinary Medicine, University of Tennessee. From Zachary JF, McGavin MD. Pathologic Basis of Veterinary Disease. 5th ed. St. Louis: Mosby/Elsevier; 2012.)

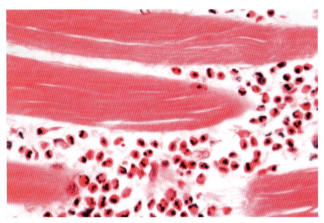

Figure 3-100 Numerous eosinophils infiltrating between myofibers in bovine *Sarcocystis*-associated **eosinophilic myositis**. H&E stain.

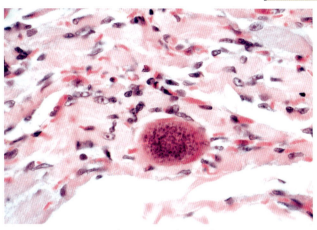

Figure 3-101 Protozoal cyst in a dog with **protozoal myositis**. This organism could be either *Neospora caninum* or *Toxoplasma gondii*. H&E stain.

eosinophils rather than muscle fibers because muscle fiber regeneration seems to be impaired or modified.

With time, fibroplasia is evident. In the chronic lesion, dense collagenous tissue is prominent and the inflammatory cell population changes from eosinophils to a smaller population of lymphocytes, plasma cells, and histiocytes.

In some cases, individual lesions may take on some of the characteristics of a *granuloma* in which central muscle fibers along with adjacent eosinophils undergo degeneration. This central necrotic mass acquires a fringe of epithelioid cells and giant cells, and fibrous tissue becomes circumferentially oriented. The central eosinophilic mass may gather calcium salts, whereas the edge of the lesion consists of infiltrating eosinophils and fibroblasts that radiate into adjacent muscle. Granulomatous lesions leave a small scar, but it is likely that the more diffuse lesions of eosinophilic myositis in cattle can disappear in time with very little residual lesion.

Eosinophilic myositis in *sheep* tends to occur in young animals <2 years of age. Lesions are comparable in distribution and type to those in cattle although the frequency of the granulomatous type of change may be higher.

Toxoplasma and Neospora myositis

In addition to *Sarcocystis*, 2 apicomplexan parasites, *Toxoplasma* and *Neospora*, produce myopathy in several species (Fig. 3-101). Both infections are dealt with more fully elsewhere (see Vol. 2, Alimentary system; and Vol. 1, Nervous system, respectively).

Toxoplasma gondii infections, particularly in puppies and kittens, or in any species of farm animal naturally immunosuppressed, or in animals on immunosuppressive therapy, may massively involve skeletal muscle fibers. *Myositis with mononuclear leukocytic infiltration, myofiber necrosis, and myofiber atrophy is accompanied by polyradiculoneuritis*. In the majority of toxoplasma infections, however, muscle lesions are rare. In muscle fibers, both tachyzoites and thin-walled cysts (bradyzoites) may be present but the former are generally transient, spherical, and nonreactive.

Neospora caninum infections occur worldwide mainly in dogs, but the organisms are also found in cats, and the disease may have originated in the latter species. *The disease is associated with abortion and perinatal mortality in cattle with nonsuppurative encephalitis, myocarditis, and periportal hepatitis in affected animals*. Neosporosis appears to have been present in the United States for >30 years and many of the organisms originally identified in tissue sections as *Toxoplasma* are now recognized as *Neospora*. The 2 organisms can be distinguished definitively by immunoperoxidase procedures. Serologic tests can detect antibodies to *N. caninum* and to *T. gondii*.

Neospora caninum has a greater tendency to produce *myositis* than *Toxoplasma* because the tachyzoites form large fusiform packets in muscle after the second division stage of meronts. When these escape from the muscle fiber in a partially immunized host, an inflammatory reaction, abundant and predominantly histiocytic and plasmacytic, separates individual fibers. There is also segmental muscle fiber degeneration, which may be a response to direct parasite invasion, but is likely the result of a local release of free radicals from inflammatory cells. At this stage, clinical signs of muscle weakness may be obvious and at autopsy, muscles over the entire body may be pale, streaky, and atrophic. Inflammatory lesions often also affect nerves and nerve roots and result in denervation atrophy.

The life cycle and source of infection for neosporosis are unknown. The only known mode of natural infection is transplacental in persistently infected bitches, with affected litters having distinctive clinical features of progressive pelvic limb weakness, muscle atrophy, and joint contracture. The disease has been produced experimentally in immunocompetent cats, but the lesions are more severe in cats given corticosteroids.

Trichinellosis

Muscle is the habitat for encysted larvae of the nematode *Trichinella* spp., which may survive there for many years (Fig. 3-102). Because animal-to-animal transmission of infection is accomplished by the consumption of infected muscle, most of the species regularly involved are carnivores or scavenger species. Humans, dogs, and a variety of wild canids, cats and wild felids, pigs, rats, mustelids, bears, polar bears, raccoons, and mice become hosts to the adult (in the small intestine) and their persistent larvae (within muscle). Other species, including horse and birds, may become infected when muscle tissue is included in their feed; horsemeat has been a natural source of trichinellosis in humans. Trichinellosis is a zoonotic disease sometimes occurring in spectacular

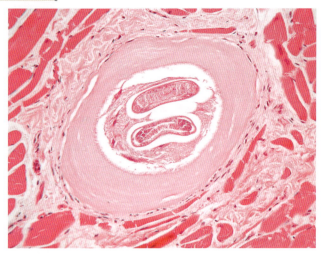

Figure 3-102 *Trichinella spiralis* larvae encysted in muscle. H&E stain. (Courtesy R. Bildfell.)

outbreaks in humans and animals. Humans become infected when they consume uncooked or incompletely cooked meat of pigs, bears, or aquatic mammals. In those regions of the world where inspection of meat is routine, the incidence of infection is very low, but even in countries such as Canada and the United States, the incidence in wild carnivores is 1-10%.

The parasitic cycle for *T. spiralis* begins with ingestion of infected meat. Gastric juices liberate the encysted larvae, which then molt twice, grow to a length of 1-4 mm as thread-like fourth-stage worms, and molt again. Maturity is reached in ~4 days after ingestion, the adults copulate, and the male dies. The ovoviviparous females penetrate via the crypts of Lieberkühn to the submucosal lymphatics, where they deposit 0.1-mm long larvae into lymph vessels. The persistence of females in the duodenum is dependent on the state of surface immunity (probably IgA antibody produced locally in the gut wall) and varies from days to 5-6 weeks. Some larvae may be passed in feces as the female moves out of the duodenal crypts. The remaining larvae migrate with the lymph, then the blood, to reach the pulmonary and systemic circulations. Those that find their way to muscle may achieve a safe haven away from developing immunity by entering a muscle fiber; those that arrive elsewhere may survive for a brief period but are soon destroyed. In a previously sensitized host, few of the ~500 larvae produced by each female are able to enter a muscle fiber in time to ensure survival.

Within the muscle fiber, the larva grows, coils, and enlarges a segment of the host muscle fiber, which is induced to develop some unusual changes as the "nurse cell." Nuclei enlarge, myofibrils are greatly reduced, the basal lamina is very greatly increased in its thickness and number of folds around the affected segment of muscle fiber, and the sarcoplasmic reticulum, which is in intimate contact with the worm, proliferates. Mitochondria in the immediate vicinity increase in number as they are reduced in size. After a month, the larvae are up to 100 μm long and coiled in a figure of 8. There is usually one per fiber. Larvae are not normally visible by naked eye inspection of muscles unless they are old and mineralized. On routine microscopic examination of muscle, larvae lie in bulging glassy segments of muscle fiber that may be loosely encircled by eosinophils, and in due course, by a scattering of lymphocytes, plasma cells, and macrophages. If the parasitized muscle segment degenerates, the larva is exposed and soon dies to become the center of a more acute inflammatory, but still predominantly eosinophilic, reaction. Segments of muscle fiber adjacent to the encysted larva may show evidence of degeneration or subsequent regenerative repair with basophilia and centrally located nuclei. In a heavy infestation, a large proportion of the muscle fibers in preferred muscle sites may be taken up with either the parasite or adjacent reactive zones. Purely physical replacement of functional muscle accounts for most of the clinical signs of infestation when they are present, although usually they are absent.

In 2-3 months, the cellular reaction subsides and the muscle fibers enclosing larvae become further modified to give the impression, on light microscopy, of a fibrous capsule. Because parasite survival can only be assured by intracellular seclusion, the "capsule" is, in reality, modified muscle cell components or, perhaps more correctly, modified satellite cells and basal lamina. Once the larvae are encysted in this way, further change, apart from muscle fiber degeneration, is usually confined to deposition of mineral in the encapsulating muscle structure, but this does not seem to affect parasite viability. *The larvae may survive >20 years*, although the average lifespan is probably a good deal less depending on host longevity and the occurrence of fiber degeneration.

Several features of this parasitism are unexplained, including the distribution of larvae within the host. Certain muscles such as the respiratory and masticatory muscles are preferentially and heavily infected while other muscles contain a reduced burden. Activity alone is not responsible because a paralyzed diaphragm is still preferentially susceptible. Concentration of larvae in preferred sites may be influenced by blood distribution, increased larval survival, the presence of some needed nutrient, or preferential shielding from normal body defense mechanisms. Heart muscle is sometimes involved, but not heavily; *the muscles most involved are tongue, masseter and laryngeal muscles, diaphragm, intercostal muscles,* and *muscles of the eye*, but no striated muscle is exempt. Because some of the selectively involved muscles are small, heavy infestation may have a significant clinical effect in the form of muscle weakness, paralysis, or reduced responsiveness. Usually parasitic infestations of muscle are asymptomatic, and this feature enhances the transfer of infection from animals to humans.

Five species of *Trichinella*, with 8 genotypes identified by DNA analysis, are parasites of muscle:

- *Trichinella spiralis* is the parasite of pigs, rodents, and humans in temperate and tropical climates, and is the most prevalent strain. It is moderately resistant to short-term freezing, and its infectivity is not reduced by freezing and thawing.
- *Trichinella nativa* is found in colder climates and is the species most often encountered in polar bears, bears, aquatic mammals, and the Inuit. Its cycle is similar in most respects to that of *T. spiralis*, but the larval form is much more resistant to freezing for long periods.
- *Trichinella nelsoni* is found in carnivores in eastern and southern Africa and also in central and eastern Europe.
- *Trichinella britovi* has been reported in southern Europe.
- *Trichinella pseudospiralis* is found in northeastern Europe and differs from the other species in its failure to encyst in muscle. The species migrates through muscle more or less continuously under experimental conditions, but appears otherwise to have a cycle similar to that of *T. spiralis*.

Cysticercosis

Many of the larval forms of tapeworms of carnivores develop and temporarily reside in the viscera or other tissues of prey species. A few have a special predilection for skeletal muscles and myocardium, and this much smaller group is dealt with here. The pathologic effects of adult tapeworms in the intestinal tract of the carnivorous host are described in Vol. 2, Alimentary system.

Taenia solium is a large tapeworm (≤8 m long) common in many parts of the world and resident in the intestinal tract of humans and sometimes other primates. The larvae (or metacestode form) usually develop in the pig or wild pig, but for this species of tapeworm humans can sometimes be host to both the tapeworm and the larval cysticercus. Gravid tapeworm segments are passed in feces, and because they are nonmotile, the 40,000 eggs in each segment tend to be concentrated over a small area. Susceptible pigs having access to infected human feces are easily infected. Eggs resist destruction for relatively long periods in soil, moist ground surfaces, or sewage sludge, and survive in flowing water for a while. Following ingestion, the outer shell is digested in the stomach releasing and activating the tiny *oncosphere*, which penetrates the intestinal blood vessels and reaches the general circulation. *Most of the larvae in the pig find their way to heart, masseter, tongue, or shoulder muscles*. When they migrate in humans, they are distributed to connective tissues, brain, and viscera. The larvae become cysticerci (*Cysticercus cellulosae*), enlarge to a cyst with a single inverted scolex, which, when mature, measure 1-2 cm and are easily visible between muscle fibers. Cysticerci are rapidly ensheathed at first in a loose, and then a denser, connective tissue capsule derived from endomysium. A few lymphocytes and a few or many eosinophils lie in the outer regions of the capsule. The cysticercus seems to avoid effective immune-mediated destruction for some time by converting elements of the complement system to inactive products, although in a strongly immunized animal the larvae are eventually destroyed, mineralized, and removed (Fig. 3-103A, B). To allow themselves growing room within developing inelastic collagenous capsules, the cysticerci create a crescentic zone of degenerative lysis (presumed to be induced enzymatically); this can often be seen in histologic sections of encysted metacestodes, as can parts of the scolices and hooks in those species that have them. *Cysticercus cellulosae* has rostellar hooks. The survival time in muscle for *C. cellulosae* is not known, but the question is usually not relevant because *pigs are normally slaughtered at a young age when virtually all cysticerci in muscle are viable*. Humans complete the cycle and become infected when they consume raw or incompletely cooked pork.

Taenia saginata is probably the most common tapeworm in humans; its larvae are in cattle, and are found in most regions of the world. Transfer of the very resistant eggs from the fecund proglottids to calves or cattle is often enhanced by contamination of open water by sewage, or by use of sewage as fertilizer on fields. It also occurs directly by contamination of animal feeds with human feces or from soiled human hands. The life cycle is similar to that described previously for *T. solium and the larval form (Cysticercus bovis) similarly preferentially infests heart and masticatory muscles*, although cysts are often widespread throughout the muscles. Histologically, the reaction to the parasite involves few eosinophils. *Cysticercus bovis* does not have rostellar hooks. Following a period of growth and development of ~10 weeks the larvae become infective. After about another 30 days the cysticerci begin to die, but some larvae may be viable 9 months after infection. Death of the larvae is probably the result of development of an immune reaction. Cattle that have acquired resistance to the invasion of oncospheres across the gut apparently do not have an enhanced capability to cause degeneration of pre-existing muscle cysticerci. Humans acquire infection when they consume inadequately cooked beef or veal.

Taenia ovis is a tapeworm commonly found in dogs and wild carnivores throughout the world that, in its larval form,

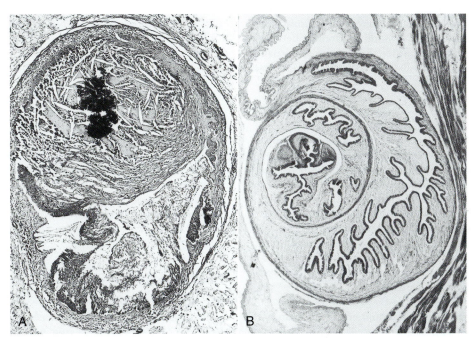

Figure 3-103 A. Degenerating and mineralizing *Cysticercus cellulosae* in the brain of a dog. **B.** *Cysticercus ovis* in the diaphragm of a sheep.

has a cysticercus (*Cysticercus ovis*) that develops in the heart and skeletal muscles of sheep and goats (see Fig. 3-103B). The cycle is similar to that for T. saginata but the larvae do have rostellar hooks, which may sometimes be an aid to histologic identification in lesions even after the cysticercus has begun to disintegrate.

Taenia krabbei is a tapeworm in *wild carnivores* in temperate and arctic climates whose larval form (*Cysticercus tarandi*) is found in reindeer, gazelle, moose, and other wild ruminants. Lesions produced in the intermediate host are similar to those seen in cattle with C. bovis, and a similar cycle is assumed.

Hepatozoonosis

Myositis caused by *Hepatozoon americanum* (initially classified as *H. canis*) was a consistent feature of 15 natural cases of infection in dogs in the southern United States. Cases have been limited mainly to the Gulf Coast area of Louisiana and Texas and from Oklahoma. The disease occurs in a variety of canids and felids in South Africa and the Middle East, and has become established in the dog and brown tick (*Rhipicephalus sanguineus*) populations in North America. Animals become infected by ingesting an infected tick or possibly another infected arthropod; sporozoites are released, invade the gut wall, and *undergo schizogony in many tissues of the host, including skeletal muscle*. Rupture of schizonts in time leads to an inflammatory reaction, but the subsequent stage, a large 250-μm, thick-walled, single-celled cyst, does not stimulate a body response.

Affected dogs (generally <6 months old) show fever, anorexia, weight loss, general body pain, and gait abnormalities, and many show respiratory signs. Concurrent disease may be needed to facilitate infection. Radiographs may show irregular periosteal proliferations. Most dogs have marked leukocytosis and a slight increase in serum creatine kinase activity. The organism in gametocyte form may be present in neutrophils, and muscle biopsy may demonstrate the cysts, or the typical pyogranulomatous reaction in response to the release of merozoites, or the schizonts themselves.

At postmortem, muscle lesions consist of *multiple acute granulomas* interspersed with rows of neutrophils between muscle fibers. Developing stages of the parasite are usually abundant. Dogs may die with *secondary amyloidosis and glomerulonephritis*.

Leishmaniasis

This disease is caused by infection with *Leishmania infantum* (*chagasi*). The disease in dogs has prominent lesions of myocarditis but may also have skeletal muscle involvement. Affected muscle has *myofiber necrosis with infiltrates of lymphocytes and macrophages*. *Leishmania* infection is most common in the Mediterranean area, Asia, and Latin America. Clinical signs of *Leishmania* myositis are muscle weakness and atrophy, and clinical severity correlated with the number of protozoal organisms. Most infiltrating cells are T cells, and muscle fibers in cases of *Leishmania* myositis were found to have MHC class I and II expression at the sarcolemma. Protozoal organisms are found within macrophages. See Vol. 3, Hematopoietic system for further information.

In dogs with symptomatic or asymptomatic leishmaniasis, *Leishmania infantum* appears to induce a mixed Th1/Th2 immune response that in the sick dog may eventually result in tissue damage via different pathogenetic mechanisms, notably granulomatous inflammation (e.g., nodular dermatitis, osteomyelitis), immune-complex deposition (e.g., glomerulonephritis), and/or autoantibody production (e.g., polymyositis). This is a compensatory but detrimental mechanism generated mainly because of the insufficient killing capacity of macrophages against the parasite in the susceptible dog. Clinical disease is typically exemplified as exfoliative and/or ulcerative dermatitis, with or without nasodigital hyperkeratosis and onychogryphosis, glomerulonephritis, atrophic myositis of masticatory muscles, anterior uveitis, keratoconjunctivitis sicca, epistaxis, and/or polyarthritis, appearing alone or in various combinations. The pathogenesis of these clinical conditions recently has been highlighted, to a greater or lesser extent. The usually subclinical conditions expressed as chronic colitis, chronic hepatitis, vasculitis, myocarditis, osteomyelitis, orchiepididymitis, and meningoencephalomyelitis, although uncommon, are of pathologic importance from a differential point of view. The leading cause of death among canine leishmaniasis patients is chronic proteinuric nephritis that may progress to end-stage renal disease, nephrotic syndrome, and/or systemic hypertension. However, even the asymptomatic proteinuria, when profuse, may be a serious problem because it predisposes to arterial thromboembolism and eventually contributes to the deterioration of body condition.

Further reading

Craig TM. Parasitic myositis of dogs and cats. Sem Vet Med Surg (Small Anim) 1989;4:161-167.

Dubey JP, Lindsay DS. Neosporosis—a newly recognized protozoan disease. J Vet Parasitol 1996;10:99-145.

Gabor M, et al. Chronic myositis in an Australian alpaca (*Llama pacos*) associated with *Sarcocystis* spp. J Vet Diagn Invest 2010;22:966-969.

Jensen R, et al. Eosinophilic myositis and muscular sarcocystosis in the carcasses of slaughtered cattle and lambs. Am J Vet Res 1986;47:587-593.

Koutinas AF, Koutinas CK. Pathologic mechanisms underlying the clinical findings in canine leishmaniasis due to *Leishmania infantum/chagasi*. Vet Pathol 2014;51:527-538.

Paciello O, et al. Canine inflammatory myopathy associated with *Leishmania infantum* infection. Neuromusc Dis 2009;19:124-130.

Panciera RJ, et al. Comparison of tissue stages of *Hepatozoon americanum* in the dog using immunohistochemical and routine histologic methods. Vet Pathol 2001;38:422-426.

Rooney AL, et al. *Sarcocystis* spp. in llamas (*Lama glama*) in Southern Bolivia: A cross sectional study of the prevalence, risk factors and loss in income caused by carcass downgrades. Prevent Vet Med 2013;pii: S0167-5877(13)00364-4.

Sykes JE, et al. Severe myositis associated with *Sarcocystis* spp. infection in 2 dogs. J Vet Intern Med 2011;25:1277-1283.

Valentine BA. Pathologic findings in equine muscle (excluding polysaccharide storage); a necropsy study. J Vet Diagn Invest 2008;20:572-579.

NEOPLASTIC DISEASES OF MUSCLE

Primary tumors of striated muscle are uncommon in domestic animals and include tumors of cardiac as well as skeletal muscle. Myogenic tumors do not arise from fully differentiated muscle fibers. In many cases, myogenic tumors are thought to originate from pluripotential mesenchymal stem cells, which accounts for the fact that they often arise in areas in which skeletal muscle is not normally present. Such stem cells can also give rise to mixed tumors containing myogenic elements as well as neurogenic, epithelial, or other mesenchymal elements. Such mixed tumors are quite rare in animals.

The cell types encountered in tumors of skeletal muscle reflect the developmental stages of embryonic and regenerating muscle. That is, *tumor cell morphology varies from mononuclear round cell resembling myoblasts, to spindle cells, to multinucleate cells resembling myotubes.* Historically, the diagnosis of skeletal muscle tumors has relied heavily on the identification of cross-striations within tumor cells. Cross-striations may be identified in elongate multinucleated cells with central chains of nuclei, the so-called "strap cells," or in ovoid cells such as the so-called "racquet cells." Cross-striations may be more readily identified following staining with phosphotungstic acid hematoxylin (PTAH). However, cells with such cross striations are often rare or nonexistent within skeletal muscle tumors, and this approach is time consuming and often frustrating. Identification by electron microscopy of primitive sarcomeric structures such as thin filaments arranged in parallel with associated electron dense Z bands has been somewhat more rewarding, but again is time consuming. More recently, given the specificity of myogenic markers and relative ease of immunohistochemical identification of muscle tumors, *immunohistochemistry has largely replaced electron microscopy and PTAH staining.* Desmin and muscle actin are proteins expressed early in skeletal muscle differentiation and are expressed by many or most skeletal muscle tumor cells. Desmin often highlights cross-striations in skeletal muscle tumors far better than the PTAH stain. These markers do not, however, differentiate tumors of skeletal and cardiac muscle origin from tumors of smooth muscle or myofibroblastic origin. Myoglobin and sarcomeric actin are specific markers of skeletal muscle differentiation that are expressed in myogenic cells. Typically, only a subpopulation of muscle tumor cells expresses these proteins, and often only the most differentiated skeletal muscle tumor cells express myoglobin. More recently, *immunostaining for the MRFs myoD and myogenin has been applied.* These markers are specific for skeletal muscle and are able to confirm even very poorly differentiated rhabdomyosarcomas.

When evaluating tumors involving skeletal muscle, the pathologist must be aware that nonmyogenic tumors infiltrating or metastatic to skeletal muscle can cause extensive damage with bizarre regenerative fibers that can mimic neoplastic cells. This is especially true of tumors with extensive sclerosis (see Fig. 3-31). These bizarre cells should not be mistaken for tumor cells. Entrapped skeletal muscle fibers within a nonmyogenic tumor also stain with immunohistochemical markers for skeletal muscle and can cause confusion.

Both benign (rhabdomyoma) and malignant (rhabdomyosarcoma) skeletal muscle tumors occur in domestic animals. As in people, rhabdomyoma and rhabdomyosarcoma often occur in young animals. Classification of these tumors, particularly rhabdomyosarcoma, has been difficult and often confusing. The classification presented here is based on the current scheme of classification of myogenic tumors in people.

Rhabdomyoma

Benign tumors of striated muscle origin are most common in the heart of pigs. The red wattle pig breed appears to be predisposed. Rare cases of cardiac rhabdomyoma have also occurred in sheep, cattle, and dogs. **Cardiac rhabdomyomas** are incidental findings most often involving the left ventricular wall. Tumors can also occur in the septum, and least commonly involve the right ventricular wall. These lesions are present in young animals, and current opinion suggests that they are most likely hamartomas or dysplastic lesions rather than true neoplasms. These lesions occur as smooth-surfaced nodular masses up to ~3 cm diameter embedded in the myocardium. They are circumscribed but nonencapsulated, and are formed by large vacuolated myocytes with pale eosinophilic cytoplasm. Mitoses are not seen. The term *purkinjeoma* has been proposed for cardiac rhabdomyoma in pigs, based on the finding in tumor cells of protein gene product 9.5, a marker for neuronal tissue and Purkinje fiber cells.

Laryngeal rhabdomyomas have been reported in dogs from 2 to 10 years of age. Tumors most often occur as nodular masses protruding into the lumen of the larynx, resulting in clinical signs of dyspnea, stridor, or altered bark. One tumor occurred in the laryngeal pharynx. Laryngeal rhabdomyoma cells are large, round, and moderately pleomorphic, and contain abundant vacuolated to granular eosinophilic cytoplasm (Fig. 3-104A). Scattered multinucleate and elongate strap cells may be seen. Intracytoplasmic glycogen may be revealed by PAS staining. Ultrastructural features include numerous mitochondria, and these tumors have been misdiagnosed as laryngeal oncocytomas. Ultrastructural identification of primitive myofilaments, often with Z-band type material (Fig. 3-104, B), and positive immunostaining for skeletal muscle markers (Fig. 3-104, C), has confirmed the striated muscle origin of these tumors. Although there are reports of invasive tumors classified as laryngeal rhabdomyosarcoma, these tumors typically exhibit minimal invasion and mitotic figures, metastasis has rarely been seen, and the vast majority of these tumors are thought to be benign and cured by wide surgical excision.

Rhabdomyoma is rare in other sites and other species. Rhabdomyoma of the skin has been reported to occur on the convex surface of the pinna in 4 white cats aged 6-7 years. These tumors were said to be made up of whorls of spindle cells with a few showing cross-striations on PTAH staining. Rhabdomyoma has been reported as a rare lesion in the skin of the trunk or legs in dogs. They are characterized histologically by large round to polygonal, eosinophilic cells with well demarcated borders but are generally not encapsulated. They stain strongly for muscle markers. A cystic rhabdomyoma attached to the diaphragm by a stalk has been reported in the mediastinum of a 2-year-old filly.

Rhabdomyosarcoma

Rhabdomyosarcomas are most often fleshy growths that occur in a variety of sites, often those normally lacking skeletal muscle. Less commonly they occur in skeletal muscle.

Rhabdomyosarcoma in people has been classified histologically as *embryonal* rhabdomyosarcoma, *alveolar* rhabdomyosarcoma, and *pleomorphic* rhabdomyosarcoma. Botryoid rhabdomyosarcoma, a tumor most common in the urogenital tract, is considered a variant of embryonal rhabdomyosarcoma. *Embryonal rhabdomyosarcoma, and the botryoid variant, are the most common forms in people and, it would appear, in animals.* Pleomorphic rhabdomyosarcoma, often thought of as being the classic and the most common form in veterinary medicine, is actually the least common type of

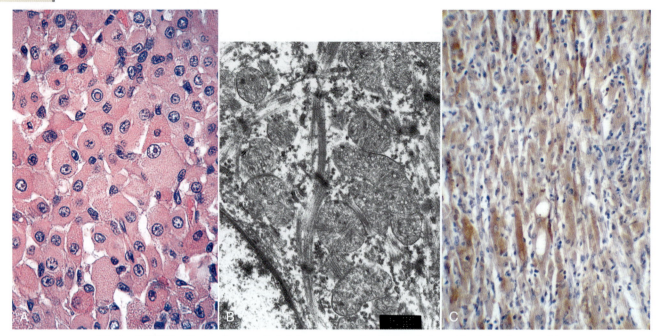

Figure 3-104 A. Canine **laryngeal rhabdomyoma** with characteristic moderately pleomorphic plump round-to-elongate cells with euchromatic nuclei and eosinophilic cytoplasm. H&E stain. B. Ultrastructural features of canine **laryngeal rhabdomyoma** demonstrating characteristic Z-band type material and associated myofilaments. Mitochondria are also prominent. Transmission electron micrograph. C. Positive myoglobin immunostaining of the cytoplasm of many cells of a canine **laryngeal rhabdomyoma**. Immunohistochemistry for myoglobin. (Courtesy D.J. Meuten.)

rhabdomyosarcoma, both in humans and animals. This diagnosis should only be made where the entire tumor is pleomorphic and myogenic differentiation has been confirmed by immunohistochemistry. The presence of any areas with embryonal morphology should be diagnosed as embryonal rather than pleomorphic. Confusion has also arisen because of the designation of pleomorphic tumors, especially those with multinucleate cells, as rhabdomyosarcoma, many of which are pleomorphic sarcomas that do not stain for muscle markers.

Embryonal rhabdomyosarcoma is composed of cells that may be either round and myoblast-like, or elongated and myotube-like ("strap cells"), and cells can be mononuclear or multinucleated. Tumors may consist entirely of one cell type or may contain a mixture of these cell types. Embryonal rhabdomyosarcoma occurs most commonly in young animals and often involves the head or neck, including the oral cavity, although occurrence at other sites is possible. The round cell form is the most common, and embryonal rhabdomyosarcoma should be considered in the differential diagnosis of any nonhistiocytic and nonlymphoid round-cell tumor of the head or neck of a young animal. The round cell embryonal rhabdomyosarcomas consist either of small cells with large central euchromatic nuclei, often with a single prominent nucleolus, and minimal cytoplasm, or of larger round cells with similar nuclei and prominent eosinophilic cytoplasm (rhabdomyoblasts); there is often an admixture of these 2 cell types (Fig. 3-105A, B). Conventional immunohistochemical muscle markers (i.e., immunostains for muscle specific proteins) are most often expressed by the better-differentiated, large rhabdomyoblasts (see Fig. 3-105B). However, immunohistochemical staining for the MRFs, myoD and myogenin, is very specific and they are expressed in the nuclei of even poorly differentiated neoplastic myogenic cells (Fig. 3-106A, B). Scattered rhabdomyoblasts may have prominent cytoplasmic vacuolation resulting in a "spider-web" cell (see Fig. 3-105A). The botryoid variant, named for its "grape-like" gross appearance (Fig. 3-107A), occurs most often in the trigone area of the urinary bladder in young large breed dogs. These tumors are composed of spindle and stellate cells within myxoid stroma, often with elongate multinucleate myotube-like cells (Fig. 3-107B, C). Rare subcutaneous myxoid forms of embryonal rhabdomyosarcoma have been recognized, which can be misdiagnosed as myxosarcoma. Although embryonal rhabdomyosarcoma is most common in dogs, this type of tumor also occurs in cats, sheep, cattle, pigs, and horses. Embryonal rhabdomyosarcoma in all species often occurs in young to young-adult individuals. There appears to be a female predominance, especially for the botryoid variant in the urogenital tract. Cytogenetic abnormalities are commonly associated with childhood rhabdomyosarcomas in people, and a similar situation has been seen in in pigs, in which a cluster of rhabdomyosarcomas in young animals was found to have a genetic basis.

Alveolar rhabdomyosarcoma is also a tumor of adolescent and young adult people. This tumor consists of sheets of uniformly small, undifferentiated round cells in which tumor cells are supported on a fibrous framework and often form alveolar-like structures because of loss of cohesiveness in the center of cell nests. Multinucleated cells can be seen, but cross-striations are rare. A solid alveolar pattern is also recognized, with sheets of small, undifferentiated round cells that resemble embryonal rhabdomyosarcoma but that lack any differentiation toward the larger eosinophilic rhabdomyoblasts. In people, this form of rhabdomyosarcoma is associated with specific chromosomal translocations resulting in the expression of fusion proteins, namely, PAX7-FOXO1 or

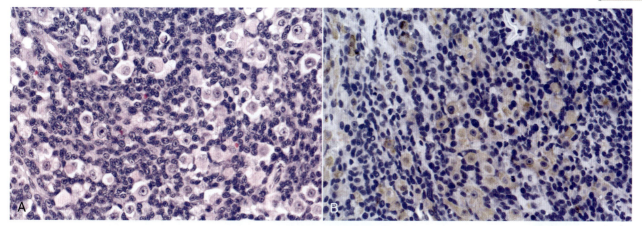

Figure 3-105 A. Embryonal rhabdomyosarcoma from a 9-year-old cat showing admixed small basophilic cells and larger rhabdomyoblasts. H&E stain. **B.** Positive immunostaining for sarcomeric actin. Note that staining is predominantly in the large rhabdomyoblasts. Immunohistochemistry for sarcomeric actin.

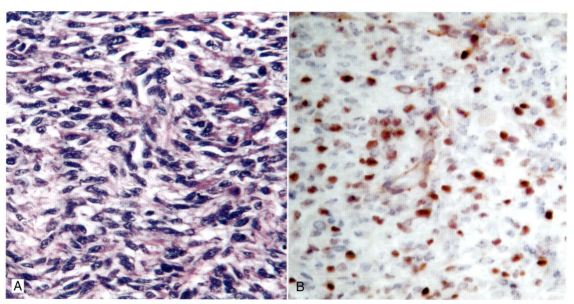

Figure 3-106 Embryonal rhabdomyosarcoma, myotubular variant. **A.** This field is composed mainly of spindle cells. H&E stain. **B.** Immunostain for myoD showing positive staining of nuclei. Immunohistochemistry for myoD.

PAX3-FOXO1. As mentioned earlier, PAX7 and PAX3 are important transcription factors involved in the development of muscle cells. It has been suggested by some investigators that this diagnosis should not be made in humans unless these translocations are present. This form of rhabdomyosarcoma carries a poor prognosis in people. It has been reported in dogs, horses, and a cow but until some similar genetic aberration is recognized, we recommend caution in making this diagnosis. Some of these neoplasms may be cell dense variants of embryonal rhabdomyosarcoma.

Virtually all rhabdomyosarcomas exhibit some degree of cellular pleomorphism. **Pleomorphic rhabdomyosarcoma** is often diagnosed, but only tumors lacking *any* areas with features of embryonal or alveolar rhabdomyosarcoma should be designated as the pleomorphic variant. In people, pleomorphic rhabdomyosarcoma is a tumor of adults, most often occurring in major muscle groups such as the muscles of the thigh. Pleomorphic rhabdomyosarcoma has been reported in dogs, cats, cows, and horses. Pleomorphic rhabdomyosarcoma consists of plump spindle cells in a haphazard arrangement that may be admixed with scattered multinucleated cells, strap cells, racket cells, and large, round rhabdomyoblasts (Fig. 3-108A, B).

Cardiac rhabdomyosarcomas occur, but are rare, with all cases to date reported in dogs. The age range of affected dogs was 14 months to 7 years. Clinical signs of cardiac failure can occur, although one tumor was found as an incidental finding. Histologic features of poor differentiation, cellular pleomorphism, mitotic activity, and local invasion warrant the diagnosis of rhabdomyosarcoma rather than rhabdomyoma.

The behavior of rhabdomyosarcoma in animals parallels that of humans, in which *aggressive local invasion and frequent metastasis* are seen. Although the data regarding pattern of metastasis is scanty in animals, metastasis to atypical sites such as to other skeletal muscle sites, to cardiac muscle, and to spinal cord have been seen.

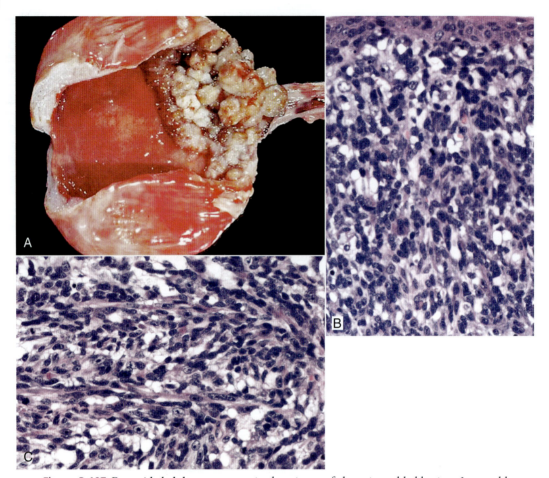

Figure 3-107 Botryoid rhabdomyosarcoma in the trigone of the urinary bladder in a 1-year-old large breed dog. **A.** The characteristic gross appearance. **B.** Predominantly mononuclear round and spindle cells immediately below the transitional epithelium. H&E stain. **C.** Primitive myotubes deeper in the neoplasm. H&E stain.

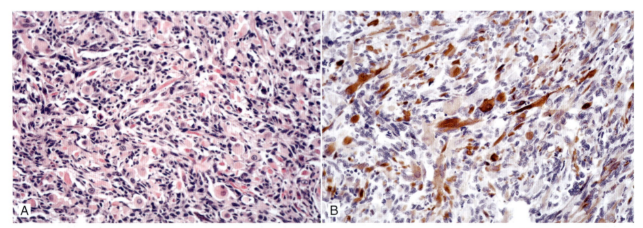

Figure 3-108 Pleomorphic rhabdomyosarcoma in muscle of the neck in a 3-year-old dog. **A.** Characteristic mixed plump and pleomorphic spindle cells and round-to-ovoid cells. H&E stain. **B.** Positive immunostaining for desmin.

Nonmuscle primary tumors of muscle

These tumors arise from supporting mesenchymal tissues of muscle. Malignant tumors are far more common than benign tumors.

- *Poorly differentiated sarcomas and giant cell sarcomas* occur within muscle, especially at the site of intramuscular vaccinations in predisposed cats. These tumors may be mistaken for rhabdomyosarcoma but do not express skeletal muscle cell markers, and are most often variants of fibrosarcoma.
- *Hemangiosarcoma* arising within skeletal muscle occurs most frequently in the dog and in the horse (Fig. 3-109A,

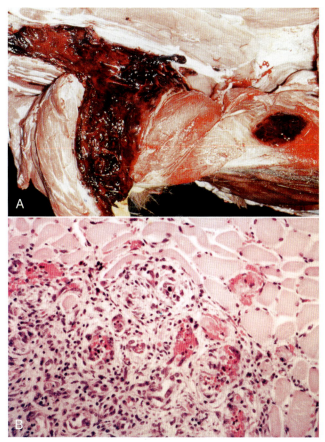

Figure 3-109 Hemangiosarcoma within the skeletal muscle of an adult horse. **A.** Gross appearance. **B.** Proliferating invasive neoplastic endothelial cells forming irregular vascular channels typical of this neoplasm. H&E stain.

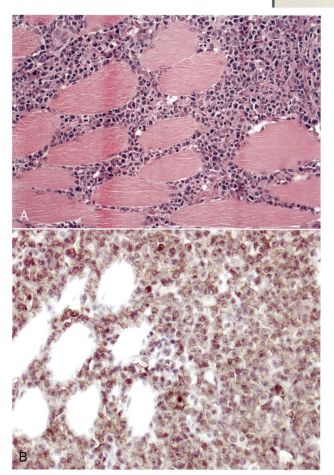

Figure 3-110 Intramuscular invasion of **lymphoma** in an adult cat. **A.** H&E stain. **B.** Immunostain for CD20 showing a homogeneous population of neoplastic B cells. Immunohistochemistry for CD20.

B). Because of the large amount of hemorrhage and scanty tumor cells, these tumors are often difficult to diagnose from biopsy specimens. Intramuscular hemangiosarcoma is often mistaken clinically for intramuscular hematoma. It is an aggressive tumor, exhibiting both local invasion and distant metastasis, such as to lung.
- *Nerve sheath neoplasms* can arise from major nerve trunks within skeletal muscle but are typically localized to intramuscular nerves without infiltration of adjacent muscle.
- *Granular cell tumor* ("granular cell myoblastoma") is a tumor that can occur in the musculature of the tongue of dogs and cats and, rarely, within cardiac muscle. Granular cell tumor consists of closely packed round cells with prominent intracytoplasmic PAS-positive, amylase-resistant granules. Ultrastructurally, these granules consist of secondary lysosomes. Although previously thought to be of skeletal muscle origin, granular cell tumor appears to be most often a tumor of neural, probably Schwann cell, origin.
- *Malignant lymphoma* may occur within skeletal muscle, but whether this represents primary intramuscular tumor or local or metastatic spread is not always certain. Infiltration of skeletal muscle by neoplastic lymphocytes must be distinguished from lymphocytic infiltration owing to immune-mediated myositis. Immunophenotyping can be helpful in making this distinction. Lymphoma cells are typically relatively homogeneous and often atypical, and surround myofibers and efface skeletal muscle architecture without obvious myofiber necrosis or "coring out" of myofibers (Fig. 3-110A, B).

Secondary tumors of skeletal muscle

The *infiltrative variant of lipoma* arising within the subcutis is characterized by prominent intramuscular invasion (Fig. 3-111A, B). This tumor, although locally invasive, does not metastasize, and wide surgical excision is generally curative. Infiltrative lipoma occurs most often in dogs and horses. Although uncommon, *subcutaneous mast cell tumors* can invade underlying skeletal muscle. *Other soft tissue sarcomas* arising in the subcutis, such as fibrosarcoma and hemangiopericytoma, can also extend into adjacent skeletal muscle. *Carcinomas* can invade or metastasize to skeletal muscle.

In general, *tumor metastasis to skeletal muscle is less common than metastasis to other organs*. However, in part this may reflect the difficulty in adequately sample such a large tissue mass. There is evidence to suggest that the microvasculature of skeletal muscle is relatively unfavorable to the establishment of metastases. Dermal melanoma of older gray horses often metastasizes to the muscle fascia, but less commonly involves the muscle itself. Skeletal muscle metastasis of canine prostatic carcinoma can result in foci of intramuscular fibroplasia, sometimes with associated chondroid differentiation, that can mimic focal or multifocal myositis ossificans (see

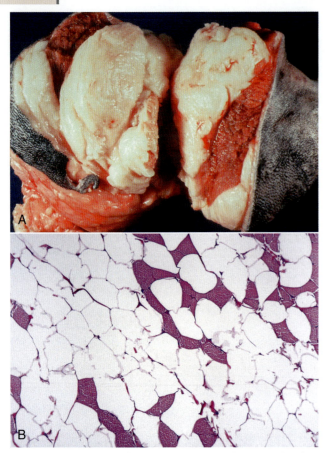

Figure 3-111 **Infiltrative lipoma** invading skeletal muscle of an adult dog. **A.** Gross appearance. **B.** Extensive infiltration of muscle by well-differentiated adipocytes. H&E stain.

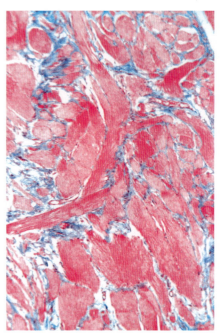

Figure 3-112 Irregular orientation of mature myofibers with associated endomysial fibrosis in a **muscle pseudotumor** from a Great Dane dog. Masson trichrome stain.

Physical injuries of muscle). Diaphragmatic muscle is often a site of intra-abdominal or intrathoracic implantation of neoplastic tissue.

Muscle pseudotumors

Muscle pseudotumors include a group of reactive lesions that can mimic neoplasia. *Localized myositis ossificans* is discussed in Physical injuries of muscle, and *musculoaponeurotic fibromatosis* in Tendons and aponeuroses. An unusual muscle pseudotumor has been seen in 2 dogs, both Great Danes, in which a localized swelling in the dorsal scapular area was found to be associated with skeletal muscle. These lesions were composed of irregularly arranged mature skeletal muscle fibers with marked cytoarchitectural alterations and associated endomysial fibrosis (Fig. 3-112). Muscle pseudotumors in humans are most often thought to be associated with muscle trauma, and a similar etiology seems logical for animals.

Further reading

Caserto B. A Comparative review of canine and human rhabdomyosarcoma with emphasis on classification and pathogenesis. Vet Pathol 2013;50:806-826.

Cooper BJ, Valentine BA. Tumors of muscle. In: Meuten DJ, editor. Moulton's Tumors of Domestic Animals. 5th ed. Ames, IA: Iowa State University Press; in press.

Hettmer S, Wagers AJ. Uncovering the origins of rhabdomyosarcoma. Nat Med 2010;16:171-173.

Jacobsen B, et al. Proposing the term purkinjeoma: protein gene product 9.5 expression in 2 porcine cardiac rhabdomyomas indicates possible purkinje fiber cell origin. Vet Pathol 2010; 47:738-740.

Parham DM, Ellison DA. Rhabdomyosarcoma in adults and children. An update. Arch Pathol Lab Med 2006;130:1454-1465.

TENDONS AND APONEUROSES

GENERAL CONSIDERATIONS

Tendons are derived from the same pool of embryonic mesenchymal cells as muscle fibers and it is very likely that although commitment occurs early, the differentiation of myoblastic and tenoblastic cells occurs relatively late. In some tendons, notably the suspensory ligaments of the limbs of the foal, the first wave of differentiation is as a muscle (the interosseous muscle) and only subsequently does further development produce a tendinous type structure. Therefore what is referred to as the suspensory ligament in horses is structurally more similar to tendon. *The basic structural units of tendons are bundles of collagen that cluster around a central elongated collection of tendon fibroblasts or tenocytes and capillaries.* Multiples of these units combine to form *fascicles* somewhat like primary muscle bundles, and fascicles in turn combine in clusters to form the *complete tendon*, which is ensheathed by a looser fibrous tissue called the *peritenon*.

Tendons are quite completely, although sparsely, supplied with blood vessels but in keeping with low nutritional requirements once the tendon is formed, relatively wide distances may separate adjacent parallel vascular channels in mature animals. Segments of long tendons may appear to be almost avascular at times, if flow volume is used as an indicator of vascularity.

At birth, tendons are cellular and vascular, as tenoblasts or tenocytes elaborate the orderly, synchronously kinked, parallel collagen bundles. The kinking provides a mechanism for absorbing stretch impact and provides an interlocking adhesive strength for adjacent fibers, which is enhanced by the presence of an amorphous, noncollagen ground substance that acts as "glue." The physical properties of tendons are largely dependent on cross-linking of collagen molecules.

TENDON AGING AND INJURY

As tendons age, they change color from pearly white to yellow-tan and may acquire an even darker brown or red-gray center. Some of these color changes are related to repeated minor episodes of capillary hemorrhage that occur even in normal, unworked horses or cattle. The distinction between normal and abnormal is often a difficult one to make, but *it is normal (in the sense of usual and harmless) for tendons to undergo focal cartilaginous metaplasia*. Osseous metaplasia in tendons, however, is distinctly pathologic.

An important issue in the process of tendon aging and injury relates to predisposing lesions. Cartilaginous metaplasia, ischemia, and local fibroblastic proliferations have been regarded as predisposing changes, but they are frequently found in normal animals. It now seems that preparatory events need not be postulated to explain most of the lesions seen. The *predilection sites for tendon damage are predictably those with anatomic weakness or that receive disproportionate stretch* forces. The subsequent changes relate to stretching of tendon collagen and vessels.

When a tendon is stretched beyond load capacity, fibrils are very likely to be pulled out of kink register and even if no fibrils break, the tendon will be subsequently weaker at that point. Such *stretch lesions* are usually accompanied by ruptured collagen fibers as well, although it may be only microscopically detectable. The sequence of events that follows involves the rupture of capillaries, release of fibrin, stimulation of tenocytes and/or peritenon cells to form myofibroblasts, and the formation of scar collagen that in many ways resembles the original tendon. In the acute stages, this process makes the tendon swollen, warm, and painful; in the chronic stage, the tendon is larger and longer than normal. Original tendon is uniquely constructed entirely of type I collagen. *When tendon repairs, the mature scar no longer consists only of type I collagen because 20-30% of the replacement tissue is type III collagen, a form of fiber less able to withstand stretch forces than type I*. It is likely that alterations in the proportions of the component glycosaminoglycans (e.g., hyaluronic acid, dermatan sulfate, chondroitin sulfate) occur after injury and during repair. The differences between a minor sprain and incomplete or even complete tendon rupture are differences in quantity, not form. In larger lesions, there is a greater chance for tendon necrosis and sequestration, and a greater chance for the formation of a fibrin clot that is not longitudinally oriented by tension. This may lead to misalignment of the scar fibrils, adhesions to adjacent sheaths, and irregular contours of the tendon. Because myofibroblastic scar tissue is capable of contracting as it matures, the result of tendon repair is not necessarily a longer tendon but, inevitably, a weaker tendon.

Degenerative suspensory desmitis occurs relatively commonly in horses. In llamas and alpacas, tendinopathy can lead to metacarpophalangeal and metatarsophalangeal hyperextension. In horses, an abnormal form of decorin with altered biologic activity and abnormal aggrecan processing has been reported in degenerative suspensory ligaments and also in connective tissue in other organs, suggesting the possibility of a systemic proteoglycan abnormality. A lower liver cobalt level and a higher serum level of zinc, molybdenum, and iron, and vitamin D concentration in summer and fall has been found in llamas and alpacas with degenerative suspensory desmitis. No evidence of inflammation, collagen or elastic defects, degenerative change, or systemic proteoglycan abnormalities has been found in affected llamas and alpacas.

PARASITIC DISEASES OF TENDONS AND APONEUROSES

Nematodes of the family *Onchocercidae* make connective tissue, vessel walls, or tendons of cattle and horses their preferred habitat. Most of these, and especially those that live in tendons, belong to the genus *Onchocerca*, although not all *Onchocerca* parasites have an affinity for tendons. Three different parasites infect domesticated cattle, *Onchocerca gibsoni*, *O. gutturosa*, and *O. lienalis*, but full investigation may eventually increase the number. Three different parasites, *O. gutturosa*, *O. reticulata*, and *O. cervicalis* infect horses. *Onchocerca gibsoni* infects cattle in Africa, Asia, and Australia. *Onchocerca gutturosa* occurs in cattle and horses in North America, Africa, Australia, and Europe. *Onchocerca lienalis* is considered to be a separate species by some and synonymous with *O. gutturosa* by others; it is not as widespread as is *O. gutturosa*, but is seen in cattle in Australia and North America. *Onchocerca reticulata* infects horses in Europe and Asia, and *O. cervicalis* infects horses worldwide. The prevalence of onchocerciasis can be very high, ranging from 20-100% of the population in endemic areas, but *infection by these connective tissue parasites has been greatly reduced by widespread use of ivermectin as an anthelmintic*.

The adult worms, <1.0 mm thick and 50-80 cm long for the female, much shorter for the male, live in tendons, tendon sheaths, or connective tissues of the brisket or abdominal wall from which site they liberate *microfilariae* over long periods. The larvae make their way to skin, where they are picked up by a blood-sucking parasite in which the next phase of development takes place.

Onchocerca gibsoni characteristically provokes and inhabits a "worm nodule" or "worm nest" on the *brisket or external surfaces of the hindlimbs that may reach 3 cm in diameter*. These fibrous lesions are important in the meat industry because the worms must be manually removed and this is time consuming if several dozen are present. The nodules may be palpable or moveable in the skin or they may be fixed to the dermis or ribs. Those in the flank are usually beneath the fascia lata and are not externally palpable. The adult worms inhabit fine tunnels in the discrete nodules of dense fibrous tissue where they form a tangled mass in a milky fluid. Female worms are just grossly visible but the smaller males are not. Sometimes old hemorrhages, or mineralized remnants of worms, are contained in the larger nodules, and microscopically many larvae also may be seen in the capsule as they exit, perhaps via lymphatic vessels. Microfilariae are rarely seen in lymph nodes or blood vessels, but these routes may be used to reach the skin where they collect in large numbers without stimulating a reaction. The intermediate blood-sucking host is probably a simulid or a culicoid insect.

Onchocerca gutturosa is most frequently located on the surface of the *ligamentum nuchae* of cattle adjacent to the thoracic vertebral spines and less frequently on the scapula, humerus, or femur. It is sometimes found in the horse. The adult worms, which are found in pairs, do not stimulate the formation of a nodule, as is the case for O. gibsoni, but lie in loose connective tissue. They apparently cause no disease or reaction and, in spite of their wide distribution around the world, they are rarely dissected out or even detected. The intermediate hosts are not all known, but simulids can transfer the infestation.

Onchocerca lienalis lies in delicate tunnels in the gastrosplenic ligament and in the splenic capsule of cattle.

Adult worms of ***Onchocerca cervicalis*** live between the fibers of the ligamentum nuchae over the shoulder or neck of the horse or in loose connective tissues nearby. A second very similar parasite, **O. reticulata**, resides at a much lower level of frequency in the tissue around tendon sheaths adjacent to the carpus or suspensory ligaments or at the fetlock where a low-grade tissue reaction is initiated by the presence of adult worms. When the worms die, they mineralize and are engulfed by a poorly defined, dense, fibrous reaction. The infestation usually goes undetected and most horses are apparently asymptomatic. The long thread-like female worm is <1 mm thick but 50-70 cm long. Larvae are hatched from eggs before their release from the uterus, and they make their way through connective tissue to the skin where they presumably travel in the dermal lymph vessels. Larvae (microfilariae), which are ~4 μm wide and 200-250 μm long, tend to aggregate in certain skin regions, particularly the skin of the ventral abdominal midline, the inner thighs, and the eyelids. Living microfilariae seem to stimulate no reaction whatever, but dead larvae are capable of stimulating a response that involves lymphocytes and eosinophils. These local nodular responses may be seen in skin accompanied by pruritus, alopecia, and scaliness, and they may be seen histologically in areas where larvae are particularly numerous. Living larvae can be quite readily detected as loosely curled structures just under the epidermis and adjacent to adnexal skin structures in histologic sections. Microfilariae of O. cervicalis and O. reticulata are transported to another horse by blood-sucking insects in which an obligatory stage of development occurs. Several different insects may be suitable hosts, but only *Culicoides* midges and mosquitoes of the *Anopheles* species have been confirmed in the role.

FIBROMATOUS DISORDERS OF TENDONS AND APONEUROSES

A number of degenerative disorders resulting in proliferation of fibrous, cartilaginous, and osseous tissue within tendons and aponeuroses are described in humans and animals. Some such disorders are inherited, whereas others are acquired. For the most part, little is known regarding the pathogenesis of these processes.

Fibromatoses *are defined as progressive, infiltrative, nonmetastasizing fibroblastic lesions.* A variety of such disorders are recognized in humans, and a similar disorder occurs in the horse. These lesions, although considered nonneoplastic by most investigators, can exhibit marked local infiltration and distortion of affected muscle.

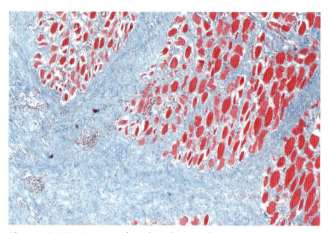

Figure 3-113 Perimysial and endomysial connective tissue dissecting between muscle bundles and myofibers in a horse with **musculoaponeurotic fibromatosis.** Foci of lymphocytes are also visible within the perimysial connective tissue. Masson trichrome stain.

Musculoaponeurotic fibromatosis (desmoid tumor) of the horse

A peculiar progressive fibrosing disorder, musculoaponeurotic fibromatosis (desmoid tumor), occurs in the horse. Although most cases involve the *pectoral region*, other sites are possible. Affected horses develop progressive distortion and induration of affected musculature because of the proliferation of fibroblasts, myofibroblasts, and subsequent fibrosis dissecting between muscle fibers and fascicles that is often accompanied by foci of lymphocytic infiltration (Fig. 3-113). Although wide surgical excision may be curative, in most cases the extent of the lesion at diagnosis precludes effective surgical intervention. Studies of a small number of horses have revealed fluid-filled pockets of apparently sterile inflammation deep within the lesion, suggesting that this disorder in horses may be a peculiar response to trauma such as from an injection or ruptured bursa.

Fibrodysplasia ossificans progressiva

Fibrodysplasia ossificans progressiva (FOP) is a progressive fibrosing and ossifying lesion of tendons and muscle-associated aponeuroses that occurs in humans and cats. This disorder was previously referred to as *myositis ossificans progressiva*, which is incorrect, because the disorder involves muscle-associated connective tissue and is not a primary myopathy (see Physical injuries of muscle). Fibrodysplasia ossificans progressiva in humans is a devastating disease of children and young adults. Progressive fibrosis and ossification of muscle-associated connective tissue, including tendons and fascia, result in eventual incapacitation. This disorder is inherited as a dominant trait.

A similar disorder occurs sporadically in young to young-adult cats. Age at diagnosis in the cat has ranged from 10 months to 6 years. To date, inheritance of FOP has not been confirmed in the cat. Clinical signs include progressive stiffness of gait, decreased joint mobility, increased bulk and firmness of muscle, and pain upon handling. Radiography and gross pathology reveal *characteristic thickening with mineralization and ossification of muscle fascia* (Figs. 3-114, 3-115). The histopathologic features are of fibroblastic proliferation within fascia with subsequent cartilage and bone formation. Early lesions may have an associated mild lymphoid infiltrate. An

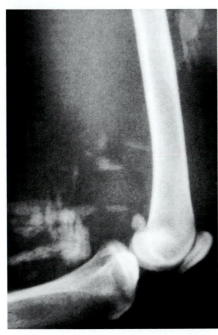

Figure 3-114 Multifocal soft tissue mineralized densities in a radiograph from a cat with **fibrodysplasia ossificans progressiva**. (Courtesy J. Carpenter.)

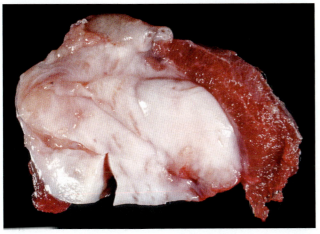

Figure 3-115 Marked thickening of the gastrocnemius muscle fascia of a young adult cat with **fibrodysplasia ossificans progressiva**. (Courtesy L. Fuhrer.)

inherited form of what was described as generalized myositis ossificans has been described in young *pigs*. The lesion in these pigs, however, was a proliferation of periosteal bone involving vertebrae, ribs, and tarsal bones, suggesting that this may be a primary bone disorder.

Further reading

Halper J. Connective tissue disorders in domestic animals. Adv Exp Med Biol 2014;802:231-240.

Scott DW, Miller WH. Parasitic diseases. In: Equine Dermatology. Philadelphia, PA: W.B. Saunders Co; 2003. p. 321-275.

Valentine BA, et al. Intramuscular desmoid tumor (musculoaponeurotic fibromatosis) in two horses. Vet Pathol 1999;36:468-470.

Yabuzoe A, et al. Fibrodysplasia ossificans progressiva in a Maine Coon cat with prominent ossification in dorsal muscle. J Vet Med Sci 2009;71:1649-1652.

For more information, please visit the companion site: PathologyofDomesticAnimals.com

CHAPTER 4

Nervous System

Carlo Cantile • Sameh Youssef

CYTOPATHOLOGY OF NERVOUS TISSUE	251
Neuron	251
Degenerative changes of the nerve cell body	252
Axon	253
Oligodendrocytes, Schwann cells, and the myelin sheath	258
Astrocytes	260
Ependymal cells	262
Microglia	262
Microcirculation	263
MALFORMATIONS OF THE CENTRAL NERVOUS SYSTEM	264
Cerebrum	266
Cerebral aplasia, anencephaly	266
Encephalocele, meningocele	267
Defects in cerebral corticogenesis	268
Disorders of axonal growth	268
Holoprosencephaly	269
Hydrocephalus	270
Hydranencephaly, porencephaly	272
Periventricular leukomalacia of neonates	274
Cerebellum/caudal fossa	274
Cerebellar agenesis, hypoplasia, and dysplasia	275
Arnold-Chiari malformation	276
Dandy-Walker syndrome	277
Spinal cord	277
Myelodysplasia	277
Spina bifida and related defects	279
Arachnoid cysts	279
Viral causes of developmental defects of the central nervous system	280
Orthobunyaviruses	280
Orbiviruses	281
Rift Valley fever virus and Wesselsbron virus	281
Pestiviruses	281
Feline panleukopenia virus	283
STORAGE DISEASES	284
Inherited storage diseases	286
Sphingolipidoses	287
Glycoproteinoses	288
Mucopolysaccharidoses	289
Glycogenoses	290
Mucolipidoses	290
Ceroid-lipofuscinoses	290
Lafora disease	292
Induced storage diseases	292
Swainsonine toxicosis	292
Trachyandra poisoning	292
Phalaris poisoning	292
Other induced storage diseases	293
INCREASED INTRACRANIAL PRESSURE, CEREBRAL SWELLING, AND EDEMA	293
LESIONS OF BLOOD VESSELS AND CIRCULATORY DISTURBANCES	296
Ischemic lesions	297
Hemorrhagic lesions	300
Microcirculatory lesions	301
TRAUMATIC INJURIES	301
Concussion	302
Contusion	302
Laceration	302
Fracture of the skull	302
Injuries to the spinal cord	303
DEGENERATION IN THE NERVOUS SYSTEM	303
Meninges	304
Choroid plexuses	304
Atrophy in the brain and spinal cord	304
Anoxia and anoxic poisons	305
Cyanide poisoning	305
Nitrate/nitrite poisoning	306
Fluoroacetate poisoning	306
Carbon monoxide poisoning	306
Hypoglycemia	306
Malacia and malacic diseases	307
Focal symmetrical poliomyelomalacia syndromes	308
Focal symmetrical encephalomalacia in swine	308
Corynetoxin poisoning	309
Polioencephalomalacia of ruminants	309
Thiamine deficiency	312
Nigropallidal encephalomalacia of horses	314
Salt (NaCl) poisoning	314
Mycotoxic leukoencephalomalacia of horses	315
Lead poisoning	316
Neurodegenerative diseases	317
Central neuronopathies and axonopathies	318
Central and peripheral neuronopathies and axonopathies	326
Peripheral axonopathies	334
Myelinopathies	336
Hypomyelinogenesis	336
Leukodystrophic and myelinolytic diseases	339
Spongy myelinopathies	342
Spongy encephalomyelopathies	346
Prion diseases	347
INFLAMMATION IN THE CENTRAL NERVOUS SYSTEM	350
Brain and infection	350
Inflammation in the central nervous system	350
Bacterial and pyogenic infections of the nervous system	353
Epidural/subdural abscess and empyema	353
Leptomeningitis	354
Septicemic lesions, septic embolism, and cerebral abscess	358
Granulomatous and pyogranulomatous meningoencephalomyelitis	362
Listeriosis	362
Histophilus somni infections (histophilosis, or H. somni disease complex)	364
Viral infections of the nervous system	365
General pathology of viral inflammation of the nervous system	366
Lyssavirus infections	367
Pseudorabies	370
Porcine hemagglutinating encephalomyelitis virus	372
Enterovirus/teschovirus polioencephalomyelitis of pigs	372
Flaviviral encephalitides	373
Alphaviruses—equine encephalitides	376
Borna disease	377
Lentiviral encephalomyelitis of sheep and goats	378

Paramyxoviral encephalomyelitis of pigs	380
Akabane viral encephalitis	381
Bovine herpesviral encephalitis	381
Bovine paramyxoviral meningoencephalomyelitis	382
Porcine circovirus 2 encephalopathies	382
Porcine encephalitis associated with PRRSV infection	383
California encephalitis virus meningoencephalomyelitis	383
Canine herpesviral encephalitis	383
Equine herpesviral myeloencephalopathy	383
Canine distemper and related conditions	384
Microsporidian infections	385
Encephalitozoonosis	385
Parasitic infections	386
Protozoal infections	386
Helminth and arthropod infestations	389
Chlamydial disease	391
Idiopathic inflammatory diseases	392
Necrotizing meningoencephalitis and necrotizing leukoencephalitis of Pugs and other small-breed dogs	392
Granulomatous meningoencephalomyelitis	393
Acute polyradiculoneuritis (coonhound paralysis)	394
Neuritis of the cauda equina	394
Steroid-responsive meningitis-arteritis (Beagle pain syndrome)	395
Shaker dog disease	395
Sensory ganglioneuritis (sensory ganglioradiculitis)	395
Postinfectious encephalomyelitis	395
Eosinophilic meningoencephalitis	396
Granulomatous radiculitis of the seventh and eighth cranial nerves of calves	396
NEOPLASTIC DISEASES OF THE NERVOUS SYSTEM	396
Tumors of the meninges	396
Meningiomas	396
Meningeal sarcomatosis	398
Tumors of neuroepithelial tissue	398
Astrocytoma	398
Oligodendroglioma	400
Oligoastrocytoma (mixed glial tumor)	400
Ependymoma	400
Choroid plexus tumors	401
Neuronal and mixed neuronal-glial tumors	401
Embryonal tumors	401
Pineal tumors	403
Hematopoietic tumors	403
Lymphoma/lymphosarcoma	403
Plasma cell tumor	403
Histiocytic sarcoma (malignant histiocytosis)	403
Non-B, non-T leukocytic neoplasm (neoplastic reticulosis)	403
Microgliomatosis	403
Tumors of the sellar region	403
Suprasellar germ cell tumors	403
Craniopharyngioma	404
Other primary tumors and cysts	404
Epidermoid cysts	404
Hamartoma or meningioangiomatosis	404
Metastatic tumors	404
Tumors affecting the CNS by extension or impingement	404
Chordoma	404
Tumors of the peripheral nervous system	404
Peripheral nerve sheath tumors	404
Peripheral neuroblastic tumors	405
Paraganglioma	406

ACKNOWLEDGMENTS

We gratefully acknowledge the foundation laid for this chapter by previous authors, including Drs. Ken Jubb, Clive Huxtable, Neil Sullivan, and Grant Maxie. We also appreciate the useful contributions and suggestions made by Drs. David Driemeier, Murray Hazlett, and members of the Veterinary Pathology Department at the Freie Universität Berlin during the current revision.

CYTOPATHOLOGY OF NERVOUS TISSUE

Nervous tissue is highly specialized and structurally complex, and neuropathology has always tended to be set apart as an arcane specialist area, to be entered only by a select few. However, the veterinary pathologist cannot escape having to deal with it frequently, and we attempt in this section to provide a contemporary basis for understanding veterinary neuropathology.

The principal cells of the central nervous system (CNS) are *neurons* and *glia*, plus cells of the meninges and blood vessels. *Macroglia* (astrocytes, oligodendrocytes, ependymal cells) are of neuroectodermal origin; *microglia* are derived from bone marrow.

Neuron

The neuron is the fundamental cell of the nervous system, and ultimately all neurologic disease must involve functional disturbances in neurons. In conventional histopathology, the term "neuron" refers to the cell body of the nerve cell that often is only a small part of the total cell volume. For the purposes of comprehending pathogenetic mechanisms, it is important to remember always that the neuron comprises both the *cell body* ("soma" or "perikaryon") and the cell processes, in particular the axon. The whole cell constitutes a structure concerned with the generation, conduction, and transmission of impulses, and in some cases, a single cell performs this task over a very long distance. For example, in a lumbar dorsal root ganglion of a horse, the cell body of a sensory neuron may project a process distally to the extremity of the hind foot and centrally to the caudal brainstem, making it without doubt the largest cell in the body. If the soma were enlarged to the size of an orange, the processes would have the dimensions of a garden hose and would be >20 km in length. Pathologic reactions within one cell may therefore be separated by considerable distance. Also, neurons function in hierarchical chains organized into anatomic systems.

The soma is the metabolic factory for the whole cell, and the great bulk of synthetic and degradative operations take place there. The axons are serviced throughout their length by a bidirectional transport system that moves components both away from and toward the soma (anterograde and retrograde transport, respectively). The transport mechanisms are fuelled by the consumption of energy along the course of the axon. Many components are moved in the anterograde direction within 25-nm vesicles by a "fast" transport system at a rate of 20-30 mm/hr. The motor for this system, intimately associated with the neurotubules, is an ATPase called *kinesin*. Larger vesicles of about 500 nm are transported retrograde by this fast pathway, and the translocator is an isoform of dynein, the ATPase that powers cilia and flagella in other types of cell.

Mitochondria are also moved by fast transport, but at a somewhat slower rate. Neurofilaments, neurotubules, and some soluble proteins move by slow transport in the anterograde direction only, at a rate of about 1-3 mm/day, and are degraded when they reach the terminus. Should the operations of the soma or the transport systems be impaired, the health of the axon will suffer and, appropriately, in most instances the largest and longest axons are most vulnerable. Equally, *when a neuron is fatally damaged, the whole cell dies*, and the consequent changes will spread over the whole extent of its domain. However, long lengths of the axon may degenerate without compromising the viability of the remainder of the cell and without inducing dramatic morphologic change in the soma, and there is often scope for adequate regeneration of the lost axonal extremity. These issues will be addressed more fully later, under Neurodegenerative diseases.

The vitality of individual neurons is sustained by their active relationship with other neurons, or other types of cells with which they interact. If a neuron dies, surviving neurons with which it has synaptic connections may regress because of lack of activation, undergo atrophy, and eventually die. This process is called *trans-synaptic degeneration*, and it will progress along specific anatomic pathways. It is useful also to realize that neurons are extremely diverse pharmacologically and biochemically; this is well illustrated by the highly selective and regionalized effects of different toxins and metabolic disturbances. The selective effects of tetanus and botulinum toxins are good examples.

During organogenesis, vast numbers of neuroblasts proliferate, and immature neurons migrate to their final destinations. As large numbers of developing neurons are superfluous, there is a need to select amongst them and eliminate the excess by apoptosis. Discrimination between those that will survive and those that are effete will depend on the transfer of trophic factors between cells, including from glia to neurons. Around the time of birth, and for variable periods afterward, the latter stages of the process may still be extant, particularly in the cerebellar cortex and paravertebral ganglia. It is probable that the signals between cells during growth and physiologic activity are the same as those, which if overloaded, may lead to neuronal injury. The margin of safety between proper levels of transmitter and too little or too much is very narrow.

The mature neuron is a postmitotic cell, and there is a net loss throughout adult life, especially during senescence. Thus, in a thorough scan of a histologic section from a senile animal, it might be expected that a few degenerate neurons will be found, even when fixation artifacts are minimal. There is, however, continuous postnatal generation of neurons in some parts of the brain and in at least some species. In species so far examined, neuroblasts generated in the dentate gyrus of the hippocampus and from the progenitor cells of the subependymal zone between the lateral ventricle and the caudate continue to migrate postnatally to the olfactory bulb. These migrations do not depend on guidance from radial glia, as in the embryonic brain. Rather, the postnatal neuroblasts migrate in a chain designated as the "rostral migratory stream," strictly delineated by rows of astrocytes. There is evidence that new neurons are generated in the olfactory bulb. Axonotomy procedures that sever the pituitary stalk in the rat and some other mammalian species are known to be followed by re-establishment of functional hypothalamic-hypophyseal connections within a few weeks. Cells with neuron-like characters appear to migrate through the neuropil of the median

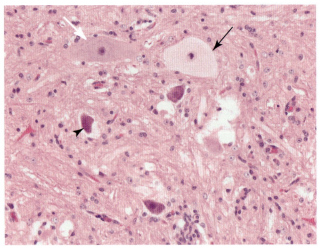

Figure 4-1 **Response of neurons to injury** in enteroviral encephalomyelitis in a pig. Normal neuron (white arrow); swollen and chromatolytic neuron (black arrow); shrunken, necrotic neuron (arrowhead).

eminence to congregate on its surface. The functional significance of these migrations and the dynamics of these populations are obscure. It is assumed that the olfactory migrants and their proliferation in situ in the bulb may have a bearing on the development of olfactory neuroblastomas.

Degenerative changes of the nerve cell body

Nuclear margination. The neuronal nucleus is usually single and centrally located (Fig. 4-1), and its *margination can be taken to indicate nonspecific degeneration*, especially when combined with loss of staining affinity. However, an eccentric nucleus can be normal in some groups of smaller neurons, and is often present in the large cells of the periventricular gray matter, such as the mesencephalic nucleus of the trigeminal nerve and the olives. These cells also tend to have a "chromatolytic" appearance.

Chromatolysis (see Fig. 4-1) is a change in appearance of the soma brought about by the *dispersal of the rough endoplasmic reticulum* (Nissl granules), and is subclassified as *central* or *peripheral* according to its locus within the cell body. Its assessment depends upon an appreciation of the prominence and distribution of Nissl granules seen normally at the particular location. There are no artifactual changes that mimic chromatolysis and, provided it is accurately identified, it can always be regarded as a lesion. A number of special stains, such as cresyl violet, will demonstrate it better than routine hematoxylin and eosin (H&E).

Central chromatolysis is best appreciated in large neurons of some of the brainstem nuclei, in the spinal motor neurons, and peripheral ganglia. The chromatolytic cells are swollen and rounded, rather than having the normal angulated appearance, and the nucleus becomes eccentric. Nissl granules clear from the central region of the cell body, leaving this zone with a smooth ground-glass appearance (see Fig. 4-76). Central chromatolysis occurs in a number of pathologic situations. It is often seen in bulbospinal motor neurons and sensory neurons whose peripherally projecting axons are injured, and especially when the injury occurs close to the cell body. The reaction follows such injury quickly, beginning within 24 hours, and becoming maximal in 1-3 weeks. When the dynamics of axonal flow are remembered, it can be appreciated that such an event will have a major feedback on the soma *(retrograde degeneration)*. In effect, the cell must rearrange its metabolism to adapt to its changed circumstances, and organize for a regenerative effort, involving the reconstruction of an axonal segment greater in volume perhaps than its surviving volume. In this context, *central chromatolysis has been termed the* **axon reaction,** *and represents an anabolic adaptive response.* In this reaction, the nucleus becomes extremely eccentric, and develops a prominent nucleolus and a basophilic cap of RNA on its cytoplasmic aspect. The Nissl substance disperses, and the cytoplasm becomes rich in free ribosomes, lysosomes, and mitochondria. There may also be some increase in the number of neurofilaments. All these changes reflect a shift in metabolic activity, with a switch toward increased synthesis of structural cellular proteins, and a marked decline in synthesis of transmitters. With completion of successful axonal regeneration, the chromatolytic soma returns to normal, sometimes passing through a densely basophilic phase in which it is packed with Nissl granules.

In some circumstances following axonal injury, central chromatolysis may proceed to cell death or permanent atrophy, and this is usually the case in neurons whose axons project entirely within the CNS. *In general, the closer to the cell body is the axonal lesion, the more likely is the cell to die*. Those cells destined to die have swollen achromatic cytoplasm depleted of organelles.

Central chromatolysis is also induced in more overtly neuronopathic conditions, most notably the numerous motor neuron degenerations described in various species, and it is a feature of the pathology of perinatal copper deficiency in the sheep and goat. Similarly, it is a striking feature in autonomic ganglia in equine and feline dysautonomias. In all such cases, the affected cells often proceed to necrosis and dissolution (Gudden's atrophy). In many of these degenerative neuronopathies, the cytoplasmic alteration is the result of massive accumulation of neurofilaments in the soma (see Progressive motor neuron diseases). Nuclear margination is not as marked as in the axon reaction, and the prominent nucleolus and nuclear cap are not evident. These differences distinguish a regressive state from a regenerative one.

Peripheral chromatolysis indicates clearing of the periphery of the soma, with Nissl granules persisting around the nucleus. This change is generally associated with slight cellular shrinkage rather than swelling. It is a nonspecific lesion and can often be regarded as an early stage en route to necrosis.

In both forms of chromatolysis, microglia and astrocytes may proliferate and cover large expanses of the cell surface, thereby separating terminal boutons from the neuronal surface.

Neuronal atrophy. Loss of cytoplasmic bulk and reduction in size might be expected in situations of permanent loss of synaptic connections (e.g., trans-synaptic degeneration), as when central axons undergo Wallerian degeneration but fail to regenerate.

Acute eosinophilic (or acidophilic) degeneration. In this *characteristic acute degenerative change*, the cytoplasm of the neuronal soma becomes shrunken and distinctly acidophilic (Fig. 4-2A), and the nucleus progresses through pyknosis and rhexis to lysis, leaving the coagulated cytoplasmic remnants to undergo liquefaction without undergoing phagocytosis. The remnant "ghosts" may persist for several days. Acute

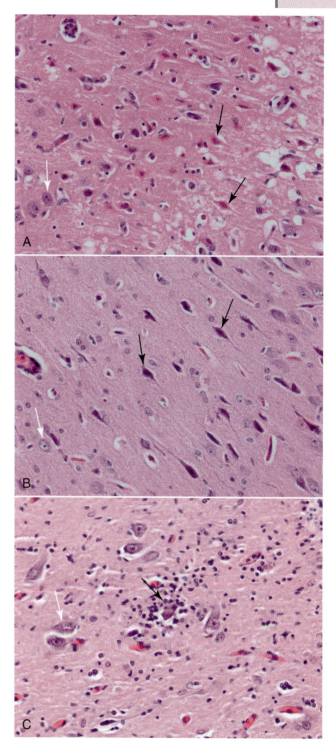

Figure 4-2 A. Early ischemic nerve cell degeneration (black arrows). Note cell shrinkage with condensed hypereosinophilic cytoplasm (pink neurons) and apoptotic nuclei. **B.** Artifactual shrunken basophilic neurons with normal nuclei *("dark neurons")* are easily misinterpreted as true necrosis. **C. Perineuronal satellitosis.** Glial cells and lymphocytes encircle a necrotic neuron (black arrow). Normal intact neurons are depicted with white arrows in all images.

eosinophilic degeneration is the morphologic reaction to ischemia, and may be also seen in the cerebral cortex in hypoxia, hypoglycemia, the encephalopathy of thiamine deficiency, and in some chemical intoxications, such as organomercurialism and indirect salt poisoning. Following seizures, it may frequently be found in the dentate gyrus of the hippocampus and the cerebellar Purkinje cells. There are usually obvious proplastic changes in astrocytes and capillary endothelia in the vicinity of the affected neurons.

This raises the concept of **excitotoxicity,** in which neuronal degeneration and death are considered to result from excessive stimulus by an excitatory neurotransmitter. This phenomenon is thought to operate particularly in those neuronal systems using glutamate as a transmitter, such as the cells in the hippocampal areas mentioned previously. Paradoxically, glutamate is potentially highly toxic to neurons, and normally is rapidly cleared by the glia following its release. Excessive release or defective clearance of glutamate from the environment of postsynaptic neurons predisposes to excitotoxicity, and such circumstances are provided by hypoxia and hypoglycemia. The pathogenesis is thought to involve ionic overloading of the cell, acute swelling, and then cell death with cytoplasmic coagulation and eosinophilia.

Neuronal necrosis may occasionally be expressed as cytoplasmic shrinkage and basophilia with nuclear dissolution (see Fig. 4-1). Shrunken basophilic neurons with normal nuclei ("*dark neurons*") are generally taken to be artifactual, and are often numerous (Fig. 4-2B).

Special stains for degenerating neurons are the amino cupric silver technique and the Fluoro-Jade stains (B and C). These stains are also helpful for distinguishing dark neurons from degenerating neurons within peracute degenerative processes in which the eosinophilic cytoplasmic alteration has not had time to develop.

Liquefactive necrosis is often at risk of being misinterpreted as autolytic change and fixation artifact, particularly shrinkage artifact. A lesion can sometimes be distinguished from an artifact by the presence or absence of significant alterations in other tissue cells, for example, the swelling of capillary endothelium or indications of glial proliferation.

Necrosis with neuronophagia. In many viral infections, the death of neurons provokes the gathering of phagocytes around the cell body **(satellitosis),** and removal by them of the debris, forming **neuronophagic nodules** (Fig. 4-2C). This is usually a response of the microglia, although satellite perineuronal oligodendrocytes may also proliferate in response to neuronal injury. Neuronophagia may also be seen in metabolic or toxigenic neuronal degenerations, but is generally not as extensive as in viral infection.

Vacuolar degeneration. Neurons in the early stages of acute injury, inflicted by viruses, toxins, or metabolic derangements, such as excitotoxicity, may develop numerous small cytoplasmic vacuoles, usually reflecting *mitochondrial swelling*. However, *artifactual peripheral vacuolation is very common,* giving the periphery of the cytoplasm a foamy web-like appearance. This is particularly so in the cerebellar Purkinje cells and large neurons of some of the brainstem nuclei.

Large neuronal vacuoles, few in number per cell, are occasionally observed in otherwise normal brains, and may be seen in the red and oculomotor nuclei of aged cattle and sheep. When they occur at high frequency in the neurons of the medulla and midbrain, they are virtually pathognomonic of *scrapie* in sheep and goats (Fig. 4-3). Widespread neuronal

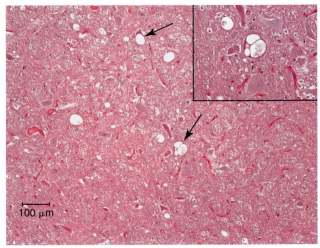

Figure 4-3 Neuronal vacuolation in scrapie in a sheep (arrows) (inset, higher magnification). (Courtesy M.J. Hazlett.)

vacuolation with single or multiple large vacuoles, unexplained as to pathogenesis, is occasionally seen in dogs and cattle with progressive neurologic dysfunction.

Vacuolar change is strikingly evident in those *lysosomal storage diseases* in which the stored material is extracted during processing, or is unstained by the routine methods. In these situations, the neuron can become dramatically bloated by the accumulation of myriad secondary lysosomes that displace the normal organelles and distend the soma with a foamy mass of apparently empty vacuoles. In most cases, the storage process involves other cell types inside and outside the nervous system, and is accompanied by additional neuropathologic manifestations (see Storage diseases).

Trans-synaptic degeneration. Loss of normal inputs can lead to atrophy or death of the affected neurons. These effects are termed trans-synaptic, because the affected neurons are synaptically related to the system that is directly damaged. When neurons die as a consequence of the removal of their targets, the phenomenon is termed *retrograde trans-synaptic degeneration,* and when neurons die following deafferentation, the phenomenon is termed *anterograde trans-synaptic degeneration.* These concepts are necessary to interpret some lesion distribution patterns. For example, loss of Purkinje cells leads to anterograde trans-synaptic degeneration of cerebellar nuclei and retrograde trans-synaptic degeneration of cerebellar granule cells.

Storage of pigments and other materials. Neurons may accumulate large quantities of **ceroid/lipofuscin** or other pigments, either as a consequence of aging, or in storage disorders involving such substances. The pathogenesis of the *ceroid/lipofuscinoses* remains unclear. There is a genetic basis in some instances, whereas in others, unspecified environmental factors may be involved. The complex storage material accumulates as granules in a manner analogous to the other lysosomal storage diseases, although a clearly defined limiting membrane is not usually apparent ultrastructurally. When the process is intense, rusty brown discoloration of the gray matter and ganglia may be evident grossly.

Neuromelanins may also accumulate excessively in those midbrain nuclei, where they are usually present in modest amounts, and extensive neuromelanosis can occur in sheep chronically poisoned by *Phalaris* spp. In extreme cases,

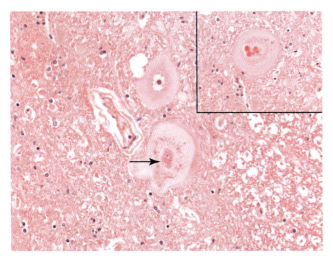

Figure 4-4 Spinal motor neuron in **motor neuron disease** in a horse. Chromatolysis, nuclear dissolution (arrow), and cytoplasmic inclusions (inset, another affected neuron). (Courtesy J. DeLay.)

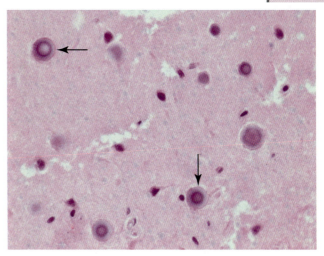

Figure 4-5 Multiple neuropilar **Lafora bodies** (arrows) in a cat. (Courtesy Armed Forces Institute of Pathology.)

the gray matter and ganglia may have macroscopic green discoloration.

Siderotic pigmentation of neurons, in which the cells become encrusted with basophilic complexes of iron, calcium, and phosphorus, may be found near contusions and hemorrhages. It is not known, however, whether the iron is derived from the hemoglobin or from intracellular iron-containing respiratory enzymes. The neurons may be otherwise normal, or their degeneration may produce small lakes of basophilic deposit. The latter are common in the neonatal cerebellar cortex.

Viral inclusion bodies. The best known is the *Negri body* of rabies, which is eosinophilic and intracytoplasmic. Herpesvirus inclusions are characteristically intranuclear, whereas those of the paramyxoviruses, such as canine distemper virus, may be intracytoplasmic or intranuclear. The use of specific immunostains has greatly facilitated the identification of viral inclusions.

Nonviral eosinophilic cytoplasmic inclusion bodies also occur. Sometimes they are an incidental finding in otherwise normal brains at sporadic locations; in cats, they can sometimes be found in the pyramidal cells of the hippocampus and lateral geniculate nuclei.

More specific inclusions have been described in people and animals in neuronal degenerative diseases. In humans, ultrastructural differences define several types of inclusion: **Hirano, Pick, Lewy, Lafora,** and **Bunina bodies.** *Hirano-like bodies,* appearing histologically as elongated eosinophilic inclusions and, ultrastructurally, as masses of beaded filaments, are reported in horses and dogs, together with other structures having some of the features of Bunina bodies. Further definition of these types of inclusions in animals is required, and their pathogenetic significance is not understood; they are a feature of equine motor neuron disease (Fig. 4-4). *Bunina bodies* are small eosinophilic inclusions of 2-5 μm, sometimes in small clusters or chains that characterize human *amyotrophic lateral sclerosis;* similar inclusions are occasionally observed in degenerative and inflammatory neurologic disease in animals.

Lafora bodies are occasionally observed in neurologic disease, but most frequently are incidental findings in aged animals. They are basophilic to amphophilic inclusions that are strongly period acid–Schiff (PAS) positive and metachromatic, 5-20 μm in size, intracytoplasmic, or in processes or free in the neuropil (Fig. 4-5). They represent an abnormality of carbohydrate metabolism, producing glucose polymers called *polyglucosans*. In the very rare *Lafora disease* (see Storage diseases), they occur in massive numbers throughout the brain within the neuronal soma, the dendrites, and less commonly the axons; they are associated with severe myoclonus epilepsy.

Mucocyte (Buscaino body) is the term applied to glassy, pale gray-blue bodies of variable size and shape, roughly the same size as neurons, seen on routinely processed and stained sections of brains. These are usually dispersed in the neuropil, typically in major white matter tracts and are considered by most to be an *artifact* of fixation and processing. They may be PAS positive, but are not always so, and there are rare reports of the accumulation of mucocytes associated with disease.

Axon

The axon acts as the solitary efferent extension of all neurons except those sensory neurons in the spinal ganglia, whose peripherally directed myelinated axons function as dendrites, in that they conduct impulses toward the cell body. Axons may branch extensively toward their terminations.

The first part of the axon is called the *initial segment*, and it has distinctive ultrastructure, related to its being the site of membrane ion channels critical for the initiation of a propagated action potential. The axoplasm contains mitochondria, endosomes, intermediate filaments (neurofilaments), microtubules (neurotubules), and secretory vesicles or granules containing neurotransmitters appropriate for the particular cell. The axoplasm will also contain soluble macromolecules such as enzymes.

Axons are sustained by their parent cell bodies and by the cells that invest them along their course. The axoplasm is devoid of ribosomes, and axoplasmic proteins are provided by the soma. Similarly, the lysosomal apparatus is limited in the axon, in terms of digestive capacity, and many obsolete materials and organelles are returned by retrograde transport to the cell body for complete degradation. The role of neurotubules in transport mechanisms has been mentioned previously, and is critically important for the maintenance of the axon. Axonal diameter is distinctly reduced at the nodes of Ranvier, and these "strictures" are probably the reason that paranodal swellings filled with transported vesicles and organelles are a feature of many axonopathies in which transport has been disturbed.

Neurofilaments are responsible for the maintenance of axonal size and geometry, and are part of the generic cytoskeletal intermediate filament family. The proteolytic destruction of neurofilaments, triggered by the influx of calcium ions, is a common pathway for the collapse and disintegration of damaged axons. Larger axons are invested in a segmental manner by a *myelin sheath*, interrupted at the *nodes of Ranvier*, and penetrated at intervals by incisures.

All this sophistication is not resolved in routine light microscopic examination of paraffin-embedded tissues. The course of axons can be highlighted by the use of silver staining techniques, which emphasize the shrinkage artifact and distortion produced by routine tissue preparation. Nonetheless, with experience, many lesions in paraffin-embedded tissue can be interpreted but, particularly for peripheral nerves, plastic embedding of specimens is far preferable.

Types of **axonopathy** have been grouped according to whether they begin in the *proximal* or the *distal* portion of the axon, and whether they involve central or peripheral axons or both. Thus, for example, one may distinguish central and peripheral distal axonopathy, or central proximal axonopathy. The principal categories of axonopathy can now be discussed in broad terms.

Wallerian degeneration *denotes the changes that follow acute focal injury to a myelinated axon*, such that distal to the injury it becomes nonviable. When the soma is uninjured, there is potential for regeneration and, in peripheral nerves, this may be complete. Should the acute injury involve death of the cell body, then Wallerian degeneration of the axon will proceed as part of the dissolution of the entire neuron. The classic scenario for Wallerian degeneration is *acute focal mechanical injury in a peripheral nerve*, which effectively transects axoplasmic flow. Within 24 hours, the distal segment begins to degenerate fairly evenly along its length *(anterograde degeneration)*. Focal eosinophilic swellings occur, often containing accumulations of degenerate organelles, and then fragmentation becomes evident by 48 hours or so. Schwann cells respond rapidly as myelin sheaths are made redundant by disintegration of the axon. Initially, myelin retracts from the nodes and then forms into *ellipsoids*, regarded originally as *"digestion chambers"* for the enzymic lysis of the axonal fragments (Fig. 4-6). The myelin itself condenses into aggregates and fragments and, together with remaining axonal debris, becomes the target of invading macrophages. Prior to this, the complex myelin lipids are progressively transformed into simpler neutral lipids over a period of 10-20 days, and this is reflected in the reaction to specific lipophilic stains. Macrophages enter the sheath and soon become filled with sudanophilic droplets. These lipid-laden cells may persist in the interstitium for many weeks. Some of the myelin debris is phagocytosed by Schwann cells themselves, and they begin to proliferate. As the debris is cleared away, proliferating Schwann cells form bands along the former course of the myelinated axons *(Büngner's bands)*. Similar Wallerian changes occur proximal to the site of injury over several internodes. If conditions are favorable at the site of injury, sprouts from the axonal stump will find their way along the Schwann cell bands and be directed to their correct destinations. In most instances, the *growing*

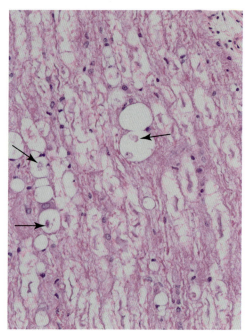

Figure 4-6 Multiple digestion chambers (arrows) containing axonal fragments and macrophages in stenotic myelopathy in a goat.

axonal sprouts advance at a rate of 2-4 mm/day, and the new axon will be invested by Schwann cell cytoplasm. Sprouting from individual axons is initially multiple and, by an unknown mechanism, one sprout is selected for the completion of regeneration. Thus a new axon may arise from a different soma than did the original. *The regenerated axon is remyelinated by Schwann cells*, although the new sheath is thinner than the original, and nodal length variable and shorter. Should axonal regeneration be prevented, Schwann cell bands persist, and endoneurial fibrosis usually develops. *Abortive regeneration can lead to a tangled clump of neurites, Schwann cells, and fibrocytes at the injury* site. This will happen after transection if too great a distance separates the severed ends of the nerve fibers.

The effectiveness of regeneration in peripheral nerves is related to the comparatively simple axon/Schwann cell relationship, the presence of a basal lamina tube around each myelinated axon, and the replicative ability and metabolic resilience of the Schwann cells.

These conditions do not apply in the central nervous system **(CNS)**, where the oligodendrocyte/axon relationship is far more complex: The oligodendrocyte is a relatively poorly regenerative cell type, there is no basal lamina scaffold, and the debris from central myelin is thought to inhibit axonal sprouting. The initial regressive changes of Wallerian degeneration are similar to those described for the peripheral nerves, although they proceed over a longer time course. This is because the involvement of hematogenous macrophages is slower and less intense in the CNS, and activated microglial cells undertake most of the work. Axonal sprouting and some remyelination can occur. However, the poverty of the regenerative response results mostly in the *permanent disappearance of the axons, myelin, and oligodendrocyte cell bodies*. Some of the myelin debris may be phagocytosed by reactive astrocytes, and their processes extend to fill the vacancy, creating a ramifying network of astroglial scar tissue. Wallerian-like degeneration in the CNS is most commonly seen in the spinal cord,

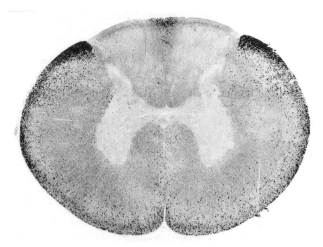

Figure 4-7 Degeneration of myelin in spinal cord in a pig with copper deficiency. Stained with Marchi technique. Note selective involvement of tracts, namely, the fasciculus gracilis and dorsal and ventral spinocerebellar tracts. (Courtesy M.D. McGavin.)

optic tract, and brainstem. Probably the best-known association is with the focal compressive myelopathies in the horse and dog (the wobbler syndromes), although this type of axonal reaction may also occur secondarily to ischemia and degenerative axonal disorders.

During the active degenerative phase, recently phagocytosed and partially digested myelin debris may be distinguished in paraffin sections by the use of the Luxol fast blue/PAS stain. Degenerate myelin is well visualized by the Marchi technique (Fig. 4-7), or by immunostaining of myelin basic protein (MBP). Normal and pathologic axons can be identified by antibodies to neurofilaments. End-stage plaques of astrogliosis may be demonstrated by traditional gliophilic stains or by the use of immunostaining for glial fibrillary acidic protein (GFAP: intermediate filament protein).

The destruction of myelin in Wallerian degeneration is known as **secondary demyelination** and is to be distinguished from **primary demyelination,** in which the axon is initially undamaged (see later).

Distal axonopathy is seen in a number of chronic intoxications and genetically determined entities. It begins with degenerative changes in the distal reaches of the affected fibers and fairly characteristically involves the largest and longest, such as the proprioceptive and motor tracts of the spinal cord, optic tract, and recurrent laryngeal and other long peripheral nerves. Implicit in this pattern is a disturbance of anterograde axonal transport, upon which the maintenance of axonal well-being depends. In general, the process begins with the formation of focal axonal swellings containing degenerate organelles. These swellings are ovoid or circular eosinophilic structures commonly referred to as **spheroids.** This may progress to axonal fragmentation and attempted regeneration that may be abortive and is succeeded by further degeneration. These changes may develop focally in the distal regions of the axon and may extend more proximally with time. Diagnostically, the key is the recognition of the pattern of degenerative changes toward the terminations of long tracts (see Cycad poisoning). The lesion is a feature of intoxication with certain of the organophosphates, for example.

Proximal axonopathy is the contrasting situation in which focal swellings and degeneration begin in the proximal axonal

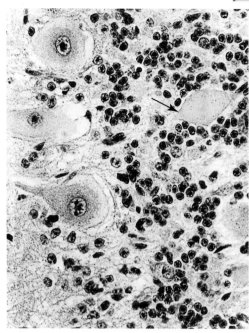

Figure 4-8 Proximal axonal enlargement—"torpedo" (arrow)—of a Purkinje cell, in mannosidosis in an Aberdeen Angus calf.

regions. It is a pattern less likely to be encountered in natural animal disease than the distal variety. It is perhaps best exemplified by the large fusiform swellings, **torpedoes,** seen on the proximal axonal segments of cerebellar Purkinje cells in the mycotoxicosis of perennial rye grass poisoning and some storage diseases (Fig. 4-8). Such lesions may develop in central or peripheral axons and be associated with genetically determined or acquired disease. Proximal axonal swellings caused by the accumulation of neurofilaments are a feature of several neurodegenerative diseases. A defect in the transport of phosphorylated neurofilaments results in the accumulation of masses of them, where they cause large, amphophilic axonal swellings. The fundamental pathogenesis remains undefined.

Axonal dystrophy is a term used to describe an axonopathic process characterized by the occurrence of *large focal swellings, often concentrated in the terminals and preterminals of long axons.* They are therefore frequently seen in and around relay nuclei in the brain, and in peripheral endings. The spheroids in axonal dystrophy can become extremely large, >100 µm in diameter, and are filled with accumulations of normal organelles, degenerate organelles, and abnormal membranous and tubular structures. In H&E sections, their appearance can be variable (Fig. 4-9A, B); some are densely eosinophilic, and either smooth or granular or vacuolated; others may be pale with central denser-staining cores; some may have a basophilic hue and evidence of focal mineralization. However, the swellings are not usually associated with any marked reaction on the part of surrounding elements and only rarely are seen to be undergoing fragmentation and dissolution. They are long-lasting, in contrast to the spheroids of acute axonal degeneration. Thinning of the myelin sheath around spheroids will occur as lamellae slip to accommodate the focal axonal enlargement (Fig. 4-10). The pathogenesis is unclear, but evidence points to a *disturbance of retrograde axonal transport.* The lesion is a common finding in the relay nuclei of the caudal brainstem in old age, and is a frequent accompaniment to neuronal storage diseases. It is the principal

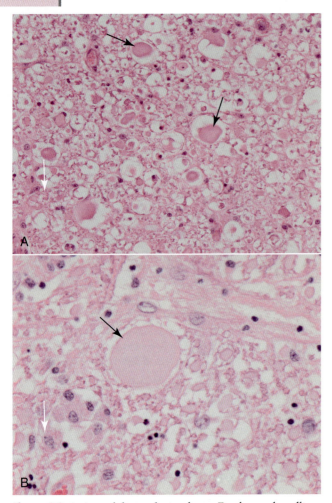

Figure 4-9 **A. Axonal dystrophy** in a horse. Focal axonal swellings with formation of spheroids (arrows). **B.** Higher magnification.

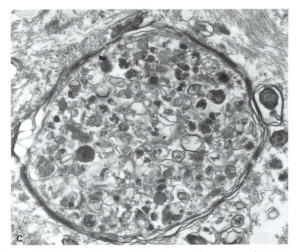

Figure 4-10 **Axonal dystrophy** in a cat with mannosidosis. Focal axonal swelling containing degenerate organelles; note thinning of myelin sheath. (Courtesy S.U. Walkley.)

feature of diseases known as **neuroaxonal dystrophies**, of which several are recorded in the veterinary literature. In several such diseases, the topography of the axonal dystrophy seems to fit the clinical deficits, but there is evidence that, in many situations, even intense development of the lesion has

no functional significance. This seems generally so in regard to axonal dystrophy in the gracilis and cuneate nuclei.

Oligodendrocytes, Schwann cells, and the myelin sheath

The **oligodendrocyte** is one of the close companion cells of the neuron in the CNS. One population of these cells occurs as satellites to nerve cell bodies and may proliferate in the event of injury to the neurons, but the role of the satellites is essentially unknown. *The role of oligodendrocytes is to provide and maintain the myelin sheaths around those axons with a diameter greater than ~1 μm.* They are accordingly located in the myelinated tracts among the fascicles of axons and are referred to as *interfascicular oligodendrocytes*. Particularly in neonates and in cases of hypomyelinogenesis or delayed myelinogenesis, distinction histologically between astrocytes and oligodendrocytes can be uncertain. Oligodendrocytes are smaller than astrocytes, nuclear density is greater, and the cells are arranged in rows between fascicles. In immature animals, nuclei of oligodendrocytes are morphologically heterogeneous, and those with large nuclei and clear nucleoplasm and not readily distinguished from astrocytes are probably immature and capable of division or synthesis of membrane myelin.

Oligodendrocytes arise from precursor cells in the subventricular zone of the developing forebrain and from the floor plate of the neural tube in the brainstem and spinal cord. These progenitors migrate extensively to settle along fiber tracts of the developing white matter, where they go through a series of maturation changes to produce myelin.

Each mature oligodendrocyte has a compact cell body of characteristic ultrastructural appearance, and a dozen or so thin processes, each of which connects the perikaryon to a segment of myelin some distance away. Each segment of myelin covers one axonal internode, and is an extended and compacted sheet of specialized oligodendroglial plasma membrane bilayers, wound concentrically and spirally around the axon, like a rolled-up newspaper. In the formation of this compacted membrane, both the intracellular and extracellular spaces are obliterated, creating the major and minor dense lines of myelin lamellae as seen with the electron microscope. In some axons, a sheath of 100 or so bilayers may be formed. A portion of intact cytoplasm remains at the innermost and outermost lamellae, known as the "inner" and "outer" tongues, respectively. Tracts of uncompacted cytoplasm course through the sheath to form the "incisures," and also occur where the myelin lamellae terminate at the paranodal region, as the "terminal loops." The lamellated myelin sheath is a relatively stable but plastic structure, whose lipid and protein components are supplied and turned over by the oligodendrocyte.

For light microscopy, myelin is well demonstrated by several special stains, with osmium tetroxide being particularly effective. Biochemically, central myelin is largely composed of cholesterol, galactocerebroside, and phospholipids, together with a number of distinctive protein constituents. The most abundant of these is the proteolipid protein (PLP), with lesser amounts of myelin basic protein (MBP), and myelin-associated glycoprotein (MAG). PLP is concentrated at the intraperiod line, MBP on the cytoplasmic face of the major dense line, and MAG at the axoplasmic-myelin interface. They probably play an important role in maintaining the stability of the sheath. Other antigens are expressed by oligodendrocytes and myelin sheath, including the transcription factor Olig2 and 2′-3′-cyclic nucleotide-3′-phosphodiesterase (CNPase).

It is thus apparent that one oligodendrocyte myelinates several axonal internodes, that the myelin sheath is part of the oligodendrocyte, and that death of the oligodendrocyte will result in the demise of all the myelin sheath segments supplied by that cell. However, destruction of one or more myelin sheath segments does not necessarily result in death of the parent oligodendrocyte, but may stimulate it to withdraw its remaining myelin. The dynamics of the oligodendrocyte population are still not absolutely clear, but it is becoming accepted that there is a system of undifferentiated reserve cells able to take on, to some extent, regenerative and reparative tasks. These cells may originate from the perineuronal satellite oligodendroglia.

Myelination occurs relatively late in the development of the CNS, and maturing oligodendrocytes invest axons with myelin by replacing an initial ensheathment of astrocytic processes. Once this is completed, most of the cells assume the characteristics of maturity, whereas some do appear to remain in a less mature state. The ability of oligodendrocytes to synthesize myelin at specific times and in specific tracts that are specific for the animal species must require signaling mechanisms that wait to be clarified.

Oligodendrocytes do not exhibit a range of reactions for the light microscopist, generally undergoing rapid lysis when injured. Acute injury may be manifested by hydropic swelling of the perikaryon. On occasion, mitotic activity and an increase in numbers may be observed when a primary demyelinating process is operating, but this seems to be very rare in veterinary pathology. Their numbers may be increased by condensation in linear rows in interfascicular gliosis. Inclusion bodies may be present in the nuclei in some viral diseases such as canine distemper. Excepting oligodendroglial tumors, damage to the cells is expressed in disordered myelin.

The process of myelination is dependent on close interaction between the axon and the myelinating cell. The two act as a unit, and signals are exchanged between them for all aspects of the process. Although the axon may survive for a long period without its myelin sheath, loss of the axon provokes immediate disintegration and removal of the myelin sheath. *This situation of axonal degeneration with secondary myelin loss is termed Wallerian degeneration*, and has been discussed above under axonopathy.

Myelination in peripheral nerves is the responsibility of **Schwann cells,** and they have a distinctly different relationship with axons to that of oligodendrocytes. Each peripheral internode is myelinated by a single cell, and the myelinated axon is invested by a basal lamina tube of Schwann cell origin, and by endoneurial collagen. Signals from Schwann cells influence the development of all components of the nerve and endoneural and epineural connective tissue and the Schwann cells themselves. Schwann cells develop from the neural crest as 2 different cell types, *myelinating* and *nonmyelinating*. This differentiation is reversible, which is consistent with the absence of precursors in mature nerves regenerating after injury. If mature Schwann cells lose contact with axons, as occurs in nerve injury, the cells undergo regression and the myelin disintegrates. The dedifferentiated cells multiply and provide growth factors that support the regrowth of axons.

The cell body of the Schwann cell directly apposes the axon. Peripheral myelin is also chemically distinct from central myelin, and this can be appreciated by the tinctorial difference between the two in appropriately stained sections of the spinal cord–spinal nerve interface. This chemical difference is reflected in antigenic differences; the major protein is termed Po and is distinct from PLP, as is the basic protein P1 from MBP. *Schwann cells are able to replicate prolifically, to phagocytose damaged myelin, and to remyelinate newly regenerated or previously demyelinated axons.* This replicative ability means that the loss of a proportion of the cells may be compensated. The peripheral myelinated axon is therefore a much more resilient structure than its central counterpart. The general principles of the axon-myelin relationship, as outlined for the CNS, still apply, however. *Destruction of Schwann cells will result in the disintegration of the dependent myelin.* Destruction of axons will cause myelin degradation, Schwann cell proliferation, and, in time, endoneurial fibrosis.

In paraffin sections of normal nerve, Schwann cells appear as ovoid nuclei closely apposed to the axon. Proliferating Schwann cells in longitudinal section often appear as bands *(Büngner's bands)* of spindle-shaped cells resembling fibroblasts. In cross-section, they form concentric whorls called *"onion bulbs."* Common incidental findings are nodular proliferations of hyaline structures attached to the inner layer of the perineurium in normal and pathologic nerves of various animals and humans. They are termed *Renaut bodies* and are composed of perineurial cells and fibroblasts immersed in an extracellular matrix, and arranged in concentric structures.

A number of diseases primarily involve the myelin sheath, and may frequently leave the myelinating cell body intact. These diseases usually require ultrastructural evaluation for adequate investigation.

In **demyelinating diseases,** the sheath is removed from the axons, leaving them naked over variable lengths and providing potential for serious slowing of impulse conduction. In peripheral nerves, the removal of myelin from randomly scattered internodes gives rise to segmental demyelination, which is best appreciated in teased fiber preparations. Demyelination is frequently carried out by macrophages that insinuate cytoplasmic processes into the intraperiod lines and strip the sheath from the axonal internode, ingesting and digesting myelin debris. In other situations, myelin appears first to be disrupted by humoral factors and undergoes splitting and vesiculation prior to phagocytosis. Myelinophagy can be identified by the use of stains such as the Luxol fast blue/PAS technique. Degenerate myelin can be visualized by the Marchi technique (see Fig. 4-7).

In the CNS, there is some scope for remyelination, but the complex arrangement and limited replicative capacity of the oligodendrocytes limits the reparative potential. Regenerated myelin sheaths are thinner than the originals, appearing to the experienced eye as being too narrow for the diameter of the axon they ensheath. Remyelinated internodes are also shorter. In the peripheral nervous system, the potential for remyelination is much more favorable. Repeated bouts of demyelination may result in "onion bulb" and Renaut body formations, and in the production of thin and irregular myelin segments.

In **hypomyelinating diseases,** myelinating cells fail, for various reasons, to provide adequate myelination during the development phase, and the affected individual suffers transient or permanent myelin deficiency, varying in extent and severity according to the particular disease (Fig. 4-11A-D). The majority of these conditions involve the CNS only (see Myelinopathies). Myelin sheaths are thin or absent, but

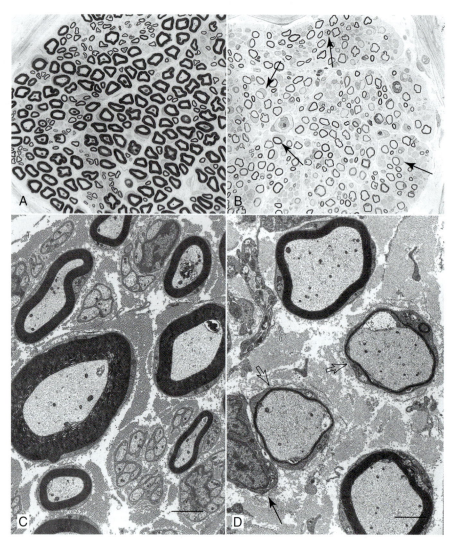

Figure 4-11 **Polyneuropathy** in a Golden Retriever. Comparison of normal (**A**) and hypomyelinated (**B**) peripheral nerve. Voluminous Schwann cell cytoplasm (arrows). **C, D.** Corresponding ultrastructure; normal (**C**), hypomyelinated (**D**). Thinly myelinated fibers (open arrow). Schwann cell nucleus (black arrow). Bar = 2 µm. (Reprinted with permission from Braund KG, et al. Vet Pathol 1989;26:202-208.)

myelinophagy is generally minimal or nonexistent. Oligodendrocytes may be few, or present in normal numbers, and may exhibit features of immaturity.

In **dysmyelinating diseases,** there is a qualitative defect in the myelin produced, and the quantity may also be reduced. A large variety of these disorders has been produced for research purposes in inbred strains of laboratory mice.

Myelinic edema *is disruption of the lamellar structure by reopening of the extracellular space along the intraperiod line.* It may occur in both central and peripheral myelin. It is caused by a number of chemical agents, for example, hexachlorophene, and leads to a spectacular state of spongy degeneration of white matter, one form of status spongiosus. With some causal agents, there are associated degenerative and reactive changes, but with other causes, there is, remarkably, no apparent response on the part of other tissue elements, including the oligodendrocytes themselves. The lesion does not necessarily cause functional disturbances even when well developed; it seems that this may depend on the number of intact lamellae left in place. It may resolve over a period of weeks, with no evidence of breakdown of the affected myelin (see Spongy myelinopathies).

Astrocytes

Astrocytes may be regarded as the interstitial cells of the CNS, as their processes occupy most of the space between and around the neuronal and oligodendroglial elements, and the perivascular and subpial zones. Astrocytes are of 2 types: the **protoplasmic** (type 1), located mainly within the cerebral gray matter, and the **fibrous** (type 2), located mainly within white matter tracts. However, astrocyte populations are heterogeneous from one brain region to another. Evidence suggests a common progenitor cell, the 011A cell, for the type 2 astrocyte and the oligodendrocyte. Indeed, there is evidence for several different functional types of astrocyte, the functional diversity reflecting diverse locational needs. Radial glial cells, which are the precursors of astrocytes, guide the migration of neurons from the subependymal generative zones to their final positions; astrocytes guide axons into their proper fiber tracts; astrocytes are important in the regulation of ionic exchanges

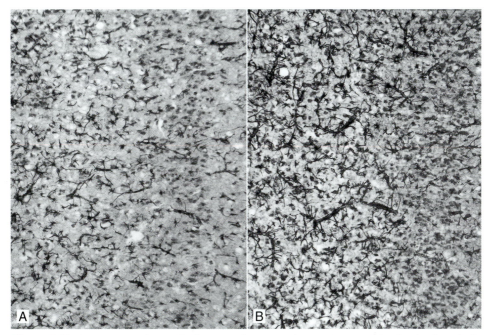

Figure 4-12 Astrocytes in the cerebral cortex of a goat with scrapie, stained by the Cajal method. A. Normal. B. Fibrous astrogliosis. (Reprinted with permission from Hadlow WJ, Race RE. Vet Pathol 1986;23:543-549.)

between cells of the nervous system; and astrocytes form functional connections by production of molecules that are tropic for other specialized cells of the nervous system.

The intercellular space of CNS tissue is a 20-nm cleft between astrocytes and the other elements, and is interrupted by loose junctions and zonulae adherentia between the former. The astrocytic perikaryon is sparse and barely evident in routine paraffin sections, and the numerous and ramifying processes are invisible. The nuclei appear, therefore, as naked and spherical, and about the size of those of small- to medium-sized neurons; they usually lack a nucleolus, but sometimes have a chromatic dot, the centrosome. Immunochemical demonstration of *vimentin* and *nestin* is used to confirm the identity of immature astrocytes, and *glial fibrillary acidic protein* (GFAP) to confirm identity of mature astrocytes, including neoplastic astrocytes. However, GFAP is not entirely specific for astrocytes. Ultrastructurally, the astrocytic cytoplasm throughout is relatively devoid of organelles and appears largely empty and watery. The chief features are bundles of intermediate filaments, clusters of glycogen granules, and a few mitochondria and lysosomes.

All capillary blood vessels in the CNS are closely invested by the expanded ends of astrocytic processes, the *end feet*. There is also a dense network of processes at the surface beneath the pia mater, the *glia limitans*. A specialized population of astrocytes occurs in the Purkinje cell layer of the cerebellum and is known as *Bergmann's glia*. These cells have long straight processes that extend out through the molecular layer to the surface.

Astrocytes and their processes are well visualized by the application of special stains, such as the Cajal method (Fig. 4-12A, B), or immunostaining for the intermediate filament GFAP. Astrocytes are considered to play an important role in the movement of cations and water, to be much involved in maintenance of conditions favorable for the electrical activity of neurons, and to be a source of cytokines and growth factors

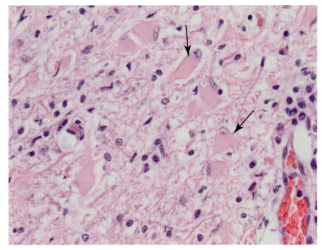

Figure 4-13 Reactive astrocytes (gemistocytes) (arrows) near malacic focus.

that support neurons and neuronal activity. Type 2 cells have a major role, in this regard, at the nodes of Ranvier, where they form a close relationship with both the axon and the terminal myelin loops. They are also involved in the detoxification of ammonia, and perhaps other metabolites.

When lethal astrocytic injury occurs, the cytoplasm swells and becomes visible, albeit faintly, and the nucleus becomes eccentric and pyknotic. Disintegration of cytoplasm and nucleus follows rapidly. Astrocytes, however, are capable of a number of reactive responses when they, or cells around them, are damaged. *A frequent response is swelling and eosinophilia of the cytoplasm, with some cells acquiring 2 or more nuclei. These plump reactive astrocytes are called* **gemistocytes** (Fig. 4-13). In a mild response, cytoplasmic swelling may be minimal, but some proliferation of both cells and processes generally occurs *(astrogliosis)*. With cessation of injury, cytoplasmic swelling regresses, but there may be a permanent residuum of extra cells and processes. Around the borders of severe lesions, such as malacic foci, the proliferation of processes may become extremely dense. Astrocytic proplasia is limited to surviving tissue, however, and postmalacic cavities cannot be filled by astrocytic processes.

Reactive astrogliosis is expected in Wallerian-like degeneration, following neuronal loss, and in sustained cerebral or spinal edema, and is a feature of many viral encephalitides in which viral infection of astrocytes is probably a prime stimulus. This is certainly the case in canine distemper, in which inclusion bodies are common in reactive astrocytes. Astrocytes are the cells primarily responsible for repair and scar formation in the brain.

In acute cerebral or spinal vasogenic edema, swollen astrocytes and their processes undergo a type of hydropic degeneration. This can only be resolved satisfactorily with the electron microscope, when the clear distention can be seen, particularly in the perivascular end feet.

An acute astrocytic reaction known as the formation of **Alzheimer type II cells** is best exemplified by the metabolic disturbance in *hepatic encephalopathy* resulting from liver failure (Fig. 4-14A, B). These reactive astrocytes are found in clusters in the gray matter. The nucleus becomes distinctly enlarged and vesicular but remains rounded; the cytoplasm swells and may become visible. This change does not involve the generation of large masses of cytoplasmic intermediate filaments, and there is a weak reaction to GFAP immunostains. It is caused by the accumulation of ammonia and other endogenous toxins, and would therefore also be expected in cases of exogenous ammonia intoxication. In some circumstances, cells suggested to be astrocytes are capable of *phagocytosis of tissue debris*, particularly myelin. This can be seen in Wallerian-like degeneration in the optic nerves when the bulk of myelinophagy may be performed by astrocytes. It has also been observed in other regions of the brain and cord.

A bizarre and rare astrocytic response is the formation of **Rosenthal fibers**; these are irregularly shaped, hyaline eosinophilic structures composed of GFAP aggregates, along with ubiquitin, heat shock proteins, and other unknown components, formed within the cell bodies and processes. The massive production of Rosenthal fibers is a feature of *Alexander disease*, an idiopathic entity described in humans, dogs, and sheep, now regarded as the only primary genetic disease of astrocytes.

Ependymal cells

Ependymocytes are columnar or cuboidal ciliated neuroepithelial cells that line the ventricular surface of the CNS, extending from the lateral ventricles to the filum terminale. They react to a variety of pathologic insults. *Atrophy, tearing,* and *discontinuity* commonly occur in chronic hydrocephalus. *Ependymitis* consists of necrosis, breaking up of the ependymal lining, subependymal inflammatory infiltration, and astrogliosis. *Rosette formation* can follow as an attempt at repairing such lesions. A particular inflammatory form, termed *granular ependymitis*, is described in equine infectious anemia and is characterized by proliferation of microscopic nodules of astrocytes not lined by ependymal cells. Ependymal cells are immunoreactive for vimentin and inconsistently for GFAP. In the **choroid plexus**, blood vessels are covered by a single layer of modified ependymal cells that secrete the cerebrospinal fluid. They can express low- and high-molecular-weight cytokeratins. The capillaries are separated from the covering epithelium by perivascular connective tissue in continuity with the pia-arachnoid. The basal lamina is immunoreactive for collagen IV.

Mention must be made of the *nests of residual glia (islands of Calleja)* that are seen beneath the ependyma of the lateral ventricles and in the dentate fascia of the hippocampus. These cells are relics of the developmental period and possibly act as a supply of replacement cells in the adult. They occur in small aggregates and often as eccentric cuffs around vessels. Generally, they are monomorphic and appear as small dark nuclei and may be mistaken for inflammatory cells.

Microglia

Microglia are derived from the mononuclear phagocyte lineage, and function as the *fixed macrophage system* of the CNS. In the normal brain and cord, they appear by routine microscopy as *inconspicuous, small hyperchromatic nuclei, often wedge shaped, and with no visible cytoplasm*. However, special staining techniques reveal extensive thin cytoplasmic processes and, with the electron microscope, dense perikaryal cytoplasm with elongated strands of rough endoplasmic reticulum and lipofuscin-like granules are characteristic. They can be labeled immunohistochemically by antibodies to CD18 and CD11d. Microglia are most frequent in the gray matter, where they may group in the vicinity of neurons, and in both gray and white matter, they are most numerous adjacent to blood vessels. During organogenesis, they are derived from blood monocytes that also give rise to the rich population of leptomeningeal and perivascular histiocytes that can migrate into the neuropil when significant vascular damage has occurred. Microglia are the primary immune effector cells of the CNS. Activated microglia at the site of injury express increased levels of major histocompatibility antigens, and, like other macrophages, microglia release inflammatory cytokines that amplify the inflammatory response by recruiting other cells to the site of injury. They may also be important in the persistence of some viral infections.

The simplest microglial response to tissue injury is a *hypertrophic reaction* in which the nucleus becomes rounded and

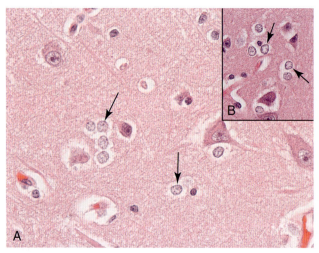

Figure 4-14 A. **Alzheimer type II astrocytosis** in equine hepatic encephalopathy. B. Inset. Alzheimer type II cells (arrows) are often arranged in pairs (cuddling cells) or clusters. (Courtesy M.J. Hazlett.)

the cytoplasm visible as a narrow, often eccentric, eosinophilic rim. In routinely stained preparations, such cells may be difficult to distinguish from astrocytes. They may also proliferate, although their ability to do so seems limited, and many of the cells in proliferative foci are probably derived from immigrant histiocytes. Focal proliferation gives rise to nodules of 30-40 or more cells, whereas diffuse proliferation creates an overall impression of increased cellularity in the microscopic field (Fig. 4-15). *Microglial nodules are very commonly a feature of viral encephalitides*, occurring in both gray and white matter, but are not specific for viral infections. Reactive microglia may develop greatly elongated and sometimes tortuous nuclei, in which case they are called *rod cells*. These, again, are often seen in viral diseases. Activated microglia release cytokines and chemokines that aid in defense against CNS infections, as well as contributing to neurodegenerative conditions.

The most vigorous response of the microglia is their *transformation to macrophages*, when they assume the morphology typical of cells engaged in phagocytosis. When ingesting myelin debris, their cytoplasm becomes foamy as they load themselves with lipid vacuoles. Often the nucleus becomes pyknotic, and they are referred to as **gitter cells, compound granular corpuscles,** or **fat-granule cells** (Fig. 4-16). In severe lesions, many of the gitter cells will have arisen from blood monocytes as well as from microglia. Lipid-laden cells may persist for months around focal lesions, but slow migration to the perivascular spaces and the meninges does take place. Some of the cells may be found at these locations after even longer periods, with the ingested lipid transformed to lipofuscin.

Microglial phagocytes are usually responsible for **neuronophagia,** in which phagocytic cells gather around fragmenting degenerate neuronal cell bodies. This response is a feature of many viral infections in which neurons die, but is uncommon in ischemic or other forms of neuronal necrosis.

Microcirculation

There are some structural peculiarities of blood vessels in the CNS that have a bearing on the development of pathologic processes. The capillaries differ from those in other tissues by being surrounded by an investment of astrocytic end feet. Also, the endothelial cells are sealed together by tight junctions, and the basement membrane divides to incorporate pericytes into the capillary wall. This arrangement in its totality creates the **blood-brain barrier** that selectively limits the entry of many molecules into the neuropil in most of the brain. The barrier is lacking in a few locales, particularly the **circumventricular organs** (CVOs) along the midline of the ventricular system. The CVOs include the vascular organ of the lamina terminalis (organum vasculosum laminae terminalis), subfornical organ, median eminence of the tuber cinereum, subcommissural organ, neurohypophysis, pineal gland (epiphysis), and area postrema (eFig. 4-1).

The distribution of brain capillaries varies considerably, but they are more abundant in the gray matter than the white. Their concentration is higher in some parts of the gray matter, such as the supraoptic and paraventricular nuclei and the area postrema, especially where neuroendocrine activity is concentrated.

Regional variations in the concentrations of capillaries do not appear to influence local pathologic processes. The capillary and venular endothelium is highly labile and responds to a variety of injuries by swelling and proliferating. However, in spite of fairly vigorous proplasia, *cerebral capillaries seem to be almost incapable of budding, so reactive neovascularization is minimal.* The formation of new capillaries is probably limited to situations where granulation tissue is derived from the mesenchyme of the meninges.

Both arterioles and venules of the CNS are thin walled, especially the latter, whose walls are composed mainly of a thin layer of fibrous tissue with very little elastica and no muscle. They are thus susceptible to injury and prone to hemorrhage and, in the cerebral white matter, leukocytes tend to sequester in them in bacterial infections. The veins are valveless and, as backflow of blood after death is usual, cerebral venous congestion can be difficult to assess.

Both arteries and veins have an outer adventitial layer of variable thickness, and a **perivascular Virchow-Robin space.** The space around veins is continuous with the subarachnoid space and is lined by an invagination of the pia-arachnoid. Around cortical arteries, however, there is an investment of leptomeninges in a single layer, an arrangement by which the intracortical perivascular space communicates with the perivascular space about arteries in the leptomeninges. Arteries that enter through the rostral perforated substance may differ from those in the dorsal cortex in that the arteries are

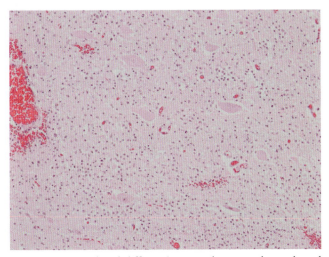

Figure 4-15 Focal and diffuse **gliosis** in the cervical spinal cord of a dog affected with rabies.

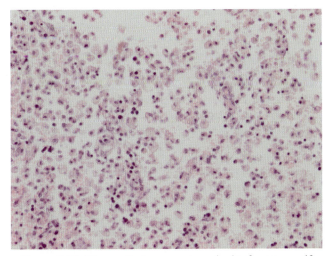

Figure 4-16 Gitter cells in a recent cerebral infarct in a calf.

surrounded by 2 leptomeningeal layers with a space between them that communicates with the perivascular space around arteries in the subarachnoid space. The varied arrangements may reflect the need to allow passage of interstitial fluid to the local lymphatics.

In diffuse inflammatory or neoplastic diseases, this space, more potential than real under normal conditions, becomes patent and accumulates reactive and invading cells. The tendency for these cells to be confined to the space gives rise to the neuropathologic term **perivascular cuffing** (Fig. 4-17A, B). The size of cuffs is usually related to the size of the space, and they may vary from one cell thick around the smallest venules to 10-12 or more cells thick around the larger vessels. *Perivascular cuffing is classically seen in inflammatory conditions*, and all classes of reactive leukocyte may be seen depending on the cause. Although most of the cells are of hematogenous origin, there is no doubt that in some diseases, enteroviral infections, for example, they may arise largely from the proliferation of adventitial cells or resident histiocytes. Lymphoid perivascular cuffing is a feature of many viral encephalitides. Some diseases too are characterized by the production of cerebral and/or spinal vasculitis, but these changes are discussed in a following section.

Further reading

Bradl M, Lassmann H. Oligodendrocytes: biology and pathology. Acta Neuropathol 2010;119:37-53.

Del Bigio MR. Ependymal cells: biology and pathology. Acta Neuropathol 2010;119:55-73.

de Olmos JS, et al. Use of an amino-cupric-silver technique for the detection of early and semiacute neuronal degeneration caused by neurotoxicants, hypoxia, and physical trauma. Neurotoxicol Teratol 1994;16:545-561.

Garman RH. Histology of the central nervous system. Toxicol Pathol 2011;39:22-35.

Graeber MB, Streit WJ. Microglia: biology and pathology. Acta Neuropathol 2010;119:89-105.

Hewett JA. Determinants of regional and local diversity within the astroglial lineage of the normal central nervous system. J Neurochem 2009;110:1717-1736.

Piña-Oviedo S, et al. Immunohistochemical characterization of Renaut bodies in superficial digital nerves: further evidence supporting their perineurial cell origin. J Peripher Nerv Syst 2009;14:22-26.

Schmued LC, et al. Fluoro-Jade C results in ultra high resolution and contrast labeling of degenerating neurons. Brain Res 2005;1035:24-31.

Sofroniew MV, Vinters HV. Astrocytes: biology and pathology. Acta Neuropathol 2010;119:7-35.

Wolburg H, Paulus W. Choroid plexus: biology and pathology. Acta Neuropathol 2010;119:75-88.

MALFORMATIONS OF THE CENTRAL NERVOUS SYSTEM

Malformations of the CNS are common in domestic animals, and their variety is perhaps greater than the variety of malformations in other tissues. There is abundant field and experimental evidence that the effects of teratogens are manifested in the nervous system with disproportionately high frequency. One explanation is that the high degree of differentiation and complexity of the CNS give it an increased susceptibility to developmental disturbances. In addition to inherited diseases, a large number of infectious and toxic environmental agents are capable of causing anomalies. The cause of malformation in an individual domestic animal fetus is seldom determined, in part because of the long time lapse between the initiating event and the fetal presentation. The most frequent sporadic anatomic abnormalities are neural tube defects, and these are initiated in a narrow time range: embryonic days 8.5-10.5 in the mouse, days 15-18 in the pig, and days 21-28 in humans.

Congenital abnormalities of the CNS consist of deviations in either the nature or velocity of the developmental process. Several main patterns of abnormal development can be recognized.

- The largest category includes those disorders with a morphologic basis that are a consequence of *failure or disorder of structural development*. Many such abnormalities are recognizable by distinctive gross changes, but others require microscopic examination.
- Some conditions appear to represent *retardation of normal development* rather than structural aberrations.
- Disturbance of the normal development may also manifest as *premature senescence or degeneration of formed tissues*, such as the various forms of neuronal abiotrophy.
- Some congenital abnormalities appear to represent *primary disturbances of function* rather than of tissue structure. The

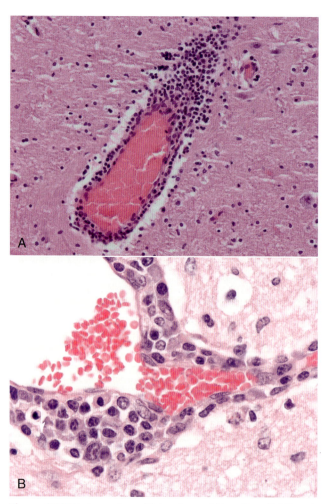

Figure 4-17 **Perivascular cuffs** in a horse (**A**) and a calf (**B**) with encephalitis. Lymphocytes and plasma cells are confined to the Virchow-Robin space. (**B** Courtesy W. Baumgärtner, V. Herder. University of Veterinary Medicine, Hannover, Germany.)

most frequently recognized functional disorders are those that arise as a consequence of inherited biochemical defects and that cause distinctive neurohistologic changes. This category is exemplified by the various lysosomal storage diseases and the leukodystrophies.
- Neither an anatomic nor a biochemical basis has yet been identified for a number of congenital neurologic diseases that often *appear to be inherited*, for example, idiopathic epileptiform conditions in various species.

The initial steps in the formation of the CNS take place early in embryogenesis. As soon as the germ layers are established, the **neural plate,** a thickened band of ectoderm, develops along the mid-dorsal line of the embryo, and is the primordium for the brain and spinal cord. Differential growth at the margins and in the mid-plane result in folding of the plate to form a *neural groove* bounded on each side by an elevated *neural fold*. The groove continues to deepen, and the neural folds meet dorsally and fuse, likely beginning at multiple sites, to form the **neural tube,** which simultaneously separates from the superficial ectoderm. Physical properties of cells and tissues both inside and outside the neural plate determine the formation of the neural tube *(neurulation)*. Cellular proliferative activity within the neural tube is concentrated within an inner subependymal or germinal layer of actively dividing neuroectodermal cells that, with differentiation and outward migration, gives rise first to neurons and later to glia.

The neural tube extends the full length of the embryo and is the progenitor of the entire CNS. **Neural tube defects** (NTD), which result from failure of a portion of the neural tube to close or from reopening of a successfully closed segment, may be cranial or spinal or concurrent in both locations. Neural tube closure is initiated at multiple sites along the craniocaudal axis. Shortly after formation of the neural tube, the rudiments of the cranium and vertebrae appear in accord with the fundamental plan of segmental organization. *Segmentation and development of the axial skeletal investment of the nervous system depend on the developmental integrity of the neural tube*. Hence, NTDs also involve malformations of overlying bony or soft tissues. The spectrum of NTDs includes anencephaly, encephalocele, spinal dysraphism, and meningomyelocele. Incomplete closure of a raphe, especially the neural tube, is referred to as *dysraphism*.

The genes controlling neurogenesis are very strongly conserved in evolution, and much effort is placed on analysis of responsible genes and gene actions in human embryos and in the many models of NTD in mutant and transgenic mice. Notwithstanding the shared gene arrays of the many mouse models and humans, only one mouse phenotype, the *curly tail mouse*, exhibits the anencephaly/meningomyelocele phenotype that is the most frequent NTD in human fetuses. The phenotype results from failure of closure of cranial and caudal neuropores, the ends of the neural tube. The *Sonic hedgehog gene (Shh)*, secreted initially from the notochord and later from the floor plate, is implicated in inducing development of the floor of the neural plate and differentiation of neurons in the ventral sections of the developing cord. Development of the dorsal roof plate of the cord, differentiation of neural crest cells, and formation of neurons within the dorsal cord are the responsibility of members of the *bone morphogenetic protein* (BMP) family derived from surface ectoderm.

The normal pattern of development of the CNS is not smoothly progressive but comprises a complicated interdependent series of growth spurts of organs and tissues. Birth does not mark a single stage in the structural development of the brain, and there is considerable species variation in the stage of CNS development at birth. *Cattle, horses, sheep, and pigs are born with nervous systems having a remarkable degree of structural and functional maturity; kittens and puppies are born with their nervous systems relatively immature*. After the nervous system is fully formed, the capacity for further production of nerve cells is lost, and subsequent development comprises mainly progressive lengthening and myelination of axons and extension of neuronal dendrites and glial processes.

For each species, neural development thus proceeds along a characteristic predetermined pathway. When mature, the nervous system possesses considerable inherent stability, but a time-linked process of decay is also part of the total system of development. Aging neurons tend to accumulate ceroid pigments that almost certainly reduce their functional efficiency. There is also a continual normal loss of neurons, and in normal animals, neuraxonal degeneration is an insignificant but not infrequent finding.

Abiotrophy designates the occurrence of intrinsic premature degeneration of cells and tissues. In the hereditary abiotrophies affecting the nervous systems of animals, such premature loss of vitality is manifested by accelerated and exacerbated degeneration of neurons and their processes.

Investigation of the etiology of neural effects is complicated by the fact that *the same type of abnormality may be produced by both genetic and exogenous causes*, and in many instances, particularly those of sporadic occurrence, the cause remains unidentified. A variety of transplacental viral infections of the fetal nervous system at critical stages of gestation may result in neurologic defects. Some viruses can produce changes, such as symmetrical cavitating lesions, that lack pathologic features that suggest antecedent infection and resemble malformations thought to be of genetic or toxic cause.

The outcome of fetal interactions with agents potentially teratogenic for the nervous system depends on the species and age of the fetus and the nature of the agent. For the various patterns of malformations, there are corresponding critical periods during which developing neural tissue is vulnerable. The teratogenicity of the agent is dependent on its cellular tropism, which is commonly directed toward immature rapidly dividing cells but which often involves specific subpopulations of these cells. Thus, time sets the stage and presents the array of vulnerability, but the agent chooses from among the parts at risk those it has special affinities for damaging.

The most common mode of action for teratogens is selective destruction of cells. Such cytolytic effects have been demonstrated with neural defects induced by *viruses* and *chemicals* as well as by *physical agents* such as hyperthermia. In the case of viruses, cellular destruction can be a direct consequence of infection but may develop as part of the inflammatory reaction. The toxicities of many drugs are mediated not by the compounds themselves but by highly reactive metabolites. If they are not detoxified, these unstable metabolites interact covalently with cell macromolecules and may kill affected cells. Cytolysis seems to be the common operative mechanism in a number of important malformations that often have gross features, such as the cavitating cerebral defects and cerebellar hypoplasia. Teratogens may sometimes act by inhibition or distortion of normal cellular development and function to produce more subtle developmental deviations, such as hypomyelinogenesis. Infection of calves with bovine viral diarrhea virus, of lambs with border disease virus, and of piglets with classical swine fever virus may provide instances of noncytolytic disturbance of fetal neural development of this type.

Some drug metabolites, rather than killing cells, result in mutations through binding to nucleoprotein. In view of the multiplicity of pathogenetic pathways that have been identified, it is not surprising that a spectrum of pathogenic effects can result from the action of one teratogen. All of the lesions may result from an exposure, or any one effect may develop either alone or in combination. Such diversity of teratogenic expression is illustrated by the wide variety of neural and extraneural defects found in kittens born to cats exposed to griseofulvin in pregnancy. *A particular abnormality may arise as an expression of many different causes, sometimes disparate in character.* The cavitating cerebral defects provide examples of this.

Several attributes of fetal neural tissue are pertinent to the interpretation of malformations. Necrosis of groups of cells occurs in normal development and may be seen in association with remodeling processes. The immature nervous system does not react to damage in the same way as adult tissue. Parts may be absorbed without a trace of connective tissue or neuroglial repair. Furthermore, severe malformations are unlikely to proceed directly from destructive processes because destruction of parts of the embryonal structure removes the inductor and inhibitor influences on neighboring cell groups. This may, in some instances, lead to arrest of normal processes and, in others, to exuberant reparative proliferation of neuroepithelium that is indicated histologically by the formation of distinctive neuroepithelial rosettes. *Thus malformations may be compounded of degeneration, necrosis, inhibition, overgrowth, and repair.* There is, at best, only a general correlation between the nature of an anomaly and the time in development when it was initiated. In retrospective studies of malformations of unknown cause, it is only possible to identify the latest time at which the malformation may have been produced, based on the normal development of the nervous system of the species in question.

In the event of infection of the developing nervous system by potentially teratogenic viruses, the outcome is determined primarily by age-related cellular susceptibility. However, the immunologic status of the fetus, particularly its capacity to produce neutralizing antibody, is likely to be important in determining the character of the neural lesions resulting from viral infection. *Lesions leading to major anomalies tend to occur prior to the fetal age at which the fetus can mount a serum neutralizing antibody response to infectious agents.* The fetal brain, especially in the early stages of development, has limited inflammatory potential, but viral-induced destruction of neural tissue in the early fetus may be accompanied by an intense macrophage reaction despite lack of immunologic maturity. Such necrotizing processes typically produce gross anatomic defects with little or no evidence of inflammation because of subsidence of the inflammatory changes. In older fetuses, cytolytic processes are reduced mainly by absence of a susceptible cell population rather than by immune mechanisms, but nonsuppurative encephalitis frequently persists as a residual lesion.

Destruction of developing neural tissue may be effected by mechanisms other than those directly cytopathic for primitive neuroectodermal cells. *Vascular damage* with consequential edema and necrosis is one such mechanism. Although the fetus is resistant to hypoxia, except if prolonged or profound, there is evidence of the potential of circulatory disturbances in the genesis of cavitating CNS malformations, such as hydranencephaly.

There are additional poorly understood pathogenetic influences that doubtless contribute to the outcome of fetal interactions with teratogens. Such factors include *maternal and fetal genotype*, and experimental evidence suggests that *pharmacogenetic differences* among fetuses of a particular species are important determinants of the results of in utero drug exposure. With viral infections, teratogenic potential may vary markedly depending on the *strain of the virus* and upon the *immune status* of the maternal host.

The detailed discussions of CNS malformations that follow are organized on an anatomic basis, from cranial to caudal.

Further reading

Copp AJ, et al. The genetic basis of mammalian neurulation. Nat Rev Genet 2003;4:784-793.

Costa LG, et al. Developmental neuropathology of environmental agents. Annu Rev Pharmacol Toxicol 2004;44:87-110.

George TM, Fuh E. Review of animal models of surgically induced spinal neural tube defects: implications for fetal surgery. Pediatr Neurosurg 2003;39:81-90.

Sarnat HB, Flores-Sarnat L. Integrative classification of morphology and molecular genetics in central nervous system malformations. Am J Med Genet A 2004;126:386-392.

Cerebrum

Cerebral aplasia, anencephaly

True **anencephaly**, which means *absence of brain*, is an exceptional event in the dog, and the term has been misapplied to cases of **cerebral aplasia**, or *prosencephalic hypoplasia*, in which the cerebral hemispheres are absent, but components of the brainstem (midbrain, pons, medulla) have formed (Fig. 4-18). Anomalies of the same general or specific pattern vary considerably from case to case in the details of their expression, various combinations of typical malformations occur, and

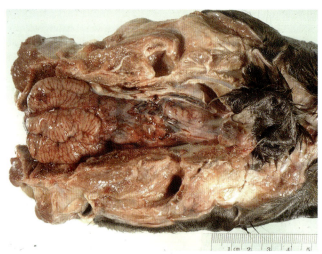

Figure 4-18 Cerebral aplasia ("anencephaly") in a foal. The cerebral hemispheres have failed to form, and only brainstem and cerebellum are present. (Courtesy Noah's Arkives, University of Georgia.)

there is considerable variability in the development of morphologic sequelae.

The primary defect in cerebral aplasia is arrest of closure of the rostral portion of the neural tube. There is, in consequence, failure of development of the cranium and, with skin lacking over the lesion, the dysplastic rudiments of neural tissue are exposed to the amniotic fluid *(exencephaly)*, leading to degeneration of neural tissue and the typical appearance of anencephaly in late gestation. Cerebral aplasia is seldom complete from the beginning because the eyes, either well developed or present as rudimentary vesicles, are present. When the eyes are rudimentary, ganglion cells and optic fibers may be missing. The cranial and neural defects are probably more or less proportionate. With severe degrees of cerebral aplasia, or true anencephaly, there may be complete failure of cranial development **(acrania)**, or there may be rudimentary development of the occipital and adjacent bones. In those cases of cerebral aplasia in which the rostral portion of the brainstem is present, there may be a greater degree of cranial development but failure of fusion **(cranioschisis)**. The base of the cranium is well developed, but there are a variety of anomalies of basal bones and no sella turcica. The neurohypophysis is absent, and the adenohypophysis is either absent or unidentifiable. Failure of development of the neurohypophysis can be responsible for the failure of the adenohypophysis to develop normally, and this in turn may be responsible for prolonged gestation of some anencephalics. The caudal extent of the neural tube defect varies greatly. There may be involvement of the cervical vertebrae or of the entire neural tube **(craniorhachischisis totalis)**; the defect is always continuous, not segmental. Even when the spinal cord is closed, it may be hypoplastic. When the cord is well developed, it is still small because of the absence of descending tracts.

In cerebral aplasia, the cerebral hemispheres are reduced to a tough formless mass of tissue on the exposed basal bones. The tissue is composed largely of blood vessels with some intermingled neural tissue and is termed the *area cerebrovasculosa*. Choroid plexuses may be recognizable, and the whole may be covered by a thin layer of squamous epithelium.

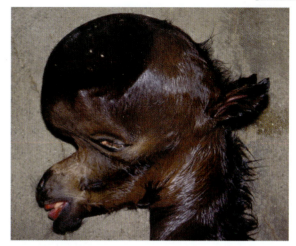

Figure 4-19 **Meningocele** in a foal. (Courtesy Noah's Arkives, University of Georgia.)

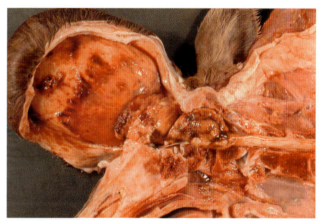

Figure 4-20 **Meningoencephalocele** in a calf. (Courtesy G. Vitellozzi.)

Further reading

Dias MS, Partington M. Embryology of myelomeningocele and anencephaly. Neurosurg Focus 2004;16:E1.

Finnell RH, et al. Pathobiology and genetics of neural tube defects. Epilepsia 2003;44(Suppl. 3):14-23.

Huisinga M, et al. Anencephaly in a German Shepherd dog. Vet Pathol 2010;47:948-951.

Encephalocele, meningocele

Encephalocele *(meningoencephalocele, cephalocele)* is protrusion of the brain through a defect in the cranium **(cranium bifidum)**. The defect is termed **meningocele** if only fluid-filled meninges protrude. In encephalocele, the brain may be either exposed or protruding. These anomalies can be inherited in pigs and in Burmese cats, and have been associated with treatment of the pregnant queen with griseofulvin, hydroxyurea, and diphenylhydantoin.

The morphogenesis of these defects is not simply a problem of defective ossification of the skull with secondary herniation of preformed intracranial tissue but, instead, *depends on a primary neural tube defect by which there is focal failure of dehiscence of the neural tube from the embryonic ectoderm* and, in consequence, focal failure of development of the axial skeletal encasement. The herniations are related to suture lines and are almost always median. They vary from 2-10 cm in diameter, and the largest diameter is always much larger than the diameter of the cranial opening. The skin forms the hernial sac, and ectopic bits of disorganized neural tissue may be attached to it; the dura mater does not form in the areas of defect. Encephalocele and meningocele usually occur in the frontal regions (Figs 4-19, 4-20), but some are occipital, and these latter tend to be located below the occipital crest. Occipital encephaloceles may also be associated with spina bifida of the upper cervical region, sometimes with enlargement of the foramen magnum and absence of the arch of the atlas. Ethmoidal meningoencephaloceles have been documented in dogs and consist in unilateral or bilateral rostral herniation of the olfactory bulb through a defect in the cribriform plate.

Further reading

Martle VA, et al. Surgical treatment of a canine intranasal meningoencephalocele. Vet Surg 2009;38:515-519.

Defects in cerebral corticogenesis

These malformations have their teratogenetic period early in fetal life following closure of the neural tube, and usually occur in association with other neural anomalies. With the establishment of the telencephalic vesicles, cortical neurogenesis begins from the germinal epithelium lining the neural tube, especially in those parts destined to become the lateral ventricles *(subventricular zone)*. Initially, cell division gives rise to similar daughter cells that also act as progenitors so that cell numbers increase geometrically. Later, the cell divisions become increasingly asymmetrical as an increasing proportion of progenitors produce postmitotic precursors of neurons. The first postmitotic neurons migrate to the subpial plate along guides produced by radial glia that extend from the periventricular zone to the cortical surface *(radial migration)*. Successive waves of migratory neurons will leapfrog the preceding waves such that the first waves will reside in the deeper layers of the cortical plate corresponding to layer 6 of the mature cortex, and the later waves will migrate to form the more superficial layers. Other populations of migrating neurons move in trajectories orthogonal to the radial glia palisade *(tangential migration)*. This mode of migration is typically adopted by cortical interneurons and Cajal-Retzius cells, which represent a transient neuronal cell type localized in the marginal zone of the developing neocortex. They are a major source of the extracellular matrix protein reelin, which is essential for the laminar development of the cerebral cortex. In any case, neurons may alternate from radial to tangential movement and vice versa during the course of their migration. Errors of proliferation of germinal neuroepithelial cells may result in microencephaly or macroencephaly; errors of migration result in various patterns of disorder affecting the cerebral gyri.

Microencephaly *refers to an abnormally small brain*. The diminution affects particularly the cerebrum. The hypoplastic brain is accommodated within the cranial cavity, which is often smaller than normal so that the cerebellum appears relatively large. The gyri are of normal size but simplified pattern, and the brainstem structures are normal. *The deficiency is of cerebral gray and white matter*. It may be an isolated defect or associated with any of a variety of other defects. Microencephaly is manifested externally by an abnormally flattened and narrowed frontal part of the cranium. The cranial bones, particularly the frontal bones, are thicker than normal. Microencephaly occurs in fetal infections by Akabane virus in lambs and calves, bovine viral diarrhea virus in calves, border disease virus in lambs, and classical swine fever virus in piglets. The condition has been produced experimentally in lambs exposed to prenatal hyperthermia.

Megalencephaly *refers to an abnormally large brain or excessive volume of the intracranial contents*. Enlargements as a result of excessive germinal cell proliferation are rare and tend to be asymmetrical with exaggerated degrees of heterotopia. When only one hemisphere is involved, the term *hemimegalencephaly* is adopted.

Cortical dysplasia *encompasses defects in the architecture of the cerebral cortex*. In its mildest expression, there is only histologic evidence of lack of the normal orderly layered appearance of the cerebral cortex. *Neuronal heterotopia* is the presence of clusters of nerve cells at a site where they are normally absent, such as subcortical white matter. This condition represents incomplete migration of neuroblasts during fetal life and is usually associated with dysplastic development of the cortex. Scattered, rather than clustered, neurons are commonly present in subcortical white matter and are not of clinical significance. *The presence of aggregations of small dark primitive neuroglial cells is a normal finding in periventricular locations and in the rhinencephalic cortex*. Heterotopia may also involve glial elements, here taking the form of aberrant nests of glial cells.

In **polymicrogyria,** *convolutions are small and unusually numerous, and the normal gyral pattern is lost in affected areas*. The lesion may be asymmetrical or patchy, abruptly demarcated from normal cortex, but its real extent may only be revealed on cut surfaces. It may be present near the margins of cavitating lesions, such as hydranencephaly. In polymicrogyria of Standard Poodles, in which a hereditary basis is suspected, lesions are consistently found in the occipital lobes. **Ulegyria** also imparts a wrinkled appearance to the cortex but arises as a consequence of scarring and atrophy in otherwise topographically normal gyri. It is a *result of laminar necrosis of the deep sulcal cortex*, which appear shrunken and atrophic, whereas the surface gyri are spared and show a characteristic "mushroom shape." It is most often caused by prolonged ischemic/anoxic injury in the perinatal period.

In **lissencephaly** (agyria), the primitive pattern of the telencephalon persists as a result of arrested migration of neuroblasts from the ventricular zone along radial glial fibers to the appropriate cortical lamina. *Convolutions are almost entirely absent*, and the brain surface may be smooth except for slight grooves in which the meningeal vessels are situated. The cerebral cortex is excessively thick. In humans with *LIS1* or *DCX* gene mutations, failure of dynein-mediated nucleus-centrosome coupling leads to abnormal neuronal migration. Lissencephaly appears to be a hereditary condition in Lhasa Apso dogs and in Churra lambs, in which it is associated with pachygyria and cerebellar hypoplasia. In cats, lissencephaly with microencephaly is described in the Korat cat breed.

Pachygyria (macrogyria) is characterized by *excessively broad brain convolutions* resulting from fewer secondary gyri and increased depth of the gray matter underlying the smooth part of the cortex. Pachygyria is a transitional malformation of the cortex, less severe than agyria but akin to it.

Further reading

Crino PB. Malformations of cortical development: molecular pathogenesis and experimental strategies. Adv Exp Med Biol 2004;548: 175-191.

Jurney C, et al. Polymicrogyria in standard poodles. J Vet Intern Med 2009;23:871-874.

Pérez V, et al. Hereditary lissencephaly and cerebellar hypoplasia in Churra lambs. BMC Vet Res 2013;9:156-166.

Tanaka T, et al. Lis1 and doublecortin function with dynein to mediate coupling of the nucleus to the centrosome in neuronal migration. J Cell Biol 2004;165:709-721.

Disorders of axonal growth

As neurons migrate from the periventricular germinal zone along radial glia, they begin to form axonal and dendritic processes. The growth and direction of growth of these processes are guided by complex cues, including molecules of the extracellular matrix, and there is an extensive literature relating to the molecular genetics that regulate these processes.

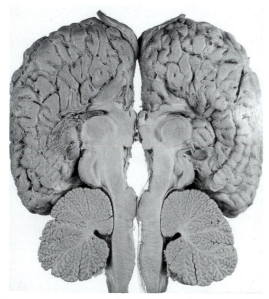

Figure 4-21 Agenesis of the corpus callosum in a horse.

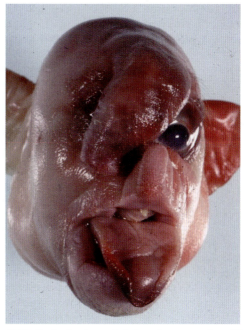

Figure 4-22 Cyclopia (synophthalmia) in a piglet. (Courtesy Noah's Arkives, University of Georgia.)

Agenesis or **hypoplasia of the corpus callosum** is an *uncommon anomaly* but is recorded in most domestic species. It is the most studied of the disorders of axonal growth in human and animal models. It may occur alone or in association with other anomalies of the brain (Fig. 4-21). The septum pellucidum is absent as a collateral defect; the leaves are separated and displaced laterally to the roof of the lateral ventricles. There is no cingulate gyrus, the interhemispheric gyri appearing to radiate from the roof of the third ventricle.

The corpus callosum is formed by the crossing over of fibers from one hemisphere to the other, a migration that begins at the lamina terminalis, which is the most rostral point of the neural tube. Dysgenesis of the prosencephalic vesicle in its midline may impair the lamina terminalis, or there may be disordered outgrowth of axons from the cerebral cortex. The migration of fibers is guided by a glial scaffold, which may be absent as the primary defect. The corpus may be entirely absent, or the commissures may be present and the corpus defective in its central part.

The development of the septum lucidum is linked to that of the corpus callosum, and its residue may form a **cystic septum pellucidum.** The cavum septi pellucidi is always present in the fetus as a midline cavity that originates within the commissural plate by tissue resorption. In the normal course, the cavity is obliterated, resulting in a glial midline raphe, but *failure of fusion of the leaflets results in a cystic fluid-filled cavity that varies from a thin slit to a rounder cavity.* The cyst is covered externally by ependyma and lined by a glial mesh. This condition occasionally accompanies defects caused by fetal infections with viruses such as those of Akabane disease, bluetongue, bovine viral diarrhea, and border disease.

Holoprosencephaly

Immediately on closure of the rostral neuropore, the rostral end of the tube enlarges to form 3 vesicles, the rostral of which, or *prosencephalon,* will become the forebrain; the intermediate vesicle will form the *mesencephalon,* or midbrain; and the caudal vesicle will form the hindbrain, or *rhombencephalon.* The dorsal wall of the rostral vesicle becomes thickened dorsally in the midline to form the commissural plate, eventually the corpus callosum, and the vesicle expands laterally to form the paired cerebral vesicles, which will become the cerebral hemispheres.

Holoprosencephaly (HPE) is a failure of the forebrain to separate normally into 2 discrete cerebral hemispheres and exists in 3 forms, depending on the severity of the malformation. The most severe expression is *alobar* HPE, in which the complete lack of separation of the 2 cerebral hemispheres is associated with absence of the olfactory bulbs and tracts (arhinencephaly), corpus callosum, septum pellucidum, and septal nuclei. This form is typically associated with facial deformities, and there may be a single eye globe (cyclopia or synophthalmia). With *semilobar* HPE, the rostral cerebral hemispheres fail to separate, but the occipital lobes are distinct. In this condition, the septal nuclei, rostral corpus callosum (genu and body), and septum pellucidum are absent, and the rostral cingulate gyri and caudate nuclei are continuous across the midline. *Lobar* HPE is the least severe variant in which only the most rostral and ventral portions of the cerebral hemispheres are nonseparated.

Cyclopia, referring to the presence of a *single large median eye,* emphasizes the most obvious and remarkable abnormality of a very complicated defect. The condition is not uncommon in domestic animals, especially pigs (Fig. 4-22), and it can be reproduced experimentally simply and in many different ways.

The causes of sporadic cases are largely unknown, but many instances in humans are the result of chromosomal anomalies. Various degrees of cyclopia are present in Guernsey and Jersey fetuses that are the subjects of *prolonged gestation.* *Veratrum californicum* is responsible for congenital cyclopian malformations that occur endemically in lambs in the western livestock grazing areas of the United States. The teratogenic agent in the plant is *cyclopamine,* a steroidal alkaloid. Induction of the cyclopian deformity in lamb fetuses is dependent on pregnant ewes ingesting *V. californicum* on day 14 of gestation. Cyclopia has also been produced experimentally in cattle and goats, with a similar narrow interval of susceptibility to maternal ingestion of *Veratrum* on or about day 14 of gestation. Cyclopamine-induced teratogenesis may result from antagonism of Sonic hedgehog gene signal transduction that is necessary for normal dorsoventral patterning of the neural tube and somites. The primary defect occurs at the neural plate stage of development and involves the rostral extremity of the notochord and the mesoderm immediately surrounding it. Failure of proper induction accounts for the changes in the skull, soft tissues of the face, and the brain. The optic defect, consisting of greater-or-lesser division of a single anlage, is probably secondary to the defects of the forebrain.

The orbits may be approximated but, typically, there is one large orbit and a single optic foramen. Several bones, including the ethmoids, nasal septum, lacrimal bones, and premaxillae, are usually absent. The globe may be absent, rudimentary, or may form a single structure of near-normal conformation, or be partially divided or completely duplicated. The nose is a proboscis or tube that does not communicate with the pharynx and that is typically situated above the median eye. The forebrain is always severely malformed; the hemispheres are not fully cleft but are present instead as a single thin-walled vesicle with a smooth surface and common ventricle and lacking olfactory nerves and tracts, corpus callosum, septum pellucidum, and fornix.

The hindbrain is usually normal. The pituitary may be displaced or absent and fetal gigantism associated with prolonged gestation (see Vol. 3, Female genital system) occurs in some deformed lambs and calves. The optic nerve is single, atrophic, or absent. The oculomotor and abducens nerves are hypoplastic or absent. There is internal hydrocephalus.

Veratrum californicum also causes embryonic death. A wide range of other defects has been produced experimentally in lambs, with abbreviation of the metacarpal and metatarsal bones being the most distinctive.

Cebocephaly (monkey face) *is anatomically comparable to cyclopia, and probably represents a less severe expression of the same basic defects.* There are 2 eyes, severely hypoplastic, in separate but approximated orbits. The nose is in the normal position, but deformed and may not protrude. There is a single, small nasal cavity or a proboscis with no communication with the pharynx. The brain appears as in cyclopia but may have a slight median sulcus.

Further reading

Koch TG, et al. Semilobar holoprosencephaly in a Morgan horse. J Vet Intern Med 2005;19:367-372.

MacKillop E. Magnetic resonance imaging of intracranial malformations in dogs and cats. Vet Radiol Ultrasound 2011;52(Suppl. 1):S42-S45.

Hydrocephalus

Hydrocephalus is characterized by abnormal accumulation of fluid in the cranial cavity. In **internal hydrocephalus,** the fluid is within the ventricular system; in **external hydrocephalus,** the fluid is in the arachnoid space; and in **communicating hydrocephalus,** the excess fluid is present in both locations. The communicating and external types of hydrocephalus, the latter to be distinguished from cerebral atrophy, are quite rare in animals. Internal hydrocephalus, which is denoted by variably dilated ventricular cavities lined by ependyma, is quite common, may be congenital or acquired, but both forms may be considered here for convenience.

Cerebrospinal fluid (CSF) is produced by the ventricular choroid plexuses by means of filtration and secretion. There are significant contributions by ependyma and extraventricular structures. Because of the permeable nature of the ependymal lining of the ventricular system, the CSF is in effect an extension of the extracellular fluid of the CNS, and its composition is affected by metabolic and pathologic changes within the brain.

The flow of CSF is from the lateral ventricle through the interventricular foramen to the third ventricle and then via the mesencephalic aqueduct to the fourth ventricle. From here, most of the fluid leaves the ventricular system and passes by way of the lateral cerebellomedullary apertures into the subarachnoid space. A small amount of CSF passes into the central canal of the spinal cord from the fourth ventricle. The greater part of the fluid flows forward into the cerebral subarachnoid spaces and basal cisterns; the balance circulates in a restricted fashion in the spinal subarachnoid space. The energy required to circulate CSF is imparted largely by the choroid plexuses through their production of fluid. The arterial pulse also contributes to CSF movement through associated variations in hemispheric volume. Venous resorption of CSF occurs where arachnoid villi form in the walls of the larger meningeal veins. Transfer of fluid is effected by hydrostatic pressure, with reflux being prevented by the valvular nature of the villi. The arachnoid villi are normally highly permeable, being able to permit the passage of red blood cells. Impedance of this resorption appears to contribute to the increased intracranial pressure of hypovitaminosis A in calves. Some outflow in dogs can occur via the cribriform plate and in cats along the subarachnoid space of olfactory, optic, and acoustic nerves, but significant outflow may possibly occur only in association with raised intracranial pressure. The spinal subarachnoid space appears to communicate freely with the lymphatic system opening in the intradural nerve roots.

Familiarity with the normal directional flow of CSF is basic to an understanding of the pathogenesis of hydrocephalus because, in most cases, it is probably of obstructive origin. Certainly, *an obstruction can be demonstrated in most instances of acquired hydrocephalus in animals.* In congenital hydrocephalus, obstruction is quite often not demonstrable, but stenotic aqueductal malformations may be found. Obstructive hydrocephalus has been induced experimentally in many species of immature laboratory animals with a range of viruses ubiquitous in animals and man. The selective destructive action of these viruses on ependymal cells, with subsequent reparative gliovascular proliferation, results in obstruction of CSF pathways, usually in the mesencephalic aqueduct. Thus far in domestic animals, viral-induced hydrocephalus of this genesis has been demonstrated only in experimental canine parainfluenza virus infection in dogs.

Hydrocephalus is "physiologic" in the early fetus when the hemispheres are largely thin-walled vesicles. *Congenital hydrocephalus exaggerates this physiologic degree of ventricular dilation.* Even in the absence of obstruction, physiologic hydrocephalus may persist or be exaggerated in instances of neural dysplasia such as, for example, in cyclopia and cebocephaly. The cavitating cerebral defects, hydranencephaly and porencephaly, are associated with internal hydrocephalus. This is likely to be an ex vacuo or compensatory hydrocephalus occurring secondary to loss of cerebral tissue as in the inherited leukodystrophies and storage diseases, but a hydrostatic component arising from deranged circulation of CSF is also possible. Hydrocephalus may accompany other neural anomalies, but chiefly, the rather rare Arnold-Chiari and Dandy-Walker malformations in which hydrocephalus is obstructive in origin and associated with abnormalities of the cerebellum and medulla.

With the exception of the few examples just given, *congenital hydrocephalus remains anatomically obvious but pathogenetically obscure*, and such cases are common. Pups, calves, foals, and piglets are chiefly affected, with a familial incidence, possibly genetic, in pigs. The defect is quite uncommon in cats.

Congenital hydrocephalus is well known in **pups**, especially those of toy and brachycephalic breeds. This should not imply that the hydrocephalus is correlative to, or a product of, brachycephaly because, within breeds, there is not much variation in the degree of the skeletal defect, and no obvious relation between it and the presence and severity of hydrocephalus. Malformation of the mesencephalic aqueduct may be a significant pathogenetic factor. The anatomic expression of the hydrocephalus also varies considerably. One lateral ventricle may be involved or both may be dilated symmetrically or asymmetrically; the third ventricle and rostral portion of the aqueduct are usually, but not always, involved; and the fourth ventricle is normal.

Sporadic cases of congenital hydrocephalus occur widely in **cattle**. Many appear to be secondary to aqueductal stenosis. An autosomal recessive gene is considered responsible for many apparently hereditary cases, but the possible roles of fetal infections and nutritional factors must be considered.

Outbreaks of congenital hydrocephalus are recorded in calves in which slit-like deformation of the aqueduct of Sylvius was associated with lateral narrowing of the midbrain, in the peripheral areas of which there was vascular proliferation and perivascular gliosis. Hydrocephalus also occurs in association with chondrodysplasias, especially of the "bulldog" type, but the primary neural defect in these is not known. Several hydrocephalic syndromes have been described in Hereford and Shorthorn cattle; features include cerebellar hypoplasia, microphthalmia, myopathy, and ocular anomalies.

Experimentally, *dietary deficiency of vitamin A* can cause congenital and neonatal hydrocephalus (Fig. 4-23), but spontaneous outbreaks occur only in cattle that have fed for prolonged periods on dry pasture or in feedlots. The hydrocephalus is ascribed to functional impairment of absorption of fluid from arachnoid villi, but there is frequently severe compression of the brain and herniations in the caudal fossa, which is expected to provide mechanical obstruction to drainage.

Hydrocephalus is uncommon in **horses**. A series of cases is described in Friesian foals, probably associated with malformation of the petrosal bone and stenosis of the jugular foramen.

Acquired hydrocephalus is fairly common in animals. It does not approach in severity the congenital defect. The causes are almost always obstructive, but minor degrees of ventricular dilation occur in association with cerebral atrophy in old dogs. Meningeal lesions that destroy the arachnoid villi can lead to external hydrocephalus. This is, however, quite rare, although it has been observed in diffuse meningeal carcinomatosis. Most diffuse meningeal lesions are inflammatory, but these are typically associated with internal rather than external hydrocephalus because meningitis tends to involve the basilar regions and the caudal fossa chiefly and there interferes with the patency of the lateral cerebellomedullary apertures. Most cases of bacterial meningitis are fatal before the changes of hydrocephalus develop unless, as frequently happens, concurrent inflammation of the choroid plexuses extends to the ependyma of the aqueduct and obstructs that channel. Even relatively chronic cases of meningitis, such as may be observed in cryptococcosis, are associated with internal rather than communicating or external hydrocephalus. Additional causes of acquired hydrocephalus are intracranial neoplasms, usually primary but sometimes metastatic, and including papillomas and carcinomas of the choroid plexus; parasitic cysts, such as hydatids and coenurids; and the late effects of chronic or healed inflammation that involve the ependyma or cause inflammatory softening or atrophy of paraependymal tissue. The pyogranulomatous ependymitis and meningoencephalitis of feline infectious peritonitis frequently results in hydrocephalus. In horses, the so-called *cholesteatomas* or cholesterol granulomas that develop in the choroid plexuses of the lateral ventricles may occlude the interventricular foramen and cause internal hydrocephalus.

Hydrocephalus does not regress. Whether it progresses or not is difficult to determine. Congenital hydrocephalus cannot be easily diagnosed in the newborn in the absence of secondary changes in the cranium, and diagnosable cases seldom live long enough for the course of the defect to be ascertained. Probably, however, congenital hydrocephalus of mild or moderate degree can remain static because, although a severe and fatal defect is common enough in puppies, *hydrocephalus in brachycephalic breeds of dogs is frequently an incidental finding at autopsy*, and the degree of ventricular dilation may be minor or moderate irrespective of the age of the animal. Acquired hydrocephalus in postnatal life tends to be progressive when of obstructive type, the course depending on the site and nature of the obstructing lesion. Compensatory (or ex vacuo) hydrocephalus occurring as a response to cerebral atrophy is static or, at the most, slowly progressive; it is never severe, except perhaps in familial lipofuscinosis of dogs.

Congenital hydrocephalus is frequently associated with malformation of the cranium. The degree of cranial malformation varies from slight doming, which may be difficult to appreciate, to enormous enlargement, which may cause dystocia. Cranial malformation is not invariable however, and many cases of congenital hydrocephalus of considerable severity may occur with a skull of normal contour. Whether cranial

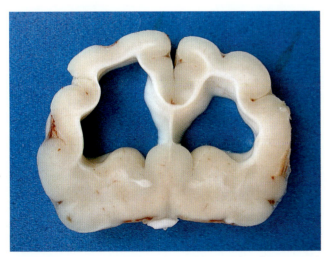

Figure 4-23 **Hydrocephalus** in a cat, a result of vitamin A deficiency.

malformation occurs or not probably depends on the time of onset of the hydrocephalus relative to the degree of ossification of the cranial bones and the development and strength of the sutures, and also on the rate at which the fluid is accumulated.

It is often difficult to be certain of the presence of minor degrees of hydrocephalus. The soft brains of the newborn collapse when removed from the skull so that dilation of ventricles may not be apparent. In older, firmer brains, asymmetry of the lateral ventricles and relative dilation of the rostral end of the aqueduct when compared with the caudal end are useful indices. *The septum pellucidum, however, is the structure most sensitive to the effects of fluid accumulation;* it may be fenestrated or may persist as an irregular lacework of connective tissue, but typically, it is absent. Even in mild hydrocephalus, there is usually atrophy in Ammon's horn readily detectable by the ease with which the piriform lobes dimple under slight pressure. With hydrocephalus of greater severity, there is ventricular dilation of corresponding degree. The lateral and third ventricles are most severely affected, and there may be no alteration in the fourth. With ventricular dilation, parenchymal atrophy affects chiefly the white matter and the cerebral cortices; ventrally, the increased pressure is buttressed by the basal ganglia. The corpus callosum is elevated and thinned, and the cerebral cortices over the vertex may be reduced to thin shells of gray matter. The floor of the third ventricle is extremely thinned, the hypophysis is atrophied, and the cerebellum is compressed and displaced caudally. In rapidly progressive internal hydrocephalus of the dog, rupture of the ependymal layer may cause the development of bilateral diverticula in the area of the internal capsule, frequently associated with hemorrhage and inflammation. These lesions have been described as *hydrocephalus associated with periventricular encephalitis.*

The extensive cranial malformation of congenital hydrocephalus can occur only if the sutures are ununited. The temporal, frontal, and parietal bones are enlarged and thin and are separated from each other by broad membranes of connective tissue in which accessory bones may form. In these severe cases, the base of the cranium is flattened, the fossae are enlarged and smoothed out, and the orbits are separated but individually reduced in size so that the eyes may protrude.

Gray matter is remarkably resistant to the effects of the pressure exerted by the fluid, but the subcortical white matter degenerates rapidly. It is edematous, the oligodendrocytes and astrocytes are reduced in number, and compound granular corpuscles can be found sometimes in short bands lying deep and parallel to the ependyma. The ependyma, tela choroidea, and meninges are usually not altered significantly.

Further reading

Sipma KD, et al. Phenotypic characteristics of hydrocephalus in stillborn Friesian foals. Vet Pathol 2013;50:1037-1042.

Thomas WB. Hydrocephalus in dogs and cats. Vet Clin North Am Small Anim Pract 2010;40:143-159.

Hydranencephaly, porencephaly

In **hydranencephaly,** there can be complete or almost complete absence of the cerebral hemispheres, leaving only membranous sacs filled with CSF and enclosed by leptomeninges. The cranial cavity is always complete, in contrast to hydrocephalus, and usually of normal conformation, although occasionally there is mild doming of the skull or thickening of the cranial bones. The dorsal, and often the caudal parts of the hemispheres, are the portions most severely defective (Fig. 4-24A-C). The leptomeninges may easily be damaged on removing the calvaria but are in their usual position and form sacs enclosing CSF,

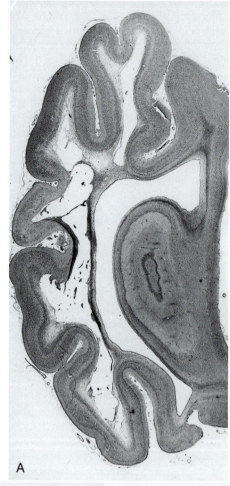

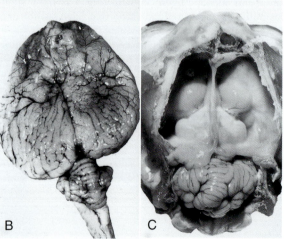

Figure 4-24 A. Hydranencephaly in a lamb with swayback. (Courtesy J. McC. Howell.) **B. Hydranencephaly** and cerebellar hypoplasia in a lamb, subsequent to intrauterine bluetongue virus infection. **C. Hydranencephaly** in a cat; meninges removed to expose the brainstem structures.

the fluid occupying the space normally occupied by parenchyma. Discrete remnants of parenchyma may be present in the meninges. When the leptomeninges are incised, it is apparent that the brainstem is of near-normal conformation with well-developed hippocampus and choroid plexuses. The rostral portion of the corpus callosum and septum pellucidum may be intact although attenuated. Cerebellar hypoplasia may be present as a concurrent defect, as may the histologic deficits of hypomyelinogenesis.

Hydranencephaly is the residual lesion of full-thickness necrosis of the cerebral hemisphere. In animals, the lesion develops in early fetal stages and before the mature arrangements of the cortex are present. The marginal tissue is dysplastic, flat, and microgyric, or the gyri have a radial arrangement from the defect. Although a diagnosis of hydranencephaly is readily made on macroscopic inspection, histologic study may provide some insight into the nature of the disease process. The membranous coverings of the remnants of the hemispheres comprise arachnoid, pia, and a thin mantle of residual cortex in normal juxtaposition. The residual cortical tissue may be lined by attenuated ependyma displaced outward with expansion of the lateral ventricles, but this ependymal lining is frequently incomplete or absent, and the cavity abuts directly on cortical tissue that may be unremarkable except for mild astrocytosis.

Hydranencephaly occurs in all species but is most common in calves, in which it occurs either sporadically or as minor epizootics. The lesion occurs similarly, although less frequently, in *lambs.* The species occurrence of hydranencephaly reflects its etiologic associations with certain viruses infecting the fetus at a critical stage of gestation. In these cases, *hydranencephaly is often part of a spectrum of neural lesions,* the expression of which depends mainly on the age of the fetus at infection. Viruses that are well established as causes of hydranencephaly tend to be either arboviruses, such as Akabane virus, bluetongue virus, Schmallenberg virus, Cache Valley virus, Chuzan virus, Aino virus, Rift Valley fever virus, and Wesselsbron virus, or pestiviruses, such as bovine viral diarrhea virus and border disease virus. In cats, hydranencephaly has been associated with feline parvovirus infection.

The pathogenesis of hydranencephaly has been clarified through studies of the cavitating encephalopathies caused by fetal viral infections, particularly bluetongue and border disease in lambs. These infections at critical periods of gestation produce *subventricular zones of necrosis* of the developing cerebral hemispheres. These zones, which may have a vascular basis, involve the neuroblasts in their outward migration and result in cavitation and deprive the cortex of its normal complement of neurons. These cavitations range in size from small cysts with only minor changes in the overlying cortex (porencephaly) to large confluent spaces with the hemispheres reduced to fluid-filled sacs (hydranencephaly). During the necrotizing process, there may be an intense macrophage response, but it is usual for this reaction to have subsided by the time the animal is born and examined.

Mechanical factors also contribute to the development of hydranencephaly. A dissecting effect associated with escape of CSF into the parenchyma may also be important because segmental loss of ventricular ependyma is an early feature of the cavitating process.

Compensatory expansion of the lateral ventricles secondary to loss of brain substance occurs, and rapid expansion of the fetal calvaria during the gestation period allows stretching and rupture of residual cortical tissue. In less severely affected areas, the outer rim of cortex overlies a band of subependymal tissue, the intervening cavity being occupied by trabecular parenchymal remnants. Rosette formations of cells that resemble ependymal epithelium may be found in the subependymal area. Accumulations of mineralized debris may be present in the meninges.

Porencephaly *is cystic cavitation of the brain evolving from a destructive process in prenatal life.* The defect typically involves the white matter of the cerebral hemispheres. An affected brain may contain a single cyst, or there may be multiple cystic lesions. The temporal portion of the cerebral hemispheres is an area of predilection, but porencephalic change may be found throughout the cerebral hemispheres, although typically sparing the basal nuclei. Occasionally, lesions are found in brainstem and cerebellum. The cysts are usually randomly located, but evidence of bilateral symmetry is sometimes apparent, particularly in well-developed lesions of the cerebral hemisphere. Rarely, cysts may communicate with ventricular cavities or with the subarachnoid space. The cysts may be apparent from the meningeal aspect as focal fluctuant areas of attenuated cerebral cortex or as superficial, clear submeningeal cysts. The cysts range in size from microscopic to several centimeters in diameter. The cysts are variable in shape, but roughly spherical or cleft-like outlines are common. On section, they are filled with clear fluid and are smooth walled, but are traversed by variable numbers of trabeculae. Less well-developed lesions may appear as gelatinous softenings.

The porencephalic cavities, particularly the larger defects, are often unremarkable microscopically, being lined by a layer of flattened glia. Apart from some mild marginal astrocytosis, they show surprisingly little evidence of reactive or inflammatory change. In other cases, there is accumulation of hemosiderin-containing gitter cells about the margins of the cyst and within the cavity. The trabeculae comprise residual brain parenchyma, usually oriented about a blood vessel. Some small lesions, evident grossly as focal gelatinous areas, appear as focal leukomalacia comprising white matter in the process of dissolution associated with accumulation of macrophages and gitter cells. Sometimes the inflammatory nature of the lesions is indicated by the presence of mild nonsuppurative meningoencephalitis with gliosis, perivascular cuffing and focal mineralization about the margins of the cysts, and mononuclear infiltration in the meninges overlying the defects.

The etiopathogenesis of porencephaly parallels, but is a less severe expression of, the pathologic process seen in hydranencephaly. Both lesions are commonly recorded in the course of outbreaks of cavitating cerebral defects and may occur together in the same brain. In the case of cavitating viral infections of the fetal brain, termination of the disease process in either porencephaly or hydranencephaly is influenced by gestational age at infection, with porencephaly tending to follow infection at a later stage than is the case with hydranencephaly.

Porencephaly is a common manifestation of prenatal infection of *lambs* with some strains of border disease virus and is seen in calves infected in utero by bovine viral diarrhea virus and Schmallenberg virus. The cystic or gelatinous transformations of the cerebral white matter that occur in some cases of copper deficiency in lambs (swayback) are porencephalic in nature. The lesion has also been induced experimentally in lambs by exposure of pregnant ewes to hyperthermia during the last ⅔ of pregnancy. In *dogs*, porencephaly and hydranencephaly have rarely been reported.

Further reading

Davies ESS, et al. Porencephaly and hydranencephaly in six dogs. Vet Rec 2012;170:179-184.

Hunter P, et al. Teratogenicity of a mutagenised Rift Valley fever virus (MVP 12) in sheep. Onderstepoort J Vet Res 2002;69:95-98.

Tsuda T, et al. Arthrogryposis, hydranencephaly and cerebellar hypoplasia syndrome in neonatal calves resulting from intrauterine infection with Aino virus. Vet Res 2004;35:531-538.

Periventricular leukomalacia of neonates

Inter-related lesions dominated by intraventricular hemorrhage, ventriculomegaly, and malacia of white matter are quite frequent in neonates. In domestic animals, the lesion has not been distinguished from hydrocephalus and hydranencephaly, which is the reason for considering it here with the malformations from which it needs to be distinguished, rather than with malacic diseases. The application of imaging technology has identified a surprising incidence of the complex in human neonates with later minimal to severe neurologic deficits. The lesions in human neonates are most frequently associated with placentitis, prematurity, and growth retardation, suggesting that placental insufficiency may be critically important. In lambs, there is an association with placentitis of toxoplasmosis, tick-borne fever, and chlamydiosis.

Periventricular leukomalacia typically refers to necrosis of white matter adjacent to the lateral ventricles that results in the formation of cysts in the cerebrum or in more extensive lesions simulating hydranencephaly or hydrocephalus ex vacuo. In animals, the lesion is not limited to the cerebrum but may extend to affect also periventricular white matter of the cerebellum, cerebellar roof nuclei, and white matter of the cerebellar folia.

Intraventricular hemorrhage may extend caudally as far as the central canal of the spinal cord causing ventricular dilation. The hemorrhage of variable severity may remain intramural in the hemispheral white matter.

Periventricular leukomalacia may allow survival in pups for several weeks. The cavitating cerebral lesion, and the cerebellar lesion, if present, is lined internally by ependyma and a thin layer of white matter. There may be local defects allowing communication with the dilated ventricle. Clustered cases are observed in kids and lambs. Affected neonates tend to be small for age, stillborn, or die immediately after delivery, although some with minor neurologic defect may survive and develop normally.

The pathogenesis of these defects is unknown. The mechanisms appear to involve the structural fragility of blood vessels in the periventricular subependymal zone and instability of blood flow in the vulnerable areas. Perivascular hemorrhages may be confined to this zone. The malacic lesion in white matter is coagulative necrosis with vacuolation of the tissue and acidophilic swollen retraction balls on axonal fragments. Microglia provide the only inflammatory cells. Cystic lesions have peripheral sprigs of capillaries and marginal and luminal macrophages expected to contain hemosiderin. In individual cases in lambs and kids, the lesions may be of different ages and, in clustered cases in these animals, some may show hemorrhage only, and some may show established cavities.

Further reading

Back SA, Rivkees SA. Emerging concepts in periventricular white matter injury. Semin Perinatol 2004;28:405-414.

Kuban K, et al. White matter disorders of prematurity: association with intraventricular hemorrhage and ventriculomegaly. J Pediatr 1999;134:539-546.

Cerebellum/caudal fossa

The cerebellum develops from the lips of the rhombencephalon in the region of incomplete closure of the neural tube. There are *2 major germinative zones*. The rostral lips give rise to precursors of the cerebellar granule cells. In their first migration, granule cell precursors cover the whole of the cerebellar pial layer at about the time of closure of the rostral neuropore. This is a germinative layer that produces a second generation of germinal cells, some of which remain as daughter cells, and others undergo lateral migration in the developing molecular layer. In a third migratory wave, postmitotic cells send axons vertically down through the molecular and Purkinje cell layers under guidance of radial glia; the cell body then moves along the axon to the maturing granular layer.

Disorder of the granule cell layer is frequently part of the disruption caused by fetal viral infections. *Focal heterotopias* are frequent in neonates, usually without clinical effect. These cells may be the origin of the medulloblastomas of young animals.

The caudal rhombic lips produce a highly proliferative neuroepithelium from which neuronal precursors migrate along several pathways to form the Purkinje cells of the cerebellar cortex; the cerebellar roof nuclei; and to the precerebellar nuclei, including the olivary, cuneate, and reticular nuclei of the medulla; and to the pontine and tegmental nuclei of the pons; axons from these nuclei project back into the cerebellum.

The cerebellum has 3 functionally distinct regions. The *vestibulocerebellum* regulates balance and eye movements. It is the oldest part of the cerebellum (paleocerebellum) and occupies the flocculonodular lobules, where it receives afferents from the vestibular nuclei. The *spinocerebellum* regulates limb and body movements, receiving somatosensory information via the spinocerebellar tracts and precerebellar nuclei, and occupies the vermis and medial aspects of the hemispheres. The lateral hemispheres, the *cerebrocerebellum*, receive input from the cerebrum via pontine nuclei and are involved in the composition of complex movements. Within these main cerebellar regions, there is further regional patterning corresponding to body parts.

Disorders of migration and survival of Purkinje cells underlie many of the cerebellar malformations, and premature loss is the most common component of the abiotrophies. Correlative changes may be present in the precerebellar nuclei and in the cerebellar roof nuclei.

Cerebellar defects are among the more important of the developmental anomalies of the CNS because of their frequent occurrence and almost invariable accompaniment by significant and distinctive clinical manifestations. They may be expressions of failure of intercellular communication and support, whereby a defect in one cell lineage may adversely affect the organizational pattern and function and viability of other cell types. *Cerebellar defects are quite common in cats and calves; relatively so in pigs, dogs, and lambs; but uncommon in foals.* Most defects of morphogenesis can be divided into 2 broad categories, and the entities are discussed later as examples of either *cerebellar hypoplasia* or *cerebellar abiotrophy (atrophy)*. This distinction into hypoplastic and atrophic types is somewhat artificial, because it is apparent that many cases are compounded by both processes.

Minor dysplastic lesions of no consequence are quite common in young animals but are fewer or less conspicuous in adults. They are most common in the flocculonodular lobules and where the cortex terminates at the peduncles. The foci are microscopic and consist of tangled islands of germinal, molecular, and granular layers with Purkinje cells distributed haphazardly. The dysplasias of the Arnold-Chiari and Dandy-Walker syndromes, of copper deficiency, and the metabolic storage disorders are discussed separately.

The name of the teratologic condition merely emphasizes the major component, in these cases the cerebellar defect. There may, however, be coincident malformations, such as agenesis of the corpus callosum or hydranencephaly. *There are always correlative changes,* this term grouping together those structural changes that occur in nuclear masses that send fibers to, or receive fibers from, the cerebellum as well as in the particular tract of fibers themselves. The term implies that there is a causal connection, the cerebellar defects being primary and the subcerebellar defects being secondary, but such an implication is less likely to be valid for the cerebellar hypoplasias than for the cerebellar atrophies. Anatomic classifications of the cerebellar hypoplasias tend to take into account the distribution and severity of correlative changes, especially those in the deep cerebellar nuclei, pontine nuclei, inferior olives and cerebellar brachia, restiform bodies, and spinocerebellar tracts. The pattern of correlative changes varies from case to case, and there is not a quantitative correspondence between the cerebellar defects and the correlative defects. There are also very wide variations in the severity of the cerebellar hypoplasias, which is reasonable if the severity is properly to be related to the time of onset, duration, and severity of the arrest of development. From these viewpoints, *anatomic classification of cerebellar hypoplasias is artificial because the defects are quantitative.*

Cerebellar agenesis, hypoplasia, and dysplasia

Cerebellar agenesis consists in *complete absence of cerebellar tissue.* The malformation is reported in Simmental calves. Selective agenesis of the cerebellar vermis or its caudal aspect is described in dogs with or without hypoplasia of the cerebellar hemispheres.

Cerebellar hypoplasia *is one of the most common congenital nervous system defects of domestic animals and is seen in all domestic species* (Figs. 4-25, 4-26). There is persuasive evidence for genetically determined occurrence of the disease in calves of various breeds, particularly beef Shorthorns, in Arabian and Arabian cross foals, and in Gotland ponies and Chow Chow dogs. The malformation is reported in several canine breeds, including Beagle, Silky Terrier, Airedale Terrier, Irish Setter, Boston Terrier, Bull Terrier, and Wire-haired Fox Terrier. A form of cerebellar hypoplasia with intraneuronal inclusions is reported from New Zealand in Cocker Spaniel dogs with progressive ataxia and seizures. A presumed inherited *cerebellar cortical dysplasia* is reported in St. Bernard puppies, characterized by loss of distinction between granule cell, Purkinje cell, or molecular layers, along with pallor and cavitation of the subcortical white matter of cerebellum and cerebrum. A

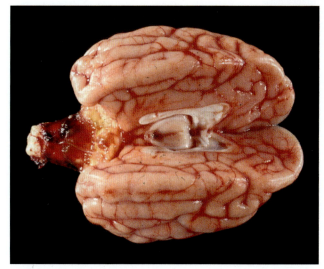

Figure 4-25 Cerebellar hypoplasia in a dog. (Courtesy Noah's Arkives, University of Georgia.)

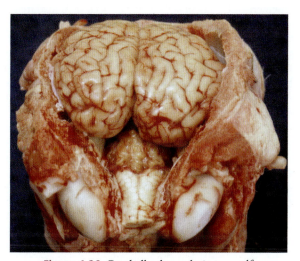

Figure 4-26 Cerebellar hypoplasia in a calf.

genetic form of hypoplasia of the cerebellum and presence of dysplastic foci, consisting of clusters of intermixed granule and Purkinje neurons has been described in Standard Poodle puppies. Cerebellar hypoplasia has been reported in piglets born to sows treated with the organophosphate trichlorfon during pregnancy, and may be detected microscopically in goat kids and lambs affected by hypocuprosis. The most prevalent and best-defined cerebellar hypoplasias are those that follow infection of the developing cerebellum by feline panleukopenia virus, bovine viral diarrhea virus, border disease virus, and classical swine fever virus. Canine parvoviral DNA has been detected in cerebellar hypoplasia in dogs. The occurrence of cerebellar hypoplasia as a consequence of viral infections of the developing nervous system is further discussed in the section Viral causes of developmental defects of the central nervous system.

Cerebellar growth patterns determine the gestational or perinatal periods during which cerebellar hypoplasia may follow the action of a teratogen and influence the nature and scope of the structural aberrations marking the hypoplastic process. The cerebellum originates as a dorsal growth of the alar plate of the metencephalon over the fourth ventricle.

Germinal cells adjacent to the fourth ventricle differentiate into neurons that migrate into the developing cerebellum to form the deep nuclei and Purkinje neurons. This differentiation occurs prior to mid-gestation. A population of germinal cells migrates to the surface of the developing cerebellum and forms a layer several cells thick. This is the external granular layer that covers the folia as they develop. In this layer, cells proliferate rapidly and differentiate into microneurons, such as basket cells, stellate cells, and granule cells, which migrate into the folium to their definitive locations. This proliferation, differentiation, and migration begins late in gestation and continues for a few weeks postnatally in most species. Normal cerebellar cytoarchitectural development, including the maturation and localization of Purkinje cells, is dependent upon these microneurons establishing orderly synaptic connections.

It is the actively mitotic germinative cells of the external granular layer that are especially vulnerable to the effects of teratogenic agents. *Feline panleukopenia virus, bovine viral diarrhea virus, and border disease virus cause selective necrosis of external granular layer cells.* That the destructive process may be augmented by vascular damage has been demonstrated for bovine viral diarrhea virus. Classical swine fever virus possibly acts through inhibition of cell division and maturation. In puppies, segmental cerebellar dysplasia may result from postnatal infection with canine herpesvirus. Because the growth behavior of the subependymal cell plate has features in common with the external granular layer of the cerebellum, residual lesions attributable to this site of infection, such as cavitating defects, may be associated with cerebellar hypoplasia, particularly in cases of viral origin.

The anatomic expressions of hypoplasia, both in the cerebellum and subcerebellar structures, are very variable in degree. In some cases, the cerebellum may appear grossly normal, the hypoplastic defects being detectable only on microscopic examination. In such cases, the defects are irregular in distribution, although there is a more or less severe loss of Purkinje cells. The granular layer is here and there narrowed and deficient in cells, but the molecular layer is normal. Correlative lesions may be present or absent and, when present, may be asymmetrical; they occur chiefly in the deep cerebellar nuclei, olives, and cerebellar peduncles. At the other extreme, the cerebellum may be represented only by a small nubbin of tissue or 2 unconnected nubbins, each related to a hypoplastic peduncle. In these severe defects, there is no folial pattern or division into lobes. Intermediate degrees of cerebellar hypoplasia are, however, the most common. It is usually possible to recognize with the naked eye that the cerebellar peduncles are diminished in size, especially the brachium pontis; that the medullary pyramids are flattened; and that the small size of the restiform bodies gives the fourth ventricle a flattened appearance. Microscopically, the cerebellar cortex is disorganized. A brief description is not possible because the pattern varies greatly from case to case and place to place in the one animal. The Purkinje cells and the cells of the granular layer are the most obviously deficient and, in those that are present, regressive changes are common.

Cerebellar atrophy (or **abiotrophy**, or **cerebellar cortical degeneration**) refers to premature or accelerated degeneration of fully formed cerebellar neurons (Figs. 4-27 to 4-29). This differs from hypoplasia, in which the cerebellum fails to form completely during development, and hence this condition will be dealt under Neurodegenerative diseases.

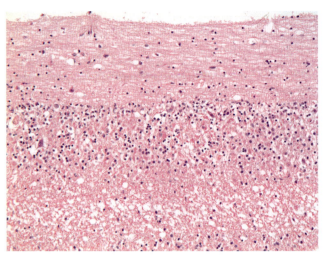

Figure 4-27 **Cerebellar abiotrophy** in a puppy; note severe hypoplasia of the granular layer with almost complete absence of Purkinje cells.

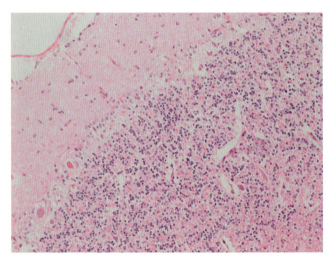

Figure 4-28 Severe loss of Purkinje cells and degeneration in **congenital cerebellar abiotrophy** in a dog.

Further reading

Chen X, et al. A neonatal encephalopathy with seizures in standard poodle dogs with a missense mutation in the canine ortholog of ATF2. Neurogenetics 2008;9:41-49.

Choi H, et al. Imaging diagnosis—cerebellar vermis hypoplasia in a miniature schnauzer. Vet Radiol Ultrasound 2007;48:129-131.

Tsuda T, et al. Arthrogryposis, hydranencephaly and cerebellar hypoplasia syndrome in neonatal calves resulting from intrauterine infection with Aino virus. Vet Res 2004;35:531-538.

Arnold-Chiari malformation

In the Arnold-Chiari malformation (Chiari type II malformation), the cerebellar vermis is herniated as a tongue-like process of tissue into the foramen magnum and cranial spinal canal, where it overlies an elongated medulla that is also displaced caudally (Fig. 4-30). The cranial nerves from the medulla alter their trajectory. The tentorium is inserted caudally toward the foramen magnum, the tentorial hiatus is shallow and wide, and the pons and occipital poles are displaced through it. The displaced occipital poles show sagittal, parallel gyri. Internal

Malformations of the Central Nervous System

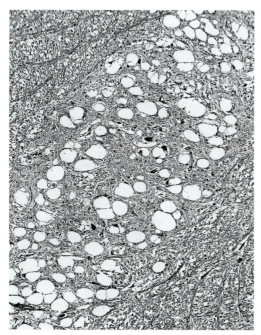

Figure 4-29 Neuronal degeneration and spongiosus, in inferior olive in a Kerry Blue Terrier with cerebellar abiotrophy.

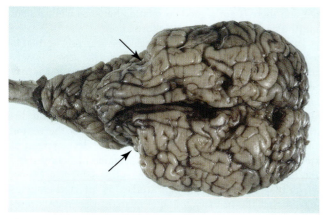

Figure 4-30 Arnold-Chiari malformation in a calf. Note coning and deformity of the cerebellum, and compression of the occipital lobes (arrows). (Courtesy Noah's Arkives, University of Georgia).

hydrocephalus may be a secondary effect, and spina bifida or meningomyelocele may be concurrent.

The caudal fossa in particular, but perhaps also the rostral fossa, is too small for the normal volume of brain tissue, suggesting that there has been failure of neurogenic induction of osseous growth. The defect is observed occasionally in calves. In the Cavalier King Charles Spaniel dog, the disease is defined as *Chiari-like malformation* and encompasses a mismatch between caudal fossa volume and the brain parenchyma within, leading to a caudal herniation of part of the cerebellum and brainstem into or through the foramen magnum. It is suggested that a smaller occiput may result from a reduced chondrocyte population in the fetus and increased number of apoptotic chondrocytes. A series of events, including dynamic alteration of CSF flow between intracranial and spinal compartments, and reduced craniospinal compliance, may lead to accumulation of fluid in the cervical spinal parenchyma and eventually the development of *syringomyelia*. Chiari-like

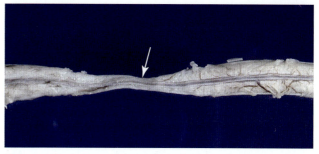

Figure 4-31 Segmental hypoplasia (arrow) of spinal cord in a calf. (Courtesy Noah's Arkives, University of Georgia).

malformation and syringomyelia is also reported in other small or "toy" dog breeds, including the French Bulldog, Griffon Bruxellois, Chihuahua, Pomeranian, Maltese Terrier, Pug, and Yorkshire Terrier.

Further reading

Driver CJ, et al. An update on the pathogenesis of syringomyelia secondary to Chiari-like malformations in dogs. Vet J 2013;198:551-559.

Rusbridge C, Knowler SP. Inheritance of occipital bone hypoplasia (Chiari type I malformation) in Cavalier King Charles Spaniels. J Vet Intern Med 2004;18:673-678.

Dandy-Walker syndrome

In the Dandy-Walker syndrome, seen in various species, *there is a midline defect of the cerebellum, with the vermis largely absent and the cerebellar hemispheres widely separated by a large fluid-filled cyst in an enlarged caudal fossa.* The roof of the cyst, which ruptures easily when the brain is removed, consists of ependyma, a disorganized layer of glial tissue, and an outer layer of leptomeningeal tissue. An expanded fourth ventricle forms the floor of the cyst. The vermal malformation is thought to be the result of a primary midline developmental defect.

Further reading

Wong D, et al. Dandy-Walker-like syndrome in a quarter horse colt. J Vet Intern Med 2007;21:1130-1134.

Spinal cord

Myelodysplasia

Myelodysplasia refers to abnormal development of the spinal cord. Segmental aplasia and hypoplasia may occur at any level of the spinal cord (Fig. 4-31), but *the lumbar region is most frequently affected.* Some cases are associated with fetal Akabane virus infection.

Perosomus elumbus, which occurs in calves and lambs, *is characterized by partial agenesis of the spinal cord.* The lumbar segment is involved, and there is failure of induction of the related vertebrae. The cranial part of the body is normal, but *the vertebral axis ends at the caudal thoracic region, and lumbar, sacral, and coccygeal vertebrae are absent.* The spinal cord ends in the thoracic region in a blind vertebral canal. The caudal part of the body remains attached to the cranial part by soft tissue only; the limbs are arthrogrypotic and their muscles atrophic. Atypically, only some lumbar segments are absent, or severely hypoplastic with absence of arches and spinal muscle, and a remnant of cauda equina may be found in the sacral region.

The most severe forms of myelodysplasia, affecting especially the potential dorsal regions of the cord, occur *in association with the forms of spina bifida* described later. Myelodysplasia, not associated with the skeletal manifestations of spina bifida but probably best included in this classification, occurs quite commonly in animals, particularly *in association with arthrogryposis in calves and lambs*. The dysplasia, which is readily detectable by the presence of *aberrant central canals* (sometimes as many as 6), chiefly involves limited lengths of the lumbar segment of the cord, but occasionally is localized to cervical or thoracic regions. *Denervation atrophy of appendicular muscle is constantly present and is the probable basis of the arthrogryptic changes.* The degree of dysplasia is quite variable, but it is characterized by aberrations of the central canal, by the absence of dorsal or ventral septa, the presence of ectopic septa and clefts, and by distortion, asymmetry, and partial duplication of the ventral and dorsal horns of gray matter. In some cases, the cord is duplicated completely within common leptomeninges and dura *(diplomyelia)* (Fig. 4-32), or within separate meningeal coverings and vertebral canals separated by a bony partition *(diastematomyelia)*.

Syringomyelia *is tubular cavitation of the spinal cord that extends over several segments* (Fig. 4-33); it is an uncommon anomaly in animals. Syringomyelia is rarely acquired and is best known as one of the lesions associated with the familial disorder of young Weimaraner dogs described later and Chiari-like malformation of Cavalier King Charles Spaniel dogs. When the cavitation involves the medulla, the defect is termed *syringobulbia*. Syringomyelia and syringobulbia may occur together.

Hydromyelia *is dilation of the central canal of the spinal cord*. It is not commonly detected but occurs in association with spina bifida and may be a precursor lesion for syringomyelia. Both hydromyelia and syringomyelia are found in the dysraphic spinal cord of arthrogryptic Charolais calves. Hydromyelia may be acquired as a consequence of obstruction of cerebrospinal fluid flow in the central canal.

A syndrome of pelvic limb gait disturbance in young **Weimaraner dogs** is a manifestation of a spectrum of myelodysplastic and dysraphic lesions, and is inherited in a co-dominant mode with variable penetrance. The trait is lethal in the homozygous state. A frameshift mutation located in exon 2 of the *NKX2-8* gene is identified. Affected animals exhibit a gait deficit from the time they begin to walk, but clinical signs in some cases may be barely noticeable. Severely affected dogs typically are unable to completely extend the hindlimbs so that their normal attitude is crouched. When walking, the hindlimbs are moved together in a "bunny-hopping" or "kangaroo-gait" fashion. Additionally, affected animals may show thoracolumbar scoliosis, depression of the sternum, and abnormal hair streams in the dorsal cervical region. There is no significant progression or regression of clinical signs with age, and there is not a good correlation between clinical signs and the degree of structural malformation.

Pathologically, the exposed spinal cord is grossly normal in size and conformation, but *a range of dysraphic defects may be present*, including anomalies of the dorsal septum, which may be absent; hydromyelia and other anomalies of the central canal, which may be absent (Fig. 4-34); duplication or displacement of the central canal; anomalies of extent and distribution of the central gray matter; anomalies of the ventral horns consisting of deficient delineation and development of medial cell groups, and aberrant collections of neurons and gray neuropil; and deficiency of the ventral median fissure, which may be total. Histologic studies on affected embryos suggest that the primary lesion is related to aberrantly positioned mantle cells ventral to the central canal in the floor-plate area.

Syringomyelia is not present until about 8 months of age and involves lumbar segments. Cavitation may be barely visible to

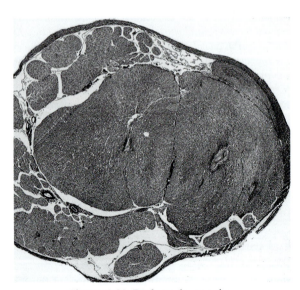

Figure 4-32 Diplomyelia in a dog.

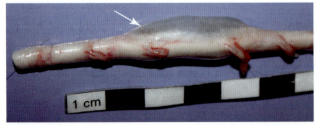

Figure 4-33 Syringomyelia (arrow) in a cat. (Courtesy J.L. Caswell.)

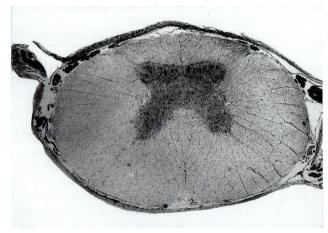

Figure 4-34 Absence of central canal of spinal cord in **dysraphism** in a dog.

the naked eye. Microscopically, the cavity is usually found in the central gray matter dorsal and lateral to the central canal. There is not much encroachment on the white matter except for that in the white commissures when the cavitation extends from one side to the other. Connection with the central canal is difficult to demonstrate but may be found in serial sections. Ependyma does not line the cavity, the walls of which are formed of frayed nervous tissue with an appearance suggesting that the cord has been squashed or torn at autopsy. The tissue around the cavity is edematous and stains poorly.

Spina bifida and related defects

Spina bifida *refers to absence of the dorsal portions of the vertebrae.* It is, however, a rather imperfect name as the various forms of the defect represent differences in degree of defective closure of the neural tube, its separation from the ectoderm, and its induction of a skeletal investment. It is convenient to divide the defect into several classes on the basis of severity: *myeloschisis, spina bifida occulta, spina bifida cystica with meningocele,* and *spina bifida with myelomeningocele* apply to the vertebral defect; *amyelia, diastematomyelia, hydromyelia,* and *dysraphism* apply to the spinal cord.

In **total myeloschisis,** *neurulation does not occur,* the neural plate remaining open. Here total means a defect that involves the whole of the vertebral axis with anencephaly an expected accompaniment. There is virtual *amyelia* (absence of spinal cord), neural tissue being present only as soft red masses in the residual groove. *Local myeloschisis* is a localized defect caused by failure of closure of the neural tube. One or more vertebral segments may be defective. The defect may occur in any portion of the vertebral axis but is expected to be lumbosacral.

The defect occurs in calves, lambs, foals, cats, and most frequently in brachycephalic breeds of dogs and is inherited as an autosomal dominant condition in Manx cats. Affected cats are heterozygotes of variable expression, whereas the homozygous state is lethal. *Sacrococcygeal agenesis* occurs in association with spina bifida in Manx cats, calves, dogs, and sheep.

Spina bifida occulta is perhaps the least rare form of the defect in animals, and it is occult because *it is not apparent except for the presence of dimpling or deeper invagination of the skin.* It may accompany defects in other remote tissues, but the defect is otherwise limited to the absence of one or more vertebral arches. The cord may be grossly normal but dysplastic microscopically, usually with diastematomyelia. The spinous processes may be bifid or absent.

In **spina bifida cystica,** a cystic swelling protrudes through the vertebral defect. Because of differential growth of the vertebral and neural axes, the cranial-caudal position of the skin and bone lesions may not correspond, especially in the caudal regions where the defects are expected to occur.

When meninges protrude (**meningocele**), the roof of the cyst is comprised of skin and condensed meninges, including dura mater. The spinal cord may be normal grossly but dysplastic segments are detected microscopically. Macroscopic lesions in the cord include partial duplication and cystic distention of the central canal that communicates with the endodural space via a cleft in the dorsal funiculi. A meningocele may contain a large accumulation of adipose tissue (**lipomeningocele**).

When meninges and spinal cord protrude (**meningomyelocele**), the cyst tends to be broad based. *Failure of dehiscence of the neural crest from surface ectoderm provides for a central area without epithelial covering.* This medullovasculosa corresponds to the cerebrovasculosa of anencephaly and consists of vascularized meninges, heterotopic cord tissue, and connective tissue. The defects in the cord include those mentioned as occurring with meningocele and, in severe cases, duplication or absence of the cord in affected segments. The tethered cord syndrome refers to attachment of the meningomyelocele that prevents the normal ascent of the spinal cord as the vertebral column grows.

A **dermoid sinus** is a congenital abnormality, inherited in Rhodesian Ridgeback dogs, in which incomplete separation of the neural tube from the overlying dorsal midline ectoderm allows persistence of a sinus connecting the skin surface to the supraspinous ligament, or it may extend as deep as the dura mater of the spinal cord. The condition is also described in Burmese cats.

Further reading

Ricci E, et al. MRI findings, surgical treatment and follow-up of a myelomeningocele with tethered spinal cord syndrome in a cat. J Feline Med Surg 2011;13:467-472.

Safra N, et al. Genome-wide association mapping in dogs enables identification of the homeobox gene, *NKX2-8*, as a genetic component of neural tube defects in humans. PLoS Genet 2013;9:e1003646.

Simpson D, et al. Dermoid sinus in Burmese cats. J Small Anim Pract 2011;52:616.

Arachnoid cysts

Spinal arachnoid cysts are characterized as CSF-filled, dorsal midline, intradural, extramedullary, single or multilobed cavitational lesions, associated with coarse arachnoid trabeculation, that result in spinal cord compression. Occasionally, cysts are located in ventral and dorsolateral locations in the cervical spinal region. The cystic cavities are separated from the compressed spinal cord by an intact pia mater and lacked an epithelial lining, and therefore the definition of pseudocyst should be more appropriate. Arachnoid cysts are observed more frequently in young Rottweilers, but there are descriptions in other canine breeds. The pathogenesis is unknown, although congenital spinal dysraphism resulting from failure of fusion of the neural crest has been suggested. Acquired arachnoid cysts may occur secondary to trauma, inflammatory changes, or subarachnoid hemorrhages, and usually show adhesions with the meninges that may result in further expansion of the subarachnoid space and compression on the spinal cord.

Intracranial arachnoid cysts (Fig. 4-35) are predominantly found dorsal to the colliculi and rostral to the cerebellum (quadrigeminal cistern). Cerebellar and/or occipital lobe compression may be associated with neurologic signs. Small and brachycephalic breeds of dog, especially the Shih Tzu, are over-represented. Reported feline cases affect young Persian cats.

Further reading

Matiasek LA, et al. Clinical and magnetic resonance imaging characteristics of quadrigeminal cysts in dogs. J Vet Intern Med 2007;21:1021-1026.

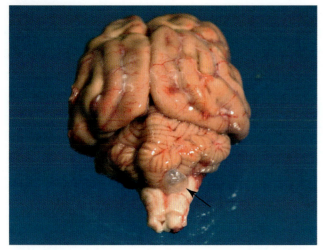

Figure 4-35 Intracranial **arachnoid cyst** in a dog (arrow). (Courtesy J.L. Caswell.)

Viral causes of developmental defects of the central nervous system

Orthobunyaviruses

Akabane virus (AKAV), a species of the genus *Orthobunyavirus*, family *Bunyaviridae*, is among the most potent of the viral teratogens of domestic animals, but the infection is otherwise asymptomatic. **Iriki virus**, a strain of AKAV, has similar pathogenic potential. Following maternal infection at critical stages of gestation, AKAV produces a range of predominantly neural abnormalities in calves, lambs, and kids, but *AKAV is best known for producing outbreaks of arthrogryposis and hydranencephaly in calves*. Epizootics of Akabane virus disease in cattle have been reported in areas of Japan, Israel, and Australia. The vector in Australia is the biting midge *Culicoides brevitarsis*, and the virus has also been isolated from mosquitoes in Japan. Buffaloes, horses, and pigs are additional vertebrate hosts. Although arthrogryposis and hydranencephaly may be the most obvious manifestations in field epizootics of **bovine** AKAV disease, a range of overlapping syndromes is observed in calves in affected herds. The pattern of fetal disease corresponds to the gestational age of the fetus at the time of infection. Infection late in gestation may cause abortion. The initial manifestation of neural abnormality in a field outbreak is the birth of incoordinate calves and, in this group, nonsuppurative encephalomyelitis is evident on histologic examination. *Microencephaly* and *cerebellar hypoplasia* occur occasionally as manifestations of late infection. *Arthrogryposis*, sometimes associated with spinal deformities, appears early in the outbreak following fetal infection at 5-6 months of pregnancy. In arthrogrypotic calves, there is loss of spinal ventral horn neurons, loss of myelin in the motor tracts of the spinal cord and in ventral spinal nerves, and denervation atrophy together with fibrous and adipose replacement of skeletal musculature.

At least some strains of AKAV have the capacity to cause *polymyositis*, particularly in the early myotubular phase of skeletal muscle development, suggesting the possible involvement of this process in the arthrogrypotic change. *Severe hydranencephaly*, manifest clinically as blindness and stupidity, is seen toward the end of the epizootic, being the result of fetal infection at 3-4 months of gestation. With increasing age of the fetus at the time of infection, the cavitating cerebral changes are less severe and grade toward *porencephaly*.

The teratogenic potential of AKAV in **sheep and goats** is qualitatively the same as for cattle. Cavitating cerebral defects, arthrogryposis, microencephaly, and agenesis or hypoplasia of the spinal cord have been produced in lambs born of ewes inoculated on days 29-48 of pregnancy. Field observations in Australian flocks suggest that, in sheep, *microencephaly* is relatively more common as a consequence of AKAV infection than it is in cattle.

Aino virus, a member of *Shuni* serogroup, can cause arthrogryposis, hydranencephaly, and cerebellar hypoplasia in bovine fetuses infected experimentally, and is suspected to be the teratogen in field cases of congenital bovine malformations in Japan.

Species **Schmallenberg virus** (SBV), a member of *Simbu* serogroup, closely related to AKAV and Aino virus, is an arthropod-borne pathogen that spread rapidly throughout the majority of European countries since 2011. SBV causes outbreaks of abortion, stillbirth and birth at term of lambs, kids, and calves with neurologic signs and/or head, spine, or limb malformations. Lesions are very similar to those induced by AKAV and include arthrogryposis, brachygnathia inferior, torticollis, kyphosis, lordosis, scoliosis, *cerebellar hypoplasia*, *hydranencephaly, porencephaly, hydrocephalus,* and *micromyelia* (Fig. 4-36A, B). Histologic lesions include lymphohistiocytic meningoencephalomyelitis in fetuses that survive infection early in gestation, glial nodules mainly in the mesencephalon and hippocampus of lambs and goats, and neuronal degeneration and necrosis mainly in the brainstem of calves. Micromyelia is characterized by a loss of gray and white matter, with few neurons remaining in the ventral horn in calves. The skeletal muscles of lambs and calves show *myofibrillar hypoplasia*. Although SBV can be detected in different regions of the CNS of aborted lambs and calves, brainstem seems to be the most appropriate tissue to maximize the likelihood of SBV detection by PCR.

Cache Valley virus (CVV), a serotype of species *Bunyamwera virus*, genus *Orthobunyavirus*, is a mosquito-borne bunyavirus that is endemic in North America. CVV is capable of infecting a variety of mammals, generally as subclinical infections, but it is occasionally teratogenic in fetal lambs. The nature and pathogenesis of the abnormalities produced are comparable to those of Akabane virus in sheep. Three other members of genus *Orthobunyavirus*—**La Crosse virus** and **San Angelo virus** (serotypes of *California encephalitis virus*), and **Main Drain virus**—also express bunyaviral tropism for fetal tissue infection and can induce lesions, including arthrogryposis, hydrocephalus, fetal death, axial skeletal deviations, anasarca, and oligohydramnios.

Further reading

Beer M, et al. "Schmallenberg virus"—a novel orthobunyavirus emerging in Europe. Epidemiol Infect 2013;141:1-8.

De Regge N, et al. Diagnosis of Schmallenberg virus infection in malformed lambs and calves and first indications for virus clearance in the fetus. Vet Microbiol 2013;162:595-600.

Herder V, et al. Salient lesions in domestic ruminants infected with the emerging so-called Schmallenberg virus in Germany. Vet Pathol 2012;49:588-591.

Wernike K, et al. Schmallenberg virus—two years of experiences. Prev Vet Med 2014;116:423-434.

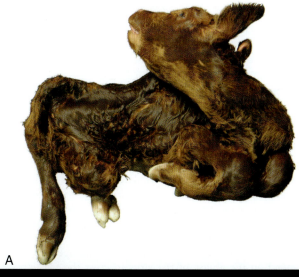

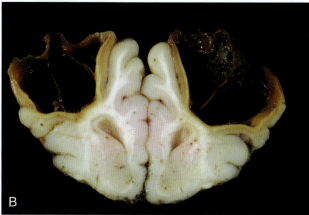

Figure 4-36 **A.** Arthrogryposis. **B.** Bilateral **porencephaly** in a calf infected with Schmallenberg virus (Courtesy W. Baumgärtner, V. Herder. University of Veterinary Medicine, Hannover, Germany).

Orbiviruses

Hydranencephaly and porencephaly have been reported in lambs and calves whose dams received a live-attenuated bluetongue vaccine or contracted species **Bluetongue virus** (BTV, genus *Orbivirus*, family *Reoviridae*) infection during pregnancy (see Fig. 4-24B). The type of congenital anomaly found depends on the fetal age at the time of infection with BTV. Lambs infected with bluetongue vaccine virus at 50-55 days gestation develop severe necrotizing encephalopathy and retinopathy, which at birth is manifested as *hydranencephaly and retinal dysplasia*. Infection of lambs at 75 days gestation causes multifocal encephalitis and selective vacuolation of white matter that is manifested as porencephalic cysts in the newborn; ocular lesions are not observed in these newborn lambs. Lesions in brains of lambs infected after 100 days gestation are confined to mild focal meningoencephalitis. BTV infection of fetal calves can cause hydranencephaly. The malformation is also recorded in calves congenitally infected during the BTV serotype 8 epizootic in Europe.

Chuzan virus (CHUV), a strain of species *Palyam virus*, genus *Orbivirus*, family *Reoviridae*, is transmitted by *Culicoides* spp. CHUV is infective for several ruminant species, and in Japan has been incriminated as a teratogen of fetal calves with features similar to those of *Akabane virus* infection.

Further reading

MacLachlan NJ, et al. The pathology and pathogenesis of bluetongue. J Comp Pathol 2009;141:1-16.

Rift Valley fever virus and Wesselsbron virus

These infections are considered more fully in Vol. 2, Liver and biliary system. In addition to species **Wesselsbron virus** (WESSV), there are several other mosquito-borne flaviviruses (genus *Flavivirus*, family *Flaviviridae*) in South Africa, including species **West Nile virus** and **Banzi virus,** to which sheep are experimentally susceptible and which result in abortion, stillbirths, and neonatal deaths; anomalies include *hydranencephaly, porencephaly*, and *internal hydrocephalus*.

Rift Valley fever virus, a serotype species of genus *Phlebovirus*, and WESSV are mosquito-borne and tend to circulate together. They are both primarily hepatotropic, but the wild strain of WESSV and attenuated strains of both are neurotropic, and vaccine strains may be responsible for most outbreaks of congenital neurologic disease. The presenting features are similar to those of Akabane disease, but the high incidence of hydrops amnii and prolonged gestation is especially a feature.

The destructive changes in the CNS produced by one or other of these viruses, or both together, can be more severe than with other teratogenic viruses and result in *segmental aplasia of the cord, aplasia of the cerebellum*, and *anencephaly*. It is more usual, however, that the defects include *brachygnathia, hydranencephaly or porencephaly, hypoplasia of cerebellum and spinal cord*, and varied musculoskeletal stigmata of *arthrogryposis*.

Further reading

Hunter P, et al. Teratogenicity of a mutagenised Rift Valley fever virus (MVP 12) in sheep. Onderstepoort J Vet Res 2002;69: 95-98.

Pestiviruses

The diseases caused by species **Bovine viral diarrhea virus** (BVDV), genus *Pestivirus*, family *Flaviviridae*, are considered in detail in Vol. 2, Alimentary system and peritoneum. The ecology of BVDV depends on transplacental transmission and the establishment of immune tolerance and persistent infections. Horizontal transfer of infection occurs readily, but is seldom clinically significant. Persistently infected fetuses that survive to become pregnant transmit BVDV to the conceptus. Although viral strains differ in their pathogenicity, infection of susceptible cows during early and middle stages of gestation is likely to result in either fetal death or a variety of developmental defects, predominantly neural and ocular. Some congenitally affected calves also have erosive lesions in the upper alimentary tract and abomasum resembling those seen in adult cattle; brachygnathism also occurs.

The outcome of infection of the fetal calf is related to gestational age, advancing fetal maturity being associated with increased resistance to the virus. Infections occurring within the first 100 days of fetal life tend to be lethal, resulting in *abortion or mummification*. Although the gross pathologic changes seen in these lethal infections lack unique features, the patterns of tissue response are characteristic, but are rarely seen, as such fetuses die in utero and undergo autolysis. Necrotizing inflammation can involve a variety of tissues. The reactive changes are dominated by mononuclear, predominantly macrophage, infiltration of hepatic portal areas, myocardium, spleen, and lymph nodes, which is reflected grossly in enlargement, nodularity, and mottling of the liver and enlargement of spleen and lymph nodes. The presence of *growth-arrest lines in long bones* suggests that the fetus undergoes one or more intrauterine crises before death. Affected fetuses may have partial alopecia that spares the tail, the lower portion of the limbs, and the head, these being points of initial hair growth during fetal development. The microscopic skin changes that evolve from the initial necrotizing dermatitis and correlate with the alopecia are hypoplasia of hair follicles and cystic distention of adnexal glands.

The teratogenic effects of BVDV are manifested during the 100-170-day period. The period of susceptibility presumably varies with the strain of virus. *Cerebellar hypoplasia is the most characteristic defect* (see Fig. 4-26). Gross cerebellar changes range from more or less uniform atrophy to irregular folial atrophy and agenesis accompanied by cavitation. The hypoplastic process is compounded by the effects of necrosis of external granular layer cells and parenchymal destruction as a consequence of folial edema resulting from vasculitis. The relative contribution of these processes is quite variable, but it appears that the vasculopathy may be more prominent in older fetuses. The nature and extent of involvement of individual folia also varies considerably. The evolution of the cerebellar changes has been studied experimentally. Acute lesions are evident 2 weeks after infection. Cellular necrosis in the external granular layer is accompanied by nonsuppurative meningitis. Vasculitis, marked by endothelial proliferation and perivascular leukocytic infiltration, is associated with folial edema, and there may be focal hemorrhages in the cerebellar white matter and cortex.

Folial edema, depending on its severity, may result in total folial destruction, cavitation, or focal, often linear, areas of folial white matter deficient in myelin and axons. Where necrosis of the external granular layer predominates, the result is irregular atrophy of affected folia. Features of the atrophic process are marked depletion of granule cells, ectopia of Purkinje cells, and the presence of swollen Purkinje cell axons in the granular layer. The evolution of the cerebellar lesion in the fetal calf extends over 6 weeks, and by 10 weeks after maternal infection, inflammatory changes are not evident in the brain.

Other CNS defects that may be a consequence of fetal infection are porencephaly, hydranencephaly, microencephaly, hydrocephalus, cystic septum pellucidum, and dysmyelination. Ocular anomalies commonly accompany cerebellar defects, and include retinal dysplasia and atrophy, cataract, optic neuritis and atrophy, microphthalmia, and persistent pupillary membrane.

Infection of the fetus later than 170 days is unlikely to cause either intrauterine death or malformation. This increased resistance coincides with the fetus acquiring the capacity to produce neutralizing antibody to the virus. However, BVDV also has the capacity to induce more subtle developmental aberrations, such as *intrauterine growth retardation* and *atrophy of the thymus and lymphoid tissues.* The regressive changes in thymus and lymphoid tissues offer a morphologic basis for the immunologic suppression and tolerance phenomena associated with congenital infections with BVDV.

Further reading

Bielefeldt-Ohmann H, et al. Transplacental infection with noncytopathic bovine viral diarrhoea virus types 1b and 2: viral spread and molecular neuropathology. J Comp Pathol 2008;138:72-85.

Border disease virus. Border disease (BD) of lambs was first described from the border counties of England and Wales, and is now recognized in many countries. Affected lambs show gross tremors and long hairy birth coats ("hairy-shaker," or "fuzzy" lambs). BD is caused by species **Border disease virus** (BDV), genus *Pestivirus*, family *Flaviviridae*, which is very closely related to bovine viral diarrhea virus (BVDV) and less closely to classical swine fever virus. These viruses possess a similar host spectrum experimentally, and interspecies transmission, especially between ruminants, does occur naturally, but the clinical expression in recipients may be modified or absent. The ecology of BDV and the pathogenesis of BD depend on the ability of the virus to cross the placenta and then either to produce disease in the fetus or a state of immunotolerance and *persistent infection (PI) that allows excretion of the virus continuously in postnatal life*. Strain variations of BDV, with differing host responses depending on breed and genotype, and gestational age at which infection occurs, contribute to the varied manifestations of the disease. Congenital disease and PI are typically caused by the *noncytopathic biotype* of BDV; mucosal disease–like syndrome is caused by a *cytopathic biotype* of BDV. Sheep can also be infected naturally with BVDV types 1 and 2, and BVDV is capable of producing the BD syndrome in sheep and goats. Pigs can be naturally infected by BDV, for example, strain Frijters, which can confuse identification of classical swine fever.

Primary infection of postnatal sheep by BDV is usually subclinical, immunity develops, and the virus is eliminated. In pregnant ewes, the virus infects the fetus within the first week of exposure and is not then influenced by the immune status of the ewe.

BDV is a potential cause of a variety of developmental disorders, including *hypomyelinogenesis; cavitating cerebral defects, such as porencephaly, hydranencephaly, and cystic septum pellucidum; cerebellar dysplasia; arthrogryposis and skeletal defects; mandibular brachygnathism; and thymic hypoplasia.* The pathogenicity of the virus is most freely expressed in experimental infections, the cavitating cerebral lesions and cerebellar dysplasia being common sequelae of experimental infections but only occasionally encountered in the natural disease.

Bovine viral diarrhea virus is capable of producing the border disease syndrome in sheep and goats, and the syndrome in piglets caused by congenital infection with classical swine fever virus.

The ovine fetus is liable to significant damage if the dam is infected with BDV between days 16-80 of gestation. *The age-related immune capacity of the fetus is the important determinant of the nature of the disease produced.* In the case of infections occurring within the first half of gestation, the result may be *fetal death and abortion.* Alternatively, the fetus may survive, frequently carrying an immunologically tolerated infection. In this event, the virus persists in fetal tissues, and postnatally the lamb fails to produce specific antibody. Such PI sheep harbor the virus for prolonged periods, are chronic excretors of the virus, and readily transmit infection. Lateral spread is important in the field and, although the virus can be transmitted experimentally by a number of routes, the mode of lateral transfer of infection under natural conditions has not been identified.

Infections in the second half of gestation elicit both humoral and cell-mediated immune responses, and it is this acquisition of immunocompetence that endows the fetus with substantial resistance to infection after day 80 of gestation. In the case of infections initiated between day 90 of gestation and the early days of postnatal life, the cell-mediated immune response is expressed morphologically as *nodular periarteritis*. The periarteritis affects medium to small arterioles, particularly in the meninges and substance of the CNS, but also occurs mildly in a wide range of other tissues.

The developmental anomalies arising from fetal infection are also related to the gestational stage at which the fetus encounters the virus, but lesions produced also vary markedly according to virus strain, dose, route of infection, and host genetic factors. *Hypomyelinogenesis, the characteristic neural lesion*, is diffuse in fetuses infected early in gestation but becomes progressively milder and more restricted to higher, later myelinating regions of the CNS in infections initiated later in gestation. The occurrence of porencephaly and cerebellar dysplasia has been confined to infections initiated at days 45-72 of gestation. The development of the cutaneous lesion requires that infection be initiated before day 80 of gestation.

Hypomyelinogenesis and clinical tremors may substantially resolve during the first few months of life, notwithstanding that the animals have persistent replicating infection, suggesting that the normal processes of myelin deposition have been delayed or that cellular injury has been slowly repaired. The virus does infect myelinating oligodendroglia, astroglia, and glial progenitor cells, and it is reasonable to assume a direct effect on the differentiation or maturation of oligodendroglia. The virus is able to induce apoptosis of neural cells through both intrinsic and extrinsic pathways. However, the virus also infects many non-neural cells, including thyroid epithelium. There are no morphologic changes in the thyroid epithelium, but reduction in circulating thyroid hormone levels may contribute to delayed maturation.

The cavitating cerebral defects and cerebellar dysplasia arise from inflammatory destruction of developing neural elements, possibly secondary to vasculitis. These lambs may have severe locomotor and behavioral abnormalities and defects of vision, the latter probably of central origin rather than the result of focal retinal dysplasias that may be present. They are serologically positive but not persistently infected.

The *abnormality of birth coats* occurs in fetuses infected before ~90 days of gestation. There are no cytologic changes in the papillae that can be ascribed to direct viral action. The primary follicles revert to a more primitive type, are enlarged, and produce heavily medullated fibers that are most prominent after ~3 weeks. There are fewer secondary follicles, and their development is retarded.

BDV infection also interferes with prenatal and postnatal development of skeleton, musculature, and viscera. Tissues most affected are those that have their main growth spurt in the fetal period. *Growth-arrest lines in long bones* suggest periods of interrupted intrauterine development.

Lambs that are persistently infected at birth remain so, but not all show neurologic signs. Growth and viability may be depressed. Some PI sheep develop oculonasal discharges and respiratory distress or severe diarrhea and die in 2-4 weeks with inflammatory lymphoproliferative lesions in many organs. In the brain, these reactions occur particularly in the choroid plexuses and periventricular substance. Proliferative metaplastic changes in the intestinal mucosa affect mainly the cecum and colon, the hyperplastic glands penetrating the muscular mucosa. *The delayed disease has features resembling those of mucosal disease of cattle*, which is considered to be caused by superinfection by a different strain of BVDV or by minor mutation of homologous virus in animals that are persistently infected.

Infection by BDV is widespread in **goats,** but disease attributable to this virus is not. The characteristics of the natural and experimental disease are similar to those in sheep, but spontaneous neurologic disease is not a feature. The fetal goat may be much more susceptible to infection than the fetal lamb; a high incidence of fetal death, mummification, and abortion is reported.

Both vaccine and certain low-virulence field strains of species **Classical swine fever virus** (CSFV, hog cholera virus) are teratogenic for the fetal piglet. The disease is discussed in detail in Vol. 3, Cardiovascular system. Fetuses are susceptible to infection regardless of the immune status of the sow. The apparent induction of immune tolerance results in the delivery of chronically infected piglets lacking antibody. The gestational interval during which fetal piglets are susceptible to the teratogenic effects of CSFV extends at least from days 10-97 of gestation, but the occurrence of malformation is favored by infection around day 30. The most characteristic anomalies involve the nervous system. The combination of *hypoplasia and dysplasia of the cerebellum and CNS hypomyelinogenesis*, most severe in the spinal cord, comprises one form of the *congenital tremor syndrome* of piglets. *Microencephaly* is also a rather characteristic sequel. The mechanism by which these lesions evolve is compatible with a persistent neural infection resulting in selective inhibition of cell division. Additional effects noted in affected litters include fetal mummification, stillbirth, pulmonary hypoplasia, nodularity of the liver, ascites, anasarca, cutaneous purpura, arthrogryposis, and micrognathia.

Further reading

Monies RJ, et al. Mucosal disease-like lesions in sheep infected with Border disease virus. Vet Rec 2004;155:765-769.

Paton DJ, Greiser-Wilke I. Classical swine fever—an update. Res Vet Sci 2003;75:169-178.

Toplu N, et al. Neuropathologic study of border disease virus in naturally infected fetal and neonatal small ruminants and its association with apoptosis. Vet Pathol 2011;48:576-583.

Feline panleukopenia virus

This disease is discussed in detail in Vol. 2, Alimentary system and peritoneum.

Species **Feline panleukopenia virus** (FPLV), genus *Parvovirus*, family *Parvoviridae*, is pathogenic to the cerebellum of kittens before and shortly after birth, at which time the cerebellum is growing and differentiating rapidly. FPLV has tropism for cells that have a high mitotic rate, and its site of action is the external germinal layer of the cerebellum. The formation of *intranuclear inclusion bodies* is an early feature of the infection; they disappear by day 14 of infection. The infected cells are destroyed and with them the growth potential of the cerebellum; hence *cerebellar hypoplasia* results. The Purkinje cells, which are postmitotic but immature, are also affected and the virus is able to replicate in them, although inclusion bodies do not form. The nuclei of the Purkinje cells show vesicular ballooning, eosinophilia, and condensation of the membrane. One or more large vacuoles form in the cytoplasm. Some Purkinje cells undergo coagulative necrosis.

In view of the tropism of FPLV for rapidly replicating cells, a wide spectrum of abnormalities might be expected to result from infection of kittens in utero. The virus will cross the placenta and produce generalized infection of the fetus as indicated by the distribution of inclusion bodies. The subependymal cell plate shares growth behavior with the external granular layer of the cerebellum and *hydranencephaly* may be attributable to damage at this site of infection. In visceral organs, only slight degrees of renal hypoplasia have been observed in infected kitten fetuses.

Further reading

Poncelet L, et al. Identification of feline panleukopenia virus proteins expressed in Purkinje cell nuclei of cats with cerebellar hypoplasia. Vet J 2013;196:381-387.

Sharp NJ, et al. Hydranencephaly and cerebellar hypoplasia in two kittens attributed to intrauterine parvovirus infection. J Comp Pathol 1999;121:39-53.

STORAGE DISEASES

As most storage diseases involve neurons and neurologic impairment, they are discussed here. Within all cells, except mature erythrocytes, normal catabolism directs a steady stream of endogenous macromolecules into vesicular compartments for degradation to simple molecules that may be reused or excreted. These essentially autophagic pathways, through which each cell recycles its own constituents, may also receive endogenous and exogenous molecules from the extracellular milieu, taken up by endocytosis or phagocytosis.

Storage states, or disorders, are characterized by the accumulation of material(s) resistant to or exceeding the capacity of the machinery of intracellular digestion, disposal, or transport. Hemosiderosis and some types of hepatic lipidosis are common examples of the storage of physiologically normal substances resulting from the overloading of essentially normal, biochemically competent cells. A storage disease, by contrast, can be regarded as a storage process with a primary pathologic basis within the storing cells, and with potential for the perturbation of their function. The implication is that the catabolic machinery of the cells is fundamentally incompetent. This is generally demonstrable, but it is difficult to provide a neat definition that clearly distinguishes this situation in all circumstances.

Practically all cell types are potentially vulnerable to storage induction, but those most vulnerable are long-lived postmitotic cells, such as neurons and cardiac myocytes. Cells in dynamic renewal systems, such as enterocytes, scarcely have the chance to become involved before their time is over.

The lysosomal apparatus provides the machinery for a great deal of intracellular degradation; most storage diseases involve intralysosomal accumulation and are hence termed **lysosomal storage diseases.** The 40 or so lysosomal acid hydrolases are capable of digesting completely the complex macromolecules synthesized for cell membranes, organelles, secretory products, and so forth. This enzymic destruction must be sequestered away from the rest of the cell, and is carried out in vesicles provided with an ion pump in their limiting membranes that maintains an acidic interior, or lysosol, for the optimal activity of the hydrolases.

Newly synthesized lysosomal enzymes are carried from the trans-Golgi region within primary lysosomal vesicles, and are delivered to substrate-containing vesicles (endosomes, heterophagosomes, autophagosomes, secretory vesicles) by fusion of vesicle membranes. The end products of digestion, which are simple lipids, amino acids, and sugars, are transported from the vesicular lysosol back into the cytosol. There may be small quantities of indigestible residues that, in cells such as hepatocytes, may be extruded by a process of exocytosis.

The lysosomal hydrolases tend to be *"exoenzymes,"* sequentially breaking linkages at the ends of large molecules, but unable to act on linkages within them. This means that if the sequence is blocked at some point, further digestion cannot proceed. Should the digestive sequence be impaired, the cell will steadily accumulate a mass of vacuoles containing undegraded substrate. One type of molecule will be the major stored substance, but often the stored material will be somewhat heterogeneous, as the enzymes are linkage specific rather than substrate specific. Thus *the morphologic hallmark of lysosomal storage disease is the presence of distended cells, crowded with vacuoles bounded by single membranes containing the stored material;* these vacuoles react enzyme-histochemically for acid phosphatase or other lysosomal hydrolases. They represent the adaptive hypertrophy of the lysosomal apparatus. In some cases, the morphology and histochemical reactivity of the stored substance may fairly clearly indicate its nature, for example, glycogen. Lectin histochemistry may also be useful for characterizing stored material, exploiting the avid carbohydrate-binding properties of these agglutinating proteins in combination with a visualizing system.

Lysosomal digestion can be impaired in several ways. The most relevant here is *deficient activity of a specific lysosomal hydrolase because of a* **genetic defect.** This is the basis of the inherited lysosomal storage diseases in humans and animals, most of which are transmitted as autosomal recessive, and some as X-linked, traits. The deficiency in activity may come about via a total absence of enzyme protein caused by a mutation of the nuclear gene that produces no mRNA or produces mRNA leading to a defective or unstable enzyme, via a defective post-translational modification of the lysosomal enzyme, or via the absence of a specific activator protein required by some enzymes for the initiation of activity. These activators are small-molecular-weight, heat-stable proteins that function as detergents. They may interact with either the enzyme or its substrate. In the category of defective enzyme protein, one could also include the rare mechanism in which the enzyme lacks the specific molecular tag required to direct it, following its synthesis, to the lysosomal compartment; it is therefore immediately excreted from the cell, and the lysosomes remain deficient in that enzyme activity.

In most *autosomally inherited conditions,* the gene dose effect results in heterozygous individuals being generally phenotypically normal, but usually having demonstrably subnormal tissue activity of the particular enzyme in question. Tissues of homozygous affected individuals will contain swollen vacuolated cells, and chemical analysis reveals large amounts of the stored substance, and variable amounts of other metabolically related substances. *Multisystem involvement is likely to occur*, with storage being evident in many cell types in many organs. The cells and tissues most affected will be those most active in turning over the substrate in question, but usually the fixed and mobile macrophages are also prominently involved. This is because they avidly accumulate substrate from tissue fluids and plasma. The process begins in utero and in many cases is well developed at birth, although clinical impairment may be mild at that time. The age of onset and speed of progression of disease can vary, probably on the basis of the amount of residual enzyme activity, and often involving the ratio between various isoenzymes. In several human entities, subtypes are described on this basis.

As pointed out previously, the in vitro tissue activity of the enzyme involved can usually be demonstrated to be negligible. However, if there was, for example, *deficiency of an activator protein*, the in vitro assay of tissues for the subject enzyme might reveal paradoxically high levels of activity, reflecting the hypertrophy of the lysosomal apparatus. The enzyme, however, would be inactive in vivo in the absence of the activator protein. In addition, and especially if the assay involves synthetic substrates, various isoenzymes may give the impression of adequate activity in vitro, which has no relation to the in vivo situation. In spite of this, assay of enzyme activity in skin fibroblasts or peripheral blood leukocytes has been diagnostically useful in many genetic storage diseases, identifying both homozygous and heterozygous individuals. Molecular genetic methods can be expected to play an increasingly important role in this area.

In an alternative mechanism of storage, *an exogenous toxin may specifically inhibit a lysosomal enzyme*, and temporarily induce a state analogous to a genetic enzyme deficiency. This is the established basis of at least one plant intoxication, "locoism," and is suspected in others. The morphologic and chemical characteristics are typical, but tissue activity of the subject enzyme may be quite high when it is separated from the inhibitor and assayed.

In a final general mechanism, *substrate that is resistant to a normal and intact enzymic battery may enter degradative pathways*. This may be an exogenous substrate, or a modified endogenous substrate. By this mechanism, several amphophilic drugs, such as chloroquine, have been found to induce storage diseases by complexing with endogenous molecules to produce indigestible products. Theoretically, this mechanism could also have a genetic basis, by which an indigestible substrate is produced.

The lysosomal basis of some storage diseases is uncertain, and *non-lysosomal entities*, such as several of the glycogenoses, are clearly defined. Further, although many storage diseases have been defined in molecular terms, some have not, and in most cases, the basis of cellular dysfunction is far from clarified. There is more involved than simply the mechanical crowding out of other organelles. In most instances, the storage process seems to have little primary cytotoxic effect. It seems rather that the induction of secondary and tertiary metabolic and structural effects is responsible for functional disturbances.

In many of the **neuronal storage diseases,** the process is multisystemic, and all neurons are involved, including those of the retina and peripheral ganglia, together with cells in most other organs. But neither of the 2 preceding conditions is invariable. When neurons are involved in storage disease,

clinical signs of neurologic impairment eventually become evident, but, in general, this does not correlate with significant neuronal death, and the mechanisms of dysfunction are still largely unresolved. Regional neuronal death begins at an early stage in a few storage diseases and is progressive; it probably contributes significantly to functional disturbance at the end stage of many storage diseases.

In the face of a progressive storage process, neurons have no recourse but to accumulate storage vacuoles until they, or the animal, die. It seems probable that there is some limited capacity to discharge some of the stored load by exocytosis but, *in general, intractable constipation is inevitable as long as enzymic activity is deficient*. In spite of this, the cell limits the sites of storage to the soma and some of the larger dendritic stems. As a result, the soma becomes greatly distended and the cell outline rounded and swollen, rather than angular (Fig. 4-37A, B). However, even within the soma, storage may be somewhat polarized, often adjacent to the axon hillock; differing planes of section may suggest that some neurons are not affected, particularly if examined early in the course of the disease. The multitude of storage vacuoles crowds and displaces other organelles, and the neuron takes on a chromatolytic and foamy appearance. Glial, endothelial, and perithelial cells are generally similarly affected.

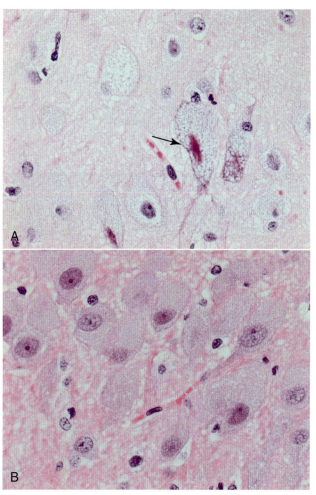

Figure 4-37 A, B. Swollen, vacuolated, and degenerating (arrow) neurons in a **lysosomal storage disease** (mucopolysaccharidosis type III) in a dog.

In several ganglioside storage diseases, certain populations of neurons, particularly in the pyramidal system of the cerebral cortex and thalamic relay nuclei, undergo a form of *focal hypertrophy* to generate more "storage space." These cells develop large swollen compartments between the axon hillock and the initial axonal segment, dubbed *"meganeurites."* In addition, cells in these regions may sprout *aberrant dendritic spines*, whether or not they have meganeurites. The spines arise from the axon hillock and from meganeurites and form synaptic contacts. The origin of the presynaptic elements of these contacts has not been determined, but such abnormal neuronal connections could well contribute to malfunction. They may be permanent in the induced storage diseases in which otherwise the stored material may be catabolized and removed if the toxic inhibition of the enzymes is removed. These changes, dramatic as they are, cannot be appreciated without the use of special techniques, most notably the Golgi impregnation method. In addition, focal swellings may develop along the course of axons, appearing as eosinophilic spheroids, similar to those described for axonal dystrophy (see Fig. 4-9). They are often very prominent in some nuclear groups, exhibiting a tendency to form in the terminal presynaptic regions of axons, but they can be seen anywhere in the white matter and also in the peripheral nerves. They do not contain specific storage material, but are crowded with degenerate organelles and/or abnormal tubules and vesicles. They probably reflect a secondary effect of the storage process on retrograde axonal transport. The functional significance of this secondary axonal dystrophy is not resolved, but it is a prominent pathologic feature in many storage diseases.

Further reading

Futerman AH, van Meer G. The cell biology of lysosomal storage disorders. Nat Rev Mol Cell Biol 2004;5:554-565.

Skelly BJ, Franklin RJM. Recognition and diagnosis of lysosomal storage diseases in the cat and dog. J Vet Intern Med 2002;16: 133-141.

Warren CD, Alroy J. Morphological, biochemical and molecular biology approaches for the diagnosis of lysosomal storage diseases. J Vet Diagn Invest 2000;12:483-496.

Inherited storage diseases

Virtually all the inherited storage diseases of animals are proven or assumed to be lysosomal in nature. This applies to all those to be described later, with the exceptions of the canine glycogenoses analogous to types 3 and 7 glycogenoses in humans. They are classified into broad groups, according to the class of macromolecule whose degradation is defective. As many of these diseases were first described in humans, the catalog is replete with eponyms, mostly derived from the names of the eminent people who provided those first descriptions. Within the broad groups, individual entities are defined by the nature of the dominant storage material, which reflects the specific enzymic deficit. Not all the storage diseases documented in humans have been found to have analogues in domestic animals, but the list is growing, and the prevalence of inbreeding makes it likely that this will continue. *The general clinical characteristic is the onset of progressive neurologic impairment at a young age.*

In the descriptions of pathology that follow, variations in the patterns of lesions are likely to surface as more cases are described. A useful practical distinction can be made between those diseases in which the vacuoles appear empty in both paraffin and resin sections (Fig. 4-38A), and those in which they contain residual material (Fig. 4-38B). The former reflect water-soluble substrates leached out during processing, and point to certain diseases (see later, Sphingolipidoses, and Glycoproteinoses).

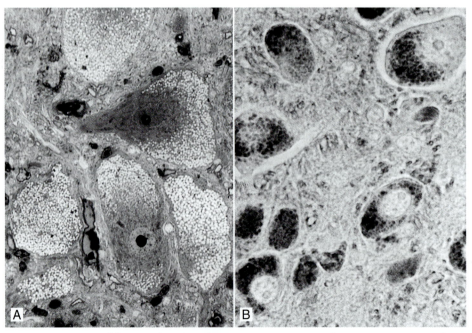

Figure 4-38 Neuronal lysosomal storage disease. **A.** Resin section showing "empty" vacuoles in **bovine mannosidosis**. (Courtesy R.D. Jolly.) **B.** Dense granules, Sudan black positive, in **gangliosidosis** in a German Short-haired Pointer dog. (Courtesy E. Karbe.)

Sphingolipidoses

Sphingolipidoses are lysosomal storage diseases caused by a genetic defect in catabolism of *glycosphingolipids*, which are important normal components of cell membranes.

In general, **gangliosidoses** are characterized clinically by the *onset at an early age of discrete head and limb tremors and dysmetria*. Worsening locomotor deficits and mentation terminate eventually in blindness, somnolence, seizures, and quadriplegia. Data indicate *autosomal recessive inheritance*.

In **GM_1 gangliosidosis** (generalized gangliosidosis), deficiency of *β-galactosidase* leads to accumulation of GM_1 ganglioside and some oligosaccharides. GM_1 gangliosidosis has been documented in cats (domestic shorthair, Korat, Siamese), dogs (Alaskan Husky, Beagle, English Springer Spaniel, Portuguese Water dog, Shiba), Friesian cattle, and sheep (Coopworth-Romney, Romney, Suffolk).

In **GM_2 gangliosidosis**, GM_2 ganglioside accumulates because of deficient lysosomal degradative activity of *hexosaminidase*, which exists as a dimer in 2 forms, αβ (hexosaminidase A, Hex A) or ββ (hexosaminidase B, Hex B), or of an *activator protein* (AB variant). Globoside may also accumulate. A defect in the α subunit results in deficiency of Hex A and causes Tay-Sachs disease (B variant) in people. A missense mutation in the gene that codes for Hex A occurs in Jacob sheep and in Japanese Chin dogs. In people, a different variant of Tay-Sachs disease (B1 variant) has been recognized, in which a stable but enzymatically inactive α subunit is produced. Sandhoff disease (O variant) is caused by deficiency in the β subunit affecting both Hex A and B. This variant has been documented in domestic shorthair, Japanese, and Korat cats; in German Short-haired Pointer, Golden Retriever, Toy Poodle, and Japanese Spaniel dogs; and in Yorkshire pigs. A mutation of the GM_2 activator protein has been described in cats.

Neuronal storage in gangliosidoses is manifested in routine paraffin sections as marked distention of the soma, with *foamy, faintly eosinophilic cytoplasm* (Fig. 4-39A). The stored material is strongly PAS-positive in frozen sections, and is evident in plastic sections as 1-3 μm osmiophilic granules. Ultrastructurally, these are seen as *characteristic membranous cytoplasmic bodies*, consisting of concentric membranous whorls with a periodicity of about 5 nm (Fig. 4-39B). Vacuolated macrophages may also be found around blood vessels in the CNS, and storage also occurs in glial cells. Axonal spheroids may be reasonably numerous. Gliosis, demyelination, and neuronal loss are not apparent until end stage. In those instances where hepatic storage occurs, hepatocytes and Kupffer cells contain large, empty vacuoles, the site of storage of a water-soluble glycopeptide.

GM_1 gangliosidosis in Suffolk sheep is associated with a dual enzyme deficiency, with βl-galactosidase deficiency being profound (5% residual activity), and α-neuraminidase deficiency less so (20% residual activity). Progressive ataxia in affected lambs first becomes evident at 4-6 months of age. Histologically, there is intense storage in most central and peripheral ganglionic neurons, and in the kidney, liver, and lymph nodes, and in cardiac Purkinje fibers. Stored material in neurons stains PAS and Luxol fast blue positive, but Sudan black negative. Axonal spheroids are frequent in cerebral and cerebellar white matter.

Glucocerebrosidosis (glucosylceramidosis) has been described in the Sydney Silky Terrier, and is the counterpart to *Gaucher disease* of humans. It results from deficient activity *of glucocerebrosidase*, which catalyzes the conversion of glucocerebroside to ceramide. The former is derived from the catabolism of gangliosides.

Storage in the dog is expressed in macrophages in the hepatic sinusoids and lymph nodes, and in neurons in some parts of the brain but, interestingly, not in Purkinje cells and not in the spinal cord. Swollen cells have weakly eosinophilic cytoplasmic vacuoles, which are PAS-positive in the macrophages but PAS-negative in neurons. Degenerating neurons

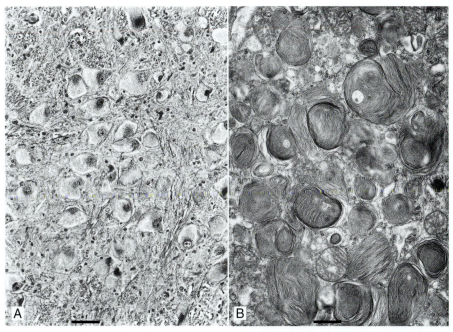

Figure 4-39 GM_1 **gangliosidosis** in a Portuguese Water dog. **A.** Pale swollen neurons. Bar = 63 μm. **B.** Storage bodies showing concentric lamellae or parallel stacks of membranes. Bar = 0.6 μm. (Reprinted with permission from Saunders GK, et al. Vet Pathol 1988;25:265-269.)

occur in the cerebral and cerebellar cortices, and Wallerian degeneration in related white matter.

Ultrastructurally, the macrophage storage material has a *characteristic twisted branching tubular structure*, and the cells in the human disease are known as *Gaucher cells*. In neurons, the storage granules are either lamellated membranous cytoplasmic bodies, resembling the zebra bodies of mucopolysaccharidoses, or bilamellar wisps. In Gaucher variants in humans, storage may not occur in neurons.

Sphingomyelinosis has been recognized in Siamese, domestic shorthair, and Balinese cats; Miniature Poodle dogs; and a Hereford calf, and is regarded as the counterpart of *Niemann-Pick disease* in people, of which there are several variants. In types A and B, deficient activity of *sphingomyelinase* results in storage of sphingomyelin, cholesterol, and gangliosides in most neurons, and in macrophages in the liver, spleen, lymph nodes, adrenals, bone marrow, and lungs. The type C variant is caused by defective activity of a cholesterol transporter, Niemann-Pick C1 (NPC1) protein, or in the soluble lysosomal cholesterol-binding NPC2 protein. In animals, most cases are analogous to human type A; type C is described in cats and Boxer dogs. A mutation in the *NPC2* gene is reported in cats.

At autopsy, there is enlargement and pallor of the liver, splenomegaly, and gray nodules in the lungs. Microscopically, the visceral organs mentioned are packed with foamy macrophages, and the neurons are distended by masses of light gray, 1-2 μm autofluorescent granules. In frozen sections, the reactivity of vacuoles to oil-red-O and PAS stains is variable.

Type C Niemann-Pick disease is also characterized by numerous axonal spheroids in many areas of the neuraxis. Ultrastructurally, neuronal storage granules are concentric multilamellar structures or dense bodies.

Galactosialidosis, which results from combined deficiency of β-galactosidase and α-neuraminidase enzyme activity, is reported in a Schipperke dog. A similar combined enzyme deficiency in inbred Suffolk sheep resembled GM_1 gangliosidosis phenotypically.

Galactocerebrosidosis *(galactosylceramide lipidosis, globoid cell leukodystrophy, Krabbe disease)*, the result of deficiency of *galactocerebrosidase*, is a member of this group, but involves storage in macrophages rather than neurons. It is discussed later under Myelinopathies.

Further reading

Hasegawa D, et al. Clinical and molecular analysis of GM2 gangliosidosis in two apparent littermate kittens of the Japanese domestic cat. J Feline Med Surg 2007;9:232-237.

Martin DR, et al. Mutation of the GM2 activator protein in a feline model of GM2 gangliosidosis. Acta Neuropathol 2005;110:443-450.

Porter BF, et al. Pathology of GM2 gangliosidosis in Jacob sheep. Vet Pathol 2011;48:807-813.

Sanders DN, et al. GM2 gangliosidosis associated with a HEXA missense mutation in Japanese Chin dogs: a potential model for Tay Sachs disease. Mol Genet Metab 2013;108:70-75.

Saunders GK, Wenger DA. Sphingomyelinase deficiency (Niemann-Pick disease) in a Hereford calf. Vet Pathol 2008;45:201-202.

Tamura S, et al. GM2 gangliosidosis variant 0 (Sandhoff-like disease) in a family of Toy Poodles. J Vet Intern Med 2010;24:1013-1019.

Zampieri S, et al. Characterization of a spontaneous novel mutation in the NPC2 gene in a cat affected by Niemann Pick type C disease. PLoS ONE 2014;9:e112503.

Glycoproteinoses

This group includes diseases in which there is *defective degradation of the carbohydrate component of N-linked glycoproteins*. These carbohydrate moieties are rich in mannose, N-acetyl glucosamine, and fucose, and in particular diseases, this is reflected in the storage residues that are detectable in the urine.

α-Mannosidosis has been the most economically important of the inherited storage diseases of animals, as it once occurred at high frequency in some populations of Angus cattle and the derivative Murray Grey breed. It is also recorded in the Galloway breed. The characterization and study of the disease in New Zealand led to effective carrier detection and certification schemes for its elimination, and the incidence declined significantly. Inheritance is autosomal recessive, and affected calves have retarded growth, increasingly severe ataxia, and behavioral changes. The disease reaches end stage by about 18 months of age.

Because of the synthesis of a defective enzyme protein, such individuals have *deficient lysosomal α-mannosidase* activity in virtually all cells except hepatocytes. All but the final mannose molecule of the glycans destined for digestion by this enzyme are alpha linked. As a result, mannose/N-acetylglucosamine oligosaccharides accumulate in storage vacuoles that appear empty by light microscopy (see Fig. 4-38A), as the material is extracted during tissue processing. Ultrastructurally, the vacuoles are seen to contain sparse membranous fragments and some floccular material (Fig. 4-40).

Neuronal storage is widespread and severe, but neuronal loss is not conspicuous until the terminal stages. Axonal spheroids are numerous in both gray and white matter, but especially in the cerebellar roof nuclei, the caudal brainstem proprioceptive nuclei, and on the proximal parts of Purkinje cell axons. The striking extent of storage in secretory epithelia, such as in pancreas and kidney, endothelia, fixed macrophages, and fibrocytes, is best appreciated in plastic-embedded sections.

α-Mannosidosis has also been described in Persian, domestic shorthair, and longhair cats. In the first 2 breeds, kittens are clinically affected very early in life, having retarded growth, facial dysmorphism, ataxia, tremor, and hepatomegaly. Intense and universal neuronal storage is accompanied by

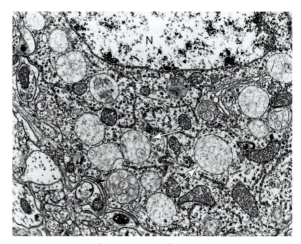

Figure 4-40 Cortical neuron in **feline mannosidosis**; storage vacuoles (arrows) contain either sparse floccular material or membranous arrays. Nucleus (N). (Courtesy S.U. Walkley.)

hypomyelination in the cerebrum, and widespread occurrence of axonal spheroids. Extensive storage in other tissues is as described for the bovine disease.

In the domestic longhair cat, nervous signs are reported to be milder and more slowly progressive, and there are no ocular abnormalities, hepatomegaly, myelin deficiency, or pancreatic acinar cell involvement. However, intense loss of Purkinje cells is evident, and there is great diversity in the morphology of the storage cytosomes, with many membranous cytoplasmic bodies in caudal brainstem nuclei.

β-Mannosidosis has been described in the Anglo-Nubian goat, and in Salers cattle. The final mannose residue of the glycoprotein glycans is beta linked to N-acetylglucosamine; its hydrolysis normally follows that of the alpha linkages described previously. Deficiency of *β-mannosidase* leads therefore to the storage of disaccharides or trisaccharides containing one molecule of mannose.

The disease has been most comprehensively documented in Nubian goats; inheritance is autosomal recessive. Clinical signs are severe at birth, affected kids having small palpebral fissures, facial dysmorphisms, domed skulls, joint contractures, intention tremors, and deafness. They are generally unable to stand and, even with intensive care, will survive for only a few months.

Grossly, there is dilation of the ventricles and hypomyelination of the cerebrum and cerebellum. The latter may be the result of congenital hypothyroidism, caused by storage-mediated interference with thyroid function, and it accounts for the congenital syndrome. Microscopically, neuronal vacuolation is ubiquitous and axonal spheroids numerous, especially in the internal capsule, cerebellar white matter, and basal ganglia. Vacuolated macrophages occur around some blood vessels in the brain, and there may be focal mineralization in the cerebellum and cerebrum. Large focal swellings filled with neurofilaments are sometimes present in the proximal axons of spinal motor neurons, and spheroids are numerous in sensory endings in mucous membranes and conjunctivae. Intense storage in most other tissues is similar to that described for α-mannosidosis, as is the ultrastructure of the storage vacuoles.

α-L-fucosidosis occurs in the English Springer Spaniel. As the result of deficient activity of *α-L-fucosidase*, water-soluble, fucose-containing compounds are stored as glycosylasparagines. Autosomal recessive inheritance is established, and the disease has a somewhat delayed clinical onset, with wasting, ataxia, and proprioceptive deficits beginning at about 6 months of age, and becoming severe by about 2 years. A striking gross lesion is marked swelling, up to 10-mm diameter, of the cervical portion of the vagus nerves, the cervical nerves, and dorsal root ganglia, the result of edema, fibroplasia, and accumulation of vacuolated endoneurial macrophages.

As in mannosidosis, storage is intense in most tissues, cells becoming distended with apparently empty vacuoles. In the CNS, it is present in all neurons and in astrocytes and microglial cells; there are numerous perivascular accumulations of vacuolated macrophages. Axonal spheroids are present in the cerebellar white matter. In the thickened nerves, there is heavy infiltration of macrophages and the accumulation of myxoid perineurial ground substance.

Mucopolysaccharidoses

This group of diseases is defined by *defective catabolism of glycosaminoglycans (GAG, mucopolysaccharides)* and has major expression in the skeleton and connective tissues. These diseases are therefore also discussed in Vol. 1, Bones and joints. Glycosaminoglycans—dermatan sulfate, heparan sulfate, keratan sulfate, and chondroitin sulfate—are long-chain complex carbohydrates, and many enzymes are involved in their degradation. As a result, 11 are entities defined in humans, each one as the result of deficient enzymatic activity of a specific lysosomal hydrolase; 5 have been reported in domestic animals, and in 4 of these, there is major involvement of neurons. General features include facial and skeletal dysmorphisms, degenerative joint disease, corneal clouding, thickening and distortion of heart valves, and thickening of the leptomeninges. Large quantities of heparan and dermatan sulfates are excreted, and are detectable, in the urine.

In animals, deficiency of **α-L-iduronidase** has been observed in the domestic shorthair cat and the Plott Hound, Rottweiler, and Boston Terrier and is regarded as the counterpart of *mucopolysaccharidosis type I* (**MPS I**) in man, variants of which include the *Hurler and Scheie syndromes*. The macroscopic features described previously are subtended by intense storage in fibroblasts, fixed macrophages, chondrocytes, myocytes, and pericytes in most organ systems. Glandular epithelial cells are consistently less affected than mesoderm-derived cells. The involvement of chondrocytes is associated with dysplasias of endochondral ossification, and with degeneration of articular cartilage.

Neuronal storage is universal, but neuronal loss is not conspicuous. Storage vacuoles are ultrastructurally pleomorphic; they may appear largely empty, or to contain sparse flocculi to granular amorphous material, or lamellar membranous structures termed *zebra bodies*. The latter appear to be lipid in nature, and probably represent induced secondary storage of sphingolipids. There is thus a somewhat variable reaction to tissue staining for GAG and lipid. There is some suggestion that affected cats may have a high incidence of cranial meningiomas.

Mucopolysaccharidosis type II (*Hunter syndrome*) is reported in a dog with coarse facial features, macrodactylia, unilateral corneal dystrophy, generalized osteopenia, and progressive neurologic deterioration. Epithelial cells, endothelial cells, and histiocytes contain intracytoplasmic vacuoles and electron-lucent flocculi to lamellar membrane-bound storage material. PAS-positive intracytoplasmic material is evident in multiple neurons, and biochemical assays identify a deficiency in **iduronate-2-sulfatase** activity in cultured dermal fibroblasts.

In the Nubian goat, **N-acetylglucosamine-6-sulfatase deficiency** gives rise to a counterpart of human **MPS III**, *Sanfilippo disease*. Clinical features encompass delayed ability of the neonate to stand and walk, persistently ataxic gait, marked bowing of the forelimbs, and corneal clouding. Gross changes include dwarfism, kyphoscoliosis, scapular hypermobility, and cartilaginous and bony abnormalities. Two main types of lysosomal storage bodies occur microscopically. The primary storage material is *heparan sulfate*, which appears as lucent flocculent material in lysosomes in arterial smooth muscle and cardiac myocytes, fibroblasts, macrophages, hepatocytes, Kupffer cells, and chondrocytes. Neurons, in contrast, are packed with PAS-positive multilamellar bodies representing secondary storage of *gangliosides* induced by interference with neuraminidase activity. Mucopolysaccharidoses IIIA and IIIB are reported in several dog breeds (see Fig. 4-37A, B); MPS IIID is described in goats.

In Siamese and domestic shorthair cats, Miniature Pinschers, Miniature Schnauzers, Chesapeake Bay Retrievers, Welsh Corgis, and a Miniature Poodle-like dog, **arylsulfatase-B deficiency** produces a counterpart to human **MPS VI** *(Maroteaux-Lamy syndrome)*. The disease has the same general features as described previously, but neuronal storage does not occur. Storage in peripheral blood neutrophils is detected as metachromatic cytoplasmic granules.

A **β-glucuronidase-deficient MPS** has been described in dogs and cats, and is considered analogous to human **MPS VII** *(Sly disease)*. The general features of the clinical disease are as described previously, and there is excessive urinary excretion of chondroitin-4-sulfate and chondroitin-6-sulfate. There is *widespread neurovisceral storage*, with cytoplasmic inclusions appearing largely empty or containing sparse granular or lamellar material.

Further reading

Haskins M, Giger U. Lysosomal storage diseases. In: Kaneko JJ, et al., editors. Clinical Biochemistry of Domestic Animals. 6th ed. New York: Elsevier; 2008. p. 731-749.

Jolly RD, et al. Mucopolysaccharidosis type VI in a Miniature Poodle-type dog caused by a deletion in the arylsulphatase B gene. N Z Vet J 2012;60:183-188.

Yogalingam G, et al. Identification of a mutation causing mucopolysaccharidosis type IIIA in New Zealand Huntaway dogs. Genomics 2002;79:150-153.

Glycogenoses

A number of enzymes are involved in the catabolism of glycogen, but only one of these, *α-1,4-glucosidase*, is a lysosomal enzyme. The lysosomal pathway degrades any glycogen that finds its way into autophagic vacuoles, whereas the other pathways are more related to metabolic mobilization of glycogen. In humans, 8 different glycogen storage diseases have been identified, with the lysosomal type being classified as **type II**, *Pompe disease*. As the storage process is very widespread in this disease, it is also referred to as *generalized glycogenosis*. In most other types, storage is concentrated in liver and muscle.

α-1,4-glucosidase deficiency has been well documented in Shorthorn and Brahman beef cattle. The disease has autosomal recessive inheritance, and at least 3 disease-associated mutations occur. Affected calves have severe clinical signs by about 1 year of age. The most damaging effects are produced in the skeletal and cardiac muscle; weakness and congestive cardiac failure are clinically dominant, and cardiomegaly and hepatomegaly evident at autopsy. There is *widespread glycogen storage*, much of which occurs in typical lysosomal storage vacuoles, but some of which is intracytoplasmic. Swollen, vacuolated cells contain diastase-sensitive, PAS-positive material, which is ultrastructurally typical of glycogen. Vacuolar myopathy and cardiomyopathy are prominent; *neuronal storage is universal and severe* and is accompanied by glial storage, with numerous axonal spheroids in the vestibular and cuneate nuclei, terminal fasciculus gracilis, and throughout the spinal cord gray matter (see Fig. 4-8). Mild Wallerian degeneration may be present in the lateral and ventral columns of the spinal cord and in some peripheral nerves.

Type II glycogenosis has also been documented in the Lapland dog, and suspected on morphologic grounds in the domestic cat and Corriedale sheep.

Glycogenosis **type Ia** *(Von Gierke disease)* is associated with **glucose-6-phosphatase deficiency** and is reported in related canine toy breeds and crossbred Maltese and Beagle dogs. Puppies have evidence of excessive glycogen accumulation in liver, kidney, and myocardium, and show tremors, weakness, and neurologic signs when hypoglycemic.

Amylo-1,6-glucosidase deficiency is recorded in the German Shepherd dog, Akita, and Curly-coated Retriever as a counterpart of glycogenosis **type III** *(Cori disease)*. Cytoplasmic glycogen storage occurs in liver, muscle, and myocardium, and in neurons and glia in the brain and spinal cord.

Amylopectinosis (glycogen storage disease **type IV**, *Andersen disease*) is reported in a mixed-breed dog and in a family of young Norwegian Forest cats as the result of an inherited (autosomal recessive) deficiency of the glycogen-branching enzyme. PAS-positive granular to globular intracytoplasmic storage material is present in neurons throughout the CNS and peripheral nervous system, liver, and myocardium. Glycogen-branching enzyme deficiency is a fatal autosomal recessive myopathy of Quarter Horses and Paint Horses. Abnormal polysaccharide can be also identified in neural tissue. Other myopathic forms are reported in Charolais cattle, associated with **myophosphorylase deficiency** (glycogen storage disease **type V**), and in the English Springer Spaniel dog, in which storage of an amylopectin-like polysaccharide is associated with **phosphofructokinase deficiency** comparable to **type VII** glycogen storage disease in people.

Further reading

Dennis JA, et al. Genotyping Brahman cattle for generalised glycogenosis. Aust Vet J 2002;80:286-291.

Johnstone AC, et al. Myophosphorylase deficiency (glycogen storage disease Type V) in a herd of Charolais cattle in New Zealand: confirmation by PCR-RFLP testing. N Z Vet J 2004;52:404-408.

Kishnani PS, et al. Canine model and genomic structural organization of glycogen storage disease type Ia (GSD Ia). Vet Pathol 2001;38:83-91.

Mucolipidoses

Mucolipidosis describes a disease with the features of both sphingolipidoses and mucopolysaccharidoses. **Mucolipidosis II (ML II)**, also called *I-cell (inclusion-cell) disease*, is a lysosomal storage disease caused by deficient activity of *N-acetylglucosamine-1-phosphotransferase*. The condition is inherited as an autosomal recessive in domestic shorthair cats. Affected kittens fail to thrive and have behavioral dullness, facial dysmorphia, and ataxia. Diffuse retinal degeneration leads to blindness. Storage lysosomes containing oligosaccharides, mucopolysaccharides, and lipids are most common in bone, cartilage, skin, and other connective tissues; a few cerebral cortical neurons have lipid inclusions, and some sciatic nerve axons are affected.

Ceroid-lipofuscinoses

With advancing age and senility, intracytoplasmic granules of the autofluorescent lipopigment, **lipofuscin,** accumulate in neurons, fixed phagocytes, macrophages, and muscle cells. This *"wear and tear" pigment* is familiar to all pathologists, and has a characteristic histochemical profile and ultrastructure; the irregularly shaped granules have a high-density component punctuated with vacuoles of low density. For many years, in the group of diseases known as the "ceroid-lipofuscinoses," it has been assumed that a similar pigment is stored in lysosomes. However, other compounds, such as the hydrophobic lipid-binding protein subunit c of mitochondrial ATP synthase and sphingolipid activator proteins (SAPs) A and D, may predominate; hence at least some of these conditions might better be termed **proteinoses.**

In animals, neuronal ceroid-lipofuscinoses (NCL) of proven or presumptive **inherited** nature have been described in Siamese and domestic shorthair cats; South Hampshire, Borderdale, Ramboulliet, Merino, and White Swedish Landrace sheep; Devon, Beefmaster, and Holstein cattle; Nubian goats; horses; and many breeds of dog, including English Setter, Chihuahua, Dachshund, Saluki, Dalmatian, Blue Heeler, Border Collie, Tibetan Terrier, Australian Cattle Dog, Labrador Retriever, Poodle, Pit Bull Terrier, Staffordshire Terrier, Irish Setter, and crossbred. In general, *although storage may be widespread in several organs, it is most damaging in neurons of the cerebral cortex, retina, and cerebellar Purkinje system.* Thus there is frequently extensive cellular loss and atrophy in these regions, and correlating dementia, blindness, and ataxia. Macroscopically, atrophied areas may have a distinctly brown tinge. Microscopically, the storage granules are brightly autofluorescent under ultraviolet light; pale brown-red or colorless with H&E; weakly acid fast, magenta with PAS; and intensely positive with Luxol fast blue. Ultrastructurally, they appear as *membrane-bound cytosomes* up to 15 nm in diameter, irregular in outline, and with a variety of forms (Fig. 4-41). Some have membranous material arranged as *"curvilinear bodies" and "fingerprint bodies,"* which are considered characteristic. Others may have *laminated stacks of membranes* akin to zebra bodies, membranous stacks, or dense granular deposits.

The variation in features of NCL is illustrated by comparing the disease in various species and breeds. In Devon cattle, the major clinical deficit is profound blindness at about 14 months of age, with death usually resulting from misadventure by about 2 years. There is severe retinal atrophy but only mild loss of neurons from the cerebral and cerebellar cortices. A single base duplication in the bovine gene *CLN5* has been identified. In Tibetan Terriers, blindness is again the dominant sign, but the onset is delayed to middle life and is accompanied terminally by stupor. In the Border Collie and some other dog breeds, there are gait and visual deficits by 18-24 months of age, accompanied by increasing aggression and dementia. Retinal lesions are mild, and blindness is central in origin. Neuronal loss and gliosis are particularly severe in the cerebellar Purkinje cell layer, and significant in the limbic system. In the American Staffordshire Terriers and crossbreds, storage primarily affects Purkinje cells and thalamic nuclei.

The pathogenesis of at least some forms of NCL may involve a defect in mitochondria rather than a defect in lysosomal catabolism, and may involve accumulation of hydrophobic protein. The NCL in South Hampshire sheep has been thoroughly studied. The brains of affected lambs grow normally until 4 months of age, and then undergo atrophy (Fig. 4-42). Half of the material stored in lysosomes is the lipid-binding protein subunit c of mitochondrial ATP synthase. NCL in Merino sheep is also a subunit c–storing disease, clinically and pathologically similar to NCL in South Hampshire sheep. The NCL in both breeds (OCL6 form) apparently results from a mutation at the same gene locus in chromosomal region OAR7q13-15, and both breeds are potential animal models for the human late infantile variant *CLN6*. The molecular genetics are being characterized in several canine breeds with NCL. Mutation in the *CLN8* gene has been found in English Setters, in the *CLN5* gene in Border Collies, in the *CLN6* gene in Australian Shepherds, in the cathepsin D gene in American Bulldogs, in the *ATP13A2* gene in Tibetan Terriers, in the *TPP1* gene (the ortholog of human *CLN2*) in Miniature Dachshunds, and in the *PPT1* gene in a Dachshund. In adult American Staffordshire Terriers, mutation in the *arylsulfatase* G gene is associated with a form of NCL.

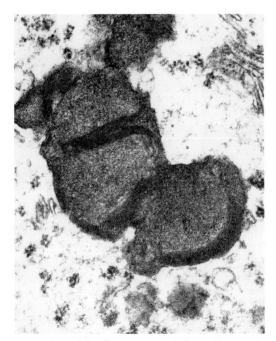

Figure 4-41 Ceroid lipofuscinosis in a Tibetan Terrier. Granular and membranous storage body in a Purkinje cell. (Courtesy J.F. Cummings.)

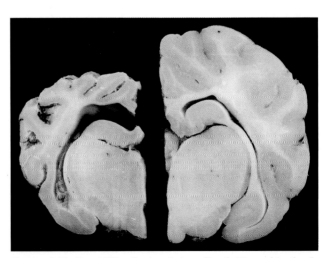

Figure 4-42 Ceroid lipofuscinosis in a South Hampshire lamb. Marked cerebral atrophy at 4 months; control on the right. (Courtesy R.D. Jolly.)

Further reading

Abitbol M, et al. A canine arylsulfatase G (ARSG) mutation leading to a sulfatase deficiency is associated with neuronal ceroid lipofuscinosis. Proc Natl Acad Sci U S A 2010;107:14775-14780.

Awano T, et al. A frame shift mutation in canine TPP1 (the ortholog of human CLN2) in a juvenile Dachshund with neuronal ceroid lipofuscinosis. Mol Genet Metab 2006;89:254-260.

Houweling PJ, et al. Neuronal ceroid lipofuscinosis in Devon cattle is caused by a single base duplication (c.662dupG) in the bovine CLN5 gene. Biochim Biophys Acta 2006;1762:890-897.

Katz ML, et al. A missense mutation in canine CLN6 in an Australian Shepherd with neuronal ceroid lipofuscinosis. J Biomed Biotechnol 2011;2011:198042.

Nakamoto Y, et al. Neuronal ceroid-lipofuscinosis in longhaired Chihuahuas: clinical, pathologic, and MRI findings. J Am Anim Hosp Assoc 2011;47:64-70.

Wöhlke A, et al. A one base pair deletion in the canine ATP13A2 gene causes exon skipping and late-onset neuronal ceroid lipofuscinosis in the Tibetan terrier. PLoS Genet 2011;7:e1002304.

Lafora disease

A counterpart to the autosomal recessive human **Lafora disease (LD)** has been recorded in Basset Hounds, Poodles, Beagle dogs, and Miniature Wire-haired Dachshunds. In the latter breed, the genetic defect is a triplet repeat disorder. The disease has also been described in a cat. Progressive myoclonus epilepsy is associated with *widespread intraneuronal storage of a complex polyglucosan*, which appears as characteristic *Lafora bodies* (see Fig. 4-5). They are most numerous in Purkinje cells, and neurons of the caudate, thalamic, and periventricular nuclei. They are non–membrane-bound spherical structures with a central basophilic core and a peripheral halo of radiating filaments. They are strongly PAS positive and are found in both perikaryon and dendrites; they vary greatly in size, ranging up to 15-20 μm. Human LD is caused by mutation in the *EPM2A* gene that encodes for laforin and the *EPM2B* gene that encodes for malin. Lafora bodies are occasionally found incidentally in otherwise normal brains and spinal cords, especially in older animals.

Further reading

Lohi H, et al. Expanded repeat in canine epilepsy. Science 2005;307:81.

Induced storage diseases

Numerous types of storage process have been successfully produced experimentally, and there is a group of naturally occurring disorders related to the ingestion of plants, in which induced storage disease is proven or suspected.

Swainsonine toxicosis

Swainsonine, *an indolizidine alkaloid*, is the active principle of several species of toxic plants that have caused considerable problems for all classes of grazing livestock. These include poison pea (*Swainsona* sp.) of Australia, locoweeds (*Astragalus, Oxytropis* sp.) of North America, broomweed *(Sida carpinifolia)* and *Turbinia cordata* of Brazil, and shrubby morning glory *(Ipomoea carnea)* of Mozambique. Endophytic fungi, such as *Embellisia*, that grow on locoweed can induce the same toxicity. As a *potent inhibitor of lysosomal α-mannosidase,* swainsonine induces a form of **α-mannosidosis** that is a close copy of the genetic disease of cattle and cats. Continued ingestion of toxic material over a period of 4-6 weeks and more results in failure to thrive, and, ultimately, ataxia, proprioceptive deficits, and behavioral abnormalities ("locoism" in North America, "pea-struck" in Australia). Postmortem examination during, or within a short time after, exposure to the plant reveals microscopic and ultrastructural lesions identical to those of genetic α-mannosidosis. Within 2 weeks of last exposure, much of the storage disease resolves, but axonal spheroids may persist in large numbers in areas such as the cerebellar roof nuclei and caudal brainstem. Swainsonine-induced mannosidosis has been experimentally compared in the cat with genetic mannosidosis, to determine the reversibility of changes such as meganeurite and aberrant synapse formation in higher neurons. Clinical recovery may or may not occur following cessation of exposure, and the persistence of secondary neuronal changes suggests that they, rather than the storage process, may underlie neuronal malfunction. Exposure of young growing animals is more likely to produce irreversible disease than exposure of adults.

The induced disease is, however, biochemically distinct from the genetic, as *the alkaloid also inhibits Golgi mannosidase II*, an enzyme involved in the post-translational trimming modifications of the glycan moiety of glycoproteins. As a result, abnormal proportions of different types of glycoproteins are produced, and the storage oligosaccharides are larger than those in the genetic disease. No modification of the storage disease appears to result from this difference.

In swainsonine intoxication of pregnant animals, both dam and fetus are affected, and *abortion and terata are well recognized in ovine locoweed toxicosis.* Suppressive effects on fertility are also recognized.

The wier vine *(Ipomoea calobra)* of Australia also contains **calystegine B2** (nortropane alkaloids), which induces phenotypic expression of 2 other lysosomal storage diseases in sheep and cattle, namely, **α-galactosidosis** and **β-glucosidosis**. *Ipomoea verbascoidea* of Brazil contains swainsonine and calystegines and causes **α-mannosidosis** in goats.

Trachyandra *poisoning*

Ingestion of *Trachyandra divaricata* or *T. laxa* for several weeks has been associated with severe neurologic disease and **lipofuscinosis** in sheep, horses, goats, and pigs in South Africa and Australia. The clinical syndrome is one of weakness, suggesting a neuromuscular disorder, and is often accompanied by *intense lipofuscin storage in all central and peripheral neurons* and, to a lesser extent, in macrophages of the intestinal lamina propria, hepatocytes, Kupffer cells, and renal tubular epithelium. Pigment storage may be sufficiently intense to cause macroscopic rusty brown discoloration of central gray nuclei and peripheral ganglia. The pigment granules have all the histochemical and ultrastructural features of lipofuscin. The clinical signs appear to be irreversible, and their relationship to the storage process is obscure; the basis of the storage process is unknown.

Phalaris *poisoning*

Extensive losses in sheep and cattle in Australia, New Zealand, South Africa, Argentina, California, and West Virginia have been the result of grazing *Phalaris* spp., principally *P. aquatica* and *P. arundinacea*, but also *P. minor, P. caroliniana,* and *P. angusta*. Several syndromes of *Phalaris* toxicosis affect principally ruminants but occasionally horses. Dramatic large-scale sudden mortalities occur in sheep; sudden deaths have been associated in horses; staggers syndromes of acute onset and recoverable or of chronic onset and not recoverable occur in sheep, and occasionally in cattle. Onset of staggers syndromes may be rapid on exposure to immature plants or delayed for up to several months. It is probable that resistance to the toxicosis may be produced by catabolism of toxins by adapted ruminal microflora.

There are 2 acute neurologic syndromes. *Sudden death* in sheep and horses without observable tissue changes is probably caused by cardiotoxic compounds, a mix of *methyl tryptamine* and *β-carboline indoleamines* chemically related to 5-hydroxytryptamine (serotonin). The second acute syndrome is in sheep and is referred to as a polioencephalomalacia-like syndrome, the result of edema of deep cortical gray matter laminae. Severe astrocytic edema in the cortex is similar to that seen in citrullinemia, and suggests peracute ammonia toxicity resulting from toxic impairment of urea-cycle enzymes.

The clinical onset of the staggers syndrome may be delayed for several months after exposure to toxic pasture has ceased. It is characterized by generalized muscle tremors progressing to stiffness, collapse on forced exercise, and tetanic seizures. In most cases, recovery does not occur, and apparent recovery is followed by relapses.

In cases examined early in the course of the disease, there may be no gross or microscopic lesions but, in general, pathologic changes are present. Most characteristically, there is *storage of granular pigment within neurons* of the brainstem nuclei, spinal gray matter and dorsal root ganglia, and in macrophages of the cerebrospinal fluid (CSF). A similar pigment is also present within renal tubular epithelial cells. When storage is intense, the affected gray matter and kidneys may have distinct green discoloration on gross inspection. Histologically, the pigment granules are green-brown and present in a perinuclear distribution in neurons (Fig. 4-43), although some granules may accumulate in dendrites. Ultrastructurally, the storage granules are composed of concentric membranous lamellae, sometimes interspersed with fine granular material. They are membrane bound and are considered to be lysosomal in nature. In most cases, there is also Wallerian degeneration concentrated in ventral, ventromedial, and lateral funiculi throughout the spinal cord, and in the medial longitudinal fasciculus. This distribution suggests selective damage to long descending motor tracts. Severely affected areas may also have intense diffuse astrogliosis. Intense reactive astrogliosis may also be seen in ventral spinal cord gray matter, along with mild neuronal loss.

Other induced storage diseases

Solanum poisoning and **Gomen disease** are discussed later under Central neuronopathies and axonopathies.

Further reading

Armién AG, et al. Spontaneous and experimental glycoprotein storage disease of goats induced by *Ipomoea carnea* subsp *fistulosa* (Convolvulaceae). Vet Pathol 2007;44:170-184.

Binder EM, et al. *Phalaris arundinacea* (reed canarygrass) grass staggers in beef cattle. J Vet Diagn Invest 2010;22:802-805.

Dantas AF, et al. Swainsonine-induced lysosomal storage disease in goats caused by the ingestion of *Turbina cordata* in Northeastern Brazil. Toxicon 2007;49:111-116.

Mendonça FS, et al. Alpha-mannosidosis in goats caused by the swainsonine-containing plant *Ipomoea verbascoidea*. J Vet Diagn Invest 2012;24:90-95.

INCREASED INTRACRANIAL PRESSURE, CEREBRAL SWELLING, AND EDEMA

Normally, only a narrow space separates the brain from the dura mater. Both the dura and skull are unyielding so that only a relatively small increase in the volume of the intracranial contents is permissible without increasing intracranial pressure. When the pressure is increased, something has to yield. The following refers particularly to the brain, but the principles apply equally to the spinal cord, especially in cases of trauma.

The causes of increased intracranial pressure are many and varied. One component of almost all of them is edema. **Brain edema** is an increase in water content of brain tissue. Brain tissue is ~75% water, a little more for gray matter and a little less for white matter. The edema may be more or less localized and geographically related to local lesions, or it may be diffuse. In addition to the pathogenetic mechanisms to be discussed here, acquired hydrocephalus and vitamin A deficiency in young animals can be responsible for increased intracranial pressure. In vitamin A deficiency, there is increased secretion of CSF by the choroid plexus and decreased absorption by arachnoid villi, effects that may be quickly repaired by administered vitamin. Also important in domestic animals is impaired growth and remodeling of cranium and vertebrae that leads to disproportion between the volume of the growing nervous system and volume of the cranial cavity and spinal canal.

The local lesions that may result in **local edema** of the brain or spinal cord include neoplasms, inflammations, parasitic cysts, focal necrosis of various causes, trauma, hemorrhages of parenchyma and meninges, and space-occupying lesions of the meninges that cause pressure on the brain. In each example, the edema may be mild or extensive and may contribute more than the primary or inciting lesion to the clinical signs, and to the swelling of the brain or spinal cord and increase of intracranial pressure.

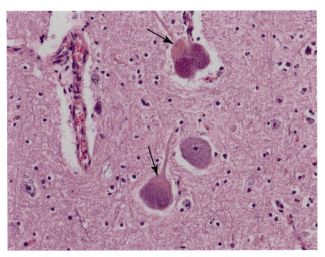

Figure 4-43 *Phalaris* sp. poisoning of an ox. Pigment granules in neuronal cytoplasm (arrows).

Generalized cerebral edema and swelling of the brain also occurs in relation to a variety of *systemic conditions*. Some degree of swelling can be anticipated as a *postmortem change*, especially in the brain of young animals, and is probably to be related to the imbibition of fluid in autolysis. Cerebral edema with swelling occurs with diffuse *meningitis*; moderately so in the diffuse *viral encephalitides, acute bacterial toxemias,* such as clostridial enterotoxemia; and *chemical intoxications,* such as lead and organomercurial poisoning; and quite severely in the pathologic syndrome of sheep and cattle known as *polioencephalomalacia*. Generalized edema of moderate degree is expected in the many metabolic and toxic conditions that are characterized by disturbances of cellular osmoregulation, in particular, disturbances that interfere with intracellular and extracellular concentrations of sodium and potassium; the acute-onset neurologic disease that occurs in *salt poisoning* of pigs and in *water intoxication* in young ruminants given water *ad libitum* after a period of deprivation would be in this category.

There are differences between gray and white matter in their susceptibility to edema, and different areas of gray substance or of white differ in their vulnerability. The considerations of edema here recognize several types of edema but are limited for descriptive purposes to the cytotoxic and vasogenic varieties. **Congestive brain swelling** is an increase in volume, especially in capillaries and postcapillary venules, as a result of loss of autoregulation of arterial input. In vivo imaging techniques can identify this edematous pattern, but it is not easily evaluated at postmortem because of the valveless character of intracerebral veins. **Interstitial edema** that affects the central white matter in hydrocephalus and the spinal cord in hydromyelia and syringomyelia is considered with those diseases; the edema is a result of acutely raised intraventricular pressure. Hypo-osmotic edema follows a reduction of serum osmolality, usually as a result of fluid administration or ingestion.

A distinction is maintained here between **cytotoxic edema** and **vasogenic edema,** notwithstanding that the endothelial barrier between blood and brain may be functionally deranged in each type. *Intracellular* or **cytotoxic edema** depends on direct or indirect noxious injury to cells and interference with the mechanisms that control cell volume. For cells in non-nervous tissues, the swelling would represent hydropic change, the movement of water from interstitial tissues into cell cytoplasm. In nervous tissue, however, there is no significant interstitial tissue or intercellular space. The intercellular space in the brain is not more than 10-20 nm. There is a layer of material that stains as glycoprotein or glycosaminoglycan on cell membranes, but there is doubt as to whether it is the counterpart of other interstitial gels. The net increase in water in the brain in cytotoxic edema must represent a movement from plasma, and the regulatory mechanisms must therefore reside in the capillary endothelium and the glial cells. The basic disturbance is in osmoregulation, which depends mainly on the efficiency of the sodium/potassium pump and ATP as an energy source. It is usually seen in toxic and metabolic disorders.

In cytotoxic edema, the swelling mainly involves endothelial cells, then astrocytes, and subsequently neurons and oligodendrocytes. Simple swelling of astrocytes is the most obvious structural change in gray matter. Swelling of the astrocytes involves the nucleus and processes. Glycogen granules accumulate in the watery protoplasm. If mild edema persists, the astrocytes react as described in an earlier section. If the edema is severe, the astrocyte nucleus is much enlarged, the chromatin is dispersed against the nuclear membrane, and the processes are voluminous. Death of acutely swollen astrocytes may not be accompanied by changes in the adjacent neuropil. Neurons may swell as a brief prelude to lysis. Satellite oligodendroglia are generally spared.

However, in cytotoxic edema, oligodendrocytes in white matter degenerate. The nucleus is swollen and less dense than normal; the nucleolus is hypertrophied, and the cytoplasm is enlarged and often visible in routine material. Changes in oligodendroglial processes that are wrapped as myelin are difficult to evaluate histologically except in those instances of specific cytotoxic edema in which there is splitting of the intraperiod line and the accumulation of water in intermyelinic clefts.

Vasogenic edema *is the term used to distinguish the extracellular accumulation of fluid from cytotoxic edema*. The basis of vasogenic edema is injury to vascular endothelium of sufficient severity to allow leakage or permeation of plasma constituents, including plasma proteins, if the injury is sufficient. The fluid spreads between cells in response to hydrostatic pressures in the cerebral circulation and those in the tissue. Vasogenic edema is a common complication of traumatic, inflammatory, neoplastic, and hemorrhagic lesions of the nervous system. In cats with renal failure, a *hypertensive encephalopathy*, characterized by severe brain edema and cerebral arteriolosclerosis, develops as a consequence of prolonged systemic increase of blood pressure. Vasogenic edema is not a conspicuous change in gray matter, because the dense tangle of neuropil resists the passage of fluid. There are exceptions, such as in the periventricular nuclei, where vasogenic edema occurs rather selectively in thiamine deficiency. The structure of white matter offers less resistance to the passage of edema fluid of this origin, and the comparison between the susceptibility of gray and white matter can be seen readily with local lesions near their junction in the cortex. The long fiber tracts, such as the spinal cord, internal capsules, and optic tracts, tend to be spared. The density and disposition of these tracts probably exert a considerable influence on the spread of edema about local lesions as, for example, the corpus callosum seems effectively to prevent spread from one hemisphere to the other.

The histologic appearances are similar to those in cytotoxic edema with the addition of dissecting changes along fiber tracts. The white matter is loosely textured, the myelinated fibers being spread apart. The spaces created may be clear or they may, depending on the degree of permeability, contain homogeneous proteinaceous fluid (Fig. 4-44). Plasma droplets that stain brightly with PAS are frequently present in perivascular clefts (Fig. 4-45).

Diffuse cerebral edema that is mild or moderate may be difficult to recognize grossly. More severe degrees are readily recognized although easily overlooked. *The brain is swollen, pale, soft, and wet*, and, because of its softness, the cerebral hemispheres tend to droop over the edges of the parietal bones when the calvaria is removed. With these severe and rapid swellings, the course is short, and there may not be signs of displacement or flattening of the gyri. When the swelling is less severe, and of longer duration, the brain may be relatively firm and dry, the gyri are pale or a faint yellow color, and the brain is displaced caudally so that it appears unusually elongate. The displacement is most obvious where it involves

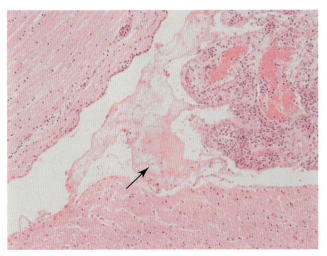

Figure 4-44 **Vasogenic edema** (arrow) secondary to vasculitis.

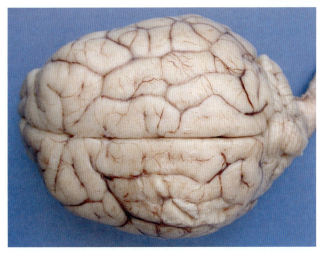

Figure 4-46 **Cerebral edema** with flattening of cerebral gyri in a dog.

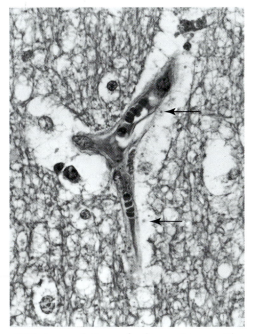

Figure 4-45 Accumulation of clear **edema** with protein droplets (arrows) around a vessel in a pig with mulberry heart disease.

the cerebellum and medulla (Fig. 4-46). With moderate displacement, the caudal surfaces of the cerebellar hemispheres are depressed by contact with the occipital bones. When the displacement is of greater degree, the medulla and caudal portion of the vermis are herniated through the foramen magnum. The displaced vermis is flattened and lies like a tongue over the medulla (so-called *lipping of the cerebellum*). The rhomboid fossa is flattened. The rostral portion of the vermis is pressed against the rostral medullary velum and may occlude the opening of the cerebral aqueduct to cause internal hydrocephalus. Such changes are usually accompanied by hemorrhage and ischemic necrosis. The brainstem is displaced caudally, and this is especially evident in the displacement of the corpora quadrigemina well into the caudal fossa. Perhaps

because the tentorium rather closely embraces the brainstem in animals, herniation of the cerebral cortex through the tentorial space into the caudal fossa *(subtentorial herniation)* is seldom observed. It may, however, be observed in cerebral edema of long standing in horses and cattle, especially if the brain is fixed in situ so that the pressure grooves produced by the free edge of the tentorium are retained. Impaction of tissue in the tentorial space interferes with the flow of CSF from the caudal to the rostral fossa and contributes to hydrocephalus.

Displacements in the rostral fossa in diffuse cerebral swelling are of lesser degree and significance. The nerves may be stretched and flattened, but pareses are seldom observed. The vasculature must be compromised in all cases. Occasionally, there is thrombosis of the superior sagittal sinus with venous infarction in the dorsal cortex, ischemic necrosis in the caudomedial surface of the occipital lobe referable to compression of the caudal cerebral arteries, and pontomedullary hemorrhage referable to stretching and occlusion of penetrating vessels in this area *(Duret hemorrhages)*.

Localized edematous changes reach their most extensive development in the centrum semiovale of the cerebrum and in the deep white matter of the cerebellum surrounding local lesions in these areas. The edematous area may be recognized by the swelling, which may be greater in volume than that produced by the primary lesion and have a soft, depressed, and damp or watery appearance on the cut surface. The extent of the edema cannot be appreciated on gross inspection because the margins are indefinite, and the same difficulty in delineating the edematous area is experienced at microscopy. When the lesion is of prolonged duration, the extent of the edematous areas can be appreciated a little better by yellow discoloration that develops.

The combination of edema with a local lesion may displace the brain in one or more directions. Caudal displacement through the caudal fossa may occur as it does in diffuse swelling. The displacements may be more local, involving lateral shifts of the base of the brain or medial displacement of one hemisphere so that the falx cerebri is displaced laterally or the cingulate gyrus is herniated beneath the free margin of the falx *(subfalcine herniation)* and the lateral and third ventricles are depressed.

LESIONS OF BLOOD VESSELS AND CIRCULATORY DISTURBANCES

Diseases of blood vessels are considered in detail in Vol. 3, Cardiovascular system. This section deals with some special features of cerebrospinal circulation and the lesions, usually ischemic or hemorrhagic, which result from vascular injury.

The blood supply to the brain is derived from the *internal carotid and vertebral arteries*, these sources anastomosing under the brainstem and at the *circle of Willis*. The major cerebral vessels, derived from the carotid and vertebral arteries, anastomose quite freely in the pia-arachnoid, but once an artery or arteriole penetrates the substance of the brain, it becomes an *end artery*, although there are some anastomoses at the capillary level. Although these anastomoses can be demonstrated readily, even those of arteriolar size in the meninges are probably of little value. Under normal circumstances, the cerebral arteries have rather set fields of supply. If one vessel is occluded, some collateral circulation develops, but it does not take over more than the periphery of the area of supply of the occluded vessel. In the brain, there may be influences governing collateral circulation in addition to those operating in other tissues, but the basic considerations still apply. The development of collateral circulation will be influenced by the anatomic arrangements of vessels, the volume of ischemic tissue, the rate at which the vascular occlusion develops, the size of the occluded vessel, and, importantly, the quantity of blood flow, which is referable to the state of the systemic circulation, and the quality of blood flow, which is referable to such matters as the oxygen tension and viscosity of plasma. For complete cessation of blood flow in an area of brain, it is probably not necessary that there be complete occlusion of the corresponding artery because flow is expected to cease, especially in peripheral twigs, while the intravascular pressure is still greater than zero. For this reason, ischemic injury in the brain localized to the field of distribution of one or other major cerebral artery may result from occlusion of a carotid vessel. Extracranial anastomoses between the major arterial vessels are, however, effective in the event of vascular occlusion occurring proximal to the circle of Willis.

Arteries entering the substance of the brain are relatively small and arise at right angles from the parent vessels in the pia-arachnoid. There are abrupt changes in caliber when the meningeal vessels divide, and this provides an entrapment mechanism for large emboli. The vessels that enter the brain are progressively attenuated to capillaries in both gray and white matter, but many capillaries loop back into the cortex from near the gray-white junction. Many small emboli lodge at the gray-white junction (Fig. 4-47), although expansion of the embolic or metastatic lesions is predominantly in the white matter.

The *arterial supply to the spinal cord* is derived from the vertebral artery in the cervical region and from radicular arteries in the lumbar region anastomosing as the ventral spinal artery. There is some doubt as to the direction of flow in cervical, thoracic, and lumbar portions of the spinal artery, and it is possible that there is a border zone in the caudal cervical and cranial thoracic region that is particularly vulnerable to ischemia if flow is impaired in the vertebral artery or the caudal portions of the ventral spinal artery.

In the spinal cord, the central gray matter is supplied by branches of the ventral spinal artery that enter the ventral sulcus, and lesions of these branches affect the gray matter of the cord rather selectively. The white matter is supplied by an anastomotic complex in the meninges that produces many small vessels that penetrate directly as end vessels and are susceptible to compression or hypotension.

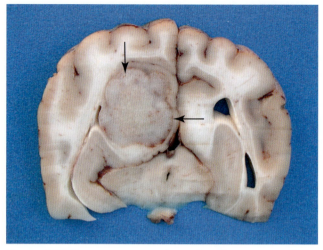

Figure 4-47 Tumor metastasis (arrows) at the junction of gray and white matter in a dog.

Cerebral veins have abundant and useful anastomoses. Untoward effects are not expected to follow occlusion of single veins because absence of valves permits reflex flow. The venous sinuses of the dura mater empty into the jugular veins, but they also communicate freely through the bones with extracranial veins. Because of these communications, the effects of obstruction of a dural sinus may be relatively slight, unless there is venous stagnation of the head or venous stagnation within the cranium produced by cerebral swelling or occlusion of more than one major sinus. The venous system of the spinal cord is freely anastomotic and drains partly via the radicular vessels and partly through denticles of ligamentum denticulatum, which is attached to the dura mater, to the paravertebral plexuses. Congestive myelopathy may occur in the cervical spinal cord, and epidural hemorrhage may occur at C6-C7 in horses subject to hyperextension or hyperflexion of the neck. These vessels are also valveless and allow very free communication up and down the spinal canal such that an embolus arising in caudal veins may bypass the caudal vena cava in passing to the lungs. These arrangements of veins may assist in temperature and pressure control in spinal and cerebral vessels. The arrangements have disadvantages. Infiltrating neoplasms may extend from extradural positions to the cord along the venules. Vertebral abscess or osteomyelitis in young pigs, cattle, and sheep may develop at or near T3-T4 in relation to azygos vein entry. In the cranial cavity, infections may extend from the face to the basal meninges. In cattle, sheep, and dogs, pyogranulomatous processes that are occasionally found in the hypothalamic-hypophyseal region are introduced in migrating intravenous foreign bodies that enter the cranial cavity in veins passing through the ophthalmic foramen.

Disturbances in the cerebrospinal vasculature with impaired blood flow may be composed of obstructive and hemorrhagic lesions, or they may be part of global cerebral ischemia with failure of adequate total perfusion. Diseases associated with abnormality of the circulating blood, such as the anoxias, hypoglycemia, and hyperviscosity, are discussed later with neurodegenerative diseases.

Ischemic lesions

The outcome of vascular obstructions depends on the type and size of the vessel obstructed, the degree and duration of ischemia, and the relative vulnerability of the tissues to anoxia. The injury may vary in severity from a temporary functional disturbance to the other extreme of infarction and necrosis. *Neurons and oligodendroglia are the most sensitive of the neural structures to ischemia, astrocytes are moderately resistant, and microglia and the blood vessels are quite resistant and may survive in small areas in which all else dies.* Gray matter, with its high metabolic rate and dependence on oxygen, is more sensitive than is white matter, but there are regional differences in the sensitivity of gray matter.

Obstructive lesions of cerebrospinal vessels are not commonly observed in animals, and ischemic changes may be absent even when the vessels are profoundly altered. On the other hand, lesions which are regarded as being of ischemic type are quite commonly observed in the absence of demonstrable vascular occlusion. These cases tend to be individual in their occurrence and without particular pattern.

Global ischemia is occasionally observed in animals suffering cardiac arrest under anesthesia, and in neonatal "barking foals and piglets." Purkinje cells, the hippocampal cortex, and neurons of the cerebral cortex are the most sensitive of all, and, within the cerebral cortex, the deeper laminae are more sensitive than the superficial laminae. Necrosis is accentuated over boundary zones at the margins of distribution of the rostral, middle, and caudal cerebral arteries. Similar regional susceptibility can be demonstrated in the cerebellar cortex. The deeper laminae of the cortex may be selectively destroyed in ischemia, producing a distribution of necrosis that is known as **laminar cortical necrosis.** Lesions are expected to be symmetrical but may not be. In severe and prolonged global ischemia, necrosis may involve all of the cortex and other nuclei, such as globus pallidus and lateral thalamus. The sensitivity to necrosis parallels that in severe hypoglycemia except that hypoglycemic injury spares the cerebellar Purkinje cells. The assumption that the injury is a result of anoxia and energy deficit does not recognize the complex biochemical perturbations set in train by cellular anoxia. In dogs with hypothermic circulatory arrest, apoptosis develops as early as 2 hours after injury and is most severe in the granule cells of the hippocampal dentate gyrus. Necrosis evolves more slowly and is most severe in amygdala and pyramidal neurons in Ammon's horn.

Feline ischemic encephalopathy is recognized in mature cats, and results from aberrant migration of *Cuterebra* larvae in the brain. Although larval migration tracks may be present, the ischemic lesions may be the result of toxin-induced vasospasm. The extent and distribution of degeneration vary from case to case. Milder lesions occur in superficial cortical laminae as multiple foci. More severe or extensive lesions tend to be in the distribution area of the middle cerebral artery and may be bilateral but asymmetrical (Fig. 4-48). In surviving animals, there is marked atrophy of the affected hemisphere. In some cases, there may be ischemic lesions in the brainstem.

Ischemic and hemorrhagic cerebral lesions occur in the **neonatal maladjustment syndrome of foals,** also known as the "barker" or "convulsive foal" syndrome, which is discussed with congenital atelectasis in Vol. 2, Respiratory system. The nature of the circulatory derangement is not understood, but the lesions are presumed to reflect hypoxic brain damage and variably delayed reflow. Hypoxic/ischemic encephalopathy has been also associated with placental insufficiency in a foal.

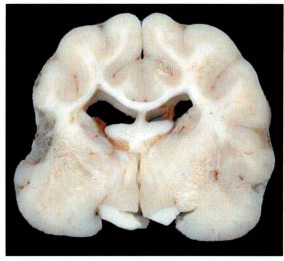

Figure 4-48 Unilateral focal loss of gray matter from the left parietal cerebral cortex, in **feline ischemic encephalopathy.**

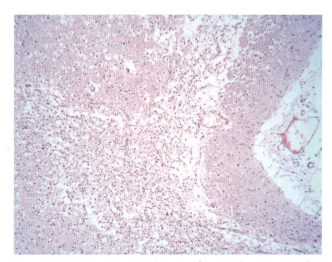

Figure 4-49 Polioencephalomalacia of cerebral cortex in a foal with neonatal maladjustment syndrome.

There is ischemic laminar necrosis of the cerebral cortex (Fig. 4-49), sometimes accompanied by necrosis in the paired gray nuclei of the midbrain and brainstem, and by multiple small hemorrhages. In some foals affected by this neonatal syndrome, there is minimal ischemic necrosis but instead a profuse distribution of small perivascular and petechial hemorrhages in the cerebrum, cerebellum, and brainstem.

Degenerative vascular disease of arteriosclerotic type is not important in animal disease. *Atheroma* occurs in some hypothyroid dogs. *Siderosis* of the walls of the arterioles occurs commonly as a change associated with advancing age in horses. The calcium and iron salts may be deposited in amounts capable of converting the vessels to rigid pipes (Fig. 4-50). The patency of the vessels is well maintained. There is no thrombosis, and vascular stenosis probably proceeds slowly enough for adaptive circulatory changes to occur because small areas of softening, presumably ischemic, are unusual.

Hyaline necrosis in meningeal vessels, which is observed in swine with hepatosis dietetica, is not usually associated with secondary lesions. The hyaline necrosis in meningeal vessels in pigs with organomercurial poisoning is associated with severe

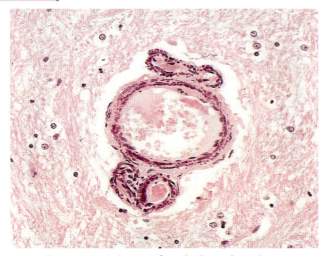

Figure 4-50 **Siderosis** of cerebral vessel in a horse.

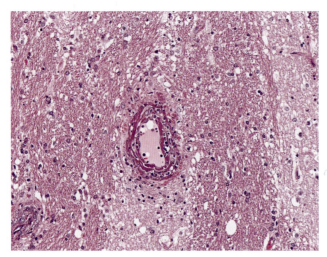

Figure 4-51 Necrosis and inflammation of vessels in the brainstem of a pig with **edema disease**. (Courtesy M. Pumarola.)

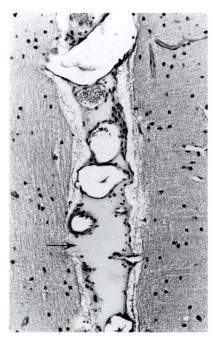

Figure 4-52 **Vascular leakage** (arrow) in the leptomeninges of the cerebellum of a sheep with annual ryegrass toxicity. (Courtesy J. McC. Howell.)

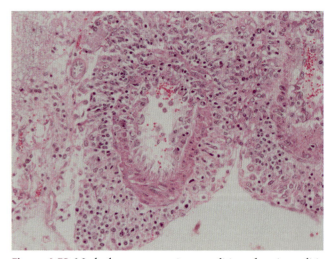

Figure 4-53 Marked **nonsuppurative vasculitis and perivasculitis** in a cow with malignant catarrhal fever.

cerebral injury that may be, in part, the result of reduced perfusion. *Amyloid degeneration* of meningeal and intracerebral vessels occurs in aged dogs, and the thickenings of the meningeal arteries may be visible grossly. Senile argyrophilic plaques that contain amyloid deposits may be associated with the vascular lesions. The systemic distribution of amyloid is minimal. Petechial hemorrhages occur in relation to the diseased vessels in about 50% of cases and, exceptionally, there is massive hemorrhage.

Cerebrospinal angiopathy is an important cause of neurologic disease in pigs. It occurs in the alimentary enterotoxemia known as **edema disease** of pigs with similar lesions in vessels of brain and other tissues (Fig. 4-51). The lesions are described in detail in Vol. 2, Alimentary system and peritoneum. In groups of older pigs, arteritis or periarteritis can develop and may represent a chronic or persistent expression of the acute angiopathy.

Vascular permeability changes provide a basis for **annual ryegrass toxicosis** (Fig. 4-52). The disease is discussed later with neurodegenerative diseases.

Cerebrospinal vasculitis, affecting both arterioles and veins, occurs in infectious diseases, genetic disorders, presumed autoimmune diseases, and neoplastic and paraneoplastic conditions of cattle, pigs, dogs, horses, and occasionally sheep. *Polyarteritis* (periarteritis nodosa) appears to have some predilection for the cerebral arteries, especially in the pig, and for the spinal arteries in the dog, in which it is cited as **steroid-responsive meningo-arteritis.** Vasculitis is a rather specific feature of classical swine fever, sporadic bovine encephalomyelitis, malignant catarrhal fever (Fig. 4-53), and mycotic diseases (Fig. 4-54). The agents of these diseases have no predilection for neural tissue, and parenchymal degeneration, which is sometimes observed, is secondary to occlusion of vessels; this occlusion, in turn, is secondary to inflammatory lesions of the vascular adventitia. Adventitial proliferations and perivascular infiltrates are common to many of the encephalitides, both bacterial and viral, and focal softenings of the brain and cord in these inflammatory diseases can

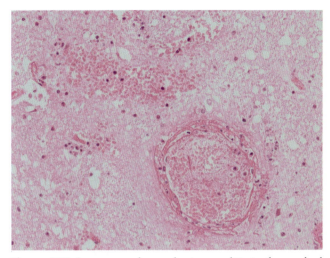

Figure 4-54 Severe **necrohemorrhagic vasculitis** in the cerebral cortex of a cow with a mycotic infection.

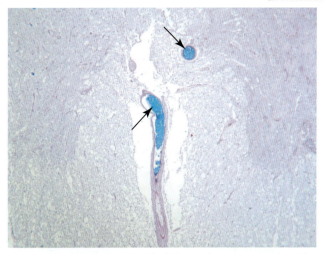

Figure 4-56 **Cartilaginous emboli** (arrows) causing spinal myelomalacia in a dog. Alcian-PAS stain.

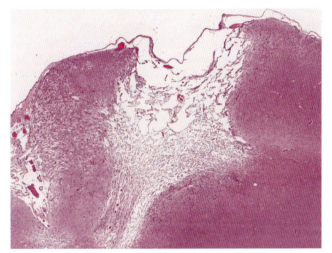

Figure 4-55 **Residual cyst** in cerebral cortex, the result of carotid thrombosis and ischemic infarction in a dog. (Courtesy M. Pumarola.)

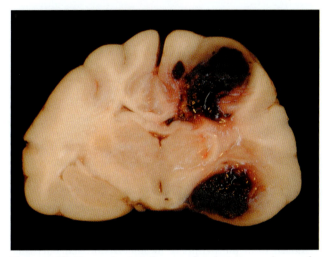

Figure 4-57 **Hemorrhagic infarcts** and **malacia** in cerebrum of a cat secondary to neoplastic thromboembolism from a metastatic pulmonary carcinoma. (Courtesy K. Dietert, Freie Universität, Berlin).

frequently be related to occlusive vasculitis. The occlusive lesions are not solely related to the acute phase of inflammation, but adventitial fibrosis and vascular stenosis may be prominent in the healed phase of encephalitis and may lead eventually to ischemic damage and softenings.

Thrombosis and embolism in the cerebrospinal arterioles is very seldom observed in animals. Thrombosis of an internal carotid vessel or ventral spinal artery may accompany atrial and aortic thrombosis (Fig. 4-55), especially in cats. Bone marrow emboli form after trauma and fractures, most commonly in dogs. *Emboli composed of fibrocartilage or nucleus pulposus* occur in spinal arteries and veins in most species, and cause hemorrhagic and ischemic infarcts of sudden onset (Fig. 4-56; also see Vol. 1, Cardiovascular system). Any segments of the spinal cord may be affected, and rarely the brainstem and cerebellum. *Bacterial thrombi* may develop in a variety of bacteremic diseases, such as erysipelas, shigellosis, pasteurellosis, and the septicemias caused by *Histophilus*, *Streptococcus*, and the coliforms. Abscessation develops rapidly about these bacterial colonies, but in the early stages, perivascular zones of softening may be observed.

Perhaps the least morphologic expression of arteriolar obstruction is death of neurons in a narrow zone of cortex representing the central portion of a field of distribution of a single arteriole. In the early stage, there is *acute ischemic necrosis* of neurons and oligodendroglia. These cells are shrunken with hypereosinophilic cytoplasm and pyknotic nuclei, but are not visible until ~8 hours after the vascular injury. There is no softening in these minimal lesions, but they are readily visible at low power as sharply demarcated narrow zones of pallor. At higher magnification, swollen axons and prominent capillaries are also observed, and the affected zone is seen to be unusually cellular, this being due in the early stages to microgliosis and later to astrogliosis.

Obstruction of an artery results typically in *territorial infarction*, and infarcts involve both gray and white matter. The localization of an infarct depends on the arterial system involved. For example, most cerebellar infarcts in dogs and cats develop within the region supplied by the rostral cerebellar artery or one of its main branches. In the early stages, affected areas swell, and the involved gray matter may be hemorrhagic (Figs. 4-57, 4-58). Obstruction of an **arteriole**

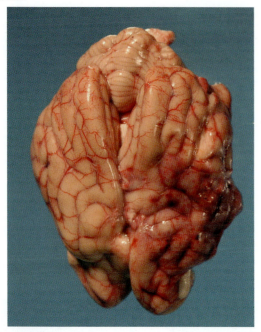

Figure 4-58 **Hemorrhagic infarct** in cerebral cortex secondary to thrombosis in a dog. (Courtesy J.L. Caswell.)

leads to a *lacunar infarct*. Frequently, the vascular obstruction cannot be demonstrated histologically. At the center of an infarct, there is coagulative and liquefactive necrosis, and around the periphery, there is a zone of minimal ischemic injury with the characters mentioned previously. Many capillary vessels survive, partly because of their relative insensitivity to anoxia and partly because they benefit first from the collateral circulation that develops. Surviving vessels show endothelial and adventitial proliferation, and the astrocytes around the margin of the lesion react. The necrotic tissues are removed from the periphery by liquefaction and microglial phagocytosis, and a cyst remains (see Fig. 4-55). The cyst contains fluid, and distended microglia, so-called *compound granular corpuscles*, may be found in it for very long periods. The wall of the cyst is ragged and irregular and is formed by reactive astrocytes. When the defect extends to the meninges, it may be partially filled in by proliferated leptomeningeal tissue.

Obstruction of cerebrospinal veins is the result either of pressure or inflammation with thrombosis, although rarely, it may be caused by neoplastic invasion and permeation of the dural sinuses. *Thrombophlebitis* is usually bacterial, and the associated meningitis is more conspicuous and important than the venous thromboses; isolated venous obstructions are not of much significance.

Intracranial thrombophlebitis can be due chiefly to retrograde spread of inflammation from an extracranial primary focus, but thrombophlebitis of this type is uncommon. Such primary foci may occur in the orbital or nasal cavities, the paranasal sinuses, or the middle ear. Intracranial inflammations have little tendency to cause thrombosis of the dural sinuses. In verminous infestations of the brain, especially those caused by *Strongylus* larvae in horses, there is some tendency for the larvae to migrate to the superior sagittal and transverse sinuses and to cause thrombosis of these. Spinal thrombophlebitis results from ascending infections from docking wounds in lambs and from bite wounds of the tails of pigs.

Noninflammatory thrombosis of the cranial dural sinuses occurs chiefly in the superior sagittal sinus. It occurs in polioencephalomalacia of cattle, in which it is probably secondary to severe and prolonged swelling of the brain. Sinus thrombosis may also be observed following head injuries, even those not accompanied by lacerations.

Venous infarcts differ from arterial infarcts by the more extensive hemorrhage in the affected areas and by the diffusion of blood into the adjacent subarachnoid space. The superficial veins are engorged, and the congested area is edematous and swollen. The hemorrhages are perivenular and petechial or larger, and are present in the gray matter and, to a lesser extent, in the white matter. The subsequent course and reaction are similar to those following arterial obstruction, and the residual lesion is a depressed and shrunken or cystic area that is dark brown-yellow. A *hemorrhagic myelomalacia* may occasionally develop in young horses that have been anesthetized in dorsal recumbency. A possible pathogenesis regards the compression of the venous drainage of the spinal cord by the abdominal viscera.

Hemorrhagic lesions

Hemorrhages in the central nervous system (CNS) may be *traumatic or spontaneous* and may be restricted to the meninges or the parenchyma or involve both. Hemorrhages accompanying periventricular leukomalacia in neonates are discussed previously. The causes are, in general, the same and are of much variety. They can be broadly grouped into those affecting the integrity of the vessel wall and those that reduce the coagulability of the blood. Care is necessary in deciding whether observed extravasations are significant because they can be produced readily as *artifacts at postmortem*. Quite extensive spread of blood into the basal meninges commonly occurs from the venous sinuses when the head is removed at the atlanto-occipital junction, and into the spinal meninges when the spinal column is transected. Hemorrhages of petechial size in the parenchyma can be largely avoided as artifacts if the brain or cord is fixed before slicing. The microscopic distinction of antemortem from postmortem hemorrhages can also be difficult because, apart from minor degenerative changes of the parenchyma, terminal hemorrhages provoke very little reaction, even on the part of the microglia.

Spontaneous hemorrhages in the brains of animals are almost invariably of petechial or slightly larger size occurring in the hemorrhagic diatheses, especially the symptomatic purpura of septicemic infections (see Vol. 3, Hematopoietic system). Such hemorrhages occur typically from capillaries as well as small venules and are found in meninges and brain. There is no specificity in the geographic distribution of purpuric hemorrhages except in *infectious canine hepatitis* in which intracranial hemorrhage, although not consistently present, has a predilection for the brainstem, thalamus, and caudate nuclei. In *focal symmetrical encephalomalacia* (see Vol. 2, Alimentary system and peritoneum), the lesions are grossly visible only when hemorrhagic; they are regularly bilateral and symmetrical and have a rather specific pattern in which the internal capsules, dorsolateral thalamus, cerebral aqueduct, and pons may all be involved. Hemorrhages also characterize *thiamine deficiency in dogs and cats* and have a specific distribution and symmetry, being regularly present in the inferior colliculi and less consistently present in the mammillary bodies and other periventricular nuclei. Multifocal hemorrhages in the brain and spinal cord may develop in dogs infected with *Angiostrongylus vasorum*.

Isolated hemorrhages or hematomas are quite rare in animals. They may result from vascular malformations *(hamartomas)* or tumors *(cavernous hemangiomas)*. The hemorrhages may extend to the ventricles and induce hydrocephalus, or involve the central canal of the cord to produce hematomyelia.

Meningeal hemorrhages, both epidural and subdural, are common in lambs and calves that have required obstetric assistance and probably reflect hemodynamic disturbances in dystocia. Hemorrhages of similar distribution occur in calves born unassisted from cows exposed to the coumarins of moldy sweet clover.

Microcirculatory lesions

A range of changes affecting the microcirculation in the nervous system may not produce ischemia or hemorrhage. They are associated with extravasation of formed or fluid elements, are not disease specific in their character, although their distribution may be specific, and result from degenerative changes, especially in capillaries and venules. Sludging of leukocytes is frequently observed in venules of cerebral and cerebellar hemispheres in diseases causing leukocytosis, including a range of infectious diseases with neutrophil leukocytosis and the rather rare intravascular lymphoma. Sludging of white cells is frequent in East Coast fever caused by *Theileria parva*, and sludging of red cells infected by *Babesia bovis* and possibly other protozoa; the pathogenesis of sludging may not be the same as for falciform malaria, in which adhesion seems to be important in pathogenesis. Viral infections, such as classical swine fever and canine adenovirus, are frequent causes of capillary hemorrhage.

Diapedesis of red cells is a common event in sudden death of many causes and is frequently mimicked in postmortem trauma. The interval between diapedesis and death may be too short for reactive changes, visible by light microscopy, to develop in the vessels. With some delay, swelling of endothelial cells and their nuclei develops. The hemorrhages may be from arterioles, with the red cells remaining in the perivascular space. Diapedesis from capillaries and small venules depends on disruption of endothelium and astrocytic processes and, depending on relative pressures, the red cells may spread in the intercellular spaces.

Diapedesis of red cells occurs in periventricular nuclei in thiamine-deficiency encephalopathy, and in the brainstem in concussion, contrecoup injury, and in hypomagnesemia in sheep and cattle. The white matter of the cerebral and cerebellar hemispheres is susceptible to diapedesis. The hemorrhages are sometimes large enough to be visible as petechiae in diverse conditions, including infectious purpuras, anoxia, fat, and other microembolism, in diseases associated with erythrocyte sludging, and in disseminated intravascular coagulation.

Leakage of plasma, usually from small venules, may occur in any part of the CNS. It is seen most frequently surrounding areas of traumatic injury or in the conditions noted previously that lead to erythrocyte diapedesis. The plasma will contain some fibrinogen, and polymerized fibrin in its usual form may be demonstrated around the vessels. It is more usual, however, for the fibrin to be in its unpolymerized or molecular form, and the plasma both within and outside the vessels to be transformed into a homogeneous gel that stains brightly by the PAS technique. The plasma gel may appear as capillary plugs or as perivascular droplets that appear to incite very little reaction.

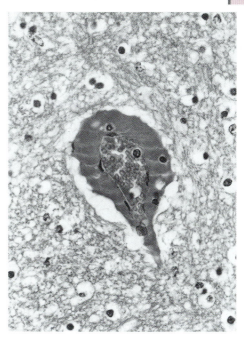

Figure 4-59 Accumulation of proteinaceous fluid around vessel in a sheep with **focal symmetrical encephalomalacia.**

Vascular injury that allows diapedesis of plasma will also allow passage of serum or protein filtrate (Fig. 4-59). In fields of injury, the differences in levels of permeability change may be evident from the protein content of transudate. Although plasma will routinely stain because of its fibrinogen content, the amount of protein in serum may be too low for preservation and staining (see Fig. 4-45). The perivascular changes occur especially about capillaries and venules in the white matter and have the characteristics described previously for vasogenic edema. Prolonged survival or recovery may leave *focal glial scars* as residue (see Fig. 4-15).

Further reading

Blue ME, et al. Brain injury in canine models of cardiac surgery. J Neuropathol Exp Neurol 2014;73:1134-1143.

Brown CA, et al. Hypertensive encephalopathy in cats with reduced renal function. Vet Pathol 2005;42:642-649.

Garosi LS. Cerebrovascular disease in dogs and cats. Vet Clin North Am Small Anim Pract 2010;40:65-79.

Schock A, et al. Cerebral segmental polyarteritis of unknown aetiology in sheep. J Comp Pathol 2009;140:283-287.

Wessmann A, et al. Brain and spinal cord haemorrhages associated with *Angiostrongylus vasorum* infection in four dogs. Vet Rec 2006;158:858-863.

Wilcox AL, et al. Hypoxic/ischemic encephalopathy associated with placental insufficiency in a cloned foal. Vet Pathol 2009;46:75-79.

TRAUMATIC INJURIES

Trauma to the head and vertebral column are of importance because of the effects that such injuries have on the contained brain and spinal cord. Both the brain and spinal cord are well protected from external injurious forces by the bony encasements. The more-or-less rounded shape of the skull favors glancing blows and the lateral diffusion of lines of force, the diploe and sutures are capable of absorbing considerable amounts of shock, and the internal system of bony ridges directs lines of force to the base of the skull. The spinal column is well protected by the surrounding soft tissues, by its own highly cancellous structure, system of ligaments, and intervertebral disks. The nature of acquired injuries is quite varied and is determined by many factors, including the relative vulnerability of the soft tissues, the direction in which the injurious force is applied, the physical rigidity of the bones, the ability of the part to move in response to the applied force, and the mass and velocity of the force.

Concussion

Concussion is a transient loss of consciousness and reflex activity following a sudden injury to the head. Full recovery is expected, and it is assumed that in mild cases there is no morphologic injury. In experimental animals, however, degenerative changes are found in the nuclear masses of the brainstem, and these are probably responsible for the clinical features. Following single injuries, chromatolysis develops in many of the larger neurons of the brainstem, and, in a proportion of affected cells, the degeneration is progressive. With repeated episodes of concussion, affected neurons have a wider distribution that includes the cerebral cortex, and the proportion of cells irreversibly injured is increased. These changes in the brainstem and reticular formation occur if the impact forces are substantial and the brain is subject to rapid acceleration/deceleration; in these cases, direct injury in the hemispheres is to be expected. The mildest degrees of concussion produce no visible structural damage when examined with the light microscope, but there is some experimental evidence that plasma substances, including proteins, may be transported in vesicles through the endothelial cells, and the brain and cord may lose their capacity for autoregulation of blood flow in local areas of static injury.

Although the dynamics of the disturbances in neurons that are responsible for the concussion are unclear, some of the physical qualities of the reaction between the head and the applied force have been elucidated. The vibrations that travel back and forth in the brain from the point of impact appear not to be important. If the head is firmly immobilized, quite a considerable force may be suddenly applied to it with relatively minor effect, the force of the blow **(coup)** being absorbed by the skull. Force of much lesser magnitude will cause concussion if the head is capable of moving in response to the blow. The principle to be obtained from these observations is that *a degree of acceleration or deceleration is necessary to produce concussion*, neural injury being caused by displacement of the cranium relative to its contents. The brain of an adult animal is normally a little smaller than the cranial cavity and, being suspended in the cavity, is capable of slight independent movement. If the head is freely movable and struck a heavy blow, it moves away from the point of impact and collides at the area of impact (coup) with the brain, which is momentarily static. As the brain moves suddenly within the skull toward the point of impact, leptomeningeal blood vessels may be torn as the brain pulls away from the skull **(contrecoup)**, and *the contrecoup injury may be greater than the coup injury*. In young animals, the brain closely fits the cranial cavity, so relative displacement of the whole brain is expected to be minimal. However, the brain is plastic, so sudden acceleration or deceleration leads to internal deformation. Displacements and transient deformations of the brain result in neuronal changes and unconsciousness, probably through the effect of shearing strains on neurons, axons, dendrites, synapses, and blood vessels, as well as direct pressure effects when the brain is displaced across bony ridges.

Contusion

In contusion, the architecture of the nervous tissue is retained, but there is hemorrhage into the meninges and about the blood vessels in the parenchyma. Contusions may be diffuse or focal injuries, although often those coexist.

The pathogenetic factors in diffuse contusions are generally the same as those operating in causing concussion, but the applied force, the displacements, and the induced shearing and direct forces are all of greater magnitude. Typically in diffuse injuries, *some of the most severe hemorrhages occur on the surface of the brain opposite the point of impact.* Hemorrhages of this distribution are known as *contrecoup*, and their development depends on the sudden movement of the brain to the point of impact *(coup)*, with tension and tearing of pial and cortical vessels opposite the point of impact, and with direct or rotational displacement of brain over bony prominences, where the vessels become exposed to tensile and shear forces.

Focal contused injuries develop typically at the point of impact, and the mechanism of development is somewhat different from that of the diffuse injuries. In focal injuries, movement of the head is not sufficient to cause significant displacement of the brain. Instead, the applied force, usually with relatively high velocity and relatively low mass, causes fracture or deformation of the skull at the point of impact. The deformation of the skull may only be transient but sufficient to cause bruising of the tissue immediately beneath.

Laceration

Laceration is a traumatic injury in which there is disruption of the architecture of the tissue. The mechanics of lacerations are, in general, the same as those of contusion. Penetrating injuries are analogous to, but more severe than, those that result in focal contusions. Lacerations may also occur with blunt injuries of the type that cause displacement of the brain. In such cases, contrecoup lacerations occur typically on the surfaces of gyri, where these are displaced over bony prominences. Shear forces developed during deformation or molding of the brain may be adequate to cause deep hemorrhages and even the cleavage of the gray from the white matter over small areas of the cortex.

Lacerations caused by penetrating injuries are always liable to *secondary infections*, especially when fragments of skin and soft tissue and spicules of bone from the internal plates are displaced into the brain. In the absence of infection, repair takes place in the manner that is usual for defects of nervous tissue. The detritus of blood and nervous tissue is removed by microglia and meningothelial macrophages. If the defect is small, an astrocytic scar forms, but usually a cyst remains, lined by proliferated astrocytes. Adhesions between the glial tissue and pia mater produce meningo-cerebral scars that are notably epileptogenic.

Fracture of the skull

Fractures of the skull can be important in terms of the concurrent injuries to the underlying meninges and brain and because they can provide a pathway of infection to the sinuses, meninges, and brain. They are indicative of injuries produced by considerable force and, when the inner plates are fractured, of contusion or laceration of the underlying brain. Fractures of the base of the skull may involve the middle ear and allow the escape of cerebrospinal fluid (CSF) and the entrance of infection. Frontal fractures involving the cribriform plate may allow CSF to escape into the nasal cavity.

Fractures of the skull are usually quite easy to detect by virtue of the displacement of bone and meningeal hemorrhage. Some, however, may be difficult to detect. This applies especially to fissures that develop during transient deformation of the skull and to impacted basilar fractures, such as occur in horses that rear backward and strike the nape of the neck and occiput. With these fractures, hemorrhages may be scant and basilar fractures are revealed only when the dura is carefully dissected away.

Injuries to the spinal cord

It is possible for direct injuries to the spinal cord to occur without obvious injury to the vertebrae. Such spinal injuries are necessarily lacerations caused by penetrating foreign bodies. Wandering parasites as causes of traumatic injury are discussed later. Much more common are indirect injuries to the cord acquired in the course of vertebral luxations or fractures with dislocation. *The most common of indirect injuries to the cord are produced by extruded nucleus pulposus in dogs, and by compression of the cervical cord in the syndrome known as "wobbler"* (see Vol. 1, Bones and joints).

Vertebral subluxations are the result of trauma, but *fracture dislocation* may be pathologic as well as traumatic, and frequently is in swine and ruminants when the fracture occurs through an area of vertebral osteomyelitis or osteochondrosis. The injuries to the cord occur chiefly at the time of accident and are due mainly to the stresses to which the cord is subjected and partly to impediment to the blood supply. Cumulative injury may occur, especially in dislocations when continued pressure on the cord or stretching of the cord over bony prominences causes intermittent ischemia.

Subluxations are largely restricted to the cervical column, where there is relative mobility of the ligaments. In the thoracic and lumbar spine, comparable forces are more likely to cause fracture because of the brevity of the ligaments. The fractures may involve only a lamina, the odontoid process, or an articular process, and therefore be difficult to detect. *Fracture dislocations of the vertebral column occur chiefly in the caudal cervical region and about the thoracolumbar junction*. Most injurious are those fractures that involve the vertebral body because there is usually displacement of a fragment caudodorsally into the spinal canal. Both in luxation and fracture displacement, pressure may be exerted over several segments of cord by epidural and endodural blood clots (Fig. 4-60).

Traumatic injuries to the spinal cord may be slight enough to be satisfactorily recoverable, or they may, at the other extreme, cause transection and an extensive length of necrosis. Early contused lesions cause swelling of the cord over 1 or 2 vertebral segments. The swelling may be easier to palpate by gently stroking the cord than to appreciate by inspection. Later, the cord is shrunken at the level of injury, and this also may be best detected by palpation. In the swollen zone, dark points of hemorrhage may be detected on section, and these occur usually in the central gray matter and at its junction

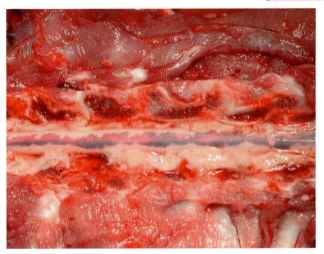

Figure 4-60 Extensive **subdural hemorrhage** of the spinal cord in a calf, caused by physical trauma.

with the white. If the demarcation of gray from white matter is obscured, it can be expected that softening of some degree is present. Cores of softening may be recognizable grossly, and the fact that they are extending up and down the cord from the point of injury is explained as tracking of exudate, especially serum or edema fluid, along the fiber tracts and the path of least resistance. Because the meninges are usually intact, the amount of local swelling is limited.

With severe compression, the cord may be entirely necrotic at the point of injury and over several segments. *Necrosis is probably the result of vascular injury*, and, for the same reason, isolated segments of necrosis may occur apart from the main injury. When the cord is necrotic, it is initially swollen, but after a lapse of some weeks, the dura forms a narrowed, collapsible tube containing debris.

Microscopically, in the mildest injuries, there is swelling of axons and myelin sheaths. The injured axons become beaded, but they are possibly not irreversibly injured unless fragmentation follows the beading, because functional recovery can follow minor and transient paralytic injuries. Where the axons are severed, there is bulbous swelling of the retracted ends. Degenerative neuronal changes consisting of the clumping of Nissl substance and central chromatolysis are constantly present. Ultimately, there is some loss of neurons. When softening occurs, the sequence of changes is the same as occurs in any neural lesion with loss of substance. The hemorrhage is usually slight and perivascular, but it may enter the central canal and pass along it for a considerable distance.

In long-standing spinal injuries, adhesions may be found between the meninges and between the dura mater and periosteum. In the injured zone of cord, there may be loss of fibers and myelin sheaths with astrogliosis or, in the more severe injuries with loss of substance, there may be cysts, pial-glial or collagenous scars, or the cord may be converted to a thin sclerotic band.

DEGENERATION IN THE NERVOUS SYSTEM

Foregoing sections dealing with cytopathology and the effects of circulatory disturbances and trauma are discussions of changes that are largely degenerative. The same will be true of many sections in later parts of this chapter because neural injury, regardless of cause or severity, is characterized chiefly by degeneration. Discussed in this section are those lesions and diseases of the CNS that are expressed as degenerations of nervous tissue.

Meninges

Age changes in the meninges may advance to such a degree as to be pathologic. *Collagenous and osseous metaplasia* occurs commonly in the cranial dura mater of dogs and cats. The process begins in the frontal region and extends to the temporal and occipital areas. The plaque-like thickenings of the surface meninges tend not to extend to the basal or cerebellar meninges. Ossification, which is detectable as small intradural plaques, follows hyalinization of the connective tissues and may or may not be preceded by mineralization. The dura adheres firmly to the periosteum. Perhaps by an independent process, *spherical mineralized nodules* form in the basal dura beneath the medulla in some aging dogs. Histologically, these nodules show a whorled pattern of fibroblastic cells often enclosing small concretions known as **psammoma bodies.**

Hyalinization of dural collagen occurs also in the spinal dura mater with aging and may be preliminary to the osseous metaplasia of the dura observed frequently in large breeds of dogs. The latter condition is referred to as **ossifying pachymeningitis** but, in spite of the frequency of the dural change, little is known of its pathogenesis or effects. *Dural ossification* is found in older age groups of some large breeds and varies in its expression from multiple separate plaques to rigid ossification over several segments of the cord. The changes are best developed in the lumbar region but may involve much of the spinal dura. The basic change appears to be degenerative and metaplastic rather than inflammatory. Locomotor dysfunction in affected animals is more likely to be attributable to concurrent spondylosis and degenerative/reactive changes in joints. The plaques consist of lamellar bone that is mature in appearance and that from the earliest stages contains cancellous spaces and active bone marrow.

Degenerative changes in leptomeninges are less well identified than those in the dura and are limited to collagenization and hyalinization. They are not functionally significant, but the opacities produced, especially the focal thickening in arachnoid granulations in old animals, can be misinterpreted as inflammatory change.

Choroid plexuses

With advancing age, there is *hyaline degeneration of the connective tissues of the choroid plexuses*, especially those of the lateral ventricles. The basement membranes of the capillaries are also involved. The hyaline tissues may become mineralized.

Cholesteatosis of the choroid plexuses in the form of tumor-like nodules, usually termed *cholesteatomas* or *cholesterol granulomas*, occurs in 15-20% of old horses. They are more frequent in the plexuses of the fourth ventricle than in the lateral ventricles, but those in the lateral ventricles are the more important because they may attain large size and, by obstructing the interventricular foramen, cause hydrocephalus leading to dilation and pressure atrophy of the walls of the ventricles (Fig. 4-61A).

The development of cholesteatosis appears to be related in some manner to chronic or intermittent congestion and edema with congestive hemorrhages in the choroid plexuses. During an edematous episode, the plexuses are slightly swollen, yellow, and soft. The interstitial tissues are edematous and

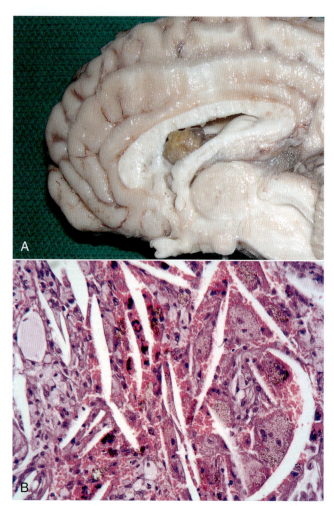

Figure 4-61 A. Cholesterol granuloma in the choroid plexus of the right lateral ventricle of a horse. (Courtesy F. Del Piero.) B. Microscopically, a **cholesterol granuloma** is composed of acicular cholesterol clefts, epithelioid macrophages, lymphocytes, and plasma cells.

infiltrated lightly by macrophages containing lipid and hemosiderin. The crystals of cholesterol are deposited in the tissue spaces and apparently act as foreign bodies to stimulate low-grade productive inflammation (Fig. 4-61B).

The affected plexus is swollen, and small areas or the whole of it may be occupied by the cholesterol granulomas. These are firm but crumbly, gray nodules with a gleaming, pearly appearance on cut surface. The crystals can be expressed from the cut surface by slight pressure.

Atrophy in the brain and spinal cord

The most spectacular atrophy of the cerebrum occurs in cases of congenital lipofuscinosis and of progressive internal hydrocephalus. **Senile atrophy** of the brain and cord is frequently obvious but seldom severe in animals. The atrophy is most marked when it is associated with the combined influences of senility and marasmus, and it occurs more frequently in sheep than in other species. The pachymeninges are thickened, and those of the cranium are partially adherent to the periosteum. The leptomeninges are thickened, tough, and granular. The brain is reduced in volume and weight and may be discolored a darker gray-yellow. The convolutions are narrowed and wrinkled, and the sulci are shallow and widened. Both brain and cord are much firmer than is normal. The ventricles are moderately dilated. Histologically, the neurons, especially of the cortex, are shrunken, distorted, and dark staining, and their numbers are depleted. The amount of Nissl substance is reduced, and the neuronal nuclei stain diffusely. Lipochromes are increased in amount, and satellitosis is prominent; macrophages laden with lipochrome are present in the perivascular spaces. There is a diffuse increase in glial fibers, which is responsible for the increased firmness of the tissue. The gliosis is most prominent about Virchow-Robin spaces, and there is a general tendency for protoplasmic astrocytes to transform into fibrous ones. The Virchow-Robin spaces are dilated, and some may be visible to the naked eye. The media of the vessels contain increased amounts of collagen.

Focal atrophy of the brain and cord is the result of slight but long-continued pressure. The loss of function is often disproportionately large as the result of acute pressure lesions compared with the extent of pathologic change. The reverse is often true in chronic pressure, and function may be retained to a surprising degree. Hydrocephalus is common as a cause of chronic pressure, and other sources of pressure are space-occupying lesions of the meninges or bony vault.

The pathogenesis of the changes produced by chronic pressure is unclarified. Because the immediate effects of pressure are more likely to be felt by veins than by arteries or solid tissue, the atrophic changes are usually attributed to venous stasis and edema. More acute pressure effects grade into circumstances and consequences discussed under trauma. Whatever the mechanism, myelin is the most vulnerable component of the tissue and undergoes slow progressive degeneration. There is also slow progressive atrophy and loss of neurons, especially of the Purkinje cells when pressure is exerted on the cerebellum, the neurons of the deeper laminae when pressure is exerted on the cerebrum, and of the ventral horn cells in the spinal cord. The degenerating myelin is replaced by glial fibers.

Segmental cerebellar atrophy is common in pigs following a variety of nervous diseases. The rostral vermis and adjacent portions of the lateral lobes are affected, these being within the distribution of the rostral cerebellar artery. There is no acute change but, instead, a gradual loss of granule and Purkinje cells with secondary changes in the white matter and reactive gliosis. The lesion is asymptomatic.

Anoxia and anoxic poisons

The neuropathologic effects of anoxia are seldom observed in animals or perhaps seldom looked for. Because most cases die acutely, there may be very little to see. The pathologic effects of anoxia, not only in the CNS, but in general, are expressions of "vulnerability," a property which differs from organ to organ and between parts and cells of one organ. *The components of the nervous system are vulnerable in a rather fixed order*, which is neuron, oligodendroglia, astroglia, microglia, and blood vessels, in that diminishing order of sensitivity. The neurons are not a uniform population, and there are regional differences in their susceptibility to anoxia, those of the cerebral cortex and the Purkinje cells being the most sensitive. Within the cerebral cortex, the neurons of the deeper laminae are more sensitive than those in the superficial laminae. Beneath these levels, there is a gradient of susceptibility through the geniculate bodies, hypothalamus, thalamus, paleocortex, and caudate nucleus. The various patterns of vulnerability are relative; they are established largely by experiments in animals and are subject to some variation, depending in part on the experimental species and on the type of anoxia induced. They do, nevertheless, emphasize the problem of selective vulnerability at the cellular level. There are, in addition, broader regional differences in vulnerability to anoxia, such as those that allow parts of the cerebral cortex to be necrotic while adjacent parts survive intact and that allow the same agent or anoxic insult to cause leukomalacia on some occasions and poliomalacia on other occasions. The basis of these regional differences in vulnerability, and the apparent differences in the patterns of degeneration following different types of anoxia, is still to be established.

The pathologic effects of anoxia on nervous tissue are of 2 types, which are to some extent differences in degree. The least clear morphologic expression is *selective neuronal necrosis*. The neuronal necrosis is typically of the ischemic type, and it is followed by glial repair. Greater degrees of anoxia, sufficient to kill astroglia as well as neurons, result in *softening*. These are the expected changes in anoxic anoxias, such as might occur with cardiac arrest or periods of apnea in grand mal epilepsy.

As a response in some episodes of anoxia, such as may be induced, for example, in the histotoxic variety of cyanide poisoning, the degeneration and necrosis may affect the white matter with only minimal changes in the gray. The reason for this is not known. The malacic changes in the white matter of the cerebral hemispheres are preceded by edema, which suggests that local circulatory disturbances contribute to its development. Clearly, the attribution of selective vulnerability on the basis of local metabolic demand for oxygen is inadequate, and a fuller explanation will probably require, in addition, consideration of vascular architecture, the autoregulation of blood pressure and flow, and local metabolic factors in the maintenance of myelin and axons.

Cyanide poisoning

The anoxia produced by cyanide is classified as *histotoxic* because the action of the poison is to *inhibit intracellular respiratory enzymes*. The cyanides are particularly rapid in their action, and death usually occurs from a few minutes to an hour after the onset of clinical signs. In the most acute cases, the clinical course occupies only a few minutes and is characterized by dyspnea, drooling, trembling, and recumbency; it terminates in convulsions. The *blood is bright red* because of its high degree of oxygen saturation. In cases that survive for an hour, the clinical signs are the same with, in addition, vomiting (especially in pigs), nystagmus, and cyanosis. In these cases, the blood is often dark because of anoxemia.

The morbid changes are those associated with anoxia. Because most cases survive for 0.5-1 hour, the blood is dark and does not clot and the tissues are dark. There is congestion in the lungs and hemorrhages of dyspneic type in the tracheal mucosa. Ecchymoses of the epicardium are usual. In pigs, there is pulmonary edema and hydropericardium, and there may be capillary hemorrhages deep in the myocardium by the coronary grooves. Severe pulmonary edema is present in some dogs.

Descriptions of lesions in the nervous system of animals in cyanide poisoning are largely limited to experimental observations in dogs and cats. In many natural cases of the poisoning, there is no significant alteration in the brain. The degenerative lesions in the brain in experimental poisoning may involve predominantly the gray matter or the white. When in gray matter, there is patchy necrosis and laminar loss of cells in the cerebral cortex, and necrosis in the head of the caudate nucleus, paleocortex, substantia nigra, and thalamus. There is edema in the cerebral white matter, sometimes in the absence of cortical change. On the other hand, single graded exposures of rats may produce the principal lesions in white matter, especially in the corpus callosum. In this species, there are gradients of injury in the callosum reflecting gradients of susceptibility, the most severe degeneration occurring in the caudal core of the callosum. The gradients are attributed to regional differences of blood supply, which are expected to reinforce the histotoxic anoxia of cytochrome oxidase inhibition by cyanide. The earliest change described in the callosal lesion is axonal swelling producing a spongy appearance by light microscopy; alterations of myelin and oligodendrocytes are second in time.

Plants containing toxic levels of hydrocyanic acid bound as glucosides are common and widespread and are the usual source of cyanide poisoning. The compounds are in general the β-glycosides of α-hydroxynitriles and are activated by endogenous glucosidases in the plant, or in other plants, or by ruminal microorganisms. For these reasons, cyanide poisoning occurs chiefly in ruminants. Toxin generation of this type does not occur at the low pH of the monogastric stomach, but a lethal amount may be absorbed from the large bowel if there has been a large intake of toxigenic material.

Both sheep and cattle are capable of detoxifying cyanide in the liver to form *thiocyanate*. *Thiocyanate* itself is toxic but in a manner different from that of cyanide; if thiocyanate is present in low concentrations over prolonged periods, it is goitrogenic. The cyanide concentration in a stated species of plant varies considerably with stage and rate of growth and with the fertility of the soil. Plants that are growing rapidly contain the highest concentrations of the glucosides, especially if the growth phase follows one of retardation caused, for example, by wilting, frostbite, or close grazing. The glucosides are regarded as being metabolic byproducts.

Plants of many species contain cyanogenetic glucosides, but only a few are important in this regard. The majority of cyanogenetic plants are usually harmless, either because of low palatability or low concentration of the glucosides. The important cultivated toxic plants are the sorghums (*Sorghum* spp.), and the star grasses (*Cynodon* spp.). Those of the cherry family are also potently cyanogenetic. Linseed concentrates can be dangerous, especially if eaten in large quantities.

Chronic cyanide intoxication is not recorded, but extended periods of grazing the cyanogenetic sorghum and Sudan grass may lead to ataxia in cattle and horses, cystitis and urinary incontinence, and abortion in mares. Attempts to link the clinical syndrome to cyanogenetic compounds in the plants are inconclusive, and a causal association with cyanides seems unlikely. There is axonal degeneration and demyelination at all levels of the cord but most prominent caudally in ventral and lateral funiculi. Ataxic syndromes occur in sheep grazing *Sorghum* spp. may involve large numbers of animals in syndromes that differ from those in horses and cattle. Urinary incontinence does not occur. There is limb paresis with knuckling, incoordination and disturbance of equilibrium, and head and body tremors. Pregnant ewes may produce stillborn, weak, or arthrogrypotic lambs. Whereas the lesions in horses and cattle are of Wallerian type in the spinal cord, those in sheep are of an axonopathy with proximal spheroids in the major nuclei of the brainstem and ventral horns of the spinal cord.

Nitrate/nitrite poisoning

Ruminants are also vulnerable to *phytogenous nitrates*, when intraruminal microbial conversion of nitrates to nitrites exceeds the rate of conversion of the latter to ammonia. The nitrate sources again include many crop plants as well as weeds; plant nitrate concentrations are influenced by soil nitrogen level, and physiologic stresses on the plants, such as water stress and herbicide damage. Occasionally, high nitrate concentration in drinking water is the problem. *Absorbed nitrites convert hemoglobin to methemoglobin*, which imparts a *dark "chocolate" color* to the blood, and causes dyspnea, cyanosis, weakness, tremors, collapse, and coma. There are no gross or histologic brain lesions. The condition is discussed more fully in Vol. 3, Hematopoietic system.

Fluoroacetate poisoning

Fluoroacetate is toxic by virtue of its ability to form fluoroacetyl–coenzyme A, which potently inhibits the Krebs cycle enzymes cis-aconitase and succinate dehydrogenase, thereby paralyzing cellular respiration. Herbivores are usually poisoned by ingesting *fluoroacetate-containing plants*, although other animals may be affected by accident or design by being exposed to sodium fluoroacetate formulated as a *pesticide*. The clinical signs are of the same general character as those described previously, but in the dog, frenzied hyperactivity is reported. As with cyanide, the myocardium is highly vulnerable, and multifocal necrosis may be seen. Fluoroacetate poisoning is discussed in Vol. 3, Cardiovascular system.

Carbon monoxide poisoning

This is rarely observed and is discussed in the interests of completeness. Carbon monoxide has an affinity for hemoglobin that is several hundred times the affinity of oxygen for hemoglobin. The carboxyhemoglobin produced prevents oxygen exchange and causes anoxic anoxia. The anoxia is reinforced by a histotoxic component resulting from the affinity of carbon monoxide for iron-containing respiratory enzymes.

Carboxyhemoglobin and, therefore, the blood and tissues of poisoned animals are *bright pink*. All organs are congested, but especially the brain, in which the veins and capillaries are much dilated. The dilated vessels are observed especially in the white matter, and hemorrhages occur from them. Acute fatalities are not expected to be associated with neural lesions. Survival is expected to be followed by complete recovery, but there may be residual lesions of anoxic type, especially neuronal loss.

Carbon monoxide poisoning is reported occasionally in animals in confined quarters that are heated by petroleum fuels. Most of the reported instances are in pigs, and poisoning is associated with a high level of stillbirth and neonatal mortality. Following experimental exposure, patchy or extensive leukomalacia may be present in the hemispheres in the newborn.

Hypoglycemia

It is useful to extend the classification of anoxia to include hypoglycemia, which causes a *disturbance of intracellular respiration*. Oxygen is available to the nervous tissue, but, in the absence or reduction of the amount of substrate, the oxygen is not used.

Hypoglycemia may occur as a result of a functioning *tumor of the pancreatic islets* or as a response to insulin overdosage in the treatment of diabetes. It is also part of the metabolic disturbance of *ketosis in cows* and *pregnancy toxemia in ewes*, and arguments have been advanced for regarding the irreversibility of pregnancy toxemia as being the result of hypoglycemic encephalopathy. Piglets in the first week of life readily develop hypoglycemia if there is dietary restriction from any cause. Effective gluconeogenesis does not develop in piglets until about the seventh day of life, and during this first week, their glycemic levels are rather precise reflections of dietary intake. In spite of the severe convulsions and deep coma that occur in hypoglycemia, conspicuous changes do not occur in the brain. It is probable that biochemical disturbances in the neurons precede histologic signs of degeneration by a considerable period. For this reason, acute hypoglycemic death is not expected to produce cerebral lesions. When the period of coma is prolonged, it is probable that all neurons are to some extent altered, but the differentiation of hypoglycemic from autolytic and nonspecific changes can seldom be made with confidence. Although classified with the anoxias, hypoglycemia does not produce the ischemic type of neuronal degeneration characteristic of the usual sorts of anoxia. There is, instead, a tendency for the severe type of neuronal degeneration to occur, characterized by rapid and complete chromatolysis, disappearance of the cytoplasmic margins, and then fading of the cytoplasm, with pyknosis, eccentricity, and fading of the nucleus. Cerebrocortical lesions tend to have a superficial laminar preponderance and generally involve caudate nuclei and putamen, CA1 and CA3-4 regions of the hippocampus, and dentate gyrus, which is usually spared in hypoxic-ischemic injury. Cerebellar cortex, cerebellar nuclei, and brainstem tend to be spared compared with hypoxic-ischemic injury.

Malacia and malacic diseases

Necrosis of individual elements of nervous tissue is described previously under Cytopathology of nervous tissue. **Encephalomalacia** and **myelomalacia** refer to necrosis in the brain and cord, respectively. *Malacia means grossly observable softening*, and is used interchangeably with that term to signify necrosis of tissue in the CNS. When neurons and neuroglia degenerate and die as part of the primary response, the term *malacia* is applicable.

The *sequence of events* in softening or malacia is specific only for the tissue. The morphologic changes in necrosis, in the removal of dead tissue, and in healing are the same regardless of the insult. The insults can be varied, and *malacia, alone or as part of another change, is one of the most common lesions in the brain and cord*. It is discussed in the sections dealing with vascular accidents and trauma, it occurs in many instances of encephalomyelitis, is discussed elsewhere in these volumes as a lesion of mulberry heart disease, of antenatal bluetongue virus infections in lambs, and of clostridial enterotoxemia in lambs that escape apoplectic death and live for some days. Malacic lesions are probably the basis of most cases of hydranencephaly.

Although the nature of the malacic process is not specific for cause, there is some specificity in the localization of lesions and in their particular pattern of distribution. These features may allow the recognition of known associations or causes, such as the nigropallidal distribution of lesions in horses poisoned by yellow star thistle, and the focal symmetrical lesions of the internal capsule in lambs with clostridial enterotoxemia. Although these and some other associations have been determined, the pathogenesis of the lesions and the problems of selective injury to certain parts of the brain remain to be resolved.

The sequence of changes in malacic foci is approximately the same in all cases and is outlined later. The rapidity of change is quite variable and depends on the species and age of the animal, the location of the necrosis, the volume of tissue affected, and the inciting cause. The speed of resolution is also affected by the quality of vascular perfusion in adjacent nervous tissue, whether the necrosis is ischemic or hemorrhagic, and on the time over which the cause acts.

The malacic process, once initiated, appears to proceed very rapidly in the fetal and immature nervous system, and to leave cystic structures and hydranencephaly without much evidence of continuing reaction at the time these animals are available for postmortem examination (see Fig. 4-24). The reasons for the rapidity of change in immature nervous tissue are not clear, but contributing factors may involve the paucity of myelin that is difficult to remove, the paucity of mature mesenchyme in meninges and about vessels, and the plasticity of vascular arrangements in the developing brain. The rapidity of change in gray matter is generally greater than in the white. Autolytic liquefactive changes depend on continued enzymatic activity that, in turn, depends on availability of oxygen either by diffusion from surrounding tissue or by reflow in the local vessels. Small foci of necrosis are expected to resolve more quickly than large ones. Malacic lesions in the neocortex, where diffusion from collateral vessels is available, are expected to resolve more rapidly than those in the paleocortex, where the vascular supply is more strictly of the end-artery type. Some causes of malacia, such as vascular occlusion, act promptly and the pathologic changes are directly consequential. The cause may act continuously over a period, as in leukoencephalomalacia of horses, and the changes may be incremental. The process, once established, may itself initiate progressive change, as in traumatic injury to the cord, in which swelling within the confines of the meninges assists the spread of edema and vascular response beyond the site of the original injury.

A malacic lesion that develops acutely may not, in the absence of hemorrhage, be demonstrable before about the twelfth hour of onset. The early change is in texture, with the affected part being soft, and in color, with the affected part being gray. Within 2-3 days, the malacic foci begin to disintegrate, the softness is more evident, and the surrounding tissue is swollen by edema, and pale in gray matter or yellow in white matter. Subject to the earlier qualifications, *the necrotic area eventually liquefies and a cyst remains*. The cyst may be loculated or traversed by vascular strands that have survived the episode.

Histologically, in acute episodes, there is reduced staining affinity by about 12 hours. The cellular elements show the changes described previously. The early active response involves circulating neutrophils, which may enter in large numbers, but this response is replaced in 3-4 days by macrophages. The first appearance of macrophages is about blood vessels; their peak activity occurs in about 2 weeks, but a few will survive for a very long time. Astrocytic gliosis replaces or surrounds the resolved necrotic area.

In the specific syndromes to be discussed later, the degenerative changes tend to be restricted to, or to affect principally, either the gray matter or the white matter. Softening of gray matter is known as **poliomalacia**, and softening of white matter is known as **leukomalacia**; each may be qualified as to whether cerebral (encephalo-) or spinal (myelo-). The diseases to be described later are specific, but malacia is not exclusive to them. Necrosis of cerebral cortex is rare in horses, except in the neonatal "barker syndrome" (see Fig. 4-49). In ruminants, poliomalacia is, in the early stages, expected to respond to thiamine, but it also occurs in lead poisoning, water intoxication, and other ill-defined circumstances. Lead also causes poliomalacia in dogs. Convulsive episodes in dogs, some associated with distemper, may leave malacic changes, especially in the parietal and temporal cortex. Metronidazole intoxication of dogs and cats can result in brainstem leukomalacia. In pigs, polioencephalomalacia is usually caused by salt poisoning, but individual cases occur in meningitis or without other association. The isolated case of malacia can be difficult to explain. Idiopathic necrosis and malacia of the hippocampus and piriform lobe in cats is reported from Europe as a cause of seizures. In this condition, known as **feline hippocampal necrosis** or **complex partial cluster seizures with orofacial involvement,** lesions are restricted to the hippocampus and in some cases are bilaterally symmetrical. In advanced cases, hippocampal sclerosis and atrophy can be observed. The pathogenesis is unclear, but toxic environmental factors are suggested.

Focal symmetrical poliomyelomalacia syndromes

This disease, as described from Kenyan **sheep,** is characterized by focal softening of the gray matter of the spinal cord, most consistent and severe in the cervical enlargement. A similar syndrome occurs in parts of West Africa. There is no information on the cause or pathogenesis, although the distribution of necrosis in relation to the cross-section of the cord and the irregular segmental involvement of the gray matter, especially in the cervical region, are consistent with a *vascular component* in the pathogenesis. Lesions of similar distribution and character are occasionally met with in dogs and cats with inflammatory or thrombotic occlusion of the ventral spinal artery. Affected sheep suddenly develop flaccid or spastic paresis that always involves the forelimbs and sometimes the hindlimbs as well. There are no cerebral signs. Affected animals are lambs or up to 18 months of age. There are no gross lesions to be observed except in cases of long standing, in which some brown discoloration may be noted in the malacic areas. Microscopically, there are bilateral lesions of remarkable symmetry in the ventral horns of the spinal cord. The dorsal horns are spared, as is a narrow rim of gray substance around the periphery of the ventral horns, and the commissural gray matter. The affected areas undergo dissolution with the usual reaction on the part of the microglia. At a later stage, proliferating capillaries in small numbers crisscross the microcavitations, and the astrocytes at the margins proliferate. The malacic foci are found in the cervical and lumbar enlargements as "skip" lesions involving a few segments and, when the necrosis is extensive, similar foci may be found in the medulla.

A similar syndrome has been responsible for heavy losses in native sheep in Ghana and Ivory Coast. All ages are affected but mainly adult ewes. Clinical progression is rapid, from initial stumbling to ataxia and recumbency, opisthotonos and nystagmus, and ultimately flaccid paralysis. There are microscopic changes of cytotoxic edema, especially affecting oligodendrocytes widely in the nervous system and also perivascular astrocytes and capsule cells of spinal ganglia. Foci of spongy degeneration and malacia, bilateral but not always symmetrical, are of patchy distribution and most frequent in the spinal

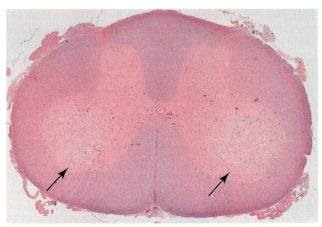

Figure 4-62 Focal symmetrical poliomyelomalacia involving ventral horns (arrows) of cervical spinal cord in a pig with selenium toxicity. (Courtesy M.J. Hazlett.)

intumescence, cerebellar roof nuclei, and large nuclei of the brainstem.

Encephalomyelomalacia of similar character is reported in young individual **goats** in California. The lesions are bilaterally symmetrical and affect particularly the lumbar and cervical enlargements and the inferior colliculi. Other brainstem nuclei are inconsistently involved. The similarity of these malacic lesions to those which can be produced experimentally by nicotinamide antagonists has been noted.

Focal symmetrical poliomyelomalacia of pigs is clinically and pathologically similar to the spontaneous poliomalacias of sheep and goats. The presenting signs are spinal with ataxia progressing to forelimb or hindlimb paresis or quadriplegia in a few days. In field cases, malacic foci are found, symmetrically in the ventral horns of the cervical and lumbar enlargements. The malacic foci are visible grossly as yellow-brown areas of softening or gray depressed areas of liquefaction. The histologic changes are typical of malacia (Fig. 4-62). There is heavy loss of neurons, and endothelial and glial proliferation in older lesions. Similar changes may be present in pontine and medullary nuclei.

Affected animals may show changes associated with *selenium toxicoses*, including scurfiness of skin, hair loss, and separation of horn at the coronet. Dietary selenium, whether as sodium selenite added to rations or the feeding of selenium-accumulator plants, reproduces the syndrome, although there is some inconsistency in the lesions produced, with degeneration being more frequent in the nuclear masses of the medulla and brainstem. *Astragalus bisulcatus*, a selenium-accumulator plant, will cause concurrent polioencephalomalacia. The mechanism of neurotoxicity of selenium is obscure, but may occur through the generation of reactive oxygen species during reaction of thiols, and is expected to be influenced by other nutritional and metabolic interactions.

Focal symmetrical poliomyelomalacia, the lesion limited to the sacral and lumbar enlargements, is described in **Ayrshire calves.** The malacia affects the ventral horns, sparing the dorsal horns and the central gray matter. The cause is not known.

Focal symmetrical encephalomalacia in swine

Aeschynomene indica is a common weed in irrigated rice fields and may be fed with rice and screenings of broken rice. Signs of neurologic disorder develop in a few days. Lesions are restricted to the brain, are symmetrical, and involve especially the vestibular and cerebellar roof nuclei, nuclei of the midbrain, and the paleocortex. They include edema and hemorrhage, followed by necrosis, infiltration with gitter cells, and endothelial hypertrophy and hyperplasia. The toxic factor is unknown, but pathogenesis may depend on primary damage to microvasculature.

Corynetoxin poisoning

This condition is a severe and frequently fatal tremorgenic syndrome ("annual ryegrass toxicosis") in ruminants, horses, and pigs caused by the ingestion of several plant genera (*Lolium*, *Polypogon*, and *Agrostis*) colonized by a nematode (*Anguina agrostis*) and a bacterium (*Rathayibacter toxicus*). The distribution of the disease is governed in part by the distribution of annual ryegrasses in winter rainfall areas, although the disease can occur in other areas by the use of transported fodder. Corynetoxin-producing *R. toxicus* is transported onto the host plants by nematode larvae and then ingested by animals. The nematode *A. agrostis* emerges from fallen galls following first autumn rains, migrates into the growing points of the ryegrass seedlings, and later penetrates the florets to produce galls. The nematodes are harmless to animals but may carry on the cuticle the bacterium that will proliferate in the gall, forming a yellow slime. The active principle, *corynetoxin*, is closely related to the tunicamycin antibiotics produced by some strains of *Streptomyces*. Indeed, tunicamycin-like metabolites have been detected in mycotoxicosis in pigs. Corynetoxins and tunicamycins inhibit lipid-linked N-glycosylation of glycoproteins, which compromises cell membrane integrity. Significant livestock losses in Australia and South Africa result from exposure during summer grazing to parasitized annual ryegrass (*L. rigidum*), annual beard grass (*P. monspeliensis*), and blown grass (*A. avenacea*). In the United States, a similar neurologic syndrome has been described in sheep and cattle fed *Festuca nigrescens* (chewings fescue) infected with *A. agrostis* and a *Rathayibacter*-like organism.

The toxicosis is characterized clinically by neurologic signs and high mortality. Pregnant ewes may abort. The pathogenesis of abortion has not been examined, but the occurrence of hemorrhages in various organs, pulmonary edema, and swelling of endoplasmic reticulum of hepatocytes indicates systemic intoxication, notwithstanding the prominence of neurologic signs.

The clinical signs, which are severe, include excitability, aggression in cattle, disturbances of gait, and convulsions. The clinical course may be <12 hours. Gross changes include pulmonary edema and a pale swollen liver, and occasionally, there are hemorrhages in various organs.

Microscopic changes in nervous tissue are subtle, especially following routine fixation by immersion, which may not preserve transudates. Tracer injections show widespread alterations to cerebrovascular permeability in the brain and meninges, indicating endothelial damage and disruption of the blood-brain barrier. The perivascular transudate resembles plasma (see Fig. 4-52) in staining properties, and may be present as perivascular lakes or droplets that stain strongly with PAS stain. Only occasionally can fibrin be demonstrated, but extravasation of red cells from capillaries may be present in neuropil. Astrocytes are swollen with acidophilic cytoplasm, and there may be widespread necrobiosis of oligodendroglia in the cerebral gray matter.

The capillary endothelium shows ultrastructural evidence of injury. Endothelial cells are swollen and electron lucent; the cisternae of rough endoplasmic reticulum are distended; mitochondria are swollen, with disorganization of cristae; and capillary lumina sometimes contain platelet aggregations. The changes are best seen in cerebellar cortex and meninges. Neuronal change is minimal, but there may be patchy loss of Purkinje cells and scattered small foci of malacia.

Further reading

Casteignau A, et al. Clinical, pathological and toxicological findings of an iatrogenic selenium toxicosis case in feeder pigs. J Vet Med A Physiol Pathol Clin Med 2006;53:323-326.

Finnie JW. Review of corynetoxins poisoning of livestock, a neurological disorder produced by a nematode-bacterium complex. Aust Vet J 2006;84:271-277.

Pakozdy A, et al. Complex partial cluster seizures in cats with orofacial involvement. J Fel Med Surg 2011;13:687-693.

Polioencephalomalacia of ruminants

Polioencephalomalacia (PEM) as used in practice applies especially to softenings restricted to the cerebrocortical gray matter of laminar distribution. The lesion may alternatively be designated as "cerebrocortical necrosis" or "laminar cortical necrosis." Necrosis of this distribution is the basis of the well-recognized syndrome of cattle, sheep, and goats known as PEM. It is also the lesion of salt poisoning in swine, is occasionally observed in lead poisoning of cattle, and is described among the residual neurologic lesions of cyanide poisoning. Apart from these known associations or causes, laminar cortical necrosis is observed sporadically in swine, dogs, and cats.

The disease, PEM of sheep, goats, and cattle and other managed ruminants, is similar in its clinical and pathologic aspects in the several species, but the course in sheep and goats is, as a rule, shorter, with fewer survivors from the stage of overt brain swelling. Merino sheep appear to be much more resistant than other breeds.

The incidence is highest in sheep in the age group from weaning to 18 months, but sporadic cases occur in older animals. This general statement of incidence applies to pastured animals as well as to those in feedlots or barns. It is a disease of young cattle, the age incidence depending on the population exposure. As originally described in Colorado, affected animals are mainly 1-2 years of age but, elsewhere, the incidence is highest in younger stock of 3-8 months of age. The severity of the disease is rather less in pastured than in feedlot or housed cattle and sheep. Its least clinical expression, occasionally observed in outbreaks in sheep, is blindness and dullness, a tendency to head press against obstacles, and cessation of feeding. There are no ocular abnormalities in this, or in any other grade of the disease, and the blindness is cortical. Animals showing these mild signs usually recover completely in the course of several days. If they are killed for examination, malacic changes may be found to be minimal or absent, but there is widespread neuronal necrosis of ischemic type in the deeper laminae of the cerebral cortex. Animals affected more severely may remain on their feet and show, in addition to the noted signs, muscular tremors, especially of the head, and intermittent opisthotonos; if they survive, they become partially decorticate and remain blind and stupid.

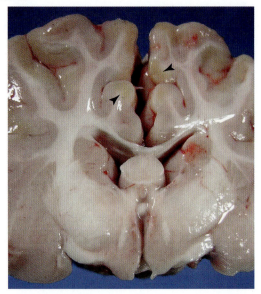

Figure 4-63 Polioencephalomalacia in a cow. Softening and yellow discoloration of affected cortical areas (arrowheads).

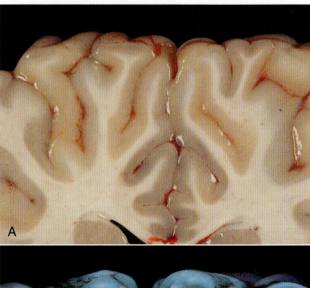
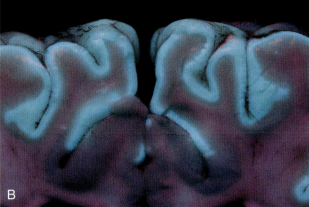

Figure 4-64 Polioencephalomalacia in an ox. A. Pallid areas of degeneration involving particularly the gyri. B. Marked bilaterally symmetrical autofluorescence of the cerebral cortex under ultraviolet light. (Courtesy K.G. Thompson.)

In severe cases of PEM, the animals are recumbent. There is twitching of the face, ears, and eyelids, intermittent grinding of teeth, drooling, and bulbar paralysis in some. Opisthotonos is present, and some animals are convulsive. In the early stages, the neurologic signs are intermittent, but later they become more constant with persistent opisthotonos and nystagmus. Flaccidity is usual, although there may be transient periods of spasticity, and clonic convulsions are intermittent. Death occurs in coma after a course of one to several days. These signs are entirely referable to the nervous system; other systems are undisturbed except for the very occasional case in which massive hemoglobinuria after excess water intake precedes the onset of neurologic signs.

The **lesions** are qualitatively the same in all cases, but they differ in their degree and in the ease with which they may be detected, this depending on severity and duration. Young animals usually die more rapidly than old ones and may show cerebral edema and swelling only. The swelling affects the cerebral hemispheres, which are pale, slightly soft, and droop over the cut edges of the cranium. In these cases of short course, there may be no obvious displacement of the brain. When the fresh cortex is sectioned, it usually shows a laminar paleness ~0.5-1 mm wide, following the contour of the gray matter at the junction between gray and white. This change may be most easily visible in the gyri rather than in the depths of the sulci (Figs. 4-63, 4-64A). Its extensiveness varies considerably from case to case but remains within the boundaries of the supply area of the middle cerebral and caudal cerebral arteries. In the rostral distribution of these vessels, the lesions are patchy but are more extensive caudally toward and over the caudal poles of the hemispheres. The dorsal surfaces of the hemispheres are involved, and the distribution is approximately symmetrical. In either fresh or formalinized material, *the gross lesions of cortical necrosis autofluoresce under ultraviolet light* because of the presence of lipid metabolites in macrophages, or of high-molecular-weight collagen-like material (Fig. 4-64A, B).

In cases that survive for several days, the necrosis becomes more and more obvious. The brain is grossly swollen, and, almost without exception, it is displaced caudally with herniation of the medulla and cerebellum into the foramen magnum. The dorsum of the hemispheres is palpably quite soft, and the normal turgidity of the brain is gone. The surfaces of the gyri are a characteristic yellow-brown, and the normal adhesion of leptomeninges to the gyral surfaces may not be present. On the cut surface of the cerebrum, there will be areas of minimal change resembling those described previously. The necrotic zones can usually be appreciated to be narrow and pale or yellow instead of gray, and they are friable and shrink away from the cut surface. Lines of cleavage between the gray and the white matter can be discerned. These are present especially over and extending down the sides of the gyri but seldom extend around the depths of the sulci. In some cases, yellow foci of softening can be found in the herniated portion of the cerebellar vermis. Hemorrhage is insignificant and usually not apparent in the cerebrum and cerebellum, but hemorrhagic foci of softening may be found in the collicular region, thalamus, and caudate nuclei. In some cases, there is thrombosis of the dorsal longitudinal sinus.

Animals that survive for 2 weeks or longer are decorticate over more or less extensive areas. The white cores of the gyri are largely intact and project nakedly or with an irregular covering of softened friable gray matter. Over some gyri, the gray matter is intact. The subarachnoid space is widened, and the meninges droop over the enlarged sulci. Subpial cysts may

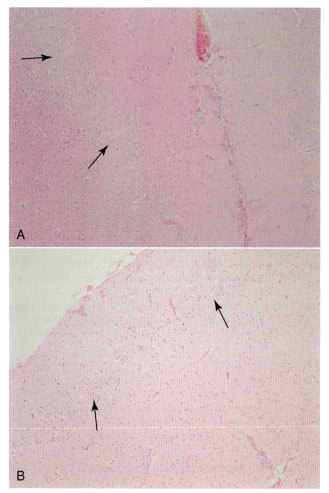

Figure 4-65 A, B. Polioencephalomalacia in an ox. Pallid areas of laminar cortical necrosis and degeneration (arrows).

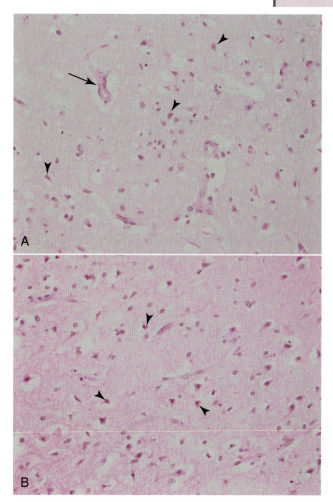

Figure 4-66 A, B. Polioencephalomalacia in an ox. Higher magnification of Figure 4-65. Affected neurons are shrunken, acidophilic (pink neurons), and surrounded by a clear space (arrowheads). Regional capillaries are hypertrophied and have swollen endothelium (arrow).

be evident where the devastation is not complete, and the meninges are adherent. The brain is smaller than normal and not displaced, the lateral and third ventricles are dilated, and there is an excess of cerebrospinal fluid.

The **microscopic changes** are of the same type in all affected parts but vary in distribution and severity. The least change is one of laminar necrosis of neurons affecting especially the deeper laminae. *The malacic areas are laminar* (Fig. 4-65A, B). The deepest laminae are consistently involved. Frequently, the superficial lamina is involved. The softened laminae do not necessarily overlie one another, although there is usually considerable overlapping. When 2 distinct laminae of necrosis overlie one another, they frequently merge in the depths of the sulci to produce necrosis of the total width of the gray stratum. Necrosis of the superficial lamina is first recognizable as a rather uniform sponginess. The layer then disintegrates, and the middle laminae, if intact, are separated from the pia by a moat of gitter cells in which vessels are very sparse. The leptomeninges are thickened and contain many activated histiocytes.

In affected areas, the neurons are shrunken, acidophilic, and surrounded by a clear space (Fig. 4-66A, B); in 2-3 days, many are converted to eosinophilic globules without nuclear remnants. Healing, if it occurs, is with intense astrogliosis.

The middle laminae may remain structurally intact for considerable periods. The neurons therein die acutely, but the glia are rather persistent. The vessels are prominent, with swollen proliferating endothelial and adventitial cells and a perivascular clear space.

There is *early edema and neuronal necrosis in the deepest laminae*, and the edema extends to the adjacent white matter, giving the zone a pale washed-out, fibrillary appearance in sections (see Fig. 4-65A, B). There is demyelination in the edematous white matter, but the glia survive fairly well, and the astrocytes react and swell. The microglia become active and concentrate in the deep laminae, which disintegrate to cleave overlying cortical remnants from the subjacent white matter.

The macroscopic lesions observed in the cerebellum and subcortical areas are typical foci of softening. Microscopic changes of less severity are more common. They occur in the herniated portion of the vermis and consist of acute degeneration of Purkinje cells with more or less extensive cytolysis in the granular layer.

The chronic lesions of surviving animals resemble those described earlier in ischemic infarcts. The dead tissue is removed by microglia. In zones where the gray matter has been entirely necrotic, the pia may be separated from the white matter by a clear space or be in contact with the white and partially adherent as a glial-pial scar formed by connection with the proliferated astrocytes that line the defect. Where the superficial laminae have remained intact, elongate cystic spaces lined by astrocytes remain where the necrotic parenchyma has been removed.

The areas of softening quite clearly have a distribution related to the field of supply of the middle cerebral artery. When the lesion is of restricted distribution, it is related to the periphery of the field of distribution of this vessel over the dorsal cerebral cortex and, when the lesion is more extensive, it covers more of the field of supply of this vessel, but necrosis is seldom found ventral to the caudal ectosylvian fissure. The cortex rostral to the transverse sulcus and in the field of supply of the rostral cerebral artery escapes significant injury. Necrosis may be observed in the distribution area of the caudal cerebral artery, but only when the swelling and displacement is severe, a fact suggesting that necrosis in this distribution is secondary to tentorial herniation with compression of the caudal vessels against the free edge of the tentorium.

Degenerative changes in periventricular nuclei of type and distribution typical of thiamine deficiency in other species are present in some cases of PEM, and their histologic appearances suggest that their development precedes the cortical necrosis. This observation applies also to the experimental disease produced by amprolium (thiamine antagonist).

The **cause** of PEM in ruminants is often unknown, as the lesion of PEM lacks etiologic specificity. Sporadic cases and outbreaks are observed in animals given access to water after a period of deprivation, suggesting that these cases may be expressions of *water deprivation–sodium ion toxicosis* developing in the manner discussed later for salt poisoning in swine. It has been observed in sheep eating the nardoo, *Marsilea drummondi*, and associated with the *thiaminase* present in that fern. The disease has been produced experimentally with analogues of thiamine with impaired activity, and by the feeding of rhizomes of bracken fern, which are known to contain thiaminase.

Deficiency of thiamine or a disturbance in its metabolism is implicated in PEM. Thiamine, if administered early, may lead to prompt clinical recovery. Calves examined early in the course of the disease may have elevated blood pyruvate, reduced blood transketolase, and reduced levels of thiamine in liver and brain. Cerebral edema and laminar necrosis have also developed in lambs and calves given the coccidiostat amprolium. Thiaminolytic enzymes can be found in rumen contents in some cases of PEM, and it is accepted that they are produced as exoenzymes of some rumen microbes as a consequence of imbalances between thiamine-producing and thiamine-destroying bacteria (e.g., *Bacillus thiaminolyticus*, *B. aneurinolyticus*, *Clostridium sporogenes*). Degradation of thiamine may reduce the amount available and simultaneously produce analogues of the vitamin. The thiamine-responsive disease is sporadic.

Sulfur compounds have emerged as important causes of morbidity. Sulfite, an intermediate in the reduction of sulfate, can cleave thiamine into pyrimidine and thiazole constituents, thereby rendering it inactive. Diets and drinking water containing high levels of sulfates can increase the incidence of PEM in cattle, and in sheep fed diets high in sulfur. Sulfur compounds, mainly sulfur dioxide, used to color meat can precipitate a thiamine deficiency syndrome in dogs and cats. The sources of sulfur to ruminants are varied. There is a high incidence of PEM in cattle in feedlots, especially when they are fed diets based on molasses, which can be high in sulfur. Inappropriate use of ammonium sulfate for urine acidification in feedlot cattle and sheep is recorded. The high incidence of the disease in animals fed sugar beet pulp and the occasional outbreak in cattle fed thiocyanate-containing *Brassica* plants may be ascribed to high sulfur content. Groundwater in many areas has a high content of calcium sulfate. The National Research Council (NRC) recommended dietary sulfur level for ruminants is <0.3%, the maximum tolerated intake is 0.4%, and water sulfate concentrations >2,000 ppm are associated with the occurrence of PEM. The molecular pathogenesis of sulfur-related PEM is unclear, as is its relationship to thiamine activity and to the malacic lesions in the corpus striatum not seen in thiamine-responsive disease.

Further reading

Cebra CK, Cebra ML. Altered mentation caused by polioencephalomalacia, hypernatremia, and lead poisoning. Vet Clin North Am Food Anim Pract 2004;20:287-302.

Niles GA, et al. The relationship between sulphur, thiamine and polioencephalomalacia—a review. Bov Pract 2002;36:93-98.

Thiamine deficiency

Thiamine (vitamin B_1) is a *dietary requirement of carnivores*. Herbivores are capable of synthesizing their own requirements, the synthesis being microbial and taking place in the rumen, and probably in the large intestine of horses. Experimental deficiency can be produced in calves and lambs, but only when they are very young and before they have established a useful ruminal flora; neurologic signs, including ataxia, cerebellar tremors, and convulsions, occur in these experimental deficiencies (see also Polioencephalomalacia of ruminants). Horses are poisoned by eating bracken fern and horsetail (*Equisetum arvense*), both of which plants contain a *thiaminase*. The plants are unpalatable, but poisoning may occur when they are included in pasture hays. The disease in horses is characterized by incoordination, which may be severe and lead to recumbency and bradycardia. Affected animals respond rapidly to thiamine. The nervous system has never been suitably examined for lesions.

Thiamine deficiency has been produced in most domestic species and in others. It has been an important natural disease in foxes and cats and continues to be of some importance in mink. In these carnivorous species, the deficiency is induced by a *thiamine-splitting enzyme naturally present in many species of fish*. Metabolic analogues of thiamine are known and have been used experimentally to produce the deficiency, but there are no known naturally occurring competitive analogues. Processed foods for dogs and cats can easily be made deficient in thiamine as the vitamin is susceptible to heating at 100° C or above in a medium of neutral or alkaline pH. The feeding to cats and dogs of meat that has been exposed to sulfur dioxide to preserve the fresh appearance can lead to thiamine deficiency; *thiamine is destroyed by sulfates*.

The syndrome, originally described as *Chastek paralysis*, produced by thiamine deficiency in foxes and mink, is comparable to that in cats and may develop in 2-4 weeks of being fed the deficient diet. The onset of neurologic signs is indicative of severe depletion of thiamine; the clinical and pathologic consequences of marginal deficiency are not known. Initially, there is reluctance to eat, and drooling and anorexia may be present for up to 1 week before distinct clinical signs occur. Neurologic signs first consist of ataxia, incoordination, pupillary dilation, and sluggish pupillary reflexes. Convulsions are easily induced and are characterized by strong ventroflexion of the head. At this stage, animals usually respond rapidly and fully to thiamine, but there may be residual mild ataxia. After 2-3 days of neurologic signs, animals pass into an irreversible phase of semicoma, opisthotonos, continual crying, and spasticity.

The *lesions of thiamine deficiency in carnivores* pass through the sequence of vacuolation of neuropil, vascular dilation, hemorrhage, and necrosis. These changes are occasionally observed in the middle laminae of the occipital and temporal cortex as poliomalacia, but *the areas of remarkable vulnerability are in the periventricular gray matter*. The periventricular lesions are always bilaterally symmetrical. The only consistency in the pattern of the lesions in the periventricular system is the involvement of the caudal colliculi. Next to the caudal colliculi, lesions are most commonly found in the medial vestibular, red and lateral geniculate nuclei, but they may be found in any of the periventricular nuclei. In contrast with Wernicke encephalopathy in man, with which the disease in carnivores can be compared, cats and foxes only irregularly develop hemorrhages in the mammillary bodies.

The initial morphologic change is *vacuolation in nuclei of special susceptibility*. This is easiest to detect in the lateral geniculate bodies, caudal colliculi, and red nuclei (Fig. 4-67). The vacuolation develops in cats at about the time they become susceptible to the induction of convulsions and at about the time that alterations in the permeability of the blood-brain barrier become demonstrable. This altered permeability, which may result from free-radical injury, is limited to those nuclear masses that are known to be vulnerable to injury in this deficiency. The case may not progress beyond this stage but, instead, pass to recovery. In the event of recovery, *intense astrogliosis* develops and remains to indicate the past presence of thiamine deficiency. With the development of vacuolation, it is also possible to recognize vascular dilation, especially affecting venules and especially in the susceptible nuclei. *Hemorrhage* occurs from both capillaries and venules, consistently in fatal cases. The hemorrhages may be large enough in the colliculi and vestibular nuclei to be visible to the naked eye (see Fig. 4-67A, B).

Thiamine deficiency appears to affect most severely the relay systems from the eye and ear, but the histogenesis of the changes is vague. Phosphorylated thiamine is the coenzyme, *cocarboxylase*, and it participates probably in all oxidative decarboxylations as well as in some other metabolic transformations. It is a cofactor for transketolase, α-ketoglutarate dehydrogenase, pyruvate dehydrogenase, and branched-chain α-keto acid dehydrogenase. It may also have a function in axonal conduction and synaptic transmission. In all animals in which thiamine deficiency has been produced, the deficiency is attended by an *elevation of the pyruvate levels of blood*. This is to be anticipated from what is known of the function of the vitamin, but cannot be connected in any way to the nature of the nervous signs or the nature or distribution of the neural lesions. There is decreased glucose use by the brain, and shortly before the development of lesions, the vulnerable areas suffer a burst of metabolic activity with local production of lactate, and it is possible that the focal lesions, initially, are the result of focal lactic acidosis. The bradycardia is explainable on the basis of impaired carbohydrate metabolism because

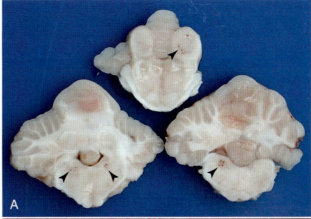

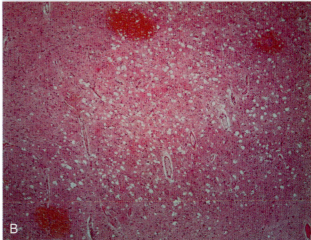

Figure 4-67 **Thiamine deficiency** in a cat. **A.** Hemorrhage in caudal colliculi and vestibular nuclei area (arrowheads). (Reprinted with permission from Mandara MT, et al. Neuropatologia e Neuroimaging. Milano: Poletto Editore, 2011.) **B.** Multifocal hemorrhages with edema in caudal colliculus.

cardiac muscle depends for its energy supplies on carbohydrate, chiefly pyruvate, and in this differs from skeletal muscle. *Myocardial degeneration* is described in the experimental disease in several species and in the spontaneous disease in cats, dogs, and foxes; focal myocardial necroses are more prominent in the right than in the left ventricle.

Although it is not possible to correlate thiamine deficiency and its lesions with the distribution and activity of pyruvate decarboxylase, there is some correlation between thiamine deficiency and the distribution of transketolase activity in the nervous system. Transketolase is a thiamine pyrophosphate–dependent enzyme active in the hexose monophosphate shunt. The enzyme is active in white matter and apparently important in the metabolism of oligodendrocytes. During progressive thiamine depletion, brain transketolase activity declines before signs of the deficiency develop, and the decline is greater than for pyruvate decarboxylase. Moreover, the decline of brain transketolase is greatest in those areas in which lesions develop in rats.

The relation of transketolase deficiency to the evolution of lesions is unclear, as is the sequence of morphologic changes. The spongy change appears to be a primary event, and vascular changes secondary. The hemorrhages are a terminal event. Fine-structural studies suggest that changes in vessels in selective areas of injury are secondary to degenerative changes in regional glia. The glial cells are edematous (swollen with clear cytoplasm), and their rupture leads to increase of extracellular spaces. Additional studies have shown early damage in the neuropil, with degenerative and hypertrophic changes, and axonal degeneration, with preservation of neurons. Increased release of glutamate in vulnerable brain structures may result in N-methyl-D-aspartate receptor-mediated excitotoxicity; apoptotic cell death may result from increased expression of immediate early genes such as *c-fos* and *c-jun*.

Further reading

Meng JS, Okeda R. Neuropathological study of the role of mast cells and histamine-positive neurons in selective vulnerability of the thalamus and inferior colliculus in thiamine-deficient encephalopathy. Neuropathol 2003;23:25-35.

Nigropallidal encephalomalacia of horses

Prolonged ingestion of yellow star thistle, *Centaurea solstitialis*, or Russian knapweed, *Centaurea repens*, produces encephalomalacia in horses. It is a disease of dry summer pastures in which the thistle, which remains green, provides most of the forage. The putative neurotoxin is *repin*, a principal sesquiterpene lactone present in aerial parts. Repin appears to cause glutathione depletion, which leads to oxidative damage, mitochondrial dysfunction, and neuronal cell death.

The onset of the disease is sudden and may occur as early as 1 month after initial exposure to star thistle. The syndrome is characterized by idle drowsiness, persistent chewing movements, and difficulty in prehension, the latter apparently related to incoordination of the lips and tongue. Sensation and reflexes are normal. Death is the result of starvation, dehydration, or intercurrent disease. *Malacic lesions are consistently present in the brain and affect specifically the globus pallidus and substantia nigra*. There is some variation of the pattern, depending on whether the lesions are symmetrical or not and involve both pallidus and substantia nigra or only one of the structures. Usually, both structures are symmetrically involved. The pallidal foci involve the rostral portion of the globus pallidus, are lenticular in form, and 1-1.5 cm in size. The core of necrotic tissue in the substantia nigra is ~0.5 cm in diameter and extends from about the level of the mammillary bodies to the point of emergence of the oculomotor nerve (Fig. 4-68). The affected areas are evident as slightly bulging, yellow, gelatinous foci. The softening progresses rapidly, and in ~3 weeks, the lesion is sharply demarcated as a *pseudocystic cavity*. The microscopic changes are those ordinary in malacia and do not give a clue to the immediate pathogenesis.

Further reading

Sanders SG, et al. Magnetic resonance imaging features of equine nigropallidal encephalomalacia. Vet Radiol Ultrasound 2001;42: 291-296.

Salt (NaCl) poisoning

Salt poisoning may be a *direct and immediate* result of excessive ingestion of salt, or it may be *indirect and delayed*, developing only after several days of excessive salt intake and restricted water intake. These 2 types of salt poisoning are

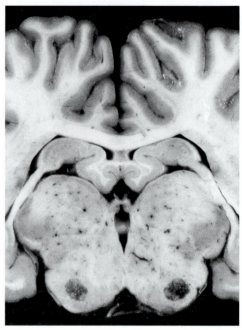

Figure 4-68 Bilaterally symmetrical foci of malacia in substantia nigra in **nigropallidal encephalomalacia** in a horse.

pathogenetically dissimilar, and neither will occur if animals are always provided with free access to water of low saline content.

Direct salt poisoning is largely a problem of salinity of drinking water. Excessive saline content of fodder is not a concern, except in terms of palatability, if an abundance of fresh water is available; for example, sheep may take rations containing up to 13% sodium chloride for prolonged periods without ill effects. This high tolerance for salt in fodder is used to restrict food intake during periods of scarcity and also to encourage water intake in the control of urolithiasis.

The salinity of drinking water is important, not only in terms of the concentration of sodium chloride or total salts, but also in terms of what salt and what acid radicals are present. It is difficult to provide figures for acceptable salinity of drinking water for livestock because of the variations in the proportions and concentrations of the various salts present, but the usual recommendation is that the concentration of sodium chloride or total salt should be <1.7% for sheep, <1.0% for cattle, and <0.9% for horses, and preferably not more than one half of these concentrations.

Acute, direct salt poisoning occurs chiefly in cattle, especially if they are very thirsty when first given access to saline water. Poisoning may also occur in cattle if they are given free access to salt supplements after a prolonged period of salt restriction, such as occurs in cattle grazing on mountain pastures. *Clinical signs in cattle are referable to the alimentary tract and nervous system*, and include vomiting, polyuria, diarrhea, abdominal pain with paresis, knuckling of the fetlocks, and blindness. Death may occur in 24 hours.

At autopsy, there is severe congestion of the mucosa of the abomasum and excessive, dark, fluid intestinal content. The alimentary changes are probably in large measure the result of osmotic disturbances in the gut, but the neurologic signs are unaccounted for. Also unexplained is the development of moderate anasarca in animals that survive for some days.

Indirect salt poisoning is a neurologic disease. There are circumstantial reasons for believing that it occurs in cattle and sheep and that it is occasionally responsible for PEM in these species, but *the disease is proven to occur only in swine*. Toxicity is related to the sodium ion; the clinical and pathologic features of this disease are not duplicated in any other.

Apparent blindness and deafness initiate the clinical syndrome in indirect salt poisoning in swine. The animal is oblivious to its environment and cannot be provoked to squeal. There is head pressing suggestive of increased intracranial pressure, arching, or pivoting, and these signs usually lead to the convulsive syndrome. The convulsions are very characteristic in their pattern and in the regularity of the time intervals in which they recur. They begin as tremors of the snout and rapidly extend as clonic spasms of the neck muscles with jerky opisthotonos that causes the pig to walk backwards and sit down. The animal passes into lateral recumbency and generalized clonic convulsions.

The lesions of this intoxication are restricted to the brain. There is moderate cerebral edema but no displacement. The basic changes in the brain are laminar loss of cortical neurons and laminar (middle laminae) malacia. These are the changes described earlier for PEM of cattle and sheep. The specificity of the lesion is given by the *abundance of eosinophils that are infiltrated into the meninges and Virchow-Robin spaces*. This particular lesion and its frequent relation to excessive intake of salt have been recognized for many decades, but until the cause was established, the syndrome was designated as "eosinophilic meningoencephalitis" on account of the relatively pure infiltrations of eosinophils that were found. Eosinophils tend to infiltrate in the meninges and perivascular spaces in the brains of pigs with other cerebral lesions, such as the leukomalacia of mulberry heart disease and various encephalitides, but *the combination of laminar change and cerebral eosinophilia is pathognomonic of salt poisoning*.

The amount of salt in the diets of pigs varies considerably, but toxicity does not occur if plenty of water is available. The critical level of salt in the fodder is approximately 2% when water intake is restricted. Signs of poisoning may occur when the water supply is replenished after a period of restriction.

Although excessive intake of salt over a period of several days sets the stage, which is reflected in elevated plasma levels of sodium and chloride, the disease is precipitated by water so that it may equally well be regarded as a *form of water intoxication*. Beyond this, the pathogenesis of the lesions remains obscure. It is noteworthy that they are anoxic in character and distribution.

Further reading

Senturk S, Huseyin C. Salt poisoning in beef cattle. Vet Hum Toxicol 2004;46:26-27.

Mycotoxic leukoencephalomalacia of horses

A neurologic syndrome occurs in horses fed moldy corn for ~1 month or longer. The neurologic signs are of fairly sudden onset and consist of drowsiness, impaired vision, partial or complete pharyngeal paralysis, weakness, staggering, and a tendency to circle. The course is from a very few hours to about a month, but death usually occurs on day 2 or 3. Recovery from clinical signs apparently does not occur; chronic cases with static signs are dummies.

The mycotoxin responsible is *fumonisin B1*, a product of *Fusarium verticillioides (Fusarium moniliforme)* and *F. proliferatum*, which grow on corn (maize) in warm moist conditions, circumstances in which outbreaks of the disease occur. Sporadic cases occur in circumstances involving moldy fodder. The neurologic disease occurs in donkeys and mules as well as in horses.

The neurologic signs described in the spontaneous disease are related to the encephalomalacia, which may be caused by fumonisin-induced microcirculatory damage as well as impairment of cardiovascular function. Fumonisin is also a competitive inhibitor of sphingosine N-acetyltransferase, leading to the accumulation of sphingosine and blocking the synthesis of sphingolipids. In the experimental disease and a small proportion of spontaneous cases, nervous signs may include mania rather than neurologic deficit; these dramatic cases may be icteric, and the nervous signs are those usual in the horse in acute hepatic failure. In natural and experimental cases, there may be *hepatic lesions* varying greatly in severity. The hepatic lesions, when present, are similar to those produced in other species by aflatoxin (see Vol. 2, Liver and biliary system).

The lesion usually described is *necrosis of the white matter of the cerebral hemispheres* (Fig. 4-69). The surface of the brain may be unaltered on inspection, but palpable softness may be detected in the cortex overlying large areas of leukomalacia. Grossly, there is no cerebral edema or brain swelling, although the overlying gyri might be slightly flattened and discolored. The foci of softening may be of microscopic dimensions, but usually they are readily visible on the cut surface. The softenings occur at random in the white matter of the cerebral hemispheres. They may be bilateral but are not necessarily symmetrical. The malacic foci are soft, pulpy, gray depressions distinct by virtue of numerous small hemorrhages in a peripheral zone of a few millimeters' breadth. Depending on the duration, there may be diffuse, yellow, edematous swelling of the adjacent white matter.

In small foci, and probably initiating them all, there is severe edema of the white matter. The white matter is spread apart by fluid, and the myelin sheaths, axons, and glia disintegrate to form a structureless, acidophilic, semifluid mass to which the microglia react. The edematous change is not confined to the cerebrum but is reported to occur in all parts of the spinal cord. Foci of softening also occur in the brainstem

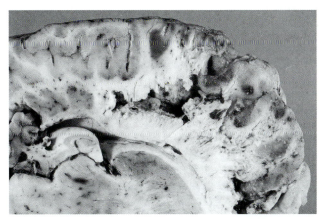

Figure 4-69 Irregular malacia and hemorrhage in cerebral hemisphere in a horse with **mycotoxic leukoencephalomalacia**. (Courtesy T.M. Wilson.)

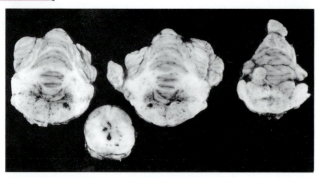

Figure 4-70 Focal hemorrhage and malacia in brain stem of a horse with **mycotoxic leukoencephalomalacia**. (Courtesy T.M. Wilson.)

and spinal cord, but here, in contrast with the brain, the necrosis affects the gray matter chiefly (Fig. 4-70).

Microscopically, *the areas of malacia are widely distributed and irregular in their form*, mainly in the white matter but a few small foci may be seen in the cortex. The irregular cavitations tend to surround and follow the course of the blood vessels, and there is edematous separation of tissue extending from the periphery of the cavitations. Cellular infiltrations, mainly of eosinophils but with some plasma cells, are present in the walls of vessels, in the perivascular spaces, and lightly in the edematous parenchyma. The adventitia of the vessels, especially in the brainstem, may be remarkably thickened. There is abundant lipofuscin pigment in macrophages.

Further reading

Smith GW, et al. Cardiovascular changes associated with intravenous administration of fumonisin B1 in horses. Am J Vet Res 2002;63: 538-545.

Lead poisoning

Lead is perhaps the most consistently important poison in farm animals. Poisoning is common and fatal in cattle; is less common but fatal in sheep; is occasionally observed in horses, dogs, and cats; and is rare in swine. The disease in cattle is probably always acute, whereas that in horses is virtually always chronic. The signs are almost exclusively neurologic even though the amount of lead deposited in nervous tissue is relatively small.

The usual sources of lead for cattle are *paint* and *metallic lead in storage batteries*. Adult cattle are most frequently poisoned at pasture by licking paint or putty cans from rubbish dumps. Calves are usually poisoned when from boredom or allotriophagia they lick painted pens, troughs, and so forth. Metallic lead does not reliably produce poisoning in ruminants under experimental conditions but frequently does so naturally, perhaps because the metal, when well weathered, contains soluble salts on its surface. Lead, chronically ingested, does accumulate in the tissues of ruminants, but it is not a cumulative poison in these species. Under conditions of chronic assimilation in ruminants, large amounts of lead may be stored in tissues, including the brain, without causing lesions or clinical disease. Cows have been shown to tolerate 2 g of lead daily for as long as 2 years without apparent harm. Sheep may accumulate large amounts of lead in the course of grazing over abandoned lead-mining areas that have been converted to pasture; the severe osteoporosis that may develop cannot be attributed to the accumulated lead, but may be related to copper deficiency.

The situation in horses is largely the reverse of that in ruminants because, in horses, lead poisoning is usually chronic. This probably represents, in part, species susceptibility, but is in part because of the manner of exposure in that horses are usually poisoned by prolonged inhalation of fumes from lead smelters or by prolonged ingestion of pastures contaminated by such effluent; such pasture exposure of course also occurs in cattle. Contaminated pastures may contain as much as 100-200 mg Pb/kg foliage.

Lead poisoning may occur in circumstances additional to those cited previously. Boiled linseed oil contains lead, and it is occasionally mistakenly used as a laxative for animals. Dogs have been poisoned by drinking gasoline that contains tetraethyl lead. Lead pipes may yield significant amounts of lead to soft water. Lead arsenate, widely used as an orchard spray, is commonly responsible for poisoning of cattle and sheep, but the signs and lesions refer largely to activity of the arsenate.

Lead is usually obtained by ingestion, but only a small proportion of the ingested dose is absorbed, something of the order of 1-2%, even of a soluble salt such as lead acetate. The limitation of absorption is due largely to formation of insoluble complexes in the alimentary tract. Absorbed lead is slowly excreted in bile, milk, and urine, and is deposited in tissues, especially in liver and kidneys in acute poisoning and in bones in chronic poisoning. The turnover of deposited lead is slow but continuous with gradual elimination in bile and urine; the half-life of lead in blood can range from months to years.

The *relative neurotropism of lead* is not well explained. Most metals exert their most deleterious effects at the sites of absorption and elimination, but lead largely spares these and affects nervous tissue with a high degree of specificity. Lead exerts toxicity by a number of mechanisms, including binding to calcium- and zinc-binding proteins, by random hydrolysis of nucleic acids, and by inducing RNA catalysis through activation of ribosomal 5S RNA, a natural leadzyme.

The various species differ in their sensitivity to lead, and the **clinical syndromes** produced also differ somewhat, although they are always chiefly neurologic. There seems to be remarkably little correlation between the doses of lead that will produce experimental poisoning and the very small amounts that induce toxicity naturally. Young animals are relatively more susceptible than adults.

The acute poisoning in *cattle* usually leads to death in 12-24 hours. Calves stagger, develop muscle tremors, and rapidly become recumbent. Convulsions are intermittent until death, and between convulsions, there is opisthotonos, muscular tremors, champing of the jaws, and hyperesthesia to touch and sound. Adults show less tendency to early recumbency. In these there is frenzy, head pressing, and apparent blindness, with death in convulsions. When the poisoning is less acute, cattle may survive for 4-5 days. They are dull and apathetic, apparently blind, and without appetite. There may be drooling, intermittent grinding of teeth, and hyperesthesia, but dullness and immobility predominate. Ruminal agony is fairly constant, and dark fetid feces may be passed terminally. Death occurs quietly or in convulsions or from misadventure. The manifestations of lead poisoning in sheep are similar to those of the subacute syndrome in cattle.

The disease in *horses* is paralytic. When horses ingest large amounts of lead, they develop severe depression and general paralysis, sometimes with clonic convulsions and abdominal pain. In chronic poisoning, usually known as *chronic plumbs*, the characteristic signs are those of specific nerve pareses affecting chiefly the cranial nerves and expressed particularly as laryngeal and pharyngeal paralysis. The clinical manifestations in dogs are also neurologic, but their pattern is not characteristic. There is anorexia, emaciation, mental irritability, muscular tremors, ataxia, and intermittent convulsions.

Specific **lesions** are not observed in lead poisoning in cattle. In cases that survive for 4-5 days, the ruminal contents may be foul because of immotility and the lower gut may contain a small volume of dark fetid feces, the color attributed to lead sulfide. There is no gastroenteritis, and any clinical signs of colic are probably related to nervous dysfunction. There may be mild degenerative changes in the parenchymatous organs, but these cannot be attributed to lead.

There is moderate brain swelling, but probably never severe enough to cause displacement and not often severe enough to be appreciated grossly. Even microscopically, the cerebral edema is not easy to appreciate or to distinguish from early autolytic change. The capillaries and venules are congested, and there may be petechial hemorrhages. The prominence of capillaries in the gray matter is due largely to congestion, but there may be some endothelial swelling and proliferation to make them more conspicuous. Neuronal changes are equivocal. In some subacute cases in which the course is prolonged for several days, there may be *laminar cortical necrosis*. The best explanations of laminar necrosis are still based on ischemia-anoxia, implying that lead is not directly neurotoxic in terms of neuronal injury. Indeed, lead tends not to accumulate in nervous tissue. The capillary alterations may therefore be of considerable functional importance and probably precede the swelling of glia. The capillary changes are best seen in thick sections stained by a Nissl stain and in the cerebellum better than in the cerebrum. In the cerebellum, the vascular lesion in the molecular and Purkinje layer is often accompanied by astrogliosis and microgliosis.

The histologic basis of the paralytic changes in lead poisoning in *horses* probably has the same basis as the peripheral neuropathy of chronic plumbs in man, in which the paralysis affects those muscles that are used most constantly and is caused by segmental degeneration of axons and myelin in the distal parts of motor fibers. In humans, the peripheral neuropathy of lead poisoning is purely motor.

In *dogs*, there is edema of the white matter of the brain and cord. Degenerative changes in myelin sheaths occur almost universally but are somewhat less severe in heavily myelinated tracts such as the optic tract, corpus callosum, and peduncles than in lightly myelinated areas, such as the deep white matter of the cerebellum and cerebrum. There is spongy degeneration in the subthalamus, head of the caudate nucleus, and deep cortical laminae, with extensive loss of neurons in such areas. Reaction on the part of astrocytes and microglia is slight.

Mild degenerative changes occur in the liver and kidneys of dogs chronically poisoned with lead, and can be overlooked in routine examinations. Most conspicuous is enlargement and vesiculation of the nuclei in the convoluted tubules. *Irregular, acid-fast, intranuclear inclusion bodies can be found in the renal tubules* in some cases. These inclusions are irregularly present in cases of lead poisoning, but when present, they have diagnostic value. They may develop in any species poisoned, but in dogs, they must be distinguished from the brick-like, acidophilic inclusions that can be present in the nuclei of renal tubules and hepatic cells. These inclusions are also acid fast, but have no specificity for lead poisoning and are present in the nuclei of apparently healthy dogs. In cattle, the degree of tubular epithelial degeneration is slight in most cases, but there is often a surprising degree of mitotic activity, and there may be severe nephrosis with extensive fibrosis in young calves.

The **diagnosis** of lead poisoning is necessarily chemical because lesions are either absent or nonspecific. Because of the variability of pathogenetic factors and species susceptibility discussed previously, precise figures cannot be given for the concentration of lead in tissues that can be regarded as indicating lead poisoning. As little as 4-7 μg lead/g liver has been found in horses dying of chronic intoxication. In cattle, levels of lead (on a wet-weight basis) of 40 μg/g or more in the kidney and 10 μg/g or more in the liver are accepted as confirmatory of lead poisoning.

Further reading

Bischoff K, et al. Declines in blood lead concentrations in clinically affected and unaffected cattle accidentally exposed to lead. J Vet Diagn Invest 2012;24:182-187.

Knight TE, Kumar MS. Lead toxicosis in cats—a review. J Feline Med Surg 2003;5:249-255.

Lemos RA, et al. Lead poisoning in cattle grazing pasture contaminated by industrial waste. Vet Hum Toxicol 2004;46:326-328.

Neurodegenerative diseases

There are some significant neurologic diseases in which dramatic clinical disturbances are not matched by equivalent morphologic alteration in nervous tissue. For example, *toxins that interfere with synaptic function can have fatal consequences*, yet leave neurons normal in appearance to routine examination. **Botulism, tetanus,** and **strychnine toxicosis** are well-known examples. In the latter 2 conditions, the release of spinal motor neurons from the inhibitory influence of "Renshaw cells" (inhibitory neurons) leads to the extensor spasms and hyperesthesia that characterize them. The activity of the inhibitory neurotransmitter glycine is blocked—in the case of tetanus by presynaptic blockade of its release and in the case of strychnine by postsynaptic blockade of its receptors. An inborn metabolic equivalent of these poisonings is *hereditary myoclonus*, in which there is an absence of glycine receptors on spinal motor neurons. The disease may occur in Poll Hereford calves, Peruvian Paso horses, Labrador Retriever dogs, and Merino lambs. In the Hereford disease, the calves are born normally, but suffer severe tetanic spasms on stimulation, are unable to stand, and are nonviable.

A distinctive locomotor disturbance in Australian sheep (Coonabarabran staggers, "cathead" staggers) has been associated with grazing of the zygophyllaceous plant *Tribulus terrestris*. The clinical disease is characterized by asymmetrical atrophy of pelvic limb extensor muscles, and irreversible asymmetrical paraparesis or tetraparesis without ataxia. There are no significant structural lesions in the nervous system. Evidence has been presented to suggest that the syndrome is caused by β-carboline alkaloids acting on dopaminergic upper motor neurons in the nigrostriatum. The long-term nature of the deficits may be the result of the ability of such compounds to form adducts with DNA sequences of genes associated with the synthesis of dopamine. Locomotor disturbances have also been documented in sheep and cattle grazing other zygophyllaceous plants in North America and Africa.

A large number of plant intoxications cause acute neurologic disease without morphologic alterations; **tremorgenic mycotoxicoses** are discussed later.

Inherited **spasticity syndromes** are described in cattle as "spastic paresis" and "spastic syndrome" and in Scottish Terriers as "Scotty cramp." Various inherited **myotonic syndromes** are referred to in Vol. 1, Muscle and tendon. The common **tetanic/paretic syndromes** that accompany hypocalcemia and hypomagnesemia are not associated with significant neural lesions.

This section will deal with noninflammatory diseases in which there is selective neuronal degeneration, involving either neurons in their entirety (**neuronopathies**) or restricted to axons (**axonopathies**). In reality, this division is somewhat arbitrary, as the axon is a wholly dependent part of any neuron, but the concept is useful for the classification of various diseases. *Neuronopathy* refers to degenerative changes and loss of neurons in specific neuroanatomic structures or in functionally related neuronal populations in different areas of the central nervous system (multisystem neuronal degeneration). *Axonopathy* is distinguished in 2 major morphologic patterns: (1) fragmentation of the axon and secondary demyelination (Wallerian-like degeneration), and (2) formation of axonal swellings (spheroids) in the white matter or in the gray matter when the dystrophic process occurs at the preterminal portion of the axon.

In general, when entire neurons or just their axons are lost in these circumstances, there are reactions by adjacent tissue elements but, as there is often minimal tissue loss overall, the predominant pathologic change is microscopic. At the end stage of severe chronic diseases, macroscopic atrophy may become evident (see Cytopathology of nervous tissue).

The diseases have been grouped into 3 categories of neuronopathies and axonopathies: "central," "peripheral," and "central and peripheral," according to the distribution of the lesions in the central and peripheral nervous systems. The choice of category for a particular disease is based on the predominant pattern of morphologic change seen in a typical case, and the criteria are not absolute. There will inevitably be some overlap and the naming and lesion topography of each may not necessarily be fully justified or complete. Some of the diseases are rare, and, because they are inherited, are highlighted by research workers aiming to use them as experimental model systems. New entities are progressively being identified. Sampling of the nervous system in diseases such as these should be as comprehensive as possible. The pattern and extent of lesions are important criteria in the diagnosis of known diseases, and in the documentation of new ones.

Further reading

Blignaut DJ, et al. Congenital reflex myoclonus in two Merino cross lambs in South Africa. Vet Rec 2011;169:24-31.

Osweiler GD. Mycotoxins. Vet Clin North Am Equine Pract 2001;17: 547-566.

Central neuronopathies and axonopathies

Cerebellar cortical degeneration. This group of diseases, also termed **cerebellar atrophy** or **abiotrophy,** refers to *premature or accelerated degeneration of formed neurons, presumably caused by some intrinsic metabolic defect*. The Purkinje cells appear particularly susceptible to spontaneous degeneration; there may be secondary depletion of granule cells, but other cortical layers are normal. In some conditions, *primary cerebellar granule cell degeneration* is recognized. Other forms are characterized by *combined degeneration of cerebellar cortical neurons and other systems*. Cerebellar atrophy occurs in dogs, cats, lambs, cattle, foals, and Yorkshire and Large White piglets.

Progressive *cerebellar cortical degeneration* is common in **dogs** and frequently an autosomal recessive mode of inheritance is suspected. In Finnish Hounds, a missense mutation in the *SEL1L* gene has been associated with an early-onset progressive cerebellar ataxia. Abiotrophic defects have been recorded in a variety of breeds, including Airedales, Gordon Setters, Rough-coated Collies, Border Collies, Beagles, Australian Kelpies, Bernese Mountain dogs, Irish Setters, Labrador Retrievers, Lagotto Romagnolos, Rhodesian Ridgebacks, Samoyeds, Old English Sheepdogs, English Bulldogs, Portuguese Podencos, Chow Chows, Scottish Terriers, Staffordshire Terriers, and Pit Bull Terriers. Clinical signs may have an early onset with rapid progression, as in Beagles, Samoyeds, and Irish Setters, or a later onset with slow progression, as in Old English Sheepdogs, Gordon Setters, American Staffordshire Terriers, and Pit Bull Terriers. The cerebellum may be normal in size and shape or slightly diminished in size and somewhat flattened. Microscopically, there is degeneration and loss of Purkinje cells and transneuronal retrograde degeneration of granule cells (see Fig. 4-27). The Purkinje cells degenerate, being either shrunken and hyperchromatic or pale, swollen and vacuolated (see Fig. 4-28); most disappear, leaving empty baskets and a fenestrated ground layer. In severely affected areas, there is gliosis in the molecular layer and proliferation of Bergmann astrocytes. The atrophic process may show evidence of regional predilection. In Gordon Setters, the dorsal portions of the median lobe and vermis are most severely affected, whereas in Collie dogs, selective involvement of the rostral folia of the vermis is reflected in macroscopic diminution of this area. Collateral changes in the subcerebellar nuclei are minor, but in this regard, it may be pertinent that affected dogs are usually euthanized shortly after the defect becomes apparent. In Scottish Terriers, the degeneration is significantly more pronounced in the dorsal portion of the vermis, and there is a conspicuous accumulation of polyglucosan bodies in the ventral half of the vermis. In some American Staffordshire Terriers and crossbreds, Purkinje cell degeneration is associated with intracytoplasmic accumulation of ceroid lipofuscin. An unusual disorder in Bernese Mountain dogs is characterized by progressive cerebellar and hepatic disease. Histologically, lesions are characterized by degeneration and depletion of Purkinje cells and vacuolation, degeneration, and nodular regeneration of liver tissue.

Primary degeneration of granule cell layer *(cerebellar granuloprival degeneration)*, with sparing of the other cerebellar cortex layers, has been reported in several canine breeds, including Brittany Spaniel, Italian Hound, Lagotto Romagnolo, Beagle, Border Collie, Bavarian Mountain dog, Australian Kelpie, and Labrador Retriever.

Nonprogressive cerebellar ataxia noted at 2 weeks of age is reported in Coton de Tuléar dogs. The disease, also known as **Bandera's neonatal ataxia**, is caused by a mutation of the *GRM1* gene, which encodes metabotropic glutamate receptor 1. A distinct, presumably immune-mediated, later-onset cerebellar ataxia of Coton de Tuléar puppies with granule cell degeneration also has been described.

Hereditary striatonigral and cerebello-olivary degeneration occurs in the *Kerry Blue Terrier* and *Chinese Crested dog*. Pedigrees of affected dogs indicate autosomal recessive inheritance. In Chinese Crested dogs, the disease is associated with a mutation of a gene which is homologous to the human *PARK2* gene. Mutations in human PARK2 cause autosomal recessive juvenile parkinsonism, which has clinical and pathologic similarities to this canine disease. Clinical signs begin between 9 and 16 weeks of age and are characterized by ataxia and dysmetria. *The inherent defect is neuronal degeneration*, and the brain changes follow a definite anatomic and temporal pattern of development. Degeneration and loss of Purkinje cells in the cerebellar cortex is evident at the onset of clinical signs. Subsequently, there is sequential involvement of the olivary nuclei, caudate nuclei and putamen, and finally the substantia nigra. In the cerebellar cortex, chromatolytic degeneration and loss of Purkinje cells is attended by astrocytosis involving Bergmann's glia and depletion of granule cells. In the cerebellar white matter and contained nuclei, there is status spongiosus and axonal swelling. Changes in the olivary nuclei, basal nuclei, and substantia nigra tend to be symmetrical and initially (see Fig. 4-29) feature neuronal degeneration, axonal swelling, spongiosus and fibrous astrocytosis, with progression to malacia, and cavitation. Olivary neurons undergo chromatolysis, whereas in the remaining nuclear structures, the nerve cells accumulate intracytoplasmic eosinophilic granules and undergo ischemic change.

Macroscopic evidence of the disease process in the cerebellum is limited to a modest degree of folial atrophy but, with progression of the condition, involvement of the basal and brainstem nuclei is manifest grossly by bilateral focal malacic lesions. Gross lesions are most severe in the caudate nucleus, which, after 7-8 months of clinical illness, may be reduced to numerous microcystic cavities. *It is proposed that the cerebellum and basal nuclei are the primary areas of involvement*, with the lesions in the olivary nucleus and substantia nigra being attributed to trans-synaptic neuronal degeneration along glutaminergic neurotransmission pathways.

Striatonigral and cerebello-olivary degeneration is not the sole cerebellar abiotrophy in which accompanying extracerebellar lesions may be found. Olivary nuclei may be affected in the Bernese Mountain dog, the cerebral cortex in the Miniature Poodle, and spinal Wallerian degeneration may be found in Rough-coated and Border Collies and in Merino sheep. In the Swedish Lapland dog, there is a neuronal abiotrophy involving Purkinje cells; however, the effects of this are overshadowed by motor neuron degeneration, and the disease is discussed later with others of that group.

A form of **olivopontocerebellar atrophy** has been reported in adult **cats**. The disease is characterized by loss of cerebellar cortical neurons, pontine nuclei, and olivary complex. Ubiquitinated nuclear inclusions, as characteristic of the human disease, are absent.

Late-onset progressive spinocerebellar degeneration is recognized in Brittany Spaniels between 7 and 14 years of age. Clinically, the disease is characterized by excessive hypermetria of the thoracic limbs ("saluting disease"), cerebellar ataxia, and intention tremors. Lesions include diffuse loss of Purkinje cells with massive neurofilament accumulation in degenerating neurons, and bilateral neuronal degeneration in the dorsal horns of the spinal cord and in the gracilis and cuneate nuclei, together with secondary axonal degeneration in the spinal cord.

Sporadic cases of various forms of juvenile and adult-onset cerebellar degeneration have been reported in **cats**. A **feline hereditary cerebellar cortical atrophy** has also been reported.

Cerebellar atrophy in **lambs,** which are commonly known as *daft lambs*, is reported from England and Canada. It is not restricted to any breed but is presumed to be inherited. The dams are normal. Affected lambs show signs of cerebellar dysfunction at birth, which include abnormalities of muscle tone, disorders of equilibrium, and tremors. The cerebellum is, however, normal in size and gross form. The histologic changes affect primarily the Purkinje and Golgi cells, and these especially in the median lobe. Degeneration and loss of these cells leave some empty baskets and a replacement astrogliosis. In the early stages of degeneration, the Purkinje and Golgi cells are shrunken and hyperchromatic or swollen and pale with cytoplasmic vacuolation. They ultimately undergo lysis and disappear, leaving a spongy zone between the granular and molecular layers. There is, simultaneously, a diminution in the population of granule cells. Regressive changes with gliosis may be apparent in the deep cerebellar nuclei and olives. A similar "daft lamb disease" has been described in newborn Corriedale and Drysdale lambs. A slowly progressive cerebellar disease, first manifested at 4-7 weeks of age, affects Wiltshire sheep in New Zealand. Cerebellar abiotrophy *(Yass ataxia)* occurs in fine-wool Australian Merino sheep aged 3-6 years. Lesions are diffuse vacuolation, shrinkage, and loss of Purkinje cells.

Bovine familial convulsions and ataxia is a heritable disorder of purebred and crossbred Aberdeen Angus cattle in the United Kingdom and New Zealand, and crossbred Hereford in Australia. The clinical syndrome is characterized by intermittent episodic seizures in newborn and young calves and by the gradual development of ataxia with spasticity and hypermetria in calves surviving bouts of seizures extending over 2-3 months. The distinctive microscopic change is Purkinje cell axonal swelling in the cerebellar granular layer. There is also degeneration and loss of Purkinje cells. An apparently similar disorder has been described in Charolais cattle in the United Kingdom, and a form with later onset of cerebellar signs has been reported in Angus cattle and their crossbred in Australia. A cerebellar cortical degeneration, almost exclusively affecting the Purkinje cells, has been described in Holstein calves in Brazil.

Cerebellar abiotrophy occurs in **horses,** particularly Arabian and part-Arabian horses, as well as in the Swedish Gotland pony and the American Miniature horse, and is an inherited, likely autosomal recessive, condition. In Arabian horses, the disease has been associated with a lowered expression of MUTYH, a DNA-repairing enzyme. Head tremors and ataxia develop in affected Arabian foals between birth and 6 months of age, as a result of loss of Purkinje cells and granule cells from the cerebellar folia. An additional finding in an American Miniature horse was degeneration of dorsal accessory olivary and lateral (accessory) cuneate nuclei and focal necrosis in the putamen.

Gomen disease is a cerebellar degeneration and ataxia of *horses in New Caledonia*. Some folial atrophy in the cerebellar vermis may be evident on gross examination. Microscopically, there is thinning of the cerebellar molecular layer and loss of Purkinje and granule cells. There is also considerable deposition of a pigment resembling lipofuscin in many of the surviving Purkinje cells as well as in the neurons of the brain and spinal cord. This material is also present in macrophages seen in areas where Purkinje cells are missing. The cause is unknown, but is thought to be an environmental toxin.

Further reading

Brault LS, et al. Mapping of equine cerebellar abiotrophy to ECA2 and identification of a potential causative mutation affecting expression of MUTYH. Genomics 2011;97:121-129.

Flegel T, et al. Cerebellar cortical degeneration with selective granule cell loss in Bavarian mountain dogs. J Small Anim Pract 2007;48:462-465.

Huska J, et al. Cerebellar granuloprival degeneration in an Australian kelpie and a Labrador retriever dog. Can Vet J 2013;54:55-60.

Kyöstilä K, et al. A SEL1L mutation links a canine progressive early-onset cerebellar ataxia to the endoplasmic reticulum-associated protein degradation (ERAD) machinery. PLoS Genet 2012;8: e1002759.

Urkasemsin G, et al. Mapping of Purkinje neuron loss and polyglucosan body accumulation in hereditary cerebellar degeneration in Scottish terriers. Vet Pathol 2012;49:852-859.

Zeng R, et al. A truncated retrotransposon disrupts the GRM1 coding sequence in Coton de Tuléar dogs with Bandera's neonatal ataxia. J Vet Intern Med 2011;25:267-272.

Multisystem neuronal degeneration of Cocker Spaniel dogs. In this condition, reported from Switzerland, **red-haired Cocker Spaniel** dogs of both sexes develop slowly progressive neurologic signs from about 6 months of age. The clinical picture is dominated by behavioral changes, disorders of gait and balance, tremors, and sometimes seizures. Ultimately, the severity of signs necessitates euthanasia. The cause remains undefined, but a genetic basis seems likely.

Neuropathologic changes are bilaterally symmetrical and involve loss of neurons, predominantly in the septal nuclei, globus pallidus, subthalamic nuclei, substantia nigra, tectum, medial geniculate nuclei, and cerebellar and vestibular nuclei. The neuronal loss is accompanied by gliosis and axonal spheroids. In addition, the white matter of the fimbriae of the fornix, central cerebellum, corpus callosum, thalamic striae, and subcallosal gyri have intense gliosis, axonal spheroids, loss of myelin, and perivascular macrophages.

Neuronal inclusion-body diseases. An acute neurologic disease of **Japanese Brown cattle** is described from the island of Kyushu, in which there is hyperexcitability, fever, profuse sweating, and usually sudden death. The cause is unknown, but cases recorded have all been in females.

There are no gross lesions of significance, but a large percentage of affected cattle have single, or sometimes multiple, *eosinophilic cytoplasmic inclusion bodies in large neurons of the midbrain, pons, and medulla*. The inclusions are mostly in the axon hillock region, are oval in shape and about 18 μm in greatest diameter. Ultrastructurally, they appear as sequestrations of degenerate mitochondria, with associated aggregations of rough endoplasmic reticulum and lipofuscin bodies. Neuronal cytoplasmic inclusions have been demonstrated in the CNS of humans dying with multi-system atrophy.

Neuronal intranuclear inclusions are reported in a **horse** suffering from progressive ataxia and motor deficiencies. The inclusions are composed of aggregates of filaments and fine granules, mainly in neurons of the brainstem and spinal cord. The disease shares some similarities with the analogous disease in humans.

Further reading

Pumarola M, et al. Neuronal intranuclear inclusion disease in a horse. Acta Neuropathol 2005;110:191-195.

Compressive optic neuropathy. Compression of optic nerves in the optic foraminae is a well-known manifestation of vitamin A deficiency in the calf and pig, resulting from stenosis of the foraminae. In poisoning by plants of the genera *Stypandra* and *Helichrysum* and by halogenated salicylanilides, the foraminae are of normal size.

These conditions are discussed fully under myelinopathies, but one usual feature of their pathology is *intense Wallerian degeneration of the optic nerves and tracts*, which may be the result of swelling and compression of the nerves within the optic canals. The acute phase of the lesion would be expected to show severe ischemic necrodegenerative changes involving all the nervous tissue elements localized within the optic canals, with acute axonal degeneration extending along the optic nerves, through the chiasm, and into the optic tracts of the midbrain. Retrobulbar segments of the optic nerves should be minimally affected. With the passage of time, the site of compression should exhibit malacic alterations, gitter cell infiltration, and astrogliosis, whereas the progression of Wallerian changes in the optic nerves and tracts should lead to extensive loss of myelinated axons and oligodendrocytes, with reactive astrogliosis. In the long term, retrograde degenerative changes lead to the loss of retinal ganglion cells and their axons, retinal atrophy, and gliosis.

Severe atrophy of optic nerves, in addition to compression of the cerebral hemispheres, cerebellar herniation, and craniofacial lesions, are described in *inherited osteopetrosis of Red Angus calves*.

Further reading

O'Toole D, et al. Neuropathology and craniofacial lesions of osteopetrotic Red Angus calves. Vet Pathol 2012;49:746-754.

Organomercurial poisoning. Mercurial compounds are cumulative poisons. The syndromes produced by the organic and inorganic salts are quite different, but the differences are probably not qualitative.

The toxicity of the organic salts depends on their solubility, and the syndrome produced depends on the size and chronicity of dosage. Poisoning by inorganic salts is expected to be by ingestion, but percutaneous absorption is possible. *Poisoning by inorganic mercury is quite rare in animals*. Acute toxicity following ingestion is characterized by severe abdominal pain, vomiting, and diarrhea caused by the coagulative effect of mercury in the lining of the gut. Death may occur in a few hours. If the animal survives the initial episode, death may occur several days later from nephrosis with uremia. At this stage, there may be ulcerative colitis because of the concentration of mercury in the colonic mucosa, by which route it is in part eliminated. Chronic cumulative poisoning probably does not occur in animals.

Mercurialism in animals is usually caused by the organic salts, such as ethyl mercury phosphate and mercury p-toluene sulfonanilide, which are applied to seed grains for the purpose of controlling fungal diseases of the germinating plants. Toxicity may not be manifested if the treated grain is consumed for a short period only. Chronic mercurialism occurs chiefly in swine and is occasionally observed in cattle, but is most unusual in other domestic species. The manifestations are almost solely neurologic. Mechanisms of organomercurial toxicity include inhibition of protein synthesis, disruption of microtubules, disturbance of neurotransmitter function, oxidative stress, and triggering of excitotoxicity mechanisms.

"Minamata disease" is a mercurialism of cats, birds, and man in the Minamata Bay area of Japan, associated with the eating of fish and shellfish from the bay. The fish contain large amounts of organomercurials, which probably spilled into the bay with industrial effluent. Similar environmental disease occurs in other countries.

The **clinical syndrome** of mercurialism in cattle closely resembles that of lead poisoning, but the signs, which are of sudden onset, may not occur for several weeks after the first of continuous exposures. Because degeneration of the conducting system of the heart is common, cardiac irregularities are to be expected. Signs may occur in swine as early as 15 days after being fed treated grain. There is loss of appetite, wasting, dullness, blindness, severe weakness, and incoordination, progressing rapidly until the animal can no longer stand. The dullness passes to coma, which may last for several days with intermittent episodes of clonic-tonic convulsions. Both swine and cattle may be moderately uremic.

Gross **lesions** are minimal. In both swine and cattle, the kidneys may be moderately swollen, pale, and wet, and in pigs there is often hydropericardium. Poisoned cattle have mild to moderate cerebral swelling and displacement. The cerebral cortices are soft and pale, and occasionally there is juxtasagittal venous infarction. The pallor of the cortex is visible on the cut surface so that there may be no clear distinction between gray and white matter; this change is irregular in distribution. Where the gray matter is distinct from the white, a narrow pallid band separating them may be visible. In swine, the dead white color of the cortex is often striking, especially when it is emphasized by the ischemia that may be present. The appearance of the 2 hemispheres may be different, that uppermost being pallid and ischemic and that of the side on which the animal is lying having congested meningeal veins. The brain is swollen and the gyri are flattened, although this is difficult to appreciate in pigs in which swelling is never severe.

Microscopically, there is *acute renal tubular injury* and *degeneration of the Purkinje network in the heart*. Degenerative changes are consistently present throughout the nervous system in both cattle and swine. They differ quantitatively from case to case but are qualitatively the same. The lesions are rather more rapidly catastrophic in cattle than in swine. There is *acute neuronal degeneration* of ischemic type and largely of ischemic distribution, the neurons of the middle laminae of the cerebral cortex being extensively injured. However, shrunken, acidophilic neurons can be found at all levels of the brain and cord and, with time, there is extensive cell loss from all cortical laminae. Moderate gliosis accompanies the neuronal degeneration and is expected to be most prominent in those areas of the cortical gray matter that, on gross inspection of the cut surface, are pallid. The *gliosis* is in part astrocytic and in part microglial. Compound granular corpuscles are not formed, the reactive microglia being prominently rod shaped. There is edema in the subjacent white matter. In swine, the edema leads in time to demyelination, but in this species, there is no softening.

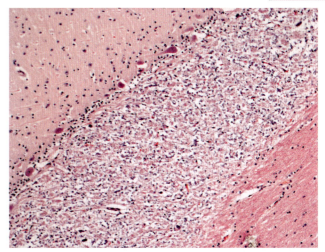

Figure 4-71 Organomercurial poisoning in an ox. Purkinje cell necrosis and degeneration in granular layer of cerebellar cortex. (Reprinted with permission from Mandara MT, et al. Neuropatologia e Neuroimaging. Milano: Poletto Editore, 2011.)

In cattle, the edema of white matter is more severe, and, in the multiform layer and middle laminae, frequently produces a spongy degeneration, which may be visible grossly. This occasionally leads to laminar necrosis in cattle.

In both cattle and swine, *fibrinoid necrosis of the media of leptomeningeal arteries* is quite characteristic. The change probably occurs in all cases, affecting both cerebral and spinal vessels, but it is well marked in a few cases only. Swine are more prone to the vascular lesions than are cattle. Accompanying the vascular lesions, there is an outpouring of much fibrin into the meningeal spaces.

Organomercurials appear rather selectively to damage the *granule cells of the cerebellum* in all species (Fig. 4-71). Cattle are more sensitive to this degeneration than are swine. In swine, the Purkinje cells remain fairly intact, but in cattle, they are often lost from about the tips of the folia. The degeneration of Purkinje cells is accompanied by microgliosis in the molecular layer and may be a response to swelling and pressure rather than a direct response to mercury.

Perhaps because the course is usually short in cattle, the spinal neurons are only mildly injured. In swine, there is often extensive ischemic necrosis of individual relay neurons. This, together with peripheral neuropathy, accounts for paralytic phenomena in swine. There is axonal degeneration and demyelination in peripheral nerves, the degenerative changes being more severe when the course is prolonged.

Further reading

Sanfeliu C, et al. Neurotoxicity of organomercurial compounds. Neurotox Res 2003;5:283-305.

***Solanum* poisoning.** Several of the many hundreds of species of the plant genus *Solanum* (family *Solanaceae*; nightshade family) are toxic to livestock by a variety of means. The disease of cattle in southern Africa, known colloquially as *maldronksiekte*, is associated with grazing *Solanum kwebense*. Affected animals show little abnormality at rest, but when moved, exhibit head tilt, muscle tremors, incoordination, and convulsions.

The brain at autopsy may show gross evidence of cerebellar atrophy, uniformly affecting all lobes. Histologically, there is diffuse loss of Purkinje cells, gliosis in the molecular layer, and atrophy of both molecular and granular layers. Surviving Purkinje cells are swollen, with strongly acidophilic cytoplasm, which contains numerous small "empty" vacuoles. Neurons elsewhere in the brain may show similar but far less intense vacuolation. Lamellated lipid material is stored in endoplasmic reticulum or lysosomes. Morphologically, the vacuolation is suggestive of a lysosomal storage process and, ultrastructurally, there are membranous cytoplasmic inclusions similar to those seen in the sphingolipidoses. The lectin-binding pattern is consistent with a glycolipid storage disease.

Similar signs and lesions in cattle have been associated with the grazing of *S. bonariensis* in Uruguay, *S. dimidiatum* in the United States, *S. fastigiatum* in Brazil, and in goats grazing *S. cinereum* in Australia and *S. viarum* in the United States.

Further reading

Porter MB, et al. Neurological disease putatively associated with ingestion of *Solanum viarum* in goats. J Am Vet Med Assoc 2003;223:501-504.

Van der Lugt JJ, et al. Cerebellar cortical degeneration in cattle caused by *Solanum kwebense*. Vet J 2010;185:225-227.

Romulea poisoning. Australian sheep grazing *Romulea rosea* (onion grass or Guildford grass)–infested pastures show limb paresis, fine head tremor, incoordination, and loss of equilibrium. Lesions include loss of Purkinje cells, gliosis, scattered vacuoles, and occasional swollen axons.

Further reading

Bourke CA, et al. Cerebellar ataxia in sheep grazing pastures infested with *Romulea rosea* (onion grass or Guildford grass). Aust Vet J 2008;86:354-356.

Cycad poisoning. The primitive palm-like plants of this family (genera *Cycas, Zamia, Bowenia, Macrozamia*) occur in tropical and subtropical environments, and have been associated with the intoxication of both people and animals. Cycad toxicity is proposed as a cause of the amyotrophic lateral sclerosis–parkinsonism–dementia complex in humans. The seeds and young fronds of cycads contain the toxic glycosides, *cycasin* and *macrozamin*, and, following ingestion, the hepatic metabolism of the aglycone, *methylazoxymethane*, may cause neuronal apoptosis and acute zonal hepatic necrosis.

In tropical Australasia, chronic exposure of cattle is associated with a neurologic syndrome known as "Zamia staggers." The syndrome is characterized by pelvic limb ataxia that may become severe. Pathologically, there is distal axonopathy in the spinal cord. The ascending fasciculus gracilis and dorsal spinocerebellar tracts have axonal degeneration most intense in the cervical segments, while the same is true of descending ventrolateral tracts (Fig. 4-72A-C). Typical Wallerian changes lead eventually to loss of myelinated axons and reactive astrogliosis.

Demyelination of the spinal cord and caudal brainstem following ingestion of *Xanthorrhea* spp. (grasstree, yacca) produces a distinctive type of incoordination, affected cattle lurching to one side, swinging laterally, and falling heavily to the ground.

Further reading

Albretsen JC, et al. Cycad palm toxicosis in dogs: 60 cases (1987-1997). J Am Vet Med Assoc 1998;213:99-101.

Yasuda N, Shimizu T. Cycad poisoning in cattle in Japan—studies on spontaneous and experimental cases. J Toxicol Sci 1998;23(Suppl. 2):126-128.

Tremorgenic neuromycotoxicoses. *Perennial ryegrass staggers* is a common mycotoxicosis in parts of Australia, New Zealand, and Europe, and is occasionally reported in the United States and southern Africa. Sheep, cattle, and horses may be affected. It occurs in the summer and autumn on dry, short pastures of *Lolium perenne*, and clinical signs appear 5-10 days following exposure. Animals develop fine head tremors and head nodding and weaving at rest and, if forced to move, have a stiff-legged, incoordinate gait, and are inclined to collapse in tetanic spasms, from which they recover quickly. There is low mortality, and total recovery will take place within 3 weeks of removal from toxic pasture. The disease is caused by indolic *lolitrems* produced by the endophytic fungus *Neotyphodium (Acremonium) lolii*. The toxins are known collectively as *tremorgens*.

There are no gross lesions in lolitrem toxicosis, and microscopic change is limited to the occurrence of fusiform enlargement of the proximal axons of some cerebellar Purkinje cells. These axonal swellings are known as *torpedoes* and represent a proximal axonopathy, but their relationship to the clinical signs is unclear, and they have not been reported in any other tremorgenic diseases. The axonal lesions are best demonstrated by the use of silver staining techniques, such as the Holmes method.

Other tremorgenic neuromycotoxicoses are described, in which lesions may be absent. *Claviceps paspali*, the ergot of *Paspalum*, produces tremorgenic paspalitrems that cause intoxication in cattle, occasionally in sheep, and rarely in horses. Tremorgenic mycotoxin intoxication occurs in dogs from penitrem A or roquefortine produced by *Penicillium* spp. and ingested in moldy food, and in horses consuming mycotoxins in dallis grass.

Further reading

Osweiler GD. Mycotoxins. Vet Clin North Am Equine Pract 2001;17:547-566.

Young KL, et al. Tremorgenic mycotoxin intoxication with penitrem A and roquefortine in two dogs. J Am Vet Med Assoc 2003;222:52-53.

Equine degenerative myeloencephalopathy. Equine degenerative myeloencephalopathy (EDM) is a *chronically progressive syndrome of symmetrical ataxia of unknown cause in equids* of several breeds and strains, including zebras. Predisposing factors include *vitamin E deficiency, hereditary predisposition*, inadequate exposure to green pasture, and possible exposure to wood preservatives or insecticides. A role for copper deficiency has not been substantiated. A familial hereditary pattern is recognized for Appaloosa, Standardbred, Paso Fino, and Lusitano horses with EDM.

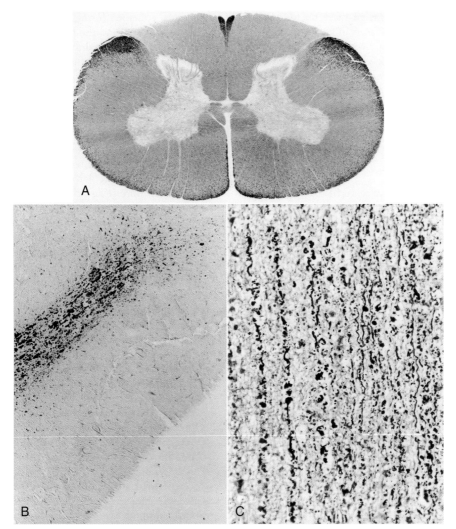

Figure 4-72 **Cycad poisoning** in an ox. (Courtesy M.D. McGavin and Pathologia Veterinaria.) **A.** C8. Symmetrical degeneration of myelin in fasciculus gracilis and dorsal spinocerebellar tracts as a result of distal "dying back" axonopathy. Marchi technique. **B.** Cerebellum. The black degenerated fibers in the white matter are part of the dorsal spinocerebellar tract. Marchi technique. **C.** Thoracic cord. Longitudinal section of fasciculus gracilis. Degenerated (black) and normal (gray) axons. Guillery axon stain.

The average age of horses at initial presentation is ~6 months, but may be as much as 24 months. The clinical presentation is dominated by disturbances of general proprioception and upper motor neuron function referable to the spinal cord, and thus closely resembles focal compressive myelopathy of the mid-cervical region. However, no skeletal or other gross lesions can be demonstrated.

Pathologically, there is evidence of *ongoing Wallerian degeneration and post-Wallerian astrogliosis in all funiculi throughout the spinal cord*, but concentrated in the ascending dorsolateral (spinocerebellar) and descending ventromedial (motor) funiculi of the cranial cervical and mid-thoracic segments. The changes are often most severe in the thoracic segments. Similar but mild changes are present in myelinated tracts of the caudal medulla and caudal cerebellar peduncles.

When well established in the thoracic cord segments, the process leads to considerable loss of myelinated axons and dense reactive astrogliosis that also involves the adjacent glia limitans. In some cases, the destructive process seems to reach an end point, with dense gliosis but little or no active Wallerian change. Chromatolytic and necrotic neurons, and axonal spheroids, can be found in Clarke's column (the nucleus of the dorsal spinocerebellar tract), which is located just dorsolateral and immediately adjacent to the central canal of the cord between the first thoracic and mid-lumbar segments. The disease involves total destruction of many neurons in this system, and macrophages containing a lipoidal pigment can also be found in this location. Lipofuscin pigment accumulation is also prominent in endothelial cells and neurons. Disruption of axonal transport likely plays a crucial role in the pathogenesis of dystrophic axons in EDM.

The origin of the degenerating descending axons in the ventromedial tracts is uncertain, and there have been no reports of neuronal degeneration in the midbrain nuclei likely to be the source of these fibers. It is possible that the descending tract lesion is purely an axonopathy. Axonal spheroids and vacuoles have also been described in the medial and lateral cuneate and gracilis nuclei of the caudal brainstem. These are the relay nuclei receiving the long ascending proprioceptive tracts of the spinal cord. However, even though this disease occurs in young horses, the changes in these nuclei may be nonspecific as they are commonly seen in a variety of situations, including animals with no overt clinical neurologic disease. In contrast to compressive cervical myelopathy (the wobbler syndrome), *there is simultaneous involvement in multiple cord segments of ascending* **and** *descending tracts.* This excludes focal compression of the cord as an etiologic factor. There is no obvious pathogenetic link between the various neuronal systems involved.

Further reading

Finno CJ, et al. Equine degenerative myeloencephalopathy in Lusitano horses. J Vet Intern Med 2011;25:1439-1446.

Sisó S, et al. Abnormal synaptic protein expression in two Arabian horses with equine degenerative myeloencephalopathy. Vet J 2003;166:238-243.

Axonal dystrophies. Diseases in which the pathology is characterized by axonal dystrophy, as described under Cytopathology of nervous tissue (see Figs. 4-9, 4-10), have been described in sheep, horses, dogs, and cats.

One of the earliest axonal dystrophies documented occurred in **Suffolk sheep.** In this disease, described in California, lambs normal at birth develop progressive ataxia at 1-6 months of age. The lambs eventually become recumbent after a course of 10-12 weeks. It is virtually certain that the disease is inherited and appears to be a recessive trait. There are no specific gross changes, and *the diagnostic histologic lesion is the presence of numerous axonal spheroids*, in and adjacent to several gray matter areas. The consistently affected areas are as follows: the entire spinal gray matter, with spheroids in greatest numbers at the base of the dorsal horns, in Clarke's column, and in the intermediolateral nuclei; the caudal brainstem nuclei, gracilis, cuneate, accessory cuneate, inferior olivary, lateral reticular, and lateral vestibular; the cerebellar roof nuclei, with the exception of the dentate; and the rostral colliculi and lateral geniculate nuclei. The spheroids are the focally swollen terminations of sensory axons, and represent a genuine axonal dystrophy. The pattern of lesions indicates the involvement of 2 sensory systems, one visual and the other proprioceptive and possibly exteroceptive, and the clinical signs could be accounted for by perturbation of the latter.

An identical condition has been described in **Coopworth, Romney,** and **Perendale sheep** in New Zealand, whereas in Australia, a disease in **Merino sheep** has been reported as an axonopathy, although the lesions described are consistent with axonal dystrophy. In this disease, as reported from localized areas of eastern Australia, sheep aged 1-4 years develop severe caudal gait abnormalities that are progressive and irreversible. Axonal spheroids are present in large numbers, predominantly in myelinated tracts in the midbrain and hindbrain and throughout the spinal cord, being more abundant in the dorsal funiculi than the ventral. Wallerian changes are mild. In the brain, areas of predilection are the cerebellar peduncles, transverse pontocerebellar fibers, dorsolateral thalamic tracts, cuneate fasciculus, median longitudinal fasciculus, and corticospinal tracts. Rather than being concentrated at terminal regions, the spheroids appear to be multiple along the course of individual axons. The cause remains undefined but seems likely to be a heritable defect. A distinct form has been described in **Merino sheep** with progressive ataxia at 3.5-6 years of age. Lesions are corticocerebellar abiotrophy and segmental spheroid formation in the white matter of the brain, spinal cord, and the peripheral nerves.

In horses, neuroaxonal dystrophy is thought by some investigators to be a localized form of equine degenerative myeloencephalopathy. Affected breeds include Morgans, Haflingers, and Quarter Horses. In the **Morgan horse,** a clinical syndrome of pelvic limb dysmetria and incoordination is accompanied by intense axonal dystrophy in the accessory cuneate nuclei. Breeding experiments suggest a familial component, but no definitive inheritance pattern has been demonstrated.

In **Haflinger horses,** a report describes an ataxia syndrome first evident at about 4 months of age, with ataxia in the pelvic limbs more severe by about 2 years of age. A familial hereditary basis is proposed. Neuroaxonal dystrophy was evident as numerous spheroids in the nuclei gracilis, cuneate, solitary tract and intermediomedialis, and in Clarke's column. These changes were accompanied by astrogliosis and lipofuscin pigmentation of neurons and macrophages, and significantly reduced serum tocopherol values. Mutations in the α-tocopherol transfer protein gene are not responsible for the development of the disease in the American Quarter Horse.

Canine diseases classified as axonal dystrophies have been described in a growing list of breeds, including Rottweilers, Collie Sheepdogs, Chihuahuas, English Cocker Spaniels, Jack Russell Terriers, and Papillons.

In the **Rottweiler,** neuroaxonal dystrophy is a *familial progressive sensory ataxia*, with a pattern of occurrence suggestive of autosomal recessive inheritance. Abnormal expression of various proteins leads to severe disruption of axonal transport in dystrophic axons. Neurologic signs may be expressed before 12 months of age, often being first noticed as abnormal clumsiness. With time, there is steadily progressing ataxia and distinct hypermetria, particularly in the forelimbs, in which there is also toe-dragging and knuckling. Mild head tremor and incoordination may also become evident. By 4-6 years of age, nystagmus, crossed-extensor reflexes, and a positive Babinski sign may be present, but dogs remain alert and responsive. Strength and conscious proprioception are maintained throughout, and the signs are related mainly to a disturbance of unconscious proprioceptive input to the cerebellum.

At autopsy, there may be mild patchy cerebellar atrophy, and the optic nerves appear small. The characteristic histologic feature is the presence of *massive numbers of axonal spheroids* (see Fig. 4-9A, B) in the nerve root entry zone of the dorsal horn throughout the spinal cord; in the vestibular, lateral, and medial geniculate, and sensory trigeminal nuclei; and in Rexed's laminae of the spinal cord. Fewer spheroids are present in the inferior olivary, trochlear, and oculomotor nuclei, and in the spinal cord ventral horn. Occasional spheroids are found in the globus pallidus, hippocampus, thalamus, hypothalamus, caudate nucleus, and reticular substance. In the cerebellum, lesions are concentrated in the vermis. Spheroids are present in the granular layer, white matter, and roof nuclei. There is some loss of Purkinje and granule cells.

Affected **Collie Sheepdogs** have progressive ataxia and gait abnormalities first apparent at 2-4 months of age. The disease is strongly suspected to be inherited as an autosomal recessive trait. The lesions are purely microscopic and confined to the deep cerebellar and vestibular areas. Many axonal spheroids are present in the central cerebellar white matter and adjacent roof nuclei, and in the lateral vestibular nuclei. Wallerian degeneration is minimal and the cerebellar cortex unaffected.

In the **Chihuahua** and **Papillons,** affected animals are normal until about 7 weeks of age, when there is sudden onset of tremor and gait disturbances. The pathogenesis remains undefined. Large numbers of axonal spheroids are present in the white matter of the internal capsule, cerebellum, lateral geniculate nucleus, rostrodorsal thalamus, acoustic tubercle, olivary nuclei, and the corticospinal and spinothalamic tracts.

In the **Scottish Terrier,** a central axonopathy associated with whole body tremor and ataxia at the age of 10-12 weeks has been described. Dystrophic axons are prominent in the brainstem, thalamus, cerebellum, and cerebral white matter. In the spinal cord, axonal damage involves the lateral and ventral columns.

In **English Cocker Spaniels** with primary metabolic vitamin E deficiency and retinal pigment epithelial dystrophy, axonal spheroids are found in the sensory relay nuclei of the brainstem.

In the **cat,** several axonal dystrophies have been reported. A γ-aminobutyric acid (GABA)ergic neuroaxonal dystrophy occurs in *feline Niemann-Pick disease type C*, an autosomal recessive lysosomal storage disease. An *autosomal recessive hereditary condition* has been as described in domestic shorthaired cats in association with an unusual lilac coat color. Clinical signs first become evident at 5-6 weeks of age as head bobbing. In the ensuing 8-10 weeks, there is progressively worsening ataxia, and possibly visual impairment and vestibular deficits. The process may then stabilize, and animals may survive to adulthood, but are poorly grown. Gross neuropathologic change is confined to slight cerebellar atrophy, most obvious in the caudal vermis. Histologically, there are numerous spheroids in the inferior olivary and lateral cuneate nuclei. Lesser numbers of spheroids are in the lateral midbrain tegmentum, lateral and rostral ventral thalamic nuclei, and the cerebellar vermis. An additional feature is diffuse swelling of axons in the above locations and in the medial lemniscus, medial longitudinal fasciculus, central tegmental tract, and spinal nerve dorsal roots. Neuronal loss and gliosis can be found in the inferior olivary and lateral thalamic nuclei, and in the Purkinje and granule cell layers in the cerebellar vermis. Spheroids and neuronal loss are also evident in the spiral ganglion and organ of Corti in the inner ear.

Further reading

Finno CJ, et al. Pedigree analysis and exclusion of alpha-tocopherol transfer protein (TTPA) as a candidate gene for neuroaxonal dystrophy in the American Quarter Horse. J Vet Intern Med 2013;27:177-185.

Jolly RD, et al. Segmental axonopathy of Merino sheep in New Zealand. N Z Vet J 2006;54:210-217.

Resibois A, Poncelet L. Purkinje cell neuroaxonal dystrophy similar to nervous mutant mice phenotype in two sibling kittens. Acta Neuropathol (Berl) 2004;107:553-558.

Multisystem axonal degeneration. This section includes neurodegenerative conditions characterized by *Wallerian-like degeneration of the white matter of the CNS*, as described under Cytopathology of nervous tissue. Diseases have been reported in dogs, cats, and cattle. *Inherited central axonopathy* has been described in **Smooth-haired Fox Terriers, Jack and Parson Russell Terriers,** and **Ibizan Hounds.** Degenerative changes of spinocerebellar tracts of the cervical spinal cord are associated with presence of spheroids in the central auditory pathways. A missense mutation in the *CAPN1* gene, which encodes an intracellular calcium-dependent cysteine protease (a member of the calpain family), has been identified in Parson Russell Terriers.

In **Labrador Retriever** axonopathy, there is extensive involvement of the spinal cord and cerebellum, in addition to aplasia or hypoplasia of the corpus callosum and loss of olivary neurons.

The first clinical sign of *progressive degenerative myeloencephalopathy* of **Brown Swiss cattle**, known colloquially as *weaver syndrome,* is slight ataxia, appearing at 5-8 months of age and worsening progressively over the ensuing 12-18 months. At the advanced stage, there is severe truncal ataxia and pelvic limb dysmetria, with distinct proprioceptive deficits. This terminates in recumbency with its secondary complications. The condition is inherited as a simple autosomal recessive trait; the weaver gene is closely associated with a microsatellite locus for milk production on bovine synteny group 13.

The major and primary lesion is in the spinal cord white matter. At all stages of the disease, there is *active axonal degeneration, with both axonal lysis and spheroid formation*. Axonolysis imparts an appearance of status spongiosus to affected white matter, and advanced lesions have myelin loss and moderate gliosis. The axonopathy is present in both ascending and descending tracts at all levels of the cord, but is most severe in the thoracic segment. The process may begin in the thoracic segment and extends anterograde and retrograde from this site. Ultrastructural changes indicate disturbed axoplasmic transport and subsequent axonal degeneration. Mild axonal lesions of a similar character occur in the brainstem, but are inconsistent in their location. However, a consistent additional lesion is degeneration and loss of Purkinje cells from the cerebellar cortex.

A series of cases of *congenital axonopathy* of **Friesian/Holstein calves** is described from Australia, in which animals were recumbent from birth and exhibited spastic paresis and a variety of other neurologic signs. The characteristic microscopic lesion is *active Wallerian degeneration in all funiculi throughout the spinal cord,* especially at the periphery. Similar changes are evident in the cerebellar peduncles, the median longitudinal fasciculus, spinocerebellar and rubrospinal tracts, and in the roots of cranial nerves III, V, VII, and VIII. In a few cases, mild degeneration occurs in the midbrain and some peripheral nerves. The Wallerian changes are accompanied by a very mild glial response, and it is likely that the disease begins in utero shortly before birth. The pathogenesis is unknown, and an autosomal recessive trait is suspected.

Inherited progressive spinal myelopathy of **Murray Grey** calves breed in Australia may afflict animals at birth, or not become expressed until ~12 months of age. The clinical syndrome is one of spinal ataxia, manifested as incoordination of the pelvic limbs and lateral swaying of the hindquarters at rest. A consistent sign is collapse of one hindlimb, with a tendency to fall to one side. These pelvic limb deficits are progressive and lead to increasing impairment. A similar condition is reported in **Simmental** calves.

The characteristic lesions are microscopic only, symmetrical, and consistently occur in the *lateral and ventral funiculi throughout the spinal cord*. There is an axonopathy associated with deficit of myelin in the lateral funiculi beneath the dorsal root entry zone, and in ventral funiculi adjacent to the ventral median fissure. In some cases, the fasciculi gracilis and cuneatus are also involved. The process appears to involve ballooning degeneration of myelin sheaths, which may impart a distinctly spongy appearance to the lesion. The progressive loss of myelin is not accompanied by large numbers of myelinophages, and Wallerian degeneration is minimal. There is substantial astrogliosis and thickening of the glia limitans.

In the brain, similar lesions may be found in the spinocerebellar tracts, tectospinal tracts, and medial longitudinal fasciculus. Some neurons undergoing central chromatolysis are present in ventral spinal gray matter, Clarke's column, the red nuclei, lateral vestibular nuclei, reticular formation, and cerebellar roof nuclei.

A translationally silent variant in the mitofusin 2 gene *(MFN2)* is associated with a form of degenerative axonopathy in Tyrolean Grey cattle.

Further reading

Drögemüller C, et al. An unusual splice defect in the mitofusin 2 gene (MFN2) is associated with degenerative axonopathy in Tyrolean Grey cattle. PLoS ONE 2011;6:e18931.

Forman OP, et al. Missense mutation in CAPN1 is associated with spinocerebellar ataxia in the Parson Russell Terrier dog breed. PLoS ONE 2013;8:e64627.

Rohdin C, et al. New aspects of hereditary ataxia in smooth-haired fox terriers. Vet Rec 2010;166:557-560.

Central and peripheral neuronopathies and axonopathies

Organophosphate poisoning. The toxicity of organophosphates (OPs) is based on their ability to phosphorylate and inactivate a number of esterases for which they can act as substrates. The acute inactivation of acetylcholinesterase is a well-known effect, exploited for pesticidal and anthelmintic purposes. Our concern here is with *delayed neurotoxicity* that follows 2-25 days after exposure and that involves the inactivation of esterases within neurons. Inactivation of esterases tends to be irreversible, and recovery depends upon synthesis of new enzyme, and this will vary with the compound and the particular enzyme(s) inactivated. There is also wide individual and species variability in sensitivity to neurointoxication. OPs are derivatives of phosphoric, thiophosphoric, and dithiophosphoric acids, and are used not only as poisons but also in industrial applications in hydraulic systems, as high-temperature lubricants, and as plasticizers. Delayed neurotoxicity, which may be induced by OPs that have no acute effect on acetylcholinesterase, is particularly a property of the *arylphosphates*, the best known being *triorthocresyl phosphate* (TOCP).

The clinical presentation is characterized by the onset of ataxia, weakness and proprioceptive deficits, and ultimately paralysis. Severe dyspnea and loss of vocalization are often present in cattle and pigs, and hypomyelinogenesis is described in piglets and laryngeal nerve degeneration in horses given organophosphate anthelmintics.

The pathology and pathogenesis of delayed OP intoxication have been studied quite thoroughly. OPs are not cumulatively toxic, but a single threshold dose will induce central and peripheral distal axonopathy. *Multifocal degenerative changes develop in distal regions of axons,* with accumulations of organelles in the regions of proximal paranodes producing marked swellings. Axonolysis then follows, and there may be cycles of attempted regeneration and further degeneration. In peripheral nerves, these changes are most intense in the intramuscular segments, and involvement of the recurrent laryngeal nerves makes *aphonia* a prominent sign in many cases. In the CNS, axonal degeneration is focused at the distal extremities of the long descending and ascending spinal tracts. The picture is dominated by axonal swellings, microcavitation, and secondary myelin loss. Neuronal chromatolysis can be observed in the brainstem and spinal cord.

Further reading

Coppock RW, et al. A review of nonpesticide phosphate ester-induced neurotoxicity in cattle. Vet Hum Toxicol 1995;37:576-579.

Coyotillo poisoning. The coyotillo or buckthorn shrub, *Karwinskia humboldtiana*, is indigenous to the southwestern United States, Mexico, and Central America, and its fruits are toxic to many species, including humans. The neurotoxin present in the fruit is *tullidinol*. Goats are most commonly affected, and intoxication is first manifested as hyperesthesia, which is followed by ataxia, gait abnormalities, and weakness, with signs developing over a couple of weeks. If the polyneuropathy is mild, recovery may occur.

Pathologically there is a *severe, predominantly motor, distal peripheral axonopathy* that appears to be the major pathologic event, although there is significant segmental demyelination as well. Denervation atrophy becomes apparent in skeletal muscle. In the CNS, numerous swellings may develop in the proximal axons of cerebellar Purkinje cells, appearing in the granule cell layer and the folial white matter. Swollen axons may also be found in the lateral and ventral funiculi of the spinal cord.

Further reading

Munoz-Martinez EJ, et al. Depression of fast axonal transport in axons demyelinated by intraneural injection of a neurotoxin from *K. humboldtiana*. Neurochem Res 1994;19:1341-1348.

Mesquite toxicosis in small ruminants. Various species of mesquite *(Prosopis)* are widespread on rangeland in the southwestern United States, Mexico, and Central and South America. Goats are more likely to be exposed, given their browsing habits. Ingestion of the leaves, pods, and seeds of *Prosopis glandulosa* (honey mesquite) and *P. juliflora* (velvet mesquite) can cause mandibular tremors, tongue protrusion, drooling, dysphagia, and weight loss resulting from selective toxicity to cranial nerve nuclei. Histologic lesions consist of fine vacuolation of the perikaryon of neurons in the trigeminal nuclei and occasionally the oculomotor nuclei. Wallerian degeneration occurs in the mandibular and trigeminal nerves, with resultant denervation atrophy of muscles that they innervate.

Further reading

Tabosa IM, et al. Neuronal vacuolation of the trigeminal nuclei in goats caused by ingestion of *Prosopis juliflora* pods (mesquite beans). Vet Hum Toxicol 2000;42:155-158.

Washburn KE, et al. Honey mesquite toxicosis in a goat. J Am Vet Med Assoc 2002;220:1837-1839.

Aspergillus clavatus **toxicosis.** An acute clinical syndrome of cattle and sheep has been reported from several countries associated with a mycotoxicosis caused by *Aspergillus clavatus*. Most outbreaks are caused by fungal growth on industrial organic waste or stored products or by plants grown in hydroponics. The fungus is known to produce a variety of toxic metabolites, including patulin, kojic acid, cytochalasins, and tremorgenic mycotoxins. The toxic syndromes observed in animals are suggested to result from synergistic action of these toxins. The clinical syndrome is dominated by acute onset of drooling and ataxia that progresses to recumbency and death. The neuropathology is characterized by *acute central chromatolysis of neurons* in the red and vestibular nuclei, and in spinal ventral horn gray matter and ganglia. Some neurons contain intracytoplasmic vacuoles. Wallerian degeneration and myelin edema are evident in all tracts of the spinal white matter.

Further reading

McKenzie RA, et al. *Aspergillus clavatus* tremorgenic neurotoxicosis in cattle fed sprouted grains. Aust Vet J 2004;82:635-638.

Sabater-Vilar M, et al. Patulin produced by an *Aspergillus clavatus* isolated from feed containing malting residues associated with a lethal neurotoxicosis in cattle. Mycopathologia 2004;158: 419-426.

Arsenic poisoning. Animals may be poisoned by arsenic by ingestion or percutaneous absorption, the toxic dose by the latter route being considerably less than the toxic oral dose. The commonest sources of arsenic are fluids used as insecticides and herbicides. Most arsenical dips and sprays for animals contain sodium arsenite and, after these operations, a considerable but nontoxic amount of arsenic is absorbed through the skin. Percutaneous absorption is increased if the animals are hot at dipping and kept hot afterward, and if they are not allowed to dry quickly. Absorption is rapid through shear wounds and through hyperemic skin, such as of the thighs and scrotum of rams in the breeding season. Local high concentrations of arsenic on the skin also cause local acute dermatitis.

Herbicides of most importance are those containing *sodium arsenite*, *lead arsenate*, and *arsenic pentoxide*, and poisoning occurs usually when animals get access to recently contaminated pasture. A variety of mistakes and accidents commonly expose animals to these compounds. Paris green (cupric acetoarsenite), used as poison for grasshoppers and other parasites of plants, is occasionally responsible for poisoning. Ore deposits frequently contain large amounts of arsenic, and chronic arsenical poisoning can occur when pasture and drinking water are contaminated by the exhaust from smelters.

The toxicity of arsenicals varies considerably, depending on the solubility of the salt and, in the case of organic arsenicals, on the rate at which the arsenic is released from organic bondage. The syndromes of arsenic poisoning differ according to acuteness or chronicity and also according to whether the arsenic is organic or inorganic, but these latter differences are probably not qualitative. One, and perhaps the main, *mechanism of action of arsenicals is combination with, and inactivation of, sulfhydryl groups*, resulting in general depression of metabolic activity. The organs most susceptible to metabolic decline are the brain, lungs, liver, kidney, and alimentary mucosa. In poisoning by inorganic arsenic, the pattern of signs and lesions is the same regardless of the route of absorption, thus indicating that, although alimentary tract signs may dominate the clinical disturbance, they are part of the systemic intoxications. In poisoning by organic arsenic, which is observed in pigs, the signs are referable entirely to the nervous system.

The ingestion of very large amounts of a soluble **inorganic arsenical** may result in death in <24 hours. There is profound depression and peripheral circulatory collapse; at postmortem in such cases, there are usually no lesions, or at most, slight edema of the abomasum.

With poisoning of lesser severity, 1-2 days lapse between the ingestion of arsenic and the onset of clinical signs. The onset is sudden, with acute abdominal distress, nervous depression, circulatory weakness, and, after some hours, terminal diarrhea and convulsions. Some cases may survive for several days and show additional neuromuscular signs of tremor and incoordination. In chronic poisoning, the signs are nonspecific, being those of unthriftiness, capricious appetite, and loss of vigor. Pregnant cows may abort. Visible mucous membranes and the muzzle may be hyperemic and inflamed.

Lesions produced by *acute poisoning by inorganic arsenicals* can be largely explained on the basis of *vascular injury*. There is splanchnic congestion with petechial hemorrhages of serous membranes. The mucosa or submucosa of the stomach or abomasum is intensely congested, and the abomasal plicae are usually thickened by edema fluid. There are intramucosal and submucosal hemorrhages of patchy distribution, and these lead quickly to more or less extensive ulceration of the stomach and intestine. The intestinal content is very fluid and may contain shreds of mucus and detritus. There is mild, usually fatty, degeneration of the parenchymatous organs, sometimes with hepatocellular necrosis and edema of the kidney. Lesions in the brain develop in the course of 3-4 days and consist of moderate diffuse cerebral edema and petechiation. The hemorrhages, which are of capillary type and apparently the result of necrosis of the walls of these vessels, are distributed throughout the white matter.

The anatomic changes in *chronic arsenical poisoning* have the same distribution as in the acute poisoning. The stomach and gut remain mildly congested, edematous, and ulcerated, and there are prominent fatty changes in the heart, liver, and kidneys. Neural lesions may not be found in the CNS except for those changes that are secondary to peripheral neuropathy. In both sensory and motor components of peripheral nerves, there is degeneration of myelin and axons.

The application of arsenic to the skin may cause acute and chronic dermatitis if cutaneous circulation is poor, but if the circulation is good, the arsenic tends to be absorbed and to cause systemic rather than local toxicity. Dermatitis, when it develops, is characterized by intense erythema, necrosis, and sloughing; the residual ulcerative lesions are indolent.

Organoarsenical phenylarsonic acid derivatives are commonly used as feed additives for swine, for growth promotion and the control of enteric disease. Poisoning is thus largely confined to this species, and is caused by accident or careless management; however, the margin of safety can be quite low when arsanilic acid is used to control swine dysentery. Two syndromes are recognized, caused by p-aminophenylarsonic acid **(arsanilic acid),** and 3-nitro-4-hydroxyphenylarsonic acid **(3-nitro).**

In *arsanilic acid poisoning*, there is usually acute onset of cutaneous erythema, hyperesthesia, ataxia, blindness, vestibular disturbances and, terminally, muscular weakness. There are no gross neural lesions, but microscopically, mild edema of the white matter may be present in the brain and spinal cord, and a few shrunken and degenerate neurons in the medulla. Extensive Wallerian degeneration frequently develops in the optic and peripheral nerves, but may not be present in spite of severe clinical signs.

In *3-nitro poisoning*, there is a syndrome of repeated clonic convulsive seizures following exercise, with progression to paraplegia, but no blindness. Pathologically, there is Wallerian-like degeneration in the spinal cord characterized by fragmentation and loss of axons and complete destruction of myelin sheaths, associated with glial proliferation. The lesion is intense in the dorsal proprioceptive and spinocerebellar tracts of the cervical segment and, as the toxicosis progresses, in the lateral and ventral funiculi of the lumbar spinal cord. Optic and peripheral neuropathy are mild.

Further reading

Neiger R, et al. Bovine arsenic toxicosis. J Vet Diagn Invest 2004;16: 436-438.

Neonatal copper deficiency (swayback, enzootic ataxia). It is generally accepted that maternal/fetal copper deficiency is a major factor in a characteristic neurologic disease of lambs, goat kids, and piglets. The syndrome has been most studied in the lamb, and the terms *"swayback"* and *"enzootic ataxia,"* used to describe the signs shown by affected animals, are entrenched as names for the disease. The provision of adequate copper supplementation of pregnant animals at risk can effectively eliminate the disease in their offspring, and treatment of affected animals with copper may produce some remission of signs. Supplementation of unaffected lambs at risk has also been claimed to be effective in prevention. Other manifestations of copper deficiency, such as "steely wool," osteoporosis, and hypopigmentation of black wool, could be expected in affected sheep flocks.

The bioavailability of and physiologic requirement for copper are influenced by many factors, and a functional deficiency state is often determined by overall availability rather than actual copper intake. Thus there may be *absolute primary deficiency*, or *conditioned secondary deficiency*, brought about by reduced absorption from the gut, reduced availability in tissues, or enhanced excretion. The interactive roles in copper metabolism of soil and dietary molybdenum, sulfate, iron, and zinc are important. *Molybdenum* is a prime antagonist for copper and, in the presence of adequate sulfate, limits the capacity to absorb copper from the gut and the capacity to store absorbed copper in the liver. This antagonism is unique to ruminants and is provided by the formation in the rumen of *thiomolybdates*, a series of anions in which sulfur progressively substitutes for oxygen in the molybdate ion. Copper complexed to thiomolybdate forms insoluble complexes that are poorly absorbed; this is primarily an effect of maximally substituted tetrathiomolybdate; lesser substituted thiomolybdates may be absorbed and be responsible for reducing copper availability at the local tissue level.

Iron is an antagonist to copper, although the mechanism is not known. Experimental exposure of ruminants to high intakes of iron induces severe hypocupremia, but a role for iron in naturally occurring copper deficiency syndromes is not of known importance.

Copper is required for the catalytic activity of enzymes that are essential for neural function and include tyrosinase for melanin synthesis, cytochrome oxidase for electron transport in mitochondrial respiration, copper/zinc superoxide dismutase for antioxidant activity, dopamine hydroxylase for catecholamine synthesis, and ceruloplasmin for iron homeostasis. Other copper-containing enzymes, such as lysyl oxidase, are important in animal disease, but anomalous relationships between copper analyses and actions and the occurrence of prenatal and neonatal disease suggest that there are as yet unidentified enzymes or functions required for developing lambs and kids.

Species and breed differences, pregnancy, plant/soil relationships, fiber content of the diet, and seasonal conditions will govern nutritional requirements. Aspects of copper metabolism differ significantly between sheep and goats. It is also possible that undefined factors may bear significantly on metabolic availability. In spite of this, the copper content of CNS tissue in affected neonates tends to be consistently below normal values, and represents the most reliable tissue assay. It is also true that some individuals with similarly low copper values can be clinically normal, although this holds more for goat kids and piglets than lambs. As the ability to metabolize copper is not impaired, tissue concentrations in affected animals may return to normal fairly rapidly after dietary correction, with concentration in the liver recovering more rapidly than in the CNS.

The effects of copper deficiency on the CNS occur in utero and during early neonatal life. Despite intensive investigation, the biological role of copper in the developing nervous system remains unclarified and contentious. Copper is a component of the enzymes cytochrome oxidase and superoxide dismutase, and of the protein ceruloplasmin. Interference with the functions of these has variously been proposed as the molecular basis of the disease via suppression of mitochondrial respiration and phospholipid synthesis or via damage inflicted by superoxide radicals. It should be added that lambs with no clinical signs have been found to have neuronal degenerative lesions, and lambs with clinical signs have minimal lesions.

Clinical swayback in lambs occurs in a congenital form and a delayed form, also called "enzootic ataxia" in which, after being normal at birth, lambs suddenly develop signs at any time between 1 week and several months of age. The clinical signs are characterized by severe ataxia progressing to recumbency and death. Congenital cases may be blind and unable to stand.

Some lambs with *congenital swayback* have an extensive structural lesion grossly evident in the *cerebral white matter*, but all have some degree of the neuronal degenerative changes described later for the delayed disease. The former lesion is bilateral and symmetrical gelatinous softening or cavitation (Fig. 4-73; see Fig. 4-24A), which may be restricted to the

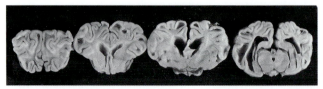

Figure 4-73 Bilaterally symmetrical cavitation of cerebral white matter in **swayback** in a lamb. (Reprinted with permission from Innes JRM, Saunders LZ. Comparative Neuropathology. New York: Academic Press, 1962.)

occipital pole or may involve the entire corpus medullare, sparing only a thin rim of white matter adjacent to gray. Histologic and ultrastructural descriptions of the gelatinous lesion are meager, but marked edema with mild fibrillary astrogliosis and a paucity of myelin can be expected. Some myelin degradation products are usually present, but never in great quantity, and gitter cells are sparse. It seems likely that many axons are initially spared, but that rapid dissolution of all elements leads to cavitation. The pathogenesis of this lesion remains obscure; it seems that both hypomyelination and demyelination may be involved, but the basis of the tissue lysis is unexplained.

Although lambs with *delayed swayback* do not have lytic lesions in the cerebral white matter, they consistently have changes in both gray and white matter in other parts of the neuraxis. Most investigators consider that these changes largely develop and progress after birth, but this is not absolute, as pointed out previously. Extensive Wallerian degeneration is concentrated in dorsolateral and ventromedial tracts throughout the spinal cord. *The pattern of tract degeneration is suggestive of a distal axonopathy.* In addition, conspicuous degenerative changes are present in neurons in the red, lateral vestibular, medullary reticular, and dorsal spinocerebellar nuclei in Clarke's column, and in the spinal motor neurons, particularly in the intumescences (see Fig. 4-1). Many such neurons are undergoing central chromatolysis, and some have nuclear rhexis and lysis. A few may be undergoing neuronophagia. Swollen neurons have been shown by immunocytochemistry to contain masses of phosphorylated neurofilament epitopes. Sites of neuronal loss are marked by fibrous astrogliosis.

Wallerian degeneration may be apparent in ventral spinal nerve exit zones and rootlets, and in peripheral nerves (see Fig. 4-6), although this finding has not been highlighted as much as in goat kids. The pattern of axonal changes is consistent with the degenerating axons being those arising from the nuclei where neurons are also degenerate. Opinion favors the hypothesis that the lesions represent primary neuroaxonal degeneration with secondary myelin loss, although the myelin has been shown to be qualitatively abnormal and therefore theoretically unstable.

A very small number of lambs may have a *cerebellar lesion*, or *cerebrocortical necrosis*, as described later for goat kids. A further variant reported in lambs with delayed swayback is the occurrence of *acute cerebral edema* that is sometimes unilateral and involves both gray and white matter. Small gelatinous or cystic foci may be present at the corticomedullary junction. The pathogenesis is unexplained.

There is no unifying explanation for the spectrum of changes found in swayback, nor for the molecular mechanisms relating to the role of copper. It has been proposed that the spectrum reflects a critical level of copper deficiency, cytotoxic at particular times when different regions of the developing brain/spinal cord are undergoing growth spurts. It has also been suggested that the lesions reflect oxidative damage concentrated in particular vascular fields.

In **goat kids,** the clinicopathologic spectrum is similar, but has different emphasis. The great majority of reports describes delayed swayback, with a high incidence of cerebellar degeneration/dysplasia, and of peripheral motor axon degeneration. The cerebellar changes include necrosis and dystopia of Purkinje cells, depletion of internal granule cells, and Wallerian degeneration in folial white matter. The lesions tend to be multifocal and may involve vermis and hemispheres or be restricted to the vermis. In a very few cases, congenital swayback is reported in kids, and in only 2 individuals were cerebral gelatinous and cavitating changes found. An additional variant reported in both lambs and kids is the occurrence of diffuse cerebrocortical necrosis.

Lesions in **piglets** have the same general character in regard to Wallerian changes as described previously for delayed swayback, but chromatolytic neurons are not evident. A swayback-like disease has also been documented in adult captive *red deer*, but the role of copper is uncertain.

Further reading

Alleyne T, et al. Cytochrome-c oxidase isolated from the brain of swayback diseased sheep displays unusual structure and uncharacteristic kinetics. Mol Chem Neuropathol 1998;34:233-247.

Waggoner DJ, et al. The role of copper in neurodegenerative disease. Neurobiol Dis 1999;6:221-230.

Progressive axonopathy of Boxer dogs. This progressive disorder is inherited as an autosomal recessive trait, and begins in early life. Defects in slow axonal transport are involved in the pathogenesis of this condition; myelin lesions may then occur in response to primary axonal changes, and represent adaptive remodeling to alterations in axonal caliber and metabolism.

Clinical signs first become apparent at about 2 months of age and progress fairly rapidly until 12 or 18 months, when they may either become static or advance very slowly. The dominant clinical sign is *hindlimb ataxia*, with proprioceptive deficits, hypotonia, areflexia, and neurogenic muscle atrophy often being evident.

Degenerative lesions have been described in the spinal cord, caudal brainstem, optic nerves, spinal and cranial nerves, and major autonomic nerve trunks. *Morphologic changes are most obvious in the spinal cord and caudal brainstem*, and their intensity seems to parallel the clinical progression. Axonal spheroids develop in the spinal cord and are concentrated in the ventral and ventrolateral funiculi in the cervical and thoracic segments. A few axons undergoing Wallerian degeneration are also evident, but are always in a minority. Myelin sheaths are thinned around the spheroids, as would be expected, but attenuated sheaths may also occur around axonal segments not obviously swollen. Vacuolation of myelin segments is also a feature. These white matter changes have no obvious tract distribution. In the gray matter, spheroids are found in many nuclei of the caudal brainstem, and to a small extent in the spinal cord. However, from the diencephalon forward, there are virtually no gray matter lesions. Axonal swellings and myelin vacuolation are prominent in the optic nerves in the area of the chiasm.

In spinal nerve roots, there are, early in the disease, focal axonal swellings and a range of myelin abnormalities, including vacuolation, thinning, and segmental loss. With time, the involvement of ventral roots is appreciably more severe than dorsal roots. As the disease advances, such changes progress distally down the nerves, but axonal degeneration is accompanied by regeneration, and denervation of muscle is not significant. Changes of a similar character have been described in cranial nerves and large autonomic trunks.

Further reading

Griffiths IR, et al. Progressive axonopathy: an inherited neuropathy of boxer dogs. An immunocytochemical study of the axonal cytoskeleton. Neuropathol Appl Neurobiol 1989;15:63-74.

Degenerative radiculomyelopathy of adult dogs. This idiopathic condition is a slowly progressive, irreversible, adult-onset disease, characterized by paraparesis, weakness, and truncal ataxia. The disease predominantly affects large-breed dogs, and particularly **German Shepherd dogs**. Other breeds include **Rhodesian Ridgebacks, Pembroke Welsh Corgies, Boxers, Chesapeake Bay Retrievers, Siberian Huskies,** and **Bernese Mountain dogs**. The condition is not completely defined, but may be hereditary, and some studies suggested that the neurodegeneration is associated with an altered immune-mediated response. Vitamin E deficiency seems unlikely to be involved. A transitional mutation in the superoxide dismutase 1 *(SOD1)* gene is demonstrated in some breeds.

Histologically, degenerative myelopathy is characterized by *axonal swelling and fragmentation, associated with myelin degeneration and gliosis*. Lesions mainly involve the dorsolateral and ventromedial funiculi, in addition to the cerebellar peduncles, and sometimes other brainstem structures, including the trapezoid body and olivary nuclei. Although lesions appear as bilateral lesions, frequently they are distributed randomly and asymmetrically. In longitudinal sections of the spinal cord, the axonopathy and secondary degeneration of the myelin sheath are discontinuous. Axonal degeneration and demyelination are most intense in the thoracic segments. In the advanced stages of the disease, lesions extend to the cervical and lumbar segments, and peripheral nerve axonopathy and denervation muscle atrophy develop.

In German Shepherds dogs, the disease is known as *chronic degenerative radiculomyelopathy*, indicating the involvement of the dorsal nerve roots by the degenerative process. This may explain the frequent clinical finding of loss of patellar reflexes.

Further reading

Awano T, et al. Genome-wide association analysis reveals a SOD1 mutation in canine degenerative myelopahty that resembles amyotrophic lateral sclerosis. Proc Natl Acad Sci U S A 2009;106:2794-2799.

Kamishina H, et al. Detection of oligoclonal bands in cerebrospinal fluid from German Shepherd dogs with degenerative myelopathy by isoelectric focusing and immunofixation. Vet Clin Pathol 2008;37:217-220.

March PA, et al. Degenerative myelopathy in 18 Pembroke Welsh Corgi dogs. Vet Pathol 2009;46:241-250.

Shelton GD, et al. Degenerative myelopathy associated with a missense mutation in the superoxide dismutase 1 *(SOD1)* gene progresses to peripheral neuropathy in Pembroke Welsh corgis and boxers. J Neurol Sci 2012;318:55-64.

Giant axonal neuropathy of the German Shepherd dog. This uncommon disease is a *distal axonopathy* in which disorderly clumps of neurofilaments accumulate toward the extremities of long axons, and their most distal regions eventually degenerate completely. The *neurofilamentous accumulations create the very large argentophilic axonal swellings* that give the disease its name.

The clinical onset is at ~15 months of age, and there is progression to paraparesis, ataxia, and megaesophagus within a few months. The disease is apparently inherited in an autosomal recessive manner.

In the CNS, the giant swellings are found in the cranial regions of the ascending fasciculus gracilis and the dorsal spinocerebellar tracts, and in the caudal regions of the descending lateral corticospinal tracts. In the peripheral nervous system, they are found in both myelinated and unmyelinated large fibers in the more distal regions of the major nerves of the limbs and the recurrent laryngeal nerves. Small focal axonal swellings are also scattered through various regions of the brain from the cerebral cortex back to the caudal brainstem, and on to the dorsal and intermediate gray columns of the cord. Some Wallerian changes accompany the small swellings in these areas.

Further reading

King RH, et al. Axonal neurofilamentous accumulations: a comparison between human and canine giant axonal neuropathy and 2,5-HD neuropathy. Neuropathol Appl Neurobiol 1993;19:224-232.

Progressive motor neuron diseases. There is a group of neurodegenerative diseases, described in several species, which have a common clinical and pathologic theme, and which can therefore be dealt with together. They are characterized by *progressive degeneration and loss of motor neurons of the spinal cord, brainstem, and motor cortex, and different forms can be distinguished by their major anatomic site of degeneration*. In the human counterpart known as *amyotrophic lateral sclerosis*, neuronal loss involves upper and lower motor neurons, whereas in *progressive spinal muscular atrophy*, lower motor neurons of the spinal cord and brainstem are affected. Diseases with this basic theme have been described in several dog breeds, domestic shorthaired cats, various breeds of horses, Yorkshire and Hampshire pigs, and in Brown Swiss, Danish Red, Piedmont, and Holstein-Friesian calves.

The clinical presentation is dominated by progressive lower motor neuron paralysis that usually ends in tetraplegia and muscle atrophy. The pathologic findings are dominated by denervation atrophy of pelvic and pectoral muscle groups, and by regressive changes in spinal motor neurons. Other neurons in the motor hierarchy may be afflicted, including the pyramidal cells of the motor cortex. In some instances, neurons in the brainstem and peripheral ganglia are also involved. In the earlier stages of neuronal degeneration, there may be chromatolytic swelling of the soma, with reduced basophilia, and fading of the nucleus, which tends to remain centrally located. In many of the diseases, the swollen cell bodies are often crowded with abnormally phosphorylated neurofilaments. Eosinophilic inclusions may be present in the cytoplasm, usually representing clustered remnants of normal organelles trapped among arrays of neurofilaments (see Fig. 4-4). In some cases, these inclusions may be found to have the characteristics of Hirano, Lewy, or Bunina bodies described in human neuropathology. The neuronopathy progresses eventually to neuronal death on a cell-by-cell basis, with individual neurons in different stages of the process at any one time. Ultimately, there may be considerable neuronal loss, with residual gliosis, and Wallerian change in motor nerves and spinal white matter. Neurogenic muscle atrophy is also conspicuous.

These diseases are considered to be primary metabolic dysfunctions of the nerve cell body; most have an apparently *genetic basis* and an early-age onset. Hereditary spinal muscular atrophy in calves may result from a missense mutation in the *FVT1* gene encoding 3-ketodihydrosphingosine reductase. The inherited disease in cats is associated with a deletion in the *LIX1* gene, probably involved in RNA metabolism of motor neurons.

A series of **horses** is reported from the northeast United States in which the epidemiology strongly suggests an environmental cause. The condition is also present in Europe. Horses particularly at risk are those that for long periods do not have access to green pasture. Vitamin E status is deficient, which suggests that the lesion is a result of free *radical injury*. Muscle biopsy shows preferential damage to type 1, high-oxidative fibers, reflected in wastage, especially of postural muscles. The presence of lipofuscin pigments in vascular endothelium and in the retinal pigment epithelium in some affected horses supports the concept of *vitamin E deficiency*. It should be noted also that the neuronal lesions in congenital copper deficiency have many of these features (see Fig. 4-1). Variations on the basic theme are provided in terms of the age of onset and speed of progression of signs, the extent and pattern of frank neuronal degeneration, involvement of nuclei in the midbrain and hindbrain, and the presence of Wallerian degeneration in the spinal white matter and peripheral nerves.

Probably the most comprehensively described condition is **hereditary spinal muscular atrophy of Brittany Spaniels,** and it will serve as a generic example. In the Spaniels, there is *autosomal dominant* inheritance and 3 phenotypic variants: chronic, intermediate, and accelerated. The latter (resembling **Werdnig-Hoffman disease** of children) leads to quadriplegia at about 3 months of age, the others over several years, if at all. At the end stage, there is pronounced denervation atrophy of pectoral and pelvic muscle groups, as well as of the tongue and masseter muscles.

The neuropathology is marked by degenerative change in spinal motor neurons, focused in the intumescences, with similar involvement of the hypoglossal and trigeminal motor nuclei. Particularly in the accelerated, homozygous variant, there are numerous pale, swollen, and chromatolytic motor neurons, with occasional cells undergoing fragmentation and necrosis. Swollen neurons are depleted of ribosomes, and a few are packed with neurofilaments (Fig. 4-74). Most characteristically, large argentophilic swellings are present in the proximal segments of many axons close to the affected cell bodies. These have been shown by electron microscopy to be *tangles of disorganized neurofilaments* (Fig. 4-75A). All these changes are much less evident in the more chronic, heterozygous forms of the disease, and clinical weakness is only mild in many cases. Although it is established that there is a defect in the metabolism of neurofilaments as they move from the cell body into the proximal axon of individual neurons, it is not yet clear that this is the primary molecular lesion. Some studies have shown that there is growth arrest of spinal motor neurons, and initially, affected pups have a greater than normal number of these cells, with a shift to a smaller cell size. Ventral root axons undergo atrophy, which may be followed by loss of entire neurons. A similar condition affects **Rottweiler** dogs.

In the **Swedish Lapland dog,** the pattern of lesions is different, there being degeneration of spinal motor neurons only in the lateral aspects of the intumescences; neuronal degeneration also occurs in spinal ganglia and cerebellar Purkinje cells,

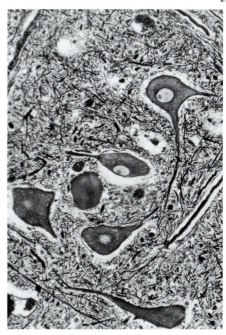

Figure 4-74 Proximal axonal swelling packed with neurofilaments in a spinal motor neuron of a Brittany Spaniel with **motor neuron disease.** Silver impregnation. (Courtesy L.C. Cork.)

but not in brainstem nuclei. The disease has been termed *neuronal abiotrophy*, and is included here because of the dominance of denervation atrophy of muscle in the clinical presentation. The atrophy is concentrated in the more distal muscle groups of the limbs, in keeping with the topography of degenerate spinal motor neurons. Any cerebellar deficits are probably over-ridden by the lower motor neuron impairment.

In the **English Pointer** dog, a strikingly different autosomal recessive motor neuron disease has been described in which weakness and muscle atrophy become obvious at about 5 months of age and severe by about 9 months. There is, correspondingly, severe distal degeneration of peripheral motor nerves and denervation of muscle. However, rather than the changes described previously, spinal motor neurons are filled with *cytoplasmic lipid inclusions* reminiscent of those seen in the gangliosidoses and mucopolysaccharidoses, and in some drug-induced conditions. No significant loss of motor neurons is apparent, and similar inclusions are present in the hypoglossal and spinal accessory nuclei, but not elsewhere.

Focal, asymmetrical spinal motor neuron degeneration with acute onset and a rapid course is described in **German Shepherd** pups. The affected neurons are within the cervical spinal cord intumescence, and exhibit peripheral chromatolysis or vacuolation. There is secondary denervation and wasting of forelimb muscles.

Progressive lower motor neuron disease has also been reported in **Saluki, Griffon Briquet Vendéen, Doberman, Collie Sheepdog, Pug, Dachshund,** and **Fox Terrier** pups. A form of motor neuron depletion associated with diffuse spinal cord axonopathy has been described in **Golden Retrievers**.

Further reading

da Costa RC, et al. Multisystem axonopathy and neuronopathy in Golden Retriever dogs. J Vet Intern Med 2009;23:935-939.

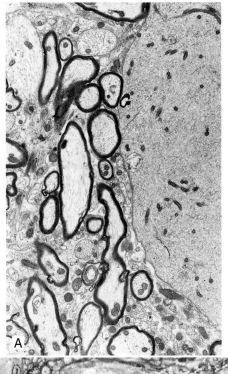

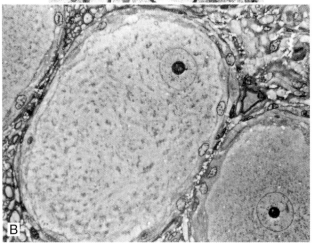

Figure 4-75 A. Proximal axonal swelling packed with neurofilaments in a spinal motor neuron of a Brittany Spaniel with **motor neuron disease**. (Courtesy L.C. Cork.) **B.** Swollen neuron in a spinal ganglion of a "shaker calf"; Nissl substance is dispersed by neurofilamentous masses. (Courtesy C.G. Rousseaux.)

Fyfe JC, et al. An approximately 140-kb deletion associated with feline spinal muscular atrophy implies an essential LIX1 function for motor neuron survival. Genome Res 2006;16:1084-1090.

Krebs S, et al. A missense mutation in the 3-ketodihydrosphingosine reductase FVT1 as candidate causal mutation for bovine spinal muscular atrophy. Proc Natl Acad Sci U S A 2007;104: 6746-6751.

Neurodegeneration of horned Hereford calves. The term "shaker calf" refers to a presumably inherited disease in which newborn horned Hereford calves are unable to stand without assistance and develop generalized fine tremors and profound muscular weakness. Although they often die in the neonatal period because of secondary complications, some, after a short period of apparent remission, show relentlessly progressive spastic paraparesis, but remain alert and may survive for some months. The disease is presumed to be inherited on the basis of pedigree analysis. The fundamental metabolic defect remains to be characterized.

The pathology is characterized by dramatic swelling of the cell bodies and processes of neurons throughout the spinal cord. Swelling is caused by the *accumulation of masses of neurofilaments* that impart a faintly fibrillar, amphophilic appearance in routine sections. This lesion involves ventral horn motor neurons, sensory neurons of the substantia gelatinosa, Clarke's column, and the intermediolateral (sympathetic) nuclei. Neuronal necrosis is minimal, although the site of occasional cell loss can be found as nodules of reactive glia. Some Wallerian degeneration is evident in ventral spinal nerve roots and the ventromedial spinal white matter.

The neuronal lesion is also present in the major motor nuclei of the brainstem, the reticular formation and the cerebellar Purkinje cells, and to a slight degree in the lateral geniculate nucleus and layer V of the frontal cortex. Some affected cells are evident in peripheral ganglia (Fig. 4-75B), including the myenteric plexus, and in the retinal ganglion cells.

Further reading

Sillevis Smitt PA, de Jong JM. Animal models of amyotrophic lateral sclerosis and the spinal muscular atrophies. J Neurol Sci 1989;91: 231-258.

Neuropathy in Gelbvieh calves. A familial, and likely hereditary, condition has been reported in Gelbvieh calves that had developed hindlimb ataxia and paresis, and were found histologically to have peripheral neuropathy and proliferative glomerulopathy; skeletal muscle degeneration was prominent in some cases. Degeneration was severe in peripheral nerves, dorsal and ventral spinal nerve roots, and less marked in dorsal fasciculi of the spinal cord.

Further reading

Panciera RJ, et al. A familial peripheral neuropathy and glomerulopathy in Gelbvieh calves. Vet Pathol 2003;40:63-70.

Central and peripheral axonopathy of Rouge-des-prés calves. A presumably inherited central and peripheral axonopathy of Rouge-des-prés calves is characterized by degeneration of the dorsolateral and ventromedial funiculi of the spinal cord and in the peripheral nerves. Spheroids are also observed in lateral vestibular and thoracic nuclei.

Further reading

Timsit E, et al. Clinical and histopathologic characterization of a central and peripheral axonopathy in Rouge-des-prés (Maine Anjou) calves. J Vet Intern Med 2011;25:386-392.

Progressive neuronopathy of the Cairn Terrier. Progressive neuronopathy occurs only in Cairn Terriers and is suspected to be inherited. This multisystem chromatolytic degeneration clinically resembles globoid cell leukodystrophy, from which it can be differentiated clinically by the exercise-induced deterioration of neurologic signs in progressive neuronopathy. Animals of both sexes develop hindlimb weakness, tetraparesis, ataxia, head tremor, and loss of reflexes at 5-7 months of age.

Both central and peripheral chromatolysis of neurons are evident, and occur in Clarke's column and dorsal and ventral horn cells in the spinal cord, in sensory ganglia, and in the cuneate, lateral cuneate, glossopharyngeal, vagus, reticular, lateral vestibular, mesencephalic trigeminal, red, and cerebellar roof nuclei. Wallerian degeneration is present in lateral and ventral funiculi of the cord, to various degrees, and also in dorsal and ventral spinal nerve roots.

Ultrastructural studies on one case suggested that the chromatolytic change was associated with depletion of ribosomes and increased numbers of mitochondria in perikarya, and that Wallerian degeneration was probably secondary to the metabolic disturbance in the cell body. This case was also marked by onset of signs at 11 weeks of age, bouts of cataplectic collapse, and thoracolumbar myelomalacia.

Primary hyperoxaluria in the cat. In this inherited metabolic disorder in cats, profound *deficiency in the activity of D-glycerate dehydrogenase* is associated with L-glyceric aciduria, hyperoxaluria, and the heavy deposition of oxalate crystals in the renal tubules. This leads to *oxalate nephrosis* and renal failure before 1 year of age.

An accompanying neuronal lesion occurs in the form of large swellings in the proximal axons of spinal motor neurons, ventral roots, intramuscular nerves, and the dorsal root ganglia. These swellings are caused by *neurofilamentous accumulations*, and are accompanied by some Wallerian degeneration in peripheral nerves. There is no obvious metabolic link between the neuronal lesions and the other biochemical disturbances, and the syndrome may represent a dual genetic defect.

Peripheral and central distal axonopathy in Birman cats. A suspected inherited distal axonopathy is described in Birman kittens with slowly progressive posterior ataxia. Lesions are characterized by degeneration of axons in the lateral pyramidal tracts of the spinal cord, the fasciculi gracili of the dorsal column in the cervical spinal cord, and the cerebellar vermian white matter. In the peripheral nervous system (PNS), degenerating nerve fibers are localized in the sciatic nerves but not in the spinal nerve roots.

Further reading

McKerrel RE. Primary hyperoxaluria (L-glyceric aciduria) in the cat: a newly recognized inherited disease. Vet Rec 1989;125:31-34.

Moreau PM, et al. Peripheral and central distal axonopathy of suspected inherited origin in Birman cats. Acta Neuropathol 1991;82:143-146.

The dysautonomias. The term dysautonomia denotes a profound failure of both sympathetic and parasympathetic functions across several organ systems. Domestic animals affected include horses **(equine grass sickness)**, cats **(Key-Gaskell syndrome)**, and dogs. Other species include sheep, rabbits, and hares. *Clostridium botulinum* type C is thought to play a role in equine dysautonomia and perhaps in the feline syndrome, which may hence be toxico-infectious forms of botulism.

Particularly in the **cat,** it is considered that there is a single episode of injury to neurons, with acute degeneration and subsequent reparative reactions if the animal survives for a number of weeks. There is a good correlation between the clinical signs and the extensive destruction in autonomic ganglia, and *autonomic denervation would account for the major functional disturbances*. The occasional expression of mild proprioceptive and lower motor neuron deficits may be explained by the lesions in dorsal root ganglia and spinal motor neurons, respectively.

The clinical onset in cats is acute and, in a few cases, may resolve after many months, but many animals die or require euthanasia early in the course. Onset is marked by dilated pupils, prolapsed nictitating membrane, dry mucous membranes, megaesophagus, constipation, vomiting, and dehydration.

In the **dog,** the most severe and consistent loss of autonomic neurons occurs in the pelvic, mesenteric, and ciliary ganglia. Minimal changes are reported in the CNS. Differential diagnoses in dogs include ganglioradiculitis (sensory neuronopathy).

In **horses,** the clinical picture is primarily the result of neurogenic obstruction of the alimentary tract, with various parts of the tract involved to differing degrees, with distinct acute, subacute, and chronic forms. Clinical differential diagnosis can be exceedingly difficult. Ileal biopsies and immunohistochemical evaluation of synaptophysin can be used for antemortem diagnosis. The outcome is usually fatal; some chronic cases may recover with intensive care. High levels of heavy metals in the herbage and abundance of *Ranunculus* spp. in the pasture have been associated with the development of the disease.

Neuropathology is similar in all species. In the acute phase, *extensive chromatolysis and death of ganglion cells* is present throughout the peripheral autonomic ganglia (Fig. 4-76), with axonal degeneration in autonomic nerve fibers. There is also neuronal degeneration in the nuclei of cranial nerves III, V, VII, and XII; the dorsal motor nucleus of the vagus; and the nucleus ambiguus. Some neuronal degeneration may be found in dorsal root ganglia, and in the ventral horn and intermediolateral areas of the spinal gray matter. In later phases of the

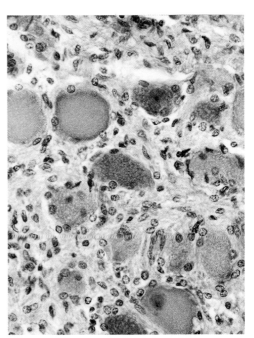

Figure 4-76 Central chromatolysis in ganglionic neurons of a horse with grass sickness.

disease, depletion of neurons at the above sites is evident, with reactive and proliferative changes on the part of non-neuronal elements.

Further reading

Michl J, et al. Metabolomic analysis of *Ranunculus* spp. as potential agents involved in the etiology of equine grass sickness. J Agric Food Chem 2011;59:10388-10393.

Milne EM, et al. Evaluation of formalin-fixed ileum as the optimum method to diagnose equine dysautonomia (grass sickness) in simulated intestinal biopsies. J Vet Diagn Invest 2010;22:248-252.

Waggett BE, et al. Evaluation of synaptophysin as an immunohistochemical marker for equine grass sickness. J Comp Pathol 2010;142:284-290.

Sensory and autonomic neuropathies in the dog. Sensory and autonomic neuropathies are reported in an increasingly long list of various dog breeds. Many of these diseases are suspected inherited autosomal recessive, whereas others are sporadic. A small number of **English Pointer** pups from a particular mating developed a syndrome of acral mutilation and analgesia. The size of spinal ganglia was reduced, with reduced numbers of neurons, and reduced fiber density in the dorsolateral fasciculus of the spinal cord (Lissauer's tract). These clinical and morphologic findings are consistent with a *specific deficit in nociceptive pathways*. It is suggested that the presumably genetically based disorder involves both hypoplasia of the system and continued degeneration postnatally. A similar condition is known in **German Short-haired Pointers** and **English Springer Spaniels,** in which analgesia and acral auto-mutilation is associated with neural loss in the dorsal root ganglia and loss of unmyelinated fibers.

In **Long-haired Dachshunds, Jack Russell Terriers,** and **Border Collies,** proprioceptive, nociceptive, and urinary deficits are associated with a *distal degenerative axonopathy*. Cutaneous nerves have marked loss of large myelinated fibers, and degenerative changes in both myelinated and unmyelinated fibers. In the spinal cord, there is axonal degeneration in the fasciculus gracilis, of greatest intensity at its distal extremity in the cervical region.

Progressive myelopathy and neuropathy causing progressive ataxia in littermate **New Zealand Huntaway** dogs is described as a *central-peripheral distal axonopathy,* in which there is degeneration of axon and myelin in sensory, proprioceptive, and motor tracts of the spinal cord and to a mild degree in some peripheral nerves. In **Swedish Golden Retrievers,** a similar disease is characterized by progressive axonopathy of sensory and motor axons of both the PNS and CNS, predominating in CNS sensory afferents. The deletion in the mitochondrial *tRNA^{Tyr}* gene is the causative mutation for this disease.

In dogs of **various breeds,** there are reports of diffuse ganglioneuritis, with destruction of primary sensory neurons and subsequent Wallerian degeneration and axonal loss in peripheral nerves in the spinal dorsal funiculi, spinal tract of the trigeminal nerve, and solitary tract. These cases are mentioned here, as the *extensive axonal degeneration* is the more likely lesion to be routinely noted, and its pattern should immediately draw attention to the primary involvement of dorsal root ganglia. The pathogenesis of this ganglioneuritis is not known but may be similar to that of Guillain-Barré syndrome, a post-infectious syndrome in people.

Further reading

Baranowska I, et al. Sensory ataxic neuropathy in Golden Retriever dogs is caused by a deletion in the mitochondrial *tRNA^{Tyr}* gene. PLoS Genet 2009;5:e1000499.

Jäderlund KH, et al. A neurologic syndrome in Golden Retrievers presenting as a sensory ataxic neuropathy. J Vet Intern Med 2007;21:1307-1315.

Vermeersch K, et al. Sensory neuropathy in two Border collie puppies. J Small Anim Pract 2005;46:295-299.

Peripheral axonopathies

Lesions involving single peripheral nerves are termed **mononeuropathies**. They are usually the result of focal compression or contusion by trauma, tumor masses, or similar lesions, and involve centrifugal Wallerian degeneration about the lesion. Other causes include vascular diseases, such as thromboembolic disease and fibrocartilaginous embolism. If several nerves are randomly involved in such a way, the term **mononeuropathy multiplex** may be applied. **Polyneuropathy** describes bilaterally symmetrical involvement of several nerves, and carries the implication of a systemic disturbance.

From the clinical point of view, most peripheral polyneuropathies occur in association with polyneuritis or demyelination, but in this section, our focus is on **noninflammatory axonopathies**. Intense Wallerian degeneration of peripheral motor axons will, of course, accompany degeneration of the ventral spinal motor nerve cell bodies, as occurs in the motor neuron diseases previously discussed. Similarly, in the very rare primary sensory polyneuropathies, peripheral sensory fibers will degenerate, but the degeneration will also extend, with the central projections of these cells, into the dorsal funiculi of the spinal cord. In some intoxications—for example, delayed organophosphate—peripheral neuropathy will be accompanied by central axonopathy, as has been illustrated previously. All the foregoing emphasizes the unity of the nervous system and the inconsistencies involved in deciding where neurons begin and end, but nonetheless certain diseases have a clear central or peripheral focus.

Noninflammatory peripheral polyneuropathies have been regularly identified in *dogs* over the last decades. They are generally to be regarded as *distal axonopathies* of the spinal neurons. Some neuropathies are termed *inherited* when a familial link between affected dogs is demonstrated, whereas, in other cases, the term *sporadic* is adopted. Motor axon involvement means that *weakness* and *denervation muscle atrophy* is the typical clinical presentation. In dogs and horses, *laryngeal paralysis and/or megaesophagus* are observed in some cases. It should be remembered too that, with advancing age, subclinical degenerative changes are to be expected in peripheral nerves and spinal roots.

Equine laryngeal hemiplegia. The clinical manifestations of this common and well-recognized disease are the consequence of *denervation atrophy of the intrinsic muscles of the left side of the larynx*. The resultant inability to adduct the arytenoid cartilage and the vocal fold leads to partial obstruction of the airway on inspiration, and inspiratory stridor on exertion, referred to as *roaring*.

The underlying lesion is *idiopathic degeneration of the left recurrent laryngeal nerve,* suggested to result from progressive degeneration of large myelinated axons, which increases in intensity toward the distal extremities of the nerve. During active degeneration, localized axonal swellings result from paranodal and internodal accumulations of granular dense bodies and degenerate mitochondria, although numerous atrophied axonal segments have also been described. Loss of axons is indicated by the presence of Büngner's bands, which may contain fragments of axonal and myelin debris, and permanent axonal loss is reflected in considerable endoneurial fibrosis. Some axonal regenerative activity may be apparent. There is also evidence of recurrent demyelination and remyelination, considered to be secondary to axonal degeneration.

The cause of this axonopathy remains unknown. Young, tall male horses with long necks seem predisposed, and there is a high incidence in Thoroughbred and draft breeds. *Mechanical factors* operating on the left recurrent laryngeal nerve have been proposed, such as stretching of the anchored nerve, or pressure exerted where it reflects around the aorta. However, subclinical involvement of the right recurrent nerve seems to be the rule. Studies of clinically normal horses have revealed bilateral neuropathy with more severe denervation of the laryngeal adductor muscles compared to the abductors, and this pattern also holds true for horses with laryngeal hemiplegia. The factors determining progression of the subclinical disease, the mechanism for the preferential adductor involvement, and the reason for the greater severity on the left side are unexplained.

One study suggested that similar distal degenerative changes also occur in the long axons of the hindlimbs, but only a few horses were sampled. Such a finding implies a *systemic metabolic or toxic disorder*, producing a polyneuropathy with maximal expression in the left recurrent laryngeal nerve. In New Zealand, laryngeal hemiplegia in association with stringhalt has occurred in seasonal outbreak form in horses grazing the plant *Hypochaeris radicata* (false dandelion, flatweed). Laryngeal paralysis has occasionally been reported in cases of intoxication with *lead*, or *organophosphates*, as part of widespread axonopathy.

No convincing evidence of lesions in the CNS is available at present, although they have been sought in the nucleus ambiguus from which the recurrent laryngeal axons arise. It has been claimed that axonal spheroids in the lateral cuneate nucleus are more numerous in horses with laryngeal paralysis, but the significance of this is unclear. Such lesions are common and generally nonspecific, and it is difficult to see how they could be related pathogenetically to the rather different lesions in the motor axons supplying the larynx.

Equine stringhalt. Stringhalt is the name given to a clinical condition of horses characterized by *extreme exaggerated flexion of the hindlimbs*. It has been recognized for many years to occur in *sporadic* and *epizootic* forms, the latter associated with the grazing of certain plants, notably *Hypochaeris radicata*. Stringhalt may develop subsequent to trauma to the dorsum of the metatarsus. Various degenerative changes have been reported in the spinal cord and peripheral nerves in stringhalt. Selective loss of large-diameter myelinated fibers in peripheral nerves in horses with Australian stringhalt is consistent with distal axonopathy leading to neurogenic muscle atrophy.

Equine suprascapular neuropathy. Mononeuropathy of the suprascapular nerve in the horse has been designated for many years by the old clinical term *"sweeney."* The nerve is prone to injury at its site of reflection around the wing of the scapula, and in many cases, *trauma* at this site is probably the initiating cause. Evidence has been advanced to suggest, however, that *entrapment of the nerve* by a tendinous band may lead to degeneration in the absence of additional trauma. In cases of sufficient severity, axonal degeneration, demyelination, and endoneurial fibrosis will be associated with denervation of the spinatus muscle and chronic lameness.

Motor neuropathies in small animals. Inherited and sporadic neuropathies are often described according to the main clinical signs that they produce. Laryngeal paralysis can be part of a generalized polyneuropathy complex. Canine inherited motor neuropathies with laryngeal paralysis are reported in **Dalmatians, Alaskan Malamutes, Bouvier des Flandres, Rottweilers, Leonbergers, Italian Spinones,** and **Pyrenean Mountain dogs.** Clinical laryngeal paralysis is accompanied by denervation atrophy of laryngeal muscles, and Wallerian degeneration of the distal recurrent laryngeal nerves. Generalized forms without laryngeal involvement are described in **Great Danes, German Shepherd dogs, Rottweilers,** and **Bouvier des Flandres.**

Lesions are characterized by chronic axonal degeneration. Myelin ovoids and foamy macrophages may be seen in properly processed peripheral nerve biopsy, sometimes associated with regenerating clusters. Nerve fiber loss and endoneurial fibrosis are common findings in dogs and cats with chronic peripheral neuropathy. With neuropathic disease, myofibers show angular atrophy, and fiber-type grouping if denervation has been followed by reinnervation. Replacement of muscle fibers by fatty tissue and pyknotic nuclear clumps are evident in end-stage disease.

In the **Bouvier** breed, autosomal dominant inheritance has been proposed for a unilateral or bilateral condition with onset at an early age. In this breed, laryngeal paralysis is attributed to an abiotrophic process in nucleus ambiguus in the medulla. Gliosis and neuronal atrophy have been recorded in vagal nuclei in **Siberian Huskies.** In **Dalmatian** dogs, the laryngeal paralysis-polyneuropathy complex is a generalized axonopathy with dying back of laryngeal and peripheral nerves. Neurogenic atrophy of muscles, including those of the larynx, is reported in related **Leonberger** and **Saint Bernard** dogs with a spontaneous distal, symmetrical polyneuropathy. A deletion in the *ARHGEF10* gene is associated with a severe juvenile onset of the disease in both breeds.

Descriptions of inherited or breed-associated polyneuropathies in **cats** are rare. Specific examples include a presumed congenital axonal neuropathy in young **Snowshoe cats,** and a chronic polyneuropathy with demyelinating and remyelinating features in young **Bengal cats.**

Metabolic neuropathies. Clinical polyneuropathy has been associated with **diabetes mellitus** *in the dog and cat* and is well recognized in people. In the cat, hindlimb weakness, poor postural reactions, depressed patellar reflexes, and plantigrade stance are described. Axonal conduction velocity is reduced in the sciatic and ulnar nerves. Clinical remission often follows therapeutic management of the diabetic state.

The pathogenesis of diabetic neuropathy remains uncertain, but it is generally accepted that there is *distal axonopathy* with cycles of degeneration/regeneration and accompanying demyelination/remyelination. The distal degeneration may be the result of impairment of axonal transport mechanisms secondary to reduced availability of glucose for the neuron. Lesions include axonal atrophy of myelinated and unmyelinated fibers, demyelination and, in some animals, intra-axonal accumulation of glycogen.

A peripheral neuropathy has also been associated with *canine hypothyroidism, hypoglycemia,* and *insulinoma*.

A series of cats has been described with a *genetically based deficiency of lipoprotein lipase activity* and a resulting severe *hyperchylomicronemia*. Among other manifestations, there is a high incidence of *mononeuropathy multiplex*, with clinical palsies related to various peripheral and cranial nerves, including instances of Horner's syndrome. Neurologic deficits are related to multiple focal red/brown nodules in the perineurium of nerve trunks, which are organizing hematomas associated with a xanthomatous/granulomatous component. Xanthomatous masses extend between nerve fascicles and appear to compress and distort them, inducing Wallerian degeneration to various degrees of severity. The xanthomas arise from phagocytosis of cholesterol esters by macrophages. These lesions are generally located in loci where trauma is likely and also occur commonly at the emergence of spinal nerve roots.

"Kangaroo gait" of lactating ewes. This condition was first reported from New Zealand, and subsequently from the United Kingdom. There is a low flock incidence, and only ewes in lactation or up to 1 month postweaning are affected. The clinical syndrome is consistent with *bilateral radial nerve palsy*, and there is a characteristic bounding gait during attempted rapid movement. In most cases, there is gradual clinical improvement and eventual recovery. The cause is not known. There have been limited studies of pathology. Extensive Wallerian degeneration with regeneration has been described in the radial nerve trunks of chronically affected ewes, but in some acutely affected animals, no radial nerve lesions could be demonstrated. In one study, there were additionally reported spongy change in the neuropil, dorsal root ganglionopathy, and neuronal degeneration in the hippocampus and cervical spinal cord, although these findings were variable. A similar disease occurs in sheep grazing fenugreek *(Trigonella foenum-graecum)* in Australia. Acute lesions are edema in the brain and spinal cord, and chronic lesions are Wallerian degeneration of peripheral nerves.

Further reading

Bensfield AC, et al. Recurrent demyelination and remyelination in 37 young Bengal cats with polyneuropathy. J Vet Intern Med 2011;25:882-889.

Bourke C. Are ovine fenugreek *(Trigonella foenum-graecum)* staggers and kangaroo gait of lactating ewes two clinically and pathologically similar nervous disorders? Aust Vet J 2009;87:99-101.

Ekenstedt KJ, et al. An ARHGEF10 deletion is highly associated with a juvenile-onset inherited polyneuropathy in Leonberger and Saint Bernard dogs. PLoS Genet 2014;10:e1004635.

Granger N. Canine inherited motor and sensory neuropathies: an updated classification in 22 breeds and comparison to Charcot-Marie-Tooth disease. Vet J 2011;188:274-285.

Matiasek LA, et al. Axonal neuropathy with unusual clinical course in young Snowshoe cats. J Feline Med Surg 2009;11:1005-1010.

Myelinopathies

Myelin sheaths in the central or peripheral nervous system may be the focus of various disease processes, but simultaneous central and peripheral involvement is rare. This is not surprising when one considers the fundamental differences between them. As previously noted, myelin breakdown and removal in Wallerian degeneration will follow as a **secondary** consequence of axonal degeneration. On the other hand, in some inflammatory diseases, macrophages acting within the orchestration of the immune system will strip myelin from axons, leaving the latter intact for a time at least. In this context, antibodies or inflammatory mediators may bind to and destabilize the structure of the myelin lamellae, causing disruption of the sheath and provoking its phagocytosis. Such **primary demyelination** occurs, for example, in the CNS in canine distemper, and in the peripheral nerves in "coonhound paralysis."

Attention in this section is on *noninflammatory diseases in which some disorder of myelin formation, maintenance, or stability is the primary event.* It should be remembered that the myelin sheath is a specialized extended process of oligodendrocyte or Schwann cell plasma membrane, and myelinopathies are therefore part of the cytopathology of these cells. Within the complex category of myelinopathies, we will discuss *leukodystrophies*, or disorders of myelin synthesis or maintenance; *hypomyelinogenesis*, which may be at one end of the spectrum of leukodystrophy; and *spongy degeneration* or spongiform myelinopathies.

Hypomyelinogenesis

The great majority of the hypomyelinogeneses are restricted to the CNS, and they have been described in most domestic species, with the notable exception of the horse. Although in many cases a genetic basis has been demonstrated or strongly implied in hypomyelinogenesis, several viruses have been implicated, and the possibility of toxic or nutritional factors should be kept in mind. A common theme is sex-linked inheritance and affected males.

Myelinogenesis begins sometime after the middle of gestation and continues in the postnatal period for various times depending on the species. It is more advanced at birth in those species in which the young are able to stand and walk soon after, for it correlates with the overall maturity of the nervous system.

The process requires a complex unfolding of events to be successful. In the first place, there must be differentiation of competent myelinating cells in sufficient number, and they must migrate to, recognize, and contact the target axons appropriately. Second, the axon itself must send a specific signal to the myelinating cell to initiate its investment. The diameter of the axon dictates whether or not it is myelinated and how thick the sheath will be. The threshold size is about 1 µm in the CNS and 2 µm in the peripheral nerves. Finally, the molecular components of the myelin must be produced and delivered to their correct sites in the membrane. One or several of these processes may be perturbed to give rise to diseases characterized by hypomyelinogenesis.

Myelination does not occur synchronously throughout the nervous system, but in a distinctly regional sequence. Thus lesions of this type may involve some tracts more than others, or completely spare some tracts. There may be complete absence of myelin, or an inadequate amount of myelin that may be either chemically normal or abnormal. For the latter case, the term *dysmyelination* has been coined but, as these conditions are characterized by a reduced quantity of myelin, **hypomyelination** is a suitable generic term. As would be expected, such diseases are manifested early in life, and a very common and dominant clinical feature is the onset of a severe generalized tremor syndrome. This has led to the use of names such as *congenital "tremor," "shaker,"* or *"trembler"* to describe the clinical state. The severity of the clinical signs can vary from life threatening to mild.

The deficiency of myelin may in some instances be permanent with unchanged clinical signs, whereas in others, it seems that myelination may be delayed, but eventually proceeds to the extent that clinical deficits resolve. In general, the pathologic picture is dominated by a paucity of myelin with little or no evidence of the breakdown and removal of previously formed sheaths. There may be other accompanying structural defects, notably cerebellar hypoplasia, particularly when a teratogenic virus is the cause.

When routine morphologic evaluations are being made on very young animals, reference should be made to age-matched controls. In the dog, for example, very little myelin is normally present prior to 2 weeks of postnatal age, whereas in sheep, myelination begins at about day 50 of gestation. The investigation of such conditions makes use of traditional stains for myelin and axons, plastic-embedded sections for light and electron microscopy, and immunostaining techniques for marker antigens, such as myelin basic protein. There needs to be some familiarity with the normal morphologic features of early myelination. Some of these are mentioned in the disease descriptions that follow.

Canine hypomyelinogenesis. A number of canine hypomyelinogeneses have been documented, and several provisional conclusions can be made. All but one of the diseases involves the central myelin only, and it appears that they are not pathogenetically identical and can be divided into 2 broad groups according to severity. The most severe are those described in the Samoyed, Springer Spaniel, and Dalmatian breeds.

In the **Samoyed,** severe generalized tremors become apparent at about 3 weeks of age, with a predominance of males being affected. Inability to stand leads to severe incapacitation and a high mortality rate. A genetic basis is suspected. It has been suggested that a central pathogenetic event is *retardation of gliogenesis,* with oligodendrocytes failing to differentiate fully. Profound hypomyelination is suggested, on gross inspection of the brain, by a lack of contrast between gray and white matter throughout the CNS. The sparing of the peripheral nervous system is well appreciated macroscopically by comparing the myelin-deficient optic nerves to the other cranial nerves, in particular the adjacent oculomotor nerve.

By routine light microscopy, there is normal peripheral myelin but *almost total absence of central myelin, and diffuse microgliosis.* Silver stains suggest axons to be present in normal number. Electron microscopy reveals a few axons to have thin and poorly compacted myelin sheaths, the presence of numerous astroglial processes, and a large number of microglia. Oligodendrocytes are greatly reduced in number and appear immature. Axons, by contrast, are normal in number and morphology but the great majority are devoid of a myelin sheath.

In the **Springer Spaniel,** severe generalized tremor in male pups is evident at 10-12 days of age *("shaking pups").* The condition is inherited as an *X-linked recessive,* and abnormal oligodendrocyte differentiation and severe myelin deficiency are caused by the shaker pup *(shp)* mutation of the myelin proteolipid protein *(Plp)* gene. Central hypomyelination is profound but less severe in the spinal cord than in the brain and optic nerves. In contrast to the Samoyed, microgliosis is not prominent, but in other respects, the gross and histologic features are similar. The electron microscope, however, resolves some further differences. For example, some thin myelin sheaths are present that have lamellae of normal configuration. Some axons have a few internodes sheathed, many of which are shorter than would be expected for the axonal caliber, and many of which are single units terminating as "heminodes." Although some immature oligodendrocytes are evident, so too are normally mature ones. In animals ≥2 months of age, there are also hallmarks of the early stages of normal myelination that persist well beyond their usual period of the first month of life. These include such features as large amounts of oligodendrocyte cytoplasm in lateral loops, and outwardly terminating lateral loops. In addition, many oligodendrocytes have lysosomal digestive vacuoles thought to relate to the degradation of abnormal myelin components.

The disease in the **Dalmatian** is reported in a male pup that developed severe tremors in the neonatal period and was destroyed at 8 weeks of age. Profound deficiency of central myelin was accompanied by reduced numbers of oligodendroglia, with a few axons having extremely thin and poorly compacted sheaths.

Disorders of lesser severity are described in the Chow Chow, Weimaraner, Bernese Mountain dog, and in 2 crossbred ("Lurcher") dogs.

Affected **Chow Chow** dogs have marked impairment from 2 weeks of age, but progressive improvement leads to a virtual absence of clinical deficits by the end of the first year of life. At all stages, the animals remain ambulatory, bright, and responsive, in spite of a pronounced hypermetric gait with a distinctive "rocking horse" motion when trying to initiate movement. Tremors and head bobbing are exacerbated by excitement and disappear at rest. It has not been possible to establish a definite heritable basis for this disease, but it is suggested to be the result of a genetically determined delay in oligodendrocyte maturation.

In pups examined at ~3 months of age, no gross lesions are reported, but profound hypomyelination is evident histologically in the CNS. This is particularly so in the cerebral subcortical white matter, cerebellar folia, ventral half of the cerebral peduncles, optic tracts, and the peripheral zones of the ventral and lateral funiculi of the spinal cord. By contrast, the cerebellar peduncles and fasciculus proprius of the spinal cord are relatively well myelinated. Electron microscopy reveals mostly thin myelin sheaths in the least-affected areas, and mostly naked axons in the worst-affected areas. Oligodendrocytes are present in normal numbers and generally appear morphologically normal, although stellate cells containing intermediate filaments may be found.

In older dogs in clinical remission, the brain is well myelinated apart from some mildly deficient foci in subcortical white matter and corpus callosum. However, myelin deficiency is still marked in the lateral and ventral funiculi of the cord, which also has a few degenerate axons. Ultrastructurally, these areas contain a few well-myelinated or thinly myelinated axons separated by masses of astrocytic processes. Indications of immaturity are provided by poorly compacted sheaths and some massively oversized sheaths that fold away from the axon in redundant loops.

The **Weimaraner** syndrome is closely similar to the above but has only been studied pathologically in the early phase. The tremor syndrome, in evidence at 3 weeks of age, seems to resolve by a year. A heritable basis has been proposed but not confirmed, and delayed oligodendrocyte differentiation suggested as the underlying defect. Pups autopsied at 4-5 weeks of age have no gross abnormalities, but histologic staining reactions suggest myelin deficiency, and this is particularly obvious at the periphery of the lateral and ventral funiculi of the spinal cord. This contrasts with the relatively well-myelinated dorsal columns. Oligodendrocytes are reduced in number. Ultrastructurally, there is considerable evidence of myelin immaturity as described previously. Astrocytic fibers are prominent and oligodendrocyte morphology seems normal.

The **Bernese Mountain dog** "trembler pup" has a fine head and limb tremor that subsides with sleep and improves substantially by 9-12 weeks of age. An autosomal recessive mode of inheritance has been proposed. There are no gross lesions, and hypomyelination is concentrated in the spinal cord, where axons are thinly sheathed by morphologically normal myelin. Oligodendrocytes in this case appear to be increased in numbers and morphologically normal. **Lurcher** pups were reported to have unmyelinated and thinly myelinated axons in the peripheral sections of the lateral funiculi of the spinal cord. The changes are subtle and not readily apparent unless plastic-embedded sections are used. These animals are of interest as they are crossbred, making a genetic cause a more remote possibility.

Congenital hypothyroidism caused by a mutation in the thyroid peroxidase gene leads to hypomyelinogenesis in **Rat Terriers**. A form of leukoencephalopathy associated with canine parvovirus 2 infection, possibly facilitated by a genetic predisposition, has been described in **Cretan Hound** puppies. An autosomal recessive disease characterized by diffuse astrocytic hypertrophy of the white matter of the brain occurs in **Gordon Setter** puppies.

Hypomyelination has been reported only rarely in **Siamese cats**.

The sole reported occurrence of **peripheral hypomyelination** in domestic animals involves the **Golden Retriever** breed. Two littermates, one male and one female, had ataxia, weakness, a crouched stance, and pelvic-limb muscle atrophy at about 2 months of age. Peripheral nerve samples revealed axons of all calibers to be thinly myelinated and Schwann cells to be increased in number and hypertrophied (see Fig. 4-11). There were no indications of demyelination.

Porcine hypomyelinogenesis. Syndromes of **congenital tremor** (CT, myoclonia congenita, dancing pig) are well recognized in pigs. CT has been classified on the basis of the presence (type A) or absence (type B) of myelin deficiency in the central or peripheral nervous system; CT type A has been subdivided into 5 subtypes, AI-AV. The various forms of CT are similar clinically; affected piglets may bounce on their digits, and have rhythmic whole-body tremors that worsen with excitement and cease with sleep.

CT type AI is caused by transplacental infection in the middle trimester with classical swine fever virus, which causes significant hypomyelinogenesis in addition to other neural lesions in the fetus, most notably cerebellar hypoplasia. The cerebellar changes may be focal and are most likely to be detected in sagittal sections of the vermis and hemispheres. The myelin lesion is generally similar to that seen in lambs with border disease.

CT type AII may be the result of porcine circovirus 2 infection, but the role, if any, of this virus remains controversial.

CT type AIII occurs in Landrace or Landrace crossbreds, and is inherited as an *X-linked recessive* trait, afflicting male neonates, and caused by a mutation in the proteolipid protein gene *Plp*. There is myelin deficiency throughout the CNS, but it is most obvious in the spinal cord, cerebellum, and cerebral gyri. Oligodendrocyte numbers are reduced; many small- and medium-sized axons are unmyelinated or only thinly so. Large-diameter axons appear normally myelinated.

CT type AIV occurs in the British Saddleback breed; there is an *autosomal recessive* inheritance mode. Hypomyelination is present throughout the neuraxis, with axons of all sizes affected. Many sheaths are poorly compacted and vacuolated. Oligodendrocytes are numerous, and many appear immature ultrastructurally, and sometimes contain cytoplasmic intermediate filaments. Still others contain autophagosomes and dense bodies. The neuropil also contains excessive astrocytic fibers and lipid-laden macrophages. These findings, together with biochemical evidence of myelin degradation, suggest that newly formed myelin is unstable and is rapidly broken down.

CT type AV occurs in piglets of sows exposed to the organophosphate *trichlorfon* between days 45 and 63 of pregnancy.

CT type B is idiopathic, and lacks structural or neurochemical defects.

Ovine and caprine hypomyelinogenesis. Border disease in lambs has become the model for the several pestivirus-induced myelin disorders of animals. Border disease virus can cause transplacental infection, which, if on or after day 50, has the potential to produce a range of terata. In the classic syndrome, newborn lambs are often referred to as *"hairy shakers,"* the result of the combination of generalized tremor and hairy birth coat. There is *diffuse hypomyelination in the CNS*, which is especially prominent in the spinal cord, particularly the more caudal regions. Some myelination is present, but has ultrastructural features of immaturity, in that lamellae remain uncompacted and axons retain the angulated profiles they normally acquire just before myelination and lose soon after. There are also compact sheaths abnormally thin for axonal diameter, and intramyelinic and periaxonal vacuoles.

Although glial cell numbers may appear normal by light microscopy, there are, in fact, reduced numbers of mature oligodendrocytes and increased numbers of microglia. Many microglia are packed with lipid droplets, the origin of which does not appear to be degraded myelin. It is suggested that maturation of oligodendrocytes is delayed, and that although the time of onset of myelination is close to normal, its rate is greatly reduced. The blockade of glial maturation may be the result of virus-induced fetal hypothyroidism; abundant viral antigen can be found in the thyroid and pituitary gland, and circulating thyroxin is significantly depressed.

Severe hypomyelinogenesis is a feature of neonatal goat kids with **β-mannosidosis**. Hypothyroidism has been proposed as the underlying mechanism, as a consequence of the lysosomal storage disease.

Bovine hypomyelinogenesis. Myelination in calves proceeds between gestational week 20 and postnatal week 8. A spectrum of terata and spinal hypomyelinogenesis similar to that in piglets and lambs may develop in calves infected with bovine viral diarrhea virus (BVDV) in utero after day 100 of gestation. Hypomyelination can also be specifically attributed to BVDV-2 infection.

A condition commonly referred to as congenital tremor occurs in several bovine breeds. In **Jersey** cattle, an autosomal recessive hereditary cerebellar ataxia with nonsymmetrical hypomyelination in the cerebellum, medulla oblongata, and midbrain has been reported. Similar syndromes have been described in **Angus, Shorthorn, Hereford,** and **Shorthorn crossbreeds**. In **Holstein-Friesian** calves, severe degenerative lesions of spinal cord and brain white matter have been reported.

Congenital *bovine spinal dysmyelination* in **American Brown Swiss** cattle and crossbreeds is characterized by congenital recumbency with spasticity and opisthotonos. The myelin lesions affect the dorsomedial, dorsolateral, and ventromedial columns of the spinal cord and are associated with axonal degeneration. The disease is caused by a missense mutation in the *SPAST* gene, whose human ortholog is associated with hereditary spastic paraplegia.

Further reading

Chae C. A review of porcine circovirus 2-associated syndromes and diseases. Vet J 2005;169:326-336.

Pettigrew R, et al. CNS hypomyelination in Rat Terrier dogs with congenital goiter and a mutation in the thyroid peroxidase gene. Vet Pathol 2007;44:50-56.

Porter BF, et al. Hypomyelination associated with bovine viral diarrhea virus type 2 infection in a longhorn calf. Vet Pathol 2010;47:658-663.

Schaudien D, et al. Leukoencephalopathy associated with parvovirus infection in Cretan hound puppies. J Clin Microbiol 2010;48:3169-3175.

Thomsen B, et al. Congenital bovine spinal dysmyelination is caused by a missense mutation in the *SPAST* gene. Neurogenetics 2010;11:175-183.

Yaeger MJ, et al. An autosomal recessive, lethal, neurologic disease of Gordon Setter puppies. J Vet Diagn Invest 2000;12:570-573.

Leukodystrophic and myelinolytic diseases

This section will address those diseases characterized by degeneration and loss of myelin, not as a result of, or in association with, inflammation but caused by some failure of myelinating cells to sustain and maintain their sheaths in an intact and ordered condition. The implication is that sheaths are initially formed, but then deteriorate, leaving their axons intact for a time at least. The use of terminology in this area is of course somewhat arbitrary. For our purposes, **primary demyelination** is taken to imply the removal from around intact axons of structurally and chemically normal myelin, usually by macrophages and often in an inflammatory setting. The term **leukodystrophy** is applied to *diseases with a heritable basis, early onset in life, lack of inflammation, bilateral symmetry of lesions, selective involvement of white matter areas, and in which some inherent qualitative defect in myelin (dysmyelinogenesis) leads to its dissolution and removal*. **Myelinolysis** refers to the initial disruption of myelin structure by extensive decompaction of lamellae as a prelude to its breakdown and removal, and as such could be involved in many processes. There is room for considerable overlap and liberal interpretation of definitions. The diseases discussed in this section will not include any that could easily be classified as demyelinating, in the sense indicated previously, or as malacic in the sense indicated elsewhere in this chapter, in spite of the propensity for focal softening and even cavitation in some of the leukodystrophies.

Globoid cell leukodystrophy. This disease, also known as *galactocerebrosidosis, galactosylceramide lipidosis,* and *Krabbe disease,* has been documented in the **Cairn Terrier** and **West Highland White Terrier,** in which a mutation of the *GALC* gene has been demonstrated. Other dog breeds include **Miniature Poodle, Bluetick Hound, Bassett Hound, Beagle, Irish Setter,** and **Australian Kelpie**. The disease is also described in the **domestic cat,** and **polled Dorset sheep**. It is the result of a genetically determined deficiency, usually autosomal recessive, in the activity of lysosomal *galactocerebrosidase*, and as such falls within the *sphingolipidosis group of lysosomal storage diseases*. However, it has special characteristics that make it more appropriate to be discussed as a leukodystrophy, and it was so named before the lysosomal defect was recognized. Neurologic impairment begins at an early age and progresses rapidly to a fatal conclusion. The enzymic deficit blocks the catabolism of the galactocerebrosides (galactosylceramides). These compounds are major components of myelin, and the disorder thus principally affects the metabolic well-being of oligodendrocytes and Schwann cells.

Early in the disease, during active myelination, the myelinating cells store galactocerebroside within lysosomes. However, the enzyme is also involved in the breakdown of other metabolites, most notably galactosylsphingosine (psychosine), which is also normally synthesized by oligodendrocytes. This substance is highly cytotoxic to oligodendrocytes when it accumulates, and causes their extensive degeneration and death. Myelination ceases and formed myelin degenerates. During this process, macrophages accumulate to ingest the degenerate myelin but are also unable to degrade galactocerebroside. They give rise to the distinctive, swollen, PAS—positive "globoid cells," which form large cuffs around blood vessels in the central white matter, and are also found in the leptomeninges and in the endoneurium of peripheral nerves (Fig. 4-77). The subcortical white matter and the fasciculus proprius of the cord are unaffected. The peripheral nerve involvement is useful for premortem diagnosis by nerve biopsy. At end stage, the pathology of the disease is marked by the presence of these cells, together with diffuse demyelination, axonal loss, and dense astrogliosis in the brain and spinal cord.

Cavitating leukodystrophy. Reported only in **Dalmatian** dogs from Norway, this form of leukodystrophy has a probable autosomal recessive inheritance and a clinical onset at around 3-6 months of age. A similar disease has been reported in

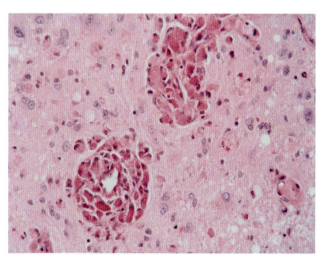

Figure 4-77 Macrophages, filled with degenerate PAS-positive myelin products, aggregating around vessels in **globoid cell leukodystrophy** in a dog.

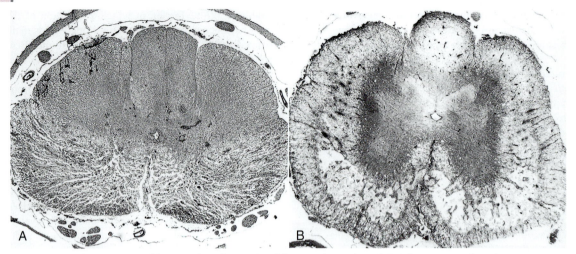

Figure 4-78 Afghan myelopathy. A. Caudal cervical spinal cord. B. Thoracic spinal cord.

Labrador Retrievers. The signs are progressive and variable, and include either gait deficit or visual impairment or both. The former begins as pelvic and then thoracic limb ataxia and dysmetria, with eventual paraparesis. Mental status remains unimpaired throughout.

The neuropathology is characterized by *bilateral, symmetrical, focal areas of intense loss of myelin* in the centrum semiovale, corpus callosum, internal capsule, caudate nucleus, occipital lobes, optic nerves, and thoracic cord white matter adjacent to the ventral horns. The subcortical white matter is unaffected. Initially axons remain intact. The myelin destruction appears to begin with lamellar vesiculation, followed by phagocytosis, and gitter cells are abundant. Fibrous astrogliosis becomes prominent around advanced plaques. The intensity of the process is variable, but lesions are usually visible macroscopically in the central cerebral white matter, appearing as gray depressed areas or, in advanced cases, as cavitations. In some animals, the brain is small and the lateral ventricles enlarged.

Necrotizing myelopathy. The initial reports of the disease in **Afghan Hounds** described acute necrotizing myelomalacia, but subsequent studies indicated a mechanism involving *florid myelinolysis and cavitation*, but essentially sparing axons. It has an apparent recessive inheritance, pre-adult onset, symmetry of lesions, and is noninflammatory, all of which allow for classification as a leukodystrophy. The fundamental pathomechanisms remain undefined. The age of clinical onset is between 3 and 12 months, and caudal ataxia and weakness progress rapidly to paraplegia in a few days. Within 2 weeks, there is thoracic limb weakness and phrenic paralysis. A similar syndrome is reported in **Miniature Poodles** and **Kooiker** dogs.

The lesions (Fig. 4-78A, B) are focused in the *thoracic spinal cord*, where cribriform and spongiotic changes are present in all funiculi (see Fig. 4-78B) and are grossly discernible as discoloration and softening or cavitation. Caudally, the lesions extend into the lumbar segments, but only in the ventral funiculi; they extend cranially to the mid-cervical level in the dorsal and/or ventral funiculi (see Fig. 4-78A). In some cases, there may be lesions in the superior olivary nuclei. The sparing of axons is reflected in the paucity of distal Wallerian degeneration in tracts ascending or descending through the lesions.

Light and electron microscopic examination has revealed initial vacuolation of myelin by splitting of lamellae at the

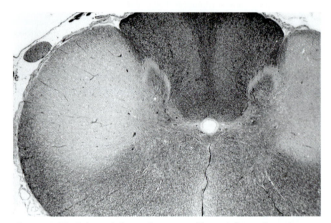

Figure 4-79 Bilateral demyelination of lateral funiculi in the cervical spinal cord in **Rottweiler leukoencephalomyelopathy**. (Courtesy R.F. Slocombe.)

intraperiod line and expansion of the extracellular space. Fragmented and degenerate myelin is phagocytosed by gitter cells, leaving surviving axons and reactive astrocytes within microcavities. The cavities are traversed by blood vessels associated with delicate glial strands. Some focal axonal swelling and disintegration are evident, but myelinolysis following vacuolation is the dominant change.

Leukoencephalomyelopathy. Some difficulties arise in classifying this disease of **Rottweiler** and **Leonberger** dogs as a true leukodystrophy, as the onset is delayed until after 12 months of age. However, there is the probability of autosomal recessive inheritance, and the lesions involve progressive noninflammatory symmetrical myelin degeneration and removal. Clinically, there are slow, but relentlessly progressive, ataxia, hypermetria, and paresis of all limbs, especially the forelimbs, and ultimately severe proprioceptive loss.

The principal locus of the disorder is the *cervical spinal cord*, which on gross inspection may have extensive dull white discoloration of the dorsal and lateral funiculi. Histologic examination reveals lesions to be present in these funiculi, and also in the deep cerebellar white matter and in other regions of the cord. Lesions are marked by significant loss of myelin (Fig. 4-79), with preservation of most axons, either naked or thinly myelinated, and fibrous astrogliosis. There is some evidence that vesicular degeneration of myelin is an early change. In the cervical cord, there may additionally be focal microcavitation deep within the affected areas, edema, numerous gitter cells, and vascular prominence. A narrow rim of intact white matter usually survives immediately deep to the glia limitans. These severe changes may on occasion extend into the thoracic cord and pyramidal tracts.

A unique form of *myelinolytic leukodystrophy*, mainly located in cerebellum and spinal cord, has been reported in crossbred **Maltese/Shih Tzu** puppies. Lesions are characterized by massive infiltration of nonmetachromatic macrophages similar to globoids cells, but not arranged around the vessels. Marked astrocytosis of the white matter precedes myelin breakdown.

Fibrinoid leukodystrophy (Alexander disease). This rare and unusual *myeloencephalopathy*, analogous to Alexander disease in humans, has been reported in the **Scottish Terrier, Labrador Retriever, Miniature Poodle, Bernese Mountain dog,** and **Merino sheep.** The clinical signs of **progressive** tetraparesis and ataxia are associated with spongy white matter lesions, astrocytic gliosis, and accumulation of eosinophilic refractile bodies *(Rosenthal fibers)* within the processes of astrocytes disposed around blood vessels, subpial, and subependymal areas.

Progressive ataxia of Charolais cattle. This disease appears to represent a progressive inability on the part of some oligodendrocytes to maintain the paranodal extremities of their myelin domains; it may represent *oligodendroglial dysplasia*. The disease is presumably genetically determined, but has been reported in three-quarter crossbred animals. Both sexes may be affected, and clinical signs become evident between 8-24 months of age.

The clinical spectrum involves increasing ataxia and dysmetria, head tremor, and some tendency to aggressive behavior. The mental status remains bright and alert. Affected females often urinate in a series of short spurts. The clinical signs progress slowly but steadily, and the animals can be expected to become recumbent by 3 years of age at the latest.

There are no specific gross lesions, but the microscopic findings are distinctive and unprecedented, and are located mainly in the cerebellar white matter and peduncles, the internal capsule, corpus callosum, optic tract, lateral lemniscus, median longitudinal fasciculus, pontine decussation, and ventral and lateral funiculi of the spinal cord. In these white matter tracts, there are *multifocal, granular eosinophilic plaques* ~30 μm in diameter (Fig. 4-80). The plaques are traversed by axons and stain with many, but not all, of the features of normal myelin. There is no sign of myelin degradation or phagocytosis. Immediately around the plaques, there appears to be an increased number of astrocytes and oligodendrocytes. Some very minor axonal degeneration may be found in some plaques and in normal white matter. It has been concluded that early plaques can be distinguished from old ones. Electron microscopy reveals them to be complex. The ultrastructure suggests great disorder at the myelin paranodes, with relatively normal internodal regions. New plaques reveal axons encompassed, near abnormally long nodes of Ranvier, by hypertrophied oligodendrocyte tongues and processes within a thin myelin sheath. Old plaques contain demyelinated axons (some of which are swollen), surrounded by disorganized myelin lamellae and masses of oligodendrocyte processes. Each plaque may represent the territory of one oligodendrocyte, and reflect its failure to maintain normal paranodal

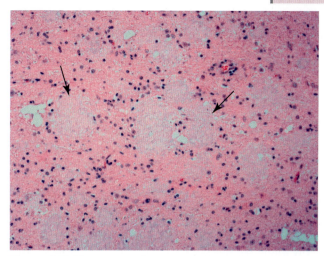

Figure 4-80 Plaques in white matter (arrows) in **progressive ataxia** of Charolais cattle.

myelin loops, in the course of which massive hypertrophy of its processes occurs.

Similar lesions have been described in **Bullmastiff dogs** with slowly progressive ataxia, spastic tetraparesis, and diffuse, action-related, whole-body tremor.

Multifocal symmetrical myelinolytic encephalopathy of Simmental, Limousin, and Aberdeen Angus calves. Reports from Australia, New Zealand, the United States, Canada, and the United Kingdom describe similar diseases in calves of these breeds, in which *spongy vacuolation of white matter progresses focally to lysis and cavitation*, but with the initial sparing of many axons and nerve cell bodies. In Limousin calves, such foci are present in the cerebellar peduncles and optic chiasm. In Simmental calves and Simmental crosses, lesions involve the internal capsule, caudate nucleus, putamen, periaqueductal white matter, lateral cuneate nucleus, and inferior olive. The distribution extends more widely in Aberdeen Angus and, in some cases, will include the spinal gray matter. In Limousins and Aberdeen Angus, blindness and dysmetria appear at about 1 month of age, and some animals develop seizures and opisthotonos, whereas others remain stable. In Simmentals, the clinical onset is between 5 and 8 months of age. There is progressive ataxia, weight loss, and eventual dullness and emaciation, with death usual by 12 months of age. The pathogenesis of these diseases is uncertain; similarities exist with Leigh disease of humans, and familial syndromes in **Australian Cattle dogs** and **Alaskan Huskies.**

Feline spinal myelinopathy. An adult-onset condition involving progressive noninflammatory myelin loss in the spinal cord has been reported in cats in California. The pathomechanism is undefined. Myelin deficiency develops in the absence of significant axonal degeneration, and is accompanied by astrogliosis. The lesions occur in all funiculi, and are most intense in the thoracic and lumbar segments.

Demyelinating neuropathy. Demyelinating peripheral neuropathies result from Schwann cell or myelin protein abnormalities. In **Miniature Schnauzers,** the disease is characterized by formation of *tomaculae*, which represent *abnormally focally folded myelin sheaths*. A form of *congenital hypomyelinating neuropathy* has been recognized in **Golden Retrievers.**

In **Tibetan Mastiffs,** a recessively inherited condition known as *hypertrophic neuropathy* is considered to reflect a primary metabolic defect of Schwann cells, with failure to maintain myelin during axonal elongation in postnatal growth. The CNS is not involved. The clinical onset is consistently between 7 and 10 weeks of age. There is rapid progression of generalized weakness with hyporeflexia, slowed nerve conduction velocity, and ultimately tetraplegia in many cases.

In peripheral nerves and their spinal roots, there are changes consistent with *demyelination, remyelination, and endoneurial fibrosis.* Thus many axons are denuded, whereas some have a thin sheath; proliferating Schwann cells form onion bulbs, and endoneurial collagen is prominent. Axonal degeneration is not a feature. The most characteristic features are revealed ultrastructurally. Schwann cell cytoplasm contains *dense accumulations of 6- to 7-nm filaments*, occurring at sites where the myelin sheath has separated along the major dense lines, and in the adaxonal cytoplasm. There are also anomalous incisure patterns within the sheaths, with many incisural openings staggered through the entire thickness of the sheath.

Further reading

Fletcher JL, et al. Clinical signs and neuropathologic abnormalities in working Australian Kelpies with globoid cell leukodystrophy (Krabbe disease). J Am Vet Med Assoc 2010;237:682-688.

Kessell AE, et al. A Rosenthal fiber encephalomyelopathy resembling Alexander's disease in 3 sheep. Vet Pathol 2012;49:248-254.

Oevermann A, et al. A novel leukoencephalomyelopathy of Leonberger dogs. J Vet Intern Med 2008;22:467-471.

Salvadori C, et al. Clinicopathological features of globoid cell leucodystrophy in cats. J Comp Pathol 2005;132:350-356.

Schock A, et al. Multifocal symmetrical necrotising encephalopathy in Simmental cross cattle in Scotland. Vet Rec 2008;162:694-695.

Sisó S, et al. A novel leucodystrophy in a dog. J Comp Pathol 2005;132:232-236.

Vanhaesebrouck AE, et al. Demyelinating polyneuropathy with focally folded myelin sheaths in a family of Miniature Schnauzer dogs. J Neurol Sci 2008;275:100-105.

Spongy myelinopathies

There is a group of diseases in which the dominant pathologic feature is *dramatic vacuolation of myelin that often occurs without any overt indication of large-scale myelin breakdown or phagocytosis.* There is still the familiar problem, however, of deciding how to categorize some diseases that have overlapping features of myelin vacuolation and myelin degeneration, and it is acknowledged that some of the conditions described later could be placed elsewhere.

Myelin vacuolation is one of several different morphologic changes encompassed by the term **"status spongiosus"** of nervous tissue (Fig. 4-81). Although producing a striking light microscopic picture when well developed, electron microscopy is required for its fine definition (Fig. 4-82A-C). Histologic changes suggestive of this lesion are a fairly common postmortem artifact.

Vacuolation of myelin may come about in several ways, the most frequent of which involves *separation of lamellae along the intraperiod line*, thereby reopening the extracellular space originally obliterated within the spiraling processes of the myelinating cell. This mechanism can produce vacuoles within the sheath at multiple levels and multiple loci along an internode. In experimental situations, this type of vacuolation has been associated with an increase in tissue water and

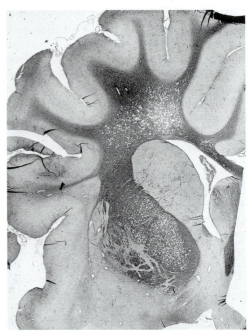

Figure 4-81 Status spongiosus of central cerebral white matter in spongiform myelinopathy in a silver fox. (Reprinted with permission from Hagen G, Bjerkas I. Vet Pathol 1990;27:187-193.)

electrolytes, consistent with simple edema, and accounts for the brain swelling that may occur in severe cases. The vacuoles therefore contain no stainable material. A variety of associated functional disturbances has been described but, remarkably, the lesion may have little functional impact, even when quite intense and prolonged. It seems likely that the myelin lesion is one facet of a complex metabolic disturbance, whose ramifications vary according to basic causes. In humans, the classic disease of this type is *Canavan disease*, with congenital and infantile forms caused by an autosomal recessive trait, and a rare juvenile form with no demonstrable familial association.

Vacuolation may also arise by separation of lamellae at the major dense line, reopening the intracellular compartment of the myelinating cell, or by ballooning of the periaxonal space. Depending on the particular disease, the vacuolation of the myelin may or may not be accompanied by structural changes in other elements of the tissue, including the myelinating cell bodies, and, in general, these are more likely to occur if vacuolation has been prolonged. In some instances too, prolongation of the process is associated with a reduced quantity of myelin. In those cases where there is no indication of myelin degradation, its steady withdrawal by the normal catabolic pathways with concurrent suppression of synthesis is implied.

The spongy myelinopathies of animals fall into 2 broad groups: those that are **idiopathic,** and those that have a defined **metabolic** or **toxic** basis.

Idiopathic spongy myelinopathies. This group is documented in a small number of case reports involving calves, pups, and kittens, and most are suspected to have a heredofamilial basis. Several conditions involving newborn **Hereford** calves have been described over the years, with some conflicting and confusing aspects. Earlier reports proposed a condition, dubbed "hereditary neuraxial edema," to be a single entity with a variable clinical and pathologic expression; the pathogenesis of several of these conditions has been unraveled, including *inherited congenital myoclonus* and *branched-chain*

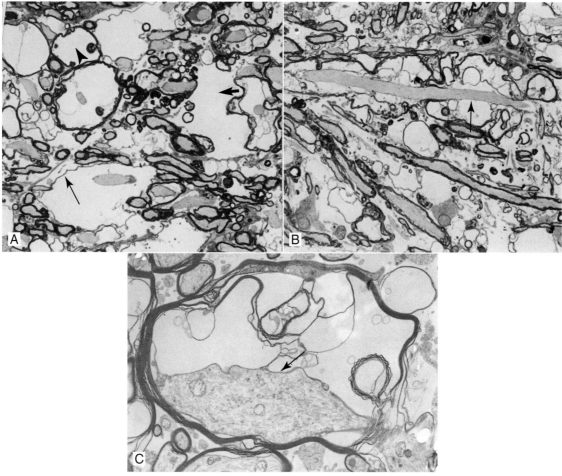

Figure 4-82 Spongiform myelinopathy in a silver fox. **A.** Note thin and dilated myelin sheath around normal axon (small arrow), empty myelin-bound vacuole (arrowhead), and expanded extracellular space (large arrow). **B.** Disrupted myelin around normal axon (arrow). **C.** Electron micrograph demonstrating periaxonal vacuolation and split myelin lamellae around normal axon (arrow). (Reprinted with permission from Hagen G, Bjerkas I. Vet Pathol 1990;27:187-193.)

ketoacid dehydrogenase deficiency (BCKD). The former is recognized in several countries in newborn polled Herefords that have violent myoclonic muscle spasms that prevent them from standing. There are no structural lesions, but biochemical studies have revealed an absence of glycinergic receptors on spinal inhibitory neurons. The functional disturbance is thus analogous to strychnine poisoning and is equally fatal. BCKD is discussed later.

From New Zealand, a disease of **horned Hereford** calves has been named *congenital brain edema*. Newborn calves are unable to stand after birth and have coarse tonic muscle contractions. Vacuolation of myelin is diffuse, extends into the gray matter, and is accompanied by elevated brain water content. Hydropic degeneration of astrocytes and expansion of the extracellular space are detectable ultrastructurally. There is also considered to be a deficiency of myelin.

In Britain, a very similar picture is recorded in **polled Hereford** calves. There may remain an entity in Hereford calves, severely neurologically impaired at birth, in which myelin vacuolation is extensive in the CNS, is confined to the white matter, and is not associated with hypomyelinogenesis. For the time being, such cases could be classified as hereditary neuraxial edema in the absence of any demonstrable metabolic disturbance suggestive of BCKD or other aminoacidopathies.

In **Samoyed** pups, a generalized tremor syndrome occurs in the first few weeks of life, with a severe and ultimately fatal outcome. Myelin vacuolation is diffuse throughout the CNS, and there is no change in any other tissue element.

Labrador Retriever pups are described to have initial episodes of extensor rigidity, tremor, and dorsal flexion of the neck at 4-6 weeks of age, and then progressive dysmetria. Intense vacuolation of myelin is confined to the white matter in the CNS, but occurs to a mild degree in peripheral nerves as well. Throughout the CNS, the myelin lesion is accompanied by fibrous astrogliosis and prominence of capillary blood vessels. A similar condition with a familial pattern *(canine spongiform leukoencephalomyelopathy)* is recognized in **Shetland Sheepdogs** and **Australian Cattle dogs.** Clinical signs usually start at 3 weeks of age and include progressive seizures and dysphagia. Spongiform degeneration is most prominent in the cerebellum and corona radiata. The disease is associated with a missense mitochondrial DNA mutation in cytochrome *b*.

In a **Silky Terrier** pup, a myoclonic syndrome is described, with vacuolation of myelin occurring in the brain but not the spinal cord, together with the presence of Alzheimer type II astrocytes. A form of hereditary spongiform leukoencephalomyelopathy is described in **Border Terrier** puppies. In **Egyptian Mau** kittens, there is progressive ataxia and hypermetria; vacuolar change extends from white into gray matter throughout the CNS. Spongiform CNS myelinopathy has been reported in a group of related **African dwarf goats** and in adult **Ragdoll cats**.

Spongy myelinopathy of silver foxes. A hereditary nervous disease occurs in farmed silver foxes in Norway. The presenting sign is hindlimb ataxia appearing between 2-4 months of age, and progressing over the next 4-8 weeks, after which time clinical improvement seems to occur.

No gross lesions are present, and histologically, there is *symmetrical myelin vacuolation* affecting white matter of the cerebrum, cerebellum, brainstem, and spinal cord (see Fig. 4-81). The extent and severity of vacuolation vary from case to case. In long-standing cases, vacuolation seems to resolve to a large extent, with residual intense astrogliosis.

Ultrastructurally, early features of the disease include intramyelinic vacuolation resulting from lamellar separation at the intraperiod line, large cytoplasmic vacuoles in oligodendrocyte cytoplasm, demyelination, expansion of extracellular space, and astrocytic hypertrophy (see Fig. 4-82A-C). Late in the disease, there is evidence of remyelination in gliotic areas.

Toxic/metabolic spongy myelinopathies

Hepatic and renal encephalopathy. Endogenous intoxications associated with hepatic and, to a lesser extent, renal failure, are recognized to induce brain lesions of this type, the former quite frequently, the latter less so.

The familiar clinicopathologic term, *hepatic encephalopathy*, designates a complex autointoxication, in which accumulations of ammonia and other metabolites reflect the inability of the liver to carry out its normal detoxifying role. This may in turn reflect reduced liver mass, portosystemic shunting, or both. Excess ammonium is metabolized by astrocytes to glutamine, which induces osmotic changes with development of cytotoxic edema. *The neural lesions of hepatic encephalopathy are several and variable.*

Clinical evidence of nervous dysfunction may be accompanied by extensive and well-developed *spongy vacuolation of myelin* (Fig. 4-83), which tends to be most intense at the junction of the cerebral cortex and adjacent white matter, and often around the deep cerebellar nuclei. The lesion is to be expected in ruminants with subacute or chronic phytotoxic or mycotoxic liver injury, and in small animals with developmental portosystemic shunts or acquired liver disease. In sheep, copper toxicosis may lead to massive myelin vacuolation. There may also be *Alzheimer type II astroglial cells* (see Fig. 4-14) although, with the notable exception of the horse, this is generally less a feature in animals than in humans. In the horse, hepatic encephalopathy is characterized by the presence of Alzheimer type II cells, with no significant myelin vacuolation.

Although myelin vacuolation may be induced experimentally with ammonia alone, the syndrome is *not simple ammonia intoxication*, but may also involve perturbed monoamine neurotransmission, imbalance between excitatory and inhibitory amino acid neurotransmission, and accumulation of an endogenous benzodiazepine-like substance. Moreover, systemic infection, inflammation and associated cytokines, as well as a lipopolysaccharide endotoxin, are involved in the development of brain edema in acute hepatic encephalopathy.

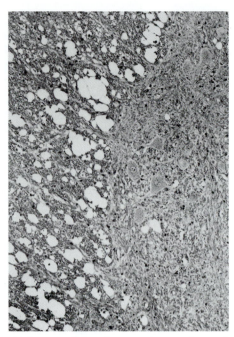

Figure 4-83 Intramyelinic edema and spongiform change surrounding spinal gray matter in **hepatic encephalopathy** in a sheep.

Branched-chain α-ketoacid decarboxylase deficiency. This disease, also known as **maple syrup urine disease,** has been described in Hereford, polled Hereford, and polled Shorthorn calves, and is inherited as an *autosomal recessive* character. This mutation causes *deficiency of the mitochondrial branched-chain α-ketoacid dehydrogenase (BCKD) complex*. Deficiency of BCKD leads to the accumulation of the branched-chain amino acids leucine, isoleucine, and valine and their respective ketoacids: ketoisocaproic, keto-β-methylvaleric, and ketoisovaleric acids. The molecular mechanism of the intoxication remains to be precisely defined, but probably involves toxic metabolites.

The disease may be expressed in utero, and calves become dull and recumbent by 2-4 days of age, and finally develop opisthotonos. The urine in many cases has the smell of maple syrup, the characteristic that gave the disease its common name in affected children. Branched-chain amino acids are found to be in abnormally high concentrations in plasma, cerebrospinal fluid, and tissues.

Pathologically, there may be gross evidence of brain swelling expressed as flattened cerebral gyri and, histologically, *severe spongy vacuolation of myelin in the CNS*. The spongiotic change is pronounced in the large myelinated tracts of the cerebral hemispheres and cerebellum (Fig. 4-84), and in myelinated tracts abutting brainstem nuclei and spinal gray matter. Most of the spinal white matter is not affected. In cases that survive for a week or more, a modest number of axonal spheroids may be found in affected white matter. The brain water content is elevated, and the electron microscope reveals splitting of myelin lamellae at the intraperiod line.

Hexachlorophene toxicosis. Hexachlorophene is a polychlorinated phenolic compound with useful topical antiseptic properties, and is sometimes given orally against *Fasciola hepatica*. Intoxication has usually been associated with repeated application to the skin of very young animals, in which absorption is rapid, and systemic accumulation may cause effects within several days. The clinical features of

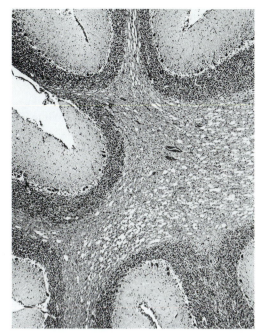

Figure 4-84 Status spongiosus in the central cerebellar white matter of a calf with **maple syrup urine disease.**

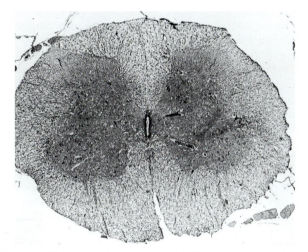

Figure 4-85 Intramyelin edema and diffuse spongiform change in the spinal cord white matter of a dog with **hexachlorophene poisoning.**

severe intoxication are shaking, shivering, excitement, tonic-clonic convulsions, and terminal coma.

The major lesion is *spongy vacuolation of central and peripheral myelin* (Fig. 4-85), with lamellar splitting at the intraperiod line, and no associated degenerative or reactive changes. This lesion may persist for many weeks, even after clinical signs have abated. Under experimental conditions, vacuolation of the retinal photoreceptor outer segments is also evident, but this has not been a reported feature of accidental intoxication.

Halogenated salicylanilide toxicosis. The halogenated salicylanilides are long-acting anthelmintics used in sheep and goats, and include closantel and rafoxanide. Accidental overdosing has led to intoxication expressed as ataxia, depression, and blindness, which may be permanent. The response appears to be inconsistent, and unknown predisposing factors are possibly involved.

Microscopically, there is *spongy vacuolation of myelin in both the CNS and peripheral nerves*, without any accompanying reaction or degeneration. The lesion in the brain is most intense in the brainstem. This change may persist for several weeks. Acute degenerative changes may be found in the optic nerves and in the retinal ganglion cell layer, where hemorrhage has also been described. The syndrome has some similarities to stypandrol poisoning, described later.

Stypandra toxicosis. The binaphthalene tetrol, **stypandrol,** is the toxic principle of the Australian liliaceous *Stypandra* sp. ("blindgrass") and also of the Asiatic *Hemerocallis* sp., hence the alternative name **hemerocallin.** Ingestion of toxic strains of such plants by grazing mammals or birds has an acute effect, usually manifested as moderate depression and blindness, although a high dose may produce prostration and death.

In acutely affected animals, *myelin vacuolation* caused by lamellar splitting at the intraperiod line is extensive throughout the CNS, and may persist for many weeks or even months, without apparent functional effect. Blindness, however, tends to be permanent and is associated with Wallerian degeneration of the optic nerves and tracts, and degeneration of retinal photoreceptors. Degeneration of the optic nerves may be the result of compression within the optic canals secondary to swelling caused by the myelin edema, and there may be a separate direct toxic effect on the photoreceptors.

Tylecodon toxicosis. *Tylecodon wallichii* is the cause of **krimpsiekte,** a neurotoxicosis of small ruminants in South Africa. The toxic principle is **cotyledoside,** a neurotoxic bufadienolide that can produce either acute or chronic poisoning, the latter probably as a cumulative effect of the toxicosis. Affected animals assume a posture with back arched, display torticollis, and then prolonged paralysis. Edema and formation of large vacuoles are particularly prominent in the optic radiations and thalamic white matter. A similar syndrome has been reported in small ruminants poisoned by *Ornithogalum toxicarium* in Namibia.

Helichrysum toxicosis. The many species of the plant genus *Helichrysum* are widely distributed, and distinct syndromes of toxicity in ruminants occur in Australia and South Africa: *Helichrysum blandowskianum* in Australia (woolly everlasting daisy) produces acute hepatic necrosis, presumptive hepatic encephalopathy, and spongiform change in the white matter of the brainstem, with a high mortality rate; *H. argyrosphaerum* in South Africa is associated with paresis, paralysis, and permanent blindness.

Intense spongy vacuolation of myelin in the brain is sufficient to cause grossly visible swelling of the optic nerves and chiasm, and gelatinous swelling of the periventricular white matter and corpus callosum. Focal hemorrhages may occur in the optic nerves and chiasm. Microscopically, the spongiform myelin lesion in the optic nerves is accompanied by Wallerian degeneration, suggesting compression within the optic canals. Myelin vacuolation is less severe in the spinal cord and peripheral nerves. The syndrome has similarities to stypandrol toxicosis.

Diplodia toxicity (diplodiosis). Diplodiosis is a mycotoxicosis of cattle and sheep grazing on maize lands toward the end of the growing season in various countries in southern Africa and in Argentina. The causative fungus is *Diplodia maydis.* The fungus is extremely fetotoxic and causes neonatal mortality in lambs of ewes ingesting the toxin during late pregnancy. The spongy change is caused by separation of myelin along the intraperiod line and may progress to lysis of myelin.

Bromethalin toxicity. Diffuse white matter spongiosus is described in dogs and cats given a single oral dose of this highly neurotoxic rodenticide.

Further reading

Comito B, et al. Adult-onset spongiform leukoencephalopathy in 2 Ragdoll cats. J Vet Intern Med 2010;24:977-982.

Jayakumar AR, et al. Role of cerebral endothelial cells in the astrocyte swelling and brain edema associated with acute hepatic encephalopathy. Neuroscience 2012;218:305-316.

Li FY, et al. Canine spongiform leukoencephalomyelopathy is associated with a missense mutation in cytochrome b. Neurobiol Dis 2006;21:35-42.

Martin-Vaquero P, et al. A novel spongiform leukoencephalomyelopathy in Border Terrier puppies. J Vet Intern Med 2012;26:402-406.

Spongy encephalomyelopathies

The term "**status spongiosus**" applies to a variety of lesions in which the microscopic appearance of the neural tissue is transformed by numerous vacuoles or microcavities. As discussed previously, one form of this state results from the vacuolation of myelin, and is the most common. This section will discuss diseases in which the change results from either the *swelling of astrocytes* or the *vacuolation of neurons and neurites*. Astrocytic swelling may occur nonspecifically in, or adjacent to, any area of neural tissue acutely injured by trauma, or ischemia, or in which vascular permeability is disturbed. In the absence of such circumstances, its occurrence suggests some direct toxic or metabolic influence upon the astrocytes themselves. It can thus be a feature in hepatic encephalopathy. Spongy vacuolation of neurons and their processes may occur to a limited degree as an incidental change in the red nucleus and nuclei of the caudal brainstem, and also as an artifact of fixation. It needs to be interpreted against this background, and is usually considered in the context of the diagnosis of scrapie and related conditions. It is distinctly different from the foamy vacuolation seen in the lysosomal storage diseases.

Organic acidurias. *Citrullinemia* is a fulminating neurologic affliction of newborn **Holstein-Friesian calves** that results from a blockade of urea cycle metabolism caused by *deficiency of arginosuccinate synthetase*. The enzyme deficiency leads to hyperammonemia and citrullinemia, and is caused by an *autosomal recessive* genetic defect. Increased cross-breeding and screening of sires for the defect have reduced its prevalence to insignificant levels.

Calves are affected within the first week of life, the clinical features being depression, head pressing, stupor, convulsions, terminal coma, and death. There are no gross neural lesions, but microscopically, there is mild to moderate spongy vacuolation of the deep laminae of the cerebral cortex. *The spongy change is the result of astrocytic swelling.* Hydropic astrocytes have enlarged vesicular nuclei, but their cell bodies and processes are vacuolated and give rise to the spongiform appearance of the neuropil, the creation of perineuronal spaces, and the enlargement of pericapillary spaces. The astrocytic reaction is believed to represent a stress on these cells in their attempts to detoxify ammonia. Astrocytes play a major role in ammonia detoxification via use of glutamine synthetase and glutamate dehydrogenase activities. In spite of the marked degenerative changes in astrocytes, other elements of the tissue remain morphologically normal, but neuronal function is obviously grossly disturbed. Affected calves also have pale yellow-ochre discoloration of the liver, which is correlated microscopically and ultrastructurally with hydropic degeneration of hepatocytes.

Organic acidurias have also been described in dogs. In **Staffordshire Bull Terriers** and **West Highland White Terriers**, a mutation in the *L-2-hydroxyglutaric acid dehydrogenase gene* causes accumulation of L-2-hydroxyglutaric acid in the organic fluids, and is associated with marked spongy degeneration of the gray matter of cerebral and cerebellar cortices, thalamus, and brainstem. *Methylmalonic and malonic aciduria* has been reported in a **Labrador Retriever** with brain atrophy and spongy degeneration.

Multifocal spongy encephalomyelopathy. A disease was originally described in **Bullmastiffs** as *familial cerebellar ataxia with hydrocephalus*, but the main pathologic feature is spongy vacuolation of several gray matter nuclei. Clinical signs emerge between 6 and 9 weeks of age, and include ataxia and visual impairment, and a number of other variable deficits. An autosomal recessive genetic defect has been proposed.

Macroscopically, there is moderate to severe dilation of the ventricular system. Microscopically, bilaterally symmetrical spongy vacuolation and gliosis are evident in all 3 deep cerebellar nuclei, the posterior colliculi, and, to a lesser extent, the lateral vestibular nuclei. The vacuolation is accompanied by axonal spheroids, but nerve cell bodies appear normal. Some of the vacuoles appear to involve myelin sheaths, but the lesions are essentially confined to the gray matter, and the cytologic basis of the vacuolation is not precisely defined.

Similar vacuolating lesions of these gray matter areas have been described in **Saluki** dogs.

An autosomal recessive *cerebellar ataxia* is described in **Malinois puppies** of 2 months of age. Lesions are marked bilateral spongy degeneration of the cerebellar nuclei and vacuolization of the cerebellar granule cells and foliate white matter. Scattered vacuoles and spheroids are detectable throughout the brainstem.

A spongy degeneration of unknown etiology and characterized histologically by *neuronal vacuolation, myelopathy, and laryngeal neuropathy* is recognized in **Rottweiler** dogs. The condition usually starts at 8 weeks of age and is characterized clinically by progressive laryngeal paralysis, tetraparesis, and cerebellar ataxia. Vacuolated neurons are prevalent in the cerebellar nuclei, nuclei of the extrapyramidal system, dorsal nerve root ganglia, myenteric plexus, and other ganglia of the autonomic nervous system. Axonopathic lesions are present in all funiculi of the spinal cord, and dying back neuropathy affects the recurrent laryngeal nerve. An analogous condition has also been reported in **Rottweiler-cross, Boxer,** and **mixed-breed dogs.**

A presumed *hereditary polioencephalomyelopathy* of **Australian Cattle dogs** is characterized histologically by neuronal, neuropilar, and astrocytic vacuolation, particularly in the ventral horn of the cervicothoracic spinal cord, cerebellar, and brainstem nuclei. An autosomal recessive trait affecting the astrocytic mitochondria is suspected.

Alaskan Husky dogs can develop a hereditary familial encephalopathy *(Alaskan Husky encephalopathy)* similar to Leigh syndrome in humans and to the multifocal symmetrical myelinolytic encephalopathy of Simmental calves described previously. Clinical signs usually start before 1 year of age and include seizures, ataxia, blindness, and behavioral abnormalities. Lesions are more prevalent in the basal nuclei, thalamus, midbrain, pons, and medulla oblongata, and include bilateral symmetrical malacia, status spongiosus, gemistocytic astrocytosis with marked intracytoplasmic vacuolation, gliosis, vascular hyperplasia, and mild infiltration of mixed inflammatory cells, with relative neuronal sparing. Similar but milder lesions occur in the cerebellar ventral vermis and the base of cerebral sulci. Neuronal sparing and marked astrocytic vacuolation suggests a role for astrocytes in the pathogenesis of this condition. A mutation in the thiamine transporter 2 gene *(SLC19A3)* is associated with the disease in Alaskan Huskies. Nearly identical lesions occur in *subacute necrotizing encephalopathy* of **Yorkshire Terriers.**

Spongy changes in the brainstem associated with gliosis and extensive spheroid formation in cerebellar nuclei, and necrosis of the caudate nuclei have been described in **Kuvasz** puppies.

In **cats,** spongy degeneration of unknown causes is reported in sporadic cases. Lesions are described as spongy degeneration throughout the cerebral and cerebellar cortices, or limited to the substantia nigra and other nuclei of the brainstem. Spongiosis of cerebellar and vestibular nuclei, associated with intraneural accumulation of phosphorylated neurofilaments and intense apoptosis, has been described in a Persian kitten. In a familial disease of Birman kittens, spongy degeneration involves the cortex of the pyriform lobe, thalamus, caudal colliculi, cerebellar peduncles, and is associated with diffuse myelopathy.

Neuronal vacuolar degeneration of Angora goats. A scrapie-like neuronopathy is described in young Angora goats in Australia (where scrapie is not present), and is presumed to be genetically determined. Animals become ataxic at about 3 months of age, and progress to severe paresis. No significant gross lesions are present, but there is spectacular vacuolation of large neurons in the red nucleus and other brainstem nuclei, and in the spinal motor neurons. Some Wallerian changes are present in the brainstem, spinal cord, and peripheral nerves.

Congenital status spongiosus of Gelbvieh-cross calves. A diffuse, bilaterally symmetrical status spongiosus with Alzheimer type II cells throughout the white matter of the brain has been described in Gelbvieh-Red Angus calves. Affected animals are unable to stand, and have constant whole-body tremors when stimulated. Genetic and biochemical analyses indicate that the disease is distinct from maple syrup urine disease.

Further reading

Baiker K, et al. Leigh-like subacute necrotising encephalopathy in Yorkshire Terriers: neuropathological characterisation, respiratory chain activities and mitochondrial DNA. Acta Neuropathol 2009;118:697-709.

Geiger DA, et al. Encephalomyelopathy and polyneuropathy associated with neuronal vacuolation in two Boxer littermates. Vet Pathol 2009;46:1160-1165.

Kleiter M, et al. Spongy degeneration with cerebellar ataxia in Malinois puppies: a hereditary autosomal recessive disorder? J Vet Intern Med 2011;25:490-496.

Penderis J, et al. L-2-hydroxyglutaric aciduria: characterisation of the molecular defect in a spontaneous canine model. J Med Genet 2007;44:334-340.

Salvadori C, et al. Neuronal vacuolation, myelopathy and laryngeal neuropathy in a mixed-breed dog. J Vet Med A 2007;54:445-448.

Salvadori C, et al. Spongiform neurodegenerative disease in a Persian kitten. J Feline Med Surg 2007;9:242-245.

Vernau KM, et al. Genome-wide association analysis identifies a mutation in the thiamine transporter 2 (SLC19A3) gene associated with Alaskan Husky encephalopathy. PLoS ONE 2013;8:e57195.

Prion diseases

Prions ("prion" is a combined form of "proteinaceous" and "infectious") are believed to be the cause of fatal neurologic diseases in humans and several other mammalian species. Prion diseases *(prionoses)* are characterized by chronic progressive fatal neurologic manifestations, with both sensory and motor deficits and spongiform encephalopathy, and result from accumulation of an abnormal isoform (PrP^{Sc}, Sc refers to scrapie) of the host prion protein (PrP). The gene *(PRNP)* encoding the prion protein is highly conserved in animals and humans. Transmissible prion diseases result from infection with an external PrP^{Sc} and accumulation of host-produced PrP^{Sc}, and are called **transmissible spongiform encephalopathies** (TSEs) to differentiate them from prion diseases originating from genetic mutation, for example, familial Creutzfeldt-Jacob disease (CJD) in humans. The prion protein is widely distributed in tissues but concentrated in nervous tissue where normal prion protein (PrP^c, c is for cellular) is a glycolipid-anchored glycoprotein located on the surface of neuronal plasma membranes; its exact function in mammals is unknown. PrP^{Sc} is not only membrane anchored, but it can also be demonstrated in lysosomes using immunohistochemistry and electron microscopy. PrP^{Sc} almost never triggers an immune response.

Prion diseases in animals include *scrapie* of sheep and goats, *bovine spongiform encephalopathy* (BSE), *chronic wasting disease* (CWD) of deer and elk, *transmissible mink encephalopathy* (TME), *feline spongiform encephalopathy* (FSE), and *exotic ungulate encephalopathy* of captive wild ruminants. Human prion diseases include *kuru*; CJD, which has 4 types—sporadic CJD, familial CJD, iatrogenic CJD, and variant CJD (vCJD); *Gerstmann-Straussler-Scheinker disease* (GSS); and *fatal familial insomnia* (FFI). The inherited prion diseases of humans are all of dominant inheritance, and all are associated with coding mutations of the *PRNP* gene. Interest in the TSEs has increased greatly for several reasons. First, the discovery that these diseases may result from an infectious protein agent that is lacking nucleic acids contradicted the central dogma of modern biology that all living organisms use nucleic acids to reproduce. Second, the appearance of BSE in Great Britain and other parts of the world, and its presumed relationship to vCJD, triggered both scientific and public interest in these diseases. Despite extensive work on prions, our understanding of their pathogenesis and etiology is incomplete.

The *protein-only hypothesis* is currently the most accepted hypothesis for the pathogenesis of prion diseases. This hypothesis states that (1) PrP^{Sc} is the etiologic agent of TSEs and other prion diseases; (2) the transformation of α-helical PrP to its misfolded β-pleated sheet isoform, the PrP^{Sc}, requires either a genetic predisposition or requires the help of unknown protein cofactors (protein X) that act as a molecular chaperone for this conversion; (3) PrP^{Sc} triggers the PrP gene *(PRNP)* to produce more PrP^{Sc} (self-replicating protein); and (4) PrP^{Sc}

can be infectious itself and can be transmitted to other hosts and cause disease (transmissible protein). There is a species barrier to transmission of the TSE agent, but it is not complete. Less accepted theories for the etiology of prion diseases include the virion or virus hypothesis, and the autoimmunity/allergic hypothesis, which states that TSEs could be autoimmune diseases resulting from ingestion of feedstuffs contaminated with certain bacteria, for example, *Acinetobacter* spp., that show molecular mimicry between bacterial components and CNS tissue. *Spiroplasma mirum*, a cell-wall–deficient bacterium, has also been proposed as a trigger for TSEs.

The mechanism by which PrP^{Sc} causes nerve cell degeneration is complicated, and several mechanisms have been proposed, including (1) mechanical destruction of nerve cell membranes from the excessive accumulations, (2) lysosomal accumulation of PrP^{Sc} may trigger apoptosis by release of cathepsin D into cytosol, and (3) PrP^{Sc} may be a direct neurotoxin. There are multiple strains of prions in scrapie of sheep, the strains distinguished by biological properties in defined strains of mice determined especially by incubation periods and lesion profiles, and the nature and patterns of neuropathologic changes. In sporadic disease in humans, different strains or types of the agent are beginning to be related to clinical phenotypes, and in some of the diseases in animals, additional to scrapie, there is evidence for strain variation. The agent of BSE is exceptional in being, so far, monotypic. Prions have unusual resistance to physical and chemical agents, and this unusual resistance makes inactivation of prion infectivity very difficult.

The pathogenesis of these diseases is further complicated by genetic variation among hosts, whereby homozygosity at particular codons is known to confer susceptibility to the natural or experimental disease and heterozygosity confers survival advantage, although this is expressed mainly as prolonged incubation time. In heterozygotes, the outcome of exposure may be further modified by other polymorphisms. For example, sheep carry 2 alleles of the *PrP* gene and 5 different allelic variants. Sheep breeds that are homozygous for the variant VRQ/VRQ (valine (V) at codon 136, arginine (R) at codon 154, and glutamine (Q) at codon 171) are the most susceptible to scrapie, whereas sheep with the ARR (alanine [A]) variant are most resistant and do not develop overt disease.

The transmission of prions between individuals or species in spontaneous disease remains a mystery, except for kuru, for which there is strong evidence for ritualistic cannibalism, and vCJD for which there is compelling evidence of oral transmission from BSE. It is noteworthy that all cases of vCJD and kuru are homozygous for methionine at *PRNP* codon 129. The oral route is probably important for BSE, vCJD, and TME. The mode of transmission of scrapie and CWD remains unclear. The origin of BSE is not well understood. The most accepted hypothesis is that BSE came from a mutated scrapie prion that contaminated ruminant feed.

There are *no gross abnormalities* in the brain other than those expected in older animals with a wasting disease. Some elements of the histologic picture are consistently present but variable in their neuroanatomic distribution and degree of expression. The most consistent pattern involves the medulla oblongata (particularly at the level of the obex); however, immunohistochemical-positive labeling of PrPSc was observed also in the brainstem and cerebral cortex of cattle with natural and experimental clinical cases of BSE. Currently, the medulla oblongata is the anatomic predilection site for detection of PrPSc.

Inflammatory change is absent. *Spongiform change is an important identifying feature*. It consists of small rounded vacuoles in the neuropil, sometimes extending into neurites. The vacuoles in the neuropil may become confluent. The extracellular space is normal. The vacuoles are of variable distribution in cerebral gray matter and may be diffuse or clustered. The pathogenesis of the spongiform change is not known.

Neuronal vacuolation has long been the identifier for scrapie. It is a feature of the natural and experimental prion diseases of animals noted previously. The vacuolation may occur in the soma, perikaryon, or neurites, but may not be accompanied by the spongy change described previously. The empty vacuoles may be single, multiple, or in chains. Loss of neurons is difficult to assess and neuronophagia is absent. Descriptions of abnormal numbers of dark neurons may not be significant.

Astrocytic hypertrophy and hyperplasia varies in severity. Astrocytic nuclei may be paired or densely packed and may be without increase of fibers. Astrocytosis usually involves gray matter affected by spongiform change and may spread to adjacent white matter.

Although frequent and readily detected in kuru and in vCJD of humans, *amyloid plaques are sparse or absent in the classic TSE*. They may be difficult to demonstrate in H&E-stained sections but are well demonstrated with Congo red and especially the PAS method. The pathogenic prion isoform is subject to limited proteolysis to produce a smaller molecule, PR P27-30, which is protease resistant and deposited as intraneural amyloid in neurons and neuropil and around neurons and blood vessels.

Electron microscopic examination of detergent extracts of infected brain reveals characteristic fibrils, termed *"scrapie-associated fibrils"* (SAF), which have PrP^{sc} as their major component. In many cases, plaques of this material may be present in the neuropil, as histochemically detectable amyloid deposits, and it can be detected more sensitively by specific immunostaining as "scrapie immunoreactive amyloid." Cerebrovascular amyloidosis is also usually demonstrable in ovine scrapie.

Scrapie was the first prion disease to be recognized and described, about 1732 in the United Kingdom, and is endemic worldwide, except in Australia and New Zealand, where it has been eradicated. The precise route of transmission is unclear, but the disease spreads in an infectious-like pattern with rapid lateral communicability in a contaminated field. Infection mostly occurs around the time of birth, and probably via ingestion, but the question of vertical modes of transmission remains unclarified. The likelihood of ewe-to-lamb transmission is highly significant, in that a ewe could give birth to and infect several lambs before showing clinical signs. The scrapie agent can infect goats sharing the pasture with affected sheep; natural spread to species other than goats grazing the same pasture is not reported.

As discussed previously, sheep breeds differ in their susceptibility to scrapie. The morbidity of the natural disease is low, except in some closed stud flocks, and clinically affected animals are usually in the 2- to 5-year age group. There is a long incubation period, and the disease, once clinically manifest, is progressive and ultimately fatal in 10 days to several months. The agent proliferates initially in the lymphoid tissues and lower intestine, but may take up to 2 years to reach the nervous system. A further 2 years may lapse before clinical signs appear. The methods of spread of the agent between both cells and organ systems are still enigmatic, although there is good evidence that the nervous system is first infected via the splanchnic nerves, which carry the agent to the thoracic spinal cord. Once within the central nervous system, the presence of the agent seems to be of no consequence until it reaches "clinical target areas," where the expression of PrP^{Sc} in select neurons could presumably lead to progressive dysfunction.

Both clinical signs and pathologic changes are somewhat variable but, in general, affected sheep are initially alert but excitable, tremble when excited, and may have seizures. Later, paresthesias may appear, manifested as agitated rubbing against posts and trees, and nibbling at the feet and legs when lying down, behavior that gave rise to the colloquial name "scrapie." Self-trauma can cause extensive loss of wool and abrasions of the skin. There is also progressive dysmetria and emaciation, and finally paralysis and death.

Apart from emaciation and self-trauma, there are no significant gross lesions, and no inflammatory changes. The most characteristic finding is the presence of *large intraneuronal vacuoles* in the medullary reticular, medial vestibular, lateral cuneate, and papilliform nuclei. The neuronal vacuolation may, however, be present throughout the brainstem and spinal cord. The vacuoles contain no stainable material and may considerably distort and displace the normal organelles. Although the vacuolated neurons do not generally appear degenerate in any other way, shrunken and apparently degenerate neurons may be found in mesencephalic, medullary, and deep cerebellar nuclei, and in the intermediolateral nucleus of the spinal cord. In late stages, neuronal loss may be evident, as well as diffuse fibrillary astrogliosis present mainly in the mesencephalon and the molecular layer of the cerebellum. These lesions are bilaterally symmetrical, and the cerebral cortex is rarely involved (see Fig. 4-12A, B). *Spongy vacuolation of the neuropil* in gray matter is the result of vacuolation of neuronal processes, but it is seldom a feature of the natural disease in sheep.

Bovine spongiform encephalopathy (BSE) causes cattle 3-6 years of age to become apprehensive, hyperesthetic, and dysmetric. The animals display fear and aggressive behavior, with progressive gait disturbances leading to frequent falling. Eventually, frenzied episodes or recumbency necessitate euthanasia. The origin of the rogue prion is still undetermined; however, ingestion of feed contaminated with infectious prion is the most likely origin for BSE. This contamination may have come from bone and meat meal from scrapie-infected sheep carcasses; however, the BSE agent is different biologically than any of the known scrapie strains. Another source suggested is feed contamination with the remains of humans infected with CJD. Sporadic and genetically determined TSEs have not been detected in cattle. BSE is basically a food-borne epidemic; lateral or vertical transmission is highly unlikely. *The pathologic features of BSE resemble those of scrapie.* Scrapie-associated fibrils and immunoreactive amyloid are demonstrable. *Vacuolation of neuronal cell bodies and processes* is particularly prominent in the dorsal vagal, medullary reticular, vestibular, solitary, spinal trigeminal, and red nuclei, and is accompanied by moderate degrees of *spongiform change in neuropil*. The severity of neuropil and neuronal somatic vacuolation varies independently among anatomic locations, and the latter is sometimes accompanied by ceroid-lipofuscin granules.

Occasional necrotic neurons and axonal spheroids may be present, as may mild astrogliosis.

In addition to the classic BSE described previously, at least 2 types of atypical BSE have been found in cattle. Atypical BSEs are thought to be caused by atypical BSE prions that either have higher molecular mass fragments than classic BSE and are called *"H-type"* BSE, or have lower molecular mass and are called *"L-type"* BSE. In contrast to the classic BSE prion that is highly expressed in the obex, relatively few deposits of atypical BSE prions are found in the obex region, but many more occurred in the more rostral structure of the brain, namely, in the thalamus and the olfactory bulb. The L-type BSE is characterized by the presence of PrP^{Sc}-positive amyloid plaques in the brain, and therefore it has been termed *bovine amyloidotic spongiform encephalopathy* (BASE).

Transmissible mink encephalopathy (TME) has caused high levels of morbidity and mortality in ranch mink in North America and northern Europe, including Finland and Russia. The source of TME infection was not determined, but contamination of feed materials by the scrapie agent was suggested. The agent was experimentally pathogenic to a variety of wild carnivores, sheep, cattle, and primates. Neuronal vacuolation is sparse in this disease, which exhibits *spongy degeneration and astrocytosis* of parallel intensity. Neuronal vacuolation is mainly in brainstem. The lesions are especially well developed in the neocortex and amygdala, corpus striatum, caudodorsal thalamus, and medial geniculate bodies. The pathologic profile may differ between countries, perhaps because of strain differences of the agent or genotype of the captive mink.

Chronic wasting disease (CWD) of cervids affects mule deer (*Odocoileus hemionus*), white-tailed deer (*Odocoileus virginianus*), Rocky Mountain elk (*Cervus elaphus nelsoni*), moose (*Alces alces*), and perhaps other cervids in several states in the United States and in western Canada. Although CWD was first diagnosed in the 1960s in captive cervids, it is now prevalent and possibly increasing among free-ranging and wild susceptible species and is considered to be the only TSE that occurs in free-ranging animals. The source of infection is unknown, but the disease is likely spread horizontally by ingestion of material contaminated with the CWD agent. CWD PrP^{Sc} is widespread not only in the CNS but also in various lymphoid tissues, including gut-associated lymphoid tissue (GALT). The presence of PrP^{Sc} in GALT led to the presumption that PrP^{Sc} could be shed in feces, causing pasture contamination and a health hazard to other animals or humans. Affected animals show slow progressive weight loss, dullness and depression, polydipsia, and polyuria. Deer may show swallowing difficulty and esophageal dilation. Spongiform change, neuronal vacuolation, gliosis, and amyloid deposition are especially well developed in the olfactory tubercle, cortex hypothalamus, and vagal nuclei. Amyloid plaques are more frequently demonstrated in deer than in elk.

Feline spongiform encephalopathy (FSE) has been observed in domestic cats and captive felids in zoos. FSE was likely transmitted to captive felids by ingestion of BSE-infected cattle carcasses, and to domestic cats by ingestion of pet food contaminated with the BSE agent. The lesion pattern emphasizes the spongy change in deep laminae of cerebrum, the corpus striatum, thalamus, medial geniculate body, and cerebellar cortex. Neuronal vacuolation occurs mainly in medullary neurons but is not pronounced.

Transmissible spongiform encephalopathy of captive wild ruminants: Several zoo members of the family *Bovidae*, for example, nyala, Arabian oryx, and a bison, developed TSE at the time of the BSE epidemic in the United Kingdom in association with ingestion of BSE-contaminated meat and bone meal.

Spongiform encephalopathy in nonhuman primates: Lemurs and a rhesus macaque in France developed TSE naturally. The disease was likely a food-borne infection from ingestion of primate food containing BSE-contaminated beef.

Laboratory **diagnosis** of TSEs can be achieved by immunohistochemistry or by rapid tests, such as ELISA or Western blot.

Further reading

Baylis M, Goldmann W. The genetics of scrapie in sheep and goats. Curr Mol Med 2004;4:385-396.

Collinge J. Prion diseases of humans and animals: their causes and molecular basis. Ann Rev Neurosci 2001;24:519-550.

DeArmond SJ. Discovering the mechanisms of neurodegeneration in prion diseases. Neurochem Res 2004;29:1979-1998.

Seuberlich T, et al. Atypical transmissible spongiform encephalopathies in ruminants: a challenge for disease surveillance and control. J Vet Diagn Invest 2010;22:823-842.

Takemura K. An overview of transmissible spongiform encephalopathies. Anim Health Res Rev 2004;5:103-124.

INFLAMMATION IN THE CENTRAL NERVOUS SYSTEM

Brain and infection

Organs defend against invading infectious organisms either by innate or adaptive immunity. Innate immunity is composed of resident components, for example, pulmonary alveolar macrophages, or recruited components, for example, neutrophils. Unlike parenchymatous organs, the brain depends solely on resident innate immunity to recognize and clear pathogens. In other words, under normal non-disease conditions, the brain does not rely either on adaptive immunity or the recruited components of innate immunity for defense. Innate immunity in the brain is diverse and composed of structural units, for example, blood-brain barrier (BBB), plus cellular and chemical components.

The structural units that separate vulnerable brain cells from the blood stream are the **BBB** and the **blood-cerebrospinal fluid barrier (BCSFB)**, which is present at the choroid plexuses. The BBB is made up of endothelial cells lining the blood capillaries, pericytes embedded in the capillary basement membranes, and the foot processes of astrocytes. The endothelial cells of the BBB differ from other body endothelial cells, first by having significantly fewer endocytotic vesicles, thereby limiting the amount of transcellular flux, and second, they are connected by both *adherens junction* (e.g., cadherin) and *tight junction proteins*; the latter significantly reduce paracellular flux. Also, BBB endothelial cells are rich in several transport systems that selectively transport essential nutrients to the brain or harmful material back into the blood (efflux transport proteins). One of the most important efflux proteins is *P-glycoprotein*. Inhibition of P-glycoprotein increases the tissue invasiveness of *Listeria monocytogenes*. In addition to these protective properties of the BBB, the CSF side of the BCSFB is also rich in tight junctions, which restricts movement to the CSF. *The ability of organisms to breach these barriers determines their neurotropism*. Neurotropic viruses and bacteria have developed several strategies to breach or to cross these barriers. For example, several neurotropic viruses bypass the BBB and invade the brain via axons (e.g., rabies virus); intracellular bacteria (e.g., *Mycobacterium bovis*) invade the brain as Trojan horses, hidden in infected leukocytes; and finally, some bacteria have a direct cytotoxic effect on the endothelial cells of the BBB (e.g., *Histophilus somni*). The cellular part of the brain's innate immunity is composed of perivascular **dendritic cells, microglia,** and **astrocytes.** These cells are rich in *pattern recognition receptors*, which bind directly and nonspecifically to *pathogen-associated molecular patterns*. For example, all 3 cell types are rich in *macrophage mannose receptor*, which is a lectin receptor that recognizes "nonself" sugars on the cell wall of gram-negative and gram-positive bacteria, parasites, and yeasts. Microglia cells also express several *tool-like receptors*, for example, TLR2 and TLR6, which have a major role as bridges between innate and adaptive immunity. Activated microglia express several receptors important for phagocytosis, for example, CR3 and CR4; recognition of pathogens is followed by phagocytosis, largely by microglial cells and to a lesser extent by astrocytes. Finally, glial cells release several *cytokines* and *antimicrobial peptides*, for example, interleukin-1β, tumor necrosis factor-α, and the antimicrobial peptide *cathelicidin*. Inflammation of the brain starts once an infectious agent overcomes the resident innate immunity and recruiting begins of different components of adaptive immunity (leukocytes and humoral immunity), which are more specific and more effective but also more destructive.

Further reading

Neudeck BL, et al. Intestinal P glycoprotein acts as a natural defense mechanism against *Listeria monocytogenes*. Infect Immun 2004; 72:3849-3854.

Inflammation in the central nervous system

Inflammation of the brain is **encephalitis,** of the spinal cord, **myelitis;** of the ependyma, **ependymitis;** of the choroid plexus; **choroiditis;** and of the meninges, **meningitis,** qualified as **leptomeningitis** when it involves the pia-arachnoid and as **pachymeningitis** when it involves the dura. This is the area of neuropathology that is of most veterinary importance because it embraces many of the transmissible highly fatal infections of animals, because even the sporadic infections are common, and because there is always a pressing need for the pathologist to separate the inflammations into general or specific etiologic categories. Most of the specific infectious diseases to be described in this chapter are caused by agents that demonstrate a remarkable or specific neurotropism. These are, however, only a segment of the list of agents that commonly, occasionally, or rarely involve the CNS (Table 4-1); neurologic lesions are also discussed with systemic infections elsewhere in these volumes.

Inflammatory processes in the CNS are basically the same as those in other tissues, but they derive some specific features from the special responsiveness and anatomic arrangements of the CNS. It is important to recognize the criteria of inflammation in the CNS and then to presume from that, as far as is possible, the nature of the infecting organisms because

Table • 4-1

Infectious agents/diseases inducing inflammatory changes in the nervous system

Species	Canine	Feline	Porcine	Bovine	Equine	Ovine/caprine	Camelid	Remarks on brain lesions
Viral disease/agent								
Akabane virus	N	N	N	Y	N	S	SC	
Bovine herpesvirus 1	N	N	N	Y	N	N	N	
Bovine herpesvirus 5	N	N	N	Y	N	N	N	
Borna disease virus	Y	Y	N	Y	Y	Y	S	
Bovine paramyxovirus (unclassified)	N	N	N	S	N	N	N	
Canine adenovirus 2	S	N	N	N	N	N	N	Multiple hemorrhages, particularly in brainstem/caudate nuclei
Canine distemper virus	Y	N	N	N	N	N	N	
Canid herpesvirus 1	Y	N	N	N	N	N	N	Necrotizing meningoencephalitis, which is most severe in cerebrum and brainstem
Canine parvovirus 2	S	N	N	N	N	N	N	Vasculitis-induced lesions
Classical swine fever virus	N	N	Y	N	N	N	N	Vasculitis-induced lesions
Equine encephalitis viruses (EEEV, WEEV, VEEV)	SC/S	N	S	SC	Y	SC	?	
Equid herpesvirus 1 (EHV-1) and EHV-4	N	N	N	N	Y	N	N	EHV4 rarely causes encephalitis
Equid herpesvirus 9	?	?	?	?	?	?	?	Natural disease only reported in deer
Encephalomyocarditis virus	?	?	Y	S	S	?	S	Infection in some species (e.g., bovine) may be limited to myocarditis
Equine infectious anemia virus (EIAV)	N	N	N	N	S	N	N	Multifocal to diffuse encephalomyelitis is a rare manifestation of EIAV infection; may also cause lymphohistiocytic periventricular leukoencephalitis
Feline immunodeficiency virus	N	S	N	N	N	N	N	Nonsuppurative encephalomyelitis in some naturally infected cats; secondary *Toxoplasma* or feline infectious peritonitis virus infections
Feline leukemia virus	N	S	N	N	N	N	N	Noninflammatory degenerative myelopathy
Feline infectious peritonitis virus	N	Y	N	N	N	N	N	Fibrinopyogranulomatous periventriculitis, meningitis, and perivasculitis; chronic leukoencephalitis; segmental myelitis; choroiditis
Hemagglutinating encephalomyelitis virus (HEV)	N	N	Y	N	N	N	N	
Highlands J virus	N	N	N	N	S	N	N	

Continued

Table • 4-1

Infectious agents/diseases inducing inflammatory changes in the nervous system—cont'd

Species	Canine	Feline	Porcine	Bovine	Equine	Ovine/caprine	Camelid	Remarks on brain lesions
Japanese encephalitis virus	SC	N	Y	SC	SC	SC	?	
La Crosse virus	S	N	N	N	N	N	?	
Lentivirus encephalomyelitis	N	N	N	N	N	Y	N	
Louping ill virus	Y	?	Y	Y	Y	Y	Y	
Malignant catarrhal fever	N	N	S	Y	N	SC	?	
Nipah virus	Y	Y	Y	S	Y	Y	?	
Porcine arterivirus	N	N	Y	N	N	N	?	
Porcine circovirus 2	N	N	Y	N	N	N	?	
Porcine paramyxovirus (unclassified)	N	N	S	N	N	N	N	
Porcine rubulavirus	N	N	S	N	N	N	N	
Pseudorabies virus	Y	Y	Y	Y	S	Y	?	
Rabies virus	Y	Y	S	Y	Y	S	Y	
Porcine teschovirus (Teschen disease)	N	N	Y	N	N	N	N	
Tick-borne encephalitis virus	Y	?	?	?	?	?	?	
West Nile virus	Y	Y	SC	SC	Y	S	Y	
Protozoal diseases								
Acanthamoeba encephalitis	S	?	?	?	?	S	?	
Babesiosis	S	S	S	Y	S	Y	Y	Sludging of parasitized RBCs in blood capillaries
Neospora caninum	Y	N	N	Y*	S	S	Y	*In bovine encephalitis, is only observed in aborted fetuses or very young calves infected in utero
Neospora hughesi	N	N	N	N	Y	N	N	
Sarcocystis canis	S	N	N	N	N	N	N	
Sarcocystis neurona	N	S	N	N	Y	N	N	
Theileriosis	S	N	N	Y	S	Y	Y	
Toxoplasmosis	Y	Y	Y	SC/S	SC	Y	Y	
Bacterial diseases								
Listeria monocytogenes	S	S	S	Y	Y	Y	Y	
Histophilus somni	N	N	N	Y	N	Y	?	
Chlamydial and rickettsial diseases								
Chlamydophila pecorum	?	?	?	S	?	?	?	

EEEV, eastern equine encephalitis virus; *VEEV*, Venezuelan equine encephalitis virus; *WEEV*, western equine encephalitis virus.
?, No refereed papers about species susceptibility to natural infection.
N, The species is not susceptible to natural infection.
S, The species is susceptible to natural infection but overt disease is reported only sporadically.
SC, The species is susceptible to natural infection but the disease occurs subclinically without neurologic signs.
Y, The species is susceptible to natural infection and overt disease is reported regularly.

opportunities to intervene clinically are brief, and the time frame for clinical intervention is less than required for definitive microbiologic identificatoin.

The problem is not only one of why and how the CNS, of known high vulnerability to infection, is so frequently spared in systemic diseases; it is also one of why and how it is infected hematogenously. There is presently no better knowledge of why 4 out of 5 cases of Glasser's disease will have meningitis than why 1 of 5 will not, even though in the one case the pathologic syndrome is otherwise fully developed.

Infections that, in other organs or tissues, may be inconsequential and even asymptomatic frequently cause death or permanent disability when they involve the nervous system. There are several contributing factors, the most important of which is the *indispensability of most portions of the CNS*. The nervous tissue cannot reconstitute itself, but it may, if the lesion develops slowly, manage a considerable degree of functional compensation. Vascular responses may be more of an impediment than a help in the reaction to inflammation, because they lead consistently to edema and brain swelling that spreads the consequences of the inflammation far from the active focus. Vascular proliferation and fibrous tissue encapsulation may develop only when the inflammatory reaction involves the meninges and the larger blood vessels because these are the only source of reticulin and collagenous tissue. Investigation continues into how viruses spread in nervous tissue; bacteria and fungi can spread rapidly and extensively in the fluid of the ventricular system and meninges. Spread of infection from the ventricular fluid to the periventricular veins occurs readily across the ependyma, and spread from the meninges to the brain, or vice versa, can occur via the Virchow-Robin spaces. The special drainage of CSF is such that exudate rich in fibrin and cells is drained very poorly.

The structure of nervous tissue and meninges limits the anatomic types of inflammation that may occur. **Fibrinous inflammation** is confined to the meninges and larger perivascular spaces. Fibrin is usually indicative of a bacterial infection, but there are exceptions. Fibrinopurulent, largely fibrinous, exudate is caused by the mycoplasmas; fibrinous exudation is typical of the meningeal reaction in malignant catarrhal fever of cattle, and it is occasionally observed in organomercurial poisoning of swine and cattle. **Hemorrhagic inflammation** is not common, except as examples of symptomatic purpura in infections such as porcine erysipelas and infectious canine hepatitis and in the infarcts of embolic infections. Hemorrhage is characteristic of helminthic infections, but these lesions are perhaps better regarded as traumatic malacias. **Suppurative or granulomatous inflammation** is the usual response to bacterial or mycotic infections. Viral infections are characterized by **nonsuppurative inflammation,** which is described in more detail later; it is typically composed of neuronal degeneration, perivascular cuffing by mononuclear cells, and focal or diffuse glial proliferations.

Applying these broad criteria, there is seldom much difficulty in deciding on the class of the infecting agent. *There is occasionally some difficulty in distinguishing between the reactions to degeneration and to viral infections*. Although suppuration does not occur in either of these processes, early infiltration of neutrophils occurs in acute degenerations, such as the malacias, and a few neutrophils can be found migrating in affected gray matter in the first stages of many cases of viral encephalomyelitis. Acute demyelinating processes are associated with, and probably stimulate, perivascular cuffing. The cuffs tend to be quite distinct from those in viral infections by being relatively very thick (up to 10 or more cells thick) and to be composed of pure populations of lymphocytes. *If there are proliferated adventitial cells with plasma cells or other leukocytes mixed in the cuffs of lymphocytes, then the cuffs are likely to be a response to infection*. Only 3 diseases in animals are caused by viruses and characterized by demyelination, and these, namely, canine distemper, leukoencephalomyelitis of goats, and visna of sheep, have their own distinguishing characteristics. A possible fourth is so-called "old dog encephalitis." Glial responsiveness occurs in a variety of degenerative and viral lesions, but *glial nodules are characteristic only of an infectious process*, usually viral but occasionally rickettsial or bacterial.

Bacterial and pyogenic infections of the nervous system

Epidural/subdural abscess and empyema

The brain and spinal cord are protected against direct penetration of infection by the skeletal encasement and by the dura mater; the dura is almost impermeable to inflammatory processes. However, infection of the epidural space or the bony encasement with pyogenic bacteria, and occasionally fungi can occur and may lead to localized *abscessation* or to the collection of suppurative material in the epidural or subdural space without forming a discrete abscess (*epidural or subdural empyema*). Infection may be hematogenous from *distant sites of infection* (e.g., septic valvular endocarditis, lung abscess), *direct extension* (e.g., osteomyelitis, middle ear and tympanic bullae, eye, paranasal sinuses, ethmoid cells), *trauma* (e.g., bite wounds, especially in cats), *foreign bodies* (e.g., grass awns, wooden sticks), or by *direct incidental injection* (e.g., contaminated spinal needle). Most cranial epidural abscesses arise by direct extension from one of the paranasal sinuses. Spread from the middle ear and through the cribriform plate is usually directly to the leptomeninges and brain. Occasionally, epidural suppuration is observed to have tracked from a retropharyngeal or nodal abscess through cranial foramina. Epidural suppuration about the base of the brain usually does not become encapsulated.

Tail biting in pigs, docking of lambs, and tail fracture in cats are common etiologies for spinal epidural abscesses that develop either secondary to local venous bacterial invasion or by direct extension from septic osteomyelitis. In cattle, spinal epidural abscesses are usually secondary to osteomyelitis of the vertebral bodies, are more prevalent at the lumbosacral area, and are usually caused by *Trueperella pyogenes* or *Fusobacterium necrophorum* (Fig. 4-86). Migrating grass awns can cause osteomyelitis and epidural abscess in the thoracolumbar regions in dogs. Common bacterial etiologies for epidural abscess or empyema in dogs and cats include *Streptococcus, Staphylococcus, Brucella, Pasteurella,* and *Fusobacterium*, and in horses include *Actinobacillus* and *Streptococcus*.

Clinical signs vary according to the area affected, and can range from mild pain and restlessness to blindness and ataxia. Epidural abscessation at the lumbosacral area in ruminants may lead to circling, which can be confused with encephalitic listeriosis. Spinal epidural abscesses usually cause compression malacia of the cord, if the osteomyelitis from which they originate does not first lead to pathologic fracture with displacement.

Subdural abscessation is seldom observed, but can result from local penetration, perhaps most frequently from the

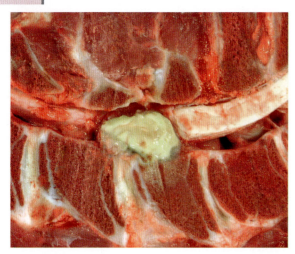

Figure 4-86 Subdural/intradural abscess at the level of the fifth cervical vertebra in a calf. (Courtesy S. Plog, Freie Universität, Berlin.)

paranasal sinuses. Extension can occur from epidural abscesses, or, because subdural suppuration is prone to cause local phlebitis, it may give rise to epidural suppuration. Subdural infection is liable to spread widely via the veins or after penetrating the outer layer of the arachnoid. Spread is also permitted by the slowness with which leptomeningeal fibrous tissue develops to encapsulate the reaction.

Leptomeningitis

Leptomeningitis can be classified according to *etiology* (e.g., bacterial, mycotic), according to *duration* (e.g., acute, chronic), and according to the *type of exudates* (e.g., fibrinous, purulent). Classification by type of exudate is very useful, not only because it indicates the expected histologic lesions, but also clinically because it indicates the possible etiology. *Purulent meningitis* is by far the most common meningitis in domestic animals, especially neonates. *Serocellular meningitis* is described later with viral inflammation. *Hemorrhagic meningitis* occurs in septicemic anthrax and very seldom in other septicemias. Purely *fibrinous meningitis* occurs in malignant catarrhal fever, chlamydiosis, and seldom in anything else. *Mycoplasma bovis* is a rare cause of fibrinous meningitis in calves. *Granulomatous meningitis* occurs in systemic infections of this type, such as tuberculosis and cryptococcosis. The nonsuppurative inflammations of the leptomeninges are described with the diseases of which they may be part. They are mentioned here to draw attention to the wide variety of infectious agents that may localize in and produce inflammation of the leptomeninges. We have also mentioned or discussed purulent leptomeningitis with the many specific diseases of which it can be part, but dwell on the purulent process here because it is common, lacks specificity, and is suitable for a "type" description. Noninfectious causes of meningitis include idiopathic or unknown forms described later in the section of idiopathic inflammatory diseases.

Purulent leptomeningitis may arise by direct extension from an adjacent structure. Extension from an epidural abscess or inflammation may result in diffuse leptomeningitis but, in most of the few cases of this origin, the leptomeningitis is local and overshadowed by the brain abscess that usually forms. Leptomeningitis may arise by local extension from a brain abscess, either by direct permeation or by spread in the Virchow-Robin spaces. Such an origin is observed frequently in listeriosis and in association with very large cerebral abscesses, but most cerebral abscesses, which are usually small, track inward to the white matter rather than out to the meninges. The reverse sequence in which meningitis spreads to the brain and cord is not unusual in granulomatous infections but is distinctly unusual in suppurative infections, and when it occurs, it consists of invasion of the surface of the brain by neutrophils (Fig. 4-87A) rather than of abscessation.

Both purulent meningitis and cerebral abscesses are usually of hematogenous origin, but they are seldom concurrent, and one usually finds meningitis alone or abscessation alone. There are occasional exceptions, including thromboembolic lesions and leptomeningitis complicated by choroiditis. Septic emboli are prone to localize in the brain but may localize in meningeal vessels (Fig. 4-87B). Although those in meningeal vessels may lead to diffuse suppurative meningitis, they are usually quickly walled off and prevented from spreading (Fig. 4-87C, D). In the other exception, that of choroiditis concurrent with leptomeningitis, encephalitis or cerebral abscesses may develop because choroiditis leads to exudation into the CSF, and the ependyma is not a strong barrier to infection. Even this combination of pathologic processes is unusual, and, when choroiditis is complicated by ependymitis and suppurative encephalitis (Fig. 4-87E), there is usually little or no meningitis. Whether encephalitis develops by spread of meningitis may be largely a question of time, but it is not unusual for animals with purulent meningitis to survive for a week, and sometimes much longer. There is ample time for the inflammation to spread throughout the cranial and spinal meninges—and to the brain if it were going to do so—but it seldom does, and *there is seldom anatomic justification for the common diagnosis of suppurative meningoencephalitis.*

In the section on inflammatory diseases of joints and synovial structures, attention is drawn to the frequent concurrence of polyarthritis with choroiditis and leptomeningitis in fibrinopurulent infections. Erysipelas, in which arthritis is a typical lesion, is an exception in that it may produce septicemic and embolic lesions in the brain, but it does not cause suppurative meningitis. Several bacteria, such as streptococci and *Escherichia coli*, cause bacteremia and suppurative meningitis in neonates, resulting in an important clinical entity, especially in ruminants and pigs, called **neonatal bacterial suppurative meningitis** (NBSM). Streptococcal NBSM in calves, lambs, and piglets (but not in foals), frequently has a combination of polyarthritis, purulent leptomeningitis, choroiditis, and in calves only, endophthalmitis (Fig. 4-88A, B). In pigs, *Streptococcus suis* types 1 and 2 (see Vol. 1, Bones and joints) cause NBSM that is usually accompanied by polyserositis; *S. suis* meningitis is suppurative in the acute stage (Fig. 4-89A, B), and lymphoplasmacytic in pigs that survive. *Streptococcus pneumoniae* usually produces fulminating septicemia in calves characterized only by very acute splenitis but, if the course of this infection is less fulminating than usual, polyarthritis and meningitis can be found. *E. coli*, another cause of NBSM of protracted course, commonly causes well-developed meningitis and polyarthritis in neonatal calves and lambs, but even in fulminating infections, the mild changes of early inflammation can be found in these structures. On the other hand, both coliform and streptococcal infections in calves and piglets may avoid the joints and meninges and localize instead in the choroid plexuses and spread from there to the ventricles and brain, or localize in the brain alone. The coliforms and

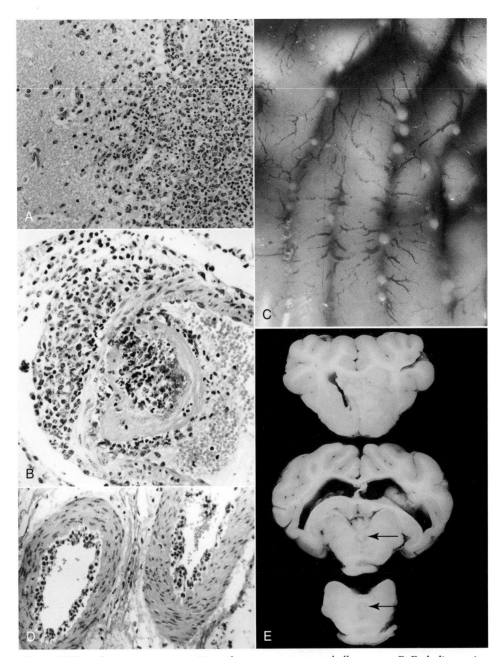

Figure 4-87 A. Suppurative meningitis with extension into cerebellar cortex. **B. Embolic meningeal arteritis** from streptococcal endocarditis in a pig. **C.** Miliary **meningeal abscesses** in a calf, caused by *Trueperella pyogenes*. **D. Meningeal arteritis** with leukocytes beneath endothelium in coliform meningitis in a calf. **E.** Frontal sections to show periventricular abscess, early hydrocephalus, and occlusive ependymitis of the aqueduct (arrows) secondary to **streptococcal choroiditis** in a pig.

streptococci behave differently in calves with respect to the eyes; a combination of synovial, meningeal, and intraocular localizations is almost invariably of streptococcal origin (and the lesions can be well developed within 12 hours of birth, or even at birth according to farmers); the coliforms can, but only seldom do, cause endophthalmitis.

Mannheimia haemolytica and *Pasteurella multocida* are usually regarded only as causes of fibrinous pneumonia and hemorrhagic septicemia, but they are responsible for localized infections in other locations, including the meninges, in ruminants. When polyarthritis is present in septicemic or pulmonary pasteurellosis, *fibrinosuppurative leptomeningitis* can also be anticipated. Isolated cases and limited outbreaks of pasteurellosis that is entirely meningeal are observed in cattle and sheep, usually young ones. The course is asymptomatic until meningitis develops.

Once infectious agents gain access to the leptomeninges, there is little resistance to spread in the meningeal spaces, and the inflammatory process becomes more or less diffuse in most cases. When the inflammatory process, excepting some that are granulomatous, remains localized, it is probable that only the inflammatory reaction, and not the infection, reaches the meningeal spaces. CSF is an excellent culture medium for many bacteria, and these spread rapidly in the fluid, assisted

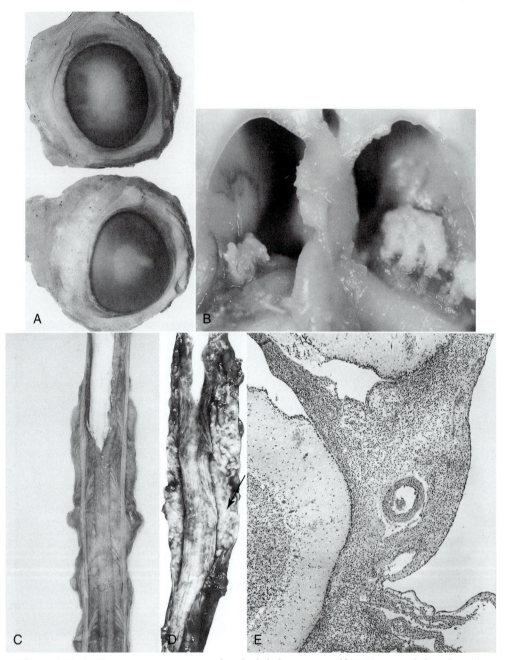

Figure 4-88 **A. Hypopyon** in streptococcal endophthalmitis in a calf. **B.** Horizontal slice through lateral ventricles to show **streptococcal choroiditis** and acquired hydrocephalus. **C. Spinal leptomeningitis** in a calf, caused by *Escherichia coli*. (The dura is incised and reflected full length, the congested leptomeninges are incised at top.) **D. Spinal meningitis** in a dog; dura reflected to expose exudate (arrow). **E. Fibrinopurulent exudate** in leptomeninges in a pig, caused by *Haemophilus parasuis*.

to some slight extent by normal flow so that, although meningitis may appear grossly to have a limited distribution, its true distribution can be determined only microscopically.

The apparent gross distribution of meningitis varies somewhat with the cause. Thus in listeriosis, the process is confined largely or entirely to the meninges covering the medulla oblongata and upper cord, and in Glasser's disease and in malignant catarrhal fever, the exudate is concentrated over the cerebellum and occipital poles of the cerebrum. In pyogenic meningitis, the basal meninges show the most obvious changes.

In the first day or so of suppurative meningitis before exudation is clearly recognizable, the meninges may be faintly opaque and hyperemic. After a few days, the appearance of the brain and cord is typical. The basal cisterns that accumulate the most exudate are filled with creamy pus or with gray-yellow fibrinopurulent exudate. The extreme exudation in these cisterns is due in part to their large size but in part also to sedimentation of particulate exudate. The exudate is in the arachnoid spaces, and there is little if any on the outer surface of this membrane (see Fig. 4-88D). The arachnoid appears stretched. *It is easy to overlook even copious exudates*

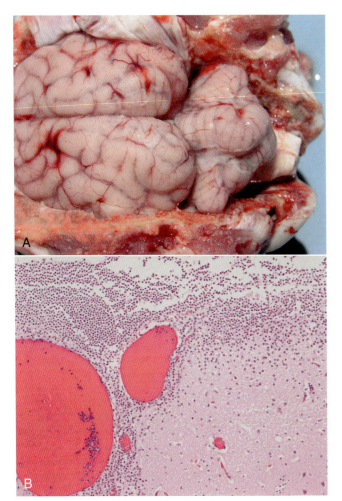

Figure 4-89 Purulent streptococcal meningitis in a pig. **A.** Gross image of suppurative meningitis. **B.** Massive exudation of neutrophils in meninges, with infiltration of neuropil. (Courtesy D. Driemeier.)

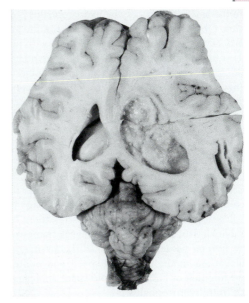

Figure 4-90 Necrobacillary abscess arising in **choroiditis** in an ox; swelling of hemisphere and caudal displacement with coning of cerebellum.

because their color is not very different from that of the brain. A useful clue is that even the largest basilar vessels and the trunk of the oculomotor nerve are partially or completely buried and obscured by exudate, and the filling-in of basal sinuses and grooves obliterates the normal topography. Over the hemispheres, the exudate is usually confined to the fissures, where the arachnoid space is wide, and spares the surfaces of the gyri, where the arachnoid space is narrow. There is seldom frank pus over the hemispheres except in cases of unusually long survival.

The severe degree of exudation described previously is what is usually seen in animals. In very acute or early cases, the exudation may be considerably less, and detectable only as congestion and cloudiness of the basal meninges extending toward the convexity of the hemispheres as fine gray sleeves about the arteries and veins. On careful inspection by naked eye, almost every case of purulent meningitis can be detected, but the microscope may be necessary to confirm some cases.

The brain is swollen in every acute case of pyogenic meningitis, and the swelling is frequently severe enough to cause displacement with coning of the cerebellum. The pathogenesis of the edema and swelling is not known. The edema affects the white matter. It is possible that obstruction of the meningeal orifices of Virchow-Robin spaces by exudate and stasis of flow of meningeal fluid may contribute to the edema. The brain itself is normal except for softness and swelling and the rare cortical infarcts in the cerebrum or cerebellum.

Choroiditis commonly complicates leptomeningitis. It is usually quite obvious when it affects the plexuses of the fourth ventricles, but that affecting the plexuses of the lateral ventricle is not apparent until the ventricles are opened, although it may be expected if cloudy fluid escapes from the third ventricle when the infundibular process is opened. The CSF is cloudy, flakes of exudate overlie the plexuses and float in the fluid, and smeary sediments of pus lie on the walls of the ventricles (see Fig. 4-88B). The exudate may be impacted in the aqueduct, occluding it and leading to ependymitis. Internal hydrocephalus then develops rapidly.

Microscopically, purulent meningitis does not differ in its character from pyogenic inflammation in other loose tissues, such as the lung. A few mononuclear cells are mixed with a very large number of neutrophils in the arachnoid spaces (see Fig. 4-88E). The amount of fibrin in the exudate varies. There may be some infiltration for a short distance along the Virchow-Robin spaces about veins (see Fig. 4-89A, B). The pia mater as a rule remains intact, and it is only in exceptional cases that some microbial activity is observed in the adjacent parenchyma, or the pia is eroded to allow neutrophils to invade the surface of the brain. When the choroid plexuses are involved, they are swollen and infiltrated with leukocytes, many of them mononuclear. The plexus epithelium is eroded and covered by fibrin and cells. The ependyma is also eroded, there is edema of subependymal tissues, and the surrounding veins are infiltrated.

Internal hydrocephalus is a sequel to ependymitis and occlusion of the aqueduct, as a result of which the lateral and third ventricles are dilated (Fig. 4-90). This condition is a complication of choroiditis, but hydrocephalus may also be a sequel without choroiditis being present. The medullary foramina are frequently occluded as a result of inflammation in the tela choroidea so that CSF cannot escape from the ventricular system to the arachnoid spaces; the hydrocephalus is noncommunicating. Obstruction to the flow of fluid in the arachnoid spaces may occur as a result of brain swelling, with impaction in the tentorial incisure, heavy deposits of exudate in the arachnoid space, or as a result of meningeal adhesions and thickenings in chronic inflammations. The hydrocephalus of this pathogenesis is communicating.

Chronic pyogenic leptomeningitis is rarely observed in animals. The process may sterilize itself or be sterilized by antimicrobials, but much of the injury is established in the early stages of the process, and once the diagnosis is evident clinically, *death is the expected outcome.* The early injury is exaggerated by the persistence of exudate even after the infection is controlled because there is no free drainage from the meningeal spaces. Healing occurs only after there has been considerable destruction of the meningeal framework with repair by fibrous tissue. Meningeal adhesions may produce cystic loculations in the arachnoid space, and obliterate the medullary foramen or basal arachnoid space and cause lingering death from hydrocephalus.

In a purulent process, *leptomeningeal vasculitis commonly* occurs. The expected sequelae of venous or ischemic infarcts are seldom observed even in those few cases with vasculitis in which thrombi can be found. This apparent discrepancy is probably the result of the rate at which the vascular obstructions develop and on the type and size of vessel. Cases in which suppurative thrombophlebitis of the sagittal or transverse sinuses, or both, can be readily observed may not have venous infarcts in the brain. Thrombosis in the afferent circulation usually involves the smallest of meningeal vessels and usually develops at a rate that allows collateral circulation to develop. Inflammation of larger arteries (see Fig. 4-87D) in which the endothelium is dissected from the intima by leukocytes has not been observed to lead to thrombosis.

Septicemic lesions, septic embolism, and cerebral abscess

The brain responds in septic or endotoxemic shock by releasing or controlling the release of several proinflammatory and anti-inflammatory cytokines; this major biochemical role is not always associated with a morphologic change in the CNS. *The CNS is injured to some extent in every episode of septicemia or sustained bacteremia.* The simplest and most common type of injury is inflicted on the venules, especially those of the cerebral white matter and, to a lesser extent, those of the cerebellar white matter. Injury of this type is not of much significance. There is sludging of leukocytes and probably of erythrocytes in these vessels, associated usually with degenerative and reactive changes in the endothelium. In the symptomatic purpuras, it is frequently possible to find the site of diapedesis in the brain, but not in other organs. Associated with endothelial injury, there is often leakage of plasma into the perivascular space and, given time, adventitial proliferation and infiltration of a few lymphocytes or other leukocytes into the Virchow-Robin spaces. Commonly, the injury is more severe, the vessel wall is totally necrotic in its cross-section, and in these lesions, a few bacteria may be demonstrable (Fig. 4-91).

Septic embolism in the CNS may be a complication of active endocarditis; the bacteria are usually gram positive. The bacteria implicated most commonly are *Erysipelothrix rhusiopathiae* in pigs, streptococci in all species, and *Arcanobacterium pyogenes* in cattle.

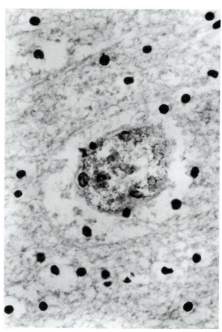

Figure 4-91 Necrosis of cerebral venule in *Escherichia coli* septicemia in a calf.

The toxigenicity and pathogenicity of many infections by gram-negative bacteria in septicemic phase seem to depend largely on the number of organisms present, as has been demonstrated in sheep for septicemic pasteurellosis caused by *Mannheimia haemolytica*. In septicemic pasteurellosis of sheep, in infection of foals by *Actinobacillus equuli*, in infections of sheep and cattle by *Histophilus somni*, and in some coliform infections of calves, the blood literally swarms with bacteria because common to these infections is massive and widespread bacterial embolism. These are the principal infections in which bacterial embolism occurs in the CNS without there being a demonstrable primary focus, such as endocarditis, pneumonia, or an abscess. The problem of cerebral embolism in these infections is not solely one of quantitative factors determined by the height of the bacteremia; qualitative factors of unknown nature are also involved.

Septic thromboemboli and **bacterial emboli** lodge in the small cerebral vessels but, whereas thromboemboli tend to lodge particularly in small arterioles, bacterial emboli lodge in capillaries and venules. Consequences depend on the vessels involved, although the consequences are not particularly significant because abscessation occurs in either location. *Arterial emboli frequently cause ischemic infarcts, and venous and capillary emboli cause hemorrhagic infarcts.* The venular lesions also extend rapidly to involve large veins, whereas local spread in arteries does not occur.

Cerebral abscesses may arise in embolism, by direct implantation in wounds, or by direct invasion of the brain from an adjacent structure. Leptomeningitis rarely leads to abscessation, whereas choroiditis commonly leads to periventricular abscess. Abscesses in the spinal cord are seldom sought or observed; they may be hematogenous via arteries or veins (Fig. 4-92), and rarely do they enter through the dura.

Abscesses of hematogenous origin may occur anywhere in the brain, but there are 2 areas of remarkable predilection: the hypothalamus and the cerebral cortex at the junction of gray and white matter (Fig. 4-93A, B). *Listeria monocytogenes* is an exception because it always demonstrates an affinity for the reticular formation in the brainstem. There may be only one abscess in the brain, or they may be multiple, especially when the result of bacterial embolism. Multiple abscesses of septic thromboembolic origin tend often to be localized in one area of the brain. Some care is necessary in specifying the origin of multiple adjacent foci of suppuration because the *production of satellites*, each of which may be larger than the primary, is a natural attribute of brain abscesses.

Abscesses arising by direct invasion of the brain may develop in any location. There are 2 common sites of invasion, namely, the *cribriform plate and inner ear*, and 2 somewhat less common, namely, the *hypophyseal fossa and the paranasal sinuses*. Hypothalamic abscesses are observed occasionally in cattle and dogs. At least some of those in dogs are caused by minute foreign bodies migrating with phlebitis through the orbital fissure or foramen rotundum and carrying actinomycetes. The importance of the cribriform plate and internal ear in the development of cerebral abscess is because of the frequency with which infections occur in those locations, that in neither site is there an actual or potential epidural space to protect the brain, and because nerves and vessels enter and leave through both.

Frontal abscesses of sinus origin occur occasionally in cattle as a complication of dehorning wounds, but abscesses in this site occur most commonly in sheep in which sinusitis, especially in the ethmoid cells, develops as a suppurative complication of myiasis *(Oestrus ovis)*. *A. pyogenes* is the organism usually present. The olfactory bulb is destroyed and the first ventricle is opened, infection then spreading to the substance of the hemisphere. There is little tendency to spread into the meninges from the point of entry or to invade the cortical gray matter, although both layers are usually secondarily involved by expansion of the abscess later.

Abscesses commonly develop at about the *cerebellopontine angle* as complications of suppurative otitis media. These are usually problems of pharyngitis, infection spreading via the Eustachian tube to the middle ear and from there to the brain, either by erosion of the bulla or extension along natural foramina.

Cerebellopontine abscesses are rarely, if ever, observed in horses in spite of the frequency of pharyngitis in this species. This exemption of horses may be because of the diversion of exudates from the Eustachian tube to the guttural pouches. Otogenic cerebral infections are very seldom observed in dogs. Those observed have come via the auditory meatus rather than the Eustachian tube, and the cerebral reaction is nonspecifically granulomatous, usually without pus. Otitis media caused by *Pasteurella multocida* is fairly common as a complication of chronic cases of upper respiratory infection in cats

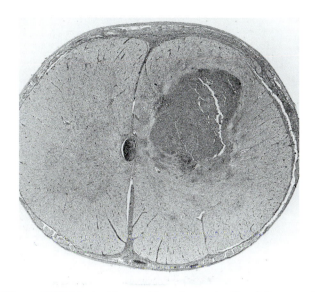

Figure 4-92 **Meningitis,** tracking abscess in dorsal horn, and ependymitis, complicating a docking wound in a lamb.

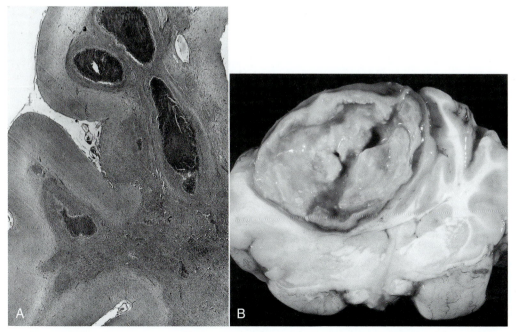

Figure 4-93 **A.** Hematogenous **abscesses** in cerebrum in a pig. **B. Abscess** distorting left cerebral hemisphere in a goat. *Pasteurella multocida* and *Fusobacterium necrophorum*.

and, when the infection extends to the cranial cavity, it produces diffuse purulent leptomeningitis and not, as expected, a cerebellopontine abscess. Most otogenic infections occur in sheep and swine; a few are observed in cattle, and in each species, the outcome is an abscess of the brain.

Otic infections are commonly bilateral so that otogenic abscesses may be also. The usual organism in these abscesses is *Trueperella pyogenes* alone or mixed with *Pseudomonas aeruginosa*, *P. multocida*, and mixed cocci. Affected pigs usually have several other chronic debilitating infections at the same time so that several animals in the herd may have otogenic abscesses. This pattern of infection in calves is uncommon and sporadic. In sheep on the other hand, the disease may be observed in limited outbreaks, and there is an association with grazing on rough, dry, mature summer pastures. The reasons for this association are unknown.

Established abscesses are found much more commonly in the white matter than in the gray, in spite of the fact that they usually begin in the gray. There is no suitable explanation for this tendency to track into white matter, but once within white matter, they do permeate along fiber tracts (Fig. 4-94). As a result of this activity, satellite abscesses are to be expected, sometimes chains of them. Connecting purulent tracts may be very thin and difficult to find.

An abscess may begin as an intense accumulation of neutrophils in and around a thrombosed vessel (Fig. 4-95A), or in a focus of septic encephalitis in which neutrophils lightly infiltrate a zone of early softening. The principal differences between a cerebral abscess and an abscess in some other location are the vulnerability of the surrounding nervous tissue to edema, which can destroy it, and the slowness with which encapsulation occurs (Fig. 4-95B). The meninges and larger blood vessels are the only sources of fibroblastic tissue for encapsulation.

In the *early stages*, the abscess cavity contains a liquefying center, and the margins are irregular and poorly defined even microscopically. The surrounding brain tissue is edematous and infiltrated by neutrophils. The microglia and vessels are fairly resistant and reactive in a narrow peripheral zone, but the neurons and neuroglia degenerate. Most abscesses develop rather slowly and later become encapsulated. The capsule seems often to be formed more by condensation of vessels around an expanding focus than by proliferating fibroblastic tissue, but both contribute; the result is an irregular capsule thicker on the meningeal than on the ventricular aspect. Most capsules are very distinct and 1-3 mm wide. Their distinctness is the result of the paucity of reticulin or collagen spreading

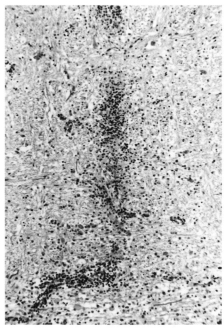

Figure 4-94 Spreading tract in suppurative (streptococcal) encephalitis in a pig.

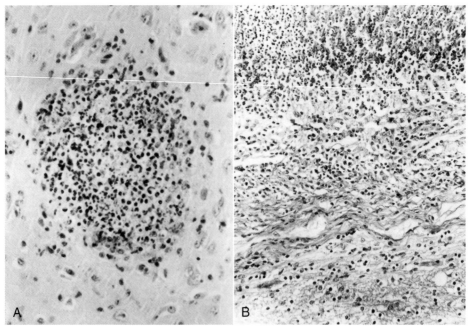

Figure 4-95 A. Early **cerebral abscess** from septic embolus in a pig. **B.** Structure of wall of **cerebral abscess.** Abscess (above) is separated from normal brain by a thin capsule.

out into the surrounding parenchyma or into the abscess cavity. In old abscesses with shrinkage, the core may separate from the capsule, and the capsule may separate extensively from the surrounding cerebral substance. The surrounding tissue is discolored yellow because of edema, the edematous zone often being much larger than the abscess itself. The *microscopic structure of the wall of a chronic abscess* does not differ much from case to case except in the thickness of the capsule. A narrow zone of histiocytes or gitter cells faces the neutrophilic debris. The next zone is a laminated layer of collagenous fibers between which are rows of gitter cells laden with debris. The outer zone is vascular, the vessels being large and usually nonreactive. The surrounding nervous tissue is severely edematous, with degeneration of myelin and fibers. Astrocytes are swollen and reactive about encapsulated abscesses, but it takes a long time for their fibrils to begin to intertwine with capsular reticulin. The veins are heavily cuffed by lymphocytes.

When abscesses are multiple, death is the outcome after a short course. When they are isolated, they may permit prolonged survival. The course is usually short with medullary abscess, even when small, because it, or more usually the edema it provokes, interferes with vital centers. Abscesses in the hypothalamus or cerebrum may track through the white matter to the ventricles to produce pyencephaly that is quickly fatal (Fig. 4-96A-D). Large abscesses ultimately expand to the meninges to produce adhesive meningitis. Many abscesses act as space-occupying lesions by virtue of their size or the edema they provoke or both. The consequences of space occupation depend on the site and size of the lesion.

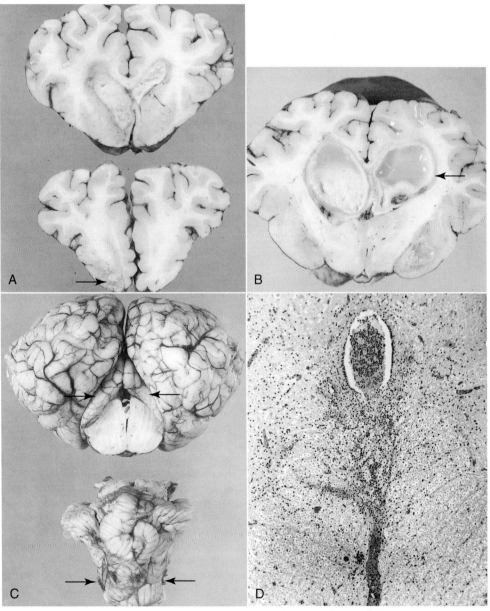

Figure 4-96 Pyencephaly in a calf. **A.** Pus in lateral ventricles (above) and left olfactory ventricle (arrow, below). **B.** Dilation of lateral ventricles by fibrinopurulent exudate (arrow). **C.** Brain swelling with cerebellar coning and hemorrhage (arrows, below) and subtentorial herniation of hemispheres (arrows, above). **D.** Inflammatory exudate in the aqueduct.

Further reading

Fecteau G, et al. Septicemia and meningitis in the newborn calf. Vet Clin North Am Food Anim Pract 2009;25:195-208.

Feng Y, et al. *Streptococcus suis* infection: an emerging/reemerging challenge of bacterial infectious diseases? Virulence 2014;5:477-497.

Smith JJ, et al. Bacterial meningitis and brain abscesses secondary to infectious disease processes involving the head in horses: seven cases (1980-2001). J Am Vet Med Assoc 2004;224:739-742.

Granulomatous and pyogranulomatous meningoencephalomyelitis

Granulomatous to pyogranulomatous meningoencephalomyelitis is observed in many systemic mycotic (e.g., blastomycosis, cryptococcosis) or algal (e.g., prototheocosis) diseases, which are described elsewhere in this book. Granulomatous inflammation can also be caused by bacteria (e.g., *Mycobacterium bovis, Nocardia* spp.) (Fig. 4-97), and migrating helminths or arthropod larvae (see later). The diagnosis and differentiation among these etiologies requires culture or demonstration of the causative pathogen using histochemical or immunohistochemical stains.

Listeriosis

Listeriosis is caused by **Listeria monocytogenes**, a gram-positive, facultative anaerobic bacillus that is ubiquitous in the environment and can multiply in diverse environmental conditions. It can grow in a temperature range of 4-45° C and at a pH range of 5-9. It is remarkably viable in the external environment, being able to survive in dried media for several months and in suitably moist soil for ~1 year. The organism is commonly isolated from tissues of normal animals, including tonsils and other gut-associated lymphoid tissue, and in large numbers from the feces of ruminants. *L. monocytogenes* has more than 11 serotypes; almost all animal infections are caused by serotypes 1/2a, 1/2b, and 4b.

Listeriosis is of worldwide distribution, possibly excepting the tropics. The organism has been isolated from diseased mammals and birds of many species and produces septicemia, meningitis, and abortion in humans. In domestic animals, the disease is most important in ruminants. *L. monocytogenes* is an intracellular pathogen of macrophages, neutrophils, and epithelial cells. Important virulence factors include the surface protein *internalin*, which internalizes with *E-cadherin*, an adherens junction protein, to overcome the intestinal, placental, and blood-brain barriers. However, the role of E-cadherin in the intracerebral spread and the distribution of microabscesses is yet to be determined. The organism also relies on another virulence factor, *cholesterol-binding hemolysin*, to lyse phagocytic cell phagosomes and escape to the cytoplasm. The organism proliferates in the host cell cytoplasm, and many migrate against the cell membrane to form protrusions that can then be taken up by other cells. It is one of the few organisms known to co-opt the host cell contractile actin to facilitate cell-to-cell transfer.

Listeriosis behaves as 3 separate diseases or syndromes. They seldom overlap, so that each syndrome probably has a separate pathogenesis. *The 3 recognized syndromes are infection of the pregnant uterus with abortion, septicemia with miliary visceral abscesses, and encephalitis.* Additional syndromes of clinical significance in ruminants include conjunctivitis, possibly from contaminated silage dust, endocarditis, and mastitis. The uterine infection is discussed with Diseases of the pregnant uterus (see Vol. 3, Female genital system). Aborting ruminants are not usually ill, and abortion is usually late in gestation. The uterine infection is probably hematogenous, and the bacteremic phase is asymptomatic, and localization occurs only in the uterus. Infection of the uterine contents can be established quite readily by oral exposure of pregnant animals and by intravenous inoculation.

Septicemic (systemic) listeriosis occurs in aborted fetuses and neonatal lambs, calves, and foals up to 1 week of age and in others that are several months of age, and is characterized by multisystemic bacterial colonization and multifocal multisystemic areas of coagulative necrosis or microabscess formation. The necrotic areas or microabscesses are miliary in distribution, very numerous in the liver, but much less numerous in the heart and other viscera, and characterized by tissue lytic necrosis with infiltration of neutrophils and fewer macrophages. Neonates generally become infected in utero.

Listerial encephalitis occurs almost solely in adult ruminants; its pathogenesis is partially understood. Listerial encephalitis may be sporadic or occur in outbreaks in which the morbidity may be 10% or higher. Outbreaks are usually associated with *heavy feeding of silage*, with disease most likely occurring in winter and early spring when the animals are indoors. This association of outbreaks of cerebral listeriosis with silage feeding is a circumstantial observation, but the association is so common that silage is fed as a calculated risk and removed from the ration when the first case occurs. The association with silage may indicate an acquired susceptibility of the animals or the provision of a growth medium that leads to heavy infection pressure. The organism will multiply in spoiled silage that is incompletely fermented and with a pH of 5.5 or above. Ingested *Listeria* is likely to breach the oral mucosal barrier through pathologic or physiologic wounds, for example, erupted teeth wounds. *After invading the oral mucosa, the bacteria invade the trigeminal nerves and travel centripetally via axons to the brain.* Listeria can also breach the blood-brain barrier under experimental conditions; however, the specific distribution of listerial encephalitis in the natural disease is inconsistent with a hematogenous infection. In animals,

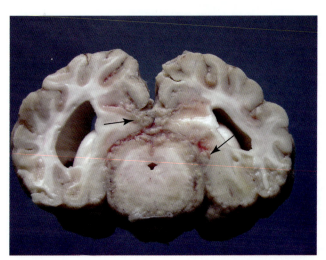

Figure 4-97 Granulomatous meningoencephalitis in bovine tuberculosis. Affected areas are malacic and filled with partially liquefied caseous material (arrows). (Courtesy D. Driemeier.)

Listeria has a remarkable affinity for the brainstem, the lesions being most severe in the medulla and pons and less severe rostrally in the thalamus and caudally in the cervical parts of the spinal cord. Intravenous or oral dosing of pregnant ruminants will regularly produce intrauterine infection but seldom produce intracranial infection and probably never produce encephalitis of the specific distribution. Bacteremias with localization in the CNS regularly cause meningitis, choroiditis, and cerebral abscesses, which is what *L. monocytogenes* does, but only as an experimental hematogenous infection. When a pregnant animal dies of encephalitic listeriosis, the uterine contents are usually sterile.

Conjunctivitis and keratitis follow experimental conjunctival exposure, but this should not imply that the endophthalmitis of the natural disease is produced by local invasion. Rhinitis is clinically apparent in many cases of encephalitic listeriosis, but histologic evidence does not support the idea that the olfactory nerves are a route of invasion of the brain. The position with respect to other cranial nerves and the internal ear has not been examined.

The *neurologic signs* and lesions of listeriosis in the various ruminants are qualitatively the same, differing only in severity. The signs are combinations of mental confusion and depression, head pressing, and paralysis of one or more medullary centers. Characteristically, there is deviation of the head to one or other side without rotation of the head; when such an animal moves, it does so in circles, hence the name *"circling disease."* There is frequently *unilateral paralysis of the seventh nerve*, causing drooping of an ear, eyelid, and lips. There may also be paralysis of the masticatory muscles and of the pharynx. *Purulent endophthalmitis*, which is usually unilateral, is often present and has caused listeriosis to be confused with malignant catarrhal fever. The course of the disease in sheep and goats is a few hours to 2 days; survival occurs but usually with neurologic handicaps.

Listeriosis in *swine* is comparable to the disease in ruminants, but is relatively rare. Outbreaks of encephalitis may be observed with lesions of usual distribution in the brainstem. Alternatively, there may be abortion and neonatal death. The usual expression of the disease is visceral with miliary abscesses in the liver and heart.

The patterns of listeriosis in *other domestic species* appear to follow the general scheme but are rarely observed. The encephalitic form in adult horses, the septicemic form in foals, and abortions in mares are reported. Several cases of encephalitis caused by *L. monocytogenes* are reported in dogs.

Gross lesions are usually not observed in the brain in listerial encephalitis. Occasionally, the medullary meninges are thickened by green gelatinous edema, and gray foci of softening may be found in the cross-section of the medulla. The initial lesions are parenchymal; involvement of the meninges, which is almost constant, is secondary to the parenchymal lesions. Mild meningitis commonly affects the cerebellum and cranial cervical cord, and less commonly is found in patches over the cerebrum and down the spinal cord. *The characteristic parenchymal lesion is a microabscess.* It may begin in a tiny collection of neutrophils (Fig. 4-98A), but more usually begins in a minute focus of microglial reaction. The glial nodules may persist as such, the cells taking on the characters of histiocytes, but the tendency is always for the nodules to be infiltrated by neutrophils and for their centers to liquefy (Fig. 4-98B). The focal lesions do not expand much, but suppurative foci may streak through the white matter. Apparently, the organism is not highly toxigenic because the parenchyma surrounding the glial nodules and focal abscesses may be little changed. Commonly however, the white matter is edematous and rarefied. Such areas may be large and lightly, but diffusely, infiltrated by neutrophils and hypertrophied microglia. Focal softening occurs and may coalesce. They are related to vessels that are occluded by inflammatory and thrombotic changes.

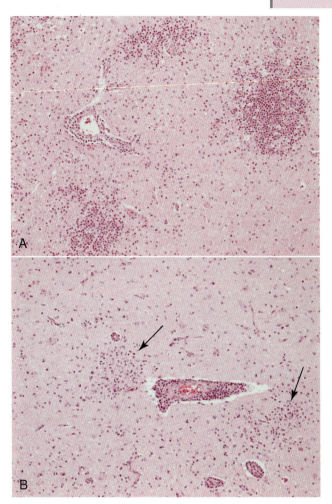

Figure 4-98 Listeriosis. **A.** Suppurative encephalitis with **microabscessation**. **B.** Microglial reaction with small foci of **suppuration** (arrows) in a sheep.

Acute vasculitis with exudation of fibrin occurs in the white matter in relation to suppurative foci. The vasculitis is secondary to drainage in the Virchow-Robin spaces from the primary parenchymal foci. It is in this manner that the meningeal infiltrates develop. Perivascular cuffing is heavy. The cuffs are composed mainly of lymphocytes and histiocytes with a few admixed neutrophils and eosinophils; granulocytes predominate in some cases.

Confirmation of the *diagnosis* is by culture, which is usually difficult and needs special procedures. Demonstrating gram-positive intramonocytic or intraneutrophilic bacilli in tissues in association with the aforementioned lesions is pathognomonic for listerial encephalitis.

Further reading

Disson O, et al. Targeting of the central nervous system by *Listeria monocytogenes*. Virulence 2012;3:213-221.

Gyles CL, et al. Pathogenesis of Bacterial Infections in Animals. 3rd ed. Oxford, UK: Blackwell Publishing; 2004. p. 99-107.

Madarame H, et al. The distribution of E-cadherin expression in listeric rhombencephalitis of ruminants indicates its involvement in *Listeria monocytogenes* neuroinvasion. Neuropathol Appl Neurobiol 2011;37:753-767.

Histophilus somni *infections (histophilosis, or* H. somni *disease complex)*

Histophilus somni (formerly *Haemophilus somnus*) is the only species of the genus *Histophilus*, family *Pasteurellaceae*, and encompasses bacteria isolated from cattle and previously described as *Haemophilus somnus*, as well as ovine isolates formerly referred to as *Histophilus ovis* and *Haemophilus agni*. *H. somni* is a fastidious gram-negative coccobacillus, and a facultative anaerobic organism that is considered normal flora of the male and female bovine genital tract and, to lesser extent, the bovine nasal cavity. Calves are infected by carrier cows in the first months of life, and they in turn disseminate the infection in feedlots. The mechanism, site, and circumstance by which the bacteria invade the bloodstream are not known, but it is possible that organisms in genital discharges or aerosolized urine invade via the respiratory tract. Infection, especially the respiratory form, is usually preceded by stress factors such as transportation.

These bacteria have virulent and avirulent strains. Important *virulence factors* include lipo-oligosaccharide (LOS), immunoglobulin Fc binding proteins, inhibition of oxygen radicals, and intracellular survival. The mechanism of vasculitis in *H. somni* infection is complex, but it can be partially explained by the effect of LOS on endothelial cells. LOS triggers apoptosis of bovine endothelial cells in vitro by caspase-3 activation. This effect is associated with the production of reactive oxygen and nitrogen intermediates. Another proposed mechanism for the vascular damage induced by *H. somni* is the activation of platelets by the bacteria and its LOS. Platelets activated by *H. somni* initiate endothelial apoptosis via caspases 8 and 9, induce endothelial cell cytokine production and adhesion molecule expression, and promote endothelial cell production of reactive oxygen species (ROS), which further enhances apoptosis. Cerebral blood vessels are particularly vulnerable to damage by the organism, but vasculitis can develop in most organs.

Histophilus somni causes a *septicemia* that may result in acute death, or it may localize in one or several organs causing subacute or chronic, fatal or nonfatal disease. The septicemic phase of the disease is brief, and accompanied by fever and stiffness. In some cases, the infection is controlled at this stage without localization, but often it leads to cerebral vasculitis with acute thrombosis, hemorrhage, and necrosis (Fig. 4-99A, B).

Histophilus somni can infect several bovine organ systems and cause infectious thrombotic meningoencephalitis (ITME), otitis externa, pneumonia, laryngitis/tracheitis, myocarditis, abortion, metritis/infertility, arthritis, mastitis, orchitis, and conjunctivitis. *Vasculitis with secondary thrombosis is the hallmark of the infection.* Bacterial embolism does not occur but may be simulated microscopically by intravascular proliferation of bacteria at sites of thrombosis. Thus the former name "thromboembolic meningoencephalitis" is inaccurate.

Septicemia caused by *H. somni* develops in cattle of various ages maintained under various management systems, but in

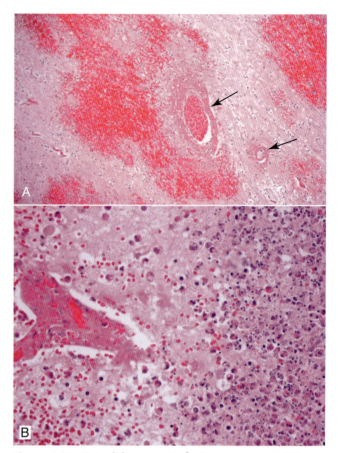

Figure 4-99 *Histophilus somni* infection in an ox. **A.** Hemorrhage and vasculitis (arrows) in cerebral cortex. **B.** Acute hemorrhage with severe suppurative encephalitis. (Courtesy J.L. Caswell.)

North America, the disease is more prevalent in young growing cattle in feedlots. It is most common in early winter, shortly after susceptible animals are moved there from pastures. Infection occurs in a large proportion of animals, but disease occurs in a minority. *H. somni* induces conditions in sheep identical to the bovine disease, that is, septicemia, ITME, abortion, and so forth. *H. somni was isolated from the nasal secretions of healthy adult goats; however, the fulminant disease has not been reported in this species.*

Cerebral localization produces a variety of neurologic signs, and without treatment, affected animals become comatose and die within 1-2 days. The cerebral lesions are distinctive, and are visible in a large majority of untreated cases. The CSF is cloudy and may contain pus and fibrin. *Scattered throughout the brain and spinal cord are multiple foci of hemorrhage and necrosis* (Fig. 4-100). These foci may be 1-30 mm in diameter, and range from the bright red of recent hemorrhage to dark red-brown in older lesions. They have near-random distribution throughout the brain, but there may be some predilection for the thalamus and junction of the gray and white matter of the cerebral cortex. Meningitis is usually visible grossly and is most easily identified over the hemorrhagic foci. In animals that survive for a day or more, diffuse purulent leptomeningitis involves the basilar portions of the brain, and in these animals, the older parenchymal lesions may have begun to soften.

The *histologic lesions* are similar in all organs but are usually most severe in the brain and consist of *intense vasculitis with*

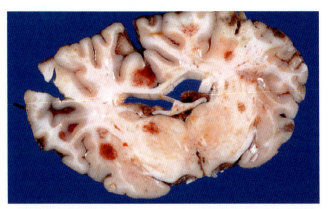

Figure 4-100 *Histophilus somni* infection in an ox. Multiple areas of hemorrhage and necrosis in brainstem and cerebral cortex. (Courtesy J.L. Caswell.)

thrombosis and extension of the inflammation into the surrounding parenchyma, with or without infarction (see Fig. 4-99A, B). Small venules (thrombophlebitis) are primarily affected, with thrombi often containing colonies of bacteria. The inflammatory response is neutrophilic, and cerebral lesions are quickly converted to abscesses.

Although cerebral vascular localization is a common and most dramatic result of the septicemia, *petechiation and evidence of inflammation are often visible throughout the body*, even in animals that die from fulminating disease. Foci of inflammation are easiest to identify in the renal medulla, skeletal muscle, lung, and laryngeal mucosa, but may also be visible in myocardium, intestine, and urinary bladder. Subacute to chronic disease develops commonly in some organs, especially joints, lungs, and heart, and is an important manifestation of *H. somni* infections.

In the acute disease, there is excess fluid in many *joints*, particularly the atlanto-occipital, where the capsule is distended by fluid that contains fibrin and sometimes blood. The synovial membranes and connective tissues around the affected joints are edematous and petechiated. The organism is sensitive to antimicrobials, and the course of the disease is often modified by therapy. The joints of animals that have survived several days contain thick mats of fibrin and pus, and the periarticular tissues are browned by old hemorrhage. Erosion of articular cartilages is rare.

Histophilus somni has been isolated from cattle with a variety of types of *pneumonia*, and its role in the bovine respiratory complex is discussed in the chapter on respiratory diseases. Pneumonia is an uncommon feature of the acute encephalitic form of the disease, but the lung can be involved as part of widespread vasculitis. *Ulcers of the larynx* occur in other diseases of feedlot animals, but, like atlanto-occipital arthritis, they are a regular enough feature of *H. somni* infection to serve as a valuable clue to the diagnosis and prompt a search for lesions in the brain. Similarly, *retinal hemorrhages* are grossly visible in a percentage of animals, and are of diagnostic assistance clinically and when gross brain lesions are absent.

A major manifestation of *H. somni* infection in some parts of North America, especially in western Canada, is *myocardial localization* following asymptomatic septicemia. Infarction, myocarditis, or abscess formation may result, and can lead to cardiac failure with or without mural and valvular endocarditis. In many animals, myocardial abscesses are found only when the myocardium of animals with chronic pneumonia or pleuritis is incised. Abscesses are most common in the left ventricular free wall, particularly in the papillary muscles.

Histophilus somni causes sporadic disease involving many other organs, including the ear, mammary gland, and those of the male and female genital tracts. It can also colonize the pregnant uterus and produce fetal disease and abortion (see Vol. 3, Female genital system). The reported cases have not involved animals with cerebral localization, and may result from asymptomatic septicemia or transcervical invasion.

Further reading

Corbeil LB. *Histophilus somni* host-parasite relationships. Anim Health Res Rev 2007;8:151-160.

Kuckleburg CJ, et al. Endothelial cell apoptosis induced by bacteria-activated platelets requires caspase-8 and -9 and generation of reactive oxygen species. Thromb Haemost 2008;99:363-372.

Siddaramppa S, Inzana TJ. *Haemophilus somnus* virulence factors and resistance to host immunity. Anim Health Res Rev 2004;5:79-93.

Viral infections of the nervous system

Viral infections of the central nervous system are common, usually as part of systemic infections rather than examples of a specialized affinity for nervous tissue. Several viruses are neurotropic; however, only a few are neurovirulent, that is, a virus that multiplies in neural tissue and is able to induce lesions.

The **routes of invasion** of the nervous system available to viruses are *via nerves*, including the olfactory tracts, and *hematogenous*. Centripetal spread in axons does not depend on viral replication in axons, but passage is provided by the mechanisms of fast axoplasmic transport. Invasion by the olfactory route is theoretically simpler because olfactory receptors extend into and beyond the olfactory epithelium, and a cuff of arachnoid extends through the cribriform plate to the olfactory submucosa. This arrangement would allow viruses to spread along nerves without first penetrating to the submucosa or, having penetrated to the submucosa, to reach the CSF directly. This may be the route taken by bovine herpesvirus 1, porcine teschovirus, and pseudorabies virus in young pigs. The olfactory route could be used following intranasal exposure or following hematogenous seeding of the olfactory epithelium or mucosa.

For most viruses, spread to the CNS is *hematogenous* after multiplication in some other tissue and the development of viremia of sufficient magnitude and duration. Viruses are susceptible to removal from blood by histiocytes, but viremia can be sustained if the viruses are small, associated with cells of blood, or replicated in endothelium or lymphatic tissues. Some viruses, such as canine distemper virus, infect vascular endothelial cells, whereas others infect surrounding glia, suggesting transport across endothelium in pinocytotic vesicles. Invasion across the choroid plexus is not impeded by the fenestrated endothelial cells there but would require active infection of the epithelium and ependyma. There are areas of selective permeability to indicator dyes in the brain, such as the tuber cinereum and area postrema, but there is no evidence that these are selectively used by viruses.

The means by which viruses *spread in nervous tissue* are not known. Rapid dissemination can occur in the CSF, but some viruses, such as rabies virus, extend rapidly through the parenchyma. The rate of spread of rabies virus, assuming cell-to-cell growth and transmission, is probably more rapid than its generation time would permit, and permeation of the limited extracellular spaces of the brain by large viruses seems unlikely.

Separation of the specialized cells of the CNS into neurons, oligodendrocytes, astrocytes, and ependymocytes understates the diversity of cell populations in the brain and cord. Different cell populations may show different susceptibilities to infection by different viruses. Thus pseudorabies virus is nonselective in the destruction of cells in the rostral cortex of piglets, feline panleukopenia virus selects rapidly proliferating cells of ependyma and cerebellar cortex, and porcine teschovirus 1 appears to affect particularly the spinal motor neurons.

Degeneration of neurons, reactivity of the glia, and perivascular reactions are the general hallmarks of viral infection of the CNS, and imply a sequence of viral cytopathogenicity and reaction to cellular degeneration. However, viruses that produce manifestations deviating from this rather simple system are many. Classical swine fever virus and bluetongue virus at a suitably early fetal stage of development may produce **malformations** characterized by degeneration of tissue without reaction; later when the animal is immunologically competent, these viruses may produce ordinary encephalomyelitis. Feline panleukopenia virus causes cerebellar hypoplasia in the neonate but is without effect at a later stage of development.

Some viruses may produce *persistent tolerated infection* without clinical signs or lesions. At the other end of the spectrum is rabies virus, which can cause death with minimal cytopathic effect and reaction, or no morphologic change at all. Some virus infections are characterized by long latency and slow attrition, visna/maedi of sheep being the standard example expressed as either degeneration or chronic inflammation. *Transformation of nervous system cells by viruses* can be demonstrated in vitro, and a variety of tumors of the nervous system can be produced by viruses in experimental animals, but they have, as yet, no natural counterpart. The contribution of an immunologic response to both the progress and morphology of encephalomyelitis is very difficult to determine.

General pathology of viral inflammation of the nervous system

Viral infections of the CNS typically induce **nonsuppurative inflammation,** a term that includes quite a variety of quantitative and qualitative changes. The changes are not specific for viral infections, being produced in some bacterial infections, such as salmonellosis in swine; in the rickettsial infection, "salmon poisoning," of dogs; and probably in other rickettsioses. Nor are the lesions qualitatively the same in all viral infections, a fact that is of considerable usefulness in differential diagnosis. The differences are due in part to inherent characters of the agents, routes of invasion, patterns of localization, success of viral replication and release, duration and degree of cellular injury, and host defense reactions. As well as the differences, there are also the very considerable similarities that allow them all to be included with the "nonsuppurative encephalomyelitides."

The distribution of lesions in different viral infections is a reflection of the varied affinities of the viruses, and is useful in differential diagnosis but only generally applicable. The distributions of lesions or of inclusion bodies are only very rough guides to the distribution and activity of the virus.

Perivascular cuffing, or accumulation of cells in the adventitia of vessels and in the perivascular Virchow-Robin space, is almost constant in encephalitis, and, when present, is usually the most striking microscopic change. The accumulated cells are usually leukocytes, but in some diseases, there may be very few hematogenous elements recognizable, the cuffs being composed instead of histiocytic cells that appear to have proliferated in situ from adventitial elements. These latter frequently fragment to resemble degenerate neutrophils if the postmortem interval is prolonged. Injury to the vessel wall proper is not constant, but when it occurs, it may affect the arteries as a hyalinizing or fibrinoid change. This is characteristic of malignant catarrhal fever (see Fig. 4-53), for example, and occurs also in equine encephalitis. The endothelium may be selectively injured in classical swine fever and infectious canine hepatitis. The lesions associated with equid herpesvirus infection may be limited to quite subtle endothelial swelling and proliferation in small blood vessels. When, in inflammation, the perivascular cuffs are large enough to disorganize the wall of the vessel and compress it, the endothelium frequently shows signs of swelling and proliferation, and there may also be altered adhesiveness so that leukocytes and red cells tend to stick to it. Thrombosis is incidental and very seldom observed, but compression of the vessels probably accounts for the ischemic parenchymal softenings that occur.

Infiltrating cells are predominantly lymphocytes, and they accumulate in the perivascular spaces (see Fig. 4-17A, B). The earliest cells in the perivascular spaces may be neutrophils; in acute lesions, some of these can be found wandering in parenchyma or grouped in dense clusters. They soon disappear but may be found later for a short time in areas that soften. Lymphocytes remain in the cuffs and are admixed after a week or so with an increasing number of plasma cells and macrophages. A few eosinophils may also be found in pigs. Perivascular cuffing is not specific for viral infections. It is also a reaction to degeneration of neural tissue.

Glial reactions occur if the parenchyma is injured, even though the injury may not be appreciable, but the reaction may be absent in those infections that selectively involve the vessel walls. In inflamed areas, the oligodendroglia degenerate. Astrocytes degenerate or react depending on how strictly and severely they are injured; the stimuli for astrocytic reaction were discussed previously in this chapter. *The gliosis that is so frequently a feature of nonsuppurative encephalomyelitis is almost solely microglial. The gliosis may be diffuse or focal but is commonly both* (see Fig. 4-15). Diffuse gliosis may be more apparent than real if resulting more from hypertrophy than from proliferation of these glia. Focal gliosis may occur anywhere in the parenchyma and may be related to small vessels and injury to microvasculature. When there are more than a dozen or so cells in such foci, some of the cells are likely to be lymphocytes, and occasionally there are a few plasma cells. The microglia in the center of a focus are frequently degenerate. There are 2 specifically named forms of microgliosis. "*Neuronophagic nodules*" are foci of microglia about degenerating neurons (see Fig. 4-2D); "*glial shrubbery*" is an accumulation of these cells in the molecular layer of the cerebellum in relation to degenerating Purkinje cells (Fig. 4-101).

Neuronal changes must be the principal determinants of the outcome of the infection. The distribution of neuronal degeneration is to some slight extent specific, but the extensiveness is nonspecific and varies considerably. The morphologic features of the degenerate cells are nonspecific. As a rule,

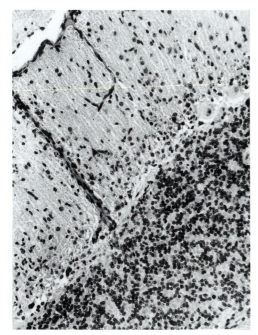

Figure 4-101 Encephalitis in **louping-ill** in a sheep. Destruction of Purkinje cells and gliosis in the molecular layer of the cerebellum ("glial shrubbery").

the more severe degrees of neuronal degeneration are caused by viruses that are highly neurotropic, such as rabies virus, but the severity of neuronal degeneration is not a dependable "lead" in differential diagnosis. The fact that rabies virus can be lethal without morphologic change in the CNS raises the possibility that other viruses may cause severe encephalopathy without inflammatory change. *The usual form of neuronal degeneration is central chromatolysis*, which may extend to completion, with the cell then swollen, pale, and devoid of a nucleus. This is typical of the axonal reaction to injury, but the axons are intact. Many neurons appear as if coagulated, being shrunken, rounded, isolated, and staining darkly with eosin. The nucleus is pyknotic or has disappeared. The coagulated neuron stimulates the formation of the neuronophagic nodule, but not all necrotic neurons elicit the reaction. Usually, intact neurons can be found adjacent to degenerate ones.

Lesions in white matter occur consistently even though many viruses are supposed to be specifically tropic for gray matter. Cuffing reactions are to be expected even if degeneration is limited to adjacent gray matter. *Microgliosis* is focal rather than diffuse, and the nodules are small. Some degree of *disintegration of myelin* is inevitable, but conspicuous demyelination is a feature only of canine distemper, lentivirus leukoencephalitis of goats, and visna. Demyelination associated with viral diseases may be the result of direct infection of melanin-forming cells, that is, oligodendroglia, as in infection with canine distemper virus, or may be a bystander lesion caused by injury from inflammatory cytokines associated with viral infection.

Meningitis is seldom severe except in local distributions, and these tend to overlie parenchymal lesions. Some agents, of which typical examples are those of sporadic bovine encephalomyelitis and malignant catarrhal fever, have a selective affinity for meningeal structures in the CNS. Others, such as canine distemper virus, share the affinities so that leptomeningitis is part of the primary response. In the more purely neurotropic infections, such as rabies, the meningitis, or more precisely the meningeal infiltration, is due probably to drainage of products of reaction via the Virchow-Robin spaces from the brain or cord. The reacting cells in the meninges are of the same type as those in the brain, and they float freely in the arachnoid spaces.

No virus is known to be tropic for peripheral nerves in the sense of selectively producing direct lesions in them. Degenerative changes occur fairly early in the end plates and terminal parts of axons when the central cell body is destroyed. Foci of microglia and lymphocytes occur in the nerve roots quite commonly. Inflammation of the paravertebral ganglia, and especially the trigeminal (Gasserian) ganglia, is characteristic of rabies and of Teschen disease and related infections in pigs, but the frequency and distribution of this lesion in other viral encephalomyelitides and in other ganglia is unknown.

Inclusion bodies may form in neurons, neuroglia, or microglia and other mesenchymal cells. Inclusion bodies in the nervous system are usually acidophilic. They may be found only in neurons as in rabies, in glia, or in both. They may be cytoplasmic, nuclear, or both. Intranuclear inclusions, which must be distinguished from altered nucleoli, have considerable specificity; somewhat less reliance can be placed on intracytoplasmic inclusions. Cytoplasmic viral inclusions must be distinguished from normal inclusions.

Lyssavirus infections

Rabies is caused by the species **Rabies virus** (RABV), genus *Lyssavirus*, family *Rhabdoviridae*. The RABV glycoprotein (RVG), which is a trimeric and surface-exposed viral coat protein, is responsible for RABV neurotropism by binding to several neural tissue receptors, including the neuronal cell adhesion molecule (NCAM), and the p75 neurotrophin receptor (p75NTR). Evolutionary studies based on genes encoding the surface glycoprotein suggest that *RABV evolved first in bats*, possibly in vampire bats much more widely distributed than at present, and only later became adapted to terrestrial carnivores. There is a single major antigenic type with minor variations that allow epidemiologic surveillance. The genus *Lyssavirus* has 7 *genotypes* that are defined by phylogenetic analysis. Type 1 is the classic rabies virus of animals and vampire bats, and of all other bat lyssaviruses in North America. Type 2 (Lagos bat virus), type 3 (Mokola virus), and type 4 (Duvenhage virus) are African genotypes. Types 5 (EBLV-1) and 6 (EBLV-2) are European bat lyssavirus 1 and 2, respectively, and type 7 (Ballina virus) is the Australian bat lyssavirus. The 7 genotypes may further be allocated into *2 major phylogroups* based on pathogenicity for mice and cross-neutralization. Phylogroup 1 includes genotypes 1, 4-7, and phylogroup 2 includes genotypes 2 and 3. Excepting Mokola virus, bats may be the preferential vector species for genotypes 2-7. Non-rabies lyssaviruses (e.g., Lagos bat virus, Duvenhage virus, Mokola virus), can cause neurologic disease identical to rabies in humans and animals.

Rabies virus has 2 biotypes: "fixed" virus and "street" virus. *Fixed RABV*, which is the basis of vaccine strains, is a laboratory biotype stabilized in its properties by serial intracerebral passage. It is highly neurotropic, is not secreted in saliva, and does not produce Negri bodies. *Street RABV* is the feral biotype that circulates in enzootics and epizootics. In addition to neurotropism, it is tropic for salivary glands, in which it reaches high concentration, and possibly in other mucus-secreting epithelia, and produces Negri bodies.

The establishment of infection ordinarily depends on inoculation of the virus into a wound, such usually being inflicted by the bite of a rabid animal. Contamination of a fresh wound by infected saliva or tissues is much less dangerous. The virus replicates in myocytes around a bite wound for a short period of time, and then buds from the plasma membrane. Viral particles invade the local neuromuscular junction through conjugation of the rabies virus glycoprotein (RVG) with the nicotinic acetylcholine receptor, and then invade neurotendinous spindles and ascend to the CNS and paravertebral ganglia via axoplasmic flow. Viral replication in the CNS is followed by centrifugal spread to major exit portals, such as the adrenal gland, nasal mucosa, and salivary glands; the virus is secreted with the saliva for a few days prior to the appearance of clinical signs. The incubation period is variable from weeks to months.

Although there are species differences in susceptibility, rabies is one disease to which *all mammals are susceptible*. The disease can be regarded as one of carnivores because it is almost always transmitted naturally only by bites. Man and herbivores are dead-end hosts. There are exceptions to the rule that RABV is transmitted by a bite. *Oral infection* can occur in diverse species, and the application of modified RABV in "baits" uses this potential; *aerosol infection* can occur, as in dense congregations of colonial bats in bat caves, probably as droplet infection from salivary secretions; and a variety of aberrant circumstances may provide transfer opportunities for infectious virus, as has been reported for *corneal transplants*.

Reservoir hosts vary from time to time and from region to region. The principal reservoir vectors are foxes and skunks in the United States and Canada, with the raccoon of importance on the Atlantic seaboard; foxes and dogs in northern Canada; foxes moving from east to west in Europe; wolves in eastern Europe and Iran; jackals in India and Northern Africa; the mongoose and genet cat in South Africa; and the mongoose in the Caribbean. *Sylvatic vectors* are responsible for most transmissions to man and domestic animals in countries where dog populations are controlled. Oral vaccination of wild carnivores, by using vaccine-laden baits, and routine vaccination of dogs have led to almost complete elimination of canine-transmitted rabies in developed countries. Rarely, vaccination of severely stressed animals with vaccines containing modified-live virus may induce postvaccinal rabies. In tropical areas where domestic and feral dogs are not controlled, these animals are the principal hazards for man and livestock.

Bats present a special epidemiologic problem. Fructivorous and insectivorous bats as well as vampires are capable of transmitting RABV. Vampire bats inhabit South and Central America, extending into northern Mexico and are, historically, responsible for a high incidence of rabies in mammals, especially cattle but including humans. When clinically affected, vampire bats manifest the disease as the furious form and show unnatural daylight activity.

The **clinical course** of rabies is usually acute, from 1-2 days, but can be as long as 10 days. It is seldom that a clinical diagnosis of rabies can be made with confidence. The terms *"furious rabies"* and *"dumb rabies"* place emphasis on particular features within a spectrum of behavioral changes and are inappropriate for noncarnivorous animals. *Aberrant behavioral patterns* can be recognized in affected animals during epizootics. The period of salivary excretion of virus before the onset of neurologic signs is expected to be not more than a few days, vampire bats possibly excepted, and the duration of clinical disease to be a few days only. Once expressed clinically as neurologic disease, *rabies is almost invariably fatal;* recovery with or without neurologic deficit is quite rare but has been observed in several species following experimental exposure. Progressive infection and clinical disease do not inevitably follow exposure; up to 25% of feral populations may have specific antibodies as evidence that the infection provoked an immune response without progression to neurologic disease.

Specific gross lesions are not present at autopsy, but self-inflicted wounds and foreign bodies in the stomach of a carnivore should raise suspicion. The **histologic lesions** of rabies, when present, are *typical of nonsuppurative encephalomyelitis, with ganglioneuritis and parotid adenitis.* Inflammatory changes are usually present, but they may be very mild or absent. To some extent at least, the severity of lesions reflects the duration of the clinical disease. In the CNS, inflammatory and degenerative changes are most severe from the pons to the hypothalamus and in the cervical spinal cord, with relative sparing of the medulla. This relative sparing of the medulla appears to apply to all domestic species. The most severe lesions of the disease are generally found in dogs, whereas other species, especially ruminants, which are highly susceptible, may show little more than an occasional vessel with a few cuffing lymphocytes and a few very small glial nodules (*Babès' nodules* in this disease), and this in spite of having numerous Negri bodies. These reactive phenomena probably reflect largely the degree of neuronal degeneration, and this may be remarkably slight in herbivores and remarkably severe in dogs.

The reaction is typically one of *perivascular cuffing and focal gliosis*. The cuffs are one to several cells thick and composed solely of lymphocytes (Fig. 4-102A); ring hemorrhages confined largely to the perivascular space are common about cuffed vessels. Hemorrhages are occasionally severe enough to be visible grossly in the spinal cord of horses and cattle (Fig. 4-102B). The Babès' nodules are composed of microglia, and they occur in both white and gray matter. The nodules vary greatly in size, some containing only 6 or 7 cells and some containing 100 or more. Diffuse as well as focal gliosis (see Fig. 4-15) occurs in areas of gray matter such as the pons and in the spinal cord, both horns of the latter being involved.

Neuronal degeneration in carnivores may be very extensive and quite out of proportion to the observed reactive changes, but may be very slight in pigs and herbivores. Neuronal and/or gray matter neuropilar vacuolation *(rabies-induced spongiform encephalopathy)* is reported to occur in experimental and natural rabies. The specificity of the neuronal changes and of the whole pathologic picture depends on the *inclusion bodies of Negri. These* are always *intracytoplasmic* and are present most commonly in the hippocampus of carnivores and in the Purkinje cells of herbivores. Fixed RABV does not produce Negri bodies, and street RABV fails to do so in up to 30% of cases. Neurons of any distribution may contain inclusion bodies, but they tend to be scarce where the inflammatory reaction is severe. Indeed, Negri bodies may be found only in neurons that are otherwise histologically normal; they are not present in degenerate neurons. They have also been found, but rarely, in ganglion cells of the adrenal medulla, salivary glands, and retina. Although the number of Negri bodies has little relation to the length of the incubation period, there is a relation to the duration of the clinical disease. They may not be found if the animal is killed instead of being allowed to die.

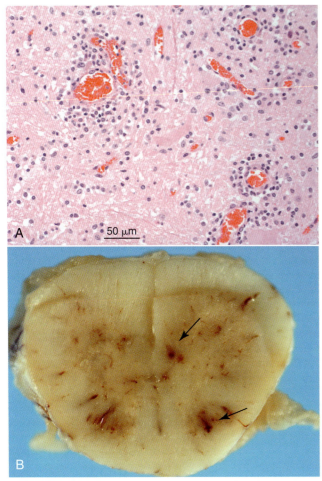

Figure 4-102 Rabies. **A.** Perivascular cuffs and focal gliosis in a horse. **B.** Hemorrhage in gray matter of spinal cord (arrows). (Courtesy M.J. Hazlett.)

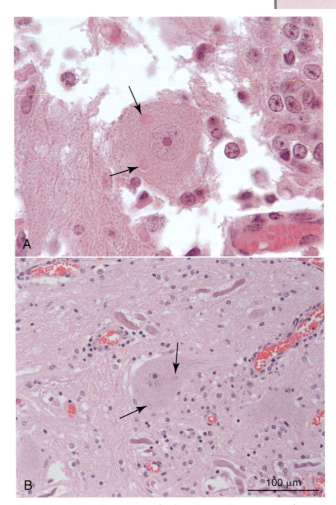

Figure 4-103 Rabies. Negri bodies (arrows) in neuronal cytoplasm of a goat (**A**) and a horse (**B**). (Courtesy M.J. Hazlett.)

They are produced consistently in white mice, the usual test animal.

Negri bodies are round or oval structures, usually ~2-8 μm in diameter (Fig. 4-103A, B). They are plastic, their shape being molded to their environment. Those in the dendrites, seldom observed except in Purkinje cells, are oval, and those in the cell body are usually rounded. There may be one or more per cell, and affected cells are otherwise only little changed. The inclusions are surrounded by a clear thin halo. Nonspecific homogeneous inclusions may be found in the pyramidal cells of the hippocampus in cats, skunks, and dogs. There may be several such inclusions per cell, but each is minute, not measuring >1.5 μm. In old sheep and cattle, larger neurons, especially of the medulla and cord, may contain nonspecific inclusions. These have a dust-like distribution, are usually numerous, and are brightly acidophilic, angulated, and ~1.0 μm in size. Nonspecific inclusions that are indistinguishable from Negri bodies by light microscopy occur in the lateral geniculate neurons in cats. *Fluorescent antibody techniques are required for positive identification* and are essential in the rare chronic cases that may not yield virus on mouse inoculation.

If there is no *ganglioneuritis* in the paravertebral ganglia, then the possibility of the animal having rabies is very remote. If there is ganglioneuritis, it may be part of rabies or something else. Pigs, for example, get ganglioneuritis in the Teschen group of infections. Inflammatory changes in the trigeminal (Gasserian) ganglion in rabies may be present without inflammatory or neuronal changes being clearly evident in the brain. The ganglionic changes are of the same character as those in the brain, namely, acute degeneration of ganglion cells, proliferation of capsule cells, and microglial nodules.

The natural transmission of RABV depends on virus being present in the saliva and therefore in the salivary glands. Fixed virus has no affinity for the salivary glands, and none is present in some cases of infection with the street virus. Degenerative changes are reported in the epithelium of the mandibular salivary gland, but not in the parotid, in dogs.

The **diagnosis** of rabies is made by using fluorescent antibody labeling by performing a direct fluorescent antibody (DFA) test on fresh or fixed tissue, or by virus isolation in cell culture. Immunohistochemistry performed on paraffin-embedded formalin-fixed tissues is considered to be a sensitive and reliable diagnostic technique. In situ hybridization, electron microscopy, and PCR-based testing may also prove useful.

Further reading

Badrane H, et al. Evidence of two Lyssavirus phylogroups with distinct pathogenicity and immunogenicity. J Virol 2001;75:3268-3276.

Calisher CH, et al. The other rabies viruses: the emergence and importance of lyssaviruses from bats and other vertebrates. Travel Med Infect Dis 2012;10:69-79.
Coertse J, et al. A case study of rabies diagnosis from formalin-fixed brain material. J S Afr Vet Assoc 2011;82:250-253.
Hatanpaa KJ, Kim JH. Neuropathology of viral infections. Handb Clin Neurol 2014;123:193-214.
Koyuncu OO, et al. Virus infections in the nervous system. Cell Host Microbe 2013;13:379-393.
Warrell M. Rabies and African bat lyssavirus encephalitis and its prevention. Int J Antimicrob Agents 2010;36(Suppl. 1):S47-S52.

Pseudorabies

Pseudorabies is also known as Aujeszky's disease, mad itch, infectious bulbar paralysis, and porcine herpesvirus infection. The causative agent, species **Suid herpesvirus 1** (SuHV-1; pseudorabies virus, PRV), genus *Varicellovirus*, subfamily *Alphaherpesvirinae*, family *Herpesviridae*, is unusual for a member of that group in its relative lack of host specificity and by being spread laterally as well as vertically in swine. A number of strains have been identified that exhibit a wide range of virulence. Pseudorabies virus is capable, as are other members of the family *Herpesviridae*, of establishing latent infection. Trigeminal ganglion, olfactory bulb, and tonsil are the most consistent sites of latency of PRV. In these organs, viral DNA can be detected in the absence of infectious virus. The pig is the only natural host, but the common domestic species are naturally susceptible; there are very few reports in horses and goats. Progressive infections do not occur in humans. The disease is reported worldwide, except for Canada and Australia. Natural infections occur in rats and mice and various species of wildlife and on fur farms. Of the laboratory animals, the rabbit is the most susceptible and is preferred for identification of the virus because of the fairly consistent development of intense local pruritus following subcutaneous inoculation. Guinea pigs are less susceptible and may resist subcutaneous inoculation but succumb to intracerebral and, occasionally, to intraperitoneal inoculation.

The virus is maintained in enzootic areas in wild and domestic swine, for which it is highly contagious but usually asymptomatic, and probably in brown rats. *Transmission* can occur by ingestion, but the usual method of spread between pigs is thought to be by contact of infective secretions with nasal mucosa or abraded skin. Animals are susceptible to intranasal inoculation, and regardless of the route of infection, the *virus can be found in nasal secretions*. The virus may also be present in saliva and urine. It is also present in blood, but this is of no significance for epidemiology or transmission. The infection will occur in pigs by contact very readily and probably by direct nose-to-nose transmission, but it does not appear to be contagious between individuals of other species, and they probably acquire their infection by contact with swine or, possibly, rats. Pigs may harbor virus for many months in tonsils and nasopharyngeal secretions after exposure, but in other domestic species, the virus is fairly strictly neurotropic, and therefore is not excreted unless given experimentally in large doses. Ingestion of *infected pig meat* is the usual source of infection for dogs and cats. Cattle and sheep may become infected by direct contact with carrier swine or by aerosol exposure, but there is strong circumstantial evidence implicating contaminated feed.

The *pathogenesis* of the infection following local inoculation is well established for the rabbit and is probably comparable in other species. The virus causes a local reaction at the site of inoculation if percutaneous and then spreads centripetally along the related nerve to the spinal cord; it then spreads outward again along other peripheral nerves as other segments of cord are progressively invaded by spread within the CNS. Because of the progressive advance of infection along the cord, death may occur before demonstrable amounts of virus reach the brain and before lesions have time to develop there. Intracerebral inoculation produces encephalitis, and virus spreads to the cord and centrifugally along peripheral nerves to an extent that depends on survival time. Because the virus also circulates in the blood, there is some possibility but no evidence that it invades the brain directly, the evidence instead suggesting that it localizes in viscera and invades the nervous system along autonomic nerves. Following nasal or intraocular exposure, the virus spreads along the related nerves. The route of invasion following ingestion is by retrograde transneuronal infection. Transplacental infections occur in pigs causing abortion in about 50% of sows pregnant in the first month, and the delivery of macerated, mummified, and normal fetuses when infection occurs at later stages of gestation. The virus is reported to be present in the semen of carrier boars.

The *signs and course* of pseudorabies in pigs are very variable. Most cases are of mild febrile illness without pruritus or nervous signs, and with recovery expected in a week or so. Sows may subsequently produce mummified litters. Age is a very important factor governing the severity of the disease in swine; the mortality rate in nursing pigs and young weaners may be very high. Very young sucklings do not show specific nervous signs but rapidly become prostrate and die in 12-24 hours. In slightly older piglets, incoordination progresses rapidly to paralysis with muscular twitchings, tremors, and convulsions. Some pigs showing severe signs of encephalitis recover. Experimental peripheral inoculation will produce asymptomatic meningitis and encephalitis in swine, the inflammatory lesions being severe. The disease in older pigs is often characterized by fever, rhinitis, and coughing. There may be generalized pruritus in natural cases but it is not severe, being expressed usually by rubbing of the nose or head. Fetal resorption, mummification, stillbirths, and abortions are reported frequently.

The characteristic clinical sign of pseudorabies in animals other than pigs is *intense cutaneous irritation* developing at the point of inoculation or at the terminal distribution of a nerve trunk that passes the point of inoculation. This does not occur until the virus reaches the related segment of cord. Dogs may become frenzied, and besides the intense pruritus (mad itch), there may be jaw paralysis and drooling reminiscent of rabies. The clinical course in these species, which always ends in death, is frequently acute (a few hours) and never longer than 1 week. Pseudorabies may occur in sporadic, although significant, outbreaks in sheep and cattle. The mortality rate is very high. Death may occur without signs of illness or within 1-2 days of the onset of clinical signs. There is fever, and the itching may be on any part of the body but is most frequently about the head or hindlimbs. Other neurologic signs are variable but constantly present.

There are *no specific gross lesions* of pseudorabies. At the site of cutaneous infection, there is acute serofibrinous inflammation, ballooning degeneration, and epithelial necrosis with rare intranuclear inclusions. Self-trauma resulting from intense itching may exacerbate these lesions. The intense pruritus at the site of inoculation is likely caused by stimulation of regional sensory nerves by viral spread and multiplication. Gross changes are seen mostly in young pigs. There may be necrosis of tonsils and sometimes of the trachea and esophagus. Rhinitis with patchy epithelial necrosis is common. The lungs may be edematous. Tiny foci (1-2 mm) of hemorrhagic necrosis typical of alphaherpesviral infection may be seen in liver, spleen, lung, intestines, adrenals, and placenta.

The **histologic lesions** reflect the neurotropic and epitheliotropic nature of the virus. Lesions are similar in all susceptible species; however, epitheliotropic lesions are more commonly seen in young, aborted, or stillbirth piglets and rarely seen in ruminants or carnivores, where the brain lesions are more common. In brain, the gray matter especially is affected, but death may occur before there are clear indications of neuronal degeneration or inflammatory reaction in the brain. With naturally acquired infections, the inflammatory changes are *nonsuppurative*. In addition, focal gliosis and lesions typical of neuronal degeneration (neuronophagia and satellitosis) are usually present (Fig. 4-104A, B). There is severe ganglioneuritis in paravertebral ganglia. The specificity of the reaction in the brain depends on the development of *acidophilic intranuclear inclusion bodies in neurons and astroglia* (Fig. 4-104C). These inclusion bodies occur in all species, including pigs; fixation in a mercurial fixative is helpful for their demonstration. Inclusions in swine are *solid and amphophilic*, but in other species, the inclusions are granular and often small and multiple in an affected nucleus. By any route of infection, piglets tend to develop panencephalitis with most severe lesions in the cerebral cortex, brainstem, spinal ganglia, and basal ganglia of the brain (see Fig. 4-104B); in other domestic species, the distribution of lesions in the CNS is local to, and determined by, the route of exposure. Lymphoplasmacytic inflammation with neuronal degeneration of the gastric myenteric plexi is also described.

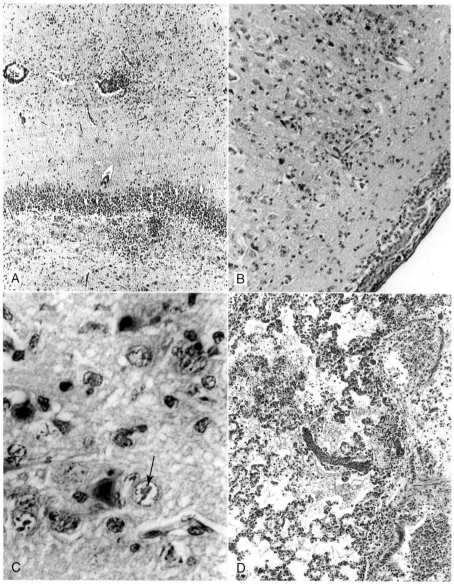

Figure 4-104 Pseudorabies in a pig. **A.** Perivascular cuffing, focal and diffuse gliosis in dentate gyrus. **B.** Meningitis and necrosis of cells in cerebrum. **C.** Neuronal necrosis and irregular inclusion bodies in nuclei (arrow). **D.** Necrotizing bronchopneumonia.

Epitheliotropic lesions include the presence of tiny areas of coagulative or lytic necrosis in the liver, tonsils, lung, spleen, placenta, and adrenals, with the presence of the characteristic intranuclear inclusions. Pulmonary lesions may be mild or severe. Edema and mild cellular infiltration may be diffuse, and there may be focal or confluent necrotizing, hemorrhagic pneumonia (Fig. 4-104D). Hemorrhage and necrosis is present in lymph nodes, and foci of necrosis may be found in tonsils, liver, spleen, and adrenal. Necrotizing vasculitis is described in natural infections in sheep and experimentally in piglets. In aborted or stillborn piglets, which are suitable for examination, there is usually no evidence of encephalitis, but foci of necrosis may be found in liver and other parenchymatous tissues, together with focal bronchiolar necrosis and interstitial pneumonia.

Rapid **diagnosis** can be achieved by fluorescent antibody tests on frozen sections of tissue, for example, tonsils, liver, or brain. Isolation in eggs or tissue culture is also available.

Further reading

Müller T, et al. Pseudorabies virus in wild swine: a global perspective. Arch Virol 2011;156:1691-1705.

Pomeranz LE, et al. Molecular biology of pseudorabies virus: impact on neurovirology and veterinary medicine. Microbiol Mol Biol Rev 2005;69:462-500.

Porcine hemagglutinating encephalomyelitis virus

The species *Porcine hemagglutinating encephalomyelitis virus* (HEV), a member of genus *Coronavirus*, family *Coronaviridae*, can be isolated from the respiratory tract of normal pigs, and is present worldwide. Other porcine coronaviruses include transmissible gastroenteritis virus, porcine epidemic diarrhea virus, porcine deltacoronavirus, and porcine respiratory coronavirus. HEV is a group 2 species coronavirus antigenically related to bovine coronavirus, human coronavirus OC43, and murine hepatitis virus. The pig is the only natural host for HEV. Although there is serologic evidence of wide distribution in many swine-raising areas, clinical disease is rare because most piglets receive protective levels of colostral antibodies to HEV. Disease occurs in piglets 1-3 weeks of age and follows a clinical course of about 3 days to 3 weeks. The mortality rate is very high and survivors are usually unthrifty.

Following exposure, replication of virus occurs in the epithelium of nose, tonsil, lung, and small intestine, with spread to the CNS along peripheral nerves rather than hematogenously; viremia is not important in the pathogenesis. Viral antigen is detectable in alimentary ganglia during the incubation period of the disease. It is first demonstrable in the brain in trigeminal and vagal sensory nuclei, with later rostral spread in brainstem. Viral replication occurs in the myenteric plexus of the stomach, and involvement of the autonomic system probably can explain the predominant clinical signs of vomition and constipation.

Two *clinical syndromes* are recognized. Neurologic signs occur in 4- to 7-day-old piglets in some outbreaks and consist of stilted gait, hyperesthesia, progressive paresis, and convulsions in some cases. Clinical signs in 4- to 14-day-old piglets are dominated by anorexia and vomiting, and this syndrome is called *"vomiting and wasting disease."*

Lesions in the CNS may be found in some affected piglets that do not show clinical signs of nervous disease. The frequency with which inflammatory change is found is quite variable. Lesions when present are those of *nonsuppurative encephalomyelitis* affecting particularly the gray matter of medulla and brainstem. In such cases, there is inflammation of the trigeminal, paravertebral, and autonomic ganglia. The gastric myenteric plexi are occasionally infiltrated with a few lymphocytes and plasma cells.

Diagnosis of HEV is problematic. Serology on acute and convalescent sera may help in detecting acute infection. Isolation of HEV can be attempted from brainstem of acutely ill piglets. Differential diagnoses of nervous conditions with high mortality in piglets include pseudorabies, classical swine fever, polioencephalomyelitis (Teschen disease), bacterial meningitis, streptococcal septicemia, and hypoglycemia.

Further reading

Hirano N, et al. Spread of swine hemagglutinating encephalomyelitis virus from peripheral nerves to the CNS. Adv Exp Med Biol 1998;440:601-607.

Pensaert MB. Hemagglutinating encephalomyelitis virus. In: Straw BE, et al., editors. Diseases of Swine. 8th ed. Ames, Iowa: Iowa State University Press; 1999. p. 151-157.

Vijgen L, et al. Evolutionary history of the closely related group 2 coronaviruses: porcine hemagglutinating encephalomyelitis virus, bovine coronavirus, and human coronavirus OC43. J Virol 2006; 80:7270-7274.

Enterovirus/teschovirus polioencephalomyelitis of pigs

Encephalomyelitis of pigs caused by porcine enteroviruses occurs in many countries and is distinguishable only by a study of the agents. Porcine enteroviruses are ubiquitous but are limited in their pathogenicity to swine. **Porcine enterovirus** A (PEV-A) and porcine enterovirus B (PEV-B) are in the genus *Enterovirus*, family *Picornaviridae*. Porcine enteroviruses serotypes 1-7 and 11-13 have been reclassified as species **Porcine teschovirus** 1-7, 11-13, genus *Teschovirus*, family *Picornaviridae*. Infection by one enterovirus/teschovirus serotype does not confer protection against infection by another.

Infection is most commonly acquired by pigs after weaning as a result of waning maternal immunity and mixing of pigs from different sources; however, most infections are asymptomatic. Infection follows the fecal-oral route and indirectly through contaminated fomites. Initial replication occurs in the tonsils and the intestinal epithelium, especially of ileum and colon; the enteric phase is not clinically significant or accompanied by tissue change. The enteric phase is followed by viremia and then invasion of the CNS. Viremia by some serotypes may lead to localization in the pregnant uterus and death of fetuses.

Infection with virulent virus may produce nervous signs as soon as 6 days after exposure. The virus is present in large amounts in tonsils and cervical lymph nodes by 24 hours, and in the mesenteric nodes and feces by 48 hours. The disease has 2 clinical forms: the highly fatal and severe form (**Teschen disease**) and a less virulent milder form (**Talfan disease,** poliomyelitis suum, benign enzootic paresis, Ontario encephalomyelitis, polioencephalomyelitis). Teschen disease, first recognized in 1929 in Teschen, Czech Republic, is caused by highly virulent **porcine teschovirus 1** and is limited mostly to Europe, but sporadic epizootics occur in Africa. Talfan disease, caused

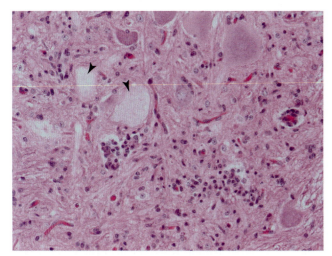

Figure 4-105 Nonsuppurative poliomyelitis with neuronal degeneration and chromatolysis (arrowheads) in **enteroviral encephalomyelitis** in a pig.

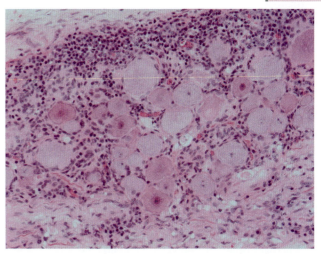

Figure 4-106 Ganglioneuritis in enteroviral encephalomyelitis in a pig. (Courtesy National Institute of Animal Health, Ibaraki, Japan).

by infection with less virulent strains of the virus, is more common than Teschen disease and occurs worldwide. Teschen disease is of high morbidity and high mortality affecting all age groups and expressed clinically as convulsions, opisthotonos, nystagmus, and coma. Death commonly occurs in 3-4 days. Survivors may have residual paralysis. Talfan disease is characterized by lower morbidity and mortality, and the clinical signs are expressed as paresis and ataxia that seldom progresses to complete paralysis. The infection is asymptomatic in the absence of neurologic signs, and up to 95% of exposed pigs develop latent or inapparent infections.

The *pathologic changes* in these syndromes are the same, although minor differences in severity and distribution of the lesions are reported. There are no gross changes. The histologic changes are those of *nonsuppurative polioencephalomyelitis* extending throughout the cerebrospinal axis from the olfactory bulbs to the lumbar cord. Any series of cases of each of the syndromes provides a continuous spectrum of severity and distribution of the lesions. Lymphocytic meningitis is mild in the cerebral meninges and usually overlies areas of parenchymal injury in the cerebrum. In weaners and older animals in which the course is more prolonged than in very young pigs, intense lymphocytic meningitis develops over the cerebellum, usually in conjunction with inflammatory lesions in the underlying molecular layer (Fig. 4-105). Cerebellar meningitis is very slight if the course of the disease is 4-5 days or less so that, although emphasized in reports of Teschen disease, it is not a feature in very young animals, in which the course is short. The most severe lesions occur in the brainstem from the hypothalamus through the medulla and decrease in intensity and diffuseness down the spinal cord. There is relative sparing of the cerebral and cerebellar cortices, but the deep substance of the cerebellum is consistently and often severely involved. Lesions in the spinal cord in each syndrome are largely confined to the gray matter, particularly the ventral horns, but may selectively involve the dorsal horns in very young pigs. Cord lesions are those of nonsuppurative myelitis and the motor neurons, particularly in gray matter of the ventral horns, experience different stages of neuronal degenerative and necrotic changes (neuronal swelling, chromatolysis, satellitosis, and finally neuronophagia). Lesions are consistently present in the dorsal root ganglia, and especially the trigeminal ganglia (Fig. 4-106).

Diagnosis can be achieved by virus isolation or immunohistochemistry.

Further reading

La Rosa G, et al. Validation of rt-PCR assays for molecular characterization of porcine teschoviruses and enteroviruses. J Vet Med B Infect Dis Vet Public Health 2006;53:257-265.

Pogranichniy RM, et al. A prolonged outbreak of polioencephalomyelitis due to infection with a group I porcine enterovirus. J Vet Diagn Invest 2003;15:191-194.

Flaviviral encephalitides

The genus *Flavivirus* of the family *Flaviviridae* contains several important viruses that cause encephalitis in domestic and wild animals. Some of these viruses are emerging as very important not only for animal health but also for public health as they are highly zoonotic. The viruses of veterinary importance in this genus belong either to the *tick-borne virus group* or the *mosquito-borne virus group*. Viruses of both groups are maintained in a cycle involving ticks or mosquitoes, respectively, as invertebrate vectors, and wild vertebrate hosts as reservoirs. In most cases, infections of humans and/or domestic animals are incidental, and are not important for viral transmission or maintenance in the environment.

Diseases caused by tick-borne flaviviruses. Important veterinary viruses in this group include louping ill virus and tick-borne encephalitis virus; these 2 viruses are very closely related, and may have originated from a common ancestor. The group also includes several other viruses—Langat virus, Kyasanur Forest disease virus, Omsk hemorrhagic fever virus, and Powassan virus (POWV)—that are primarily of importance in humans. POWV causes severe encephalitis in humans in the United States, Canada, and Siberia, but induces encephalitis in animals only under experimental conditions.

Louping ill (ovine encephalomyelitis). Louping ill is a tick-borne viral encephalomyelitis of sheep caused by species ***Louping ill virus*** (LIV), which has been enzootic in England,

Scotland, and Northern Ireland for more than a century and has been reported in Norway. The disease is named after the leaping (or louping) demonstrated by the diseased sheep. A similar disease has been reported in Spain, Greece, and Turkey, affecting sheep or goats, but because the etiologic viruses are different by nucleotide sequencing from LIV, each was considered a subtype of LIV but assigned different names: Spanish sheep encephalomyelitis virus and Greek goat encephalomyelitis virus. Cattle, horses, goats, and deer pastured with affected sheep sometimes contract the disease, and nonfatal human infections are known. The virus causes fatal encephalomyelitis in red grouse *(Lagopus scoticus)*. Outbreaks in piglets have followed the feeding of raw meat from lambs, and a case has been described in a dog.

The tick responsible for transmission in Great Britain is *Ixodes ricinus*, the castor-bean tick. Other species of *Ixodes*, and perhaps other arthropods, are potential vectors. *I. ricinus* is parasitic on a variety of mammals in addition to sheep and on birds; however, the most significant wildlife host is the red grouse. Larval and nymphal ticks acquire the virus when feeding on infected sheep, and transmit the infection to new hosts in the succeeding nymphal and adult phases. Because of its natural mode of transmission, louping ill is most prevalent in early summer and early autumn when the ticks are active. After infection, the virus propagates in regional lymph nodes, proceeds to viremia, and then enters the CNS via the hematogenous route. Alternatively, the virus may localize indirectly from the blood in nasal structures and enter the brain via the olfactory nerves. Under experimental conditions, a number of factors may facilitate entry of virus into the brain, and facilitation is apparently given in natural cases by concurrent tick-borne fever, a rickettsiosis also transmitted by *I. ricinus*, and known to impair humoral and cellular defense mechanisms.

Although tick transmission is the usual mode of infection, the disease can be contracted in humans, monkeys, and mice by inhalation of infective droplets, but this route is not thought to be important naturally. Rabbits and guinea pigs are not susceptible even by intracerebral inoculation.

Louping ill is a systemic infection and, although it remains so, the disease is mildly febrile but otherwise of no consequence. When it invades the CNS and produces signs of encephalitis, the mortality rate is very high. The morbidity in endemic areas is quite low, and the disease is largely confined to either naive lambs or to older lambs and yearlings whose colostral immunity is not reinforced by natural exposure. The viremic phase of louping ill is clinically silent or a febrile phase with dullness. Recovery may occur in a couple of days and leave solid immunity. If neurologic signs are to develop, they do so at about day 5 and are characterized by incoordination, tremors, cerebellar ataxia, and terminal paralysis.

There are no gross lesions. The disease is an *acute polioencephalomyelitis*. There is mild leptomeningitis corresponding to areas of inflammation of the parenchyma. Inflammation of the cerebellar leptomeninges may be quite severe when the cerebellar cortex is acutely affected (see Fig. 4-101). The inflammatory lesions are more obvious than in most viral encephalitides, but are of the usual type, although unusually large numbers of neutrophils may be present in very severe cases, and largely restricted to gray matter, although cuffing and focal gliosis occur in the white matter. Neuronal degeneration may be severe and neuronophagia prominent. Some degree of selective vulnerability of the Purkinje and Golgi cells of the cerebellum is generally accepted and, although it can be demonstrated in many cases, its detection probably depends to a large extent on the duration of active infection. The spinal lesion is poliomyelitis affecting particularly the ventral horns. Inclusion bodies have not been observed in sheep, but acidophilic, intracytoplasmic inclusions in neurons of the brainstem and cord are reported in experimentally affected monkeys and mice. IHC is available, and viral antigen can be identified easily, especially in the Purkinje cells of the cerebellum and their dendritic processes.

Encephalitis caused by tick-borne encephalitis virus. *Tick-borne encephalitis virus* (TBEV) is a serious human threat that causes thousands of cases of encephalitis every year in endemic areas in Europe and Asia. Several wild and domestic animals are susceptible to infection, but the infection is frequently subclinical; however, TBEV is pathogenic for dogs and horses and is able to cause fatal meningoencephalitis. The virus is transmitted to humans and animals mainly by *I. ricinus* or *Ixodes persulcatus*. Humans can also become infected through consumption of milk from infected ruminants. Most infected dogs seroconvert without developing TBE, but the peracute disease in dogs has a high fatality rate. Affected dogs are usually euthanized because of associated severe convulsions, tremors, and ataxia. The histologic lesions are those of severe necrotizing lymphoplasmacytic and histiocytic meningoencephalomyelitis with severe glial nodule formation affecting mostly the basal ganglia, thalamus, mesencephalon, neuroparenchyma surrounding the fourth ventricle, and the medulla oblongata. The disease in horses is seldom fatal and causes clinical signs that range from mild ataxia to sudden cramps, epileptic attacks, and paralysis of neck and shoulder muscles.

Further reading

Hubálek Z, et al. Arboviruses pathogenic for domestic and wild animals. Adv Virus Res 2014;89:201-275.

Klaus C, et al. Tick-borne encephalitis virus (TBEV)—findings on cross reactivity and longevity of TBEV antibodies in animal sera. BMC Vet Res 2014;10:78.

Lasala PR, Holbrook M. Tick-borne flaviviruses. Clin Lab Med 2010;30: 221-235.

Diseases caused by mosquito-borne flaviviruses. The important veterinary viruses in genus *Flavivirus*, family *Flaviviridae*, in the mosquito-borne Japanese encephalitis virus group, include species *West Nile virus* (WNV) and *Japanese encephalitis virus*. Also included are *Murray Valley encephalitis (MVE) virus, Kunjin encephalitis virus (KEV)*, and *St. Louis encephalitis virus*. MVE and KEV are indigenous to Australia and Oceania. KEV is a strain of WNV and can cause a disease that is clinically and pathologically identical to WNV. MVE is a rare but potentially fatal disease that occurs particularly in horses, with lesions ranging from mild lymphohistiocytic leptomeningitis to severe nonsuppurative polioencephalomyelitis.

West Nile virus encephalomyelitis. *West Nile virus* (WNV) was first discovered in 1937 in the West Nile district of Uganda. In 1999 it was introduced into New York City, where it caused a massive outbreak in animals and humans. During the period 1999-2004, the virus spread rapidly to most of the United States and southern parts of Canada. It has been suggested that the virus was imported from the Middle East, given the genetic similarity between strains isolated in the

Middle East and New York. The virus is now distributed throughout the world, and fulminant disease is reported in humans, horses, and birds from all continents. The virus is divided genetically into 2 lineages: lineage 1 WNV is present in North America and some other parts of the world; lineage 2 is restricted to enzootic areas in Africa. Lineage 2 WNV strains are either nonpathogenic or occasionally cause mild human and equine disease. Some clades in lineage 1 (e.g., clade 1a) are highly virulent and are believed to be responsible for the recent outbreaks in North America. The virus has a wide host range, but is maintained in the environment mainly by a bird-mosquito-bird cycle. Wild birds, especially corvids, that is, crows, are the main amplifying hosts. Wild birds usually develop prolonged viremia, and the virus is distributed in almost every organ. In contrast, the viral antigen in infected horses, which is by far the most susceptible species of domestic animal, is sparse and limited to the CNS. Infection between birds or between birds and mammals or reptiles is mainly via mosquitoes. Mosquitoes of the *Culex* spp. are the main maintenance vectors. The virus is also found in other vectors, such as ticks, but the biological importance of these vectors is yet to be determined. Rare methods of virus transmission include direct contact with infected materials and ingestion. Transplacental WNV transmission is only reported in human.

The *pathogenesis* of the encephalitis induced by WNV is not completely understood; however, after the virus is injected by an infected mosquito, it propagates in keratinocytes, cutaneous dendritic cells, regional endothelial cells, and fibroblasts; viremia develops; and the virus reaches the brain hematogenously. CNS entry through peripheral neurons (retrograde axonal transport) could contribute to WNV neuroinvasion.

Equids, especially horses, are very susceptible to the infection. In naive areas, the first signs of WNV are the marked increase in cases of equine encephalitis and increased numbers of wild bird mortalities, especially in corvids. WN fever is a seasonal disease, related to the time of the year of mosquito activity, that is, summer and fall. When naive horses are infected by the virus, mortality can reach up to 50% of affected horses, and clinical signs range from weakness and anorexia to severe acute ataxia or recumbency. However, the mortality rate decreases dramatically in the following seasons. Gross lesions are usually absent, but a few cases may have acute areas of hemorrhage or malacia affecting the thoracic and/or lumbar spinal cord. *Histologic lesions* are present mainly in the brainstem and thoracolumbar spinal cord, and to a lesser extent in cerebral cortex and cervical cord. The cerebellum is usually spared. *Lesions are those of nonsuppurative encephalomyelitis, gliosis, and glial nodule formation with occasional neuronal degeneration and necrosis* (Fig. 4-107A, B). Lesions are more pronounced in the gray matter. The glial nodules usually contain a few neutrophils amid the glial cells. Areas of hemorrhage and malacia are present in severe cases, especially in brainstem and the ventral horn of the thoracic and lumbar spinal cord. Axonal swelling and spheroid formation is frequent. The severity of lesions is greatly variable between outbreaks, and frequently the severity of clinical signs is not correlated with the severity of lesions. In most cases, the lesions are mild and confined to thin cuffs of a few blood vessels in the brainstem. Extraneural lesions, for example, hepatitis and myocarditis, which occur in avian WNV infection, do not occur in equine WNV infection.

The information about clinical signs and lesions in nonequine domestic species other than birds is very limited.

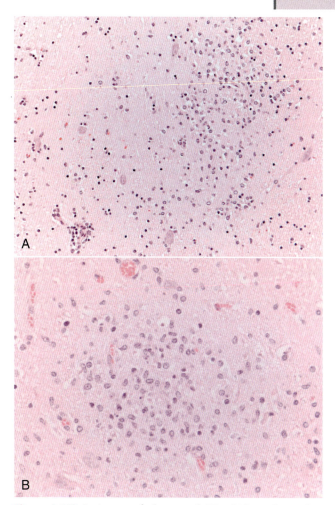

Figure 4-107 Brainstem of a horse with **West Nile viral encephalomyelitis. A.** Perivascular cuffs composed of lymphocytes and plasma cells are usually thin. **B.** Glial nodules are common and usually contain only a few neutrophils. (Courtesy M.J. Hazlett.)

Ruminants, canids, felids, and swine are far less susceptible to the disease than are horses or birds. These species are susceptible to the infection and develop very short viremia with subclinical disease; histologic lesions are very similar to those described in horses.

Diagnosis of WNV infection can be achieved by detection of WNV antigen in the brain by using PCR or IHC. WNV antigen in many cases can be very sparse, which makes the interpretation of IHC difficult. Positive IHC staining in most cases is limited to sparse axonal immunostaining.

Further reading

Angenvoort J, et al. West Nile viral infection of equids. Vet Microbiol 2013;167:168-180.

Mann BR, et al. Molecular epidemiology and evolution of West Nile virus in North America. Int J Environ Res Public Health 2013;10:5111-5129.

Samuel MA, et al. Axonal transport mediates West Nile virus entry into the central nervous system and induces acute flaccid paralysis. Proc Natl Acad Sci U S A 2007;104:17140-17145.

Terry RL, et al. Inflammatory monocytes and the pathogenesis of viral encephalitis. J Neuroinflammation 2012;9:270.

Japanese encephalitis. *Japanese encephalitis virus* (JEV) is found through much of eastern, southern, and southeastern Asia, Papua New Guinea, and the Torres Strait of Northern Australia, where the agent causes endemic disease with dramatic annual epidemics. In humans, there is a high ratio of subclinical to overt infections, with a case fatality rate of 10-15% and a high incidence of residual neurologic deficits in survivors. Transplacental infection followed by abortion occurs in humans, and this is also the most serious expression of the disease in *pigs, the domestic species most importantly infected.*

The virus is maintained through mosquito-bird or mosquito-pig cycles. The virus is transmitted mainly by the mosquito, *Culex tritaeniorhynchus*, but other species of this genus and of the genera *Aedes* and *Armigeres* may be important as the virus is known to be vertically transmitted through some of them. *Ardeid water birds (e.g., herons and egrets) are the main maintenance reservoirs.* Many species of animals and birds are susceptible to mosquito-borne infection and develop antibody responses in timing with suitable climatic and habitat cycles. The pig is a very important domestic animal in many of the endemic areas, and it is the most important amplifier host for the virus, developing sustained viremia of sufficient titer to infect feeding mosquitoes and indeed is probably the preferred host for *C. tritaeniohynchus*. Infection of humans and horses is incidental and both species are considered to be dead-end hosts.

Most horses, pigs, and cattle in endemic areas possess neutralizing antibodies against the virus. Intranasal and intracerebral inoculation can produce fatal encephalitis in calves, but natural cases of encephalitis in this species are quite rare. Among animals infected naturally with the virus, *only horses and donkeys develop clinical encephalitis.* There are no clinical signs of encephalitis in pigs, but pregnant susceptible sows may produce *stillborn piglets.* Infected stillborn and neonatal pigs may show hydrocephalus, cerebellar hypoplasia, and hypomyelinogenesis and anasarca; histologic changes are restricted to the nervous system and may include *nonsuppurative encephalitis.* The lesions in these neonatal and stillborn piglets probably reflect the timing of infection in relation to the development of immune competence. Diffuse nonsuppurative encephalitis occurs in the brain and cord of piglets up to 6 months of age, but in the cerebellum, it affects rather selectively the molecular and Purkinje layers. The histologic pattern of Japanese encephalitis in pigs appears similar to that of Teschen and related diseases. In boars, the virus induces orchitis.

Severe epidemics of encephalitis have occurred in horses in Japan. The incubation period in horses ranges from 4-14 days, and case fatality is 5-15%. Lesions are confined to the CNS, are more prevalent in the cerebral hemispheres, and include extensive perivascular lymphoplasmacytic cuffing, gliosis, and areas of malacia with hemorrhage. The lesions in quality and distribution are the same as those produced by the eastern and western equine encephalitis viruses. Inclusion bodies are not reported in the Japanese disease. *Diagnosis is best achieved by detection of viral RNA by using PCR.*

Further reading

Katayama T, et al. Nonsuppurative encephalomyelitis in a calf in Japan and isolation of Japanese encephalitis virus genotype 1 from the affected calf. J Clin Microbiol 2013;51:3448-3453.

Alphaviruses—equine encephalitides

Several members of the genus *Alphavirus*, family *Togaviridae*, cause either overt or subclinical encephalitis in horses or other animals. They all require an arthropod vector (frequently mosquitoes) for transmission.

Eastern, Western, and Venezuelan encephalitis in horses. Species **Western equine encephalitis virus** (WEEV), **Eastern equine encephalitis virus** (EEEV), and **Venezuelan equine encephalitis virus** (VEEV) are all in the genus *Alphavirus*, family *Togaviridae*. Horses were originally regarded as the primary hosts of the EEVs, but horses are actually accidental and unfortunate hosts; birds for the American viruses (eastern and western type) or rodents for the Venezuelan virus are the most common vertebrate reservoir hosts, and mosquitoes are the principal vectors. Horses and humans, in both of which species the disease is of very considerable importance, are now known to be, in terms of transmission and often literally as well, dead-end hosts in which the titer of virus in blood is ordinarily too low to be a source of infection for mosquitoes.

Not all birds are capable of acting as reservoir hosts. Red-winged blackbirds, cardinals, sparrows, cedar waxwings, and the captive Chinese pheasant are highly susceptible to infection and nearly always die. Many other species, including adult domestic fowl and turkeys, are not sickened by the infection, although fatalities can be produced in the young of these species.

EEEV is endemic along the North American Atlantic course, in the Caribbean, Central America, and along the northeastern coast of South America. The virus cycles between water birds and the mosquito, *Culiseta melanura*, which feeds on birds and does not feed on large mammals. Horses are likely to get infected by other mosquitoes, *Aedes sollicitans* and *A. vexans*, which feed on both horses and birds.

WEEV is present mostly in the valleys of western North American states, where the cycle is between wild birds, especially passerines, and the mosquito, *Culex tarsalis*. This mosquito feeds readily on animals, and human and animal cases occur regularly.

VEEV has 2 major different strain groups, the enzootic strains that are avirulent and cycle between *Culex* spp. mosquito and small rodents in the Caribbean areas, and the epizootic strains that are virulent to human and horse, found mainly in Venezuela, Colombia, and Peru, and circulate between several mosquito species and horses, which produce high-titered viremia sufficient to infect the vector mosquitoes. Outbreaks of EEE and WEE occur in seasonal patterns related to the time of the year when mosquitoes are active. VEE outbreaks usually occur in a cyclical pattern approximately every 10 years.

Once infected, mosquitoes are known to remain so for life, and there is evidence that the virus is capable of multiplying in the insects. Arthropods other than mosquitoes may also be of some, but lesser, importance. The virus has been found in chicken mites (*Dermanyssus gallinae*), chicken lice (*Menopon pallidum, Eomenocanthus stramineus*), and assassin bugs (*Triatoma sanguisuga*). The spotted-fever tick, *Dermacentor andersoni*, is capable of transmitting the infection stage to stage and hereditarily. Transmission by aerosolization is reported only in humans; laboratory workers are at high risk of infection by aerosols.

Although humans and horses are the principal mammalian victims, other species are susceptible. Pigs readily develop asymptomatic infections, but a few outbreaks have been reported in this species with histology typical of EEE. Pigs are not of significance for natural propagation of the virus because they do not develop significant viremia. Calves are susceptible to intracerebral inoculation but recover in 2 weeks. Guinea pigs and white mice are highly susceptible, rabbits are less so, and sheep, dogs, and cats are refractory.

The 3 viruses are similar in their pathogenesis. After the mosquito bite, the virus replicates in the regional blood vessels and lymph nodes, viremia develops, followed by secondary replication in lymph nodes and muscles. A second viremia then develops and is followed by brain invasion via the blood. In the CNS, the virus replicates in neurons, glial cells, and blood vessels. The virus causes neuronal necrosis, likely via stimulation of apoptosis.

Young horses are more susceptible than the old. Initially, there is viremia with fever and depression, usually unnoticed. The animal may then recover, or the virus may invade the CNS, by which time the fever has subsided. The neurologic signs are characterized by derangements of consciousness and terminal paralysis. There may be early restlessness with compulsive walking, often in circles. There is central blindness. The animal becomes somnolent and assumes unnatural postures. At this stage, the course may remain static, and the animal lives as a "dummy," or paralysis may develop, often first affecting cranial nerves but later general and flaccid. *The signs are largely cortical, and the cortex is the principal site of the lesions.* The course, if fatal, is usually 2-4 days.

There are no gross changes. The microscopic changes are limited almost exclusively to *gray matter* (see Fig. 4-2D). When the course is short, 1 day or less, the reaction is largely on the part of neutrophils. These infiltrate the gray matter diffusely and may be found in foci suggestive of malacia. There is early microglial reaction to produce rod cells. Endothelial cells, especially of veins are swollen, and hyaline or granular thrombi are common in these vessels. Necrotizing vasculitis with thrombosis and cerebrocortical malacia can be present in severe cases. There are narrow cuffs of lymphocytes and neutrophils (Fig. 4-108), with perivenous hemorrhage and edema. After a couple of days, the neutrophils disappear, the cuffs are composed of lymphocytes, and there are both focal and diffuse microglial proliferations as in the standard nonsuppurative reactions. Neuronal degeneration and neuronophagia are common findings. Intranuclear inclusions similar to those in Borna disease may be present, but may be very difficult to identify.

The most severe lesions are in the cerebral cortex, especially the frontal, rhinencephalic, and occipital areas, with lesions of lesser intensity in the pyriform lobes. Severe lesions are also present in thalamus and hypothalamus. From the thalamus caudally, the intensity of inflammation diminishes but reveals no selectivity for particular nuclear masses. The cerebellum is less severely injured than other portions, although inflammatory changes may be found in the deep nuclei and spottily in the cortex. Mild changes occur in both dorsal and ventral horns of the cord, but their distribution is irregular. The trigeminal ganglia are not affected. The encephalomyelitis in the Venezuelan type may be purely nonsuppurative. Extraneural lesions are common in humans and birds but are rare in susceptible domestic mammals. Small intestinal lesions in a horse with EEE include multifocal myonecrosis and lymphomonocytic infiltration in the muscular layer and focal mild perivascular lymphocytic infiltration in the submucosa. Myocarditis is not uncommon in pigs suffering from EEE. Horses infected with VEEV can occasionally have some nonspecific extraneural lesions, such as myeloid depletion in bone marrow and lympholysis in spleen and lymph nodes.

Other **Alphavirus** encephalitides. **Highlands J virus** of America's east coast, **Getah virus** of southeast Asia, and **Semliki Forest virus** of the Americas are all equine pathogens that are able to induce at least a febrile disease. All of these viruses are maintained in the environment by a mosquito-bird-mosquito cycle. Several mammals and birds seroconvert to these viruses; however, overt disease is rare. Highlands J virus was reported as the cause of encephalitis in 2 horses. Getah virus does not induce encephalitis, but clinical signs and lesions have some similarities to equine viral arteritis.

Further reading

Greenlee JE. The equine encephalitides. Handb Clin Neurol 2014;123:417-432.

Mackenzie JS, et al. Emerging flaviviruses: the spread and resurgence of Japanese encephalitis, West Nile and dengue viruses. Nat Med 2004;10(Suppl. 12):S98-S109.

Steele KE, Twenhafel NA. Review paper: pathology of animal models of alphavirus encephalitis. Vet Pathol 2010;47:790-805.

Zacks MA1, Paessler S. Encephalitic alphaviruses. Vet Microbiol 2010;140:281-286.

Borna disease

Borna disease, named after the village of Borna in Germany, is caused by species **Borna disease virus** (BDV), genus *Bornavirus*, family *Bornaviridae*. The virus exists worldwide in many vertebrates but most commonly infects horses, sheep, cattle, cats, dogs, and ostriches. The traditional endemic area is central Europe, but antibodies to the virus are found in horses outside Europe, including the United States and Japan. The mortality rate may be high (>80% in horses, 5-40% in sheep); surviving horses may be asymptomatic carriers, or may suffer relapses of disease. The virus has a controversial link to several human neuropsychiatric illnesses. In experimental hosts (tree shrews, rats), infection with BDV not only produces pathoanatomic changes, that is, nonsuppurative encephalitis, but also behavioral changes and learning deficits.

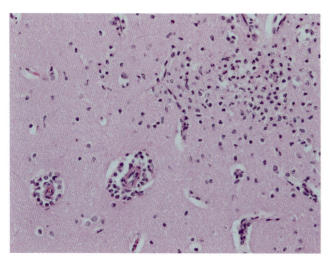

Figure 4-108 Lymphoplasmacytic and neutrophilic necrotizing encephalitis in cerebrum in **equine encephalitis** in a horse.

The virus replicates in the nucleolus of the host cell without cytopathic effect, persistently infects cells, and induces brain lesions by *immune-mediated mechanisms*. In Lewis rats, acute (4-8 weeks postinfection) BDV infection is followed by massive infiltrates in the brain of CD4+ Th1, CD8+ T, and natural killer (NK) cells with a predominance of Th1 cytokines that favors cell-mediated immunity. In the chronic stage (beyond 15 weeks of infection), the aforementioned cellular infiltrates significantly decrease, and the predominant cytokines are of Th2 type, favoring the shift to a humoral immune response; the resultant antibodies are not protective and have no significant effect on the disease. Because of this unique feature, infection of neonatal or immunocompromised animals does not lead to disease or to encephalitis.

The epidemiology of Borna disease, including reservoir, methods of transmission, and infection, remains obscure. BDV is considered to be a true neurotropic virus, with a particular predilection for neurons of the limbic system. Inflammation of the olfactory bulbs at the early stages of natural infection in humans suggests an intranasal route of infection, followed by transaxonal migration to the olfactory bulb. Vertical transmission in horses and rats with life-long persistent infection is also suggested. The high prevalence of BDV on farms lacking proper rodent control and hygiene suggests a small wild rodent, such as the shrew, to be a possible reservoir.

Clinically, the disease occurs sporadically or in clusters; however, severe outbreaks are described in different species. The incidence of disease in horses and sheep peaks between March and June and in cats between December and March. *Equids and sheep are the most susceptible animals*, but natural disease is reported in many domestic species, including, but not limited to, cattle, alpacas, cats, dogs, and ostriches. Most infections in horses remain subclinical, and BDV-specific antibodies are frequently found in clinically healthy horses. The incubation period is not <4 weeks and introduces a clinical syndrome that is purely neurologic but of varied course, death occurring in 1-3 weeks. The mortality rate in diseased horses is 90-100%. Recurrent episodes at time of stress occur in surviving animals. Clinical signs include pharyngeal paralysis, hyperesthesia, standing in awkward positions, circling, muscular tremors, and spasms; blindness is common. Drowsiness and flaccid paresis develop terminally.

There are no gross lesions. The distribution of lesions in Borna disease differs from that in other equine encephalomyelitides and parallels closely the distribution of viral antigen, as displayed by immunohistochemistry, and the distribution of infectivity, as determined by titration in cell cultures. Virus and lesions are present mostly in the gray matter of olfactory bulbs (early stage), hippocampus (Fig. 4-109), limbic system, basal ganglia, and brainstem. The dorsal cerebrum and the cerebellum are relatively spared. Lesions may be present in optic nerves and retina. Histologic lesions are those of *nonsuppurative encephalomyelitis* with predilection for the aforementioned areas. Perivascular cuffs can be dramatically thick (>7-cell layer), and usually there are neuropilar clusters of lymphocytes and plasma cells. Other lesions include neuronophagia and focal gliosis. The presence of inclusion bodies (Joest-Degen bodies) is fairly pathognomonic; these are mainly in nuclei, especially in the hippocampus, and are very occasionally cytoplasmic. They stain well and red with Giemsa, and have a clear halo. Commercial PCR and immunohistochemistry kits are available for diagnosis.

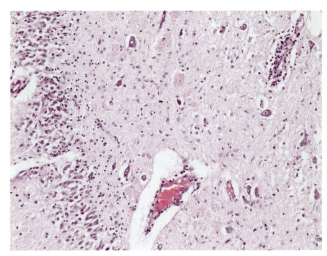

Figure 4-109 Nonsuppurative encephalitis and gliosis in the hippocampus of a horse with **Borna disease.**

Borna disease virus has been proposed as the cause of a chronic, slowly progressive neurologic disease affecting *cats* of all ages, sexes, and breeds. The disease is known clinically as *staggering disease*, and clinical signs include ataxia, paraparesis, and tetraparesis. Behavioral change is not a constant finding. BDV infection markers (BDV-specific antibodies and/or BDV RNA) were found in many cats suffering from staggering disease. Lesions are more prevalent in the gray matter of brainstem and in dorsal and ventral horns of the thoracic and/or cervical spinal cord segments. Lesions include mild to moderate lymphoplasmacytic cuffing with neuronophagia and neuronal degeneration and astrogliosis. Severe Wallerian degeneration is usually present in ventral and lateral columns of the cervical and thoracic spinal cord.

Further reading

Kinnunen PM, et al. Epidemiology and host spectrum of Borna disease virus infections. J Gen Virol 2013;94(Pt 2):247-262.

Okamoto M, et al. Borna disease in a dog in Japan. J Comp Pathol 2002;126:312-317.

Richt JA, et al. Borna disease in horses. Vet Clin North Am Equine Pract 2000;16:579-595.

Wensman JJ, et al. Borna disease virus infection in cats. Vet J 2014;201:142-149.

Lentiviral encephalomyelitis of sheep and goats

The species **Caprine arthritis encephalitis virus** (CAEV) of goats and **Visna-maedi virus** (VISNA) of sheep, in the genus *Lentivirus*, family *Retroviridae*, are small-ruminant lentiviruses (SRLV). CAEV is the causative agent of caprine arthritis-encephalitis of goats and VISNA is the causative agent of the visna-maedi disease complex of sheep; at least some strains of the SRLV are transmissible between sheep and goats. In both natural hosts, *4 clinical and pathologic syndromes are recognized*, namely, **mastitis, arthritis, interstitial pneumonia** (maedi, or ovine progressive pneumonia), and **encephalomyelitis** (visna of sheep). Within endemic situations, any one or combination of the 4 syndromes may be present and, when in combination, 1 syndrome usually predominates.

Once infected, the virus is never eliminated and, while present, it is active even though there may be no clinical sign of neurologic deficit. Typically for this type of virus infection, the virus is highly cell associated and replicates only slowly, infection persists for the life of the animal, the incubation period before seroconversion may be several months and before clinical disease may be months or years, the clinical disease is progressive, and the lesions are dominated by active mononuclear inflammatory cells. The pathogenesis and epidemiology of the various conditions are described in detail in Vol. 2, Respiratory system. Described later are the gross and histologic lesions and clinical signs found in the encephalomyelitis form of these diseases.

The encephalomyelitis form in sheep is called **visna** (Icelandic for wasting). As a natural disease, visna occurs in sheep of both sexes, but clinical signs are seldom, if ever, observed in animals <2 years of age. Disease onset is insidious. The earliest sign may be barely perceptible caudal ataxia and fine trembling of the lips. The first sign to be noticed may be extensor paralysis of the hindlimbs. Once paralytic signs are evident, a fatal outcome appears certain. There is no fever and no sign of cerebral dysfunction, and death results from starvation or secondary infection. The incidence of visna is relatively low. The course of the infection can be followed fairly well by routine examination of the CSF for lymphocytosis.

Normal sheep are expected to have $\leq 0.005 \times 10^9$ cells/L ($\leq 5/mm^3$) of CSF; in visna, cell numbers, chiefly lymphocytes, can be markedly elevated. After intracerebral inoculation, there is a latent period of up to 8 weeks, after which the CSF cell count begins to increase. The cell count may remain high for several months without other signs of disease. Thereafter the animal may recover, as indicated by a drop in the CSF cell count, or the cell count may remain high, paralysis develops, and death follows.

The disease in the brain is chronic and demyelinating. There are no gross neural changes in this disease, and the histologic change is one of *patchy demyelinating encephalomyelitis*. The distribution of lesions, involving principally the white matter, is unlike the distribution produced by other neurotropic viruses. There is a mild to severe mononuclear type of cerebrospinal meningitis. The parenchymal lesion may be well established by 1-2 months, and these early lesions are intensely inflammatory, with perivascular cuffing and gliosis. They reveal clearly that the process begins in, and immediately beneath, the ependyma diffusely throughout the cerebrospinal axis. In this early stage, the myelinated fibers in the inflammatory foci remain remarkably intact; the gray matter of the cord is irregularly but often intensely affected by a nonsuppurative reaction even 2-3 months after inoculation. In the paralytic and terminal stages of the disease, the periventricular destruction of white matter in the cerebrum and cerebellum is extensive, and in some sections of the brain, especially in the cerebellum, almost every bit of white matter is destroyed, leaving the gray matter free.

Destruction of myelinated fibers in the spinal cord is patchy and not caused by progressive spread of the pericentral inflammation. The demyelinated plaques are characteristically peripheral and triangular in shape, with a base on the pia mater. Although dorsal and lateral tracts are most frequently involved, there is no selectivity for particular fiber tracts and no symmetry. The degenerating foci are almost malacic in their severity, and the plaques contain numerous reactive microglia and astroglia. Spinal nerve roots share in the degenerative process. Germinal centers may form in the choroid plexus. In areas of intense inflammation, liquefactive foci of necrosis occur in the white matter, and the loss of myelin is expected to be of Wallerian type. In the spinal cord, evidence of remyelination can be found, indicating that oligodendrocytes are not target cells and that demyelination may be primary.

Caprine arthritis-encephalitis (CAE) appears to be widely distributed, but the expression of the infection is highly variable, and many infected goats show little or no clinical disease. Clinical disease of the nervous system affects kids 2-4 months of age and is frequently fatal. Animals that develop the early nervous disease or have early inapparent infections tend to develop synovitis and periarthritis in adulthood (see Vol. 1, Bones and joints).

The clinical signs of CAE are referable to motor spinal dysfunction without signs of cerebral disease. Onset is indicated by hindlimb lameness and ataxia with paresis that progresses over several weeks to paralysis. The inflammatory lesions in the CNS may remain active for several years in goats that survive (Fig. 4-110A, B). In the early clinical phase of the disease, changes are widely distributed in the white matter of the brain and cord, particularly in the subependyma and beneath the pia in the cord. The distribution and character of the lesions in the nervous tissue in the goat are, in general, similar to those in visna of sheep. There is, however, less tendency for the periventricular lesions to progress to gross cavitation of cerebral white matter. Instead, there is a tendency for the inflammatory and myelinoclastic areas to increase in number and severity caudally from the mesencephalon. As in

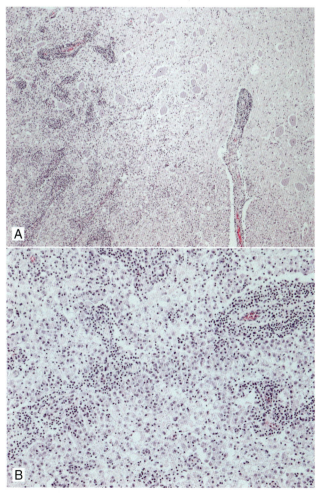

Figure 4-110 Caprine arthritis-encephalitis. **A.** Leukomyelitis. **B.** Detail of perivascular reaction.

visna, the spinal cord changes are discontinuous and, where present, involve the myelin in subpial plaques or in one or more quadrants of the cord. The extent of perivascular infiltration by mononuclear cells (see Fig. 4-110B) is also greater in kids than in sheep. In addition to the encephalomyelitis, mastitis, and arthritis seen in CAE, interstitial pneumonia occurs in some natural and experimental cases (see Vol. 2, Respiratory system).

The clinical *diagnosis* of the 4 lentiviral syndromes in sheep and goats is usually confirmed antemortem by ELISA, and at autopsy by IHC and/or PCR testing.

Further reading

Larruskain A, Jugo BM. Retroviral infections in sheep and goats: small ruminant lentiviruses and host interaction. Viruses 2013;5:2043-2061.

Minardi da Cruz JC, et al. Small ruminant lentiviruses (SRLVs) break the species barrier to acquire new host range. Viruses 2013;5:1867-1884.

Murphy B, et al. Tissue tropism and promoter sequence variation in caprine arthritis encephalitis virus infected goats. Virus Res 2010;151:177-184.

Shah C, et al. Direct evidence for natural transmission of small-ruminant lentiviruses of subtype A4 from goats to sheep and vice versa. J Virol 2004;78:7518-7522.

Paramyxoviral encephalomyelitis of pigs

Porcine rubulavirus encephalomyelitis (blue eye disease). Blue eye disease is caused by **Porcine rubulavirus** (La Piedad–Michoacan-Mexico virus), genus *Rubulavirus*, family *Paramyxoviridae*. The disease is characterized by encephalomyelitis, interstitial pneumonia, reproductive failure, and corneal opacity. The virus is endemic in the central and west-central regions of Mexico, and outbreaks have been recorded in Mexico since 1980. In pregnant sows, the infection may be subclinical or responsible for *fetal death, mummification, and stillbirths*, and for the occasional appearance of corneal opacity in the sow. Piglets up to 2 weeks of age are most susceptible, with up to 50% morbidity and very high mortality. The clinical signs are of encephalomyelitis leading to death within 2-4 days, although subclinical infections are also frequent and may be manifested only by corneal opacity.

The lesion is a typical *nonsuppurative encephalomyelitis* affecting mainly gray matter of the thalamus, midbrain, and cortex. Inclusion bodies have not been demonstrated. Anterior uveitis is mild, the inflammatory cells congregating in the iridocorneal angle and the corneoscleral junction. The corneal opacity is the result of edema, which will resolve if the animal survives.

In mature male pigs, experimental exposure will result in epididymitis in almost all exposed and in a lesser number with orchitis and testicular atrophy. Interstitial pneumonia is part of the description.

Further reading

Mendoza-Magaña ML, et al. Blue eye disease porcine rubulavirus (PoRv) infects pig neurons and glial cells using sialo-glycoprotein as receptor. Vet J 2007;173:428-436.

Rivera-Benitez JF, et al. Respiratory disease in growing pigs after Porcine rubulavirus experimental infection. Virus Res 2013;176:137-143.

Nipah virus encephalitis. Nipah encephalitis, an emerging disease characterized by severe and rapidly progressive encephalitis, is caused by species **Nipah virus** (NiV), genus *Henipavirus*, a novel genus in the family *Paramyxoviridae*. This genus also contains Hendra virus. Both are newly emerging viruses that can cause fatal encephalitis and pneumonia in humans and several animal species. The first severe outbreak of NiV encephalitis in humans occurred in 1998 near Ipoh, Malaysia, primarily among pig farmers and their families; the outbreak was preceded by an outbreak of encephalitis and pneumonia affecting pigs on many local farms. The *fruit bat (flying fox)* of the *Pteropus* species was later confirmed to be the natural reservoir host of NiV. Bats shed virus in their urine and saliva, which contaminates fruit that falls into pig pens and is eaten by pigs; bats in these trees also urinate directly on pigs. Initial human infection occurred in pig farmers by direct contact or aerosolization from infected pens. Pig-to-pig or pig-to-domestic-animal infections occur by direct contact with infected pig or mechanically by contact with contaminated utensils or feed. Direct transmission from bats-to-human or from human-to-human is controversial.

Pigs are the animals most susceptible to infection, but natural infection is reported in horses, cats, goats, and dogs; these species were infected by direct contact with infected pigs. Morbidity rates in pigs are ~10%, with case mortality rates of <15%. The incubation period is estimated to be 1-2 weeks. The virus targets 2 systems, the CNS and the respiratory system. The virus overcomes the blood-brain barrier through infection of brain endothelial cells. Clinical signs are those of acute dyspnea (labored and harsh respiration, open-mouth breathing, severe cough) and acute nervous signs (trembling, seizures, or tetanus-like spasms). Abortion may occur to pregnant sows.

The lung is diffusely edematous with patchy acute hemorrhage. Meningeal blood vessels are severely congested. The histologic hallmark is *necrotizing vasculitis affecting arterioles, venules, and capillaries*, with the presence of binucleated or multinucleated syncytial cells attached to the endothelium of affected blood vessels. Blood vessels undergo fibrinoid degeneration and leukocytoclastic vasculitis. Affected blood vessels are present most commonly in lung, brain, renal glomeruli, and lymphoid organs. Other pulmonary lesions include moderate lymphoplasmacytic bronchointerstitial pneumonia with mild necrotizing bronchiolitis and mild to moderate filling of alveoli with neutrophils, even in the absence of significant secondary bacterial infection. Severe lymphocytic and neutrophilic meningitis with mild lymphoplasmacytic encephalitis and occasional gliosis are consistent findings. Because of vasculitis, large areas of hemorrhage and infarction are common in affected organs. Occasionally, *eosinophilic intracytoplasmic and intranuclear inclusions* are present in neurons and syncytial endothelial cells. Syncytial cells can also be found attached within lymphatic vessels and to pulmonary alveolar septa.

The laboratory *diagnosis* of NiV infection is made through serology, histopathology, immunohistochemistry, electron microscopy, PCR, and/or virus isolation.

Further reading

Erbar S, Maisner A. Nipah virus infection and glycoprotein targeting in endothelial cells. Virol J 2010;7:305.

Hooper P, et al. Comparative pathology of the diseases caused by Hendra and Nipah viruses. Microbes Infect 2001;3:315-322.

Mackenzie JS, Field HE. Emerging encephalitogenic viruses: lyssaviruses and henipaviruses transmitted by frugivorous bats. Arch Virol Suppl 2004;18:97-111.

Other porcine paramyxoviral encephalitides. An outbreak of respiratory disease (necrotizing bronchointerstitial pneumonia) and encephalitis was recorded in a large pig farm, affecting all ages. The etiologic agent was a previously unknown, as yet unclassified, paramyxovirus different than the other known porcine paramyxoviruses. CNS signs were characterized by recurring episodes of distress, head pressing, tremors, and hindlimb ataxia. No gross lesions were observed in brain. CNS lesions were lymphocytic perivasculitis and diffuse gliosis.

Further reading

Janke BH, et al. Paramyxovirus infection in pigs with interstitial pneumonia and encephalitis in the United States. J Vet Diagn Invest 2001;13:428-433.

Akabane viral encephalitis

Akabane disease is caused by species *Akabane virus* (AKAV) of the Simbu virus group, genus *Bunyavirus*, family *Bunyaviridae*. Iriki virus, a strain of AKAV, causes similar disease. The group also contains **Aino virus,** which causes congenital disease identical to that caused by AKAV. As mentioned earlier in this chapter, AKAV is a common cause of congenital CNS defects in infected bovine fetuses; however, the virus has also been associated with nonsuppurative meningoencephalomyelitis in adult cows and young calves. Histologic lesions are more prominent in brainstem, pons, medulla oblongata, and the spinal cord ventral horn. Lesions are those of lymphohistiocytic cuffing with multifocal gliosis, neuronal necrosis, and occasional neuronophagia with microglial cells.

Further reading

Oem JK, et al. Bovine epizootic encephalomyelitis caused by Akabane virus infection in Korea. J Comp Pathol 2012;147:101-105.

Bovine herpesviral encephalitis

Bovine necrotizing meningoencephalitis caused by *Bovine herpesvirus 5*. Species ***Bovine herpesvirus 5*** (BoHV-5), the cause of bovine necrotizing meningoencephalitis, is antigenically related to *Bovine herpesvirus 1* (BoHV-1), the cause of infectious bovine rhinotracheitis. Both viruses are neurotropic, undergo latency in the trigeminal ganglia, and can be reactivated by natural or experimental stress; however, BoHV-1 rarely causes encephalitis. Both of these herpesviruses are in family *Herpesviridae*, subfamily *Alphaherpesvirinae*, genus *Varicellovirus*. Outbreaks of severe BoHV-5 necrotizing meningoencephalitis have occurred most frequently in South America, but the disease has been observed in other countries, including the United States. Infection is by direct contact, aerosolization, or by indirect contact through contaminated food and water, or by semen. Following intranasal inoculation, BoHV-5 reaches and invades the brain through the olfactory pathway. BoHV-5 envelope glycoproteins E (gE), gI, and Us9 convey viral neurovirulence and neuroinvasiveness by affecting anterograde viral spread via the olfactory pathway.

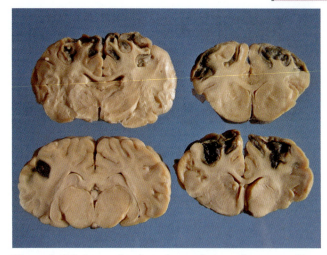

Figure 4-111 Areas of malacia, hemorrhage, and necrosis affecting the gray matter of the rostral cerebrum, mostly in a bilaterally symmetrical pattern in **bovine necrotizing meningoencephalitis** caused by bovine herpesvirus 5. (Courtesy D. Driemeier.)

BoHV-5 encephalitis occurs as a sporadic disease or sometimes as outbreaks in calves and yearlings. The morbidity in herds may be as high as 50%, but is usually much lower; few recognizably sick animals survive. The incubation period is 1-2 weeks, followed by anorexia, apathy, circling, jaw chomping, and finally paddling and recumbency. These clinical signs may be associated with mild to severe rhinitis. BoHV-5 antibodies have been found in sheep and goats; however, natural disease has not been reported in these species.

Gross lesions are usually absent; however, in the severe form of the disease, bilaterally symmetrical areas of malacia, hemorrhage, and necrosis are described in the gray matter of the rostral cerebrum (Fig. 4-111). The hallmark histologic lesion is *severe cytonecrotizing nonsuppurative meningoencephalitis with marked gliosis* (Fig. 4-112A, B). Lesions are more commonly present in the gray matter of the rostral cerebrum, including olfactory bulb, and to a lesser extent in the cerebellum and diencephalon. Perivascular cuffs can be markedly thick (more than 6 layers of lymphocytes, plasma cells, and fewer histiocytes). Necrotic neurons are usually swollen, have lost their angularity, are basophilic, and have pyknotic nuclei. Typical *intranuclear alphaherpesviral inclusions* are occasionally present in degenerate neurons and astrocytes (Fig. 4-112C). Trigeminal ganglioneuritis, neuronophagia, and satellitosis are commonly present. Necrotic or malacic areas can take the laminar cortical necrosis pattern of bovine polioencephalomalacia; however, the latter syndrome is not associated with the severe perivascular cuffing present in BoHV-5 encephalitis. Vasculitis affecting the cerebral microvasculature is only described in rabbits experimentally infected with the virus. The histologic lesions are fairly pathognomonic; however, confirmation of the diagnosis by PCR is recommended.

Further reading

Al-Mubarak A, Chowdhury SI. In the absence of glycoprotein I (gI), gE determines bovine herpesvirus type 5 neuroinvasiveness and neurovirulence. J Neurovirol 2004;10:233-243.

Del Médico Zajac MP, et al. Biology of bovine herpesvirus 5. Vet J 2010;184:138-145.

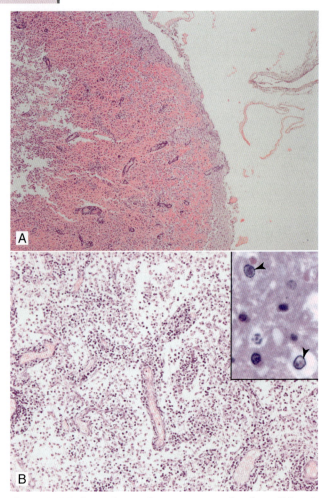

Figure 4-112 Severe hemorrhagic necrosis and malacia (**A**) with perivascular lymphocytic and plasmacytic cuffing (**B**) affecting the external cortical layers of the rostral cerebrum in **bovine necrotizing meningoencephalitis** caused by bovine herpesvirus 5. Intra-astrocytic intranuclear herpesviral inclusions (inset in **B**, arrowheads). (Courtesy D. Driemeier.)

Elias F, et al. Herpesvirus type-5 meningoencephalitis and malacia: histological lesions distribution in the central nervous system of naturally infected cattle. Pesq Vet Bras 2004;24:123-131.

Bovine meningoencephalomyelitis caused by *Bovine herpesvirus 1*. Nonsuppurative encephalomyelitis caused by species ***Bovine herpesvirus 1*** (BoHV-1, infectious bovine rhinotracheitis virus) is reported worldwide. BoHV-1 causes multiple and diverse conditions in cattle, such as abortion, infectious bovine rhinotracheitis, infectious bovine vulvovaginitis, and balanoposthitis. Some BoHV-1 serotypes are neurovirulent and are able to induce encephalitis. Marked upper respiratory disease typically precedes or occurs concurrently with the encephalitis. The pathogenesis and clinical signs are similar to those described for BoHV-5. Histologic lesions are those of *nonsuppurative encephalomyelitis with occasional intranuclear herpetic inclusions*. The massive neuronal necrosis and gliosis described in BoHV-5 are not usually seen in association with BoHV-1. BoHV-1 encephalitis is more prevalent in calves; however, sporadic cases can affect adult cattle, particularly in the Near and Middle East.

Further reading

Penny CD, et al. Upper respiratory disease and encephalitis in neonatal beef calves caused by bovine herpesvirus type 1. Vet Rec 2002;151:89-91.

Rissi DR, et al. Necrotizing meningoencephalitis in a cow. Vet Pathol 2013;50:926-929.

Malignant catarrhal fever. Malignant catarrhal fever (MCF) is a fatal multisystemic lymphoproliferative and inflammatory disease affecting many ruminant species. The details of MCF, including the lesions associated with its encephalomyelitic form, are described in Vol. 2, Alimentary system and peritoneum.

Nonsuppurative meningoencephalitis is reported in "malignant catarrhal fever" in *swine* in Europe, resulting from infection with ovine herpesvirus 2. *Caprine herpesvirus 2*, a gammaherpesvirus, does not cause overt disease in goats, but causes fatal goat-associated MCF in certain species of deer.

Further reading

Callan RJ, Van Metre DC. Viral diseases of the ruminant nervous system. Vet Clin North Am Food Anim Pract 2004;20:327-362.

Bovine paramyxoviral meningoencephalomyelitis

Sporadic cases of nonsuppurative meningoencephalomyelitis caused by paramyxovirus are rarely reported. The causative virus is restricted to the European continent and is not classified within the *Paramyxoviridae* but is distinct from the other bovine paramyxoviruses, such as *Bovine parainfluenza virus 3*. The disease should be differentiated from the sporadic bovine encephalitis caused by *Chlamydophila* spp.

Further reading

Theil D, et al. Neuropathological and aetiological studies of sporadic nonsuppurative meningoencephalomyelitis of cattle. Vet Rec 1998;143:244-249.

Porcine circovirus 2 encephalopathies

Species ***Porcine circovirus 2*** (PCV-2), the cause of porcine postweaning multisystemic wasting syndrome, produces nonsuppurative or granulomatous encephalitis with gliosis under experimental conditions, either alone or in association with porcine parvovirus. The PCV-2 antigen has been identified in brain in these cases, demonstrating neurotropism of the virus under experimental conditions. The role of PCV-2 in encephalitis associated with natural infection is controversial. PCV-2 antigen has been detected in brains of pigs with naturally occurring encephalitis but always in association with other pathogens that can cause encephalitis alone and under natural conditions (e.g., porcine reproductive and respiratory syndrome virus or *Streptococcus suis*). Also, the PCV-2 antigen was demonstrated in neonatal pigs in association with naturally occurring congenital tremor type A2 (see Porcine hypomyelinogenesis); however, the exact role of PCV-2 in this condition is yet to be determined.

Further reading

Bukovsky C, et al. Studies on the aetiology of non-suppurative encephalitis in pigs. Vet Rec 2007;161:552-558.

Stevenson GW, et al. Tissue distribution and genetic typing of porcine circoviruses in pigs with naturally occurring congenital tremors. J Vet Diagn Invest 2001;13:57-62.

Porcine encephalitis associated with PRRSV infection

Species **Porcine reproductive and respiratory syndrome virus** (PRRSV) is neurovirulent, especially in young pigs and can cause encephalitis under natural conditions, often in association with other PRRSV syndromes (e.g., interstitial pneumonia; see Vol. 2, Respiratory system).

California encephalitis virus meningoencephalomyelitis

Several serotypes of species *California encephalitis virus* of genus *Orthobunyavirus*, family *Bunyaviridae*, usually cause only asymptomatic infections, but are capable of causing encephalitis. These include La Crosse virus (LACV), snowshoe hare virus (SSHV), and Jamestown Canyon virus.

La Crosse virus is maintained in the environment and transmitted between susceptible hosts by *Aedes triseriatus* mosquitoes. Chipmunks *(Tamias striatus)* and squirrels *(Sciurus carolinensis)* are the principal amplifying vertebrate hosts. Other wild mammals, such as foxes *(Vulpes fulva* and *Urocyon cinereoargenteus)* and woodchucks *(Marmota monax)*, may also contribute to virus maintenance. LACV causes encephalitis and secondary neurologic deficits in humans, particularly school-aged children. A few cases have been reported in dogs in Florida and Georgia (United States). The most predominant clinical signs in these dogs were seizures and head tilt. Gross lesions were usually unremarkable, but areas of malacia may be present in cortex. Histologic lesions are predominantly in the cerebral cortex and characterized by *histiocytic and lymphoplasmacytic meningoencephalitis*, with fairly thick cuffs and multifocal necrotizing panencephalitis. The necrotic areas in the acute stage are histiocyte and neutrophil rich. The lesions of this disease are similar to those seen in idiopathic granulomatous meningoencephalomyelitis (GME), described later.

Antibodies to **snowshoe hare virus** have been found in a wide range of wild and domestic mammals, but overt disease is very rare. Encephalitis in association with SSHV was reported in 2 horses from Canada, but the diagnosis was made based on detection of seroconversion; one horse recovered, and the pathologic changes found in the second case were not described.

Further reading

Goff G, et al. Roles of host species, geographic separation, and isolation in the seroprevalence of Jamestown Canyon and snowshoe hare viruses in Newfoundland. Appl Environ Microbiol 2012;78: 6734-6740.

Tatum LM, et al. Canine LaCrosse viral meningoencephalomyelitis with possible public health implications. J Vet Diagn Invest 1999;11: 184-188.

Canine herpesviral encephalitis

Species **Canid herpesvirus 1** can cause an acute, highly fatal disease of neonates. Puppies after the age of 3 weeks are resistant to infection. The incidence is low, and the disease is only diagnosed at autopsy. Hypothermia predisposes to disease in neonates, in which the infection would otherwise be asymptomatic. Infection at birth is followed by cell-associated viremia and viral replication in vascular endothelium. This tropism is reflected in large hemorrhages at postmortem, most apparent in renal surface, adrenal, and serosa of gastrointestinal tract. Focal necroses occur in parenchymatous organs, and inclusion bodies may be demonstrated in these foci. *Nonsuppurative meningoencephalitis* is most severe in cerebellum and brainstem. It may be accompanied by necrosis, especially in the cerebellar cortex. Vascular endothelial hypertrophy and hyperplasia is accompanied by mononuclear infiltrates. There may be inflammatory changes in the retina, peripheral nerves, and ganglia.

Further reading

Muñana KR. Encephalitis and meningitis. Vet Clin North Am Small Anim Pract 1996;26:857-874.

Equine herpesviral myeloencephalopathy

Species **Equid herpesvirus 1** (EHV-1) and **Equid herpesvirus 4** (EHV-4) are antigenically related but distinct species in the genus *Varicellovirus*, subfamily *Alphaherpesvirinae*, family *Herpesviridae*. Both viruses are widespread in horses, have significant economic impact on the equine industry, and are responsible for several clinical conditions, including respiratory disease, pulmonary vasculotropic disease, enteric disease, abortion, and neurologic disease, known as *equine herpesviral myeloencephalopathy* (EHM). EHM *is an important neurologic disease* characterized clinically by ataxia, paresis, and paralysis, and caused mainly by EHV-1 and incidentally by EHV-4. Almost all recent outbreaks have been associated with EHV-1 infection. Increased numbers of EHM-outbreaks have been attributed to strains of the virus that are neurovirulent or neuropathogenic. The neuropathogenic strains have a single point mutation in the polymerase-coding gene of EHV-1. This mutation is commonly known as the *neuropathogenic versus non-neuropathogenic mutation*. This mutation results in variation of a single amino acid of the DNA polymerase, such that "non-neuropathogenic" strains have asparagine (N752) and neuropathogenic strains have aspartic acid (D752).

Other members of equine alphaherpesviruses that are pathogenic but do not cause neurologic disease include *Equid herpesvirus 3* (equine coital exanthema virus) and *Equid herpesvirus 8* (Asinine herpesvirus 8), which induces interstitial pneumonia in donkeys. *Equid herpesvirus 9* (Gazelle herpesvirus) causes severe encephalitis experimentally in several species of domestic animals; the natural outbreak of fulminant encephalitis has been reported in a herd of Thomson's gazelles that were in close association with zebras. The natural reservoir for EHV-9 is unknown, but zebras or other equids have been suspected.

Most horses are seropositive to EHV-1 and EHV-4 but are asymptomatic, and vaccination does not necessarily confer protection from neurologic manifestations. Both viruses contain at least 13 glycoproteins, which are important virulence factors for attachment, entry to the host cell, and cell-to-cell dissemination. The natural spread of EHV-1 is through direct horse-to-horse contact, by inhalation of nasal aerosols from infected horses, or through direct contact with an infected aborted fetus or placenta. EHV-1 replicates first in upper respiratory tract epithelium and local lymph nodes, and then induces T-cell and monocyte-associated viremia that ends with invasion of endothelial cells of the CNS and pregnant uterus. This leukocyte-associated viremia protects the virus from humoral immunity. *The virus is endotheliotropic, epitheliotropic, and neurotropic, but not neurovirulent.* The replication of virus in endothelial cells of the CNS leads to initiation of the inflammatory cascade that ends in *thrombo-occlusive necrotizing vasculitis.* The resultant myeloencephalopathy is the result of destruction of CNS tissue secondary to vasculitis. The vasculitis is either caused by direct viral cytotoxic effect or by an immune-mediated (Arthus-type reaction) mechanism. A similar mechanism is responsible for EHV-1–induced abortion and pulmonary vasculotropic disease. There are no genetic or antigenic differences between the EHV strains isolated from neurogenic cases versus abortigenic or respiratory cases.

EHV-1 and EHV-4 have life-long latency in T cells and in neural tissue such as trigeminal ganglia. Latent virus can be reactivated experimentally after very high doses of corticosteroids and naturally after stress (such as castration). In contrast to the extensive studies on EHV-1, the pathogenesis of EHV-4 infection is poorly documented.

The disease occurs sporadically, but in several recent outbreaks, most affected horses either died or were euthanized. The disease is common in late winter and spring, which is also the time of greatest prevalence of EHV-1 abortion outbreaks. The incubation period is 6-10 days and usually occurs in association with abortion and/or respiratory disease but can occur without preceding signs. All ages are susceptible, but *pregnant mares and mares nursing foals are over-represented.* Clinical signs start with fever and mild rhinitis. Neurologic signs are variable and depend on the part of the CNS affected by vasculitis; however, common clinical signs include variable degrees of symmetrical ataxia and paresis that are more severe in pelvic limbs. Fecal and urinary incontinence are common, and clinical signs may end in hemiplegia or paraplegia. Gross and histologic lesions are sequelae to vasculitis. Gross lesions are not always present, but small (0.2-0.5 cm), random, multifocal areas of hemorrhage may be present throughout the meninges, brain, and spinal cord (Fig. 4-113). In severe cases, multifocal necrohemorrhagic or malacic areas (up to 1.5 cm in diameter) can be present, especially in the white matter of spinal cord or the white or gray matter of the brain. *The characteristic histologic lesions are nonsuppurative necrotizing vasculitis and thrombosis,* with greater prevalence in the meningeal and parenchymal blood vessels of the brainstem and spinal cord. Perivascular edema, hemorrhage, focal areas of malacia, and infarction are present adjacent to the affected blood vessels. Occasionally, axonal swelling and mild nonsuppurative trigeminal ganglionitis are present. Extraneural lesions include uveal vasculitis and optic neuritis, especially in foals, and testicular and epididymal vasculitis in stallions.

Further reading

Dunowska M. A review of equid herpesvirus 1 for the veterinary practitioner. Part B: pathogenesis and epidemiology. N Z Vet J 2014;62:179-188.

Ma G, et al. Equine herpesviruses type 1 (EHV-1) and 4 (EHV-4)—masters of co-evolution and a constant threat to equids and beyond. Vet Microbiol 2013;167:123-134.

Reed SM, Toribio RE. Equine herpesvirus 1 and 4. Vet Clin North Am Equine Pract 2004;20:631-642.

Canine distemper and related conditions

Canine distemper is discussed in detail in Vol. 2, Respiratory system. Three neurologic conditions are discussed here: multifocal distemper encephalomyelitis in mature dogs, postvaccinal distemper, and old dog encephalitis.

Multifocal distemper encephalomyelitis in mature dogs. This rare chronic progressive disease occurs when species **Canine distemper virus** infects dogs at 4-8 years of age. This disease is not preceded by the classic form of canine distemper, and signs of systemic illness are often absent or transient. Clinical signs have a slow progressive course and include weakness of the pelvic limbs, generalized incoordination, but no seizures or personality changes, and occasionally head tremors. Lesions are restricted to the CNS and are most prevalent in the cerebellum and white matter of the spinal cord, as demyelinating leukoencephalomyelitis. The cerebral cortex is frequently spared. This distribution differentiates this condition from an extremely rare condition, old dog encephalitis, wherein the cerebral cortex is constantly affected. The lesions are those of *multifocal necrotizing nonsuppurative encephalitis* with rare canine distemper intranuclear intraastrocytic inclusion bodies, and demyelination in the internal capsule and corona radiata. Axonopathy appears to precede demyelination.

Postvaccinal canine distemper encephalitis. This condition occurs in young dogs 1-3 weeks after vaccination with attenuated canine distemper virus vaccines and is characterized by an acute to subacute clinical course (1-5 days). The acute course is characterized by clinical signs reminiscent of the furious form of rabies, including aggressive behavior and attempts to attack. It is not completely clear why some dogs develop this condition post-vaccination. Immune stimulation by other canine viruses (e.g., species *Canine parvovirus*) at the time of vaccination was suggested. The lesions are not well documented; however, lesions are always restricted to the CNS and are reminiscent of the natural disease, but distinguished by the relative sparing of the white matter.

"Old dog" encephalitis. "Old dog" encephalitis (ODE) is rather rare. Most cases occur in dogs past middle age, but it

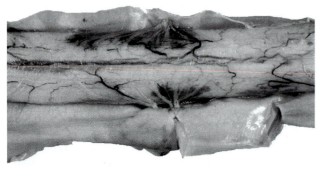

Figure 4-113 Acute spinal cord hemorrhage in a horse with **equine herpesviral myeloencephalopathy.** (Courtesy R.F. Slocombe.)

has been observed in dogs as young as 1 year of age. The disease is of insidious onset and is characterized by circling, swaying, and weaving. Compulsive walking with pushing against fixed objects is typical, but there is neither paralysis nor convulsions. The disease progresses over 3-4 months to coma or termination.

ODE is caused by species *Canine distemper virus* (CDV), apparently as a consequence of long-term subclinical, persistent infection: CDV appears to persist in a replication-defective state. ODE does not appear to be simply a progression of the encephalomyelitis of canine distemper. Virus can be isolated from affected animals only by explantation of affected brain and then only with difficulty, and the disease is not transmissible by direct inoculation. Inclusion bodies are readily found in some cases, and their structure is identical with paramyxovirus nucleocapsids of CDV in nervous tissue. Antigen that responds to fluorescent antibody prepared against CDV is abundant in cells of the gray matter, and serum antibody titers can be very high.

Lesions are confined to the brain, which appears slightly reduced in size. The ventricles are moderately dilated. Lesions are diffusely distributed throughout the cerebral cortex, thalamus, and midbrain. The reaction is nonsuppurative, qualitatively always the same but varying in degree. The most obvious change is cuffing, and the cuffs are remarkable for their large size and the purity of the lymphocytic populations in them. Plasma cells are present in small numbers. The infiltrating cells are confined to the Virchow-Robin space and seldom spread into the parenchyma. The large cuffs occur in both gray and white matter but are most common at the junction of these 2 zones. Focal gliosis does not occur in this disease, but there is some proliferation of astrocytes about vessels and neurons. There is uniform and rather diffuse atrophic sclerosis of the cerebral white matter, which gives an impression of gliosis, but astrogliosis is not prominent. There is some demyelination, producing typical punched-out areas in the white matter, and distorted myelin sheaths in the heavily myelinated tracts are quite extensive when specially stained. Lymphocytes may be found in the choroid plexuses, where they are inserted into the brain, and about vessels, where they enter the parenchyma.

Nerve cells, especially in Ammon's horn and the pons, reveal chromatolysis with only a few remnants of Nissl substance in the periphery of the cytoplasm. The chromatolytic cytoplasm is slightly acidophilic. The neuronal nuclei in the forebrain are remarkably swollen in most of the altered nerve cells. In occasional nuclei, there is pink inclusion-like material. Neuronophagia does not occur. The astrocytic nuclei are remarkably swollen, have an irregular outline, and may contain traces of pink deposit in the nucleoplasm. In a proportion of cases, possibly those of longest duration, prominent *intranuclear and cytoplasmic eosinophilic inclusion bodies* may be found easily.

Further reading

Amude AM, et al. Atypical necrotizing encephalitis associated with systemic canine distemper virus infection in pups. J Vet Sci 2011;12:409-412.

Headley SA, et al. Molecular detection of Canine distemper virus and the immunohistochemical characterization of the neurologic lesions in naturally occurring old dog encephalitis. J Vet Diagn Invest 2009;21:588-597.

Lempp C, et al. New aspects of the pathogenesis of canine distemper leukoencephalitis. Viruses 2014;6:2571-2601.

Ulrich R, et al. Transcriptional changes in canine distemper virus-induced demyelinating leukoencephalitis favor a biphasic mode of demyelination. PLoS ONE 2014;9:e95917.

Microsporidian infections
Encephalitozoonosis

Encephalitozoon *(Nosema)* cuniculi is a microsporidian organism capable of establishing infection in a wide variety of mammalian species, particularly if they are immunocompromised. It is rarely a zoonotic infection. Microsporidia are *obligate intracellular eukaryotic organisms* that are most closely related to *fungi* at the genomic level.

Endemic infection is common in colonies of laboratory rodents in which the clinical consequences are mild, but the pathologic changes may confuse other studies. Among domestic species, the disease is of interest in carnivores, especially farmed foxes in which serious mortalities occur, and occasionally in dogs and mink. The incidence of subclinical infection is not known, but a serologic survey of an unselected population of asymptomatic stray dogs identified 10-15% to be seropositive.

The organism develops in vacuoles in cells of many tissues, especially endothelial cells, but is most easily found in brain and kidney in acute active infections. In chronic infections, the organisms can be sparse or impossible to find in microscopic sections, although it seems that animals once infected remain permanently so and excrete the organism mainly in urine.

Clinical disease occurs in dog and fox pups; the organism is shed in urine and feces of affected animals. In both hosts, transplacental infections appear to be important, but oral transmission, as by ingestion of infected rabbit carcasses, may occur.

Tissue changes in encephalitozoonosis are most prominent in brain and kidney, but the organism selectively parasitizes vascular endothelium, and the *segmental vasculitis* that results is responsible for lesions in many tissues. Gross lesions may be limited to the kidneys as severe, nonsuppurative interstitial nephritis. Organisms are abundant in sections of kidney early in the disease, but they are difficult to find at later stages. They are especially numerous in the epithelium and lumen of tubules, in glomerular capillaries, and in the interstitium, and are present in small vessels and in the media and adventitia of intrarenal arteries. Fibrinoid necrosis affects some glomeruli, and the arterial lesions resemble those of periarteritis nodosa. Focal hepatic necrosis and nonsuppurative portal infiltrations are associated with organisms in hepatocytes and Kupffer cells and with nodular vasculitis in the triads. Focal myocardial necrosis and inflammation are frequently associated with vasculitis.

The lesions in the nervous system are those of *widespread nonsuppurative meningoencephalomyelitis*. The severity of lesions varies unpredictably in different parts of the nervous system, reflecting the random localization of the organism and the irregular distribution of inflammatory vascular change. Focal gliosis and microscopic granulomas surround small vessels (Fig. 4-114). About larger vessels showing segmental fibrinoid change, mononuclear cells form cuffs involving the adventitia and perivascular space and eventually assume an epithelioid cell appearance. There is astrocytosis in the surrounding parenchyma. The vascular lesions in the meninges

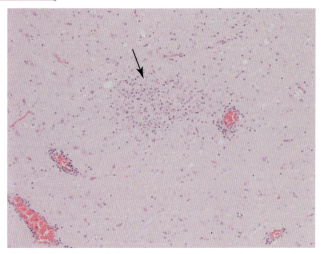

Figure 4-114 Encephalitozoonosis. An area of focal astrogliosis and granulomatous encephalitis (arrow) with narrow lymphoplasmacytic perivascular cuffs.

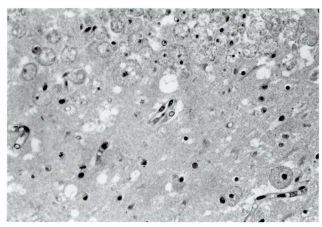

Figure 4-115 Amebic encephalitis in a dog; large numbers of amebae are present in this field, with only minimal reaction. (Courtesy R.F. Slocombe.)

in the acute disease resemble those of polyarteritis nodosa and become dominated by sclerotic changes in the chronic disease in which perivascular cuffing and granulomatous reactions persist.

Puppies that survive the early clinical disease may remain stunted and develop progressive renal disease. It is possible that encephalitozoonosis, as for any sporadic disease, is underdiagnosed, especially in chronic infections in which the organism is difficult to demonstrate. Immunohistochemical methods help to identify sparse organisms and to distinguish them from similar organisms, particularly *Toxoplasma* and *Neospora*.

Further reading

Snowden KF, et al. *Encephalitozoon cuniculi* infections in dogs: a case series. J Am Anim Hosp Assoc 2009;45:225-231.

Wasson K, Peper RL. Mammalian microsporidiosis. Vet Pathol 2000;37:113-128.

Xiang H, et al. New evidence on the relationship between Microsporidia and Fungi: a genome-wide analysis by DarkHorse software. Can J Microbiol 2014;60:557-568.

Parasitic infections
Protozoal infections

The cerebral complications of infections by protozoa, such as *Babesia*, *Theileria*, *Trypanosoma*, and *Toxoplasma*, are discussed elsewhere in these volumes. ***Acanthamoeba***, a free-living ameba, can produce granulomatous meningoencephalitis in dogs as part of an opportunistic generalized infection (Fig. 4-115).

From time to time and in individual cases, pathologists observe *sporozoan parasites* in neural tissues of fetuses, neonates, and adults and lesions presumed to be the consequence of their presence. There are, however, difficulties in specific identification of the parasites and in attribution of pathogenicity. The syndromes considered here are reasonably defined but are subject to revision as the parasites are identified and their life cycles clarified.

Further reading

Kent M, et al. Multisystemic infection with an *Acanthamoeba* sp in a dog. J Am Vet Med Assoc 2011;238:1476-1481.

Equine protozoal myeloencephalitis. *Equine protozoal myeloencephalitis (EPM) is caused* mainly by ***Sarcocystis neurona***, an apicomplexan protozoan parasite; however, identical disease is reported in association with **Neospora caninum** and ***N. hughesi***. Opossums (*Didelphis* spp.) are the definitive host for *S. neurona*, and they are infected by eating intermediate host tissues that contain infective tissue cysts. *S. neurona*–induced EPM is restricted to the Americas in the geographic range of the opossum. Natural intermediate hosts (e.g., armadillos, sea otters, raccoons, skunks, cats) are infected by ingestion of food or water contaminated by sporocysts shed in opossum feces. Horses are assumed to be dead-end hosts, but may also act as intermediate hosts.

Exposure to *S. neurona* is widespread among horses, but the prevalence of the classic progressive disease is much lower. A seropositive horse is positive for exposure but not necessarily for the presence of the disease. However, the presence of seropositivity and the clinical signs of weakness and acute ataxia usually indicate active disease. Infection with *S. neurona* has no age predilection. Most EPM cases caused by *S. neurona* infection appear in the summer and fall. Affected horses are presented with ataxia, limb weakness, lameness, and rarely seizures.

Gross lesions are present only in severe cases, and range from multifocal acute hemorrhage to the presence of discrete multifocal gray to dark yellow areas primarily in cross-sections of fixed brainstem, obex, pons, and cervical and thoracic cord. The histologic lesions are usually moderate to severe and characterized by multifocal areas of necrosis, malacia with aggregation of gitter cells, gliosis, and infiltration of large numbers of lymphocytes, histiocytes, plasma cells, and fewer eosinophils and neutrophils with severe involvement of the meninges (Fig. 4-116A-C). The blood vessels in these areas have swollen, activated endothelium with thick perivascular cuffs of mononuclear cells and occasional eosinophils. Also, and particularly in cord sections, there is axonal swelling or loss besides the appearance of spheroids and some digestion chambers. In chronic cases, the inflammation can be diameter, and contain a few basophilic ovoid merozoites 5 μm × 1.5 μm. The stage infective to the definitive host, that is, sporocysts, can be found in tongue and other skeletal muscles. The *S. neurona* sporocyst is round (50-100 μm) or elongate (500 μm long and 40 μm wide), and contains a number of bradyzoites.

In intermediate hosts, the sarcocysts tend to develop in muscle rather than the CNS. However, EPM-like disease can occur in other *S. neurona* intermediate hosts, including the cat and dog, and this disease should be considered in the differential diagnosis of inflammatory encephalomyelitis in this species. Both *N. hughesi* and *N. caninum* can cause identical EPM lesions in horses. The complete life cycle and methods of transmission for *N. hughesi* have not been determined. *N. hughesi* tachyzoites are crescent shaped, approximately 5 × 2 μm. Definitive *diagnosis* of EPM in a live horse is challenging. Detection of *S. neurona* or *N. hughesi* antibodies in serum and cerebrospinal fluid by an immunoblot test is available. Positive results indicate exposure, but do not necessarily indicate that the horse has EPM. The postmortem diagnosis depends on finding characteristic lesions, especially in the presence of the characteristic protozoal stages. Immunohistochemistry kits for *S. neurona* and *N. caninum* are available commercially.

Further reading

Bisby TM, et al. *Sarcocystis* sp. encephalomyelitis in a cat. Vet Clin Pathol 2010;39:105-112.

Dubey JP, et al. *Sarcocystis neurona* schizonts-associated encephalitis, chorioretinitis, and myositis in a two-month-old dog simulating toxoplasmosis, and presence of mature sarcocysts in muscles. Vet Parasitol 2014;202:194-200.

Pusterla N, et al. Comparison of prevalence factors in horses with and without seropositivity to *Neospora hughesi* and/or *Sarcocystis neurona*. Vet J 2014;200:332-334.

Reed SM, et al. Accurate antemortem diagnosis of equine protozoal myeloencephalitis (EPM) based on detecting intrathecal antibodies against *Sarcocystis neurona* using the SnSAG2 and SnSAG4/3 ELISAs. J Vet Intern Med 2013;27:1193-1200.

Neosporosis. *Neospora caninum* is an apicomplexan coccidian parasite that is a major pathogen of cattle, in which it causes abortion, and for dogs. Other species, such as goats, sheep, deer, and horses, can be infected occasionally. Dogs are the primary definitive host, and they are also considered as an intermediate host. Other canids, for example, coyotes *(Canis latrans)*, may also be important definitive hosts. *N. caninum* has 3 infectious stages: tachyzoites, tissue cysts, and oocysts. Tachyzoites and tissue cysts are found both in intermediate hosts and the definitive host. However, oocysts are only present in the definitive host. Tachyzoites have been found in neurons; reticuloendothelial cells; hepatocytes; muscle cells, including myocardium; and bovine placenta. Tissue cysts have been found in the CNS, muscles, and retina. The exact modes of transmission are not well understood. Dogs become infected by ingesting tissues contaminated with tissue cysts, and then shed oocysts in their feces. Cattle and other intermediate hosts become infected by ingesting sporulated oocyst-contaminated food, water, or soil. However, the principal route for infection in cattle is transplacental (vertical) transmission.

N. caninum does not cause significant clinical disease in adult **cattle;** however, it causes *abortion in both dairy and beef*

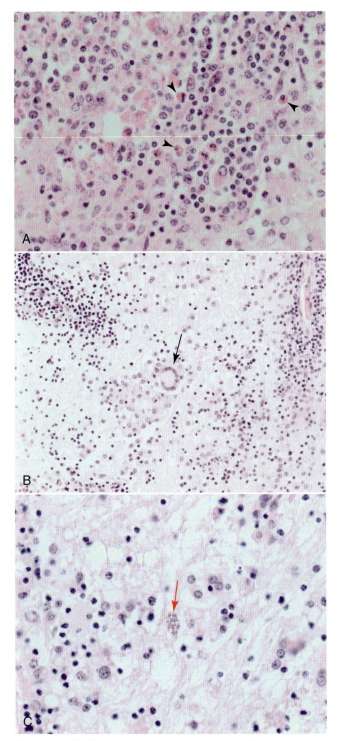

Figure 4-116 Equine protozoal myeloencephalitis. **A.** Severe mixed inflammatory cell encephalitis with variable numbers of eosinophils (arrowheads). **B.** Multinucleated giant cells (black arrow). **C.** Rare intralesional ***Sarcocystis neurona*** merozoites (red arrow).

predominantly histiocytic with occasional eosinophils and multinucleated giant cells.

Finding *S. neurona* merozoites or schizonts can be a challenge, and serial sections must be examined in most cases. *S. neurona* schizonts are almost always present near areas of inflammation and necrosis, schizonts are oval or irregularly round, have very thin walls (<0.5 μm), are up to 20 μm in

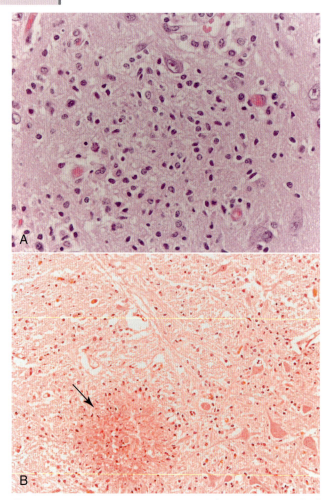

Figure 4-117 Neosporosis. A. Lesions of neosporosis in fetal bovine brains may consist only of focal gliosis, or, **B,** may occur as multifocal areas of neuropil necrosis (arrow) encircled by glial cells and rarely giant cells. *Neospora caninum* cysts are rarely seen.

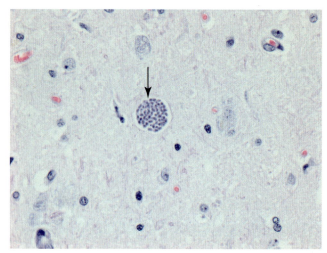

Figure 4-118 *Neospora caninum* **cyst** (arrow) in the brain of a dog.

cows, particularly at mid-term, although cows can abort at any time from 3 months to term. Infected fetuses may die in utero, be mummified, stillborn, or born alive with or without clinical signs. Extraneural lesions in bovine fetuses include *lymphocytic, plasmacytic, and to a lesser extent, histiocytic, hepatitis, pancarditis or myocarditis, myositis, and placentitis.* Cotyledonary necrosis may be associated with the placentitis. Intralesional *N. caninum* tachyzoites are occasionally present in the aforementioned organs. Tachyzoites appear in groups, either intracellular in neurons, endothelium, or epithelial cells, or extracellular. Tachyzoites are spindle shaped, 4-7 × 2 μm. Tissue cysts are primarily present in the CNS and rarely in skeletal muscles. Cyst diameter is up to 107 μm, with wall thickness of 1-4 μm, and containing numerous bradyzoites 8 × 2 μm.

The most frequent and almost pathognomonic CNS lesion in *bovine fetuses* is the presence of *multifocal discrete foci of necrosis* (~100-300 μm diameter), particularly in the brain and to a lesser extent in the cord (Fig. 4-117A, B). The necrotic areas are fairly well circumscribed, have necrotic centers and are surrounded by a rim of glial cells and macrophages. In advanced lesions, the necrotic area may be completely replaced by macrophages and a few glial cells, which make the lesions appear as discrete granulomas. The recognition of *N. caninum* tachyzoites and tissue cysts in aborted fetal brain or other fetal tissue is usually difficult on H&E stain, and immunohistochemistry must be performed to confirm the diagnosis of neosporosis. Other CNS lesions include mild nonsuppurative meningoencephalomyelitis. Fetal anomalies are not common in association with *Neospora* abortion.

Infection in **dogs** is transmitted either horizontally or vertically (transplacental). Dogs of any age can be affected and the infection can be generalized affecting any organs, including the skin, or can be localized. Infection in adult dogs is usually subclinical. Infection in young congenitally infected dogs is severe and characterized pathologically by encephalomyelitis and myositis/polyradiculoneuritis and clinically by hindlimb paresis that is followed by paralysis. CNS lesions are those of *necrotizing granulomatous, lymphoplasmacytic, and occasionally eosinophilic meningoencephalomyelitis* with diffuse gliosis, occasional axonal swelling, digestion chamber formation, and intralesional *N. caninum* tachyzoites and cysts (Fig. 4-118). These lesions are widely distributed in the brain and cord; however, in the cortex, the gray matter is affected predominantly. Lesions associated with the neuritis/polyradiculoneuritis is frequently severe, mostly affecting pelvic limbs, and characterized by severe lymphohistiocytic and occasional eosinophilic inflammation with associated secondary degenerative and necrotizing changes either in muscles or nerves, with intralesional tachyzoites and rare cysts.

Experimental infection of pregnant **ewes** and **does** produces a disease that is identical pathologically to that observed in cattle; however, natural disease is rare.

The epidemiology and methods of transmission of *N. caninum* and other *Neospora* in **horses**, for example, *N. hughesi*, are not completely understood. Transplacental infection is suggested but not completely confirmed. *N. caninum* has been isolated from a few aborted fetuses. *N. caninum* and *N. hughesi* are alternative causes of equine protozoal myeloencephalitis.

Further reading

Cabral AD, et al. Diagnosis of *Neospora caninum* in bovine fetuses by histology, immunohistochemistry, and nested-PCR. Rev Bras Parasitol Vet 2009;18:14-19.

Dubey JP. Review of *Neospora caninum* and neosporosis in animals. Korean J Parasitol 2003;41:1-16.

MacKay RJ, et al. Equine protozoal myeloencephalitis. Vet Clin North Am Equine Pract 2000;16:405-425.

Moreno B, et al. Occurrence of *Neospora caninum* and *Toxoplasma gondii* infections in ovine and caprine abortions. Vet Parasitol 2012;187:312-318.

Saey V, et al. Neuritis of the cauda equina in a dog. J Small Anim Pract 2010;51:549-552.

Toxoplasmosis. *Toxoplasmosis is one of the most common protozoal diseases affecting humans and animals* and is caused by **Toxoplasma gondii.** Diseases caused by *T. gondii* are very similar in clinical presentation and pathology to those caused by *N. caninum*. Felids are the only definitive host and they also can act as an intermediate host. Other intermediate hosts include humans and other mammals. *T. gondii* has 3 infectious stages: *tachyzoites, tissue cysts, and oocysts*. Tachyzoites and tissue cysts are found in both intermediate and definitive hosts; however, oocysts are only present in the definitive host. Tachyzoites and tissue cysts are present more commonly in neural tissue and muscles, but can be present in virtually any tissue. Felids become infected by ingestion of tissues contaminated with tissue cysts, and shed oocysts in their feces. Human and other intermediate hosts, including felids, can become infected by ingesting sporulated oocyst-contaminated food, water, or soil. Transplacental transmission is important in cats, goats, and sheep.

The extraneural pathology of toxoplasmosis is discussed elsewhere in these volumes. The nervous system lesions, including polyradiculoneuritis, are identical to those described for neosporosis; however, *the tissue cyst has a thinner wall (<0.5 μm), is 5-70 μm in size, and contains several bradyzoites 0.7-1.5 μm. Tachyzoites are 2-6 μm in size*. The encephalitic form of toxoplasmosis is most likely to occur in immunosuppressed dog and cats or kittens. Toxoplasmosis in pigs is generalized and can cause devastating disease with lesions, including nonsuppurative encephalomyelitis with intralesional *T. gondii* stages.

Further reading

Dubey JP. Toxoplasmosis—a waterborne zoonosis. Vet Parasitol 2004; 126:57-72.

Halonen SK, Weiss LM. Toxoplasmosis. Handb Clin Neurol 2013;114: 125-145.

Sarcocystis canis encephalitis. A rare and generalized disease affecting dogs mostly in North America is caused by *S. canis* and characterized histologically by multisystemic vasculitis, hepatitis, and necrotizing lymphohistiocytic encephalitis in association with the presence of intralesional *S. canis* schizonts and merozoites (schizonts are $5-25 \times 4-20$ μm and contain 6-40 merozoites of $5-7$ μm $\times 1$ μm in size).

Further reading

Dubey JP, et al. Clinical *Sarcocystis neurona, Sarcocystis canis, Toxoplasma gondii,* and *Neospora caninum* infections in dogs. Vet Parasitol 2006;137:36-49.

Helminth and arthropod infestations

Nothing is known of what motivates and directs the migration of larval parasites. Those that migrate somatically are apt to go astray, and this appears especially likely when they wander in an alien host. Aberrant pathways include the nervous system with such frequency as to suggest that nematodes have a special propensity for wandering in the CNS. Whether this is indeed the case remains to be proven, but parasitic migrations in nervous tissue are more likely to be symptomatic than aberrant migrations in other tissues, and there is an impressive list of parasites that have been found in brain or cord.

Cestodes. Adult cestodes live almost exclusively in the small intestines of the final host; however, certain larval stages can infest the brain of the intermediate host. **Coenurus cerebralis,** the larval stage of **Taenia multiceps,** which infests the small intestines of dogs and wild carnivores, is fairly common in the brains of sheep in Europe, less common in other herbivores, and rather rare in horses and humans. About 40% of pigs harboring **Cysticercus cellulosae** (the larval stage of the human tapeworm **Taenia solium**) have cysts in the meninges and brain as well as in the muscle, and the same species has been identified in the brains of dogs. Possibly, **Cysticercus bovis** (the larval stage of human tapeworm **Taenia saginata**) and other cysticerci will invade nervous tissue with comparable frequency. Apparently, hydatids are seldom found in brain.

Nematodes. The term **cerebrospinal nematodiasis** is applied to nervous diseases resulting from aberrant nematode larval migrations. The few nematodes that produce the syndrome with any frequency are discussed later.

Parastrongylus (Angiostrongylus) cantonensis is a metastrongylid lungworm whose only known definitive host is the rat. It is widely distributed in the warm Pacific regions, but its distribution is much more limited than that of the gastropod intermediate hosts and the rat. The parasite resides in the pulmonary arteries of rats; eggs lodge as emboli in alveolar capillaries and the larvae, which hatch in about 6 days, and follow the tracheal-intestinal route to the exterior. First-stage larvae actively penetrate terrestrial and aquatic slugs and snails, which act as intermediate hosts. Transport hosts for third-stage larvae include frogs, crabs, and prawns. In addition to the rat, dogs, humans, and occasionally other species are infected by eating intermediate or transport hosts and, possibly, directly by ingestion of infective larvae that have emerged from intermediate hosts. Ingested larvae enter and are dispersed by the circulation to many tissues, but predominantly to brain, kidney, and muscle. Molting larvae in the brain produce a mild to severe inflammatory reaction before re-entering the venous circulation for return to the pulmonary arteries. Aberrant infections are important in humans and dogs, and are reported in horses and macropods. The human disease, eosinophilic meningoencephalitis, is usually mild and without sequelae, but infection in dogs can be accompanied by ascending paralysis. Larvae that enter the brain in dogs are probably inhibited in their development and destroyed there (Fig. 4-119). The lesions are granulomatous, randomly distributed in the cord and brain and are most frequent and severe in the cord. Rarely, degenerate parasites are present in the granulomas, but apparently viable worms in the tissue are not accompanied by an inflammatory reaction. Eosinophils infiltrate the granulomas but are more numerous in affected meninges.

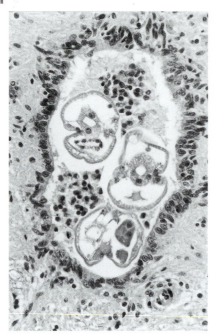

Figure 4-119 Larvae of *Parastrongylus* sp. in central canal of spinal cord in a dog.

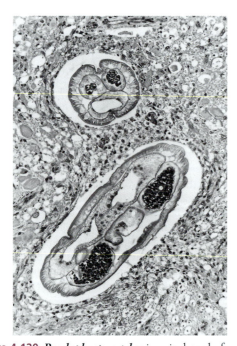

Figure 4-120 *Parelaphostrongylus* in spinal cord of a sheep.

Parelaphostrongylus (Pneumostrongylus) tenuis is a metastrongylid parasite of white-tailed deer, *Odocoileus virginianus*, in North America. The intermediate hosts are terrestrial slugs and snails. Ingested larvae reach the spinal cord of the deer in ~10 days. They develop for up to 1 month in the dorsal horns of the cord at all levels and then migrate into the meningeal spaces. Some penetrate the dural veins and sinuses and mature. Eggs or larvae are carried in venous blood to the lungs. The larvae do very little to the cord in white-tailed deer, but the reaction is more severe in other species, including red deer, elk, moose, and sheep (Fig. 4-120). *Elaphostrongylus panticola* and *E. rangifera* of deer in northern Europe and Russia

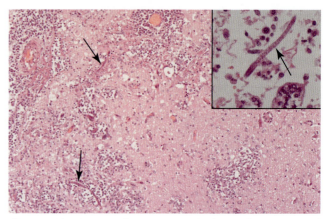

Figure 4-121 Severe inflammation in the brain of a horse caused by ***Halicephalobus gingivalis*** *(Micronema deletrix)* (arrows). Inset: parasite (arrow) with cellular reaction. (Courtesy M.J. Stalker.)

have a life cycle similar to that of *P. tenuis*, but infections are usually subclinical. ***Elaphostrongylus cervi*** cerebrospinal nematodiasis has been recorded in goats grazing the same area as infected red deer.

When larvae of ***Elaeophora schneideri***—a filarial parasite discussed in Vol. 3, Cardiovascular system—develop in the leptomeningeal arteries of various cervids, sheep, and goats, they can cause ischemic necrosis of brain tissue.

Setaria digitata is normally found as an adult in the peritoneal cavity of cattle and buffalo in Asia (see also Vol. 2, Alimentary system and peritoneum). Microfilariae can be carried to aberrant hosts, such as horses, camels, sheep, and goats, by mosquitoes, and larvae wandering in the brain and spinal cord are responsible for the neurologic disease known as *kumri* (lumbar paralysis) in Asia. The migrating larvae apparently cause little or no damage in the natural host. The location of the lesions is variable, as are the clinical signs produced. Characteristically, the neurologic signs are ataxia, weakness, or paralysis. The severity of the signs varies from slight weakness to quadriplegia, depending on the number and location of the wandering parasites; however, affected animals may remain bright and alert. The CNS lesions produced are fundamentally traumatic, and lead to microcavitation, as described later.

Halicephalobus gingivalis *(Micronema deletrix)* is a free-living nematode that is accidentally, but rarely, a parasite; this nematode is characterized by a rhabditiform esophagus. Massive intracranial invasion is reported in horses. The syndrome is acute and of short duration. There are focal arachnoid hemorrhages and patchy meningeal thickenings. Only parthenogenetic female worms and larvae are found among the specimens in the brain, most easily in perivascular spaces (Fig. 4-121). Depending on the area of the CNS affected, lesions are granulomatous and eosinophilic meningoencephalitis, myelitis, polyradiculitis, or even cauda equina neuritis-like lesions. Parasitic granulomas in the kidney and gingiva may accompany the cerebral invasion. Little is known about the life cycle and method of transmission of this nematode. Oral ingestion or wound contamination then hematogenous distribution is suggested. Also, transmission from infected dam to her foal through milk is described in one case.

Gurltia paralysans, found in the spinal veins of cats, is reported to be responsible for a high incidence of paralysis in this host, and *Angiostrongylus vasorum* has caused hemorrhagic malacia in the brains of dogs. Aberrant hosts can develop severe cerebrospinal nematodiasis when they incidentally ingest the eggs of *Baylisascaris procyonis* (raccoon ascarid) or *B. columnaris* (skunk ascarid).

Larval worms may also migrate aberrantly in the CNS of their natural hosts. *Stephanurus dentatus* quite frequently invades the spinal canal and may even encyst in the meninges in pigs. *Strongylus* spp. occasionally invade the brains of horses. Ascarids have a propensity for wandering in the brain of alien hosts and occasionally do so in their natural hosts.

Trematodes. Trematodes apparently have little tendency to invade nervous tissue. *Troglotrema acutum* may invade the brain from its normal habitat in the paranasal sinuses. The eggs of the lung flukes, *Paragonimus* spp., have been observed in the brains of dogs, possibly arriving there as emboli.

Arthropods. The only larval arthropods of interest are *Hypoderma bovis*, which normally migrates through the spinal canal, and *Oestrus ovis*, which may invade the brain from the nasal sinuses.

Cuterebra spp. (larva of a rodent or rabbit bot) in an abnormal host, that is, cat and to a lesser extent dog, can undergo aberrant migration and has been reported in many organs, including the eyes and CNS. Adult *Cuterebra* are nonparasitic and are seldom observed. Lesions in the brain are characteristic and indicative of vascular compromise and direct toxicity by toxin released from the larvae. These lesions include superficial laminar cerebrocortical necrosis, cerebral (particularly at the olfactory bulbs and peduncles) and subependymal malacia and infarction, and finally larval migratory track lesions that are characterized by focal necrosis, hemorrhage, and infiltration of eosinophils, lymphocytes, plasma cells, and fewer neutrophils. Most of the track lesions are present in caudate nucleus or thalamus. Cuterebral larval migrans in the feline brain is thought to be the cause of *feline ischemic encephalopathy*.

The few parasites specifically mentioned are the most important in terms of neuropathology. Occasionally, helminth larvae are discovered accidentally but rarely identified in sections of brain or cord, and it is somewhat more common to find lesions typical of those produced by migratory parasites without being able to locate the parasite. Some parasites, such as *Elaphostrongylus*, usually remain in the CNS, whereas others, such as ascarids and strongyles, can be expected to keep moving. Finding the parasite is therefore largely a matter of luck, even when it is sought very early after the onset of clinical signs.

The lesions produced in nervous tissue by migratory larvae are mainly *malacic* and, although random, are fairly distinctive in their pattern. *Coenurus cerebralis* produces, in the invasion phase, purulent meningoencephalitis and later acts as a space-occupying lesion, but other invading parasites produce mainly traumatic lesions with very little inflammatory reaction except for a few eosinophils. The lesions produced by nematodes are sometimes grossly visible as *hemorrhagic foci or narrow, slightly tortuous tracks*. Brown, hemorrhagic discoloration depends on the parasite hitting a vein or arteriole, and it appears that some worms have a tendency to migrate along veins. There may be only one or several such tracks in the CNS, and they occur quite at random. Microscopically, the lesion is an irregular focus or pathway of traumatic malacia into which some hemorrhage may have occurred. There may be slight cellular infiltration in the adjacent meninges or nerve roots. The track is liquefied, and its margins not sharp, and apart from lymphocytes, gitter cells, and a few eosinophils, there is no significant reaction in the damaged tissue or in the adjacent vessels. The disruption, which is not selective in the tissues destroyed, leads to *microcavitation*. The disrupted axons, swollen, tortuous, and as globose fragments, persist for some time in the microcavitations. Gemistocytic astrocytes may be present in older lesions.

Further reading

Alberti EG, et al. *Elaphostrongylus cervi* in a population of red deer (*Cervus elaphus*) and evidence of cerebrospinal nematodiasis in small ruminants in the province of Varese, Italy. J Helminthol 2011;85:313-318.

Gavin PJ, et al. Baylisascariasis. Clin Microbiol Rev 2005;18:703-718.

Glass EN, et al. Clinical and clinicopathologic features in 11 cats with *Cuterebra* larvae myiasis of the central nervous system. J Vet Intern Med 1998;12:365-368.

Jung JY, et al. Meningoencephalitis caused by *Halicephalobus gingivalis* in a thoroughbred gelding. J Vet Med Sci 2014;76:281-284.

LeVan IK, et al. High elaeophorosis prevalence among harvested Colorado moose. J Wildl Dis 2013;49:666-669.

Lunn JA, et al. Twenty two cases of canine neural angiostrongylosis in eastern Australia (2002-2005) and a review of the literature. Parasit Vectors 2012;5:70.

Mahmoud OM, et al. An outbreak of neurofilariosis in young goats. Vet Parasitol 2004;120:151-156.

Mitchell KJ, et al. Diagnosis of *Parelaphostrongylus* spp. infection as a cause of meningomyelitis in calves. J Vet Diagn Invest 2011;23:1097-1103.

Suja MS, et al. Cerebral cysticercosis mimicking rabies in a dog. Vet Rec 2003;153:304-305.

Tieber LM, et al. Survival of a suspected case of central nervous system cuterebrosis in a dog: clinical and magnetic resonance imaging findings. J Am Anim Hosp Assoc 2006;42:238-242.

Chlamydial disease

Sporadic bovine encephalomyelitis (SBE) occurs in calves <6 months of age, and is caused by **Chlamydophila pecorum.** Identical disease is also reported caused by infection with *C. psittaci*. *C. pecorum* also causes a wide range of other conditions in calves, including polyarthritis, metritis, conjunctivitis, and pneumonia. The disease occurs in the United States, Japan, Europe, and Australia; the agent probably has a worldwide distribution, and most infections are asymptomatic. Encephalomyelitis is reported to occur naturally only in cattle and buffalo. As a rule, SBE is indeed sporadic, affecting only a few animals in a herd; however, outbreaks of the disease with morbidity of 25% are described. Transmission appears to be by direct contact. The clinical syndrome is not particularly characteristic. It is composed of moderate fever and signs of catarrhal inflammation of the respiratory tract. There is some stiffness, weakness of the hindlimbs with staggering and knuckling of the fetlocks, and muscle tremors. There is some dullness; signs of excitement are not present. Death occurs in a few days to a few weeks.

The organism has a tropism for blood vessels, mesenchymal tissue and serous membranes, which make *vasculitis and polyserositis the hallmark of lesions*. Encephalitis is secondary to vascular damage. The gross morbid change that suggests a diagnosis of SBE is serofibrinous inflammation of serous membranes and synoviae. This is most consistently *peritonitis*, and in ~50% of fatal cases, there is also *pleuritis and pericarditis*. The meninges appear congested and edematous and occasionally are covered with a few fibrin tags. Microscopically, there is a rather *severe and diffuse meningoencephalomyelitis*. The leptomeningitis is most severe about the base of the brain. The reactive cells are almost solely histiocytes and plasma cells, with only a few neutrophils. These cells infiltrate the meninges and perivascular spaces and mix with reactive adventitial cells of the vessel walls. The vascular endothelium proliferates secondary to lesions in the vascular walls, and ischemic changes may occur in the parenchyma. Reactive microglial nodules are widespread in the brain.

Cell culture of *Chlamydophila*, the gold standard diagnostic tool, is being displaced by detection by PCR. Elementary bodies produced by this organism occur in the cytoplasm of mononuclear cells in the exudates in the meninges and from serosal membranes and in microglia of nodules, but they are not numerous, and their demonstration by special stains or immunohistochemistry is not usually rewarding.

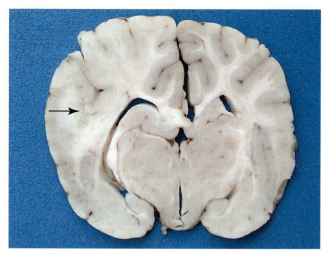

Figure 4-122 Malacic focus in lateral cerebral hemisphere (arrow) in **canine necrotizing meningoencephalitis**.

Further reading

Jee J, et al. High prevalence of natural *Chlamydophila* species infection in calves. J Clin Microbiol 2004;42:5664-5672.

Jelocnik M, et al. Molecular and pathological insights into *Chlamydia pecorum*-associated sporadic bovine encephalomyelitis (SBE) in Western Australia. BMC Vet Res 2014;10:121.

Idiopathic inflammatory diseases

Necrotizing meningoencephalitis and necrotizing leukoencephalitis of Pugs and other small-breed dogs

Canine necrotizing meningoencephalitis (NME), formerly "Pug dog encephalitis," is an idiopathic disease affecting mainly Pug dogs, but also reported rarely in the Maltese, Pekingese, Shih Tzu, and Chihuahua. A similar condition, but with lesions more prevalent in the white matter, is reported in the Boston Terrier, Chihuahua, and Yorkshire Terrier (distinct from *Yorkshire Terrier necrotizing encephalopathy*, which affects brainstem), named necrotizing leukoencephalitis (NLE). The cause of NME and NLE is unknown; several etiologic agents have been suggested as causes, including alphaherpesvirus, but none has been confirmed. An autoimmune reaction against canine brain tissue has been suggested as a possible mechanism. A wide age range is affected. Generalized convulsions and their aftermath dominate the clinical picture, which may include lethargy, ataxia, and progression to coma. The clinical signs refer essentially to cortical disease that progresses rapidly over a few weeks, but which may extend to several months.

The lesions are particularly in the cerebral cortex, and are bilateral but asymmetrical, often confluent over large areas, and extend to the adjacent white matter with relative sparing of the deeper periventricular tissue. The geography of the lesions therefore helps to distinguish this disease from other encephalitides of the dog. Grossly, localized swellings in the cerebrum contribute to asymmetry, and malacic foci may be seen as typical yellow areas of softening (Fig. 4-122) or, in cases of longer duration, as tiny cystic cavities.

The histologic changes are necrotizing and with an affinity for the hemispheres. Numerous foci of meningitis, characterized by infiltrations of lymphocytes, plasma cells, and

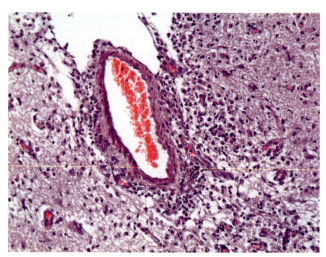

Figure 4-123 Meningeal arteriole surrounded by mixed mononuclear infiltrate in **canine necrotizing meningoencephalitis**.

monocytes (Fig. 4-123), diminish caudally and may be absent in the caudal fossa and spinal cord. These infiltrates breach the pial barrier and destroy the superficial cortex to an extent and severity that is unusual. The evidence of cerebral necrosis extends from selective neuronal necrosis to areas of malacia, the latter especially in chronic cases. Vascular endothelium in the cortex is reactive and associated with edema, occasional petechiae, and diffuse accumulation of mononuclear cells in parenchyma and vascular cuffs.

The differential features of this meningoencephalitis, in addition to its nonsuppurative nature, are the malacic degenerations and predilection for the cerebral cortex. This condition must be differentiated also from granulomatous meningoencephalomyelitis (GME). The inflammatory infiltrate in GME contains more histiocytes, which in the chronic stage transform to epithelioid cells that can form discrete cohesive sheets or granuloma-like lesions. Also, in GME, the reaction is predominantly in the white matter and is distributed in almost all parts of the CNS. In contrast, the reaction in NME is mostly in the cortical gray matter.

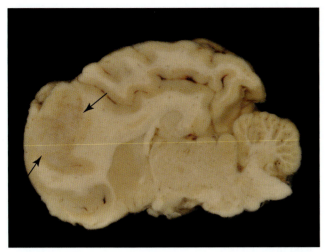

Figure 4-124 Poorly demarcated gray mass in the frontal lobe (arrows) of a dog with **granulomatous encephalitis** (Courtesy A. Ostrowski, Freie Universität, Berlin).

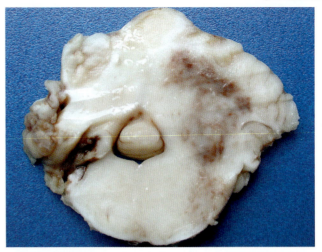

Figure 4-125 Malacia of cerebellum secondary to infarction in a dog with **granulomatous encephalitis**.

Further reading

Cantile C, et al. Necrotizing meningoencephalitis associated with cortical hippocampal hamartia in a Pekingese dog. Vet Pathol 2001;38:119-122.

Miyake H, et al. Serum glial fibrillary acidic protein as a specific marker for necrotizing meningoencephalitis in Pug dogs. J Vet Med Sci 2013;75:1543-1545.

Park ES, et al. Comprehensive immunohistochemical studies on canine necrotizing meningoencephalitis (NME), necrotizing leukoencephalitis (NLE), and granulomatous meningoencephalomyelitis (GME). Vet Pathol 2012;49:682-692.

Granulomatous meningoencephalomyelitis

Granulomatous meningoencephalomyelitis (GME) is a sporadic disease of the CNS of dogs. GME appears to have a worldwide distribution and to occur mostly in *young to middle-aged dogs of small breeds*, for example, terriers and toy breeds; however, the disease can occur in any breed and in an age range of 6 months to 12 years. The cause of GME is unknown; several infectious causes have been suggested but not confirmed to be the cause of this condition. Based on the predominance of CD3+ T cells and major histocompatibility complex (MHC) class II antigen-positive macrophages, an immune-mediated mechanism has been proposed.

Variations in the distribution and extent of the lesions result in a variety of clinical signs. Spinal lesions may be associated with ataxia, paresis, or paralysis. Lesions in the brainstem frequently produce signs of vestibular dysfunction. Changes of behavior, forced movement and circling, depression, and convulsions occur with supratentorial lesions. Macroscopic lesions, if evident, consist of gray-white discoloration of the white matter of the brain or spinal cord (Fig. 4-124), and in those cases in which the cellular aggregations become confluent, there may be irregular areas of malacia (Fig. 4-125).

The histologic changes are patchy in distribution. There may be very few foci, or they may be disseminated, or they may be localized to one area and confluent, or there may, in the same animal, be both confluent and disseminated distributions. *The essential histologic feature is perivascular aggregation of cells rather selectively in the white matter.* The minimal lesion

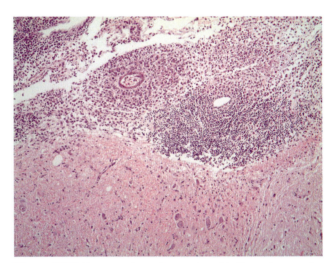

Figure 4-126 Dense perivascular meningeal infiltrate in **granulomatous encephalitis** in a dog.

is cuffing of vessels by lymphocytes and plasma cells with small eccentric clumps of macrophages. The macrophages increase in number and may come to comprise the cuff, appearing as discrete granulomas, which, depending on the plane of section, may appear to be in the parenchyma. Occasional mitoses are present in these cells. Transformation to epithelioid cells occurs later. The perivascular aggregates expand in concentric arrangements and displace surrounding parenchyma (Fig. 4-126). Where the cuffing response is severe, edema and necrosis may occur in the adjacent white matter, leading to a spillover of mononuclear cells into the parenchyma and to the usual reactive changes. Large malacic foci are unusual. In cases of prolonged duration, confluence of lesions occurs and reparative responses include the deposition of abundant reticulin and collagen in perivascular arrangements. Involvement of meninges is patchy and often related to lesions of white matter directly underlying.

Cytologic characterization of the cell aggregates can be difficult. In many, and perhaps most, cases, the cells are easy to classify, being well differentiated as lymphocytes, monocytes, plasma cells, and histiocytes (Fig. 4-127A, B). Granulocytes may be present but are not numerous, and histiocytes

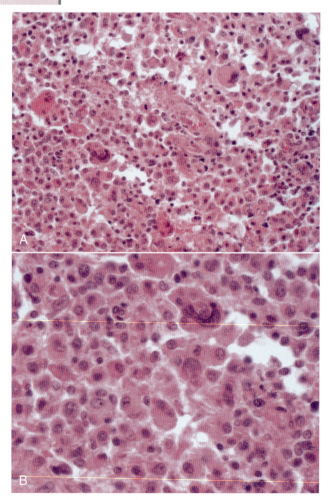

Figure 4-127 A, B. Detail of cellular infiltrate in brain in **granulomatous encephalitis** in a dog. (Courtesy A. Ostrowski, Freie Universität, Berlin.)

often show epithelioid transformation and may form small syncytial masses. There may also be, in some cases, large immature cells of reticulohistiocytic type in which mitoses may be few or many. Differentiation between GME and brain malignant histiocytosis (BMH) can be problematic occasionally; BMH is frequently part of a multisystemic tumor and rarely occurs in isolation. Also, the absence of cellular atypia and the predominance of perivascular orientation should favor the diagnosis of GME.

Further reading

Park ES, et al. Comprehensive immunohistochemical studies on canine necrotizing meningoencephalitis (NME), necrotizing leukoencephalitis (NLE), and granulomatous meningoencephalomyelitis (GME). Vet Pathol 2012;49:682-692.

Talarico LR, Schatzberg SJ. Idiopathic granulomatous and necrotising inflammatory disorders of the canine central nervous system: a review and future perspectives. J Small Anim Pract 2010;51: 138-149.

Acute polyradiculoneuritis (coonhound paralysis)

Acute canine polyradiculoneuritis (ACP), or polyradiculoneuropathy, affects primarily dogs, occasionally cats, and rarely horses, and has many similarities to Guillain-Barré syndrome (GBS) in humans. The condition was named coonhound paralysis to reflect the fact that some affected dogs had been bitten or scratched by raccoons, although cases may have no known exposure to raccoons. Within 7-10 days, ascending flaccid paralysis, starting in the hindlimbs and progressing cranially to involve the forelimbs, leads to quadriplegia and rapid atrophy of muscle. There are no cerebral signs. Some dogs die of respiratory paralysis, but most will recover slowly if nursing is adequate. Dogs that have recovered appear to have increased sensitivity to subsequent exposure but may survive several bouts of paralysis. The disease has been transmitted using pooled saliva of raccoons, but the cause has not been identified; an autoimmune mechanism and microbial triggers, such as *Toxoplasma*, have been suspected. Similar to GBS in humans, anti–GM_2 ganglioside antibodies have been found in ACP dogs.

Lesions are found in the *ventral roots of spinal nerves and in peripheral nerves*. Mononuclear and plasma cells infiltrate around venules, but the extent of the infiltrate is variable and not correlated with the course of the illness or the severity of nerve degeneration. There is primary and Wallerian degeneration afflicting ventral roots in particular, with axonal reaction in motor neurons and atrophy of denervation in muscle. This idiopathic polyradiculoneuritis is the most common inflammatory condition of peripheral nerves in dogs.

Further reading

Holt N, et al. Seroprevalence of various infectious agents in dogs with suspected acute canine polyradiculoneuritis. J Vet Intern Med 2011;25:261-266.

Rupp A, et al. Anti-GM2 ganglioside antibodies are a biomarker for acute canine polyradiculoneuritis. J Peripher Nerv Syst 2013;18: 75-88.

Neuritis of the cauda equina

Neuritis of the cauda equina of **horses** is a polyneuritis in which the presenting signs are referable to the sacrococcygeal nerves and include perineal anesthesia, tail paralysis, urinary incontinence, fecal retention, weakness, atrophy of coccygeal muscles and, in long-standing cases, atrophy of the muscles of the hindlimbs. The neuritis is progressive. The cause is unknown, but the nature of the reaction suggests immune mediation, which may follow viral infection. The condition has been compared to experimental allergic neuritis in laboratory animals. *Halicephalobus gingivalis* is reported as a novel cause of cauda equina neuritis in one horse.

Although the pathologic changes emphasize the *sacral and caudal spinal nerve roots*, there may simultaneously be asymmetrical pareses of other nerves, producing isolated limb pareses, and paresis or paralysis referable to cranial nerves. The lesions in these other nerves are similar in character to, but much milder than, those in caudal nerve roots. Inflammatory changes are present in sensory and some autonomic ganglia, but changes in the spinal cord are limited to those that reflect peripheral nerve injury.

The gross changes affect in particular the extradural parts of the sacral and coccygeal nerves and may extend through the intervertebral foraminae into the adjacent muscle. The roots are thickened and fusiform and usually discolored by recent or old hemorrhage. The intradural segments of affected nerves are discolored but not usually enlarged.

Microscopically there is *granulomatous inflammation with extensive* fibrosis. The thickening and discoloration are attributable to hemorrhage, proliferation of epineural tissue, and inflammatory cell infiltrates. The infiltrating lymphocytes, plasma cells, and macrophages are frequently disposed as to form granulomas, often with central epithelioid and giant cells; granulocytes do not feature in the infiltrates. Degenerative and regenerative changes are present in the myelin and axons of affected roots and appear to be more closely associated with endoneurial and perineurial fibroplasia than with leukocytic infiltrates.

Further reading

Johnson JS, et al. Radiculomeningomyelitis due to *Halicephalobus gingivalis* in a horse. Vet Pathol 2001;38:559-561.

Steblaj B, et al. Occurence of cauda equina neuritis symptoms after epidural catheter placement and drug delivery in a horse. Vet Anaesth Analg 2013;40:653-655.

Steroid-responsive meningitis-arteritis (Beagle pain syndrome)

Steroid-responsive meningitis-arteritis (SRMA) is a *polyarteritis of possible immune-mediated origin, affecting mainly small- to medium-sized leptomeningeal and myocardial arteries*, but arteries in many organs can be affected. The autoimmune response may be enhanced through the action of various signaling proteins (transforming growth factor-β1, interleukin-6, and vascular endothelial growth factor) and pattern recognition receptors (toll-like receptors). Beagles, especially those in laboratory-bred colonies, are at high risk, but the disease is reported in Boxers, German Shorthaired Pointers, Nova Scotia Duck-tolling Retrievers, and rarely in other breeds.

Affected dogs have fever, hyperesthesia, severe pain on manipulation, cervical rigidity, and anorexia. The clinical course of SRMA is usually acute, but a chronic form exists. Gross lesions are minimal, but areas of subarachnoid hemorrhage may be present along the brainstem and the spinal cord, especially the cervical part. Histologically, small- to medium-sized leptomeningeal arteries, especially of the brainstem and spinal cord, and, to a lesser extent, heart and cranial mediastinum, have moderate to severe perivascular and transmural infiltrates of lymphocytes, plasma cells, histiocytes, and fewer neutrophils. Occasionally, neutrophils predominate. Also, there is severe fibrinoid necrosis, thrombosis, and occasionally periarterial fibrosis. Mild lymphocytic and histiocytic leptomeningitis is also a constant finding.

Distinct from SRMA, an unusual case of idiopathic vasculitis resembling *isolated angiitis of the CNS* in humans has been reported in a mixed-breed dog. The necrotizing vasculitis, with cuffs of mixed cell types, including multinucleated giant cells, resulted in localized cerebral necrosis.

Further reading

Maiolini A, et al. Interleukin-6, vascular endothelial growth factor and transforming growth factor beta 1 in canine steroid responsive meningitis-arteritis. BMC Vet Res 2013;9:23.

Tipold A, Schatzberg SJ. An update on steroid responsive meningitis-arteritis. J Small Anim Pract 2010;51:150-154.

Shaker dog disease

Shaker dog disease is an idiopathic condition characterized clinically by *tremors* that worsen after stress or excitement. The condition was described first affecting solely young adult white-haired small dogs (little white shakers), but now is recognized in dogs of any size or coat color. A shaker puppy syndrome reported in Cretan hound puppies was caused by a leukoencephalopathy and concurrent parvovirus infection. Histologically, *mild diffuse, nonsuppurative encephalomyelitis* is present. No myelin disease is present.

Further reading

Schaudien D, et al. Leukoencephalopathy associated with parvovirus infection in Cretan hound puppies. J Clin Microbiol 2010;48:3169-3175.

Yamaya Y, et al. A case of shaker dog disease in a miniature Dachshund. J Vet Med Sci 2004;66:1159-1160.

Sensory ganglioneuritis (sensory ganglioradiculitis)

Sensory ganglioneuritis (sensory neuronopathy) is a rare idiopathic disease of adult dogs, characterized by *nonsuppurative inflammation of dorsal root (sensory) spinal ganglia and cranial sensory ganglia*, with degeneration and necrosis of sensory neuronal cell bodies and proliferation of ganglionic satellite cells. The cause may be a cell-mediated immune mechanism. Secondary to sensory ganglion neuronal injury, Wallerian degeneration develops in the dorsal funiculi (fasciculus cuneatus and fasciculus gracilis), and the affected areas appear grossly as white V-shaped or triangular areas throughout the entire length of the spinal cord. Similar but milder lesions can be present in sympathetic ganglia, peripheral nerves, myenteric plexi, motor roots, and the spinal tract of the trigeminal nerve. Breed or sex predilection have not been observed. Clinical signs are variable and include generalized sensory ataxia, depression, or absence of spinal reflexes; facial hypoalgesia/paresthesia; megaesophagus; and dysphagia. Masticatory muscle atrophy is observed in a few dogs in association with this condition and is attributed to loss of motor fibers as they course through the trigeminal ganglion.

Further reading

Funamoto M, et al. Pathological features of ganglioradiculitis (sensory neuropathy) in two dogs. J Vet Med Sci 2007;69:1247-1253.

Postinfectious encephalomyelitis

Neurologic disease that follows, after a variable period, common viral infections or vaccination exposure is well known in children as post-infectious or postvaccinal encephalitis, or acute disseminated encephalomyelitis. The common pathologic basis is a *demyelinating inflammatory process dominated by mononuclear inflammatory cells with a distinctive perivenous distribution*. Examples that meet the criteria have occurred in relation to rabies vaccination in dogs when such vaccines were prepared in neural tissue, and the pathologic process is the same as that in experimental allergic encephalomyelitis. The histologic changes are widely distributed in the brain and cord and affect mainly the white matter. Perivascular infiltrates of lymphocytes, plasma cells, and monocytes/macrophages widely distend the space and spread into the surrounding parenchyma. Proliferation of adventitial cells may be prominent. Although much descriptive emphasis has been given to demyelination, this is restricted to the perivascular areas of infiltration and to surrounding areas showing the usual degenerative and reactive changes.

Further reading

Martella V, et al. Lights and shades on an historical vaccine canine distemper virus, the Rockborn strain. Vaccine 2011;29:1222-1227.

Eosinophilic meningoencephalitis

Recognized causes of eosinophilic meningoencephalitis include nematode and protozoan parasites. **Idiopathic eosinophilic meningoencephalitis** has been reported in dogs, with Rottweilers and Golden Retrievers over-represented, and one cat. The condition is characterized clinically by behavioral changes, such as inappropriate urination and lack of response to commands. In severe cases, episodes of sternal or lateral recumbency without loss of consciousness are described. Clinical pathology findings are mild to moderate peripheral blood eosinophilia and CSF pleocytosis with predominance of eosinophils. Grossly, there is thickening and green discoloration of the meninges. Histologic changes are those of eosinophilic and granulomatous meningitis of the cortex and cerebellum, and the underlying neural parenchyma appears pallid, occasionally spongiotic, and has mild eosinophilic and histiocytic cuffing with rare areas of axonal swelling and neuronal degeneration. Spinal cord lesions are poorly documented. The condition is usually responsive to steroid treatment, suggesting an immune-mediated mechanism.

Further reading

Olivier AK, et al. Idiopathic eosinophilic meningoencephalomyelitis in a Rottweiler dog. J Vet Diagn Invest 2010;22:646-648.

Williams JH, et al. Review of idiopathic eosinophilic meningitis in dogs and cats, with a detailed description of two recent cases in dogs. J S Afr Vet Assoc 2008;79:194-204.

Granulomatous radiculitis of the seventh and eighth cranial nerves of calves

This is a rare condition affecting young calves and characterized clinically by facial paralysis and pathologically by the presence of multifocal granulomas affecting mainly the roots of cranial nerves VII and VIII. The etiology is unknown; however, *Mycoplasma bovis* was suggested as a cause because some affected calves had concurrent mycoplasmal otitis media.

Further reading

Van der Lugt JJ, Jordaan P. Facial paralysis associated with space occupying lesions of cranial nerves in calves. Vet Rec 1994;134: 579-580.

NEOPLASTIC DISEASES OF THE NERVOUS SYSTEM

Primary and secondary neoplastic diseases of the CNS are reported in all domestic animals, but are best characterized in dogs and cats with a reported prevalence of 4.5% and 2.2%, respectively. Neoplasms derived from virtually every cell type in the nervous system are recorded.

The tumors may be *congenital*, and these do not differ in their characteristics from similar tumors in adult animals, with the possible exceptions of *medulloblastoma*, which is thought to be derived from the residual cells of the external granular layer of the cerebellum; *craniopharyngiomas*, which are thought to arise from remnants of Rathke's pouch, which forms the adenohypophysis; *chordoma*, which is thought to arise from remnants of notochord; *intracranial teratoma*, which is probably derived from germ cells; and *cystic epidermoid tumors*, which are thought to result from the inclusion of surface ectodermal cells at the time of closure of the neural groove. The relatively high incidence of primary tumors in Boxers, English Bulldogs, Boston Terriers, and Golden Retrievers may indicate a hereditary predisposition, which these breeds also have for endocrine neoplasia. The introduction of computerized tomography (CT) and magnetic resonance imaging (MRI), in addition to the use of immunohistochemistry, has improved our understanding of CNS tumors in various domestic animals and has helped in reaching more accurate diagnoses. However, up to 26% of neuroectodermal brain tumors are undifferentiated. Neoplasms of the CNS rarely metastasize to extraneural tissue, and their clinical importance depends on their destructive effect on host neural tissue and the resulting neurologic deficits. Generally, primary tumors show a slowly progressive growth pattern, whereas highly malignant and metastatic tumors frequently have a more acute progression.

The conventional tumors of the CNS are discussed here and classified according to the current histologic classification published by the Armed Forces Institute of Pathology (AFIP—as of 2011, the Joint Pathology Center) in cooperation with the World Health Organization (WHO). Tumors of the pituitary and nonchromaffin paraganglia are discussed in Vol. 3 Endocrine system.

Tumors of the meninges

These include the only tumor arising from meningothelial cells, **meningioma,** and those arising from non-meningothelial cells, such as meningeal sarcomatosis, leiomyoma, leiomyosarcoma, and hemangioblastoma.

Meningiomas

Meningioma is the most common type of intracranial tumor in the cat, in which it may be multiple in 17% of cases, and is one of the commonest of the intracranial and intraspinal tumors in man. It is relatively common in dogs (30-50% of intracranial tumors) but very rare in ruminants and horses. It rises within the meninges, usually in close association with the dura, and grows expansively, compressing but seldom invading the brain (Fig. 4-128). Those in humans are presumed, by virtue of their site and structure, to arise from arachnoidal cap cells, which form the outer layer of the arachnoid mater, and the arachnoid villi. A rare variant of meningioma is the **paranasal meningioma** (Fig. 4-129), which arises from meningeal arachnoid cells that are trapped within or outside bone during development of the skull, and is reported in horses and dogs. The meningiomas observed in animals conform in histologic type to those observed in humans.

Meningiomas are globular, ovoid or tuberous, sometimes plaque-like, well circumscribed, and have a smooth surface.

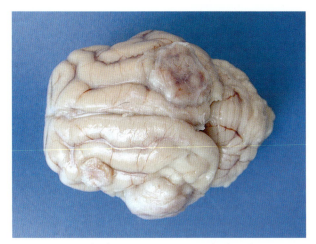

Figure 4-128 Multiple **meningiomas** attached to dura mater in a cat.

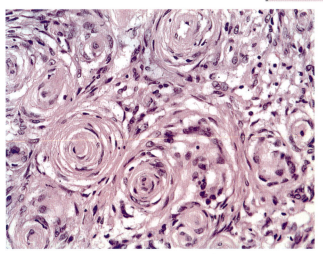

Figure 4-130 Histologic appearance of a **psammomatous meningioma**.

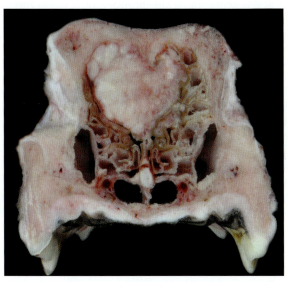

Figure 4-129 Paranasal meningioma in a dog. (Courtesy A. Breithaupt, Institute of Veterinary Pathology, Freie Universität, Berlin.)

They are gray; sometimes yellow, on cut surface; firm; and may be gritty. Feline meningiomas are more easily separated from the brain parenchyma than are the canine ones, which are usually more interdigitated into the brain parenchyma. Common locations include the cerebral convexity and the basilar meninges, and in cats, the tela choroidea of the third ventricle. Meningiomas display both mesenchymal and epithelial-like features showing spindle cell morphology with deposition of collagenous stroma, or polygonal cell morphology with presence of intercellular junctions and occasionally secretory activity.

Canine meningiomas are currently classified following the criteria of the human WHO system (2007). Grade I meningiomas include different histologic subtypes and are classified by their predominant pattern. Meningothelial and transitional subtypes are the most common grade I meningiomas. The **meningotheliomatous** or **epithelioid meningioma** is diffusely cellular with the cells in sheets or lobules of different size, separated by thin collagenous septa. The cells are large with abundant finely granular pale cytoplasm without a distinct margin, and the nuclei are spherical or ovoid, and may show pseudoinclusions formed by intranuclear invaginations of the cytoplasm. The **psammomatous meningioma** has the same general features as the foregoing, but the cells are arranged in whorls (Fig. 4-130). In the center of a whorl, lamellar hyaline tissue forms, derived possibly from cells, stroma, or a blood vessel. As the hyaline focus expands, it tends to be impregnated with salts of calcium and iron to form *psammoma bodies*. The **fibrous** or **fibroblastic meningioma** is similar to fibroblastic tumors elsewhere, showing bundles of spindle cells with collagen deposition. The **transitional** or **mixed type** has features of both epithelioid and fibroblastic meningioma with formation of whorls and psammoma bodies. **Angiomatous** or **angioblastic meningiomas** are highly vascular with prominent endothelial cells in formed vessels and lining vascular clefts. The vessels are surrounded by spindle cells giving a distinct resemblance to hemangiopericytoma. **Microcystic meningioma** is characterized by tumor cells with elongated processes and cytoplasmic and interstitial vacuolation. **Myxoid meningioma** is similar to myxoma elsewhere. There may be some difficulty in separating hemangioma from highly vascular meningiomas; both contain endothelial cells, pericytes, and stromal cells, the latter of uncertain parentage.

Grade II meningiomas include chordoid and atypical subtypes. **Chordoid meningioma** forms cords and trabeculae of eosinophilic epithelioid cells in a basophilic matrix. **Atypical meningiomas** show hypercellularity, necrotic areas, loss of whorls and fascicles, and more than 4 mitotic figures per 10 HPF.

Grade III meningiomas belong to the papillary and anaplastic variants. **Papillary meningiomas** are rare in dogs and composed of meningothelial cells arranged in papillary structures supported by fibrovascular cores. **Anaplastic (malignant) meningiomas** show distinct features of malignancy, including more than 20 mitotic figures per 10 HPF and/or obviously malignant cytologic characteristics such that tumor cells resemble carcinoma, sarcoma, or melanoma.

Granular cell meningiomas resemble granular cell tumors that occur elsewhere. They are included here because they do occur over the cerebral convexity, neurohypophysis, and spinal nerve roots of dogs, and the notion is attractive that some, at least, of the tumors are derived in common with cells of nerve sheaths and other neural crest mesenchyme. The tumors are usually small and well circumscribed but not well encapsulated. The cells are large and rounded; the cytoplasm clear, apart from fine granules that may be few or numerous; and the nuclei small and rounded. The cytoplasmic granules are acidophilic and PAS-positive. Delicate stroma, in which amyloid may be deposited, separates the cells individually or in small groups. Stigmata of anaplasia are absent.

The incidence of canine meningiomas is 56% grade I, 46% grade II, and 1% grade III. Extracranial meningiomas, which occur mainly in the paranasal region and orbit, are anaplastic and locally aggressive. In cats, meningiomas consistently have a uniform histologic pattern, with whorls, collagen deposition, focal mineralization, and cholesterol clefts. They are consistent with grade I tumor. Meningiomas stain positively for vimentin and negative for synaptophysin and glial fibrillary acidic protein (GFAP). Staining for cytokeratin, neuron-specific enolase (NSE), and S-100 usually yield positive results but with sparse to moderate expression. Canine meningiomas of various histologic patterns are frequently immunopositive for CD34 and E-cadherin and have early loss of tumor suppressor genes *NF2*, *4.1B*, and *TSLC1*. Anaplastic meningiomas overexpress doublecortin and nuclear β-catenin.

Meningeal sarcomatosis

Meningeal sarcomatosis is a rare condition reported only in dogs and characterized by diffuse infiltration of the leptomeninges, especially of the lumbar spinal cord, by pleomorphic neoplastic mesenchymal cells. Tumor may extend along the entire cerebrospinal axis from medulla to sacral cord. Neoplastic cells are present usually circumferentially in the subarachnoid space and may invade the subpial parenchyma of the spinal cord and, to a lesser extent, the brain. Individual cells are pleomorphic, where the main neoplastic cells are large irregularly round cells (35-80 μm) with abundant cytoplasm and large round to ovoid hyperchromatic nuclei (20-65 μm). Neoplastic cells usually have a high mitotic rate and up to 3-fold anisokaryosis. In addition, several lymphoid, plasmacytoid, and histiocytic cells are present amid the neoplastic cells. A few multinucleated giant cells and intact neutrophils may also be present. The neoplastic large cells stain positively for vimentin. They usually stain positive, but with sparse to moderate expression, for CD18 and actin. They stain negatively for lymphocyte markers, S-100, cytokeratin, and GFAP.

Tumors of neuroepithelial tissue

Astrocytoma

Astrocytoma is the most common primary intracranial tumor (Fig. 4-131A-E). Astrocytomas are found most commonly in dogs (about 17% of all primary nervous system tumors), but are reported also in cats, cattle, horses, and pigs. They may occur in the brain or spinal cord but are more prevalent in cerebral hemispheres, thalamus, hypothalamus, and midbrain. In dogs, astrocytomas are common in brachycephalic breeds but can occur in any breed. Astrocytomas have no age predilection, but are more prevalent in middle-aged or older dogs. The gross appearance varies, depending largely on the degree of malignancy. Sometimes these tumors can be difficult to detect grossly, especially when they involve white matter or grow slowly. They are gray to white and, because of their firmness, may be more readily palpable than visible. Their presence may be suspected only by deviation of some architectural feature (see Fig. 4-131B, D). Larger and more malignant tumors are prone to vascular accidents and necrosis, and they are then easy to see (see Fig. 4-131E), but the margins are never discrete, especially not when they are surrounded by edematous tissue. The extent of the tumor is always much greater than can be appreciated grossly.

Histologically, these tumors are very diverse and are classified as *low-grade astrocytoma* (well differentiated), *medium-grade astrocytoma* (anaplastic), and *high-grade astrocytoma* (glioblastoma). Most astrocytomas exhibit positive immunostaining for GFAP, nestin, S-100 protein, and vimentin. The staining pattern for GFAP varies from sparse to abundant.

Low-grade astrocytoma (WHO grade I) appears as an unencapsulated expansile and subtly invasive mass that replaces pre-existing tissues and has low to moderate numbers of bland, round to oval cells. In most cases, the neoplasm appears as an increased population of fibrous astrocytes that individually are not clearly malignant (see Fig. 4-131A). Variants of this neoplasm include **fibrillary astrocytoma** (neoplastic cells have scant cytoplasm but abundant fibrillary processes and filaments), **protoplasmic astrocytoma** (neoplastic cells have scant cytoplasm and few short processes and filaments), **pilocytic astrocytoma** (neoplastic cells are bipolar, elongated [piloid or hair-like] astrocytes and have few Rosenthal fibers). The **subependymal giant cell astrocytoma** originates from the subependymal tissue of lateral or fourth ventricles and is composed of spindloid to polygonal large eosinophilic cells arranged in short interlacing streams and irregular nests.

In **medium-grade astrocytoma** (WHO grade II), the population is denser, and the nuclei are a little larger and darker and show slight but definite variations in size and shape but no mitoses. The cells are diffusely infiltrating and recognizable as astrocytes, showing GFAP and vimentin immunoreactivity. The walls of the vessels may be slightly thickened. In **gemistocytic astrocytoma**, neoplastic cells have abundant acidophilic cytoplasm and eccentric oval to round nuclei (see Fig. 4-128C).

Anaplastic astrocytomas (WHO grade III) show nuclear atypia, mitotic figures, and high proliferative index.

In **high-grade astrocytoma** (WHO IV grade), or *glioblastoma* (formerly glioblastoma multiforme), hemorrhage and necrosis are expected, and the adventitial and endothelial cells of the vessels proliferate, forming glomeruloid blood vessels. Generally, only a few cells are recognizable as astrocytes. Neoplastic cells have a tendency for pseudopalisading around necrotic areas. Pleomorphism, giant nuclei, and multinucleated giant cells are common. Mitotic figures are common and atypical. Canine glioblastomas overexpress epidermal growth factor receptor (EGFR), platelet-derived growth factor-α (PDGFR-α), and insulin-like growth factor binding protein 2 (IGFBP-2).

Rare variants reported in dogs include astroblastoma, giant cell glioblastoma, gliosarcoma, and **gliomatosis cerebri**. This latter form is a diffuse infiltrating disease of dogs, predominantly of brachycephalic breeds, and humans, characterized by an *infiltrative cell type reminiscent of astrocytes* rather than by the formation of a distinct tumor mass. The infiltrates involve the brain, often bilaterally but asymmetrically, with discontinuous areas also in the spinal cord. There is no tumor "mass," rather diffuse enlargement of affected regions, the cells insinuate among normal structures that remain intact with only slight damage to axons and neurons. Where the infiltrates

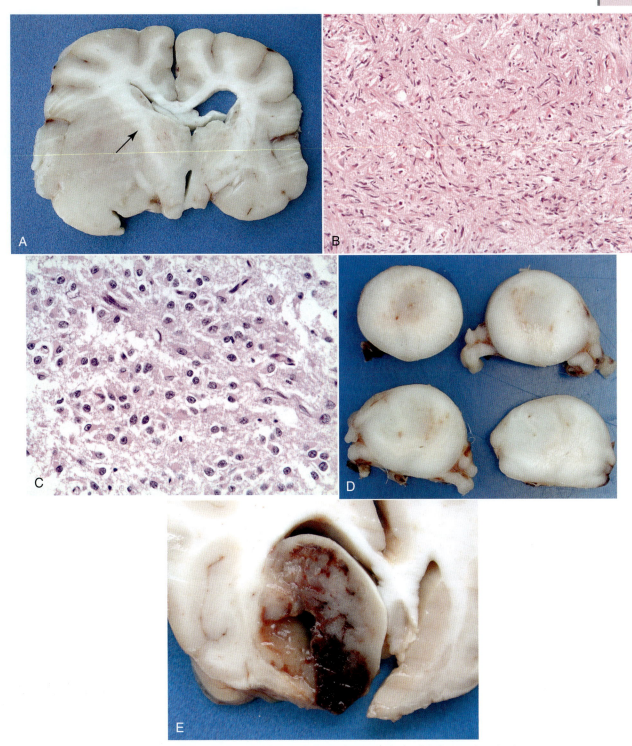

Figure 4-131 A. Astrocytoma in piriform lobe in a dog. Note lack of definition but displacement of internal capsule (arrow) by the homogeneous tumor. **B. Fibrous astrocytoma** in a dog. **C. Gemistocytic astrocytoma** in a dog. **D. Astrocytoma** of spinal cord in a dog. **E. Hemorrhagic astrocytoma** of basal nuclei area in a dog.

involve the molecular layer of the cerebrum or the deep white matter, they spread in veils on leptomeninges and ependyma. Gliomatosis cerebri is composed mainly of cells reminiscent of fibrillary astrocytic cells with elongated and hyperchromatic nuclei, but there are also oligodendrocytes, cells of transitional character, and small unclassified cells (Fig. 4-132). The origin of the neoplastic cells in the canine cases is still controversial, as they do not stain with glial markers such as GFAP. The pattern of infiltration is unexplained, but involves participation of cell adhesion molecules.

Gliosarcoma is a rare tumor composed of highly anaplastic glial cells with abundant sarcomatous components. Positive GFAP staining should differentiate this tumor from other spindle cell tumors, for example, fibrosarcoma.

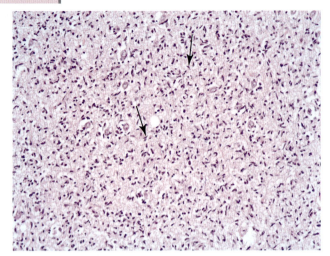

Figure 4-132 Gliomatosis cerebri appears as an increase in the cellularity of cerebrocortical white matter resulting from diffuse infiltration of neoplastic cells (arrows) that do not form a discrete mass or efface the pre-existing tissue (Boxer dog).

Oligodendroglioma

This is the easiest of the glial tumors to recognize even when growing rapidly. This tumor is reported in dogs, especially in brachycephalic breeds and rarely in cats, cattle, and horses. Grossly, it usually appears well demarcated, being gray, translucent, soft, and almost fluctuating (Fig. 4-133A). Most commonly, it arises in the frontal, olfactory, temporal, and piriform lobes. The tumor is densely cellular with almost no stroma. The nuclei are remarkably uniform and like those of normal oligodendroglia in size and shape. The cytoplasm does not stain, but its membrane does, so that the nucleus seems to lie in a clear polyhedral or rounded halo (honeycomb cell pattern) (Fig. 4-133B). These tumors occur in white matter, and those near the third ventricle may contain areas distinguishable as astrocytoma or ependymoma. Blood vessels may proliferate, especially at neoplasm margins to form glomeruli-like vessels. Mucinous degeneration and cyst formation may occur in these tumors and mineralization may occur in some of them. In the **anaplastic variant** (WHO grade III), there are multifocal hemorrhagic and necrotic areas, prominent neovascularization, nuclear atypia, and CSF dissemination of the neoplastic cells. A diffuse subarachnoid dissemination of the entire spinal cord and brainstem, analogous to human *leptomeningeal oligodendrogliomatosis*, has been described in dogs. Oligodendrogliomas are consistently immunoreactive to Olig2 and do not stain with GFAP; however, the neoplastic cells are usually intermingled with some astrocytes that readily stain with GFAP.

Oligoastrocytoma (mixed glial tumor)

This glial neoplasm is composed of both neoplastic astrocytes and oligodendroglia.

Ependymoma

Ependymomas are neuroglial tumors derived from the ependymal lining cells of the ventricles and central canal of the spinal cord. Most arise about the third ventricle. They are gray and fleshy but may be dark from hemorrhage if they project into a ventricle. They are more prevalent in dogs (2% of all neuroepithelial tumors), but are reported in cats, horses, and cattle.

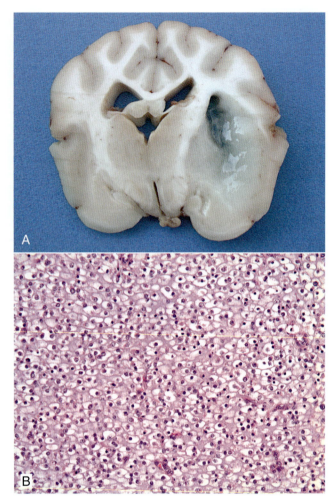

Figure 4-133 A. Oligodendroglioma involving right side of cerebral hemisphere and piriform lobe in a dog. **B.** Histologic pattern of oligodendroglioma.

The tumors are usually densely cellular, and those arising about the third ventricle may be difficult to distinguish from undifferentiated pituitary tumors. The nuclei are small, dark, and regular, and the cytoplasm has no distinct boundaries. Pseudorosettes form around blood vessels (Fig. 4-134), and are characterized by a GFAP immunoreactive perivascular nuclear-free zone. True rosettes are also present and appear as tubular cavities lined by cells of epithelial appearance. The cells forming true rosettes are bound together by desmosomes, have basally located nuclei, and have surface cilia anchoring phosphotungstic acid hematoxylin (PTAH)-positive blepharoplasts. A **papillary variant** does exist and is characterized by branching papillary stroma covered by recognizable, usually ciliated, ependymal cells. Ependymomas of the spinal cord may be more papilliferous than those in the brain, with tumor cells attached to fronds that are supported by a delicate stroma and embedded in mucinous intercellular stroma. A **clear cell variant** resembling oligodendroglioma is occasionally reported in dogs and cats. Myxopapillary, tanycytic, extraventricular ependymomas, and subependymomas are also reported. **Malignant ependymoma** (WHO grade III) is characterized by increased cellular atypia and mitoses.

Most canine ependymomas stain negatively for GFAP; however, feline and equine cases are reported to stain positively for this marker. Most ependymomas show slight positive

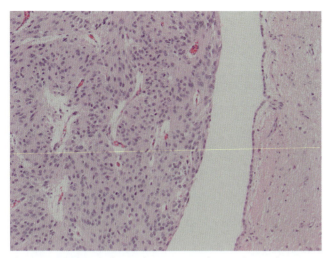

Figure 4-134 Typical pseudorosettes and true rosette formation in an **ependymoma** in a dog.

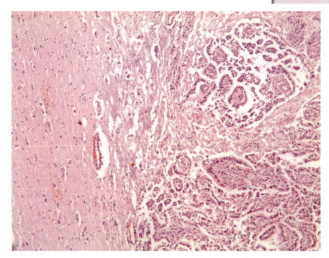

Figure 4-136 Invasion into the periventricular white matter of a dog by a **choroid plexus carcinoma**.

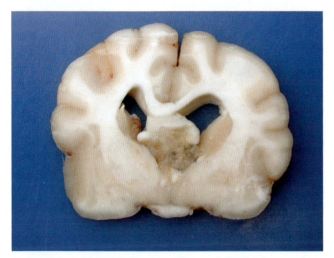

Figure 4-135 **Choroid plexus papilloma** of the third ventricle in a dog.

staining for vimentin and cytokeratin. Human ependymomas stain strongly with anti–epithelial membrane antigen antibody (EMA); however, information about immunoreactivity of domestic animal ependymomas to EMA is not available.

Choroid plexus tumors

This is rare, reported in cats, horses, and cattle, and occurs with higher frequency in dogs comprising 7-10% of all primary tumors of the CNS. The tumor can be located in the lateral ventricles, the third ventricle (Fig. 4-135), but more frequently in the fourth ventricle. The mass has a red-gray lobular or granular appearance and is often associated to secondary obstructive hydrocephalus. Histologically, choroid plexus papilloma (WHO grade I) has branched papillary structures lined by cuboidal or columnar epithelial cells arranged in a single layer, with a rich stroma of connective tissue and blood vessels (Fig. 4-136). There is frequent mineralization and formation of psammoma bodies. According to cellular atypia, local brain invasiveness, and dissemination to the brain and spinal cord subarachnoid space, the tumor can be classified as carcinoma (WHO grade III). Choroid plexus tumors express epithelial markers, for example, cytokeratin AE1/AE3, and focally GFAP.

Neuronal and mixed neuronal-glial tumors

These tumors of adult animals are composed of neurons and/or neurons admixed with glial cells.

Olfactory neuroblastomas (esthesioneuroblastoma). This rare malignant tumor arises from primitive neurosensory cells present in the olfactory mucosa. They are uncommon but have been identified in various animal species, mainly dogs and cats. The olfactory epithelium is unique among neuronal structures in that the basal cells retain the ability to divide and differentiate to become sustentacular cells or bipolar neurosensory cells. The tumors are locally aggressive and may penetrate the cribriform plate. The dense cellular population is homogeneous, arranged in sheets or clusters but also forming true and pseudorosettes (Flexner-type rosettes and Homer-Wright–type pseudorosettes). They may be palisaded on trabeculae, oval in shape with scant cytoplasm. Cytoplasmic processes may form an abundant, delicate fibrillary matrix. The detection of type C retroviral particles identified with feline leukemia in spontaneous olfactory neuroblastomas of cats is of interest. Neoplastic cells stain with different degrees of reactivity for both neuronal and epithelial immunohistochemical markers, for example, NSE and cytokeratin, respectively. Cells also express microtubule-associated protein-2 (MAP-2).

Gangliocytomas. These are extremely rare tumors that are reported in dogs, a cow, and a horse. They appear to have a predilection for the thalamus. The tumor is composed of cells reminiscent of large ganglion cells or mature pyramidal cells. Neoplastic cells do not stain with glial markers but show different reactivity with neuronal markers, such as NSE, synaptophysin, neuron-specific nuclear protein (NeuN), and neurofilaments.

Ganglioglioma. This is another rare bicellular tumor composed of neoplastic neuronal cells and neoplastic astrocytic cells. They have the same immunohistochemical staining pattern as gangliocytomas, but the astrocytic cells stain with GFAP.

Embryonal tumors

These tumors arise from primitive or progenitor cells present in the nervous system and are capable of differentiating into different lineages, including glial or neuronal cell lines.

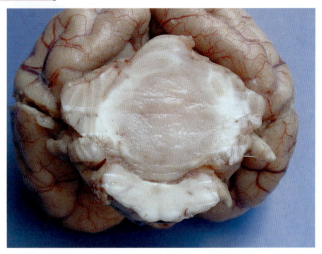

Figure 4-137 Medulloblastoma of the cerebellar vermis in a dog. (Reprinted with permission from Mandara MT, et al. Neuropatologia e Neuroimaging. Milano: Poletto Editore, 2011.)

Medulloblastoma (cerebellar primitive neuroectodermal tumor). Medulloblastoma, well-known in children, is rare in animals, but occurs in the young of several species (Fig. 4-137), mainly calves and dogs. There is no such cell as a "medulloblast," the name invented for this tumor of unknown parentage. It is currently thought to arise from undifferentiated cells found in neonatal life beneath the cerebellar pia mater and thought to be the precursors of the cerebellar cortex. These tumors grow rapidly and are usually located in the cerebellar vermis. Histologically, they are densely cellular with scant stroma and few vessels (Fig. 4-138A). The cells are small and classically "carrot shaped" with oval or elongate nuclei and the cytoplasm tapering at one pole. They are also supposed to produce small perivascular palisades and pseudorosettes (Fig. 4-138B). These classic features are not always present, and then there is nothing by which this tumor can be identified except its location in the cerebellum. The term medulloblastoma should be limited to those embryonal tumors originating in the cerebellum. Tumors of this histologic appearance in other sites in the brain of calves or other species are called *primitive neuroectodermal tumor*, not medulloblastoma. Medulloblastomas stain positively for different neuronal markers, including NSE and synaptophysin, and some show positive staining for GFAP.

Neuroblastomas. These tumors are rare and occur in any part of the CNS. Histologic criteria to distinguish them from other cellular neurogenic tumors are not satisfactory and identification must depend on other means. They are thought to arise from primitive neuroepithelial cells with differentiation toward postmitotic neuroblasts. The histologic appearances are similar to those of medulloblastoma, consisting of masses of small rounded cells that resemble lymphocytes, with hyperchromatic nuclei and scant cytoplasm. The presence of rosettes and pseudorosettes is helpful. Neoplastic cells stain positively with neuronal markers and negatively with glial markers such as GFAP.

Thoracolumbar spinal tumor of young dogs (spinal nephroblastoma). These are single intradural extramedullary or intramedullary masses occurring between the tenth thoracic and second lumbar segments in young, large-breed dogs. Affected animals are presented with signs of cord compres-

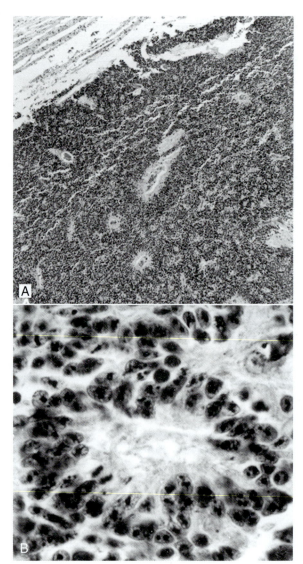

Figure 4-138 Histologic patterns of **medulloblastoma** in a calf. Pseudorosettes are visible in (**A**) and are detailed in (**B**), as circular groupings of dark tumor cells around a central pale area containing neurofibrils. (Courtesy M.D. McGavin.)

sion. The tumor likely originates from the renal primordium, a renal ectopic embryonic remnant from which diverse nephron cell types are derived, present at this area. For this reason, this tumor can be regarded as a non-neuroepithelial ectopic embryonal tumor. The histologic appearance is of glandular areas intermingling with cellular areas. The glandular areas consist of rosettes and tubules, the latter tortuous, branching, and sometimes papilliferous, with infoldings reminiscent of embryonic glomerular capsules (Fig. 4-139). The cellular areas contain densely packed cells of blastema appearance with ovoid clear nuclei and indistinct cytoplasm. Some streaming is evident, but muscle fibers are not present. In some of these tumors, glomerular structures can be recognized with confidence as can tubular cross-sections strongly suggestive of distal renal tubules. Presumably, these tumors arise from ectopic embryonic remnants, but notably the kidneys do not contain neoplasm, although nephroblastomas are well recognized in dogs. From time to time, undifferentiated tumors of embryonic type and possibly derived from remnants of pronephros are seen in the cervical region of dogs and sheep.

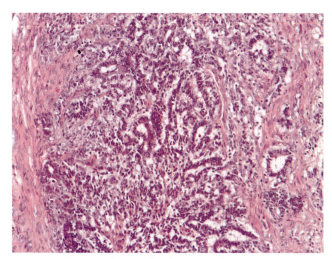

Figure 4-139 Neoplastic cells showing tubular structures with infoldings in **spinal nephroblastoma** in a dog.

These tumors stain positive for cytokeratin and negative for glial and neuronal markers.

Pineal tumors

These tumors are extremely rare. The benign variant is called *pineocytoma*, and the malignant variant is called *pineoblastoma*. They are described in horses, cattle, and dogs. The diagnosis is based on the site of the tumor and its replacement of the pineal body. Other positive identifying characteristics are absent. Microscopically, there is a resemblance to medulloblastoma. The tumor may extend into midbrain and thalamus. Teratomatous tumors with characteristics of the gonadal teratomas are not described in the pineal gland of animals. Specific markers for tumors in animals are not reported.

Hematopoietic tumors

Hematopoietic tumors, such as lymphosarcoma, multiple myeloma, and histiocytic sarcoma, that originate in extraneural locations can metastasize to the CNS as part of their multisystemic metastasis; however, in the following section, we will describe those hematopoietic tumors that originate primarily in the CNS. The use of a panel of cell-specific antibodies is often necessary for diagnostic immunohistochemical confirmation of these tumors.

Lymphoma/lymphosarcoma

Primary CNS lymphomas are reported mainly in cats and dogs and sporadically in ruminants. They are mostly intraparenchymal and have an angiocentric (perivascular) pattern in contrast to lymphosarcomas metastatic from extraneural areas that are usually arranged diffusely in the meninges. Most primary CNS lymphomas in dogs are of B-cell type, whereas T- and B-cell phenotypes are more frequent in feline lymphoma. Histologically, they follow the same morphology as extraneural lymphomas/lymphosarcomas. Variants include **intravascular lymphoma,** which is characterized by massive proliferation of lymphoblasts within the lumen of small vessels, causing thrombosis and hemorrhagic infarction of the nervous tissue.

Plasma cell tumor

A primary intracerebral intraparenchymal plasma cell tumor has been reported in a dog. An identical tumor was reported in a cat, but the diagnosis of primary neural plasma cell tumor was not confirmed because of an incomplete postmortem examination.

Histiocytic sarcoma (malignant histiocytosis)

Primary histiocytic sarcoma of the CNS occurs in some canine breeds, including the Bernese Mountain dog and Golden Retriever. The tumor is characterized by marked infiltration and destruction of the neuroparenchyma by extremely pleomorphic large cells, often multinucleated, and with abundant cytoplasm. Atypical mitoses are commonly observed. Neoplastic cells stain positively for lysozyme and vimentin.

Non-B, non-T leukocytic neoplasm (neoplastic reticulosis)

This controversial malignant neoplasm has a histologic resemblance to canine granulomatous meningoencephalitis (GME). The term "reticulosis" came into use because of aggregation of reticular fibers around neoplastic cells. Many cases diagnosed previously as reticulosis have been reclassified as lymphoma and a few as histiocytic tumors. The tumor may be single or multiple and can occur in any part of the CNS but is more prevalent in the cerebral white matter. The exact histogenesis of the neoplastic cells is yet to be determined; however, the neoplasm is composed histologically of angiocentric large (25-50 µm) round cells reminiscent of histiocytes and numerous non-neoplastic lymphocytes and macrophages. Multinucleated giant cells may predominate. Neoplastic cells usually show atypia and a moderate mitotic rate. The neoplastic cells stain positively with CD18 and negatively for lymphocyte markers, proving a leukocytic but nonlymphoid origin. The neoplasm has been reported in dogs and rarely in cats, cattle, and horses. The differentiation between neoplastic reticulosis and GME (formerly called inflammatory reticulosis) is difficult. The predominance of neoplastic histiocytic-like cells, cellular atypia, and high mitotic rate should favor the diagnosis of neoplastic reticulosis.

Microgliomatosis

The histogenic origin of the neoplastic cell in this rare neoplasm is controversial. The neoplasm diffusely infiltrates the cerebral white matter and brainstem with cells reminiscent of microglial cells. The infiltration, in some cases, can be limited to meninges or can be perivascular. In any case, this is a non–mass-forming neoplasm, and the brain is almost unremarkable grossly. The neoplastic cells do not cause significant destruction of the pre-existing tissue. Neoplastic cells stain negatively for GFAP. There is strong overlap between microgliomatosis and gliomatosis cerebri. In human microgliomatosis, most neoplastic cells stain for CD18 and other monocyte/macrophage lineage markers. Similar studies on the immunohistochemical markers expressed by canine microgliomatosis are not available.

Tumors of the sellar region

Common tumors of the sellar region are pituitary adenomas and carcinomas. They usually compress and extend to the hypothalamic region. Pituitary tumors are discussed in Vol. 3, Endocrine glands.

Suprasellar germ cell tumors

Germ cell tumors are presumed to arise from ectopic embryonic germ cells which, intended for the developing gonad, may become widely distributed. They are responsible for a spectrum of tumors in humans, usually in the midline and according to histologic features designated as *seminoma, choriocarcinoma, entodermal sinus tumor,* and *teratoma.* They are revealed early in life, and the preferred locations in the cranial cavity are in the pineal region or in the hypothalamus above the sella. These are rare tumors in dogs. Their location and growth pattern is similar to that of pituitary adenomas, and some may be misdiagnosed as craniopharyngioma.

The reported canine cases in Doberman and Rottweiler were suprasellar and classified on the basis of location, admixture of distinct cell types and patterns, and positive immunochemical staining for α-fetoprotein. Sheets and nests of cells resembling seminoma were admixed with areas of vacuolated hepatoid cells, glandular formations similar to those in gonadal teratomas, and occasional foci of squamous epithelium.

Craniopharyngioma

Craniopharyngiomas are thought to arise from remnants of Rathke's pouch, which forms the adenohypophysis. Aberrant differentiation of Rathke's epithelium is common in dogs, expressed in cystic structures lined by respiratory-type epithelium. The craniopharyngioma, in contrast, consists of clumps of epithelial cells palisaded on collagenous stroma. Keratinization may be present to form pearls, as in well-differentiated squamous carcinoma. Degenerative foci contain cholesterol crystals and blood pigments. Neoplastic cells are positive for cytokeratin.

Other primary tumors and cysts
Epidermoid cysts

Epidermoid cysts in the brain are confined to the fourth ventricle and environs. They are rare, probably represent surface ectoderm misplaced at the period of closure of the neural groove, and are described only in humans, dogs, a horse, and a kitten. The cystic structure is lined by squamous epithelium, and the cavities contain keratinaceous debris. In young dogs, they may develop to several centimeters in diameter. The clinical signs are determined by the location of the tumor.

Hamartoma or meningioangiomatosis

Hamartoma or meningioangiomatosis is a rare benign lesion, best regarded as a malformation or hamartoma producing circumscribed plaques on the surface of the brainstem and cervical spinal cord. Blood vessels are in excess in the lesions and are cuffed by proliferating cells that are considered to be meningothelial. The lesion does extend into the underlying neural substance, which shows mixed degenerative and reactive changes.

Metastatic tumors

Secondary tumors can frequently metastasize from extraneural tissue to the CNS. The most common examples include canine hemangiosarcoma (29% of metastatic tumors), histiocytic sarcoma, carcinoma (12%, including mammary, lung, and thyroid), lymphoma (12%), and malignant melanoma of dogs and rarely other species. Metastases retain the histologic characteristics of the primary tumor and are typically well demarcated and distinct from the adjacent nervous tissue that often shows vascular and degenerative changes.

Leptomeningeal carcinomatosis consists of a focal, multifocal, or diffuse infiltration of the leptomeninges of the brain or spinal cord, or both, by malignant cells originating from an extraneural solid tumor. Intestinal, mammary, and cutaneous squamous cell carcinomas comprise the majority of solid tumors spreading to the leptomeninges in dogs and cats.

Tumors affecting the CNS by extension or impingement

There are several tumors that do not arise directly from the CNS, but arise from structures adjacent to the CNS and sometimes impinge on the CNS, for example, vertebral osteosarcomas, nasal carcinomas, and chordomas.

Chordoma

Chordomas are rare tumors in animals, with the exception of mink and European ferrets. In ferrets, they are usually present at the tip of the tail. In humans, dogs, and cats, they are slow-growing persistent tumors mainly of the sacrococcygeal region, with some occurring in paraspinal and cranial regions. On the basis of histologic characters, *the tumor is presumed to arise from notochordal remnants.* Grossly, they are gelatinous, gray, friable, and lobulated. Histologically, the lobules are not encapsulated but are well defined by bands of connective tissue. The principal cell types (physaliferous cells) are large, clear, and vacuolated, with a botanical appearance and some resemblance to cartilage (Fig. 4-140). The cytoplasm contains large clear vacuoles with distinct boundaries. At the periphery of the lobules, there are smaller, stellate cells with eosinophilic cytoplasm; mitotic figures are rare in these, but they may be the germinative cells. There may be islands of bone or cartilage. Mucinous substance can be demonstrated in the cytoplasmic vacuoles of the larger cells and between the cells; the smaller peripheral cells may contain PAS-positive granules. Differentiation from mucinous chondrosarcoma can be difficult without assistance of immunochemical methods. Chordomas will stain immunohistochemically for cytokeratin, but chondrosarcomas will not. Chordomas also stain positively for vimentin and S-100.

Tumors of the peripheral nervous system
Peripheral nerve sheath tumors

Tumors of the peripheral nerves can originate from Schwann cells, fibroblasts, or perineural cells. They are rare in most

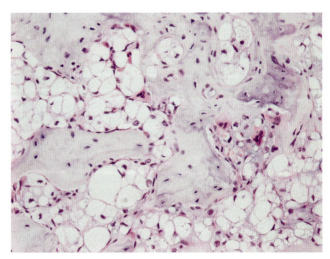

Figure 4-140 A **chordoma** in the tail of a ferret is composed of large, clear vacuolated principal cells (physaliferous cells) in association with chondro-osteoid metaplasia.

domestic animals, except for dogs and cattle. Tumors include the *benign forms* (schwannoma, neurofibroma, perineurioma) or the *malignant form* (malignant peripheral nerve sheath tumor).

Schwannomas may be largely solitary infiltrating lesions at any site on a nerve trunk. Those distant from the CNS are not encapsulated or well defined, are difficult to dissect cleanly, and have an ordinary fibrous appearance and texture. Schwannomas of nerve roots tend to be well-defined fusiform tumors. They probably arise from a single nerve and extend proximally and distally in conjunction with the nerve but external to it. In this way, they may extend through the intervertebral foraminae and extend also to involve other nerves that have a plexus arrangement, such as the brachial plexus. They may arise within and remain within the dura mater, and such tumors may be globose rather than fusiform and soft and discolored from hemorrhage. Expansive intradural growth may be slow and compress the brain or cord. Any cranial or spinal nerve root may be the site of growth, but in the dog, in which they are not rare, the brachial plexus is most frequently involved. In the thoracic region and on the acoustic or trigeminal nerve, the tumors tend to originate within the dura.

The histologic appearance of schwannoma is characterized by 2 dominant patterns referred to as Antoni A and Antoni B. *Antoni A arrangements* are repetitive and give the tumor its character. Uniform, fusiform cells are arranged as bands, herring bones, whorls, or palisades (Verocay bodies) (Fig. 4-141A). *Antoni B tissue* is degenerative and may predominate in some sections. It is loose and myxoid, sometimes hyalinized and may be sparsely cellular (Fig. 4-141B). Microcysts may be present in areas of myxoid change. Cartilaginous and osseous metaplasia occur infrequently. Blood vessels are often prominent but ill formed. The basal lamina bordering each neoplastic Schwann cell is immunoreactive to laminin and collagen IV.

Neurofibroma is composed of a mixed population of neoplastic cells, including Schwann cells, perineural cells, and fibroblasts within variable amounts of collagen fibers and mucoid matrix. The nuclei of the neoplastic cells are typically oval or fusiform, often curved, and generally smaller than those of schwannoma. **Neurofibromatosis** of cattle is a multicentric form of schwannoma. It is common in abattoir material from old animals but has been observed in very young calves. The skin may be affected, but the lesions are usually restricted to deeper nerves of the thoracic wall and viscera. The brachial plexus, intercostal nerves, hepatic autonomic plexus, epicardial plexus, and autonomic nerves of the mediastinum are those most frequently affected in various collective patterns. Sympathetic ganglia, especially the stellate and others of the thorax, are also frequently involved. Affected nerves are thickened, firm, and gray, and may bear yellow-gray nodules. Affected ganglia may be enlarged to several centimeters and appear lobulated on section.

Perineurioma is a rare canine peripheral nerve sheath tumor composed of neoplastic spindle cells arranged in concentric patterns around a central, variably myelinated axon. The cells are immunoreactive for laminin.

The malignant variant (**malignant peripheral nerve sheath tumor**) (Fig. 4-142) is more invasive grossly and occasionally metastasizes to the lung and other organs. The tumors consist of closely packed cells with oval or elongate nuclei that give an impression of interlacing streams not supported or guided

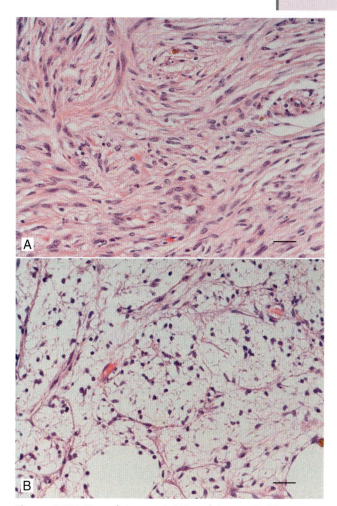

Figure 4-141 Typical Antoni A (**A**) and Antoni B (**B**) patterns in a **schwannoma** of a dog. (Courtesy W. Bergmann, Utrecht University.)

by reticulin or collagen. Frequently, they invade the surrounding tissue. The neoplastic cells stain strongly for vimentin and usually stain positively but with variable intensity with S-100, GFAP, nerve growth factor receptor, and myoglobin. They stain negatively with α–smooth muscle actin, which stains hemangiopericytoma and rhabdomyosarcoma positively.

Peripheral neuroblastic tumors

These rare tumors include **peripheral neuroblastoma, ganglioneuroma,** and **ganglioneuroblastoma.** These subtypes originate from the cranial and spinal ganglia and from sympathetic ganglia of the autonomic nervous system and reflect a spectrum of differentiation of progenitor cells, ranging from tumors with predominant undifferentiated neuroblasts to those consisting of quite differentiated neuronal cell bodies. They have been reported in cats, pigs, cattle, dogs, and horses. They can be solitary or multicentric. In the more primitive form, neuroblastoma, the tumor is composed of sheets of round to oval cells with scant cytoplasm, round hyperchromatic nuclei with finely stippled chromatin, and indistinct nucleoli. True rosettes (Homer-Wright) or pseudorosettes are observed. The few ganglioneuromas observed in cattle have developed in relation to the abdominal sympathetic plexuses. Ganglioneuroma is composed of ganglion cells and glial cells. Ganglioneuroblastoma is composed of poorly to fairly well

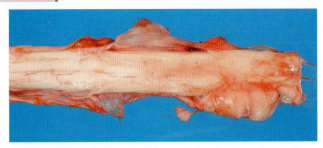

Figure 4-142 Malignant spinal nerve sheath tumor (**neurofibrosarcoma**) in a dog. (Courtesy J.L. Caswell.)

differentiated ganglion cells with more atypia and high nuclear-to-cytoplasmic ratio. The degree of differentiation of these tumors varies considerably, and they are a mixture of ganglion cells, Schwann cells, and nerve fibers. The ganglion cells show different degrees of differentiation from primitive neuroblasts to some that are remarkably mature.

Paraganglioma

This rare neuroendocrine tumor originates from extra-adrenal paraganglion chief cells associated with autonomic nervous system ganglia. The histologic picture resembles chemodectoma described in Vol. 3, Cardiovascular system. The neoplastic cells stain positive for neuroendocrine markers, such as synaptophysin and chromogranin.

Further reading

Brewer DM, et al. Spinal cord nephroblastoma in dogs: 11 cases (1985-2007). J Am Vet Med Assoc 2011;238:618-624.

Brosinski K, et al. Olfactory neuroblastoma in dogs and cats—a histological and immunohistochemical analysis. J Comp Pathol 2012;146:152-159.

Dickinson PJ, et al. Expression of the tumor suppressor genes *NF2, 4.1B,* and *TSLC1* in canine meningiomas. Vet Pathol 2009;46:884-892.

Higgins RJ, et al. Spontaneous canine gliomas: overexpression of EGFR, PDGFRα and IGFBP2 demonstrated by tissue microarray immunophenotyping. J Neurooncol 2010;98:49-55.

Ide T, et al. Immunohistochemical characterization of canine neuroepithelial tumors. Vet Pathol 2010;47:741-750.

Ide T, et al. Expression of cell adhesion molecules and doublecortin in canine anaplastic meningiomas. Vet Pathol 2011;48:292-301.

Louis DN, et al. The 2007 WHO classification of tumours of the central nervous system. Acta Neuropathol (Berl) 2007;114:97-109.

Kovi RC, et al. Spinal meningeal oligodendrogliomatosis in two Boxer dogs. Vet Pathol 2013;50:761-764.

Petersen SA, et al. Canine intraspinal meningiomas: imaging features, histopathologic classification, and long-term outcome in 34 dogs. J Vet Intern Med 2008;22:946-953.

Ramos-Vara JA, et al. Immunohistochemical detection of CD34, E-cadherin, claudin-1, glucose transporter 1, laminin, and protein gene product 9.5 in 28 canine and 8 feline meningiomas. Vet Pathol 2010;47:725-737.

Snyder JM, et al. Canine intracranial primary neoplasia: 173 cases (1986-2003). J Vet Intern Med 2006;20:669-675.

Snyder JM, et al. Secondary intracranial neoplasia in the dog: 177 cases (1986-2003). J Vet Intern Med 2008;22:172-177.

Song RB, et al. Postmortem evaluation of 435 cases of intracranial neoplasia in dogs and relationship of neoplasm with breed, age, and body weight. J Vet Intern Med 2013;27:1143-1152.

Stoica G, et al. Canine astrocytic tumors: a comparative review. Vet Pathol 2011;48:266-275.

Sturges BK, et al. Magnetic resonance imaging and histological classification of intracranial meningiomas in 112 dogs. J Vet Intern Med 2008;22:586-595.

Westworth DR, et al. Choroid plexus tumors in 56 dogs (1985-2007). J Vet Intern Med 2008;22:1157-1165.

Woolford L, et al. Ventricular and extraventricular ependymal tumors in 18 cats. Vet Pathol 2013;50:243-251.

 For more information, please visit the companion site: PathologyofDomesticAnimals.com.

CHAPTER 5

Special Senses

Brian P. Wilcock • Bradley L. Njaa

EYE	**408**
GENERAL CONSIDERATIONS	408
Ocular fixation	408
DEVELOPMENTAL ANOMALIES	409
Review of early ocular organogenesis	409
Defective organogenesis	410
Anophthalmos and microphthalmos	410
Cyclopia and synophthalmos	410
Cystic eye and retinal nonattachment	411
Coloboma	412
Defective differentiation	413
Anomalies of mesenchyme	413
Defects primarily in anterior chamber mesenchyme	415
Incomplete atrophy of posterior segment mesenchyme	417
Anomalies of neuroectoderm	419
Anomalies of surface ectoderm	421
Ocular adnexa	423
Eyelids	423
Lacrimal system	423
Conjunctiva	424
CORNEA	427
Corneal edema	428
Corneal cutaneous metaplasia	429
Corneal wound healing	429
Corneal dystrophies and deposits	433
Corneal lipid and crystalline dystrophies	433
Corneal deposits secondary to metabolic disease	433
Corneal deposits secondary to injury	434
Corneal degeneration	434
Keratitis	436
Pannus keratitis	438
Herpetic keratitis of cats	438
Feline eosinophilic keratitis	438
Mycotic keratitis	439
Infectious bovine keratoconjunctivitis	440
Infectious keratoconjunctivitis (contagious ophthalmia, pinkeye) of sheep and goats	440
LENS	441
Ectopia lentis	441
Cataract	442
UVEA	445
Uveitis	446
The vocabulary of uveitis	446
The significance of uveitis	447
The histologic classification of uveitis	448
Bacterial endophthalmitis	449
Mycotic endophthalmitis	449
Protozoal endophthalmitis	451
Parasitic endophthalmitis	451
Viral endophthalmitis	452
Canine adenovirus	452
Feline infectious peritonitis–associated uveitis	453
Bovine malignant catarrhal fever–associated uveitis	453
Idiopathic immune-mediated uveitis	453
Equine recurrent ophthalmitis (periodic ophthalmia)	455
Idiopathic lymphonodular uveitis of cats	456
Idiopathic lymphocytic uveitis in dogs	456
Uveodermatologic syndrome in dogs (Vogt-Koyanagi-Harada syndrome)	456
Lens-induced uveitis	457
Glaucoma	459
The histologic lesions of glaucoma	460
Lesions causing glaucoma	462
RETINA	465
Overview of retinal histopathology	467
Retinal separation	467
Retinal degeneration	468
Inherited photoreceptor dysplasias and degenerations in dogs	469
Other examples of inherited photoreceptor degenerations and dysplasias	469
Inherited retinal degeneration and dysplasia in cats	469
Noninherited retinal degenerations	470
Light-induced retinal degeneration	470
Nutritional retinopathy	470
Hypovitaminosis A	470
Taurine-deficiency retinopathy	471
Toxic retinopathies	471
Miscellaneous retinopathies	472
Retinitis	474
OPTIC NERVE	475
SCLERA	476
ORBIT	477
OCULAR NEOPLASIA	478
Eyelid and conjunctival neoplasms	479
Squamous cell carcinoma	479
Meibomian adenoma	480
Other adnexal and conjunctival tumors	481
Melanotic tumors of the eye	482
Tumors of ocular neuroectoderm	485
Other primary intraocular tumors	486
Feline post-traumatic sarcoma	486
Spindle cell tumor of blue-eyed dogs	486
Optic nerve tumors	487
Primary orbital neoplasms	487
Tumors metastatic within the globe and orbit	488
EAR	**488**
GENERAL CONSIDERATIONS	488
INTERNAL EAR	488
Hearing and the internal ear	491
Hearing impairment	491
Congenital hearing impairment	491
Acquired deafness	493
Traumatic causes of deafness	493
Internal ear neoplasia	404
Peripheral vestibular disease	494
Horner and Pourfour du Petit syndromes	494
MIDDLE EAR	495
Hearing and the middle ear	496
Developmental disease of the middle ear	496
Otitis media	496
Middle ear parasites	498
Non-neoplastic and neoplastic disease	498

Inflammatory aural polyps	498	External ear parasitism	505
Tympanokeratoma (cholesteatoma)	499	Otoacariasis	505
Mucoperiosteal exostoses	499	External ear ticks	506
Temporohyoid osteoarthropathy	500	External ear nematodes	507
Middle ear epithelial neoplasia	500	External acoustic meatal neoplasia	507
Jugulotympanic paragangliomas	500	Feline ceruminous cystomatosis	507
EXTERNAL EAR	500	Ceruminous gland neoplasms	507
Hearing and the external ear	501	Other external acoustic meatal neoplasms	508
Developmental disease of the external ear	501	**Histologic preparation and examination**	508
Otitis externa	502		
Dermatologic diseases of the external ear	503		
Pinnae	503		
Pinnal tumor-like growths and neoplasia	504		

EYE

Brian P. Wilcock

GENERAL CONSIDERATIONS

The role of the veterinary pathologist in the diagnosis of ocular disease is usually restricted to histologic examination. Gross pathology of the eye is the realm of the clinical ophthalmologist.

The reluctance of many pathologists to embrace ophthalmic pathology stems from the disappointing quality of sections made from formalin-fixed globes processed by routine methods, from unfamiliarity with ocular anatomy and histology, and from fear of the complex terminology shared by clinical ophthalmology and ophthalmic pathology. At least equally daunting is the need to be familiar with the ever-growing list of specific ocular syndromes, the correct identification of which has huge significance in terms of therapy and prognosis. There are many examples in which a perfectly adequate description and general morphologic diagnosis will nonetheless fail to communicate the appropriate prognostic or therapeutic information, simply because the clinician reading the report cannot make the connection between the histologic description and the specific clinical syndrome as outlined in clinical reference texts.

Ocular fixation

The eye undergoes very rapid postmortem/postenucleation change that not only obscures subtle degenerative lesions but also mimics genuine developmental or degenerative diseases. Even with a globe obtained within minutes of death or surgical removal, improper handling of the specimen frequently results in a section of poor quality. The globe can be speedily and gently removed by grasping the third eyelid with forceps and applying traction to the globe while making a circumferential incision at the fornix. Blunt curved scissors inserted through this incision may be used to sever the extraocular muscles and optic nerve, and allow the globe to be removed from the orbit. All orbital fat and extraocular muscles should be gently removed from the sclera to permit rapid penetration of fixative to the retina.

The choice of fixative depends upon the disease suspected and upon the type of examination to which the eye will be subjected. *Formalin* has the advantage of ready availability, ease of shipment, little danger of overfixation, and adequate preservation of color and macroscopic detail for photography. Also, it permits localization in the bisected globe of lesions identified ophthalmoscopically, and the use of electron microscopy should such examination be warranted by the findings of light microscopy. However, formalin penetrates the sclera slowly, and there are postmortem changes, including retinal detachment, even in globes fixed immediately after death or surgery. Injection of formalin into the vitreous (0.25 mL for a dog or cat, 2.0 mL for a horse) greatly improves retinal fixation and helps prevent the almost inevitable retinal detachment that follows routine formalin fixation. Rapid-penetrating fixatives, such as *Zenker's, Davidson's, or Bouin's,* are preferred for globes in which preservation of histologic detail, especially retinal detail, is paramount. All render the globe and its refractive media opaque and less suitable for macroscopic assessment and photography than does formalin, but they also make the globe more rigid and therefore much easier to trim in preparation for histologic processing. All require strict attention to the duration of fixation.

> **Key Points**
>
> Considering ease of use, quality of fixation, and product safety, Davidson's fixative is the best overall ocular fixative.

In all domestic animals, *the preferred section for histology is made from a mid-sagittal slab that includes pupil and optic nerve,* thereby allowing examination of both tapetal and nontapetal fundus in the same section. **Attempting to slice the fixed globe with a scalpel blade is perhaps the single biggest contributor to sections of poor quality.** *The optimal cutting instrument is a new disposable microtome blade.*

Because there is no easily accessible instruction manual on how to obtain a good histologic section, those details are included here.

- The fixed globe, free of extraocular muscles and eyelids, is opened by a smooth sagittal incision beginning adjacent to the optic nerve and ending with the cornea.
- The correct 6:00-12:00 o-clock orientation, needed to capture tapetal and nontapetal fundus, is insured by making the incision at right angles to the orientation of the posterior ciliary artery (Fig. 5-1A).
- The open globe is then inspected for macroscopic lesions.
- A second cut, parallel to the first, is made from the cornea backward through the retina (Fig. 5-1B).

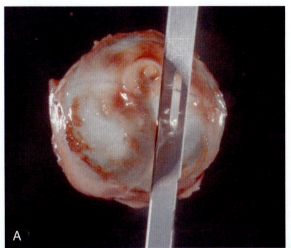

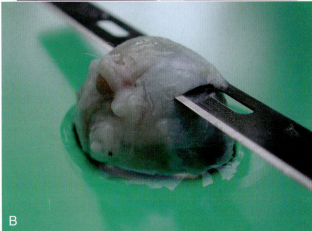

Figure 5-1 Trimming a fixed eye. A. The first incision is made from back to front, perpendicular to the posterior ciliary artery and just adjacent to the optic nerve. **B.** The second cut, made from front to back to avoid detaching the retina, is parallel to the first and far enough to the periphery to miss the lens.

- That second cut should be far enough to the periphery to leave the already bisected lens undisturbed, for a second cut through the lens will surely dislocate it.
- The resulting slab should be lifted carefully into a thick processing cassette or a tissue bag.
- Even though the piece of tissue is as much as 1 cm thick, it is hollow and thus presents no difficulty in terms of automated tissue embedding procedures.

Key Points

Habitually poor sections?

By far the most common reason for poor histologic sections is trimming the fixed globe with a scalpel blade. Switching to a disposable microtome blade will make a huge difference. The second most common reason is trying to make your specimen thin enough to fit in a regular tissue cassette for processing. Whenever possible, use deeper embedding cassettes (or tissue bags) that allow you to avoid hitting the lens with your second cut as described previously.

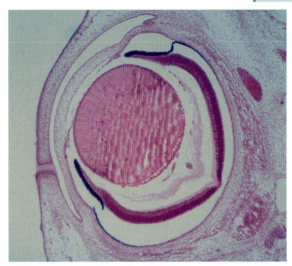

Figure 5-2 Canine embryo at 34 days of gestation. Lids fused, cornea fully formed. Large lens surrounded by complete vascular tunic derived caudally from hyaloid artery and rostrally from the future pupillary membrane. The iris is not yet formed.

DEVELOPMENTAL ANOMALIES

Ocular developmental defects are common in domestic animals, particularly in purebred dog breeds in which extensive line-breeding has been used to increase the predictability of the phenotype.

Anomalies are usually multiple, which reflects the stepwise induction and interdependence of the various parts of the developing eye. Without proper consideration of ocular embryology, any discussion of the lesions found in anomalous eyes threatens to be just a catalog of observations rather than a roadmap to understanding that such lesions are all predictable results of a relatively small number of errors in organogenesis. It is also important to recognize the differences in normal ocular structure among the various species, and the different rates at which mature form is attained. For example, the retina of carnivore eyes continues to develop for ~6 weeks postnatally, whereas that of ruminants and horses is mature at birth. Thus a condition such as retinal dysplasia is necessarily an in utero event in ungulates, but may be in response to early postnatal injury in carnivores. In the globes of carnivores, the terms congenital and developmental are therefore not synonymous.

Review of early ocular organogenesis

The primary optic vesicle is an evagination of the forebrain that, with differential growth of brain and surface ectoderm, becomes separated from the presumptive diencephalon by the *optic stalk*. The apposition of primary optic vesicle to overlying surface ectoderm induces a focal ectodermal thickening, the *lens placode*. The placode grows to form a primitive *lens vesicle*. It is the developing lens that orchestrates the invagination of the optic vesicle to form the bilayered *optic cup* and bring the lining neuroectoderm into the apposition that provides the future photoreceptor and pigment epithelial layers. Surrounding the optic cup is a mass of *mesenchyme*, derived from neural crest, which will form the vascular and fibrous tunics of the eye (iris and ciliary body stroma, corneal stroma and endothelium, choroid and sclera) under the induction of the differentiating neuroectoderm (Fig. 5-2). *Ocular adnexa and muscles* form independently and seem not to require normal development of the globe, as evidenced by the presence of normal lacrimal gland, lids, and extraocular muscles in most cases of severe microphthalmos.

Further reading

Cook CS. Embryogenesis of congenital eye malformations. Vet Comp Ophthalmol 1995;5:109-123.

Cook CS. Ocular embryology and congenital malformations. In: Gelatt KN, editor. Veterinary Ophthalmology. 5th ed. Ames, Iowa: Blackwell; 2013. p. 3-38.

Samuelson DA. Ophthalmic anatomy. In: Gelatt KN, editor. Veterinary Ophthalmology. 5th ed. Ames, Iowa: Blackwell; 2013. p. 39-170.

Defective organogenesis

Failure of the eye to attain even the stage of optic cup is a rare occurrence and is usually of unknown cause. The defect is usually bilateral but asymmetrical, and the severity of the defect relates to the stage of organogenesis at which the insult occurred. Failure of formation of the primary vesicle, or its early and complete regression, is *true anophthalmos* and is very rare. Failure of optic vesicle invagination gives rise to the very rare *congenital cystic eye*. Incomplete invagination results in *congenital retinal nonattachment*. Failure of division (or subsequent fusion) of the optic primordium as it grows from the telencephalon results in very rare true *cyclopia*. More prevalent is *synophthalmos*, a single dysplastic midline globe that microscopically will have duplication of at least some intraocular structures to indicate either partial separation of the optic vesicles or subsequent fusion.

Anophthalmos and microphthalmos

Anophthalmos, total absence of ocular tissue, is a very rare lesion, and almost all cases described are more correctly termed *severe microphthalmos* because some vestige of eye is found in serially sectioned orbital content. The usefulness of distinguishing between the two is questionable, and *many authors have adopted the term "clinical anophthalmos" for all such cases*. Concurrent anomalies of skeletal and central nervous systems are common.

Macroscopic examination of orbital content usually reveals a normal lacrimal gland and vestigial extraocular muscles. The globe is usually recognized as an irregular mass of black pigment, with structures such as cornea or optic nerve variably recognizable (Fig. 5-3A, B). Histologically, there is almost always a mass of pigmented neuroectoderm, reminiscent of ciliary processes, and some effort at retinal differentiation. There is frequently some remnant of lens, a finding that suggests regression of an embryonic globe that had reached at least the stage of optic cup. One or more plates of cartilage, presumably derived from third eyelid analogue, are common.

Mild and moderate microphthalmos is much more common, and may occur by several different mechanisms. Primary microphthalmos results from inadequate growth of the primary optic vesicle or early optic cup, and is usually accompanied by a variety of other intraocular anomalies as well as a small palpebral fissure. The size of the palpebral fissure is determined by the size of the optic vesicle during its contact with the fetal surface ectoderm, so those examples of microphthalmos accompanied by a small palpebral fissure can be ascribed to very early interference with optic vesicle

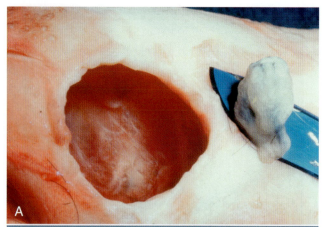
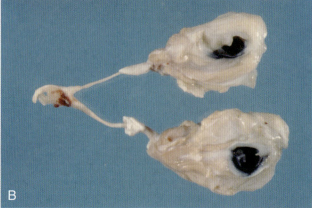

Figure 5-3 A. Secondary microphthalmos. The miniature globe lies within a normal orbit, implying secondary microphthalmos. **B.** Even when tiny, such globes always retain at least some pigmented uveal tissue.

formation. A separate mechanism for primary microphthalmos is failure to establish or maintain intraocular pressure, probably stemming from incomplete closure of the optic (embryonic) fissure. In those globes, lenticular and retinal growth is not affected, and so those structures become disproportionately large when contrasted to the stunted growth of choroid, anterior uvea, and sclera. Virtually all globes with primary microphthalmos have multiple ocular anomalies, including anterior segment dysgenesis, persistent embryonic vasculature, and cataract, and not just "miniaturization."

Most examples of clinically diagnosed sporadic microphthalmos are probably not primary developmental anomalies, but responses by the fetal or neonatal globe to traumatic or other injuries that result in a cessation of development or even regression. This is particularly true in carnivores, in which the globe continues to develop for several weeks after birth and is thus susceptible to interference by penetrating trauma or neonatal infections.

Cyclopia and synophthalmos

Damage to the prosencephalon prior to the outgrowth of the optic vesicles may result in improper separation of paired cranial midline structures, including eyes. *Cyclopia is a fetal malformation characterized by a single median orbit containing a single globe*. Most specimens have some duplication of intraocular structures, such as lens, iris, or hyaloid vessels, and are thus more properly considered *incomplete separation or early*

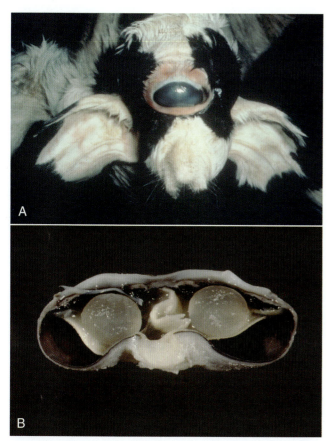

Figure 5-4 A. Synophthalmos. Typical "cyclopian" calf with multiple facial anomalies. **B.** Duplication of lens and a midline septum indicate synophthalmos rather than cyclopia.

fusion (synophthalmos) (Fig. 5-4A, B). Some specimens have 2 dysplastic globes within a single orbit. Severe cranial anomalies invariably accompany cyclopia and synophthalmos, including absent or deformed ears, a median proboscis, cranioschisis, cleft palate, and brain anomalies ranging from microcephaly to hydranencephaly and hydrocephalus.

Cyclopian-like malformations have been reported in sheep, chickens, and dogs, and as inherited defects in cattle, but the most thoroughly documented cases are in sheep grazing alpine pastures rich in the legume *Veratrum californicum*. Fresh and dried plants contain 3 steroidal alkaloids—jervine, cyclopamine, and cycloposine—capable of damaging the developing neural groove of the fetal lamb. Ewes eating the plant on gestational day 15 have lambs with the cyclopian malformation, for it is at that time that the neural groove has formed and the first cranial somites are forming. A similar syndrome has been produced in kids and calves by maternal feeding of the plant on day 14 of gestation. Ingestion of the alkaloids before day 15 in sheep may cause fetal death but no anomalies, and exposure soon after day 15 may cause various skeletal abnormalities but not cyclopia.

In naturally occurring outbreaks, affected lambs have deformities ranging from cyclopia with microcephaly to relatively normal lambs with harelip and cleft palate. Prolonged gestation is common in the case of severely malformed fetuses.

Cystic eye and retinal nonattachment

Failure of apposition of the optic vesicle to the cranial ectoderm results in failure of lens induction, which in turn removes

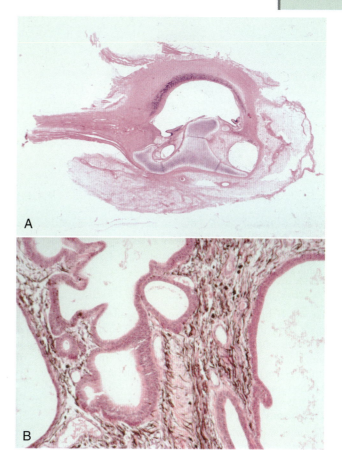

Figure 5-5 Cystic globe in a foal. **A.** There is no lens, no attempt at invagination, and no neurosensory differentiation. The cartilage plate is probably derived from the third eyelid. **B.** Cystic globes have just a single layer of neuroectoderm, indicating a failure of involution of the optic vesicle.

the major stimulus for invagination of the optic vesicle to form the optic cup. *Persistence of the primary optic vesicle is seen as a cystic eye* (Fig. 5-5A, B), consisting of a scleral sheet lined by neuroectoderm of variable neurosensory and pigmentary differentiation. The absence of lens and of bilayered iridociliary epithelium distinguishes this rare lesion from the more common dysplastic eye of secondary microphthalmos.

Incomplete invagination of the optic vesicle allows persistence of the cavity of the primary optic vesicle and prevents attachment of the presumptive neurosensory retina to the developing retinal pigment epithelium (RPE). *In the postnatal globe, retinal nonattachment cannot easily be distinguished from acquired retinal separation.* In each instance, the retina is extensively folded and may have improper differentiation of neuronal layers. The diagnosis of retinal nonattachment is assisted if there is also lack of apposition between the 2 layers of neuroectoderm covering the anterior uvea (destined to be iridal and ciliary epithelium) and if retinal rosettes are evident. In addition, because nonattachment is an early and fundamental error in organogenesis, such eyes usually lack a lens and probably will be microphthalmic with multiple anomalies.

A syndrome of multiple ocular anomalies reflecting a less profound defect in the formation of the optic cup has been reported in Rocky Mountain horses. The defects are always bilateral and are characterized primarily by the presence of multifocal defective adhesion between the inner and outer

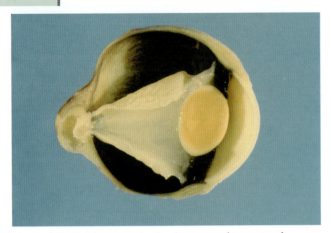

Figure 5-6 **Coloboma and scleral ectasia** adjacent to the optic disc, accompanied by retinal separation, in Collie eye anomaly. Bouin's fixative.

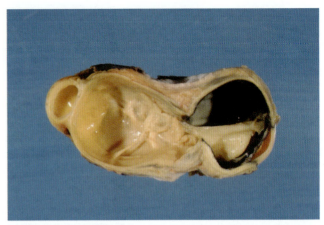

Figure 5-7 **Retrobulbar cyst** formed by coloboma and massive scleral ectasia in a calf. The globe is small, and the retina is completely separated.

layers of the optic cup. These are manifested as numerous cysts involving the posterior iris, ciliary body, and peripheral retina. Less frequent anomalies, such as iris hypoplasia and megalocornea, are probably secondary manifestations of improper maturation of the neuroectoderm at the anterior lip of the optic cup.

Coloboma

The mildest and latest defect in organogenesis results from failure of complete fusion of the lips of the optic (embryonic) fissure, a slit-like but normal channel in the floor of the optic cup and stalk through which the vasoformative mesoderm and stromal mesenchyme enter the globe. Failure of closure of the fissure may occur anywhere along its length, but the channel persists most frequently as a notch-like defect of the caudal pole at, or just ventral to, the optic disc. Its exact location can vary substantially. Such defects are known as colobomas ("congenital missing parts"). When they occur as the result of a failure of closure of the most posterior portion of the optic fissure, they are known as "typical" colobomas, and are lined by an outpouching of dysplastic neuroectoderm. If the defect is sufficiently large, the outpouching of neuroectoderm induces a similar bulge in the sclera, termed **scleral ectasia** (Fig. 5-6). Occasionally, such ectasias are so large as to form a **retrobulbar cyst** as large as the globe itself (Fig. 5-7). Regardless of size, the lining of the scleral coloboma is formed by neuroectoderm that bulged through the defect in the optic cup. Abortive neurosensory differentiation within the cyst wall is common and permits definitive identification of the retrobulbar cyst as being a coloboma. Segmental defects in the development of uvea or sclera occurring in sites other than the optic fissure are known as "atypical" colobomas and have a separate pathogenesis related to improper induction of uveal and scleral maturation by defective neuroectoderm (Fig. 5-8A, B).

Colobomas occur in all domestic species, but are especially frequent in Collie dogs as one manifestation of Collie eye anomaly, and in Australian Shepherd dogs with merle ocular dysgenesis syndrome. In Collies (and less frequently in Border Collies and Shetland Sheepdogs), they usually arise within or just adjacent to the optic disc. They appear to arise as focal defects in the induction of sclera and choroid that normally is stimulated by the RPE that is forming from the outer layer of the optic cup.

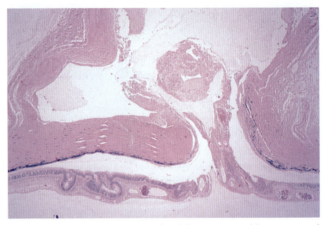

Figure 5-8 **Coloboma.** Atypical coloboma created by segmental aplasia of retina, choroid, and sclera.

Because the exact location of the embryonic fissure is somewhat variable, it is difficult to determine how many examples of coloboma are the result of delayed closure of that normal embryologic structure, and how many represent some more fundamental defect in the proper interaction of RPE and the developing periocular mesenchyme destined to form choroid and sclera. Proper maturation of the RPE and in particular, the normal acquisition of pigmentation, appears to be critical to the induction of normal mesenchymal migration and maturation. Failure by the developing RPE to induce proper mesenchymal maturation results in such varied anomalies as choroidal hypoplasia, segmental or diffuse iris, and ciliary hypoplasia (known clinically as **iris coloboma**), and even microphthalmia. Because of its frequent association with the merle dilution defect in the coat color of dogs, the general syndrome is known as merle ocular dysgenesis and is particularly prevalent in Australian Shepherd dogs. It is similar, but not identical, to Collie eye anomaly. The same defect occurs, with much less frequency, in color-dilute (incompletely albinotic) horses, cattle, non-merle dogs, and cats. In Charolais cattle, colobomas of (or near) the optic disc are inherited as an autosomal dominant trait with incomplete penetrance. The lesion is bilateral but not necessarily equal in severity.

Defective differentiation

Subsequent to formation of the optic cup, ocular differentiation involves continued differentiation of neuroectoderm into retinal and uveal neuroepithelium, and induction of primitive periocular neural crest mesenchyme to form the sclera and uvea. The normal development of RPE from the neuroectoderm of the posterior half of the optic vesicle, and of iridociliary epithelium from the anterior lip of the involuting optic cup seems to be a prerequisite for these differentiations to occur.

It is traditional to present specific ocular anomalies as they relate to structures of the adult eye, and thus as anomalies of cornea, iris, lens, retina, and so on. This approach correlates well with the clinical examination of the eye but provides no understanding of the fundamental pathogenesis of the anomaly. *Here we will organize these "later" anomalies (occurring after the stage of optic cup formation) on the basis of the presumed pathogenesis: defective migration, proliferation, or remodeling of ocular mesenchyme, defective maturation of neuroectoderm, and defective development of ectoderm.*

Further reading

Onwochei BC, et al. Ocular colobomata. Surv Ophthalmol 2000;45:175-194.

Ramsey DT, et al. Congenital ocular anomalies of Rocky Mountain horses. Vet Ophthalmol 1999;2:47-59.

Zhao S, Overbeek PA. Regulation of choroid development by the retinal pigment epithelium. Mol Vis 2001;7:277-282.

Anomalies of mesenchyme

After formation of the optic cup and separation of the lens vesicle, the periocular mesenchyme undergoes a complex series of migrations, differentiations, and atrophies that determines the final structure of the vascular and fibrous tunics of the globe. At the anterior edge of the optic cup, one or more waves of mesenchymal invasion form corneal endothelium, corneal stroma, and the anterior half of the transient perilenticular vascular network, including the pupillary membrane. The posterior half of this perilenticular vascular tunic is formed by invasion of mesodermal endothelial cell precursors and supporting perivascular mesenchyme through the optic fissure to form the extensive but transient *hyaloid artery system* (see Fig. 5-2). Another mesenchymal wave accompanies the ingrowth of the neuroectoderm at the anterior lip of the optic cup to form the iris stroma, although it is unclear which layer acts as the primary inducer. Its peripheral portion later atrophies to form the porous *filtration angle* of the anterior chamber, a process that may not be completed in carnivores until 6-8 weeks after birth. The choroid and sclera are induced by the developing RPE to form from the mesenchyme surrounding the caudal half of the optic cup.

Anomalies of mesenchyme may result from defective ingrowth or differentiation, as with choroidal and iris hypoplasia, incomplete atrophy of the tunica vasculosa lentis or hyaloid artery system, or incomplete remodeling of the filtration angle to cause primary glaucoma.

Choroidal hypoplasia. *This is a relatively common lesion in the eye of dogs* by virtue of its prevalence in the Collie breed as the hallmark of Collie eye anomaly, and a very similar syndrome occurs in Border Collies and Shetland Sheepdogs. It is also seen in a variety of dog breeds in association with genes for color dilution (merle, dapple, and harlequin), especially Australian Shepherd dogs. *The hypoplasia is thought to result from induction failure by a defective RPE or by the more anterior neuroectoderm destined to form iridociliary epithelium.* The basic defect is not clearly established but may be related to defective pigmentation, a suggestion supported by the prevalence of iris and choroidal hypoplasia in white animals of all species, especially those with blue irises. Other anomalies linked to the choroidal hypoplasia/hypopigmentation include optic nerve coloboma; microphthalmos and, with the merle ocular dysgenesis, cataract and segmental iris hypoplasia. Some degree of retinal dysplasia is also common. At least in theory, all of these defects are predictable outcomes of improper mesenchymal induction by a defective, inadequately pigmented neuroectoderm lining the primitive optic cup. Even in otherwise normal (nonwhite) animals with a blue iris, there is usually hypoplasia of the tapetum and choroid (classified by ophthalmologists as a so-called "subalbinotic fundus").

Collie eye anomaly. *Collie eye anomaly (CEA) is a common congenital inherited disease of smooth and rough Collies and in Collie-related breeds*, first reported in 1953 and at one time estimated to have affected 90% of North American Collies. During the period 1975-1979, CEA was still present in >70% of 20,000 Collies examined in a voluntary screening program. Prevalence in Europe and the United Kingdom is lower (30-60%). *The basic defect, patchy to diffuse choroidal hypoplasia, is inherited as an autosomal recessive trait*, but the numerous associated defects are more unpredictable in their familial pattern. The CEA-associated genetic mutation is reported as an intronic 7.8-kb deletion in the canine *NHEJ1* gene that is detectable in homozygotes and heterozygotes by PCR testing.

The ophthalmoscopic findings include one or more of retinal vessel tortuosity, focal to diffuse choroidal and tapetal hypoplasia, optic nerve coloboma, and retinal separation with intraocular hemorrhage. Other observations that are occasionally made in eyes of affected dogs are enophthalmos, microphthalmos, and corneal stromal mineralization. The disease is always bilateral but not necessarily equal. Even the mild, visually insignificant lesion of focal choroidal hypoplasia is genetically significant.

Macroscopic examination of the bisected globe reveals abnormal pallor of the posterior segment of the globe. If the globe is transilluminated, the sclera and choroid are focally or diffusely more translucent than normal. The pallor and translucency imply choroidal hypoplasia. Within or adjacent to the optic disc, there may be a colobomatous pit of variable size, the lining of which is continuous with the retina. Accompanying the larger type of pit is a bulge in the overlying sclera, called **scleral ectasia** or **posterior staphyloma**. If there is retinal separation, it is usually complete, with the only sites of attachment being at the abnormal optic disc and at the ora ciliaris. In such cases, there may be extensive intravitreal hemorrhage and retinal tears. Almost all Collie eyes with retinal separation have large optic disc colobomas. Detachment from the ora ciliaris (so-called *retinal disinsertion*) may also occur, leaving the folded retina on the floor of the globe (Fig. 5-9).

The fundamental histologic lesion found in all affected eyes is choroidal hypoplasia (Fig. 5-10A, B). It is always diffuse, despite ophthalmoscopic observation of a lesion that may

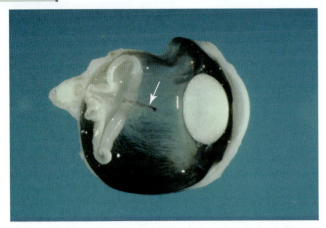

Figure 5-9 **Retinal separation from the ora ciliaris in Collie eye anomaly.** There is a coloboma at the optic disc. Choroid and sclera are so thin as to be transparent. The pigmented strand (arrow) extending from optic disc toward the lens is a remnant of hyaloid artery.

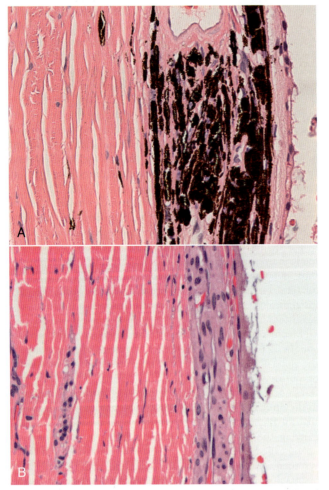

Figure 5-10 **A. Normal canine choroid and sclera** 1 mm dorsal to the optic disc. **B. Choroidal hypoplasia** in Collie eye anomaly at the same location and magnification as **A**.

appear only to be focal within the dorsal temporal quadrant of the fundus. The choroid is thin and poorly pigmented, and the tapetum is thinner than normal or even absent. Retinal pigment epithelium is poorly pigmented, even in nontapetal fundus, and may be vacuolated. Because the choroid and tapetum in the normal dog do not reach adult thickness until ~4 months postpartum, age-matched control eyes are essential if over-interpretation of normal choroidal immaturity is to be avoided.

Histologic examination of eyes with optic disc colobomas reveals the bulging of dysplastic neuroectoderm, continuous with retina, into the pit in the nerve head. The neuroectoderm may show jumbled differentiation into ganglion cells, photoreceptor rosettes, glial cells, or pigment epithelium. Rosettes are common in the neurosensory retina adjacent to affected discs or embedded in the optic disc itself. In some specimens, there are degenerative retinal lesions overlying severely hypoplastic choroid. Edematous clefts are seen in the nerve fiber layer, and ganglion cells may be severely vacuolated.

Other retinal lesions include retinal folds and detachment. The folds are seen on histologic section as tubes of fully differentiated retina cut in cross-section or tangentially, and are thought to represent folds in a neurosensory retina that at least temporarily has grown in excess of the space available for it within the optic cup. These folds correspond to the clinically detectable vermiform streaks in the fundus, and gradually disappear as the dog (and eye) matures, allowing the growth of scleral shell to catch up with that of retina. Presumably, it is a similar growth imbalance, but in the opposite direction, that causes retinal separation in ~10% of eyes with this syndrome. In this situation, a retina that is too small attempts to stretch from optic disc to ora ciliaris by the shortest route, rather than following the curvature of the scleral shell.

Focal fibroblastic metaplasia and mineralization are occasionally seen in the subepithelial corneal stroma of dogs with Collie eye anomaly, but a similar defect is seen in anomalous eyes of other breeds; a genetic link to the Collie eye defect is not established. Tortuosity of retinal veins, a controversial clinical lesion sometimes considered part of Collie eye anomaly, has no described histologic counterpart.

The earliest lesion of this anomaly is defective differentiation of primitive RPE to form rosette-like structures near the optic disc. Proper differentiation of both pigment epithelium and neurosensory retina requires obliteration of the lumen of the primary optic vesicle, which allows the 2 neuroectodermal layers to come into apposition. Whether the earliest lesion of Collie eye anomaly results from inherently defective differentiation of pigment epithelium or from imperfect apposition of the 2 neuroectodermal layers has not been resolved, but the central role of the pigment epithelium in determining ocular morphology suggests that the primary defect is in maturation of the presumptive RPE. Anomalous development of choroid and sclera, including coloboma, is not seen in fetuses up to 45 gestational days, but is seen in neonates. This suggests that the defect is in choroidal maturation rather than in initial induction.

Another manifestation of mesenchymal maldevelopment in Collie eye anomaly, rarely noted clinically, is delayed atrophy and remodeling in the anterior chamber. The filtration angle may be closed, iris stroma may be attached to the corneal endothelium by a mesenchymal bridge, and remnants of anterior perilenticular mesenchyme are unusually prominent. Pigmentation of iridal neuroectoderm is sparse. As these neonatal anterior segment lesions are not seen later in life (8-20 weeks) when puppies are examined ophthalmoscopically, it is presumed that they reflect only a minor delay in mesenchymal remodeling.

Eye

Developmental Anomalies

Defects primarily in anterior chamber mesenchyme

Hypoplasia of the iris *is a rare defect that may occur alone or in conjunction with multiple ocular defects.* It is relatively most frequent in horses, where it may be inherited and associated with cataract and conjunctival dermoids. The defect presumably results from incomplete inward migration of the anterior lip of the optic cup, with resultant lack of a neuroectodermal scaffold to guide the subsequent migration of mesenchyme destined to form the iris stroma. The hypoplasia is usually severe and most cases are clinically described as *aniridia*. Histologic examination of such eyes usually reveals the vestigial iris as a triangular mesenchymal stump covered posteriorly by normal-appearing pigmented epithelium (Fig. 5-11A). The trabecular meshwork within the filtration angles may be malformed, but the ciliary apparatus is usually normal. The lens often is cataractous (Fig. 5-11B) and sometimes ectopic or hypoplastic. Glaucoma has been described as a sequel in horses (but not in other species), but it should be an expected sequel in severely affected eyes in any species because of the inevitable concurrent trabecular hypoplasia.

Hypopigmentation of the iris may be unilateral or bilateral. When the loss of pigment is patchy in one or both irises, it is known as *heterochromia iridis*. The pigmentation may be diffusely absent in the iris stroma but present in the posterior iris epithelium *(subalbinotic)*, or absent in both stroma and epithelium *(true albinism)*. The iris is normal except for absence of visible pigment granules in the cytoplasm of otherwise normal stromal melanocytes and epithelial cells. Tapetum and, less reliably, choroid of affected eyes usually are hypoplastic as well as poorly pigmented.

Incomplete atrophy of the anterior chamber mesenchyme is relatively common in dogs and occurs occasionally in other domestic species. During organogenesis, waves of mesenchyme migrate between the surface ectoderm and the anterior rim of the optic cup. Some of the ingrowing mesenchyme forms corneal endothelium and stroma, whereas other portions of mesenchyme form the iris stroma and trabecular meshwork (Fig. 5-12A). Some of that mesenchyme occupies the anterior chamber and, as it matures, it forms a fibrovascular sheet stretching across the face of the lens and developing iris, known as the *pupillary membrane*. Its vascular component creates the anterior portion of an embryonic perilenticular vascular plexus, known as the *tunica vasculosa lentis* (Fig. 5-12B). Both the pupillary membrane and the tunica vasculosa lentis normally disappear late in gestation or in the early postnatal period. Failure of this anterior chamber fibrovascular mesenchyme to atrophy results in the very common anomaly of **persistent pupillary membrane** (persistence of the tunica vasculosa lentis alone is discussed later).

Atrophy of the pupillary membrane is frequently incomplete at birth, and, in dogs, persistent remnants are common up to ~6 months of age. These insignificant and usually bloodless strands

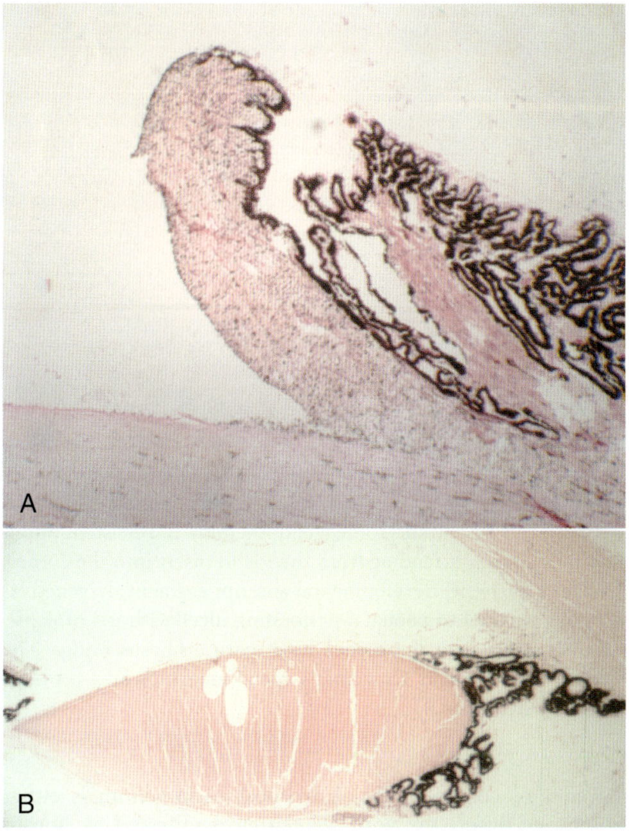

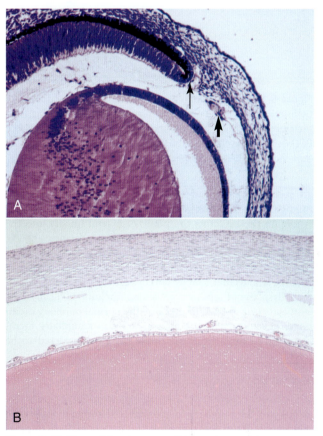

Figure 5-11 A. Iris hypoplasia with hypoplasia of the trabecular meshwork in a dog. The ciliary processes have developed normally. **B. Iris hypoplasia,** congenital cataract, and dysplasia of ciliary processes in a piglet. The adherence of ciliary processes to the lens represents an arrest in remodeling rather than improper development.

Figure 5-12 Normal development of the canine anterior segment. A. Normal 34-day canine embryo. The bilayered neuroectoderm at the anterior lip of the optic cup (thick arrow) will soon migrate inwardly to induce the formation of iris. Blood vessels at that lip (thin arrow) are growing inwardly to form the anterior half of the tunica vasculosa lentis. **B.** Normal anterior vasculosa lentis (pupillary membrane) in a neonatal dog.

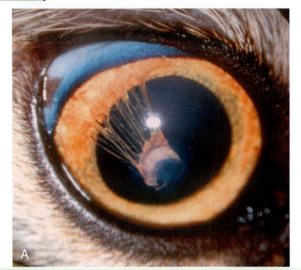

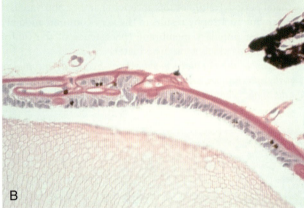

Figure 5-13 Persistent pupillary membrane. A. Central crescentic insertion of the persistent pupillary membrane in a dog is on the anterior pole of the lens, where it has induced a focal cataract. **B.** Dysplastic development of the anterior lens capsule as a consequence of adherence of persistent pupillary membrane.

are seen as short, thread-like protrusions from the area of the minor arterial circle (iris collarette), and they may insert elsewhere on the iris, cross the pupil, or extend blindly into the anterior chamber. Persistent pupillary membranes achieve clinical significance in 2 ways. First, the size and number of strands crossing the pupil may be such that vision is obstructed. Second, strands that contact lens or cornea are associated with focal dysplasia of lens or corneal endothelium, clinically seen as opacity (Fig. 5-13A, B). Because the normal pupillary membrane never contacts the cornea, strands of pupillary membrane that extend from iris to cornea are considered to be minor versions of anterior segment dysgenesis (see later).

Histologic descriptions are mainly from studies in *Basenji dogs*, in which persistent pupillary membrane occurs as an autosomal recessive trait of variable penetrance. In this breed, atrophy of the pupillary membrane is abnormally slow even in dogs free of the defect in adult life, and remnants in puppies up to 8 months of age are common. The membranes are seen as thin endothelial tubes, invested with a thin adventitial stroma, extending from vessels in the iris stroma near the collarette (Fig. 5-14). The tubes are usually empty, but in severely affected eyes may contain erythrocytes, and the adventitia may contain melanin. The tubes weave in and out of the plane of section en route to corneal, iridic, or lenticular insertions.

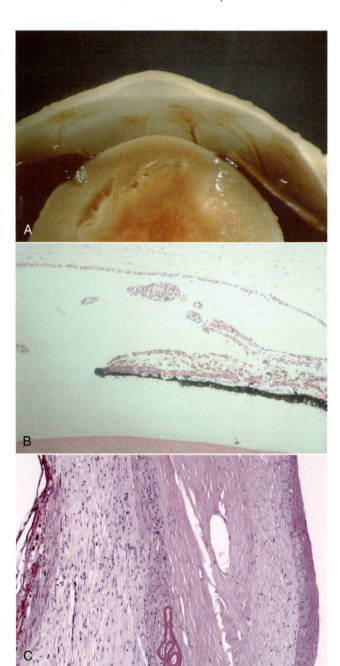

Figure 5-14 Anterior segment dysgenesis. A. Improper development of the tunica vasculosa lentis creates slender adhesions between the iris and the corneal endothelium. **B.** Persistent pupillary membranes extending from the iris to insert into the cornea. **C.** This (apparent) developmental anterior segment dysgenesis is actually a sequel to neonatal perforating ulcer with iris prolapse. The iris is fused to the cornea by a mature fibrous bridge. The presence of a coiled Descemet's membrane indicates previous corneal perforation.

At sites of corneal insertion, corneal endothelium is either absent or dysplastic, with the latter manifested as fibrous metaplasia. Descemet's membrane is malformed or absent in the areas of attachment, and there is associated deep stromal corneal edema to account for the clinically observed, minute gray stromal opacities. *Contact with the lens is accompanied by similar epithelial and basement membrane dysplasia, resulting in one or more epithelial, subcapsular, or polar cortical cataracts.*

Much less common than persistent pupillary membrane are those defects grouped under the general category of **anterior segment dysgenesis** (or **anterior segment cleavage syndrome**). This group includes multiple anomalies of cornea, lens, and anterior uvea that stem from disordered development of anterior segment mesenchyme and/or improper separation of the developing lens from the overlying cornea. Such eyes are commonly microphthalmic and usually have microphakia, cataract, and congenital corneal opacities at sites of congenital anterior synechiae. The most severe cases have fusion of iris with corneal stroma without observed corneal endothelium or Descemet's membrane, and thus have no detectable anterior chamber (see Fig. 5-14). *Most examples of this severe form in dogs and cats probably result from perinatal corneal perforation from trauma or from progression of suppurative bacterial keratoconjunctivitis (ophthalmia neonatorum) rather than from in utero maldevelopment.* The result is iris prolapse and incorporation of the iris into the developing cornea, which in turn results in obliteration of the anterior chamber. Because the globe of dogs and cats continues to develop for many weeks after birth, this is yet another example of how difficult it can be to precisely distinguish primary developmental disorders from those resulting from postnatal trauma or inflammation.

Maldevelopment of the filtration angle (goniodysgenesis) occurs as a solitary, prevalent, inherited anomaly in dogs, and in severely anomalous eyes of animals of any species. The defect results from incomplete atrophy of mesenchyme that normally fills the fetal iridocorneal angle. The defect is much more common in dogs than any other species. In the most severe cases, the trabecular meshwork may appear as a solid mesenchymal mass indistinguishable from the adjacent iris stroma. This rare lesion, known as *trabecular hypoplasia*, is a cause for truly congenital glaucoma (Fig. 5-15A, B). It is often accompanied by iris hypoplasia and other anomalies involving anterior chamber maturation. Much more commonly, the error in remodeling is less profound, and the lesion is seen as a continuous sheet of iris stroma (therefore resembling an abnormally solid pectinate ligament) that separates the anterior chamber from a relatively normal trabecular meshwork. This more common lesion is usually referred to as *pectinate dysplasia* (Fig. 5-15C). For a more complete discussion, see Glaucoma.

Incomplete atrophy of posterior segment mesenchyme

Incomplete atrophy of posterior segment mesenchyme may result in the mild and common lesion of **persistent hyaloid artery**, or in the much rarer but clinically more significant lesions of **persistent posterior perilenticular vascular tunic** with or without concurrent persistence of the primary vitreous. There is a tendency in clinical literature to group all of these defects under the umbrella of **persistent hyperplastic primary vitreous**, but histologically, there is quite a wide range in the nature of the defect. Only the most severe qualify as true persistent hyperplastic primary vitreous.

The hyaloid artery and its branches are formed from mesenchyme and pre-endothelial mesoderm that enter the optic cup through the optic fissure prior to its closure. The vessel traverses the optic cup from optic disc to lens, where it ramifies over the posterior lens surface (posterior tunica vasculosa lentis). It joins with the vascular portion of the pupillary membrane (anterior tunica vasculosa lentis) to form a

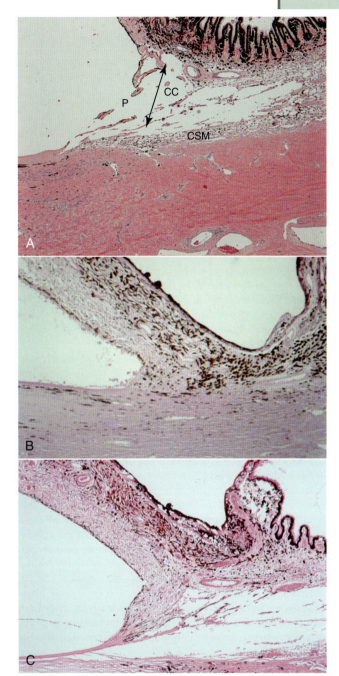

Figure 5-15 Goniodysgenesis. **A.** Normal feline filtration angle. *CC*, ciliary cleft; *CSM*, corneoscleral trabecular meshwork; *P*, pectinate ligament.. **B. Trabecular hypoplasia**, with little maturation of the embryonic mesenchyme destined to form pectinate ligament and trabecular meshwork. **C.** More common **pectinate dysplasia**, in which a solid sheet of iris-like mesenchyme extends from the termination of Descemet's membrane into the iris stroma, with no obvious pectinate ligament. Other portions of the trabecular meshwork are relatively normal.

complete perilenticular vascular tunic. *As with its anterior chamber counterpart, the hyaloid system undergoes almost complete atrophy before birth.* Persistence of some vestige into adult life is common and clinically insignificant. In ruminants, the most common remnant is *Bergmeister's papilla*, a cone of glial tissue with a vascular core that extends from optic disc for a few millimeters into the vitreous (Fig. 5-16). In calves up to

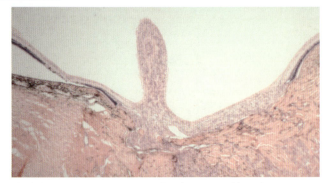

Figure 5-16 Bergmeister's papilla, the minimal histologic presentation of persistent hyaloid artery.

~2 months of age, the vestigial hyaloid system may still contain blood. In carnivores, it is the pupillary membrane that normally persists for several weeks postnatally. Bloodless remnants of the anterior termination of the hyaloid artery on the posterior lens capsule are known as *Mittendorf's dot*; it is a harmless anomaly, common in dogs and ruminants up to several years of age.

Much less common is undue persistence and even hyperplasia of the anterior end of the hyaloid system **(posterior tunica vasculosa lentis)**. The normal tissue is a combination of blood vessels and perivascular mesenchyme. Surrounding the hyaloid system is some primitive collagen, poorly characterized extracellular matrix, and a few macrophages. The combination of blood vessels and surrounding stroma is known as the *primary vitreous*. At least theoretically, *anomalous retention of the hyaloid artery and/or primary vitreous could therefore be separated into distinct entities of persistent hyaloid, persistent posterior tunica vasculosa lentis, persistent primary vitreous, and persistent hyperplastic primary vitreous*. Of these, the one most frequently reported (perhaps just because it is the most spectacular and significant) is **persistent hyperplastic primary vitreous**. In people, this rare anomaly is typically unilateral and is accompanied by microphthalmos, microphakia, retinal detachment, shallow anterior chamber, and embryonic filtration angles. The many reports of this anomaly in dogs have described a unilateral or bilateral retrolental vascular or fibrovascular network, usually without any other reported anomalies other than the expected posterior polar cataract. Such lesions are better described as *persistent posterior tunica vasculosa lentis*. In Doberman Pinschers, Bouviers, and Staffordshire Bull Terriers, the classification as hyperplastic primary vitreous is more credible. In these breeds, the defect is inherited and forms a spectrum that includes persistent pupillary membrane, cataract, lenticonus, and microphthalmos as well as persistence of variable amounts of primary vitreous and posterior tunica vasculosa lentis (Fig. 5-17A-C). The defects are detected as early as gestational day 30, at which time hyperplasia of posterior tunica vasculosa lentis is already obvious. Posterior polar cataracts and preretinal membranes are observed by day 37. The one report of 2 cases in cats was not supported by histopathology, and its correct classification remains unknown.

Further reading

Cook CS. Experimental models of anterior segment dysgenesis. Ophthalmic Ped Genet 1989;10:33-46.

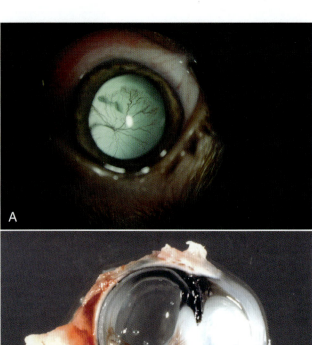

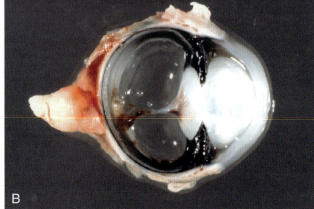

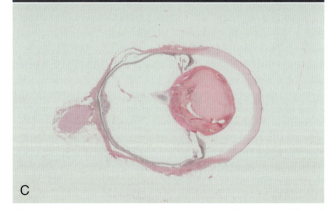

Figure 5-17 Persistent primary vitreous syndrome. **A.** Clinical photograph of persistent hyaloid artery and posterior tunica vasculosa lentis. **B.** The same globe with the persistent hyaloid artery ramifying over the posterior lens capsule. The lens is misshapen (posterior lentiglobus) and has anterior subluxation. **C.** Histologic section of the same globe. Note the retinal folding, cartilaginous metaplasia, and the posterior lenticonus that allow this to be classified as persistent hyperplastic primary vitreous.

Crispin SM. Developmental anomalies and abnormalities of the equine iris. Vet Ophthalmol 2000;3:93-98.

Gemensky-Metzler AJ, Wilkie DA. Surgical management and histologic and immunohistochemical features of a cataract and retrolental plaque secondary to persistent hyperplastic tunica vasculosa lentis/persistent hyperplastic primary vitreous (PHTVL/PHPV) in a Bloodhound puppy. Vet Ophthalmol 2004;7:369-375.

Mizukami K, et al. Collie eye anomaly in Hokkaido dogs: case study. Vet Ophthalmol 2012;15:128-132.

Parker HG, et al. Breed relationships facilitate fine-mapping studies: a 7.8-kb deletion cosegregates with Collie eye anomaly across multiple dog breeds. Genome Res 2007;17:1562-1571.

Pearl R, et al. Progression of pectinate ligament dysplasia over time in two populations of Flat-Coated Retrievers. Vet Ophthalmol 2013;18:6-12.

Williams DL. A comparative approach to anterior segment dysgenesis. Eye (Lond) 1993;7(Pt 5):607-616.

Anomalies of neuroectoderm

Included under this heading are anomalies of retina, optic nerve, and of neuroepithelium of iris and ciliary body. Of these, *retinal anomalies are by far the most frequent and most significant.*

Retinal dysplasia. Retinal dysplasia *is a general term denoting abnormal retinal differentiation characterized by jumbling of retinal layers and by glial proliferation.* In clinical practice, the term has been used incautiously to include genuine retinal dysplasia, postnecrotic retinal scarring of the developing retina, and retinal folding. Genuine retinal dysplasia results from failure of proper apposition of the 2 layers of the optic cup or from failure of proper induction of retinal maturation by an inherently defective RPE. Those examples clinically classified as retinal dysplasia that reflect disordered wound healing of developing retina, or just folding of retina with no jumbling, should not be considered examples of true retinal dysplasia. *True retinal dysplasia is thus very rare.*

Those examples of retinal dysplasia in which the only abnormality is **retinal folding** are by far the most common, and are seen primarily in dogs. The anatomic location, ophthalmoscopic appearance, and effect on vision vary from breed to breed but tend to be uniform within each breed, a fact used by clinical ophthalmologists when attempting to distinguish inherited dysplasias from those occurring as isolated anomalies or as sequelae to in utero infections. Most examples probably reflect inequity in growth rate between the retina and the outer layer of the optic cup (choroid and sclera). In such cases, the folds may be transient and disappear as continued choroidal and scleral growth eventually create a globe large enough to accommodate the retina. At least in Collies (and other related breeds with syndromes similar to Collie eye anomaly), *the retinal lesion is probably secondary to defective signaling from the RPE,* as are most of the other defects that make up Collie eye anomaly (Fig. 5-18).

Retinal folding that may not depend on retinal:scleral growth imbalance is seen in English Springer Spaniels. Changes are seen as early as gestational day 45 and always by day 55. Focal infolding of the neuroblastic layer away from the RPE and focal loss of the junctions between the neuroblasts (the outer limiting membrane) are the early changes, followed by overt focal retinal separation and extensive retinal folding. In all breeds in which this type of dysplasia has been adequately studied, it is inherited as a simple autosomal trait.

Retinal dysplasia as a sequel to **retinal necrosis** can occur as a sequel to a wide variety of viral and physical-chemical insults to the embryonic eye; naturally occurring examples are almost exclusively viral. Because the carnivore retina continues to develop for ~6 weeks after birth, the opportunity is great for postnatal injury in puppies and kittens to produce retinal maldevelopment. Retinal maturation is most rapid in central (peripapillary) retina and progressively less toward the periphery, so that occasionally dysplastic lesions may be

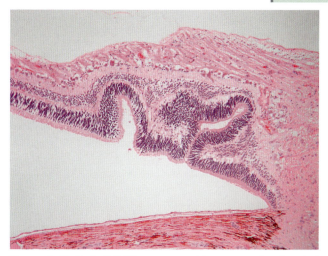

Figure 5-18 **Retinal folding,** presumably as a result of retinal redundancy that may eventually self-correct as the scleral shell grows to accommodate the retina. Retinal histologic organization is normal, distinguishing this from true retinal dysplasia.

encountered only in peripheral retina, suggesting a viral (or other) injury quite close to the 6-week-old limit for dysplasia of this pathogenesis. Mature retina will scar but will not develop lesions of dysplasia because it lacks neuronal proliferative capacity.

The specific viruses implicated in domestic animals are bovine viral diarrhea virus in cattle, bluetongue virus in sheep, herpesvirus in dogs, and both parvovirus and leukemia virus in cats. The histologic lesion is similar for all diseases, with variation in lesions caused by the same virus in one species as great as the variation caused by different viruses in different species. *The most significant clue suggesting viral rather than genetic cause is the presence of residual inflammation and postnecrotic scarring in retina, optic nerve, and, perhaps subtly, in choroid.* Injured RPE undergoes one or more of reactive hyperplasia, migration into injured retina as discrete pigmented cells in areas of scarred retina, or metaplastic formation of multilayered fibroglial plaques in place of normal simple cuboidal epithelium (Fig. 5-19A-C). Disorganization of nuclear layers and rosette formation are seen as in other types of dysplasia.

Infection of calves with bovine viral diarrhea virus between 79 and 150 days of gestation is the most frequently encountered and thoroughly studied retinal dysplasia of known viral etiology. Work with other viruses has been too limited to allow definition of the susceptible period in fetal development or of the full range of resultant lesions. The limited descriptions of the other viral-induced retinal lesions suggest that the sequence of events is probably quite similar for all such agents.

The initial ocular lesion is nonsuppurative panuveitis and retinitis with multifocal retinal and choroidal necrosis. The acute inflammatory disease gradually subsides over several weeks, and most cases of spontaneous abortion or neonatal death retain scant vestige of previous inflammation. Those ocular structures already well differentiated at the time of the endophthalmitis (cornea, uvea, optic nerve) may undergo atrophy and scarring or be left virtually untouched. Other tissues, such as retina, are actively differentiating and exhibit a combination of the above atrophy and scarring as well as abortive regeneration and arrested differentiation. RPE in most examples (bluetongue virus being an apparent exception) is infected and

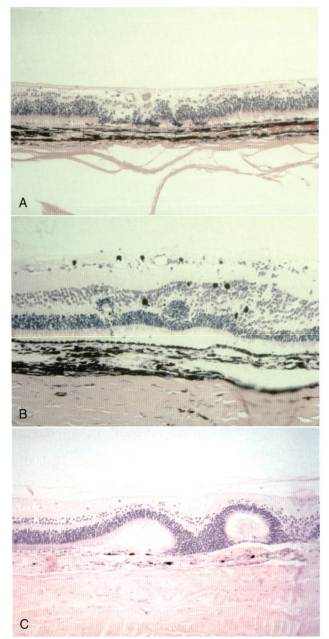

Figure 5-19 Retinal dysplasia. **A.** Postnecrotic retinal "dysplasia" caused by bovine viral diarrhea virus (BVDV) infection of a calf. Multifocal loss of outer nuclear layer and photoreceptors and the paucity of ganglion cells result from in utero viral infection. Blending of inner and outer nuclear layers reflects loss of neurons from both the inner and outer nuclear layers. **B.** Pigment-laden cells from retinal pigment epithelium (RPE) have migrated into the disorganized retina in a puppy surviving canine distemper. **C.** Focal chorioretinal scar with loss of outer nuclear layer and fibrous metaplasia of adjacent RPE in a calf with prenatal BVDV infection.

subsequently injured. *The result is a patchy alternation of abortive retinal regeneration, hyperplastic pigment epithelium, and postnecrotic glial scarring* (Fig. 5-19C). The lesions are usually more severe in nontapetal retina and are bilateral but not necessarily symmetrical. It seems reasonable to speculate that those naturally occurring cases in which the dysplasia is confined to peripheral retina represent late viral infection when only peripheral retina is still differentiating.

Because the virus has affinity for other neural tissues, *all calves with retinal dysplasia induced by bovine viral diarrhea virus also have cerebellar atrophy, and some have hydrocephalus or hydranencephaly.* A similar association with hydrocephalus and other brain anomalies has been described for feline panleukopenia virus infection in cats, bluetongue virus infection in sheep, and in a possibly hereditary syndrome in white Shorthorn and Hereford cattle. In the latter 2 instances, the involvement of virus could not be excluded based upon published information.

Experimental irradiation of neonatal puppies (and, presumably, kittens) results in retinal necrosis and scarring virtually indistinguishable from postviral retinal dysplasia.

True retinal dysplasia, not associated with exogenous infection or teratogen, is rare. *It is characterized by retinal folds, retinal rosettes, patchy to diffuse blending of nuclear layers, loss of retinal cells, and glial scars.* The folds and rosettes are the histologic counterparts of the vermiform streaks seen on the fundus with the ophthalmoscope. The hallmark of retinal dysplasia is the rosette, composed of a central lumen surrounded by 1-3 layers of neuroblasts. The 3-layered rosette is the most common in naturally occurring cases in animals, and shows more or less complete retinal differentiation. Most such rosettes are probably retinal folds cut transversely and, as mentioned previously, should not be considered true dysplasia if no additional lesions are present. The lumen contains pink fibrils resembling photoreceptors and is bounded by a thin membrane resembling the normal outer limiting membrane. One- and 2-layered rosettes are encountered infrequently and consist of a lumen surrounded by undifferentiated neuroblasts.

True retinal dysplasia occurs in combination with chondrodysplasia in several dog breeds, but particularly in Labrador Retrievers and Samoyeds. Cataract and persistent hyaloid remnants may accompany the retinal lesion. In Labradors, all the defects are the result of a single gene, with recessive effects on the skeleton and incompletely dominant effects on the eye.

Optic nerve hypoplasia. *Hypoplasia is the most common anomaly of the optic nerve.* The defect may be unilateral or bilateral, and usually occurs in eyes with other anomalies and particularly in eyes with retinal dysplasia. *In most instances, the so-called "hypoplasia" is more likely to be atrophy* as the inevitable result of the destruction of ganglion cells in glaucomatous, viral, toxic, genetic, or idiopathic retinal disease (Fig. 5-20). The only clear example of an alternative pathogenesis is that associated with *maternal deficiency of vitamin A in cattle*, in which atrophy of the developing optic nerve results from failure of remodeling of the optic nerve foramen and subsequent stenosis. A similar lesion occurs in *pigs*, but in that species, hypovitaminosis A seems more indiscriminately teratogenic, and optic nerve hypoplasia is accompanied by diffuse ocular dysplasia and multiple systemic anomalies. Hypoplasia is a relatively frequent clinical diagnosis in *toy breeds of dogs*, without apparent visual defects (and thus rarely receives histologic examination). Most examples are probably hypomyelination of the optic disc, which results from premature halt of myelinated nerve fibers at, or posterior to, the lamina cribrosa. The opposite, with myelin extending too far into the nerve fiber layer of the peripapillary retina, is also seen in dogs and is a frequent but insignificant occurrence in horses.

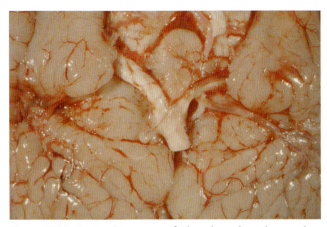

Figure 5-20 **Optic chiasm** in a foal with unilateral secondary (degenerative) microphthalmos. Small left optic nerve caused by prenatal atrophy following ganglion cell destruction.

Inherited optic nerve hypoplasia is documented in one strain of laboratory mice, although it may accompany inherited retinal dysplasia or multiple inherited anomalies in any species. Histologic examination of affected eyes reveals few, if any, ganglion cells and a thin and moth-eaten nerve fiber layer.

Further reading

Grahn BH, et al. Inherited retinal dysplasia and persistent hyperplastic primary vitreous in Miniature Schnauzer dogs. Vet Ophthalmol 2004;7:151-158.

Narfstrom K. Hereditary and congenital ocular disease in the cat. J Feline Med Surg 1999;1:135-141.

O'Toole D, et al. Retinal dysplasia of English springer spaniel dogs: light microscopy of the postnatal lesions. Vet Pathol 1983;20:298-311.

Percy DH, et al. Lesions in puppies surviving infection with canine herpesvirus. Vet Pathol 1971;8:37-53.

Uchida K, et al. Congenital multiple ocular defects with falciform retinal folds among Japanese black cattle. Vet Pathol 2006;43: 1017-1021.

Anomalies of surface ectoderm

From fetal surface ectoderm are derived corneal epithelium, lens, lacrimal apparatus, and the epithelial portions of the eyelids and associated adnexa. Seldom are anomalies of the extraocular structures the subject of histopathologic study inasmuch as they are clinically obvious and of significance only if they result in corneal irritation, impaired vision, or unacceptable appearance.

Excessively large or small palpebral fissures are part of current fashion in some dog breeds. *Micropalpebral fissure frequently leads to entropion* as the lid margin curls inward, and resultant corneal abrasion necessitates surgical correction. Congenital entropion also occurs as sporadic flock epizootics in lambs, but whether this is a structural deformity or the result of eyelid spasm is unclear. Entropion associated with microphthalmos occurs in all species. Other eyelid defects include colobomas, which are focal to diffuse examples of eyelid agenesis, and delayed separation of the eyelid fusion, which is the normal state during organogenesis.

Disorders of cilia are very common in dogs, but uncommon in other species. Congenital defects include one or more of ectopic cilia, misdirected but otherwise normal cilia (**trichiasis**), the occurrence of a second row of cilia from the orifice of normal or atrophic Meibomian glands (**distichiasis**), and excessively large cilia (**trichomegaly**). In each instance, the significance of the anomaly depends on the presence or absence of corneal irritation.

The lacrimal gland and its ducts develop from an isolated bud of surface ectoderm and, although anomalies must surely exist, they have not been investigated. *Failure of patency of the lacrimal puncta* occurs in dogs and horses and manifests as excessive tearing. Ectopic or supernumerary openings have been reported in dogs and in cattle.

Corneal anomalies. Primary corneal maldevelopment is rare in all species. The category may be expanded to include *corneal dystrophies*, defined as bilateral, inherited, and usually central corneal opacities that, despite their typically adult onset, presumably have a congenital basis. These rare lesions will be discussed with degenerative diseases of the adult cornea.

Corneal anomalies may be ectodermal or mesenchymal, and may affect one or more of corneal size, shape, or transparency. **Microcornea** refers to a small but histologically normal cornea in an otherwise normal globe. A small cornea occurring in a microphthalmic globe is expected and does not merit a separate description. Mild microcornea of no clinical significance is reportedly common in certain dog breeds. **Megalocornea** has not been reported in domestic animals, except in predictable association with congenital buphthalmos.

Dermoid is a congenital lesion of cornea or conjunctiva characterized by *focal skin–like differentiation*, and as such is properly termed a **choristoma**. They occur in all species. There is one report of a geographically high prevalence of multiple, and sometimes bilateral, dermoids as an inherited phenomenon in Polled Hereford cattle in the American Midwest, but ordinarily they seem to occur as single, random anomalies of unknown pathogenesis. Defective induction (skin instead of corneal epithelium) by the invading corneal stromal mesenchyme is the most popular speculation.

The *degree of differentiation varies*, but most consist of stratified squamous keratinized and variably pigmented epithelium overlying an irregular dermis containing hair, sweat glands, and sebaceous glands. Very rarely, cartilage or bone is seen. The degree of adnexal differentiation varies widely but may approach that of normal skin (Fig. 5-21). At the edge of the dermoid, the dermal collagen reorients to blend with the regular stroma of cornea, and the epidermis transforms itself to corneal epithelium. Surgical removal may be for cosmetic reasons, or may be required if dermoid hairs irritate cornea, or if the position of the dermoid interferes with vision. In most instances of corneal dermoid, the choristoma is attached to the surface of a corneal stroma of normal thickness, so excision of the dermoid should not risk perforation of the globe.

Congenital corneal opacities are usually caused by anomalous *formation of the anterior chamber, particularly anterior segment dysgenesis and persistent pupillary membranes.* Adherence of anterior chamber structures to the corneal endothelium results in focal absence of the corneal endothelium and disorganization of adjacent corneal stroma. Grossly, the affected cornea has deep stromal opacity caused by stromal edema or fibrosis in the area of the defective endothelium. Pigment, originating from adherent uveal strands, may be found in the corneal stroma. The opacity may be diffuse or focal, depending on the extent of uveal-corneal adhesion. Many examples probably reflect sequels to early neonatal

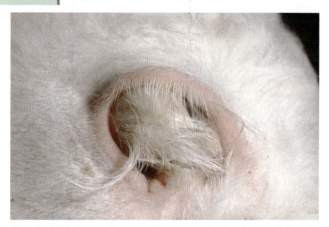

Figure 5-21 Corneal dermoid in a calf. Notch-like defect in lower lid is a coloboma.

corneal perforation that resulted in iris prolapse and subsequent anterior synechiae rather than true developmental disorders, but that distinction can be very difficult to make when looking at globes enucleated many weeks or months after the original event.

Diffuse, congenital corneal opacity occurs in Holstein-Friesian cattle in England and Germany. The histologic lesion is diffuse corneal edema, but its pathogenesis is unknown. The cornea remains permanently opaque.

Corneal opacity caused by noncellular depositions occurs in dogs and is usually of adult onset despite an apparently genetic basis. The exception is multifocal, subepithelial deposition of basophilic, PAS-positive material in the corneas of puppies with Collie eye anomaly or other mesodermal dysgeneses. The material is of unknown origin and may be the histologic counterpart of the transient, multifocal, subepithelial opacities seen quite commonly in 2-3 week-old puppies whose eyes are otherwise normal and thus unavailable for histologic examination.

Anomalies of lens. The lens may be abnormally small, abnormally shaped, ectopic, or cataractous. Of these, *only ectopia and cataract are common.*

Aphakia *is the congenital absence of the lens, and it may be primary or secondary.* It is claimed that primary aphakia is possible only in a rudimentary globe because of the central role of lens in the induction of invagination of the primary optic vesicle. Any globe with the structure of optic cup, regardless of how dysplastic, must have had a lens early in organogenesis, and its absence later must be the result of degeneration. This assumption is an extrapolation from work done many years ago in chicken embryos; although no work has been published to refute this contention, there is no work in mammals to confirm it. In the one report of aphakia in modern literature that includes histologic examination, several other puppies had small lenses, and all had invaginated optic cups with iris and retina. There was no conclusion about the nature of the injury to the developing eyes or the timing of such injury.

Microphakia, *or congenitally small lens,* is reported in dogs, calves, and cats, but is nonetheless rare. Because the development of the lens is so intrinsic to proper ocular development, almost all reports describe the defect in association with ectopia lentis, microphthalmos, and anterior chamber mesenchymal anomalies. Such lenses are spherical and almost always are cataractous.

Lenticonus and **lentiglobus** *are rare defects of lens shape* characterized by an abrupt change in capsular configuration so that the lens acquires a conical or globular protrusion. The defect is usually polar and, in animals, usually posterior. From scattered and very old descriptions, it is difficult to define the "typical" histology of such lesions or their pathogenesis. The defect usually appears as a focal overgrowth of cortical lens fibers covered by thin posterior lens capsule and retained posterior epithelium. Of 4 relatively recent descriptions, all of canine eyes, all had congenital cataract, but only in one did the cataract involve the protruding lens fibers themselves. Other ocular lesions reported include hyperplasia of tunica vasculosa lentis, rupture of the lens protrusion, and dysplasia of ciliary epithelium. At least in Doberman Pinscher dogs, the posterior lentiglobus or lenticonus accompanying hyperplastic tunica vasculosa lentis appears to be an acquired defect caused by the abnormal fibrovascular elements adherent to the lens.

Congenitally ectopic lenses occur in all species, but are relatively common only in dogs and horses. *Much more common than congenital luxations are spontaneous luxations in adult dogs,* which may be associated with acquired lesions of the zonule. The reason for the particular susceptibility of small terriers is related to the widespread prevalence of a mutation within the *ADAMST17* gene that is involved in the remodeling of structural proteins in many different tissues, including the lens zonules (see further under Ectopia lentis).

Congenital cataract occurs in most severely anomalous eyes, but may occur as an isolated ocular lesion. When cataract is present in eyes with multiple anomalies, it usually results from persistence of some part of perilenticular vasoformative mesoderm, but may also result from intraocular inflammation or toxic degeneration. Persistence of pupillary membrane or hyaloid system frequently results in multiple epithelial defects and subcapsular opacities at the sites of mesodermal contact with the lens.

In dogs, congenital primary cataracts are frequently hereditary but, as with corneal and retinal diseases, most hereditary cataracts are not detectable until later in life. Subtle, nonprogressive nuclear or cortical opacities are common but clinically insignificant in dogs and are of unknown pathogenesis. Primary, and usually diffuse, cataract is the most common ocular anomaly of horses. The pathogenesis is unknown, but there is usually no other ocular lesion. Congenital cataract is rare in cattle, swine, sheep, and goats. In cattle, hereditary congenital cataract occurs in Holstein-Friesians and in Jerseys and is thought to be an autosomal recessive trait. It is also seen as an infrequent result of fetal infection with bovine viral diarrhea virus.

There is a single report of bilateral, complete cataracts in a litter of Persian kittens, but there are no examples in swine or small ruminants except in association with multiple ocular defects.

The pathology of congenital cataract is the same as acquired cataract, and is discussed later. It may be nuclear, cortical or capsular, focal or diffuse, stationary or progressive, depending upon the timing and pathogenesis of the original injury.

Further reading

Brudenall DK, et al. Bilateral corneoconjunctival dermoids and nasal choristomas in a calf. Vet Ophthalmol 2008;11:202-206.

Hubmacher D, Apte SS. Genetic and functional linkage between ADAMTS superfamily proteins and fibrillin-1: a novel mechanism influencing microfibril assembly and function. Cell Mol Life Sci 2011;68:3137-3148.

Müller C, et al. Analysis of systematic and genetic effects on the prevalence of different types of primary lens opacifications in the wild-boar-colored wirehaired Dachshund. Berl Munch Tierarztl Wochenschr 2008;121:286-291.

Nafstrom K, Dubielzig R. Posterior lenticonus, cataracts and microphthalmia in the Cavalier King Charles Spaniel. J Small Anim Pract 1984;25:669-677.

Samuelson DA, et al. Prenatal morphogenesis of the congenital cataracts in the miniature schnauzer. Lens Res 1987;231-250.

Ocular adnexa

The adnexa include eyelids, nictitating membrane, and lacrimal and accessory lacrimal glands. Developmental, degenerative, inflammatory, and neoplastic diseases of these structures are commonly encountered in clinical practice, but only the neoplasms and proliferative inflammatory lesions are regularly submitted for histologic examination.

Eyelids

Developmental anomalies and acquired diseases of the eyelid are very common in clinical practice, but almost none of these are submitted for histologic assessment. The exceptions are eyelid neoplasms and proliferative nodules that have not responded to routine medical therapy, and those are the examples emphasized here.

Blepharitis is inflammation of the haired skin of the eyelid. In most cases, the blepharitis is only part of a more generalized skin disease, such as atopy, demodicosis, or pemphigus, and such examples will not be considered here. Inflammatory lesions more or less unique to the eyelid include hordeolum, chalazion, and idiopathic granulomatous marginal blepharitis.

External hordeolum or **stye** is *suppurative adenitis of the adnexal glands of Zeis or Moll.* **Internal hordeolum** is *suppurative inflammation of the Meibomian gland.* They are mentioned here only because they are part of traditional eyelid pathology and will be mentioned in clinical texts, but receiving histology samples from such lesions is extremely infrequent.

Chalazion is *sterile granulomatous inflammation in response to the leakage of Meibomian secretion into the surrounding dermis.* Although it can theoretically occur in response to any type of injury to the Meibomian gland, almost all cases are found adjacent to Meibomian adenomas. The histologic lesion is distinctive, consisting of an accumulation of lakes of free lipid and numerous large foamy macrophages and multinucleated cells around the abnormal Meibomian gland. The macrophages contain distinctive refractile intracellular slender elongated slit-like unstained spaces that we assume represent secretory material unique to Meibomian glands. Similar lipid-rich granulomatous inflammation is seen in response to the leakage of secretion from sebaceous adenomas elsewhere in skin, but these slit-like clear spaces are not seen in anything other than Meibomian adenomas (Fig. 5-22A, B). In cats, those examples with particularly prominent free lipid accumulation were originally described as idiopathic lipogranulomatous conjunctivitis (see later), but current opinion is that it is just a feline version of chalazion.

Idiopathic granulomatous marginal blepharitis is a uniquely canine lesion. The macroscopic lesion varies from a single nodule to a series of coalescing nodules that create

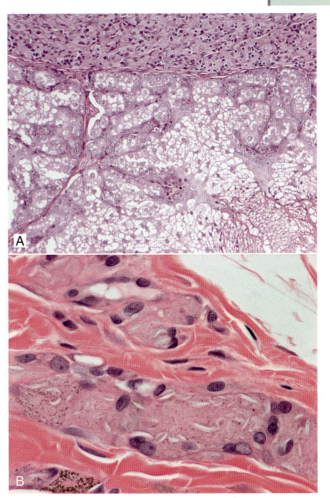

Figure 5-22 Chalazion. **A.** Leaking Meibomian adenoma surrounded by foamy macrophages. **B.** The macrophages contain characteristic unstained slit-like inclusions of unknown chemical composition, unique to chalazion.

virtually diffuse thickening of one or both eyelid margins. *The histologic lesion is a coalescence of suppurating granulomas in the subconjunctival tissue of the eyelid margin, without any proven association with adnexal structures and without any identifiable etiologic agent.* The granulomas often form around a clear central lipid vacuole, with or without neutrophils at the interface between the vacuole and the surrounding macrophages. The lesion bears considerable similarity to cutaneous sterile pyogranuloma syndrome and other idiopathic granulomatous panniculitis syndromes, all of which are equally mysterious in terms of pathogenesis. *The lesions differ from those of chalazion in that the latter does not form discrete granulomas, does not involve neutrophils, and is always found adjacent to Meibomian glands.*

Lacrimal system

Acquired disease of the lacrimal system is probably quite common in dogs if one includes keratoconjunctivitis sicca (see Keratitis) and eversion of the gland of the third eyelid.

Dacryoadenitis is *inflammation of the lacrimal gland,* and may result from involvement in orbital cellulitis or orbital trauma, spread from severe intraocular inflammation, incidental involvement in systemic diseases, such as malignant catarrhal fever, feline infectious peritonitis, and canine distemper; or apparently specific immunologic assault. Specific dacryoadenitis caused by a coronavirus is extremely common in laboratory rats in which acute necrotizing inflammation of lacrimal, Harderian, and salivary glands results in eventual fibrosis and squamous metaplasia of affected glands. Residual lesions in mildly affected rats are multiple lymphoid aggregates in the glandular interstitium. Similar changes are often seen in dogs with keratoconjunctivitis sicca, and in the absence of demonstrated viral cause, are assumed to represent autoimmune lacrimal adenitis. The analogous lesion in people with Sjögren syndrome is associated with influx of numerous T-helper cells into the gland, but no studies have yet been published to prove this immune pathogenesis for canine lacrimal adenitis and atrophy. However, the efficacy of cyclosporine, which acts primarily by suppression of T-helper cells, in reversing canine lacrimal adenitis provides evidence for such a pathogenesis.

Similar inflammation affects the histologically similar gland of the third eyelid, and it is probably true that the third eyelid can be used to monitor the presence of disease within the main orbital lacrimal gland and the response to cyclosporine therapy.

Protrusion of the nictitans gland is quite common in dogs, and is thought to reflect a congenital laxity in the connective tissue anchoring the gland to the cartilage of the third eyelid. Because the resultant eversion is unsightly and resembles a neoplasm, these lesions frequently are excised even though the membrana nictitans may be normal except for overlying conjunctival inflammation from exposure and abrasion. Because this gland sometimes supplies a significant proportion of total lacrimal secretion, its surgical removal may be followed by keratoconjunctivitis sicca in dogs that have less than optimal function of the primary lacrimal gland. In dogs with keratoconjunctivitis sicca, the gland may suffer the same lymphocytic interstitial adenitis, fibrosis, and atrophy as affects the lacrimal gland itself.

Lacrimal duct cysts are seen clinically as focal accumulations of clear watery fluid causing cystic distention of the lacrimal canaliculi or lacrimal sac embedded within the conjunctival lamina propria near the medial canthus. Microscopically, there is cystic distention of a canaliculus, lacrimal sac, or proximal lacrimal duct lined by stratified squamous or pseudostratified cuboidal-to-columnar epithelium, depending on the exact location of the cyst. There may be residual lymphocytic inflammation and proprial fibrosis to suggest previous inflammation that may have caused duct obstruction either with exudate or via stricture. The surgical specimen seldom contains the exact site of obstruction, and in most cases, the cause for the obstruction remains speculative.

Conjunctiva

At the orifice of the Meibomian glands, the epidermis of the lid undergoes abrupt transition to the pseudostratified columnar mucous membrane typical of the palpebral conjunctiva. Goblet cells increase in number from the lid margin to the fornix, but ordinarily are absent in that portion of conjunctiva that extends from the fornix to the corneoscleral junction (bulbar conjunctiva). The number of goblet cells within the palpebral conjunctiva is regionally variable and also varies by species, so that any diagnoses based on an assumption of increased or decreased goblet cell numbers must be made with great care. Lymphoid aggregates are normal in the subepithelial connective tissue, particularly below the bulbar conjunctiva and the bulbar (inner) aspect of the nictitating membrane. These aggregates are more prominent in the conjunctiva of horses than other domestic species. Whether this increased prominence is normal or a reflection of increased antigenic stimulation of the conjunctiva in the dusty environment of many horse stables is unknown. The palpebral conjunctiva parallels the eyelid skin as it is directed toward the orbital rim, but then reverses direction at the fornix (also known as the conjunctival cul-de-sac) and transforms into the stratified squamous nonkeratinized epithelium of the bulbar conjunctiva heading toward the cornea. The transition from conjunctival to corneal epithelium overlies the transition from sclera to corneal stroma known as the **limbus.** It is an important structure clinically because it is the origin for most of the inflammation, pigmentation, scarring, and vascularization that characterize most severe corneal diseases. The limbus is not a precise line but a region characterized by transition from conjunctival to corneal epithelium, and by transition from the disorganized and vascularized connective tissue of the sclera to the nonvascular and highly regimented stroma of the cornea. There is often a slight thickening of the conjunctival epithelium at this transition zone, which is the site of the permanent replicative population of germinal cells important in normal corneal epithelial turnover and especially important in the healing of corneal wounds.

The general pathology of the conjunctiva is similar to that of other mucous membranes, but those reactions are also similarly "stereotypic" and seldom contain any histologic clues as to exact etiology or pathogenesis. *It is therefore rare for conjunctival biopsies to contain any specific etiologic information.* The diagnostic utility of conjunctival biopsies is further limited by the fact that most samples are not taken until the disease is chronic and all reasonable medical therapies have failed.

Acute conjunctival injury, whether physical, chemical, or microbial, results in hyperemia and severe edema. Evacuation of goblet cells and cellular exudation from the very labile conjunctival vessels add to the excessive lacrimation caused by any ocular irritation. With increasing severity of insult, the ocular discharge progresses from serous to mucoid and perhaps purulent.

Chronic injury results in various combinations of epithelial hyperplasia, disappearance of visible goblet cells, lymphofollicular hyperplasia, and squamous metaplasia progressing to keratinization. Lymphoid hyperplasia may be so marked as to result in grossly visible white nodules that may require surgical or chemical removal to reduce irritation of the adjacent cornea (clinically known as lymphofollicular conjunctivitis). Such *lymphoid hyperplasia is best considered a nonspecific response to any chronic antigenic stimulation, and it carries no etiologic specificity.* Conjunctivitis frequently accompanies other ocular disease, notably keratitis, uveitis, and glaucoma. Conversely, conjunctival inflammation may spread to the cornea, uvea, and orbit, although only secondary corneal involvement is common. The discussion later is directed at those diseases that cause conjunctivitis as the major clinical presentation, rather than examples of conjunctivitis that are simply bystander effects of inflammation in other parts of the globe.

The causes of primary **conjunctivitis** *include every class of noxious stimulus, including allergy and desiccation. As mentioned previously,* conjunctival biopsy is rarely performed until all therapeutic measures have failed. Also as mentioned previously, because conjunctiva seems to have such a limited range in histologic reaction, regardless of the nature of the initial injury, and also because such biopsies are usually delayed until the disease is chronic, it is rare for either histology or cytology to provide any real insight into the etiology of conjunctivitis. The etiologic significance of the lists of bacterial, fungal, and even viral agents mentioned in clinical textbooks should be considered with considerable skepticism in light of the normal bacterial and mycotic flora, and the high prevalence of conjunctival carriage of several viral agents in clinically normal animals.

Conjunctivitis occurs in a wide variety of multisystem diseases, such as canine distemper, Rocky Mountain spotted fever and ehrlichiosis, equine viral arteritis and babesiosis, bovine viral diarrhea, malignant catarrhal fever, classical swine fever, African swine fever, and others. Conjunctivitis accompanies most viral and allergic diseases of the upper respiratory tract. Only those diseases in which conjunctivitis is particularly prominent are discussed here.

Infectious bovine rhinotracheitis (IBR) in **cattle** is usually accompanied by serous to purulent conjunctivitis, which can be confused clinically with *infectious bovine keratoconjunctivitis* ("pinkeye") caused by *Moraxella bovis* (discussed later). However, corneal involvement with IBR is uncommon and is never the central suppurating ulcer typical of infectious keratoconjunctivitis. In an unpredictable number of animals, multifocal white glistening nodules, 1-2 mm in diameter, may be seen on the palpebral or bulbar conjunctiva. They appear as early as 3 days after instillation of bovine herpesvirus 1 into the conjunctival sac, and represent hyperplastic lymphoid aggregates. Overlying conjunctiva may be ulcerated and the defect filled with fibrin. IBR is discussed in Vol. 2, Respiratory system; Vol. 2, Alimentary system and peritoneum; and Vol. 3, Female genital system.

Conjunctivitis in **dogs** is most often a manifestation of allergy, desiccation, or mechanical irritation. Confirmed examples of infectious conjunctivitis are rare except as part of some of the systemic diseases mentioned previously.

In **cats**, however, most examples of *primary conjunctivitis* are probably caused by infectious agents. The agents most often incriminated are felid herpesvirus 1 (FHV-1, feline rhinotracheitis virus) and *Chlamydophila felis* (formerly *Chlamydia psittaci*). The diagnosis is usually made based upon clinical characteristics, the presence of other clinical signs, and demonstration of the infectious agent via PCR, immunofluorescence assay (IFA), or culture. Histologic lesions are not etiologically specific, and demonstration of the specific infectious agent in histology or cytology samples (even with the aid of immunofluorescence) is seldom possible because the smears or biopsies are taken too late in the course of the disease.

Felid herpesvirus 1 causes a combination of conjunctivitis, keratitis, and upper respiratory disease when it first infects young cats, but it may cause conjunctivitis alone as a recurring infection in older cats that had recovered from the initial disease. The disease caused by the initial infection (usually in kittens 8-12 weeks of age, but occasionally in naive older cats) is much more severe than the conjunctivitis and/or keratitis associated with recurring disease in older cats. Infection of conjunctival and corneal epithelium results in cellular necrosis, transient suppurative or fibrinopurulent conjunctivitis, and then a more chronic lingering lymphocytic-plasmacytic conjunctivitis with squamous metaplasia. The etiologic specificity in the form of intranuclear eosinophilic herpetic inclusions is usually seen only in the first week of disease, a time at which clinicians are most unlikely to take biopsies. Many cats become lifelong carriers, with virus persisting in the trigeminal ganglion and periodically returning to the conjunctiva and/or cornea via retrograde axonal migration. The conjunctivitis seen in older cats is the result of unpredictable reactivation of latent infection, but is generally a mild and histologically nonspecific lymphocytic-plasmacytic conjunctivitis. A reliable etiologic diagnosis is difficult because of the poor sensitivity of virus isolation and immunofluorescence, and false positives related to the high prevalence of subclinical carriers.

Chlamydophila felis usually causes unilateral conjunctivitis in cats of any age, without any other associated disease. The conjunctivitis is initially neutrophilic, but rapidly becomes a nonspecific mixed infection with subepithelial neutrophils, macrophages, lymphocytes, and plasma cells. Early in the disease (between days 3 and 14), typical intracytoplasmic inclusion bodies can be seen, and their detection is enhanced by immunofluorescent staining. Because the clinical signs are characteristic and disease is easily treated with tetracycline, histologic assessment is rarely required. In cases that are resistant to therapy, the disease is usually chronic and histologically nonspecific by the time biopsy is eventually done.

Parasitic conjunctivitis. Parasitic conjunctivitis is relatively common worldwide and may be caused by members of the genera *Thelazia, Habronema, Draschia, Onchocerca,* and several members of the family *Oestridae*. Of these, only *Thelazia* is truly an ocular parasite; the others cause eyelid, conjunctival, or orbital disease incidentally in the course of larval migration.

Members of the genus ***Thelazia*** are thin, rapidly motile nematodes 7-20 mm in length that inhabit the conjunctival sac and lacrimal duct of a variety of wild and domestic mammals worldwide. Their prevalence is much greater than the prevalence of conjunctivitis, suggesting that their number must be greater than usual before signs of conjunctival irritation are observed. The species most commonly associated with conjunctivitis in domestic animals are *T. lacrymalis* in horses; *T. rhodesi, T. gulosa,* and *T. skrjabini* in ruminants; *T. callipaeda* in carnivores and humans; and *T. californiensis* in many species, including dog, cat, bear, coyote, deer, and man. Female worms are viviparous, and larvae free in lacrimal secretions are consumed by flies of the genus *Musca*, in which they develop for 15-30 days. The third-stage infective larvae migrate to the fly's proboscis and are returned to the conjunctival sac as the fly feeds.

Ocular habronemiasis results from deposition of larvae by the fly intermediate host, usually *Musca domestica* or *Stomoxys calcitrans*, in the moisture of the medial canthus of horses. Larvae of *Habronema muscae, H. microstoma,* or *Draschia (Habronema) megastomum* are the culprits. The burrowing larvae cause an ulcerative, oozing lesion ~0.5-1.0 cm in diameter at the medial canthus, which becomes progressively more nodular as a granulomatous reaction to the larvae mounts. Mineralized granules may be found within the lesion along with caseous debris, liquefaction, and viable larvae. The histologic lesion is similar to that of cutaneous habronemiasis, namely, chronic eosinophilic and granulomatous inflammation surrounding live or dead larvae and eosinophils (Fig. 5-23).

Ocular onchocerciasis results in the formation of granulomas and suppurating granulomas around fragmented or viable adult filarids within the sclera and subconjunctival lamina

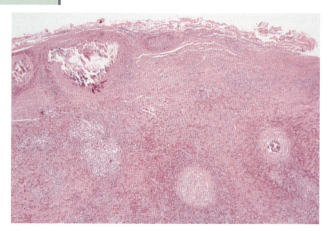

Figure 5-23 Conjunctival habronemiasis. Only rarely would fragments of larvae be detected within the center of these eosinophil-rich mineralizing granulomas.

propria of dogs. Dogs are considered abnormal hosts for this parasite, which is much more commonly found in horses, cattle, and other ungulates. In horses, the infection causes a more diffuse eosinophilic and granulomatous conjunctivitis and peripheral stromal keratitis with a character similar to that in skin. Adults and microfilariae can be identified within the reaction. Microfilariae of *Onchocerca* are routinely encountered within conjunctival lamina propria and almost never cause histologic lesions or clinical signs.

Ophthalmomyiasis. A syndrome of periocular and even intraocular invasion by *fly larvae* occurs in various species, including humans. Its various manifestations are known collectively as ophthalmomyiasis. Specific *oculovascular myiasis*, "*uitpeuloog*," or "*gedoelstial myiasis*" is a disease of domestic ruminants and horses caused by invasion and migration of larvae of **Gedoelstia** spp. of the family *Oestridae*. The *Gedoelstia* are parasites of the blue wildebeest and hartebeest, the larvae being deposited in the eye, rather than in the nares, as is the habit of *Oestrus ovis*. The most important member of the genus in terms of frequent aberrant parasitism in domestic species is *G. hassleri*, which in its natural antelope host migrates to the nasal cavity via the vascular system, cerebral meninges, and subdural space. The parasitism is not clinically significant in the antelope, but in domestic species that are aberrant hosts, severe ocular and neural disease occurs, sometimes on a large scale. The disease is seasonal and occurs particularly in domestic ruminants in contact with wildebeest.

The ocular lesions vary from *transient mild conjunctivitis to destructive ophthalmitis* with orbital or periorbital edema or abscessation affecting one or both eyes. Neurologic signs of varied pattern are common in sheep, partly caused by the larvae directly and partly by thrombophlebitis marking their route of invasion. Thrombosis may be very extensive, may involve the jugular vessels and endocardium, and may cause sudden death when coronary vessels are affected.

Larval migration may be into the conjunctival sac, orbital tissues, or into the eye itself. In the last instance, *ophthalmomyiasis interna*, the globe is often destroyed by the larval penetration. However, a syndrome of relatively harmless larval migration in the subretinal space or within vitreous has been reported in people. The characteristic subretinal linear tracks may be accompanied by focal retinal separation, preretinal and subretinal hemorrhage, and focal proliferations of retinal pigment epithelium. Two reported cases in cats had similar subretinal tracks, hyperplasia of pigment epithelium, and retinal hemorrhages. In one, the live motile larva was detected either on the face of, or just within, the retina. Subsequent examination failed to detect the larva, and the eye lesions resolved except for the subretinal tracks and pigment clumps.

The penetration is usually by a single larva despite numerous eggs or larvae within the conjunctiva. The larva may die within the globe or continue its migration by uneventful exit from the globe via sclera, optic nerve, or vessel adventitia.

Ophthalmomyiasis interna anterior has also been reported in a cat in association with infection with a first instar larva of **Cuterebra** spp. Severe anterior uveitis resolved after prompt surgical removal of the larva, but retinal degeneration and blindness ensued.

Immune-mediated conjunctivitis. Presumed allergic conjunctivitis occurs in all species but is most likely to be investigated in dogs (most examples of conjunctivitis in cats are assumed to have an infectious pathogenesis). Rarely is a specific allergen identified and, like its counterparts in allergic skin diseases, the diagnosis is based upon the failure to demonstrate infectious or mechanical causes, response to corticosteroid therapy, and sometimes a convincing association with environmental changes. Biopsy is rarely warranted, but when taken during the acute disease may show epithelial changes ranging from erosion to hyperplasia to squamous metaplasia, with eosinophils around dilated subepithelial blood vessels and percolating throughout the epithelium. Eosinophils are much more likely to be identified in cats than in dogs, a species difference that is also true of allergic skin disease in general. More chronic lesions, which are the more usual to be biopsied, have squamous metaplasia, lymphocytic-plasmacytic subepithelial infiltrates, and the formation of lymphoid nodules.

There are a few histologically distinctive examples of conjunctivitis that are assumed to represent immune-mediated disease, mostly because they respond only to aggressive immunosuppressive therapy. In some dogs with chronic conjunctivitis (perhaps particularly German Shepherd dogs), the infiltrate sometimes becomes particularly plasmacytic, diffuse, and thick in a fashion resembling an interface dermatitis. The bulbar surface of the third eyelid is the favorite location, and many believe this lesion (sometimes referred to as "*plasmoma*") to be the conjunctival variant of pannus keratitis.

Cats and horses may develop a severe **eosinophilic conjunctivitis** that is thought, by some, to be a conjunctival counterpart of the eosinophilic keratitis syndrome. Lesions may be unilateral or bilateral, and, at least in cats, there is almost always a concurrent ulcerative marginal blepharitis. Histologic changes include ulceration, epithelial hyperplasia, squamous metaplasia, and a heavy lymphocytic infiltration with a large proportion of eosinophils. The role of felid herpesvirus 1 in the pathogenesis of eosinophilic conjunctivitis and keratitis in cats remains controversial, with strongly conflicting results in different studies. For further details, see Feline eosinophilic keratitis.

Ligneous conjunctivitis is a distinctive clinical and histologic entity, thus far confirmed only in dogs. It appears to be a close clinical and histologic counterpart for the human disease of the same name. The clinical disease is bilateral and characterized by marked "wooden" thickening and opacity of the palpebral conjunctiva and conjunctiva of the third eyelid. Histologically, the conjunctival lamina propria is thickened by

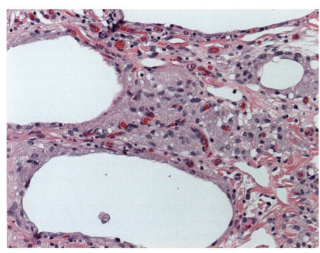

Figure 5-24 Feline lipogranulomatous conjunctivitis. Lipid lakes and foamy macrophages indistinguishable from canine chalazion.

massive deposition of hyalinized fibrin and a diffuse scattering of mononuclear leukocytes. The defect is seen in dogs with congenital (and probably inherited) plasminogen deficiency, resulting in the excessive persistence of fibrin that is presumably being generated as part of almost any type of inflammatory disease. The specificity of the diagnosis does not reside in the character of the inflammation, but in the abnormal persistence of the fibrin once it is generated. Only one report included postmortem evaluation of other tissues, and there were similar fibrin deposits below other mucous membranes, as well as in epicardium and endocardium. Conjunctival lesions can be successfully treated with topical plasminogen.

Feline lipogranulomatous conjunctivitis is probably the feline counterpart of canine chalazion. The lesion occurs almost exclusively in the lamina propria of the palpebral conjunctiva adjacent to the margin of either the upper or lower eyelid. The histology is very repeatable, consisting of a nodular accumulation of clear lipid lakes intermingled with large foamy macrophages and a few small or mononuclear leukocytes (Fig. 5-24). Although the original report contained no mention of adjacent Meibomian lobules, the similarity between this entity and canine chalazion is impossible to ignore (see Fig. 5-22B).

> **Key Points**
>
> Almost every enucleated globe will have lymphocytes and plasma cells diffusely and/or in nodules within the bulbar and palpebral conjunctival lamina propria. We have no idea of the normal reference range for leukocytes in this location, and therefore distinguishing normal resident leukocytosis from pathologic lymphocytic-plasmacytic conjunctivitis is completely subjective.

Further reading

Dugan S, et al. Clinical and histologic evaluation of the prolapsed third eyelid gland in dogs. J Am Vet Med Assoc 1992;201:1861-1867.
Hillstrom A, et al. Evaluation of cytologic findings in feline conjunctivitis. Vet Clin Pathol 2012;41:283-290.
Horak IG. Parasites of domestic and wild animals in South Africa. XLVI. Oestrid fly larvae of sheep, goats, springbok and black wildebeest in the Eastern Cape Province. Onderstepoort J Vet Res 2005;72:315-320.
Labelle AL, et al. Canine ocular onchocercosis in the United States is associated with *Onchocerca lupi*. Vet Parasitol 2013;193:297-301.
Mason SL, et al. Ligneous membranitis in Scottish terriers. Vet Rec 2012;171:160.
Pusterla N, et al. Cutaneous and ocular habronemiasis in horses: 63 cases (1988-2002). J Am Vet Med Assoc 2003;222:978-982.
Wieliczko AK, Płoneczka-Janeczko K. Feline herpesvirus 1 and *Chlamydophila felis* prevalence in cats with chronic conjunctivitis. Pol J Vet Sci 2010;13:381-383.

CORNEA

The cornea of domestic mammals is a horizontal ellipse of modified skin varying from 0.6-2.0 mm in thickness among the various species. In general, the larger and older the animal, the thicker is the cornea. It has 3 histologic layers; physiologically, there is a fourth and most superficial layer of precorneal tear film, but that is not visible histologically. The most superficial layer is 10-15 layers of *stratified squamous nonkeratinized epithelium* sitting on a thin basal lamina. That epithelium has limited regenerative capacity, forms a hydrophobic barrier via tight junctions between the horizontal cell membranes, and is anchored to the underlying stroma by hemidesmosomes with anchoring fibrils that penetrate through the basal lamina and into the superficial stroma. That epithelium has a turnover time of approximately 2 weeks, and the germinal basal cells are continuously replenished by centripetal migration of cells from the permanent replicative population that resides in the bulbar conjunctiva at the limbus.

The middle layer, and always the thickest layer, is the *corneal stroma*. It resembles modified sclera, with the collagen fibers being particularly thin and regular, stretching the entire diameter of the cornea without interruption and lying parallel to the corneal surface. The stromal fibrocytes, known as *keratocytes*, are inconspicuous. There are no blood vessels, and there are no visible leukocytes within the normal corneal stroma. Innermost is a single layer of flattened cuboidal epithelial cells known as the *corneal endothelium*. It makes a basement membrane that becomes progressively thicker throughout life, known as *Descemet's membrane*. That membrane separates the corneal endothelium from overlying stroma (Fig. 5-25A). Further details of corneal histology and biology will be introduced later as they become relevant to lesion interpretation.

Understanding corneal disease requires a firm grasp of corneal embryology, physiology, and microscopic anatomy. Without this understanding, corneal disease simply becomes a list to be memorized and diagnosed only if the lesions match pictures and descriptions already contained in various textbooks. This is not fruitful because the range of diseases is seemingly infinite, and the lesions hardly ever match perfectly with published photographs! *Fortunately, there are only 3 fundamental concepts required to truly understand 95% of all corneal diseases.*

1. The cornea begins its embryologic life as skin, and seems to harbor a secret desire lifelong to return to being skin! It is able to survive postnatally as an avascular, cell-poor, transparent cornea only because it is afforded a moist and

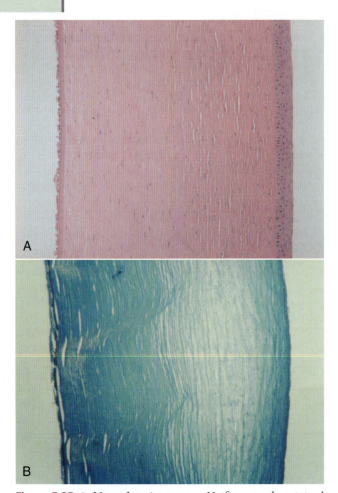

Figure 5-25 A. Normal canine cornea. Uniform, nonkeratinized epithelium without pigmentation or rete ridges. Stroma is poorly cellular. The clefts among the stromal fibers are unavoidable formalin fixation artifacts. **B. Central corneal edema** from abrasion of the corneal endothelium by a luxated lens. Masson trichrome stain.

sheltered environment thanks to the constant protection and support offered by the eyelids, the tear film, and the orbital bones. If there is any lapse in the ability of these structures to properly protect and nurture the cornea, it will slowly revert to being skin by becoming keratinized, pigmented, and vascularized.

2. When subjected to an injury that overwhelms the structural and functional protection offered by the tear film, eyelids, and orbit, the cornea has only 2 fundamental responses: acute and severe injury that results in epithelial or stromal death seen clinically as ulceration, or mild and chronic injury permitting the cornea to adapt via cutaneous metaplasia to become histologically and functionally skin-like and therefore much more resistant to further injury.

3. Because the cornea has no resident blood vessels or leukocytes, it cannot undergo true inflammation, and so *there is no such thing as primary "keratitis."* Almost all lesions interpreted clinically as keratitis are actually the result of corneal injury and repair. Only in the event of cutaneous metaplasia, with the acquisition of blood vessels, can the cornea undergo true inflammation.

The cornea exists in a privileged environmental niche, bathed in the nurturing and antimicrobial saline of the tear film and protected from other irritation by the movable eyelids. Within this protected niche, the cornea does therefore not require the protective attributes of skin (keratinization, leukocytes, blood vessels) to protect itself from the harsh external environment. If there is rapid deterioration in any component of this protective environment, the cornea is most likely to respond with ulceration and subsequent wound healing. If, on the other hand, the shift is of gradual onset, then the more likely response is adaptive metaplasia in which the cornea reaches into its embryologic cutaneous heritage and becomes skin-like.

Corneal injury may result from physical or chemical trauma, microbial agents, increased intraocular pressure and, rarely, from inborn errors of metabolism. Specific features of some of these injuries will be discussed later, but the general reactions to most corneal injuries are presented here.

Corneal edema

The essential clinical attribute of the cornea is its clarity, and it is the loss of clarity that is the most obvious indicator of corneal disease. The clarity results from several highly specialized anatomic and physiologic features: an unusually regular, nonkeratinized, and nonpigmented surface epithelium; an avascular, cell-poor stroma composed of very thin collagen (mostly type I) fibrils arranged in orderly lamellae separated by a critical distance to allow the uninterrupted passage of light (62–64 nm); and a high degree of stromal dehydration maintained by the presence of epithelial tight junctions, endothelial tight junctions, and a Na^+-K^+–dependent ATPase pump in the cell membrane of the corneal endothelium (see Fig. 5-25A).

Corneal edema occurs rapidly following injury and results from imbibition of lacrimal water through damaged corneal epithelium, absorption of anterior chamber water at a site of corneal endothelial damage, or failure of electrolyte (and thus water) extrusion by the corneal endothelial electrolyte pump (a mechanism for corneal edema, which is fluid leakage from ingrowing corneal blood vessels, as discussed later). If the epithelial or endothelial defect is focal, the resultant edema is limited to the stroma adjacent to the defect. The edematous cornea is clinically opaque, and may be up to 5 times its normal thickness. At least experimentally, edema subsequent to endothelial damage tends to be more severe than edema secondary to epithelial injury. Edematous stroma stains less intensely than normal, and collagen lamellae are separated into a fine feltwork of pale-staining fibrils by excessive hydration of the glycosaminoglycan ground substance (principally keratan sulfate, dermatan sulfate, and chondroitin sulfate). These sulfated glycosaminoglycans have different water-binding capacities, and differences in glycosaminoglycan distribution within different layers of the corneal stroma may explain why corneal edema is sometimes more obvious at one level of the stroma than others (Fig. 5-25B). Percolation of stromal fluid into the epithelium results in the intercellular and intracellular edema known as bullous keratopathy.

Edema may also accompany corneal vascularization in response to severe corneal injury or in response to angiogenic growth factors produced elsewhere in the globe (e.g., uveitis or intraocular neoplasia) that simply "overflow" to stimulate the corneal ingrowth of the blood vessels at the limbus. Other examples of corneal edema are seen in glaucoma, lens luxation, and anterior segment anomalies. In the former, it is assumed that the high aqueous pressure drives fluid into the hydrophilic corneal stroma to a degree that overcomes the endothelial ion pump that dehydrates the stroma under normal conditions. In lens luxation, there is mechanical abrasion of corneal endothelial cells, and in anterior segment anomalies (such as persistent pupillary membranes or congenital anterior synechiae), there are focal developmental defects in endothelial continuity.

Persistent corneal edema seems to predispose to stromal vascularization and fibrosis, but numerous experimental models show that edema itself is not the stimulus. Instead, it is probably the accompanying infiltration of neutrophils through corneal epithelial defects or from peripheral neovascularization that provide most of the angiogenic and fibroblastic cytokines. Damaged epithelium and stromal fibroblasts are alternative sources. A natural example of virtually permanent corneal edema, without accompanying vascularization, occurs in several dog breeds (most frequently in Boston Terriers, Dachshunds, Chihuahuas, and German Shepherd dogs) with corneal endothelial dystrophy. The disease in all breeds is of adult onset, with slowly progressive, bilateral, and apparently spontaneous degeneration of corneal endothelial cells accompanied by ineffective repair in the form of fibrous metaplasia. When the number of viable endothelial cells decreases to <50% of normal, persistent bilateral diffuse stromal edema ensues (for more details, see Corneal dystrophies and deposits).

> ### Key Points
> Fixation of cornea in isotonic fixatives such as 10% formalin results in unavoidable artifactual osmotic edema that is seen as clear clefts separating adjacent stromal collagen fibers. Distinguishing this from genuine edema can be almost impossible, and it is wise to rely on clinical descriptions more than histopathology for the detection of acute corneal edema.

Corneal cutaneous metaplasia

Injury to the corneal surface that exceeds the homeostatic ability of that epithelium, resulting in corneal ulceration, is described later. Less drastic change to the local environment that results in sublethal injury to the surface epithelium (qualitative or quantitative inadequacy of tears, irritation from misdirected eyelashes or from entropion, or exophthalmos) will result in adaptive cutaneous metaplasia. As mentioned previously, even the adult cornea retains an embryonic capacity to revert to skin if it is deprived of its normal nurturing environment. *The chronically irritated epithelium therefore undergoes reactive hyperplasia with the appearance of rete ridges, melanin pigmentation, and surface keratinization.* The adjacent stroma undergoes dermis-like irregular fibroplasia and acquires vascularization via capillary migration from the limbus. These changes, although they enable the cornea to survive in a hostile environment and to combat the inflammatory stimulus, also deprive it of its transparency (Fig. 5-26A, B).

Corneal cutaneous metaplasia is probably not an in situ transformation of corneal stroma and epithelium. Instead, it probably represents a failure of corneal transformation by the permanent replicative population of scleral fibroblasts and conjunctival epithelium that constantly replenish the corneal stroma and epithelium.

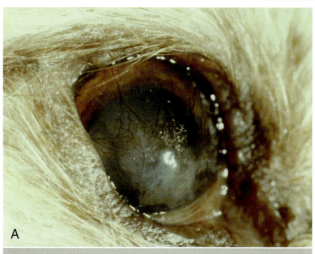
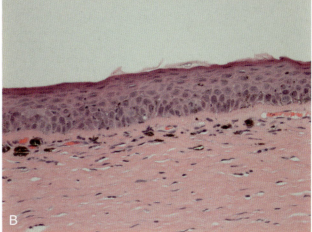

Figure 5-26 Corneal cutaneous metaplasia. A. Dog with stromal vascularization and scarring in response to chronic keratoconjunctivitis sicca. B. Corneal keratinization, epithelial and stromal pigmentation, thickened basement membrane, and superficial stromal vascularization. Chronic keratoconjunctivitis sicca.

> ### Key Points
> Virtually every enucleated globe will have corneal lesions of some type. The most common are peripheral stromal fibrovascular ingrowth as part of corneal wound healing or in response to intraocular inflammatory disease, and corneal ulceration or cutaneous metaplasia in response to acute or chronic corneal desiccation.

Corneal wound healing

Virtually every globe submitted by a veterinary practitioner for histologic assessment will have some type of corneal injury, varying from acute ulceration to more chronic manifestations of post-ulcerative wound healing. These lesions may be intrinsic to the primary ocular disease or may be purely secondary to conditions such as glaucoma, endophthalmitis, or exophthalmos. A thorough understanding of corneal injury and wound healing is essential to properly interpret the clinical and diagnostic significance of the corneal lesions.

Corneal ulceration represents a loss of the surface epithelial barrier. It causes rapid osmotic imbibition of the tear film water, resulting in corneal edema. Neutrophils are absorbed as well, usually just in small numbers appropriate to the physiologic debridement and sterilization of the injured tissue. Neutrophils are also important contributors to the initiation of the wound healing process. Excessive or abnormally persistent recruitment of neutrophils, however, carries the risk of initiating excessive stromal lysis as a reflection of bystander injury. Such excessive recruitment is usually a reflection of secondary bacterial infection and is discussed further in the sections dealing with keratitis.

The mechanisms of healing of corneal wounds vary with the severity of the injury, and involve an extremely complex interaction of epithelium, stroma, and innumerable cytokine growth factors derived from tear film, infiltrating leukocytes, and resident epithelium and stroma. Only the major elements will be described here, with an emphasis on histologically detectable events rather than on chemical mediators.

The most pragmatic classification of corneal injuries is to distinguish septic from nonseptic injuries, and then to subdivide nonseptic injuries into superficial versus deep, and transient versus persistent or recurrent. Even these distinctions are not ironclad because nonseptic injuries may become secondarily infected, and shallow injuries may progress to involve deeper stroma. Nonetheless, it is helpful to impose some sense of order on this potentially chaotic picture to facilitate understanding.

Shallow and transient nonseptic defects involving epithelium alone, or epithelium and superficial stroma, heal by epithelial sliding, followed after ~24 hours by mitosis (Fig. 5-27A). One

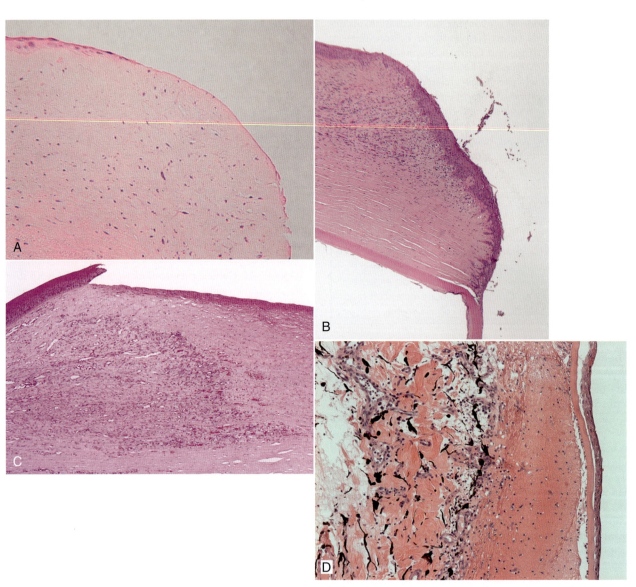

Figure 5-27 Corneal wound healing. A. Recent shallow uncomplicated ulcer healing by local epithelial sliding. Note the osmotic stromal edema and the expected sparse accumulation of neutrophils from the tear film, **B.** In this deep ulcer, the proliferating epithelium has migrated down the edges of the wound to reach Descemet's membrane. Note the accompanying stromal granulation tissue originating from the limbus. **C.** Coordinated migration from the limbus by epithelium and granulation tissue attempting to heal a stubborn corneal ulcer. **D.** The migrating corneal epithelium is using a remnant of Descemet's membrane and a prolapsed iris as a scaffold for migration following corneal perforation.

cannot claim that the initial depth alone is the deciding factor, because even very deep wounds will sometimes heal just with epithelial sliding and eventual mitotic rebuilding, as long as the epithelium is satisfied with the quality of the underlying stroma. The sliding begins within a few hours, initially from wing cells from the immediately adjacent, viable cornea. Migration by basal cells rapidly follows. The sliding is preceded by lysis of the hemidesmosomes. Adhesion of the sliding epithelium is initially to adhesion molecules such as fibronectin and laminin deposited along the exposed stromal surface. Reformation of the hemidesmosomes and their anchoring filaments may take weeks or even months, during which time epithelial adhesion remains precarious. Healing of shallow, uninfected corneal ulcers by sliding epithelium is rapid, ~1 mm per day; restoration of the basal lamina and hemidesmosomes may take up to ~6 weeks.

Persisting or reoccurring shallow ulcers that cannot be healed just by sliding, and replication of adjacent corneal epithelium may require the recruitment of cells from the conjunctival epithelium at the corneoscleral junction, which is the site of the permanent replicative population. Such cells, when recruited for corneal wound healing, may retain a conjunctival phenotype that includes pigmentation and a tendency to form rete ridges. The exact chemical signaling that determines whether the migrating epithelium retains a conjunctival phenotype or becomes truly corneal is not known, but epithelium that is migrating into an environment of persistent desiccation or superficial irritation will typically remain "conjunctival," and is often referred to as *cutaneous metaplasia* (see Fig. 5-26). The regenerating epithelium always seems to produce its own new basement membrane even if pre-existing basement membrane still seems available, so thickening of the basement membrane is one of the histologic clues by which we identify recurrent ulceration. If the injurious stimulus disappears, the conjunctival character of the epithelium slowly fades, being replaced within 4-6 weeks by a normal corneal epithelial configuration. Epithelial adhesion to the underlying stroma remains fragile for 6-8 weeks until the hemidesmosomal attachments of epithelium to basal lamina and stroma can rebuild. In the interim, the cells adhere to a mixture of fibrin and fibronectin derived from the inflamed conjunctival vessels via the tear film or from the injured cornea itself. In many cases, the only evidence of previous shallow ulceration is a thickened basal lamina resulting from secretion by the regenerating epithelium, and gentle undulation of the normally flat epithelial-stromal interface.

Injuries involving substantial stromal damage may be a direct result of the severity of the initial injury, but more often, it is the result of neutrophil-mediated stromal lysis in those corneal injuries that were initially, or later became, septic. Sometimes this neutrophil-mediated stromal lysis (known clinically as keratomalacia) develops even in the absence of detectable sepsis. Shallow defects in the superficial stroma may become filled by a thickened plaque of epithelial cells that create an *epithelial facet*. Deeper defects that include more than the outer third of stroma will usually require rebuilding of the damaged stroma before epithelial sliding and regeneration can occur, but this is not invariable. The quality of the stroma seems to be more important than the quantity of stroma when it comes to determining whether wound healing will occur just by epithelial sliding, or whether the stroma itself must be rebuilt as a prelude to successful epithelial healing. Even very deep corneal ulcers sometimes heal almost exclusively with epithelial sliding and subsequent replication, with no apparent effort to rebuild the stroma (Fig. 5-27B). What determines the exact pattern of wound healing is probably the mixture of cytokine growth factors produced in response to corneal injury. The list of growth factors and their origins seems almost endless, and the confusion is perpetuated by our inability to accurately transfer in vitro experimental information into an in vivo clinical situation. The activity of these various cytokines depends on when the cytokine is introduced, how much of it is present, and what other cytokines are present within the environment. The major cytokines involved in corneal wound healing, their most common functions, and the usual cells of origin are listed in Table 5-1. What follows is a greatly simplified version of these events.

Within a few hours of the insult, neutrophils enter the wound via the tear film. They migrate into the stroma and control bacterial contamination, degrade damaged collagen, and stimulate both fibroplasia and vascularization via production of various cytokines, especially basic fibroblast growth factor derived from injured epithelium, stromal neutrophils, and injured stromal fibroblasts themselves. Viable stromal cells (keratocytes) adjacent to the wound undergo fibroblastic

Table 5-1

Cytokine mediators of corneal wound healing

Event*	Cytokine trigger	Sources
Superficial stromal apoptosis	IL-1	Injured corneal epithelium, injured keratocytes, tear film
Corneal epithelial flattening, sliding	EGF, HGF	Tear film, corneal epithelium
Stromal myofibroblastic differentiation	PDGF	Epithelial basement membrane, leucocytes
	TGF-β	Tear film
Influx of leucocytes	MCAF	Keratocytes stimulated by IL-1 or TNF-α
	TNF-α	Injured epithelium
Stromal lysis	IL-1 upregulates local proteases	Keratocytes, corneal epithelium, tear film
	MCAF attracts leucocytes	Injured keratocytes
	TNF-α attracts leucocytes	Injured epithelium

EGF, epidermal growth factor; *HGF*, hepatocyte growth factor; *IL-1*, interleukin-1; *MCAF*, monocyte chemotactic and activating factor; *PDGF*, platelet-derived growth factor; *TGF-β*, transforming growth factor-β; *TNF-α*, tumor necrosis factor-α.
*Listed in order of occurrence following shallow corneal mechanical injury.

metaplasia and secrete large amounts of sulfated ground substance, particularly chondroitin sulfate. Most of the new stroma is produced by fibroblasts recruited from the limbus. Their ingrowth is always accompanied by a similar ingrowth of new blood vessels (Fig. 5-27C). This ingrowth begins ~4 days after substantial corneal injury, and migrates from the limbus centrally at a maximal rate of ~1 mm per day. This 4-day lag time is, presumably, a period of grace in which small or shallow defects can heal with epithelial regeneration alone, without the visual impairment that inevitably follows stromal fibroplasia. Once the epithelium seals the defect, there is immediate cessation of neutrophilic influx and, presumably, a similarly abrupt drop in the production of fibroblastic/angioplastic stimulatory cytokines. *The scarring and vascularization that are the manifestations of stromal rebuilding are permanent*, even though the fibrous tissue gradually becomes less cellular, the collagen fibrils reorient to resemble more closely the parallel arrays of normal stroma, and the ground substance gradually reverts from an embryonic configuration dominated by chondroitin sulfate to the normal predominance of keratan sulfate. Complete restitution of normal stroma, however, never occurs, although the residual scar may be subtle and better detected by clinical examination than by histology. Undesirable though such scarring may be, it is certainly better than the alternative of ineffective corneal healing and inevitable corneal rupture.

Healing of a corneal perforation involves the same events as does healing of a deep corneal ulcer, but there are some added challenges and complications. The cut edges of Descemet's elastic membrane retract from the wound, and the transcorneal gap is initially plugged with fibrin and, sometimes, by prolapsed iris. The migrating corneal epithelium seems so focused on sealing the defect that it will sometimes use that temporary scaffold as a substrate on which to slide (Fig. 5-27D). If the gap is not closed by suturing or by a provisional matrix supplied by fibrin and/or iris stroma, there is the risk that the surface epithelium will grow downward along the cut surface of the stroma and into the anterior chamber. Its migration will be inhibited only by contact with viable corneal endothelium. If it does not encounter that endothelium, there is nothing to stop the epithelium from growing as a layer of stratified squamous epithelium all over the inside of the globe. Obstruction of the filtration angle inevitably causes glaucoma.

As with the surface epithelium, the corneal endothelium at the deep edge of the perforation attempts to bridge the defect by sliding over the fibrin scaffold to restore endothelial continuity. Replacement by mitosis begins within ~24 hours in some experimental models, but *the replicative capability of the corneal endothelium in adult animals of most domestic species is very limited, and repair occurs by endothelial sliding and hypertrophy*. So potent is this capability that normal stromal dehydration can be maintained even in the face of a 50% reduction in endothelial cell density (in dogs, ~25,000 cells/mm^2). The cut ends of Descemet's membrane make no apparent effort at regrowth, but rather, the endothelium gradually secretes a new membrane that may eventually fuse with the old or remain separated from it by a layer of fibrous tissue.

The sequence of epithelial sliding and regeneration, remodeling stromal fibrosis, and endothelial repair is not uniformly successful. There are many variations on this stereotypic theme because there are so many different variables related to initial causation and to secondary complications (especially

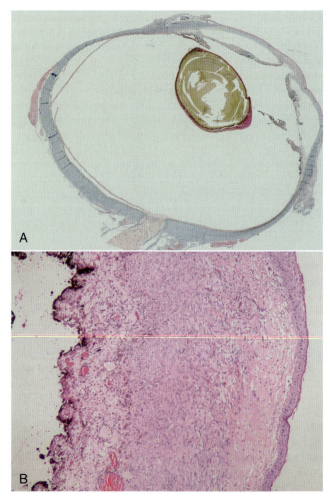

Figure 5-28 Anterior synechiae. **A.** Permanent focal anterior synechia as a sequel to iris prolapse following corneal perforation in a steer with *Moraxella bovis* infection. Masson trichrome stain. **B.** The iris is firmly adherent to the deep border of the scarred cornea, thereby obliterating the anterior chamber.

sepsis). This influences the exact intermingling of all the chemical and cellular ingredients involved in this wound healing. Large gaping wounds commonly fill with a mixture of prolapsed iris and fibrin that will usually resolve into permanent iridocorneal adhesions known as *anterior synechiae* (Fig. 5-28A). The migrating corneal epithelium will commonly use the iris as a "substitute stroma," growing across its surface to seal the corneal defect while leaving the iris permanently incorporated into the corneal stroma (Fig. 5-28B). Perforating injuries that disrupt Descemet's membrane and corneal endothelium stimulate repair of that endothelium as described previously, but in many cases, there is also a plaque of fibrous tissue that forms in the deep stroma and in the anterior chamber adjacent to that injury. The fibroblasts, most of which are probably derived from stromal keratocytes but which may also evolve via endothelial fibroblastic metaplasia, tend to grow along the posterior surface of Descemet's membrane to form what is known as a *retrocorneal fibrous membrane*. Eventually, the corneal endothelium may regain continuity on the posterior surface of this membrane, secrete a new Descemet's membrane, and result in a cornea with 2 separate Descemet's membranes separated by persistence of this retrocorneal fibrous membrane.

Corneal dystrophies and deposits

Deposits of various lipids and minerals may occur within the corneal stroma or basement membrane zone as part of an inborn metabolic error (corneal dystrophies), secondary to excessive circulating levels of these lipids and minerals, or secondary to corneal injury. Such deposits are clinically obvious and are relatively common in clinical practice, but they are neither common nor obvious in samples submitted for histologic assessment. With the exception of corneal endothelial dystrophy (which is very different from all the others), only rarely do they cause significant visual impairment, and they are almost never the cause for ocular enucleation or evisceration. They are occasionally encountered in globes removed for other reasons, and they are included here only for completeness.

Corneal dystrophies are bilateral, inherited (but not necessarily congenital) defects in structure or function of one or more corneal components not triggered by injury or systemic disease. They are subclassified as epithelial, stromal, or endothelial, but as a group they are poorly understood, and the current classifications are based mostly on clinical parameters. They are all uncommon, and almost all examples have been described in dogs. The list grows daily, with more than 30 different breeds affected. The least infrequent are the stromal dystrophies characterized by the deposition of lipids and/or minerals within an otherwise normal-appearing stroma. The deposition of mineral or lipid secondary to inflammatory disease or systemic metabolic abnormality should not be interpreted as corneal dystrophy (corneal dystrophies are considered separately later).

True corneal dystrophies are clinically obvious, and they are diagnosed based on clinical characteristics and especially based on the breed of dog affected. They are not usually significant to visual function and are of concern only because they are unsightly and inherited. *It would be rare for a pathologist to receive any type of biopsy specimen except as part of a research study.* Only a few of the most common or most classic examples are presented here.

Corneal lipid and crystalline dystrophies

Corneal stromal crystalline dystrophies are by far the most common dystrophies that are seen in clinical practice. They include a wide range of breed-specific lipid and/or mineral deposits within the corneal stroma, with the exact age of onset, location, and clinical appearance being relatively specific in each breed and therefore allowing fairly reliable clinical diagnosis. Specimens are rarely available for histologic assessment because the disease does not cause blindness and is not associated with any systemic abnormality. In most, the chemical nature of the deposit and character of the corneal stromal metabolic abnormality have not been determined. They are seen as accumulations of cholesterol crystals within and among corneal stromal collagen fibers, or as deposits of mineral within the very superficial stroma or basement membrane. They are usually bilateral and symmetrical, and initially they are not associated with inflammation or repair. It is claimed that some will eventually trigger corneal injury with resultant scarring and vascularization, but there are virtually no histologic studies, and it is very difficult to be certain whether such cases are true dystrophies or are occurring secondary to some other type of corneal injury.

Corneal endothelial dystrophy occurs in Boston Terriers, Chihuahuas, Dachshunds, German Shepherd dogs, and several other dog breeds, and causes slowly progressive bilateral corneal edema in mature dogs. The edema usually begins adjacent to the lateral limbus and may initially be unilateral and unaccompanied by other clinical signs. Later, epithelial fluid bullae may rupture to cause painful corneal ulcers and associated inflammation. Despite the persistent stromal edema, fibrosis and vascularization do not occur unless rupture of epithelial bullae initiates keratitis. *The primary lesion is spontaneous necrosis of corneal endothelium, followed by hypertrophy, fibroblastic metaplasia, and sliding of viable endothelium.* A marked progressive decrease in overall endothelial cell density eventually causes severe bilateral corneal edema. The reason for the endothelial cell death is unknown. Focal irregularities in Descemet's membrane occur in areas of endothelial loss, presumably a result of new basement membrane production by adjacent endothelium making a futile effort at regeneration.

A rare, juvenile-onset, genetically transmitted *endothelial dystrophy in Manx and domestic shorthair cats* is manifest as bilateral, progressive central epithelial and stromal edema. Fluid accumulates within superficial stroma and within the epithelium. Primary morphologic abnormalities are not described in the Manx, but in shorthairs there is irregularity and vacuolation of corneal endothelium.

Corneal deposits secondary to metabolic disease

Deposition of mineral, lipid, or pigment within the cornea may occur secondary to chronic corneal injury or to systemic metabolic disease in any species. The most frequent of these is peripheral stromal deposition by lipids in animals with hyperlipidemia associated with Cushing's disease, diabetes mellitus, hypothyroidism, or excessive dietary lipid intake. Most of these animals have documented hyperlipidemia, and the deposition of these lipids within cornea is just accidental "overflow" from the limbal blood vessels. Such depositions may initially be noninflammatory, but in most instances, they are accompanied by substantial secondary inflammation and vascularization. Histologically, there is disruption of normal corneal architecture by superficial stromal deposition of cholesterol crystals, accompanied by nonseptic granulomatous inflammation, fibrosis, edema, and vascularization (Fig. 5-29).

Much less prevalent than secondary corneal lipidosis is stromal or basement membrane mineralization in animals with hypercalcemia. Most examples of stromal or basement

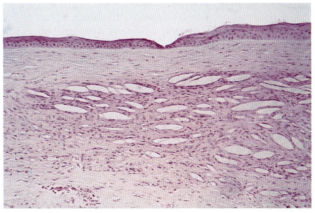

Figure 5-29 Lipid keratopathy. Clefts of cholesterol within the corneal stroma trigger mild nonseptic granulomatous inflammation.

membrane mineralization are reflections either of a primary corneal dystrophy or of dystrophic mineralization secondary to stromal injury (see later).

Corneal deposits secondary to injury

Corneal melanosis often accompanies *chronic corneal irritation in dogs* and less frequently in other species, particularly horses. The pigment is found in the basal layer of the corneal epithelium and in the superficial stroma. *It is the result of progressive ingrowth of new germinal cells that have retained pigment from the bulbar conjunctiva.* The clinical name, "pigmentary keratitis," is inaccurate because the disease is not inflammatory. The corneal epithelium is invariably hyperplastic and often has the other features of *corneal cutaneous metaplasia*, such as rete ridge formation, keratinization, and abnormally thick basement membrane. There is usually evidence of chronic stromal inflammation, including vascularization. Deeper focal corneal stromal pigmentation without evidence of epithelial cutaneous metaplasia occurs infrequently, associated with previous iris prolapse that has contributed uveal melanin to the corneal stromal scar.

Hemosiderin will be found within corneal endothelial cells subsequent to anterior chamber hemorrhage or within stromal macrophages if there has been hemorrhage into the corneal stroma itself. Similar pigment may occur following implantation of corneal foreign bodies containing iron or other metals.

Vascularization is often present, but its pathogenesis is unknown. It appears that corneal vascularization can predispose to stromal lipidosis in animals with hyperlipemia, but it is also true that some animals with primary corneal lipidosis will develop secondary inflammation and vascularization.

Mineral deposition occurs primarily in the anterior stroma and the epithelial basement membrane. Predisposing corneal changes include desiccation, anesthesia, edema, or inflammation. *There are many methods for inducing deposition of calcium salts, but stromal edema seems to be the common denominator in almost all cases.* The edema may result from corneal epithelial desiccation (exposure keratitis), uveitis, corneal trauma, or chemical injury. Hypercalcemia from vitamin D toxicity or hyperparathyroidism exacerbates the mineralization and is essential to lesion development in some experimental models.

An unidentified corneal deposition is often seen in canine eyes suffering from multiple anomalies, particularly those involving uvea. Similar deposits are seen, with less regularity, in the horizontal mid-portion of the cornea of many normal puppies. Fine basophilic PAS-positive linear deposits are associated with the epithelial basement membrane or superficial stroma. There is some disarray of superficial stromal fibers but no inflammation. The nature and pathogenesis of the deposit are unknown, but most disappear after a few months.

Corneal degeneration

"Corneal degeneration" is a vague term sometimes used to describe those corneal lesions characterized by *noninflammatory loss of epithelial or stromal viability*. Diseases such as keratoconjunctivitis sicca and pannus keratopathy are sometimes considered primary degenerative lesions, but their principal manifestation is inflammation, and they are discussed under the section Keratitis.

The only degenerative, noninflammatory, acquired corneal lesions presented here are corneal sequestrum in cats and horses, and canine persistent erosion syndrome. All 3 diseases probably have a similar pathogenesis, but for the moment,

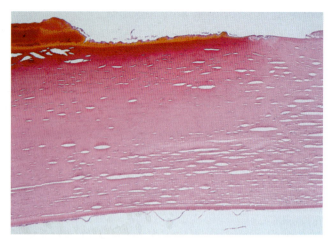

Figure 5-30 Feline corneal sequestrum with the characteristic orange-brown discoloration of the dead stroma.

they will be listed as 3 different diseases because they continue to be listed as separate diseases in clinical textbooks.

Feline corneal sequestrum *is recognized clinically as a discrete orange-brown discoloration of the central cornea, affecting one or both eyes*. Persian and Himalayan cats are more frequently affected than other breeds. Histologically, *the lesion is noninflammatory necrosis of stromal keratocytes, accompanied by pallor, hyalinization, and slight orange discoloration of the affected stroma*. The discoloration may be absent in very early cases (Fig. 5-30). The overlying epithelium may be ulcerated or intact, but in those cases with an intact epithelium, there is virtually always histologic evidence of previous ulceration. In older lesions, the periphery of the sequestrum may be marked by a zone of reactive mononuclear leukocytes and, perhaps, a few giant cells. The pigment is derived from porphyrins within the tear film, absorbed into the cornea as part of corneal edema that follows ulceration. *The sequestrum will eventually slough, and the defect heals by granulation* (although most lesions are treated by excision before that stage is reached).

The pathogenesis remains controversial. In flat-faced Persian and Himalayan cats, the pathogenesis probably involves corneal ulceration secondary to desiccation because of facial configuration. In non-Persian cats, there is a loose statistical association with herpesviral infection, and *it is reasonable to propose that corneal sequestrum is an uncommon sequel to any corneal ulceration in cats*. As will become clearer later, the brown discoloration is unique to cats and, for a long time, caused us to overlook the histologic similarity between the feline disease and similar histologic entities in horses and dogs. Not all feline cases acquire the characteristic brown pigmentation, and indeed, some examples are virtually indistinguishable from canine and equine persistent ulcers described later.

Canine persistent (recurrent) ulcer syndrome was first described in Boxer dogs (hence the old name "*Boxer* ulcer"). Although Boxers and related breeds may be predisposed, similar persistent or recurrent erosions are encountered in a wide variety of breeds. The recently proposed name of *spontaneous chronic corneal epithelial defects* (SCCED) is unfortunate because the defect is not primarily epithelial, and in many cases, it is not spontaneous but secondary to anything causing superficial corneal ulceration.

The clinical syndrome is distinctive, characterized by a shallow central corneal erosion with scant edema and (at least initially) no vascularization. The lesion refuses to heal, or repeatedly re-ulcerates, because of poor adhesion of the epithelium to the underlying stroma. The defect appears not to be in epithelial healing per se, because sliding and mitotic activity are normal in affected dogs, and all of the adhesion molecules and growth factors seem to be present. Keratectomy specimens reveal poorly adherent hyperplastic epithelium at the ulcer margins, usually with multiple clefts separating epithelium from stroma even in areas distant from the obvious ulcer. The basal lamina is usually not visible with light microscopy, and the epithelium appears to be attempting to adhere to a thin zone of hypocellular, pale-staining stroma that could correctly be interpreted as a very shallow sequestrum qualitatively similar to what was described previously in cats (Fig. 5-31A, B). *The observation of pyknotic and lytic keratocyte nuclei within this superficial zone suggests that the basic defect is degeneration of the superficial stroma*, so that epithelial hemidesmosomes and anchoring collagen fibrils attempting to reform after ulceration have no substrate in which to anchor. Very chronic cases usually acquire superficial stromal granulation tissue appropriate to any chronic ulceration, but its onset is much delayed in comparison to infectious or traumatic ulcers. The fact that epithelial adhesion and wound healing will be successful following the use of any technique that either removes the superficial sequestrum or punches multiple holes through it to allow deeper stromal granulation tissue to reach the wound healing surface strongly supports the notion that the barrier to wound healing lies in the presence of the devitalized stroma itself (Fig. 5-31C).

Corneal sequestrum in horses is less frequent and less well characterized than in dogs or cats. It is histologically identical to what occurs in dogs, although it seems often to be more complicated and disguised by superimposed fungal infection.

A unifying hypothesis for all 3 diseases is beginning to emerge. Studies of normal corneal wound healing have documented that degeneration of the most superficial stroma, detectable only with electron microscopy, is a normal response to corneal epithelial injury. It appears that these clinical syndromes of "persistent/recurrent ulceration" do not reflect ulceration of any specific pathogenesis, nor the persistence of the ulcerative stimulus. Instead, they seem to represent exaggeration and undue persistence of a normal superficial stromal degeneration that occurs with any superficial corneal injury. The persistence of this dead stroma prevents proper restitution of hemidesmosomal adhesion, but we still do not know why some superficial injuries trigger this excessive stromal degeneration.

Key Points

The syndrome of persistent/recurrent ulceration and corneal sequestration in any species is not a specific disease with a specific etiology and pathogenesis. Such lesions more likely reflect an unexplained exaggeration or persistence of the normal superficial stromal degeneration that occurs as a prerequisite for wound healing following superficial corneal ulceration of virtually any pathogenesis.

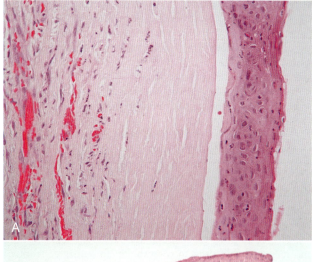
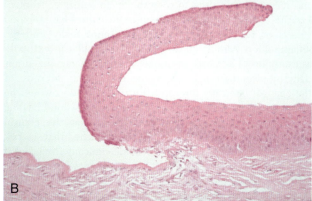
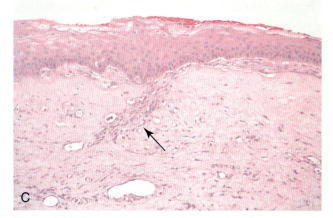

Figure 5-31 Canine persistent ulcer. A. Dysplastic, strongly regenerative epithelium is unable to adhere to the underlying superficial stroma. Note the superficial stromal acellularity indistinguishable from sequestrum. **B.** A clinically characteristic, non-adherent epithelial flap at the edge of a persistent ulcer. Note the very thin hypereosinophilic superficial stromal sequestrum. **C.** A "spot weld" of granulation tissue (arrow) penetrates the sequestrum as a result of successful surgical keratotomy. The epithelium can now adhere to a layer of granulation tissue on top of the sequestrum.

Further reading

Burling K, et al. Effect of topical administration of epidermal growth factor on healing of corneal epithelial defects in horses. Am J Vet Res 2000;61:1150-1155.

Cooley PL, Wyman M. Indolent-like corneal ulcers in three horses. J Am Vet Med Assoc 1986;188:295-297.

Crispin S. Ocular lipid deposition and hyperlipoproteinaemia. Prog Retin Eye Res 2002;21:169-224.

Hempstead JE, et al. Histopathological features of equine superficial, nonhealing, corneal ulcers. Vet Ophthalmol 2014;(Suppl. 1):46-52.

Maycock NJ, Marshall J. Genomics of corneal wound healing: a review of the literature. Acta Ophthalmol 2014;92:e170-e184.

Netto MV, et al. Wound healing in the cornea: a review of refractive surgery complications and new prospects for therapy. Cornea 2005;24:509-522.

Sanchez RF, et al. Canine keratoconjunctivitis sicca: disease trends in a review of 229 cases. J Small Anim Pract 2007;48:211-217.

Stepp MA, et al. Wounding the cornea to learn how it heals. Exp Eye Res 2014;121C:178-193.

Yu FS, et al. Growth factors and corneal epithelial wound healing. Brain Res Bull 2010;81:229-235.

Keratitis

Corneal inflammation is called **keratitis** *and has traditionally been divided into epithelial, stromal (interstitial), and ulcerative keratitis.* It is time to abandon this arbitrary classification, and it is probably time to re-evaluate the entire concept of keratitis as a primary disease. Because the cornea has no blood vessels or resident lymphocytes, it cannot really undergo inflammation. Almost all diseases listed in clinical textbooks as examples of keratitis are in fact diseases characterized initially by ulceration or by cutaneous metaplasia, and most of the changes clinically interpreted as inflammation would be better interpreted as essential parts of normal wound healing or adaptive metaplasia. The problem is that the clinical nomenclature of keratitis is so firmly entrenched that we risk having our histologic diagnoses become clinically irrelevant if we use terminology that strays too far from what is in the clinical textbooks.

Keratoconjunctivitis sicca is probably the most frequent example of the imprecision of clinical terminology, because this disease is not inflammatory. Corneal desiccation of any pathogenesis (from breed-related exophthalmos, from defective eyelid structure or function, from exophthalmos related to orbital masses, or from ocular enlargement secondary to glaucoma) is profoundly damaging to the cornea, but the specific terminology of keratoconjunctivitis sicca is ordinarily reserved for those examples of corneal desiccation resulting from defects in the quantity (and very rarely, in the quality) of the tear film. Keratoconjunctivitis sicca, as a specific disease entity, is encountered more commonly in **dogs** than in any other species, with an overall prevalence in North America of ~1%. Most cases are chronic, progressive, and idiopathic. The reason for greater than expected prevalence in certain breeds (English Bulldog, Lhasa Apso, Shih Tzu, West Highland White Terrier, and others) is unknown. Because the disease is amenable to medical or surgical management, few specimens are available for histologic examination until the very chronic stages. At this time, the lacrimal gland is atrophic with interstitial lymphoid infiltration and fibrosis, but provides no clue as to the initial lesion. The ability of certain immune modulators, notably cyclosporine, to reverse the disease points to some kind of immune-mediated phenomenon, perhaps autoimmunity causing a progressive destructive lymphocytic interstitial sialoadenitis.

The corneal changes vary with the severity and rapidity of onset of lacrimal deficiency. In acute disease with marked lacrimal deficiency, clinical signs of ulcerative keratitis may occur. The corneal epithelium is thinned, has numerous hydropically degenerate cells, and may suffer full-thickness ulceration. The accompanying stromal changes, including eventual vascularization and fibrosis, are those of ulcerative keratitis. More commonly in dogs, however, the desiccation is not absolute (at least initially), and the epithelial response is protective **cutaneous metaplasia** without prior ulceration. Keratinization, marked hyperplasia with rete ridge formation, and pigmentation are commonly seen. Stromal inflammation and vascularization are usually superficial, resulting in a lesion very similar to pannus keratitis. Squamous metaplasia may also occur in the bulbar conjunctiva. The conjunctivitis that clinically is the earliest lesion of keratoconjunctivitis sicca is rarely available for histologic examination.

The lesions following corneal desiccation from any other pathogenesis (in histology specimens, most commonly related to incomplete eyelid closure in dogs with ocular enlargement from glaucoma) resemble those of any other acute superficial ulceration, with the notable exception that the ulceration is not usually accompanied by edema or any substantial neutrophilic infiltration simply because there is no tear film to contribute the fluid or the neutrophils.

Most examples of **ulcerative keratitis** are more correctly thought of as corneal ulceration triggering purely secondary inflammation as part of normal wound healing or in response to purely opportunistic infection taking advantage of the loss of the epithelial barrier. The most common causes are desiccation or trauma, but there are a few very specific bacterial and viral pathogens that seem capable of colonizing and injuring even the normal cornea. *Regardless of cause, the loss of epithelium initiates a predictable series of corneal reactions caused by absorption of water and neutrophils from the tear film, local production of inflammatory mediators and cytokines, and opportunistic microbial contamination of the wound.* Imbibition of water causes superficial stromal edema below the ulcer and is followed by migration of neutrophils from the tear film and, later, from the limbus. The leukocytes, although somewhat protective against opportunistic pathogens, also add their collagenases, proteases, and stimulatory cytokines to the wound and thereby may inadvertently contribute to its progression. Epithelial and stromal repair proceeds as already described for corneal wound healing, but the repair fails in those cases in which microbial contamination is well established or in which the cause of the initial ulceration has not been corrected. Common examples of the latter are found in dogs in which corneal trauma by misdirected cilia or facial hair, or desiccation resulting from lacrimal gland dysfunction (keratoconjunctivitis sicca), persists.

The usual role of bacteria and fungi in the pathogenesis of corneal ulceration is opportunistic. However, these opportunists contribute significantly to the perpetuation and worsening of the lesion. Proteases and collagenases of microbial, leukocytic, or corneal origin progressively liquefy corneal stroma, a process termed **keratomalacia** (Fig. 5-32). Ulcers contaminated by *Pseudomonas* and *Streptococcus* spp. are particularly prone to rapid liquefaction because of the potent collagenases and proteases produced by these organisms. *Pseudomonas* ulcers have been extensively investigated because of the devastating liquefaction of cornea that commonly accompanies this infection. The bacteria themselves produce numerous proteases and other toxins that may be important in the establishment of the early infection, but most of the characteristic stromal malacia results from the action of proteases originating from leukocytes, reactive corneal epithelium, or injured stroma. The stroma contains a variety of proenzymes (for collagenases, elastases, gelatinases, and other stromal lysins) that are cleaved by the *Pseudomonas* toxins to produce

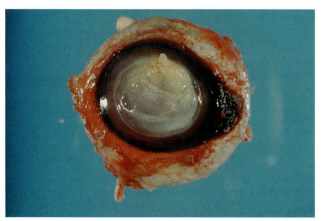

Figure 5-32 **Keratomalacia** in a horse with secondary *Pseudomonas* keratitis.

the active enzymes. Which toxins are produced, and in what quantities, is very strain dependent. The stepwise degradation of stroma is seen histologically as a featureless eosinophilic coagulum, which occurs with progressive septic ulcers regardless of the species of bacterium. Neutrophils may encircle the liquefying focus as a thick wall of live and fragmented cells. The resulting localized suppurative keratomalacia is called a *ring abscess*, although that terminology is rarely used today. It is seen more commonly in cattle than any other species, perhaps because of the prevalence of untreated, contaminated corneal ulcers in that species and the prevalence of septic corneal perforation.

The sequelae of ulcerative keratitis involve cornea, conjunctiva, and uvea. *The ulcer itself may heal with vascularization and scarring proportional to the severity of the initial lesion. It may persist as a stubborn but nonprogressive lesion, or it may progress to involve more of the stroma and epithelium.* Stromal liquefaction that reaches Descemet's membrane results in its forward bulging known as a **descemetocele.** Descemet's membrane, although resistant to penetration of the microbial agents themselves, is apparently permeable to inflammatory mediators and microbial toxins that diffuse into the anterior chamber. These chemicals, combined with a vasoactive sensory neural reflex from irritated cornea, are responsible for the anterior uveitis that accompanies virtually all cases of deep corneal ulceration.

In the case of corneal perforation, the iris flows forward to plug the defect *(iris prolapse)* and may subsequently become incorporated into the corneal scarring. This outcome creates an acquired **anterior staphyloma,** meaning a focal defect in the ocular fibrous tunic (i.e., cornea) that becomes lined by uvea (Fig. 5-33A-C). The distinction from a firmly incorporated anterior synechia is just semantics.

The conjunctiva is involved in almost all instances of keratitis, either as a victim of the same injury or as the nearest vascularized tissue capable of mounting an inflammatory response to the corneal injury. Hyperemia, cellular exudation, and lymphofollicular hyperplasia are common as the conjunctiva responds to the diffusion of inflammatory mediators of microbial, leukocytic, and tissue origin.

There are some instances in which the lesions are found primarily within the stroma. Examples of bacterial or fungal keratitis in which the organisms were implanted into the stroma by penetrating injury may cause chronic suppurative

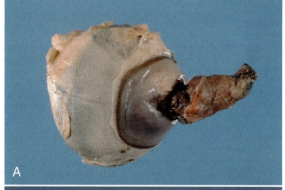

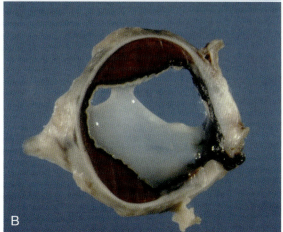

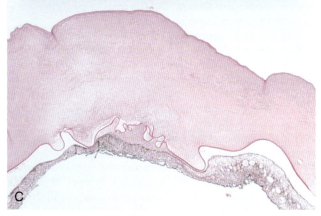

Figure 5-33 **Corneal perforation. A.** Iris prolapse as a sequel to a melting corneal ulcer (suppurative keratomalacia) in a steer. **B.** Iris prolapse and dissecting choroidal hemorrhage following massive head trauma in a dog. **C.** Corneal scarring, ruptured Descemet's membrane, and anterior synechia as sequels to corneal perforation. PAS stain.

keratomalacia with negligible involvement of superficial stroma or epithelium. Alternatively, deep ulcerative septic keratitis may heal superficially, yet persist deep within the stroma. In either of these 2 situations, the deep lesion is referred to as *stromal abscess*.

Midstromal corneal vascular ingrowth from the limbus is a very common lesion in response to vascular endothelial growth factors elaborated in the course of chronic uveitis of virtually any cause. It appears to be a purely accidental lesion with no obvious purpose, but it does serve as a valuable and permanent histologic marker for previous or ongoing intraocular inflammatory disease. Its liability as a marker for subacute or chronic intraocular inflammation is probably not absolute, because similar midstromal vascularization can probably occur in response to growth factors liberated from detached retina or intraocular neoplasms (see The significance of uveitis).

Although most examples of clinically diagnosed keratitis are consequences of corneal injury by trauma or desiccation, there are a few specific examples of true keratitis initiated by niche-adapted infectious agents or presumed immune mechanisms. These are presented here.

Pannus keratitis

Pannus keratitis (chronic superficial keratitis) *is an idiopathic superficial stromal keratitis seen most frequently in German Shepherd dogs and phenotypically similar breeds.* Its prevalence and severity are directly correlated with altitude, suggesting that *sunlight exposure* is part of the pathogenesis. The clinical disease is distinctive. The early lesion is seen in dogs of either sex, usually in early middle age, as a vascularized opacity growing into the corneal stroma from the limbus. The ingrowth is bilateral although not always of simultaneous onset, and most frequently originates from the ventrolateral limbus. There is no ulceration, but pigmentation is often marked. The untreated lesion eventually infiltrates the entire cornea, converting the superficial stroma to an opaque membrane resembling granulation tissue. At one time, superficial keratectomy was the recommended therapy, and histologic specimens were quite often available. Today, most cases are treated with potent immunosuppressive therapy, and the need to perform a keratectomy to restore vision is rare indeed.

The histologic appearance varies with the duration of the lesion. *The initial lesion is superficial stromal infiltration of mononuclear cells, especially plasma cells.* Subsequently, there is progressive vascularization and fibroplasia in the superficial third of the stroma, accompanied by epithelial hyperplasia and pigmentation that may include the stroma. The deep stroma is never affected.

The pathogenesis of the condition is unknown, but an immune reaction to altered corneal epithelial antigens is hypothesized. Its response to aggressive corticosteroid or cyclosporine administration supports this hypothesis, as does its striking histologic similarity to discoid lupus and other lupoid dermatoses. Despite the similarity, immunofluorescence tests for intraepithelial or basement membrane immunoglobulin are negative, and there is no actual proof that this disease has an autoimmune pathogenesis, even though that is often stated in clinical literature. Infectious agents are not consistently isolated. A histologically similar lesion of the bulbar conjunctiva of third eyelid occurs in the same breed (so-called *"plasmoma"*) and may reflect the same mysterious pathogenesis.

Herpetic keratitis of cats

Feline herpetic keratitis, caused by felid herpesvirus 1, is seen either as the sole ocular lesion or in concert with conjunctivitis. Clinical signs associated with herpesviral infections in cats include conjunctivitis, keratitis, rhinotracheitis, and, in neonates, systemic disease with encephalitis and necrosis in visceral organs. Acquired immunity alters the manifestations of the disease and results in different lesions predominating in different age groups. *Keratitis is most common in adult cats* and seems to result from activation of latent infection during concurrent immunosuppressive disease or corticosteroid therapy. Concurrent mild respiratory disease may be present, but *in adults, the disease is often purely corneal and may even be unilateral.* In contrast, *the infection in adolescent cats causes nonspecific bilateral erosive conjunctivitis without keratitis.* Intranuclear inclusions are numerous within cells prior to sloughing, and leukocytes are sparse until ulceration permits opportunistic contamination. Upper respiratory disease is almost always present.

The corneal lesions fall into 2 very different categories: *shallow transient erosions and ulcers* that represent the direct cytopathic effect of acute viral infection, and *more severe stromal keratitis* that is probably an immune response to viral antigen in persistent or recurring infections. The typical acute superficial corneal lesions are multifocal minute corneal erosions and ulcers that have a tendency to coalesce into branching dendritic ulcers. Early in the disease, typical herpesviral inclusions may be seen with histology, and herpesviral antigen can be demonstrated with immunofluorescence or other techniques. Severe or recurrent lesions in immunosuppressed cats may result in underlying stromal keratitis with lymphocytic infiltration, persistent edema, and vascularization.

There is much more written about the clinical features and clinical diagnosis of herpesviral keratitis than there it is about its pathology, simply because most cases are never subjected to histologic evaluation. By the time a sample of conjunctiva or cornea is taken for histologic assessment in cases that have been therapeutically resistant, histologic detection of inclusion bodies is futile, and immunofluorescence is usually negative. Virus can usually be detected with PCR, but interpretation of that result is almost impossible because of the high prevalence of carriage in asymptomatic, healthy cats. For the same reason, attempts to link persistent herpesviral infection with feline corneal sequestrum or feline eosinophilic keratitis have been less than convincing.

Feline eosinophilic keratitis

Another uniquely feline ocular lesion, feline eosinophilic keratitis is seen clinically as unilateral or bilateral proliferative, "fluffy" white superficial stromal keratitis. There is no breed, age, or sex predilection, and no proven association with other ocular or systemic disease. Because the diagnosis is made by cytologic evaluation of superficial scrapings or (occasionally) by histologic examination of surgical keratectomy specimens, this disease is more likely to be seen by pathologists than most other corneal disorders. Scrapings of the surface of the lesion reveal numerous eosinophils and fewer mast cells and other mononuclear leukocytes. Eosinophils may be less conspicuous on histologic examination of keratectomy specimens, perhaps because most seem determined to emigrate through the epithelium and into the tear film rather than remain within the tissue. Instead, the stromal lesion is a *mixture of macrophages, plasma cells, fibroblasts and, unpredictably, mast cells and at least a few eosinophils.* The latter are least frequent in older lesions, either because of time alone or because older lesions are more likely to have received a lot of corticosteroid therapy. A characteristic lesion, not present in every case, is a dense granular eosinophilic coagulum along the surface of the keratectomy specimen. It seems to consist of free eosinophil granules (Fig. 5-34). No bacterial or fungal agents have been seen. Although there are histologic similarities to cutaneous eosinophilic ulcer and linear granuloma, no statistical association has been proven, and the lack of understanding even of the

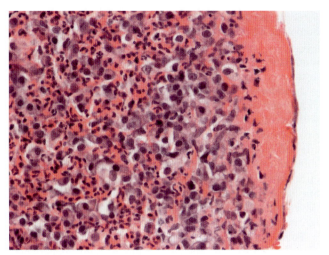

Figure 5-34 **Eosinophilic keratitis in a cat.** The corneal stroma is filled with a mixture of eosinophils and plasma cells, and is covered by a coagulum of eosinophil granules.

cutaneous eosinophilic lesions makes such attempted comparisons of very limited value. Although much speculation exists about the relationship between persistent herpesviral infection and eosinophilic keratitis, there is no proven etiologic link.

Mycotic keratitis

Mycotic keratitis is a term used for 2 fundamentally different diseases. The first, which we will consider to be "true" mycotic keratitis, is a destructive, suppurative, ulcerative, and deep stromal keratitis most commonly seen in horses, but occasionally encountered in all domestic species. The offending fungus is usually a member of the normal conjunctival flora, and its role in the disease is always that of opportunistic contaminant. *Aspergillus* is the most frequent isolate, but cases caused by other common conjunctival fungi, such as *Alternaria, Penicillium,* and *Cladosporium,* are not rare. Most cases are probably iatrogenic, occurring in animals in which a corneal ulcer, laceration, or penetrating wound had been treated with long-term antibiotics and/or corticosteroids. The latter is a particularly common villain in this context. Horses seem particularly prone to mycotic keratitis, perhaps related to the mold-laden, dusty environment in which many horses are housed; only rarely does the lesion occur in dogs or cats. Because virtually all stabled horses have fungi as part of their conjunctival flora, seeing hyphae within the corneal stroma is required for the diagnosis. Isolation from a corneal swab or shallow scraping is not adequate.

Because the disease is much more prevalent in horses than any other species, most of the description is derived from equine cases. The histologic changes in other species, however, are very similar to what occurs in horses. There appears to be a difference in the typical lesion seen in temperate climates and what occurs in horses in very warm and humid environments. In the latter, there are cases in which the fungi are found throughout the cornea and are easily identified by even shallow scraping. That is not the case in those examples of the disease diagnosed in cooler climates, which I will consider the "typical" disease.

The typical early lesion is deep ulcerative keratitis with suppurative keratomalacia. Some chronic lesions are exclusively

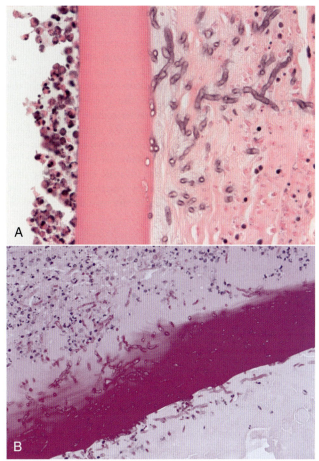

Figure 5-35 **Equine mycotic keratitis. A.** The fungi typically are found within and adjacent to Descemet's membrane, accompanied by karyorrhectic neutrophils and stromal malacia. **B.** The fungi permeate Descemet's membrane and dangle within the anterior chamber, but never actually colonize the inside of the globe.

stromal because of successful epithelial and superficial stromal healing of the initial penetration (or perhaps because therapy eliminated the infection in the superficial stroma). For whatever reason, the typical equine eye enucleated for mycotic keratitis has an intense neutrophil-rich deep stromal keratitis with several characteristic features: neutrophils are karyorrhectic, inflammation is most intense immediately adjacent to Descemet's membrane, and frequently there is lysis of the normally resistant Descemet's membrane with spillage of the corneal inflammation into the anterior chamber. *Fungi are numerous within the malacia of the deep stroma and within Descemet's membrane itself,* but rarely, if ever, are seen within the anterior chamber (Fig. 5-35A, B). When they occur within the anterior chamber, they are always anchored to the nearby Descemet's membrane. Despite ample opportunity, there has never been a reported case of disseminated intraocular mycosis as a sequel to mycotic keratitis. Fungi are sparse or absent within the superficial half of the stroma, which explains why corneal scrapings or even keratectomy specimens may fail to reveal the agent. The reason for the apparent targeting of Descemet's membrane is not known, but the presence of the tropism even in untreated eyes suggests that it is a genuine tropism and not just persistence of a previously generalized stromal infection in the site least likely to be reached by topical fungicides.

In horses in tropical and near-tropical climates (many reports come, e.g., from Florida), the fungi are more diffusely distributed within the cornea and are thus more easily captured by routine cytology or culture swabs. Although the distribution of the lesion within the cornea is also more diffuse, its fundamental lytic character remains the same.

The other disease that is also given the name "*mycotic keratitis*" is a very different entity in which *corneal sequestra in dogs, cats, or horses have become contaminated with opportunistic fungi*. In sharp contrast to genuine mycotic keratitis described previously, *there is no inflammatory reaction*. The fungi are easily found on scraping, leading to the mistaken impression that this is true mycotic keratitis.

> **Key Points**
>
> Most claims that any specific infectious agent is a cause for corneal disease are not proven. In almost all cases, the infectious agent is purely opportunistic, even though it may make a very significant contribution to disease progression, as in mycotic keratitis, or postulcerative corneal infections with *Pseudomonas* or *Streptococcus*.

Infectious bovine keratoconjunctivitis

Infectious bovine keratoconjunctivitis ("pinkeye") vies with squamous cell carcinoma as the most important disease of the bovine eye. It occurs worldwide, is most prevalent in summer because of the increase in fly vectors, and has a clinical expression that ranges from initial conjunctivitis and ulcerative keratitis to iris prolapse, glaucoma, and phthisis bulbi. The prevalence of severe sequelae reflects inadequate management of the disease rather than any special virulence of this agent as compared to other infectious causes of keratitis in other species.

The disease behaves as an infectious epizootic within a susceptible population, frequently affecting >50% of the cattle at risk within 2 weeks of the initial clinical case. Shedding of virulent organisms by a carrier animal is thought to be the usual route of introduction into a previously unexposed group, although a role for various mechanical or biological vectors is also assumed.

Moraxella bovis has been confirmed as the most important causative agent, and the only one for which Koch's postulates have been fulfilled. Concurrent infection with other agents, such as *Mycoplasma bovoculi, Mycoplasma conjunctivae, Acholeplasma laidlawii,* and bovine herpesvirus, may contribute to lesion severity. Earlier skepticism about the virulence of *M. bovis,* based upon the unreliability of reproduction of the disease, isolation of the organism from apparently healthy cattle, and failure of isolation from some overtly affected cattle, has been overcome by detailed information on the pathogenesis of the disease. *It is now clear that virulence of M. bovis is associated with hemolytic, leukocytolytic, piliated strains that predominate only in the eyes of affected cattle*. Pathogenic isolates of *M. bovis* express a calcium-dependent transmembrane pore-forming cytotoxin. Nonpiliated, nonhemolytic strains predominate in healthy cattle and are probably part of the normal conjunctival flora. The use of immunofluorescence has demonstrated *M. bovis* in many of the naturally occurring cases for which the results of culture were negative. In naturally occurring outbreaks, the number of isolations of hemolytic *M. bovis* falls to almost zero as the outbreak wanes, but a few chronically affected carriers remain as the most important source of virulent bacteria for outbreaks of disease in the next summer.

In addition to variation in the virulence of different strains of *M. bovis*, sunlight, dust, and, perhaps, concurrent infection with infectious bovine rhinotracheitis virus (bovine herpesvirus 1) increase the severity of the disease. Calves are usually affected more severely than cattle >2 years of age, although absolute resistance to infection seems fragile. The protective effect of serum antibody against the disease is controversial. Specific immunoglobulin A (IgA) is found in tears of infected calves, and there is substantial evidence that locally produced IgA is strongly protective.

Following experimental inoculation of virulent *M. bovis* onto the cornea, pilus-mediated adhesion and production of bacterial cytotoxin result in microscopic ulceration in as little as 12 hours. Initial adhesion is to older surface epithelium ("dark cells") and results in the development of microscopic pits in the cell surface. *Moraxella* is found within degenerate epithelial cells, but it is not known whether invasion is necessary for subsequent cellular destruction. *In field epizootics, the earliest lesion is bulbar conjunctival edema and hyperemia, followed in 24-48 hours by the appearance of a shallow central corneal ulcer*. The ulcer is a small (<0.5 cm) focus of epithelial necrosis that may appear as erosion, vesicle, or full-thickness epithelial loss. In untreated animals destined to develop the full clinical expression, the ulcer enlarges, deepens, and frequently attracts enough neutrophils to qualify as a *corneal abscess*. Stromal liquefaction ensues, probably as a result of neutrophil lysis, which is itself initiated by *Moraxella*-derived leukotoxins. By the end of the first week, there is extensive stromal edema and vascularization extending from the limbus. As with any severe ulcerative keratitis, the subsequent progression or regression of the lesion varies with each case as modifications by therapy, opportunistic bacterial and fungal contamination, trauma, inflammation, and immunity interact. Keratomalacia frequently leads to forward coning of the weakened cornea *(keratoconus)*. In most instances, whether treated or not, the cornea heals by sloughing of necrotic tissue and filling of the defect by granulation tissue. Re-epithelialization may take up to a month, leaving a cornea that is slightly coned and variably scarred. The scarring often is scant and interferes little with vision in spite of the severity of the primary lesion.

Less satisfactory sequelae, although not common in relation to the overall disease prevalence, are still relatively common. Sterile anterior uveal inflammation may result in focal or generalized adherence of iris to cornea (anterior synechia) or lens (posterior synechia). Descemetocele may progress to corneal rupture, which in turn may lead to phthisis bulbi or resolve by sealing with prolapse of the iris. Synechia and staphyloma may lead to impairment of aqueous drainage and thus to glaucoma.

Infectious keratoconjunctivitis (contagious ophthalmia, pinkeye) of sheep and goats

Epizootics of conjunctivitis and keratitis in sheep and goats share many of the features of the bovine disease: summer prevalence, rapid spread, and exacerbation by dust, sunlight, and flies. Feedlot lambs seem particularly susceptible. Unlike bovine keratoconjunctivitis, the range of clinical signs and proposed causes suggests that there may in fact be several different diseases. Many agents including bacteria, mycoplasmas, chlamydiae, and rickettsiae have been suggested as causes, but various mycoplasmas and *Chlamydophila psittaci* may be the most important agents. The lesions caused by *Mycoplasma mycoides* var. *capri* in goats and *Mycoplasma conjunctivae* var. *ovis* in sheep are similar but usually milder than those caused by *Moraxella bovis* in cattle. This is particularly true of goats, in which deep corneal ulceration is uncommon.

Keratoconjunctivitis associated with *C. psittaci* is usually predominantly conjunctivitis. Initial chemosis and reddening are followed by massive lymphofollicular hyperplasia in bulbar conjunctiva and nictitating membrane. Keratitis may occur, but ulceration is seldom prominent. Animals with conjunctivitis may have concurrent polyarthritis from which chlamydiae can be isolated.

Further reading

Dean E, Meunier V. Feline eosinophilic keratoconjunctivitis: a retrospective study of 45 cases (56 eyes). J Feline Med Surg 2013;15:661-666.

Gould D. Feline herpesvirus-1: ocular manifestations, diagnosis and treatment options. J Feline Med Surg 2011;13:333-346.

Hamilton HI, et al. Histological findings in corneal stromal abscesses of 11 horses: correlation with cultures and cytology. Equine Vet J 1994;26:448-453.

Hartley C. Aetiology of corneal ulcers assume FHV-1 unless proven otherwise. J Feline Med Surg 2010;12:24-35.

Lassaline-Utter M, et al. Eosinophilic keratitis in 46 eyes of 27 horses in the Mid-Atlantic United States (2008-2012). Vet Ophthalmol 2014;17:76-81.

Ledbetter EC, et al. Characterization of fungal keratitis in alpacas: 11 cases (2003-2012). J Am Vet Med Assoc 2013;243:1616-1622.

Massa KL, et al. Usefulness of aerobic microbial culture and cytologic evaluation of corneal specimens in the diagnosis of infectious ulcerative keratitis in animals. J Am Vet Med Assoc 1999;215:1671-1674.

Pate DO, et al. Immunohistochemical and immunopathologic characterization of superficial stromal immune-mediated keratitis in horses. Am J Vet Res 2012;73:1067-1073.

Reed Z, et al. Equine keratomycoses in California from 1987 to 2010 (47 cases). Equine Vet J 2013;45:361-366.

Sanchez RF, et al. Canine keratoconjunctivitis sicca: disease trends in a review of 229 cases. J Small Anim Pract 2007;48:211-217.

Scott EM, Carter RT. Canine keratomycosis in 11 dogs: a case series (2000-2011). J Am Anim Hosp Assoc 2014;50:112-118.

Voelter-Ratson K, et al. Equine keratomycosis in Switzerland: a retrospective evaluation of 35 horses (January 2000-August 2011). Equine Vet J 2013;45:608-612.

Wada S, et al. Ulcerative keratitis in thoroughbred racehorses in Japan from 1997 to 2008. Vet Ophthalmol 2010;13:99-105.

Williams LB, Pinard CL. Corneal ulcers in horses. Compend Contin Educ Vet 2013;35:E4.

LENS

The lens is a flattened sphere of epithelial cells suspended in the pupillary aperture by a large number of transparent elastin-like fibers known as *lens zonules*. These originate from the lens capsule near the equator, and fuse with the nonpigmented ciliary epithelium along the lateral surfaces of the ciliary processes or in the valleys between adjacent ciliary processes. *The range of histologic reaction of lens to injury is very limited because of the simplicity of its structure and physiology, and its lack of vascularity.*

The lens is entirely epithelial. Outermost is a *thick, elastic capsule*, which is the basement membrane produced by the underlying germinal epithelial cells. The capsule is thickest at the anterior pole and becomes progressively thinner over the posterior half of the lens. The capsule in the neonate is thin, but it thickens progressively throughout life.

Below the capsule is a layer of simple cuboidal *lens epithelium* that, in all but fetal globes, is found below the capsule of only the anterior half of the lens. The apex of these cells faces inward toward the lens nucleus. At the equator, these germinal cells extend into the lens cortex as the *nuclear bow*, an arc of cells being progressively transformed from cuboidal germinal epithelium to the elongated spindle shape of the mature *lens fibers*. The bulk of the lens is composed of onion-like layers of elongated epithelial cells anchored to each other by interlocking surface ridges, grooves, and ball-and-socket protuberances. These elongated fibers contain no nucleus and few cytoplasmic organelles, relying almost entirely on anaerobic glycolysis for energy. Because the lens cannot shed aging fibers as does skin or intestine, these cells are compacted into *the oldest central part of the lens, the nucleus*. The continuous accumulation of these old desiccated fibers with altered crystalline protein results in the common but visually insignificant *aging change of nuclear sclerosis.*

Although in many ways similar to cornea in structure and function, the optical clarity of lens rests not with the regularity of its fibers but in its high percentage of cytoplasmic soluble crystalline protein and paucity of light-scattering nuclei or mitochondria. The lens is ~35% protein, the highest of any tissue, and >90% is of the soluble crystalline variety. Insoluble high-molecular-weight protein (albuminoid) is found in the nucleus and cell membranes. Opacity of lens is associated, at least in some cases, with decreasing concentrations of crystalline and increasing albuminoid protein, the latter insoluble in water and optically opaque. *Many of the insults that result in degeneration of lens ultimately interfere with its nutrition.* Because it is avascular in the postnatal animal, *the lens relies entirely upon the aqueous for the delivery of nutrients and removal of metabolic wastes.* Glaucoma, ocular inflammation, metabolic disorders, and various toxins share the common feature of altering the amount or quality of lenticular nutrition by altering the flow or composition of the aqueous humor.

Ectopia lentis

The only lenticular defects of importance in domestic animals are those affecting location, configuration, and clarity. Those affecting configuration are usually developmental defects and are discussed earlier. **Dislocations of the lens** may be congenital or acquired, and the latter include spontaneous dislocations and those secondary to trauma and glaucoma. *Apparently spontaneous dislocations* are encountered most frequently in middle-aged (3-8 years) terrier dogs in which an inherited predisposition to bilateral zonular rupture exists. Particularly in various terrier breeds, there is a widespread inherited mutation in the *ADAMST17* gene, which codes for a metalloproteinase that is important in the remodeling of various structural matrix proteins, including those involved in the formation and maintenance of lens zonules. The pathogenesis of the defect has been best studied in the Tibetan Terrier, in which the zonules develop in a dysplastic, reticulate fashion that precedes luxation by several years. *Traumatic dislocation* is usually via blunt trauma, notably automobile accidents. The dislocation may be partial *(subluxation)* or complete *(luxation)*, and in the latter instance, the free lens may damage corneal endothelium or vitreous, causing edema and liquefaction, respectively. Such lenses may be surgically removed but seldom receive histologic examination. Anterior luxation frequently results in glaucoma, perhaps caused by anterior prolapse of the vitreous into the pupil. Lens luxation is inexplicably uncommon in cats. It is seen in middle-aged cats as unilateral and usually anterior luxation. One-third of cases occur in eyes with no other observed lesion; the remainder occur in eyes with pre-existent uveitis or glaucoma, or a history of trauma.

Further reading

Gould D, et al. *ADAMTS17* mutation associated with primary lens luxation is widespread among breeds. Vet Ophthalmol 2011;14: 378-384.

Oberbauer AM, et al. Inheritance of cataracts and primary lens luxation in Jack Russell Terriers. Am J Vet Res 2008;69:222-227.

Cataract

Cataract is the most common and most important disorder of the lens. Cataract means lenticular opacity, and is usually prefixed by adjectives relating to location, maturity, extent, suspected cause, and ophthalmoscopic appearance. Of these adjectives, only those of location and, to some extent, maturity are useful in histologic description. *The simple structure of the lens results in a stereotyped reaction to injury that provides few clues to pathogenesis.* Unless permitted by invasion through a capsular tear, inflammation cannot occur within the avascular and totally epithelial lens.

The main challenge facing the pathologist looking at a histologic section of lens is whether any of the microscopic changes are genuine or not. The lens is difficult to section, and artifacts such as fiber disruption and capsular tearing are almost unavoidable. *Histologic changes that distinguish genuine cataract from fixation or sectioning artifact are (in order of overall utility): detection of Morgagnian globules, bladder cells, lens epithelial hyperplasia, posterior migration of lens epithelium, and mineralization* (Fig. 5-36A, B).

Morgagnian globules *are bright pink spherical globules of denatured lens protein*. They are distinguished from artifactual fragmentation of lens fibers because the latter form jagged rectangular fragments, not spheres. With more advanced liquefactive change, fluid lakes appear between fibers, presumably the result of complete liquefaction of fibers. Some of the clefts are probably the result of osmotic fluid imbibition by the cataractous lens. The osmosis results from protein denaturation into more numerous, smaller peptides and from degeneration of the capsular epithelium in which resides the Na^+-K^+–dependent ATPase osmotic pump critical to normal lens hydration.

In advanced cataracts, the degenerate fibers may liquefy to the extent that their low-molecular-weight end products diffuse through the semipermeable capsule, resulting in the spontaneous clearing of the opaque lens typical of the *hypermature cataract*. Histologically, such lenses consist of a dense, eccentric residual nucleus in a lake of proteinaceous fluid

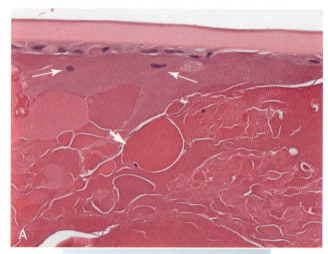

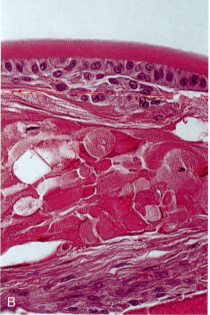

Figure 5-36 Cataract. **A.** Liquefaction of cortical lens fibers, Morgagnian globules (wide arrow), reactive hyperplasia of capsular epithelium, and nucleated bladder cells (thin arrows). **B.** Plaque of reactive hyperplasia and fibrous metaplasia of the anterior lens capsule with underlying bladder cells creating an anterior polar cataract.

surrounded by a wrinkled capsule. The adjacent uvea will usually have a moderately severe lymphocytic-plasmacytic infiltration in response to unidentified inflammatory mediators present in that leaking lens fluid. The lesion/process is known as *phacolytic uveitis* (see later).

Bladder cells are claimed to reflect abortive efforts at new fiber formation by lens epithelium. Such efforts are apparently never successful, and the hydropic degeneration of such cells results in the formation of *large foamy nucleated cells called bladder cells*, because of their bloated, fusiform shape.

Epithelial hyperplasia or **fibroblastic metaplasia** is the usual histologic counterpart of anterior subcapsular cataract, and is usually seen following focal trauma, or adherence of the iris or of persistent pupillary membranes to the anterior surface of the lens. *Initial epithelial degeneration or necrosis is followed by hyperplasia and sometimes by fibrous metaplasia.*

The resultant *epithelial plaque* lies just under the anterior lens capsule. The innermost epithelial layer may remain basilar in type rather than fibroblastic. Each epithelial layer, even if metaplastic, secretes a new basement membrane that separates each layer from the adjacent layers. This characteristic feature is best seen with PAS stains. The end result is a focal plaque formed by multiple, sandwiched layers of flattened epithelium and basement membrane at the anterior pole of the lens. Remnants of adherent iris or pupillary membrane, including pigment, may complicate the histologic appearance.

Posterior migration of lens epithelium is a common change in chronic cataracts. Although it seems to occur more slowly than the changes of Morgagnian globule or bladder cell formation, it is equally reliable (when present) as a histologic indicator of cataract formation. The flattened cuboidal epithelial cells migrate from the equator to line the posterior capsule. Usually, they will also undergo stratification and sometimes fibroblast-like metaplasia. This re-establishment of the fetal morphology is seen most commonly with any chronic cataract in young animals, whose epithelial cells perhaps retain greater migratory ability. Adjacent cortical fibers are usually degenerate (Morgagnian globules, bladder cells, and clefts of granular proteinaceous fluid).

Deposition of calcium salts occurs quite frequently within cataracts of any type, and provides no clue as to pathogenesis.

The sequence of histologic change in cataract is the same regardless of cause, and thus diagnosis of cause can be made only in light of patient data or concurrent disease. In dogs, for example, familial cataracts may be congenital or of later onset. Specific examples may typically occur alone or with other ocular lesions, and occur at an age, in a location, and with a progression sufficiently characteristic to allow presumptive diagnosis of a breed-specific syndrome. Cataract also occurs secondary to glaucoma, endophthalmitis, ocular trauma, and anterior segment anomalies, and observation of these latter defects permits presumptive diagnosis of the pathogenesis of the accompanying cataract.

Cataract may result from exposure of the lens to a wide variety of physical and chemical insults, such as solar or other irradiation, cold, increased intraocular pressure, toxins, nutritional excesses and deficiencies, nearby inflammation, and direct trauma. The list of potential cataractogenic chemical toxins grows daily and includes food additives, chemotherapeutic agents, and byproducts of ocular inflammation. The pathogenesis of the cataract is not determined for more than a few such insults, but a common denominator seems to be the ability to upset the precarious balance between substrate supply and enzymic activity within the almost exclusively anaerobic lens. This imbalance results in degeneration of fibers, accumulation of nonmetabolized substrate, or production of abnormal metabolites. The latter 2 classes of products may be cytotoxic or osmotically active, thus drawing water into the critically dehydrated lens and causing opacity.

Most cataracts in people and animals are not identified as being caused by a single insult, but are assumed to represent the result of years of accumulated and perhaps synergistic cataractogenic activity of environmental, dietary, and inborn insults. *The majority of cataracts seen in veterinary practice fall into 1 of 3 categories: inherited, postinflammatory, and idiopathic.* In reality, the large group of inherited cataracts in dogs is of unknown pathogenesis, although extrapolation from knowledge of similar cataracts in rodents and man suggests that inborn errors of lenticular metabolism are at fault. Postinflammatory cataracts result from injury to lenticular epithelium by adjacent inflammation, interference with aqueous production, composition and flow, and accumulation of toxic bacterial, leukocytic, and plasma byproducts in the lenticular environment. Adherence of iris to lens (posterior synechia) inevitably causes a focal subcapsular cataract.

Other than these broad categories, there are a few naturally occurring examples of cataract about which there is some understanding.

Diabetic cataract develops in ~70% of spontaneously diabetic dogs, but is rare in diabetic cats. The opacity is bilateral and begins in the cortex at the equator. Progression to complete cortical opacity usually occurs within a few weeks. The pathogenesis of the cataract has traditionally been ascribed to the excessively high level of glucose within the aqueous. Glucose is normally the major energy source for lens fibers, with most of it used to fuel the Embden-Meyerhof pathway of anaerobic glycolysis. When the rate-limiting enzyme of this pathway, hexokinase, is saturated with glucose, the backup of glucose is shunted to alternative metabolic pathways. Chief among these is the *sorbitol pathway*, activated in the rabbit lens by glucose concentrations of >5 mmol/L (>90 mg/dL). In this pathway, the excess glucose is converted by an aldose reductase to the polyalcohol, sorbitol, which is then slowly reduced to a D-fructose, a ketohexose. Because this second reaction is much slower than the first, *sorbitol may accumulate to very high concentrations within the lens and osmotically attracts water even to the point of hydropic cell rupture.* Under experimental conditions at least, the early cataract may be reversed if aqueous sugar levels are reduced to normal, but the later cataract is irreversible.

However, osmotic events alone are not enough to explain all of the structural and metabolic changes in sugar-induced cataracts. The efficacy of antioxidants in ameliorating such cataracts, the nature of intralenticular biochemical alterations, and detection of increased intralenticular oxidants all point to some kind of oxidative damage as an additional promoter of cataract.

Galactose-induced cataracts probably have the same complex and incompletely understood pathogenesis as the diabetic cataract and are seen in orphaned kangaroos and wallabies raised on cow's milk, as well as in a host of experimental models. Because marsupial milk is much lower in lactose than bovine milk, the enzymically ill-equipped neonate develops osmotic diarrhea from undigested lactose and galactose in the intestine, and some excess galactose enters the aqueous humor. The lens, deficient in the enzymes needed to use the galactose by converting it to glucose-6-phosphate for anaerobic glycolysis, shunts the galactose via aldose reductase to its polyalcohol, *dulcitol*, which acts osmotically, as does sorbitol, to disrupt lens fibers.

Cataract reported in puppies and wolf cubs fed commercial milk replacer, or in kittens on feline milk replacer, has been attributed to *deficiency of arginine*, although in several case reports, the specific dietary error was not identified. Cataract caused by **dietary deficiency** of any of several sulfur-containing amino acids, zinc, or vitamin C occurs in farmed fish, and many models of nutritional cataract exist in various laboratory animals.

Various forms of **irradiation** cause cataract. The lens absorbs most of the ultraviolet (UV) and short-wavelength visible blue light that would otherwise damage the retina. At least in people, the chronic exposure to such irradiation is thought to be important in the pathogenesis of senile cataract. **Sunlight-induced cataract** has been described several times in farmed fish, but not yet for other domestic animals as a naturally occurring phenomenon. Absorption of UV or near-UV wavelengths by lens epithelium nucleic acids or lenticular aromatic amino acids results in photochemical generation of free radicals and peroxidative damage to numerous structural components of the lens.

A similar pathogenesis probably explains the development of cataract in animals irradiated as part of cancer therapy. In one study, 28% of dogs receiving **megavoltage X-radiation** for nasal carcinoma developed *diffuse cortical cataract* within 12 months of irradiation. In people, the risk of cataract is dose related, and reaches virtual certainty with dosages of 800-1,500 centigrays (cGy) or rads, whereas rodents require at least twice that dosage. The dogs in the study cited previously received 3,680-5,000 cGy. Antioxidants such as vitamin E or C, or hypoxia, are significantly protective against several models of light or other irradiation-induced cataract, providing further support for the common denominator of oxidative stress in the pathogenesis of such cataracts.

The aminoglycoside antibiotic and anthelmintic **hygromycin B** has been shown to induce *posterior cortical and subcapsular cataracts* in sows, but not boars, fed the drug continuously for 10-14 months. The effect is dose dependent and perhaps even cumulative. Pigs fed the same therapeutic daily dose, but consuming the drug on an 8-week-on/8-week-off basis in accordance with the manufacturer's recommendations, do not develop cataracts. The pathogenesis of the cataract is unknown, but a partial inhibition of hygromycin-induced cataracts in vitro by addition of vitamin E suggests that peroxidative damage to lens fiber membranes may be important. *Deafness* in pigs, and also dogs, caused by hygromycin B is discussed in the section Ear.

Traumatic lens rupture results in a spectrum of change much different from the changes of cataract described previously. First, massive release of more or less native lens protein at the time of rupture may cause severe perilenticular nonsuppurative endophthalmitis ~10 days after the initial trauma (see **Lens-induced uveitis**). Second, the capsular rent permits leukocytes to enter the lens to speed the dissolution of lens fibers. Fibroblastic metaplasia of lens epithelium may result in cartilage or even bone within the lens. *Even after total destruction of the lens fibers, the durable capsule will be found somewhere in the anterior or posterior chamber as a curled eosinophilic mass*, often encapsulated in fibrous tissue probably derived from surviving lens epithelium or from injured ciliary epithelium. Such remnants distinguish lenticular rupture with subsequent dissolution from true developmental aphakia.

Cataract surgery is nothing more than planned traumatic lens rupture, and it is therefore not surprising that we sometimes encounter the same sequence of events as seen with accidental rupture. The main difference is that, with cataract surgery, the lens is already degenerate, and the material that may be released following surgical incision of the capsule is not capable of inducing the same magnitude of inflammatory and proliferative reaction. Nonetheless, *complications of cataract surgery and prosthetic lens implantation are quite common in dogs*, the only species in which the surgery is performed on a regular basis. In most instances, the lens capsule remains

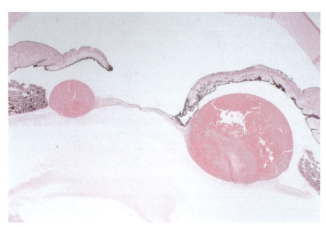

Figure 5-37 **Soemmering ring cataract** created by circumferential regrowth and maturation of residual lens epithelium following previous cataract surgery or, occasionally, naturally occurring lens rupture.

within the globe, and the degenerate lens material is removed by aspiration. The artificial lens is then implanted within the pre-existent capsular "bag." Any lens epithelium left behind after removal of most of the cataractous lens forms the nidus for potential regrowth of lens fibers, usually at the periphery of the lens capsular bag. This forms a circumferential ring of new (but inevitably cataractous) lens fibers known as a *Soemmering ring cataract* (Fig. 5-37). This postoperative proliferation may also use the implanted prosthetic lens (or, in its absence, the lens capsular bag) as the growth substrate, not only causing postoperative opacity but also posing the threat of causing glaucoma via pupillary occlusion or peripheral anterior synechia in a fashion very similar to that commonly seen with pre-iridal fibrovascular membranes. Some degree of postoperative epithelial/fibroblastic proliferation is normal in all such eyes, but the amount can be minimized by religious "vacuuming" of the inner surface of the lens capsule to remove all possible germinal epithelium.

Adhesion of pigmented or nonpigmented cellular material to the anterior lens capsule is a valuable histologic clue. *Pigmented epithelium adherent to the lens capsule is a reliable marker for previous posterior synechia*, even if this synechia has been reversed by surgical or pharmacologic intervention or has been accidentally broken during trimming of the globe. Similarly, fibrous or fibrovascular membranes along the anterior lens capsule most often are derived from previous posterior synechia (but they can represent complications of phacoclastic uveitis, pre-iridal fibrovascular membrane, or persistent pupillary membrane). They are significant causes for pupillary obstruction and secondary glaucoma.

Further reading

Collinson PN, Peiffer RL Jr. Pathology of canine cataract surgery complications. N Z Vet J 2002;50:26-31.

Pfahler S, et al. Prevalence and formation of primary cataracts and persistent hyperplastic tunica vasculosa lentis in the German Pinscher population in Germany. Vet Ophthalmol 2014;doi:10.1111/vop.12167; [Epub ahead of print].

Williams DL, et al. Prevalence of canine cataract: preliminary results of a crosssectional study. Vet Ophthalmol 2004;7:29-35.

UVEA

The uvea is the vascular tunic of the eye. It is derived from the primitive neural crest mesenchyme surrounding the primary optic cup (only the vascular endothelium is mesodermal). Its posterior differentiation into *choroid* is guided by the developing retinal pigment epithelium (RPE), but its differentiation anteriorly into *iris and ciliary body* is probably orchestrated mostly by lens. The presumptive anterior uveal mesenchyme accompanies the infolding of the neuroectoderm at the anterior lip of the optic cup to form the stroma of the iris and ciliary processes. That portion of anterior periorbital mesenchyme not accompanying these neuroectodermal ingrowths remains to form the ciliary muscle and trabecular meshwork. Posteriorly, it forms the choroid and sclera. In all domestic mammals except the pig, the choroid undergoes further differentiation to produce the *tapetum lucidum* dorsal to the optic disc. Defects in development of the RPE (including its cranial specialization as iridal and ciliary epithelium) inevitably result in defective induction or differentiation of the adjacent uvea.

The mature uvea includes iris, ciliary body, and choroid, the last divided into vascular portion and tapetum lucidum. The filtration angle is shared by the iris, ciliary body, and sclera. Its diseases are discussed in the section Glaucoma.

The **iris** is the most anterior portion of the uveal tract. It is a muscular diaphragm separating anterior from posterior chamber, forming the pupil and resting against the anterior face of the lens. The bulk of the iris is stroma of mesenchymal origin, with melanocytes, fibroblasts, and endothelial cells its major constituents. There is neither epithelium nor basement membrane along its anterior face, but rather a single layer of tightly compacted fibrocytes and melanocytes. *The iris stroma is thus in free communication with the aqueous,* a fact of great importance when we consider the secretion or absorption of inflammatory mediators and growth factors in the anterior half of the globe.

The posterior surface of the iris is formed by the double layer of neuroectoderm from the anterior infolding of the optic cup. The 2 layers are heavily pigmented and are apposed apex to apex, with the basal aspect of the posterior epithelium facing the posterior chamber, and separated from it by a basement membrane. The basilar portion of the anterior epithelium, in contrast, is differentiated to form the smooth muscle fibers of the *dilator muscle* of the iris. These fibers lie along the posterior aspect of the iris stroma immediately adjacent to the epithelium. The *constrictor muscle* is found deeper within iris stroma but only in the pupillary third to quarter of the iris. The iris epithelium is rather loosely adherent between layers and between adjacent cells of the same layer, so that *cystic separation* occurs quite commonly. Numerous spaces reminiscent of bile canaliculi lie between adjacent cells and communicate freely with the aqueous humor of the posterior chamber (Fig. 5-38).

The **ciliary body** extends from the posterior iris root to the origin of the neurosensory retina. Like iris, it consists of an inner double layer of neuroepithelium and an outer mesenchymal stroma. The epithelial cells are oriented apex to apex and are separated from the posterior chamber and vitreous by a basal lamina. Only the outer epithelial layer is pigmented. The ciliary body is divided into an anterior *pars plicata* and a posterior *pars plana,* the latter blending with retina at the *ora ciliaris retinae*. The pars plicata consists of a circumferential

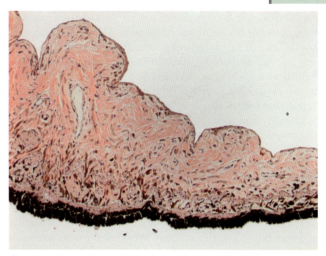

Figure 5-38 Normal feline iris. There is prominent normal pigmentation along the anterior border layer, but no tight junctions to prevent free exchange of mediators between iris stroma and aqueous humor. The normal iris contains no leukocytes.

ring of villus-like epithelial ingrowths supported by a fibrovascular core, called *ciliary processes*. External to the ciliary processes, the mesenchyme forms a ring of smooth muscle, the *ciliary muscle,* responsible for putting traction on the lens zonules and effecting the changes in lens shape necessary for visual accommodation in mammals (other vertebrates may use different and remarkably effective mechanisms). The muscle in domestic animals, particularly ungulates, is poorly developed, and accommodation is thought to be minimal in these species. The lens zonules anchor in the basal lamina of the nonpigmented ciliary epithelium, particularly of the pars plana and within the crypts between ciliary processes. The precise location of this anchoring is highly variable among species.

The **choroid** is the posterior continuation of the stroma of the ciliary body. The posterior continuations of the inner and outer layers of ciliary epithelium are retina and RPE, respectively, with the transition made rather abruptly at the ora ciliaris retinae. *The choroid consists almost entirely of blood vessels and melanocytes,* except for the postnatal metaplasia to tapetum dorsal to the optic disc. The choroid is thinnest peripherally, thickest at the posterior pole, blends indistinctly with sclera externally and is separated from the RPE internally by a complex basal lamina called *Bruch's membrane.*

Many portions of the uveal tract in carnivores continue to develop for at least several weeks after birth, and many of the uveal anomalies, such as goniodysgenesis or choroidal hypoplasia, probably represent developmental errors in postnatal remodeling and maturation, rather than being truly "congenital."

The **general pathology of uvea** includes *anomalous or incomplete differentiation, degeneration, inflammation, and neoplasia*. Anomalies have been previously discussed, and uveal neoplasms are considered in the section on Ocular neoplasia.

Uveal degenerations, except as a sequel to uveitis, are poorly documented. *Idiopathic atrophy of the iris* is described in Shropshire sheep as a bilateral defect obvious by 1-2 years of age. About 25% of the iris is converted to full- or partial-thickness holes; those of partial thickness are spanned by a posterior bridge of iris epithelium. The eye is otherwise normal except for rudimentary corpora nigra. The pathogenesis of the apparently spontaneous atrophy is unknown. Similar atrophy is extremely common in *old dogs*, particularly those of smaller breeds (Poodles, Chihuahuas, Miniature Schnauzers). It is also seen in *old cats*, although much less frequently than in dogs. In both species, the pathogenesis is unknown, and there are no published descriptions of the microscopic lesions.

Uveal cysts probably form as the result of fluid accumulation between the 2 layers of the posterior iris or ciliary epithelium. Such cyst formation is *common in old dogs* and less common in old cats. These cysts may be seen clinically as one or more translucent black cysts attached to the posterior iris or freely floating in the aqueous. Whether the cysts are truly degenerative, or represent residual lesions of fluid exudation from an undetected anterior uveitis, is unknown. Cyst formation as a sequel to uveitis is predisposed by the intrinsic anatomy of the iridociliary epithelium. The 2 layers are apposed, apex to apex, as a manifestation of the involution of the optic vesicle to form the optic cup. It is exactly the same anatomic relationship as between the retina and the RPE, where there are also no actual adhesions. In the event of inflammatory serous effusion, the fluid easily leaves the anterior uveal blood vessels, but the tight junctions between the cells forming the inner layer of the iridociliary epithelium initially may prevent fluid exudation into the aqueous humor. The subepithelial buildup of that fluid results in cystic separation of the inner and outer layers of the iridociliary epithelium (Fig. 5-39A, B).

A breed-specific syndrome of *iris cyst formation associated with the development of glaucoma* has been reported in Golden Retrievers and Irish Wolfhounds. In the Retrievers, there is concurrent lymphocytic anterior uveitis, although that uveitis is often barely perceptible when the globe is finally submitted for histologic examination. Whether the subtlety of the inflammation is genuine or just a result of aggressive anti-inflammatory therapy prior to enucleation is unknown. The exact relationship between the uveitis, the cyst formation, and the glaucoma has not been clarified.

Uveitis

Uveal inflammation is common and may result from ocular trauma, noxious chemicals, infectious agents, neoplasia, or immunologic events. In addition, corneal injury may cause hyperemia and increased permeability of anterior uveal vessels either by percolation of bacterial toxins or inflammatory mediators into the aqueous, or by stimulation of a vasoactive sensory reflex via the trigeminal nerve. The uvea may be the initial site of inflammation, as in localization of infectious agents, or may become involved as the nearest vascular tissue capable of responding to injury of the lens, cornea, or ocular chambers. *Conversely, the uvea seldom undergoes inflammation without affecting adjacent ocular structures.* The pathogenesis of uveitis can be arbitrarily divided into 3 broad categories: those examples associated with the hematogenous localization of infectious agents within the uveal tract, diseases resulting from the uveal response to infectious or noninfectious irritants within the ocular chambers, and "autoimmune" uveitis that results from a failure of immune tolerance or from immune mimicry by some infectious agent.

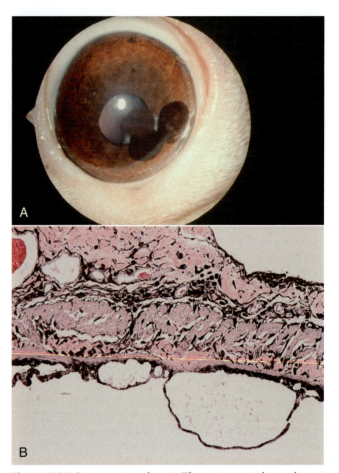

Figure 5-39 Iris cysts in a dog. **A.** These pigmented, translucent cysts can be confused with uveal melanocytomas. **B.** These cysts most commonly result from serous exudate from an inflamed iris accumulating between the inner and outer layers of the iridociliary epithelium. Tight junctions between adjacent epithelial cells prevent its diffusion into the posterior chamber.

The vocabulary of uveitis

The vocabulary of uveitis is complex:
- **Anterior uveitis** describes inflammation of iris and ciliary body.
- **Posterior uveitis** involves ciliary body and choroid, with **panuveitis** occasionally used to designate diffuse uveitis.
- **Chorioretinitis** describes inflammation of choroid and, usually less severely, overlying retina.
- **Endophthalmitis** is inflammation of uvea, retina, and ocular cavities, with **panophthalmitis** reserved for inflammation that has spread to involve all ocular structures, including sclera.

The usefulness of such terminology is doubtful when one considers the vascular unity of the uvea and its intimate association with other ocular tissues. Disagreement between clinical assessment of the extent of the uveitis and histologic evaluation is common; most cases diagnosed clinically as anterior uveitis would be designated as endophthalmitis by histologic assessment. *By convention, the choice of diagnostic classification is strongly influenced by clinical severity, with anterior uveitis the mildest, and panophthalmitis the most severe lesion.*

The significance of uveitis

Uveitis is clinically significant as a cause for ocular pain, but most cases of uveitis reaching a pathologist are because the uveitis is a manifestation of systemic disease, or because the bystander effects of uveitis led to glaucoma or to blindness from retinal detachment. Some of these vision-threatening bystander effects result from the accumulation of exudates (as with exudative retinal detachment), but most result from the later organization of exudates and proliferative events of wound healing within ocular cavities. Not all of the changes associated with uveitis are equally devastating, but they are all worthy of histologic recognition and description when looking at these globes.

Corneal changes include edema and peripheral stromal hyperemia *(ciliary flush).* The edema results from corneal endothelial damage or from increased permeability of limbic blood vessels responding to inflammatory mediators released from the adjacent uvea. In the former instance, damage may be the direct result of the agent causing uveitis, as occurs in infectious canine hepatitis or feline infectious peritonitis. It may also occur as a result of an immune response to endothelial cells containing antigens of these infectious agents, to cross-reaction between microbial and corneal endothelial antigens (immune mimicry), or as a nonspecific response to the presence of the chemical byproducts of inflammation within the anterior chamber. Similar byproducts mediate the acute inflammatory response in the nearby limbic and conjunctival vasculature, leading to edema in the peripheral corneal stroma. Hyperemia of this limbic network also results in *the circumferential peripheral corneal stromal hyperemia, resembling a brush border, which is a clinical hallmark of anterior uveitis.* In eyes with chronic uveitis, corneal edema may also result from glaucoma or from anterior synechia. Persistent edema may lead to stromal fibrosis, vascularization, bullous keratopathy, and the risk of ulceration. *Limbic hyperemia may give way to corneal midstromal vascularization.* This last lesion is extremely common and is a reliable indicator of current or previous uveitis. It is presumed to be an "accidental" and apparently purposeless response to the percolation of angiogenic cytokines from the nearby uveal inflammation.

The accumulation of fibrin, leukocytes, and erythrocytes in the aqueous may result in plugging of the filtration angle and subsequent glaucoma. The infrequent observation of this sequel suggests either unusual potency of the fibrinolytic system within the aqueous, or the inability of exudates to plug more than the most ventral portion of the circumferential angle. Much more common is the organization of inflammatory exudates upon the surface of iris or ciliary body. Adherence of iris to lens **(posterior synechia)** is more common than adherence to cornea **(anterior synechia)** because of the normally intimate association of the lens and iris. If the posterior synechia involves the circumference of the iris, the pupillary flow of aqueous is blocked, posterior chamber pressure rises, and the iris bows forward **(iris bombé)** and may actually adhere anteriorly to the cornea (Fig. 5-40). Glaucoma results from pupillary block, peripheral anterior synechia, or both. In severe and prolonged anterior uveitis, there may be development of a **pre-iridal fibrovascular membrane** on the iris face (Fig. 5-41A), which may span the pupil to cause pupillary block. Alternatively, this fibrovascular membrane may extend to cover the face of the pectinate ligament and cause neovascular glaucoma (Fig. 5-41B). This membrane may contract on the face of the iris, resulting in infolding of the pupillary border to adhere to

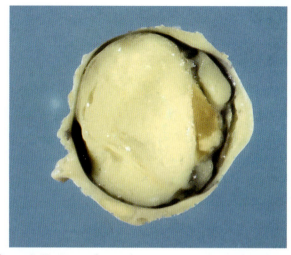

Figure 5-40 Circumferential posterior synechia and iris bombé. Iris bombé develops only as a result of complete pupillary obstruction.

the anterior **(ectropion uveae)** or posterior **(entropion uveae)** iris surface (Fig. 5-41C) (see additional discussion under Lesions causing glaucoma).

Atrophy of iris may follow severe and necrotizing inflammation, and some examples can be distinguished from idiopathic and senile atrophy by the observation of residual lesions of the previous uveitis, such as lymphoid aggregates, focal synechiae, and uveal hyalinization.

The ciliary body suffers the same range of chronic lesions as does the iris. Deposition of PAS-positive hyaline material along the lumenal surface of the ciliary epithelium is particularly frequent in horses. It appears to be deposited in the cytoplasm of the nonpigmented epithelium, and may represent aberrant basement membrane. It is not fibrin; in many instances, it has the staining properties of amyloid. Organization of exudate within the posterior chamber or vitreous results in *a retrolental fibrovascular membrane, called a* **cyclitic membrane,** which stretches around the ciliary body and across the back of the lens. Vitreous is almost always liquefied as a result of the severe uveitis, and continued contraction of fibrin in the posterior chamber and vitreous causes a **tractional retinal separation.** Histologic examination of most cyclitic membranes reveals a fibrovascular retrolental membrane incorporating lens into its anterior face and a folded, degenerate retina in its posterior surface.

The residual lesions of chronic choroiditis include focal lymphoid aggregates and scarring. Tapetum usually remains unaffected. As choroiditis severe enough to evoke these lesions will almost invariably have involved retina and RPE, the residual scar will involve these structures. *Chorioretinal scars are seen as focal fibrous chorioretinal adhesions* in place of normal RPE. Because these scars prevent the involved retina from separating as part of processing artifact, they frequently appear as "spot welds" along an otherwise artifactually detached retina. RPE may be hypertrophic or hyperplastic, particularly if retina has been chronically separated by choroidal effusion. The fibroblast-like cells forming the scar may be derived from retinal Muller cells, choroidal fibroblasts, or metaplasia of RPE, the last being the major source.

Cataract *is a common sequel to uveitis,* either as a result of uveal adhesions to lens surface, altered aqueous flow with

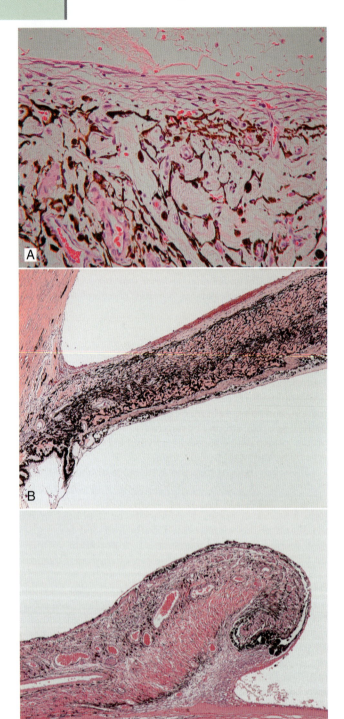

Figure 5-41 Pre-iridal fibrovascular membrane. A. Activation, budding, and migration of iris vascular endothelium and fibroblasts create this potentially devastating membrane of granulation tissue on the anterior surface of the iris. **B.** The migrating pre-iridal membrane crosses the face of the pectinate ligament to create obstruction of aqueous outflow and secondary glaucoma. **C.** Eventual contraction of the pre-iridal membrane "shrink wraps" the iris, a phenomenon seen clinically as a permanently dilated pupil or a scalloped pupillary margin.

lenticular malnutrition, exposure to injurious inflammatory byproducts, or increased aqueous pressure in postinflammatory glaucoma.

Phthisis bulbi *describes a hypotonic, shrunken, structurally disorganized eye that is the end stage of severe ophthalmitis.* Phthisis is seen most commonly as a sequel to severe prolonged suppurative septic ophthalmitis from corneal perforation. Cornea and sclera are thickened by fibrosis and leukocytic infiltration, and ocular content is barely recognizable. Mineralization and even ossification may occur, but cartilage is absent (unlike congenitally dysplastic globes). *A shrunken, end-stage eye that contains ocular structures with at least recognizable orientation is properly termed* **atrophia bulbi**. The term is seldom used, but atrophia is much more common than true phthisis bulbi.

Further reading

Esson D, et al. The histopathological and immunohistochemical characteristics of pigmentary and cystic glaucoma in the golden retriever. Vet Ophthalmol 2009;12:361-368.

Townsend WM, Gornik KR. Prevalence of uveal cysts and pigmentary uveitis in Golden Retrievers in three Midwestern states. J Am Vet Med Assoc 2013;243:1298-1301.

The histologic classification of uveitis

There is no truly satisfactory method for classifying uveitis. It does little good to classify it based upon the exact etiology or pathogenesis, because that approach suffers from the "catch-22" that you need to know what the disease is before you can read about it! The clinical classification as anterior versus posterior uveitis is essentially irrelevant when looking at histologic sections, because virtually all uveitis would be histologically classified as endophthalmitis. In the end, what seems most practical, at least for an audience of pathologists, is to initially classify uveitis on the basis of exudate type, with subdivision based upon histologic or other evidence of pathogenesis (lens-induced, traumatic, etc.) or etiology as appropriate.

Uveitis is thus classified as serous, suppurative, granulomatous, or lymphocytic-plasmacytic. The usefulness of such classification in predicting causes decreases as the lesion ages and as the events of host immune response blend with the initial inflammation. Furthermore, the reaction may differ among different compartments within the same globe. In general, the highly mobile neutrophils (if present) will be found mostly within the ocular chambers. The less mobile but longer-lived lymphocytes, plasma cells, or macrophages will usually predominate within the uveal tissue itself. As is true in other tissues, such as joint and uterus, this may give rise to conflicting terminology, depending upon whether the disease is being diagnosed by aspiration cytology of chamber fluid or histologic assessment of the solid tissue.

Acute serous uveitis involves the usual sequence of protein-rich fluid exudation, sometimes with fibrin, followed by emigration of neutrophils. In the iris, the protein-rich fluid readily percolates through the loose stroma to enter the anterior chamber as the clinically observed **aqueous flare**. The ciliary processes are usually distended by inflammatory stromal edema, perhaps a consequence of the initial inability of the serous exudate to pass through the tight intercellular junctions of the ciliary epithelium. Choroid exhibits the most convincing vascular engorgement as well as edema, with the latter frequently seeping through the RPE to cause **serous retinal separation.** Because such mild uveitis is not likely to result in removal of the globe, observation of serous uveitis is usually restricted to globes enucleated for other reasons, such as severe ocular trauma, neoplasia, or corneal ulceration.

Suppurative uveitis *usually reflects a bacterial pathogenesis. It is usually bilateral when it is a reflection of hematogenous localization*, such as in the neonatal septicemias of calves, foals, and pigs. When unilateral, it is more often a reflection of penetrating ocular trauma with implantation of bacteria into the globe. Neutrophils also predominate in acute mild neurogenic uveitis associated with corneal epithelial injury and in the acute phase of phacoclastic uveitis. In very mild examples, they are found marginated along the endothelium of iris and ciliary venules, in perivascular adventitia, adherent to ciliary processes, and in the filtration angle. Neutrophils rapidly degenerate within the aqueous to assume an unsegmented globular morphology. Clumps may adhere to the corneal endothelium as **keratic precipitates,** or settle ventrally within the anterior chamber as **hypopyon.** The hypopyon may, in histologic section, seem to be plugging the filtration angle, but only rarely would such exudate cause glaucoma, because only rarely would such exudate be able to occlude a significant part of the circumferential filtration angle. Fibrin exudation may accompany the suppurative inflammation, but fibrinolysis is very efficient within the anterior chamber, and glaucoma rarely results.

Granulomatous uveitis is characterized by the conspicuous presence of epithelioid macrophages and, occasionally, giant cells. As is true of granulomatous disease elsewhere, only rarely is the exudate purely granulomatous, and most involve substantial participation by neutrophils. Ocular localization of some species of dimorphic fungi or of algae, helminths, or mycobacteria may cause granulomatous endophthalmitis, as may lens rupture (phacoclastic uveitis) and the Vogt-Koyanagi-Harada–like syndrome in dogs.

Lymphocytic-plasmacytic uveitis *is by far the most common histologic type of uveitis encountered in enucleated globes.* The leukocytes that are resident within the uveal tissue are dominated by lymphocytes and plasma cells, with or without the formation of actual lymphoid aggregates and nodules. It may occur simply as a chronic form of what was initially a suppurative uveitis, but is more frequently seen as the typical manifestation of immune-mediated uveitis, viral infection, phacolytic uveitis, or uveitis secondary to intraocular neoplasia.

Specific examples of uveitis/endophthalmitis follow.

Bacterial endophthalmitis

Bacteria may enter the eye hematogenously or via penetrating wounds. Those arriving hematogenously cause their initial lesion in ciliary body or, less frequently, in choroid. Those arising via penetration usually incite the initial reaction in anterior chamber, particularly if the penetration is via perforation of an ulcerated cornea. Most are suppurative, and their extent and severity vary with the size of inoculum, virulence of the agent, and host response and its duration.

The list of organisms capable of causing endophthalmitis is long. *It is probably true that any bacterium capable of bacteremia or septicemia can cause endophthalmitis.* Particularly prominent are the streptococci and coliforms in neonatal septicemia. The failure to detect ocular lesions in such animals is more often the result of the brief, fatal course of the disease than of specific ocular resistance. The ocular lesion may be very mild, better detected by opacification of the plasmoid aqueous in Bouin's or Zenker's fixative than by histologic examination. Histology may reveal only edema of ciliary processes with a few neutrophils along the capillary endothelium or enmeshed in filaments among ciliary processes. The well-known bovine *Histophilus somni* bacteremia, infectious thrombotic meningoencephalitis, is often seen as focal rather than diffuse chorioretinitis.

Exceptions to the generalization that bacterial endophthalmitis is suppurative occur if infection is caused by bacteria that, in other tissues, incite lymphocytic or even granulomatous inflammation. *Ocular tuberculosis* is largely of historical interest. It occurred as part of generalized systemic disease, and the typical tubercles were most numerous in the choroid. *Mycobacterium tuberculosis* var. *bovis* was the usual isolate except in cats where the human strain was common. In cats, ocular tuberculosis may also occur as keratoconjunctivitis without uveal involvement.

Brucella canis may cause chronic lymphocytic endophthalmitis that is probably immunologically mediated. Agglutinating titers for *B. canis* antigen in aqueous exceed those of serum, and the ocular lesions are similar to those of equine recurrent ophthalmitis.

Listeria monocytogenes often causes endophthalmitis in association with meningoencephalitis in ruminants (see Vol. 1, Nervous system). The condition is unilateral, and the pathogenesis is obscure.

Uveitis caused by the rickettsias of *Rocky Mountain spotted fever* and *ehrlichiosis* are discussed under Retinitis.

Mycotic endophthalmitis

Fungi may affect the eye as causes of keratitis, orbital cellulitis, or endophthalmitis. Only rarely do the fungi causing keratitis or orbital infection penetrate the fibrous tunic to cause intraocular disease. However, hematogenous uveal localization is rather common in the course of systemic mycoses caused by *Cryptococcus neoformans* and *Blastomyces dermatitidis* and, less regularly, with *Coccidioides immitis* and *Histoplasma capsulatum*. In immunodeficient animals, one might expect occasionally to detect endophthalmitis as part of generalized disease caused by saprophytic fungi such as *Aspergillus* or *Candida*; these same agents will occasionally cause endophthalmitis in conjunction with penetrating plant foreign bodies. The frequency with which endophthalmitis accompanies systemic mycosis is unknown and probably varies with the specific agent, the species affected, and whether the disease is in an endemic area or is a sporadic occurrence. Hematogenous ocular mycosis is found almost exclusively in dogs, except for cryptococcosis, which is more common in cats. *Blastomyces* and *Cryptococcus* are more likely to invade the eye in the course of generalized infection than are *Coccidioides* or *Histoplasma*, and occurrence in nonendemic areas is strongly linked to prolonged systemic corticosteroid therapy. Involvement is bilateral but not necessarily equal. Blastomycosis, cryptococcosis, and coccidioidomycosis are discussed Vol. 2, Respiratory system, and histoplasmosis in Vol. 3, Hematopoietic system.

Blastomycosis *is the most frequently reported cause of intraocular mycosis in dogs*. It is rare in cats. Between 20-26% of dogs with the systemic disease are blind or have grossly observed ocular lesions, suggesting that intraocular

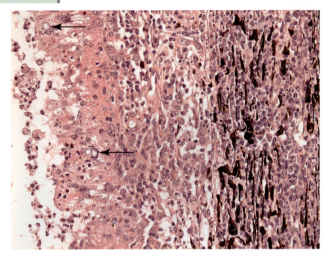

Figure 5-42 **Blastomycosis.** The lesions range from suppurative to pyogranulomatous endophthalmitis, usually with prominent subretinal exudation as seen here. The number of fungi is highly variable, here showing the typical thick refractile capsule and broad-based budding (arrows).

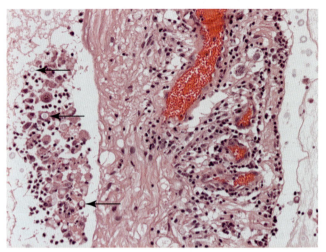

Figure 5-43 **Cryptococcosis.** Large numbers of yeast with characteristic unstained mucinous capsules (arrows) are embedded in a preretinal and subretinal granulomatous exudate. The number of organisms is typically much larger than seen with blastomycosis, and the cellular reaction is usually less dramatic.

involvement would be recognized more often if histologic examinations were routinely done. The clinical ocular disease is severe diffuse uveitis, frequently with retinal separation.

The histologic appearance is of diffuse pyogranulomatous or granulomatous endophthalmitis with retinitis, exudative retinal separation, and, commonly, granulomatous optic neuritis. Choroiditis is often more pronounced than is the anterior uveitis. The greatest accumulation of leukocytes often is in the subretinal space enlarged by exudative retinal detachment. The causative diagnosis depends upon the demonstration of the spherical-to-oval, thick-walled yeasts in vitreous aspirates or in the histologic section. They are usually most numerous in the subretinal exudate, but are rare in anterior chamber or in retina itself (Fig. 5-42).

The organisms are free or within macrophages, are 5-20 μm in diameter, and show occasional *broad-based budding*. Extremes in sizes may result in yeasts from 2-30 μm diameter. The eye may, in addition, have the full spectrum of corneal, lenticular, and glaucomatous sequelae expected of any severe uveitis. Panophthalmitis with orbital cellulitis is seen in about ⅓ of enucleated globes.

Cryptococcosis is similar to blastomycosis in that *the lesions are predominantly within retina, choroid, and optic nerve.* However, infection of the eye may arise either hematogenously or by extension from the brain via optic nerves, and lesions are often conspicuously lacking in cellular host reaction. *Large collections of poorly stained pleomorphic yeasts, surrounded by wide capsular halos, impart a typical "soap-bubble" appearance to the histologic lesions* (Fig. 5-43). The yeasts vary in size, but most are 4-10 μm in diameter. Round, oval, and crescentic forms are seen. In some animals, however, a granulomatous reaction mimicking that of blastomycosis can be found. In such lesions, the organisms typically are scarce.

The frequency with which **Coccidioides immitis** infects the eye appears to be low (~2%), despite the prevalence of generalized infection in endemic areas. The ocular lesion resembles blastomycosis in that *pyogranulomatous reaction occurs around fungal spherules.* The reaction is predominantly purulent around newly ruptured spherules, gradually

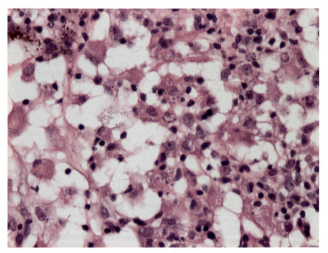

Figure 5-44 **Histoplasmosis.** Although lesions are similar to those of blastomycosis, the reaction tends to be more purely choroidal, less suppurative, and with much larger numbers of small intracellular organisms surrounded by a thin clear halo.

becoming granulomatous as the released endospores mature. The lesion tends to be more destructive than other mycoses, usually spreading to involve sclera and even episclera in a suppurative panophthalmitis.

Histoplasma capsulatum is a common cause of generalized mycosis in dogs but is rare in other domestic species. It has a predilection for lymphoid tissue and other tissues rich in phagocytes, such as lung and liver, and it is perhaps this preference that accounts for the paucity of ocular involvement in spontaneous disease. In dogs and cats, infiltrative choroiditis or panuveitis occurs and is dominated by plasma cells and by macrophages filled with the organisms (Fig. 5-44). Retinal separation, plasmoid vitreous, and optic neuritis also develop. The reaction tends to target the choroid, and to be less destructive than either blastomycosis or coccidioidomycosis.

Encephalitozoon may induce periarteritis within the uvea and retina as it does elsewhere.

Prototheca are not fungi, but they are most easily confused with *Cryptococcus* and *Blastomyces*, and histologic lesions are certainly similar to those occurring in mycotic endophthalmitis. They are *colorless saprophytic algae* capable of causing enteric, cutaneous, mammary, or generalized granulomatous disease in a variety of mammalian species. Ocular lesions have been described only in dogs with the disseminated form of the disease. *The lesions are bilateral and may vary from lymphocytic-plasmacytic to granulomatous panuveitis with optic neuritis and exudative retinal separation.* The host response is usually quite mild. The lesions resemble ocular mycosis, particularly cryptococcosis, and are distinguished only by the observation of the pleomorphic algae. In histologic section, the algae are free or within phagocytes. The organisms are spherical to oval, from 2-20 μm in diameter, with a refractile, PAS-positive, and argyrophilic cellulosic cell wall. Each cell consists of granular, weakly basophilic cytoplasm surrounding a central nucleus. *Prototheca* reproduces by asexual multiple fission, so that multiple daughter cells form within a single cell wall. One or 2 cycles of nuclear division without cytoplasmic cleavage may produce transient multinucleated cells before eventual cytoplasmic division results in up to 8 daughter cells. Each daughter cell acquires a capsule, resulting in a parent cell crisscrossed by septations that represent the cell walls of maturing daughter cells. Rupture of the parent cell wall releases the unicellular autospores. Collapsed, crumpled, and seemingly empty cell walls are visible in histologic section. There is no budding, as with *Blastomyces* and *Cryptococcus*.

Those canine isolates that were definitively identified were *Prototheca zopfii*. An enteric route of entry is probable inasmuch as necrotic enteritis is a feature of the disease (see Vol. 2, Alimentary system and peritoneum). Immunodeficiency may be a prerequisite for dissemination of the organism. Lesions are found in many visceral organs, skin, and lymph nodes in most cases. The reaction is granulomatous but is usually minimal in comparison to the large number of organisms.

Protozoal endophthalmitis

Although ocular lesions have been reported in infections caused by protozoa of the genera *Toxoplasma*, *Leishmania*, *Besnoitia*, and *Trypanosoma*, only *Toxoplasma* specifically causes intraocular lesions, although many cases diagnosed as toxoplasmosis were probably caused by *Neospora*. Most of the others cause keratoconjunctivitis that occasionally extends to anterior or generalized uveitis in which the causal agent may be found.

Toxoplasmosis affecting the eye is, as elsewhere, much more frequently suspected than proven, and clinical diagnoses greatly outnumber those confirmed by histopathology. *The histologic lesion is usually in retina, uvea, or extraocular muscles, and varies from focal, acute coagulative necrosis to granulomatous or lymphocyte-rich inflammation.* The organisms are seen most easily as intracellular pseudocysts during acute disease or as true cysts during remission. The more noxious merozoites are found only with difficulty as 7-9 μm crescentic, basophilic bodies within phagocytes or free amid necrotic debris.

The histologic changes of ocular toxoplasmosis have received various interpretations, and valid differences probably exist between species and between individuals of differing immune status. In man, the disseminated disease is usually congenital, and the ocular lesion is multifocal necrotic retinitis in which free or encysted *Toxoplasma gondii* are found. There may be lymphocytes and plasma cells in adjacent choroid. In human adults, the ocular lesion is predominantly a lymphocytic-plasmacytic choroiditis, suggesting that the pathogenesis is related more to a host immune response to the previously encountered, ubiquitous antigen than it is to local infection.

Lesions analogous to human congenital toxoplasmosis occur in *young cats* as multiple foci of retinal necrosis. Choroiditis may be present and is lymphocytic-plasmacytic, and anterior uveitis is seen in only 20-30% of such cases. *Much more common than this classic retinochoroiditis, however, is lymphocytic-plasmacytic anterior uveitis with serologic evidence of active Toxoplasma infection.* The role of toxoplasmosis in feline anterior uveitis is controversial (see Idiopathic lymphonodular uveitis of cats). Retrospective histologic studies list the majority of such cases as idiopathic and are presumed to be immune mediated, with antigen or antigens unknown. In the several large published studies, there has not been a single case confirmed by observation of merozoites or cysts in the eye; even serologic evidence in these studies pointed to toxoplasmosis in only 1-2% of cases. In contrast, one study reported evidence of anterior uveal production of *Toxoplasma*-specific antibody in 32 of 69 cats with anterior uveitis, and another report confirmed that anterior uveitis is indeed the most frequent manifestation of toxoplasmosis in cats, seen in 60% of cats with confirmed toxoplasmosis. Nonetheless, evidence remains less than conclusive about the role of *T. gondii* in the prevalent and enigmatic syndrome of anterior uveitis in this species. It may be that the local production of *Toxoplasma* antibody in cats with uveitis is merely the result of nonspecific recruitment of *Toxoplasma*-sensitized lymphocytes into the chronically inflamed uvea, and that lymphoid aggregates in such eyes are producing a whole range of antibody quite irrelevant to the original cause of the uveitis.

The situation in other species is not clear, but the prevalence of ocular lesions seems quite low. Lymphocytic cyclitis and multifocal necrotic retinitis are most frequently described and are usually seen together. *Multifocal choroiditis*, not necessarily adjacent to retinal lesions, is lymphocytic-plasmacytic in most species but granulomatous in sheep. A more common lesion is severe myonecrosis in extraocular muscles associated with free and encysted *Toxoplasma*. Toxoplasmosis is discussed in more detail in Vol. 2, Alimentary system and peritoneum.

Parasitic endophthalmitis

Many parasites are found incidentally in the eye, including *Echinococcus* in primates and *Cysticercus* in swine; multifocal ischemic chorioretinitis and optic neuritis in elk, caused by occlusive vasculitis caused by microfilariae of *Elaeophora schneideri*; and uveitis associated with fortuitous localization of larvae of *Toxocara canis* or other ascarids, *Angiostrongylus vasorum*, *Dirofilaria immitis*, and *Onchocerca cervicalis*. In addition, adults of *Setaria* spp. are occasionally found within the eye of horses. The long thread-like worms are seen floating within the aqueous, and the uveitis that results seems to be the result of mechanical irritation. The only specific intraocular parasitism is seen with the lens fluke of fish (*Diplostomum spathaceum*), which, after penetrating the skin, seeks the lens with remarkable speed and specificity. The principal lesion is cataract induced by the intralenticular presence of hundreds of larvae awaiting ingestion by fish-eating birds for completion of their life cycle, but infected fish may have larvae arrested in many other ocular or extraocular locations.

Chronic mild anterior uveitis is reported to accompany ectopic localization of immature *D. immitis* within aqueous and vitreous cavities of canine eyes. Studies of pathology are sparse, but endophthalmitis is reported in which anterior synechiae, subretinal exudate, and early cyclitic membrane may accompany the numerous vitreal and subretinal larval nematodes.

Ocular onchocerciasis affects people and horses. The *human* disease is endemic in Africa and Central America and is one of the most frequent causes of blindness in the world. The microfilariae of the causal agent, *Onchocerca volvulus*, are transmitted by *Simulium* spp. flies, and affect the skin, eyelids, and corneas of children and young adults. The microfilariae are found throughout the eye, but the lesion of greatest visual significance is diffuse, sclerosing, superficial stromal keratitis complicated by anterior uveitis with synechiae and eventual glaucoma.

Equine onchocerciasis has some similarities. The parasite, *O. cervicalis*, is of worldwide distribution, and surveys from the United States document the prevalence of dermal infection in horses as varying from 48-96%. About ½ of the infected horses have microfilariae in conjunctiva or sclera. The microfilariae enter the eye only incidentally in the migration from the ligamentum nuchae to the subcutis. The ocular sites of greatest concentration are the peripheral cornea and the lamina propria of the bulbar conjunctiva near the limbus. The microfilariae in the cornea are associated with superficial stromal keratitis resembling the disease of humans, albeit much milder. Some of the horses also have anterior uveitis typical of equine recurrent ophthalmitis, prompting theories that *Onchocerca* is one cause of this disease. The microfilariae can be recovered from the conjunctiva and eyelids of horses with uveitis, keratoconjunctivitis, and eyelid depigmentation, but are recovered with equal frequency from horses with no ocular disease and no microscopic reaction to the worms.

Ocular manifestations of **visceral larva migrans** in people are associated with larvae of *Toxocara canis* or, perhaps more frequently, of the raccoon roundworm *Baylisascaris procyonis*. The unilateral granulomatous fundic lesions are caused by a single wandering larva, and are relatively common in children but have rarely been described in nonhuman subjects despite the rather common occurrence of ascarid-induced granulomas in canine kidneys, lungs, or livers. The paucity of reports may not reflect the actual prevalence of disease in specific canine populations. One large survey of working sheepdogs in New Zealand recorded a 39% prevalence of lesions attributed to visceral larva migrans, contrasted to a 6% prevalence in similar dogs living in urban environments. *The active lesions were lymphocytic and granulomatous uveitis, nonsuppurative retinitis, and peripapillary nontapetal retinal necrosis.* Inactive lesions involved chorioretinal scars and multifocal chronic retinal separations in dogs older than 3 years. Larvae most compatible with *T. canis* were seen in sections of some acutely affected eyes. The high prevalence in these dogs was tentatively ascribed to the feeding of uncooked frozen mutton that may have contained *T. canis* larvae as part of a dog-sheep-dog life cycle. A report of similar lesions in Border Collies in the United States was associated with the feeding of raw pork.

Ocular disease may also result from the intraocular migration of *fly larvae*. This syndrome, termed *internal ophthalmomyiasis*, is discussed with diseases of conjunctiva.

Further reading

Callegan MC, et al. Bacterial endophthalmitis: epidemiology, therapeutics, and bacterium-host interactions. Clin Microbiol Rev 2002; 15:111-124.

Hollingsworth SR. Canine protothecosis. Vet Clin North Am Small Anim Pract 2000;30:1091-1101.

Maenz M, et al. Ocular toxoplasmosis past, present and new aspects of an old disease. Prog Retin Eye Res 2014;39C:77-106.

Massa KL, et al. Causes of uveitis in dogs: 102 cases (1989-2000). Vet Ophthalmol 2002;5:93-98.

Panciera RJ, et al. Ocular histopathology of ehrlichial infections in the dog. Vet Pathol 2001;38:43-46.

Trivedi SR, et al. Feline cryptococcosis: impact of current research on clinical management. J Feline Med Surg 2011;13:163-172.

Viral endophthalmitis

The fuzzy distinction between infectious uveitis/endophthalmitis and immune-mediated disease is most obvious when dealing with viral causes of endophthalmitis, even though it is probably also a major factor in mycotic and parasitic diseases. The distinction is therefore arbitrary, and *discussed later are those diseases that are probably best classified as immune-mediated endophthalmitis for which the antigen is identified as viral.*

Canine adenovirus

Canine adenovirus 1 (infectious canine hepatitis virus) is the best-documented cause of virally induced, immune-mediated uveitis in domestic animals. At least in North America, many years of widespread vaccination have reduced it to a virtually historical disease in domestic dogs. The systemic disease is discussed in Vol. 2, Liver and biliary system. During the acute viral stage of the disease, viral replication within endothelium and stromal phagocytes of the uvea results in a primary mild nonsuppurative uveitis that usually is clinically undetected. Inoculation of field virus into the anterior chamber of dogs and foxes may result in viral inclusion bodies within corneal endothelium and subsequent edema, but edema is not a feature of the active stage of naturally occurring disease. During the convalescent phase of the disease, or 6-7 days after vaccination with a modified live virus, a small percentage of dogs develop anterior uveitis, endothelial damage, and corneal edema ("blue eye") that is a manifestation of type III hypersensitivity to persistent viral antigen, in which complement fixation attracts neutrophils. The proteases of neutrophils are responsible for the cell injury.

The histologic lesion is bilateral but not usually of equal intensity, thus clinically apparent disease may be unilateral. *Corneal edema results from diffuse hydropic degeneration of corneal endothelium and secondary stromal edema.* In a small percentage of affected dogs, the damage is so persistent as to cause interstitial keratitis and permanent fibrosis. Whether this sequel results from unusually persistent antigen, unusually severe endothelial damage or age-dependent variation in endothelial regenerative ability is unknown. *Intranuclear inclusion bodies* of adenovirus type may be seen in a few degenerate endothelial cells. There is accompanying anterior uveitis, with lymphocytes and plasma cells around vessels in the iris and ciliary body; in the filtration angle; and adherent to cornea as keratic precipitates. Choroidal involvement is mild or absent. Sequelae such as synechia or angle obstruction with debris are infrequent, occurring in <5% of affected eyes. In most dogs, whether recovering from natural or vaccine-induced infection, the ocular reaction subsides within 3-4 weeks.

Feline infectious peritonitis–associated uveitis

The coronavirus of feline infectious peritonitis (FIP) causes diffuse uveitis that is probably immune mediated (see Vol. 2, Alimentary system and peritoneum). The frequency of ocular lesions is unknown because the eyes are not regularly examined in cats with the disease. Estimates based upon clinical examination range from ~10% in an outbreak to 50% of unselected clinical cases. *Most cats that die of the disease have ocular involvement as detected by coagulation of aqueous with acidic fixatives (indicating increased aqueous protein).* The histologic evidence for inflammation in some eyes may be subtle indeed, and such eyes usually reach postmortem without clinically detected uveitis. Conversely, some cats develop severe uveitis attributed to this virus by clinical, serologic, or histologic evaluation, without concurrent evidence of the disease elsewhere.

The typical histologic lesion, as is the case elsewhere in the body, varies with time and location. Leukocytic infiltration is most extensive in the ciliary body and adjacent limbic sclera, and is usually a rather even mixture of neutrophils, lymphocytes, plasma cells, and macrophages. In some eyes, the infiltrate is purely histiocytic. The inflammatory cell population often becomes more purely lymphoid in the choroid and more neutrophilic in the anterior chamber. Perivascular lymphocytic-plasmacytic aggregates are common in retrobulbar connective tissue and in the optic nerve sheath, and in the retina. In the retina, the accumulations are larger and are more likely to involve a true phlebitis than is the case with the subtle perivascular retinitis that is a frequent and nonspecific accompaniment to most forms of anterior uveitis (Fig. 5-45). Sequelae to the uveitis are rarely seen, either because the cats are in the late stages of the disease when ocular lesions are examined or because euthanasia halts its progression. Retinal separation with serous subretinal exudate is occasionally observed. The presence of large globular accumulations of macrophages and neutrophils adherent to the corneal endothelium *(keratic precipitates)* is an important clinical hallmark of the disease, and is useful histologically as well. Neutrophilic endothelialitis with severe corneal edema may also occur.

The histologic lesions of FIP within the globe are not absolutely specific, and so the gold standard for the diagnosis is immunohistochemical demonstration of coronaviral antigen within uveal leukocytes.

Bovine malignant catarrhal fever–associated uveitis

The presence of severe uveitis is an important clue in the clinical differentiation of malignant catarrhal fever from other bovine systemic disorders, particularly from mucosal disease. The histologic lesions within the eye resemble those elsewhere in the body: *arterial necrosis and perivascular and intramural lymphocytic accumulations.* The presence of mitotic figures among the lymphoid cells is distinctive. The arteritis usually is most obvious in the iris, but may be seen affecting arterioles or venules in the retina, choroid, meninges of optic nerve, or even peripheral cornea. There is *marked corneal edema with a ring of peripheral corneal stromal vascularization,* clinically seen as a dark red circumferential brush border of straight vessels in the perilimbal cornea. Blood vessels in the conjunctiva and even in the newly vascularized cornea may be targets for the disease, so that the edema and hemorrhage of vessel injury are added to the nonspecific lesions of conjunctivitis and peripheral keratitis that accompany uveitis of any cause in all species.

Infiltration of lymphocytes among corneal endothelial cells is associated with patchy necrosis of that layer, which may also contribute to the corneal edema. A layer of mononuclear leukocytes enmeshed in fibrin often is adherent to the aqueous face of the corneal endothelium.

Even the very early lesions are lymphocytic. In vessels, the first changes involve subendothelial and adventitial lymphocytic and lymphoblastic accumulation, with little necrosis. Despite long-standing speculation for an immune-complex pathogenesis for the vasculitis, proof is lacking. Deposition of immunoglobulin or complement is not a significant feature of the vascular lesion within the eye, and a T-cell–dependent, type IV immune pathogenesis has been suggested.

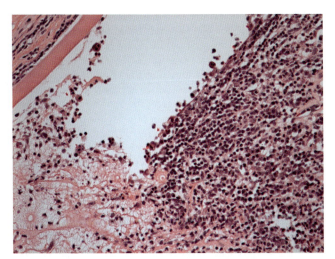

Figure 5-45 **Feline infectious peritonitis (FIP).** The simultaneous presence of a fibrinonecrotic, suppurative, and plasmacytic endophthalmitis is characteristic of FIP, but not always seen. Ocular lesions are so variable that a firm diagnosis virtually always requires immunohistochemistry to demonstrate the coronaviral antigen within the lesion.

Further reading

Kipar A, Meli ML. Feline infectious peritonitis: still an enigma? Vet Pathol 2014;51:505-526.
Li H, et al. Malignant catarrhal fever: inching toward understanding. Ann Rev Anim Biosci 2014;2:209-233.
O'Toole D, Li H. The pathology of malignant catarrhal fever, with an emphasis on ovine herpesvirus 2. Vet Pathol 2014;51:437-452.
Stiles J. Ocular manifestations of feline viral diseases. Vet J 2014; 201:166-173.

Idiopathic immune-mediated uveitis

There is no clear histologic distinction between idiopathic immune-mediated uveitis and uveitis traditionally ascribed to a specific causative agent. Except for rapidly progressing bacterial uveitis following hematogenous localization or penetrating injury, *virtually all uveitis probably has an immune component superimposed on initial nonspecific inflammation.* Even traumatic uveitis probably permits unusually large amounts of endogenous ocular antigens to overwhelm immune tolerance and induce uveitis. Types III and IV hypersensitivity have been induced in various laboratory animals by using tissue-specific antigens of photoreceptor, uveal, lens, and corneal origin. *Lens-induced uveitis* and *uveodermatologic syndrome (Vogt-Koyanagi-Harada syndrome)* are naturally occurring examples of uveitis induced by endogenous ocular antigens. Strong cross-reactivity between *leptospiral antigens* and equine corneal endothelium (immune mimicry) serves to further obscure the distinction between infectious and immune-mediated ocular disease.

Included in this section are those diseases that are exclusively or predominantly immune mediated, and for which the triggering antigen has not been proven to be an infectious agent. *In general, all are characterized by chronic, lymphocytic-plasmacytic panuveitis, in which the infiltrating leukocytes form lymphoid aggregates and perivascular cuffs.* Clinically, they are either continuously progressive syndromes or subject to periodic irregular clinical exacerbations and remissions. This is by far the most common histologic pattern of uveitis in cats and in horses (Fig. 5-46). It is relatively less common (although still prevalent) in globes submitted from dogs simply because of the prevalence of other patterns of uveitis, such as lens-induced uveitis and uveitis associated with systemic mycoses.

Understanding the pathogenesis of all uveitis, but particularly those examples with a presumed immune pathogenesis, requires an understanding of the unique immune status of the globe, a phenomenon commonly referred to as "immune privilege."

Immune privilege refers to a combination of structural and functional mechanisms by which the globe seeks to avoid the bystander consequences of inflammation, as occur in most other tissues. Because the function of the globe is so dependent on very precise anatomic relationships and the clarity of ocular media, events of serous effusion, bystander cellular necrosis, and accumulation of exudates are much more damaging within the globe than in most other tissues.

The elements of this immune privilege include the absence of lymphatic drainage within the globe, a relative paucity of intraocular major histocompatibility complex (MHC) II antigen-presenting cells, intrinsic production of anti-inflammatory and immune-inhibitory cytokines within the aqueous and vitreous, the almost complete absence of intraocular resident leukocytes, and anterior chamber–associated immune deviation. This *"immune deviation"* begins with the continuous presence of immunomodulating cytokines within the aqueous, vitreous, and subretinal space (notably but not exclusively transforming growth factor-β [TGF-β]) that alter endogenous and exogenous intraocular antigens interacting with antigen-presenting cells resident within the trabecular meshwork and elsewhere in the uvea. Those antigen-presenting cells then leave the globe, enter the spleen, and specifically induce a population of splenic lymphocytes that will return to the globe as immune effector cells with very specific functional limitations. These splenic-origin B cells, natural killer (NK) cells, and CD4+ or CD8+ T lymphocytes have impaired complement-fixing ability, little ability to induce a delayed hypersensitivity reaction, yet unimpaired antigen-specific cytotoxicity and production of non–complement-fixing antibody. In short, the immune response to intraocular antigenic challenge is specifically altered to limit those types of immune responses that typically have a lot of "collateral damage," and to favor those very precise cytotoxic responses that typically have little bystander injury.

Anterior segment immune deviation seems designed to dampen the significance of the "day to day" leakage of autoantigens and low-level exogenous antigens into the globe and is a critical component of immune tolerance to retinal and lens antigens. **It is not effective** if there is a break in the blood-eye barrier that allows large amounts of exogenous antigen into the globe, or if there is any intraocular disease that counteracts the immunosuppressive effect of the constitutive intraocular cytokines or increases the release of autoantigens. Failure of anterior segment immune deviation therefore allows entry into the globe by immunocytes capable of activating complement and triggering delayed-type hypersensitivity reactions that are unacceptably damaging to the globe. Without proof, we assume that most of the clinical and histologic manifestations of "idiopathic" lymphocytic uveitis are manifestations of a failure in this immune deviation.

The usual histologic features of idiopathic (presumed immune-mediated uveitis) in all species include perivascular lymphocytic-plasmacytic aggregates in iris stroma, in the ciliary body, and, less obviously, in the choroid and even the retina. In long-standing cases (which are most likely to receive histologic examination), the aggregates may be very large and resemble lymphoid follicles. As in other tissues, amplification of the immune response results in recruitment of lymphocytes that are not necessarily specific for the inciting antigen. The polyclonal nature of these lymphocytes is probably important in the typically recurrent nature of uveitis in all species. Once established in the eye, these cells respond to a diverse range of circulating antigens that enter the eye through a blood-eye barrier at least temporarily disrupted by the inflammation. *It is thus possible, or even probable, that* **chronic, recurrent lymphonodular uveitis,** *which is the classic histologic pattern for "idiopathic" uveitis seen in all species, results not from persistence of a single triggering antigen, or repeated exposure to the same antigen, but from ongoing impairment of immune deviation and permeability of the blood-eye barrier that allows both exogenous and endogenous antigens easy access to the intraocular environment.*

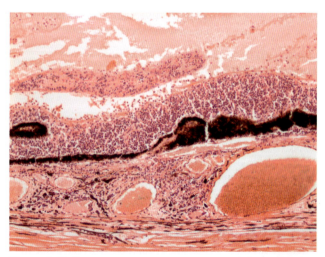

Figure 5-46 Equine recurrent uveitis. Neutrophilic-to-lymphocytic pars planitis is a characteristic lesion.

Specific examples of idiopathic lymphonodular uveitis or endophthalmitis are discussed later, and include equine recurrent uveitis, idiopathic lymphonodular uveitis of cats, canine lymphocytic uveitis, canine uveodermatologic syndrome (Vogt-Koyanagi-Harada–like syndrome), and lens-induced uveitis.

Equine recurrent ophthalmitis (periodic ophthalmia)

This is a worldwide and important cause of blindness in horses and mules. The blindness results from repeated attacks of anterior uveitis occurring at unpredictable intervals and with increasing severity. With each attack, there is increasing involvement of the posterior uvea, retina, and optic nerve, and increasingly frequent sequelae of cataract, lens luxation, synechiae, retinal separation, and interstitial keratitis. Despite the frequent observation of posterior synechiae, glaucoma is rarely reported. It is speculated that aqueous drainage in horses relies less on the trabecular meshwork and more on uveal resorption than is true of dogs or cats. The disease may initially be unilateral but eventually affects both eyes. Blindness is usually a late sequela, but may occur early in the disease if exudative choroiditis causes retinal separation.

Gross lesions of the acute disease are typical of anterior uveitis in any species: serous conjunctivitis, chemosis, circumcorneal ciliary hyperemia, corneal edema, and plasmoid aqueous and vitreous, with fibrin and leukocytes in the aqueous. Clinically, such animals are often systemically ill, as detected by fever, decreased appetite, and depression. Lacrimation and photophobia are usually marked. Subsequent attacks tend to become increasingly severe, and resolution of the gross lesions between attacks is less complete. Such horses, during the quiescent period, may have one or more of the following: peripheral corneal vascularization with fibrosis and persistent edema, irregular thickening and pigmentation of iris, multiple posterior synechiae, patchy residual uveal pigment on lens capsule, and peripapillary retinal hyperreflectivity suggesting retinal scarring.

The microscopic lesions depend on the stage of the disease and represent a continuum from anterior uveitis to endophthalmitis with retinal scarring, or even phthisis bulbi. The earliest lesion is anterior uveal inflammation that is transiently neutrophilic but rapidly becomes predominantly lymphocytic. Ciliary processes are most obviously affected. Edema, fibrin, and leukocytes distend the stroma, and leukocytes and fibrin lie in the anterior chamber and in the filtration angle. Neutrophilic-to-lymphocytic pars planitis is fairly common (see Fig. 5-46). In the eyes of horses with a history of several attacks of uveitis, the exudate in these acute flare-ups of the disease is almost purely lymphocytic-plasmacytic and is found about vessels of the choroid, retina, and optic nerve as well as the anterior uvea. Peripheral corneal vascularization, both from conjunctival and limbic ciliary vessels, becomes increasingly prominent and extends further toward the center of the cornea. Edema accompanies the newly formed vessels. The chorioretinitis may be sufficiently exudative to cause multifocal retinal separation. As these severe uveal lesions regress during clinically quiescent periods, they leave behind characteristic residual changes. Relatively early in the disease, there is the development of perivascular lymphoid aggregates in the iris and ciliary body that persist and may even form true lymphoid nodules (Fig. 5-47). The ciliary processes may remain thickened by fibrous organization of stromal edema, and a hyaline membrane often seems to cover the ciliary epithelium. This

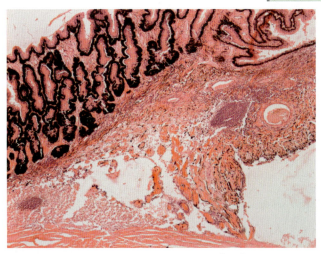

Figure 5-47 Equine recurrent uveitis. As the disease matures, large lymphoid nodules typically form within the iris stroma, trabecular meshwork, and ciliary body.

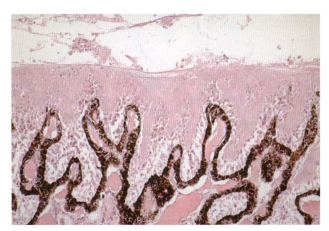

Figure 5-48 Equine recurrent uveitis. Deposition of amyloid-like material within the apical cytoplasm of the inner nonpigmented ciliary epithelium, unique to this disease.

material, in fact, lies within the apical cytoplasm of the non-pigmented ciliary epithelium. In most respects, it resembles amyloid (Fig. 5-48). Small blood vessels persist along corneal stromal lamellae, and there is subtle fibrous disorganization of the stroma, the result of previous edema. Peripapillary chorioretinal scarring is seen as focal retinal photoreceptor loss, jumbling of layers, and gliosis. Adjacent retinal pigment epithelium may be hypertrophic or hyperplastic, and a focal cluster of lymphocytes in the nearby choroid is common.

Choroidal vessels are unusually thick walled because of edema or fibrin, the latter probably analogous to the hyalinization described in several reports. Increased vascular permeability persists even in quiescent periods, with loss of the blood-aqueous barrier demonstrated by fluorescein angiography. Whether or not this vascular alteration participates in the perpetuation of the uveitis is unknown, but it is known that such alterations predispose to localization of circulating immune complexes and subsequent type III hypersensitivity–induced inflammation.

Focal retinal detachments may reattach by fibrous organization of subretinal exudate or may progress to total separation with a barely recognizable retina adherent to the posterior lens capsule. Gliosis and lymphocytic aggregates may be found within the proximal optic nerve. Scarring in optic disc and adjacent retina often is clinically obvious and may occur in horses with no other lesions of uveitis, leading to speculation that it is not really linked to, or at least not specific for, equine recurrent uveitis.

The causes and pathogenesis of recurrent equine ophthalmitis remain controversial. The most compelling single candidate for an etiologic agent is *Leptospira interrogans* serovar *pomona*, which can induce the syndrome after experimental introduction of bacteremia by subcutaneous inoculation. Leptospiral antigens or DNA have been repeatedly demonstrated within the globe of 50-70% of horses with classic clinical and histologic changes of equine recurrent uveitis. The problem, however, is that not all cases can be blamed on this agent. Various studies in various parts of the world have implicated other leptospiral serovars; various other bacterial, viral, protozoal, and other infectious agents; or even reaction to endogenous antigens. For most, the evidence is not compelling. Over the years, interest in pursuing the cause of the initial uveitis has faded as our collective interest in understanding the recurrent and progressive nature of this disease has focused more on the probability that the persistent disease is not caused by persistence of leptospiral or other infection as much as by the triggering of autoimmunity by impairment of anterior segment immune deviation or increased production of autoantigens. There is cross-reactivity between leptospiral antigens and equine corneal endothelial, lenticular, and retinal antigens. Horses with recurrent uveitis have intravitreal antibody and CD4+ T cells directed against numerous retinal antigens, and at least some of those antigens will stimulate uveitis when injected into the equine vitreous. They also have an increase in MHC II antigen-presenting cells within the choroid. The predominant cells within the anterior uvea of horses with chronic equine recurrent uveitis are CD4+ T cells, implying a Th1 inflammatory reaction. All of this points to the probability that the initial uveitis substantially alters the character of the intraocular environment so that immune privilege no longer exists, and the globe becomes susceptible to the potentially injurious effects of a wide range of endogenous and exogenous antigens unrelated to what caused the initial uveitis. At least in the case of leptospirosis, some of the persisting inflammation may represent humoral and cellular reaction to retinal and other autoantibodies that cross-react with leptospiral glycoproteins.

Idiopathic lymphonodular uveitis of cats

This is by far the most frequent histologic pattern of uveitis in cats, and vies with diffuse iris melanoma as the most common cause of glaucoma in this species. These eyes are enucleated and thus become available for histologic evaluation because of the glaucoma. The mechanism by which the uveitis causes the glaucoma is unknown.

The intraocular lesions are essentially identical to those seen with recurrent uveitis of horses, except there is no deposition of amyloid-like material within the ciliary epithelium. Perivascular accumulations of lymphocytes and plasma cells are seen throughout the uvea and, with less regularity, around small vessels in the retina. The iris tends to have the greatest accumulation, and the lymphocytic-plasmacytic perivascular aggregates may become so large as to be clinically visible. Formation of actual lymphoid follicles may occur in chronic and severe cases (Fig. 5-49). The nodules and follicles may also

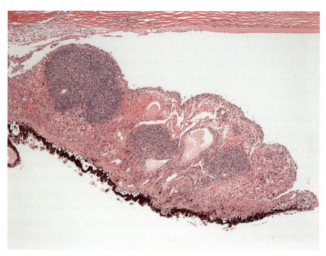

Figure 5-49 **Lymphonodular iritis** and secondary glaucoma in a cat. The lymphoid nodules occur within the iris and ciliary body, but the trabecular meshwork remains open, and the pathogenesis for the glaucoma is unknown.

occur within the trabecular meshwork and within the ciliary body, but choroidal involvement is usually quite subtle.

The syndrome is presumed to be immune mediated, but the identity of the antigen or antigens is unknown. Its initial clinical presentation is usually unilateral, but the other globe is considered "at risk" for developing subsequent uveitis. There has been no study to document the actual risk. The pattern of serologic reactions in cats with this lymphonodular uveitis is no different than the general population, except perhaps to *Toxoplasma* (see Protozoal endophthalmitis, previously). That debate continues, but it seems clear that the syndrome is not associated with the presence of a histologically detectable infectious agent within the globe (at least by the time those globes are available for histologic assessment). Studies using immunohistochemistry and PCR to detect infectious agents have been similarly inconsistent, conflicting, and therefore inconclusive. Much of the confusion probably stems from the mistaken belief that the fairly uniform histologic picture must therefore be predictive of a single and repetitive etiology. As suggested previously with equine recurrent uveitis, it is likely that the pathogenesis for the recurring disease is different from the cause for the initial episode of uveitis.

Idiopathic lymphocytic uveitis in dogs

The histologic lesions are, in general, similar to those described previously for cats and horses: *lymphocytic-plasmacytic panuveitis that tends to be more severe in the anterior uvea than in the choroid.* Some cases develop lymphoid nodules and even follicles within the anterior uveal stroma. The disease is bilateral but not necessarily of uniform severity. Unlike the situation in cats, it rarely is associated with glaucoma. The main differential diagnosis is phacolytic uveitis, and indeed, in some cases the distinction is impossible.

Uveodermatologic syndrome in dogs (Vogt-Koyanagi-Harada syndrome)

Despite the exotic-sounding name, *this disease is relatively frequent in those areas in which the most susceptible breeds (Akitas, Siberian Huskies, Samoyeds) are popular.* The clinical syndrome of facial dermal depigmentation and severe bilateral uveitis is distinctive, although many dogs examined for the uveitis are not noted to have skin lesions. The canine syndrome closely parallels the human disease, except for the encephalitis that is the least-frequent part of the human syndrome and has not been confirmed in dogs. The human disease is most prevalent in people of Asian, Latin, or Mediterranean descent; the predilection in dogs for the Japanese Akita is an interesting but unexplained parallel.

The histologic lesion is a destructive granulomatous endophthalmitis with abundant dispersal of melanin (Fig. 5-50A). The melanin-laden retinal pigment epithelium seems to be especially susceptible. Retinal detachment and destructive granulomatous inflammation are seen in advanced cases. The lesion is distinguished from the more prevalent systemic mycotic diseases by the predilection for pigmented tissues within the eye, lack of visceral involvement, and by the distinctive skin lesions, if they are present (see Vol. 1, Integumentary system). Most cases submitted for histologic assessment are chronic and have been heavily treated, and so histologic lesions are rarely "textbook." They usually are dominated by uveal scarring with dispersal of pigment from previously-injured pigmented neuroectoderm (Fig. 5-50B).

The pathogenesis of the human disease is thought to involve cell-mediated immune reaction to uveal (or epidermal) melanin.

Further reading

Deeg CA. A proteomic approach for studying the pathogenesis of spontaneous equine recurrent uveitis (ERU). Vet Immunol and Immunopathol 2009;128:132-136.

Faber NA, et al. Detection of leptospiral species in the aqueous humor of horses with naturally acquired recurrent uveitis. J Clin Microbiol 2009;128:132-136.

Gilger BC. Equine recurrent uveitis: the viewpoint from the USA. Equine Vet J Suppl 2010;37:57-61.

Sapienza JS, et al. Golden retriever uveitis: 75 cases (1994-1999). Vet Ophthalmol 2000;3:241-246.

Taylor AW. Ocular immune privilege. Eye 2009;23:1885-1889.

Zipplies JK, et al. Miscellaneous vitreous-derived IgM antibodies target numerous retinal proteins in equine recurrent uveitis. Vet Ophthalmol 2012;15(Suppl. 2):57-64.

Lens-induced uveitis

Uveitis in response to leakage of lens material is seen in all species, but is most frequent by far in dogs. The term lens-induced uveitis encompasses 2 very different syndromes—phacolytic and phacoclastic uveitis—that differ markedly in clinical severity, histopathology, and pathogenesis.

Phacolytic uveitis is a *mild lymphocytic-plasmacytic anterior uveitis that occurs in response to the leakage of denatured lens protein through an intact lens capsule, which occurs regularly in the course of maturation of cataracts toward total liquefaction.* Some degree of phacolytic uveitis is assumed to occur in virtually all animals with cataract. It is most significant as a cause of postoperative complications and reduced overall success of cataract surgery in dogs, and routine preoperative and postoperative anti-inflammatory medication to reduce the severity of phacolytic uveitis has had a major impact on the success of canine cataract surgery. The inflammation is generally mild and is readily controlled by routine anti-inflammatory therapy, so the pathologist is likely to encounter this lesion only as an

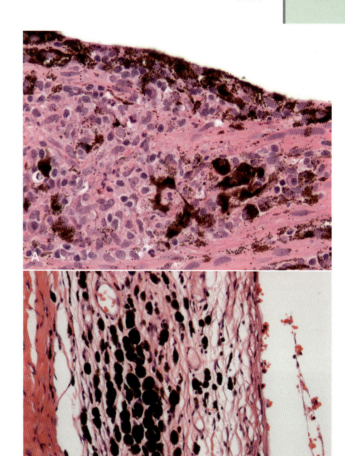

Figure 5-50 Uveodermatologic syndrome (Vogt-Koyanagi-Harada–like disease). **A.** Destructive granulomatous inflammation is targeting the pigmented neuroectoderm along the posterior surface of the iris. **B.** Chronic, treated uveodermatologic syndrome with postinflammatory destruction of choroidal architecture, dispersal of pigment, and disappearance of the retinal pigmented epithelium.

incidental finding in eyes with cataracts that were enucleated for reasons unrelated to the uveitis. The lesion is qualitatively identical to that described for idiopathic ("immune-mediated") uveitis, and so one cannot prove that an anterior mild lymphocytic uveitis in a specific globe is necessarily phacolytic.

The pathogenesis of phacolytic uveitis is assumed to represent an immune response to crystalline lens proteins leaking into the aqueous humor in amounts sufficient to overwhelm immune tolerance. That may explain why phacolytic uveitis is paradoxically more severe in dogs with early cataracts than in those with hypermature, extensively liquefied lenses in which denaturation of lens protein may have rendered it less antigenic.

Phacoclastic uveitis is, *at least histologically, a more complicated disease that follows rupture of a normal lens in an unknown percentage of cases.* The rupture is usually from corneal penetration by a thorn, quill, bullet, or cat claw, and thus usually is of the anterior capsule. It can also occur, albeit rarely, in dogs with rapidly-progressing diabetic cataracts even when the capsule seems to be intact. The clinical syndrome is distinctive: corneal perforation and mild traumatic uveitis that are successfully managed by conventional therapy, followed by the sudden reappearance of a severe, intractable uveitis 10-14 days after the initial injury. Poor response to medical therapy and the eventual development of glaucoma or phthisis bulbi prompt enucleation.

The macroscopic changes in the bisected globe are diagnostic. The lens is flattened in its anteroposterior dimension, and there frequently is a wedge of opacification extending from the anterior capsule toward the nucleus. Usually, there is posterior synechia, iris bombé, and the various other lesions as seen in any severe uveitis (Fig. 5-51A, B).

The histologic lesions vary considerably depending on duration and, probably, on the amount of lens protein that escaped through the rupture site. Ophthalmologists will use the size of the rupture and their estimate of the amount of lens material lost into the anterior or posterior chamber to predict whether phacoclastic uveitis is likely to ensue, and thus whether prophylactic lens removal and irrigation of the anterior chamber is likely to be required. The anecdotal observation that the amount of lens material entering the anterior chamber seems to be important in predicting whether phacoclastic uveitis will develop or not is certainly in keeping with the theoretical pathogenesis for this disease that is related to the overwhelming of normal immune tolerance for small amounts of lens protein.

The lesions of phacoclastic uveitis are complex and reflect the direct effects of trauma, immunologic reaction to massive release of lens protein, reparative proliferation of metaplastic lens and/or iridociliary epithelium, the intraocular implantation of bacteria at the time of initial trauma, and lesions attributable to eventual secondary glaucoma. It is worth mentioning that some, and perhaps most, of these globes have at least some participation by bacterial infection that occurs concurrently with the original penetrating injury. How much that infection contributes to the histopathology described later remains unknown. Most samples reaching a pathologist are from animals that have been treated extensively with antibiotics, but it is still possible that previous septic inflammation was the significant contributor to the persisting histologic changes. Examples in which the intraocular lesions are dominated by suppurative intralenticular inflammation mixed with numerous bacteria (rather than by perilenticular granulomatous inflammation or by uncontrolled lens epithelial proliferation as described later) have been published under a separate name of "septic implantation syndrome."

The simplest and presumably earliest lesion of phacoclastic uveitis occurs at the site of capsular perforation. The edges of the capsule are retracted and coiled outward, and a wedge of neutrophils and liquefied lens material extends from the perforation toward the nucleus. The inflammation outside of the lens is usually distinctly perilenticular and involves a mixture of neutrophils and macrophages in the anterior and posterior chambers, and a lymphocyte-dominated reaction within the uveal stroma (Fig. 5-52).

Older lesions, which predominate in most globes by the time they are enucleated, are dominated by perilenticular proliferative changes of wound repair. There is proliferation and fibroblastic metaplasia of lens epithelium adjacent to the perforation, which escapes from the lens to ramify over the lens surface and frequently incorporates the lens, ciliary processes, and iris

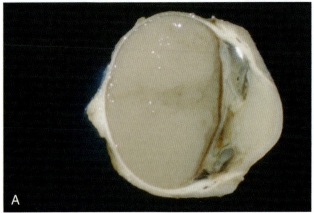
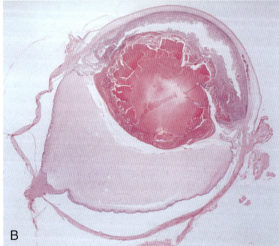

Figure 5-51 **Phacoclastic uveitis. A.** Bisected globe with coagulated aqueous and vitreous typical of uveitis, anteroposterior collapse of the lens with capsular rupture, and posterior synechia with probable pupillary block. **B.** Rabbit globe with lens rupture secondary to infection with *Encephalitozoon cuniculi*. The anterior lens capsule has shredded, and the lens is surrounded by a robust mixed leukocytic accumulation. The vitreous is filled with coagulated protein typical of endophthalmitis.

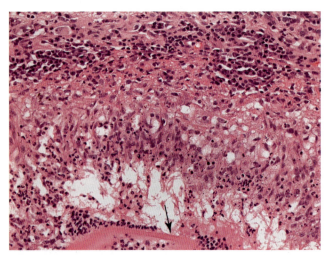

Figure 5-52 **Acute phacoclastic uveitis.** Lens capsular remnant (arrow) is surrounded by a lamellar accumulation of neutrophils, macrophages, and then finally by lymphocytes and plasma cells. This lamellar and strictly perilenticular orientation by these 3 layers is characteristic.

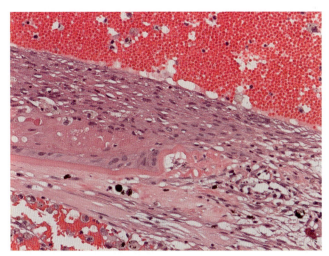

Figure 5-53 **Chronic phacoclastic uveitis.** Severed ends of anterior lens capsule are retracted and frayed. Lens epithelial cells have migrated through the defect and have undergone fibroblastic metaplasia, creating the risk of pupillary block and secondary glaucoma.

leaves into a large fibrous mass that obstructs aqueous outflow. Metaplasia of ciliary epithelium or recruitment of fibroblasts from uveal stroma may contribute to the proliferation (Fig. 5-53). Many such specimens contain little evidence of inflammation other than fibroplasia, probably because of very extensive anti-inflammatory therapy that is, in hindsight, useless against the proliferative events that doom the eye to glaucoma or phthisis.

Phacoclastic uveitis is an important complication of cataract surgery in which fragments of lens cortex or epithelium may be left in the eye. These initiate the same inflammatory and proliferative reaction as described previously, and the complications are as refractory to conventional anti-inflammatory therapy as is the naturally occurring disease. Iatrogenic phacoclastic uveitis has now become uncommon thanks to improvements in surgical technique as cataract surgery in dogs has become more routine.

The immune pathogenesis of phacoclastic uveitis has been extensively studied, but with no universally accepted conclusion. The current theory is that the release of massive amounts of lens protein overwhelms the anterior chamber–associated immune deviation (ACAID)-dependent tolerance to small, physiologic amounts of lens crystalline antigen. The return of lens-sensitized lymphocytes from the spleen into the perilenticular uvea then initiates both the pyogranulomatous perilenticular inflammation and the proliferative events of healing that, unfortunately, doom the eye. This pathogenesis, if true, explains the typical delay between injury and reaction, and why rapid surgical removal of the lens is preventive. It may also explain the unpredictability of phacoclastic uveitis, especially following small perforations in puppies, which seem often to heal uneventfully. Even in adult dogs, the disease in unpredictable, so owners' questions about the risk of phacoclastic uveitis as the justification for surgical removal of a perforated lens cannot be answered with certainty. One study found lens removal shortly after perforation prevented serious complications in 6 of 7 dogs thus treated, whereas 5 of 6 dogs treated with aggressive medical therapy lost the eye to complications of uveitis. A more recent study with larger numbers of dogs concluded, however, that prophylactic removal of the ruptured lens was unnecessary in the vast majority of cases. That later study, however, specifically excluded globes with massive lenticular trauma and was unable to measure the actual size of the capsular tears or the amount of lens protein lost.

Two interesting variations on what is basically a canine scheme are seen in rabbits and cats. *Rabbits* suffer what appears to be spontaneous lens capsule rupture of a previously normal lens. The response is well-contained perilenticular granulomatous inflammation very similar to human phacoanaphylactic uveitis. The rupture is associated with the intralenticular presence of *Encephalitozoon*, and it is assumed that the organisms penetrate and thus weaken the posterior lens capsule. *Cats* occasionally develop lesions similar to those in dogs, but also develop a unique feline primary intraocular pleomorphic sarcoma that may arise from metaplastic lens epithelium or from other transformed epithelial elements in the reparative reaction (see Feline post-traumatic sarcoma). There are 2 reports of similar sarcomas following lens rupture in rabbits.

Further reading

Bell CM, et al. Septic implantation syndrome in dogs and cats: a distinct pattern of endophthalmitis with lenticular abscess. Vet Ophthalmol 2013;16:180-185.

Collinson PN, Peiffer RL Jr. Pathology of canine cataract surgery complications. N Z Vet J 2002;50:26-31.

Paulsen ME, Kass PH. Traumatic corneal laceration with associated lens capsule disruption: a retrospective study of 77 clinical cases from 1999 to 2009. Vet Ophthalmol 2012;15:355-368.

Thach AB, et al. Phacoanaphylactic endophthalmitis: a clinicopathologic review. Int Ophthalmol 1991;15:271-279.

Zeiss CJ, et al. Feline intraocular tumors may arise from transformation of lens epithelium. Vet Pathol 2003;40:355-362.

Glaucoma

Glaucoma is a pathophysiologic state characterized by an increase in intraocular pressure sufficient to cause functionally significant injury to the optic nerve and retina. Although such increases of pressure may theoretically result from increased production or decreased removal of aqueous, only the latter is known to occur. Glaucoma is not a single disease entity, and the increase in intraocular pressure may result from many different mechanisms and combinations of mechanisms. The lesions in glaucomatous eyes include those related to the pathogenesis of the glaucoma and those resulting from the glaucoma itself. Because most globes submitted for histologic assessment have chronic glaucoma, the lesions that occur secondary to the glaucoma often predominate and serve to obscure the primary lesions.

Glaucoma occurs most commonly in dogs, less commonly in cats and horses, and is rarely documented in other species. The long-term medical and surgical control of glaucoma remains problematic despite extensive treatment with many different therapeutic modalities. Because most affected eyes eventually require enucleation or evisceration, *glaucoma is one of the most frequent ocular conditions submitted for histologic evaluation.*

The most logical way to deal with this complicated disease syndrome is to present the lesions in exactly the same way as

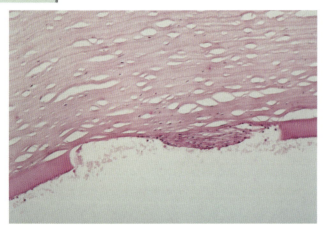

Figure 5-54 Recent corneal stria with no evidence of endothelial migration or reconstitution of Descemet's membrane.

one would encounter them when examining a histologic section: to look first at the various lesions that confirm the presence of glaucoma, and only then specifically direct your attention at those changes that might explain the pathogenesis for that particular example of glaucoma.

The histologic lesions of glaucoma

Lesions that develop as a result of glaucoma vary with the duration and severity of the glaucoma and the distensibility of the globe, and affect virtually all parts of the globe. *Enlargement of the globe* (**buphthalmos** or **megaloglobus**) occurs most readily in young animals or in those species with thin scleras, such as cats and laboratory animals. In the cornea, increased aqueous pressure injures the corneal endothelium, resulting in *diffuse edema and eventual fibrosis and vascularization*. If buphthalmos occurs, corneal stretching results in rents in Descemet's membrane, visible clinically as **corneal striae** (Fig. 5-54). These are relatively most frequent in horses and least prevalent in cats with glaucoma. Failure of lids to cover the enlarged globe permits *corneal desiccation and eventual ulceration* with all its sequels. If the ocular enlargement has developed only slowly, the cornea may have time to undergo adaptive keratinization and even cutaneous metaplasia. *Cataract is usual*, presumably the result of stagnation of aqueous humor and subsequent lens malnutrition. Iris and ciliary body undergo bland atrophy, most obvious as thinning and flattening of ciliary processes. Collapse of the ciliary cleft and trabecular meshwork itself is frequent and makes evaluation of these structures for possible goniodysgenesis very difficult. *Migration of corneal endothelium across the face of the pectinate ligament and onto the surface of the iris is commonly seen*, but we do not know whether it is part of the pathogenesis of glaucoma, or just a result of that glaucoma.

The retinal lesions are characteristic. Atrophy begins in nerve fiber and ganglion cell layers (Fig. 5-55A), making glaucoma the only naturally occurring cause of inner retinal atrophy other than the rare instances of traumatic or neoplastic disruption of optic nerve. *Loss of nerve fibers unmasks the normally inconspicuous Muller fibers*, a lesion that may be more easily seen and more confidently interpreted than the loss of the nerve fibers or ganglion cells per se (Fig. 5-55B). This is particularly true in cats, in which the ganglion cells persist with considerable tenacity under circumstances that would, in dogs, have progressed to a very obvious atrophy. With increasing duration or severity, the inner nuclear layer and its axons and dendrites also atrophy, resulting in thinning of the inner nuclear layer and the blending of this layer with the outer nuclear layer as the plexiform layers (the axons and dendrites of the nuclear layer cells) rarify.

In dogs with high-pressure glaucoma, there is sometimes *full-thickness retinal atrophy* that even includes damage to the retinal pigment epithelium (Fig. 5-55C). Although the cause is unknown, it may be that the very high pressure causes collapse of the choriocapillaris, resulting in ischemic damage to those tissues supplied by this delicate but essential capillary layer. This appears to be a uniquely canine susceptibility, in that the glaucomatous retina of other species rarely if ever shows full-thickness atrophy.

In all species, the dorsal half of the retina is less severely affected than ventral retina. The basis for this sparing remains speculative, but it may be related to the anatomy of the lamina cribrosa and the ease with which increased intraocular pressure compresses axons as they exit through that scleral sieve.

The pathogenesis of the selective ganglion cell loss in glaucoma remains controversial, and there is probably more than one mechanism. The loss may be the result of in situ apoptosis triggered by exposure to elevated retinal and vitreal levels of excitatory amino acids (especially glutamate), a response to pressure-associated ischemic injury, or a result of loss of axoplasmic flow secondary to pressure-induced injury to the optic nerve as it traverses the lamina cribrosa. It is clear that the ganglion cell injury is not directly correlated with the magnitude of the increase in intraocular pressure.

Excavation ("cupping") of the optic disc *is a pathognomonic lesion when present*, but its absence does not rule out the diagnosis. It occurs by at least 3 mechanisms, any (or all) of which may explain the cupping in an individual eye. Particularly in animals with a thin sclera and lamina cribrosa, the elevation of pressure may cause rapid posterior bowing of the lamina, resulting in visible cupping without apparent nerve atrophy. This is frequently seen in cats and rabbits, but not in ungulates with their thick, rigid lamina. In all species, cupping also occurs by axonal loss from the optic nerve. The pathogenesis for that axonal degeneration is either direct compression of axons or ischemic injury. It has been suggested that the posterior bowing of the lamina cribrosa contributes to the axonal injury by mechanical pinching of axons or blood vessels as they pass through the distorted lamina (Fig. 5-56). This cupping is distinguished from coloboma by the absence of dysplastic neuroectoderm lining the defect and by the presence of inner retinal atrophy. The cup sometimes is filled with fibrillar, PAS-positive material thought to represent degenerate vitreous.

The lesion predisposing to glaucoma may be the result of *antecedent ocular disease*, particularly intraocular neoplasia and anterior uveal inflammation with posterior or anterior synechiae. Such cases are termed **secondary glaucoma. Primary glaucoma** describes those cases without evidence of prior ocular disease and, in practical terms, is *synonymous with malformation of the filtration angle*. Primary glaucoma is seen almost exclusively in dogs, and vies with neoplasia as the most frequent cause of glaucoma in dogs.

Because the pathogenesis of glaucoma so frequently involves developmental or acquired distortion of the filtration angle, a description of that structure is appropriate here.

The **filtration apparatus** is a series of mesenchymal sieves that occupies the iridocorneal angle, and extends

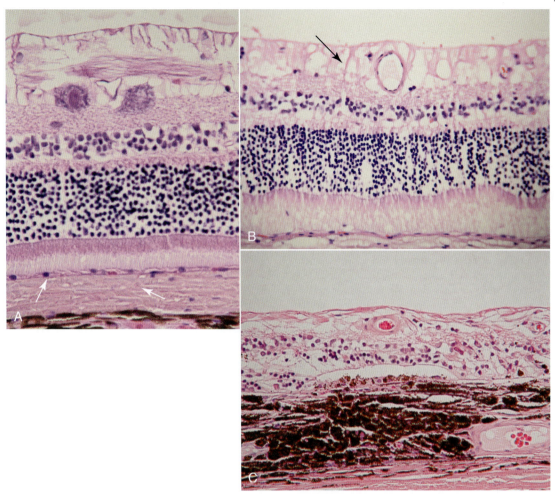

Figure 5-55 Retinal changes in glaucoma. A. Normal canine retina with retinal pigment epithelium (RPE) (left arrow) and tapetum (right arrow). B. Traditional glaucomatous atrophy with disappearance of the nerve fiber layer to expose the normally inconspicuous Muller fibers (arrow), disappearance of ganglion cells, but sparing of the inner and outer nuclear layers and photoreceptors. C. Full-thickness retinal atrophy in a dog with high-pressure glaucoma. The neurons of the inner and outer nuclear layers have almost completely disappeared. There are no photoreceptors, and the retina adheres directly to the choroid in areas where the RPE has been destroyed. Only where the RPE persists does the retina undergo the usual artifactual detachment.

circumferentially around the globe. These sieves appear to form by rarefaction of the same mesenchyme that forms iris stroma, and its rarefaction continues (at least in carnivores) for several weeks after birth. This area of perforated mesenchyme is the **ciliary cleft,** bordered externally by sclera, posteriorly by the muscles of the ciliary body, and internally by the iris stroma and anterior chamber. Its anterior border, at least in dogs, extends for about a millimeter into the deep peripheral corneal stroma just external to Descemet's membrane. Its border with the anterior chamber is marked by the **pectinate ligament,** which is visible clinically as a series of cobweb-like branching cords (carnivores) or a fenestrated sheet (ungulates) stretching from the termination of Descemet's membrane to the anterior portion of the iris root. They consist of collagenous cords covered by a very thin endothelium, with a thin intervening layer of basement membrane–like material. The endothelium is continuous with the corneal endothelium, and the collagenous core is continuous with corneal stroma.

Aqueous humor percolating through the pectinate ligament into the ciliary cleft must then pass through mesenchymal sieves consisting of collagenous cords covered by phagocytic and pinocytotic endothelium, called the **trabecular meshwork.** The large, open network of cords occupying most of the ciliary cleft is the uveal trabecular meshwork; anterior and external to it is a more compressed network called the corneoscleral trabecular meshwork. Ordinarily, aqueous humor produced by the ciliary processes passes through the pupil, through the pectinate ligament, and then through the uveal and corneoscleral trabecular meshworks en route to the *scleral venous plexus* that will return the aqueous to the systemic circulation (Fig. 5-57). Improper development or acquired obstruction of any part of this drainage pathway may result in glaucoma, but one must remember that *the ciliary cleft extends 360 degrees around the iridocorneal angle. Blockage of most of it is required for the development of glaucoma,* and this assessment is virtually impossible with 2-dimensional histologic examination. It is quite common to encounter dog eyes

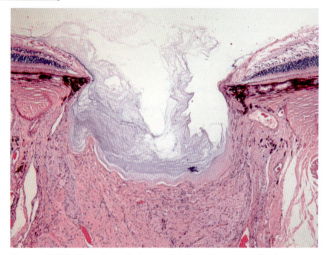

Figure 5-56 Cupping of the optic disc. Posterior displacement of the lamina cribrosa and destruction of the axons populating the optic disc create deep cupping in a dog with chronic glaucoma. The excavation now contains degenerate vitreous, and the surviving optic nerve has profound gliosis.

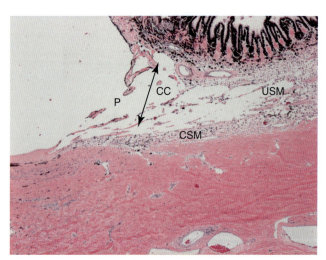

Figure 5-57 Normal feline filtration angle. CC, ciliary cleft; CSM, corneoscleral trabecular meshwork; P, pectinate ligament; USM, anterior border of uveoscleral trabecular meshwork.

with maldeveloped filtration angles in both the dorsal and ventral portions contained in a routine sagittal histologic section, yet with no evidence of glaucoma. Examination of the circumference of the angle with a dissecting microscope or scanning electron microscope in such cases often reveals the maldevelopment to be segmental and thus not a cause for glaucoma.

Differences exist among species in the finer details of angle structure and in the degree to which alternative routes of aqueous outflow are used. The horse, for example, has very thick pectinate fibers, and an inconspicuous corneoscleral trabecular meshwork and scleral venous plexus. As implied by these histologic features, *the horse uses alternative routes of aqueous outflow* (into iris stroma and especially posteriorly through ciliary muscle and into choroid) that are much more important than similar routes in dogs or cats. In contrast, the *cat* has extremely delicate pectinate fibers, a very large, open ciliary cleft, a conspicuous scleral venous plexus, and minimal (~3% of aqueous outflow) reliance on alternative outflow pathways. In dogs, alternative drainage routes account for 15-25% of all outflow. The existence of these alternative routes may explain the absence of glaucoma in some eyes (especially in horses) in which the angle changes would ordinarily have resulted in glaucoma, and may even explain the presence of glaucoma in eyes with apparently normal angles but lesions affecting portions of these other potential drainage routes.

Key Points

The terminology used to describe the filtration apparatus is potentially confusing:

The **filtration angle** is simply the geometric angle created by the junction of the iris with the peripheral cornea and sclera.

The **ciliary cleft** is the triangular space bordered internally by the base of the iris, externally by the peripheral sclera, posteriorly by the ciliary body, and anteriorly by the anterior chamber that is created by rarefaction of the neural crest mesenchyme that previously created the iris and ciliary body.

The **trabecular meshwork** is the actual tissue that occupies the ciliary cleft as a result of that late developmental rarefaction. It is a meshwork of permeable channels lined by trabecular epithelial cells and collagen that carry aqueous humor either outwardly into the scleral venous plexus or posteriorly into draining choroidal veins. This is the only one of these 3 often-confused terms that actually refers to **tissue**.

Lesions causing glaucoma

Primary glaucoma is most frequently encountered in dogs. Although, theoretically, primary glaucoma may have no visible angle lesion (which is frequently the case in humans), *in dogs there is almost always a readily detected maldevelopment*. The one exception is primary open-angle glaucoma in Beagle dogs, in which there is no visible antecedent lesion. The broad term **goniodysgenesis** encompasses all developmental defects of the filtration angle, of which 2 types account for most canine cases. *The most prevalent is continuation of mature iris stroma across the most anterior face of the trabecular meshwork to insert into the termination of Descemet's membrane.* Some consider this an example of **dysplasia of the pectinate ligament,** alternatively known as **imperforate pectinate ligament.** The band is much thicker than pectinate ligament and lacks the appropriate perforation to allow the drainage of aqueous humor. The trabecular meshwork posterior/exterior to this broad mesenchymal band often seems normal, although that is quite variable (Fig. 5-58A). It is seen as a *breed-related and thus presumably inherited defect* in Bouvier des Flandres, Basset Hounds, American Cocker Spaniels, Dandie Dinmont Terriers, Siberian Huskies, Samoyeds, Chows, and numerous other breeds. The defect, and the resultant glaucoma, is occasionally seen in mixed-breed dogs. The pectinate dysplasia is usually bilateral but not necessarily of equal extent, perhaps explaining why the glaucoma is often present initially only in one eye. The prevalence of pectinate dysplasia is much higher than the prevalence of glaucoma, and even in dogs with very extensive dysplasia that should seemingly eliminate almost all aqueous drainage, the onset of glaucoma is not until several years of age. It is not unusual to have cases in which clinically detected glaucoma was delayed until 8-10 years of age. Age-related changes in outflow resistance within the alternative routes of aqueous outflow have been postulated as the explanation, as

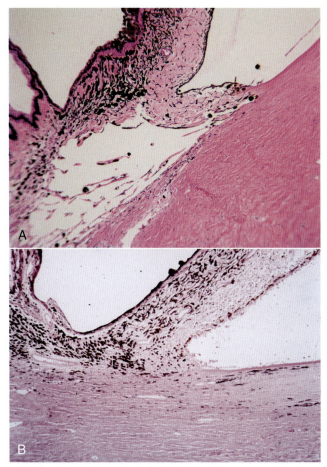

Figure 5-58 **Goniodysgenesis predisposing to primary glaucoma. A. Trabecular dysplasia** represents premature cessation of mesenchymal remodeling, resulting in a persisting spur of iris stroma in place of what should be the pectinate ligament. **B. Trabecular hypoplasia** represents an earlier cessation of mesenchymal remodeling, resulting in virtually no development of the trabecular meshwork. Some cases have concurrent iris hypoplasia or other manifestations of anterior segment dysgenesis, but not here.

have changes to the angle configuration related to age-related forward movement of the lens. These remain as theories.

Importantly, there appears to be little direct correlation between the severity of the goniodysgenesis and the actual risk of developing glaucoma, its age of onset, or its severity. The extent to which this is true seems to vary by breed, and perhaps the best generalization is that dogs with structurally (i.e., as evaluated by gonioscopy) normal filtration angles have no increased risk of glaucoma, although those that have at least some developmental abnormality are at increased risk. *Continuing to breed dogs with abnormal angles increases the prevalence of glaucoma within that line.* It may be that the goniodysgenesis that is visible clinically and histologically is not the direct cause for the glaucoma, but a marker for some other defect in trabecular development that is the real cause of the glaucoma. Alternatively, the goniodysgenesis may simply act to greatly diminish the reserve capacity in aqueous outflow so that these individuals become susceptible to developing secondary glaucoma under circumstances that would not cause glaucoma in a dog with a truly normal aqueous outflow pathway. Anecdotally, many of these dogs seem to develop glaucoma subsequent to episodes of mild uveitis or ocular trauma that might cause some additional degree of aqueous outflow obstruction simply by accumulation of red cells, fibrin, or leukocytes.

The second major type of goniodysgenesis is seen as a more fundamental arrest in the maturation of the trabecular meshwork such that the ciliary cleft is filled with tissue resembling primitive anterior uveal mesenchyme (Fig. 5-58B). This may occur in conjunction with iris hypoplasia or anterior chamber cleavage syndromes (therefore with concurrent lesions, such as congenital cataract or microphakia, persistent pupillary membranes, or other perilenticular vascular maldevelopment), but it may exist as an isolated defect termed **trabecular hypoplasia**. It has no known familial predilections. Such animals usually have truly congenital glaucoma, in contrast to the adult onset that characterizes the more common breed-associated glaucomas. It is important to note that the remodeling of the trabecular meshwork in dogs and cats continues for several weeks after birth so that one should avoid overinterpreting apparent angle solidification in very young carnivores.

> **Key Points**
>
> The most common causes of secondary glaucoma in **dogs** are pre-iridal fibrovascular membrane, anterior lens luxation, and direct obliteration of the trabecular meshwork by anterior uveal melanocytoma. In **cats**, the most common causes are diffuse iris melanoma and idiopathic lymphonodular uveitis.

Secondary glaucoma in dogs *occurs most commonly as the result of the development of a pre-iridal fibrovascular membrane.* Such membranes reflect nothing more than the development of granulation tissue along the anterior border layer of the iris in response to increased levels of fibroblastic and angiogenic growth factors within the aqueous humor. Because the anterior border of the iris has no tight junctions, such growth factors are readily absorbed into the iris, where they stimulate microvascular and fibroblastic proliferation and migration from within the iris stroma. Ordinarily, a thin membrane of granulation tissue would have little functional consequence, but within the unforgiving environment of the globe this membrane can be devastating. Most commonly, it migrates across the face of the pectinate ligament to create the equivalent of a peripheral anterior synechia and thus secondary glaucoma (Fig. 5-59). Alternatively, it may extend from the pupillary margin of the iris to the lens capsule, creating either posterior synechia or outright pupillary block; the pupillary margin of the iris normally floats along the surface

> **Key Points**
>
> Although most pre-iridal membranes are fibrovascular membranes triggered by increased circulating vascular endothelial growth factor, we occasionally encounter "other" pre-iridal membranes created by corneal endothelial overgrowth, by migrating lens epithelium following lens rupture, by fibrous metaplasia of injured iridociliary epithelium, or by metastatic stromal sarcoma. Essential for a diagnosis of pre-iridal fibrovascular membrane is the observation of vascular budding and endothelial migration from within the iris stroma.

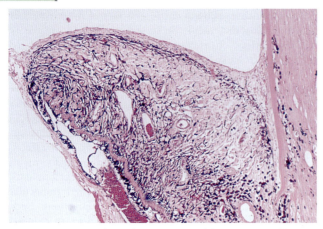

Figure 5-59 Secondary glaucoma caused by **pre-iridal fibrovascular membrane** covering the face of the pectinate ligament, creating the equivalent of peripheral anterior synechia.

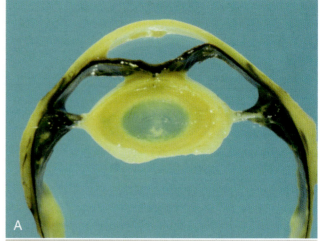

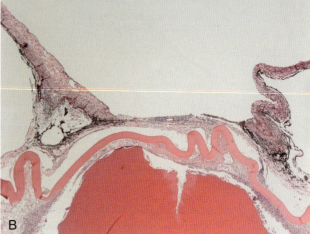

Figure 5-60 Secondary glaucoma. **A.** Posterior synechia followed by iris bombé, indicating complete pupillary block. Bouin's fixative. **B.** Wrinkled lens capsule indicating hypermature cataract or adjacent lens capsular rupture, along with posterior synechia and pupillary block.

of the lens, so iridolenticular adhesion from pre-iridal fibrovascular membrane or even just fibrin alone is always a risk. The most common stimuli for the development of pre-iridal fibrovascular membranes are retinal detachment, intraocular neoplasia (particularly iridociliary tumors), corneal angiogenesis, and chronic uveitis. All result in increased circulating levels of vascular endothelial growth factor within the aqueous humor.

Less prevalent than pupillary block caused by pre-iridal fibrovascular membrane (at least in histologic specimens) is posterior synechia caused by fibrinous effusion from the iris in the course of any anterior uveitis. With pupillary block of any cause, the continued production of aqueous humor in the presence of pupillary obstruction results in characteristic forward bowing of the iris known as *iris bombé* (Fig. 5-60A). Subsequent to the development of *iris bombé*, the glaucoma is therefore caused not only by the initial pupillary obstruction but also by peripheral anterior synechia as the forward bulging of the iris effectively seals the iridocorneal angle. Anterior synechia occurring independently of iris bombé is an occasional cause of secondary glaucoma. Because the iris does not normally contact the cornea, anterior synechia unrelated to iris bombé is frequent only as a consequence of corneal perforation, in which case the iris flows forward as an iris prolapse to seal the defect and may then adhere diffusely to the corneal endothelium (Fig. 5-60B).

Other frequent causes of secondary glaucoma in dogs include occlusion of the trabecular meshwork by anterior uveal melanocytoma, or pupillary obstruction by vitreal prolapse that occurs subsequent to anterior lens luxation of any cause. Rarely, lens swelling with cataract (intumescent cataract) seems to occlude the pupil. Posterior migration by corneal endothelium to cover the anterior face of the pectinate ligament and iris is seen quite frequently and may represent an important mechanism for the development of secondary glaucoma, even though the cause for the endothelial migration is usually not obvious. It may be particularly important as a trigger for the still unexplained delayed onset of glaucoma in adult dogs with lifelong goniodysgenesis. The causes of secondary glaucoma in **cats** are very different from what we see in dogs. Greater than 80% of glaucoma in cats can be attributed to 1 of 2 diseases: diffuse iris melanoma and chronic idiopathic lymphonodular uveitis. The former causes glaucoma by direct obstruction of the trabecular meshwork. The mechanism by which idiopathic lymphonodular uveitis triggers glaucoma remains a mystery. It is not by traditional mechanisms such as posterior synechia, which is remarkably rare in cats.

In **horses**, the presence of pre-iridal fibrovascular membranes across the pectinate face is the most frequent cause, although the stimulus for the membrane development is unknown in most reported cases. Many horses with glaucoma have a clinical history of previous uveitis, but histologic assessment of the glaucomatous globe usually reveals very little evidence of that inflammation and no obvious connection between the inflammation and the development of glaucoma. In those horses with glaucoma in which the membrane had not apparently crossed the pectinate ligament, glaucoma may have been caused by obstruction of alternative uveal routes of aqueous outflow, which are more important in horses than in dogs or cats.

Further reading

Bauer BS, et al. Immunohistochemical evaluation of fibrovascular and cellular pre-iridal membranes in dogs. Vet Ophthalmol 2012; 15(Suppl. 1):54-59.

Binder DR, et al. Expression of vascular endothelial growth factor receptor-1 and -2 in normal and diseased canine eyes. Vet Ophthalmol 2012;15:223-230.

Curto EM, et al. Equine glaucoma: a histopathologic retrospective study (1999-2012). Vet Ophthalmol 2014;17:334-342.

Esson D, et al. The histopathological and immunohistochemical characteristics of pigmentary and cystic glaucoma in the golden retriever. Vet Ophthalmol 2009;12:361-368.

Jacobi S, Dubielzig RR. Feline primary open angle glaucoma. Vet Ophthalmol 2008;11:162-165.

Kallberg ME, et al. Endothelin-1, nitric oxide, and glutamate in the normal and glaucomatous dog eye. Vet Ophthalmol 2007;10(Suppl. 1):46-52.

McLellan GJ, Miller PE. Feline glaucoma—a comprehensive review. Vet Ophthalmol 2011;14(Suppl. 1):15-29.

Papaioannou NG, Dubielzig RR. Histopathological and immunohistochemical features of vitreoretinopathy in Shih Tzu dogs. J Comp Pathol 2013;148:230-235.

Pearl R, et al. Progression of pectinate ligament dysplasia over time in two populations of Flat-Coated Retrievers. Vet Ophthalmol 2015;18:6-12.

Reilly CM, et al. Canine goniodysgenesis-related glaucoma: a morphologic review of 100 cases looking at inflammation and pigment dispersion. Vet Ophthalmol 2005;8:253-258.

Sandberg CA, et al. Aqueous humor vascular endothelial growth factor in dogs: association with intraocular disease and the development of pre-iridal fibrovascular membrane. Vet Ophthalmol 2012;15(Suppl. 1):21-30.

Scott EM, et al. Major breed distribution of canine patients enucleated or eviscerated due to glaucoma following routine cataract surgery as well as common histopathologic findings within enucleated globes. Vet Ophthalmol 2013;16(Suppl. 1):64-72.

Scott EM, et al. Early histopathologic changes in the retina and optic nerve in canine primary angle-closure glaucoma. Vet Ophthalmol 2013;16(Suppl. 1):79-86.

Strom AR, et al. Epidemiology of canine glaucoma presented to the University of Zürich from 1995 to 2009. Part two: secondary glaucoma (217 cases). Vet Ophthalmol 2011;14:121-126.

Wood JL, et al. Relationship of the degree of goniodysgenesis and other ocular measurements to glaucoma in Great Danes. Am J Vet Res 2001;62:1493-1499.

RETINA

When involution of the primary optic vesicle brings into apposition the anterior and posterior poles, the anterior (innermost) neuroectodermal layer undergoes mitotic replication and subsequent specialization to form the *9 layers of the neurosensory retina*. The outermost neuroectoderm remains as a relatively unspecialized simple cuboidal layer, the *retinal pigment epithelium (RPE)*. Although it is traditionally considered the tenth retinal layer, its structure, function, and reaction to injury are unlike those of neurosensory retina, and it is best discussed separately. *In this discussion, retina refers only to the neurosensory retina.*

In the fixed, bisected globe, the retina is seen as a thin, opaque membrane lining the posterior half of the globe between vitreous and choroid. It joins the darkly pigmented pars plana of the ciliary body at an abrupt transitional point called the *ora ciliaris retinae*. In all but the best-preserved specimens, the retina is separated artifactually from the RPE and adjacent choroid, remaining adherent only at the ora ciliaris and at the optic disc.

Histologically, the neurosensory retina begins abruptly at the ora ciliaris as a multilayered continuation of the inner layer of the ciliary epithelium. In dogs and sometimes in horses, the layers here are poorly defined and photoreceptors sparse. The peripheral retina is only about half the thickness (100 μm) and has half the photoreceptor density (250,000/mm^2) of the central retina, with fewer nuclear and plexiform elements and a thin innermost nerve fiber layer.

The retina consists of 3 structural components: neurons, glia, and vasculature. The neurons are the functional elements and transmit the photoactivated electrical impulse from photoreceptor process to occipital cortex. *The photoreceptor is the raison d'être of the entire globe.* It is a sensory, apical cytoplasmic process of the neurons forming the outer nuclear layer. These processes, called **rods or cones** based upon their shape and ultrastructural composition, extend from the outer nuclear layer toward the choroid. They are enveloped by a glycosaminoglycan interphotoreceptor matrix, and interdigitate with apical processes of the RPE, but no actual adhesions exist between the 2 layers. Within the outer segment of the photoreceptors are stacks of collapsed, disc-like spheres that contain the photoactive chemicals. The discs within rod outer segments are constantly produced basally and shed apically at the rate of 80-100 discs per day, with an outer segment turnover time of 6 days in dogs. Effete disc debris is engulfed and degraded by the RPE. Such turnover has not been demonstrated in the outer segment of cones, which have stacks of lamellae formed by infoldings of the plasma membrane. In addition, cones appear to be of many different types within a single retina. It is probably the ratio of different cones sensitive to different wavelengths of light that permits the visual cortex to discriminate color. *In general, fish, amphibia, reptiles, and birds have excellent color discrimination. Ungulates can distinguish yellows, blues, and, variably, green and red. Carnivores have very limited color perception, as far as can be determined.*

Other retinal layers are best described in terms of function (Fig. 5-61). The photoelectric stimulus originating in the photoreceptor outer segment is transmitted through the outer

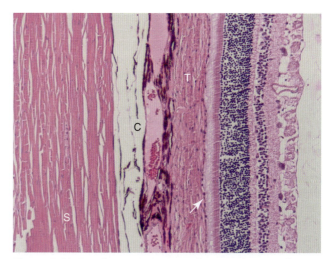

Figure 5-61 Histologic counterpart of a normal canine fundus. From inside out: normal retina, retinal pigment epithelium (arrow), tapetum (T), choroid (C), and sclera (S).

nuclear layer and along the axons of the photoreceptor nuclei to the bipolar and horizontal neurons of the *inner nuclear layer. The* accumulation of outer nuclear layer axons and inner nuclear layer dendrites forms the *outer synaptic or plexiform layer.* The inner nuclear layer contains the nuclei of the bipolar, horizontal, amacrine, and glial (Muller) cells. The bipolar cells receive impulses from the photoreceptors and relay them to ganglion cells. The bipolar cells also stimulate the horizontal cells, which transmit the impulse horizontally to excite adjacent bipolar cells. Amacrine cells counterbalance the bipolar cells in that their stimulation releases an inhibitor of ganglion cell excitation. The glial cells are primarily structural support cells, whose processes traverse the retina to form the retinal scaffold, and their anterior and posterior terminations fuse to form the inner and outer limiting membranes. The axons of the bipolar and amacrine cells, dendrites of ganglion and horizontal cells, and glial processes form the thick *inner synaptic or plexiform layer.* The *ganglion cell layer* is the thinnest and innermost of the neuronal layers. Large, granular neurons form a single and often sparse layer, supplemented by a few astrocytes, which become bilayered in the area centralis to accommodate the marked increase in photoreceptor density. The *density of ganglion cells predicts, in a general way, visual acuity.* They are most closely packed in animals requiring fine visual discrimination (most birds, predatory fish, many reptiles). In contrast, they are sparse in ungulates who do not feed by sight but who flee at anything that moves. Their axons form the *nerve fiber layer* that gradually increases in thickness toward the optic disc. In most animals, the fibers are not myelinated until they reach the optic disc. The nerve fiber layer is separated from the vitreous by an *internal limiting membrane* formed by the terminations of the Muller fibers and a true basal lamina.

The organization of the **retinal vasculature** is an important variable in ophthalmoscopic examination, both because vascular abnormalities are frequent signposts of disease and because normal species variation can erroneously be diagnosed as disease. Carnivores, ruminants, and swine have large venules and smaller arterioles radiating from the optic disc to the peripheral retina. The horse has ~60 thin, short vessels extending from the disc for ~5 mm into surrounding retina. In dogs and cats, the major vessels lie within the deep half of the nerve fiber layer and the ganglion cell layer. In ruminants and pigs, the vessels are very superficial and bulge into the vitreous, covered only by a thin layer of nerve fibers and basal lamina. The retinal vessels form an end-artery circulation that supplies the inner layers of the retina. The photoreceptors and outer nuclear layers are avascular and receive nutrients primarily by diffusion from choroid. Such dependence cannot be absolute (except in horses) because degeneration of these outer layers is surprisingly slow (weeks to months) following retinal separation. In contrast, occlusion of a retinal vessel results in focal infarction of the inner retina within <1 hour.

The blood vessels also participate in the *blood-eye barrier,* similar to that already described for the uvea. The tight endothelial junctions and junctions between adjacent retinal pigment epithelial cells conspire to create a retina that is immunologically isolated from non-ocular tissues in a manner similar to that described for the uvea. Like the uvea, such a barrier is likely not absolute, and the various retinal antigens are likely to be neither totally sequestered nor absolutely unique to the retina. Saline extracts of retina yield the retinal S antigen, and the interphotoreceptor retinoid-binding protein is another antigen that may be important in the initiation or perpetuation of degenerative (see Retinal degeneration) or inflammatory retinopathies.

The **retinal pigment epithelium** extends from the ora ciliaris to the optic disc as the posterior continuation of the outer layer of ciliary epithelium. It forms a simple cuboidal epithelial layer that is separated from the choroid by a complex basal lamina, *Bruch's membrane.* The apical border interdigitates with the photoreceptors, with an average of ~30 photoreceptors contacting a single pigment epithelial cell, but forms no junctional complexes. The inclusion of the adjective "pigmented" is something of a misnomer in domestic species except the pig, inasmuch as the epithelium overlying the tapetum contains no cytoplasmic pigment granules. This seemingly insignificant layer plays a major role in embryologic induction of the eye as previously described, and also plays a crucial role in the nurturing of the photoreceptors throughout life. The pigment epithelium engulfs and degrades obsolete rod and cone outer segments, absorbs light to protect photoreceptors, synthesizes and degrades part of the glycosaminoglycan matrix enveloping photoreceptor outer segments, and participates in the vitamin A–rhodopsin cycle. Which of these functions are most essential for photoreceptor health is still unclear.

The **ocular fundus** *is a clinical term describing those ophthalmoscopically visible portions of the posterior globe, excluding vitreous.* The fundus is commonly divided into dorsal tapetal and ventral nontapetal fundus, with the optic disc usually at the junction of the two. The retina, although almost transparent, does absorb some incident and reflected light to dull somewhat the fundus reflection ophthalmoscopically. Areas of retinal atrophy absorb less light and are seen as areas of increased tapetal reflectivity. Preretinal or subretinal exudates, conversely, increase light absorption and are seen as focal fundic opacities. Developmental or acquired absence of tapetum allows black choroidal pigment to be seen. More severe choroidal lesions may be seen as red choroidal vasculature or even pink sclera obscured by variable amounts of residual pigment. Particularly in dogs, cats, and horses, selective breeding has made hypoplastic variations in amount and pigmentation of choroid and tapetum normal for particular breed or color varieties.

The **general pathology of the retina** is often said to resemble that of the brain. Although this is undoubtedly true inasmuch as retina is merely an extension of the brain, the prevalence of such lesions as malacia, nonsuppurative perivascular cuffing, and proliferative microgliosis within the retina is very low compared to the brain. Although no actual data are published, *most animals with encephalitis do not, in fact, have concurrent retinitis. Retinal inflammation is most often the result of spread from choroid or across the vitreous from anterior uvea.* Degenerations are much more common than inflammations and are not usually accompanied by inflammatory reaction. The mature mammalian retina has no capacity for regeneration of entire neural cells, although photoreceptor outer segments and glia may be replaced if destroyed in the course of degenerative or inflammatory disease. Even the fetal retina has poor regenerative capacity, as evidenced by the prevalence of retinal dysplasia following prenatal or neonatal retinal injury. Retinal repair is by proliferation of inner layer astrocytes that eventually form a dense glial scar. Occasionally, the astrocytes proliferate along the vitreal face of the retina, forming a preretinal fibroglial membrane. Similar subretinal membranes are seen with chronic detachments and originate from RPE or Muller cells. The RPE retains mitotic ability. When injured, these cells respond with hypertrophy, hyperplasia, and fibrous metaplasia. The presence of pigment in the neuroretina is frequent in instances of retinal atrophy, most probably derived from migration of retinal pigment epithelial cells into the adjacent retina.

Autolytic changes are visible within retina within 30 minutes of death, and within a few hours are of sufficient magnitude to interfere with the diagnosis of retinal degenerations. The earliest histologic change is pyknosis of a few nuclei in outer and inner nuclear layers, and loss of uniform density of the photoreceptor layer. Progressive dissolution of the photoreceptor outer segments results in retinal separation. Nuclear layer pyknosis and ganglion cell chromatolysis are widespread within 4-6 hours. *By 12 hours, retinal separation is complete and the extensively folded retina, with autolytic photoreceptors, may mimic genuine retinal separation.* The extensive pyknosis within both nuclear layers distinguishes the two, being absent in antemortem separation (see later for other criteria). By 18 hours after death, the retina is represented by a barely separable bilayer of pyknotic nuclei suspended in a pale, eosinophilic foamy matrix representing fragmented nerve fiber and plexiform layers.

Overview of retinal histopathology

The large amount of information about the causation and clinical features of the various retinal diseases is intimidating and serves to obscure the *fundamental simplicity of retinal histopathology*. The vast majority of retinal lesions fall into 3 categories: *inflammatory disease* as part of endophthalmitis; *photoreceptor degeneration* from inherited metabolic disease, detachment, or toxicity; and *inner retinal atrophy* (particularly ganglion cells) as a result of glaucoma. The angst over retinal histopathology can be further reduced by recognizing that many diseases of different pathogenesis share the same histologic appearance. For example, there are dozens of inherited photoreceptor diseases of dogs, yet they all look histologically identical. Most are even ultrastructurally identical. Furthermore, photoreceptor degeneration resulting from inherited retinopathy looks histologically identical to atrophy resulting from excessive exposure to light, from chemical toxicity, and even from retinal separation.

> **Key Points**
>
> By far the most common clinically significant retinal lesions encountered in surgically enucleated *canine* globes are glaucomatous atrophy and photoreceptor degeneration secondary to retinal detachment.
>
> The most common retinal lesions in *feline* enucleated globes are glaucomatous atrophy and mild lymphocytic perivascular retinitis occurring in sympathy to idiopathic lymphonodular anterior uveitis.

Retinal separation

The retina is firmly attached in the globe only at the ora ciliaris and at the optic disc. *When the retina separates, it does so by cleaving photoreceptors from their interdigitations with the RPE.* Separation may occur as the result of accumulation of inflammatory exudates, transudates, tumor cells, or helminths

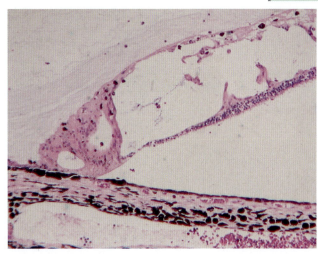

Figure 5-62 **Peripheral microcystoid retinal degeneration**, a normal aging change in dogs that represents the risk of creating peripheral retinal holes and predisposing to rhegmatogenous retinal detachment.

between RPE and photoreceptors, by contraction of a cyclitic membrane, or by the subretinal leakage of liquefied vitreous through retinal tears. Such tears may result from orbital trauma or from progression of peripheral cystic retinal degeneration. The latter is relatively common in man but not in domestic animals despite the frequent occurrence of microcystoid retinal degeneration in the peripheral retina of dogs (Fig. 5-62) and, less often, of horses.

The diagnosis of retinal separation in fixed specimens is complicated by the ease with which retinal separation can be induced by delayed fixation or improper handling of globes. The credibility of the diagnosis is greatly enhanced by the presence of subretinal exudates or cyclitic membranes, but in their absence, the diagnosis rests upon the observation of photoreceptor outer segment degeneration, hypertrophy and hyperplasia of pigmented epithelium, and the development of marked edema in inner nuclear, ganglion cell, and inner plexiform layers (Fig. 5-63A-C). Hypertrophy of the RPE is the most rapid change, occurring within a few hours of separation. The edematous changes are visible with the light microscope as early as 3 days following experimentally induced separation in owl monkeys. Coalescence of the edema creates a virtual cleavage of inner from outer retina, called retinoschisis. The cleavage is spanned by the radial Muller fibers, which seem the only anchors holding the retina together. Photoreceptor degeneration is slower to appear under the light microscope, with loss of outer segments (probably the most subtle change that can be unequivocally diagnosed with routine light microscopy) visible by ~14 days after experimental saline-induced "exudative" retinal detachment. It is probably much faster than that when the exudate is full of noxious byproducts of cell necrosis and inflammation, but no precise figure is available. Inner segments and the cell bodies of the outer nuclear layer are almost unaffected and may remain so for months, suggesting that their maintenance is not so intimately linked to the pigment epithelium as is the case with the outer segments. This temporal hierarchy of change permits reasonably accurate aging of retinal separations, sometimes a necessary or at least interesting assessment in eyes enucleated after numerous clinical examinations or manipulation. The outer retinal

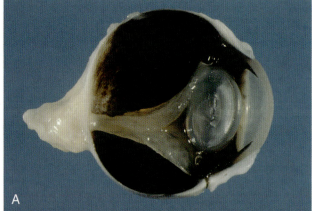
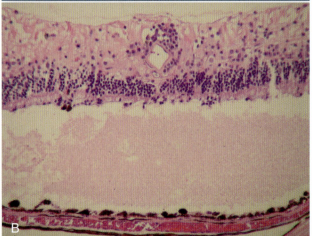
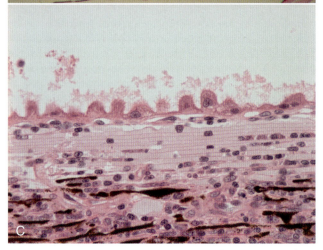

Figure 5-63 Retinal detachment. A. Complete "morning glory" retinal detachment. **B.** Lymphocytic retinitis causing serous retinal detachment with resulting hypertrophy of the retinal pigment epithelium (RPE) and ischemic atrophy of photoreceptors. **C.** Higher magnification of hypertrophy of the RPE secondary to a lymphocytic choroiditis causing exudative retinal detachment.

lesions are apparently not ischemic inasmuch as there is very little necrosis and no similarity to the lesion induced by retinal artery occlusion. Perhaps the outer layers can survive by diffusion of oxygen and nutrients from the subretinal fluid or from vascularized inner layers, and indeed, the speed of photoreceptor atrophy varies with the height of the separation. An exception is seen in horses, inasmuch as the horse retina

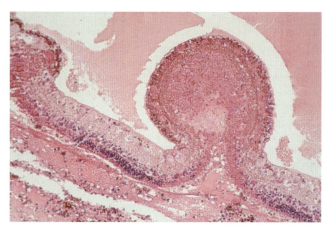

Figure 5-64 Focal traumatic retinal separation causing retinal infarction following head trauma in a horse.

depends almost entirely on choroidal diffusion for oxygenation. Separation in this species results in rapid, full-thickness retinal infarction (Fig. 5-64). A very frequent lesion in horses is focal, linear, or multifocal chorioretinal glial scarring with pigment migration and fibrous metaplasia of RPE, a lesion that is probably a healed infarct following traumatic separation or thromboembolic disease.

Further reading

Grahn BH, et al. Chronic retinal detachment and giant retinal tears in 34 dogs: outcome comparison of no treatment, topical medical therapy, and retinal reattachment after vitrectomy. Can Vet J 2007;48:1031-1039.

Komaromy AM, et al. Hypertensive retinopathy and choroidopathy in a cat. Vet Ophthalmol 2004;7:3-9.

Strobel BW, et al. Retinal detachment in horses: 40 cases (1998-2005). Vet Ophthalmol 2007;10:380-385.

Retinal degeneration

Retinal degenerations include a long list of important noninflammatory retinal diseases, but only a small portion of these are likely to be seen in routine diagnostic submissions. The largest group is bilateral inherited photoreceptor disease in dogs of many different breeds. Although clinically important, especially when screening for retinal disease in breeding programs, globes with inherited retinal degenerations and dystrophies are rarely sampled for routine histopathology. In turn, routine histopathology does not discriminate among the many different diseases included within this broad group. Such discrimination requires genomic evaluation, electron microscopy, or in vivo functional assessment. For this reason, this important group of clinical diseases is given only brief discussion here, and interested readers can consult the Further reading section for guidance to more exhaustive discussions elsewhere.

Additional common examples of retinal degeneration, listed more or less in order of prevalence within a diagnostic caseload, include glaucomatous retinal atrophy, photoreceptor atrophy secondary to retinal detachment, and hypertensive retinopathy. Uncommon examples of retinal degeneration include light-induced retinopathy, various toxic retinopathies, and a few examples of nutritional retinopathy.

Retinal degenerations, as encountered histologically, can be divided into those examples specifically targeting the photoreceptors (inherited retinal atrophies, retinal detachment, light-induced retinopathy, and most toxic and nutritional retinopathies) and those causing panretinal degeneration (glaucoma and vascular hypertension). Those examples caused by glaucoma or retinal detachment are usually unilateral; all the rest are bilateral.

Inherited photoreceptor dysplasias and degenerations in dogs

Formerly grouped under the broad but imprecise umbrella of progressive retinal atrophy (PRA), these diseases are now more correctly divided into photoreceptor dysplasias and degenerations that differ in terms of the usual age of onset (juvenile vs. adult), the exact cells that are targeted (rods only, cones only, or a combination), the mode of inheritance (most are autosomal recessive), the molecular pathogenesis, and (when known) the defective gene. In broad terms, the photoreceptor dysplasias are those diseases in which the degenerative changes are detectable prior to the cessation of postnatal photoreceptor maturation; photoreceptor degenerations are those diseases with later onset (and sometimes much later). Histologically, almost all are seen as bilateral progressive atrophy of the photoreceptors. A few are nonprogressive, and a few are purely biochemical diseases with no histologic counterpart. Most of the diseases initially target rods and are therefore seen initially as night blindness (sometimes as early as 2-3 months of age). The rate of progression to complete blindness is highly variable, depending on the exact disease syndrome. The degenerative changes progress from initial disappearance of photoreceptors to eventually involve thinning and then disappearance of the outer nuclear layer and eventually even the inner nuclear layer. There are a few examples that typically are nonprogressive, especially those with preferential cone dysplasia.

Biochemical changes detectable via electroretinography always precede histologic lesions, and many of these diseases can now be detected by genomic analysis that offers a huge advantage of pre-breeding identification of carrier animals in addition to those destined to be clinically affected. Constantly expanding lists of the affected breeds, the specific biochemical abnormalities underlying the photoreceptor dysplasia or degeneration, and the availability of various diagnostic tests can be found in any of the clinical ophthalmology textbooks listed in the Further reading section. The latest lists contain >100 breeds, and, quite clearly, a detailed description of the retinopathy for each of these breeds is beyond the scope of this text. These lists, like all published lists of genetic diseases, suffer from not necessarily reflecting what are sometimes dramatic geographic or temporal variations in overall prevalence within the breed, and in some cases, the presence of a breed on that list may reflect just a single kennel "outbreak" that has perhaps unfairly stigmatized the entire breed. Once a breed is placed on "the list," it seems there is no mechanism for it ever to be removed!

Other examples of inherited photoreceptor degenerations and dysplasias

Examples of inherited photoreceptor dysplasias and degenerations that do not follow the usual general description include cone dysplasia, canine multifocal retinopathy, and RPE dystrophy.

A specific **cone dysplasia** is seen in Alaskan Malamutes, Gordon Setters, and German Shorthaired Pointers. These dogs develop day blindness as early as 2-3 months of age, but that disease is nonprogressive, and rods do not become affected. The ocular fundus is normal on clinical inspection, but these dogs have profoundly abnormal electroretinograms. Because rod function remains normal, these dogs are not blind, and such globes are virtually never available for histologic assessment.

Canine multifocal retinopathy is an inherited disease originally described in Great Pyrenees, but subsequently has been seen in a number of other breeds. Puppies <6 months of age are presented with acute multifocal serous detachment that may occasionally involve detachment of RPE from the underlying choroid. These cystic detachments may slowly enlarge over the next few months, remain unchanged, or even regress. The pathogenesis is unknown, but the defective gene has been identified.

Retinal pigment epithelial dystrophy (formerly known as central PRA) is today a relatively rare disease that initially targets the RPE, but, of course, destruction of the RPE will inevitably result in secondary degeneration of the photoreceptors that depend on the RPE for their well-being. It is a poorly understood syndrome that probably reflects more than one disease, and it has wide geographic variation in terms of prevalence. At least historically, England was always the country with greatest prevalence, and the disease had by far the greatest relative prevalence in Briards. Its current prevalence is unknown, but thought to be much lower than when first reported 30 years ago. The failure by the defective RPE to engulf and enzymatically degrade effete photoreceptor material results in a gradual buildup of intracellular lipopigments throughout life. Associated with the pigmentary accumulation, the epithelial cells hypertrophy. Photoreceptor outer segments adjacent to hypertrophic pigment epithelium degenerate. As the lesion progresses, hypertrophy and hyperplasia of RPE give rise to dysplastic pigmented cell clumps. Within such clusters, there may be an eosinophilic, hyaline, PAS-positive concretion resembling drusen. This material, rather frequent in ophthalmic specimens from people with a variety of degenerative retinal or choroidal diseases, is a concretion of excess basal lamina produced by the RPE. The eventual histologic lesion in affected dogs is a *monolayer of hypertrophic, lipochrome-rich pigment epithelial cells with multifocal hyperplastic clumps*. Retina has atrophy of photoreceptors and outer nuclear layer, and some irregular gliosis. Pigment-laden cells may invade the retina.

The mode of transmission is autosomal recessive in those breeds for which it is known. An interesting speculation, based upon morphologic similarities, is that the disease represents a defect in vitamin E metabolism within pigment epithelium.

Inherited retinal degeneration and dysplasia in cats

Inherited retinal dysplasias and degenerations have been reported as sporadic occurrences in a variety of cat breeds, but only in the *Abyssinian breed* has the syndrome been adequately studied. In this breed, there are 2 different diseases: *early-onset rod-cone dysplasia*, and *late-onset retinal degeneration* affecting rods much sooner than cones. The early-onset dysplasia is inherited as an autosomal dominant trait. It is histologically and ultrastructurally similar to the disease in Irish Setter dogs, and a similar defect in the activity of cyclic guanosine monophosphate (cGMP) phosphodiesterase has been reported. Affected cats are blind by a few months of age.

The late-onset retinal degeneration is inherited as an autosomal recessive, and affected cats progress slowly to blindness by 5-10 years of age. The earliest structural changes are in rod outer segments in peripheral retina, with jumbling of the rod discs and patchy blunting of the photoreceptors themselves. Only after many years is there histologically detected diffuse photoreceptor loss.

Non-inherited retinal degenerations

Sudden acquired retinal degeneration is *an enigmatic, rapidly progressing photoreceptor degeneration that is histologically identical to the inherited progressive retinal atrophies. Blindness occurs very rapidly (over a period of a few days to a few weeks). Affected dogs are adult or even elderly, and the disease can affect any breed or crossbreed.* The fundoscopic lesion is bilaterally symmetrical and diffuse across the retina, but histologic studies of the early lesions are very few. The cause is unknown, but the presence of the retinal disease is linked to systemic signs of polyuria, polydipsia, and elevated serum cholesterol and alkaline phosphatase. Some, but not even the majority, of the affected dogs have adrenal cortical hyperfunction. How this malfunction causes the irreversible retinopathy, if indeed it does, is unknown. Results of studies to demonstrate circulating anti-retinal autoantibodies have been contradictory and inconclusive.

Further reading

Downs LM, et al. Genetic screening for PRA-associated mutations in multiple dog breeds shows that PRA is heterogeneous within and between breeds. Vet Ophthalmol 2014;17:126-130.

Narfstrom K, et al. Characterization of feline hereditary retinal dystrophies using clinical, functional, structural and molecular genetic studies. Vet Ophthalmol 2011;14(Suppl. 1):30-36.

Light-induced retinal degeneration

Light of various wavelengths has a variety of injurious effects on cornea, lens, or retina that vary with the wavelength, duration, and intensity of the light.

The effects also vary with a large but poorly understood group of animal variables that include ocular pigmentation, habitat, previous experience with photoperiod, nutrition, body temperature, age, and, most obviously, species. The wavelength of light has the greatest effect; short wavelengths in the *ultraviolet (UV) and blue range* (up to ~475 nm) have the greatest energy per photon and are the most damaging. Fortunately, most of these wavelengths are absorbed by cornea and lens, so that their lethal effects on retina are seldom seen. They may cause corneal epithelial injury or cataract, although these effects are apparently rare in domestic animals (see Cataract).

In people, accidental exposure to light from arc welding, solar eclipses, or ophthalmic examination or operating equipment (including lasers) creates the potential for rapid injury from mechanical disruption or heat. Although such damage is certainly possible in other animals, most naturally occurring lesions result from the additive effects of much less intense UV and short-wavelength visible light because of unnatural photoperiods. Animals with poorly pigmented eyes, and those adapted for nocturnal vision, are most susceptible. Susceptibility also increases with age and with temperature.

The initial lesion is disruption of rod outer segment discs, with eventual destruction of all photoreceptors and their nuclei. Because the lesion is identical to most inherited, nutritional, and toxic retinopathies, *the diagnosis is made on the circumstantial evidence of abnormally bright light, abnormally long-light photoperiod, or a rapid change in photoperiod.* Most instances occur with rodents or fish kept in continuous fluorescent light. Albino rodents or deepwater fish are, predictably, the most susceptible.

The mechanism by which visible light of moderate intensity damages the retina is still incompletely understood, and different experimental models give rise to different theories. Most studies use blue light in the 400-475 nm range, which, unlike shorter UV wavelengths, is not filtered out by the cornea or lens. The most popular theory is that of light-induced oxidation of the very abundant polyunsaturated long-chain fatty acids of the rod discs, with the generation of free radicals to then cause cell membrane damage. This theory gains support from studies showing a protective effect by vitamin C or E, and enhanced injury under conditions of retinal hyperoxia.

Nutritional retinopathy

Nutritional causes of retinal degeneration include deficiencies of *vitamins C, A, or E*, and the amino acid, *taurine*. Retinal atrophy and cataracts have been seen in fish with a dietary deficiency of vitamin C. The lesions were thought to be light induced, with the fish unusually susceptible because of the deficiency in the antioxidant effects of the vitamin. The ocular lesions of vitamin E deficiency resemble those of retinal pigment epithelial dystrophy and were referred to briefly under that heading. Pups fed severely deficient diets develop night blindness within ~6 weeks, and an extinguished electroretinogram suggestive of diffuse photoreceptor damage. These last 2 effects are not seen in naturally occurring central retinal atrophy. Retinopathy has been described in primates and dogs fed rations deliberately and severely deficient in vitamin E. *Lipofuscin,* seen as eosinophilic cytoplasmic inclusions, accumulated to excess in the pigment epithelium, and was followed by hypertrophy of the pigment epithelium and degeneration of photoreceptor outer segments. Eventually, there was full-thickness central retinal atrophy and some small foci of retinal separation. Retinal degeneration with ceroid-lipofuscin accumulation in the retinal pigment epithelium has also been noted in vitamin E–deficient horses, but did not appear to cause visual impairment.

Hypovitaminosis A

Retinopathy caused by hypovitaminosis A is seldom encountered except in growing cattle or swine kept in confinement and fed a ration deficient in the vitamin over months or years. Grains other than corn (maize) are very poor sources of vitamin A, and the level in corn falls markedly with prolonged storage. Green pasture is very rich in carotene, which is converted to vitamin A by intestinal epithelium. Hay that is excessively dry, leached by rain, cut late in the year, or stored for prolonged periods is a much less adequate source. In most pastured animals, the liver reserves are sufficient to prevent clinical signs of deficiency for at least 6 months and often up to 2 years. Young, rapidly growing animals have greater requirements and smaller stores of the vitamin and are thus more susceptible than adults.

Hypovitaminosis A affects bone remodeling and causes epithelial cell atrophy and defects in synthesis of rhodopsin. Ocular lesions can result from each of these 3 defects.

As previously discussed, *maternal deficiency of vitamin A causes blindness in offspring resulting from defective remodeling of optic nerve foraminae and subsequent ischemic or pressure atrophy of the nerve.* In piglets, there may be massive ocular dysplasia and such anomalies as cleft palate, skeletal deformities, hydrocephalus, epidermal cysts, genital hypoplasia, and anomalous hearts. Optic nerve atrophy is preceded by optic disc swelling (papilledema), and followed by atrophy of nerve fiber and ganglion cell layers. This sequence of events may occur if very young animals are on deficient diets, with the optic nerve changes being caused in part by stenosis of optic foramen and in part by increased cerebrospinal fluid pressure that itself results from atrophy and metaplasia of arachnoid villi. The papilledema precedes optic nerve necrosis and is reversible. The corneal lesions of hypovitaminosis A have received scant attention and are seldom seen in natural outbreaks.

The acquired ocular effect of hypovitaminosis A involves photoreceptor outer segments. The ophthalmoscopic lesion is multifocal retinal atrophy and scarring in animals with slow or absent pupillary light reflex and apparent blindness. The histologic lesion is patchy-to-diffuse photoreceptor atrophy that first affects the rod outer segments. Night blindness is thus the initial complaint and is often the chief complaint about a deficient herd. Eventually, the atrophy affects all photoreceptors and their nuclei, and may progress to full-thickness atrophy with scarring. The lesions have been produced in all domestic species on specially formulated diets, but naturally occurring retinal lesions are almost restricted to cattle with chronic deficiencies.

The pathogenesis of the photoreceptor atrophy demonstrates the structure-function interdependence of retinal cells. Vitamin A is converted to retinene and then to the glycoprotein rhodopsin. Rhodopsin is stored as a component of the lamellar discs of the outer segment. Light initiates a physicochemical change in rhodopsin, resulting in a cascade of events culminating in the hyperpolarization of the outer segment membrane. The resultant electrical impulse is transmitted to bipolar cells, ganglion cells, and then to brain. *Deficiency of vitamin A necessarily results in a deficiency of rhodopsin.* The corresponding ultrastructural lesion is swelling, then fragmentation of lamellar discs that can be reversed by therapy with vitamin A, unless inner segments have also been affected. Regeneration simulates normal development and requires ~2 weeks to rebuild outer segments completely. Vitamin A is discussed further in Vol. 1, Bones and joints.

Taurine-deficiency retinopathy

Retinal degeneration caused by taurine deficiency is seen only in cats, although taurine is the predominant free amino acid in the retina of other species. Among domestic mammals, only the cat seems unable to synthesize taurine from cysteine in amounts adequate for retinal function. Taurine is considered a dietary essential for cats, and its deficiency results in *characteristic central retinal atrophy* and in *myocardial failure* (see Vol. 3, Cardiovascular system). Changes in commercial diets, and better recognition of the risk of diseases related to taurine deficiency, have almost eliminated this disease.

The ocular lesion of taurine deficiency was first detected in cats fed semi-purified diets in which casein was the only protein. After several months, such cats developed focal retinal atrophy adjacent to the optic disc, which progressed to generalized retinal atrophy. Supplementation with taurine halted but did not reverse the lesion, presumably because photoreceptor nuclei or inner segments already had been damaged. The clinical and histologic features of this newly recognized nutritional retinopathy were virtually identical to those that had already been recognized in an idiopathic, naturally occurring disease of cats called *"feline central retinal degeneration."* It is assumed that the 2 diseases are actually the same, although that may not be true in every single instance. At least some of the cases of idiopathic central atrophy were associated with the feeding and of dry dog food, which (for a cat) is deficient in taurine.

The clinical lesion is a *focal lesion of tapetal hyper-reflectivity* that is bilateral, dorsolateral to the optic disc, and is usually unassociated with visual impairment. *The histologic lesion is photoreceptor degeneration,* initially targeting cone outer segments but eventually affecting rods as well. The rods of the peripheral retina are the last to degenerate. Taurine also seems essential for membrane integrity of the tapetal reflective rodlets, so that dissolution of the membrane surrounding these crystalline intracytoplasmic inclusions is another characteristic lesion. Less clear is the association of taurine deficiency with diffuse retinal atrophy in cats.

Familial atrophy occurs in Abyssinian and Persian cats, but most cases are of unknown cause. Continued deficiency of taurine leads to diffuse retinal atrophy and thus might be responsible.

Toxic retinopathies

Experimental toxic retinopathies have been caused by many chemicals and toxic plants, but only a few toxic plants cause important diseases of domestic animals.

Bracken fern *(Pteridium aquilinum)* causes progressive retinal degeneration in sheep in several areas of Great Britain. The common name "bright blindness" refers to pupillary dilation and tapetal hyper-reflectivity of the severely affected sheep. The disease has been seen only in flocks grazing hills rich in bracken fern, and has been reproduced by prolonged feeding of the fern to sheep. A similar syndrome has been noted in cattle during long-term exposure to the fern. The lesion is usually seen in middle-aged or older sheep as bilateral and initially central tapetal hyper-reflectivity. Diffuse involvement follows. *The histologic lesion is nonspecific, consisting of photoreceptor outer segment degeneration progressing to depletion of all retinal layers.*

Blindness is one of the features of intoxication with **locoweed** *(Astragalus* and *Oxytropis* spp.) in the United States; **darling pea** *(Swainsona* spp.) and **blind grass** *(Stypandra* spp.) in Australia; and **selenium indicator plants** worldwide.

Astragalus and *Swainsona* cause a *neurovisceral lysosomal storage disease* analogous to genetically transmitted mannosidosis (see Vol. 1, Nervous system). All members of the genus *Swainsona* contain an indolizidine alkaloid, swainsonine, which is a potent inhibitor of lysosomal mannosidase. At least some *Astragalus* spp. contain a similar alkaloid. Chronic ingestion of the plant occurs in cattle, sheep, and horses forced to eat the plants on dry pastures where nothing more palatable is available. Affected animals develop behavioral abnormalities and defects of gait and vision. The histologic lesion consists of widespread cytoplasmic vacuolation in most organs because of the intralysosomal accumulation of mannose-rich oligosaccharides. Onset of clinical signs may require several months of heavy *Swainsona* ingestion, but ultrastructural vacuolation is seen within a few days. The ocular lesion is, as elsewhere in the central nervous system, vacuolation of neuronal cytoplasm, and, later, axonal degeneration. The vacuolation is readily reversible upon cessation of ingestion of the plant and seems not to be the lesion responsible for clinical signs. The axonal degeneration is not reversible and is probably the more important lesion. Whether blindness is retinal or central in origin is unknown.

Poisoning with *Stypandra* spp. occurs in sheep and goats on dry pastures in southwestern Australia. The plant is among the first to reappear after autumn rains end the drought, and is eaten if nothing better is available. Acute intoxication is frequently fatal. Animals surviving the acute stage become blind and ataxic. In retina, there is diffuse photoreceptor atrophy and patchy hyperplasia of retinal pigment epithelium (RPE). Axonal degeneration is found within the optic nerve and elsewhere within the central nervous system.

The colloquial term *"blind staggers" refers to chronic intoxication of sheep and cattle with plants known to accumulate organic selenium selectively.* Affected animals wander aimlessly, become weak and ataxic, and are finally paralyzed prior to death. There is some question as to whether blindness is genuine or merely the result of stupor. Ocular lesions are not described. The syndrome of blind staggers does not occur in experimental selenium toxicity, and it is possible that the syndrome is of much more complex pathogenesis than simple selenium toxicity. Plants of the genera *Astragalus* and *Oxytropis* are selenium accumulators as well as sources of swainsonine-like alkaloids.

Mycotoxicosis associated with the consumption of *Corallocytostroma* sp. fungus on Mitchell grass is reported to cause "black soil blindness" in cattle in Australia. The disease presents as rapidly progressive blindness and death. The histologic lesion is not described.

Photoreceptor degeneration has been described in cats treated with the antibiotic **enrofloxacin**. Initial reports suggested that this was an idiosyncratic reaction because the toxicity occurred after administration of the drug at recommended dosages. Subsequent analysis suggests that this is a direct toxicity that occurs when the retina is exposed to unusually high levels of this widely used antibiotic, even when administered at the daily recommended dosages (subsequently revised). Retinotoxic levels are likely to be reached when the drug is given by rapid intravenous infusion or when given to cats with impaired renal or liver function that may not properly metabolize and eliminate the drug. *Toxicity is thus most likely to be seen in old cats receiving prolonged therapy.* Similar retinal toxicity is likely to be shared by other fluoroquinolone antibiotics. Most cats had clinically obvious visual impairment within a few weeks of drug administration, and the blindness was permanent in most cases.

Miscellaneous retinopathies

Retinal lesions are found in a number of metabolic disorders and systemic states. Best known among these is diabetes mellitus, but retinal lesions are found also in any of the neuronal storage diseases, coagulation disorders, anemia, disseminated intravascular coagulation, hyperviscosity syndrome, hypertension, and following excessive exposure to oxygen or light.

Diabetes mellitus is *the major cause of blindness in people in North America. The cause of the blindness is chorioretinal vascular disease with subsequent retinal degeneration.* The characteristic lesions are seen only in patients with diabetes of 10-15 years duration. Even though virtually all chronic diabetics develop some retinal lesions, <10% become blind. Blindness is strongly predictive of the development of fatal diabetic nephropathy. Lesion development is not prevented by insulin replacement. Other ocular lesions include cataract, rubeosis iridis, glycogen-induced vacuolation of iris epithelium, and massive thickening of the ciliary basal lamina. The corneal epithelium may be unduly fragile, and tear production may be reduced.

The retinal lesion in people is mostly the result of microvascular disease. Loss of retinal pericytes, development of microaneurysms, thickening of capillary basal lamina, and retinal hemorrhages constitute the early, degenerative phase of the retinopathy. This is followed by a proliferative phase in which more capillary aneurysms, arteriolar-venular shunts, and neovascularization occur as the presumed responses to retinal ischemia. The neovascularization is initially bland and confined to the retina, but later there is extension into preretinal vitreous with accompanying fibroplasia (retinitis proliferans). Hemorrhages and hyalinized collections of leaked plasma are common in the retina.

In nonprimates, the naturally occurring retinopathy is seen only in dogs and, even then, infrequently. This low frequency may be due to the fact that affected dogs do not live long enough for the retinal disease to develop. In dogs deliberately made diabetic and kept for up to 6 years, microvascular lesions typical of human diabetes occur. Pericyte loss is accompanied by capillary aneurysms, reactive endothelial proliferation, and perivascular plasmoid exudates or hemorrhages.

Other types of **ischemic retinal injury** are much more frequent in domestic animals than is diabetic retinopathy. *Undoubtedly, the most frequent examples are associated with vascular hypertension in cats and, less frequently, in dogs.* Ischemic retinopathy as a consequence of disseminated intravascular coagulopathy (DIC), of *tumor metastasis*, or of *bacteremia* is fairly common, with the prevalence varying greatly with species. *Perhaps the most common example of ischemic retinal injury is that resulting from retinal detachment.* The blood vessels of the choriocapillaris supply oxygen and other nutrients to the photoreceptors and outer nuclear layer, hence retinal detachment inevitably results in gradual outer retinal ischemic/malnutritive atrophy.

Hypertensive retinopathy is in most cases associated with *chronic renal failure.* At least 60% of dogs with chronic renal failure are hypertensive. Dogs and cats are most frequently affected. In cats, hypertensive retinopathy is also claimed to be associated with hyperthyroidism, but a study of 100 hyperthyroid cats did not provide any evidence for that anecdotal association.

The macroscopic ocular lesions include retinal or preretinal hemorrhage, retinal edema, and retinal detachment because of serous effusion from injured choroidal blood vessels. *The histologic lesions are primarily in retinal and choroidal vessels,* which have lesions varying from fibrinoid necrosis of tunica media to medial hypertrophy with adventitial fibrosis (Fig. 5-65). Changes that are probably secondary to vessel damage include localized retinal necrosis, exudative retinal separation with resultant atrophy of photoreceptors and hypertrophy of RPE, and intraretinal hemosiderin deposition. Usually, there

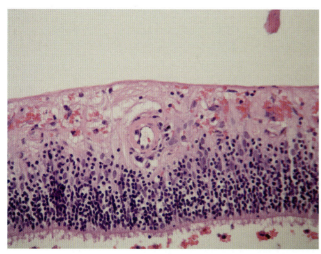

Figure 5-65 **Systemic vascular hypertension** causing fibrinoid necrosis of small arteries within the retina, resulting in hemorrhage and necrosis.

is ischemic necrosis of RPE, which allows for the leakage of hypertensive edema fluid from the choroid into the subretinal space, which would normally be prevented by the tight junctions between adjacent RPE cells. Vascular lesions and associated necrosis may also occur in anterior uvea. Eyes that are eventually enucleated or obtained at necropsy may have a variety of other lesions that probably occur secondary to chronic retinal detachment and chronic intraocular hemorrhage. Most notable among these is pre-iridal fibrovascular membrane and its resultant hyphema or neovascular glaucoma.

The early lesions, likely to be seen only under experimental conditions, are the result of exaggerated autoregulatory vasoconstriction in response to systemic hypertension. Sustained vasoconstriction leads to ischemic necrosis of the deprived retina, RPE, or choroid, as well as necrosis of vascular endothelium distal to the constricted precapillary sphincters. The histologic consequences are focal retinal necrosis, and leakage of plasma or even erythrocytes through damaged endothelium. This leakage causes intramural fibrinoid change in the vessels and edema or hemorrhage in adjacent retina.

Retinal infarction, usually seen as a combination of hemorrhage and liquefaction, occurs subsequent to retinal vessel thrombosis (especially in detached retinas), occlusion by tumor emboli, or vasculitis associated with immune disease or a few infectious diseases (Fig. 5-66A, B). The most likely to be encountered are thrombotic meningoencephalitis of cattle, and Rocky Mountain spotted fever or ehrlichiosis in dogs. In addition to the vascular lesions themselves, which may have specific characteristics associated with the individual diseases, the retinal lesions vary from focal hemorrhage to areas of hemorrhagic liquefactive necrosis or healed lesions of chorioretinal scarring.

Similar retinal scarring has been seen in horses following massive but sublethal blood loss, as in surgery or from nasal hemorrhage subsequent to severe cranial trauma. Affected eyes have multifocal retinal atrophy and hyperpigmentation. Similar lesions may also result from focal retinal separation. In horses, such separation carries a high risk of causing focal retinal infarction because they have such limited intrinsic retinal vasculature (see Fig. 5-64).

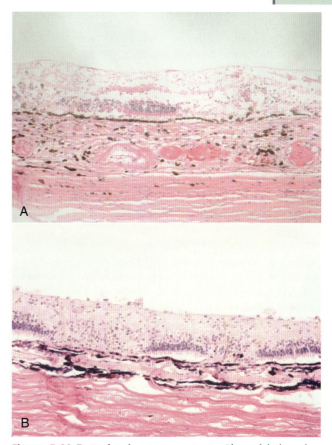

Figure 5-66 **Retinal ischemic necrosis. A.** Choroidal thrombophlebitis with secondary retinal infarction in a horse with purpura hemorrhagica. **B.** Postnecrotic scarring causing multiple adhesions between the damaged retina and previously injured choroid.

Retinal hemorrhages are seen in a variety of primary clotting disorders, in thrombocytopenia of any cause, and in degenerative or inflammatory vascular disorders. Retinal hemorrhages also recur in cats with profound anemia of any cause; the mechanism is unknown. The lesions heal with scarring if the cat survives the anemia, suggesting that the hemorrhage is only the most visible manifestation of multifocal and probably ischemic retinopathy.

Many of the **neuronal storage diseases** cause retinal lesions identical to those in the brain. The list of those with described ocular lesions probably reflects those in which the eyes have been examined rather than a true reflection of those diseases in which ocular lesions do, or do not, occur. Those interested should consult a useful, referenced table in the text by Slatter (see Further reading).

Senile retinopathy *is characterized by microcystoid degeneration,* which is very common in dogs from middle age onward (see Fig. 5-62). A similar lesion is found occasionally in horses. The lesion affects peripheral retina adjacent to ora ciliaris and for a variable distance posteriorly. There is formation of small cystic spaces within inner nuclear and plexiform layers, fusion of inner and outer nuclear layers, pigment cell accumulation, and haphazard atrophy and mingling of nuclei in a manner simulating peripheral retinal dysplasia. If the cysts rupture, there is the risk that liquefied vitreous may slip through the resulting hole and cause rhegmatogenous retinal detachment. For some unknown reason, this is most commonly seen in small dogs (especially Shih Tzu), in which the detachment of

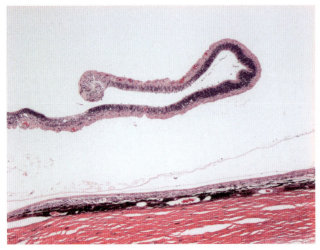

Figure 5-67 **Retinal separation** from the ora ciliaris (retinal dialysis) as a sequel to peripheral microcystoid retinal degeneration and subsequent rhegmatogenous detachment. The coiled and smoothly rounded edge of the retina at the site of the break distinguishes this from purely artifactual detachment occurring during sectioning of the globe.

the retina triggers pre-iridal fibrovascular membrane and secondary glaucoma (Fig. 5-67).

Multifocal coalescing peripheral retinal atrophy is very frequent in very old dogs and horses, but is of no apparent visual importance.

Further reading

Herring IP, et al. Longitudinal prevalence of hypertension, proteinuria, and retinopathy in dogs with spontaneous diabetes mellitus. J Vet Intern Med 2014;28:488-495.

Maggio F, et al. Ocular lesions associated with systemic hypertension in cats: 69 cases (1985-1998). J Am Vet Med Assoc 2000;217:695-702.

Mason CS, et al. Congenital ocular abnormalities in calves associated with maternal hypovitaminosis A. Vet Rec 2003;153:213-214.

McLellan GJ, et al. Clinical and pathological observations in English cocker spaniels with primary metabolic vitamin E deficiency and retinal pigment epithelial dystrophy. Vet Rec 2003;153:287-292.

Slatter D. Retina. In: Slatter D, editor. Fundamentals of Veterinary Ophthalmology. 3rd ed. Philadelphia: WB Saunders; 2001. p. 419-456.

Retinitis

Retinitis as the sole ocular lesion is rare, but may occur in animals with neurotropic virus infections, with toxoplasmosis, and with thrombotic meningoencephalitis of cattle (Fig. 5-68). In the latter disease, however, it is more usual to find the typical thrombotic, inflammatory lesions in choroid as well as retina. Their character is identical to the lesions in the brain. The multifocal chorioretinal scars expected as sequelae are seldom seen, perhaps because cattle with neurologic and ocular lesions almost inevitably die. The prevalence of the ocular lesion, useful as an aid in the clinical diagnosis, is estimated at 30-50% in animals with the septicemic form of the disease, and as high as 65% in experimentally infected calves.

Multifocal viral retinitis with the same histologic features as the respective brain lesions occurs in animals with classical

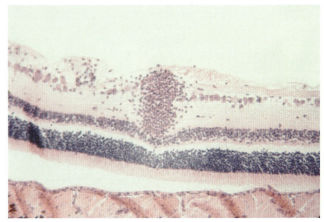

Figure 5-68 **Retinal suppurative thrombophlebitis** in a steer with thromboembolic meningoencephalitis.

swine fever, rabies, Teschen disease, Borna disease, pseudorabies in pigs, canine distemper, and scrapie (a prion disease). Undoubtedly, the list is incomplete, and is probably limited only by the rarity with which retinas receive histologic evaluation in animals dying with systemic viral, bacterial, and protozoal diseases. *The ocular lesions associated with canine distemper will be described here in some detail as the archetypal example of viral retinopathy;* other aspects of canine distemper are discussed in Vol. 2, Respiratory system.

Retinal and optic nerve lesions occur in most dogs with naturally occurring **canine distemper**. The lesions most often are degenerative rather than inflammatory, although some of the degenerative changes may have been sites of inflammation earlier in the disease course.

Acute lymphocytic-plasmacytic chorioretinitis and optic neuritis are found in ~25% of dogs submitted for laboratory confirmation of the disease. Random perivascular cuffing, edema, focal exudative retinal separation, and hypertrophy of RPE are present. Eosinophilic intranuclear inclusion bodies occur in ganglion cells or astrocytes in 30-40% of the cases, which is the only etiologically specific change in what is an otherwise nonspecific picture shared by many systemic infections.

The more prevalent lesions are multiple random foci of retinal degeneration and scarring. These usually affect the full thickness of retina, and are most likely sequelae to the previous undetected retinitis. Such foci often contain numerous melanin-laden cells, probably derived from migration of adjacent, injured RPE. Occasionally, only the outer nuclear layer and photoreceptors are missing, probably a sequel to focal exudative retinal detachment.

Optic nerve lesions of one type or another are present in all dogs with ocular lesions. Nonsuppurative neuritis, astrocytic scarring, and demyelination similar to that in brain are the 3 most frequent changes. In those dogs suffering only the demyelinating disease, the ocular lesions may be inapparent, or there may be demyelination of optic nerve and ganglion cell degeneration.

Other infectious examples of retinitis in dogs include **Rocky Mountain spotted fever** (RMSF, *Rickettsia rickettsii*) and **canine ehrlichiosis** (*Ehrlichia canis*). The clinical and histologic ocular lesions are virtually identical and occur in a high percentage (80% for RMSF) of dogs with active infection. Most of the lesions result from injury to vascular endothelium parasitized by the rickettsiae; multifocal hemorrhage, edema, and vascular necrosis occur in all parts of the eye. *Multifocal retinal hemorrhage, perivascular retinal edema, and necrosis of endothelium in retinal venules and arterioles are the characteristic retinal changes.* Although often listed along with other agents as a cause of anterior uveitis or endophthalmitis, most naturally occurring infections have clinical signs attributable only to the vascular injury rather than a genuine uveal inflammation. There is one report of unusually severe uveitis occurring 14-28 days after experimental infection with *R. rickettsii*, following the disappearance of all other signs of the acute systemic disease. Dogs thus affected had neutrophilic and lymphocytic destructive vasculitis, assumed to represent a type III immune reaction to parasitized endothelium.

Visceral larva migrans from *Toxocara canis* has been linked to granulomatous endophthalmitis and chorioretinitis in dogs. It is likely that many of these cases were actually caused by the raccoon roundworm *Baylisascaris procyonis* (see Parasitic endophthalmitis).

Further reading

Dubey JP, et al. *Sarcocystis neurona* schizonts-associated encephalitis, chorioretinitis, and myositis in a two-month-old dog simulating toxoplasmosis, and presence of mature sarcocysts in muscles. Vet Parasitol 2014;202:194-200.

Panciera RJ, et al. Ocular histopathology of ehrlichial infections in the dog. Vet Pathol 2001;38:43-46.

OPTIC NERVE

The optic nerve is a white fiber tract of brain formed by the outgrowth of ganglion cell axons from the eye through sieve-like perforations in posterior polar sclera, called the *lamina cribrosa*. The axons travel within a preformed neuroectodermal tube formed by the primary optic stalk to reach the optic chiasm and then the lateral geniculate body. The neuroectoderm lining the optic stalk induces the surrounding mesenchyme to form the 3 meningeal layers, similar to and continuous with those of brain itself. Later differentiation of neuroectoderm produces astrocytes and oligodendroglia that, together with the ganglion cell, axons, and fibrovascular septa from pia mater, form the substance of the optic nerve. The *optic disc* is the intraocular portion of the nerve and is the only portion available to ophthalmoscopic examination. It is formed by the convergence of ganglion cell axons prior to their exit via the lamina cribrosa. The axons of the nerve fiber layer are unmyelinated, and at what point (relative to lamina cribrosa) the axons become myelinated determines the ophthalmoscopic appearance of the optic disc. Histologically, the disc is unmyelinated in most domestic species except the dog, contains abundant glia, and may have a small paracentral excavation—*the physiologic cup*—from which Bergmeister's papilla originates. A few pigmented cells are commonly seen, as are small neuroblastic clusters, both probably minor anomalies of retinal differentiation but of no significance.

There is considerable variation in the normal histology of the optic nerve among animals of different species and ages. Optic disc myelination has already been mentioned. The lamina cribrosa is formed by heavy fibrous trabeculae in horses, dogs, and cattle and is therefore more obvious than in cats and laboratory animals. Fibrous septa within the nerve are prominent in cattle and horses, and their similarity to the axons in hematoxylin and eosin sections may mask a pathologic paucity of nerve fibers. The fibrous tissue reportedly increases with age.

The general pathology of the optic nerve shares features of both retinal and neural disease. Because it is in direct continuity with both structures via its axons, and with brain via the perineural cerebrospinal fluid, it is common for optic nerve to be affected by diseases of either retina or brain. Thus optic neuritis is expected in at least a proportion of animals suffering with inflammation of retina or neural white matter, and optic nerve atrophy inevitably follows loss of ganglion cells. Fortuitous hematogenous localization of infectious agents or tumor cells may occur in optic nerve as anywhere else. The optic nerve is occasionally the site of origin for meningiomas and various glial tumors that are clinically significant.

In general, lesions of the optic nerve are found as more or less incidental findings when examining globes removed for other reasons, such as glaucoma, endophthalmitis, or neoplasia. Clinical abnormalities affecting the optic disc or optic nerve are quite common, but only rarely would such globes be removed for histologic assessment.

> **Key Points**
>
> Optic nerve disease is hardly ever the reason for enucleation, and most optic nerve lesions are considered "incidental" findings in globes with more prominent disease in the retina or uvea. The most common optic nerve lesion by far is glaucomatous atrophy and cupping, involving a mixture of axonal necrosis, gliosis, and posterior mechanical displacement of the optic disc.

Papilledema *is hydropic swelling of the optic disc.* It may result from extraocular events that cause an increase in cerebrospinal fluid pressure within the optic nerve or from local vascular leakage. The former is usually associated with retrobulbar tissue masses, but is also seen with intracranial neoplasms and with hypovitaminosis A. Ocular hypotony may cause optic disc edema as a result of decreased tissue hydrostatic pressure. Serous inflammation within the nerve also results in papilledema. Papilledema is a common clinical diagnosis that rarely is available for histologic examination.

Optic neuritis *is a term sometimes used rather broadly to describe both inflammatory and degenerative diseases of the nerve.* Optic neuritis is seen clinically as swelling, hyperemia, and focal hemorrhage within the optic disc. Affected animals, usually dogs or horses, are blind when the lesion is bilateral. Although described as a clinical entity not associated with other ocular lesions, the vast majority of cases of "clinical" optic neuritis are not confirmed histologically may, of course, accompany any case of retinitis or endophthalmitis.

The pattern of inflammation within the nerve may provide clues to the pathogenesis of the neuritis. Perineuritis, or optic nerve leptomeningitis, is typical of meningeal spread of bacterial meningitis from the brain. Toxoplasmosis and cryptococcosis frequently cause multifocal and nonselective lesions within the extraocular nerve, as does canine distemper. Optic neuritis originating as endophthalmitis is usually restricted to the optic disc. Feline infectious peritonitis is frequently associated with perineuritis and optic neuritis in which the mononuclear aggregates are around blood vessels in the meninges and in the extensions of the meninges into the nerve. Optic neuritis may also be prominent in equine recurrent uveitis and in dogs with the syndrome of granulomatous meningoencephalitis.

Chronic optic neuritis, like its counterpart in the brain, is characterized by focal gliosis, astrocytic scarring, and secondary axonal degeneration. The loss of axons may be partially masked by the increased prominence of glia and pial septa.

Degeneration of the optic nerve *may be a sequel to trauma, optic neuritis, glaucoma, and chronic, severe retinal atrophy of any cause.* Initiation of gliosis and fibrosis may eventually make the chronic degenerative lesion indistinguishable from that of chronic inflammation. The most frequently diagnosed example is that following *trauma* to one or both nerves in dogs, horses, or cats with head trauma. The gross lesion may be avulsion, laceration, or contusion. Injury to the nerve may be instantaneous, as caused by tearing or complete severance, or may result from vascular injury with slightly delayed ischemic necrosis. In severed nerves, there is disintegration of the distal axons back to the lateral geniculate body. The proximal portion of each affected axon dies back to the ganglion cell, which eventually also dies. The inner nuclear layer remains unaffected, a useful criterion to distinguish traumatic, "die back," ganglion cell atrophy from that of glaucoma.

Degeneration of optic nerve also occurs in calves *deficient in vitamin A*, and in ruminants ingesting *male fern* or *hexachlorophene*. Ingestion of male fern, *Dryopteris*, on pasture or as a taenicidal extract, causes papilledema and subsequent optic nerve demyelination when ingested in large amounts. Retina may be unaffected early, but ganglion cell atrophy occurs eventually. Hexachlorophene administered to calves or sheep as an anthelmintic causes edema and then atrophy and gliosis of optic nerve.

Proliferative optic neuropathy is an unusual lesion of horses. Anecdotal descriptions are numerous, but histologic descriptions are few. The lesion is a raised, gray mass on the surface of the optic disc, unassociated with visual deficit. *The mass is composed of spherical mononuclear cells with hyperchromatic, eccentric nuclei and foamy eosinophilic cytoplasm.* Some of these cells are also found within extraocular optic nerve. The cytoplasmic content may be stored lipid, but its origin is not known. The described lesion bears much resemblance to the proliferation of myelin-laden macrophages that occurs in and on optic nerves injured by trauma or ischemia. Also, the distinction between the proliferative optic neuropathy and gliomas or granular cell tumors described in various reports is unclear.

Further reading

Godin AC, et al. Retinal and optic nerve degeneration in cattle after accidental acrylamide intoxication. Vet Ophthalmol 2000;3:235-239.

Scott EM, et al. Early histopathologic changes in the retina and optic nerve in canine primary angle-closure glaucoma. Vet Ophthalmol 2013;16(Suppl. 1):79-86.

SCLERA

The **limbus** *marks the transition from the avascular, nonpigmented, and very orderly cornea to the vascularized, pigmented, and interwoven fibrous tissue that identifies sclera.* It is also the site of transition from corneal epithelium into bulbar conjunctiva. The sclera forms the posterior ⅔ of the fibrous tunic of the eye, blending with choroid on its inner aspect and orbital fascia exteriorly. Its thickness increases with age and varies considerably among domestic species. In cattle and horses, it is thickest at the posterior pole (2.2 mm in cattle, 1.3 mm in horses) and thinnest at the orbital equator (1.0 mm in cattle, ~0.5 mm in horses). In dogs and cats, it is much thinner, ~0.3 mm at the posterior pole and 0.1 mm at the equator, varying somewhat with age and globe size. In carnivores, however, there is a circumferential ring of thickened (1 mm) sclera at the limbus in which is buried the venous plexus receiving aqueous drainage. The sclera is perforated by numerous vessels and nerves, the most notable of which are the optic nerve and limbic scleral venous plexus.

The optic nerve fibers exit the globe through extensive scleral fenestrations called the **lamina cribrosa.** Diseases of the sclera are few in comparison to diseases of other ocular structures. Most are inflammatory and arise by extension from within the globe or from orbital cellulitis. *The efficiency with which the sclera resists inflammatory spread is evidenced by the infrequency of panophthalmitis as opposed to endophthalmitis, and the even greater infrequency of intraocular involvement resulting from orbital inflammation.* When the sclera is involved in inflammatory disease originating within the eye, its initial involvement is seen histologically as leukocytes in perivascular adventitia that is in direct communication with the choroid. A similar phenomenon is seen in scleral extension of choroidal neoplasms, in which collars of tumor cells surround scleral vessels but show little inclination to infiltrate directly into scleral and connective tissue.

Nodular granulomatous episcleritis (NGE) or sclerokeratitis *is the most prevalent disease of dogs that is primarily scleral.* It is a proliferative, nodular lesion of the episclera or conjunctival lamina propria that has been variously termed nodular fasciitis, nodular scleritis or episcleritis, fibrous histiocytoma, proliferative keratoconjunctivitis, conjunctival granuloma, and Collie granuloma.

The clinical spectrum includes lesions that are unilateral or bilateral, nodular or multinodular, and episcleral or conjunctival. It is not yet clear how many different diseases are actually existent under what is currently a broad clinical umbrella of "nodular episcleritis." Regardless, the histologic lesions seem to be relatively uniform and are certainly more uniform than the clinical presentation. By far the most prevalent macroscopic lesion submitted for histologic assessment is a firm, painless, moveable, nodular swelling, 0.5-1.0 cm in diameter, below the bulbar conjunctiva at, or just posterior to, the limbus. Infiltrative extension of the mass into the peripheral corneal stroma is accompanied by edema and vascularization. Other common locations include the third eyelid and elsewhere within the lamina propria of the bulbar conjunctiva.

Histologically, the lesion is a proliferative, nonencapsulated mixture of histiocytic cells, spindle cells, plasma cells, and lymphocytes (Fig. 5-69A, B). The spindle cells may be fibroblasts, histiocytes, or a mixture of both. The spindle cells are haphazardly arranged, and, despite a fibrous appearance to the section, surprisingly little collagen is demonstrated by special stains, except in coarse septa that may dissect the mass into irregular lobules. Reticulin, however, is abundant. The lymphocytes are found loosely throughout the mass but are usually most numerous near the periphery. Characterization of the lymphocytes or histiocytes via immunohistochemistry

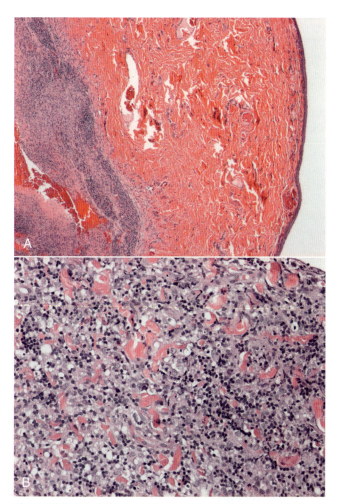

Figure 5-69 Nodular granulomatous episcleritis. **A.** Discrete, expansile nodule of intermingled histiocytes and lymphocytes within the deep conjunctival lamina propria or episclera. **B.** Characteristic intermingling of histiocytes and lymphocytes with very few plasma cells or granulocytes, and with no formation of granulomas or lymphoid follicles.

has not yet yielded any useful information in terms of understanding the pathogenesis or providing guidelines for further subclassification.

Important histologic features distinguishing NGE from an early lesion of idiopathic necrotic scleritis (see later) are the absence of collagenolysis and the absence of discrete granulomas. When present in peripheral cornea, the above cell mixture affects stroma but spares the epithelium and an adjacent zone of subepithelial stroma.

The lesions of NGE show a substantial range in the proportion of the various leukocytes as well as in clinical presentation, and it may be that this disease will eventually be divided into several different entities to better explain this variation. At the moment, however, we have insufficient evidence to justify any subclassification based on histopathology, immunohistochemistry, or clinical behavior. This clinical and histologic syndrome is unique, and suggestions that NGE might be a conjunctival or scleral manifestation of cutaneous histiocytosis or cutaneous sterile pyogranuloma syndrome have no basis, and dogs with NGE do not usually have any histologically similar skin lesions.

> **Key Points**
>
> **Nodular granulomatous episcleritis** (NGE) illustrates very well the problems that arise when a perfectly accurate description and morphologic diagnosis are not further accompanied by a specific syndrome diagnosis. A diagnosis of "nodular nonseptic mixed lymphocytic and granulomatous conjunctivitis" or "focal lymphocytic and granulomatous episcleritis" may be accurate from a histologic perspective and yet be worthless as a final diagnosis because clinicians will not be able to translate that morphologic diagnosis into a clinically useful diagnosis of NGE.

Necrotizing scleritis (idiopathic necrotic scleritis) *is a rare lesion seen in dogs as a poorly delineated inflammatory and proliferative lesion of the anterior sclera.* The disease incites a much more inflammatory reaction and progresses much more rapidly than does NGE. *The lesion consists of coalescing scleral granulomas centered on remnants of denatured, refractile collagen.* Eosinophils sometimes are numerous, and most lesions contain at least modest numbers of lymphocytes (Fig. 5-70A). The exact histologic appearance varies with the stage of disease and is probably greatly influenced by what therapy has been used prior to biopsy or enucleation, but at least some degree of collagenolysis and some hint of granuloma formation are requirements for the diagnosis. The lesion tends to rapidly spread circumferentially and posteriorly to involve the entire sclera, and involvement of uvea and even retina with necrosis and granulomas eventually occurring (Fig. 5-70B). The disease usually begins unilaterally, but most cases eventually are bilateral. Response to anti-inflammatory therapy is poor unless that therapy is very aggressive, and so an unusually high percentage of eyes with this disease eventually become available for histologic assessment. No etiologic agent has been seen.

> **Key Points**
>
> **Nodular granulomatous episcleritis (NGE) versus necrotic scleritis?**
> **NGE** affects the loose connective tissue of the episclera or conjunctival lamina propria, does not involve collagenolysis, and usually creates a discrete nodule.
> **Necrotic scleritis** arises within the dense connective tissue of the sclera itself, has collagenolysis as a highly conserved feature, and is always invasive.

ORBIT

Diseases of the orbit are few and relatively uncommon in domestic animals except for those resulting from trauma and, in dogs, from neoplasia. Systemic diseases of bone, muscle, blood vessels, and nerves may incidentally affect orbital components. Orbital fat fluctuates with nutritional status, contributing to the enophthalmos of malnourished animals. Ordinarily, however, orbital disease arises by extension of inflammatory lesions from the mouth, paranasal sinuses, or from penetrating wounds through periorbital soft tissue. Extension from intraocular inflammation is surprisingly rare, a tribute to the barrier offered by the sclera. Conversely, orbital disease rarely invades the globe. Metastatic orbital neoplasia is rare except for lymphoma of cattle and cats. Direct invasion by malignancies arising in the

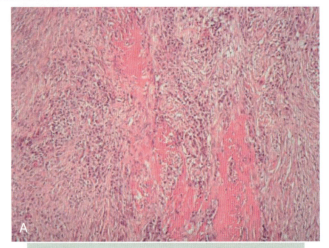

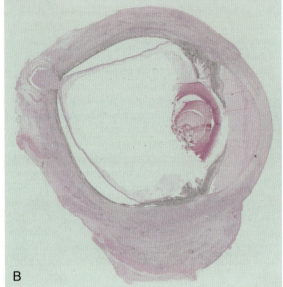

Figure 5-70 Idiopathic necrotic scleritis. **A.** Granulomatous and lymphocytic inflammation with prominent collagenolysis. Neutrophils and eosinophils may be present, especially in early and untreated lesions. **B.** Rapid progression throughout the sclera to encircle the globe is characteristic.

mouth, facial bone, nasal cavity, or sinus is more common. Although theoretically the orbit may suffer from primary neoplasia of any of the bony or soft tissues within it, such occurrences are infrequent. Of these, optic nerve meningiomas, ill-defined spindle cell sarcomas, and lacrimal gland tumors in dogs are the most common (see Ocular neoplasia).

Orbital cellulitis *is the term commonly used to describe pyogenic orbital inflammation.* The cause is usually bacterial, and the pathogenesis involves penetrating injury or direct extension from nearby inflammation of paranasal sinuses, molar tooth socket, or periorbital soft tissue. Only rarely does uncontrolled endophthalmitis spread through the sclera into the orbit. Bacteremic localization within the orbit is seldom detected, except perhaps for *Streptococcus equi* infection in young horses.

Orbital myositis *occurs as a specific syndrome in dogs, affecting the extraocular muscles.* It affects primarily young dogs of large breeds, and is not associated with masticatory or generalized myositis. The histologic changes are identical to immune-mediated masticatory myositis, with multifocal random interstitial lymphocytic myositis, muscle fiber necrosis, and subsequent fibrosis. Antibodies against type 2M muscle fibers have been demonstrated in affected dogs.

Orbital inflammation most frequently results from *penetrating foreign bodies*, whether by direct penetration or particle migration from conjunctival sac or pharynx. Horses seem particularly prone. Aberrant localization by nematode parasites (*Dirofilaria immitis, Angiostrongylus, Onchocerca,* spp., *Ancylostoma caninum*) or *Diptera* larvae is reported.

Postoperative conjunctival inclusion cysts are the result of intraorbital migration of bulbar conjunctiva left in place at the time of enucleation. This represents improper surgical technique. The epithelium migrates into the orbit, creates a cyst, and continues to enlarge as the conjunctival epithelium continues to produce its normal tear film secretion. The cyst creates a tumor-like mass requiring surgical excision. Histologically, the epithelium looks like normal bulbar or palpebral conjunctiva with variable numbers of goblet cells.

Further reading

Denk N, et al. A retrospective study of the clinical, histological, and immunohistochemical manifestations of 5 dogs originally diagnosed histologically as necrotizing scleritis. Vet Ophthalmol 2012;15:102-109.

Grahn BH, Sandmeyer LS. Canine episcleritis, nodular episclerokeratitis, scleritis, and necrotic scleritis. Vet Clin North Am Small Anim Pract 2008;38:291-308.

OCULAR NEOPLASIA

Although the eye is the site of a wide range of primary and metastatic neoplasms, only a few are of sufficient prevalence or importance to justify discussion here. Pathologists get a very biased view of the relative importance of neoplasia overall within the world of veterinary ophthalmology simply because virtually every globe containing a neoplasm is going to be submitted for histologic assessment. *At least in dogs and cats, which are the species from which we are most likely to receive histologic specimens for assessment, neoplasia is second only to glaucoma as a cause for enucleation.*

Primary ocular tumors may arise from the eyelids and adnexa, from optic nerve, or from within the globe. Those arising within the globe may originate from any of the tissues, but only those from uveal melanocytes and iridociliary neuroectoderm are anything other than rare. *Most primary intraocular tumors have negligible potential for metastasis.* Dogs and cats are most frequently affected; primary intraocular neoplasms are inexplicably rare in other domestic species.

Metastatic ocular neoplasia is reported rather infrequently, but it is common when sought. Multicentric lymphoma in cats, dogs, and cattle regularly involves the eye, although, in cattle, the retrobulbar tissue is preferred over the eye itself. *With the exception of malignant lymphoma, carcinomas are reported more frequently than sarcomas.* This probably reflects the greater metastatic potential of carcinomas in general, rather than any specific difference in ocular tropism. Uveal vessels are the usual sites of lodgment, and ocular disease may result from vessel occlusion, or from inflammation in response to tumor antigen, or to necrosis of either tumor or damaged host tissue.

Further reading

Baptiste KE, Grahn BH. Equine orbital neoplasia: a review of 10 cases (1983-1998). Can Vet J 2000;41:291-295.

Grahn BH, et al. Classification of feline intraocular neoplasms based on morphology, histochemical staining, and immunohistochemical labeling. Vet Ophthalmol 2006;9:395-403.

Labelle AL, Labelle P. Canine ocular neoplasia: a review. Vet Ophthalmol 2013;16(Suppl. 1):3-14.

Eyelid and conjunctival neoplasms
Squamous cell carcinoma

Squamous cell carcinoma arises from the conjunctival epithelium of the limbus, third eyelid, or eyelid in cattle, horses, cats, and dogs, in that order of frequency. **Bovine** ocular squamous cell carcinoma is one of the most common and most economically significant neoplasms of domestic animals. Its relative rarity in dogs is peculiar and unexplained. The disease in horses and cattle usually arises within the conjunctiva, whereas in cats, it is primarily a disease of the haired skin of the eyelid margin. The prevalence of the disease in all species is related primarily to exposure to ultraviolet (UV) radiation and to lack of pigment in lids and conjunctiva. Its geographic prevalence is therefore directly correlated with altitude and inversely correlated with latitude, as well as with the prevalence of animals with poor periocular pigmentation. In cattle, in which this disease is of greatest significance, the prevalence is highest in the "white faced" Hereford breed and in the high-altitude regions of the Canadian and American West. It also occurs in other breeds of cattle, as well as Indian water buffalo, sheep, and cattalo. Variation in prevalence in different lines of Herefords, even in the same region, has led to speculation that other genetic factors within the breed, other than facial pigmentation, may influence susceptibility. The question of etiology has been further widened by demonstration of papillomaviruses in some of the papillomatous precursor lesions that eventually transform into squamous cell carcinoma. Similar papillomaviruses, as well as being the causative agents of cutaneous warts, have been demonstrated in bovine alimentary papillomas in Scotland, and viral DNA persists in the squamous cell carcinomas that arise from these papillomas in cattle grazing pastures that contain bracken fern. It remains to be determined whether or not there is any relationship between a viral component of the ocular carcinoma and the fact that, in many cases, the tumor regresses after immunotherapy. *At least at the moment, no viral particle or viral genome has been consistently demonstrated in ocular squamous cell carcinomas in any species.* Environmental co-carcinogens, such as those in bracken fern, have not yet been implicated in the induction of ocular tumors.

The tumor in all species develops through a series of premalignant stages, called epidermal plaques and papillomas, before proceeding over months or years to carcinoma in situ and to invasive carcinoma. Spontaneous regression of the precancerous lesions may occur with an estimated frequency of 25-50%. At least in cattle, plaques are much more common (~6:1) than papillomas or outright carcinomas. The *epidermal plaque* is characterized by marked acanthosis, with variable presence of keratinization, dyskeratosis, and epidermal downgrowth into the subconjunctival connective tissue. Invasion through basal layer or basement membrane is not seen. *Papilloma* also

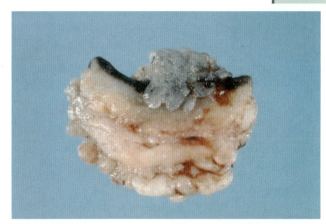

Figure 5-71 **Papillary squamous cell carcinoma** protruding from the third eyelid of a horse.

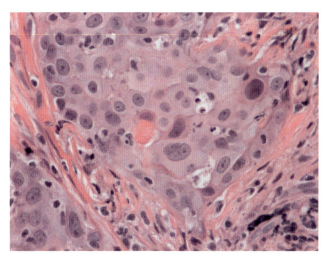

Figure 5-72 **Classic histologic features of mature squamous cell carcinoma,** including jumbled maturation, premature keratinization, and especially invasion by stratum spinosum–like epithelium.

involves acanthosis but, in addition, there is marked parakeratosis and hyperkeratosis with papillary projections supported by a vascularized connective tissue core. Papillomas may be up to 3 cm in diameter, pedunculated or sessile, and are often ulcerated (Fig. 5-71). *Carcinoma in situ* arises by focal or multifocal transformation of increasingly dysplastic cell nests in the deep layers of plaques or papillomas. *Fully developed carcinoma* has squamous cell invasion across the basement membrane. Tumor invasion is almost always accompanied by *intense lymphocytic-plasmacytic infiltration*, presumably the host response to tumor antigen. It is assumed that it is this response that is responsible for regression of some of the precursor lesions, although spontaneous regression of fully developed carcinoma is rare. Stimulation of immune-mediated rejection by intralesional inoculation of antigenic tumor extracts or nonspecific lymphocyte stimulants induces partial or total regression of small tumors.

Histologically, ocular squamous cell carcinoma resembles similar tumors in other sites and ranges from well-differentiated carcinomas with keratin pearl formation to anaplastic carcinomas with marked nuclear size variation and mononuclear tumor giant cells (Fig. 5-72). *Metastatic or invasive potential*

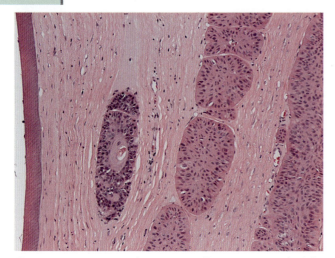

Figure 5-73 **Conjunctival squamous cell carcinoma** invading the peripheral cornea of a horse.

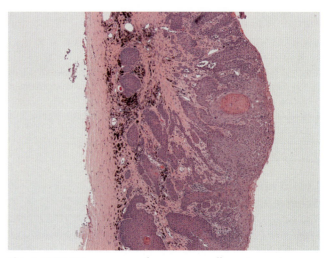

Figure 5-74 **Primary corneal squamous cell carcinoma** in a pug with pre-existent corneal cutaneous metaplasia.

has not been correlated with histologic criteria, but there is a correlation between site of origin and subsequent behavior. Most surveys in cattle identify the bulbar conjunctiva of the limbus as the most frequent site of origin, estimated at ~70% of all occurrences. Some surveys consider nictitating membrane as next most frequent, with palpebral conjunctiva of the true eyelid as third. Other reports claim nictitans origin to be uncommon, and eyelid tumors to be as common as those of limbic origin. Tumors arise only very rarely from the cornea because of the limited mitotic capability of that tissue. Apparent corneal tumors are almost always extensions from tumors arising at the limbus. Tumors arising at the limbus are confronted by the dense and poorly vascularized connective tissue of sclera and peripheral cornea, which retards metastasis to extraocular sites. Invasion of corneal stroma and sclera occurs slowly, but intraocular invasion is very uncommon (Fig. 5-73). Tumors arising from the nictitans extend to the root of the membrane and then to the cartilage and bone of the orbit and internal nares. *Metastasis probably will eventually occur in all instances,* with parotid lymph node the initial site. Wide dissemination to thoracic and abdominal organs has been reported and is probably limited only by the limited longevity of the target animals.

Squamous cell carcinoma of the **equine** eye is much less thoroughly documented, but is quite common. In contrast to cattle, *the preferred site is the edge of the third eyelid, followed by limbic bulbar conjunctiva.* This targeting is, again, inversely correlated with the presence of protective melanin pigmentation, and is positively correlated with those factors causing increased exposure to UV radiation. In some reports, heavy draft horses are predisposed, but all breeds may be affected. The mean age of affected horses is ~9 years. Bilateral involvement is seen in 15-20%. The same range of precancerous lesions occurs in horses as in cattle. Prognosis is strongly influenced by therapy, but even the untreated neoplasm is slow to metastasize, and even then it is usually only to local lymph nodes. Retrospective studies document 10-15% of equine ocular squamous cell carcinomas to have regional or distant spread, but the data do not consider duration of the disease prior to therapy.

In **cats**, *ocular squamous cell carcinoma most frequently affects the skin of the eyelids.* White cats are particularly susceptible, and squamous cell carcinomas in these animals may occur simultaneously or sequentially on eyelids, ear pinnae, nose, and lips. The early lesion is one of sunlight-induced epithelial necrosis, and even the early neoplasm may be ulcerated and inflamed to a degree that may mask its neoplastic character and delay appropriate therapy. Growth tends to be circumferential around the lid margins, resulting in a palpebral fissure bordered by a thickened, red, and ulcerated tumor. Metastasis to local lymph nodes occurs late in the course of the disease.

In **dogs**, *squamous cell carcinoma infrequently involves the eye.* Proliferative eyelid or conjunctival growths in dogs are much more likely to be Meibomian adenomas, viral and nonviral papillomas, or nodular granulomatous episcleritis. In one study of 202 canine eyelid neoplasms, squamous cell carcinoma accounted for only 2% of lesions. Primary corneal squamous cell carcinomas can arise within the hyperplastic epithelium of corneas transformed by chronic low-grade irritation into corneal cutaneous metaplasia. Most reported cases have been in brachycephalic breeds predisposed to chronic pigmentary keratitis (Fig. 5-74).

Further reading

Giuliano EA. Equine periocular neoplasia: current concepts in aetiopathogenesis and emerging treatment modalities. Equine Vet J Suppl 2010;37:9-18.

Newkirk KM, Rohrbach BW. A retrospective study of eyelid tumors from 43 cats. Vet Pathol 2009;46:916-927.

Meibomian adenoma

Meibomian adenoma is the most common ocular neoplasm of dogs, accounting for at least 70% of eyelid tumors. It is inexplicably rare in cats, and virtually nonexistent in other domestic species. It is comparable in many respects to sebaceous adenomas found elsewhere in the skin. However, these tumors originate specifically from Meibomian gland and not from other eyelid sebaceous glands, and have several distinctive histologic features that distinguish them from "ordinary" sebaceous adenomas. The similarities, however, are stronger than the differences. Like sebaceous adenomas elsewhere, they are

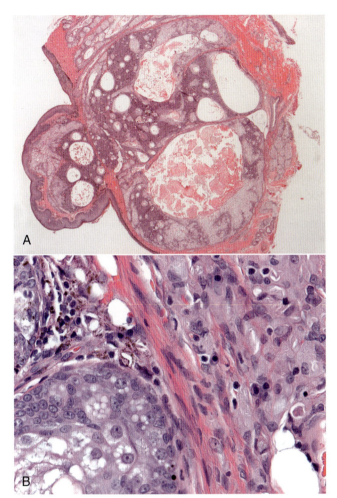

Figure 5-75 Meibomian adenoma. A. Purely expansile mixture of germinal basal cells and mature sebaceous cells occupies the tarsal plate at the eyelid margin, inducing a characteristic squamous papilloma in the overlying epithelium. **B.** Almost all Meibomian adenomas are surrounded by foamy macrophages typical of chalazion.

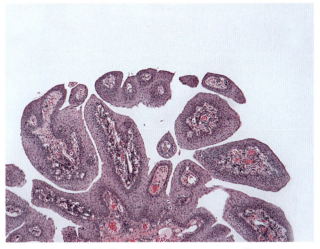

Figure 5-76 Conjunctival squamous papilloma.

formed by a purely expansile population of sebaceous lobules populated by variable proportions of germinal basal cells and more mature sebaceous cells (Fig. 5-75A). There is no prognostic significance to the wide range in the relative proportions of these 2 populations, and therefore no justification for dividing these very common tumors into Meibomian adenoma versus Meibomian epithelioma (the latter referring to those tumors with a "higher" proportion of basal cells). Behavioral malignancy is exceedingly rare. Features that are distinctive for Meibomian adenoma that are not seen in sebaceous adenomas elsewhere include the presence of lipid lakes and foamy macrophages around the periphery of the tumor, and papillary hyperplasia of the squamous epithelium at the eyelid margin overlying the tumor (Fig. 5-75B). Both of these secondary phenomena may actually be more prominent than the tumor itself. The accumulation of macrophages and lipid is known as *chalazion*. The macrophages may form multinucleated giant cells, and they contain distinctive clear split-like cytoplasmic inclusions that are unique to chalazion and not seen in the granulomatous reaction that may occasionally surround sebaceous adenomas found elsewhere in skin.

Other adnexal and conjunctival tumors

A wide range of neoplasms has been reported to occasionally affect the conjunctiva or adnexa of domestic animals. Most examples are reported primarily in dogs, and they are discussed in order of overall prevalence in that species.

Melanocytoma *is probably the second most common tumor of the eyelid in dogs.* It will occasionally occur in cats and in gray horses. In dogs, it is a typical cutaneous benign melanoma, identical to what occurs so frequently anywhere else in skin. In cats, they are also similar to those tumors occurring elsewhere in skin, and more than half are both histologically and behaviorally malignant. It is important to note that the behavior of melanocytic tumors associated with the eye is greatly influenced by exact anatomic location, so these comments are applicable only to those melanomas arising in the haired skin of the eyelid.

Other melanomas arising from conjunctiva and limbus are described later in the section on melanocytic tumors of the eye.

Conjunctival papilloma usually arises from bulbar conjunctiva as a series of slender protruding stalks of conjunctival lamina propria covered by bland, often pigmented, stratified squamous epithelium with no cytologic atypia and no ballooning degeneration, as is typical of viral papillomas (Fig. 5-76). Viral papillomas associated with canine oral papillomavirus, identical to those affecting the mouth, will occasionally occur in any portion of conjunctiva.

Conjunctival vascular tumors *represent a continuum from subepithelial preneoplastic telangiectasia to hemangioma and hemangiosarcoma.* They arise with equal frequency in the temporal (lateral) bulbar conjunctiva and along the leading edge of the third eyelid, suggesting that sunlight is important in their pathogenesis. Their prevalence increases dramatically in geographic regions with a lot of sunlight. They usually arise in the very superficial subepithelial vascular plexus. *There is virtually no metastatic risk* regardless of cytologic and histologic criteria of malignancy, but postoperative recurrence is common, probably because of de novo tumors forming from precancerous lesions elsewhere in the irradiated conjunctiva (Fig. 5-77). Behaviorally malignant examples seem more prevalent in horses, where more than half of the reported cases are solid hemangiosarcomas with very aggressive local infiltration and, usually, distant metastasis. They are easily mistaken

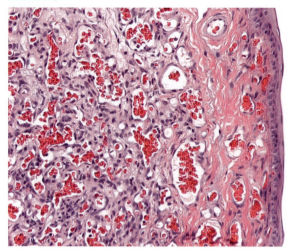

Figure 5-77 Primary conjunctival hemangioma affecting the leading edge of the third eyelid in a dog. Most of these are sunlight induced and may be multifocal and/or bilateral.

for fibrosarcomas because they have such poor channel formation and so little blood. Indeed, some of these might arise from lymphatic endothelium. There is much speculation, but no proof, that sunlight is important in their causation.

Mast cell tumors, with the same histologic range as those arising elsewhere in skin, may occur in the conjunctiva of dogs. Their biological behavior seems to correlate with the histologic grading validated for mast cell tumors in the skin. Most are well-differentiated, low-grade tumors. In cats, mast cell tumors more commonly arise within the haired skin of the eyelid, and in fact, they are the most common tumor of the feline eyelid.

Adenocarcinoma of the gland of the third eyelid occurs as a nodular swelling in very old dogs (mean age 11.5 years). They occur, albeit very rarely, in cats. *They are locally infiltrative, recur after attempted resection, but are cured by complete removal of the third eyelid.* Only chronically neglected cases metastasize to lung after a very protracted local expansion. Histologically, these are tubular carcinomas with abundant squamous metaplasia. They should not be confused with the prominence of the gland that occurs with prolapse of the gland ("cherry eye") or with lymphocytic interstitial adenitis.

Lymphoma may have several ocular manifestations, the most frequent of which are diffuse uveal metastases as part of generalized lymphoma in dogs or cats, or as retrobulbar tumor in cattle. It may occasionally occur as a conjunctival disease as part of generalized lymphoma or as a mucocutaneous manifestation of epitheliotropic lymphoma. There are several reports of conjunctival or third eyelid lymphoma occurring in horses and in cats as an apparently isolated lesion that can be cured by local excision, suggesting that they have actually arisen in those locations.

Further reading

Dreyfus J, et al. Superficial corneal squamous cell carcinoma occurring in dogs with chronic keratitis. Vet Ophthalmol 2011;14:161-168.
Fife M, et al. Canine conjunctival mast cell tumors: a retrospective study. Vet Ophthalmol 2011;14:153-160.
McCowan C, et al. Conjunctival lymphoma: immunophenotype and outcome in five dogs and three cats. Vet Ophthalmol 2014;17:351-357.
Pirie C, Dubielzig R. Feline conjunctival hemangioma and hemangiosarcoma: a retrospective evaluation of eight cases (1993-2004). Vet Ophthalmol 2006;9:227-231.
Pirie C, et al. Canine conjunctival hemangioma and hemangiosarcoma: a retrospective evaluation of 108 cases (1989-2004). Vet Ophthalmol 2006;9:215-226.
Schobert C, et al. Feline conjunctival melanoma: histopathological characteristics and clinical outcomes. Vet Ophthalmol 2010;13:43-46.

Melanocytic tumors of the eye

Melanocytic tumors affecting various portions of the globe and its adnexal structures are of such importance that they deserve a special section. The exact anatomic location exhibits a powerful influence on their prognosis. In brief, canine melanocytic tumors arising from the *eyelid margin* are benign tumors analogous in structure and function to ordinary dermal melanocytomas. Those arising from *conjunctiva* more closely resemble oral melanomas and are more likely to be histologically malignant, locally invasive, and prone to postoperative recurrence. Those arising specifically at the *limbus* are benign expansile lesions that are histologically indistinguishable from more common benign anterior uveal melanocytomas. Finally, benign *choroidal* melanocytomas occur only infrequently but are histologically and behaviorally identical to more common anterior uveal melanocytomas. The appearance and behavior of conjunctival and limbal melanocytic tumors in cats are very similar to those in dogs, but almost all intraocular melanocytic tumors in cats represent a specific histologic and behavioral entity known as *diffuse iris melanoma*.

In **horses,** one encounters cutaneous melanocytomas in the skin of the eyelids, primarily in gray horses. There are a few reports of benign anterior uveal melanocytomas, and one report of a locally invasive, histologically malignant conjunctival melanoma.

Melanomas arising in the conjunctiva *often are histologically and behaviorally malignant.* Conjunctival melanomas may appear as well-pigmented tumors of bland, plump melanocytes with little anisokaryosis or mitotic activity, or as cytologically malignant tumors with marked anisocytosis, anisokaryosis, hyperchromasia, and even multinucleation. Primary conjunctival melanomas often are poorly melanotic. The most reliable histologic criterion in such cases is the observation of intraepithelial nests of tumor cells. Local recurrence and spread after excision are more frequent than metastatic spread, but there are not enough reported cases to provide reliable statistics.

Limbal (epibulbar) melanocytoma *is a histologically and behaviorally benign tumor* of the melanocytes normally found in an oblique line (the limbus) that demarcates corneal stroma from the sclera. The tumor is composed of large plump melanocytes with a central nucleus and abundant cytoplasmic pigment, identical to the cells that populate more common benign anterior uveal melanocytomas. Mitotic figures are absent, and nuclear variation is minimal. The tumor grows outwardly as a protruding spherical nodule, hence the alternative name of *epibulbar melanoma*. There may be nodular expansion into peripheral cornea, but virtually never into the uvea or anterior chamber. **Anterior uveal melanocytoma** *is by far the most frequent intraocular tumor in dogs.* The typical tumor arises from stromal melanocytes of the iris root or adjacent ciliary body, and is composed of variable proportions of lightly pigmented spindle cells and heavily pigmented plump melanocytes identical to those of limbal melanomas. The spindle cells are assumed to be the proliferative population, and the plump cells probably represent the mature, end-stage melanocytes with a storehouse of cytoplasmic pigment (Fig. 5-78A-C).

The diagnosis itself presents no problem, but offering an accurate prognosis is more complex. About 15% of all canine anterior uveal melanocytomas are histologically malignant, and ⅓ of these (or ~5% of all uveal melanocytomas) have been confirmed to be behaviorally malignant by virtue of extraocular metastases. *This small group of genuine malignancies can be predicted by mitotic index.* Histologically, malignant tumors are dominated by the spindle cells rather than the plump cells, are more lightly pigmented, have much more anisokaryosis and more mitotic figures than the benign tumors. Of these, mitotic index is the most reliable predictor of behavior. Benign tumors have virtually no mitotic figures. Those confirmed as behaviorally malignant have 3 or more (usually many more!) mitoses in 10 high-power (400×) microscopic fields; conversely, not all tumors with high mitotic index are destined for metastasis.

Even these benign melanocytomas are eventually significant to the eye, spreading trans-sclerally and circumferentially within the globe. *Glaucoma* from occlusion of ciliary cleft is probably the eventual fate of all eyes with this neoplasm.

Feline multifocal uveal melanocytoma *is a rare tumor of cats* that looks histologically identical to the canine uveal melanocytomas. They are sufficiently different from the much more common diffuse iris melanoma of cats to justify a separate classification. There is no published information about metastatic risk. They seem to arise as multiple foci randomly throughout the uveal tract, expanding inwardly to create multiple nodules within the ocular cavities, and sometimes outwardly as space-occupying scleral nodules.

Equine anterior uveal melanocytomas occur most often in gray horses, many quite young (<8 years of age). Most involve anterior uvea and are histologically similar to the benign uveal melanocytomas of dogs. None has metastasized. Although almost all intraocular melanocytic tumors of cats are diffuse iris melanomas, one will occasionally encounter focal or **multifocal melanocytomas** similar to those of dogs. Other than having a more unpredictable site of origin within the uveal tract, they seem histologically and behaviorally identical to their more common canine counterparts.

Choroidal melanocytomas account for ~80% of all human ocular melanomas, but are rare in other species. The few cases described in dogs were discovered as incidental findings on fundoscopic examination, and grew very slowly. They seem very similar to the benign melanocytomas of limbus or anterior uvea: well pigmented, cytologically bland, and cause clinical signs only by their slow expansion to cause retinal detachment or compression of optic nerve. There is a single report of systemic metastasis from a tumor that looked histologically benign.

Clinically insignificant **iris nevi** or **freckles** occur in dogs as nonprogressive pigmented spots. Their only significance is to cause unnecessary enucleation. Histologically, the lesions are well-circumscribed clusters of bland melanocytes adjacent to the anterior border layer of the iris.

Feline diffuse iris melanomas are unique. The usual clinical presentation is of patchy iris hyperpigmentation that very slowly progresses to diffuse iris hyperpigmentation and thickening over several years. *The eventual outcome is virtually always glaucoma.* Histologically, these tumors begin as a proliferation of hyperchromatic, hyperpigmented melanocytes along the anterior border layer of the iris (Fig. 5-79A). *Over an interval that may be as long as 3-5 years, these cells diffusely infiltrate the stroma of the iris and the ciliary cleft, and then the overlying*

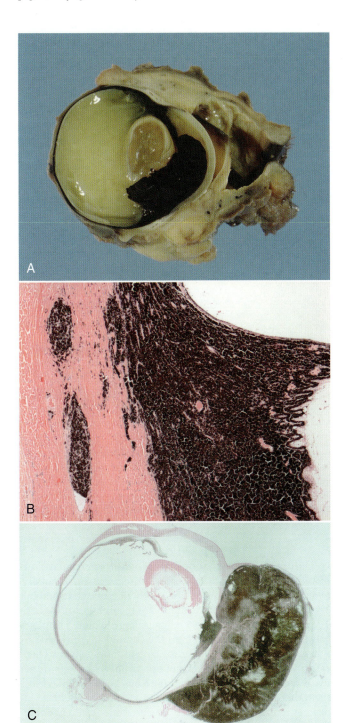

Figure 5-78 Canine uveal melanocytoma. **A.** Classic presentation as a solitary, heavily pigmented mass originating from the iris and expanding to fill half of the anterior chamber. **B.** Heavily pigmented, cytologically benign epithelioid melanocytes obliterate the trabecular meshwork and extend outwardly to surround blood vessels of the anterior sclera, but this is not predictive of metastatic spread. **C.** If left long enough, most will grow outwardly to cause a discrete protruding limbal mass.

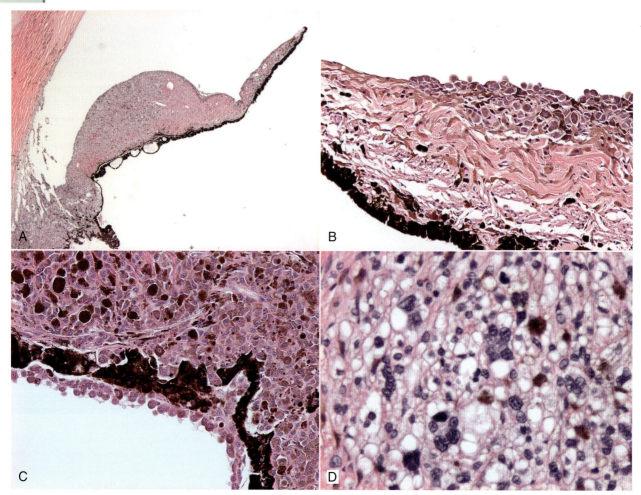

Figure 5-79 Feline diffuse iris melanoma. **A.** Low power illustrates the classic, very diffuse thickening of the iris that typically does not create a tumor "mass." Progression to this point may have taken many years. **B.** Early diffuse iris melanoma, originating (as usual) from the anterior border layer of the iris. **C.** More advanced diffuse iris melanoma with obliteration of iris architecture, including even the heavily pigmented posterior iris epithelium. **D.** The tumor cells are notoriously pleomorphic, often with poor pigmentation, multinucleation, anisokaryosis, and cytoplasmic ballooning.

sclera, peripheral cornea, and ciliary body. The tumor cells are notoriously pleomorphic, and are apt to be misdiagnosed by those pathologists not aware of this disease as malignant lymphoma or anaplastic metastatic malignancy. Tumor cells vary from spindle-shaped cells to multinucleated epithelioid cells (Fig. 5-79B-D). Pigmentation often is light, and the cytoplasm may be foamy and eosinophilic. Balloon cells with foamy cytoplasm and very distinct cell boundaries are frequent in some tumors. The accurate prediction of tumor behavior is compromised, in all published studies, by the low percentage of affected cats available for follow-up. Metastasis has been correlated with large tumor size and intrascleral spread. There remains a substantial gap between the prevalence of clinically significant metastatic disease and the presence of metastatic foci as detected by imaging or postmortem. It appears that the tumor foci within lung or other distant sites usually grow just as slowly as did the primary uveal tumor, and these cats rarely develop clinical signs of metastatic spread. There is no proof that early enucleation influences the risk of metastatic spread or the risk of metastatic disease.

Diffuse uveal melanocytosis *is included here because it is histologically indistinguishable from a diffuse uveal melanocytoma.* The syndrome was originally described as a bilateral but asymmetrical massive pigmentation of the uveal tract of Cairn Terrier dogs that seemed to be causing glaucoma. Histologically, the anterior uvea and even the choroid are thickened by a heavy, diffuse accumulation of large plump cells histologically indistinguishable from those of ordinary canine anterior uveal melanocytoma. The syndrome has been described in a few other breeds in association with glaucoma, but the syndrome remains controversial because one can encounter equally heavy pigmentation in clinically normal globes from breeds that typically have very heavy pigmentation, such as Kerry Blue Terriers, Scottish Terriers, black Labradors, and others. *The causal relationship between the pigmentation and glaucoma therefore remains somewhat controversial.* Some would prefer to refer to the disease as "canine diffuse uveal melanosis," or even as diffuse uveal melanocytoma. Original claims that these accumulating cells are abnormal melanocytes have been challenged by recent electron microscopy, indicating that the majority of the accumulating cells are melanin-laden macrophages. That is perhaps not surprising, and it does not rule out the possibility that this is indeed a melanocytic proliferative disorder that, over time, has had a lot of leakage of melanin and thus a lot of macrophage recruitment.

> **Key Points**
>
> **Canine ocular melanocytic tumors: location, location, location!**
> Histologically identical and completely benign melanocytomas originate in the skin at the eyelid margin, deep within the limbus, in the anterior uvea, and occasionally within the choroid.
> Locally invasive and potentially metastatic melanomas occur most commonly in bulbar conjunctiva, occasionally in other conjunctival locations, and rarely within the anterior uvea.

Further reading

Hyman JA, et al. Canine choroidal melanoma with metastases. Vet Ophthalmol 2002;5:113-117.

Labelle AL, Labelle P. Canine ocular neoplasia: a review. Vet Ophthalmol 2013;16:3-14.

Moore CP, et al. Conjunctival malignant melanoma in a horse. Vet Ophthalmol 2000;3:201-208.

Tumors of ocular neuroectoderm

These tumors include iridociliary epithelial tumors from mature anterior uveal neuroectoderm, and medulloepithelioma and retinoblastoma from embryonic neuroectoderm.

Iridociliary epithelial tumor (iridociliary adenoma, iridociliary carcinoma) is by far the most common of this group. Most examples are well-differentiated papillary or tubular adenomas arising from the nonpigmented inner layer of ciliary or iris epithelium (Fig. 5-80A). There are certainly examples in which the histologic and cytologic character is more primitive, but metastasis is so rare (if indeed it exists at all) that there is *no justification for diagnosing any of these tumors as iridociliary carcinomas.* Most originate from the pars plicata, but occasionally, the histologic evidence points to origin from posterior iris epithelium. The tumor cells usually resemble mature ciliary epithelium and usually have very little associated stroma. Nuclei are basilar, regular, and are surrounded by eosinophilic cytoplasm (Fig. 5-80B). The tumor cells are not pigmented, although melanophages are occasionally seen within tumor stroma. *They make an abundance of basal lamina,* oriented, as in normal ciliary epithelium, toward the inside of the eye. Its abundance, easily seen with PAS reagent, is useful in distinguishing ciliary tumors from carcinomas metastatic to the eye. Examples that have little tubular or papillary organization, or a more primitive cytologic character, may be difficult to recognize as being of iridociliary epithelial origin. They almost always retain abundant basement membrane production that can be accentuated with PAS staining. *The cells also stain for vimentin, S-100, and neuron-specific enolase, which makes them unique among tumors that otherwise look epithelial.* Such additional staining may occasionally be necessary to distinguish primitive iridociliary epithelial tumors from metastatic carcinomas.

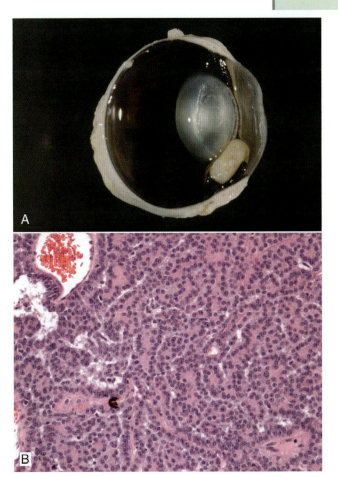

Figure 5-80 Iridociliary adenoma. **A.** Typical, discrete expansile white tumor growing into the posterior chamber. **B.** Orderly cord-like proliferation of mature cuboidal cells reminiscent of normal iridociliary epithelium. PAS stain will further accentuate the basement membranes, which are usually very prominent, helping to distinguish this tumor from the occasional well-differentiated metastatic carcinoma.

Even small iridociliary epithelial tumors may cause hyphema or glaucoma, attributed to this tumor's strong propensity to induce pre-iridal fibrovascular membranes. This is, presumably, the result of absorption through the porous anterior border layer of the iris of fibrovascular growth factors produced by the tumor cells in an effort to ensure their own survival. Iridociliary tumors are more likely to induce such neovascularization than is any other ocular disease.

Medulloepitheliomas and retinoblastomas *arise from the primitive neuroectoderm of the optic cup.* Only those examples that show at least focal maturation into recognizable photoreceptors are classified as retinoblastomas; the others, more or less by default, are classified as medulloepitheliomas. *This retinal differentiation is classically in the form of photoreceptor-like neuroblasts clustered around a central lumen. The apical portions of these neuroblasts are linked by terminal bars reminiscent of the outer limiting membrane of retina, and often have at least a hint of photoreceptor differentiation with positive staining for retinal S antigen.* Retinoblastoma is the second most frequent neoplasm of children, yet a critical review of the veterinary literature reveals only a few credible diagnoses of this tumor.

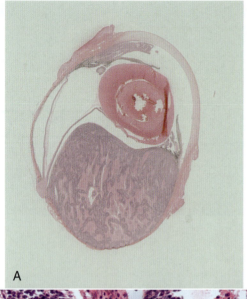
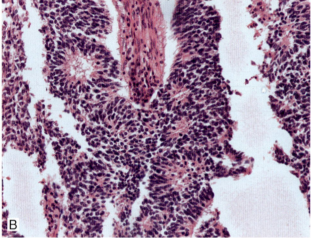

Figure 5-81 Medulloepithelioma in a 9-year-old dog. **A.** Low-power view of this long-standing, purely expansile tumor originating from embryonic neuroectoderm. **B.** Differentiation into primitive retinal rosettes illustrates the pluripotential neuroectodermal origin.

Conversely, *medulloepitheliomas* are rare in children, but many examples have been observed in animals, mainly in the *horse*, in which these are probably the *most common primary intraocular tumors*. Medulloepitheliomas may originate from any portion of embryonic neuroectoderm and may show differentiation into any neuroectodermal derivative, that is, retina, ciliary epithelium, vitreous, or neuroglia (Fig. 5-81A, B). The typical neoplasm is a loose network of branching cords of small basophilic neuroblasts resembling those of embryonic retina. Mitotic figures are numerous. The neuroblasts may form cords reminiscent of ciliary processes, or form primitive rosette-like structures around a lumen of fibrillar hyaluronic acid matrix reminiscent of vitreous. Many tumors also contain foci of cartilage, skeletal muscle, or brain tissue and are classified as *teratoid medulloepitheliomas*. Metastases are very rare, despite many of these being classified histologically as "malignant."

Further reading

Aleksandersen M, et al. Malignant teratoid medulloepithelioma with brain and kidney involvement in a dog. Vet Ophthalmol 2004;7: 407-411.

Regan DP, et al. Primary primitive neuroectodermal tumors of the retina and ciliary body in dogs. Vet Ophthalmol 2013;16(Suppl. 1): 87-93.

Other primary intraocular tumors

Feline post-traumatic sarcoma

This syndrome seems almost unique to cats, but there are 2 recent case reports in rabbits. This description is based on the disease as it occurs in cats. As the name implies, eyes subjected to trauma, especially penetrating injury, are prone to develop pleomorphic spindle cell sarcomas that destroy the globe and have substantial risk of metastasis. The interval between injury and observed tumor varies from 5 months to 11 years. Those skeptical about claiming such neoplasia to be the result of an injury 10 years previously prefer to call these tumors "primary ocular sarcomas," although such lag times are common in experimental models of carcinogenesis. The risk for injured eyes to develop sarcoma is unknown. Almost all recorded cases have perforated lenses. Most of these tumors appear to be fibrosarcomas, but some have a mixed epithelial-mesenchymal phenotype, and elaborate basement membrane–type matrix as well as express vimentin strongly. Based on immunopositivity for collagen type IV and crystallin alpha A, at least some of these tumors are of lens epithelial origin. Of relevance to ocular surgeons is the development of sarcomas in cat eyes receiving prosthetic lens implants, presumably viewed by the eye as just another form of unwanted lenticular trauma.

The tumor itself varies from fibrosarcoma to osteosarcoma to giant cell tumor, varying even within the same eye. The tumor tends to first surround the lens, then to line the inside of the eye, and finally to extend via scleral venous plexus or optic nerve to involve the orbit (Fig. 5-82A, B). *The inclination to "line the globe" is a repeatable feature that is useful in distinguishing primary ocular sarcoma from rare metastatic sarcomas.* Most cases are presented with advanced disease, and follow-up data to document the prevalence of metastasis are scant. Available evidence documents a metastatic risk of at least 60%, and, in many cases, there is remarkably rapid development of post-enucleation neurologic signs attributable to invasion of brain via the optic foramen.

Spindle cell tumor of blue-eyed dogs

A locally invasive spindle cell tumor tentatively identified as schwannoma, based on immunohistochemical reactivity, occurs within the iris of blue-eyed dogs (or in blue portions of dogs with multicolored irises). Most cases have been in Australian Shepherd dogs. The histologic features are identical to low-grade spindle cell tumors anywhere else. There is a single report of metastatic spread.

Further reading

Duke FD, et al. Metastatic uveal schwannoma of blue-eyed dogs. Vet Ophthalmol 2013;16(Suppl. 1):141-144.

Zarfoss MK, et al. Uveal spindle cell tumor of blue-eyed dogs: an immunohistochemical study. Vet Pathol 2007;44:276-284.

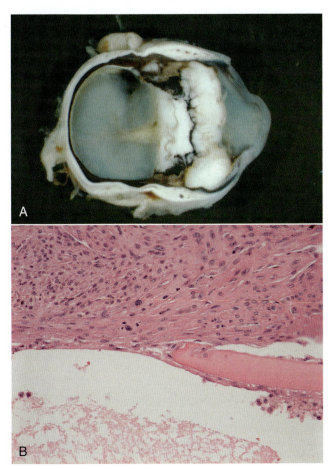

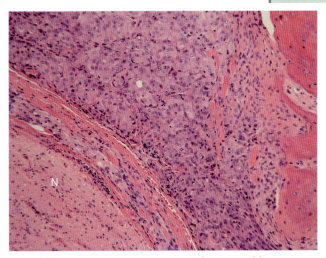

Figure 5-83 Optic nerve meningioma. These resemble meningiomas elsewhere, although often exhibiting particularly prominent "squamous" metaplasia as seen here. The osseous metaplasia is common. Almost all examples have perineural expansile growth limited to the interior of the cone created by the extraocular muscles, a growth habit so distinctive that these tumors can be diagnosed quite reliably with advanced imaging. N, optic nerve.

Figure 5-82 Post-traumatic sarcoma in a cat. A. Ruptured lens is surrounded by dense white proliferative tissue. B. Lens epithelium escaping through a rupture in the anterior lens capsule creates a proliferative plaque of pleomorphic fibroblast-like cells with hyperchromasia and nuclear gigantism.

Optic nerve tumors

Although the optic nerve and adjacent retina can presumably develop all of the neoplasms of the central nervous system (excepting those from tissues such as ependyma that are not present in the eye), documented examples are few indeed. Most are reported as individual case reports prior to the era of immunohistochemical markers that would have permitted more precise classification.

Optic nerve meningioma *has a distinctive macroscopic and histologic appearance.* It has been described only in dogs, although it will probably be seen in other species as we begin to look. The tumor probably arises from meningeal rests of arachnoid cells that project through the dura mater of the optic nerve into the orbital connective tissue. Tumors arising from these cells create a conical soft tissue mass that surrounds the optic nerve, but usually remains within the cone created by the extraocular muscles. Limited extension into the choroid or posterior vitreous through the optic nerve occurs only occasionally; more often, there is infiltration into the muscle and fat of the orbit. Most often, *the histologic appearance is of large stellate mesenchymal cells that can be confused with epithelial cells.* They have abundant glassy eosinophilic cytoplasm, and may or may not form the *characteristic swirling pattern* typical of central nervous system meningiomas in general (Fig. 5-83). Myxoid, chondroid, or even osseous metaplasia is quite common. Metastasis appears to be extremely infrequent.

Tumors published as **optic nerve astrocytomas** or as less specific "gliomas" were, in retrospect, *more likely to be examples of proliferative optic neuropathy* with the accumulation of reactive astrocytes and macrophages.

Primary orbital neoplasms

Tumors may be primary within the orbit, or arise by extension from adjacent structures or by hematogenous localization. They usually produce deviation or protrusion of the globe with secondary desiccation keratitis. Only those arising as primary tumors within the orbit are considered here. After saying that, *it is not always easy to decide whether the tumor is indeed primary or not*, and the decision is often made only after failure to find any credible primary tumor elsewhere. Of the primary orbital tumors reported in dogs and in horses, *sarcomas are much more prevalent than epithelial tumors.* The sarcomas are a bewildering array of locally infiltrative spindle cell tumors of unknown origin, with the abundance of diagnoses probably reflecting the diversity of pathologists' opinions rather than actual proof of histologic identity. Metastasis is rare, but their infiltrative growth habit in this difficult site makes eventual elective euthanasia a frequent outcome.

Among the primary sarcomas, the only ones deserving specific consideration because of a distinctive histologic appearance are *multilobular osteochondrosarcomas* and *optic nerve meningiomas.* The latter were described in the preceding section. The **multilobular osteochondrosarcomas** arise from the aponeuroses between adjacent bones of the orbit, and are identical in appearance and behavior to this tumor arising elsewhere in the canine skull.

Most primary epithelial tumors of the canine orbit are **lacrimal adenocarcinomas,** *which are locally invasive, recur after attempted resection, but which apparently have little metastatic potential.* In truth, there is so little follow-up information about these uncommon tumors that any statement about metastatic risk is premature. Both adenoma and nodular hyperplasia occur, but seem much less frequent than the malignant tumors. Tumors infiltrating the orbit from the nearby *zygomatic salivary gland* are similar histologically and behaviorally to lacrimal adenocarcinomas. They can sometimes be distinguished on the basis of location alone, but it is also helpful that the zygomatic gland is a mixed salivary gland with a prominent mucinous component that may be retained in well-differentiated tumors. The lacrimal gland is purely serous.

Primitive neuroepithelial tumors of unknown origin are occasionally seen in young dogs and in horses. They are composed of nests, cords, and rosette-like structures formed by small hyperchromatic neuroblastic cells with a very high mitotic index. Very rapid spread throughout the orbit and into brain occurs in affected dogs, but the extremely sparse information on these tumors in horses (4 cases in 2 reports) suggest that they may be much less aggressive in horses than in dogs.

Tumors metastatic within the globe and orbit

The list of tumors that may be found as metastatic localizations within the globe or orbit is the same as any list of metastatic neoplasms in general. Any estimates of prevalence are unreliable because the globe is not routinely investigated in animals dying from disseminated malignancy. *Most of the reported cases are carcinomas,* simply because carcinomas are more likely to undergo hematogenous dissemination than are sarcomas, with the round cell "lymphoreticular" malignancies being a notable exception. In dogs, the most common are probably transitional cell carcinomas and mammary carcinomas, whereas, in cats, mammary adenocarcinoma and bronchial adenocarcinomas are probably the most prevalent. Across all species, however, malignant lymphoma is undoubtedly at the top of the list both as an intraocular and as an orbital metastatic tumor.

Further reading

Bell C, et al. Diagnostic features of feline restrictive orbital myofibroblastic sarcoma. Vet Pathol 2011;48:742-750.
Mombaerts I, et al. What is orbital pseudotumor? Surv Ophthalmol 1996;41:66-78.
Regan DP, et al. Clinicopathologic findings in a dog with a retrobulbar meningioma. J Vet Diagn Invest 2011;23:857-862.

EAR

Bradley L. Njaa

GENERAL CONSIDERATIONS

Although dogs and cats and other animals have been used as model systems for human otic disease, much of the published information on these studies has laid dormant, rarely referenced in the veterinary literature. In recent decades, the importance of and better understanding of otic disease and anatomy has expanded with the inclusion of various diagnostic modalities, such as advanced imaging techniques, behavioral studies, histologic investigations, and the use of brain auditory-evoked responses (BAER) as well as newer more sophisticated measures of hearing. This has led to an expanding repository of ear-related publications in domestic animal species that include a renewed understanding of a wide range of conditions that include deafness as a discerning clinical feature, an expanding list of causes of peripheral vestibular disease, middle ear conditions related to vestibulocochlear and/or facial nerve deficits, and an ever-expanding group of dermatologic, pinna-associated conditions.

Part of the dearth of reports on the pathology of the ear in the veterinary literature may be the result of the perception that hearing remains secondary or tertiary to the senses of sight and smell, which are considered of greater functional importance in domestic animals. Yet, prevention of predation and the advent of domestic animals functioning as working companions for the hearing-impaired necessitate a greater understanding of otic anatomy as well as function and dysfunction. Of equal or greater significance is the requisite time and effort required to properly prepare and process internal and middle ear portions for histologic examination. Because the ear is a complex amalgam of an osseous encasement, articulated sound-transducing ossicles, delicate sensory epithelium, complex innervation, fluid-filled and air-filled compartment interfaces, and skin-covered auricular cartilage and bone, a typical "complete" autopsy frequently excludes gross examination and rarely progresses to histologic evaluation. Even when all signs point to cochlear, vestibular, or middle ear maladies, many publications, regrettably, exclude or merely include limited investigation.

To follow is a discussion of the pertinent anatomic features of the various compartments and structures of the ear, as well as methods to aid and encourage processing and investigation. This highly specialized sensory organ will be divided into its 3 functional domains: internal, middle, and external ear. Although this compartmentalization is anatomically and functionally useful, conditions with domain overlap will be clarified in the text. This section is not exhaustive but highlights the majority of conditions reported in domestic animals.

INTERNAL EAR

Originating as bilaterally symmetrical embryonic ectoderm placodes at the level of the myelencephalon, internal ear primordia invaginate to form the otic vesicle (otocyst) around day 22 post fertilization in the dog (corresponding days for various species: 15, cat; 17, pig; 18, sheep; 23, cattle; 21, horses). The ectoderm will become the endolymphatic compartments, and the surrounding mesenchyme-derived cartilaginous otic capsule eventually becomes the bony labyrinth of the ossified petrous portion of the temporal bone.

The **bony labyrinth** (the space within the petrous portion of the temporal bone housing the membranous labyrinth) of the internal ear can be divided into 3 interconnected compartments: the rostral cochlea, the middle vestibule, and the caudal semicircular canals. (*Auris interna* means "internal ear," and is more correct than the more commonly used inner ear.) The perilymph-filled space of the cochlea comprises the *scala vestibuli* and *scala tympani*, which connect at the apical end via the *helicotrema*, surround the *vestibular sacculus and utriculus* and the 3 *semicircular canals* subdivided by numerous fine trabeculae, and finally communicate via the perilymphatic duct near the base of the cochlea with the subarachnoid space. Perilymph is a distillate of serum with similar ionic characteristics.

The **membranous labyrinth** is an endolymph-filled, epithelial-lined, otic vesicle–derived, ductular system that

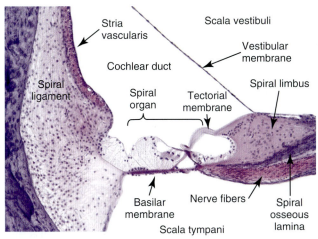

Figure 5-84 The **normal membranous and bony labyrinth** from a healthy cat. The vestibular membrane extends from the outer spiral ligament to the inner spiral osseous lamina, forming the partition between the cochlear duct and scala vestibuli. The basilar membrane is a flexible membrane that spans between the spiral osseous lamina and spiral ligament, forming the partition between the cochlear duct and scala tympani. The spiral organ rests atop the basilar membrane and outer portion of the spiral osseous lamina. (Courtesy G. Pagonis, Massachusetts Eye and Ear Infirmary.)

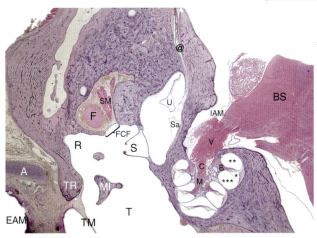

Figure 5-85 A mid-modiolar section through the cochlea, vestibule, tympanic cavity, and external acoustic meatus of a **normal cat.** *, cochlear duct; **, scala tympani; ***, scala vestibuli; @, endolymphatic sac; *A*, auricular cartilage; *B*, basal turn of the cochlea; *BS*, brainstem; *C*, cochlear branch of the vestibulocochlear nerve; *EAM*, external acoustic meatus; *F*, facial nerve; *FCF*, facial canal foramen; *IAM*, internal acoustic meatus; *M*, modiolus; *MI*, malleus and incus; *R*, epitympanic recess; *S*, stapes; *Sa*, sacculus; *SM*, stapedius muscle; *T*, tympanic cavity; *TM*, tympanic membrane; *TR*, tympanic ring; *U*, utriculus; *V*, vestibulocochlear nerve. (Courtesy G. Pagonis, Massachusetts Eye and Ear Infirmary.)

includes the cochlear duct rostrally, which connects basally to the sacculus via the reuniens duct. The utriculosaccular duct is a narrow connection between the utriculus and sacculus from which the endolymphatic duct (Fig. 5-84) extends through the vestibular aqueduct of the petrous portion of the temporal bone into the dura mater of the caudal cranial fossa. Finally, the modestly dilated ampullae of each semicircular canal that houses the sensory portion is connected directly with the utriculus.

Sandwiched between the scala vestibuli and scala tympani is the triangular *cochlear duct* (scala media) encased in a bony *otic capsule*. Spiraling rostrally and ventrally from the vestibule, these melded cavities wind around a central osseous axis known as the *modiolus*. The number of turns is species dependent: sheep, 2.25; horses, 2.5; cat, 3; dogs, 3.25; cattle, 3.5. Within the central modiolar bony cavity lies the cochlear portion of the *vestibulocochlear nerve*. The *spiral osseous lamina* is a bony shelf of the modiolus that is morphologically similar to the thread of a screw and through which courses the spiral ganglion and nerve fibers that innervate the sensory cells of the spiral organ (organ of Corti) (Fig. 5-85). The cochlear duct ends blindly at the apex in the cupula; however, in this region, the scala vestibuli and scala tympani meet via the helicotrema. Toward the basal end, the scala vestibuli is connected to the *vestibular window* (oval window) that houses the stapes, whereas the scala tympani terminates in the cochlear window (round window) across which is a thin membrane. Basally, the cochlear duct also ends bluntly but maintains a small ductular connection with the sacculus via the reuniens duct.

The stria vascularis aligns along the inner surface of the spiral ligament of the cochlea located along the outer edge of the cochlear turns (see Fig. 5-84). It spans from the spiral prominence adjacent to the basilar membrane to the *vestibular (Reissner's) membrane*. True to its name, it is richly vascularized and composed of at least 3 functional layers: *marginal cells, intermediate cells, and basal cells*. Marginal cells are mitochondria-rich, otic vesicle–derived epithelial cells that line the inner edge of the stria. Specialized apical membrane channels represent the source for potassium found in high concentration in endolymph. Intermediate cells are neural crest–derived melanocytes that play a critical role in recycling potassium retrieved through a complex network of critical membrane pumps and epithelial and mesenchymal cells interconnected by gap junctions. Thus certain breed-associated hearing dysfunction conditions in animals with phenotypic pigment alterations are related to defective intermediate cell function in the stria vascularis. Finally, the basal cells maintain a barrier via tight junctions between the intrastrial space and the perilymph.

Endolymph is a unique extracellular fluid because its predominant cation is potassium, and its electrical potential is positive by 90 mV relative to the perilymph. Maintenance of this high electrical and ionic potassium potential requires a properly functioning stria vascularis. Part of the maintenance requires competent tight junctions anchoring the apical domains of the epithelium that line the cochlear duct. Any loss of this energy-costly electrical potential gradient or failure to maintain high ionic potassium will result in hearing impairment, vestibular dysfunction, or both.

Spanning between the osseous spiral lamina and the spiral ligament is the *basilar membrane*, upon which sits the spiral organ and which separates the cochlear duct from the scala tympani (Fig. 5-86). Specialized *sensory hair cells* and supporting cells complexly align to form this unique sensory structure. The spiral limbus is a thick tuft of interdental cells that overlays the osseous spiral lamina, which terminates toward the modiolus near the modiolar terminus of the vestibular membrane. Extending from the surface of the spiral limbus is a

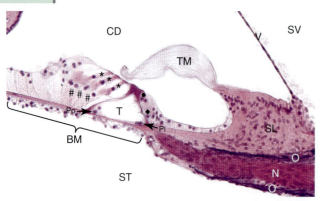

Figure 5-86 Both inner and outer hair cells are the **sensory cells of the spiral organ** from this healthy cat with normal hearing. Sound energy is transformed into fluid waves in the scala vestibuli as a result of oscillating movements of the stapes in the vestibular window. Scala vestibular fluid waves result in deflection of the basilar membrane in the region of the cochlea corresponding to the resonant frequency of the incoming sound, causing hair cell apical stereocilia to deflect, depolarize, and transmit to the auditory portions of the brainstem and auditory cortex. *, outer hair cells; #, outer phalangeal cells; •, inner hair cells; ♦, inner phalangeal cells; *BM*, basilar membrane; *CD*, cochlear duct; *N*, nerve fibers; *O*, osseous spiral lamina; *Pi*, inner pillar cells; *Po*, outer pillar cells; *SL*, spiral limbus; *ST*, scala tympani; *SV*, scala vestibuli; *T*, inner tunnel; *TM*, tectorial membrane; *V*, vestibular membrane. (Courtesy G. Pagonis, Massachusetts Eye and Ear Infirmary.)

gelatinous structure, the *tectorial membrane*, which overlays the hair cells of the spiral organ. This membrane comprises collagen proteins (types II, V, IX, XI), produced by the cells of the developing spiral organ that eventually regress, and various glycoproteins (otogelin, α-tectorin, β-tectorin) produced by limbal cells, resulting in a striated mosaic in which outer hair cell stereocilia are embedded.

Sensory hair cells are specialized epithelium with apical stereocilia that alter membrane polarization in response to fluid-wave–induced deflection or bending. Inner hair cells form a single row of cells that are closest to the osseous spiral lamia of the modiolus (see Fig. 5-86). Depending on the species, 3-5 rows of outer hair cells overlie the basilar membrane, all extending the length of the cochlea and representing 75-80% of the sensory cell population in the cochlea. Between the inner and outer hair cells is the *inner tunnel* (tunnel of Corti) formed by the *inner and outer pillar cells*. These cells align such that they have interlocked heads nearest the tectorial membrane but broader feet that are in contact with the basilar membrane, forming a triangular tunnel. These cells contain networks of microtubules conferring a region of rigidity. The inner edge of the inner pillar cell is in close apposition to the spiral osseous lamina and is the functional fulcrum for basilar membrane deflection. Outer hair cells align adjacent to the outer pillar cells and have basal support from *outer phalangeal cells* (Deiters' cells) containing structural microtubules and microfilaments that provide rigidity. Outer phalangeal cells fittingly have a phalangeal process that provides support to outer hair cells through apical tight junctions. Several other epithelial and supporting cells function in part to facilitate potassium recycling through gap junctions and also via tight junctions to maintain the electrical and potassium potential in endolymph.

Spiral ganglion cells are the cell bodies of bipolar neurons located within the spiral osseous lamina of the modiolus that provide afferent innervation to the cochlea. Nerve fibers extend through the habenula perforata of the spiral osseous lamina to synapse with the hair cells. From 10-30 afferent nerve fibers synapse with the inner hair cells, and in all mammals, inner hair cells synapse with 90-95% of afferent cochlear nerve fibers. Conversely, very few afferent nerve fibers make contact with outer hair cells, with one nerve synapsing groups of 10-20 outer hair cells. However, numerous efferent nerve fibers from the trapezoid nuclear complex synapse with the outer hair cells.

The caudal ⅔ of the petrous portion of the temporal bone is for *peripheral vestibular function*. Both the sacculus and utriculus are endolymph compartments within the vestibule that contain sensory maculae oriented in vertical and horizontal planes, respectively. Sensory cells are hair cells, types I and II, similar to those in the spiral organ, with the addition of a single kinocilium. Overlying the macular hair cells is the otolithic membrane composed of *otoconia* or *otoliths* embedded in a glycosaminoglycan matrix. Otoconia are organic crystals composed of calcium carbonate and various other inorganic elements. Degeneration of otoconia via aging, disease, or intoxication can lead to peripheral vestibular dysfunction.

Semicircular canals connect directly with the utriculus, each oriented perpendicular to each other, representing 3 spatial planes: anterior (vertical), posterior, and lateral (horizontal) canals. The lateral canal connects to the utriculus at both ends, one ampullated, one not, whereas only the ampullated ends of both the anterior and posterior canals attach to the utriculus, but the nonampullated ends join to form a common crus that communicates with the utriculus. Ampullated connections are dilated regions composed of the osseous ampullae representing the bony labyrinth of the vestibular system and the endolymph-filled membranous labyrinth. The sensory structures in the membranous labyrinth are semilunar cristae that contain apical hair cells overlaid by a gelatinous cupula. Nerve fibers of the vestibular portion of cranial nerve (CN) VIII penetrate the maculae cribrosae to synapse with the hair cells.

Sensory cells are *hair cells, types I and II*, similar to those in the spiral organ, with the addition of a single *kinocilium* per cell in addition to numerous stereocilia. The kinocilium is the only apical appendage that is a true cilium with appropriate microtubule arrangements. Stereocilia are in descending lengths moving from the kinocilia. Central to the maculae is the *striola*, which represents an axis in which hair cells reverse their orientation; kinocilia are polarized away from the axis. Bending of apical hair cell bundles toward the kinocilium is excitatory, whereas movement away from the kinocilium is inhibitory.

The *vestibulocochlear nerve* enters the internal acoustic meatus of the petrous portion of the temporal bone along with the *facial nerve*. The cochlear portion of CN VIII courses rostrally and enters the central core of the modiolus of the cochlea, whereas the vestibular portion of the vestibulocochlear nerve courses caudally, with branches innervating the utriculus, sacculus, and 3 ampullated cristae. The facial nerve courses through the facial canal, exiting through the stylomastoid foramen caudal to the osseous external acoustic meatus and dorsal to the tympanic bulla, with the chorda tympani coursing through the middle ear and crossing the medial surface of the tympanic membrane and a stapedial branch that innervates the stapedius muscle.

Further reading

Evans HE, de Lahunta A. The ear. In: Evans HE, de Lahunta A, editors. Miller's Anatomy of the Dog. 4th ed. St Louis: Elsevier; 2013. p. 731-745.

Hearing and the internal ear

Tympanic membrane vibrations from sound energy produce inward movements of the stapes into the perilymph of the scala vestibuli. Because the bony labyrinth scalae form a singular closed fluid compartment connected to the cochlear window at the terminal end of the scala tympani, the magnitude of the inward deviation of the stapes is matched by the outward bulging of the cochlear window. An extremely thin vestibular membrane separates the scala vestibuli from the cochlear duct, and stapes movements cause fluid waves in the scala vestibuli to directly transmit to the cochlear duct with minimal deviation. However, the flexible basilar membrane that forms the base of the cochlear duct pivots in response to the fluid wave.

Extending the full length of the cochlear duct, the basilar membrane is narrow and thick at the base of the cochlea, becoming wider and thinner toward its apex. *This progressive basilar membrane variation corresponds to how the ear is tuned to sound;* high-frequency sounds are detected in the basal turns of the cochlea and low frequencies toward the apex. In other words, low-frequency sound energy travels through the perilymph of the scala vestibuli toward the apex and only deflects the portion of the basilar membrane with a corresponding resonant frequency, whereas higher-frequency sounds vibrate the basilar membrane in the more basilar portion of the cochlea. The length of the basilar membrane then determines the frequency range of sound detection for any particular species. Similarly, cochlear hair cells and associated ganglion cells are tonotopically organized such that these neurons and hair cells are "tuned" to the resonant frequency based on their location in the cochlea and their corresponding dorsal region of the ectosylvian gyrus in the auditory cortex, where high-frequency sound detection is rostral and lower-frequency sound detection is more caudal.

Sound detection within the internal ear begins as fluid waves deflect the basilar membrane corresponding to the sound frequency. Fluid vibrations cause stiff stereocilia to pivot at their narrowed points of the connection with the apical plasma membrane. Specialized tip links, composed of cadherin 23 and protocadherin 15, connect tips of stereocilia that progressively decrease in height to lateral membrane transduction channels of taller adjacent stereocilia. Tension or relaxation of the tip link–related deflection of stereocilia toward or away from their taller neighbors results in opening or closing of the transduction channels. Open channels favor rapid "downhill" influx of K^+ and Ca^{2+} into the hair cell cytoplasm because of the extremely high K^+ ionic content and the strong electrical potential gradient between endolymph and intracellular fluid.

The basolateral membrane of inner hair cells is coupled to numerous afferent synapses. Up to 200 synaptic vesicles containing glutamate congregate near these synaptic ribbons. Depolarized inner hair cell neurotransmitters released at synaptic ribbons bind to glutamate receptors and produce postsynaptic action potentials. This translates into detection of sound in the auditory cortex as well as the important reflex arc for the acoustic reflex.

Outer hair cells have a fraction of the afferent nerve fibers relative to inner hair cells but receive significant efferent innervation. Fluid-wave deflections lead to depolarization of outer hair cells as described previously, but are directly related to tectorial membrane movement within which outer hair cell apical stereocilia are embedded. Unique to the outer hair cells is the ability to lengthen and shorten through voltage-dependent conformational change of a membrane protein, prestin, related to binding or release of chloride anions. This size variation is termed *electromotility*, whereby outer hair cells are essentially small cellular motors that fluctuate their linear length. Inner hair cells and vestibular hair cells lack this electromotility. Functionally, *outer hair cells are part of a feedback loop*. Sound-induced afferent neural traffic to the brainstem trapezoid nuclei return efferent signals to modify outer hair cell shape and responsiveness, serving to amplify or dampen sound detected by inner hair cells and help acoustically tune incoming sound to the appropriate region of the cochlea.

Further reading

Pickles JO. An Introduction to the Physiology of Hearing. 4th ed. Bingley, UK: Emerald Group Publishing; 2014. p. 25-153.

Hearing impairment

The complex physiology of hearing briefly presented previously highlights several potential avenues for dysfunction. Globally, *hearing dysfunction is congenital or acquired*. Further, hearing dysfunction is subclassified as *sensorineural or conductive*. Dysfunction or disease of the cochlea and its neural connections broadly defines sensorineural hearing impairment, whereas anatomic and functional impairment of the ossicular chain, tympanic membrane, and external acoustic meatus encompass conductive hearing dysfunction.

Congenital hearing impairment

Storage diseases. A number of lysosomal storage diseases are reported in domestic animals. **Mucopolysaccharidoses (MPS)** represent a group of mostly autosomal recessive hereditary diseases that comprise a range of defects in glycosaminoglycan metabolism. **MPS I** is reported in dogs and cats, and disease is related to *deficiency of α-L-iduronidase*. Internal ear lesions in dogs include vacuolation of the intermediate cells and perivascular macrophages in the stria vascularis, basilar membrane mesenchymal cells, fibroblasts of spiral ligament and limbus, scala tympani lining cells, vestibular membrane cells, spiral ganglia, and macrophages within the cochlear nerve. Additionally, ossicular osteocytes and chondrocytes are markedly enlarged relative to cytoplasmic vacuoles, and there is bony deformation. Finally, the middle lamina of the tympanic membrane is thickened because of vacuolated macrophages. Brain auditory-evoked responses (BAER) testing confirms that hearing impairment is sensorineural and retrocochlear (beyond the inner ear in neural pathways and nuclei).

MPS II is the only X-linked disease related to iduronate-2-sulfate sulfatase deficiency and associated with deafness in people. It was reported in a male Labrador Retriever; however, hearing was not assessed and ears were not examined.

MPS VII has been reported in dogs from accumulation of glycosaminoglycan residues with terminally β-linked glucuronic acid. *Deficiency of lysosomal enzyme β-glucuronidase* is associated with external, middle, and internal ear lesions. External ear canals were markedly stenotic and tympanic membranes thickened, related to mononuclear infiltration and hyperkeratosis. Auricular ossicles have enlarged, vacuolated osteocytes and chondrocytes, and are encased in mesenchyme along with marked, chronic otitis media with macrophage and lymphocyte infiltration. The mucoperiosteum was markedly thickened. In aggregate, these restrictive middle ear lesions result in conductive hearing loss. Internal ear changes included vacuolar changes in marginal and basal cells of the stria vascularis, fibroblasts of spiral limbus, and spiral ligament and scala tympani lining cells. No cochlear lesions were observed.

β-Mannosidosis has been thoroughly described in Nubian goats and Salers calves because of *congenital lysosomal β-mannosidase deficiency*. Pinnae are bilaterally abnormally positioned and shaped. Tympanic bullae are smaller in both, depicting abnormal luminal projections in goats with a thickened mucoperiosteum that contains vacuolated fibroblasts. Most of the mesenchymal and epithelial cells of the scala and cochlear ducts, including the spiral organ as well as spiral ganglia, were abnormal because of distorting cytoplasmic vacuoles. Vacuolated macrophage infiltration was reported only in the Nubian goats. BAER testing confirmed sensorineural deafness in the goats, whereas testing in the calves depicted normal peaks temporally delayed. Initial descriptions of the disease in veterinary species preceded its eventual identification in people by several years.

Further reading

Hordeaux J, et al. Histopathologic changes of the ear in canine models of mucopolysaccharidosis types I and VII. Vet Pathol 2011;48:616-626.

Render JA, et al. The ocular and otic pathology of bovine β-mannosidosis. J Vet Diagn Invest 1992;4:96-98.

Suzuki K, Suzuki K. Lysosomal diseases. In: Graham DI, Lantos PL, editors. Greenfield's Neuropathology, vol. 1. 7th ed. London: Arnold; 2002. p. 653-735.

Hereditary deafness. Certain pigmentary phenotypes of hair coat and eye color have been linked to deafness. Pigmented neural crest–derived intermediate cells are considered important for the stria vascularis to function normally. Classic early investigation of deaf Collies and Dalmatians in 1948 determined *diminished pigment in strial intermediate cells*. The spectrum of lesions often involves both the cochlea and sacculus and is thus termed **cochleosaccular degeneration** or *Scheibe-type deafness*. Cochlear lesions include cochlear duct collapse with a vestibular membrane that remains intact; stria vascularis atrophy in all turns, with loss of capillaries and diminished melanin; abnormal texture or location of the tectorial membrane; degeneration of pillar cells, hair cells, and potentially phalangeal cells; and cochlear nerve and ganglion cell atrophy that lags behind hair cell degeneration (Fig. 5-87). Saccular collapse ranges from partial to complete and is most pronounced in close proximity to the cochlear window. The macular neuroepithelium of the sacculus degenerates, as does the saccular nerve. However, maculae and cristae of the utriculus and semicircular ampullae, respectively, remain morphologically normal.

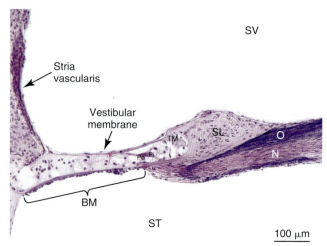

Figure 5-87 A young deaf puppy with **sensorineural deafness**, depicting complete collapse of the cochlear duct. The vestibular membrane is in close apposition to the markedly atrophic stria vascularis. Pillar cells are present but severely atrophic. The spiral organ is complete distorted with loss of outer and inner hair cells and jumbling of the phalangeal cells. The tympanic membrane is in an abnormal location and smaller than normal. Pillar cells are intact but also markedly atrophic. *BM*, basilar membrane; *N*, nerve fibers; *O*, osseous spiral lamina; *SL*, spinal limbus; *ST*, scala tympani; *SV*, scala vestibuli; *TM*, tectorial membrane. (Courtesy G. Pagonis, Massachusetts Eye and Ear Infirmary.)

Cochleosaccular degeneration is confirmed in *blue-eyed white cats*, as well as various *dog* breeds: Australian Cattle dogs, Australian Sheepdogs, Border Collies, Bull Terriers, Norwegian Dunkers, West Highland White Terriers, Great Danes, Great Pyrenees, Louisiana Catahoula Cattle dogs, Old English Sheepdogs, Maltese, and Dachshunds. This mechanism is presumed in *alpacas and llamas* with pure white hair coats and blue irides, proven deaf by BAER, however, not yet confirmed with histopathology. Functionally, defective or inadequate strial intermediate cells translate into failure to maintain normal endolymph necessary for proper mechanotransduction of fluid waves into sound recognition.

A different form of deafness known as **neuroepithelial degeneration** has been reported in Dobermans, a Rottweiler, and "nervous Pointer dogs." In Dobermans, all cochleae examined histologically displayed *progressive degeneration of the spiral organ*. Most dramatic were shrunken outer hair cells, with loss of or abnormal stereocilia becoming splayed, fused, or clubbed. Beginning in the middle turn by 11 weeks, most outer hair cells degenerate, and the defect is filled by the expanded surface of phalangeal processes of outer phalangeal cells. Steadily, inner hair cells and pillar cells were lost followed by loss of nerve fibers and spiral ganglia. Lesions were not observed in stria vascularis or vestibular membranes. Similarly, severe *bilateral spiral organ and spiral ganglion degeneration* is reported in the Rottweiler, with spiral ganglion changes occurring earlier and being more severe than in Dalmatians. Also, inner hair cells were more severely affected than outer hair cells. The cochlear duct did not collapse. Likewise, nervous Pointer dogs have lesions confined to the spiral organ and spiral ganglion, with the apical turn preferentially spared. The most severely affected depicted an estimated 70-90% loss of neurons in the basal turn. Abnormalities are not identified in the stria vascularis.

Deafness in Paint horses has been investigated, and BAER testing confirms a strong correlation with particular phenotypes. One group has confirmed that most deaf horses have splashed white or splashed white-frame blend coat patterns. All horses had extensive white markings to the head, most commonly designated as bald, apron, or bonnet face. Similarly, all horses had prominent white markings involving 2 or more limbs. Every deaf horse had at least 1 partially heterochromic iris, with most having 2 blue irides and partial nonpigmentation of palpebral skin. Endothelin B receptor *(EDNBR)* gene mutations were confirmed in 31 of 34 deaf horses. *EDNBR* gene mutation is also associated with the overo lethal white foal syndrome.

Otosclerosis is a hereditary disorder of endochondral ossification of the otic capsule in people, with no comparable animal model. Bony remodeling and new bone formation in the otic capsule is most clinically evident as conduction hearing dysfunction when the vestibular window is involved. The excess bone results in ankylosis of the stapediovestibular joint, which prevents ossicular transmission of sound energy to the internal ear. Speculation exists for an infectious etiology related to measles infection in people.

Further reading

Aleman M, et al. Brainstem auditory evoked responses in an equine patient population: part I—adult horses. J Vet Intern Med 2014; 28:1310-1317.

Magdesian KG, et al. Evaluation of deafness in American Paint horses by phenotype, brainstem auditory-evoked responses, and endothelin receptor B genotype. J Am Vet Med Assoc 2009;235:1204-1211.

Strain G. Deafness prevalence and pigmentation and gender associations in dog breeds at risk. Vet J 2006;167:23-32.

Acquired deafness

Otitis interna or *labyrinthitis* is most commonly linked to concurrent otitis media (eFig. 5-1). Bacteria are most commonly cultured from the inflamed tympanic cavity or from the cranial cavity following penetration through the internal acoustic meatus. The cochlear window in cats was investigated as the most plausible region for spread of middle ear infection to the internal ear. Initially, permeability was increased, but with chronicity, the permeability decreased. In swine, suppurative otitis media most commonly caused by β-hemolytic streptococci resulted in neutrophilic infiltration of the cochlea, sacculus, and utriculus, but lacked widespread infiltration into the osseous labyrinth.

Canine distemper virus has been implicated as a cause of labyrinthitis that likely penetrates the membranous labyrinth via a hematogenous route. Inclusion bodies are observed in the cells in the middle and internal ear. Rarely, fungal infections, such as *Cryptococcus* spp., have been associated with feline labyrinthitis. A single case of disseminated canine protothecosis with BAER-confirmed deafness reported abundant *Prototheca zopfii* in the cochlea, along with a prominent plasmacytic infiltrate. Reported disruptions to the spiral organ were likely artifacts related to tissue processing. The end stage of chronic bacterial labyrinthitis in people is formation of granulation tissue, followed by fibrosis and ossification, termed *labyrinthitis ossificans*, which to date has not been confirmed in domestic animals.

Further reading

Paulin J. Otitis interna induced by *Cryptococcus neoformans* var. *grubii* in a cat. Vet Pathol 2013;50:260-263.

Presbycusis. *Age-related hearing loss*, also called presbycusis, is defined in dogs as rapid, progressive loss of middle- and high-frequency hearing starting at 8-10 years of age. Lesions are typically mixed, including sensory, neural, and metabolic changes. Sensory changes include a radial gradient loss of the first and second rows of outer hair cells preferentially affecting the basal as well as middle cochlear turns. Inner hair cells are lost but much less severely. Primary loss of afferent nerves and loss of ganglion cells defines the neural changes. Finally, stria vascularis is thinner in all cochlear turns because of shrunken intermediate cells and marginal cell vacuolation. Cochlear nuclei are affected as well, with nerve cell loss, astrogliosis, and ubiquitin deposition in all dogs >10 years of age. BAER testing confirms hearing impairment; however, degree of hearing dysfunction and severity of cochlear duct lesions are not correlated. *Presbycusis is considered the cumulative effect of environmental noise, hereditary factors, concurrent disease, and exposure to ototoxic agents.*

Similarly, BAER testing has confirmed partial deafness in a group of non-Paint, older horses with an age range of 17-22 years compared with a younger group of 5-8 year-olds. Analysis of the waves and latencies supported possible high-frequency cochlear dysfunction, implying mechanisms similar to those observed in dogs with presbycusis. This hearing impairment was not appreciated based on clinical and behavioral assessment, although these tests are subjective and can be unreliable.

Further reading

Ter Haar G, et al. Effects of aging on inner ear morphology in dogs in relation to brainstem responses to toneburst auditory stimuli. J Vet Intern Med 2009;23:536-543.

Wilson WJ, et al. Use of BAER to identify loss of auditory function in older horses. Aust Vet J 2011;89:73-76.

Traumatic causes of deafness

Acoustic trauma. Based on studies in the cat, the most vulnerable portions of the internal ear to acoustic trauma include the spiral organ, spiral ligament and limbal fibrocytes, and spiral ganglion cells. Injury to the spiral organ begins as loss of outer and/or inner hair cells, followed by complete loss of the spiral organ. Loss of spiral ganglion cells may be "secondary" to the "primary" loss of hair cells or can occur independent of hair cell loss. Only in extreme explosive instances is there corresponding injury to auditory ossicles or rupture of the tympanic membrane.

Radiation. Irradiation injury to the internal ear includes early changes and late changes. *Early changes* include loss of outer hair cells of the basal cochlear turn, preferential loss of type II hair cells in the periphery of maculae and cristae, and severe degeneration of cochlear neurons. *Late reactions* include degenerative changes to spiral and annular ligaments; rupture of the cochlear duct, leading to spiral organ degeneration; and osteoradionecrosis. Necrotic bone is characterized by empty lacunae, osteolysis, loss of bone marrow, and reparative fibrosis, and is prone to injury and fracture.

Ototoxicity. Most of the compounds known to be ototoxic were initially discovered in people and further investigated in animals as models. Interestingly, *most ototoxic compounds are also nephrotoxic* because of common molecular mechanism of the internal ear and kidney in addressing fluid and ionic homeostasis. In most instances, toxic compounds exert their toxic effects as irreversible injury to hair cells in the spiral organ, the utricular and saccular maculae, and cristae of the semicircular canals in aggregate or with more anatomic specificity (eFig. 5-2). In cats, *amikacin* exerts its effects almost exclusively on the cochlear hair cells, whereas *gentamicin* more specifically caused hair cell damage to vestibular maculae. However, histologic studies confirm that gentamicin will also lead to loss of outer hair cells of the basal turn of the cochlea as well as preferential loss of type I hair cells of the cristae ampullares and striolar region of the utricular and saccular maculae. *Cisplatin* not only damages the outer hair cells but also may induce degeneration of the stria vascularis. *Chlorhexidine* can damage both inner and outer hair cells of the spiral organ and is much more toxic in cats than dogs. *Salicylates* and loop diuretics, such as *furosemide*, typically induce more temporary effects by disrupting membrane conductance. In the case of loop diuretics, edema and degeneration of the stria vascularis are documented.

Further reading

Oishi N, et al. Ototoxicity in dogs and cats. Vet Clin North Am Small Anim Pract 2012;42:1259-1271.

Internal ear neoplasia

The vast majority of neoplasms that cause internal ear signs are cranial nerve (CN) associated. Acoustic nerve sheath neoplasms have been reported in dogs and cattle, either arising in CN VIII or extending from one of the nearby cranial nerves, with *schwannomas* most commonly originating in the trigeminal nerve in dogs. Penetration into the internal ear may occur via the internal acoustic meatus or lytic necrosis of the petrous portion of the temporal bone as cranial nerve neoplasms expand and compress. A cranial nerve *hamartoma* involving CN VIII has been reported in a single dog.

Intracranial *meningiomas* are the most commonly reported tumor in dogs, leading to vestibular signs. The expansile growth and compression of portions of the brain and ear important for vestibular function are the reason for clinical signs of dysfunction. *Lymphosarcoma* of multiple CNs has been reported in a Persian cat with associated vestibular signs.

Further reading

Holland CT, et al. Unilateral facial myokymia in a dog with an intracranial meningioma. Aust Vet J 2010;88:357-361.

Ottinger T. Malignant acoustic schwannoma in a dog. J Vet Diagn Invest 2009;21:129-132.

Peripheral vestibular disease

Peripheral vestibular disease is defined as vestibular signs related to *dysfunction of CN VIII (vestibular nerve) and the internal ear*. Clinical signs of unilateral loss of equilibrium and vestibular ataxia include head tilt, circling, and leaning or falling toward the affected side; that blindfolds worsen the ataxia, and abnormal nystagmus being horizontal or rotatory, with the quick phase directed away from the affected side. Bilateral disease results in a more crouched posture, greater exaggeration of head movements when following an object from side to side, and a lack of normal and abnormal nystagmus. Inflammatory lesions confined to the middle ear may produce vestibular signs because of altered middle ear temperature.

Doberman Pinschers, Beagles, English Cocker Spaniels, German Shepherd dogs, Akitas, and Asian cat breeds (Siamese, Tonkinese, Burmese) develop vestibular disease early in life, in which spontaneous nystagmus is usually absent and central compensation over time lessens signs. Congenital vestibular disease in Doberman puppies is autosomal recessive. Rolling, falling, circling, and head tilt were recognized as early as 10 weeks of age, but because of central compensation, signs improved with age. Sensory hair cells of the maculae and crista ampullares were morphologically unaffected; however, otoconia were abnormal in shape and size, with the presumed mechanism resulting from an underlying functional or biochemical defect in the vestibular system. Deafness, however, results from progressive loss and abnormalities of outer hair cells and inner hair cells.

Unilateral, acute-onset vestibular signs in geriatric dogs are most often diagnosed as *benign idiopathic canine peripheral vestibular disease*. The genesis of this syndrome is unknown but presumed localized to the vestibulocochlear nerve, sensory maculae, and cristae, or a combination. Because most dogs recover spontaneously, it has not been investigated histologically.

Otitis media/interna is one of the most common causes of vestibular disease in dogs and cats, and is reported sporadically or as epizootics in neonatal and young livestock. Signs may include drooping ears, head tilt, or circling. In cases of acute vestibular signs with concurrent signs of otitis (externa, media, interna, or combination), the index of suspicion for intracranial extension of otitis media/interna should be high.

Neoplasia impinging on or arising within the vestibulocochlear nerve will lead to recognizable vestibular signs.

Horner and Pourfour du Petit syndromes

Sympathetic innervation of the eye is a complex pathway involving central, preganglionic, and postganglionic neurons. In the cat, preganglionic neuronal axons, originating from T1-T5, converge on the cranial cervical ganglion in close proximity to the tympanic bulla. Postganglionic neuronal axons pass through the tympanic bulla along the ventral surface of the petrous portion of the temporal bone and possibly join the tympanic plexus, a group of parasympathetic preganglionic axons of the glossopharyngeal nerve. In small animals, *otitis media* can lead to sympathetic postganglionic neuronal axon dysfunction, leading to the hallmark signs of *Horner syndrome*, namely, miosis, enophthalmos, narrowing of the palpebral fissure, and protrusion of the third eyelid. Horner syndrome associated with otitis media is more commonly seen in cats than dogs. Otitis media in horses and other farm animals does not affect these sympathetic postganglionic neurons, likely reflecting anatomic differences. Rarely, an association with flushing of the tympanic bullae in anesthetized cats can lead to presumed hyperactivity to the postganglionic sympathetic neurons, clinically manifesting as mydriasis, widening of the palpebral fissure, and exophthalmos. This clinical triad is referred to by some as *Pourfour du Petit syndrome*.

Further reading

Boydell P. Iatrogenic pupillary dilation resembling Pourfour du Petit syndrome in three cats. J Small Anim Pract 2000;41:202-203.

Kent M, et al. The neurology of balance: function and dysfunction of the vestibular system in dogs and cats. Vet J 2010;185: 247-258.

Rossmeisl JH. Vestibular disease in dogs and cats. Vet Clin North Am Small Anim Pract 2010;40:81-100.

MIDDLE EAR

Rostrally, the pharyngeal portion of the embryonic endodermal tube expands laterally to form the first pharyngeal pouch. Bilaterally, this pouch expands between the first 2 pharyngeal or branchial arches. The pharyngeal pouch and surrounding mesenchyme develop into the nasopharynx, auditory tube, tympanic cavity, and, in horses, the guttural pouch. During the same time frame, ectoderm extends medially between the first and second pharyngeal arches toward the pharyngeal pouch to form the first pharyngeal groove or cleft. This ectodermal-lined invagination becomes the external acoustic meatus (EAM), and the apposition between the first pharyngeal pouch and groove forms the tympanic membrane. Mesenchyme from the first arch forms the *malleus, incus, tensor tympani muscle, tensor veli palatini muscle, and malleus ligament*, and these muscles are innervated by the trigeminal nerve, whereas the *stapes and stapedius muscle* are derived from the second arch, with the stapedius muscle innervated by the facial nerve.

Anatomically and functionally, the **tympanic membrane** borders the middle and external ear. It is normally very thin and composed of 3 layers: epidermis contiguous with the external ear, middle stroma, and epithelium that lines the middle ear cavity. Its surface area is variable, ranging from 41 mm^2 in cats to 63.3 mm^2 in dogs. Most of the tympanic membrane consists of the *pars tensa*, which is stretched tightly across the bony tympanic ring that is incomplete dorsally, corresponding to the smaller, looser membrane *pars flaccida*. Embedded medially in the pars tensa is the manubrium of the malleus, and in this region, the tympanic membrane stroma is thickened and contains blood vessels.

The head of the **malleus** articulates with the body of the **incus** to form the incudomalleolar joint. Dorsally, this articulation, along with the short crus of the incus, is anchored within the epitympanic recess by ligamentous attachments forming a fulcrum, allowing the malleus and incus to function as a lever arm. Arising from the neck of the malleus is the muscular process of the malleus that represents the attachment site for the tensor tympani muscle, which originates from its muscular fossa in the rostral medial pyramidal portion of the petrous portion of the temporal bone. Directed medially from these 2 ossicles toward the stapes is the long crus of the incus. At the end of the long crus is the *lenticular process*, a tiny cup-shaped bony appendage that articulates with the head of the stapes to form the incudostapedius joint.

The **stapes** is the roughly triangular bone anchored by its annular ligament in the vestibular window of the petrous portion of the temporal bone. Its base has a convex surface that closely apposes a thin diaphragm. This interface represents the anatomic and functional transition between the middle and internal ear. The base of the stapes is in direct communication with the perilymph of the scala vestibuli of the basal portion of the cochlea. The facial canal (Fallopian canal) initially branches from the internal acoustic meatus, following a path that resembles a Z-shape, with the facial nerve emerging caudal to the EAM through the stylomastoid foramen. Midway through the canal, the facial nerve is exposed to the tympanic cavity, lacking a complete bony shell known as the facial canal foramen (see Fig. 5-85). Through this opening emerges the tendon of the stapedius muscle that attaches to the head of the stapes. The stapedius muscle originates from the stapedius muscular fossa, a shallow depression within the facial canal.

Tympanic cavities represent the middle ear air-filled compartments. Ventrally, this cavity is demarcated by the typically bulbous bony appendage known as the *tympanic bulla*. Tympanic bullae in cattle, goats, camelids, and pigs are septate, composed of numerous air-filled compartments with numerous interconnected bony septa. In dogs, cats, and sheep, tympanic bullae are large, typically singular, air-filled cavities surrounded by bone. In both the dog and cat, there is a central bony cleft, known as the *septum bulla*, which is incomplete in the dog and nearly complete in the cat. The horse has the shallowest bullae of all domestic species, and they are difficult to visualize externally. Short bony clefts span the bullae and subdivide them into several small, dished, bony cavities resulting in a partially septate tympanic cavity.

At birth, the tympanic ring is fully formed with a tympanic membrane stretched across its opening (eFig. 5-3). The middle ear compartment is filled with primordial mesenchyme. In altricial animals, such as cats and dogs, hearing is dysfunctional until ~10 days of age, related to the middle ear cavity mesenchyme, a functionally stenotic but patent EAM, and undeveloped tympanic bullae. Over time, the bullae become aerated and expand; the mesenchyme regresses and contributes to the middle ear lining and allows aeration of the middle ear cavity, and the luminal diameter of the EAM expands.

The tympanic cavity is one of the only anatomic locations in which a mucous membrane closely apposes bone with a normally thin, loose intervening stroma representing merged propria-submucosa and periosteum. Thus this mucosal epithelium and subjacent fused periosteum is frequently referred to as the *mucoperiosteum*. The mucoperiosteal epithelium varies from respiratory epithelium continuous with the auditory tube and nasopharynx; to cuboidal; to flattened, lining ventral portions of the tympanic bulla, inner surface of the tympanic membrane, and auditory ossicles. Variation exists in the location and percentage of mucoperiosteum that comprise respiratory epithelium among species. Normally, the mucoperiosteal stroma is a thin, loose mesenchyme sandwiched between tympanic bone and the mucosal epithelium. There is debate in the literature regarding the presence of glands in the mucoperiosteum. When observed in dogs and cats, they may be observed in proximity to the opening of the auditory tube. They have also been found in a small region dorsal to the tympanic membrane with close proximity to the auditory tube opening. Invaginations of the mucoperiosteum are observed but are most often associated with previous or ongoing, chronic otitis media.

The middle ear originates from the first pharyngeal pouch directly communicating with the primitive nasopharynx. This connection is maintained through the **auditory tube** *(Eustachian tube)*. Maintained closed at rest, the auditory tube in most species receives structural support through elastic cartilage. The tubal lining is pseudostratified, ciliated columnar epithelium, richly endowed with goblet cells, that is contiguous with the nasopharynx. In horses, thin-walled diverticula form, extending medially, ventrally, and dorsally, and are called **guttural pouches.** In the lateral wall of the pharyngeal opening of the auditory tube, diffuse to nodular aggregates of lymphocytes are found in ruminants and horses. Follicle-associated epithelium overlies these lymphoid aggregates known as *tubal tonsils* and contains M cells with apical microvilli. Dogs and cats reportedly do not possess tubal tonsils.

Yawning and swallowing result in contraction of the tensor veli palatini and the levator veli palatini muscles. Primarily through the actions of the tensor veli palatini, the auditory tube opens. Opening serves the important function of altering the pressure in the middle ear. Impaired auditory tube ventilation of the middle ear plays a role in the development of middle ear effusion and middle ear inflammation.

Further reading

Njaa BL, et al. Practical otic anatomy and physiology of the dog and cat. Vet Clin North Am Small Anim Pract 2012;42:1109-1126.

Hearing and the middle ear

The ossicular chain—malleus, incus, and stapes—functions to couple sound energy collected by the external ear into fluid waves in the cochlea. The malleus has its longest appendage, the manubrium, embedded in the pars tensa of the tympanic membrane; is firmly articulated with the incus; and is anchored dorsally in the epitympanic recess. The long crus of the incus articulates with the head of the stapes via its terminal lenticular process. Sound-induced tympanic membrane vibrations result in piston-like oscillation of the stapes anchored in the vestibular window by the stapedial annular ligament.

Inherent to transducing sound energy from air (low impedance) to cochlear fluid (higher impedance) is the need for *impedance matching*; otherwise, much of the sound energy would be reflected. Impedance transformer function of the middle ear is achieved in 3 ways. First, tympanic membrane surface area is far greater than the surface area of the foot plate of the stapes in the vestibular window, ~20:1 in the cat. Second, the long crus of the incus is much shorter than the manubrium of the malleus, resulting in a lever action that increases the force at the stapes, ~2:1 in the cat. The net effect is a maximal middle ear amplification of 43 in the cat. Third, air in the tympanic cavity provides stiffness with respect to sound vibrations across the tympanic membrane. As external sound frequencies decrease, the stiffness or acoustic impedance of the middle ear increases. Thus low-frequency sounds are more apt to be reflected away rather than transduced into cochlear waves and sound detection. However, as the volume of the middle ear cavity increases, the stiffness decreases in an inverse relationship. Therefore animals with larger tympanic bullae have reduced stiffness and a greater ability to hear a lower range of sound frequencies.

Any condition that impairs this mechanical transduction of air vibrations to cochlear fluid waves can lead to hearing impairment known as **conduction hearing loss.** Diminished middle ear volume, through accumulated mucoid fluid, inflammatory exudate, fibrosis, neoplasia, or a combination, leads to altered range of detected sound frequencies. Inflammation of the tympanic membrane, *myringitis*, increases middle ear stiffness, impairing hearing. Chronic otitis media may restrict auditory ossicle movement or result in bony lysis and conduction hearing loss.

The middle ear muscles, tensor tympani and stapedius, are innervated by the branches of the trigeminal and facial nerves, respectively. Their motor neurons are located in the brainstem close to the auditory centers. In aggregate, these 2 muscles act on the auditory ossicles, making them stiffer in response to loud noises or high-energy sound. This increases the reflection of low-frequency sound at the tympanic membrane and vestibular window and reduces the magnitude of sound energy transmitted to the internal ear. These muscles also contract in anticipation of a loud self-vocalization, resulting in local attenuation of the sound energy at the internal ear. This is known as the *acoustic reflex* and is an important mechanism for protecting the cochlea from exposure to high-amplitude pressure waves.

Further reading

Adams JC, Liberman MC. Physiology and pathophysiology. In: Merchant SN, Nadol JB, editors. Schuknecht's Pathology of the Ear. 3rd ed. Shelton, Conn: People's Medical Publishing House–USA; 2010. p. 97-140.

Developmental disease of the middle ear

Otognathia has been described in sheep and cattle and is defined as *a complete pharyngeal fistula that forms near the base of the ear.* Also referred to as a *rudimentary or ectopic mouth*, these are lined by mucous membranes and are either blind or continuous with the pharynx. The genesis of this is a rupture or permanent fistula that forms through the membrane formed when the first pharyngeal pouch and groove become apposed. In affected sheep, all had concurrent palatoschisis. In the calf, fistulae were contiguous with the auditory tube and external acoustic meatus.

Ciliary dyskinesis is a rare developmental disorder reported in dogs in which cilia are dysfunctional. Clinical signs are related to immotile or dyskinetic cilia. Dogs typically develop chronic and persistent rhinitis and bronchopneumonia at a very early age resulting from dysfunctional mucociliary clearance. Otitis media occurs in some cases, also related to impairment of normal mucociliary clearance via the auditory tube.

Otosclerosis is a term specifically used for *endochondral ossification of the otic capsule*. This disorder is reported only in people and is one of the most common causes of conduction hearing loss.

Several of the *storage diseases* have middle ear pathology (see Developmental disease and the internal ear).

Further reading

Edwards DF, et al. Primary ciliary dyskinesia in the dog. Prob Vet Med 1992;4:291-319.

Otitis media

The tympanic cavity is a nasopharyngeal diverticulum arising from the first pharyngeal pouch that maintains a muscle-controlled opening via the auditory tube. Tubal lining cells normally provide a functioning mucociliary apparatus important for clearance. Additional defense mechanisms are in place to keep otitis media from developing. Resident lymphocytes produce secretory immunoglobulin A (IgA). Tubal epithelium produces surfactants rich in phosphatidylcholine and surfactant protein-A (SP-A). Surfactant proteins are collectins of the innate immune system functioning by opsonizing bacteria, viruses, fungi, and allergens. Surfactants also reduce the local surface tension, facilitating opening of the auditory tube. Local production of antimicrobial peptides, such as β-defensin 3, is one means of mucosal defense against tubal colonization by pathogenic bacteria.

Normally maintained closed, the auditory tube functions to adjust the pressure of the tympanic cavity. Through muscular contraction by the tensor veli palatini, innervated by a branch of the trigeminal nerve, and the levator veli palatini, innervated by a branch of the vagus nerve, the auditory tube opens. The mucosal lining is contiguous with the respiratory epithelium of the nasopharynx rich in ciliated, columnar epithelial cells, and goblet cells. Numerous surfactant phospholipids are produced to decrease the surface tension and facilitate tubal opening.

Possible predisposing factors for auditory tube dysfunction include craniofacial defects, ciliary dyskinesis, shortened soft palates, auditory tube obstruction by inflammation or neoplasia, and nerve or muscular dysfunction of the 2 auditory tube muscles.

Inflammation of the tympanic cavity can be categorized into **acute or chronic otitis media.** In acute disease, tympanic cavities and bullae are filled with suppurative exudate consisting mostly of degenerate neutrophils. The surrounding mucoperiosteum is thickened as a result of edema within the loose stromal layer, and the mucosal epithelium may be eroded or ulcerated. Auditory ossicles may undergo bony erosion related to the proteolytic activity of suppurative inflammation.

Chronically, the edematous mucoperiosteum begins to form polypoid projections and folds resulting in the formation of *pseudoglands* (eFig. 5-4). The mucoperiosteum also becomes infiltrated by lymphocytes and plasma cells that may form discrete lymphoid nodular aggregates. With time, the stroma thickens because of fibroplasia. Underlying bony changes vary from erosion to marked thickening, to regions of invaginating spicules. Reversal lines become numerous and prominent with continued remodeling. The surface mucosal epithelium becomes hyperplastic, and frequently there is goblet cell hyperplasia.

> ### Key Points
>
> **Middle ear submucosal glands**
> Submucosal glands in the mucoperiosteum are readily identified in the rostral middle ear in proximity to the auditory tube opening in cats and dogs, but are poorly documented in other species. In otitis media in most species, redundant, edematous mucoperiosteum forms small polypoid projections that become folded and form pseudoglands lined by pseudostratified columnar epithelium mixed with goblet cells as well as possibly ciliated epithelium.

Luminal diameter is compressed related to mucoperiosteal expansion related to proliferation of fibrovascular connective tissue along with the formation of granulation tissue.

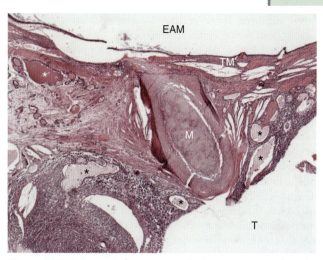

Figure 5-88 Myringitis from a cat with chronic otitis media. The tympanic membrane (TM) is markedly thickened by fibrosis, lymphoplasmacytic infiltration, and abundant, embedded pseudoglands (*). This infiltration and expansion also extends to the mucoperiosteum, resulting in a decreased functional volume of the tympanic cavity (T). The external acoustic meatus (EAM) is relatively free of exudate. *M,* manubrium of the malleus.

Aggregates of acicular clefts are very common in chronic otitis media. The source of these crystals is likely membrane cholesterol from inflammatory cells or hemorrhage. *Cholesterol granulomas* may develop. The mucoperiosteal response to chronic otitis media is to form granulation tissue that is variably inflamed, edematous and polypoid, and frequently has embedded cholesterol clefts. Therefore tympanic cavity cholesterol granulomas may simply represent a morphologic hallmark of chronic infection rather than a distinctive disease.

Auditory ossicles may become encased in and restricted by this fibroplasia. This can be most prominent in the vicinity of the tympanic membrane, where the normally very thin tympanic membrane becomes markedly thickened because of expansion of the middle stromal layer with changes described previously and infiltrated by mixtures of inflammatory cells, known as **myringitis** (Fig. 5-88). Thickening may also occur on the external surface related to concurrent otitis externa (eFig. 5-5). Chronically, they may undergo bony remodeling with exostoses and potential for ossicular chain dysfunction resulting in conductive hearing impairment. Suppurative otitis media in pigs, caused by β-hemolytic streptococci, was associated with bony lysis of the auditory ossicles and reduction of the tympanic membrane to scarred remnants.

In animals with septate bullae (cattle, pigs, goats, camelids), these bony partitions are frequently lysed by the proteolytic effects of the proliferative bacteria and suppuration. Severe infections may manifest as a draining tract in the ventrolateral neck corresponding to spread into the soft tissue surrounding the bullae. Large abscesses up to 4 cm in diameter were reported in pigs with suppurative otitis media that spilled from the lytic bullae into the surrounding soft tissue and musculature. This has been referred to by some as *para-aural abscesses.*

In dogs, otitis media is typically a sequela of chronic otitis externa, frequently associated with tympanic membrane rupture. At the time of diagnosis, tympanic membranes are rarely ruptured; however, they have a remarkable ability to rapidly reseal via epithelial migration. Conversely, several studies in cats have confirmed that otitis externa is not a major contributing factor, and infections mostly likely ascend the auditory tube. An ascending pathogenesis is presumed for otitis media of piglets and calves. Experimentally induced otitis media in pigs frequently became bilateral, presumably as a result of spread through auditory tubes. Atrophic rhinitis has been associated with a higher frequency of otitis media in pigs.

Bacterial pathogens are most commonly implicated in otitis media in any species. Often, cultured bacteria represent commensal organisms that have become pathogenic or bacterial pathogens that may have arrived hematogenously. In livestock species, *Mycoplasma bovis*, *Streptococcus* spp., *Trueperella pyogenes*, *Mannheimia haemolytica*, *Pasteurella multocida*, *Histophilus somni*, and various enterococci are pathogens commonly isolated in otitis media. The pathogenesis of *Mycoplasma bovis* otitis media in calves has been linked to infection during nursing and colonization of tonsils. In dogs and cats, many bacteria have been cultured, including *Staphylococcus* spp., *Streptococcus* spp., *Escherichia coli*, *Pseudomonas aeruginosa*, and *Proteus* spp.

Rarely, fungal infections such as *Aspergillus* spp. may cause otitis media in production animals such as camelids. The mycotic organisms *Cryptococcus neoformans*, *Blastomyces dermatitidis*, *Histoplasma capsulatum*, *Sporothrix schenkii*, and *Coccidioides immitis* are capable of causing otitis media, but only rare reports have confirmed their presence in the middle ear.

Otitis media with effusion (OME) refers to a condition in people with minimal clinical signs and presumed auditory tube dysfunction. In dogs and guinea pigs, auditory tube occlusion can result in lesions with similarities to OME, including *increased mucoperiosteal goblet cells and copious amounts of tenacious, mucoid contents in the tympanic cavity*. Initially referred to as primary secretory otitis media (PSOM), in which Cavalier King Charles Spaniels were over-represented, more recent evidence points to a disease entity that is mostly silent clinically and therefore has greater similarities with OME. The tympanic membrane becomes opaque without evidence of rupture, and the pars flaccida may bulge laterally into the external acoustic meatus. Brachycephalic conformation has been associated with the development of OME. Dogs with OME also have confirmed hearing impairment based on brain auditory-evoked responses testing, comparable to dampening of sound energy associated with fitting a foam ear plug in the external acoustic meatus.

Guttural pouch disease. Horses have some of the longest auditory tubes of any domestic species. Guttural pouches are thin-walled diverticula that are contiguous with and extend off the auditory tube. Suppuration of the auditory tube diverticula is referred to as *guttural pouch empyema*, most often caused by *Streptococcus* spp. infection. The wall and mucous membrane of the guttural pouch is greatly thickened, and lumina are greatly expanded by exudate. This same exudate may be grossly visible in the nasopharyngeal auditory tube openings or fill tympanic cavities associated with otitis media. Chronic exudate may become inspissated and form *chondroids* that may be present in 20% of cases. Chondroid formation in guttural pouch empyema has been associated with greater concurrent retropharyngeal swelling and pharyngeal narrowing.

Further reading

Friend EJ, et al. Progression of otitis media with effusion in the Cavalier King Charles Spaniel. Vet Rec 2013;172:315-316.

Gosselin VB, et al. A retrospective study of 29 cases of otitis media/interna in dairy calves. Can Vet J 2012;53:957-962.

Juhn SK, et al. The role of inflammatory mediators in the pathogenesis of otitis media and sequelae. Clin Exp Otorhinolaryngol 2008;1:117-138.

McGuire JF. Surfactant in the middle ear and eustachian tube: a review. Int J Pediatr Otorhinolaryngol 2002;66:1-15.

Sula MM, et al. Histologic characterization of the cat middle ear: in sickness and in health. Vet Pathol 2014;51:951-967.

Middle ear parasites

Mammomonogamus auris (formerly *Syngamus auris*) is a strongylid nematode parasite localized to the nasopharynx, auditory tube, and middle ear that occurs exclusively in cats from the Asian Pacific region. Most cats are asymptomatic but may display head shaking. Typically a unilateral disease, male and female nematodes are permanently joined in union; 1-8 worm pairs may infect a single tympanic cavity. *These nematodes are able to freely move between the middle ear and nasopharynx*. During otic examination, the red color of the parasitic pair gives the appearance of an erythematous tympanic membrane with worm movement in the middle ear. The tympanic membrane may tinctorially normalize because of the paired parasites suddenly exiting the middle ear through the auditory tube. The life cycle is not fully understood, although the tympanic membrane is always intact, and therefore the external ear is not considered a portal of entry.

Further reading

Tudor EG, et al. *Mammomonogamus auris* infection in the middle ear of a domestic cat in Saipan, Northern Mariana Islands, USA. J Feline Med Surg 2008;10:501-504.

Non-neoplastic and neoplastic disease
Inflammatory aural polyps

Inflammatory aural polyps are masses that frequently plague young cats but are also diagnosed in dogs and much less frequently in horses. Regardless of species, these polypoid growths are composed of fibrovascular stromal cores with variable edema and usually contain mixtures of inflammatory cells that include scattered to aggregated lymphocytes, plasma cells, macrophages, and neutrophils (eFig. 5-6). Superficially, these are covered by epithelium that may constitute squamous epithelium, respiratory epithelium, or a combination. Ulceration is nearly always a feature.

Site of origin likely includes the middle ear mucoperiosteum, possibly the auditory tube mucosa, and the external ear epidermis and dermis. Differentiating between the former two is likely an academic exercise. In both cases, they will likely have a mixed epithelial covering, and because they are associated most often with middle ear inflammation, nearly always contain pseudoglands lined by respiratory epithelium replete with goblet cells, a histologic feature also observed in middle ear–derived polyps in people. The presence of pseudoglands is common in otitis media, and their presence should not be confused with an underlying glandular tumor. Conversely, polyps arising from the EAM should not contain pseudoglands, but may include ceruminous or sebaceous glands.

> **Key Points**
>
> **Defining origin of inflammatory aural polyps**
> Polypoid masses collected from the external auditory meatus may originate from the middle ear mucoperiosteum or the external ear dermis. The surface epithelium is highly variable, often ulcerated, and most often contains an inflamed, edematous core. Pseudoglands within the core or extending to the surface confirm the middle ear/auditory tube origin.

Clinical signs depend on final location of the polyp. Middle ear inflammatory polyps may remain in the middle ear; evert through the auditory tube into the nasopharynx, where they are often called *nasopharyngeal polyps*; or perforate the tympanic membrane and partially fill the EAM, where they are often called *aural polyps*. Polyps derived from the EAM may penetrate into the middle ear through the tympanic membrane or remain and grow within the external ear canal. Polyps confined to the middle ear may remain clinically silent or may be associated with facial nerve dysfunction. Signs of external ear extension include otomiasmic otorrhea (otoblennorrhea), otalgia, erythematous ear canals, and head shaking.

Tympanokeratoma (cholesteatoma)

Cholesteatoma, a misnomer that has lingered for centuries, is used to describe a *proliferative, keratinizing growth that arises in the middles ears of dogs* and people associated with otitis media. These cystic formations likely arise in and gradually destroy the middle ear as a consequence of expansion at the expense of the middle ear and chronic otitis media (Fig. 5-89). The most plausible pathogenesis in dogs involves chronic, recurrent otitis media with some impairment of the auditory tube and pressure equalization, leading to the formation of retraction pockets associated with the tympanic membrane. Continued enlargement leads to compression and erosion of both soft and bony tissue. Because these are keratinizing structures arising almost exclusively from the tympanic membrane, a more appropriate term proposed is tympanokeratoma.

Grossly, the tympanic cavity is filled with pasty material variably associated with concurrent middle ear exudate and loss of grossly recognizable auditory ossicles. Their histologic appearance is rather underwhelming, given the destructive consequence of their growth, consisting of luminal contents of variably sized, nucleated and non-nucleated, keratin surrounded by a variably thick layer of squamous epithelium, and further surrounded by granulation tissue and evidence of chronic otitis media. The surrounding granulation tissue may be embedded with numerous acicular cholesterol clefts.

Mucoperiosteal exostoses

Representing bony proliferation arising from the mucoperiosteum of the incomplete septum bullae of one or both tympanic bullae in dogs, mucoperiosteal exostoses (formerly *otolithiasis*) are morphologically very similar to stalagmites and stalactites (Fig. 5-90). However, the major difference from their cavernous cousins is their broad, bony ends. These pedunculated, bulbous bony masses are frequently observed in bullae of older dogs at the time of autopsy, without historical or gross evidence of otitis media. The pathogenesis for mucoperiosteal exostoses is unknown; however, based on gross postmortem examination, it does not appear to result from dystrophic mineralization of inflammatory polyps. Mucoperiosteal exostoses have not been reported in domestic cats; there is a single report of this condition found in archived samples from African lions.

Mucoperiosteal exostoses were originally reported as otolithiasis associated with otitis media in a single dog based on radiographic imaging. Use of the term otolith for this condition is discouraged because it most commonly refers to crystals present in the matrix overlying the maculae of the vestibular apparatus, also called otoconia (see Internal ear).

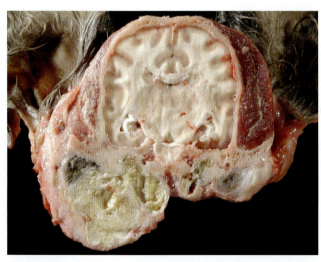

Figure 5-89 A Miniature Schnauzer with **tympanokeratoma** (cholesteatoma) of the right ear. The laminated, yellow-green keratin causes marked expansion of the right tympanic bulla as well as erosion of the petrous portion of the temporal bone. (Courtesy D. Reel, University of Tennessee.)

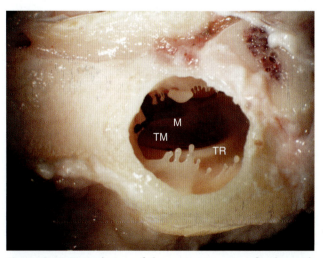

Figure 5-90 Ventral view of the tympanic cavity of a dog with **mucoperiosteal exostoses** arising from the inner edge of the septum bulla. The bulla has been opened to allow visualization of these bony proliferations. In the background, the tympanic ring (TR) is observed as well as the tympanic membrane (TM) and manubrium of the malleus (M).

Temporohyoid osteoarthropathy

Temporohyoid osteoarthropathy (THO) is an uncommon condition affecting *horses*. The hyoid apparatus is made of several bones and articulations, and the stylohyoid bone is the largest, articulating proximally with the styloid process of the petrous portion of the temporal bone forming the *tympanohyoid synchondrosis*. It is speculated that one of its functions is to dampen the hyoid apparatus during tongue movements. Inflammation or degeneration of this joint can lead to bony proliferation that manifests as head shaking, resentment to a bit, ear rubbing, difficulty chewing, and pain at the base of the ear. Unilateral or bilateral fusion of this joint may be associated with reduced clinical signs but an increased susceptibility to fracture, either through the petrous portion of the temporal bone or midshaft through the stylohyoid bone. The vestibulocochlear and facial nerves leave the cranial cavity through the internal acoustic meatus of the petrous portion of the temporal bone. In close proximity are the vagus, glossopharyngeal, and hypoglossal nerves. Additionally, the facial nerve courses through the facial canal in the petrous portion of the temporal bone. Because of proximity, fracture through the petrous portion of the temporal bone will lead to vestibular and facial nerve dysfunction and, less commonly, signs related to vagal, glossopharyngeal, and hypoglossal nerve dysfunction.

The pathogenesis of this lesion likely involves more than one mechanism. Disease observed in older horses is more likely related to degenerative joint disease of the tympanohyoid synchondrosis. Histologic changes that were noted to increase with advancing age included extension of osteophytes from the petrous temporal bone, typically enveloping the stylohyoid head, and rarely, bridging of the joint and chondro-osseous replacement of fibrocartilage. The close proximity to the shallow tympanic bulla supports the idea that inflammation related to otitis media is a viable mechanism for THO, likely limited mostly to younger horses.

Deafness, based on brain auditory-evoked responses (BAER) testing, in a small group of horses with THO has been reported. BAER abnormalities suggested peripheral sensorineural dysfunction, although conductive hearing impairment could not be excluded. Bony remodeling of the stylohyoid, temporohyoid, and tympanic bulla, and presumptive internal acoustic meatal narrowing, is observed with imaging. It is presumed that these bony changes compress CN VIII, leading to demyelination and axonal drop out. Histopathologic confirmation is lacking.

Middle ear epithelial neoplasia

Papillary adenomas of the middle ear have been reported in dogs and a cat. Originally described as arising from the respiratory epithelium of the auditory tube, it is likely that these could originate from other regions of the tympanic cavity related to a mucoperiosteum region lined by respiratory epithelium. In one instance, the site of origin was presumed to be the medial surface of the tympanic membrane. Neoplastic cells were cuboidal to columnar epithelial cells with minimal nuclear variation and low mitotic activity supported by thin, fibrovascular stromal stalks.

Middle ear malignancies include adenocarcinomas of glandular epithelium, adenocarcinomas of undetermined origin, and squamous cell carcinoma. Each may arise from the portion of the mucoperiosteum normally lined by the appropriate originating epithelium. Sites of origin may also include the guttural pouch epithelium, external ear canal, or oral cavity. At the time of diagnosis, animals may display evidence of facial paralysis, vestibular disease, and Horner syndrome. **Meningeal carcinomatosis** has been reported in cats, and meningeal spread may also be associated with concurrent bacterial meningitis and brain or brainstem abscesses in close proximity to the internal acoustic meatus.

Epithelial cysts have been identified in the guttural pouch of young horses. Lined by pseudostratified epithelium with associated propria-submucosal lymphoplasmacytic infiltrates, these can result in dyspnea. **Squamous cell carcinomas** have also been rarely reported to arise from the guttural pouch of older horses. Vestibular and facial nerve dysfunction as well as nasal discharge are the first signs of disease. Neoplasia may extend into the oropharynx, into the tympanic cavity and through the petrous portion of the temporal bone into the calvaria, as well as through the mandible and into the regional lymph node. Pulmonary metastasis has rarely been reported.

Jugulotympanic paragangliomas

Jugulotympanic paragangliomas have rarely been reported, and only in dogs, most commonly affecting male dogs of no specific breed. They arise from the extra-adrenal paraganglia located at the base of the skull, including paraganglia of the jugular bulb, the tympanic branch of the glossopharyngeal nerve, and the vagus and facial nerves. At the time of diagnosis, dogs exhibit signs that include head tilt toward the affected side, facial nerve paralysis, Horner syndrome, as well as other cranial nerve signs, dependent on location. These masses typically occupy the tympanic cavity and cause expansion and erosion of the tympanic bulla. The auditory ossicles as well as the petrous portion of the temporal bone may also be eroded or infiltrated. These masses may extend into the external ear canal, nasopharynx through the auditory tube, or penetrate through the petrous portion of the temporal bone into the cranial cavity. Grossly, these masses range from tan to red and are highly vascular. Histologically, fibrovascular stroma subdivides lobules and nests of uniform, small polyhedral to cuboidal cells that contain granular cytoplasm with small, round, euchromatic to hyperchromatic nuclei. Most tumors contain numerous vascular channels, and mitotic indices are highly variable among published accounts. Approximately $\frac{1}{3}$ of the cases are metastatic at the time of diagnosis or death.

Further reading

Banco B, et al. Canine aural cholesteatoma: a histological and immunohistochemical study. Vet J 2014;200:440-445.

Fan TM, et al. Inflammatory polyps and aural neoplasia. Vet Clin North Am Small Anim Pract 2004;32:489-509.

Pratschke KM. Inflammatory polyps of the middle ear in 5 dogs. Vet Surg 2003;32:292-296.

Readford PK, et al. Temporohyoid osteoarthropathy in two young horses. Aust Vet J 2013;91:209-212.

EXTERNAL EAR

As the branchial pouches develop, mounds of mesenchyme known as the branchial arches form. The first 2 branchial or pharyngeal arches and the intervening, invaginating first pharyngeal groove or cleft represent the *external ear primordia*. The pharyngeal groove becomes the external acoustic meatus (EAM) or external ear canal, which at birth is patent but very narrow, lined by haired epidermis. Apposition between pharyngeal pouches and grooves form bilateral tympanic membranes. A series of mesenchymal bulges forms on either side of this first pharyngeal groove, known as auricular hillocks. The tragus and rostral portion of the pinna are derived from the first pharyngeal arch, whereas the remainder of the pinna arises from the second pharyngeal arch.

In domestic animals, **pinnae** are flattened sheets of elastic cartilage covered by haired skin. In most breeds within many domestic animal species, pinnae are erect or semierect and highly mobile, able to localize and focus sound transmission as well as dissipate heat and convey mood. In other breeds, pinnae may be floppy or lop (Cocker Spaniels, certain Zebu breeds of cattle, Nubian goats) or folded (Scottish Fold cats). In dogs, ear traits have been localized to a single region on *CFA10* (*Canis familiaris* 10). Supportive elastic cartilage forms various folds that include the tragus, antitragus, helix, antihelix, and the marginal pouch (also referred to as Henry's pouch) as part of the conical opening to the EAM. This canal gradually narrows with structural support from auricular cartilage and annular cartilage, the latter overlapping with the bony flanges of the temporal bone EAM, the osseous acoustic meatus. A complex series of skeletal muscles control pinnal movements, all innervated by the facial nerve, and therefore drooping ears, especially unilateral, is an excellent indication of facial nerve paralysis.

Haired skin covers the external or convex surface of the pinna and lines the concave surface that extends into the EAM. Hair follicle numbers diminish descending the length of the EAM, and hair cover is often greater on the external pinna when compared with the inner surface. In dogs and cats, hair follicles extend the full length of the EAM, whereas in horses, hair follicles and associated adnexa abruptly stop at the junction of the cartilaginous and osseous EAM. Deeper portions of the equine EAM also abruptly depict loss of pigmentation, accumulation of superficial keratin, and marked thinning of the dermis.

Within the dermis, sebaceous glands are typically most plentiful in the superficial dermis, varying in number between species, among breeds, and depending on concurrent dermatologic conditions. Deeper adnexal glands are specialized apocrine glands called *ceruminous glands*. Cerumen, also known as "ear wax," is the aggregate mixture of watery apocrine secretion by ceruminous glands and oily holocrine secretion of sebaceous glands. In dogs, the density of sebaceous glands increases moving away from the tympanic membrane toward the external opening of the EAM, whereas the density of ceruminous glands is the reverse, being most dense in close proximity to the tympanic membrane. The external surface of the tympanic membrane is covered by a thin layer of squamous epithelium that overlays a thin stromal layer, lacking adnexa and only containing blood vessels in the stria mallearis in close proximity to the manubrium of the malleus.

Further reading

Blanke A, et al. Histological study of the external, middle and inner ear of horses. Anat Histol Embryol 2014;doi:10.1111/ahe.12151; [Epub ahead of print].

Hearing and the external ear

Sound energy is collected by the pinna and funneled down the EAM to the tympanic membrane. Localization of sound in domestic animals is achieved in at least 2 ways. First, 2 ears allow for interaural differences in terms of sound amplitude and time of arrival to auditory centers in the brain between the 2 ears. It is these time differences that help animals localize the sound source. Second, domestic animals have very mobile pinnae resulting from robust muscular control of external ear movements, allowing variation of the axis of sound collection without moving the head.

The EAM is a gradually narrowing tube that must remain patent with a very thin, highly responsive tympanic membrane at its medial terminus. Keeping the EAM clear of debris and maintenance of a thin tympanic membrane are both achieved through a process called *epithelial migration*. Progenitor epithelial cells are located along the outer rim of the pars tensa and in the region of the stria mallearis along the manubrium of the malleus. Squamous epithelium continually advances radially and linearly from the tympanic membrane surface to the external ear canal, keeping the surface of the tympanic membrane from accumulating debris. Epithelial migration is also the mechanism used to close perforations in the tympanic membrane, uniquely first bridging these defects with advancing keratin, followed by epithelial cells using the keratin as scaffolding to close the gap closely, followed by advancing granulation tissue in the middle stromal layer of the tympanic membrane.

Any condition that results in narrowing or obstruction of the external acoustic meatus may result in hearing impairment, including external ear neoplasms, external ear parasitism, or exudative otitis externa. Chronic otitis externa may lead to hearing impairment related to narrowing of the canal from fibrosis, adnexal proliferation and associated exudate, or obstruction related to the aggregate effects.

Further reading

Pickles JO. An Introduction to the Physiology of Hearing. 4th ed. Bingley, UK: Emerald Group Publishing; 2014. p. 1-15.

Tabacca NE, et al. Epithelial migration on the canine tympanic membrane. Vet Dermatol 2011;22:502-510.

Developmental disease of the external ear

Defective maturation of the first and second pharyngeal arches as well as the first pharyngeal groove can manifest as external ear defects. Defects of the pinna can manifest as *microtia* or small pinnae, which may be normal to certain breeds (La Mancha goats) as well as a bilateral or unilateral abnormality. Other defects, most commonly reported in pigs, goats, and sheep include *anotia, macrotia*, and *heterotopic otia*. Polyotia has been reported in cats (also called "4-eared" cats) as a recessive, bilateral condition with concurrent microphthalmos and undershot jaw.

A condition only reported in sheep has been termed *synotia and otocephaly*, representing the same condition. Affected lambs also had aprosencephaly (absence of telencephalon and diencephalon) and dysgnathia (lack of upper and lower jaws, tongue, and frontonasal bones). Both reported cases were nonviable, each with viable siblings. Left and right pinnae extended laterally from a central, narrow pharyngeal aperture contiguous with the esophagus. One case was confirmed to have tympanic bullae by radiographs, but neither included histologic examination.

Bilateral rostral pinnal folds that develop by 3-4 weeks of age phenotypically define Scottish Fold cats. There is no associated middle or internal ear defect; however, both heterozygous and homozygous progeny develop osteochondrodysplasia. Physeal lesions are evident in limbs and vertebrae. They have shortened distal limbs that result in compressed stature, abnormal gaits, and chronic lameness.

Temporal odontomas, also referred to as *dentigerous cysts, heterotopic polyodontia, or ear fistulas*, are cystic structures with fistulous epidermal openings that commonly form mostly unilaterally on the rostral or medial border or rostral base of the pinna in *horses*. Shaped like Erlenmeyer flasks, these congenital structures arise from failure of the first pharyngeal cleft to close, resulting in an open fistula. Neural crest ectomesenchyme improperly migrates into the first branchial arch, resulting in dental tissue arising in the incorrect location; however, teeth are not found in every case. Squamous epithelium lines these structures often with associated salivary tissue and, if teeth are present, they may be loosely or firmly adherent to the temporal bone.

External acoustic meatal stenosis has been reported as unilateral or bilateral disease related to disturbance in development of the first pharyngeal groove or cleft. Portions or all of the EAM may be missing, and a tympanic membrane may be present. Rare reports have documented abnormal brain auditory-evoked responses (BAER) testing, confirming some degree of hearing impairment.

Cropped or notched pinnae have been described in Ayrshire, Highland, and Irish Dexter cattle. Affected cattle have otic phenotypes ranging from mild to moderate notches in pinna with normal cartilage to microtic pinnae with large notches that have prominent cartilage along the upper edges. A third phenotype of short, rudimentary, deformed pinnae has also been described. BAER testing has not assessed hearing function; however, behavior analysis suggested no hearing deficits. This is an inherited dominant condition and in Highland cattle has been mapped to a conserved, noncoding region on bovine chromosome 6 (*BTA6*) downstream from the H6 family homeobox 1 *(HMX1)*.

Further reading

Brachthäuser L, et al. Aprosencephaly with otocephaly in a lamb. Vet Pathol 2012;49:1043-1048.

Koch CT, et al. A non-coding genomic duplication at the HMX1 locus is associated with crop ears in Highland cattle. PLoS ONE 2013;8:1-7. (e77841).

Smith LCR, et al. Bilateral dentigerous cysts (heterotopic polyodontia) in a yearling Standardbred colt. Equine Vet Educ 2012;24:573-578.

Takanosu M, et al. Incomplete dominant osteochondrodysplasia in heterozygous Scottish fold cats. J Small Anim Pract 2008;49:197-199.

Otitis externa

Among domestic animals, otitis externa is most commonly diagnosed in dogs and cats but rarely recognized in other genera. Otitis externa has long been considered a very complex and truly multifactorial disease related to a variety of causes that have been further subclassified into primary causes, secondary causes, predisposing factors, and perpetuating factors. The list of *primary causes* is the largest and includes allergic, immune-mediated, endocrine, epithelialization, glandular, parasitic, and viral disorders. These disorders may remain unrecognized or extremely subtle until the animal is afflicted by additional secondary causes that result in otitis externa in an already abnormal ear. *Secondary causes* are primarily bacterial and mycotic infections or alteration of the microenvironment related to medications or local traumatic effects of excessive ear cleaning. Finally, factors represent congenital or acquired alterations to the structure, function, and physiology of the ear canal, which contribute to or promote the development of otitis media. *Predisposing factors* include external ear conformation, local aural environment, concurrent systemic disease, and side effects of local treatment. *Perpetuating factors* represent acquired changes, such as narrowing of the ear canal for a variety of reasons, altered or impaired epithelial migration, inflamed glandular adnexa, or concurrent middle ear disease, to name a few. For complete lists, refer to Vol. 1, Integumentary system or the Miller reference in this section.

Histologic changes of otitis externa are as varied as the associated causes and factors. In general, there is a wide range of hyperplasia affecting the epidermis, sebaceous glands, and ceruminous glands, dependent on the associated causes. Hair follicles do not tend to increase in number but become hyperplastic. The dermis may be edematous or fibrotic, dependent on chronicity and similarly, the infiltrate is typically a combination of plasma cells, lymphocytes, mast cells, and neutrophils in interstitial to diffuse to nodular patterns. Ceruminous glands tend to become hyperplastic and larger with both luminal and periglandular inflammation, but also tend to increase in number relative to the canals of normal patients.

With increasing chronicity, the dermis of the ear canal may become more densely fibrotic. Soft tissue surrounding the auricular cartilage may undergo osseous metaplasia with cords of bone that closely appose the pre-existing cartilage or may arise from the pre-existing auricular cartilage (Fig. 5-91). The osseous portion of the EAM may develop proliferative exostoses. In dogs especially, otitis externa is a predisposing factor

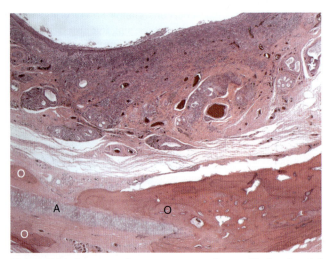

Figure 5-91 An external acoustic meatus from a Cocker Spaniel with **chronic otitis externa.** The epidermis is both hyperplastic and ulcerated with pleocellular dermatitis and ceruminous gland adenitis. Osseous metaplasia (O) is marked, either associated with pre-existing auricular cartilage (A) or in the connective tissue immediately adjacent to this cartilage.

for the development of otitis media, most likely related to perforation of the tympanic membrane. Concurrent otitis externa and otitis media can result in neurologic signs that may include facial nerve dysfunction, abnormal nystagmus, and possibly a head tilt or circling with internal ear involvement.

The net effect of these histologic changes is narrowing of the EAM, which represents a very important perpetuating factor for otitis externa. With the development of irreversible fibrosis and osseous metaplasia, the ear canal becomes increasingly stenotic, and medical management eventually becomes ineffective. Total ear canal ablation is often required, and these surgically collected tissues should be examined histologically to evaluate for possible causes or factors, because neoplasia of the external ear may initially occur as otitis externa.

Further reading

Miller WH, et al. Diseases of eyelids, claws, anal sacs, and ear. In: Miller WH, et al., editors. Muller & Kirk's Small Animal Dermatology. 7th ed. St Louis: 2013. p. 724-773.

Saridomichelakis MN, et al. Aetiology of canine otitis externa: a retrospective study of 100 cases. Vet Dermatol 2007;18:341-347.

Dermatologic diseases of the external ear

Descriptions follow of several dermatologic conditions that primarily affect the external ear, either the pinnae or the external acoustic meatus.

Pinnae

Pinnal necrosis in pigs. This is alternatively known as *porcine ear necrosis syndrome* and represents a multifactorial disease that develops in nursery pigs. Ear biting, high humidity, and possibly nutritional deficiencies are associated with development of lesions. Spirochetes have been observed within ulcerated skin lesions by some groups, whereas others have more commonly isolated *Staphylococcus* spp. The spirochete most commonly associated with these lesions was *Treponema pedis*, detected by fluorescence in situ hybridization (FISH). The lesion is a necrotizing dermatitis that includes ulceration with thick crusts as well as severe acanthosis with hyperkeratosis, and may contain intralesional spirochetes (eFig. 5-7). Underlying dermal vasculitis with mural degeneration and thrombosis has been observed.

Leishmaniasis. Cutaneous leishmaniasis is 1 of 3 forms of the disease caused by the *Leishmania* protozoan. Nodular lesions may commonly affect the head of dogs and cats when infected. A recent report documents the pinnae as the most frequent site of nodule formation in cats in northern and central Texas, with intralesional *Leishmania mexicana* being the most common species amplified by PCR. Regional species variation of these protozoa exists. Lesions consist of nodular to diffuse aggregations of macrophages with variable numbers of infiltrating neutrophils, lymphocytes, plasma cells, and mast cells. Numerous amastigotes are most commonly observed within macrophage cytoplasm. The overlying epidermis ranges from acanthotic with mixed hyperkeratosis to ulcerated. Kinetoplasts are not visualized without the aid of oil immersion objectives, and the most effective histochemical stain for confirming this organism is Giemsa.

Dermatophilosis. *Dermatophilus congolensis* is the causative organism of a superficial, pustular and crusting dermatitis. Species affected include sheep, goats, cattle, horses, cats, and rabbits. In sheep, cattle, dogs, cats, rabbits, and foxes, the face, particularly the ears, feet, and dorsum, may develop erythematous papules and pustules with crusts. Histologic features include intraepidermal pustular dermatitis, and superficial perivascular dermatitis and folliculitis. Surface crusts are typically thick and have alternating layers of keratin and suppurative exudate, referred to as palisading crusts.

Canine leproid granuloma. First reported in Boxer dogs and Bullmastiffs, it has now been reported in a number of breeds. Affected animals, typically short-coated, large-breed dogs of any age or either sex, have one to multiple, well-circumscribed, mildly painful, frequently ulcerated, firm papules, plaques, or nodules ranging from 2 mm to 5 cm in diameter. The pinna is most commonly affected, mostly on the convex surface or near the base. Pyogranulomatous inflammation in the subcutis and dermis is composed of mostly epithelioid macrophages mixed with neutrophils, plasma cells, lymphocytes, and variable numbers of multinucleated giant cells. Acid-fast bacteria are typically found in macrophages and multinucleated giant cells, ranging from slender, elongate bacilli to short beaded bacilli. Infections are thought to be the result of percutaneous inoculation of saprophytic organisms into wounds or by arthropods. Lesions are most commonly recognized during the warmest months of the year. Bacteria remain localized to the skin, with no reports of nodal or internal organ involvement. Lesions are localized, do not spread, and do not recur.

Feline proliferative, necrotizing otitis externa. Proliferative and necrotizing otitis externa is rarely diagnosed in cats and is characterized by plaques forming on the convex surface or scapha of the pinna and variably extending into the conical opening of the external acoustic meatus. Rarely, the plaques may extend to the tympanic membrane or into the middle ear. Young cats are most often affected by this disorder; however, the age range reported is 3 months to 5 years old. Lesions may be painful and are reported to regress spontaneously or persist for years. Key diagnostic microscopic features include orthokeratotic and parakeratotic hyperkeratosis overlying superficial papillomatous and follicular epidermal hyperplasia with variable neutrophilic crusts that overlay the surface and occlude affected hair follicles. Single-cell necrosis/apoptosis is present at different levels of the epidermis with prominent lymphocytic exocytosis and satellitosis of the dead keratinocytes. Confluent dead keratinocytes manifest as superficial regions of necrosis. The dermal inflammation is mixed, including neutrophils, lymphocytes, plasma cells, eosinophils, and mast cells that congregate around dilated superficial dermal blood vessels. Predominantly CD3+ T lymphocytes infiltrate the epidermis and dermis, leading to speculation that this is a predominantly lymphocyte-mediated disease in response to an instigating viral infection. A definitive cause remains undetermined, and possibilities include viral infection, food hypersensitivity, and drug eruption. Many are unresponsive to treatment; however, 2 cases reported successful resolution with the use of tacrolimus ointment, a macrolide lactone that is a potent inhibitor of T-lymphocyte–mediated cytokines.

Further reading

Conceição LG, et al. Epidemiology, clinical signs, histopathology and molecular characterization of canine leproid granuloma:

a retrospective study of cases from Brazil. Vet Dermatol 2011;22: 249-256.

Karlsson F, et al. Identification of *Treponema pedis* as the predominant *Treponema* species in porcine skin ulcers by fluorescence in situ hybridization and high-throughput sequencing. Vet Microbiol 2014;171:122-131.

Santoro D, et al. Cutaneous sterile granulomas/pyogranulomas, leishmaniasis and mycobacterial infections. J Small Anim Pract 2008;49:552-561.

Pinnal tumor-like growths and neoplasia

Aural hematoma. A single plate of auricular cartilage forms the pinna. Throughout are numerous perforations through which fibrovascular stroma penetrates. In animals with concurrent otitis externa or otitis media, chronic head shaking is a common clinical sign. Repeated, vigorous rotational shaking of the ears exerts shearing forces, especially in the regions of cartilage perforations, and the sheared edges of cartilage can lacerate penetrating blood vessels. The resultant hemorrhage leads to aural hematomas.

Aural hematomas are most commonly reported in dogs and lop-eared breeds of pigs, and less commonly in cats and ruminants. Firm, warm swellings affect the concave or scaphal surface of the pinna and typically hang abnormally because of increased weight. Histologic features include hemorrhage, cartilage fractures, splitting of cartilage plates, and granulation tissue infiltration. If left untreated, pinnae become deformed with firm to hard regions of dense fibrosis and dystrophic mineralization.

Auricular chondritis (relapsing polychondritis). Auricular chondritis is the pinnal manifestation of a rare immune-mediated disease that targets type II collagen and possibly matrilin-1 cartilage matrix proteins. In humans, this condition is also referred to as relapsing polychondritis in which other cartilaginous sites are affected, including the trachea, larynx, costae, and joints of limbs. Auricular chondritis manifests as a painful, typically bilateral pinnal thickening and distortion with curling, erythema, and alopecia primarily affecting cats <3 years of age. It has been reported in ear-tagged rodents, and there is a case report in a dog. Histologic features include distortion of the aural cartilage surrounded by lymphocytes, macrophages, multinucleated giant cells, variable numbers of neutrophils, and fibrosis. The normally basophilic hyaline cartilage is transformed to a much more eosinophilic matrix centrally. In several cases, concurrent ocular and cardiac disease was reported related to type II collagen present in the uvea and heart valves.

Equine aural plaques. One or both pinnae of affected horses manifest flattened, verrucous, circumscribed, depigmented, hyperkeratotic nodules that can affect up to 40% of the inner concave surface. These plaques are individual to coalescing, ranging from 4-20 mm in diameter and 2-4 mm above the epidermal surface. Characteristic microscopic features include abrupt, moderate to severe, acanthosis with equally abrupt loss of pigment, with variable numbers of koilocytes, and overlying hyperkeratosis. Mixtures of lymphocytes, macrophages, neutrophils, and eosinophils infiltrate the dermis.

Aural plaques are associated with *papillomavirus* based on the histologic appearance of the lesions, immunohistochemical detection of papillomavirus antigen, and PCR confirmation of 4 novel *Equus caballus* papillomaviruses (EcPV), further classified into 2 genera: *Dyoiota* (EcPV-4 and EcPV-5) and *Dyorho* (EcPV-3 and EcPV-6). Unlike most other papillomavirus infections, aural plaques are never observed in horses <1 year of age, and they do not spontaneously resolve or regress. Additionally, these pinnal lesions are primarily reported in the Northern Hemisphere and are believed to be associated with or spread by aural irritation by biting flies, especially blackflies (*Simulium vittatum, S. argus*).

Epithelial tumors. *Squamous cell carcinoma* (SCC) has long been associated with ulcerated, crusted, and bleeding lesions affecting the tips or caudal edges of the pinnae of cats. Reported as the most common neoplasm affecting the pinnae of cats and representing 2% of tumors in cats, the largest study to date determined that 95% of cases were in white or partially white cats, and the median age was 12 years. The vast majority of cases are bilateral—one reason this lesion is strongly correlated with prolonged exposure to ultraviolet radiation. Greater than 80% of pinnal SCC in cats overexpressed p53 protein. Morphologic features are typical for SCC. Complete resection of the pinna had the longest reported median survival times. The worst prognosis is reported in cats with concurrent pinnal and nasal planum involvement. Neoplasms can be locally invasive, involving other compartments of the ear or spread via lymphatics of the head and neck to the lungs.

In *sheep*, precancerous lesions involving the ear typically begin as inflamed, highly proliferative lesions that may deform the entire ear. Papillomavirus most closely related to bovine papillomavirus 2 (BPV-2) transform into squamous cell carcinoma. Australian shepherds refer to this simply as "ear cancer." Lesions may arise in regions of a previous ear-mark. An epizootic of aural papillomas was reported in a Polled Hereford herd involving one or both ears because of the presumptive spread of papillomavirus arising in the tattoo sites. Some lesions took 8 months to resolve.

Either the base of the ear or pinna represents a common site for *several epithelial growths* mostly seen in dogs and cats. These include trichoblastomas, trichoepitheliomas, sebaceous gland hyperplasia, sebaceous gland adenoma, apocrine cysts, apocrine adenomas, and basal cell carcinomas. Malignant phenotypes of these tumors may also be recognized in this location. Epitrichial sweat gland tumors are benign neoplasms that commonly affect the pinna in horses. Viral-induced papillomas may also involve the pinnae in younger dogs.

Common mesenchymal tumors of the ear. Similar to folliculosebaceous tumors indicated previously, mast cell tumors, histiocytomas, and plasmacytomas have a tendency to involve extremities, such as pinnae or the base of the ear.

Aural melanoma (Angora goats, cats). Pinnal-associated melanomas can be classified into 3 broad groups: (1) congenital melanomas (cattle, swine), (2) feline dermal melanomas, and (3) dermal melanomas of Angora goats.

Congenital neoplasms are rarely reported in domestic animals. There are even rarer case reports documenting dermal melanomas with pinnal involvement. One report documents a male, red Sindhi calf with a congenital pinnal melanoma that was discovered at birth, prompting curative pinnal amputation. One earlier report involved the root of the ear in a Japanese black bovid and 2 different cattle with left mandibular expansive masses that extended to include the ear canal or squamous temporal bone.

Congenital melanocytic neoplasms have been documented as common in swine; however, most authors report the head but do not specifically list pinnae as a predilection site.

Dermal melanocytic neoplasms frequently affect dogs, and most are benign. In cats, melanomas are far less common, reportedly accounting for 0.5% of feline cutaneous neoplasms. Based on several studies, dermal melanomas in cats most frequently involve the head, and head tumors are most often pinnal. There is conflicting evidence in the literature regarding biological behavior of these aural tumors, with 2 large studies strongly asserting that pinnal melanomas are nearly uniformly benign, whereas a third retrospective study found 12% of aural melanomas were malignant.

The final group involves *ultraviolet (UV) radiation-induced melanomas in Angora goats*. The Angora breed is described as brown-eyed, white-skinned goats with dense pale mohair except for the ears, nose, and perineum. Prevalence rates are much higher in goats that graze in low latitudes, such as northern Africa, India, New Zealand, and Australia, where there is high solar UV exposure. The anatomic sites with the least protection from UV radiation include the dorsal, convex surface of the pinnae, base of the horn, and the perineum.

Young goats in Australia were observed to develop *lentigines* (sharply circumscribed regions of epidermal hyperplasia confined to the epidermis) beginning at 3 months of age and peaking by 2 years of age. These benign proliferations remained unchanged in appearance and number between 2-3 years of age. Lentigines are considered possible but not obligate melanoma precursors.

Malignant melanomas develop in older goats, with a peak age of 4-5 years of age. They are considered by many to be highly malignant, commonly spreading via lymphatics and blood vessels to regional lymph nodes, liver, and lungs as well as other parenchymal organs. Tumors tend to be multiple, dermoepidermal, or subcutaneous and black. Microscopic features include large, anaplastic epithelioid melanocytes mixed with spindle cells that are variably pigmented. Mitotic figures are numerous and frequently bizarre.

Uncommon pinnal mesenchymal tumors. A small number of reports document uncommon causes of pinnal neoplasia in cats. *Rhabdomyoma* has been reported in a series of 4 cats as discoid, well-circumscribed, nonulcerated masses affecting the convex surface of the ear. Histologic features included whorls and bundles of spindle-shaped cells with cross-striations and rare mitotic activity. All cats were white and 6-7 years of age. Excision was curative in all cases.

Cutaneous *hemangiosarcomas* are infrequently reported in cats. With a mean age of 12.5 years, 50% of reported cases affect the pinnae. Neoplastic endothelial cells displayed variable anisokaryosis, chromatin patterns, and mitotic index. Solar elastosis, acanthosis, ulceration, and hemorrhage were reported in several cases. Most of the affected cats were white.

Rarely, *fibromas and fibrosarcomas* have been reported in cats and dogs, and a single case of a fibroleiomyoma was reported in a pig. *Sarcoids* may involve any location in horses and cats but have been reported to commonly involve the head and pinnae of cats.

Further reading

Baba T, et al. Auricular chondritis associated with systemic joint and cartilage inflammation in a cat. J Vet Med Sci 2009;71:79-82.

Gorino AC, et al. Use of PCR to estimate the prevalence of *Equus caballus* papillomavirus in aural plaques in horses. Vet J 2013;197:903-904.

Lange CE, et al. Four novel papillomavirus sequences support a broad diversity among equine papillomaviruses. J Gen Virol 2013;94:1365-1372.

Ley RD. Animal models of ultraviolet radiation (UVR)-induced cutaneous melanoma. Front Biosci 2002;7:d1531-d1534.

Torres SMF, Koch SN. Papillomavirus-associated diseases. Vet Clin North Am Equine Pract 2013;29:643-655.

External ear parasitism

Several parasites preferentially or exclusively infest the external ear of domestic and wild mammals. In other cases, only a portion of the life cycle involves the external acoustic meatus (EAM). Parasitic maladies include otoacariasis (ear mite infestations), ear ticks, and nematodes.

Otoacariasis

***Raillietia* spp.** are tiny, blood-feeding mites that parasitize the deepest portions of the EAM and external surface of the tympanic membrane affecting cattle, goats, and buffalo in the Americas, Australia, Great Britain, Europe, and the Middle East. Infestations frequently go undetected because host species display no clinical disease, or tiny mites deep in the EAM remain obscured from otoscopic view because of thick plugs of exudate. External ear lesions include mild to moderate, suppurative otitis media, mild parakeratotic hyperkeratosis, and acanthosis, with an inflamed but typically intact tympanic membrane. Infrequently, tympanic membranes become perforated with mites also infesting the tympanic cavity, and animals develop suppurative otitis media as well as suppurative bulla osteitis, resulting in signs that may include ataxia, head tilt, circling, and inability to right themselves.

In cattle and buffalo, *Raillietia auris* has been associated with transmission of a rhabditiform nematode, *Rhabditis bovis*. A link between *Raillietia caprae* infections in goats and concurrent *Mycoplasma* spp. isolated from the ears has been made, either related to acquisition through blood ingestion or possibly by transovarial or trans-stadial transmission. Finally, various other bacterial and fungal infections may be concurrently cultured from ruminants infected with *Raillietia* spp.

Described as the most common parasite associated with otitis externa in dogs and cats, **Otodectes cynotis** is associated with severe pruritus and a dark otorrhea likened to ground coffee representing cerumen, keratin, exudation, and mite waste. It is estimated that >50% of feline otitis externa is related to *O. cynotis* infestations compared with 5-10% in dogs. These mites reside deep in the EAM and instigate intense epidermal irritation (Fig. 5-92). Mites feed on lymph and whole blood, resulting in introduction of salivary antigens and sensitization. Thus intensity of pruritus may be related to an underlying immediate-type or Arthus-type reaction. Protective immunity may develop in cats. Infestations are typically bilateral, and the mites are extremely contagious, often traveling from dam to nursing young. Histologic lesions include epidermal hyperplasia with mixed hyperkeratosis and crusts. Ceruminous glands are both hypertrophied and ectatic. A mixed infiltrate is present in the dermis, including lymphocytes and macrophages. Animals may develop auricular hematomas, otitis media, and vestibular dysfunction, and convulsions may occur with severe, long-standing infestations.

There are several ***Psoroptes* spp.**; however, only *P. cuniculi* are found to preferentially infest ears of goats, sheep, horses, and rabbits. In some regions, coinfection with *Raillietia* spp.

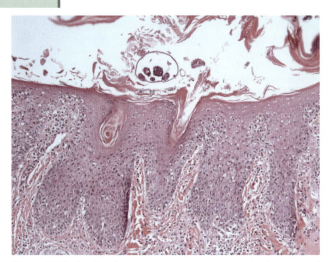

Figure 5-92 An *Otodectes cynotis* mite is present in the external acoustic meatus of a cat. The reaction includes hyperkeratosis, epidermal hyperplasia, and mostly mononuclear cell infiltration of the superficial dermis with exocytosis through the thickened epithelium.

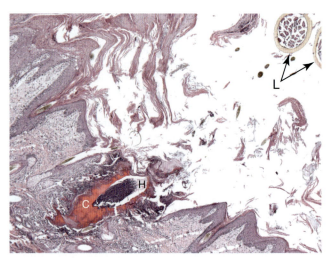

Figure 5-93 An 8-month-old calf with "**gotch ear.**" The hypostome (H) of the *Amblyomma maculatum* tick is embedded through the epidermis into the dermis surrounded by a brightly eosinophilic cone of cement (C). There is marked necrosis and suppurative dermatitis surrounding the hypostome. In the upper right corner are cross-sections through the segmented legs of this tick (L).

may occur. Surface irritation within the EAM leads to luminal cerumen, lipids, keratin, and crusts that sustain these mites and manifest as intense pruritus. Histologic changes include epidermal hyperplasia with variable hyperkeratosis and crusts, and perivascular, eosinophilic dermatitis.

***Demodex* spp.** infestations are recognized as primarily localized or generalized, noncontagious cutaneous disease resulting in folliculitis, furunculosis, and pleocellular dermatitis in reaction to intradermal mites, and often secondary pyoderma. Primary otitis is a rare, sporadic form of demodicosis that primarily causes an intensely pruritic, refractory ceruminous exudative otitis externa in dogs and cats.

Trombiculosis is a rare form of otoacariasis caused by *Neotrombicula autumnalis* (Europe) and *Eutrombicula alfredduggesi* (southeastern and south-central United States), more commonly referred to as "chiggers" or harvest mites. Parasitic larvae occasionally infest cats, dogs, horses, people, and birds, causing papulopustular dermatitis of the ears and feet, whereas adult mites are free living in soil and leaf litter. Lesions are more commonly reported in cats in autumn months. The cutaneous margin pouch, also referred to as Henry's pocket or pouch, is the preferential site for infestation. Infesting larvae are red-orange, hexapod, and much smaller than *O. cynotis*. Cats may be clinically unaffected or intensely pruritic with evidence of periaural self-trauma. This difference may also reflect a hypersensitivity reaction.

External ear ticks

***Ixodidae* ticks** are the large family of hard ticks that possess a scutum, the Latin term for their hard shield. Infestation in production animals is a global scourge with related poor weight gain, a drop in milk production, impaired immunity, anemia, or a combination. In addition, these ticks act as vectors for infectious diseases that include rickettsia, spirochetes, protozoa, and viruses.

Ixodid ticks lacerate the skin using cheliceral digits, allowing insertion of their hypostome to begin feeding. Specific cells in type II and III salivary granular acini secrete proteins and lipids that congeal around the embedded hypostome to form a cone of cement that anchors the tick to the host to allow long feeding periods. During feeding, blood drawn in through the hypostome alternates with deposition of saliva contents that include anticoagulants, anti-inflammatory factors, complement inhibitors, immune modulator defensins, and chemokine binders called evasins. Similarly, salivary glands and the midgut serve as the sources of infectious bacteria, protozoa, and viruses.

***Amblyomma maculatum*,** or the *Gulf Coast ear tick*, plagues the pinnae of livestock in the states with proximity to the Gulf of Mexico. This is a hard tick that commonly infests small rodents, but the host range includes cattle, goats, horses, mules, pigs, wild ungulates, raccoons, coyotes, foxes, dogs, and cats. Larvae and nymphs engorge on birds or small mammals, but adults attach to and engorge on the pinna of larger mammals. Infested pinnae tend to droop forward and over time will become severely deformed, resulting in an ear morphology referred by some as "gotch ear." Histologically, a brightly eosinophilic cone of cement in the dermis encircles the hypostome surrounded by marked edema and necrosis associated with large numbers of neutrophils, macrophages, lymphocytes, and variable numbers of eosinophils (Fig. 5-93). Presumptively, this intense inflammation may lead to cartilage injury and distortion.

Another group of ticks that preferentially infest the host ear are ***Rhipicephalus* spp.** The lesion described for *A. maculatum* is similar for *Rhipicephalus* spp. infestations. *Rhipicephalus appendiculatus* is known as the *brown ear tick*, which is distributed in eastern, central, and southern Africa. Large and small ruminants, horses, carnivores, and hares serve as natural hosts of this tick. Several *Ehrlichia* spp. are transmitted by these ticks, including *Theileria parva*, the cause of East Coast fever; *Ehrlichia bovis*; lumpy skin disease virus; and Nairobi sheep disease virus. *Rhipicephalus sanguineus* is one of the most widely distributed ticks, with the dog serving as the primary host and so named the *brown dog tick*.

Tick larvae and nymphs of **Otobius megnini,** also known as the *spinose ear tick,* infest deep in the external ear canals of most domestic species, most commonly reported in horses, cattle, sheep, camelids, dogs, wild large mammals, and rarely people. These are the only argasid ticks that commonly infest domestic mammals native to North and Central America. No infectious organisms are vector transmitted by O. megnini. Adults are nonparasitic, laying eggs on the ground; however, larvae access the host from vegetation and locate to the EAM. Within a few days, they molt into nymphs and remain within the canal for 1-7 months. Nymphs cause severe and constant local irritation, often confined deep in the EAM next to the tympanic membrane and hidden from otoscopic examination by thick luminal exudate. Rarely, infestations in horses have been associated with colic, muscle pain, elevated creatine kinase (CK) and aspartate aminotransferase (AST), and muscle fasciculations that resolve and return to normal once the ears are successfully treated.

External ear nematodes

Rhabditis bovis are tiny nematodes that spend their entire life cycle in the ear canals of affected cattle, transmitted by *Raillietia* spp. More commonly diagnosed in South America and India, rhabditiform otitis externa is more commonly reported in cattle breeds with long, pendulous pinnae (Gyr and Indubrasil breeds). Older cattle are more severely affected than younger animals. In addition to mite infestation, other risk factors include flies, cow dips, high ambient heat and humidity, presence of manure, and possibly the presence of large horns. Chronic, severe otitis externa is associated with bloody and otomiasmic otorrhea. Infections can also lead to distorted or occluded external ear canals, ruptured tympanic membranes, and otitis media with secondary bacterial infections. Facial nerve and vestibulocochlear nerve dysfunction may lead to drooping ears and head tilt, respectively. Up to 10% of severely affected cattle may die with morphologic evidence of microabscesses to gangrenous lesions in the medulla and cerebellum. Histologic changes of the internal ear have not been reported.

Stephanofilaria zaheeri is a nematode that preferentially localizes to the skin of the inner surface of the ear of buffalo in India. Microfilaria may be obtained from infected animals. Grossly, the ears range from normal to alopecic and congested to ulcerated with exudation, hemorrhage, and depigmentation. Microfilaria may be observed in the dermis, hair follicles, or sebaceous glands. The dermal infiltration varies from lymphocytes and macrophages to areas of cavitation associated with macrophages, eosinophils, and plasma cells centered on degenerate microfilaria.

Further reading

Angus JC. Otic cytology in health and disease. Vet Clin North Am Small Anim Pract 2004;34:411-424.

Duarte ER, Hamdan JS. Otitis in cattle, an aetiological review. J Vet Med B 2004;51:1-7.

Jimena ON, et al. Association of *Riallietia caprae* with the presence of mycoplasmas in the external ear canal of goats. Prev Vet Med 2009;92:150-152.

Klemm E, et al. Otitis externa and myringitis due to demodicosis. Acta Dermatoven APA 2009;18:73-76.

Leone F, et al. Feline trombiculosis: a retrospective study in 72 cats. Vet Dermatol 2013;24:535-537.

External acoustic meatal neoplasia

Feline ceruminous cystomatosis

Commonly referred to as *ceruminous cysts* or *ceruminous cystic hyperplasia* or ceruminous cystomatosis, these are dark black to blue to purple, multiple, nodules or vesicles with a typical diameter of 1-5 mm affecting the EAM and inner concave surface of the pinnae. One or, commonly, both ears are affected. One report determined a predilection in Abyssinian and Persian cats; however, any cat breed can be affected. These cystic growths can be progressive and may lead to obstruction of the EAM.

Ceruminous gland neoplasms

Ceruminous glands are specialized apocrine glands localized to the EAM and lower portion of the inner pinna. These glands consist of a secretory epithelium that rests atop myoepithelial cells with a surrounding basal lamina. These glands lie deep to sebaceous glands and have ducts that empty either into follicular infundibula or directly onto the epidermal surface of the external ear. Luminal contents are variably described as green-brown to orange-brown glassy, representing the apocrine secretion of ceruminous glands. This more watery secretion mixes with the holocrine, lipid-laden secretion of sebaceous glands to form *cerumen*.

Neoplasms arising from these glands are morphologically similar to apocrine gland neoplasms found elsewhere in the skin. Ceruminous gland neoplasms have only been reported in dogs, cats, a ferret, and rarely in people. Primarily with reference to dogs and cats, neoplasms are classified as adenomas, adenocarcinomas, and mixed or complex ceruminous gland tumors.

Ceruminous gland adenomas are diagnosed in both dogs and cats but are considered more common in the dog. Adenomas tend to be large and may partially or completely occlude the EAM. They most often manifest clinically as chronic otitis externa, and as a result, adenomas are most often associated with chronic, ongoing inflammation. They tend to be lobulated masses composed of cuboidal to columnar epithelial cells that form tubules or papillary proliferations. Neoplastic cells display minimal pleomorphism and rare mitotic figures. Plasma cells tend to predominate within the periglandular dermis with mixtures of neutrophils in the dermis as well as in glandular lumens. Dysplasia of pre-existing glands may be present. Several authors report the difficulty in differentiating chronic otitis externa with ceruminous gland hyperplasia, and dysplasia from ceruminous gland adenomas.

Ceruminous gland adenocarcinomas are diagnosed in both dogs and cats and are more common in cats than are adenomas. Neoplastic cells tend to be more pleomorphic with large, vesicular nuclei and a single, prominent nucleolus per nucleus. These neoplasms tend to be locally invasive and are more difficult to delineate. Mitotic figures tend to be more numerous, with one author determining that a mitotic index of ≥3/high-power field in cats was associated with poor long-term survival. Nodal metastasis has been reported to occur in a minority of cases in both dogs and cats. Pulmonary metastasis is reported more commonly in dogs compared with cats; however, overall, this is normally <10% and late in the disease.

Mixed or complex ceruminous gland tumors are morphologically similar to their counterpart in apocrine gland tumors, comprising mixtures of epithelial and myoepithelial proliferation as well as stroma that displays chondroid metaplasia, possibly with concurrent osseous metaplasia. This neoplastic phenotype has rarely been reported in ceruminous gland tumors but is commonly found with apocrine gland tumors elsewhere in the body.

Other external acoustic meatal neoplasms
Other neoplasia affecting the EAM includes carcinomas of undetermined origin, squamous cell carcinomas, and rarely a variety of other mesenchymal tumors that more commonly affect the pinnae. One study found that only malignant neoplasms involved both the EAM and the bullae in dogs and cats.

Further reading
De Lorenzi D, et al. Fine-needle biopsy of external ear canal masses in the cat: cytologic results and histologic correlations in 27 cases. Vet Clin Pathol 2005;34:100-105.

Romanucci M, et al. Aural carcinoma with chondroid metaplasia at metastatic sites in a dog. Vet Dermatol 2011;22:373-377.

Wilcock B, et al. Histological classification of ocular and otic tumors of domestic animals. In: Wilcock B, et al., editors. World Health Organization International Histological Classification of Tumors of Domestic Animals. 2nd series, vol. IX. Washington, DC: Armed Forces Institute of Pathology; 2002.

Zur G. Bilateral ear canal neoplasia in three dogs. Vet Dermatol 2005;16:276-280.

Histologic preparation and examination
Laboratories that specialize in human temporal bone processing and sectioning within North America tend to use very specialized techniques and reagents that are not commonly used for routine tissue processing. Instead of formic acid–containing demineralization solutions, buffered, cold ethylenediamine tetra-acetic acid (EDTA) solutions are used to slowly removed calcium from the otic capsule, a process that takes several months as opposed to days or weeks. Paraffin-embedding is replaced with celloidin, and the process requires several steps that make use of chloroform. On average, nearly a full year after the temporal bones are collected, stained slides are available for histologic examination. The entire block is sectioned, and every tenth slide is stained. Complete assessment of all turns of the cochlea, the vestibular system, the middle ear cavity and associated structures, and the portion of external ear present encompasses more than 30 glass slides. The final product is absolutely gorgeous, with exquisite retention of detail of the spiral organ and vestibular membrane. This process is impractical for routine veterinary diagnostic laboratories.

In most veterinary histology laboratories, tissue samples are formalin fixed and paraffin embedded. In high-throughput veterinary laboratories, bony samples are often processed in decalcifying reagents that use acids to help rapidly soften bony tissues to minimize processing delays and facilitate prompt final diagnoses. Although this is likely fine for histologic examination of an external ear or middle ear, the internal ear requires more fastidious demineralization techniques. Additionally, the spiral organ and vestibular membrane are extremely delicate, prone to damage from tissue processing, and presumed to rapidly autolyze postmortem. Therefore, if examination of the internal ear is of greatest importance, rapid collection and fixation of the bony and membranous labyrinth are paramount for histologic sections to be most useful.

For dogs and cats, routine sections that include the external, middle, and internal ear compartments on a single glass slide are well documented in the Further reading section. Briefly, following formalin-fixation and proper demineralization of the otic capsule and associated temporal bone, using commercial solutions with various concentrations of formic acid, a sharp blade is positioned so that a shallow portion of the external ear, tympanic membrane, associated ossicles, tympanic cavity, and portions of the cochlea and vestibule are included in the section. The plane of section may be ventrodorsal through an opened tympanic bulla, with the blade directed through to the inner surface of the petrous portion of the temporal bone, or mediolateral, with the blade directed toward the external acoustic meatus. Either technique will allow assessment of most of the ear compartments in a single section.

Few methods are published for assessment of the internal ear of livestock species; longer periods of time are required for demineralization as well as trimming modifications related to anatomic variation between species. Whereas demineralization of feline and canine temporal bones may take 2-4 weeks, demineralization of the petrous portion of the temporal bone of a horse will take several months and numerous, regular changes of the commercial demineralization solution.

Further reading
Hordeaux J, et al. Histopathologic changes of the ear in canine models of mucopolysaccharidosis types I and VII. Vet Pathol 2011;48: 616-626.

Njaa BL, Sula MM. Collection and preparation of dog and cat ears for histologic examination. Vet Clin North Am Small Anim Pract 2012; 42:1127-1135.

For more information, please visit the companion site: PathologyofDomesticAnimals.com.

CHAPTER 6

Integumentary System

Elizabeth A. Mauldin • Jeanine Peters-Kennedy

GENERAL CONSIDERATIONS	511
Epidermis	512
Epidermal nonkeratinocytes	513
Basement membrane zone	513
Dermis	514
Dermal muscles	515
Immunologic function	515
Hair follicles	515
Sebaceous glands	517
Perianal glands	517
Sweat glands	517
Subcutis	518
DERMATOHISTOPATHOLOGY	518
Glossary: histologic terms	518
Gross terminology	524
Pattern analysis	524
Perivascular dermatitis	525
Interface dermatitis	525
Vasculitis	525
Nodular and diffuse dermatitis	526
Intraepidermal vesicular and pustular dermatitis	527
Subepidermal vesicular and pustular dermatitis	527
Perifolliculitis, folliculitis, and furunculosis	528
Fibrosing dermatitis	528
Panniculitis	528
Atrophic dermatosis	529
CONGENITAL AND HEREDITARY DISEASES OF SKIN	530
Ichthyosis	530
Nonepidermolytic ichthyosis	531
Wattles	532
Hereditary zinc deficiency	532
Epidermolysis bullosa	533
Cattle	534
Sheep	535
Goats	535
Horses	535
Dogs	536
Cats	536
Genetic acantholytic dermatoses in dogs	537
Genetic acantholytic dermatoses in cattle	537
Congenital hypotrichosis	538
Cattle	538
Dogs	539
Cats	539
Hypotrichosis associated with pigmentary alterations	539
Hypertrichosis	541
Canine dermatomyositis	541
Hereditary connective tissue disorders	542
Hereditary collagen dysplasia	543
Cattle	544
Sheep	544
Horses	544
Dogs	544
Cats	545
Abnormalities of elastic fibers	545
Congenital abnormalities of ground substance	545
Dermatosis vegetans	546
Dermoid cyst	547
DISORDERS OF EPIDERMAL DIFFERENTIATION	547
Seborrhea	548
Acne	549
Schnauzer comedo syndrome	549
Tail gland hyperplasia	549
Canine nasodigital hyperkeratosis	549
Labrador Retriever nasal parakeratosis	550
Keratoses	550
Sebaceous adenitis	551
Vitamin A–responsive dermatosis	552
Lichenoid-psoriasiform dermatosis	552
Ear margin dermatosis	553
Exfoliative dermatoses (exfoliative erythroderma)	553
Hyperplastic dermatosis of West Highland White Terriers	553
Equine coronary band dystrophy	553
Ichthyosis	554
DISORDERS OF PIGMENTATION	554
Disorders of hyperpigmentation	554
Acquired hyperpigmentation	554
Focal macular melanosis	554
Canine acanthosis nigricans	555
Acromelanism	555
Disorders of hypopigmentation	555
Leukoderma and leukotrichia	555
Hereditary hypopigmentation	555
Acquired hypopigmentation	557
Leukotrichia	557
Copper deficiency	558
PHYSICOCHEMICAL DISEASES OF SKIN	558
Physical injury to skin	559
Mechanical, frictional, and traumatic injury	559
Psychogenic injury	561
Mineral deposition in cutaneous tissues	562
Cold injury	564
Thermal injury	564
Radiation injury	566
Chemical injury to skin	566
Primary irritant contact dermatitis	566
Envenomation	568
Thallotoxicosis	568
Arsenic toxicosis	570
Mercury toxicosis	570
Cutaneous iodism	570
Selenium toxicosis	570
Organochlorine and organobromine toxicoses	571
Mimosine toxicosis	572
Gangrenous ergotism and fescue toxicosis	572
Trichothecene toxicoses	573
Vetch toxicosis and vetch-like diseases	574
Quassinoid toxicosis	574
ACTINIC DISEASES OF SKIN	575
Direct effect of solar radiation	575
Photosensitization dermatitis	577
Primary photosensitization (type I photosensitization)	578
Photosensitization resulting from defective pigment synthesis (type II photosensitization)	579
Hepatogenous photosensitization (type III photosensitization)	579
Photoaggravated dermatoses	580

NUTRITIONAL DISEASES OF SKIN 580
  Protein-calorie deficiency 581
  Fatty acid deficiency 581
  Hypovitaminoses and vitamin-responsive dermatoses 581
    Vitamin A deficiency 581
    Vitamin B deficiencies 582
    Vitamin C deficiency 582
    Vitamin E deficiency 583
  Mineral deficiency and mineral-responsive dermatoses 583
    Zinc deficiency 583
    Canine zinc-responsive dermatoses 585
  Superficial necrolytic dermatitis (hepatocutaneous syndrome) 586
ENDOCRINE DISEASES OF SKIN 587
  Hypothyroidism 587
  Hyperadrenocorticism 588
  Hyposomatotropism and hypersomatotropism 589
  Hyperestrogenism 589
  Alopecia X 589
  Canine recurrent flank alopecia 590
IMMUNE-MEDIATED DERMATOSES 590
  Hypersensitivity dermatoses 590
    Atopic dermatitis 591
    Urticaria and angioedema 594
    Cutaneous adverse food reaction 594
    Allergic contact dermatitis 596
    Insect hypersensitivity 597
    Hormonal hypersensitivity 599
    Intestinal parasite hypersensitivity 599
  Autoimmune dermatoses 600
    Autoimmune diseases characterized by vesicles, pustules, or bullae as the primary lesion 600
    Lupus erythematosus 604
  Other immune-mediated dermatoses 607
    Drug eruptions 607
    Cryopathies 608
    Graft-versus-host disease 608
    Erythema multiforme/Stevens-Johnson syndrome/toxic epidermal necrolysis 609
    Vasculitis 611
    Rabies vaccine–induced vasculitis and alopecia in dogs 612
    Canine uveodermatologic syndrome (Vogt-Koyanagi-Harada [VKH] syndrome) 613
    Plasma cell pododermatitis 613
    Cutaneous amyloidosis 614
    Alopecia areata 614
VIRAL DISEASES OF SKIN 615
  Poxviral infections 616
    Parapoxviral diseases 617
    Orthopoxviral diseases 619
    Molluscipoxviral disease 621
    Capripoxviral diseases 622
    Suipoxviral disease 625
  Herpesviral infections 625
    Bovine herpesvirus 2 diseases 625
    Bovine herpesvirus 4 diseases 626
    Equine herpesvirus 626
    Felid herpesvirus 1 627
  Retroviral infections 627
  Parvoviral infections 628
  Caliciviral infection 628
  Papillomaviral infections 628
  Miscellaneous viral infections of the skin 628
BACTERIAL DISEASES OF SKIN 629
  Superficial bacterial pyoderma 629
    Impetigo 630
    Exudative epidermitis of pigs 630
    Dermatophilosis 632
    Ovine fleece rot 634
  Deep bacterial pyoderma 634
    Staphylococcal folliculitis and furunculosis 634
    Abscesses and cellulitis 636
  Cutaneous bacterial granulomas 637
    Actinomycosis and nocardiosis 637
    Mycobacterial infections 639
    Cutaneous infections caused by slow-growing mycobacteria 639
    Bacterial pseudomycetoma 642
  Bacterial pododermatitis of horses and ruminants 642
    Proliferative pododermatitis (equine canker) 642
    Necrotizing pododermatitis (equine thrush) 643
    Necrobacillosis of cattle 643
    Necrobacillosis of pigs 643
    Necrobacillosis of sheep 643
    Contagious footrot 643
    Contagious ovine digital dermatitis 644
    Papillomatous digital dermatitis 644
    Porcine ear necrosis syndrome 645
  Skin lesions in systemic bacterial disease 645
    Bartonella 646
    Borreliosis 646
FUNGAL DISEASES OF SKIN 646
  Cutaneous fungal infections 647
    Candidiasis 647
    Malassezia dermatitis 647
    Dermatophytosis 649
  Subcutaneous fungal infections 653
    Eumycotic mycetoma 653
    Chromomycosis (phaeohyphomycosis and chromoblastomycosis) 654
    Hyalohyphomycosis 655
    Sporotrichosis 655
    Cutaneous oomycosis (pythiosis and lagenidiosis) 657
    Zygomycosis 659
    Miscellaneous fungal infections of skin 660
PROTOZOAL DISEASES OF SKIN 661
  Besnoitiosis 661
  Leishmaniasis 663
  Miscellaneous coccidian parasites 664
ALGAL DISEASES OF SKIN 665
ARTHROPOD ECTOPARASITES 666
  Flies 666
    Myiasis 668
    Sheep ked infestation 670
    Horn fly dermatitis 670
    Mosquito-bite dermatitis 670
  Miscellaneous insects 671
  Lice 671
  Fleas 672
  Mites 673
    Sarcoptic mange 673
    Notoedric mange 675
    Psoroptic mange 675
    Chorioptic mange 676
    Otodectic mange 677
    Cheyletiellosis 678
    Psorergatic mange 678
    Demodectic mange 678
    Trombiculiasis 682
    Other mite-induced dermatoses 683
  Ticks 684
HELMINTH DISEASES OF SKIN 685
  Cutaneous habronemiasis 685
  Stephanofilariasis 686

Onchocerciasis	687		Symmetrical lupoid onychitis	702
Equine cutaneous onchocerciasis	687		Laminitis	702
Bovine cutaneous onchocerciasis	688		**NEOPLASTIC AND REACTIVE DISEASES OF THE SKIN**	703
Pinworms	688		Epithelial tumors of the skin	703
Parafilariasis	688		Cysts, hamartomas, and tumor-like lesions	703
Pelodera dermatitis	689		*Cysts*	703
Miscellaneous helminths	689		*Hamartomas*	705
MISCELLANEOUS SKIN CONDITIONS	690		*Tumor-like lesions*	705
Canine juvenile cellulitis	690		Tumors of the epidermis	706
Cutaneous paraneoplastic syndromes	691		*Papillomas and papillomavirus-induced lesions*	706
Eosinophilic dermatitides	693		*Squamous cell carcinoma*	712
Feline eosinophilic granuloma complex	693		*Basal cell carcinoma*	714
Canine eosinophilic granuloma	694		*Basosquamous carcinoma*	714
Equine eosinophilic nodular diseases	694		Tumors with adnexal differentiation	714
Multisystemic, eosinophilic, epitheliotropic disease in the horse	695		*Tumors arising from hair follicles*	714
Sterile eosinophilic folliculitis and furunculosis	696		*Tumors arising from sebaceous or modified sebaceous glands*	717
Sterile eosinophilic pustulosis	696		*Tumors arising from sweat glands*	718
Eosinophilic dermatitis with edema	696		Melanocytic tumors	720
Sterile neutrophilic dermatoses	696		*Benign melanocytic tumors*	721
Auricular chondritis	697		*Malignant melanoma*	721
Follicular lipidosis	697		Spindle cell tumors	722
Follicular mucinosis (alopecia mucinosa)	697		*Benign spindle cell tumors*	722
Feline scleromyxedema	697		*Locally infiltrative and malignant spindle cell tumors*	723
Localized scleroderma (morphea) and cicatricial alopecia	698		*Other mesenchymal tumors*	726
Psoriasiform dermatitis of goats	698		Vascular tumors	726
Porcine juvenile pustular psoriasiform dermatitis	698		Histiocytic proliferative disorders	728
Miscellaneous porcine dermatoses	698		*Canine cutaneous histiocytoma*	728
Spiculosis	699		*Canine cutaneous Langerhans cell histiocytosis*	729
Sebaceous gland dysplasia	699		*Cutaneous and systemic reactive histiocytosis*	729
Perforating dermatitis	699		*Histiocytic sarcoma complex*	729
Sterile granulomas and pyogranulomas	699		*Feline progressive histiocytosis*	730
Sterile pyogranuloma syndrome	700		Mast cell tumors	730
Cutaneous xanthoma	700		Cutaneous lymphoma	733
Sarcoidosis	700		Cutaneous plasmacytoma	735
Sterile nodular panniculitis	701		Merkel cell tumor	735
			Tumors metastatic to the skin	736

ACKNOWLEDGMENTS

We gratefully acknowledge the contributions to prior editions of this chapter by Drs. Ken Jubb, Peter Kennedy, Nigel Palmer, Julie Yager, Danny Scott, Pamela Ginn, Joanne Mansell, and Pauline Rakich.

GENERAL CONSIDERATIONS

The integument serves as the anatomic boundary between the body and the ambient environment. The vast surface area of the skin puts it in constant contact with environmental irritants, pollutants, and pathogens. Unlike diseases in internal viscera, lesions in the skin are readily apparent, and thus skin disease is one of the most common reasons for veterinary consultation. Skin diseases range from minor, esthetic problems to life-threatening conditions. In companion animals, a healthy pelage (haircoat) stands as the interface between the human owner and pet. In addition to causing undo suffering, severe skin disease may interfere with the human-animal bond. In farm animals, skin diseases produce severe economic losses because of damage to wool, hides, and meat or from decreased milk production or growth rates.

The protective barrier of the skin is complex, and much of this function is provided by the *stratum corneum* (SC), the outermost layer of the epidermis. This innocuous appearing layer of terminally differentiated (dead) keratin squames maintains hydration of the body by restricting water loss. The constant shedding (desquamation) and renewal aids in the removal of surface pathogens. The SC also contains antimicrobial peptides (e.g., β-defensins, cathelicidins) and a variety of lipids that also aid in bacterial and chemical defense. Constant immunosurveillance is provided by the *skin immune system* that consists of orchestrated interactions between Langerhans cells, keratinocytes, lymphocytes, and dermal dendritic cells. Hair and melanin pigment deliver the bulk of photoprotection as well as provide thermoregulation. The epidermis is also an important site of vitamin D regulation. Sunlight acts on the epidermis to convert provitamin D3 (7-dehydrocholesterol) to vitamin D3 (cholecalciferol). In the liver, vitamin D3 is hydroxylated to 25-hydroxy D3 and in kidneys to the active form 1,25-vitamin D3. Vitamin D3 regulates epidermal differentiation and proliferation. The skin is involved in thermoregulation by virtue of the pelage, blood flow, and, in some species (e.g., equids), sweating. Last, the state of the skin is an indicator or general health and internal disease.

As dermatologic cases are more commonly presented to veterinary clinicians for examination, skin biopsies have become a routine diagnostic tool. An understanding of the pathologic processes in skin, as in any tissue, requires knowledge of normal structure and function. *As a general rule, clinicians are more adept at recognizing gross lesions than anatomic pathologists. To interpret skin biopsies, pathologists must have a* good understanding of the characteristic gross lesions and patterns manifest by diseases in the species being examined. This fact underscores the importance of the inclusion of the gross findings in the surgical pathology request. Although the architecture of the skin is conserved across most mammalian species, the pathologist must be aware of differences between species and site differences within the same species, to interpret normal versus abnormal. The dermis contributes most to the thickness of the skin. The haired skin is thickest over the dorsal surface of the body and lateral aspect of the limbs and thinnest on the ventral aspect of the trunk and medial limbs. The epidermis is naturally thicker in areas that need enhanced protection because of lack of hair and exposure to surface trauma (e.g., lips, pawpads, and nasal planum). The thinnest epidermis is found in well-protected sites (e.g., ventral abdomen, inguinal area).

The integument is composed of epidermis, dermis, adnexal structures (simple and compound hair follicles, epitrichial apocrine glands, atrichial [eccrine] glands, sebaceous glands, arrector pili muscles), and the subcutis, as well as nails, hooves, and claws.

Epidermis

The epidermis consists of a highly organized, continuously renewing squamous epithelium that is stratified into functionally distinct layers: stratum basale, stratum spinosum, stratum granulosum, and stratum corneum. The keratinocytes of the epidermis undergo a process of differentiation and proliferation that facilitates repair after external trauma and yields a hydrophobic protective barrier, the stratum corneum, which is continuously shed into the environment. The steady state of the epidermis is a balance between cell proliferation, differentiation, and desquamation. The renewal is provided by a small population of slow-cycling stem cells (~10% of cells) in the basal layer that undergo proliferation into transiently amplifying cells. The amplified cells briefly proliferate then exit the cell cycle and undergo terminal differentiation. In doing so, the cells march toward the final product—fully-cornified anucleate keratinocytes (corneocytes) that are shed into the environment. Within keratinocytes as well as other epithelial cells, keratin, an intermediate filament, forms the fibrous cytoskeleton that connects to desmosomes. Type I (acidic) and type II (basic) keratin subunits assemble into heterodimers through disulfide bonds. The type of keratin is differentially expressed in layers of the epidermis as well as body site (e.g., nonhaired skin of the pawpad and hair follicles). Keratin 5 (K5) and keratin 14 (K14) form heterodimers in basal layer keratinocytes. Commitment to differentiation in suprabasal keratinocytes is associated with induction of keratins 1 (K1) and K10. Keratin 2 (K2) is expressed in the stratum granulosum (SG).

The epidermis is a prime example of an adult tissue that undergoes continual and rapid flux. The epidermis maintains homeostasis by constant proliferation of a single inner (basal) layer of rapidly dividing progeny of stem cells. As the basal keratinocytes withdraw from the cell cycle, the transiently amplifying cells commit to terminally differentiate, detaching from the basement membrane and initiating a trek toward the skin surface.

- The **stratum basale** *(basal layer)* is the deep germinative layer of the epidermis and is composed of a single layer of cuboidal to low columnar cells resting on the basement membrane zone. The basal cells are attached to the underlying basement membrane by *hemidesmosomes* and to adjacent and overlying keratinocytes by *desmosomes*. Desmosomes are anchoring structures that mediate adhesion between cells. They have a complex structure that includes *cadherin proteins* of 2 types—desmocollins and desmogleins. These proteins have different isoforms, and they are differentially expressed in different layers of the epidermis. Whereas basal cells express a pair of desmogleins and desmocollins of simple epithelia, desmosomes of the spinous layer express more varied isoforms. These adhesion molecules are the immunologic target in several blistering autoimmune diseases.

- The **stratum spinosum** *(prickle cell layer)* is characterized by *prominent intercellular bridges that are the desmosomal attachments between cells.* The spinous appearance is due to shrinkage artifact that occurs during tissue processing. The cells are polyhedral to slightly flattened and are arranged in 1 or 2 layers in haired skin of dogs and cats and up to 4 layers in large animals. This layer is much thicker in nonhaired skin and may be up to 20 cells thick in the footpads and nasal planum.

- The **stratum granulosum** is variably apparent on light microscopy in haired skin and appears only 1-2 cells thick. In nonhaired skin, this layer is more prominent, averaging 4-8 layers in thickness. The SG is composed of flattened cells with shrunken nuclei and deeply basophilic keratohyaline granules. The granules contain a precursor of *filaggrin*, a histidine-rich interfibrillary matrix protein that *functions as a biological glue* that aggregates and aligns keratin filaments.

- The **stratum corneum** (SC) is composed of >20 overlapping layers of bland, polyhedral, anucleate cells sandwiched between layers of lipid. This inconspicuous layer is an active and tough hydrophobic barrier that regulates water movement into and out of the skin. Much of the content of the SC is lost during biopsy sampling, cutting, and processing. The *basket-weave pattern* is an artifact resulting from loss of the lipid lamellae during processing. Thickness varies by species and site, but it is generally adapted to the degree of surface trauma or friction. The SC is thickest in nonhaired areas, such as footpads and nasal planum. *Cornification (keratinization)* is the process by which keratinocytes undergo terminal differentiation from the basal layer to the highly specialized corneocyte. In doing so, keratinocytes must lose a large amount of water volume (from 70% water in nucleated layers to 15% in stratum corneum). Minor injuries to the corneal layer from tape stripping or applications of solvents will result in increased transepidermal water loss.

Several steps must occur for **cornification** to proceed normally: (1) bundling of keratin to establish the corneocyte core, (2) replacement of the cell membrane with a thick cornified envelope, (3) formation of lipid lamellar bilayers, and (4) active desquamation. Alterations in any step can lead to hyperkeratosis, clinical scaling, and decreased barrier function.

The **lipid** is derived via lipid-laden organelles, called *lamellar bodies* (also called Odland bodies, membrane coating granules, lamellar granules, keratinosomes), which are synthesized in the upper stratum spinosum. At the junction of the SG and SC, the lamellar bodies fuse with the cell membrane and expel their contents into the intercellular space. Lamellar bodies contain glucosylceramides (GlcCer), sphingomyelin, glycerophospholipids, and cholesterol sulfate, along with many modifying enzymes. During this release, enzymes modify polar "probarrier" lipids into nonpolar "barrier" lipids. The final product in the lipid bilayers of the SC contains an equimolar ratio of ceramides, cholesterol, and free fatty acids that together create a hydrophobic seal.

The **protein core** of the corneocyte provides much of the structural integrity of the stratum corneum. Profilaggrin, found in the keratohyaline granules of the SG, undergoes processing (proteolysis, dephosphorylation) to the active enzyme *filaggrin*, which cross-links the cytoplasmic keratin filaments. Transglutaminases, calcium-containing enzymes, are located within both the epidermis and hair follicles. These proteins (in particular, transglutaminase 1) catalyze the formation of the **cornified envelope** (CE) by cross-linking small protein molecules (e.g., involucrin, loricrin, cystatin A) that replace the cell membrane. The CE surrounds the protein core and provides a mechanical barrier as well as a scaffold that organizes the extracellular lipids into lamellar membranes. In the mature SC, multiple layers of corneocytes are sandwiched between layers of lipid, producing the so-called "mortar and bricks" analogy. Corneodesmosomes (desmosomes retained in the SC) are enzymatically cleaved, and keratin squames (corneocytes) are shed into the environment.

Epidermal nonkeratinocytes

Melanocytes are located in the basal layer of the epidermis and outer root sheath of hair follicles; and in hematoxylin and eosin (H&E) sections, they appear as clear cells with a small dark-staining nucleus because of shrinkage artifact. There is ~1 melanocyte per 10-20 keratinocytes. The dendritic processes can be seen with silver stains. Derived from the neural crest, melanocytes migrate into the epidermis during early fetal life. Their processes are intertwined between the surrounding keratinocytes to which they transfer melanin pigment. A melanocyte and its surrounding constellation of keratinocytes is termed the *"epidermal melanin unit."* Melanogenesis occurs in membrane-bound organelles called *melanosomes,* which originate from the Golgi apparatus. The melanosomes migrate to the tips of the dendrites and are phagocytosed by adjacent keratinocytes. Most melanin pigment in skin is in the basal layer, but in dark-skinned animals, melanin may be present throughout the epidermis. The epidermis of most dogs and cats is only lightly pigmented. Melanin is photoprotective, and exposure to ultraviolet (UV) light increases melanin production, often resulting in a cap of pigment granules over the nucleus. Skin pigmentation is affected by local inflammation because melanocytes respond to inflammatory mediators by increasing or decreasing melanogenesis and by altering melanin transfer to keratinocytes.

Langerhans cells *are bone marrow–derived dendritic cells that are functionally and immunologically related to monocyte-macrophage cells.* They appear as clear cells on routine H&E sections and may be distributed from the stratum basale to the stratum spinosum, depending on species and region of the skin. They are usually less numerous than melanocytes, however. Langerhans cells are characterized ultrastructurally by rod- or racket-shaped cytoplasmic granules called *Birbeck granules.* Birbeck granules have been identified in Langerhans cells of the pig, cat, cattle, sheep, goat, horse, and human, but not in the Langerhans cells of the dog. Langerhans cells express CD1, class II major histocompatibility complex (MHC) antigens, CD45, vimentin, and S-100. The long dendritic processes of Langerhans cells traverse the intercellular space to the granular cell layer, where *they function in immunosurveillance as antigen-presenting cells.* Langerhans cells trap antigens in the epidermis and migrate via afferent lymphatics to draining lymph nodes, where they present antigen to T cells in paracortical areas, resulting in proliferation of a population of sensitized T cells. Langerhans cells express a high-affinity receptor for immunoglobulin E (IgE) (FcεRI), which allows Fc receptor–mediated uptake of allergens. Exposure to UVB radiation decreases Langerhans cell numbers in the epidermis and interferes with their antigen-presenting capacity. Langerhans cells are involved in development of contact hypersensitivity, and increased numbers of epidermal Langerhans cells have been found in horses with insect hypersensitivity and dogs with atopic dermatitis.

A second type of clear cell in the basal layer is the **Merkel cell.** There has been a long-standing debate over whether Merkel cells originate from epidermal or neural stem cells, but current studies indicate an epidermal origin. Unlike melanocytes, Merkel cells are connected to adjacent keratinocytes by desmosomes. Merkel cells are also located in the external root sheath of hair follicles. They are identified ultrastructurally by characteristic *dense-core cytoplasmic granules.* Immunohistochemical markers include cytokeratin, neurofilaments, neuron-specific enolase, and desmosomal proteins. Merkel cells have been identified in the dog, cat, sheep, pig, monkey, various laboratory animals, birds, reptiles, and amphibians. Their density in the epidermis is variable, and they are in highest numbers in areas involved with sensory perception. Merkel cells form *Merkel cell–neurite complexes* with axons in tylotrich pads and sinus hairs that are thought to function as gentle touch receptors that initiate slow-adapting type 1 responses. Their exact function in these structures is uncertain, but they are thought not to act as sensory cells but rather to function as abutments for deformation of the mechanosensitive nerve endings. Merkel cells are also thought to have various neuroendocrine effects and to be involved in control of the hair cycle.

Basement membrane zone

The basement membrane zone (BMZ) is the structurally and biochemically complex junction between the epidermis and dermis. Both the epidermis and dermis contribute to production of the various components of the BMZ. The area is indistinct in H&E sections but visible as a thin, homogeneous band with periodic acid–Schiff (PAS) stain. It varies in thickness in different sites and is most prominent in nonhaired areas of skin and mucocutaneous junctions. In all animals except swine, the dermal-epidermal junction is straight, and the BMZ parallels the skin surface, whereas in swine and humans, the dermal-epidermal junction is thrown into undulating folds called rete ridges. *The BMZ has a crucial role in anchoring the epidermis to the dermis, and abnormalities of the BMZ result in serious and potentially fatal bullous diseases.* The BMZ also influences growth and differentiation of keratinocytes and acts as a selective barrier for passage of molecules between the epidermis and dermis.

Ultrastructurally, the BMZ is composed of (1) the **plasma membrane** of basal keratinocytes with their specialized attachment structures, *hemidesmosomes;* (2) the electron-lucent **lamina lucida;** (3) the electron-dense **lamina densa;** and (4) the subbasal **lamina fibrous zone.** Hemidesmosomes are located on the basal aspect of basal keratinocytes, and they consist of a cytoplasmic plaque that connects to the cytoskeleton and a transmembrane portion that binds to the underlying basement membrane. The *cytoplasmic plaque* is composed of a number of proteins, including bullous pemphigoid antigen 230 (bullous pemphigoid antigen 1) and plectin, which connect keratin 5 and 14 intermediate filaments to the plasma membrane. Hemidesmosomes also have a transmembrane portion that includes α6β4 integrin and bullous pemphigoid antigen 2 (type XVII collagen). The proposed ligand for α6β4 integrin is laminin 5, which is a component of the anchoring filaments of the lamina lucida, and this binding mediates the stable adhesion of keratinocytes to components of the BMZ. *Anchoring filaments* are 2-4 nm diameter filaments composed of laminin 5 (also called epiligrin, kalinin, and BM600). They pass from the plasma membrane through the lamina lucida to attach to the lamina densa. The lamina densa is composed of multiple molecules, including type IV collagen, laminin, nidogen, and several glycoproteins. The lamina densa is connected to anchoring plaques of the underlying dermis by anchoring fibrils. The subbasal lamina fibrous zone of the superficial dermis is composed of anchoring fibrils, anchoring plaques, and microfibrils. Anchoring fibrils are composed of type VII collagen and form looping arrays with one or both ends of the fibrils attached to the lamina densa, thereby anchoring the BMZ to the dermis.

Dermis

The dermis is involved in maintenance and repair of the skin and is the major component responsible for the tensile strength and elasticity of the skin. In addition, the thickness of the dermis largely determines the thickness of the skin. *The dermis is composed of collagen and elastic fibers embedded in a ground substance, blood and lymphatic vessels, nerves, and low numbers of lymphoid cells.* Except for swine, domestic animals have no dermal papillae as occur in human skin. Thus, instead of papillary and reticular dermis, the dermis is divided somewhat arbitrarily into *superficial and deep dermis* in domestic animals.

The **dermal fibers** include collagen, reticular fibers (reticulin), and elastic fibers, all of which are synthesized by dermal fibroblasts. Collagen fibers are the most abundant constituent of the dermis, and they confer tensile strength to skin. The majority of *dermal collagen is types I and III*. The superficial dermis is composed of fine, loosely arranged collagen fibers. The deep dermis consists of thick, densely arranged collagen fibers that roughly parallel the skin surface. Reticular fibers represent a special thin type of collagen III. *Elastic fibers* are inconspicuous in routine H&E sections. They can be visualized with special stains, such as orcein stain or Verhoeff–van Gieson elastin stain. They are thicker and less numerous in the deep dermis and arranged parallel to the skin surface. The elastic fibers become progressively thinner near the epidermis.

The **ground or interstitial substance** is an amorphous gel-sol that fills the space between dermal structures but allows electrolytes, nutrients, growth factors, and cells to pass through. It consists of *proteoglycans and glycoproteins*. Proteoglycans are high-molecular-weight complexes composed of glycosaminoglycans linked to proteins, and those most abundant in the dermis include hyaluronic acid and various chondroitin sulfates. Proteoglycans bind various chemical mediators and thereby function as storage matrix as well as provide lubrication and structural support. *Fibronectins* are glycoproteins involved in mediating cell-cell and cell-matrix interactions that are required for various cell functions, including cell adhesion, phagocytosis, and cell migration. The ground substance is usually not visible in normal H&E sections; however, a fine granular to fibrillar basophilic material is occasionally evident between collagen fibers. This material is especially abundant in the dermis of Chinese Shar-Pei dogs as a normal variant for this breed.

The **dermal vasculature** is arranged in 3 intercommunicating plexuses. The *deep plexus* is located at the junction of the dermis and subcutis, and it supplies branches to the *middle plexus*, which is located at the level of the sebaceous glands. It, in turn, supplies branches to the *superficial plexus*. The capillary loops parallel to the skin surface immediately beneath the epidermis arise from the superficial plexus. An unusual vascular arrangement is present in the dermis of the llama. It consists of clusters of capillary-sized, thick-walled vessels lined by plump endothelial cells distributed throughout the superficial and middle dermis. *Dermal lymphatic vessels* are inconspicuous in normal skin and only become visible when they become dilated because of increased lymphatic drainage. The skin is supplied with sensory and autonomic *nerves* that are usually associated with blood vessels.

The dermis is normally **sparsely cellular.** *Fibroblasts* are distributed in low numbers throughout the dermis. They synthesize most of the fibrillar and ground substance proteins of the dermis as well as various growth factors and cytokines. *Melanocytes* in the dermis are usually located near superficial dermal vessels. In contrast to melanocytes of the epidermis and hair follicles ("secretory melanocytes"), dermal melanocytes do not transfer their melanin to surrounding cells ("continent melanocytes"). Normal dermis also contains small numbers of perivascular *monocytes and lymphocytes*, which are indistinguishable from each other. Dermal lymphocytes are primarily T cells of the helper subtype.

Mast cells are tissue-dwelling cells that are most numerous in sites, such as the skin, that interface with the environment. Mast cell numbers in skin vary greatly, depending on body location, with numbers in cats of 4-20 per 400× field around superficial dermal blood vessels, and 4-12 per 400× field in dogs. In dogs, the highest mast cell density is in the pinnae and interdigital skin, whereas the nasal planum has the lowest density. Mast cells are concentrated around blood vessels, especially postcapillary venules. Mast cells are not present in normal epidermis. Although mast cells are evident in routine H&E sections, they are better visualized with Giemsa and toluidine blue, which stain mast cell granules metachromatically.

Mast cells are released from the bone marrow as immature precursors and migrate to tissues, where they differentiate into mature cells. The proliferation and differentiation is regulated by stem cell factor (SCF), a cytokine produced by fibroblasts and keratinocytes, as well as T-cell–derived cytokines (e.g., interleukin-3 [IL-3], IL-4, IL-9, IL-10). SCF is thought to home mast cells to the dermis as well as regulate the synthesis of mast cell mediators and secretory function. The receptor for SCF on mast cells is c-kit. Mast cells exert their effects by synthesizing and releasing a host of inflammatory mediators (e.g., histamine, proteases, cytokines). The release of mast cell granules is triggered by the interaction between allergens and allergen-specific IgE bound to a high-affinity IgE receptor (FcεRI). Degranulation of both canine and human mast cells is thought to involve breakdown of their secretory granules and solubilization of contents during exocytosis. Mast cells have laminin receptors that mediate their adhesion to the extracellular matrix. The perivascular space is rich in laminin, which contributes to the localization of mast cells to this site.

Mast cells are a heterogeneous population based on differences in histochemical, biochemical, and functional characteristics that vary between species and different tissues within a single species. Mast cell heterogeneity has been demonstrated in the skin of cattle, dogs, and sheep. A subpopulation of mast cells that does not exhibit metachromasia following formalin fixation has been demonstrated in the skin of dogs and cattle, and heterogeneity of protein content has been identified in dermal mast cells of sheep.

Mast cell granules contain an array of *preformed mediators*, but they are also capable of *synthesizing mediators* such as leukotrienes (LTC_4) and prostaglandins (PGD_2) following stimulation. Tumor necrosis factor-α (TNF-α), a potent proinflammatory cytokine, is both preformed and newly synthesized upon activation of mast cells. Mast cells have long been known to be the *critical effector cell* in initiation of acute type I hypersensitivity reactions and in protection against parasitic infections with helminths and ectoparasitic arthropods. Mast cells also function in persistent chronic inflammatory reactions, tissue repair and remodeling, pathologic fibrosis, angiogenesis, hemostasis, hematopoiesis, antibody production, protection against bacterial infections, response to neoplasms, and possibly in control of the hair cycle.

Dermal muscles

Arrector pili muscles are smooth muscles present in all haired skin. They arise in the connective tissue of the superficial dermis and attach to the connective tissue sheath of the hair follicle below the level of the sebaceous gland duct. They are situated on the obtuse angle of the hair follicle, and when the muscles contract, the hair follicles are pulled into a vertical position *(piloerection)*. This results in formation of air pockets in the haircoat, which provides insulation. Contraction of arrector pili muscles may also be involved in emptying of sebaceous glands. These muscles are largest in skin of the dorsal midline from the neck to the tail. They may be vacuolated in normal animals, especially aged dogs.

In addition to arrector pili muscles, pigs also have **interfollicular smooth muscles**. These muscles span the triad of hair follicles at a level midway between the sebaceous and apocrine glands. Their contraction draws the hair follicles together and rotates the outer follicle of the triad. The functional significance of this muscle is uncertain.

Skeletal muscles may be present in the muzzle, forehead, eyelid, and perianal regions. These muscle fibers originate from cutaneous trunci muscle that penetrates into the dermis to allow voluntary movement of the skin. Skeletal muscle fibers also are associated with the large sinus hairs of the face.

Immunologic function

The skin has been proposed to function as an immunosurveillance organ, and the term *skin-associated lymphoid tissue* (SALT), analogous to gut-associated and bronchial-associated lymphoid tissues (GALT, BALT), has been suggested to describe those cellular elements of the skin that deal with antigenic challenges at the skin surface. However, this concept has been disputed because of presumed differences in immune function between the common mucosal immune system and normal skin. The alternative name, **skin immune system (SIS)**, has been suggested as a more appropriate term to encompass the skin-specific immune response–associated cells and humoral factors present in normal skin. Key components of this system *include keratinocytes, Langerhans cells, the dermal perivascular unit, and skin-homing T cells.*

- **Keratinocytes** produce multiple inflammatory cytokines, adhesion molecules, and chemotactic factors following nonspecific stimulation, and thereby have a nonspecific proinflammatory and upregulating effect.
- **Langerhans cells** are thought to trap antigens in the epidermis, migrate out to regional lymph nodes via lymphatics, and present the antigen to T cells. Thus induction of the immune response does not normally occur within the skin itself but rather in the skin-draining lymph nodes.
- The **dermal perivascular unit** consists of the mast cells, monocytes and macrophages, tissue dendritic cells, and T cells situated around postcapillary venules. As a result of cytokines such as IL-1 and TNF-α released by injured keratinocytes, endothelial cells increase their expression of addressins intercellular adhesion molecule-1 (ICAM-1) and E-selectin and vascular cell adhesion molecule-1 (VCAM-1). These vascular endothelial molecules promote adhesion of circulating leukocytes, especially granulocytes and memory T cells.
- E-selectin is thought to act as an adhesion molecule or vascular addressin for a specific subset of **skin-homing memory T cells,** which have the ligand cutaneous lymphocyte antigen (CLA) on their surface. A circulating pool of such skin-homing T lymphocytes, identified by CLA antigen, represents the cellular basis of immunologic memory of skin.

Thus it appears that the proinflammatory, upregulating effects of keratinocytes prepare the dermis for specific immunologic activity, whereas migrating antigen-presenting Langerhans cells induce expansion of specific lymphocytes in skin-draining lymph nodes. T cells are then recruited to the skin because of binding of skin-specific adhesion molecules to the vascular addressins of dermal endothelial cells.

Hair follicles

Hair serves a number of functions, including protection, thermal insulation, social communication, and sensory perception. Arrangement and type of hair follicles vary with species, breed, individual, and body region. In general, however, hair follicle density is greatest over the dorsolateral aspect of the body and least on the ventral aspect. Hair follicles are classified as *primary or secondary*, and *simple or compound*. **Primary hairs** have a large diameter, are rooted more deeply in the dermis or subcutis, and are associated with sebaceous and epitrichial sweat glands and an arrector pili muscle. **Secondary hair follicles** are smaller in diameter, are more superficially rooted, and may be accompanied by a sebaceous gland but lack a sweat gland and arrector pili muscle. Follicles in which a single hair emerges from the follicular orifice are termed **simple follicles**, whereas those in which multiple hairs emerge from a single opening are called **compound follicles.** Each hair of the compound follicle has its own *papilla*, but at the level of the sebaceous gland opening, the follicles unite to exit from a single external follicular orifice. Horses and cattle have simple hair follicles that are evenly distributed. Swine have simple follicles that are grouped in clusters of 2-4 surrounded by dense connective tissue. In sheep, the hair-growing areas consist predominantly of simple follicles, whereas the wool-growing areas have many compound follicles and consist of clusters of 3 primary follicles and a number of secondary follicles. Goats have primary follicles in groups of 3, with 3-6 secondary follicles associated with each group. Follicular arrangement in dogs and cats consists of 2-5 large primary hairs surrounded by groups of smaller secondary hairs. The primary hairs tend to be simple, whereas the secondary hairs are compound. As many as 15 hairs may emerge from a single follicular orifice. In cats, secondary hairs far outnumber primary hairs (10-24 secondary hairs per 1 primary hair).

The hair follicle is formed by a downward invasion of the surface ectoderm *(primary hair germ)* into the underlying mesoderm of the embryo. As they grow down, the epithelial cells envelop a small group of mesenchymal cells in the underlying dermis. These mesodermal cells eventually become the **follicular papilla** that repeatedly induces and maintains growth of the hair follicle throughout the life of the individual. If the papilla is somehow damaged or destroyed, the hair follicle fails to regrow. The epithelial downgrowth eventually becomes canalized to form the hair follicle. In longitudinal section, the fully developed hair follicle consists of 3 segments:

- The **lower or inferior portion,** from the base of the follicle to the point of insertion of the arrector pili muscle
- The **isthmus,** the short section from the attachment of the arrector pili muscle to the entrance of the sebaceous duct
- The **infundibulum,** extending from the entrance of the sebaceous duct to the follicular orifice

The inferior segment can be considered temporary because it disappears during the involution stage of the hair cycle and reforms again during the active phase. In contrast, *the isthmus and infundibular portions of the hair follicle are permanent.*

The **base of the hair follicle** consists of a terminal bulbous expansion of epithelial cells, the hair bulb, with a concavity at its bottom that is occupied by the connective tissue papilla. The *bulb* is composed of the highly proliferative matrix cells and melanocytes, and they are separated from the papilla by a thin extension of the basement membrane. The *matrix cells* give rise to 6 different cell types arranged in concentric layers. The 3 innermost layers form the *medulla, cortex, and cuticle of the emerging hair.* The next 3 layers form the *cuticle, Huxley layer, and Henle layer of the inner root sheath.* These layers are further surrounded by the outer root sheath, which is an extension of the epidermis and becomes continuous with the epidermis in the upper portion of the follicle. *External to the outer root sheath* are the *glassy membrane,* corresponding to the basement membrane of the epidermis, and finally the *connective tissue sheath.* All 3 layers of the inner root sheath keratinize by means of eosinophilic trichohyaline granules and become fully keratinized and disintegrate at the level of the isthmus. The inner root sheath is responsible for providing the rigid support for the developing hair and its final shape, for instance, twisted hair follicles produce curly hairs. From the base of the hair follicle to the isthmus, the outer root sheath is covered by the inner root sheath, and it does not keratinize. In the isthmus, where the inner root sheath is no longer present, the outer root sheath undergoes trichilemmal cornification that is, without keratohyaline granules. In the infundibulum, the outer root sheath is identical to surface epidermis and undergoes keratinization with formation of keratohyaline granules.

Hair does not grow continuously but rather in *cycles* consisting of a growth phase, **anagen;** a transitional or involuting phase, **catagen;** and a resting phase, **telogen.** This cyclic activity is thought to be an adaptive response to seasonal variation in ambient temperature. The hair growth cycle varies between different species, breeds, body sites, and hair follicle type. A detailed study of the hair cycle in Beagle dogs revealed that 30% of the follicles were in anagen, 8% in catagen, and 27% in telogen. The hair cycle in the remaining follicles could not be assigned a specific stage.

In domestic animals, *neighboring hairs cycle independently of each other and are in different stages of the hair cycle at any one time.* Hair shaft length is directly related to the duration of anagen phase, which is preordained according to body region and genetics. At the onset of catagen, mitotic activity of matrix cells and melanin production by melanocytes of the hair bulb cease. The keratinocytes of the inferior segment of the follicle undergo a controlled process of involution via a burst of apoptosis. This results in the upward migration of the hair follicle and the lower follicle becoming a thin cord of epithelial cells surrounded by a fibrous root sheath. Growth of the inner root sheath stops so that the lower end of the hair shaft is surrounded by thick trichilemmal keratin. The thin cord of epithelial cells is surrounded by a thickened, corrugated glassy membrane, and as it retracts upward, it is followed by the shrunken, contracted papilla. In telogen phase, the base of the bulb is located at the level of attachment of the arrector pili muscle and is ~$\frac{1}{3}$ of its former length. The base of the hair is encased in trichilemmal keratin and surrounded completely by outer root sheath *(club hair).* A population of stem cells (secondary hair germ) remains somewhere in the permanent portion of the hair follicle. These cells eventually reform the hair follicle during the next growth cycle. In rodents, the *bulge region of the follicle* appears to be the site that contains slow-cycling relatively undifferentiated cells from which arise a population of transient amplifying cells that become the matrix keratinocytes of the new hair bulb. *The bulge region is an area on the outer root sheath at the base of the permanent portion of the hair follicle to which the arrector pili muscle attaches.* Slow-cycling stem cells have been identified in the bulge region of canine hair follicles that share features with human bulge cells.

Hair growth in many animals has been shown to be regulated by photoperiod, ambient temperature, various hormones, nutritional status, and general health. However, the exact mechanisms that control the cycle are incompletely understood. Growth and development of hair are influenced by many growth factors; these include fibroblast growth factor (FGF), epidermal growth factor (EGF), insulin-like growth factor-1 (IGF-1), transforming growth factor-β (TGF-β), and keratinocyte growth factor (KGF, same as FGF-7). Both IGF-1 and KGF are produced by the dermal papilla, and their receptors are found in the overlying anagen hair follicle matrix cells. Factors from the papilla mesenchymal cells are thought to act on a stem cell population in the permanent upper portion of the hair follicle. These competent cells respond to the signals from the papilla by growing deep into the dermis to form the full-length anagen hair follicle. Transition between anagen and catagen appears to be regulated by FGF-5.

The *histologic appearance* of the hair follicle changes considerably during the hair cycle. The hair cycle has been best characterized in the mouse because the follicles cycle together (i.e., synchronous stages of anagen, catagen, and telogen). In contrast, most companion animals have a *mosaic cycle* (i.e., hair follicles cycle into different stages independently of each other). Hair shafts are only produced in anagen. Anagen follicles have a well-developed, flame-shaped, plump dermal papilla (DP) that is capped completely by the hair bulb. The inner root sheath is fully developed. The bulb is located in the deep dermis or subcutis. A layer of columnar matrix cells lines the papilla, and melanocytes are dispersed among the matrix cells in pigmented hair follicles. Catagen, the intermediate remodeling stage, is short-lived and very difficult to assess on routine histology as it requires a perfectly sectioned follicle in a longitudinal plane. In catagen, the hair bulb is lost, and the follicular papilla devaginates. The inner root sheath is partially replaced by trichilemmal keratin. Catagen follicles have a thick glassy membrane and increased apoptotic cells. In dogs, catagen has been described as having an onion-shaped dermal papilla and a fibrous stalk that trails behind the DP. In telogen, the resting stage, the inner root sheath is replaced completely by trichilemmal cornification that anchors the club hair to the outer root sheath. The dermal papilla is located at the base of the follicle. Telogen may be further described as "haired telogen," which has retention of the hair shaft, and "hairless telogen" or "kenogen," in which a telogen follicle rests without a hair shaft.

Sinus hairs (tactile hairs, vibrissae) are highly specialized mechanoreceptors that respond to vibratory stimuli as well as static hair displacements. They are located on the muzzle (whiskers, vibrissae), face, throat, and palmar aspect of the carpus. They are thick, stiff hairs that are tapered distally. Histologically, they are composed of a large simple hair follicle surrounded by an endothelial cell-lined blood-filled sinus situated within the dermal connective tissue sheath. The sinus is supplied with numerous nerves, and skeletal muscles attach to the outer sheath of the follicle to confer some voluntary control of the hairs.

Sebaceous glands

Sebaceous glands are distributed throughout the haired skin of all mammals, with the exception of whales and porpoises, and are essential for maintaining normal skin and hair. The sebaceous glands have a long list of important functions, including production of sebum, photoprotection, thermoregulatory and repelling properties, wound healing, regulating the independent endocrine function of the skin, and the expression of vitamin D receptors and vitamin D–metabolizing enzymes. *Sebaceous glands produce sebum, an oily secretion composed of triglycerides, phospholipids, and cholesterol.* This material combines with epitrichial gland secretions to form an emulsion that coats the skin to act as a physical barrier to retain moisture and maintain normal hydration, and as a chemical barrier against microbial pathogens. In addition, the oily film coats the hair shafts to give them a glossy sheen; it also acts as a pheromone. Sebum also has proinflammatory and anti-inflammatory properties, antimicrobial activity, and transports anti-oxidants to and from the skin surface. Sebaceous glands also appear to be involved with normal hair development, because, in the absence of sebaceous glands, the hair shaft fails to separate normally from the sheath. For a more thorough discussion on all of the functions of the sebaceous glands, the reader is directed to the reference by Zouboulis et al. in the Further reading section.

Sebaceous glands consist of a solid mass of epithelial cells surrounded by a connective tissue sheath. The periphery of the gland consists of a single layer of cuboidal mitotically active cells resting on a basal lamina, analogous to basal cells of the epidermis. As the cells move inward toward the duct, they enlarge and accumulate lipid that is lost during routine processing. Sebaceous glands are *holocrine glands*, and their secretion is formed by decomposition of cells. This is brought about by release of lysosomal enzymes in cells nearest the duct, causing them to disintegrate and form sebum, which empties via a squamous epithelium-lined duct into the upper portion of the hair canal. All primary hairs and some secondary hairs have sebaceous glands. They are usually largest in areas with lowest hair follicle density, such as mucocutaneous junctions, interdigital spaces, coronet, and dorsal neck and rump. Sebaceous glands are especially numerous and well developed in the chin of cats *(submental organ)*, dorsal surface of the tail in dogs and cats *(tail gland)*, base of the horn in goats, and infraorbital, inguinal, and interdigital regions of sheep. The footpads and nasal planum are devoid of sebaceous glands, and they are rare in glabrous skin, where they empty directly to the skin surface.

Perianal glands

These are specialized secretory glands in the perianal regions, and they are commonly sites for the development of lesions.

- *Anal glands* are *specialized apocrine glands* that open directly onto anal skin via a duct at the rectoanal junction. Similar apocrine glands line the anal sacs. The anal sacs are squamous epithelial-lined cystic cavities containing odoriferous secretions, presumably with some territorial marking function. They are present in many species, including domestic and wild felids, ferrets, raccoons, mink, rodents, pigs, and canids.
- *Hepatoid glands (also called circumanal, perianal glands)* are presumed to be *modified sebaceous glands* based on histology, and are composed of small glands and nests of cells without a prominent ductular network. Islands of these glands are concentrated in the subcutis around the anus, but foci are commonly present over lateral and ventral aspects of the base of the tail, the dorsum of the tail, the dorsolumbosacral area, and prepuce. The glands are distinctive, composed of lobules of large eosinophilic epithelial cells *(hepatoid cells)* surrounded by low numbers of small basal reserve cells. Larger ducts, lined by stratified squamous epithelium, may be evident in neoplasms. These ducts are thought to regress during embryonal development, which leaves the glands largely ductless. *Hepatoid glands are best described in the dog*, and are most developed in entire males. Their function is uncertain, but they may have a role in steroid metabolism, in production of pheromones, and in territorial marking. Similar glands are also present in cats and in pericloacal glands of reptiles, where they probably have similar roles in territorial marking.

Sweat glands

Two types of sweat glands are present in the skin of mammals; they differ in origin, distribution, and possibly in the mode of secretion. These glands have been called apocrine and eccrine glands, but because of questions concerning the mechanism of the secretory process of these glands, the names *epitrichial and atrichial glands have been proposed for apocrine and eccrine glands, respectively*. **Epitrichial (apocrine) sweat glands** develop embryologically from primary hair germ, and they are distributed throughout all haired skin, usually deep to the sebaceous glands. *Epitrichial glands are associated with primary hair follicles only*, and they tend to be largest in areas with lower hair follicle density, such as mucocutaneous junctions, interdigital spaces, coronet, and dorsal midline. Sweat mixes with sebum to form the protective skin surface film. Epitrichial sweat glands function in thermoregulation only in horses and cattle. In other species, the secretion may contribute to scent that is involved in social communication. Epitrichial secretion may also provide a means of excreting waste products and secreting immunoglobulins that are present on the skin surface. They are *simple saccular or tubular glands* with a coiled secretory portion and straight duct. The secretory portion is composed of a single row of flat cuboidal to columnar epithelial cells surrounded by a single layer of myoepithelial cells situated between the secretory cells and basal lamina. *The duct empties into the pilary canal, usually above the entrance of the sebaceous duct or, rarely, directly to the skin surface.* The name apocrine refers to the mode of secretion, which was originally thought to involve pinching off (apo = off) of a portion of the cell. The existence of an apocrine secretory process has been questioned; however, ultrastructural examination of these glands in humans, pigs, horses, and dogs indicates that *several modes of secretion are involved*, including the apocrine type.

In contrast to epitrichial glands, **atrichial (eccrine) sweat glands** are derived from the embryonal epidermis rather than from the primary hair germ, and they are located only in specialized areas. They occur in the *pawpad of dogs and cats, frog of ungulates, snout of pigs, planum nasolabiale of cattle, and medial surface of the carpus of pigs (carpal glands)*. The function of eccrine glands is uncertain. The secretion may be involved with scent signaling, and in the footpad of cats, it may improve frictional capacity of the paw. Atrichial glands are histologically similar to apocrine glands, but their ducts open directly to the skin surface. There is no recent detailed examination of eccrine gland secretion to identify the mode of secretion conclusively.

Subcutis

The deepest layer of the skin is the subcutis. It is composed of lipocytes subdivided into lobules by thin bands of collagen and small vessels. The collagenous septa provide structural support by compartmentalizing the subcutis and anchoring the dermis to the fascial planes deep to the subcutis.

Further reading

de Mora F, et al. The role of mast cells in atopy: what can we learn from canine models? A thorough review of the biology of mast cells in canine and human systems. Br J Dermatol 2006;155:1109-1123.

Kobayashi T, et al. Canine follicle stem cell candidates reside in the bulge and share characteristic features with human bulge cells. J Invest Dermatol 2010;130:1988-1995.

Miller WH, et al. Structure and function of the skin. In: Miller WH, et al., editors. Muller & Kirk's Small Animal Dermatology. 7th ed. St Louis: Elsevier; 2013.

Müntener T, et al. The canine hair cycle—a guide for the assessment of morphological and immunohistochemical criteria. Vet Dermatol 2011;22:383-395.

Müntener T, et al. Canine noninflammatory alopecia: a comprehensive evaluation of common and distinguishing histological characteristics. Vet Dermatol 2012;23:206-e44.

Nishifuji K, Yoon JS. The stratum corneum: the rampart of the mammalian body. Vet Dermatol 2013;24:60-72.

Zouboulis CC, et al. Frontiers in sebaceous gland biology and pathology. Exp Dermatol 2008;17(6):542-551.

DERMATOHISTOPATHOLOGY

The pathology of the skin, more than that of any other organ, has a specialized vocabulary. Many gross and histologic changes are unique to the skin. The pathologist must communicate proper terminology of both gross and histologic lesions to interpret lesions.

Glossary: histologic terms

Acantholysis refers to a *loss of cohesion between individual keratinocytes* resulting from a breakdown of the intercellular bridges (desmosomes). **Acantholytic cells** are individualized round cells with a central nucleus that is rimmed by condensed eosinophilic cytoplasm (Fig. 6-1). Acantholysis is the hallmark of the *pemphigus complex*. It can also result from proteolytic enzymes released by neutrophils or eosinophils in an inflammatory process. In domestic animals, acantholysis is most commonly manifested within pustules and crusts of pemphigus foliaceus.

Acanthosis specifically indicates an *increased thickness of the stratum spinosum*, and is the result of hyperplasia and occasionally hypertrophy of cells of the stratum spinosum. Acanthosis, however, is *often used synonymously with hyperplasia* when referring to the epidermis.

Apoptosis refers to *individual programmed cell death*. It is usually seen in the basal layer but can be seen in any layer of the epidermis. Apoptotic keratinocytes are eosinophilic and shrunken. They are sometimes referred to as *apoptotic bodies* (colloid bodies, hyaline bodies). In general, the term Civatte body refers to an apoptotic keratinocyte in the stratum basale. The term **"dyskeratosis"** has been previously used to describe premature or abnormal keratinization of individual keratinocytes; however, apoptosis is most likely the underlying process as the histologic features are indistinguishable from each other.

Atrophy, in regard to the epidermis, is assessed by *decreased thickness of the nucleated layers*. An early sign of epidermal atrophy is the loss of the rete ridges in areas of skin, where they are normally present. *Atrophy can be difficult to interpret as the normal epidermis in the haired skin of domestic animals is naturally thin.* Atrophy is most commonly seen with hypercortisolemia (topical or systemic) and chronic ischemia.

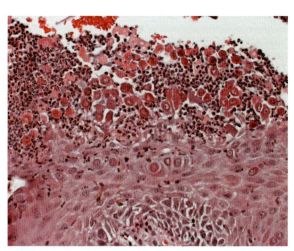

Figure 6-1 *Acantholysis* in pemphigus foliaceus. Loss of cohesion between keratinocytes leads to individualization of cells. Note that the acantholytic cells have normal nuclear morphology.

Dermal atrophy is thinning of dermal collagen fibrils resulting in decreased dermal thickness.

Ballooning degeneration of the epidermis is the result of *intracellular edema* (Fig. 6-2). It is characterized by swollen eosinophilic cytoplasm, enlarged or condensed nuclei, and a loss of cohesion, resulting in acantholysis and sometimes vesicle formation. Ballooning degeneration is a *characteristic feature of viral infections*, particularly of herpesviruses and poxviruses.

Clefts are *slit-like spaces* within the epidermis or at the dermoepidermal junction. Clefts may be caused by acantholysis or hydropic degeneration of basal cells. However, clefts may also result from handling artifacts (Fig. 6-3).

Collagen degeneration is a term that has been replaced by "**collagen flame figure**" or "**flame figure.**" Collagen flame figures are characterized by dermal deposition of amorphous eosinophilic material on collagen fibers with an infiltrate of eosinophils. The collagen fibrils have a frayed appearance. Ultrastructurally, flame figures contain degranulated eosinophils, but the collagen fibrils have a normal (i.e., not degenerate) periodicity. In chronic lesions, the eosinophil content decreases, histiocytes increase in number, and *palisading granulomas* may be formed. Flame figures may be seen in eosinophilic granuloma, insect-/arthropod-bite reactions, and other eosinophil-rich conditions, such as mast cell tumors.

Crust is a gross and histologic term that refers to consolidated, desiccated surface exudate that contains keratin, serum, cellular debris, and often microorganisms. Crusts are described on the basis of their composition: *serous* (mostly serum), *hemorrhagic* (mostly blood), *cellular* (mostly inflammatory cells), and *serocellular* (a mixture of serum and inflammatory cells). Crusts should be examined closely for dermatophyte spores and hyphae, *Dermatophilus congolensis*, and acantholytic keratinocytes, which can be indicators of superficial pemphigus.

Dermal edema is recognized by *dilated lymphatics* (not visible in normal skin), widened spaces between blood vessels and perivascular collagen *(perivascular edema)*, or widened spaces between dermal collagen fibers *(interstitial edema)*. The dilated lymphatics and widened perivascular and interstitial spaces may or may not contain lightly eosinophilic, homogeneous, proteinaceous fluid. Dermal edema is a common feature of any *inflammatory dermatosis*. Severe edema of the superficial dermis may result in subepidermal vesicles and bullae, necrosis of the overlying epidermis, and predisposition to artifactual dermoepidermal separation during handling and processing of biopsy specimens. Severe edema of the superficial dermis may result in vertical orientation and stretching of collagen fibers, producing the "gossamer" (web-like) collagen effect seen in severe urticaria.

Desmoplasia usually refers to fibroplasia and collagenous stroma induced by neoplastic processes.

Dyskeratosis is *premature or abnormal keratinization of individual keratinocytes* in the epidermis or follicular epithelium. Histologically, dyskeratotic cells are eosinophilic and shrunken, with condensed, dark-staining nuclei. Dyskeratosis may be seen in a number of dermatoses, including lupus erythematosus, erythema multiforme, and graft-versus-host disease. It can also occur in neoplastic dermatoses, especially papillomas. Dyskeratosis is a feature of the severe epidermal dysplasia that precedes the development of some squamous cell carcinomas.

Dysplasia refers to *faulty or abnormal development* of the epidermis, hair follicles, or any component of the skin. It is an abnormal but nonneoplastic change; however, it can accompany or precede neoplastic changes.

Dystrophic mineralization is the deposition of *calcium salts as basophilic, amorphous, granular material along collagen fibrils*, as in hyperglucocorticism. Dystrophic mineralization of the hair follicle basement membrane can be seen in hyperglucocorticism, in dogs receiving exogenous glucocorticoids, and as a senile change in dogs, especially in Poodles.

Epidermal mast cells are frequently seen in biopsies from cats with inflammatory dermatoses. They are found within the epidermis as well as the hair follicle outer root sheath, and are most commonly found in diseases associated with tissue eosinophilia, such as feline eosinophilic plaque and feline eosinophilic granuloma, and thus are associated with allergic skin disease in cats.

Exocytosis is the migration of *inflammatory cells and/or erythrocytes through the intercellular spaces of the epidermis.* Exocytosis of inflammatory cells is a common feature of any inflammatory dermatosis. Exocytosis of neutrophils implies an infectious process, whereas exocytosis of eosinophils suggests a hypersensitivity reaction, such as ectoparasitism and feline

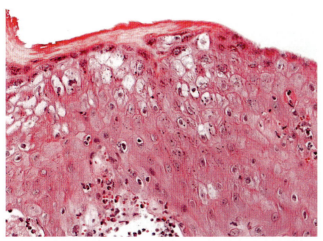

Figure 6-2 Ballooning degeneration in viral dermatitis. Keratinocytes are enlarged and pale because of marked intracellular edema.

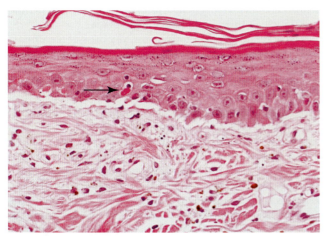

Figure 6-3 Subepidermal cleft in dermatomyositis. There is separation of the epidermis from the dermis by a clear space. Note the shrunken, darkly staining necrotic (apoptotic) keratinocytes with hypereosinophilic cytoplasm and pyknotic nuclei (arrow).

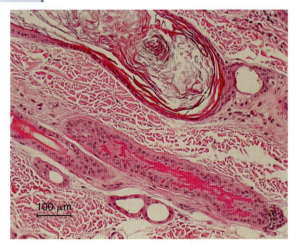

Figure 6-4 Flame follicle in canine alopecia X. The follicle has pronounced eosinophilic trichilemmal cornification. The keratin has a serrated border resembling a flickering flame.

eosinophilic plaque. Exocytosis of erythrocytes implies purpura, severe vasodilation, or trauma.

Festoons are dermal papillae devoid of attached epidermal cells that project into a vesicle or bulla. Festoons can be seen in mechanobullous disorders, such as epidermolysis bullosa or bullous pemphigoid.

Fibrinoid degeneration or **fibrinoid necrosis** typically refers to the deposition of amorphous eosinophilic material resembling fibrin in the walls of blood vessels. The fibrinoid change results in loss of structural detail and may be accompanied by necrotic cell debris or leukocytoclasia.

Fibroplasia is a reactive process and is the formation and development of fibrous tissue resulting from an increased number of fibroblasts.

Flame follicles are catagen and telogen follicles with pronounced eosinophilic trichilemmal keratin (Fig. 6-4). These can be seen in endocrinopathies, hair cycle arrest, and are also prominent in normal haired skin of plush-coated breeds of dog, such as the Nordic breeds and Pomeranians.

Follicular atrophy refers to the *gradual involution and disappearance of hair follicles* characteristic of hormonal dermatoses, follicular dysplasia, and ischemia.

Follicular dysplasia (also known as follicular dystrophy) refers to the inability to produce structurally normal hair follicles and hair shafts. Examples include black hair follicular dysplasia and color-dilution alopecia.

Follicular keratosis refers to *the distention of hair follicle infundibula by keratin.*

Folliculitis is inflammation of the hair follicle. It can further be divided into *mural folliculitis* (inflammation of the follicular epithelium) (Fig. 6-5A), *luminal folliculitis* (inflammation in the follicular lumen) (Fig. 6-5B), and *perifolliculitis* (inflammation around but not significantly impinging on the follicle) (Fig. 6-5C).

Furunculosis is *inflammation of the hair follicle that has resulted in destruction of the follicular epithelium and release of the luminal contents into the dermis, causing dermal inflammation* (Fig. 6-5D, 6-6). This can be seen in any process that is destructive to hair follicles, such as bacterial infection, dermatophytosis, demodicosis, and trauma.

Granulation tissue is the result of a reparative process characterized by neovascularization and a proliferation of fibroblasts within a proteoglycan rich matrix. It is named for the pink granular appearance of a wound bed. The blood vessels have plump endothelial cells and are oriented perpendicular to the surface of the skin. Fibroblasts and collagen fibrils are oriented parallel to the surface of the skin.

Grenz zone is a zone of relatively normal collagen that separates the epidermis from an underlying dermal alteration. The presence or absence of a grenz zone is a criterion used in the diagnosis of neoplastic conditions (e.g., plasmacytomas often have a prominent grenz zone, whereas histiocytomas abut the dermoepidermal junction).

Hamartoma is *a tumor-like malformation composed of an abnormal mixture of normal tissue elements or an abnormal proportion of a single element.* Unlike a **choristoma,** the components of a hamartoma are normal to the location. By definition, hamartomas are congenital lesions; however, they may not be detected until later in life, and the term is often used interchangeably with nevus. The term "nevus" refers to focal malformation of the skin, congenital or tardive in onset, caused by an embryonic failure of normal development. Hamartoma is the term preferred in veterinary dermatopathology; however, there are a few conditions where "nevus" is ingrained in the veterinary literature.

Hidradenitis is *inflammation of epitrichial (apocrine) sweat glands.* These glands commonly become involved secondarily in suppurative and granulomatous dermatoses. Periglandular accumulation of plasma cells is commonly seen in chronic pyoderma and acral lick dermatitis.

Horn cysts (keratin cysts) are epidermal cysts that contain concentric layers of keratin and are lined by attenuated keratinocytes. Horn cysts are features of some follicular and epithelial tumors. **Pseudohorn cysts** are keratin-filled, cyst-like structures formed by the *irregular invagination of a hyperplastic, hyperkeratotic epidermis,* having a cystic appearance because of cross-sectioning. They are seen in numerous hyperplastic or neoplastic epidermal dermatoses.

Keratin pearls (horn pearls, squamous pearls) are focal, circular, *concentric layers of squamous cells showing gradual keratinization toward the center,* often accompanied by cellular atypia and dyskeratosis. Keratin pearls are commonly seen in squamous cell carcinoma.

Hypergranulosis indicates *increased thickness of the stratum granulosum,* often accompanied by larger, more intensely stained granules. Hypergranulosis may be seen in any dermatosis in which there is epidermal hyperplasia.

Hyperkeratosis refers to *increased thickness of the stratum corneum.* It can be either **orthokeratotic** (without nuclei) (Fig. 6-7A), or **parakeratotic** (nuclei retained) (Fig. 6-7B). *Hyperkeratosis and orthokeratosis are sometimes used synonymously.* Orthokeratosis can be divided into basket weave (the normal pattern in the stratum corneum), compact, and laminated. *Basket weave orthokeratosis* is the most common form and is seen in many conditions, including hypersensitivities, endocrinopathies, and cornification disorders. *Compact orthokeratosis is a feature of long-standing surface trauma. Laminated orthokeratosis* characterizes ichthyosis. Orthokeratosis and parakeratosis are not mutually exclusive and are often seen in the same section of hyperkeratotic skin. *Diffuse parakeratosis* can be seen in many chronic dermatoses, especially zinc-responsive dermatosis, dermatophilosis, superficial necrolytic dermatitis, and thallotoxicosis.

Hyperpigmentation refers to *increased melanin within the epidermis and, often, concurrently in dermal melanophages.*

Dermatohistopathology

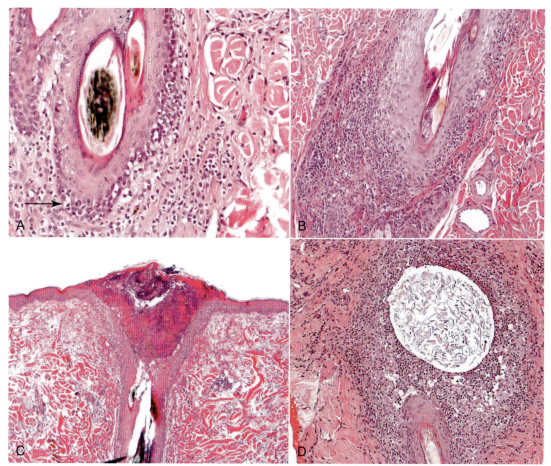

Figure 6-5 Folliculitis. **A.** Idiopathic mural folliculitis in a dog. Note the wall of the hair follicle is infiltrated by mononuclear leukocytes (arrow). **B.** Perifolliculitis and mural folliculitis in demodicosis. Note the periadnexal inflammatory infiltrate. **C.** Luminal folliculitis in staphylococcal pyoderma. **D.** Furunculosis in bacterial folliculitis. The wall of the follicle has been perforated, and follicular contents are in the dermis.

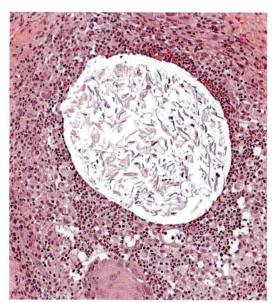

Figure 6-6 Furunculosis. Higher magnification of Figure 6-5D. Note the abundant free keratin surrounded by pyogranulomatous inflammation.

Hyperpigmentation may be focal or diffuse, and confined to the stratum basale or present throughout all epidermal layers. It is a common nondiagnostic finding in chronic inflammatory and hormonal dermatoses, as well as in some developmental and neoplastic disorders. Hyperpigmentation must always be cautiously assessed with regard to the animal's normal pigmentation.

Hyperplasia is an increase in the number of cells. In reference to the epidermis, it refers to an increased number of keratinocytes. *Epidermal hyperplasia is a common feature of almost all chronic inflammatory conditions. Acanthosis* is a term often used synonymously with epidermal hyperplasia. Epidermal hyperplasia may be further specified as *irregular* (in which the hyperplastic rete ridges are uneven in shape and height), *regular or psoriasiform* (in which the hyperplastic rete ridges are of even thickness and length), *papillated* (digitate projections of the epidermis above the skin surface), and *pseudocarcinomatous* (extreme, irregular hyperplasia that may demonstrate increased mitotic activity and branched or fused rete pegs) (Fig. 6-8). The process may resemble squamous cell carcinoma; however, there is no cellular atypia, and the basement membrane remains intact.

Hypopigmentation refers to *decreased melanin in the epidermis*. It may be associated with congenital or acquired idiopathic defects in melanization (leukoderma, vitiligo),

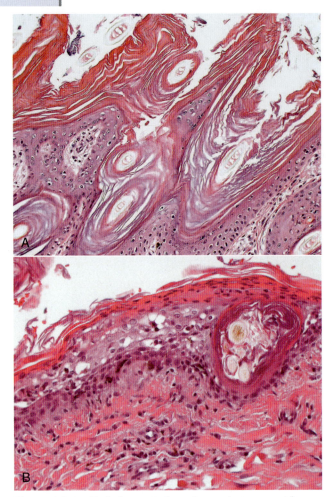

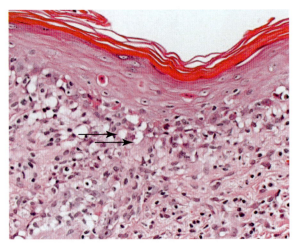

Figure 6-9 Hydropic degeneration. Clear spaces (arrows) are present within and below basal keratinocytes.

Figure 6-7 A. Orthokeratotic hyperkeratosis in nonepidermolytic ichthyosis. The stratum corneum is expanded by laminated layers of compact anuclear keratin. **B. Parakeratotic hyperkeratosis** in superficial necrolytic dermatitis. The corneal layer is expanded by nucleated corneocytes.

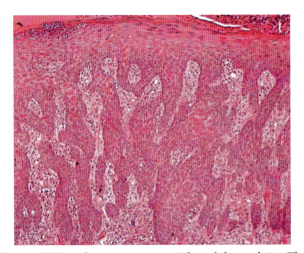

Figure 6-8 Pseudocarcinomatous epidermal hyperplasia. The epidermis has marked irregular hyperplasia with branched or fused rete pegs. The basement membrane is intact, and there is no cellular atypia.

toxic effects of certain chemicals on melanocytes (e.g., monobenzylether of dihydroquinone in rubbers and plastics), inflammatory disorders that affect melanization or destroy melanocytes, hormonal disorders, and dermatoses featuring hydropic degeneration of basal cells (e.g., lupus erythematosus).

Intracellular edema of the epidermis is characterized by increased size, cytoplasmic pallor, and, sometimes, displacement of the nucleus to the periphery of the affected cell. Intracellular edema of the epidermis may affect cells in a laminar fashion, leading to horizontal layers of edematous keratinocytes. Severe intracellular edema may result in reticular degeneration and intraepidermal vesicles. *Intracellular edema is a common feature of any acute or subacute inflammatory dermatosis.* **Hydropic degeneration** is a specific type of intracellular edema restricted to the basal layer and basal keratinocytes of the outer root sheath of hair follicles. Hydropic degeneration may result in intrabasal clefts or vesicles, or subepidermal clefts or vesicles because of dermoepidermal separation. It is characterized by clear vacuoles within basal keratinocytes, sometimes accompanied by individual keratinocyte necrosis (Fig. 6-9). **Vacuolar degeneration** is sometimes seen in conjunction with hydropic degeneration and refers to vacuoles above and below the basement membrane zone. Hydropic degeneration of basal cells can be seen in lichenoid dermatitides, drug eruptions, lupoid dermatoses, and dermatomyositis. Caution must be exercised not to confuse freezing artifact or delayed fixation artifact with intracellular edema.

Lymphoid nodules are well-circumscribed, rounded, dense, sometimes perivascular accumulations of predominantly mature lymphocytes in the deep dermis and/or subcutis. They are uncommon and *seen primarily in the cat*. They are seen most frequently in conjunction with immune-mediated dermatoses, dermatoses associated with tissue eosinophilia, and in panniculitis, such as injection-site panniculitis. They can also be seen in insect-bite granuloma (pseudolymphoma).

Mucinosis (myxedema, myxoid degeneration, mucoid degeneration) is an accumulation of dermal ground substance that appears as slightly granular, basophilic material that separates, thins, or replaces dermal collagen fibers and surrounds blood vessels and appendages in H&E-stained sections. Only small amounts of mucin are visible in normal skin. Mucin is more easily demonstrated with stains for glycosaminoglycans, such as Alcian blue and colloidal iron. Mucinous degeneration may be seen as a focal process in numerous inflammatory, neoplastic, and developmental dermatoses. Diffuse mucinosis is a feature of normal skin of the Chinese Shar-Pei dog.

Multinucleated keratinocytes can occasionally be seen in infections by viruses, such as herpesvirus, canine distemper virus, and feline leukemia virus.

Munro's microabscess is a small, desiccated accumulation of *neutrophils within the stratum corneum*.

Necrosis is the death of cells or tissues. *Necrotic keratinocytes* are identified by loss of intercellular bridges with resultant rounding up of the cell, and a normal-sized or swollen eosinophilic cytoplasm. The nucleus becomes pyknotic, cytoplasm becomes eosinophilic and homogeneous, and the cell loses its normal shape. Apoptosis is often used synonymously with individual keratinocyte death that may occur from a variety of processes. Individual keratinocyte necrosis can occur in erythema multiforme, graft-versus-host disease, and interface dermatoses. Necrosis of the epidermis or dermis may be more extensive due to physical and chemical injury, or to interference with vascular supply.

Nests (theques) are well-circumscribed clusters or groups of cells within the epidermis and/or the dermis. Epidermal nests are often seen in melanocytic neoplasms.

Panniculitis (steatitis) refers to *inflammation of subcutaneous fat*. It can occur without significant involvement of the overlying dermis and epidermis (e.g., sterile nodular panniculitis, feline nutritional steatitis), or can be involved by extension of inflammation of the dermis. Fat micropseudocyst formation and lipocytes containing radially arranged needle-shaped clefts can be seen with subcutaneous fat sclerosis and idiopathic sterile panniculitis.

Papillomatosis refers to the projection of dermal papillae and epidermis above the surface of the skin, resulting in an irregular undulating configuration of the epidermis. Papillomatosis is associated with epidermal hyperplasia and is seen with chronic inflammatory and neoplastic dermatoses.

Pautrier's microabscess is a small, focal accumulation of *abnormal lymphoid cells* in the epidermis or follicular epithelium, typical of epitheliotropic lymphoma (Fig. 6-10).

Pigmentary incontinence refers to the presence of *melanin granules free within the subepidermal dermis and within dermal macrophages (melanophages)*. It can result from any process that damages the stratum basale, especially hydropic degeneration of basal cells (lichenoid dermatoses, lupus erythematosus, dermatomyositis, erythema multiforme).

Reticular degeneration is caused by severe intracellular edema of epidermal cells. These cells burst, resulting in *multilocular intraepidermal vesicles whose septa are formed by resistant cell walls*. It may be seen with any acute or subacute inflammatory dermatosis, such as acute contact dermatitis.

Satellitosis refers to *individual necrotic keratinocytes in the epidermis surrounded by lymphoid cells (satellite cells)* (Fig. 6-11). It is a characteristic finding in erythema multiforme and occasionally is seen in other interface dermatoses.

Sclerosis (scar) is the end point of fibrosis. *Increased numbers of collagen fibers* have a thick, eosinophilic, hyalinized appearance, and the number of fibroblasts is greatly reduced.

Sebaceous gland hyperplasia refers to increased numbers of sebaceous glands and is common in chronic inflammatory conditions. Generalized sebaceous gland hyperplasia is a histologic feature seen in many chronic inflammatory conditions. Nodular aggregates of hyperplastic sebaceous glands form exophytic firm papules. These lesions are common and often multifocal in aged dogs.

Spongiform pustule of Kogoj is a multilocular accumulation of neutrophils within a sponge-like area of the stratum granulosum and stratum spinosum.

Spongiosis (intercellular edema) of the epidermis is characterized by widening of the intercellular spaces with accentuation of the intercellular bridges, giving the epidermis a "spongy" appearance (Fig. 6-12A). Severe intercellular edema may lead to rupture of the intercellular bridges and the formation of *intraepidermal vesicles* (Fig. 6-12B). Severe spongiotic vesicle formation may disrupt the basement membrane zone in some areas and form subepidermal vesicles. Intercellular edema is a common feature of acute or subacute inflammatory dermatoses. Diffuse spongiosis, which also involves the hair follicle outer root sheath, may be seen in other inflammatory disorders, including feline eosinophilic plaque or granuloma.

Squamous eddies *are whorl-like patterns of squamous cells with no atypia, dyskeratosis, or central keratinization*. Squamous eddies are features of numerous neoplastic and hyperplastic epidermal disorders.

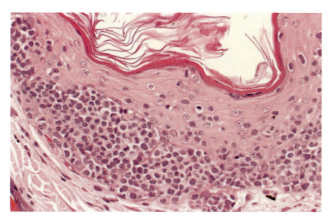

Figure 6-10 Pautrier's microabscess in epitheliotropic lymphoma. Aggregates of neoplastic lymphocytes reside within the epidermis.

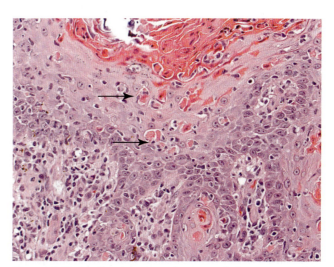

Figure 6-11 Satellitosis in erythema multiforme. Lymphocytes (arrows) surround individually necrotic (apoptotic) keratinocytes.

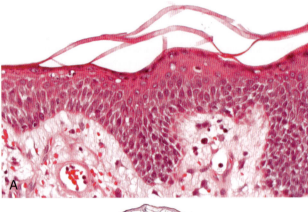

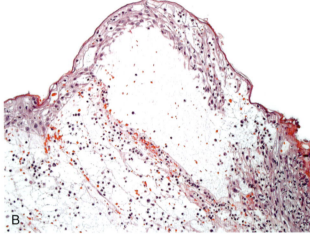

Figure 6-12 Spongiosis. A. Extracellular edema results in widening of intercellular spaces between keratinocytes. **B. Spongiosis with vesicle formation.** Marked intercellular edema has led to breakdown of intercellular bridges and vesicle formation.

Transepidermal elimination is a mechanism by which foreign or altered constituents can be removed from the dermis. This can be illustrated by the elimination of mineralized collagen across the epidermis and follicular epithelium in calcinosis cutis.

Vesicle is a *fluid-filled blister <1.0 cm in diameter. They may be subcorneal, suprabasilar, subepidermal, or immediately below the epidermis.* When these lesions contain large numbers of inflammatory cells, they may be referred to as **vesicopustules.**

Villus is a dermal papilla covered by 1 or 2 layers of epidermal cells that projects into the base of a vesicle or bulla. Villi are seen in pemphigus vulgaris and warty dyskeratoma.

Gross terminology

Bullae are *collections of fluid* within or below the epidermis >1.0 cm in diameter. They may be caused by severe intercellular or intracellular edema, ballooning degeneration, acantholysis, hydropic degeneration of basal cells, subepidermal edema, or other factors resulting in dermoepidermal separation, such as the autoantibodies in bullous pemphigoid.

Callus is a thickened, often pigmented, and hyperkeratotic plaque that occurs in areas of chronic pressure trauma or friction (e.g., elbow callus in large-breed dogs).

Comedo is a *cystically dilated, keratin-filled hair follicle.* Comedones are characteristically seen in Schnauzer comedo syndrome, some endocrine dermatopathies, and actinic dermatosis.

Dells are *small depressions or hollows* in the surface of the epidermis independent of adnexal structures. They are usually associated with focal epidermal atrophy and orthokeratotic hyperkeratosis. This term is not commonly used in veterinary dermatology.

Epidermal collarette is a special type of loose scale that is arranged in a circular pattern around a central area of erythema or hyperpigmentation. Epidermal collarettes most likely represent ruptured pustules or papules from bacterial folliculitis.

Eschar is a thick crust that forms in association with an ulcer and is tightly adherent to the skin because of the incorporation of dermal collagen (e.g., thermal burn).

Lichenification is exaggeration of the normal skin markings resulting from long-standing surface trauma or friction (e.g., axilla in chronic atopic dermatitis). Lichenified areas are often hyperpigmented.

Macules are nonraised lesions of <1.0 cm diameter in which the color differs from that of the surrounding normal skin (e.g., black macules in feline lentigo simplex). A **patch** is a macule that measures >1 cm.

Papules are solid, circumscribed, elevations in the skin that are <1 cm in diameter. Papules can be follicular (e.g., staphylococcal folliculitis) or nonfollicular (e.g., flea-bite hypersensitivity).

Plaques are solid, slightly raised elevations in the skin that are >1 cm in diameter (e.g., feline eosinophilic plaque).

Pustules can be gross or microscopic accumulations in skin that are filled with inflammatory cells, usually neutrophils or eosinophils. Grossly, pustules, as in papules, can be follicular or nonfollicular (e.g., superficial pemphigus).

Scale refers to a flat plate of stratum corneum (e.g., Golden Retriever ichthyosis). It is important to distinguish scale versus crust on physical examination.

Wheal is a firm, circumscribed, raised elevation in the skin, composed of edema and is often erythematous (e.g., equine urticaria).

Pattern analysis

Used commonly in the diagnoses of neoplasms, a system of pattern analysis is also applied to inflammatory/nonneoplastic dermatoses. *Most dermatologic lesions can be grouped into 1 of 10 histologic patterns on low magnification.* It is far more efficient for a dermatopathology trainee to use pattern recognition to generate a list of differentials than to learn by memorizing the histologic features of each disease. Unlike "tumor" biopsies, where the name of the neoplasm is given (e.g., squamous cell carcinoma), *most skin biopsies generate a morphologic diagnosis and comment that will aid the clinician in making therapeutic choices.*

The pathologist must be aware of the normal features of the species and the specific site being examined. *The specimen is initially perused at scanning magnification to determine the dermatopathologic pattern.* At higher magnification, additional features (e.g., cell type: lymphocytic, histiocytic, neutrophilic, eosinophilic, plasmacytic) will be used to narrow the differential diagnosis. *It is not unusual to see more than one pattern of inflammation in a biopsy.* For instance, it is quite common to have a hyperplastic perivascular pattern in allergic skin disease along with a superficial pustular pattern of pyoderma. It can be difficult to gauge the importance of each pattern within the biopsy. Some patterns are more specific than others; there are far fewer differentials for interface dermatitis than perivascular dermatitis.

Perivascular dermatitis

Perivascular dermatitis is the *least specific pattern of inflammation*, and it is necessary to observe the type of leukocyte involved and the epidermal changes to create a differential list. In perivascular dermatitis, *the predominant inflammatory reaction is centered on the superficial or deep dermal blood vessels, or both*. Most perivascular dermatitides involve predominantly the superficial dermal blood vessels. In the horse and cat, most perivascular dermatitis is both superficial and deep. *The primary cause of superficial perivascular dermatitis is a hypersensitivity reaction*, although chronic bacterial infections, viral infections, cornification disorders, and metabolic disease can all demonstrate this pattern at some point during evolution of the condition. Perivascular infiltrates containing *eosinophils* should first be suspected of representing dermatitis, such as ectoparasitism, food allergy, or atopy. Focal areas of eosinophilic exocytosis and necrosis (*"epidermal nibbles"*) are suggestive of ectoparasitism. Other perivascular dermatitides that may contain eosinophils include zinc-responsive dermatosis, equine multisystemic eosinophilic epitheliotropic disease, and chronic pyoderma. Perivascular dermatitis is subdivided on the basis of accompanying epidermal changes into 4 types:

- In **pure perivascular dermatitis,** there are few or no epidermal changes. The most common dermatoses in this category include acute hypersensitivity reactions and urticaria (Fig. 6-13).
- **Perivascular dermatitis with spongiosis** is characterized by various degrees of spongiosis and spongiotic vesicle formation. Severe spongiotic vesiculation may disrupt the basement membrane zone, resulting in subepidermal vesicles. The epidermis has variably severe hyperkeratosis and hyperplasia. The most common dermatoses in this category include hypersensitivity reactions, acute contact or irritant dermatitis, ectoparasitism, feline eosinophilic plaque, feline miliary dermatitis, and viral infections. When the hair follicle outer root sheath is also involved, feline allergic dermatitides, such as feline eosinophilic plaque and feline eosinophilic granuloma, are suggested.
- **Perivascular dermatitis with epidermal hyperplasia** is characterized by various degrees of epidermal hyperplasia and hyperkeratosis with little or no spongiosis. This is a common, nondiagnostic, chronic reaction pattern. The most common dermatoses in this category are chronic hypersensitivity reactions, acral lick dermatitis, and any dermatitis that has undergone chronic irritation and trauma.
- **Perivascular dermatitis with hyperkeratosis** is characterized by various degrees of either orthokeratosis or parakeratosis. The presence of parakeratosis suggests zinc-responsive dermatosis, chronic ectoparasite hypersensitivity, or *Malassezia* dermatitis.

Interface dermatitis

Interface dermatitis is characterized by damage to the basal layer of keratinocytes, such as basal cell degeneration or necrosis of keratinocytes that obscures the dermoepidermal junction. This pattern can be divided into interface cell poor (interface changes with minimal superficial dermal inflammation) or interface lichenoid (interface changes with a lichenoid band of mononuclear inflammation). Pigmentary incontinence and apoptotic bodies are commonly seen in both types.

- The **cell-poor interface pattern** can be seen in diseases such as dermatomyositis, ischemic dermatopathy, erythema multiforme, drug eruptions, graft-versus-host reactions, bovine viral diarrhea, and bovine pseudolumpy skin disease.
- The **lichenoid interface pattern** is seen with discoid lupus erythematosus, cutaneous exfoliative lupus erythematosus, vesicular lupus erythematous, idiopathic lichenoid dermatoses, lichenoid keratoses, Vogt-Koyanagi-Harada (VKH)-like syndrome (uveodermatologic syndrome), lichenoid psoriasiform dermatosis of Springer Spaniels, cyclosporine-associated lichenoid psoriasiform dermatosis, malignant catarrhal fever, and drug eruptions (Fig. 6-14). The lichenoid band of inflammation is usually lymphocytic and plasmacytic, except in VKH-like syndrome, where it is primarily composed of lymphocytes and histiocytes that contain fine melanin granules.

Caution should be exercised in differentiating interface lichenoid inflammation from lichenoid inflammation. There is controversy over these terms in the literature. To date in veterinary dermatopathology, the term "lichenoid" refers to a band of inflammation, commonly plasmacytic, closely apposed to the dermoepidermal junction, which does not necessarily involve damage to the basal cell layer, such as mucocutaneous pyoderma.

Vasculitis

Vasculitis is characterized by *inflammation targeting the walls of venules or arterioles*, resulting in at least partial destruction

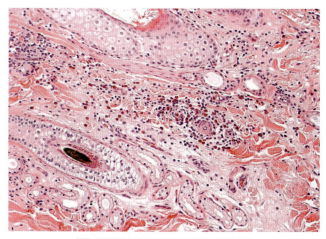

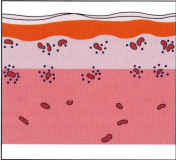

Figure 6-13 Histologic and schematic appearance of **superficial perivascular dermatitis.** *Culicoides* insect-bite hypersensitivity in a horse. Note leukocytes, in this case eosinophils, surrounding dermal vessels.

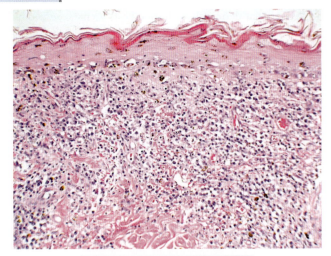

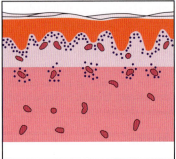

Figure 6-14 Histologic and schematic appearance of **lichenoid interface dermatitis** in chronic cutaneous lupus erythematosus. Large numbers of lymphocytes and plasma cells abut the epidermal-dermal junction. The basal layer of the epidermis demonstrates apoptosis and vacuolar degeneration of keratinocytes.

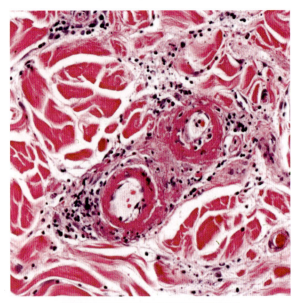

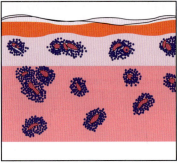

Figure 6-15 Histologic and schematic appearance of **vasculitis**. Leukocytes target vessel walls. Fibrin, erythrocytes and leukocytic debris are in the dermis and vessel walls.

of the vessel wall, sometimes with fibrin deposition (Fig. 6-15). It can be accompanied by fibrinoid necrosis, thrombosis, hemorrhage, and evidence of ischemia. Vasculitis can be immune mediated or septic. *Immune-mediated vasculitis* is due to type III hypersensitivity. The deposition of antigen-antibody complexes in vessel walls activates complement, which results in generation of factors chemotactic for neutrophils. Activation of neutrophils with release of reactive oxygen species and lysosomal enzymes then directly damages vessel walls. *Septic vasculitis* is caused by systemic infection with agents that have a predilection for endothelial cells, resulting in endothelial damage. Vasculitis can also be locally induced by bacterial antigens deposited in vessel walls.

Vasculitis can further be classified on the basis of the *dominant inflammatory cell* within vessel walls. There are neutrophilic, eosinophilic, lymphocytic, and mixed types. It should be noted that the inflammatory cell involved often reflects the stage of the disease rather than characterizing a specific disease.

- **Neutrophilic vasculitis** is by far the most common type and may be *leukocytoclastic* (associated with karyorrhexis of neutrophils resulting in "nuclear dust") or *nonleukocytoclastic*. It is seen with hypersensitivity reactions, septicemia, connective tissue disorders, equine purpura hemorrhagica, Rocky Mountain spotted fever, classical swine fever, thrombophlebitis, and as an idiopathic disorder.
- **Lymphocytic vasculitis** may be seen with dermatomyositis, malignant catarrhal fever, vaccine-induced panniculitis, and rarely in cutaneous lymphoma. It can also reflect a chronic stage of a vasculitis that was originally neutrophilic.
- **Eosinophilic vasculitis** is rare. It is seen most commonly in lesions induced by arthropod insult, drug eruptions, food hypersensitivity, equine axillary nodular necrosis, idiopathic nodular eosinophilic vasculitis in horses, feline eosinophilic granulomas, and rarely in mast cell tumors.

Nodular and diffuse dermatitis

Nodular and diffuse dermatitis is characterized by nodules, or diffuse sheet-like infiltrates of inflammatory cells, in the dermis or subcutis (Fig. 6-16). Nodular and diffuse dermatitis may be characterized by the predominant cell type present (neutrophils, macrophages, lymphocytes, eosinophils, or mixed). The inciting antigen may be an infectious agent, non-infectious material, or the inflammation may be idiopathic. **Neutrophils** predominate in dermal abscesses associated with infectious agents such as bacteria, fungi, algae, and protozoa. They can also be present in sterile lesions, as in foreign-body reactions and the sterile pyogranuloma syndrome. **Histiocytes** predominate in granulomatous inflammation, which is typically chronic. Granulomatous infiltrates containing large numbers of neutrophils are frequently called pyogranulomas. Although all granulomatous dermatitis is nodular or diffuse in pattern, not all nodular and diffuse dermatitides are granulomatous.

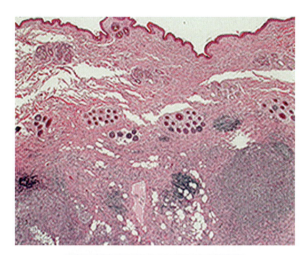

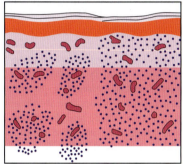

Figure 6-16 Histologic and schematic appearance of **nodular-to-diffuse dermatitis** in bacterial dermatitis. Coalescing nodules of lymphocytes, plasma cells, and macrophages obscure the deep dermis.

Granulomas are discrete foci of granulomatous inflammation. They may be subclassified as "tuberculoid" (a central zone of neutrophils and necrosis surrounded by histiocytes, epithelioid macrophages, and giant cells, in turn surrounded by lymphocytes and an outer layer of fibroblasts) or "sarcoidal" (consisting of epithelioid macrophages). *Tuberculoid granulomas* may be seen in tuberculosis, feline leprosy, atypical mycobacterial infection, and *Corynebacterium pseudotuberculosis* infections. *Sarcoidal granulomas* may be seen in sterile sarcoidal granulomas and foreign-body reactions. *Palisading granulomas* are characterized by the alignment of histiocytes, such as staves around a central focus of collagen degeneration (feline, canine, and equine eosinophilic granuloma; equine mastocytoma); parasite or fungus (habronemiasis, pythiosis, conidiobolomycosis, basidiobolomycosis, demodicosis); lipids (xanthoma); or other foreign material (e.g., calcium as in dystrophic calcinosis cutis and calcinosis circumscripta). Granulomas and pyogranulomas that track hair follicles, resulting in large, vertically oriented ("sausage-shaped") lesions, are seen in sterile granuloma/pyogranuloma syndrome of dogs and cats, or can be seen together with folliculitis because of the presence of intrafollicular antigens such as dermatophytes.

Nodular and diffuse dermatitis is often associated with certain unusual inflammatory cell types. **Foam cells** are histiocytes with vacuolated cytoplasm resulting from their contents (lipid, debris, microorganisms). **Epithelioid macrophages** are histiocytes with elongated or oval vesicular nuclei and abundant finely granular, eosinophilic cytoplasm with ill-defined cell borders. **Multinucleated giant cells** are histiocytic variants that assume 3 morphologic forms: *Langhans* (nuclei form a circle or semicircle at the periphery of the cell), *foreign body* (nuclei are scattered throughout the cytoplasm), and *Touton* (nuclei form a wreath that surrounds a central, homogeneous, amphophilic core of cytoplasm that is, in turn, surrounded by abundant foamy cytoplasm). In general, these 3 forms of giant cells have little diagnostic specificity, although the Touton variety is strongly indicative of xanthomas, and the Langhans type suggests the need for an acid-fast stain. **Eosinophils** may predominate in feline, canine, and equine eosinophilic granuloma; in certain parasitic dermatoses (habronemiasis, elaeophoriasis, parafilariasis, dirofilariasis, dracunculiasis); in furunculosis, and in hairy vetch toxicosis. Mixed cellular infiltrates are most commonly neutrophils and macrophages (pyogranuloma), or eosinophils and macrophages (eosinophilic granuloma), or a combination of the 3 cell types. **Plasma cells** are common components of nodular and diffuse dermatitis in domestic animals and are of no particular diagnostic significance. They may contain eosinophilic, intracytoplasmic inclusions that are called *Russell bodies*. These accumulations of glycoprotein are largely globulin and may be large enough to displace the cell nucleus. Reactions to ruptured hair follicles are a common cause of nodular and diffuse pyogranulomatous dermatitis in domestic animals, and any such lesion should be examined for keratinous and epithelial debris. All other nodular and diffuse dermatitides should be cultured, examined in polarized light for foreign material, and stained for bacteria and fungi. In general, microorganisms are most likely to be found near areas of suppuration and necrosis.

Intraepidermal vesicular and pustular dermatitis

Intraepidermal vesicles and pustules can be caused by intercellular edema that can be seen in any acute or subacute dermatosis, viral infections, hydropic degeneration of keratinocytes, and by acantholysis (Fig. 6-17). It can be useful to subdivide this category on the basis of the site of the vesicle or pustule within the epidermis.

- *Subcorneal pustules and vesicles* are most commonly seen in pemphigus foliaceus, pustules associated with superficial pyoderma, and eosinophilic pustules resulting from hypersensitivities.
- *Pustules and vesicles in the stratum spinosum* are most commonly seen in the pemphigus complex, viral diseases, and occasionally in hepatocutaneous syndrome.
- *Suprabasilar pustules and vesicles* are a feature of pemphigus vulgaris.
- *Intrabasilar vesicles* can be seen in lupus erythematosus, dermatomyositis, erythema multiforme, graft-versus-host disease, and toxic epidermal necrolysis.

Subepidermal vesicular and pustular dermatitis

This pattern is characterized by separation of the epidermis from the dermis (Fig. 6-18). Subepidermal vesicles and pustules may be formed through hydropic degeneration of basal cells, dermoepidermal separation, severe subepidermal edema and/or cellular infiltration, and severe intercellular edema with disruption of the basement membrane zone. Caution is warranted when examining older lesions, as re-epithelialization may result in subepidermal vesicles and pustules assuming an intraepidermal location as re-epithelialization forms a pseudobase to a vesicle. Such re-epithelialization is usually

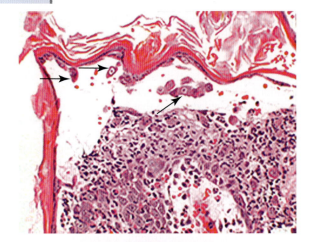
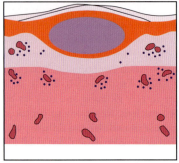

Figure 6-17 Histologic and schematic appearance of **intraepidermal vesicular/pustular dermatitis** in pemphigus foliaceus. A collection of neutrophils and acantholytic keratinocytes (arrows) is within a subcorneal pustule.

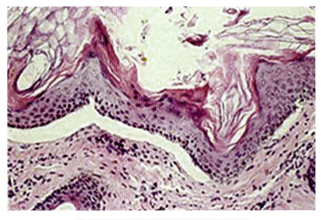
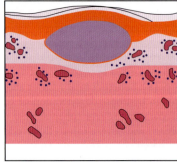

Figure 6-18 Histologic and schematic appearance of **subepidermal vesicular dermatitis** in junctional bullosa. The epidermis is separated at the dermal-epidermal junction.

recognized as a single layer of flattened, elongated basal epidermal cells at the base of the vesicle or pustule.

Perifolliculitis, folliculitis, and furunculosis

Perifolliculitis (see Fig. 6-5C) means accumulation of inflammatory cells around a hair follicle in which the inflammation does not significantly impinge on the follicular epithelium. It can be accompanied by mild follicular spongiosis. **Mural folliculitis** (see Fig. 6-5A) is characterized by inflammation that targets the wall of the follicle. **Luminal folliculitis** (see Fig. 6-5B) implies the accumulation of inflammatory cells within follicular lumina. **Furunculosis** (see Fig. 6-6) occurs when the hair follicle ruptures, releasing the contents into the dermis. *Perifolliculitis, mural and luminal folliculitis, and furunculosis usually represent a pathologic continuum, and all may be present in the same specimen.* Follicular inflammation is a common gross and microscopic finding in dogs, and is less common in other species. It can be caused by bacteria, dermatophytes, and parasites, such as *Demodex* spp., *Pelodera strongyloides*, and *Stephanofilaria* spp.

Furunculosis leads to a foreign-body reaction to free keratin. Aside from granulomatous to pyogranulomatous inflammation, it is not uncommon to find eosinophils, presumably present in reaction to released keratin. Idiopathic sterile eosinophilic folliculitides may be seen in cattle and dogs (sterile eosinophilic pustulosis). Insect stings are postulated as the cause of eosinophilic folliculitides affecting the muzzle of dogs. In cats and horses, sterile eosinophilic folliculitis may be seen in conjunction with hypersensitivity reactions (mosquito-bite hypersensitivity, atopy, food allergy, onchocerciasis, equine eosinophilic granuloma, *Culicoides* hypersensitivity, flea-bite hypersensitivity). Feline herpesviral dermatitis can also result in eosinophilic folliculitis and furunculosis.

Mural folliculitis can be seen with interface dermatitis as well as demodicosis and dermatophytosis. Less common conditions include feline degenerative mucinotic mural folliculitis and pseudopelade. The hair follicle outer root sheath may be involved in hydropic degeneration and lichenoid cellular infiltrates of lupus erythematosus, drug eruptions, erythema multiforme, and idiopathic lichenoid dermatoses.

Lymphocytic peribulbitis directed at the bulb of anagen hair follicles is characteristic of alopecia areata.

Fibrosing dermatitis

Fibrosis marks the resolving stage of an intense, destructive inflammatory reaction or signifies an ongoing, more insidious, inflammatory process. Fibrosis that is recognizable histologically does not necessarily produce a visible clinical scar. Ulcers limited to the upper portion of the superficial dermis do not usually result in scarring, whereas virtually all ulcers that extend into the deep dermis result in fibrosis and clinical signs of scarring. *Fibrosing dermatitis follows many severe insults to the dermis and is often of minimal diagnostic value.* Common causes of fibrosing dermatitis include furunculosis, equine exuberant granulation tissue, actinic dermatitis, acral lick dermatitis, scleroderma, and morphea (localized scleroderma).

Panniculitis

Panniculitis is inflammation of subcutaneous fat (Fig. 6-19). This inflammation often also secondarily involves the deep dermis. Likewise, the panniculus can be secondarily involved in deep dermal inflammation. Panniculitis may be caused by infectious agents, foreign bodies, vitamin E deficiency, trauma, pancreatic

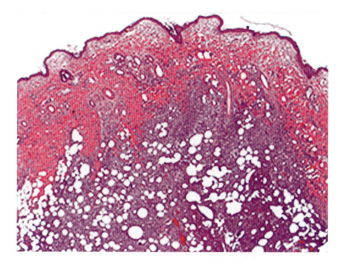

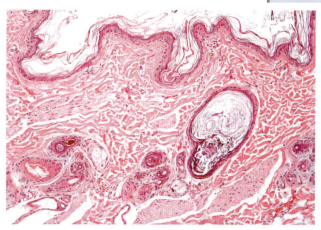

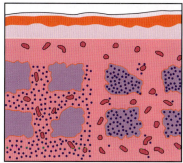

Figure 6-19 Histologic and schematic appearance of **panniculitis.** Inflammation targets the subcutaneous tissues. Note replacement of the adipose tissue with dense inflammatory cell aggregates.

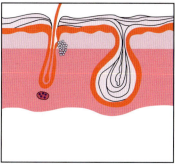

Figure 6-20 Histologic and schematic appearance of **atrophic dermatosis.** The epidermis is thinned at 1-2 nucleated cells in this layer, and follicles are reduced to small epithelial cell clusters. Sebaceous glands are inconspicuous. There is outer root sheath thinning with follicular keratosis. In the schematic, note the thin dermis, hyperkeratosis, pilosebaceous atrophy, follicular keratosis, and plugging.

disease, vasculitis, and adverse drug reaction. However, it is often sterile and idiopathic.

Panniculitis can be divided into **lobular** (fat lobules are primarily involved), **septal** (interlobular connective tissue septa are primarily involved), and **diffuse** (both anatomic areas involved) types. Septal panniculitis is often associated with vasculitis. However, all 3 patterns may be seen in a single lesion from the same patient. *The majority of inflammatory conditions of the panniculus are granulomatous or pyogranulomatous*, and the histologic appearance of panniculitis caused by an infectious agent can be very similar to sterile panniculitis.

In dogs, one form occurs in dogs at sites of previous rabies vaccination and is characterized by lobular hyaline degeneration of fat, lymphocytic vasculitis, lymphoid nodules, and sometimes mucinous degeneration.

Atrophic dermatosis

Atrophic dermatosis is usually characterized by atrophic changes in the hair follicles and adnexal structures (Fig. 6-20). *It can also refer to atrophy of the epidermis or the dermis.* Evaluation of atrophy of the epidermis and dermis should always take into account the site from which the biopsy was taken. Epidermis is normally thicker on the dorsum than the ventrum, and hair follicles and shafts are larger and closer together on the dorsum than on the ventral or glabrous skin. In addition, familiarity with the various stages of the hair follicle cycle is essential if atrophy of the follicle is to be evaluated. Atrophic dermatosis is often accompanied by some, or all, of the following features: atrophic hair follicles (telogen follicles are usually predominant), orthokeratotic hyperkeratosis, follicular keratosis, decreased numbers of hair shafts in follicular infundibula, epidermal atrophy, sebaceous gland atrophy, and dermal atrophy (this can be difficult to assess without site-matched controls). Atrophic dermatosis is rarely diagnostic for a specific condition but can suggest a group of diseases such as the *endocrine dermatoses, the most common cause of atrophic dermatosis*. It will almost always be necessary to confirm the identity of the endocrinopathy with endocrine function tests. Other causes of atrophic dermatoses include ischemia, feline acquired skin fragility, and alopecia X.

Follicular and adnexal atrophy can also be secondary, rather than the primary disease process. An example is follicular atrophy as a result of a chronic inflammatory process, such as chronic allergic dermatitis, or sebaceous adenitis. In this case, there would be histologic evidence of the chronic inflammation previously present, such as scarring or epidermal hyperplasia/hyperkeratosis and superficial dermal perivascular inflammation.

Further reading

Fitzpatrick JE, et al. Patterns in dermatopathology. In: Farmer ER, Hood AF, editors. Pathology of the Skin. New York: McGraw-Hill; 2000. p. 113-130.

Gross TL, et al. Diseases of the panniculus. In: Gross TL, et al., editors. Skin Diseases of the Dog and Cat: Clinical and Histopathologic Diagnosis. 2nd ed. Ames, Iowa: Blackwell; 2005. p. 537-561.

Miller WH, et al. Structure and function of the skin. In: Miller WH, et al., editors. Muller & Kirk's Small Animal Dermatology. 7th ed. St Louis: Elsevier; 2013. p. 1-56.

Scott DW, et al. Diagnostic methods. In: Scott DW, et al., editors. Muller & Kirk's Small Animal Dermatology. 6th ed. St Louis: Elsevier; 2001. p. 71-206.

CONGENITAL AND HEREDITARY DISEASES OF SKIN

Congenital diseases are those that are present at birth. They may be hereditary or result from other factors that were present during development in utero. Various environmental influences, such as infectious agents, nutrient imbalances, toxic chemicals and plants, and ambient temperature, present during gestation, can bring about abnormalities in the skin and hair that are present at birth but are not hereditary. Some congenital diseases are incompatible with life and result in death at birth or shortly thereafter. Congenital abnormalities of the skin may be associated with abnormalities of other tissues or organs. In contrast, although they are genetically determined, some hereditary abnormalities of skin *(genodermatoses)* are not apparent at birth and may instead be manifested later in life, that is, tardive onset. For example, color-dilution alopecia may not be evident until early adulthood. These conditions are covered elsewhere in the chapter under the appropriate section.

As developments in medical science have reduced the incidence of preventable diseases, an increasing awareness of genetic diseases has developed. New genetic disorders are being recognized at an increasing rate as the degree of diagnostic sophistication of veterinary medicine has grown. This is happening, at least in part, because knowledge from genetic disorders in humans often leads to recognition of similar diseases in animals. Once an analogous genetic disease is identified in animals, affected animals may be used to gain new knowledge regarding the genetics, pathogenesis, or treatment of the condition, thereby producing reciprocal benefits for both human and animal health.

Ichthyosis

In veterinary medicine, the term "ichthyosis" is used to describe generalized scaling that arises from congenital and/or hereditary defects in the formation of the stratum corneum (Fig. 6-21). Ichthyosis is derived from the Greek word for fish, and reflects the resemblance of clinical lesions to fish scales. In human medicine, "ichthyosis," is used for both hereditary and acquired (e.g., paraneoplastic ichthyosis) conditions. "Inherited ichthyosis" is the generic term for Mendelian disorders of cornification (MeDOC).

The literature on ichthyosiform disorders in human medicine is extensive and complex, and, not unlike veterinary medicine, molecular tests are not available for all disorders. MeDOC are characterized by an abnormal skin barrier; the resulting phenotype is a reflection of the body's response to correct the barrier defect. There have been deliberate attempts to refine the classification system and apply structure- and function-based algorithms to understand and therapeutically address the phenotypic manifestations. **Ichthyosis vulgaris,** the most common form in humans is an autosomal dominant disease characterized histologically by orthokeratotic hyperkeratosis and a decreased or absent granular layer, and ultrastructurally by retention of corneodesmosomes in the stratum corneum and small or absent keratohyaline granules. It is produced by a defect in synthesis of filaggrin. **X-linked ichthyosis,** a recessive disorder in which males have more severe disease than female heterozygotes, is caused by an absence of steroid sulfatase activity. Steroid sulfatase acts on cholesteryl sulfate, a product of lamellar bodies, which is discharged into the intercellular space and is involved in cell cohesion in the lower stratum corneum. Failure of the enzyme to inactivate cholesteryl sulfate results in persistent cell cohesion and interferes with the normal process of desquamation. The histologic features of X-linked recessive ichthyosis are orthokeratotic hyperkeratosis with a normal or hyperplastic granular layer. Keratohyaline granules are ultrastructurally normal. Neither ichthyosis vulgaris nor X-linked ichthyosis has been documented in domestic animals.

Autosomal recessive congenital ichthyoses (ARCI) is the umbrella that captures a group of inherited cornification disorders. Most of the reported veterinary disorders fall into this grouping. In humans, ARCI may manifest as 1 of 3 clinical forms: lamellar ichthyosis (LI), nonbullous congenital ichthyosiform erythroderma (CIE), and harlequin ichthyosis (HI). The phenotypes of LI and CIE are often overlapping, and some patients may switch phenotypes with age and treatment. HI is a severe disorder that is characterized by generalized severe plate-like scaling at birth and clinically a high mortality rate (Fig. 6-22). HI has been seen in a calf and a greater kudu. LI is characterized by brown plate-like scale in the absence of erythema, whereas the scale in CIE is fine and white with prominent erythema. Although LI is often associated with the transglutaminase 1 *(TGM1)* gene, it is by no means specific for a *TGM1* mutation. To date, 8 genes have been associated with ACRI: *TGM1, ABCA12, ABHD5 (CG158),* 2 lipoxygenases *(ALOXE3* and *ALOX12B),* a NIPA-like domain containing 4 *(NIPAL4* or *ICTHYIN), LIPN, CYP4F22,* and *PNPLA-1.*

The *diagnosis* of ichthyosiform disorders is based on the following: signalment, history, character and distribution of the scale, presence or absence of extracutaneous lesions, and skin biopsy analysis, perhaps including molecular testing. For breeding dogs, *molecular testing, if available, may be needed to identify carrier dogs.* A pathologist should be able to narrow the mutational causes by determining if the disorder is epidermolytic (rare but uniquely associated with keratin mutations) or nonepidermolytic (more common and less specific).

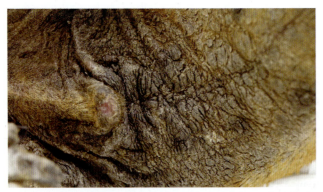

Figure 6-21 Lamellar ichthyosis in a Dachshund. Marked thickening of the skin by thick adherent brown scale.

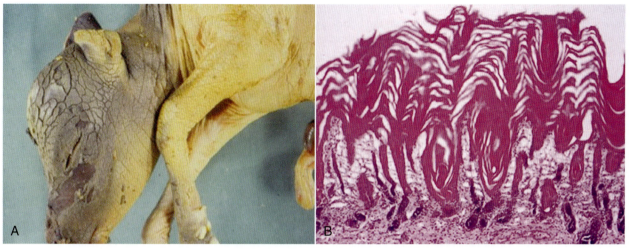

Figure 6-22 **Harlequin ichthyosis** in a neonatal calf. **A.** Generalized plate-like scaling. **B.** Diffuse and severe orthokeratotic hyperkeratosis (Courtesy R. Dunstan.)

Epidermolytic ichthyosis is also referred to as *epidermolytic hyperkeratosis*. The name "epidermolytic" is based on the presence of vacuoles and lysis of keratinocytes within the spinous and granular cell layers, which occur along with hypergranulosis and hyperkeratosis (eFig. 6-1). Unlike nonepidermolytic ichthyosis (see later), this finding uniquely corresponds to a defect in keratin formation (i.e., formation of the corneocyte core). Ultrastructurally, the keratin filaments are clumped and retracted. The biochemical basis is most often associated with a defect in the *K1* and *K10* genes. Epidermolytic ichthyosis in the Norfolk terrier is autosomal recessive and caused by a mutation in epidermal keratin *(KRT10)*. Epidermolytic ichthyosis has been sporadically described in other dogs (Rhodesian Ridgeback, Labrador cross). The affected dogs have multifocal regions of pigmented scale with alopecia and roughening of the skin.

Nonepidermolytic ichthyosis

To date, the nonepidermolytic forms of ichthyosis, which have been characterized in dogs, have been documented or presumed to be autosomal recessive traits. Nonepidermolytic ichthyosis (NI) is not necessarily recessive (e.g., X-linked ichthyosis and autosomal dominant ichthyosis vulgaris are also nonepidermolytic); however, these disorders have yet to be documented in domestic animals. Veterinary pathologists currently label these ARCI disorders by their breed predilection, a practice that may change in the future.

Golden Retriever ichthyosis is generally considered a "mild" form of scaling, and affected dogs are otherwise healthy. The clinical presentation consists of large, soft, white-to-gray adherent scale that is prominent on the trunk and may be associated with ventral hyperpigmentation (eFig.6-2). Histologically, affected dogs have diffuse lamellar orthokeratotic hyperkeratosis in the absence of epidermal hyperplasia and dermal inflammation. The granular layer is prominent and contains keratinocytes with distinct perinuclear clear spaces. Golden Retrievers are typically diagnosed at <1 year of age; however, adult-onset cases are not uncommon. Some dogs develop secondary bacterial folliculitis, which may lead to pruritus and clinical confusion with allergic skin disease. The disease may wax and wane with periodic bouts of exacerbation and remission. Golden Retriever ichthyosis is caused by a mutation in *PNPLA1* gene. The gene is thought to play a role in lipid organization and metabolism within the outer epidermis.

American Bulldogs have a similar but more severe ichthyosiform disorder. Unlike the Golden Retriever, the Bulldogs consistently develop clinical signs before weaning. Young puppies have a scruffy/disheveled haircoat when compared to the smooth coat of normal littermates. The glabrous skin is erythematous with tightly adherent light brown scale, which gives the abdominal skin a "wrinkled" appearance. In the adult dog, the entire abdomen, axilla, and inguinal regions have a red-brown discoloration (eFig. 6-3). Large white to light tan scales are distributed throughout the haircoat. *Malassezia* yeast overgrowth may be severe. The development of otitis externa, intertrigo, and pododermatitis corresponds with yeast proliferation and the onset of pruritus. The clinical presentation may be misinterpreted as nonseasonal atopic skin disease. Occasional adult dogs may have footpad hyperkeratosis. The disorder has been linked to *ICHTHYN*, and similar to the *PLPLA1* mutation in Golden Retrievers, is likely related to lipid metabolism in the epidermis. The histologic lesions are the similar but more severe than Golden Retriever ichthyosis; furthermore, yeast are often found in the stratum corneum (eFig. 6-4).

Nonepidermolytic ichthyosis in **Jack Russell Terriers** (JRTs) is caused by a loss-of-function mutation in transglutaminase 1 *(TGM1)*. TGM1 mediates calcium-dependent cross-linking of peptides (e.g., involucrin, loricrin) to form the cornified envelope—the strong exterior of the corneocyte. The phenotype in the JRT is characterized by large, thick, adherent parchment paper-like scales. This is generally more severe than the previously described disorders. The dogs develop severe *Malassezia* infections with corresponding inflammation and pruritus.

A number of **other breeds** have been diagnosed with NI on light microscopy and clinical examination (Soft-coated Wheaten Terriers, West Highland White Terriers), but further molecular characterizations have not been documented. Many cases are likely confirmed on skin biopsy and do not receive further workup.

A congenital and familial form of keratoconjunctivitis sicca with scaling has been documented in **Cavalier King Charles**

Spaniel dogs. The dogs have a syndrome that includes the following features: keratoconjunctivitis noted from the beginning of eyelid opening, a roughened/curly haircoat, scaling with abdominal hyperpigmentation, footpad hyperkeratosis, and nail dystrophy. A recessive mode of inheritance has been proposed.

Congenital follicular parakeratosis is a cornification disorder reported in Rottweiler and Labrador Retriever dogs. An X-linked dominant mode of inheritance has been suggested in **Rottweilers** because the 5 reported dogs were female, and no male relatives were affected. The clinical lesions are generalized scaling and hyperkeratotic pigmented plaques. The plaques contain thick waxy and papillated follicular fronds. In Rottweilers, the lesions follow Blasko's lines. Histologically, the epidermis is acanthotic, and hair follicles have marked papillated parakeratotic hyperkeratosis that forms conically shaped projections. Clear (lipid-laden) vacuoles are located in the thick nucleated keratin. Ultrastructural changes in 2 dogs included large keratohyaline granules, tonofilament clumps, and numerous lipid vacuoles in the stratum corneum and granulosum. In Labradors, the condition may be confused with a presumably immune-mediated adult-onset form of mural folliculitis with parakeratosis.

Hereditary footpad hyperkeratosis has been reported in Irish Terriers and in a family of Dogues de Bordeaux. All footpads become progressively hyperkeratotic, fissured, and painful. Both males and females are affected, and lesions are evident by 6 months of age. The mode of inheritance has not been determined. The histologic features are mild to moderate papillated epidermal hyperplasia and diffuse orthokeratotic hyperkeratosis.

Ichthyosis has been reported in many breeds of **cattle,** and the mode of inheritance appears to be *autosomal recessive.* Both males and females are affected. Two forms of ichthyosis have been described in cattle, *ichthyosis fetalis* and *ichthyosis congenita.* However, the underlying molecular defect(s) is unknown, and it is uncertain whether the forms are distinct diseases or merely represent variations in expression of a single abnormality. *Ichthyosis fetalis* is the more severe form, and it has been compared to the harlequin fetus form of ichthyosis in humans. Affected calves are stillborn or die shortly after birth. The skin is hairless and covered by thick scales divided into plates by deep fissures that represent normal cleavage planes of the skin. The tight, inelastic skin is everted at the mucocutaneous junctions, and the ears are usually smaller than normal. *Ichthyosis congenita* is a less severe form compatible with life in which the limbs, abdomen, and muzzle are primarily involved. The skin is dry, hard, and inflexible like old leather, and may be prominently folded. There are flat plates of hyperkeratosis in which dense mats of hairs are entrapped. The keratin plaques are separated by shallow hyperemic fissures. The condition is characterized histologically by *prominent laminated orthokeratotic hyperkeratosis of the epidermis and superficial portion of hair follicles.* The epidermal surface is wrinkled or folded and acanthosis is variable.

Further reading

Credille KM, et al. Mild recessive epidermolytic hyperkeratosis with a novel keratin 10 donor splice-site mutation in a family of Norfolk terrier dogs. Br J Dermatol 2005;153:51-58.

Elias PM, et al. Ichthyoses. Clinical, Biochemical, Pathogenic and Diagnostic Assessment. Current Problems in Dermatology. Basel: Karger; 2010;39. p. 1-29.

Grall S, et al. PNPLA1 mutations cause autosomal recessive congenital ichthyosis in golden retriever dogs and humans. Nat Genet 2012;44:140-147.

Hargis A, et al. Proliferative, lymphocytic, infundibular mural folliculitis and dermatitis with prominent follicular apoptosis and parakeratotic casts in four Labrador retrievers: preliminary description and response to therapy. Vet Dermatol 2013;24:346-354.

Helman RG, et al. Ichthyosiform dermatosis in a soft-coated wheaten terrier. Vet Dermatol 1997;8:53-58.

Mauldin EA, et al. The clinical and morphologic features of nonepidermolytic ichthyosis in the golden retriever. Vet Pathol 2008;45:174-180.

Mauldin EA. Canine ichthyosis and related disorders of cornification. Vet Clin North Am Small Anim Pract 2013;43:89-97.

Wattles

Wattles (tassels), similar to those seen in goats, occur occasionally in swine and rarely in sheep. They occur in many breeds of **swine** with no apparent sex predilection and are inherited as an autosomal dominant trait. Wattles are asymptomatic, cylindrical, teat-like structures that hang from the ventral mandibular region. They are 5-7 cm long and may be unilateral or bilateral. Histologically, they are composed of a core of fibrocartilage, surrounded by fibrous and adipose connective tissue, and covered by haired skin.

Wattles have also been reported in Dorset Down, Merino, and Karakul **sheep.** The structures in sheep are smaller than those of pigs, and they lack the fibrocartilaginous core seen in wattles of goats and pigs.

Hereditary zinc deficiency

Hereditary zinc deficiency occurs in cattle and Bull Terrier dogs and results in multisystemic disease that includes skin lesions. Animals are normal at birth and usually begin developing skin lesions at approximately 1-2 months of age, at which time growth retardation also becomes evident. Skin lesions consist of crusting, which is most prominent on the face and distal extremities, dry flaky skin, and hair color fading. A decrease in serum zinc concentration precedes clinical signs; and alkaline phosphatase, a zinc-dependent enzyme, frequently decreases in parallel with the zinc concentration. Affected animals also commonly have diarrhea. Animals with hereditary zinc deficiency have a hypoplastic thymus, and, consequently, secondary infections are common because of associated immune system dysfunction involving both humoral and cell-mediated immunity. The condition is an *autosomal recessive trait* in both cattle and dogs, and it is considered analogous to acrodermatitis enteropathica of humans. *The characteristic histologic lesion is marked diffuse parakeratotic hyperkeratosis.*

Hereditary zinc deficiency (HZD) in cattle is also called *lethal trait A46, hereditary parakeratosis, hereditary thymic aplasia,* and *Adema disease.* It affects Friesian cattle and Black Pied Danish cattle of Friesian descent in Europe, and has been reported in Shorthorn cattle in the United States. The condition normally begins with depression, diarrhea, and skin lesions when calves are 4-8 weeks of age. The skin becomes dry and flaky, and the haircoat is rough. Patches of erythema, scaling, oozing, crusting, and alopecia begin on the muzzle and then appear around the eyes, ears, and intermandibular space. Similar lesions develop later on the legs, and the skin around the stifles, fetlocks, and coronary bands becomes particularly crusty, fissured, and painful. The flanks, perianal area, and ventral abdomen may also be affected. The hair may lighten in color, a change that may be especially prominent around the eyes and resemble the spectacle lesion of copper deficiency. Affected calves are lethargic, drool, and may have difficulty suckling. They are smaller than unaffected calves of the same age. Conjunctivitis, rhinitis, bronchopneumonia, and other infections are common because of *immune dysfunction*. Untreated calves usually die 4-8 weeks after the onset of clinical disease.

This disease is associated with impaired intestinal zinc absorption caused by abnormal function of a protein belonging to a family of zinc-uptake proteins. Acrodermatitis enteropathica and HZD are associated with defects in the gene SLC39A4. Oral zinc supplementation effects a complete reversal of clinical signs and may restore thymic morphology if instituted early enough. *Intestinal malabsorption of zinc is the cause of the disorder in cattle.* Zinc is absorbed from the intestine by 2 separate pathways, that is, a transporter-dependent active system and passive diffusion, and it is the zinc-binding ligand system that is suspected to be defective. A cysteine-rich intestinal protein (CRIP) has been identified in the ligand-dependent pathway and has been suggested as being defective in this condition.

The most striking and consistent gross abnormality is *marked thymic hypoplasia*. Histologic abnormalities include *depletion of small lymphocytes* of the thymus, especially in the cortical region, and hypoplasia of the spleen, lymph nodes, and Peyer's patches. The skin lesions are characterized histologically by *perivascular dermatitis, acanthosis, pallor and vacuolation of the upper spinous and granular layers, and marked diffuse parakeratosis*. Neutrophilic exocytosis and superficial bacterial cocci may be prominent.

Lethal acrodermatitis of Bull Terrier dogs is also thought to be caused by an abnormality in zinc absorption or metabolism; however, zinc supplementation fails to produce clinical improvement. The concentrations of both serum zinc and copper have been found to be lower in affected Bull Terriers compared with control dogs, raising the question of the role of copper deficiency in the pathogenesis of the canine disease. The condition is characterized by growth retardation, progressive skin lesions, paronychia, diarrhea, abnormal behavior, bronchopneumonia, and death usually by 18 months. Some affected puppies have lighter pigmentation than their normal littermates, and this difference becomes more pronounced with age. By 2 months of age, they are obviously smaller than their normal littermates. Skin lesions usually begin by 6-8 weeks of age and consist of crusty exfoliative lesions involving the distal extremities, footpads, and mucocutaneous junctions, particularly on the muzzle and mouth (eFig. 6-5). Digits are prominently splayed, and footpads develop cracks and frond-like masses of keratin. The skin is erythematous and moist under the crusts. Interdigital pyoderma and paronychia are common. Many affected dogs also have diarrhea and exhibit abnormal behavior consisting of increased aggressiveness initially, and lethargy and decreased responsiveness later in the course of disease. Respiratory tract infections are common, and bronchopneumonia is a common cause of death.

Extracutaneous postmortem lesions consist of a *small or absent thymus* and may also include a high, arched palate and brachygnathia inferior. Histologic changes in the skin are *mild to moderate perivascular dermatitis, moderate to marked acanthosis that may be accompanied by pallor of the superficial epidermis, and marked diffuse parakeratotic hyperkeratosis* (see eFig. 6-5D). There may also be neutrophilic exocytosis, intraepidermal neutrophilic pustules, and serocellular crusts containing bacterial cocci and/or yeasts. Diagnosis is straightforward if signalment and clinical history are known. If this information is not available, differential diagnoses include superficial necrolytic dermatitis, zinc-responsive dermatosis, and generic dog food dermatosis. However, parakeratosis is less severe in these diseases, and superficial epidermal necrolysis is not a feature of lethal acrodermatitis.

Further reading

Ackland ML, Michalczyk A. Zinc deficiency and its inherited disorders—a review. Genes Nutr 2006;1:41-49.

McEwan NA, et al. Diagnostic features, confirmation and disease progression in 28 cases of lethal acrodermatitis of bull terriers. J Small Anim Pract 2000;41:501-507.

Wang K, et al. A novel member of a zinc transporter family is defective in acrodermatitis enteropathica. Am J Hum Genet 2002;71:66-73.

Yuzbasiyan-Gurkana V, Bartletta E. Identification of a unique splice site variant in SLC39A4 in bovine hereditary zinc deficiency, lethal trait A46: an animal model of acrodermatitis enteropathica. Genes Nutr 2006;88:521-526.

Epidermolysis bullosa

Epidermolysis bullosa (EB) is a heterogeneous group of mechanobullous genodermatoses that are all characterized by skin and mucous membrane blistering and ulceration in response to minor mechanical trauma. EB is caused by mutations in structural proteins that comprise the basement membrane zone and cytoskeleton of basal keratinocytes. In veterinary medicine, advances in molecular techniques have elucidated the mutations in genes that encode structural proteins: plakophilin 1 *(PKP1)*, desmoplakin *(DSP)*, keratins 5 and 14 *(KRT5 and KRT14)*, plectin *(PLEC1)*, α6β5 integrin *(ITGA6)*, laminin *(LAMA3, LAMB3, LAMC2)*, and collagen types XVII and VII *(COL17A1, COL7A)*.

Much of the older literature uses the term epitheliogenesis imperfecta (EI) to describe congenital mechanobullous conditions in many species; however, many of these conditions would be more appropriately termed epidermolysis bullosa in the current classification. Furthermore, epitheliogenesis imperfecta descriptively encompassed 2 different diseases: epidermolysis bullosa and aplasia cutis congenita. In **swine,** aplasia cutis congenita (also called epitheliogenesis imperfecta) is very rare and a clinically distinct, recessively inherited trait. The disorder arises predominantly in male piglets. Most piglets have extensive lesions and die shortly after birth. Piglets with small focal lesions may survive but are smaller than normal littermates. At least some affected piglets also have hydroureter and hydronephrosis. The defects are typically located within the caudal half of the body (Fig. 6-23), and are characterized by an absence of epidermis and sometimes loss of dermis. Piglets may have fluid-filled subcutaneous bullae. An underlying cause is not known.

Epidermolysis bullosa is divided into *3 broad groups* based on the ultrastructural level of the skin cleavage: *epidermolysis bullosa simplex* (EBS; epidermolytic epidermolysis bullosa),

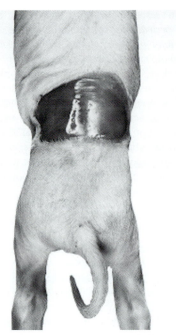

Figure 6-23 Aplasia cutis congenita (epitheliogenesis imperfecta) in a pig.

junctional epidermolysis bullosa (JEB), and *dystrophic epidermolysis bullosa* (dermolytic epidermolysis bullosa). JEB may be further classified into *Herlitz or non-Herlitz type*. Herlitz JEB is a severe (typically lethal) and generalized disease with widespread cutaneous and mucous membrane blistering. EB is further classified into >20 subtypes in humans based on clinical manifestations of skin lesions, mode of inheritance, and presence or absence of extracutaneous abnormalities, as well as ultrastructural features. The clinical presentation may range from minimal localized involvement of hands and feet to severe, life-threatening generalized blistering with extracutaneous involvement. Corneal erosions, tooth, nail, and hair abnormalities, and tracheal, gastrointestinal, genitourinary, and musculoskeletal involvement occur in various subtypes of epidermolysis bullosa in humans. In animals, epidermolysis bullosa has been reported rarely and, in most instances, has led to the death of affected individuals.

- **Epidermolysis bullosa simplex** is characterized by *cytolysis of the basal keratinocytes*, which produces intraepidermal clefting. This form of the disease is caused by fragility of the epidermal basal cells because of mutations in basal cell–specific keratins 5 and 14. These mutations result in disruption of the assembly, structure, and/or function of the keratin intermediate filaments that act as the skeleton of basal keratinocytes. Ultrastructurally, cytolysis of the basal cells is seen as intraepidermal clefting. In some forms, cytolysis is preceded by aggregation and clumping of the keratin tonofilaments that are attached to hemidesmosomes.
- In **junctional epidermolysis bullosa**, clefting occurs within the lamina lucida because of abnormalities of the anchoring filament-hemidesmosome complexes, which may be reduced in number and poorly formed or may be completely absent. Most cases of JEB are the result of a deficiency or abnormality in one of the hemidesmosome-associated proteins laminin-5, collagen XVII (also called BPAG 2 and BP180), or integrin α6β4, or the extracellular protein LAD-1, which is secreted by epidermal cells and localizes to the upper aspect of the anchoring filaments. The Herlitz type of JEB has more severe skin lesions than other types of EB. The lesions are widespread with all hooves affected, and most animals die within the first week of life. Whereas hemidesmosomes may be normal or reduced in size and number in the non-Herlitz type, they are markedly reduced or absent with an absent sub-basal dense plate in the Herlitz type of JEB.
- **Dystrophic epidermolysis bullosa** is characterized by a split in the superficial dermis below the lamina densa in the region of the anchoring fibrils, which are fewer in number and distorted or completely absent. The molecular cause of dystrophic epidermolysis bullosa is a mutation in the anchoring fibril protein, type VII collagen.

Affected animals usually develop lesions shortly after birth; however, in some cases, the disease is not evident until the animal is several months old. *Initial lesions consist of vesicles and bullae, but they quickly rupture, and only ulcers may be evident clinically.* Lesions are located in areas of the skin and mucous membranes that are most prone to frictional trauma, such as *over bony prominences of the distal extremities, footpads, lips, tongue, palate, and gingiva.* Hoof sloughing and nail dystrophy and shedding accompany skin lesions in some forms of the disease. Lesions may be induced accidentally by rough handling of an affected animal or intentionally for diagnostic purposes by gentle frictional trauma.

Histologically, most forms of epidermolysis bullosa are characterized by subepidermal clefts and vesicles with minimal inflammation (see Fig. 6-18), changes that are indistinguishable from other mechanobullous diseases (e.g., bullous pemphigoid [BP], mucous membrane pemphigoid). Even in the epidermolytic form of epidermolysis bullosa, the cleavage is usually so low in the epidermis that the vesicle appears subepidermal in routine sections. PAS staining to visualize the basement membrane zone may be helpful in determining the level of cleavage, but definitive diagnosis requires ultrastructural examination. Basement membrane antigen mapping by immunofluorescence or immunohistochemistry may be a diagnostic adjunct or alternative to electron microscopy to establish the diagnosis. In epidermolysis bullosa simplex, the PAS-positive basement membrane is at the base of the blister as are type IV collagen, laminin, and BP antigen. In JEB, the PAS-positive basement membrane, type IV collagen, and laminin are at the base of the blister, whereas the BP antigen is primarily on the blister roof. The PAS-positive basement membrane as well as all 3 basement membrane proteins, that is, type IV collagen, laminin, and BP antigen, are at the roof of the blister in dystrophic epidermolysis bullosa.

Further reading

Benoit-Biancamano MO, et al. Aplasia cutis congenita (epitheliogenesis imperfecta) in swine: observations from a large breeding herd. J Vet Diagn Invest 2006;18:573-579.

Cattle

All 3 forms of epidermolysis bullosa have been described in cattle. In **calves**, epidermolysis bullosa (termed EI) has been reported in many breeds and appears to be an *autosomal recessive trait*, and it is seen most often in herds in which there is extensive inbreeding. Both male and female calves are affected. Lesions are usually extensive and involve the extremities most commonly; however, any portion of the body may be affected as well as the squamous epithelium of the muzzle, lips, and oral cavity. Hooves and dewclaws may be missing or incompletely formed. Some affected calves also have deformed teeth and lack pinnae. Brachygnathia and atresia ani have accompanied the cutaneous abnormalities in some calves.

Epidermolysis bullosa simplex (EBS) associated with a mutation in the keratin 5 gene *(KRT5)* has been identified in the progeny of a 3-year-old Friesian-Jersey crossbred bull. Histologically, the lesions were characterized by dermoepidermal separation; electron microscopy showed that the cleavage occurred above the basement membrane zone and involved basal keratinocyte lysis.

Epidermolysis bullosa simplex has been reported in Simmental cross calves in the United Kingdom. Ultrastructural findings were typical of EBS, but no mutations were found in *KRT5* or *KRT 14*. EBS has also been described in 25 of 72 calves sired by a single Simmental bull. The condition appeared to be inherited as an *autosomal dominant trait* with high mortality. Lesions were evident in newborn calves and consisted of ulcers of the muzzle, lips, gingiva, dorsum of the tongue, and around joints of distal limbs. Calves were unthrifty, became emaciated after weaning, and developed areas of alopecia, hyperkeratosis, ulcers, and exfoliative dermatitis. Three animals kept under laboratory conditions showed gradual improvement in severity of lesions, but rough handling could still elicit lesions. Histologic changes were typical of EB and consisted of *dermal-epidermal separation unassociated with any significant inflammation*. PAS-positive basement membrane was evident on the dermal side of the cleft. In thin sections of skin, cytolysis of the basal keratinocytes was seen, but no ultrastructural examination was done to confirm the diagnosis. JEB has been described in a Gir crossbred calf.

A mechanobullous disease suspected to be *dystrophic epidermolysis bullosa* has been reported in Texas Brangus calves with a common bull in their pedigree. The calves developed ulceration of distal limbs and oral mucosa, nasolabial mucosal sloughing, and sloughing of hooves within the first few days of life. The mode of inheritance was suspected to be recessive because of extensive inbreeding. Histologically, the lesions were dermal-epidermal clefts, with the PAS-positive basement membrane remaining attached to the basal cell layer, that is, forming the roof of the bullae. Ultrastructural examination revealed that the lamina densa was attached to the basal layer of the epidermis; inadequate fixation prevented accurate evaluation of the anchoring fibrils.

A single case report of JEB was reported in a Gir-cross calf. The calf had exungulation of all hooves, oral ulcers, and widespread erosions and crusts on the body.

Sheep

Inherited junctional epidermolysis bullosa (Herlitz type) has been described in 16 German black-headed mutton sheep. The sheep died within the first week of life. Skin lesions, mostly crusted ulcers with a few intact blisters, were most pronounced over the dorsal aspects of the carpal and tarsal regions, coronary bands, hooves, and tongue. Immunohistochemistry with the antibody to laminin-5 showed reduced expression on frozen sections of skin and tongue. A frameshift mutation in *LAMC2* was documented.

A congenital bullous disease suggestive of *dystrophic epidermolysis bullosa* has been described in Suffolk and South Dorset Down lambs in New Zealand, Scottish Blackface lambs, and Weisses Alpenschaf lambs in Switzerland. Blisters that evolved into ulcers were seen at birth or within the first few weeks of life. Lesions occurred in areas with sparse hair and those prone to frictional trauma, such as the muzzle, ears, groin, coronary band, lips, tongue, gums, dental pad, and palate. Lameness and hoof separation and sloughing were common and gave rise to the colloquial name "red foot disease" in Scotland. The lambs grew poorly and were underdeveloped, and there were changes attributed to oral ulceration and reluctance to nurse. Histologic changes were typical of EB and consisted of *dermal-epidermal separation with minimal inflammation*. The PAS-positive basement membrane zone remained attached to the epithelium and formed the roof of the vesicle, suggestive of dystrophic epidermolysis bullosa. The condition has been characterized only in the Swiss Weisses Alpenschaf breed. Ultrastructural examination of skin from the Swiss lambs indicated that the splitting was below the lamina densa and that anchoring fibrils were absent or rare and rudimentary. Antigen mapping of the lesion identified laminin and type IV collagen at the roof of the cleft, which *confirms sublamina densa blistering*; and no type VII collagen, the major structural component of anchoring fibrils, could be identified. These findings are consistent with the dystrophic form of epidermolysis bullosa. The disease was found to have a *recessive mode of inheritance*.

Goats

Dystrophic epidermolysis bullosa (DEB) occurs in goats. The condition was first described in an Anglo-Nubian dairy buck from Brazil. The unaffected twin brother of this buck was bred over 5 consecutive years with the dam and produced 12 kids, 4 of which were affected with DEB, suggesting an autosomal recessive mode of inheritance. Affected kids had a positive Nikolsky sign and developed spontaneous lesions within the first week of life. Alopecia, erosions, and crusts were observed on the pinnae, ventral thorax and abdomen, and dorsal surface of the carpal and tarsal regions. The gums and lips were ulcerated. Erythema and hemorrhage of the coronary bands with detachment of the hooves was observed. Also described in humans with DEB, there was spontaneous healing with scarring of the skin lesions in most of the kids. Malnutrition and growth retardation were also noted.

Horses

The Herlitz form of JEB has been described in both male and female Belgian foals within the first week or 2 of life, in American Saddlebred horses, and in 2 French draft-breed horses. Lesions in **foals** usually involve the legs and oral cavity. The proximal esophagus may also be affected and hooves may be lacking. In some instances, teeth are malformed. Lesions consist of skin and oral mucosal ulceration, most often of the carpi, stifles, hocks, fetlocks, tongue, gingiva, and hard palate. Hoof separation and sloughing (exungulation) are common features. Extracutaneous lesions are rare, and included ocular lesions in one foal and dental dysplasia in another. The histologic lesions consist of *subepidermal clefting with minimal inflammation and PAS-positive basement membrane material evident at the base of the cleft* (see Fig. 6-18). Ultrastructurally, the separation is located within the lamina lucida, indicating that hemidesmosomes are underdeveloped. In Belgian foals, the trait is inherited as autosomal recessive. The mutation responsible—a cytosine insertion in exon 10 of the *LAMC2* gene—has also been identified in JEB phenotype horses in 2

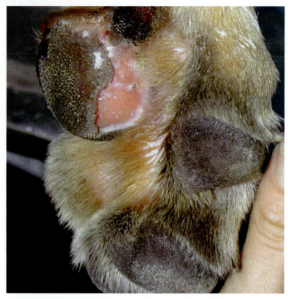

Figure 6-24 Epidermolysis bullosa in a dog. Note that the epidermis of the pawpad is easily detached, leading to extensive ulceration in areas exposed to mechanical trauma.

French draft breeds, the Breton and Comtois. In American Saddlebred horses, the mutation has been identified in *LAMA3*.

Dogs

All 3 forms of epidermolysis bullosa (EB) have been reported in dogs (Fig. 6-24). However, the initial cases reported as epidermolysis bullosa simplex in young Collies are now thought to represent a mild form of dermatomyositis with unrecognized myositis. *JEB (Herlitz type)* has been described in newborn Toy Poodle and German Shorthaired Pointer puppies via histopathology and electron microscopy. Shortly after birth, the dogs developed vesicles and bullae, and ulcers were present on the pawpads, mucous membranes, and haired skin of frictional sites. Non-Herlitz (nonlethal) JEB has been documented in a 4-year-old mongrel dog. The dog had a history of vesicles, erosions, crusts, and alopecia since birth. Lesions initially occurred on the lips and ventral abdomen and eventually progressed to involve the face, trunk, tail, and acral regions. Cutaneous atrophy and hyperpigmentation, alopecia, and nail dystrophy developed later. In skin sections from the mongrel dog, expression of laminin-5, BPAG2, the α6 subunit of integrin α6β4, and type VII collagen was similar to that of normal canine skin.

Junctional EB in German Shorthaired Pointers is autosomal recessive and has been proposed as an animal model. Affected dogs have spontaneous or traumatically induced blisters and ulcers on the footpads, pinnae, tail tip, and on pressure points on the distal limbs. Onychodystrophy or dental enamel dysplasia are not reported. The disease is associated with reduced expression of laminin 5 and is caused by a mutation in the *LAMA3* gene for the laminin α3 chain.

Dystrophic epidermolysis bullosa (DEB), associated with mutation in the gene encoding type VII collagen *(COL7A1)*, has been characterized in Golden Retriever dogs. Affected dogs have blisters and ulcers in the oral and esophageal epithelia, together with onychodystrophy and growth retardation. DEB was reported in a 4-year-old female Akita with a lifelong history of trauma-induced ulcers and scars over pressure points of limbs and on footpads. Nail dystrophy was apparent from 1 year of age. The lesions had periodic exacerbations and remissions. The histologic changes were *dermal-epidermal clefting* with minimal inflammation and PAS-positive basement membrane visible at the roof of the cleft. Ultrastructural examination indicated that the separation was beneath the lamina densa, and anchoring fibrils were in reduced numbers. Expression of type VII collagen, the major structural protein of anchoring fibrils, was normal. A *dominant mode of inheritance* was speculated in this nonlethal case of EB because the dominant form of DEB in humans is typically relatively mild.

Cats

Epidermolysis bullosa appears to be *very rare in cats*. JEB has been reported in 2 unrelated domestic shorthaired kittens. Pinnal erosions, oral ulcerations, and severe onychomadesis were described in both. Cat 1 was euthanized because of severe oral and ocular involvement; the second cat had lesions that were relatively mild and was maintained with lifelong conservative management. Immunostaining revealed decreased expression of the γ2 laminin chain in cat 1 and decreased β3 laminin chains in cat 2. Mutations were not documented but proposed to lie in the genes *LAMC2* in cat 1 and *LAMB* in cat 2.

An undetermined type of EB was reported in a 3-year-old male domestic longhaired cat in the United Kingdom. The skin condition had been evident since the cat was 3 months old; a female littermate obtained showed no skin abnormalities. The affected cat had widespread scarring, alopecia, crusting, scaling, blisters, and ulcers. Several nails had been shed, and very few whiskers were present. No lesions were evident in the oral cavity. Histologically, lesions were characterized by dermal-epidermal separation. Ultrastructural examination indicated the cleavage to be above the lamina densa and that hemidesmosomes and anchoring fibrils were fewer and less distinct when compared to skin from a normal cat. EB (termed EI) was reported in a litter of Siamese kittens with linear ulcers on the tongue.

Dystrophic EB has been described in a domestic shorthaired cat and in a Persian cat. The cats had a juvenile onset of ulcers in the oral cavity, haired skin (dorsum), footpads, and onychomadesis. Ultrastructural examination in the Persian cat demonstrated a reduced number of anchoring fibrils, and immunostaining revealed a decreased expression of type VII collagen. Histologic examination of skin biopsies showed dermal-epidermal separation progressing to ulcers. Type IV collagen was shown by immunohistochemistry to be present at the roof of the blisters. *Sublamina densa clefting* was confirmed by electron microscopic examination, and anchoring fibrils were markedly reduced in number and appeared rudimentary and filamentous in skin sections from the Persian cat. Immunofluorescent staining for collagen VII, the primary component of anchoring fibrils, was markedly reduced. A mutation in the collagen VII encoding gene *COL7A1* was suggested as the cause, because this gene is mutated in all subsets of DEB in affected human patients.

Further reading

Alhaidari Z, et al. Junctional epidermolysis bullosa in two domestic shorthair kittens. Vet Dermatol 2005;16:69-73.

Bruckner-Tuderman L, et al. Animal models of epidermolysis bullosa: update 2010. J Invest Dermatol 2010;130:1485-1488.

Foster AP, et al. Epidermolysis bullosa in calves in the United Kingdom. J Comp Pathol 2010;142:336-340.

Medeiros GX, Riet-Correa F. Epidermolysis bullosa in animals: a review. Vet Dermatol 2015;26:3-e2.

Milenkovic D, et al. A mutation in the *LAMC2* gene causes the Herlitz junctional epidermolysis bullosa (H-JEB) in two French draft horse breeds. Genet Sel Evol 2003;35:249-256.

Olivry T, Linder KE. Dermatoses affecting desmosomes in animals: a mechanistic review of acantholytic blistering skin diseases. Vet Dermatol 2009;20:313-326.

Ostmeier M, et al. Inherited junctional epidermolysis bullosa (Herlitz type) in German black-headed mutton sheep. J Comp Pathol 2012;146:338-347.

Palazzi X, et al. Inherited dystrophic epidermolysis bullosa in inbred dogs: a spontaneous animal model for somatic gene therapy. J Invest Dermatol 2000;115:135-137.

Spirito F, et al. Animal models for skin blistering conditions: absence of laminin 5 causes hereditary junctional mechanobullous disease in the Belgian horse. J Invest Dermatol 2002;119:684-691.

Genetic acantholytic dermatoses in dogs

A dominantly inherited epidermal acantholytic disease has been described in English Setters. The disease was initially compared to **Hailey-Hailey disease** (HHD) in humans, but current thought is that the disorder is more likely a form of **Darier disease** (DD) In humans, autosomal dominant mutations in genes that encode calcium pumps are responsible for both HHD (SPCA1: secretory calcium/magnesium ATPase isoform) and DD (SERCA2: sarcoendoplasmic reticulum calcium ATPase isoform 2).

Hailey-Hailey disease is an autosomal dominant hereditary skin disorder of epidermal keratinocyte cohesion. Lesions in humans consist of vesicles and bullae in flexural regions exposed to chronic frictional trauma. The histologic characteristics include suprabasilar clefting and extensive separation of keratinocytes that remain loosely in place, giving the appearance of a "dilapidated brick wall." Because of the resemblance to autoimmune pemphigus, HHD is also called *benign familial chronic pemphigus*. In contrast to HHD, the *lesions of DD are papular to verrucous and occur in seborrheic areas.* In addition to suprabasilar acantholysis, DD is characterized by dyskeratosis of the keratinocytes with formation of "corps ronds" (cells with small pyknotic nuclei, a perinuclear clear halo, and eosinophilic cytoplasm) and "grains" (compressed cells with elongated nuclei seen in the stratum corneum and granular layer) and columns of parakeratosis. In each disease, ultrastructure shows a retraction of keratin filaments from desmosomal plaques and formation of a ring of keratin around the keratinocyte nucleus.

The condition was seen in a 7-month-old male English Setter and in 2 of his female offspring, at the ages of 1 and 2 months, respectively. Lesions consisted of well-demarcated, alopecic, erythematous, hyperplastic plaques with a rough surface, occasional serous crusting, and peripheral scaling. The lesions occurred on the ventral thorax, head, and stifle. The clinical appearance of the lesions was not typical HHD, but the histologic and ultrastructural features were thought to be similar to benign familial chronic pemphigus. Microscopically, the epidermis was markedly hyperplastic, and suprabasal keratinocytes were much larger than those in the perilesional epidermis. Extensive acantholysis resulted in lacuna formation in the suprabasal and upper epidermis and the follicular epithelium along with parakeratosis and corneocyte separation (eFig. 6-6). Ultrastructurally, the changes included increased intercellular spaces, and intact desmosome-tonofilament complexes and actin filaments in early lesions. Keratin filaments retracted from the desmosomal plaques to form a perinuclear whorl. Immunohistochemical examination of various desmosomal proteins failed to demonstrate any abnormalities, and the molecular defect in these dogs was not identified. Further studies have shown that keratinocytes in lesional and nonlesional skin have depleted SERCA2 stores. Although the precise mechanism is not known, depletion of calcium stores may delay exit from the cell cycle and enhance apoptosis. Thus the clinical appearance, histologic features, and SERCA2 abnormality suggest the disease in dogs is more similar to DD than HHD.

A unique *autosomal recessive acantholytic dermatosis* has been reported in related Chesapeake Bay Retriever dogs. At birth, the dogs showed sloughing of the superficial epidermal layers upon pressure. At 3 months of age, the dogs had recurrent lesions on the mucocutaneous junctions and an abnormal haircoat with multifocal hair loss. Histologically, the puppies had suprabasilar acantholysis, which became less severe with age. The condition is associated with a *PKP1* mutation and loss of plakophilin-1 in desmosomal attachments as well as an abnormal arrangement of desmoplakin and keratins 10 and 14.

Genetic acantholytic dermatoses in cattle

A *congenital mechanobullous dermatosis of uncertain type* has been described in Angus calves in New Zealand and Murrah buffalo *(Bubalus bubalis)* calves in Brazil. In both reports, skin lesions developed in newborn calves in sites prone to trauma or were induced by trauma. Hoof separation and sloughing were also observed, and in buffalo calves, horns were frequently deformed and partially or completely separated from the underlying corium. Mucous membrane and mucocutaneous involvement was seen in the Angus calves but not in the buffalo calves. The histologic changes seen in the Angus calves were separation of prickle cells and basal cells from each other and sometimes basal cells from the underlying dermis, resulting in *suprabasilar to sub-basilar vesicles* and subsequent shedding of the epithelium. Many basal and prickle cells contained large eosinophilic cytoplasmic bodies. In the Murrah buffalo calves, the characteristic histologic alteration was *suprabasilar clefting* with detachment of the stratum spinosum from the underlying basal layer. Ultrastructural changes in affected areas of skin in the buffalo calves consisted of loss of desmosomal adhesion between the basal and prickle cell layers. The basal lamina, hemidesmosomes, anchoring fibrils, and anchoring filaments appeared normal. In the Angus calves, desmosomes were lacking or fewer than normal, and many keratinocytes contained a mass of tonofilaments arranged in whorls. Hemidesmosomes were normal. Although the clinical presentation of these cases was typical of epidermolysis bullosa, the histologic and ultrastructural features were unlike those of the common forms of epidermolysis bullosa. However, some variants of epidermolysis bullosa simplex in humans are characterized by cleft formation with acantholysis in the middle or upper epidermis, and in some instances, cells contain round clumps within their cytoplasm produced by aggregation of tonofilaments. In both reports, the condition in the calves was suspected to be inherited as an *autosomal recessive* trait.

Further reading

Olivry T, et al. Deficient plakophilin-1 expression due to a mutation in PKP1 causes ectodermal dysplasia-skin fragility syndrome in Chesapeake Bay retriever dogs. PLoS ONE 2012;7:e32072.

Congenital hypotrichosis

Congenital hypotrichosis has been described in all domestic species, but it occurs most frequently in calves. The hairlessness may be associated with congenital anomalies of other systems, such as brachygnathism, dental defects, and thymic or genital abnormalities. Many affected animals are otherwise completely healthy, but some forms of congenital hypotrichosis are associated with ill-thrift and early death. Deliberate propagation of spontaneous mutations producing hairlessness has resulted in development of *specific hairless breeds*, such as the Chinese Crested dog, Mexican Hairless dog, American Hairless Terrier, Sphinx cat, and Mexican Hairless pig, among others. The haircoat is an important protective barrier for animals, and when it is compromised, as in congenital hypotrichosis, *affected animals are predisposed to sunburn, less tolerant to temperature extremes, and more susceptible to bacterial and fungal infection.*

Hairlessness varies from partial to complete. Partial hypotrichosis is frequently bilaterally symmetrical, and the hair that is present is frequently abnormal. It is usually sparse, short and fine, or coarse and wiry, brittle, and easily broken or epilated. Histologic changes are variable, likely a reflection of the different mutations responsible for the hypotrichosis. Some affected animals have only follicular disease, whereas others have involvement of other skin appendages, in which case the condition is called *ectodermal dysplasia*.

Genetic hypotrichosis must be differentiated from various causes of nongenetic hypotrichosis. Iodine deficiency can cause goiter and hypotrichosis in piglets, lambs, and calves. Adenohypophyseal hypoplasia in Guernseys and Jerseys, and maternal ingestion of *Veratrum album* by Japanese cattle, has been associated with hairlessness in calves. In addition, alopecia of various degrees has been associated with intrauterine infection with bovine viral diarrhea virus in calves and classical swine fever virus in piglets.

Cattle

Various types of inherited hypotrichosis occur in cattle. Many breeds of cattle are affected, and the mode of inheritance varies with the particular form of hypotrichosis. Histologic features are not well characterized for all forms of hypotrichosis in cattle.

A form of **lethal hypotrichosis** occurs in Holstein-Friesian and Japanese native cattle. Calves are born almost hairless and have only small amounts of hair on the muzzle, eyelids, ears, tail, and pasterns. The condition is inherited as a simple autosomal recessive trait, and homozygous calves die within hours after birth. Histologically the skin contains normal numbers of follicles, but they are shallow, rudimentary in appearance, and do not form hairs. Sebaceous glands and arrector pili muscles appear normal; sweat glands undergo cystic degeneration.

A condition called **semihairlessness** has been reported in polled and horned Hereford calves. Calves have a thin coat of short fine, curly hair at birth and progressively develop a patchy sparse coat of coarse wiry hair that is thicker and longer on legs than elsewhere. The skin is wrinkled and scaly. Animals may not grow well and may have a wild temperament. The condition is a simple autosomal recessive trait. The histologic changes described are dysplastic hair follicles that do not produce hairs. Similar histologic features have been described in **viable hypotrichosis** reported in various breeds of cattle, including Guernseys, Jerseys, Holsteins, Ayrshires, and Herefords. Calves are born with various degrees of hairlessness. The condition appears to be inherited as a simple autosomal recessive trait in all breeds affected.

Hypotrichosis and anodontia (hypotrichosis anodontia defect, HAD) has been described in male mixed Maine-Anjou-Normandy cross calves and suspected to be a sex-linked recessive trait. Calves are born hairless and toothless and develop a fine, downy haircoat and partial dentition after several months. Affected calves also have a thick protruding tongue, defective horns, and hypoplastic testicles, and they usually do not survive beyond 6 months of age. Histologic changes include small, inactive hair follicles, deformed dermal papillae lacking a vascular network, and degenerative sweat glands. A HAD syndrome, with hypotrichosis, almost complete lack of teeth, and complete absence of eccrine nasolabial glands, has been observed in a family of German Holsteins; similar anomalies in humans are known as X-linked anhidrotic ectodermal dysplasia (ED1). This Holstein phenotype was inherited as a monogenic X-linked recessive trait and was caused by a deletion in the bovine *ED1* gene.

Hypotrichosis and incisor anodontia (hypotrichosis incisor defect, HID) has been described in Holstein-Friesian cross calves, and inheritance is suspected to be an X-linked incompletely dominant gene. Affected calves have variable areas of thin coat of fine short silky hairs usually involving the face, neck, ears, back, and inner thighs. Eyelashes, vibrissae, and tail brush are usually normal. Calves may become normal with age. Histologically, there are numerous small hairs, but large medullated hairs are absent, and only telogen follicles are evident in severely affected HID calves.

Inherited epidermal dysplasia, also called **baldy calf syndrome,** is a lethal disease of Holstein-Friesian calves that is likely inherited as a single autosomal recessive trait. The disease causes loss of condition and skin, horn, and hoof lesions that can be confused with inherited zinc deficiency. Calves appear normal at birth, but at 1-2 months of age, they begin to lose condition despite normal appetite, and develop generalized hair loss and patchy areas of scaly, wrinkled, thickened skin over the neck, shoulders, flanks, and on pressure points. Hooves are elongated, narrow, and pointed and frequently have horizontal rippling. Horns fail to develop, and ear tips are curled backward. Calves have fine slender limbs and drool. They become emaciated and usually die at 6-8 months of age. Histologic examination indicates variable atrophy of adnexa, remnants of hair follicles and sebaceous glands incorporated into the basal layer, and scattered atrophic remnants of epitrichial sweat glands.

Congenital hypotrichosis of Hereford cattle is thought to be due to a simple autosomal dominant gene. Alopecia is variable and nonprogressive. Calves have thin, pliable skin, extremely curly facial hair, and may have sparse pelage of thin soft curly, easily broken and epilated hairs, or they may be completely hairless. Some calves also have impaired hoof development. The condition is characterized histologically by hypoplastic or degenerate hair follicles with vacuolation and necrosis of Huxley's and Henle's layers and abnormally large trichohyaline granules in Huxley's layer. Most follicles contain fragmented hair shafts. Arrector pili muscles are reduced in number and frequently not associated with hair shafts. Ultrastructural examination indicates that the giant trichohyaline granules lack normal microfilament and macrofilament structures.

A condition consisting of **congenital anemia, dyskeratosis, and progressive alopecia** has also been described in polled Hereford calves in Canada and the United States. Affected calves are often small at birth and have a prominent forehead. They have a hyperkeratotic muzzle with a dirty faced appearance, and their hair is wiry and kinked or tightly curled and easily epilated. Alopecia is evident initially on the bridge of the nose and ears, and it becomes generalized but is most severe on the head, lateral neck, shoulders, and back. The skin of the face and neck is wrinkled, and hairless skin is hyperkeratotic. Affected calves also have nonregenerative anemia and fail to grow despite a normal appetite. Histologic abnormalities in the skin consist of orthokeratotic hyperkeratosis and hypergranulosis extending into the infundibular portion of hair follicles and prominent dyskeratosis (apoptosis) of individual epidermal and follicular keratinocytes. Hair follicles are normal in number, but many follicles are in telogen phase. There is degeneration of the internal root sheath and atrophy of sebaceous glands. The bone marrow is hyperplastic and characterized by ineffective erythropoiesis with maturation arrest in the late rubricyte stage.

The **"rat-tail syndrome"** is a form of hereditary congenital hypotrichosis that occurs in a small percentage of calves produced by crossing some Continental cattle breeds, for instance, Simmental with black Angus or Holsteins. The calves have short, curly, malformed, sometimes sparse hair, and a lack of normal tail switch development.

Dogs

X-linked hypohidrotic ectodermal dysplasia (XHED) has been documented in dogs and the inheritance confirmed by breeding studies. XHED is a spontaneous model for the disease in humans. Affected dogs have a triad of lesions: patterned hairlessness, an absence of atrichial sweat glands, and dental abnormalities (conically shaped teeth, anodontia). The lack of hair is apparent on the dorsal head, ventrum, and dorsal tail base (eFig. 6-7). The dogs also have absence of serous and mucinous glands in the trachea, esophagus, and bronchi. The puppies have decreased weight gain and fail to thrive. Hairless areas may have decreased adnexal density as well as partial to complete adnexal loss. XHED is caused by a mutation in ectodysplasin 1 *(ED1)*, which encodes for transmembrane proteins, with a short intracellular domain, a transmembrane domain, and a tumor necrosis factor–ligand motif. This protein is thought to control some epithelial-mesenchymal cell interactions that regulate development of the ectoderm. In humans, this disease causes significant mortality and mortality resulting from hyperthermia and respiratory infections.

A semidominant form of ectodermal dysplasia has been documented in congenitally hairless breeds (Mexican and Peruvian hairless dogs, Chinese Crested dog). The disorder has been associated with a member of the forkhead box transcription factor family *(FOXI3)*, which is specifically expressed in developing hair and teeth.

Cats

An autosomal recessive form of congenital hypotrichosis has been described in *Siamese and Birman kittens*. The Birman kittens were born virtually hairless and had short fragile wrinkled whiskers or lacked whiskers altogether. Both males and females were affected. Although initially healthy, all affected kittens in one report died by 13 weeks of age from various infections. Postmortem examination of some of the affected Birman kittens revealed *thymic aplasia and lymphoid depletion* of paracortical regions of lymph nodes, spleen, and Peyer's patches, suggesting an immunologic deficiency. Histologic examination of skin indicated reduced numbers of primary hair follicles, which were hypoplastic and devoid of hairs. Sebaceous glands were normal, but sweat glands were hypoplastic and in decreased number, and arrector pili muscles were rare.

Hereditary hypotrichosis is recognized in **piglets,** and there may be both dominant and recessive forms. The dominant form is thought to be lethal in homozygotes; it is characterized histologically by a decreased number of hair follicles, and most appear atrophic. Congenital hypotrichosis is thought to be a simple autosomal recessive trait in polled Dorset **sheep.** Alopecia is most pronounced on the face and legs. Histologic abnormalities consist of hypoplastic hair follicles containing keratosebaceous material but no hairs. Congenital hypotrichosis has been described in a Percheron, but is rare in **horses.** Congenital hypotrichosis is rare in **goats.**

Further reading

Drögemüller C, et al. A mutation in hairless dogs implicates FOXI3 in ectodermal development. Sci 2008;321:1462.

Mauldin EA, et al. Neonatal treatment with recombinant ectodysplasin prevents respiratory disease in dogs with X-linked ectodermal dysplasia. Am J Med Gen 2009;149A:2045-2049.

Hypotrichosis associated with pigmentary alterations

Generalized or regional alopecia attributed to follicular dysplasias that include histologic evidence of pigment abnormalities have been frequently described in dogs and less frequently in other species. They have arbitrarily been divided into 2 categories.

The first of these 2 categories is **color dilution alopecia,** described in color-dilute animals of breeds such as the Doberman Pinscher, Irish Setter, Dachshund, Chow Chow, Poodle, Whippet, Italian Greyhound, Boston Terrier, Chihuahua, Saluki, Yorkshire Terrier, and mongrels, in which the onset of alopecia can be tardive, generally ranging from 4 months to 3 years. Puppies are born with normal hair, but develop slowly progressive alopecia (Fig. 6-25). Pedigree analysis in color-dilute Dachshunds suggests this disorder may be inherited as an autosomal recessive trait. The histologic lesions include *misshapen, fragmented anagen hair follicles with pigment clumping in follicular epithelium, hair bulb matrix cells, hair shafts, infundibular keratin, and epidermis* (Fig. 6-26). *Melanin-containing macrophages are frequently present in the dermis around hair bulbs.* There can be some hair follicle atrophy in chronic cases; however, this is a secondary change. A condition similar to color-dilution alopecia in dogs has been described in cattle as **cross-related congenital hypotrichosis**. This has been reported in crosses involving Simmental, Gelbvieh, and Charolais cattle, most common in the Simmental-Angus and Simmental-Holstein crosses. The condition appears in calves that have color-dilute (gray or chocolate) coats. The affected hair is short, curly, and sparsely haired, leaving the white-haired areas of the coat unaffected. The histologic lesions are virtually identical to canine color-dilution alopecia. **Coat-color–linked hair follicle dysplasia** has also been described in buckskin Holstein cows (color-dilute tan-and-white Holsteins). These animals have short and clinically abnormal hair in the tan areas of the coat.

The second traditional category is **black hair follicular dysplasia** (see Fig. 6-25), seen in bicolor or tricolor black and white dogs, such as Bassett Hounds, Beagles, Bearded Collies, and mongrels, and in Holstein cattle, in which the alopecia affects only the black-haired areas of the coat, and in which onset is generally in the first few weeks or months of life. Black hair follicular dysplasia is thought to be an autosomal inherited disorder in mongrel puppies, and is thought to have a genetic component in some purebred animals such as Bearded Collies. *The histologic lesions in black hair follicular dysplasias are virtually identical to those of color-dilution alopecia.* A difference in the appearance of the melanin clumps in whole mounts of hair shafts has been suggested. In Greater Musterlanders, the hair shaft defect appears to be associated with inadequate and disorganized melanosome transfer to keratinocytes, with resultant melanin clumping (see Fig. 6-26).

There are *other follicular dysplasias associated with pigment abnormalities* that do not fall easily into these 2 categories, but have similar histologic changes. These include follicular dysplasia in the **Portuguese Water dog** that occurs in the black or red color phase of this breed. These are not color-dilute dogs, and the onset can be tardive, generally between 3 months and 5 years. **Black-and-red Doberman Pinschers** that are not phenotypically color dilute are also reported to have a follicular dysplasia that is generally confined to the caudal dorsum and that has an adult onset. An adult-onset alopecic disorder has been identified in Chesapeake Bay Retrievers (eFig. 6-8). Clinically, the hair loss occurs on the axillae, ventral thorax, flanks, ventrum, dorsum, rump, and/or the caudal part of the thighs in both male and female dogs. Histologically, the lesions resemble cyclic flank alopecia (follicular atrophy with hyperkeratosis), with occasional melanin clumping and hypereosinophilic hair shafts. Follicular dysplasia has been described in **Weimaraners,** in which affected young adults had progressive alopecia of the trunk with recurrent folliculitis/furunculosis.

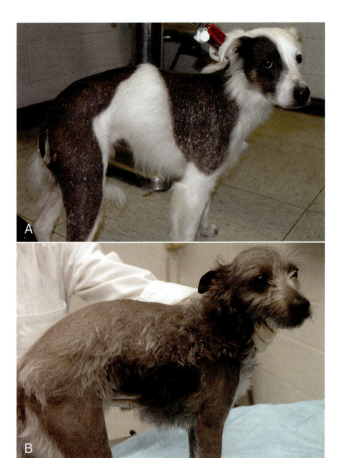

Figure 6-25 Pigmentary follicular dysplasia in 2 dogs. **A.** In **black hair follicular dysplasia,** the hair loss is confined to pigmented areas. **B.** The dog with **color-dilution alopecia** has generalized thinning hair loss.

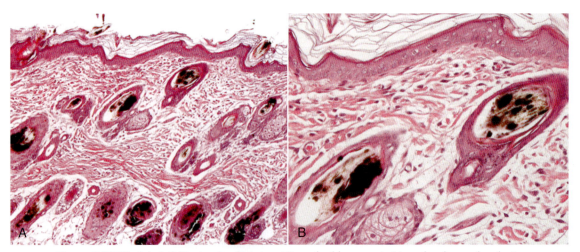

Figure 6-26 Black hair follicular dysplasia in a 12-week-old puppy. **A.** Note the clumped melanin in the hair bulbs as well as an accumulation of coarse free melanin within hair follicle infundibula and within misshapen hair shafts. **B.** Higher magnification.

In **cattle,** follicular dysplasia has been reported in black Angus and black Angus-Brahman crosses; the histologic changes are similar to those in dogs. These cattle are all black animals that are not phenotypically color dilute; however, there is adult onset of alopecia that is more commonly associated with color-dilution alopecia. In view of the dysplasias in Portuguese Water dogs, black-and-red Doberman Pinschers, and black Angus and their crosses that occur in animals not phenotypically color dilute but that can have adult onset, *it is quite possible that separation of follicular dysplasias with pigmentary alteration into color-dilution alopecia and black hair follicular dysplasia is artificial.* It is likely that these histologically similar follicular dysplasias are subtypes of a single process; however, until the mechanism underlying follicular dysplasia is characterized, the classification is somewhat arbitrary.

Further reading

Cerundolo R, et al. Adult onset hair loss in Chesapeake Bay retrievers. A clinical and histological and study. Vet Dermatol 2005;16:39-46.

Ishida Y, et al. A homozygous single-base deletion in MLPH causes the dilute coat color phenotype in the domestic cat. Genomics 2006;88:698-705.

Kim JH, et al. Color-dilution alopecia in dogs. J Vet Sci 2005;6:259-261.

Laffort-Dassot C, et al. Follicular dysplasia in five Weimaraners. Vet Dermatol 2002;13:253-260.

von Bomhard W, et al. Black hair follicular dysplasia in Large Munsterlander dogs: clinical, histological and ultrastructural features. Vet Dermatol 2006;17:182-188.

Welle M, et al. MLPH genotype—melanin phenotype correlation in dilute dogs. J Hered 2009;100:75-79.

Hypertrichosis

Congenital hypertrichosis, a condition characterized by an *excessive amount of hair,* is rare. In some instances, the abnormality involves a change in the character of the hair rather than an absolute increase in amount. Excessively long hair is inherited as an autosomal dominant trait in **Friesian cattle** in Europe. The condition results in discomfort during hot weather and decreased productivity. High environmental temperature during gestation has been associated with an unusual hairy appearance of newborn **lambs.** The lambs are small, and most do not survive to weaning; the histologic appearance of this abnormality has not been described. *Border disease* is a congenital pestiviral infection of sheep in which lambs are born weak and small, have an abnormal haircoat, and exhibit tonic-clonic spasms *(hairy shaker disease).* Instead of the normal short, fine, closely crimped birthcoat, affected lambs have a long, straight, coarse coat. The coat abnormality is due to aberrant differentiation of hair follicles that develops only when infection occurs prior to 80 days of gestation. The histologic changes include enlargement of primary hair follicles with an increased degree of medullation and a decreased number and retarded development of secondary follicles.

Canine dermatomyositis

Dermatomyositis is an idiopathic inflammatory condition of skin, muscle, and occasionally blood vessels of humans and dogs. A familial pattern of occurrence has been found in Collies, Shetland Sheepdogs (Shelties), and their crosses. It has also been described in Beauceron Shepherd, Belgian Tervuren, and Portuguese Water dogs. A similar disease, referred to as dermatomyositis-like disease, has been described in a number of other breeds. Dermatomyositis in Collies is an autosomal dominant trait with variable expressivity; and it appears to be widespread in Collies in the United States. The disease in Collies has been proposed as a model for a nonfatal form of childhood dermatomyositis, although familial cases are uncommon in humans. The condition in Shelties has been linked to chromosome 35. Dermatomyositis has been identified in Shelties in the United Kingdom. The disease has not been characterized as well in this breed; but it appears that myositis is a less prominent feature of the disease in Shelties.

Dermatomyositis must be distinguished from *vaccine-associated ischemic dermatopathy.* The latter condition tends to occur in small-breed dogs 1-5 months following rabies immunization. At sites distant from the vaccine injection site, the histologic features are indistinguishable from dermatomyositis. The histologic changes of *ischemic dermatopathy* can be categorized into 5 subtypes: (1) canine familiar dermatomyositis, (2) juvenile-onset ischemic dermatopathy (similar to canine familial dermatomyositis except for the breed predispositions), (3) focal postrabies vaccination reaction, (4) generalized vaccine-induced ischemic dermatopathy, and (5) adult-onset non–vaccine-induced generalized ischemic dermatopathy.

The cause and pathogenesis of dermatomyositis are unknown. The primary target is thought to be capillary endothelium, although histologic evidence of vessel wall inflammation is often absent. Skin and muscle lesions are a consequence of ischemia leading to atrophy of hair follicles and muscle. Variation in expression of dermatomyositis in dogs suggests that factors other than simple autosomal dominant inheritance are involved in the etiopathogenesis of the disease. Immunologic mechanisms are thought to be involved in this disease in humans, and both cell-mediated and humoral immunity have been implicated in the pathogenesis. In Collies with dermatomyositis, serum levels of circulating immune complexes were found to be increased above normal before clinical disease was evident; the onset and severity of dermatitis and myositis correlated with the serum levels of circulating immune complexes and IgG, and circulating immune complex levels decreased to normal as disease resolved. These findings suggest that the immune complexes initiated inflammation rather than resulted from it. IgG was identified as the immunoglobulin component of the immune complexes, but the identity of the antigen component was not determined. Dermatomyositis has been associated with viral, bacterial, and *Toxoplasma* infections, but infectious agents are generally not isolated from tissues of affected people. Crystalline structures, suggestive of picornaviruses, have been seen in endothelial cells of muscle from severely affected Collies. Cases in humans have also occurred following immunization, therapy with various drugs, during pregnancy, and in association with neoplasia.

Skin lesions usually develop in juvenile dogs at 7 weeks to 6 months of age. *Earliest lesions consist of small pustules, vesicles, papules, and nodules that evolve into erythematous, crusty, ulcerated, alopecic areas with hypopigmentation or hyperpigmentation* (Fig. 6-27). Lesions are most common on the pinnae, bridge of the nose, lips, periocular skin, over bony prominences of the distal extremities, sternum, and tip of the tail. Mucous membranes and mucocutaneous junctions may be transiently involved early in the course of disease. Pawpad ulceration is rare. The disease exhibits a *waxing and waning course* over weeks to months, with a variable outcome. In mildly to

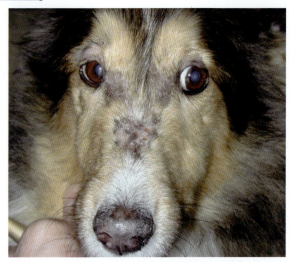

Figure 6-27 Familial canine dermatomyositis in a Shetland Sheepdog. The muzzle and periocular areas have scarring alopecia with small ulcers and hyperpigmentation and hypopigmentation.

moderately affected dogs, lesions may resolve spontaneously in 6-12 months, whereas in severely affected dogs, lesions may regress but do not usually resolve completely, and disease may be lifelong and extensive. Lesions heal with no residual scarring in mildly affected dogs; permanent alopecic, hypopigmented, or hyperpigmented disfiguring scars develop, especially on the face, in severely affected dogs. Lesions may be exacerbated by estrus, parturition, or exposure to sunlight. Although cases of adult-onset dermatomyositis have been reported, it is likely that at least some of these dogs had mild transient lesions that were overlooked when they were pups and subsequently developed more obvious disease as adults.

Myositis usually develops several weeks after dermatitis and is proportional in severity to the dermatitis. It is usually first recognized as a bilaterally symmetrical decrease in temporal muscle mass. However, because of the dolichocephalic shape of the Collie head, mild temporal or masseter muscle atrophy may be missed. *Myositis principally involves muscles of mastication and extremities below the elbow and stifle*, but it is more generalized in more severely affected dogs. Over time, active myositis is succeeded by muscle atrophy and fibrosis. Generalized symmetrical muscle atrophy, weakness, and exercise intolerance may develop in moderately and severely affected dogs. Megaesophagus may develop in some dogs.

Various additional abnormalities may accompany skin and muscle lesions in more severely affected dogs. Peripheral lymph nodes are enlarged because of reactive hyperplasia. Conjunctivitis may develop in dogs with severe periocular skin lesions or because of facial palsy and inability to blink. More severely affected dogs are small and unthrifty compared with normal or mildly affected dogs. Fever and joint swelling are noted in some dogs. Secondary bacterial pyoderma, septicemia, or megaesophagus with secondary aspiration pneumonia may develop in more severely affected dogs. Demodicosis may also be present and complicate diagnosis. Severe secondary amyloidosis with resultant renal failure has been described in one affected Collie.

Affected dogs have variable and usually nonspecific clinicopathologic abnormalities. Moderately and severely affected dogs commonly have inflammatory leukogram changes that include neutrophilia, with or without a left shift, and monocytosis. Nonregenerative anemia typical of chronic inflammation may develop in severely affected dogs. Serum creatine kinase levels in Collies with dermatomyositis were normal or only slightly increased; however, most serum muscle enzyme determinations were done in later stages of disease when active myositis may have been waning. Mild to moderate elevations in serum creatine kinase concentrations were present in several young Shelties with the disease. Occasionally, dogs have positive Coombs tests, and rarely, rheumatoid factor (RF) tests are positive.

The histologic changes in the skin are variable and may be quite subtle or nonspecific. Early lesions consist of scattered individual vacuolated or shrunken, brightly eosinophilic necrotic keratinocytes in the epidermis and infundibular portion of hair follicles. Hydropic degeneration of basal keratinocytes is often present and leads to *dermal-epidermal clefts* that develop into vesicles that contain proteinaceous fluid, erythrocytes, and inflammatory cells. Diagnostically useful artifactual dermal-epidermal separation may be induced at the margins of the section by the shearing action of the punch biopsy. Ulceration and crusting result from lesions with extensive dermal-epidermal separation. Intraepidermal pustules are uncommon. Hyperkeratosis and acanthosis are variable. In the absence of ulceration, dermal inflammation tends to be mild and consists of mixed cells either surrounding superficial dermal vessels, hair follicles, and glands or distributed in an interface pattern, or in some cases, diffusely distributed. The infiltrate includes mononuclear cells primarily, fewer neutrophils, and occasional eosinophils and mast cells. *The most consistently present histologic abnormalities are follicular atrophy and perifollicular inflammation that may be accompanied by perifollicular fibrosis* (Fig. 6-28A-C). Variable dermal fibrosis is usually evident in biopsies from dogs >6 months of age. *Muscle lesions* include multifocal interstitial and perivascular infiltrations with mixed cells; myofiber degeneration, regeneration, and atrophy; and fibrosis. *Vasculitis* is an infrequent and subtle finding in the skin, muscle, and occasionally in other tissues.

Further reading

Bresciani F, et al. Dermatomyositis-like disease in a Rottweiler. Vet Dermatol 2014;25:229-232.

Morris DO. Ischemic dermatopathies. Vet Clin North Am Small Anim Pract 2013;43:99-111.

Wahl JM, et al. Analysis of gene transcript profiling and immunobiology in Shetland sheepdogs with dermatomyositis. Vet Dermatol 2008;19:52-58.

Hereditary connective tissue disorders

The connective tissue components of the skin include collagen (primarily types I and III), elastic fibers, and ground substance composed of glycoproteins and proteoglycans. A defect in any one of these skin molecules can result in structural and functional abnormalities of the entire tissue. Inherited connective tissue disorders of skin may consist of abnormalities involving only one of these components, or there may be concurrent alterations in several components. Hereditary collagen dysplasia, the most commonly recognized connective tissue disease, is a complex group of disorders of collagen that results in decreased tensile strength of the skin and may also affect other connective tissues. Alterations in elastic fibers and ground substance may accompany some forms of collagen dysplasia, but there

Congenital and Hereditary Diseases of Skin

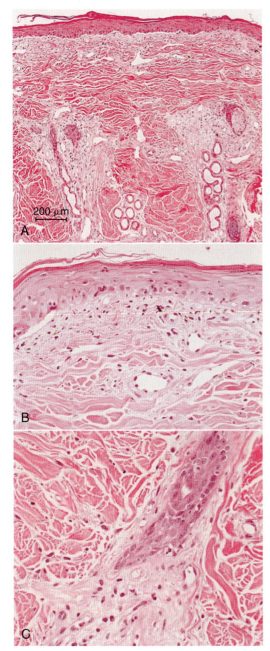

Figure 6-28 Familial canine dermatomyositis. A. Low magnification showing follicular atrophy, and orphaned adnexal structures. **B.** Higher magnification showing cell-poor hydropic, interface dermatitis with dermoepidermal clefting. **C.** An atrophic (faded) follicle is surrounded by prominent connective tissue and scattered lymphocytes and plasma cells.

are also diseases in which an abnormality of the elastic fibers or ground substance appears to be primary. *Diagnosis of many of these conditions requires ultrastructural examination and biochemical analysis to confirm the presence of structural abnormalities and to identify the molecular defect.*

Hereditary collagen dysplasia

Collagen dysplasia (dermatosparaxis, Ehlers-Danlos syndrome, cutaneous asthenia, cutis hyperelastica) has been reported in humans, cattle, sheep, horses, dogs, cats, mink, and rabbits. Collagen is the major structural protein in skin and other connective tissues, and abnormalities in its structure result in skin that is fragile, easily torn, and frequently hyperextensible and loose. In humans, Ehlers-Danlos syndrome (EDS) is divided into at least 10 types based on clinical, biochemical, and molecular genetic studies. The natural history of clinical disease and mode of inheritance vary among the different types of EDS. Joint laxity, vascular abnormalities, bowel or uterine rupture, bone abnormalities, ocular abnormalities, and periodontal disease occur in addition to the fragile skin in the various forms of human EDS. Inheritance may be autosomal dominant, autosomal recessive, or X-linked recessive. In animals, clinical disease has been restricted almost exclusively to skin abnormalities and has been characterized in only a few breeding colonies or herd outbreaks. Most instances of collagen dysplasia occur in single animals, and the molecular defect and mode of inheritance are usually not determined.

Individuals with inherited collagen dysplasia typically have a *history of frequent skin lacerations following routine handling,* such as shearing or manual restraint; normal activities, such as scratching or playing with littermates; or minor trauma. The skin wounds commonly *develop into wide gaping wounds with minimal hemorrhage.* Healing usually proceeds normally but results in *characteristic thin, pale wrinkled scars* resembling tissue paper. Extracutaneous signs, such as joint laxity and ocular abnormalities, have been reported in animals only rarely. The skin is usually soft and velvety, hyperextensible, and may hang in loose folds. In some affected animals, the skin laxity becomes progressively more pronounced with age. Severity of clinical signs is variable, even among animals with the same biochemical abnormality. This variability in clinical severity is most pronounced in sheep. One form of the disease described in sheep exhibits such severe manifestations that all lambs die or require euthanasia within the first day or 2 of life. A second milder form of collagen dysplasia is usually not recognized until later in life when sheep are handled for shearing. *In general, the disease tends to be most severe in sheep, less severe in cattle, followed by dogs and cats, and least severe in horses.*

Diagnosis of collagen dysplasia is based on typical clinical signs and demonstration of morphologic or biochemical abnormalities of the dermal collagen. In some cases, abnormalities are evident at the light microscopic level, but frequently none are found or the differences are subtle and difficult to determine except by comparison to a breed- and age-matched control. The dermis may be normal, thinner than normal, or thicker than normal because of an increased amount of ground substance. Collagen fibers may be widely separated, finer and paler than normal, and haphazardly arranged. Rarely, increased numbers of elastic fibers are seen with elastic stains. Fibroblasts are in increased numbers in the dermis of some affected animals. Abnormal collagen fibers may stain unevenly with collagen stains such as Masson trichrome. Instead of the uniform blue staining of normal collagen, the abnormal collagen may have a red core. This staining feature is not unique to collagen dysplasia, however, as uneven collagen staining also occurs with degenerative disorders of collagen.

In most cases, ultrastructural examination is required to confirm the collagen abnormality. A variety of alterations of collagen fibrils have been found. In longitudinal sections, collagen fibrils may be loosely wound and flat or helical. In cross-section, they may have several irregular thin projecting arms that give them a "hieroglyphic" appearance. This appearance is typical of dermatosparaxis of sheep and cattle and has also been described in a Himalayan cat and a dog. In other forms of the disease, the collagen fibrils are shaped normally but vary markedly in diameter from the normal range. They may all be uniformly larger or smaller, or there is a mixed population of fibrils that extend beyond the range of normal minimum and maximum diameter sizes. The fibrils frequently are loose and disorganized rather than being arranged in uniform, compact bundles.

The ultrastructural abnormalities are not specific, and biochemical analysis is necessary to determine the particular molecular defect. Collagen synthesis is a multistep process that includes extensive post-translational processing involving multiple intracellular and extracellular enzymes. Abnormalities in several of these enzymes as well as structural mutations involving the collagen chains have been identified in the various forms of collagen dysplasia in humans and animals. For unknown reasons, the same biochemical defect may produce different clinical abnormalities in different individuals and in different species.

Cattle

Collagen dysplasia in cattle is usually referred to as **dermatosparaxis,** which means "torn skin." The condition is *caused by a mutation in the gene for procollagen I N-proteinase* (also called procollagen aminopeptidase), the enzyme that excises the amino-propeptide of type I and type II procollagens. Each of the 3 polypeptide chains making up a collagen molecule have short extensions at the amino and carboxy termini. These additional propeptides make the molecules soluble, to aid in their transport out of the cell. Subsequent extracellular conversion of the procollagen to collagen requires 2 enzymes to cleave the amino- and carboxy-terminal extensions. Following cleavage of the procollagen peptides, the collagen molecules spontaneously assemble into collagen fibrils. *The defect in processing of type I procollagen to collagen results in abnormal precursor molecules with peptide extensions that inhibit formation of uniform fibers and fibers capable of producing normal cross-links.* They assemble instead into abnormal ribbon-shaped collagen fibrils lacking normal tensile strength. Dermatosparaxis in cattle is recessively inherited as is the biochemically analogous condition in humans, Ehlers-Danlos syndrome type VII C, although clinical signs are not identical.

Most affected calves have thick, wet skin that tears easily and sometimes hangs in loose folds. Associated joint laxity and soft bones have been reported rarely. Light microscopic changes consist of a thicker than normal dermis composed of sparse bundles of fine pale collagen distributed in abundant Alcian blue–positive ground substance (proteoglycans). Individual collagen fibers are smaller in diameter than in normal skin, and their arrangement appears disorganized. There may be an increase in dermal elastin and number of fibroblasts. Ultrastructural examination reveals the collagen to be arranged in loose, twisted flat, or helical ribbons rather than being organized in compact parallel arrays. In cross-section, these fibrils have irregular projecting arms that confer a "hieroglyphic" appearance.

Sheep

At least 2 forms of collagen dysplasia, called *dermatosparaxis*, have been described in sheep, that is, a *severe form in lambs* noted shortly after birth, and a *milder form* not apparent until sheep are handled as adults. The severe form has been described in Norwegian Dala sheep, Border-Leicester-Southdown crossbred sheep in Australia, and white Dorper sheep in South Africa. The condition is inherited as a simple autosomal recessive trait. Only in the Dala breed has the biochemical defect been identified, and it consists of a deficiency in procollagen aminopeptidase activity, as in bovine dermatosparaxis. In Border-Leicester-Southdown crossbred lambs, the biochemical abnormality was not determined, but it did not appear to be a procollagen peptidase deficiency because there was no increase in dermal procollagen detected. Affected lambs develop skin lacerations during birth or shortly thereafter. The skin is soft and edematous. Lambs frequently die within a few days as a consequence of wound infection and septicemia. Gross examination of the skin indicates that the dermis is moist and thicker than normal, with a jelly-like consistency. In some instances, increased friability of internal organs and joint capsules was observed. The histologic and ultrastructural abnormalities are similar to those in cattle with dermatosparaxis.

The *less severe form of dermatosparaxis* has been found in Merino sheep in Australia when adult sheep were handled for shearing. No skin hyperelasticity or joint hypermobility are associated with the skin fragility. The skin lacerations predispose affected individuals to infections and fly strike. This form is also caused by a deficiency of procollagen aminopeptidase activity. Light microscopic examination reveals a loose, more open appearance to the dermis and a significant increase in the number of dermal fibroblasts in comparison to normal skin. Most collagen fiber bundles are smaller and more lightly stained than those in normal skin. The collagen in some areas is arranged in prominent layers. Transmission electron microscopic examination shows a combination of distorted, hieroglyphic-type fibrils mixed with normal collagen fibrils.

Horses

Hereditary equine regional dermal asthenia (HERDA) is an autosomal recessive skin disorder in Quarter Horses, and predominantly those that originated from elite cutting horse bloodlines. The affected horses have hyperextensible and loose fragile skin that results in poor wound healing and disfiguring scars (eFig. 6-9). Collagen dysplasia has also been reported in a Thoroughbred gelding and an Arabian-cross filly. HERDA is not usually recognized until the animal is 6-12 months of age and develops frequent skin wounds and scarring on the legs, shoulders, and saddle area. Although histology is not diagnostic, the deep dermis contains a horizontal clearing in which the collagen fibers are thinner and shorter than normal.

Dogs

Collagen dysplasia has been described in many purebred and mixed-breed dogs. Affected dogs typically have *soft, easily torn, hyperextensible skin* (Fig. 6-29). In some cases, the skin hangs in loose pendulous folds, a feature that frequently becomes more prominent with age. Thin, white scars are typically the sequelae to skin wounds. Ocular abnormalities and joint laxity, associated problems commonly seen in humans with Ehlers-Danlos syndrome, have been reported infrequently in dogs, and bone abnormalities are rare. Several breeding studies have shown collagen dysplasia to be inherited in a simple autosomal dominant manner with complete penetrance. *The biochemical abnormality has not been identified in any cases of collagen dysplasia in dogs;* but the skin of Springer Spaniels with

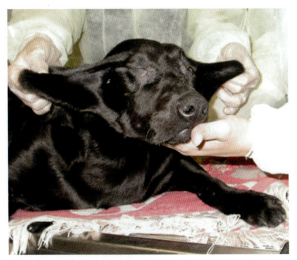

Figure 6-29 **Collagen dysplasia** in a dog. Note hyperextensible facial skin.

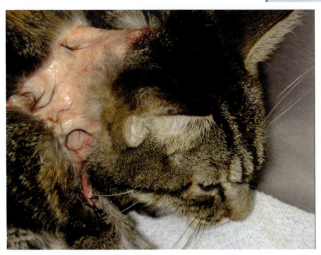

Figure 6-30 **Feline acquired fragile skin syndrome.** Note tearing of fragile skin with minimal hemorrhage.

collagen dysplasia has been found to have more uncross-linked α-chains than collagen from normal dogs.

Histologic changes may be subtle and consist of dermal thinning evident only in comparison to a section from a normal control. In other cases, a decreased amount of dermal collagen, collagen disorganization, variation in collagen staining, increased number of elastic fibers, or increased amount of extracellular matrix may be seen. The abnormal collagen fibers may stain red with trichrome stain. Ultrastructural abnormalities of the collagen consist of variation in the fibril diameter, shape abnormalities, fibril disorganization, and loose fibril packing. A mixture of normal and abnormal collagen fibers may be present.

Cats

Collagen dysplasia in cats is usually referred to as **cutaneous asthenia**, although in early reports it was called dermatosparaxis. The condition has been reported in a number of breeds; *in the majority of the cases, neither the biochemical defect nor the mode of inheritance has been identified.* In a single Himalayan cat with collagen dysplasia, the abnormality was determined to be a defect of the amino-terminal procollagen peptidase, as in dermatosparaxis of cattle and sheep. This cat could not be bred, however, and the mode of inheritance was not determined. A breeding study based on an affected male domestic shorthaired cat indicated that the condition is inherited as an autosomal dominant trait, and heterozygous individuals synthesize both normal and abnormal collagen molecules.

Cats with cutaneous asthenia have thin, soft, velvety skin that tears easily but with minimal hemorrhage. Lacerations heal to form typical white, tissue paper–like scars. In some cats, loose folds of skin develop as the cats age. No joint laxity has been described in cats with cutaneous asthenia. Histologic examination of the skin yields variable results. No dermal changes are evident in some cases, whereas in others, the dermis is thinner and collagen fibers are finer and separated by an increased amount of ground substance when compared to skin from an unaffected cat. Normal collagen fibers stain uniformly blue with Masson trichrome stain; abnormal fibers exhibit segmental red staining areas that are birefringent under polarized light. Ultrastructural examination indicates that normal and abnormal collagen fibers may be present in varying proportions. Abnormal fibers are characterized by disorganized, tangled, nonparallel packing of fibrils. Abnormal "hieroglyphic" fibrils were a feature of the affected Himalayan cat.

Skin fragility in cats has also been reported as an acquired condition associated with a number of conditions, including spontaneous and iatrogenic hyperglucocorticism, diabetes mellitus, cholangiohepatitis, hepatic lipidosis, cholangiocarcinoma, multicentric follicular lymphoma, feline infectious peritonitis, disseminated histoplasmosis, and administration of various drugs, including megestrol acetate and other progestational compounds (Fig. 6-30). Histologically, cats with acquired skin fragility have profound atrophy of dermal collagen fibers. Collagen fibers are thin and disorganized. Hair follicles are in kenogen and markedly atrophied. The epidermis and other adnexa are also often atrophic. There may be orthokeratotic hyperkeratosis. The exact pathomechanism is unknown; however, it is thought to be related to an effect of glucocorticoids on collagen production. In addition, many of the associated conditions have moderate to severe liver involvement, which suggests that hepatic dysfunction may play a role in pathogenesis.

Abnormalities of elastic fibers

An *excess of elastic fibers* was reported in several piglets of a litter of Large White X Essex pigs with multiple circular to oval shallow depressed skin lesions. The skin was abnormally elastic in these areas and seemed to be bound less tightly to the underlying subcutis. The increase in thick elastic fibers was present only in those areas in which the skin was hyperextensible, and the condition was termed **cutis hyperelastica.**

Congenital abnormalities of ground substance

Proteoglycan deficiency. An abnormality of dermal proteoglycan is a rarely documented cause of fragile skin in humans and animals. Proteoglycan is composed of a core protein and glycosaminoglycan (mucopolysaccharide) side chains, and it is the major component of the extracellular ground substance of the dermis. A 4-month-old female Holstein calf with skin fragility, soft and hyperextensible skin, and poor wound healing typical of dermatosparaxis was found to have normal collagen fibers. However, levels of dermatan sulfate proteoglycan in the dermal connective tissue were undetectable. The defect was identified as a mutation involving the gene that codes for the proteoglycan core protein. The mode of inheritance was not determined.

Cutaneous mucinosis (hyaluronosis) of Chinese Shar-Pei dogs. Cutaneous mucinosis is a dermal connective tissue disorder in which *excessive mucin accumulates in the skin*. The mucin deposition is caused by excessive production by dermal fibroblasts of the polysaccharide hyaluronan (HA). The hyaluronan accumulation is related to a higher expression of hyaluronan synthase 2 (HAS2) mRNA and HAS2 protein by dermal fibroblasts. *The inherited form of cutaneous mucinosis is considered normal in the Chinese Shar-Pei dog* and is responsible for the thick, wrinkled skin characteristic of the breed. The degree of mucin accumulation is variable. In some dogs, large lakes of mucin form nodules or cysts that may rupture and drip clear, stringy fluid.

Histologically, cutaneous mucinosis is characterized by a variable increase in dermal thickness because of excessive mucin separating collagen fibers. Mucin has great water-binding capacity and thus contains a substantial amount of water, the majority of which is removed during processing of the tissue. What remains in H&E-stained tissue sections is fine basophilic granular to fibrillar material separating dermal collagen fibers. Special stains can be used to better visualize the mucin; these include Alcian blue at pH 2.5, which stains mucin blue-green, and mucicarmine, which stains it red. Mucin stains metachromatically with toluidine blue and methylene blue. PAS stain, which stains neutral mucopolysaccharides, does not stain dermal mucin.

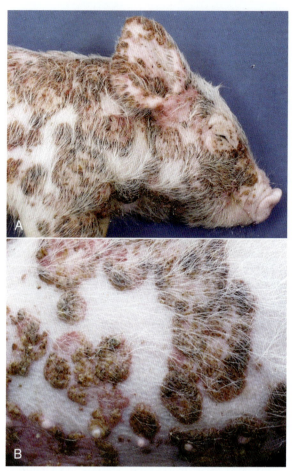

Figure 6-31 Dermatosis vegetans in a pig. **A.** Coalesced, red-black crusted plaques on the head, neck, and abdominal wall. **B.** Close-up view. (Courtesy P. Habecker.)

Further reading

Bellini MH, et al. Increased elastic microfibrils and thickening of fibroblastic nuclear lamina in canine cutaneous asthenia. Vet Dermatol 2009;20:139-143.

Crosaz O, et al. Skin fragility syndrome in a cat with multicentric follicular lymphoma. J Feline Med Surg 2013;15:953-958.

Docampo MJ, et al. Increased HAS2-driven hyaluronic acid synthesis in shar-pei dogs with hereditary cutaneous hyaluronosis (mucinosis). Vet Dermatol 2011;22:535-545.

Dermatosis vegetans

Dermatosis vegetans is an inherited disorder of young pigs characterized by vegetating skin lesions, hoof malformation, and giant cell pneumonia. The condition is a simple autosomal recessive trait of Landrace swine in Europe, Canada, and Australia. Clinically affected pigs grow slowly, become emaciated and unkempt, and usually die by 2 months of life. The economic impact of the disease may be considerable because virtually all homozygotes die before reaching slaughter age.

Skin lesions may be present at birth, but more commonly, they develop during the first 3 weeks of life, and in rare cases may not arise until 2-3 months of age. *Lesions begin as erythematous papules*, 0.5-2.0 cm in diameter, usually on the ventral abdomen and medial aspect of the thighs. They may extend up the sides and back but do not affect the head. The papules enlarge peripherally over the course of 2 or 3 days, and the center becomes depressed. At this stage, the lesions are clinically similar to pityriasis rosea. The papules enlarge to form *plaques* with a depressed center filled with characteristic gray to brown-black granular brittle material. Over a period of weeks, the lesions continue to expand and develop a dry, horny, papilloma-like appearance. They become dark brown to black, and *each crusty plaque is surrounded by a hyperemic raised border that sharply demarcates the lesions from the surrounding normal skin* (Fig. 6.31). As lesions spread peripherally, they coalesce to form extensive areas covered by black crusts. Affected piglets frequently die when lesions reach the typical papilloma-like appearance at 5-8 weeks of age. Skin lesions then begin to resolve if the pig survives.

When they occur, *foot and hoof lesions* are always present at birth. Usually more than one limb is affected, and typically all digits, including accessory digits, of an affected foot are involved. The coronary region is markedly swollen and erythematous; and the skin is covered by yellow-brown greasy material. The wall of the hoof is thickened by ridges and furrows parallel to the coronary band. Affected hooves become progressively enlarged, wider, and flatter than normal if pigs survive to 5 or 6 months. Coronary band changes, however, diminish as the pig ages.

At birth, affected piglets seem otherwise normal, but over a period of weeks they gradually decline in growth and vitality. Except for animals that die perinatally, virtually all affected pigs show signs of *respiratory dysfunction*, typically increased respiratory rate and labored respiration, several days prior to death. Affected pigs commonly develop anemia and secondary infections, especially bacterial pneumonia.

The *histologic lesions* in the skin vary according to the stage of the condition. Initially, there is superficial dermal edema, vascular congestion, and dermal infiltration with numerous granulocytes, many of which are eosinophils. Fully developed lesions are characterized by *marked orthokeratotic and parakeratotic hyperkeratosis, prominent irregular epidermal hyperplasia, intercellular edema, and intraepidermal pustules and microabscesses containing eosinophils and neutrophils*. The characteristic histologic lesion in the lung is *giant cells in alveoli*. The giant cells have been identified immunohistochemically as originating from monocytes/macrophages. In chronic cases, epithelialization and interstitial fibrosis are evident, and multinucleated giant cells may be infrequent when the condition has lasted several months. Typical pulmonary changes may be obscured by secondary infections.

Dermoid cyst

The *dermoid cyst (dermoid sinus)* is an uncommon developmental anomaly that has been reported in dogs, cats, horses, and cattle. *It is caused by defective epidermal closure along embryonic fissures, which isolates an island of ectoderm in the dermis or subcutis.* The majority of dermoid cysts occur on the dorsal midline because of incomplete separation of skin and neural tube during embryonic development; but they also occur in other locations. Although present at birth, dermoid cysts are usually asymptomatic and may not be noticed until they become distended or infected in an older animal. The cyst usually *contains hair, keratin, and sebum*, and this material may produce progressive enlargement of the structure so that it becomes clinically apparent. Cysts frequently become infected, producing clinical signs such as purulent discharge, local swelling from cellulitis, or neurologic signs secondary to meningomyelitis.

In **dogs**, dermoid cysts have been reported most commonly in the *Rhodesian Ridgeback*, a breed in which the lesion appears to be inherited as a simple recessive trait; development of a cyst is predisposed to by a dominant mutation in 3 fibroblast growth factor genes. Dermoid cysts have also been reported in several other breeds. It is unknown whether the lesion is an inherited condition in other breeds of dogs. Dermoid cysts have been associated with multiple vertebral and spinal malformations and hindlimb neurologic deficits in several dogs. The rare condition of *nasal dermoid sinus cyst* results in a discharging sinus over the external nares in dogs; the cyst may extend into the cranial vault and cause cerebral abscessation or recurrent meningitis. In one survey, all cases in *horses* were in Thoroughbreds. Several cases reported in *cattle* all involved Angus. Dermoid cysts are rare in *cats*, and both cases reported were in domestic shorthairs.

Dermoid cysts may be single or multiple. They consist of a well-circumscribed circular or tubular structure in the skin or subcutis and frequently connect to the skin surface by a small pore. A tuft of hair may protrude through this pore, and it may be surrounded by a whorl of hair. The cyst may end blindly in the subcutis; it may connect to the dorsal spinous process of vertebrae directly or by a fibrous cord; or rarely, it extends down to be continuous with the dura mater of the spinal cord. *Microscopically*, the dermoid cyst is a circular or tubular structure lined by a wall of well-differentiated, keratinizing squamous epithelium with associated small but well-developed hair follicles, sebaceous glands, and occasional epitrichial sweat glands. The hair shafts project into the cyst cavity that also contains keratin and variable amounts of sebum. Bacterial infection results in neutrophilic infiltration into the cyst. Pyogranulomatous dermatitis or cellulitis ensues when the cyst ruptures because of infection, trauma, or obstruction of the pore.

Further reading

Fleming JM, et al. Cervical dermoid sinus in a cat: case presentation and review of the literature. J Feline Med Surg 2011;13:992-996.

Hillyer LL, et al. Epidermal (infundibular) and dermoid cysts in the dorsal midline of a three-year-old thoroughbred-cross gelding. Vet Dermatol 2003;14:205-209.

Perazzi A, et al. Multiple dermoid sinuses of type Vb and IIIb on the head of a Saint Bernard dog. Acta Vet Scand 2013;55:62.

Salmon Hillbertz NH, et al. Duplication of FGF3, FGF4, FGF19 and ORAOV1 causes hair ridge and predisposition to dermoid sinus in Ridgeback dogs. Nat Genet 2007;39:1318-1320.

DISORDERS OF EPIDERMAL DIFFERENTIATION

The epidermis is stratified squamous epithelium that forms a continuously regenerating protective sheet around the body. Basal keratinocytes proliferate, then differentiate, become keratinized, and are then sloughed. *In normal canine skin, the migration from the basal to the cornified layer requires 22 days*, as measured by tritiated thymidine incorporation studies. This turnover rate is shortened in some skin diseases; for example, in seborrheic skin disease, it is 7-8 days. The basement membrane separates the epidermis from the dermis, and basal keratinocytes rest on this membrane anchored by hemidesmosomes and focal adhesions. Basal keratinocytes are the only cells in the epidermis that can undergo mitosis, and once mitosis occurs, the basal cell proceeds to undergo terminal differentiation. These postmitotic cells enter the stratum spinosum, develop intercellular attachments, desmosomes and adherens junctions, and change the keratin composition of the cytoplasmic keratin filaments. In the basal layer, keratins K5 and K14 are expressed, whereas in the suprabasal cells, K1 and K10 are expressed. The intercellular and cell substrate adhesions are complex. *Hemidesmosomes* and *desmosomes* are stable junctions that associate with cytoplasmic keratin filaments, whereas *focal adhesions* and *adherens junctions* connect to actin filaments and are transitory adhesions. *Integrins* are receptors that mediate cell-substrate adhesion, whereas *cadherins* mediate cell-cell adhesion. As the cells are pushed outward, they move into the stratum granulosum and start to make proteins that make up *keratohyaline granules*. As the cells move into the stratum corneum (SC), the cytoplasmic organelles are lost, and they become metabolically inactive. These flattened inactive keratinocytes are compacted into a keratin layer that eventually exfoliates. In this way, *the epidermis is continuously regenerating and degenerating by proliferation, differentiation, and keratinization*.

While the cells are moving outward, keratin polypeptides form and polymerize into *keratin intermediate filaments* that are epithelial specific and the major component of the cytoskeleton of epithelial cells. The keratin intermediate filaments aggregate into *tonofilaments* that connect with desmosomes, and therefore indirectly with adjacent cells. The molecular structure of keratin is very important, and genetic mutation(s) can affect keratin filament formation. There are at least 30 keratins in epithelium; K9-20 are acidic (type I), and K1-8 are basic (type II). Two different keratins (one acidic and one basic) pair to form *heterodimers*, for example K1 and K10 in suprabasal cells, and K5 and K14 in basal cells. Hyperproliferative epidermis in skin diseases expresses keratins K6 and K16, not seen in normal skin.

When the cells reach the stratum granulosum, they start to synthesize proteins, stored in keratohyaline granules, necessary to form the mechanically strong *macrokeratins* in the SC. One of these, profilaggrin, dephosphorylates to form *filaggrin*, the major molecule responsible for the glue-like aggregation of intermediate filaments. *Loricrin* is also stored in keratohyaline granules, and this polypeptide contributes to the cell envelope, an insoluble intracytoplasmic barrier. *Other proteins* involved in cell envelope formation include involucrin, cystatin A, cystine-rich envelope protein (CREP), trichohyaline, small proline-rich proteins (SPRRs), sciellin, and filaggrin. These serve as substrates for the 3 *transglutaminases* that polymerize and crosslink these proteins in the formation of the cell envelope. The granular layer also contains small lipid-rich granules—*submembranous lamellar bodies* (Odland bodies, membrane-coating granules)—that contain lipids necessary to form a permeability barrier between cells when they are secreted into the intercellular space. Keratinocytes forming the SC are dead and can be sloughed when desmosomes are broken down. Hydrolytic enzymes, such as cathepsin B–like, carboxypeptidase, and acid phosphatase, are thought to be responsible for this desmosomal degradation and subsequent keratinocyte desquamation.

In various epidermal diseases, this orderly epidermal turnover is altered. For instance, increased proliferation and/or decreased dyshesion of epithelial cells will lead to thickening of the epidermis. Nutritional factors such as amino acids, vitamins A or B, zinc, fatty acids, and copper influence proper differentiation and maintenance of the epidermis. Altered expression of different molecules and keratin mutations, and aberrations in the Notch signaling pathway, are the focus of much research.

Further reading

Hegde S, Raghavan S. A skin-depth analysis of integrins: role of the integrin network in health and disease. Cell Commun Adhes 2013;20:155-169.

Johnson JL, et al. Desmosomes: regulators of cellular signaling and adhesion in epidermal health and disease. Cold Spring Harb Perspect Med 2014;4:a015297.

Nowell C, Radtke F. Cutaneous Notch signaling in health and disease. Cold Spring Harb Perspect Med 2013;3:a017772.

Seborrhea

The term "seborrhea" dates back in the veterinary dermatology literature for more than 5 decades. Seborrheic skin disease is reported most commonly in the dog, but also occurs in horses, cats, goats, sheep, cattle, rodents, and primates. Seborrhea literally means "flow of sebum," and it has been loosely correlated with abnormal sebaceous gland function. *Seborrhea is a clinical, not histologic, term used to describe excessive scaling.* Scaling (i.e., seborrhea) is a common reaction of the skin to normalize a damaged skin barrier and can occur with almost any insult. Historically, seborrhea was subdivided into those cases with dry scale **(seborrhea sicca)** or oily/greasy scale **(seborrhea oleosa)**. The term "seborrheic dermatitis" was used to describe scaling accompanied by inflammation. In older literature, the diagnosis of "seborrhea" was based on gross skin lesions, and in general, histopathology and skin surface cytologic assessments were not included in the dermatologic workup.

Seborrhea has been divided into primary and secondary causes. The term "primary seborrhea" has been reserved for cases in which all known causes of scaling have been ruled out (e.g., ectoparasitism, metabolic diseases and endocrinopathies, allergic disease, etc.). In the 1980s, this designation was potentially useful for treatment purposes, but it antedated the discovery of numerous hyperkeratotic conditions, with sebaceous adenitis and ichthyosis being prime examples. Furthermore, the newer scientific literature has shed light onto the role of *Malassezia* and staphylococcal infections as promoters of inflammation and epidermal proliferation.

Primary idiopathic seborrheic skin disease is reported in many breeds and has been suggested to have an inherited basis; however, the breed predilections and clinical lesions overlap those of allergic skin disease. Cocker Spaniels and Springer Spaniels with purported idiopathic seborrhea have greasy, inflamed skin with hyperkeratotic plaques, comedones, and follicular casts. *Inflammatory ceruminous otitis externa* is also a constant finding. In Cocker Spaniels, cell proliferation kinetics indicate that seborrheic individuals have increased epithelial cell proliferation of the epidermis, hair follicle infundibulum, and sebaceous gland. In addition, recombinant grafting studies have shown that the hyperproliferative epidermis from seborrheic Cocker Spaniels remains hyperproliferative. These studies, although showing proliferative response, do not rule out a primary cornification disorder. Other breeds with primary, greasy seborrhea include the Basset Hound, West Highland White Terrier, German Shepherd, Dachshund, and Chinese Shar-Pei. Breeds having a dry form of primary seborrhea include the Irish Setter, Doberman Pinscher, Dachshund, and West Highland White Terrier. Primary seborrhea in German Shepherds, West Highland White Terriers, and Labrador Retrievers is often very inflammatory, lichenified, and pruritic. Seborrheic skin disease is typically more pronounced on the face, pinnae, trunk, pressure points, intertriginous areas, mucocutaneous areas, and paws. In Labrador Retrievers, the distribution is often strikingly ventral ("water-line disease"), which in the current literature would be interpreted as atopic dermatitis. Thus many cases that would have been called "primary seborrhea" in the past would now be classified as pyoderma, *Malassezia* dermatitis, sebaceous adenitis, allergic dermatitis, and so on. Therefore *"seborrhea" should be used only as a clinical descriptive, not an etiologic, term.*

The histologic features of primary seborrhea are not specific because they overlap those of allergic skin disease, *Malassezia* dermatitis, zinc-responsive dermatosis, and superficial pyoderma. Primary seborrhea has been characterized by superficial perivascular dermatitis with epidermal hyperplasia that is mild to moderate and papillated in configuration. The stratum corneum is expanded by *alternating vertical tiers of orthokeratotic and parakeratotic hyperkeratosis*. The parakeratosis is typically found overlying the shoulders of follicular ostia (*parakeratotic* "caps"). The underlying dermal papillae are often edematous, leading to spongiosis and *leukocytic exocytosis of the overlying epidermis ("papillary squirting")* (Fig. 6-32). Spongiform or Munro's microabscesses may be seen in conjunction with the parakeratosis. The perivascular

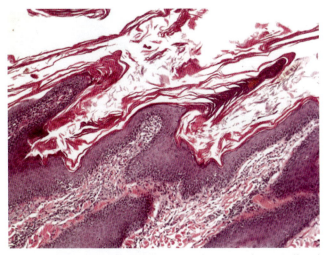

Figure 6-32 Primary idiopathic seborrhea in a dog. Papillated epidermal hyperplasia with vertical tiers of orthokeratotic and parakeratotic hyperkeratosis. (Courtesy R. Dunstan.)

inflammatory cells include variable combinations of lymphocytes, neutrophils, plasma cells, macrophages, and mast cells. The cases may have subordinate patterns of suppurative folliculitis, furunculosis, perifolliculitis, and intraepidermal pustular dermatitis.

Primary seborrhea oleosa, presumably of autosomal recessive inheritance, has been described in Persian **cats**. Severely affected kittens show lesions at 3-4 days of age, and develop progressively severe, generalized greasiness, matting of the haircoat, rancid odor, comedones, alopecia, and ceruminous otitis externa. Pruritus is absent. A milder form of the disease is recognized in 6-8 week-old kittens, with mild to moderate greasiness of the skin and haircoat. Primary seborrhea in the **horse** occurs in both dry and greasy forms, and tends to be restricted to the mane and tail. Pruritus is absent. Generalized primary seborrhea is rare in the horse.

Further reading

Mauldin EA. Canine ichthyosis and related disorders of cornification. Vet Clin North Am Small Anim Pract 2013;43:89-97.

Acne

Acne is seen in large *short-coated breeds of* **dogs,** especially Boxers, Mastiffs, German Shorthaired Pointers, English Bulldogs, Great Danes, and Doberman Pinschers. It usually occurs at 3-12 months of age with no sex predilection and occasionally persists into adult life. The *etiology and pathogenesis are unknown*, and aside from an association with puberty, there is little similarity to human acne. The lesions are thought to develop from external hair follicle trauma (rubbing of face) that results in follicular inflammation and traumatic rupture. The lesions consist of follicular *papules and pustules on the chin and lips that may ulcerate and ooze suppurative exudate.* Histologically, the lesions are characterized by suppurative folliculitis with follicular rupture and pyogranulomatous to suppurative inflammation surrounding free hair shafts. Early lesions may exhibit follicular keratosis, comedones, and variable inflammation.

Acne is common in **cats** and has no sex or breed predilections. It typically arises in mature cats with a median age of onset at 4 years, and persists for life. Acne is usually asymptomatic, although some cats may develop secondary bacterial folliculitis and furunculosis. The clinical lesions appear on the chin and lips and include comedones, papules, alopecia, crusts, and erythema. Histologically, the lesions consist of dilated sebaceous gland ducts, follicular keratosis with plugging and dilation, chronic periadnexal lymphoplasmacytic inflammation, and less commonly, luminal folliculitis and furunculosis.

Schnauzer comedo syndrome

This condition occurs only in the Miniature Schnauzer breed. Either sex may be affected, and the condition usually develops early in life. The disorder may represent *a form of inherited follicular dysplasia or a follicular disorder of cornification*. It has some resemblance to a developmental follicular dysplasia in humans termed nevus comedonicus. Clinically, the condition is characterized by multiple asymptomatic comedones over the *dorsal midline*. Occasionally, secondary bacterial folliculitis and furunculosis may develop. Histologically, there is marked orthokeratotic hyperkeratosis, dilation and plugging of hair follicles (comedones), and variable inflammation.

Tail gland hyperplasia

Many **dogs** have an oval area of skin on the dorsal surface of the tail above the fifth to seventh coccygeal vertebrae referred to as the *tail (supracaudal, preen) gland*. Microscopically, large, densely packed *perianal ("hepatoid") and sebaceous glands* characterize this area. In some dogs, especially adult to aged males, this area enlarges. The enlargement is usually firm to slightly spongy, and associated with partial alopecia, scaling, and greasiness. At this stage, the lesion is asymptomatic. Occasionally, the lesions become cystic and/or secondarily infected, or neoplastic.

In most instances, canine tail gland hyperplasia is associated with *hormonal imbalances*, especially elevated levels of blood testosterone. Histologically, the lesions are characterized by *marked hyperplasia of the perianal gland component, with a variable inflammatory response*.

The entire dorsal surface of the tail in **cats** is replete with large, densely packed sebaceous glands, which are proposed to be embryonal hepatoid glands. In some cats, especially sexually active males of the Persian, Siamese, and Rex breeds, this area becomes clinically seborrheic, whereupon a brown to black, greasy keratosebaceous material accumulates on the hairs of the skin surface. Unless secondarily infected, the condition is asymptomatic. The cause of feline tail gland hyperplasia is unknown, and the colloquialism "stud tail" is misleading, as the condition is also seen in intact females and neutered males and females. Histologically, the condition is characterized by *marked hyperplasia of sebaceous glands, with variable orthokeratotic hyperkeratosis and inflammation*.

Further reading

Ruth J. Poor haircoat in a Persian. Feline tail gland hyperplasia (FTGH). Compend Contin Educ Vet 2009;31:208-210.

Canine nasodigital hyperkeratosis

Canine nasodigital hyperkeratosis is an idiopathic disorder of cornification that is characterized by villous proliferation of *keratin on the nasal planum and/or footpads*. This disorder occurs in *aged dogs* and is not associated with inflammation, although the development of fissures may lead to secondary bacterial infections. The clinical presentation is typically diagnostic: thickening of the nose and footpads by fronds of keratin. The footpad lesions typically occur in areas that are not worn (e.g., margins of the footpad). Histologically, the corneal layer is thickened by vertical projections of anucleate (orthokeratotic) keratin.

Digital hyperkeratosis can occur as a congenital and presumed hereditary disorder in the Irish Terrier and Dogue de Bordeaux. The dogs develop severe footpad hyperkeratosis with large fronds of keratin by 5-6 months of age. Fissure formation leads to lameness and secondary bacterial infections. An autosomal mode of inheritance has been shown in the Irish Terrier.

Labrador Retriever nasal parakeratosis

This condition arises in Labradors Retrievers and their crosses at <1 year of age, and is thought to be autosomal recessive. The dogs develop thick, slightly verrucous, brown scale on the nasal planum with variable depigmentation. The disorder has characteristic histologic features: marked parakeratotic hyperkeratosis with serum lake formation with a band of lymphocytes and plasma cells in the superficial dermis. Other histopathologic findings include epidermal hyperplasia, neutrophilic and lymphocytic exocytosis, and pigmentary incontinence. Differentials include canine discoid lupus–like disease, pemphigus erythematosus/foliaceus, and idiopathic (senile) hyperkeratosis.

Keratoses

Keratoses are firm, elevated, circumscribed areas of excessive keratin production. In humans, keratoses are common and of numerous types. *Keratoses are uncommonly reported in domestic animals.* Actinic keratosis is discussed elsewhere.

Equine linear alopecia (linear keratosis) is a characteristic clinical entity. It occurs in many breeds; however, Quarter Horses seem to be predisposed. The age of onset is usually at 1-5 years. The clinical lesions are characterized by one or more *vertically oriented linear areas of alopecia, with variable crusting and scaling.* They are usually unilateral and occur most commonly on the *neck, shoulder, and lateral thorax* (Fig. 6-33A). The lesions are usually asymptomatic, and may be persistent or permanent. The *etiology of the condition is unknown* but may involve an immune-mediated attack on the wall of the hair follicle. The reason for the linearity is unknown. Histologically, the lesion is characterized by *lymphocytic or lymphohistiocytic mural folliculitis,* sometimes with follicular destruction (Fig. 6-33B, C). Multinucleated giant cells and eosinophils are variably present. Sebaceous glands can be secondarily effaced, and there is a variable amount of orthokeratotic or parakeratotic hyperkeratosis, with or without superficial perivascular nonsuppurative inflammation. Linear keratoses with a similar gross and histologic appearance have also been described in *cattle.*

Equine cannon keratosis is a clinically recognizable disease of the horse. It represents a localized form of seborrheic dermatosis, can occur at any age, and has no breed predilection. The colloquial term, "stud crud," is inappropriate as it also occurs in mares. The lesions consist of *vertically oriented, moderately well-demarcated areas of alopecia, scaling, and crusting on the cranial surface of the rear cannon bones.* The lesions are usually bilateral and persist for life. Pruritus and pain are

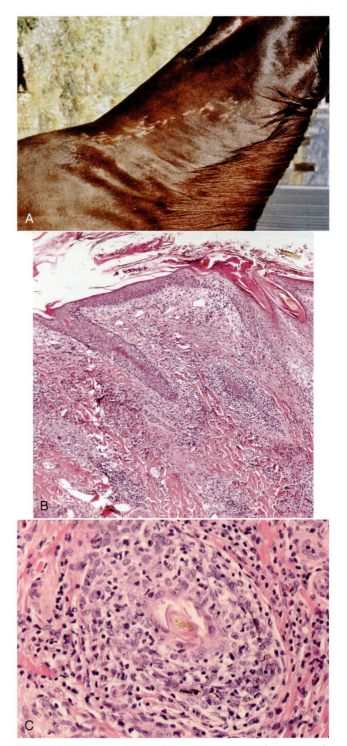

Figure 6-33 Equine linear alopecia. **A.** Linear alopecia, with crusting and scaling, on the neck of a horse. **B.** Low magnification showing a follicular orientation of the inflammatory infiltrate. **C.** Lymphohistiocytic to granulomatous mural folliculitis disrupts hair follicles. (Courtesy C. von Tscharner.)

absent. Histopathologic findings include orthokeratotic and/or parakeratotic hyperkeratosis, irregular to papillated epidermal hyperplasia, and mild superficial perivascular dermatitis featuring lymphocytes and macrophages.

Seborrheic keratoses have been recognized in dogs. The lesions are considered benign epidermal neoplasms and are very common in humans but rarely diagnosed in middle age to older dogs (mean age 9 years). They are of unknown cause, and have nothing to do with the clinical term seborrhea. The lesions may be single or multiple and have no apparent breed, sex, or site predilections. In both man and dog, the clinical lesion is an irregularly raised, variably pigmented plaque with dry to waxy scale, and a sessile or "stuck-on" appearance. Histologically, the lesions are characterized by papillated exophytic and mildly endophytic acanthosis with orthokeratotic hyperkeratosis (eFig. 6-10). This proliferation of monomorphic basaloid keratinocytes undergoes abrupt cornification and surrounds impacted, hyperkeratotic follicular ostia, which may develop into keratin horn-cysts. The lesions can be confused with viral plaques and are distinguished by the lack of hypergranulosis and papillomavirus cytopathic effect. In humans, the sudden appearance or enlargement of multiple lesions can be associated with an internal malignancy. This association has not been made in domestic animals.

Lichenoid keratoses have been reported as single or occasionally multiple wart-like papules or hyperkeratotic plaques that may be hyperpigmented on the *inner surface of the pinna in dogs*. Age, breed, and sex predilections have not been noted. Histologically, irregular to papillated epidermal hyperplasia, moderate to marked orthokeratotic and/or parakeratotic hyperkeratosis, and a lichenoid inflammatory infiltrate predominantly consisting of lymphocytes and plasma cells characterizes lichenoid keratosis.

Lichenoid reaction patterns in dogs, and rarely cats, may correspond to specific diseases (e.g., uveodermatologic syndrome, discoid lupus), but an idiopathic lichenoid reaction (**lichenoid dermatosis**) is occasionally seen in dogs and may represent a poorly characterized form of chronic cutaneous lupus erythematosus. Idiopathic lichenoid dermatosis is characterized by usually asymptomatic, *symmetrical, grouped, flat-topped papules and plaques that are variably distributed, and that develop a scaly to markedly hyperkeratotic surface*. The lesions have been described as *self-limiting*, although resolution may take several years. Histologically, these dermatoses are characterized by lichenoid interface dermatitis composed of plasma cells and lymphocytes, marked orthokeratotic hyperkeratosis and follicular keratosis, and moderate epidermal hyperplasia. Apoptotic keratinocytes can be seen primarily, although not exclusively, in the basal layer, and there is often hydropic degeneration of basal keratinocytes. If focal areas of suppurative epidermitis and/or suppurative luminal folliculitis are present, a lichenoid tissue reaction in response to staphylococcal infection should be suspected. A **lichenoid psoriasiform dermatosis** may occur in dogs on long-standing oral cyclosporine for refractory allergic skin or other conditions.

Cutaneous horns are recognized occasionally in all domestic species. Some are of unknown cause; *others originate from papillomas, basal cell tumors, squamous cell carcinomas, or other keratoses*. In cattle, sheep, and goats, cutaneous horns may arise in lesions of dermatophilosis. In the cat, multiple cutaneous horns on the footpads have been reported in association with feline leukemia virus (FeLV) infection; FeLV was isolated from the horns, and type C viral particles were seen in the lesions with the electron microscope.

Cutaneous horns may be single or multiple, and have no apparent age, breed, sex, or site predilections. The lesions are *firm, well-circumscribed horn-like projections from the skin. They may be small (1-mm diameter × 5-mm length) or quite large (3-cm diameter × 12-cm length)*. Histologically, cutaneous horns are characterized by *extensive, compact, laminated, orthokeratotic, and/or parakeratotic hyperkeratosis*. The base of the horn must be inspected for the possible underlying cause.

Linear epidermal nevi are characterized histologically by *linear hyperkeratosis with epidermal hyperplasia*. They have been reported in several species. These include linear epidermal nevi in Belgian horses, inflammatory linear verrucous epidermal nevus in dogs, and a hereditary disorder of cornification in Rottweiler dogs (see Congenital and hereditary diseases of skin). The term nevus implies a lesion present at birth and composed of mature elements, and therefore, because these linear hyperkeratotic lesions have in common an early age of onset, *they may represent linear epidermal nevi that have tardive onset*. Equine cannon keratosis is grossly and histologically similar to linear epidermal nevi but differs from the linear epidermal nevi of Belgian horses, as it can occur at any age, and is restricted to the skin of the cannon area.

Further reading

Bradley CW, et al. Clinicopathological findings of canine seborrhoeic keratosis with comparison to pigmented viral plaques. Vet Dermatol 2013;24:432-438.

Clifford C. Neoplastic and non-neoplastic tumors. In: Miller WH, et al., editors. Muller & Kirk's Small Animal Dermatology. 7th ed. St Louis: Elsevier; 2013:20. p. 829-831.

Gross TL, et al. Pustular and nodular diseases with adnexal destruction. In: Gross TL, et al., editors. Skin Diseases of the Dog and Cat: Clinical and Histopathological Diagnosis. 2nd ed. Oxford, UK: Blackwell; 2005. p. 435-440.

Jazic E, et al. An evaluation of the clinical, cytological, infectious and histopathological features of feline acne. Vet Dermatol 2006;17:134-140.

Miller WH, et al. Congenital and Hereditary Defects. In: Miller WH, et al., editors. Muller & Kirk's Small Animal Dermatology. 7th ed. St Louis: Elsevier; 2013. p. 581-582.

Miller WH, et al. Keratinization Defects. In: Miller WH, et al., editors. Muller & Kirk's Small Animal Dermatology. 7th ed. St Louis: Elsevier; 2013. p. 639-642.

Miller WH, et al. Miscellaneous Skin Diseases. In: Muller & Kirk's Small Anim Dermatol. 7th ed. St Louis: Elsevier; 2013. p. 700-701.

Peters J, et al. Hereditary nasal parakeratosis in Labrador retrievers: 11 new cases and a retrospective study on the presence of accumulations of serum ("serum lakes") in the epidermis of parakeratotic dermatoses and inflamed nasal plana of dogs. Vet Dermatol 2003;14:197-203.

Werner AH. Psoriasiform-lichenoid-like dermatosis in three dogs treated with microemulsion cyclosporine A. J Am Vet Med Assoc 2003;223:1013-1016.

Sebaceous adenitis

Sebaceous adenitis is an *uncommon skin disease of dogs* that has also been reported in the cat and rabbit. The condition has been reported in more than 50 breeds of dogs and in mongrels; however, there *are breed predilections* for the Standard Poodle, Akita, Samoyed, Vizsla, Lhasa Apso, and Havanese. In Standard Poodles and Akitas, an autosomal recessive trait is proposed. Onset of the disorder is usually in young adult to middle-aged animals. There appears to be a slight sex predilection for males in Standard Poodles, Havanese dogs, and Springer Spaniels.

The clinical lesions vary among the breeds of dogs. Longer-coated animals, as typical of the Standard Poodle, initially develop a thin coat because of loss of the undercoat, and then develop symmetrical multifocal to generalized areas of patchy alopecia and brittle to broken hairs encircled by *yellow to brown follicular casts*. Secondary bacterial infection is common. In short-coated dogs, early lesions consist of patches of scaling and alopecia that tend to appear on the *ears and dorsum*. These progress to annular areas of alopecia and scaling on the trunk and head. Early histopathologic changes are characterized by *granulomatous or pyogranulomatous inflammation targeted on the sebaceous glands and eventually destroying the gland* (Fig. 6-34A). Long-coated dogs tend to have rapid and complete sebaceous gland destruction with little residual inflammation. In short-coated dogs, the lesions are more inflammatory, and sebaceous destruction progresses slowly. Inflammation can occasionally impinge secondarily on the follicular epithelium causing folliculitis. Orthokeratotic and/or parakeratotic hyperkeratosis together with follicular keratosis can be marked. In the chronic stages, both active inflammation and sebaceous glands may be absent, and there may be perifollicular fibrosis (Fig. 6-34B). After the disappearance of the glands, the hair follicles frequently assume a "stretched out" configuration and are keratin filled. Regeneration of sebaceous glands after variable amounts of time has been reported in occasional cases.

The pathogenesis of this disease has not been fully characterized. Several possibilities include (1) destruction of the gland resulting from immune-mediated mechanisms, leading to secondary hyperkeratosis; (2) a primary keratinization defect, resulting in increased amounts of follicular keratin blocking the sebaceous duct and causing inflammation of the gland; or (3) a defect in the structure of the sebaceous duct or gland, resulting in inflammation directed at free sebum. In the predisposed breeds, such as Standard Poodles and Akita, a genetic basis seems probable together with other factors that would explain the variation in onset and progression of the disease.

Further reading

Bardagí M, et al. Histopathological differences between canine idiopathic sebaceous adenitis and canine leishmaniosis with sebaceous adenitis. Vet Dermatol 2010;21:159-165.

Bond R, Brooks H. Transverse sectioning for histological assessment of sebaceous glands in healthy dogs and canine sebaceous adenitis. J Small Anim Pract 2013;54:299-303.

Frazer MM, et al. Sebaceous adenitis in Havanese dogs: a retrospective study of the clinical presentation and incidence. Vet Dermatol 2011;22:267-274.

Hernblad Tevell E, et al. Sebaceous adenitis in Swedish dogs, a retrospective study of 104 cases. Acta Vet Scand 2008;50:11.

Vitamin A–responsive dermatosis

This disorders occurs almost exclusively in adult Cocker Spaniels, but has been reported in a Labrador Retriever and Miniature Schnauzer. True vitamin A deficiency has not been documented. Clinical lesions consist of hyperkeratotic plaques with follicular plugging and follicular casts on the ventral and lateral chest and abdomen. The dogs may have a greasy haircoat with ceruminous otitis. The histologic features are marked follicular orthokeratotic hyperkeratosis, which is more severe than the epidermal surface hyperkeratosis.

Further reading

Gross TL, et al. Diseases with abnormal cornification. In: Gross TL, et al., editors. Skin Diseases of the Dog and Cat: Clinical and Histopathological Diagnosis. 2nd ed. Oxford, UK: Blackwell; 2005. p. 165-167.

Miller WH, et al. Keratinization defects. In: Miller WH, et al., editors. Muller & Kirk's Small Animal Dermatology. 7th ed. St Louis: Elsevier; 2013. p. 630-646.

Lichenoid-psoriasiform dermatosis

This is an uncommon dermatosis that affects young English Springer Spaniels of either sex. Asymptomatic, generally symmetrical, hyperkeratotic, erythematous papules usually begin on the pinnae and groin, coalesce to plaques, and progressively involve large areas of the body, especially the ventral abdomen and prepuce. Secondary bacterial infection is common.

Histopathologic findings include *lichenoid band* of predominantly of plasma cells, with areas of *psoriasiform epidermal hyperplasia*, occasional apoptotic basal keratinocytes, and

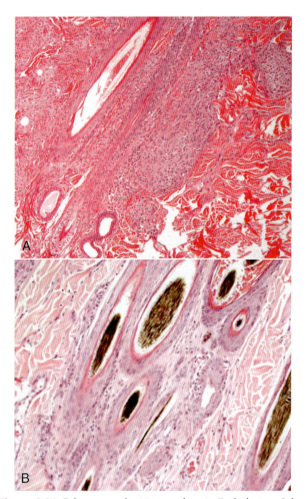

Figure 6-34 Sebaceous adenitis in a dog. **A.** Early lesion. Sebaceous glands targeted by pyogranulomatous inflammation. **B.** Late lesion. Complete sebaceous gland loss with minimal residual inflammation.

intraepidermal microabscesses (containing eosinophils and neutrophils). Although the infiltrate may obscure the dermo-epidermal junction, basal cell apoptosis is not a feature. *The histologic findings are very similar to lichenoid keratosis and must be differentiated clinically by knowledge of distribution of lesions and knowledge of the breed.*

Lichenoid psoriasiform dermatosis can also occur in any dog on long-standing cyclosporine therapy. The lesions respond to decreasing the dose or stopping the drug. An association with staphylococcal infection has been proposed for the condition.

Further reading

Favrot C, et al. Evaluation of papillomaviruses associated with cyclosporine-induced hyperplastic verrucous lesions in dogs. Am J Vet Res 2005;66:1764-1769.

Werner AH. Psoriasiform-lichenoid-like dermatosis in three dogs treated with microemulsified cyclosporine A. J Am Vet Med Assoc 2003;223:1013-1016.

Ear margin dermatosis

This is an idiopathic seborrheic disorder that is localized to the margins of the pinnae. It occurs primarily in the Dachshund, although it can be seen in other breeds with pendulous ears. There is no sex predilection, and the disorder usually begins in young adults. Waxy keratosebaceous accumulations and alopecia follow initial scaling of the ear margins. The disease is symmetrical and asymptomatic. The dermatosis may be complicated by secondary bacterial infection and fissures, at which point ulceration, oozing, crusting, pain, and pruritus may be seen. Histopathologic findings are characterized by *marked orthokeratotic and/or parakeratotic hyperkeratosis with follicular keratosis and variable mild superficial perivascular dermatitis.*

Further reading

Gross TL, et al. Canine ear margin seborrhea. In: Gross TL, et al., editors. Skin Diseases of the Dog and Cat: Clinical and Histopathological Diagnosis. 2nd ed. Oxford, UK: Blackwell; 2005. p. 167-169.

Miller WH, et al. Keratinization defects. In: Miller WH, et al., editors. Muller & Kirk's Small Animal Dermatology. 7th ed. St Louis: Elsevier; 2013. p. 642.

Exfoliative dermatoses (exfoliative erythroderma)

This refers to a cutaneous reaction pattern that can be associated with many diseases. Clinically, it is characterized by scaling and erythema that can be localized or generalized. Most cases of exfoliative dermatosis have been reported *in association with thymoma, epitheliotropic lymphoma, visceral malignant neoplasms, drug reactions, or are idiopathic*. Histopathologic findings can reflect the underlying condition and can include parakeratosis, epidermal acanthosis, variable psoriasiform epidermal hyperplasia, variable lymphocytic exocytosis, and perivascular to lichenoid dermal inflammation.

Exfoliative dermatosis resembling human large plaque parapsoriasis has been reported in a dog and a cat. The human disease, to which these cases were compared, is frequently a precursor to epitheliotropic lymphoma.

Further reading

Rottenberg S, et al. Thymoma-associated exfoliative dermatitis in cats. Vet Pathol 2004;41:429-433.

Turek MM. Cutaneous paraneoplastic syndromes in dogs and cats: a review of the literature. Vet Dermatol 2003;14:279-296.

Hyperplastic dermatosis of West Highland White Terriers

West Highland White Terriers develop a severe skin disorder that was previously referred to as "epidermal dysplasia of West Highland White Terriers." This disorder is now considered an unusually severe manifestation of allergic skin disease and *Malassezia* and/or staphylococcal infection. Most authors do not believe epidermal disorganization or keratinocyte abnormalities characteristic of dysplasia are present. Clinical signs begin at <1 year to middle age, with severely affected dogs tending to have an earlier age of onset.

Erythema and scaling with pruritus develop on the trunk, especially axillary and inguinal regions, and progress to involve the whole body. In chronic cases, the skin becomes lichenified, alopecic, hyperpigmented, and greasy. This combination of gross lesions has led to this condition being referred to as the "armadillo Westie syndrome." Histologic epidermal lesions are characterized by *irregular epidermal hyperplasia with mild to marked predominantly parakeratotic hyperkeratosis.* The base of the hyperplastic epithelium can have a scalloped appearance with crowding of basilar keratinocytes, and there is multifocal spongiosis with lymphocytic exocytosis. Superficial perivascular infiltrates include neutrophils, macrophages, lymphocytes, and plasma cells. Sebaceous glands are often markedly hyperplastic. *There is commonly secondary pyoderma and/or infection with Malassezia.* The absence of *Malassezia* organisms in histologic sections does not necessarily exclude their presence as the organisms may be lost in tissue processing. Cytologic evaluation for yeasts is a more reliable indicator of the presence and numbers of yeasts. *The lesions of hyperplastic dermatosis of West Highland White Terriers are histologically the same as lesions of chronic allergic dermatitis.*

Further reading

Miller WH, et al. Congenital and hereditary diseases. In: Miller WH, et al., editors. Muller & Kirk's Small Animal Dermatology. 7th ed. St Louis: Elsevier; 2013. p. 573-617.

Equine coronary band dystrophy

Equine coronary band dystrophy is a condition of *unknown etiology and pathogenesis*. The condition affects adult horses of any breed, but draft breeds are considered predisposed. Equine coronary band dystrophy is characterized by *marked proliferation and hyperkeratosis of the epidermis of the coronary band, and in some cases, the chestnuts and ergots.* Usually all 4 limbs are affected; however, the lesion may not encompass the entire coronary band. Clinically, the coronary band is thickened, crusty, and scaly. Cracks and fissures may develop and lead to lameness. The chestnuts and ergots are similarly affected and may be ulcerated. Histologically, the epidermis of affected areas is characterized by marked papillary hyperplasia and marked orthokeratotic to parakeratotic hyperkeratosis. There may be various degrees of neutrophilic and eosinophilic exocytosis with microabscesses, edema, and crust formation. Dermal inflammation is minimal unless secondary infection is present. *The diagnosis is made by ruling out other differential diagnoses that include pemphigus foliaceus, the hepatocutaneous syndrome, bacterial or fungal infection, selenium toxicosis, and eosinophilic exfoliative dermatitis.* The condition is chronic and treatment is palliative.

Further reading

Menzies-Gow NJ, et al. Coronary band dystrophy in two horses. Vet Rec 2002;150:665-668.

Ichthyosis

The ichthyoses are rare disorders of cornification that result in severe generalized scaling. These disorders are congenital and heritable (see Congenital and hereditary diseases of skin).

DISORDERS OF PIGMENTATION

Melanin pigments are responsible for the coloration of the hair, skin, and eyes, and also play an important role in photoprotection. Melanin is synthesized by melanocytes, which are dendritic cells originating as melanoblasts in the neural crest. Melanoblasts develop in the neural crest; migrate to peripheral sites such as skin, hair follicles, and dermis; differentiate into melanocytes; and synthesize melanosomes and melanin. Genetic mutations affecting any of these steps can lead to hereditary hypopigmentation. Many such mutations have been characterized in the murine model, but this area has been little studied in domestic animals. Many types of exogenous influences, such as inflammation, ultraviolet (UV) radiation, endocrinopathies, autoimmune diseases, and nutritional status can affect melanocytes in the skin, resulting in acquired hypopigmentation or hyperpigmentation.

Melanin synthesis in melanocytes takes place in *melanosomes*, which are round or elliptical membrane-bound organelles thought to be derived from endoplasmic reticulum and containing enzymes from the Golgi and lysosomal system. Melanosomes are designated type I through IV, according to their stage of maturation. Type I melanosomes contain no melanin and are electron lucent, whereas type IV are mature melanosomes that are electron dense and migrate to the tips of the dendritic processes to be transferred to adjacent epithelial cells. Melanogenesis in round melanosomes produces *eumelanins, the black pigments*, and in elliptical melanosomes produces *pheomelanins, red and yellow pigments*. Pigment types in horses, sheep, goats, and llamas have been analyzed. These melanin pigments arise from the common metabolic pathway of conversion of tyrosine to 3, 4-dihydrophenylalanine (DOPA) and then oxidation to DOPAquinone. *Tyrosinase*, a copper-containing enzyme, is the critical and rate-limiting enzyme in this pathway, catalyzing tyrosine to DOPA. Many gene products are sequentially important to the melanoblast and melanocyte during their development and maturation. Apart from tyrosinase, the molecular role of these gene products has not been completely characterized, but it appears that platelet-derived growth factor (PDGF), and receptors for fibroblast growth factor-2 (FGF-2), endothelin-B, and the Steel factor (cKIT) are crucial.

Cutaneous pigmentary disorders can be divided into disorders of *hyperpigmentation* and *hypopigmentation*.

Further reading

Baxter LL, Pavan WJ. The etiology and molecular genetics of human pigmentation disorders. Wiley Interdiscip Rev Dev Biol 2013;2:379-392.

Mort RL, et al. The melanocyte lineage in development and disease. Development 2015;142:620-632.

Disorders of hyperpigmentation
Acquired hyperpigmentation

Acquired hyperpigmentation of the skin (**melanoderma**) is encountered frequently. It is usually postinflammatory, a result of minor or chronic irritation, and may be accompanied by mild hyperkeratosis. *Both melanosis and hyperkeratosis are common responses to mild injuries by agents as diverse as mites and irradiation.* Hypermelanosis results from an increased rate of melanosome production, an increase in melanosome size, or an increase in the degree of melanization of the melanosome. It is usually associated with an accelerated melanocyte turnover with an increased number of melanosomes, as occurs following trauma and UV exposure. Inflammatory mediators likely play a role in stimulating melanocyte production. Activation of pre-existing immature melanocytes by sunlight, estrogen, and progesterone is thought to occur. Endothelin-1, which is produced and secreted by keratinocytes after UV irradiation, has been shown to accelerate melanogenesis. Basic fibroblast growth factor (bFGF) has been shown to be a mitogen for human melanocytes. Proliferating human epidermal cells in culture produce bFGF, perhaps illustrating the mechanism behind the hyperplastic and hyperpigmented lesions that typify many chronic dermatoses.

Acquired hyperpigmentation may also involve hair (**melanotrichia**). This is usually seen as a result of inflammatory skin disorders, especially those caused by biting insects in the horse and also has been described in white Merino sheep exposed to UV light.

Focal macular melanosis

Lentigo simplex has been reported in *cats and dogs*, and is most common in cats with orange, cream, or tricolored coats. The lesions are flat, or minimally raised, pigmented macules and usually occur on the mucocutaneous junctions of the mouth, eye, and nose, and the footpads. Lesions tend to start at <1 year of age and may increase in size and number with age. *The lesions are of no significance, except that they can be confused clinically with melanoma or pigmented hamartoma.* Histologically, lentigines are characterized by minimal to mild epidermal hyperplasia with formation of elongated rete ridges. There are increased numbers of melanocytes, particularly in the stratum basale, and usually increased melanin in basal keratinocytes. Low numbers of melanophages may be present in the underlying dermis. Papillated epidermal hyperplasia and hyperkeratosis are not present. Generalized lesions have been reported in a silver cat.

Merino **sheep** may acquire pigmented macules, particularly after shearing. *Lesions are concentrated on the back, suggesting a role for sunlight exposure.* Experimental exposure to UV light–induced lesions as early as 10 days postirradiation. Histologically, these lesions are characterized by increased numbers of epidermal melanocytes at the dermoepidermal junction and in the normally nonpigmented outer root sheath epithelium.

Canine acanthosis nigricans

Canine acanthosis nigricans *is an idiopathic dermatitis, characterized by progressive hyperpigmentation, alopecia, and lichenification.* The lesions are roughly bilaterally symmetrical and typically start in the axillae, spreading to involve proximal limbs, ventral abdomen, neck, and inguinal area. Seborrhea, *Malassezia* infection, and bacterial pyoderma are frequent complications. Histologic examination reveals hyperplastic dermatitis with orthokeratotic and parakeratotic hyperkeratosis, acanthosis, and rete ridge formation. All layers of the epidermis are heavily melanized. Spongiosis, neutrophilic exocytosis, and serous crusts may also be present. The dermal inflammatory reaction is mild, pleomorphic in cell type, and superficial perivascular in location.

The primary or idiopathic form of acanthosis nigricans occurs predominantly in Dachshunds. In view of the early age of onset (usually <1 year of age) and the strong predilection for Dachshunds, it is probable that canine idiopathic acanthosis nigricans is a *heritable disorder*. In humans, some forms of acanthosis nigricans are associated with internal malignancies, hyperinsulinemia, insulin resistance, drug administration, endocrine dysfunction, and concurrent autoimmune disease; a similar correlation has not been demonstrated in dogs. The histologic lesions of primary acanthosis nigricans are virtually identical to the common histologic changes associated with chronic pruritic dermatitides (sometimes referred to as pseudoacanthosis nigricans or secondary acanthosis nigricans) resulting from several causes, including chronic pyoderma, atopy, seborrheic dermatitis, and some endocrine disorders. *The diagnosis of primary acanthosis nigricans requires clinical correlation, together with the histologic findings, to support the diagnosis in a young Dachshund with compatible distribution of lesions.*

Further reading

Yager J, Wilcock B. Color Atlas and Text of Surgical Pathology of the Dog and Cat. St Louis: Mosby; 1994. p. 64.

Acromelanism

Acromelanism is seen in Siamese and Himalayan cats, rabbits, and mice. It is a condition in which coat color can be influenced by external temperature (high temperatures producing light hairs, low temperatures producing dark hairs) and factors affecting heat production and loss (alopecia, inflammation). *The coat color changes are usually temporary*, and the hair returns to the normal color with the next hair cycle. *These phenomena are due to a missense nucleotide substitution in tyrosinase, making the enzyme thermally unstable.*

Disorders of hypopigmentation
Leukoderma and leukotrichia

Reduction in pigmentation of the skin is **leukoderma,** and of the hair is **leukotrichia.** Leukoderma and leukotrichia may occur independently. They can result from a decrease in melanin **(hypomelanosis),** a complete absence of melanin **(amelanosis),** or from a loss of existing melanin **(depigmentation).** These events result from either an absence of the pigment-synthesizing melanocytes or from a failure of melanocytes to produce normal amounts of melanin or to transfer it to adjacent keratinocytes.

Hereditary hypopigmentation

Hereditary hypopigmentation can be divided into *melanocytopenic hypomelanosis*, characterized by the absence of melanocytes in affected areas, and *melanopenic hypomelanosis*, in which melanocytes are present but defective. The condition can be localized, focally extensive, or generalized. Melanocytopenic hypomelanosis can be extensive, as is seen in animals with Waardenburg syndromes and in piebaldism. In these cases, there is failure of melanoblasts to migrate from the neural crest into the skin, or failure to survive in the skin. Melanocytopenic hypomelanosis can also be localized, as in vitiligo, in which there is genetically programmed destruction of melanocytes. Melanopenic hypomelanosis is seen in the various forms of albinism.

Melanocytopenic hypomelanosis. Syndromes analogous to the human **Waardenburg syndrome** have been reported in cats, dogs, horses, and rabbits. *Affected animals typically have white coats and blue or heterochromatic irides, and are deaf.* In *cats*, this has been shown to be due to an autosomal dominant mutation with complete penetrance for loss of pigmentation and incomplete penetrance for deafness. In *dogs*, this syndrome has been described in breeds such as the Dalmatian, Bull Terrier, Sealyham Terrier, Collie, and Great Dane. A syndrome analogous to human Waardenburg type 4 (Hirschsprung disease) has been reported in mice with lethal spotting mutation, and in American Paint horses in which white foals from overo mares are born with aganglionic colons. These foals develop colic and die shortly after birth.

Piebaldism is also a form of genetic melanocytopenic hypomelanosis, resulting in *multifocal white patches* in which there is absence of melanocytes due to a congenital failure of melanoblasts to migrate from the neural crest to the skin, or by their inability to survive and proliferate in the skin. Piebaldism has been *seen in many species*, including horses, dogs such as the Dalmatian, cats, cattle, and rodents. The defect has been shown to be a mutation in the gene encoding c-kit tyrosine kinase receptor, or a mutation in the gene for stem cell factor, which is the receptor ligand. The c-kit tyrosine kinase receptor is associated with proliferation and survival of melanoblasts.

Literally meaning "blemish," **vitiligo** is a melanocytopenic hypomelanosis of humans and animals, which is characterized by *gradually expanding pale macules that are often symmetrical or segmental in distribution* (Fig. 6-35). Vitiligo has been described in the dog, cat, horse, cattle, and the Smyth chicken (DAM chicken), which has been used as an animal model of the human disease. The immediate cause of vitiligo is the destruction of melanocytes. It is considered to be a *genetic amelanosis inherited as an autosomal recessive trait in animals*. It is thought to be a polygenic disease necessitating simultaneous mutations in several genes, resulting in melanocyte destruction or increased risk of immune-mediated destruction of melanocytes. Theories regarding the pathogenesis of this disease include autoimmune destruction of melanocytes, a neurogenic theory involving release of a neurochemical from peripheral nerves that inhibits melanogenesis, a self-destruction theory that involves failure of protection of melanocytes against the toxic effects of melanin precursors, or a combination of factors. Circulating antimelanocytic antibodies have been detected in some studies, lending support to an immune-mediated pathogenesis.

Vitiligo in the **dog** has been described in Belgian Tervuren, Doberman Pinscher, Newfoundland, Rottweiler, German

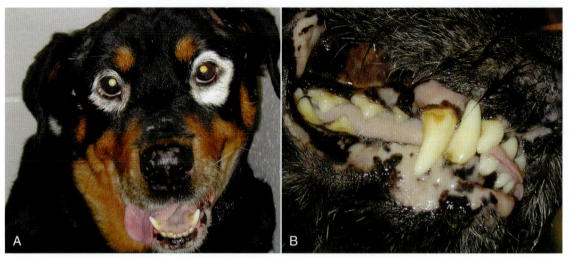

Figure 6-35 Vitiligo in a dog. **A.** Periocular leukotrichia. **A, B.** Coalescing pale macules on the skin of the lips and nasal planum.

Shepherd, Dachshund, German Shorthaired Pointer, and Old English Sheepdogs. Vitiligo in a Dachshund developed concurrently with juvenile-onset diabetes mellitus. The condition is best characterized in Belgian Tervurens (eFig. 6-11). The depigmentation in this breed occurs chiefly on the pigmented skin and mucous membranes of the face and mouth in young adult dogs. Histologic examination of affected skin shows an epithelium devoid of both pigment granules and DOPA-positive cells. Electron microscopy confirms the lack of melanocytes in the lesions; their place is taken by Langerhans or indeterminate dendritic cells. Antimelanocytic antibodies have been demonstrated in affected dogs but not in normal animals. Depigmentation restricted to the nasal planum (also called "Dudley nose," "snow nose") has been also termed "vitiligo." This is commonly seen in the Golden Retriever, Nordic breeds (Siberian Husky, Malamute), and yellow Labrador Retrievers. The etiology is not known.

Vitiligo has also been described in **horses,** and is more common in gray horses. In one form, the *Arabian fading syndrome,* affected animals develop round, depigmented macules on the lips, muzzle, around the eyes, and occasionally the anus, vulva, prepuce, and hooves. The disease can start at any age, but is more common in horses <2 years of age. Circulating antimelanocytic antibodies have been detected in some cases.

In **cattle,** vitiligo-like lesions have been described in Holstein-Friesians, in black Japanese cattle, and in water buffalo.

Siamese cats may develop vitiligo. Antibodies to an 85-kDa surface antigen of melanocytes were demonstrated in 4 cats with vitiligo. No antibodies were detected in 3 normal Siamese cats tested.

Further reading

Eizirik E, et al. Defining and mapping mammalian coat pattern genes: multiple genomic regions implicated in domestic cat stripes and spots. Genetics 2010;184:267-275.

Hauswirth R, et al. Novel variants in the KIT and PAX3 genes in horses with white-spotted coat colour phenotypes. Anim Genet 2013;44:763-765.

Kemp EH, et al. Immunological pathomechanisms in vitiligo. Expert Rev Mol Med 2001;2001:1-22.

Miller WH, et al. Pigmentary abnormalities. In: Miller WH, et al., editors. Muller & Kirk's Small Animal Dermatology. 7th ed. St Louis: Elsevier; 2013. p. 618-629.

Scott DW, Miller WH. Pigmentary abnormalities. In: Scott DW, Miller WH, editors. Equine Dermatology. 2nd ed. St Louis: Elsevier Saunders; 2011. p. 389-397.

Melanopenic hypomelanosis. The various forms of **albinism** are examples of melanopenic hypomelanosis. In albino animals and people, melanocytes are present and normally distributed but are defective in function and fail to synthesize melanin. The extent of the biochemical defect varies so that *albinism covers a spectrum from amelanosis, oculocutaneous albinism (OCA), through graded pigmentary dilution*. Oculocutaneous albinisms and pigment dilutions are inherited as autosomal recessive traits. In albino animals with white hair and skin, and translucent irides, there is a mutation in the tyrosinase gene resulting in no residual enzyme activity. A mutation resulting in residual enzyme activity produces animals born with white hair but producing blond or pigmented hair as juveniles. The skin remains white but can develop pigmented nevi. This form has been reported in a gorilla.

Chediak-Higashi syndrome in humans; Hereford, Brangus, and Japanese Black cattle; Persian cats; mink; blue and silver fox; and various other animal species is an example of *partial albinism and is inherited as an autosomal recessive trait*. Although melanin is produced, there is a mutation of the *beige* gene, which plays a major role in generating cellular organelles. This results in a membrane defect leading to the formation of giant melanosomes that are passed with difficulty to the keratinocytes. The clumping of these giant melanosomes produces the color-dilution effect. Chediak-Higashi syndrome is discussed in Vol. 3, Hematopoietic system.

Cyclic hematopoiesis (also called Grey Collie syndrome, cyclic neutropenia), a lethal hereditary disease of Collie dogs, is caused by an autosomal recessive gene with a pleiotropic effect on coat color dilution. The mutation in the *AP3* gene is responsible for defects in protein sorting processes as well as a silver-gray coat color. The abnormal hair pigmentation results from the diminished formation of melanin from its precursor tyrosine rather than from pigment clumping. The normal Collie coat color is restored in animals receiving bone marrow transplants to correct cyclic hematopoiesis. The hematologic aspects of this disease are considered in Vol. 3, Hematopoietic system.

Coat color dilution and black hair follicular dysplasia has been reported in many species. It occurs in many breeds of dog; in cats, particularly Siamese cats; horses; and cattle. The pale coat coloration is due to clumping of large melanin granules in hair follicles and sometimes in the epidermis. In cats, dilute coat color is thought to be due to an autosomal recessive trait *(Maltese dilution)*. **Color-dilution alopecia,** a tardive onset hypotrichosis associated with color-dilution traits in the dog, is discussed under Congenital and hereditary diseases of the skin.

Further reading

Benson KF, et al. Mutations associated with neutropenia in dogs and humans disrupt intracellular transport of neutrophil elastase. Nat Genet 2003;35:90-96.

Schmutz SM, Berryere TG. Genes affecting coat colour and pattern in domestic dogs: a review. Anim Genet 2007;38:539-549.

Schmutz SM, et al. A form of albinism in cattle is caused by a tyrosinase frameshift mutation. Mamm Genome 2004;15:62-67.

Acquired hypopigmentation

This follows damage to the epidermal melanin unit by various insults, including trauma, inflammation, radiation, contactants, endocrinopathies, infections, and nutritional deficiencies. In general, the severity of the injury determines whether an insult will result in hypopigmentation or hyperpigmentation. *Mild injury results in pigmentary incontinence and epidermal hypopigmentation;* however, a mild injury allows accelerated keratinocyte turnover and a subsequent increase in production of melanosomes. *Severe injury results in the death of melanocytes and no subsequent repigmentation.*

Examples of depigmenting diseases in **horses** include onchocerciasis, *Culicoides* hypersensitivity, ventral midline dermatitis, and coital vesicular exanthema. Depigmenting lesions in horses may result from contact with equipment, such as rubber bit guards or crupper straps or with feed buckets. *Monobenzone* (monobenzyl ether of hydroquinone, 4-[benzyloxy]phenol), a common ingredient in rubber, inhibits melanogenesis.

In **dogs,** hypopigmentation can occur in immune-mediated diseases, such as lupus erythematosus, drug eruptions, bullous pemphigoid, and the various forms of pemphigus. Acquired depigmentation of the lips and/or nose also occurs in dogs as a result of contact with rubber dishes or toys containing monobenzone. Microbial lesions, such as deep pyoderma, may heal with depigmentation. Depigmenting lesions have been noted also in canine leishmaniasis and in dermatophytosis caused by *Microsporum persicolor.* Epitheliotropic lymphoma often is seen with depigmenting, ulcerative lesions of skin and mucocutaneous junctions. Transient depigmentation has been reported in drug eruptions. Subcutaneous injection of corticosteroid or progesterone hormones may lead to focal hypopigmentation in the dog.

Canine uveodermatologic syndrome (Vogt-Koyanagi-Harada-like syndrome) is a depigmenting condition that partially resembles an extremely rare condition in humans. *Arctic*

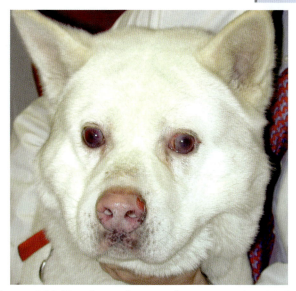

Figure 6-36 Uveodermatologic syndrome in a dog. Marked depigmentation of the nose with focal ulcer, regional corneal edema, and anterior uveitis.

breeds such as the Akita, Siberian Husky, Samoyed, and Malamute are predisposed to the condition; however, it has been reported in many breeds. The cause is unknown, although an immune-mediated attack on melanocytes, as in the human disease, is presumed. A recent study demonstrated a loss of dog leukocyte antigen (DLA) genetic diversity and suggested a role for certain DLA class II gene alleles in the pathogenesis of canine uveodermatologic syndrome. The canine lesions comprise *bilateral panuveitis* (see Vol. 1, Special senses) and *bilateral cutaneous depigmentation,* chiefly of the lips, nose, and periorbital skin (Fig. 6-36). Ocular lesions most often precede onset of cutaneous lesions. The scrotum, vulva, perianal skin, and footpads are less often affected. Leukotrichia is a common finding around the areas of leukoderma. Occasionally, depigmented lesions become ulcerated, erythematous or crusted. Histologically, the lesions are characterized by a lichenoid interface reaction pattern that is composed of histiocytes, often in aggregates, with fewer neutrophils, lymphocytes, and plasma cells (Fig. 6-37). There is pigmentary incontinence, and histiocytes often contain fine melanin granules. The basal cell layer does not have a pronounced vacuolar change and apoptotic basal keratinocytes are uncommon. This and the histiocytic nature of the inflammatory infiltrate are *major features of differentiation from discoid and systemic lupus.*

Further reading

Angles JM, et al. Uveodermatologic (VKH-like) syndrome in American Akita dogs is associated with an increased frequency of DQA1*00201. Tissue Antigens 2005;66:656-665.

Blackwood SE, et al. Uveodermatologic syndrome in a rat terrier. J Am Anim Hosp Assoc 2011;47:56-63.

Sigle KJ, et al. Unilateral uveitis in a dog with uveodermatologic syndrome. J Am Vet Med Assoc 2006;228:543-548.

Leukotrichia

Reticulated leukotrichia, colloquially known as "tiger stripe," is recognized in the Standardbred, Thoroughbred, and Quarter

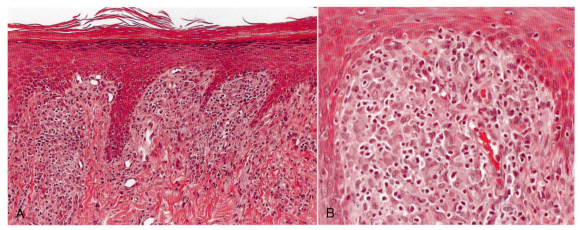

Figure 6-37 **Uveodermatologic syndrome** in a dog. **A.** Low magnification shows a slightly nodular mononuclear cell infiltrate that abuts the dermoepidermal junction. **B.** The infiltrate is composed predominantly of macrophages and fewer lymphocytes.

Horse breeds. The lesions occur predominantly in yearlings and comprise linear crusts arranged in a cross-hatch pattern on the dorsal midline from the withers to the tail. Transient alopecia and regrowth of permanently white hair follow crusting. The underlying skin has normal pigmentation. Well-documented precise descriptions of the expected histologic lesions are lacking. Some reports indicate an interface lichenoid dermatitis may be present, whereas others suggest that a mild superficial dermal mononuclear cell infiltrate and pigmentary incontinence are to be expected. The etiology and pathogenesis are unknown. **Spotted leukotrichia** occurs in the horse as multiple, often somewhat symmetrical, small circular areas of white hair. The spots occur most commonly on the rump and thorax, and Arabians have a predilection. The etiology and pathogenesis are unknown. **Hyperesthetic leukotrichia,** so-called because the lesions are extremely painful, has been reported only in Californian horses. Single or multiple crusted lesions occur on the dorsal midline and heal leaving permanently white hairs.

Leukotrichia, also termed *poliosis,* has been reported in **dogs** in association with Vogt-Koyanagi-Harada–like syndrome, tyrosinase deficiency in Chow Chows, and as an idiopathic, possibly heritable condition in a litter of Labrador Retrievers. In the last example, the condition resolved.

Leukotrichia can be associated with *alopecia areata.* Alopecia areata and alopecia universalis are discussed in more detail under Other immune-mediated dermatoses.

Further reading

Scott DW, Miller WH. Miscellaneous skin diseases. In: Scott DW, Miller WH, editors. Equine Dermatology. 2nd ed. St Louis: Elsevier; 2011. p. 436-467.

Copper deficiency

This pigmentary disorder is seen primarily in *cattle and sheep.* It has also been reported in *moose,* and experimentally in *dogs.* Copper deficiency may be simple or conditioned by other dietary substances, particularly sulfate and molybdenum. Because copper is an essential constituent of tyrosinase, there is *depressed tyrosinase activity,* and deficient animals show depigmentation of hair or wool. Affected cattle with normally

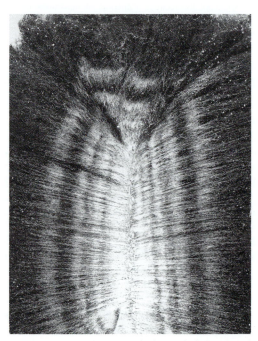

Figure 6-38 **Copper deficiency.** Black-wooled sheep with bands of achromotrichia corresponding to periods of molybdenum administration. (Courtesy W.J. Hartley.)

black coats become rusty brown and develop "spectacle" lesions round the eyes. Black sheep develop intermittent bands of light-colored wool corresponding to periods of restricted availability of copper (Fig. 6-38). The deficiency of copper also affects the physical nature of the wool or hair. In sheep, *the wool has less crimp,* prompting the colloquial name of "string" or "steely" wool. The straightness of the wool is due to inadequate keratinization, probably caused by imperfect oxidation of sulfhydryl groups in prekeratin, a process that involves copper (Fig. 6-39).

PHYSICOCHEMICAL DISEASES OF SKIN

The integument has a large surface area in direct contact with the environment and is hence extremely vulnerable to chemical and physical injuries. *Physical stresses* include

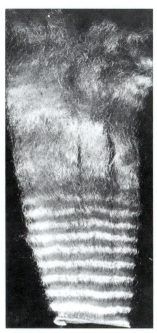

Figure 6-39 Staple from sheep that received 1.0 mg of copper per day, then 10 mg per day. Note stringiness and lack of crimp on deficient regime. (Courtesy W.J. Hartley.)

friction, pressure, vibration, electricity, high and low ambient temperatures, humidity, visible light, and ultraviolet, infrared, and ionizing radiation. Cutaneous reactions to visible light are discussed separately. *Chemical toxins* may exert their effect directly as in irritant contact dermatitis or envenomation or indirectly, as in thallium poisoning.

Physical injury to skin
Mechanical, frictional, and traumatic injury

The haircoat of most domestic animals protects from "blisters" that so commonly develop in human skin subjected to prolonged pressure or frictional contact with a hard surface. The following examples tend to occur in heavy animals with skin exposed to repeated or constant pressure, such as in animals immobilized by paralysis, or in those exposed to a physically harsh environment.

Dogs. Calluses occur when continual or repetitive pressure or friction is applied to a localized area of skin and represent a protective response of the integument to the physical injury. They tend to occur over bony prominences, particularly the hocks, elbows, lateral surfaces of the digits, and on the sternum. Callosities can develop in all domestic animal species, but are most common in dogs, particularly the giant breeds, and in pigs housed on concrete floors with inadequate bedding. They are characterized by epidermal proliferation with prominent epidermal and follicular hyperkeratosis. Dilated hair follicles may lead to furunculosis with severe suppurative to pyogranulomatous dermatitis and eventual fibrosis. Grossly, callosities are *well-circumscribed, lichenified, raised, alopecic, gray, keratinous plaques*. Ulceration may occur. The pig may also develop bursitis.

A **hygroma** *is a false or acquired bursa that develops subcutaneously over bony prominences.* Hygromas are most common in the giant breeds of dogs at pressure points such as the lateral aspect of the elbow, the greater trochanter of the femur, and the tuber coxae. Hip dysplasia in dogs can lead to elbow hygromas, as dogs develop an abnormal method of lying down that relies upon dropping to the olecranons to spare the hips. Usually pressure induces a protective callus, but in some animals, persistent decubitus ulcers or recurrent hematoma formation eventually lead to the induction of a hygroma. The gross lesion is a variably sized cystic cavity separated from the skin by loose connective tissue. The wall of the hygroma is dense connective tissue that may have a smooth or a villus inner lining. The contents are mucinous and yellow to red, depending on the degree of hemorrhage. *Histologically, the wall is composed of granulation tissue of variable maturity.* A flattened layer of fibroblasts may give the appearance of an epithelial lining. The cavity may contain clumps of fibrin. Organization of fibrin deposits at the margin of the cavity gives rise to the grossly apparent villus projections that occasionally undergo cartilaginous metaplasia.

Decubitus ulcers *are the result of ischemic necrosis that follows application of constant pressure to a localized area of skin.* Studies in Greyhounds suggest that intermittent repeated focal vascular occlusion leads to increased tissue damage from *reperfusion injury*. Thromboxane A_2 and its metabolite, thromboxane B_2, are thought to contribute to vasoconstriction and platelet aggregation. Predisposing conditions include prolonged recumbency, lack of proper bedding, improperly applied bandages or casts, poorly fitting tack, atrophy of muscle, loss of fat, malnutrition associated with systemic disease, contusions, irritation from feces or urine, and body types with large bones, thin skin, and low body fat. In large animals, postanesthetic myopathies, laminitis, and neurologic diseases are predisposing conditions. The "downer" cow is particularly prone to decubitus ulcers. *Decubitus ulcers are graded from I to IV.* In grade I, the lesion consists of focal erythema. In grade II, an ulcer extends into the subcutis. In grade III, the ulcer extends into the deep fascia, and the wound edges may be undermined. Grade IV ulcers extend to bone, have undermined edges, and possibly underlying osteomyelitis and septic arthritis.

Intertrigo *refers to localized dermatitis affecting folded areas of skin.* The combined effect of friction, heat, maceration, bacterial or yeast proliferation, and irritation by retained secretions leads to superficial inflammation. Examples in dogs include *facial, lip, vulvar, and tail fold dermatitis* of English Bulldogs and Pugs. Obesity is a predisposing factor. Body fold dermatitis is particularly common in Chinese Shar-Pei puppies. Udder-thigh dermatitis occurs predominantly in first-calf *dairy heifers.* Udder edema is a predisposing factor. Lesions are erythematous and swollen, sometimes ulcerated, and often have an unpleasant odor. Histologically, the epidermis is hyperplastic, spongiotic, and possibly eroded or ulcerated. Surface pustules, neutrophilic exocytosis, and pigmentary incontinence may be present. The dermis has a dense band of lymphocytes and plasma cells at the dermoepidermal junction. Mucocutaneous pyoderma is the primary differential.

Traumatic injury to the skin is quite common in dogs and is often associated with *compound fractures* sustained in motor vehicle accidents. Post-traumatic alopecia may occur on the lower back in cats with history of pelvic injury. *Dogfight wounds* tend to be tears rather than punctures, as occur in cats; consequently, abscesses are a less common sequel. A plethora of **foreign bodies** may penetrate the canine integument, 2 of the more dramatic examples being *foxtails* and *porcupine quills.* The external ear canal and interdigital webs are favored sites for grass awn entry and subsequent migration. Retrievers or other animals wounded with *steel shot* may develop fistulous tracts or abscesses as steel shot corrodes when embedded in tissues.

Myospherulosis is a rare form of foreign-body reaction in which endogenous erythrocytes interact with an exogenous substance, such as antibiotics or ointments, or with endogenous fat. *The lesions are subcutaneous nodules composed of sheets of large macrophages in which the cytoplasm is filled with homogeneous eosinophilic spherules.* These structures may resemble fungal organisms but are negative with fungal special stains such as periodic acid–Schiff. The spherules stain for endogenous peroxidase, thus establishing their identity as erythrocytes.

Traction alopecia has been reported in dogs. It results from low-grade local ischemia induced by traction on hairs. The traction force is applied by elastic ties or hair barrettes applied to pull the forelock hair into a topknot. The lesions are focal patches of cutaneous atrophy and alopecia that may become eroded and crusted. Histologically, the lesion is an *atrophic dermatosis*. The epidermis is thin and may occasionally show single-cell necrosis, erosion, or ulceration. The hair follicles are inactive and atrophic, pale staining, and appear "faded." Inflammation is minimal and is restricted to areas of surface ulceration.

Pyotraumatic dermatitis or "hot spot" is a common complication of flea-bite hypersensitivity or any pruritic dermatosis that leads to an *itch-scratch cycle*. It occurs most often in times of warm, humid weather. Breeds with a thick undercoat, such as German Shepherds, Golden Retrievers, Labradors, and Saint Bernards, are particularly prone to develop pyotraumatic dermatitis. Lesions are extremely painful and occur at sites of *self-trauma*. Lesions are most often seen on the cheek, neck, and lateral thigh or the dorsal rump in flea-infested dogs. In Rottweilers, lesions typically occur on cheek and neck, whereas the lesions in German Shepherd dogs occur on the rump and thighs. Grossly, the initial lesions are erythematous, exudative, sharply demarcated patches, spreading extensively if not treated. The surface may be colonized by gram-positive cocci. Alopecia and hyperpigmentation are the typical sequelae. Pyotraumatic dermatitis is characterized histologically by *epidermal ulceration*. A thick serocellular inflammatory crust covers the denuded dermis. The predominantly neutrophilic reaction tends to be restricted to the area beneath the ulcer. Folliculitis and furunculosis are not features of classic pyotraumatic dermatitis but occasionally are concurrent conditions as indicated clinically by scattered papules at the periphery of the lesion. Eosinophils and/or folliculitis were common in one series of cases.

Injection site reactions are relatively common in domestic animals. Subcutaneously administered vaccines and therapeutic drugs may be responsible. The nodules may ulcerate or fistulate and are often suspected to be neoplasms. *Histologically, the classic injection site reaction is composed predominantly of nodular aggregates of lymphocytes arranged around a central core of caseous necrosis.* Lymphocytes may form follicles. Irregular refractile or faintly basophilic granular material is often embedded in the eosinophilic debris or found within phagocytic cells. Plasma cells, macrophages, and multinucleated giant cells are also present, but in lesser numbers than lymphocytes. The strong antigenic stimulus provided by the exogenous antigen sometimes results in the formation of germinal centers. The heterogeneity of the cell population and the lack of anaplastic characteristics in the lymphoid cells may differentiate these lesions, sometimes termed *pseudolymphoma*, from genuine lymphoma.

Vaccine administration in **cats** has been linked to the development of a variety of sarcomas, including fibrosarcomas, osteosarcomas, malignant fibrous histiocytomas, chondrosarcomas, and rhabdomyosarcomas. **Vaccine-associated sarcomas** have the unique features of a *subcutaneous location, concurrent lymphocytic infiltrates, and macrophages that contain blue-gray foreign material*. The proposed mechanism involves an overzealous reparative response, followed by malignant transformation of mesenchymal cells. Antigen load and degree of inflammation present at the vaccination site are possible influencing factors. Aluminum adjuvant particles have been identified in tumor-associated macrophages; however, vaccine-associated sarcomas have also been documented to arise from the use of nonadjuvanted vaccines. Injection of killed **rabies vaccine** in **dogs** can lead to focal mononuclear vasculitis and ischemic atrophy of surrounding follicles, resulting in a focal area of alopecia and is further discussed under Immune-mediated dermatoses. **Injection-site eosinophilic granulomas** with necrotic centers developed in some **horses** within 1-3 days as a response to the use of silicone-coated hypodermic needles. The lesion is suspected to be a form of delayed hypersensitivity.

Cats. Cats are particularly prone to develop subcutaneous abscesses or cellulitis as a result of fight wounds. The cat bite produces a puncture-type wound that seals over and enables the introduced bacteria (chiefly oral flora) to multiply in the damaged tissue.

Cattle. Tail tip necrosis of feedlot beef cattle is a disease in which slatted floor housing has been shown to be an important causal factor. The pathogenesis is presumed to be *ischemia*, secondary to compression of, or blunt trauma to, the more proximal parts of the tail. Clinically, there is alopecia, scaling, and crusting. Ulceration and suppuration are frequent sequelae. In early lesions, histologic examination reveals only perivascular edema and hemorrhage. Fully developed lesions are characterized by dermal scarring, follicular atrophy, vascular wall hypertrophy, and fragmentation of extravasated erythrocytes.

Pigs. Intensive rearing systems for swine production have increased the occurrence of a variety of traumatic lesions. Those in piglets probably result from contact with *concrete floors* in farrowing crates. The carpi are the most common site affected, followed by the fetlocks and hocks. The nipples, particularly the cranial pair, are often involved, as is the tail. The lesions occur within a few hours of birth as circumscribed red macules, followed by necrosis, ulceration, and crusting. The ulcers heal over 3-4 weeks, leaving no permanent defect. The supernumerary digits of the hindlegs are subject to trauma in sows housed on concrete slats. Trauma resulting from *vices*, such as tail biting, ear biting, and flank biting, are common in growing pigs under intensive rearing systems of management. Wounds from a variety of causes, including fight wounds, often develop into subcutaneous abscesses in pigs.

Horses. Cutaneous wounds are common in horses and can be attributed largely to the flighty temperament of the species. *Exuberant granulation tissue—proud flesh—*is a relatively frequent and serious sequel to wounds of the distal limbs. Poor circulation, minimal soft tissue, lack of adequate drainage, and a tendency for excessive movement predisposes the distal limbs to the development of excess granulation tissue.

Decreased blood flow has been shown in horses with experimentally induced limb wounds as compared with wounds on the body. Furthermore, the limb wounds had lower glucose and higher lactate concentration than body wounds. These findings further support a role for decreased perfusion as well as metabolic disturbances in the development of equine exuberant granulation tissue. The gross lesion, *a tumor-like mass of red-brown tissue, must be distinguished from equine sarcoid, cutaneous habronemiasis, mycoses, pythiosis, and squamous cell carcinoma.* Histologically, immature capillaries and capillary loops arranged perpendicularly to the elongated fibroblasts and newly synthesized collagen are distinctive features. A superficial layer of granulation tissue may form in association with any of the above-mentioned conditions, and the entire lesion should be examined before a diagnosis is made.

Further reading

Declercq J. Alopecia and dermatopathy of the lower back following pelvic fractures in three cats. Vet Dermatol 2004;15:42-46.

Holm BR, et al. A prospective study of the clinical findings, treatment and histopathology of 44 cases of pyotraumatic dermatitis. Vet Dermatol 2004;15:369-376.

Miller WM, et al. Environmental skin diseases. In: Miller WH, et al., editors. Muller & Kirk's Small Animal Dermatology. 7th ed. St Louis: Elsevier; 2013. p. 659-684.

Sørensen MA, et al. Regional disturbances in blood flow and metabolism in equine limb wound healing with formation of exuberant granulation tissue. Wound Repair Regen 2014;22:647-653.

Psychogenic injury

Several conditions in animals are considered to be similar to **obsessive-compulsive disorders** in humans. In theory, stress causes an increase in the production of endorphins, creating reinforcement of the stereotypic behavior characterizing each syndrome.

Psychogenic alopecia in **cats,** a self-induced form of alopecia precipitated or exacerbated by environmental stress, is similar to the obsessive-compulsive disorder of humans, trichotillomania. Although this condition does occur, it is very rare and generally overdiagnosed. A thorough diagnostic workup is needed to rule out allergic skin disease, ectoparasitism, and other medical causes for pruritus. In a study of 18 cats with presumed psychogenic alopecia, 16 cats were identified with medical causes of pruritus, whereas only 2 cats were found to have only psychogenic alopecia, and 3 cats had a combination of psychogenic alopecia and a medical cause of pruritus. The condition can occur in any cat, but is most common in indoor cats and oriental breeds. Affected cats groom excessively, licking, and pulling at the haircoat. Psychogenic alopecia/dermatitis has *2 clinical forms.* In one, *psychogenic dermatitis,* affected cats lick and chew at a single site, creating a well-demarcated erythematous, ulcerated lesion of variable size, which usually is located on an extremity, the abdomen, or flank. The lesion grossly resembles those of eosinophilic plaque. The second, or *alopecic form,* is characterized by regional alopecia or hypotrichosis or regions of broken (barbered) hairs and normal skin. A trichogram examination of epilated hairs reveals a normal anagen to telogen ratio and fractured tips of hairs rather than tapered ends. *Microscopic examination of skin in the alopecic form is usually normal,* although wrinkling of the outer root sheath and intrafollicular and perifollicular hemorrhage may reflect the trauma applied to the hairs. Skin biopsies are helpful to identify an allergic reaction pattern in suspected cases; however, a normal biopsy cannot confirm psychogenic alopecia. The inflammatory form has no distinctive histologic features, as it is a nonspecific, ulcerative, hyperplastic, superficial perivascular dermatitis. *Differentials for the alopecic form include atopy, flea allergic dermatitis, cheyletiellosis, and Demodex gatoi infestation.* As pruritus in the cat is manifested in part by excessive grooming, any degree of perivascular eosinophilic dermatitis should be considered indicative of an underlying hypersensitivity disorder. The condition must also be differentiated from **feline acquired hair shaft abnormality,** a condition resembling *trichorrhexis nodosa* in humans. In this condition, cats with an underlying pruritic skin disease, such as flea allergic dermatitis groom excessively. Weakened hair shafts break easily and lead to alopecia. A trichogram reveals white nodes on the hair shafts corresponding to foci of frayed cortical fibers. A biopsy should show evidence of the underlying hypersensitivity condition.

Dogs also develop *psychogenic dermatitis, including foot chewing and licking, tail biting, and flank sucking.* The gross lesions may be slight, but the superficial excoriations often develop into pyoderma. **Acral lick dermatitis,** otherwise known as "lick granuloma," acral pruritic nodule, or neurodermatitis, is a relatively common disorder of large active-breed dogs younger than 5 years. Allergic skin disease may be a predisposing factor. Males are affected twice as frequently as females. The areas traumatized by persistent licking and chewing are most commonly the cranial carpus and metacarpus, followed by the radius, tibia, and metatarsus. Erythema and epidermal excoriations give rise to a single well-circumscribed, eroded or ulcerated, oval plaque. Occasionally, lesions are multiple. Secondary bacterial infection may result. Re-epithelialization of the lesion leaves a well-circumscribed alopecic plaque, often with peripheral hyperpigmentation. Histologically, the lesions have *superficial perivascular dermatitis with marked acanthosis and rete ridge formation and compact orthokeratotic and parakeratotic hyperkeratosis* (Fig. 6-40). The hair follicles are enlarged and elongate. Superficial dermal fibrosis is usually marked, and collagen fibers in dermal papillae are often arranged perpendicular to the surface

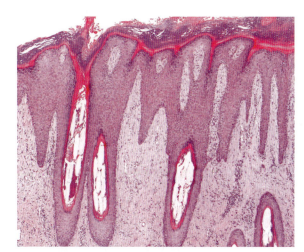

Figure 6-40 **Acral lick dermatitis** in a dog. Superficial perivascular dermatitis with marked compact orthokeratotic hyperkeratosis, and acanthosis with rete ridge formation.

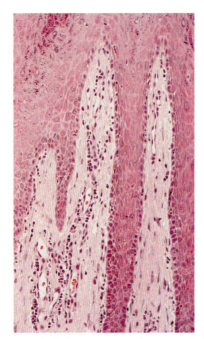

Figure 6-41 Acral lick dermatitis in a dog. Vertical alignment of collagen.

epithelium (Fig. 6-41). *This "vertical streaking" of collagen is thought to result from chronic irritation.* Perifolliculitis, folliculitis, and sometimes furunculosis are often present. Plasmacytic infiltrates often surround the sweat glands. Sebaceous glands and hair follicles appear hyperplastic.

In **horses,** the **equine self-mutilation syndrome** can be misinterpreted as a possible cutaneous disorder as horses bite, kick, or rub the flank or pectoral areas. The behavior is usually accompanied by vocalization, spinning, or rolling and is most common in *stallions*. The condition is thought to be *stress related*. There are no primary cutaneous lesions; however, secondary excoriations may be present.

A **self-destructive behavioral condition** primarily affecting **first-calf heifers** is characterized by *excessive licking of the udder and teats,* sometimes leading to teat necrosis and culling. The condition is associated with udder edema and increased levels of histamine in the udder tissue leading to pruritus.

Further reading

Beale K. Feline demodicosis: a consideration in the itchy or overgrooming cat. J Feline Med Surg 2012;14:209-213.

Shumaker AK, et al. Microbiological and histopathological features of canine acral lick dermatitis. Vet Dermatol 2008;19:288-298.

Waisglass SE, et al. Underlying medical conditions in cats with presumptive psychogenic alopecia. J Am Vet Med Assoc 2006; 228:1705-1709.

Mineral deposition in cutaneous tissues

Deposition of insoluble calcium salts within cutaneous tissues can occur as a result of injury or degeneration of skin components **(dystrophic mineralization** or calcification), secondary to calcium/phosphorus metabolic alterations **(metastatic mineralization** or calcification), as an idiopathic condition, or may occur iatrogenically. Mechanisms leading to calcium salt deposition are complex and involve such factors as the lower pH of injured tissue, mitochondrial concentration of calcium and phosphorus, and the influx of calcium into injured cells in dystrophic forms. In metastatic forms, loss of mineralization inhibitors, changing of ions into a solid phase, and phosphate ion initiation of crystal formation are implicated in salt formation. Mineralization can be *localized*, as in inflammatory foci (granulomas), in degenerative lesions (follicular cysts), or in neoplasms (pilomatricomas), or may be *generalized* as in the tissue mineralization associated with chronic renal failure.

Dystrophic mineralization has been associated with hyperadrenocorticism, diabetes mellitus, local inflammation, and tissue degeneration or necrosis. It has also been reported in association with drug injections and severe systemic disease such as leptospirosis. The most well-known form of dystrophic mineralization is **calcinosis cutis** in dogs with iatrogenic or naturally occurring hyperadrenocorticism, which is discussed in Endocrine diseases of skin.

Metastatic calcinosis is rare. It has been associated with chronic renal failure; congenital renal dysfunction, including renal dysplasia; primary hyperparathyroidism; and hypervitaminosis D. It has also been reported in dogs with systemic blastomycosis and paecilomycosis. Dogs with systemic blastomycosis treated with **amphotericin B** developed lesions that resolved over time and were *indistinguishable from calcinosis cutis of hypercortisolism.* Dogs had severe granulomatous cutaneous lesions that may have been predisposed to dystrophic mineralization, but mineralizing lesions were more extensive or separate from primary inflammatory lesions. The dogs had no clinically significant serum calcium/phosphorus abnormalities. Additional factors suspected to contribute to mineralization included mild intermittent serum calcium fluctuations, mononuclear cell production of factors leading to increased osteoclast-mediated bone resorption, and alteration of vitamin D metabolism.

Idiopathic calcinosis cutis occurs in otherwise healthy dogs <1 year of age with no history of glucocorticoid administration. These dogs have widespread lesions that spontaneously regress within 1 year.

Iatrogenic calcinosis cutis occurs secondary to percutaneous absorption of products containing **calcium chloride or calcium carbonate.** Multifocal, flat-topped, and centrally ulcerated papules and small nodules affect glabrous skin, such as the lips, axilla, and inguinal and interdigital skin. Histologically, granulomas are centered on degenerate, mineralized collagen fibers. Ultrastructural examination of experimental lesions indicated that mineral was deposited within the collagen bundles within 24 hours of initial skin contact. The main differential diagnosis was *calcinosis cutis of hyperadrenocorticism*, to which the lesions are histologically identical.

A chemically induced, iatrogenic form of calcinosis cutis has been reported in humans and a dog as a consequence of the subcutaneous administration of a **10% calcium gluconate** solution for treatment of hypoparathyroidism. In the dog, calcium salts formed on basement membranes, dermal collagen, vessel walls, and adipocyte membranes. Dermoepidermal separation, pyogranulomatous dermatitis, panniculitis, and vasculopathy ensued, leading to marked necrosis and sloughing of the skin. Concurrent hyperphosphatemia was thought to predispose to precipitation of calcium salts.

Calcinosis universalis *refers to widespread areas of calcinosis cutis* and can be seen with hypercortisolism, percutaneous absorption of calcium-containing products, or from the iatrogenic administration of calcium-containing solutions. Some forms of calcinosis cutis can be indistinguishable histologically from calcinosis cutis associated with hyperadrenocorticism. The clinical presentation, concurrent abnormalities, signalment, and history should allow distinction of the various forms of calcinosis cutis.

Cutaneous lesions include papules, plaques, and nodules that are firm, gritty, and white to yellow. Ulceration and secondary infection are common. Lesions may occur anywhere, but common sites are over the dorsal cervical region, groin, and axillae. Metastatic mineralization may occur more commonly in the pawpads of cats and dogs. Histologically, calcium salts are deposited on collagen and elastin fibers in the dermis and basement membrane zones. The basophilic stippled and fractured material is often surrounded by macrophages, multinucleated giant cells, and fibrosis. The mineralized material is eliminated transepithelially through the epidermis and hair follicles, often leading to ulceration.

Calcinosis circumscripta (tumoral calcinosis) occurs most often in *dogs, horses,* and occasionally *cats* (see also Ectopic mineralization and ossification, in Vol. 1, Bones and joints). Lesions in dogs are most often solitary but can be multiple and occur most often in large breeds <2 years of age. German Shepherd dogs are predisposed. The *skin over bony prominences of the limbs* is most often affected. The tongue and paravertebral soft tissues, pawpads, edges of the pinna in dogs with cropped ears, and cheeks of Boston Terriers are other reported sites. Calcinosis circumscripta of the dorsal thoracolumbar region at a site of previous progestogen injection has been reported in a cat. In horses, young male Standardbred horses appear to be predisposed, and lesions are most common over the lateral stifle.

The gross and histologic features of the lesion evolve over time. Initially, the lesion may be bulging, fluctuant or cystic, variably ulcerated, and contains chalky white material (Fig. 6-42). Histologically, subcutaneous to deep dermal lakes of basophilic granular material that stain with von Kossa are surrounded by mild fibrosis and a cellular zone of variable width with giant cells, large macrophages, and fewer lymphocytes and plasma cells (Fig. 6-43). Over time, the lesions become firm, progressively more mineralized, and associated with dense fibrous connective tissue bands. Inflammation may subside to some degree over time, and osseous or cartilaginous metaplasia may take place. Epidermal sequestration or transepidermal elimination of mineralized material may lead to ulceration.

The pathogenesis of calcinosis circumscripta is not known; it is likely that multiple factors are involved. Dystrophic mineralization secondary to previous tissue trauma has been proposed based on the predilection for skin covering bony prominences. This explanation is not entirely satisfactory as the lesions do not recur after surgical excision, and trauma to these sites in large dogs would be expected to be repetitive. The name "apocrine cystic calcinosis" was previously applied to calcinosis circumscripta because it has been documented to arise from degenerating, cystic apocrine (epitrichial) glands. A relationship to epitrichial glands is not evident in most cases. Lesions have also developed at sites of previous injections, or in association with surgical sites sutured with polydioxanone sutures. Cases of calcinosis circumscripta have also been reported to occur in the pawpads of dogs and cats with chronic renal failure, and in the pawpads of an otherwise healthy German Shepherd dog and in another German Shepherd

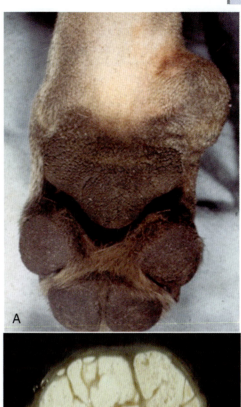
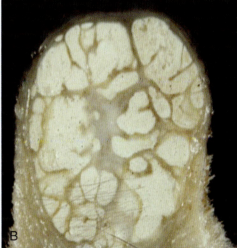

Figure 6-42 Calcinosis circumscripta in a dog. **A.** Note the swelling on the medial side of the carpus. **B.** Subgross shows lakes of chalky material. (Courtesy M. Goldschmidt.)

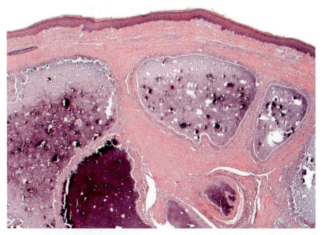

Figure 6-43 Calcinosis circumscripta in a dog. Dermal lakes of basophilic granular material are surrounded by mild fibrosis and giant cells, macrophages, and fewer lymphocytes and plasma cells.

dog with pododermatitis. Symmetrical cases that resolved spontaneously have been reported in young dogs with underlying skeletal disease, such as hypertrophic osteodystrophy. In humans, the disorder can be inherited as an autosomal recessive trait.

Further reading

Bertazzolo W, et al. Clinicopathological findings in five cats with paw calcification. J Feline Med Surg 2003;5:11-17.

Declercq J, Bhatti S. Calcinosis involving multiple paws in a cat with chronic renal failure and in a cat with hyperthyroidism. Vet Dermatol 2005;16:74-78.

Doerr KA, et al. Calcinosis cutis in dogs: histopathological and clinical analysis of 46 cases. Vet Dermatol 2013;24:355-361.

Holahan ML, et al. Generalized calcinosis cutis associated with disseminated paecilomycosis in a dog. Vet Dermatol 2008;19:368-372.

Tafti AK, et al. Calcinosis circumscripta in a dog: a retrospective pathological study. J Vet Med A Physiol Pathol Clin Med 2005;52:13-17.

Volk AV, et al. Calcinosis cutis at cytarabine injection site in three dogs receiving prednisolone. Vet Rec 2012;171:327-329.

Cold injury

Most cold-induced cutaneous lesions (frostbite) result not only from direct freezing and disruption of the cells, but more importantly from vascular injury and resultant tissue anoxia. In experimental frostbite lesions in Hanford miniature swine, vacuolation of keratinocytes was the earliest change in the epidermis, followed by spongiosis, epidermal necrosis, and separation of the necrotic epithelium from the dermis. Hyperemia and hemorrhage were also early lesions. Inflammatory changes, comprising neutrophilic infiltration and necrotizing vasculitis, occurred 6-48 hours postinjury. Thrombosis of small arterioles increased in severity up to 1 week postinjury. By 2 weeks, considerable epithelial regeneration had taken place, either as a complete replacement or as crescents beneath the necrotic epidermis.

Cutaneous injury resulting from cold is uncommon in well-nourished, healthy domestic animals. Well-acclimatized long-haired animals can tolerate temperatures of −50° C for indefinite periods. Cold injury occurs most commonly on the tips of the ears and tail of cats, the scrotum of male dogs and bulls, and the tips of the ears, tail, and teats in cattle. The teats are particularly vulnerable if cows are turned out into the cold with wet udders. Affected skin is cool, pale, and hypoesthetic. The gross lesions include alopecia, scaling, and pigmentary alterations of the skin, hair, or both. In severe cases, the ischemic necrosis results in dry gangrene and sloughing of the affected part.

Freeze branding using a branding iron cooled with dry ice or liquid nitrogen—used to identify horses permanently—causes damage to pigment-producing hair cells resulting in leukotrichia.

Further reading

Rothenberger J, et al. Assessment of microcirculatory changes of cold contact injuries in a swine model using laser Doppler flowmetry and tissue spectrophotometry. Burns 2014;40:725-730.

Thermal injury

Heat may be applied to the skin in a variety of forms and, depending on duration and intensity, will produce *mild to severe necrotizing lesions.* Longer exposure to lower temperatures is more damaging than short exposure to higher temperatures. The lowest temperature at which skin can burn is 44° C (111° F). *Dry heat causes desiccation and carbonization, whereas moist heat causes "boiling" or coagulation.* Thermal injury in domestic animals may be caused by hot liquids, steam, heating pads, hair dryers, drying cages, hot metals such as wood stoves or car engines, fires, friction from rope "scalds," electrical burns from chewing electrical wires, improperly grounded electrocautery units, or lightning strikes. Linear burns may occur on the dorsum of dogs exposed to hot water from garden hoses. This typically occurs in the warm summer months when the ambient temperature exceeds 32° C (90° F). Animals struck by lightning may show a jagged line of singed hair running down a shoulder or flank (Fig. 6-44). This finding is valuable in establishing an otherwise difficult diagnosis. Rarely, small animals incur microwave burns.

Burns are classified into 4 degrees according to depth of injury.

- **First-degree burns** *involve only the epidermis.* The heated areas are erythematous and edematous as a result of vascular reaction in the dermis, but vesicles do not form. The epithelial cells show no morphologic sign of injury, although there may be surface desquamation after a few days.
- In **second-degree burns,** *the epidermis and part of the dermis are damaged. The* cytoplasm of the epithelial cells is hypereosinophilic, and the nuclei are shrunken or karyorrhectic. Coagulative necrosis of the epidermis (Fig. 6-45) can occur in the absence of substantial dermal injury and often "wicks" down to involve the follicular epithelium (Fig. 6-46). The vascular changes are more prominent than in lesser burns, with marked dermal edema and spongiosis. Vesicles and bullae form in the epidermis, often at the dermoepidermal junction. The bullae contain serum, granular debris, and leukocytes. Healing can be complete if secondary infection does not lead to deeper injury.
- In **third-degree burns,** *the destructive effect of the heat extends full thickness through the epidermis and dermis,* causing coagulative necrosis of connective tissues, blood

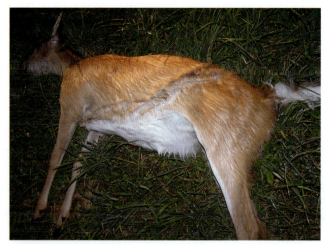

Figure 6-44 Lightning strike. A linear arrangement of singed hairs in a deer. (Courtesy J. Czech, Pennsylvania Game Commission.)

Physicochemical Diseases of Skin   565

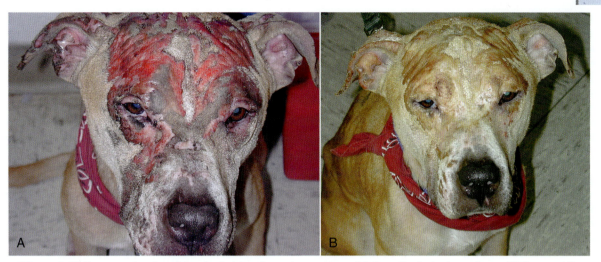

Figure 6-45 Burn on the dorsal head of a dog from the ignition of lighter fluid. **A.** Acute burn (12 hours old). **B.** Three weeks later, with scarring.

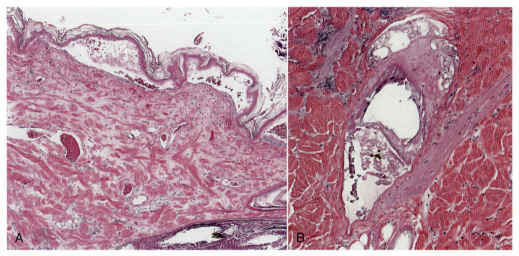

Figure 6-46 Burn. **A.** Full-thickness coagulative necrosis of the epidermis with vesiculation and loss of cell detail in the dermis. **B.** Necrosis in the dermis may be subtle; however, hair follicles and sebaceous glands are often more severely affected because of a "wicking effect." (Courtesy K. Credille.)

vessels, and adnexa. Thermal injury causes thrombosis of blood vessels and vascular leakage, leading to the coagulative necrosis of more superficial tissues. Heat of sufficient intensity or duration to penetrate this deeply usually desiccates and chars the outer epidermis. Coagulative necrosis of the dermis produces a swollen amorphous accretion of the connective tissues accompanied by an acute inflammatory reaction. Over time, histiocytes infiltrate the subcutis and fibrosis ensues. Subcutaneous vasculitis may be present. The necrotic tissue sloughs, and the defect is filled in by granulation tissue. Permanent scarring results, with loss of adnexa.

- **Fourth-degree burns** *are similar in character to those of third degree but penetrate below the dermis to and beyond the subcutaneous fascia;* their local consequences depend on what lies underneath. Heat in surface tissue is conducted to deeper tissues via the blood and lymph. The degree of injury may not be evident for several days after the insult occurred. Follicular and sweat gland damage continues for 24-48 hours. Once lesions fully develop, the progress of injury should cease, which is helpful in making the diagnosis. Histologically, thermally induced tissue damage is not sharply demarcated and should dissipate gradually with increasing depth of the biopsy. *Clinical differentials* include toxic epidermal necrolysis, erythema multiforme major, bullous pemphigoid, pemphigus vulgaris, vasculitis, trauma, and other causes of ischemia. Lesions from thermal injury sometimes have an abnormal anatomic distribution or pattern, such as drips, angles, lines, or areas of contact that may be helpful in the differential diagnosis.

Microwave burns are unique in that the lesions are sharply delineated histologically without a tapering of the degree of coagulative necrosis in the deeper tissues. The degree of injury is uniform throughout the tissue, and inflammation is minimal. The depth of damage depends on the frequency of the microwaves, with some frequencies sparing the superficial tissues and coagulating the deeper tissues. Pain perception may not occur until the damage is done and lesions may not be evident for up to 6 days. There is no surface charring, blister formation, or edema. There is thrombosis of vessels, and the tissue is mummified. Injury is due to ionizing radiation leading to heat generated from the vibration of molecules in the tissue.

Full-thickness cutaneous burns have been reported to occur in black-haired spots of Dalmatians as a result of **solar radiation.** Normally, cutaneous injury from solar radiation affects lightly pigmented sparsely haired skin rather than areas protected by pigment. *Black skin absorbs approximately 45% more solar radiation than white skin.* The absorption of visible light (400-700 nm) can result in the production of thermal energy resulting in a burn. Ultraviolet (UV) light (100-400 nm) does not penetrate into the dermis and does not produce substantial thermal energy, but has other deleterious effects (see Actinic diseases of skin). Pain, prompting moving to the shade, was likely not perceived by the dogs as the burns were multifocal, involving only black-haired areas, and Dalmatians are primarily white.

Another unique type of thermal injury, **radiant heat dermatitis,** is similar to *erythema ab igne* in humans. Tissue damage occurs from repeated exposure to moderate heat. Radiant heat dermatitis has been reported as an asymptomatic condition in dogs sleeping next to wood burning stoves or fires, or chronically exposed to heat lamps. The lesions were on the dorsolateral trunk and had a drip-like configuration. Grossly, irregular areas of alopecia were erythematous and hyperpigmented peripherally. Centrally, the lesions are scaly and depigmented. In the acute form, lesions resemble actinic dermatosis with epidermal thinning, basal cell vacuolation, and possible epidermal dysplasia. The dermis has thin fragmented or smudged collagen, increased elastin fibers, and melanin and hemosiderin deposits. There may be eosinophilic, wavy elastin fibrils in the superficial dermis ("red spaghetti of Walder"). Over time, epidermal and infundibular hyperplasia, hyperkeratosis, and dyskeratosis develop with focal spongiosis and cell necrosis. Karyomegaly of basal cells, dermal edema and mucinosis, hyperplastic sebaceous glands, dilated epitrichial glands, and mixed perivascular dermatitis may be present.

Radiation injury

Advances in the treatment of cancer in companion animals have made the possibility of **radiation-induced skin injury** more likely. Clinicians and pathologists need to be able to recognize these lesions to provide the best management options and accurate prognosis for resolution of the lesions. *The varieties of radiation modalities available have variable degrees of tissue penetration and potential for tissue injury.* Some forms of radiotherapy penetrate deeper tissues while sparing the skin, and others are more concentrated in the superficial tissues or are preferentially absorbed by specific tissues. The type of radiation therapy, source, dose, intensity, and duration of exposure dictate the range of possible side effects. Ionizing photons disrupt chemical bonds in cells, leading to injury or cell death. Some cells are not lethally damaged but sustain DNA damage to the extent that replication/replacement are not possible. The effects of radiation damage can be divided into acute and chronic forms.

Acute radiation injury to the skin is a result of damage to rapidly dividing cells. Damage is self-limiting and recovery is associated with rapid cell turnover. Clinical lesions of radiation dermatitis appear 2-4 weeks after exposure. Initially, there is erythema, pain, edema, and heat, followed several weeks later by dry or moist desquamation, depending on the degree of injury. Histologically, the lesions resemble a second-degree burn, with suprabasilar or subepidermal bullae formation, dermal edema with fibrin exudation, and a marked leukocytic infiltrate. Re-epithelialization occurs over a period of 10-60 days. The damage sustained to germinal epithelium of hair follicles and sebaceous glands leads to *alopecia* within 2-4 weeks after exposure. Hair regrowth will follow over the next several months, but damage to sebaceous glands is not reversible and leads to *permanent scaling.*

The *chronic lesions of radiation injury* are evident months to years after treatment and are primarily *due to damage to the microvasculature.* The epidermis is thin, friable, and in some areas hyperplastic, and may become neoplastic. There is hyperpigmentation and hyperkeratosis. Chronic exudative ulcers may develop but granulation tissue does not form. The dermis is fibrotic with atypical fibroblasts, telangiectasia, and possibly deep arteriolar changes. Endothelial swelling, necrosis, and thrombosis lead to occlusion and excessive endothelial proliferation, that when combined with the effects of vascular leakage, leads to vascular collapse. This condition of progressive vessel abnormalities is referred to as *obliterative endoarteritis* and is known to form a "histohematic" barrier to surrounding tissue, leading to continued anoxia and nutrient shortage.

Further reading

Holm BR, et al. A prospective study of the clinical findings, treatment and histopathology of 44 cases of pyotraumatic dermatitis. Vet Dermatol 2004;15:369-376.

Miller WM, et al. Environmental skin diseases. In: Miller WH, et al., editors. Muller & Kirk's Small Animal Dermatology. 7th ed. St Louis: Elsevier; 2013. p. 659-684.

Quist EM, et al. A case series of thermal scald injuries in dogs exposed to hot water from garden hoses (garden hose scalding syndrome). Vet Dermatol 2012;23:162-166.

Chemical injury to skin
Primary irritant contact dermatitis

Irritant contact dermatitis is caused by contact with a substance that causes direct toxic damage. An abnormal skin barrier from either physical damage to the stratum corneum (e.g., excessive moisture) or pre-existing inflammatory skin disease may enhance penetration of the offending substance. In small animals, irritant contact dermatitis is relatively uncommon. Irritant substances vary in their potency. Strong acids or alkalis induce immediate and severe tissue damage, whereas mild detergents or soaps may require repeated applications. Agents capable of causing direct cutaneous damage include acids, such as carbolic or sulfuric, alkalis, cresol tars, paints, kerosene, turpentine, antiseptics, and insecticides. An example of the last mentioned is "flea collar dermatitis" of dogs and cats. Feces and urine are also potential irritants.

Primary irritant contact dermatitis must be distinguished from allergic contact dermatitis (discussed under Hypersensitivity dermatoses). *Irritant contact dermatitis does not involve prior sensitization.* It may occur in any species, but is most frequent in the horse, cow, and dog.

The distribution of gross lesions of contact irritant dermatitis in the dog (Fig. 6-47A, B) and cat typically involves the glabrous skin of the ventral abdomen, axilla, medial thigh, perianal and perineal areas, footpads, ventral tail, chin, and inner aspect of the pinnae. An irritant reaction can occur in the ear canals of dogs being treated with topical medications for otitis. The concave pinna and vertical canal may develop

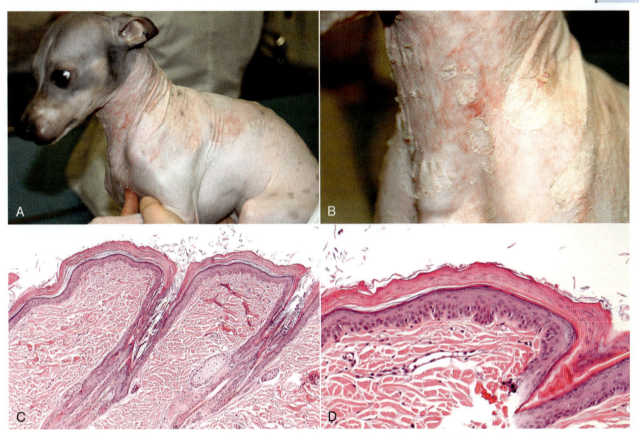

Figure 6-47 **Irritant contact dermatitis** in a hairless mixed-breed dog. **A, B.** Marked erythema and scaling on the neck and thorax caused by a sweater that was washed in irritating laundry soap. **C.** Diffuse parakeratotic hyperkeratosis with a prominent granular layer. **D.** Note the inner stratum corneum has normalized to a basketweave pattern.

transient blisters, followed by erosions and a dark red to brown discoloration and fine white scale. The haired skin is only involved if the irritant substance is in an aerosol or liquid form. Flea collar dermatitis lesions occur as a band around the neck corresponding to the position of the offending collar. In horses, lesions occur most commonly on the muzzle, lower limbs, and in areas of contact with the riding tack. Horses with diarrhea may develop severe irritant dermatitis on the soiled perineum.

The *gross lesions* consist of marked erythema, swelling, and a transient papular-vesicular stage that leads to ulceration and, in severe cases, sloughing of the affected skin. The sequelae include alopecia, scarring, and alteration in skin and hair pigmentation. In dogs, lesions often occur on the glabrous skin of the abdomen and appear erythematous with shiny adherent scale. Hyperpigmentation occurs in most species of domestic animals, but in horses, leukoderma or leukotrichia may be a permanent result of irritant contact dermatitis. Severe lesions can be considered a chemical burn. Differentials include thermal injury and allergic contact dermatitis.

The *histologic lesions* of irritant contact can be complicated by self-trauma and can be difficult to differentiate from those of allergic contact dermatitis (Fig. 6-47C, D). The histologic lesions vary depending on the caustic nature of the compound. Early lesions consist of epidermal edema with spongiotic vesicles and neutrophils or epidermal necrosis with separation from the dermis. In client-owned animals, lesions that are biopsied are typically in a chronic stage. Histologic suggestions of a chronic irritant reaction include mild acanthosis with compact parakeratotic hyperkeratosis in the presence of a granular layer. The nucleation of the keratin is subtle, which distinguishes the lesion form the robust nuclei in superficial necrolytic dermatitis or zinc-responsive dermatosis. The lesion can mimic ichthyosis, particularly if the reaction occurs in a young dog. The inflammatory infiltrate is variable in nature, probably reflecting such factors as chronicity, self-trauma, and secondary infection. *The diagnosis of irritant contact dermatitis depends largely on the history and the clinical signs, particularly the distribution of the lesions.*

In **swine,** cutaneous erythema and pruritus have been observed within 48 hours of *tiamulin* administration. The most severely affected pigs were recumbent and developed *fatal necrolytic dermatitis*. The areas most severely affected were those in contact with feces and urine. Histologic lesions included full-thickness epidermal necrosis, intraepidermal pustules, and serocellular crusting. It was hypothesized that the lesions represent a severe form of contact irritant dermatitis to tiamulin or one of its metabolites in the excreta. Skin lesions regressed when the drug was withdrawn.

An eosinophilic dermatitis was observed in pigs following heavy salting of pen floors. Lesions were present on the feet.

Further reading

Declercq J, De Bosschere H. Diesel oil-induced alopecia in two cats. Vet Dermatol 2009;20:135-138.

Kimura T. Contact dermatitis caused by sunless tanning treatment with dihydroxyacetone in hairless descendants of Mexican hairless dogs. Environ Toxicol 2009;24:506-512.

Trenti D, et al. Suspected contact scrotal dermatitis in the dog: a retrospective study of 13 cases (1987 to 2003). J Small Anim Pract 2011;52:295-300.

Envenomation

The venom of insects, spiders, other arthropods and snakes can cause mild or severe skin lesions with or without systemic signs. Effects are dependent upon composition of the venom, individual victim response, anatomic location of the envenomation, and specific characteristics of the offending organism that may be influenced by season of the year, geographic location, time since the last inflicted bite or sting, depth of injury, and so on. Different species of animals respond differently to the same venom.

Stings from *Solenopsis invicta,* the **imported fire ant,** are common in humans in South America and in most of the southern United States. The ants swarm by the hundreds, covering objects or parts of victims and simultaneously inflict numerous painful stings. The fire ant venom is primarily composed of an insoluble alkaloid (solenopsin A), shown to be cytotoxic, bactericidal, fungicidal, insecticidal, and hemolytic. Lesions in dogs have been documented and consist of initial swelling progressing to erythematous nodules within 10-20 minutes. Histologically, the sting in dogs produces a vertically oriented zone of coagulative dermal necrosis with variable epidermal necrosis. Necrosis includes the adnexa and may extend into the subcutis. Lesions resolve quickly. Severe type I hypersensitivity (anaphylaxis) reactions are possible.

Stings from **hymenopteran insects,** such as *bees, wasps, and hornets,* produce effects of a local (angioedema) or possibly systemic type I hypersensitivity reaction caused by the histamine, serotonin, and kinins in the venom (see Hypersensitivity dermatoses). Multiple-sting dermatoses lead to toxic reactions that can be fatal.

Spider bites are rarely documented definitively in animal or human patients as the initial bite goes unnoticed, and the spider is no longer recoverable by the time lesions develop. Bites occur most often on the face and extremities. Most spider bites produce localized pain, erythema, and swelling and are not of further consequence. Spiders of importance to the study of the integumentary system are those with venoms leading to *dermonecrosis and eschar formation, a condition referred to as "necrotic arachnidism."* The **brown recluse spider** (*Loxosceles reclusus*) is the spider most well known to induce dermal necrosis, although there are a number of others. Brown recluse venom contains hyaluronidase and sphingomyelinase-D, which degrade tissues. A blister with a surrounding pale halo and more peripheral erythema characterizes initial reactions documented in humans and some experimental animals. Necrosis and eschar formation occur within 5-7 days. Ulceration may be extensive. Histologically, there is hemorrhage and edema, neutrophilic vasculitis, and arterial wall necrosis. The epidermis and dermis undergo necrosis that may extend into the subcutis and underlying muscle. Panniculitis may be present. Eventually, there is dermal scarring and replacement of the subcutis and muscle by hypocellular connective tissue. Brown recluse spider bites in humans can also lead to massive hemolysis. *Differentials include other venomous bites, vasculitis, slough caused by iatrogenic injection of irritating substances, thermal burns, necrotizing fasciitis or other cutaneous infection, septic embolization, or trauma.* Compatible lesions, environmental history, and ruling out other conditions producing similar lesions can lead to the presumptive diagnosis of a spider bite.

Snakebite envenomation produces local tissue necrosis and variable systemic effects. Snake venom contains various enzymes, proteins, peptides, and kinins. Systemic effects of snake venom include paralysis, coagulation disturbances, shock, increased capillary permeability, myocardial damage, rhabdomyolysis, and renal failure. Of the 5 genera of venomous snakes, *crotaline* (rattlesnake, copperhead, cottonmouth, and others) *venom* contains the highest concentration of proteolytic enzymes. Local effects include pain, edema, hemorrhage, bullae formation, necrosis, and sloughing of tissue. Bites inflicted in the head or neck region may lead to swelling that interferes with respiration. Bites of pit vipers also introduce potentially dangerous bacteria, such as *Clostridia* spp., into the puncture wound. Bites are common in the dog, horse, and, to a lesser degree, cats, and most often are inflicted on the head or legs. The differential diagnoses are similar to those for necrotic arachnidism.

Further reading

Cullimore AM, et al. Tiger snake *(Notechis scutatus)* envenomation in a horse. Aust Vet J 2013;91:381-384.

Fitzgerald KT, et al. *Hymenoptera* stings. Clin Tech Small Anim Pract 2006;21:194-204.

Langhorn R, et al. Myocardial injury in dogs with snake envenomation and its relation to systemic inflammation. J Vet Emerg Crit Care (San Antonio) 2014;24:174-181.

Lewis N, et al. Mass envenomation of a mare and foal by bees. Aust Vet J 2014;92:141-148.

Peterson ME. Brown spider envenomation. Clin Tech Small Anim Pract 2006;21:191-193.

Thallotoxicosis

The heavy metal thallium is a potent toxin with pharmacologic actions similar to lead and mercury. Thallium salts are odorless, tasteless, colorless, and water soluble. Thallium was used extensively as a rodenticide and insecticide prior to 1963, when its sale to the general public in the United States and some other countries was banned. It continued to be used by government agencies as a pesticide and in various industries, such as the manufacture of optical lenses, jewelry, and scintillation counters. Thallium remains available from chemical supply companies; it has a restricted use as a rodenticide in Europe, and can be used without restrictions in some developing countries. Currently, thallium is used by the semiconductor industry, in optical lenses, and for cardiac perfusion imaging. A recent case of thallium toxicosis in a dog was associated with ingestion of mycoplasma agar plates in which thallium is used as a growth medium. Thallium, purchased from a chemical supply company, was also used in the malicious poisoning of a dog and human family.

Accidental or malicious thallium poisoning is rare and is due to the use of undestroyed supplies of old, but newly exposed, baits. *It occurs chiefly in dogs,* less often in cats, and is reported in sheep, cattle, and pigs. The LD_{50} for the dog is 10-15 mg/kg, and the toxin is cumulative. Absorption occurs rapidly from the gastrointestinal and respiratory tracts and skin. The toxin is disseminated widely in the body and is persistent, being very slowly excreted in bile and urine.

The mechanism of toxicity is not fully understood. There are 2 main hypotheses. The first holds that thallium exerts its toxic effect by combining with sulfhydryl groups, a mechanism common to many heavy metals and leading to disruption of mitochondrial respiratory chain enzymes. The second, which is based on the similarity of ionic radii between thallium and potassium, suggests that thallium may replace potassium in many critical biochemical functions, thus acting as a general cellular poison. The toxic effect may be, in part, the result of thallium interacting adversely with derivatives of riboflavin. Thallium can depolarize nerve cell membranes and antagonize effects of calcium on the heart.

The clinical effects depend on the dose and rapidity of administration. Signs of *acute thallotoxicosis* are evident within 12 hours of exposure and are characterized by severe gastrointestinal irritation and neurologic signs, including motor paralysis. Glossitis, stomatitis, rhinitis, and bronchitis develop. Death by respiratory failure may occur. Animals may survive the acute episode to develop the chronic syndrome or may bypass the acute disease altogether. Cutaneous, renal and neurologic abnormalities, progressive debilitation, and death characterize the *chronic syndrome.*

The *cutaneous lesions* develop 7-10 days after ingestion of thallium and principally affect frictional areas. The pattern of skin involvement in cats and dogs is characteristic, beginning at the commissures of the lips or nasal cleft, occasionally on the ear margins, and expanding over the face and head. The mucous membranes are characteristically "brick-red" and may be ulcerated. Lesions also develop on the interdigital skin, footpads, axillae, inguinal areas, perineum, and lateral extensor surfaces. The lesions are *marked erythema, scaling, alopecia, exudation, and crusting.* The layers of scale-crust exfoliate with attached hairs to leave a raw, oozing surface. The paws often become very swollen. In more chronic cases, thick scales on the footpads resemble "hard pad" disease conventionally associated with canine distemper. In less severely affected animals, *ease of depilation may be the only clinical indication of thallium poisoning.* The pathogenesis of the alopecia is not fully understood. Although thallium enters the hair, as do other heavy metals, by binding to sulfhydryl groups in the keratin, this is unlikely to be destructive to the hair follicle. Thallium may interfere with the energy metabolism of the rapidly dividing matrix cells of anagen follicles. In experimental intoxication of rats, a rapid decline in the mitotic rate is followed by necrosis of the matrix cells within 48 hours. The follicle passes into an abnormal catagen phase, followed by complete involution (telogen). However, no club attachment is formed, and the hairs are rapidly shed. If the animal survives, hair growth is resumed. Thallium also severely alters the cornification process, and both the surface and external root sheath epithelium demonstrate marked parakeratotic hyperkeratosis.

The *microscopic lesions* in the skin are dominated by *massive, diffuse parakeratotic hyperkeratosis,* which affects both surface and external root sheath epithelia. There is accompanying follicular plugging, hypogranulosis, and epidermal hyperplasia (Fig. 6-48). Neutrophil exocytosis and spongiform pustules develop in both surface and follicular epithelia. Partial or full-thickness necrosis of the surface epithelium may also occur. The dermal lesions include marked hyperemia, edema,

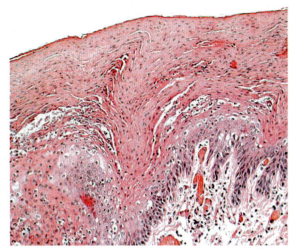

Figure 6-48 Thallium toxicity in a dog. Marked parakeratosis.

erythrocytic exocytosis and infiltration of neutrophils and mononuclear cells. There may be focal necrosis of sweat and sebaceous glands. Hair follicles are mostly in catagen or telogen. Degenerative changes are noted in anagen follicles.

Histologic lesions in *other tissues* include multifocal necrosis of myocardial and skeletal muscle fibers, nephrosis, pulmonary edema, reticuloendothelial hyperplasia, and lymphoid depletion of spleen and lymph nodes. Secondary bacterial bronchopneumonia may occur as a result of the damage to ciliated epithelia and resultant disturbance of the mucociliary apparatus. Hemorrhagic gastroenteritis occurs in acute thallotoxicosis. Focal suppurative pancreatitis has been described in several animals, but its causal relationship to thallium is not established. Ulcerative esophagitis follows dilation secondary to neuronal damage. Lesions in the central nervous system include neuronal chromatolysis, neuronophagia, and severe edema with little glial reaction. Myelinated peripheral nerves have degenerative lesions, including focal distention of myelin sheaths and swelling and occasional fragmentation of axons.

The *differential diagnoses* of acute thallium toxicity include other heavy metal toxicoses, infectious and noninfectious causes of hemorrhagic gastroenteritis, and pancreatitis. Differentials for the clinical lesions include superficial necrolytic dermatitis, zinc-responsive dermatosis, generic dog food dermatosis, toxic epidermal necrolysis, mucocutaneous candidiasis, epitheliotropic lymphoma, and autoimmune diseases, such as pemphigus vulgaris and bullous pemphigoid. The *microscopic lesions of thallium toxicosis, zinc-responsive dermatosis, and superficial necrolytic dermatitis are similar,* and confirmation requires a compatible history and demonstration of thallium in the urine by the Gabriel-Dubin colorimetric assay or in the stomach content, suspected bait, urine, liver, or kidneys by atomic absorption spectroscopy.

Further reading

Puschner B, et al. Thallium toxicosis in a dog consequent to ingestion of mycoplasma agar plates. J Vet Diagn Invest 2012;24:227-230.

Volmer PA, et al. Thallium toxicosis in a Pit Bull Terrier. J Vet Diagn Invest 2006;18:134-137.

Arsenic toxicosis

Arsenic is the metal most toxic to the skin and is found as a component of wood preservatives, herbicides, insecticides, insulation materials, paint pigments, feed additives, and some medications, and is a byproduct of some mining activities. It is a water supply contaminant in some parts of Mexico, Argentina, Chile, Taiwan, India, the United Kingdom, and the United States. Safe standards for levels of arsenic in drinking water have not been established. Arsenic is absorbed by the gastrointestinal tract and skin and is excreted in urine, bile, milk, hair, nails, and exfoliated epidermal cells. Its presence in the skin increases the skin's susceptibility to damage by UV light. Chronic arsenic exposure in humans occurs in environmental (water contamination) and industrial settings and is associated with increased incidence of visceral and cutaneous malignancies, Bowen's disease, palmar and solar hyperkeratoses, and cutaneous pigmentary disturbances. The generation of free radicals with resultant nucleic acid damage is suspected to be involved in arsenic-related carcinogenesis. Arsenic may lead to cellular proliferation through increased production of keratinocyte-derived growth factors. *Urine, hair, and liver are the tissues of choice for establishing arsenic exposure.*

Acute arsenic poisoning is an important toxicosis in domestic animals, particularly cattle and dogs, and is due to sulfhydryl group binding and inhibition of cellular metabolism. Signs and lesions are referable to the gastrointestinal tract, liver, and kidneys. Skin lesions are the result of chronic systemic low-level arsenic exposure or to direct contact. *Arsenic is an established low-grade corrosive that produces irritant contact dermatitis.* Contact lesions occur in animals sprayed or dipped in a concentrated arsenic solution or in dogs lying on heavily contaminated ground. Lesions include erythema and epidermal necrosis, leading to the formation of nonhealing ulcers. Lesions may affect oral cavity, lips, other mucocutaneous junctions, and the feet. Less is known about the effects of chronic systemic exposure of arsenic on the skin in animals; however, chronic arsenic poisoning in farm animals is associated with ill thrift and a dry, seborrheic, alopecic coat.

Further reading

Ashrafihelan J, et al. Arsenic toxicosis in sheep: the first report from Iran. Interdiscip Toxicol 2013;6:93-98.

Bertin FR, et al. Arsenic toxicosis in cattle: meta-analysis of 156 cases. J Vet Intern Med 2013;27:977-981.

Hughes MF, et al. Arsenic exposure and toxicology: a historical perspective. Toxicol Sci 2011;123:305-332.

Mercury toxicosis

Organomercurial toxicosis in domestic animals is associated chiefly with neurologic and renal disorders and is discussed in Vol. 1, Nervous system and Vol. 2, Urinary system, respectively. In chronic poisoning in **cattle,** skin manifestations, including *pustules, ulcers, hyperkeratosis, and alopecia* at the tail head are described, but their pathogenesis is poorly understood. **Horses** ingesting mercury-treated seed grain develop *total body alopecia,* followed by loss of the long hairs of mane, tail, and forelock. The hooves are not affected, and the cutaneous lesion is mild scaling. Experimental chronic methylmercury intoxication in horses produces *exudative dermatitis,* but histologic lesions are not described. Local toxic contact dermatitis follows application of mercurial containing counterirritants to the legs in horses.

Further reading

Casteel SW. Metal toxicosis in horses. Vet Clin North Am Equine Pract 2001;17:517-527.

Cutaneous iodism

Iodides have widespread use as antiseptics, expectorants, intravenous contrast agents, bronchodilators, antithyrotoxicants, and as salt or feed additives. Iodine is readily absorbed from the skin. The majority of reports of adverse effects of iodine occur as hypersensitivity reactions and not toxicoses. *Generalized seborrhea sicca* is reported in horses and cattle accidentally overdosed with iodine-containing drugs or medicated feed. In experimental toxicosis of calves, the cutaneous lesions were limited to scaly patches without alopecia. Conversely, suspected iodism in a horse produced generalized alopecia, sparing only the face, mane, and tail.

Selenium toxicosis

Selenium is a metalloid that acts as an antioxidant with toxic potential. It has chemical properties similar to sulfur. It is excreted from the body in urine, feces, and sweat and integumentary structures. Experimental studies in rodents suggest that selenium may diminish UV radiation–induced skin damage when applied topically. However, some forms are strong contact irritants and vesiculants. The toxic potential of selenium in the diet varies by the chemical form present, nature of the diet, rate of consumption, and by the species and individual animal. The mechanism by which selenium might exert its effects on the integument is not known, but conceivably, being competitive with sulfur, it modifies the structure of keratin.

Selenium is widely distributed in soils at concentrations ranging from <0.01 parts per million (ppm) to >500 ppm. Areas of high soil concentration are particularly extensive in parts of the United States (Wyoming, Montana, Utah, Colorado, North and South Dakota, Arizona, Kansas, Nebraska) and in western Canada, but also occur in parts of Australia, New Zealand, China, Ireland, Mexico, and Israel, among other countries.

Selenium toxicosis occurs in *horses, cattle, sheep, and pigs,* chiefly as a result of the ingestion of plants that have accumulated toxic levels of selenium, but occasionally as a result of accidental overdose of selenium supplements. Plants are divisible into seleniferous and nonselenifcrous species. **Seleniferous plants** can selectively concentrate selenium in their foliage and seeds as compared with nonseleniferous species grown under the same conditions. The seleniferous species are subdivided into obligate accumulators, which require high levels of selenium for survival, and facultative accumulators. The former, which include members of the genus *Astragalus, Machaeranthera,* and *Stanleya,* may accumulate >1,000 ppm selenium. Because of their high requirement for selenium, they are known as "indicator" species. Facultative or secondary selenium accumulators, such as *Aster, Atriplex, Castilleja,* and *Gutierrezia,* take up lesser amounts of selenium. Many nonseleniferous weeds, crop plants, and grasses are capable of passively accumulating selenium if growing on soils with high selenium content. Also, indicator plants increase the availability of selenium to nonseleniferous plants by converting insoluble selenites to soluble selenates and returning these to the soil. Selenium poisoning can occur whenever seleniferous plants are eaten, irrespective of levels of selenium in the soil, and it can occur whenever the levels of water-soluble selenium in the soil are high, irrespective of the botanical composition.

Seleniferous plants are not palatable, and indigenous stock learns to avoid them. Selenium poisoning occurs chiefly in newly introduced or traveling animals and in indigenous animals forced to eat the seleniferous plants in times of scarcity. Clinically, there are acute and chronic syndromes associated with the ingestion of seleniferous plants, such as *Astragalus* and *Oxytropis*. *Acute toxicity* causes severe gastrointestinal and cardiovascular signs, with mortality in some instances approaching 100%. Two different syndromes have been described as *chronic selenium poisoning*. **Blind staggers,** characterized by neurologic signs, is probably not due to selenium alone but to other toxic principles in the seleniferous plants. The second syndrome is named **alkali disease** because it was originally believed that the pH of the selenium-rich soils was a factor in its pathogenesis. Unlike blind staggers, alkali disease is reproducible in ungulates fed sublethal concentrations of selenium. The presence of internal lesions, such as nephrosis, myocardial degeneration, and hepatic fibrosis, in chronically poisoned livestock is not found in experimentally reproduced disease, suggesting that other factors are involved.

Horses and cattle chronically intoxicated with selenium become emaciated and develop partial alopecia and a general roughness of coat. Foals delivered from affected mares may have lesions. Initially, there is loss of the long hairs in the mane, forelock, and tail of horses (leading to the name bobtail disease), and loss of the long tail hairs in cattle. Sheep do not show cutaneous lesions, although, in Australia, fleece shedding has been attributed to selenium toxicity on some properties. Selenium toxicity is also suspected in alopecias of the beard and flanks of goats in the western United States. In all species, lesions commencing at the coronary band may lead to separation and shedding of the hoof or to the formation of dystrophic grooves, cracks, or corrugations that parallel the coronary band, resulting in lameness (Fig. 6-49). Lesions take months to develop. *Histologic lesions* of experimental chronic selenium toxicosis in cattle showed extensive separation of the stratum medium of the hoof with replacement by parakeratotic cellular debris. The germinal epithelium of the hoof wall was disorganized, parakeratotic, and hyperplastic. Hair follicles from the tail were atrophic with dyskeratosis and mild hyperkeratosis.

Diagnosis requires the demonstration of compatible clinical signs, progression of lesions, and identification of a dietary source of selenium with a concentration in the air-dried feed sample of >5 ppm selenium. High levels of selenium in the blood (>2 ppm) or integumentary tissues, such as hair, hoofwall, or sole (>10 ppm), should also be present. Individual animals have a variable response to selenium exposure, and some animals with high levels of selenium may not show signs of toxicosis.

Further reading

Davis TZ, et al. Toxicokinetics and pathology of plant-associated acute selenium toxicosis in steers. J Vet Diagn Invest 2012;24: 319-327.

Desta B1, et al. Acute selenium toxicosis in polo ponies. J Vet Diagn Invest 2011;23:623-628.

Raisbeck MF. Selenosis. Vet Clin North Am Food Anim Pract 2000; 16:465-480.

Organochlorine and organobromine toxicoses

Organochlorine and organobromine compounds implicated in toxicities causing, among others, cutaneous lesions, include the *highly chlorinated naphthalenes (HCNs), polybrominated biphenyls (PBBs),* and *dibenzofurans. Polychlorinated biphenyls (PCBs)* are the cause of an important industrial dermatitis of humans known as *chloracne*.

Highly chlorinated naphthalene toxicosis (X-disease, bovine hyperkeratosis), the result of exposure to tetra-, penta-, hexa-, hepta-, or octachloronaphthalenes, is largely of *historical interest*. HCNs were found to be responsible for high mortality and large economic losses in the cattle industry within the United States, Australia, New Zealand, and Germany during the 1940s and early 1950s. HCN was a common additive in many petroleum products, including those used as lubricants for farm machinery, such as feed pelleting equipment; wood preservatives; roofing paper; and building board. HCNs were a frequent feed contaminant. *These chemicals have not been used in lubricants since 1953.* Recent reports are the result of animals exposed to dumps with stores of old lubricant or abandoned machinery lubricated years ago with HCN-containing products. Percutaneous exposure produces cutaneous lesions, whereas parenteral exposure results in both cutaneous and visceral lesions. The poison is cumulative, and the disease is chronic. Lesions of HCN toxicity result from interference with the conversion of carotene to vitamin A and resemble the lesions of vitamin A deficiency. The first sign of poisoning is a fall in vitamin A levels in the plasma.

Cattle are the most susceptible species. Initial signs are increased lacrimation and drooling, depression, decreased appetite, and weight loss. Within the first few months, *hallmark cutaneous lesions of marked alopecia with nonpruritic, lichenified, deeply fissured plaques of hyperkeratotic scale are evident on the skin of the neck, shoulders and perineum.* Lesions

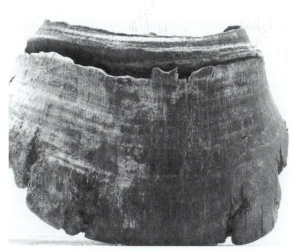

Figure 6-49 Selenium toxicosis in a horse. Hoof wall deformed by rings and grooves. (Courtesy Queensland Department of Agriculture.)

gradually generalize, sparing only the legs. Marked involvement of the skin of the medial thighs is characteristic. Horn growth may be delayed. The animal may die before the skin lesions are severe, if exposure is high. Concurrent severe secondary infections with bovine papular stomatitis virus, papilloma virus, or dermatophytes may be present. The histologic lesions are marked hyperkeratosis of surface and follicular epithelia. Internal lesions are the result of hyperplasia and squamous metaplasia of the epithelial lining of ducts and glands of the body, including liver, pancreas, kidneys, and reproductive tract. Bulls may have epididymal enlargement early in the disease process, from hyperplasia and squamous metaplasia of ducts.

Differential diagnoses include other markedly hyperkeratotic dermatopathies, such as zinc or vitamin A deficiency, dermatophilosis, dermatophytosis, or toxicosis caused by other polyhalogenated aromatic compounds. Definitive diagnosis is dependent upon identification of a source of HCN and extraction of the toxin by capillary gas chromatography and mass spectrometry. Vitamin A levels in the plasma and liver are low, but toxicosis cannot be reversed by vitamin A therapy, and the prognosis is poor.

Cutaneous lesions in **cats** exposed to wood preservatives have been ascribed to chlorinated naphthalene toxicity. The lesions include bilateral alopecia and encrustations on the eyelid and around the nostrils.

Pentachlorophenol (PCP)-contaminated wood shavings used as bedding led to chronic toxicity characterized by a *proliferative dermatitis* with crusting, scaling, and alopecia accompanied by a *multitude of systemic signs*, including peripheral edema, bone marrow hypoplasia, liver disease, and wasting in a group of horses. Gross and histologic cutaneous lesions resembled those of HCN toxicity. Wood shavings containing 4 times the maximal allowable levels of PCP/kg were traced to a lumber company using improper processing techniques. Toxicity was attributed to dibenzofuran and chlorinated dibenzo-p-dioxin isomers found as contaminants of the PCP. *Contaminants of PCP products include a large group of dioxin isomers with a wide range of toxicity that can vary by species exposed and among animals within the species.* PCP compounds are used as antiseptics, disinfectants, herbicides, fungicides, and wood and hide preservatives. The toxicity of the herbicide, Agent Orange, widely sprayed in Vietnam, is attributed to *dioxin contaminants.* The compounds enter the body via oral, dermal, or respiratory routes. High exposure leads to rapid death because of uncoupling of mitochondrial oxidative phosphorylation. Chronic toxicity is more common. The contaminants in the PCP compounds are thought to bind to aromatic hydrocarbon receptors in the cell nucleus and influence gene expression. The response may be proliferative or suppressive. Elevated levels of the compounds can be demonstrated in the liver and adipose tissue years after exposure, whereas serum levels are cleared quickly. Similar cases of dioxin isomer toxicity have been reported in *horses* exposed to riding arenas sprayed with contaminated waste oil used for dust control.

Further reading

Kerkvliet NI, et al. Dioxin intoxication from chronic exposure of horses to pentachlorophenol-contaminated wood shavings. J Am Vet Med Assoc 1992;201:296-302.

Mimosine toxicosis

Mimosine is a *toxic amino acid* found as a main constituent in the tropical to subtropical, cultivated *leguminous shrubs Mimosa pudica* and *Leucaena leucocephala* (formerly *L. glauca*). Mimosine and its metabolite, 3-hydroxy-4-(1H)-pyridone (DHP), are toxic. In ruminants, mimosine is a depilatory, whereas DHP is a goitrogen. Poisoning can be acute or chronic and is characterized by *alopecia, poor growth, oral ulcerations,* and *goiter* not prevented by iodine supplementation. Toxicity occurs in a number of countries and goes by a variety of local names: *jumbey* in the West Indies, *lamtoro* in Indonesia, and *koa haole* in Hawaii. A variation of animal susceptibility to mimosine toxicity in different parts of the world is due to the geographic distribution of ruminal bacteria capable of degrading DHP. In vitro antemortem assays for detection of DHP-degrading bacteria can be performed on feces or ruminal contents. A group of bacteria, *Synergistes jonesii*, can be inoculated into the rumen of livestock to prevent toxicity. Mimosine has been shown to reduce DNA synthesis and to block the progression of the cell cycle by chelating iron. DHP prevents iodine binding in the thyroid gland. *Mimosine toxicity occurs in horses, cattle, pigs, and sheep* and has been experimentally reproduced in cattle and laboratory animals.

Horses appear to be most susceptible and lose their hair, especially the long hair of the mane and tail. In severe cases, there is patchy loss of hair above and below the hocks and knees and on the flanks and neck. Disturbed growth at the coronet and periople may produce dystrophic rings on the hooves. There is loss of condition and weakness that perhaps is attributable to malnutrition rather than to mimosine.

Mimosine has a marked depilatory action on the fleece of **sheep.** The fleece becomes easily epilated 14 days after a single oral dose of 400-650 mg/kg body weight. DNA synthesis in the wool follicles is reduced. Mimosine toxicity causing depilation in **pigs** is reported from Indonesia and the Bahamas.

Further reading

Anderson RC. Drought associated poisoning of cattle in South Texas by the high quality forage legume *Leucaena leucocephala*. Vet Human Toxicol 2001;43:95-96.

Gangrenous ergotism and fescue toxicosis

These conditions can be considered together because the cutaneous lesions of chronic ergotism caused by *Claviceps purpurea* and those of poisoning by tall fescue, *Festuca arundinacea* or *F. eliator*, are identical.

Ergotism is the oldest known mycotoxicosis. The ergot of *Claviceps* spp. fungi is a *compacted mass of hyphae, the sclerotium*, which develops in the seed heads of many species of grasses and cereal grains and completely replaces the ovary. *Ergotism is the disease that results from ingestion of toxic alkaloids produced by the fungi.* The alkaloids are derivatives of lysergic acid and include *ergotamine, ergometrine, and ergotoxine*, which is a composite of 3 alkaloids. The quantity and spectrum of alkaloids in the ergots vary considerably with the strain of fungus, type of plant, season of the year, climatic conditions, and other regional factors. The ergots also produce a *variety of amines*, such as histamine, acetylcholine, and other nitrogenous compounds with physiologic activity.

Of the various pharmacologic effects exerted by the ergot alkaloids, the most important in the pathogenesis of

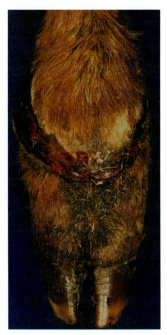

Figure 6-50 Ergotism in a bovid. Sharply demarcated ischemic necrosis of digit with foot ready to slough. (Courtesy C.L. Davis Foundation and National Northeast University.)

gangrenous ergotism is direct stimulation of adrenergic nerves supplying arteriolar smooth muscle. This produces *marked peripheral vasoconstriction*. Arteriolar spasm and damage to capillary endothelium leads to thrombosis and ischemic necrosis of tissues.

Gangrenous ergotism caused by *C. purpurea* is a disease mainly of cattle. It may occur in animals at pasture but is more common in housed animals fed infected grain. Gangrenous ergotism represents the chronic form of intoxication by ergot-producing fungi. Chronic ergotism develops after a week of feeding contaminated grain and begins with *acute lameness with redness and swelling of the extremities*. The hindlegs are more frequently affected than the forelegs. Lesions seldom extend above the fetlock (Fig. 6-50), but ischemic necrosis may extend to the mid-metatarsus. The feet become cold and insensitive, with dry necrosis and a prominent line of separation between viable and dead tissue. The necrotic tissue may slough. Ergotism also causes *dry gangrene of the tips of the ears and tail*. Gangrenous ergotism has been described in goats feeding on ergot-infected pasture. The toxicosis can be produced experimentally in sheep, but the syndrome is quite different from that in cattle, being characterized by ulceration of the tongue and of the alimentary mucosae. Sows are relatively resistant but may develop agalactia as a result of central inhibition of prolactin secretion.

Fescue toxicosis has a variable presentation, depending upon the animal species exposed. The most common manifestation, "fescue foot," is a disease of *cattle* characterized in the acute form by *dry gangrene of the extremities* commencing 2 weeks after ingestion of the tall fescue grass, *Festuca arundinacea*. This perennial grass is the most common pasture plant in the United States and is usually harmless. The endophytic fungus *Neotyphodium (Acremonium) coenophialum* infects ~75% of fescue pastures and imparts increased resistance of the plant to insects and extreme environmental temperatures. Under certain poorly understood conditions, the endophyte-infected plant is toxic. Fescue foot tends to occur with the onset of colder weather, indicating that low ambient temperatures may contribute to its development. The alkaloids, *ergonovine, ergotamine, and N-acetyl loline* are responsible for toxicity and act as *peripheral vasoconstrictors*. The acute syndrome in cattle is virtually identical to ergotism.

A chronic disease in **cattle**, known as "summer slump," refers to an increased susceptibility to heat stress seen in certain breeds of cattle in conditions of high environmental temperature combined with intake of endophyte-infected fescue. Cattle have decreased skin temperature and open-mouth breathing, suggesting defective thermoregulation. Experimental intravenous injection of alkaloids found in fescue produced lowered skin temperature, heart rate, and prolactin levels, and elevated blood pressure and respiratory rates in heifers. Ingestion of endophyte-infected fescue in **horses** does not lead to the visibly evident effects of peripheral vasoconstriction as in cattle, but experimental studies have demonstrated that peripheral vasoconstriction does occur, suggesting exposure could lead to foot or leg problems. The more commonly recognized manifestations of fescue toxicosis in the horse are *prolonged gestation, agalactia, thickened placentas, and possible abortion*. Abdominal lipomatosis associated with marked necrosis of abdominal fat and severe weight loss occurs in *domestic ruminants* and some species of wildlife consuming endophyte-infected fescue. A heritable predisposition exists in cattle.

Further reading

Belser-Ehrlich S, et al. Human and cattle ergotism since 1900: symptoms, outbreaks, and regulations. Toxicol Ind Health 2013;29: 307-316.

Riet-Correa F, et al. Mycotoxicoses of ruminants and horses. J Vet Diagn Invest 2013;25:692-708.

Trichothecene toxicoses

Macrocyclic trichothecene toxins produced by the fungus *Stachybotrys* spp. cause **stachybotryotoxicosis**. *Ulcerative and necrotizing lesions of the skin and mucous membranes* have been reported in horses, cattle, sheep, and pigs, chiefly from Russia and Eastern Europe. Initial lesions affect the lips, buccal commissures, and nostrils. Marked edema of the face may follow. Death follows development of *hemorrhagic diathesis, enteritis, and septicemia*. At autopsy, lesions in addition to the hemorrhagic diathesis include alimentary ulceration, pneumonia, renal infarcts, multifocal hepatic necrosis, and lymphadenitis. In many instances, these lesions may represent secondary mycotic or bacterial involvement.

T-2 toxin is a highly irritant trichothecene mycotoxin from *Fusarium* molds on grain, and causes cutaneous ulceration when applied locally to the skin of pigs. Experimental feeding of T-2 toxin–contaminated feed, in combination with aflatoxin, induces crusting and ulceration of the lips, snout, buccal commissures, and prepuce. The pathogenesis of the lesion is thought to be *contact irritant dermatitis* due directly to the T-2 toxin or to a urinary metabolite, HT-2 toxin. In rodent studies, topical T-2 toxin induces a cascade of events that leads to oxidative stress and subsequent apoptosis of keratinocytes, with release of tumor necrosis factor-α and interleukin-1β.

Various other trichothecene mycotoxins are also cutaneous irritants and may cause vomition or feed refusal.

Further reading

Doi K, Uetsuka K. Mechanisms of mycotoxin-induced dermal toxicity and tumorigenesis through oxidative stress-related pathways. J Toxicol Pathol 2014;27:1-10.

Vetch toxicosis and vetch-like diseases

Hairy vetch (*Vicia villosa* Roth) is a cultivated legume used as pasture, hay, and silage in most of the United States, and in other countries such as Argentina, Australia, and South Africa. Hairy vetch toxicosis in **cattle** is seen as 3 unique syndromes: (1) acute neurologic disease and hemolysis, followed by death after consumption of seeds; (2) swelling of the upper body, accompanied by herpetiform eruptions of the oral mucous membranes, respiratory distress, and death after consuming vetch pasture; and (3) a syndrome characterized by *dermatitis, conjunctivitis, diarrhea, and granulomatous inflammation of many organs*. The third syndrome is the most common form of hairy vetch toxicosis and occurs in *cattle* and, to a lesser extent, *horses* after consumption of vetch-containing pastures. The clinical syndrome begins 2 or more weeks after consumption and consists of pruritic dermatitis, diarrhea (possibly bloody), and wasting. Morbidity is low and mortality is high. Holsteins, Angus, and cattle aged 3 years or older are more often affected. Death in cattle occurs approximately 10-20 days after illness begins.

Initial lesions consist of a rough coat with papules and crusts affecting the skin of the udder, teats, escutcheon, and neck, followed by involvement of the trunk, face, and limbs. The skin becomes less pliable, alopecic, and lichenified. Marked pruritus leads to excoriations. At autopsy, *yellow nodular infiltrates disrupt the architecture of a wide range of organs*, but are most severe in myocardium, kidney, lymph nodes, thyroid, and adrenal glands. The kidney may have radially oriented cortical infiltrates that follow the vasculature. Other affected organs may include the mammary and salivary glands, liver, urinary bladder, meninges, and spleen. Histologically, *the infiltrates consist of monocytes, lymphocytes, plasma cells, multinucleated giant cells, and, in the cow, eosinophils*. The skin has similar perivascular to diffuse infiltrates, marked hyperkeratosis, and dermal and epidermal edema. This form of the disease has been induced experimentally in an Angus cow that had recovered from vetch toxicosis the previous year. Lesions were evident 11 days after feeding vetch. Death occurred even though vetch was removed from the diet at 12 days. Experimental lesions mirrored those of naturally occurring disease with the additional finding of necrosis of cutaneous apocrine glands.

Other species of *Vicia* and additional compounds are capable of inducing disease indistinguishable from vetch toxicity. **Pyrexia with dermatitis in dairy cows** is a syndrome with similarities to hairy vetch toxicity. It has been reported in the United States, England, Wales, France, and the Netherlands. Friesian dairy cows developed pruritic papular eruptions affecting the head and neck, tail head, and udder. Secondary lesions were the result of self-trauma. In another outbreak, hemorrhages were a prominent clinical sign. The episode in Wales was associated with the introduction of a new silage additive on several farms. The outbreak in the Netherlands was associated with the feeding of *di-ureido-isobutane* (DUIB) in the seed cake. This condition was reproduced in 2 cows fed a DUIB-containing diet for 1 month. Histologically, *the lesions of the Dutch outbreak also resembled those of the putative hairy vetch toxicity*. Visceral lesions resembling hairy vetch toxicity occur in dairy cows fed a diet containing *citrus pulp*; the syndrome resolves after removal of citrus pulp from the diet.

Hairy vetch toxicosis in **horses** resembles that in cattle, except for the infrequent finding of eosinophils in the infiltrate and lack of heart involvement. Conditions very similar to vetch toxicosis have been reported in horses with no vetch exposure. These cases have been variably referred to as *idiopathic granulomatous disease involving the skin, systemic granulomatous disease, generalized granulomatous disease, or equine sarcoidosis*. Organ involvement is variable. Skin lesions include scaling, crusting, and alopecia on the face or limbs, and progress to a generalized exfoliative dermatitis. Histologically, *the skin has multifocal, sometimes perifollicular to deep dermal nodules of granulomatous inflammation*. Sarcoidosis in man has a genetic basis and is thought to represent a hypersensitivity response to a persistent antigen. Equine sarcoidosis is discussed more fully under Miscellaneous skin conditions.

Toxicity from vetch seeds is known to be due to the presence of *prussic acid*. The cause of the granulomatous diseases listed above remains unclear. Nor is it certain whether they represent one entity or a common tissue reaction to a variety of insults. One proposed pathogenesis is that ingestion of vetch or another substance leads to antigen formation in the form of a hapten or a complete antigen that sensitizes lymphocytes and evokes the cell-mediated response upon repeat exposure. Factors that support this hypothesis are the resemblance of the histologic lesions to a type IV hypersensitivity response, age incidence, low morbidity, genetic influence, and possible need for repeat exposure. Lymphocyte blastogenesis and cutaneous hypersensitivity studies have not substantiated this hypothesis; however, only a few vetch antigens have been studied.

The diagnosis of vetch toxicity or vetch-like disease is a *diagnosis by exclusion*. It is made after review of the herd history, and character and distribution of the lesions. The combination of lesions is fairly distinctive.

Further reading

Iizuka A, et al. An outbreak of systemic granulomatous disease in cows with high milk yields. J Vet Med Sci 2005;67:693-699.

Saunders GK, et al. Suspected citrus pulp toxicosis in dairy cattle. J Vet Diagn Invest 2000;12:269-271.

Quassinoid toxicosis

Quassinoid compounds, such as neoquassin and quassin found in hardwood trees of the genus *Quassia (Simarouba amara)* in the family *Simaroubaceae*, have been reported to be associated with a *vesiculobullous dermatitis of the skin* around the eyes, nose, ears, anus, and lips of horses. *Wood shavings* from these plants have been incorporated in bedding, and the outbreaks have occurred in large numbers of exposed horses. Gross lesions develop within the first few days of exposure, and most often resolve within a week. Systemic signs such as anorexia and icterus accompany cutaneous lesions in some cases. Hepatopathy and nephrosis have been reported. Similar symmetrical lesions of the oral mucosa, mucocutaneous junctions, and pressure points have been reported in dogs exposed to *Simarouba* shavings.

Quassinoids have been shown experimentally to have insecticidal and anthelmintic properties, whereas their derivatives have antitumor, antiulcer, and cytotoxic activity in vitro. The mechanisms leading to toxicity are not known. Definitive diagnosis is dependent upon a compatible history, exclusion of viral diseases such as vesicular stomatitis, and exposure to other toxins, and the positive identification of plants of the *Quassia* genus in the bedding material.

Further reading

Declercq J. Suspected wood poisoning caused by *Simarouba amara* (marupa/caixeta) shavings in two dogs with erosive stomatitis and dermatitis. Vet Dermatol 2004;15:188-193.

Matsumura T. *Simarouba* poisoning in horses—Japan. Equine Dis Q 2002;10:2.

ACTINIC DISEASES OF SKIN

The radiant energy of the sun includes components that are potentially harmful to mammalian skin. This radiation is known as **actinic radiation,** and its acute effect is the well-known *sunburn* reaction. **Photosensitization** is essentially an *exacerbated form of sunburn,* caused by the activation of photodynamic chemicals in the skin by radiation of an appropriate wavelength and is discussed under the heading Photosensitization dermatitis. **Photoallergy** is distinct from phototoxicity; *it occurs when the photoproduct of an exogenous chemical acts as an antigen*. Photoallergic reactions require prior sensitization to the drug or chemical and are more clinically diverse. Photoallergies have not been documented conclusively in animals. **Skin cancers** induced or exacerbated by actinic radiation are considered with Tumors of the epidermis. The terms "actinic" and "solar" are used interchangeably; however, "actinic" is defined as ultraviolet (UV) rays from sunlight and UV lamps, whereas "solar" refers to radiation from the sun.

Direct effect of solar radiation

Solar energy is a form of nonionizing radiation composed of UV light (100-400 nm), visible light (400-700 nm), and infrared light (700 nm to 1 mm) rays. *Most of the direct photobiologic reactions in the skin are induced by high-energy light in the ultraviolet radiation UVB range (290-320 nm)*. Longer wavelengths of 320-400 nm constitute UVA and may augment UVB-mediated damage. The integument is normally protected against the deleterious effects of ultraviolet radiation by the haircoat, the stratum corneum, and melanin pigmentation. The quantity of ozone, smog, altitude, latitude, season of the year, and time of day also strongly influence the amount of UV rays reaching the skin. The greatest potential for solar-induced skin damage occurs at high altitudes and temperate latitudes during mid-summer days, and in thin, lightly pigmented, sparsely haired, sun-exposed skin. An increasing prevalence of sun-induced dermatoses and tumors has been noted in humans, coincident with *the depletion of the ozone layer and a consequent increase in the intensity of UV radiation reaching the earth's surface.* This trend may also become evident in animals. Potentially, all animals are susceptible to the acute and chronic effects of actinic radiation, but the protection afforded by the haircoat, and, to a lesser extent, stratum corneum and skin pigmentation, is normally sufficient to prevent solar-induced damage. The conditions described below typically affect animals whose anatomic defenses are poor, either by lacking skin pigmentation or hair cover.

UVB radiation stimulates light-absorbing molecules in the skin referred to as chromophores. *Chromophores include keratin proteins, melanin, carotene, nucleic acids, peptide bonds, and some amino acids*, to name a few. Light absorbed by chromophores results in electron transfers and *free radical* production. Energy dissipated from electron transfers induces chemical reactions to form altered cell components referred to as *photoproducts*, which include altered DNA molecules, enzymes, and hydrogen and disulfide bonds within proteins. Nucleoprotein is susceptible to UV radiation damage, resulting in mitotic inhibition and, if extensive enough, cell death. Sublethal damage may promote mutagenesis or carcinogenesis by the formation of thymidine dimers between pyrimidine base pairs of DNA. Pyrimidine dimer repair mechanisms normally correct DNA damage prior to cell replication; however, repeated or extensive damage may lead to failure of repair mechanisms and cell transformation. The *"sunburn cell"* associated with UV damage is a keratinocyte that has undergone apoptosis. UVB-induced keratinocyte apoptosis is a complex event that involves cytokines such as tumor necrosis factor-α and probable p53-mediated induction of apoptosis in cells sustaining substantial DNA damage. Studies in mice have shown that UVB radiation–induced apoptotic keratinocytes are replaced by hyperproliferative keratinocytes, leading to epidermal hyperplasia, suggesting that apoptosis and hyperplasia are related events. UV light also induces mutations of the p53 tumor suppressor gene in keratinocytes, contributing to a proliferative advantage to mutated cells that is found in solar-induced actinic keratoses and squamous cell carcinomas in humans. These findings indicate that UV radiation can serve as both a tumor initiator and promoter. UV radiation may also alter immunologic reactivity in favor of the growth of the tumor, through the induction of suppressor T cells and possible impairment of natural killer–cell function. UVB radiation exposure reduces the number of Langerhans cells and impairs their antigen-presenting functions. Contact hypersensitivity responses in experimental animals are reduced following UVB irradiation.

Apoptotic keratinocytes, "sunburn cells," arranged singly or in clusters or bands in the outer stratum spinosum, are a characteristic microscopic feature of acute sun-induced epithelial damage. These may be induced within 30 minutes of sun exposure. Other lesions include spongiosis, vacuolation of keratinocytes, loss of the granular layer, and, in severe burns, vesiculation. Dermal hyperemia and edema are prominent features. In mild lesions, there is a slight increase in mononuclear cells; in severe burns, there is marked vascular damage, erythrocyte extravasation, and neutrophilic exocytosis. The initial lesion of UV irradiation–induced injury consists of transient erythema, probably resulting from a direct heating effect and the photobiologic effects of UVB acting directly on dermal capillaries. The delayed erythema reaction may be due to direct damage to endothelial cells or the release of cytokines from the radiation-damaged keratinocytes. UV radiation has been shown to increase the production of keratinocyte-derived cytokines. UV light also induces adaptive responses in the epidermis, in particular epidermal hyperplasia and alterations in melanin pigmentation. An immediate pigment darkening is due to changes in existing melanin, and the delayed or

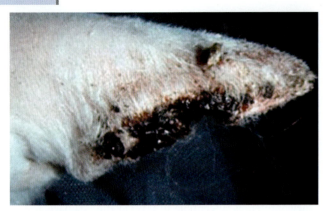

Figure 6-51 Squamous cell carcinoma on the pinna of a white cat, with erythematous, crusted patches, and plaques, likely a progression from **solar dermatitis.**

"tanning" reaction to stimulation of melanogenesis and proliferation of melanocytes. *Melanin both absorbs and scatters UV radiation and, being able to trap free radicals, is important in minimizing the deleterious effects of incident photons.* Basal keratinocytes with melanin granules forming protective caps over the nucleus have an increased distribution in sun-exposed skin. In chronically sun-damaged skin, pigment distribution can become irregular because of impaired transfer of melanin from melanocytes to keratinocytes, thereby weakening host defenses. *Long-term effects* of UV irradiation include variable degenerative changes in the dermis (solar elastosis and fibrosis), adnexa (comedones, cysts), and epidermis (solar keratosis). Lesions vary by species and among individuals within the species.

Solar dermatitis, or *sunburn,* occurs most frequently in *cats, dogs, pigs, cows, and goats.* The lesions in *cats* typically affect the tips of the ears, nose, eyelids, and lips of white, blue-eyed animals. The initial lesion is erythema followed by alopecia, scaling, and crusting. The ear tip may curl over. Lesions are exacerbated each summer, often eventuating in malignant transformation into squamous cell carcinoma (Fig. 6-51). Primary phototoxicity in swine occurs in white or light-colored *pigs.* Although any age group may be affected, the condition is most severe in suckling and weaner pigs. Occasionally, severely affected ears may slough. Light-colored *goats* and *cows* are also prone to solar dermatitis. The udders are particularly susceptible when does are turned out into strong sunlight after a winter indoors.

Solar dermatitis occurs most often in *shorthaired dogs with light pigmentation.* Breeds most often affected include Bull Terriers, Whippets, Beagles, and Dalmatians. Lesions are most often present on the ventrolateral abdomen and thorax, lateral flank, hocks, and bridge of nose in nonpigmented skin. Such lesions are probably related to the basking behavior exhibited by the animals. *Early lesions of erythema and scaling evolve into thick, lichenified, erythematous, crusted patches and plaques.* Hemorrhagic bullae may develop. The most consistent histologic finding in dogs with chronic solar dermatitis is a *narrow, hypocellular, pale-staining band of collagen along the dermoepidermal junction.* This change may be present prior to clinical signs of actinic dermatitis and may be used as an indicator of solar damage if the history, anatomic site, and breed are supportive. Other changes noted in canine sun-damaged skin include epidermal acanthosis, epitrichial gland ectasia, and follicular keratosis, resulting in follicular cyst formation and

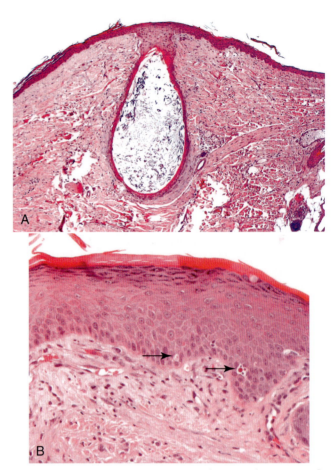

Figure 6-52 Solar dermatitis. **A.** Hyperplastic epidermis, superficial layer of pale dermal collagen, and comedone formation. **B.** A few individually necrotic keratinocytes in the lower epidermis (arrows).

possible furunculosis, particularly over pressure points (Fig. 6-52A). A layer of fibrosis often surrounds cystic follicles. A superficial perivascular mixed infiltrate of lymphocytes, plasma cells, monocytes, neutrophils, and rare eosinophils is usually present. Furunculosis leads to a marked foreign body response. Follicular changes are thought to be due to loss of support of follicles; however, elastin studies in dogs have not demonstrated degeneration of elastin fibers supporting the follicular wall. Advanced lesions may have epidermal dysplasia (Fig. 6-52B) or concurrent UV light–induced neoplasms, such as squamous cell carcinoma, hemangioma, or hemangiosarcoma. It is important to note that UV light–induced neoplasms may arise in skin devoid of other changes suggestive of actinic damage. *Actinic comedones* may also be present without lesions suggestive of actinic epidermal damage. *Differentials* are many and include other conditions resulting in comedone formation, acne, various allergies, bacterial or fungal infections, neoplasia, or a primary keratinization disorder. Restriction of lesions to nonpigmented, sparsely haired skin and a history of sun exposure should be helpful in differentiation.

Increased cyclooxygenase-2 (COX-2) expression appears to play an early role in actinic keratosis and squamous cell carcinoma in rodent studies and humans. COX-2 overexpression leads to increased expression of prostaglandin E2 (PGE_2). Activation of the COX-2/PGE_2 pathway induces cell

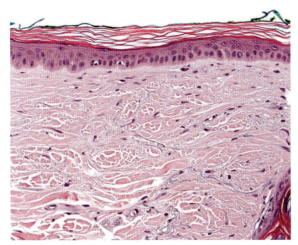

Figure 6-53 Solar elastosis. The dermis is filled with agglomerated, thick, irregular, basophilic, degenerate elastic fibers.

proliferation, inhibits apoptosis, and promotes angiogenesis and carcinogenesis. COX-2 expression has been shown in feline, canine, and equine cutaneous squamous cell carcinoma (SCC). Furthermore, use of COX-2 inhibitors may have a therapeutic role in the prevention or management of actinic keratosis and SCC.

Solar elastosis, a hallmark of chronic sun exposure in humans, has been described only rarely in *dogs, cats, sheep, and horses* and essentially represents *disorganization of dermal components caused by altered fibroblast function*. The lesions usually occur in conjunction with solar radiation–associated neoplasms, particularly SCCs. Solar elastosis appears in H&E-stained sections as *scattered or agglomerated, thick, irregular, basophilic degenerate elastic fibers* (Fig. 6-53). Silver impregnation staining techniques may be needed to demonstrate elastin changes in animals. Solar dermatitis is often present without evidence of elastosis.

Solar keratoses, common *precancerous skin lesions* in humans, occur in cats, dogs, and horses. The conjunctiva of horses with white eyelids is a common site. Histologically, the early lesions have many of the features of sunburn, including epidermal hyperplasia, spongiosis, acute dermal inflammation, and focal necrotic keratinocytes. More chronic lesions show pronounced epidermal hyperplasia with *dysplasia*, orthokeratotic and parakeratotic hyperkeratosis, perivascular mononuclear cell infiltrates, and dermal scarring, but seldom develop significant solar elastosis, as typifies human solar keratoses. *Lesions frequently progress to invasive SCC.* Solar keratoses may also develop cutaneous horns.

Further reading

Almeida EM, et al. Photodamage in feline skin: clinical and histomorphometric analysis. Vet Pathol 2008;45:327-335.

Bardagí M, et al. Immunohistochemical detection of COX-2 in feline and canine actinic keratoses and cutaneous squamous cell carcinoma. J Comp Pathol 2012;146:11-77.

Gross TL, et al. Hyperplastic diseases of the epidermis. In: Gross TL, et al., editors. Skin Diseases of the Dog and Cat: Clinical and Histopathological Diagnosis. 2nd ed. Oxford, UK: Blackwell; 2005. p. 148-151.

Hargis AM. Actinic keratosis and squamous cell carcinoma. J Small Anim Dermatol Pract 2009;2:12-24.

Photosensitization dermatitis

Photosensitization dermatitis occurs in animals when photodynamic or fluorescent pigments are deposited in sunlight-exposed skin. Photodynamic pigments absorb UV light or visible light in the action spectrum and convert it to light of a longer wavelength, usually beyond the UVB range. The energy from the absorbed light leads to tissue injury by reacting directly with molecular oxygen, producing reactive oxygen intermediates, such as superoxide anion, singlet oxygen, and hydroxyl radical. Oxygen free radicals may also be formed indirectly, as the result of calcium-dependent, protease-mediated activation of xanthine-oxidase in the skin. Release of reactive oxygen species initiates chain reactions that lead to mast cell degranulation and damage to cell membranes, nucleic acids, proteins and subcellular organelles, particularly lysosomes and mitochondria.

The photodynamic agent usually reaches the skin via the *systemic circulation*, although *percutaneous absorption* of some photodynamic agents can cause local contact photosensitization. The agent may originate externally, or it may be an endogenous substance that has accumulated to an abnormal degree as a result of metabolic dysfunction. Sources include *plant pigments and drugs* or, in the case of metabolic dysfunction, the *byproducts of hemoglobin metabolism or chlorophyll degradation products*. The 3 categories of photosensitization are classified according to the source of the agents.

- In *type I, or primary, photosensitization*, the animal *ingests plants or drugs* containing photoreactive substances that are deposited in the skin. Most exogenous sources of photoreactive pigments are found in plants, and therefore foraging animals, such as horses, sheep, cattle, and goats, are most frequently affected.
- In *type II photosensitization*, an inherent inability to properly metabolize heme pigments necessary for erythrocyte production leads to the build-up of the photoreactive pigments, *hematoporphyrins*.
- An abnormal build-up of *phylloerythrin*, a degradation product of chlorophyll, induces *type III photosensitization*. This is known also as *hepatogenous photosensitization* because it depends upon the failure of a damaged or immature liver to eliminate phylloerythrin. Type III photosensitization occurs most often in animals ingesting large amounts of green forage.
- A fourth group contains those examples of photosensitization for which the pathogenesis is presently undetermined.

The **gross lesions** are similar for all forms of photosensitization. They occur on those areas of the body most exposed to sunlight and that lack protective fleece, haircoat, or skin pigmentation. In *cattle*, any area of light-colored skin is susceptible. This is best demonstrated in broken-colored animals such as Holsteins, in which the white skin is affected, but the black is spared. The relatively hairless skin of the teats, udder, perineum, and muzzle is also affected. The ventral surface of the tongue is frequently affected in cattle if constantly exposed during licking. In *sheep*, the susceptible sites are the ears, eyelids, face, muzzle, and coronets, although the back may be affected in animals with an open fleece or that have been shorn closely. The udders and teats of dairy *goats* are predisposed. In *horses*, lesions are most common on the face, perineum, and distal extremities but may affect any white skin. Lesions in *pigs* are uncommon, and have a predilection for the ears, eyelids, udder, and back. Photosensitization is rare in *dogs* and *cats*, and causative agents remain obscure.

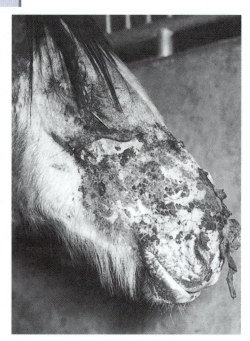

Figure 6-54 Photosensitization in a horse. Note necrosis and sloughing of skin from white areas of the face.

The initial reaction in photosensitization is erythema, followed by edema, which is more prominent in sheep than in cattle. The very marked edema of the ears in sheep causes them to droop, and swelling of the muzzle may cause dyspnea. The disease in sheep is appropriately known as "bighead" or geeldikkop, a South African term meaning "thick, yellow head"; the equivalent term in New Zealand is "facial eczema." The lesions are *intensely pruritic*, causing rubbing, scratching, and kicking at affected parts. Vesicles or bullae may develop. There is marked exudation and extensive necrosis. Affected skin becomes dry and sloughs in desiccated sheets (Fig. 6-54). Necrosis is frequently seen on the upper surfaces of the ears of sheep; the tips typically curl upward as a result of mummification or may slough entirely. There is swelling of the eyelids and excessive lacrimation. Among the more obscure manifestations of photosensitization is the convulsive reaction of some sheep and cattle, photosensitized by ingestion of St. John's wort, on contact with cold water. *Icterus* typically is associated with hepatogenous photosensitization, but hepatogenous photosensitization may occur in its absence. Economic losses in livestock can be severe due to damaged hides, weight loss, fly strikes, secondary infections, and reluctance of animals to let the young nurse damaged udders. In severe episodes of photosensitization, animals may die. This is more often the result of concomitant damage to other organs, particularly the liver, than to cutaneous damage alone. Injury to erythrocytes in cutaneous circulation may produce severe hemolysis.

Histologic lesions mirror the gross lesions with *coagulative necrosis of the epidermis* and possibly the follicular epithelium, adnexal glands, and superficial dermis. Subepidermal clefts or vesicles form, and the *dermis is edematous*. Endothelial cells of the superficial, mid, and occasionally deep dermal vessels are often swollen or necrotic. Fibrinoid degeneration of vessel walls and thrombosis may be present. Initially, inflammation is sparse, but soon the lesions are infiltrated by neutrophils. Secondary bacterial colonization is common.

Differential diagnosis should include other vesicular or necrotizing dermatopathies, including chemical or thermal burns. *Establishing the diagnosis is dependent upon anatomic distribution of lesions in nonpigmented, poorly haired, sun-exposed regions.* Lesions limited to areas of contact, such as the extremities, ventrum, or muzzle, suggests the presence of a contact photosensitizing agent. Multiple affected animals in a herd suggest exposure to a photosensitizing agent rather than a photoallergic reaction. Types I, II, and III photosensitivities can be differentiated by signalment and concurrent clinical signs, such as evidence of liver disease combined with examination of pastures and feedstuffs, and investigating photodynamic drug or chemical exposure. The *Candida albicans* inhibition assay is a simple, inexpensive, quantitative, and relatively rapid assay for screening plants and feedstuffs for potential primary contact or systemic photosensitizers. The test does not detect all phototoxins. Thin-layer chromatography techniques may be useful in identifying phototoxic compounds. Analysis of suspect vegetation for the identification and quantification of fungal spores may be needed to establish fungal organisms and associated mycotoxins as contributing factors.

Primary photosensitization (type I photosensitization)

Plants are the most common cause of primary photosensitization; hence herbivores are most commonly affected. Additional sources include *mycotoxins, molds, chemicals, and drugs. The majority of photosensitizing plants contain pigments belonging to either the helianthrone or furocoumarin family of pigments.*

The **helianthrones** include the red fluorescent pigments, *hypericin, and fagopyrin*. Some of the most commonly implicated plants include St. John's wort (*Hypericum perforatum*) and buckwheat (*Fagopyrum* spp.), and the resulting diseases are referred to as *hypericism* and *fagopyrism*, respectively. Photosensitization induced by St. John's wort affects horses, cattle, sheep, and goats. Hypericin is present at all stages of plant growth but significant amounts are consumed by livestock only when the plant is prolific or other feed is scarce. Other related plants that can lead to hypericism include goatweed, Tipton weed, amber, cammock, and Klamath weed. Photosensitization induced by buckwheat affects sheep, pigs, cattle, goats, and horses.

The **furocoumarin** family of pigments contains the photodynamic agents, *psoralens*. Photosensitization occurs in cattle, sheep, white chickens, and ducks as a result of ingestion of plants such as spring parsley (*Cymopterus watsonii*), bishop's weed (*Ammi majus*), and Dutchman's breeches (*Thamnosma texana*). The furocoumarins differ from the helianthrone-photosensitizing pigments by inducing, additionally, *corneal edema and keratoconjunctivitis*. Primary photodermatitis of pigs in Argentina occurred after consumption of feed contaminated with *Ammi majus* seeds containing the furocoumarin xanthotoxin. Furocoumarins have also been documented to form *phytoalexins* in fungus-infected parsnips (*Pastinaca sativa*) and celery (*Apium graveolens*), leading to **phytophotocontact dermatitis.** *Psoralens* adsorbed onto the skin react with UV light. These have been associated with phytophotocontact dermatitis in pigs in New Zealand. Lesions were vesicular, affecting only the dorsal aspect of the snout. Rubbing the snouts and feet of white pigs with the leaves of the fungus-infected celery and parsnips before exposing the areas to

UV light reproduced the lesions. *Cymopterus watsoni* causes phytophotodermatitis in sheep in Utah and Nevada. Lesions principally affected the nonwooled areas, such as the muzzle, lips, and udder. High lamb mortality may be incurred from mismothering. Contact photodermatitis suspected to be caused by giant hogweed *(Heracleum mantegazzianum)* occurred in dogs. Giant hogweed contains psoralens and has been documented to cause photodermatitis in man, ducks, and goats.

Texas cattle and deer develop primary photosensitization after consuming moldy leaves of *Cooperia pedunculata*. In addition to skin lesions, keratitis occurs frequently and may lead to blindness.

Ingestion of alsike clover *(Trifolium hybridum)*, also known as red clover hay, results in a primary photodermatitis referred to as *trifoliosis* in cattle, sheep, hogs, and some horses. Trifoliosis has been reported in the United States, Canada, Australia, and England. A second syndrome, referred to as *alsike clover poisoning*, is characterized by hepatic dysfunction and photodermatitis and has only been reported in the horse. The toxic mechanism is not known but is thought to be due to a toxin within the plant itself or to the presence of a mycotoxin. The variable presentations are speculated to be related to seasonal changes, stage of plant growth, and soil and environmental conditions.

A condition clinically and histologically compatible with a primary photodermatitis occurred in 12 of 30 Harrier Hounds in a kennel in New Zealand. Lesions were limited to the nonpigmented, sun-exposed skin of the tricolored hounds and resolved within a short period of time with supportive care. The hounds were fed a diet of horse and cattle meat. Although an ingested compound was suspected as the cause, no phototoxin could be identified. Similar cases have been reported in Foxhounds in England and Border Collie dogs in New Zealand. Photosensitization has been reported in a cat receiving clofazimine for the treatment of feline leprosy.

Phenothiazine photosensitization is characterized by typical cutaneous lesions and in ruminants by the additional lesions of corneal edema and keratoconjunctivitis. The secretion of the ruminal metabolite, phenothiazine sulfoxide, in tears and aqueous humor, has explained the unusual location of the lesions. Phenothiazine photosensitization occurs most commonly in *calves* but also in *sheep, swine, and birds*. Pigs develop cutaneous lesions more frequently than sheep or cattle, probably because the activating radiation is more able to penetrate the integument. The greater susceptibility of calves has been ascribed to a relatively inefficient conversion of the photodynamic sulfoxide metabolite back to phenothiazine in the liver. This conversion depends on effective mixed-function oxidase enzyme activity in the liver.

Photosensitization resulting from defective pigment synthesis (type II photosensitization)

Photosensitization resulting from *endogenous pigment accumulation* occurs because of a congenital enzyme deficiency causing abnormal heme synthesis, with the resultant blood and tissue accumulation of photodynamic agents, such as *uroporphyrin I, coproporphyrin I, and protoporphyrin III*.

Bovine congenital hematopoietic porphyria is the result of *a deficiency in uroporphyrinogen III cosynthetase*, a key enzyme in heme biosynthesis. The condition is inherited as a simple recessive trait affecting many breeds, including Shorthorn, Ayrshire, Holstein, and Jamaican cattle. It has also been reported in crossbred cattle. The disease is known as "osteohemochromatosis" and "pink tooth," both suggested by the *red-brown coloration of porphyrin pigments in dentin and bone*. The pigment is also deposited in other tissues, but the discoloration may be obvious only in lungs, spleen, and kidney, in which it is deposited in the interstitial tissue and tubular epithelium.

The pigments are *excreted in the urine;* hence the alternative names "porphyrinuria" and "hematoporphyrinuria." Affected urine is amber to brown, darkens on exposure to light, and fluoresces bright red on exposure to UV radiation. *Affected teeth and bones also fluoresce*. The anemia of bovine congenital erythropoietic porphyria is discussed in Vol. 3, Hematopoietic system.

The cutaneous lesions result from the photodynamic properties of the accumulated porphyrins, in particular the *uroporphyrins* that absorb UVA radiation. Reactive oxygen species directly induced by the porphyrins or, possibly, via activation of xanthine oxidase in the skin are responsible for the cell membrane damage. The gross cutaneous lesions are typical of photosensitization. The microscopic lesions closely resemble those of erythropoietic porphyrias in man. The chief lesions are subepidermal clefts, hyalinization of dermal capillary walls, and a minimal infiltrate of inflammatory cells. The basement membrane zone lines the base of the subepidermal cleft, in some instances covering small projections of dermal papillae (festoons). Festoons are a more prominent feature of the human lesion because dermal papillae are better developed in human skin.

Bovine erythropoietic protoporphyria is inherited as a *recessive trait in Limousin cattle* in the United States. It differs from bovine congenital porphyria in that photodermatitis is the sole clinical manifestation of the disease. Animals do not have discolored teeth, anemia, or urine porphyrin excretion. The enzyme defect is a *deficiency of ferrochelatase*, which allows protoporphyrin IX to accumulate in blood and tissues. Heterozygotes have reduced (50%) ferrochelatase activity and are clinically normal.

Porphyria of **swine** is inherited as a *dominant characteristic*. Although it mimics certain aspects of bovine erythropoietic porphyria, *photosensitization does not occur*, even in white-skinned animals. The defect in porcine porphyria is not known.

Photosensitization occurs in Siamese **cats** with excessive accumulation of uroporphyrinogen I, coproporphyrinogen I, and protoporphyrins in blood, urine, feces, and tissues. The defect is presumably a *deficiency of uroporphyrinogen cosynthetase III*, as has been established in humans and cattle.

Hepatogenous photosensitization (type III photosensitization)

The most common form of photosensitization in domestic animals occurs in conjunction with primary hepatocellular damage or, less commonly, bile duct obstruction and is due to impaired capacity of the liver to excrete the potent photodynamic agent, **phylloerythrin.** Phylloerythrin is a chlorophyll catabolite formed by microbial action in the intestinal tract and transported to the liver via the portal circulation. Hepatocytes assimilate the phylloerythrin and excrete it into the bile. One of the earliest signs of liver cell damage is a reduced ability to transport and excrete phylloerythrin. Mild renal tubular damage caused by some toxins may further inhibit the excretion of phylloerythrin. The circulating phylloerythrin accumulates in tissues, including the skin. Photodermatitis occurs provided the animal is on a chlorophyll-rich diet and is exposed to sufficient solar radiation of the appropriate wavelength. High ambient solar radiation and lack of shade are contributing factors. Photosensitization tends to occur most often when the hepatic damage is generalized, even if mild. Severe focal necrotizing lesions of the liver generally do not cause photosensitization because there is enough hepatic reserve to remove the phylloerythrin from the circulation. The cause of hepatic damage may be a plant toxin, mycotoxin, infectious agent, or chemical.

Toxic plants and mycotoxins account for most cases of hepatogenous photosensitization. A few of the many plants implicated in hepatotoxic photosensitization include lantana (*Lantana camara*), bog asphodel (*Narthecium ossifragum*), *Tribulus terrestris*, *Agave lecheguilla*, *Nolina texana*, *Cymadothea trifolii*–infested clover, *Trifolium hybridum* ("alsike clover poisoning"), and *Panicum* spp. grasses, such as kleingrass (*Panicum coloratum*). Kleingrass is a perennial grass forage crop with a toxic principle suspected to be a saponin. Cases of kleingrass induced–photosensitization are sporadic, potentially related to environmental conditions and have been reported in Australia, Africa, and Texas. Some plants work in combination; black sagebrush appears to precondition sheep to photosensitization caused ultimately by *Tetradymia* spp.

A number of reports of hepatogenous photosensitization in livestock cite a variety of common forage crops, such as alfalfa hay or silage, winter wheat, Bermuda grass pasture, crab grass, oat stubble, or various clover pastures. In the majority of cases, the toxicity was preceded by unusual climatic conditions of drought, increased rainfall, or temperature variations. In many cases, a specific toxic compound cannot be identified. A plausible explanation is the establishment of optimum conditions for the production of mycotoxins, hepatotoxins, or photodynamic agents in the damaged plant material.

Forages containing the mycotoxin *sporidesmin*, from spores of *Pithomyces chartarum*, cause **facial eczema,** an economically important hepatogenous photosensitization of sheep and cattle in Australia, New Zealand, South Africa, and the northwestern United States. *Geeldikkop*, a disease characterized by hepatogenous photosensitization, is associated with extensive losses among sheep and goats in South Africa. A hepatogenous photosensitization, secondary to a presumed genetic defect in phylloerythrin transport, has been reported in Corriedale lambs.

Hepatic dicrocoeliosis has been identified as a probable cause of photosensitization affecting a group of 14-month-old ewe lambs in Scotland. Hepatogenous photosensitization is discussed in more detail in Vol. 2, Liver and biliary system.

Further reading

Bennett S. Photosensitization induced by clofazimine in a cat. Aust Vet J 2007;85:375-380.

Campbell WM, et al. Photodynamic chlorophyll a metabolites, including phytoporphyrin (phylloerythrin), in the blood of photosensitive livestock: overview and measurement. N Z Vet J 2010;58:146-154.

Quinn JC, et al. Secondary plant products causing photosensitization in grazing herbivores: their structure, activity and regulation. Int J Mol Sci 2014;15:1441-1465.

Riet-Correa F, et al. Mycotoxicoses of ruminants and horses. J Vet Diagn Invest 2013;25:692-708.

Sargison ND, et al. Hepatogenous photosensitisation in Scottish sheep casued by *Dicrocoelium dendriticum*. Vet Parasitol 2012;189:233-237.

Photoaggravated dermatoses

In humans, several autoimmune dermatoses are exacerbated by exposure to UV light. These include pemphigus, lupus erythematosus, and bullous pemphigoid. A similar relationship has been proposed in the analogous canine diseases.

A poorly understood disease in the *horse*, **photoactivated vasculitis** affects only the white-haired extremities. The pathogenesis is not currently known. An immune-mediated vasculitis, in which immune complexes may be acting as photodynamic agents has been proposed. Percutaneous absorption of initiating agents has not been ruled out. Affected horses have normal liver function and no known exposure to photosensitizing compounds. In addition, lesions may be restricted to one white extremity, other white areas on the horse are unaffected, and the lesions do not always regress with cessation of exposure to sunlight, all indicating the lesions are *not a form of photosensitization*. The lesions often affect the heels and must be differentiated from the other manifestations of the "greasy heel" complex. The acute lesions are well demarcated, erythematous, oozing, and crusted in lesional white skin; erosion and ulceration may occur, and the affected limb may be edematous and painful. The lesions tend to occur on the lateral and medial aspects of unpigmented hindlegs. The chronic lesions are hyperkeratotic plaques. Histologically, there is dermal edema, vascular dilation and intramural inflammatory cells, leukocytoclasia with nuclear dust, microhemorrhages, and thickening of the vessel wall of the small superficial, mid, and deep dermal vessels. Thrombi may be seen occasionally. The epidermis may be eroded or ulcerated but undergoes papillary hyperplasia over time.

Further reading

Psalla D, et al. Equine pastern vasculitis: a clinical and histopathological study. Vet J 2013;198:524-530.

White SD, et al. Cutaneous vasculitis in equines: a retrospective study of 72 cases. Vet Dermatol 2009;20:600-606.

NUTRITIONAL DISEASES OF SKIN

The elasticity of the skin, the orderly maturation of the epidermis, and the quality and luster of the horny appendages are an indication of the state of the health of the animal as a whole. This applies equally to nutritional diseases and to diseases of other causes. Many systemic diseases result in cutaneous changes. The general metabolic transformations that take place in the skin are not qualitatively different from those in other tissues, but there are some quantitative differences, such as the high requirements and turnover of sulfur-containing amino acids in the elaboration of keratin. *In most metabolic disturbances and deficiencies of essential nutrients, whether from dietary lack, malabsorption, the action of antimetabolites, or the body's inability to properly absorb or use nutrients, changes will be reflected in the skin.* The molecular basis for these skin lesions is, however, poorly understood. There are only a few syndromes that occur naturally and are sufficiently clearly defined to warrant discussion here. A larger number can be produced experimentally. Cutaneous manifestations of systemic disease not known to be a result of a nutritional derangement are discussed in other, more appropriate sections of this chapter, such as Endocrine diseases of skin and Cutaneous paraneoplastic syndromes.

Protein-calorie deficiency

Starvation or protein-calorie malnutrition results in changes in the skin, the first being the *disappearance of subcutaneous fat*. Even though water intake may not be restricted, there is reduced hydration of the connective tissues of the subcutis and dermis, and the skin wrinkles and loses its elasticity. As hair is 95% protein, *hair growth and keratinization can require up to 25-30% of an animal's daily protein requirement*. Protein deficiencies are rare but can occur in cats fed primarily food formulated for dogs, in young dogs fed a low-protein diet, or in animals with increased nutrient requirements.

An early sign of starvation is the development of a *dull, dry, and often brittle haircoat*. Hypotrichosis develops as a thinning of the hair rather than baldness, and seasonal shedding may cease or be prolonged. Lesions may be symmetrical on the head and trunk and spread to the limbs. The skin may atrophy, or hyperkeratosis, hyperpigmentation, and possibly loss of hair pigmentation develop. The histopathologic findings in the skin may mimic an endocrinopathy, with severe epidermal and adnexal atrophy, orthokeratotic hyperkeratosis, and telogenization of hair follicles. In pigs, the skin often becomes hyperkeratotic and assumes a dirty, dry appearance, and the hair becomes long and shaggy. The skin of a malnourished animal has an increased susceptibility to bacterial infection and parasitic infestations and their effects. Under-nutrition of the pregnant ewe, between 115-135 days of gestation, decreases the number of secondary wool follicles in the developing fetus. Most experimental work on the effects of nutrition on hair growth has been performed in sheep, the purpose being either to improve wool production or to investigate chemical methods of shearing. Changing sheep from a low-protein to a high-protein diet led to a 33% increase in fleece production, attributed mostly to an increase in the rate of mitosis in the hair bulb. Specific amino acid deficiencies have been investigated as potential replacements for mechanical shearing as wool production is highly dependent upon levels of certain amino acids, specifically cysteine.

The effects of starvation on other organs such as liver, pancreas, bone, and bone marrow are discussed elsewhere.

Fatty acid deficiency

Fatty acid deficiency may occur in all domestic species in association with general dietary deficiency, malabsorption, or liver disease. Deficiencies may be evident in animals when the fat has either leached from a diet, has become rancid from improper or prolonged storage, or when the diet was formulated with low fat content to save cost. Animals on specially formulated low-fat diets for therapeutic reasons may develop signs of fatty acid deficiency and require specific types of supplementation. Animals on antioxidant-deficient diets may also develop signs of fatty acid deficiency. Cutaneous lesions take months to develop and begin with *diffuse scaling, loss of haircoat sheen, and alopecia*. The scaliness is initially dry but over months progresses to an oily, often pruritic stage. Otitis externa may be an accompanying lesion, and the skin is susceptible to secondary bacterial and yeast infection. Histologic lesions include *epidermal hyperplasia, orthokeratotic or parakeratotic hyperkeratosis, and hypergranulosis*. The pathologic mechanisms underlying the epidermal hyperproliferation are not well understood. Experimental studies demonstrated an increase in epidermal DNA synthesis and a decrease in prostaglandin E and F levels in the skin of essential fatty acid–deficient mice. The lower prostaglandin levels likely reflect a lack of precursor arachidonic acid. Deficiency of prostaglandin E_2 could influence epidermal cell kinetics through its effect on ratios of cyclic AMP to guanosine monophosphate (GMP). Supplementation of animal diets with balanced omega-6 and omega-3 fatty acids is thought to modulate arachidonic acid metabolism and subsequent production of leukotrienes and prostaglandins that, in turn, may influence epidermal turnover kinetics and the inflammatory response.

A seborrheic dermatosis in **cats,** characterized by dry scaly skin and alopecia, is responsive to fatty acid supplementation but is not likely to be the result of a true deficiency. Experimental essential fatty acid deprivation in cats produces dry, scaly coats. Diets containing linoleic acid and linolenic acids as the sole source of essential fatty acids also induce a seborrheic dermatosis. Cats are obligate carnivores, as they lack delta-6-desaturase, the enzyme responsible for converting these 18-carbon fatty acids to longer-chain fatty acids. Arachidonic acid is an essential fatty acid for the cat.

Hypovitaminoses and vitamin-responsive dermatoses

Cutaneous lesions may occur as manifestations of deficiencies of *vitamins A, C, and E; riboflavin; pantothenic acid; biotin; and niacin*. Most of these are described in experimentally induced deficiencies. Many of the naturally occurring hypovitaminoses are probably not the result of a single vitamin deficiency but represent the cumulative effect of several inadequacies of the diet.

Vitamin A deficiency

Vitamin A is a fat-soluble vitamin belonging to a group of compounds referred to as *retinoids*. Vitamin A is involved in cellular growth and differentiation, as well as in visual processes and reproduction. Vitamin A has a controlling effect on epithelial differentiation. *Cutaneous lesions of vitamin A deficiency are squamous epithelial hyperkeratosis and squamous metaplasia of secretory epithelia*. Vitamin A oversupplementation is teratogenic and can lead to toxicity if liver storage capacity is exceeded. Signs are manifest primarily in the skeletal system and liver, or as malformations of the fetus in pregnant animals.

Hypovitaminosis A has been reported in all species of domestic animals, although many accounts are anecdotal. It may be secondary to dietary deficiency, decreased intestinal absorption, liver disease, or toxicities such as chlorinated naphthalene toxicity of cattle. Bile and pancreatic enzymes are needed for dietary absorption of vitamin A. The cutaneous lesions of hypovitaminosis A in *cattle* are a marked scaling and crusting dermatitis; in the *pig*, follicular hyperkeratosis; and, in *cats*, scaling, follicular plugging, and alopecia. A report in the *dog* indicated thickened, hyperpigmented skin with alopecia and follicular hyperkeratosis.

Vitamin A–responsive dermatoses occur in **dogs** and almost exclusively in the Cocker Spaniel. In one syndrome, Cocker Spaniels are predisposed, probably because of a congenital abnormality of epidermopoiesis and keratinization (see Seborrhea). The condition is characterized by adult-onset

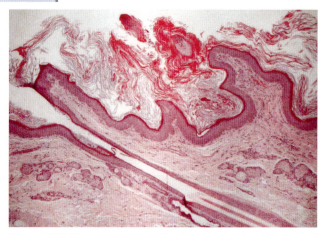

Figure 6-55 Vitamin A–responsive dermatosis. Note the marked follicular hyperkeratosis.

hyperkeratotic plaques, follicular plugging, and the formation of keratin fronds. Ventral and lateral chest and abdomen are sites of predilection. There may be accompanying ceruminous otitis externa and pyoderma. Histologically, *the predominant lesion is marked follicular orthokeratotic keratosis* (Fig. 6-55). Vertically oriented keratin casts protrude from the follicular ostia. There is mild to moderate epidermal hyperplasia and surface hyperkeratosis of the basket-weave type. Dermal inflammation is mild, mononuclear, and perivascular, unless secondary bacterial infection intervenes to produce neutrophilic folliculitis and/or furunculosis. There are rare reports of vitamin A–responsive dermatoses in other breeds of dogs. These diseases are not vitamin A deficiencies per se, in that plasma levels of vitamin A are within the normal range. The fact that therapy is effective can be attributed more to the "normalizing" effect of vitamin A (and retinoids) on cellular differentiation in the epidermis. Differentials include primary or secondary seborrhea and late-stage sebaceous adenitis. Oral supplementation with vitamin A may be needed to confirm the diagnosis.

Vitamin B deficiencies

The **B-vitamin complex** is essential to the maintenance and proper functioning of many important metabolic pathways. B vitamins are water soluble and not stored within the body, necessitating a constant dietary supply. These vitamins interact with each other, with vitamin C, and with fat-soluble vitamins. Single deficiencies of these vitamins are rare. *Deficiencies result in dry, flaky seborrhea with alopecia, anorexia, and weight loss.*

Riboflavin (vitamin B_2) deficiency is mostly a problem in *swine and chickens* fed grain rations with borderline concentrations of the vitamin. Ruminants do not become deficient because of rumen synthesis of the B-complex vitamins. Young calves, however, may develop deficiency if deprived of milk or an appropriate replacer. Animals develop hyperemia around the lips, nose, and buccal mucosa; diarrhea; weight loss; and generalized alopecia. Cutaneous lesions described in hyporiboflavinosis include scaling and ulcerative dermatitis in the pig, erythema, scaling, and dry haircoat on the ventral abdomen and hindlegs in the dog, and alopecia in the cat.

Pantothenic acid is a component of coenzyme A, an essential factor for entrance of acetic acid into the Krebs cycle. Deficiency is documented in *pigs*, but may occur in dogs and calves. Pantothenic acid deficiency in pigs produces progressive alopecia with dermatitis and ulceration, in addition to the general effects of weight loss, diarrhea, and neurologic signs. Young preruminant calves may show dermatologic signs that include alopecia, a roughened coat, and dermatitis. Leukotrichia has been described in dogs.

Biotin deficiency rarely occurs spontaneously, except in intensively reared *swine*, as the vitamin is widely distributed in feeds. Biotin is essential for proper use of fats, glucose, and amino acids. Feeding raw egg whites that contain avidin, a substance that renders biotin unavailable, may induce deficiencies. Cutaneous lesions reported in biotin-deficient pigs include *alopecia, pustular dermatitis, and cracked hooves*, causing lameness and significant economic loss. Microscopic lesions include epidermal hyperplasia, orthokeratotic and parakeratotic hyperkeratosis, epidermal necrosis and pustules, and folliculitis. A deficiency attributed, in part, to a lack of vitamin B, probably biotin, was reported in *lambs* reared artificially on reconstituted cow's milk. Alopecia was largely due to a fleece in which individual fibers were thin, weak, and straight. Histologically and ultrastructurally, the wool fibers had reduced numbers of cortical cells. Histochemical stains showed a delay in the incorporation and oxidation of sulfhydryl groups. Supplementation with B-group vitamins partially restored the fleece. Biotin deficiency reportedly causes a dry, brittle, haircoat, scaling, and leukotrichia in *dogs*. Dogs deficient in biotin may develop periocular and facial alopecia resembling the clinical lesions of systemic lupus erythematosus, discoid lupus, or other dermatoses affecting the face.

Niacin is a component of the pyridine nucleotides NAD^+ and $NADP^+$ needed for the function of a number of enzymes involved in nutrient metabolism. Deficiency occurs spontaneously in animals fed diets low in pyridoxine (vitamin B_6) and tryptophan, as all of these components are needed for pyridine nucleotide synthesis. *Pigs* fed a low animal-protein diet that is also high in corn renders niacin unavailable to the animal because of low tryptophan levels. Cutaneous lesions include alopecia and a crusting dermatitis. Niacin deficiency in *dogs* induces reddening and ulceration of the oral mucous membranes, resembling human hyponiacinosis, known as *pellagra*. Reports of canine cases from the first quarter of the 20th century indicate severe necrotizing glossitis and stomatitis, leading to the term *black tongue*.

Pyridoxine (vitamin B_6) serves as coenzyme in amino acid and protein metabolism. Deficiency produced experimentally in *cats* resulted in a dull, unkempt coat with scaliness and alopecia of the head and extremities. Histologically, hair follicles were in telogen, and there was epidermal and follicular hyperkeratosis. Because pyridoxine may be indirectly involved in zinc transport, through its effect on tryptophan metabolism, these effects might be due to alteration in the levels of zinc. Isoniazid has been reported to inactivate pyridoxine.

Vitamin C deficiency

Vitamin C (ascorbic acid) is required for the proper synthesis and structural maintenance of collagen and as a component of a number of essential enzymes. Almost all mammals synthesize vitamin C with the exception of humans, nonhuman primates, guinea pigs, Indian fruit bats, and Indian pipistrelles. Insects, invertebrates, and fish also cannot synthesize vitamin C. *Deficiencies (scurvy or scorbutus) are limited to these species of animals*, and signs are related to the inability of fibroblasts to form collagen or osteoid and are discussed in Vol. 1, Bones and joints.

Vitamin C–responsive dermatosis has been described in two 10-week-old dairy calves. The condition is characterized by nonpruritic scaling, alopecia, crusts, and easily epilated hair on the head and limbs. There may be erythema, petechiae, and ecchymoses on extremities. Severely affected calves may have systemic signs, such as depression and slow growth. Histologic changes include diffuse orthokeratotic hyperkeratosis, curlicue hairs, periadnexal hemorrhage, and vascular dilation and congestion.

Vitamin E deficiency

Vitamin E deficiency is discussed primarily in Vol. 1, Bones and joints and Vol. 2, Liver and biliary system. Steatitis or *"yellow-fat disease"* involves subcutaneous fat and may be seen clinically as a skin disease, and can result from consumption of high levels of unsaturated fatty acids and/or insufficient vitamin E. The yellowness of the fat is due to the *deposition of ceroid*. Vitamin E acts as an antioxidant to prevent lipid peroxidation. Dietary requirements vary by species and individual and with the other components of the diet. Naturally occurring vitamin E deficiency has not been reported in the dog.

Nutritional panniculitis occurs in cats, mink, foals, and swine. The disease is associated the feeding of fishmeal, fish offal, or other products with a high concentration of unsaturated fatty acids. Diets with a high content of oily fish, such as tuna, white fish, and sardines, are most often implicated; however, the condition in cats also has been associated with diets containing primarily pig's brain, liver, diets with only a small fish content, or improperly stored or outdated commercial cat food. The practice of feeding high-fish diets to cats is reported to be common in Greece. Destruction of vitamin E also occurs in food that, through improper processing or storage, becomes rancid. The disease is not, however, the result of a simple deficiency, because cats fed diets deficient in vitamin E but also lacking in unsaturated fatty acids, do not develop panniculitis. In *mink and foals*, it may be associated with degeneration of muscles, and in *swine* it may occur alone or be associated with any one or combination of ulceration of the squamous mucosa of the stomach, muscle degeneration, and hepatosis dietetica. The disease has variable mortality in *cats* after a short clinical course in which there is progressive depression, possible fever, hyperesthesia, reluctance to move, and palpable thickening and increased firmness of the subcutaneous fat, easiest to detect in the inguinal region. The changes are not confined to the subcutaneous tissues but affect all fat depots. Biopsy reveals fat that varies from gray to lemon yellow to orange and is indurated and sometimes edematous. Hematologic changes may include neutrophilic leukocytosis and anemia.

The initial histologic change is deposition of globules of ceroid in the interstitial tissue. This, together with a fishy odor, may be all that is observed in swine in which the fat is soft and gray rather than yellow. In most affected cats, *fat necrosis stimulates inflammation, which is initially neutrophilic but becomes granulomatous*. Numerous macrophages, and occasionally giant cells, ingest the ceroid pigment. Mineralization may be present. Ceroid may be found also in macrophages of the liver, spleen, and lymph nodes. In cats, the initial differential should include infectious steatitis, sterile nodular panniculitis, lupus panniculitis, or other noncutaneous diseases, such as feline infectious peritonitis, ascites of various causes, and other causes of hyperesthesia. *The clinical signs and the demonstration of ceroid, a variant of lipofuscin, which is acid fast and autofluorescent, should establish the diagnosis.*

Vitamin E–responsive dermatosis has been described in goats. Kids and adults on a selenium-deficient diet developed periorbital alopecia and generalized seborrhea. The haircoat was dull and brittle. Histologically, the lesions were orthokeratotic hyperkeratosis and mild superficial perivascular dermatitis, in which mononuclear cells predominated.

Alopecia in **calves** associated with the feeding of milk substitute was attributed, in part, to vitamin E deficiency. The calves had low levels of serum vitamin E, and the hair regrew after vitamin E therapy was initiated for concurrent nutritional myopathy.

Further reading

Blanchard PC, et al. Pathology associated with vitamin B-6 deficiency in growing kittens. J Nutr 1991;121:S77-S78.

Hensel P. Nutrition and skin diseases in veterinary medicine. Clin Dermatol 2010;28:686-693.

Miller WM. et al. Nutrition and skin diseases. In: Miller WH, et al., editors. Muller & Kirk's Small Animal Dermatology. 7th ed. St Louis: Elsevier; 2013. p. 685-694.

Niza MM, et al. Feline pansteatitis revisited: hazards of unbalanced home-made diets. J Feline Med Surg 2003;5:271-277.

Zini E, et al. Pansteatitis and severe hypocalcaemia in a cat. J Feline Med Surg 2007;9:168-171.

Mineral deficiency and mineral-responsive dermatoses

Iodine, cobalt, copper, and zinc deficiencies may lead to integumentary lesions. Iodine deficiency is discussed in Vol. 3, Endocrine glands. The effects of copper deficiency on wool and hair are referred to under Disorders of pigmentation. Cobalt deficiency causes a progressive, wasting disease in ruminants. There are nonspecific changes in the wool or haircoat, including lack of growth and increased fragility.

Zinc deficiency

Zinc is an essential trace element. Naturally occurring true zinc deficiency is rare in dogs, extremely rare in cats, and not reported in horses. Zinc-responsive dermatosis in dogs is discussed in the next section. In the integument, a substantial proportion of zinc is in the wool or the haircoat. Zinc is a component of many important metalloenzymes and is a cofactor for many others. It exerts its primary effect through zinc-dependent enzymes that regulate RNA and DNA metabolism. Zinc thus plays a role in all metabolic processes involved with tissue growth, maturation, and repair, and is involved in vitamin A metabolism and in enzymes needed for free radical scavenging. Zinc also modulates many aspects of the immune and inflammatory responses. The relationship between the changes in particular tissue enzyme activities brought about by zinc deficiency and clinical manifestations of the deficiency syndrome are not, however, well understood. Zinc is known to have an inhibitory effect on apoptotic pathways. The parakeratosis seen in cases of zinc deficiency and zinc-responsive dermatosis may be related to decreased activity of zinc-related lytic enzymes along with increased epidermal cell turnover, which results in failure of nuclear hydrolysis.

Zinc deficiency causes anorexia, alterations in food use, growth retardation, reproductive disorders, depression of the immune response, hematologic abnormalities, depression of central nervous system development, decreased wound healing, and keratinization defects in epidermis, hair, wool, and horny appendages. True zinc deficiency is of most significance in the pig.

Parakeratosis in swine. *Zinc-responsive dermatosis in swine (parakeratosis) became an important clinical entity in the 1950s, coincident with and related to the widespread introduction of dry meal feeding. The cause is not a simple deficiency.* The availability of dietary zinc is adversely affected by the presence of phytic acid in plant protein rations, a high concentration of calcium, a low concentration of free fatty acids, alterations in intestinal flora, and the presence of bacterial and viral enteric pathogens, such as transmissible gastroenteritis virus. Zinc deficiency may induce secondary vitamin A deficiency as a result of its effect on appetite and food use. Economic losses are due to depression of growth rate, but, with improved management techniques, *parakeratosis is no longer a major problem*. Parakeratosis occurs in young, growing pigs, 2-4 months of age. The initial gross lesions are erythematous macules on the ventral abdomen and medial surface of the thigh. The lesions develop into papules, which become covered with a gray-brown, dry, roughened scale-crust that may reach 5-7 mm in thickness. Deep fissures penetrate the crust and are filled with brown-black detritus, which is composed of sebum, sweat, soil, and other debris. These areas are susceptible to secondary bacterial infection, often leading to pyoderma or subcutaneous abscessation. *Lesions are roughly symmetrical and have a predilection for the lower limbs, particularly over the joints, around the eyes, ears, snout, scrotum, and tail.* In severely affected animals, lesions may become generalized. Pruritus is not a feature of parakeratosis. The dorsal surface of the tongue is "furred," and the esophageal mucosa loses its normal smooth sheen and becomes dull and white.

The microscopic lesion in the skin is marked hyperplastic dermatitis with diffuse parakeratotic hyperkeratosis (Fig. 6-56A, B). The oral mucous membranes also demonstrate hyperplastic epithelium. Acanthosis, elongation of rete ridges, and mitotic figures in the basal keratinocytes are regular features of the hyperplastic response of the epidermis. The dermal lesions in uncomplicated parakeratosis include variable vasodilation and a mild to moderate, predominantly mononuclear cell, perivascular infiltrate. With bacterial infection, there may be nodular or diffuse neutrophilic dermatitis, folliculitis, perifolliculitis, or furunculosis.

Parakeratosis in swine must be differentiated grossly from sarcoptic mange and exudative epidermitis. The former is usually intensely pruritic, and the latter usually occurs in a younger age group, and the scale-crust is greasy rather than dry. Parakeratosis is rarely fatal unless toxemia or septicemia secondary to cutaneous bacterial infection develop or because of exacerbation of intercurrent infections such as pneumonia. Affected pigs recover rapidly upon zinc supplementation.

Zinc deficiency in ruminants and camelids. Zinc-responsive dermatoses occur in **goats, sheep, cattle, alpacas, and llamas.** The condition is uncommon to rare. Characteristic dermatitis occurs in true zinc deficiency as well as an idiopathic zinc-responsive condition. Hyperkeratosis also affects the forestomachs of ruminants. Secondary infections in the skin are common. Causes of zinc deficiency include diets deficient in zinc or diets with high calcium, iron, phytates, or other zinc-chelating agents. Drinking water with excessive iron can also be a factor. In true zinc deficiency, multiple animals in a herd may be affected and show clinical signs of decreased appetite and growth, weight loss, decreased milk production, depression, stiff joints, and diarrhea. Those with idiopathic zinc-responsive disease do not have systemic signs, and, in general, only one animal is affected. The hereditary zinc deficiencies of cattle are discussed under Congenital and hereditary diseases of skin.

In ruminants, scaling, crusting, and alopecia occur in a symmetrical pattern over the face, pinnae, mucocutaneous junctions, pressure points, and distal limbs. Dull, rough, brittle haircoat may be seen. Pruritus is variable. In sheep, fleece/wool biting may be seen. Histopathologic changes include irregular to papillated epidermal hyperplasia with spongiosis, superficial perivascular to interstitial lymphoeosinophilic dermatitis, with marked diffuse parakeratotic hyperkeratosis. In **goats and**

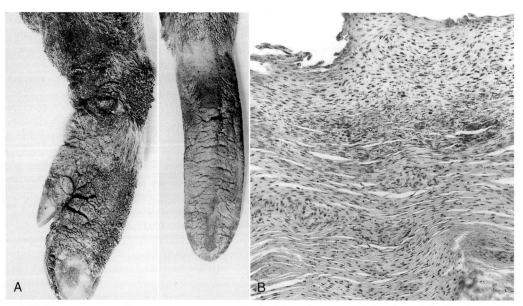

Figure 6-56 Zinc-responsive dermatosis in a pig. **A.** Marked hyperkeratosis of the skin of the foreleg and tongue epithelium. **B.** Marked parakeratotic hyperkeratosis.

sheep, there may be a mix of orthokeratotic and parakeratotic hyperkeratosis.

In **alpacas,** tightly adherent crusts are seen on the perineum, ventral abdomen, groin, medial thighs, axillae, and medial forelegs. The bridge of the nose, muzzle, and periocular region may also be affected. Pruritus is absent or mild. In alpacas, it is thought that breeding females and those with darker fleeces are more susceptible to zinc-responsive dermatosis because of a higher demand for zinc. Histopathologic findings include papillated epidermal hyperplasia with predominantly orthokeratotic hyperkeratosis, parakeratotic caps, and lymphoeosinophilic superficial perivascular dermatitis.

Zinc deficiency in horses. Experimental zinc deficiency has been reported in foals fed a zinc-deficient diet. Lesions included alopecia and scaling of the limbs, ventral abdomen, and thorax. Anecdotally, a few horses with scaling and erythema around the eyes, lips, coronets, and other pressure points; with histologic changes of epidermal hyperplasia; diffuse parakeratotic hyperkeratosis; and superficial perivascular lymphoeosinophilic dermatitis responded well to oral zinc supplementation.

Further reading

Krametter-Froetscher R, et al. Zinc-responsive dermatosis in goats suggestive of hereditary malabsorption: two field cases. Vet Dermatol 2005;16:269-275.

Nielsen FH. History of zinc in agriculture. Adv Nutr 2012;3:783-789.

Scott DW, et al. Skin diseases in the alpaca (Vicugna pacos): a literature review and retrospective analysis of 68 cases (Cornell University 1997-2006). Vet Dermatol 2010;22:2-16.

Scott DW, Miller WH. Endocrine, nutritional, and miscellaneous hair coat disorders. In: Scott DW, Miller WH, editors. Equine Dermatology. 2nd ed. St Louis: Elsevier Saunders; 2011. p. 360-377.

Canine zinc-responsive dermatoses

Naturally occurring zinc-responsive dermatoses in the dog fall under 2 syndromes:

- **Syndrome 1** *affects primarily Siberian Huskies and Alaskan Malamutes*, and rarely other breeds not of Arctic origin, such as Great Danes. The cutaneous lesions usually become manifest before the dogs are 1 year of age. Older dogs may develop lesions during times of stress, such as pregnancy, lactation, or intercurrent disease. Lesions comprise *scaling and crusting dermatitis* with a predilection for the face, particularly around the eyes, lips and nose, pressure points, and footpads (Fig. 6-57A). Lesions may be unilateral initially and progress to a bilateral distribution. Pruritus may be present. Secondary pyoderma is not uncommon. *The pathogenesis of the syndrome is not well established.* Alaskan Malamutes with chondrodysplasia have zinc-responsive spermatozoal defects and reduced zinc absorption from the intestinal tract; malabsorption may be responsible for the dermatologic disease. Lifetime supplementation of zinc is necessary to alleviate signs. A severe form of zinc-responsive dermatosis has been documented in a litter of Pharaoh Hounds. A role for oxidative stress has been shown in cases of canine zinc-responsive dermatosis. Dogs with zinc-responsive dermatosis have decreased epidermal immunoreactivity for metallothioneins, which are sulfhydryl-rich proteins that store zinc and act as free radical scavengers. The change may be indicative of low epidermal zinc levels.

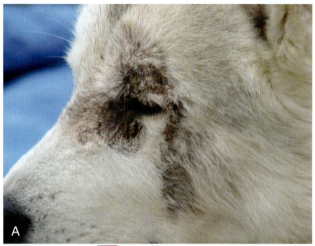
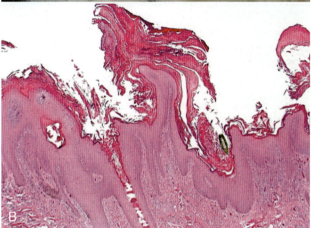
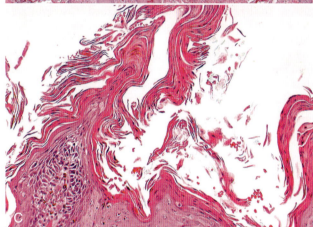

Figure 6-57 Zinc-responsive dermatosis in a dog. **A.** Hyperkeratotic plaques on muzzle and around the eyes. **B.** Papillary epidermal hyperplasia with prominent parakeratotic follicular spires. **C.** Higher magnification for parakeratotic projections from hair follicle ostia.

The epidermis of affected dogs also shows high expression levels of heat shock proteins, increased ki-67, as well an absence of caspase 3 activation.

- **Syndrome 2** *occurs in puppies of any breed and is associated with a relative deficiency of zinc, probably secondary to excessively high levels of calcium and/or phytates in the diet in rapidly growing animals.* Excessive iron in the drinking water may also contribute. In the United States, this disease has been associated with the feeding of *generic dog food*, in Britain and Sweden with the feeding of soy- and/or cereal-based diets. Recovery quickly follows restoration of a diet meeting the National Research Council standards for canine nutrition or zinc supplementation of cereal diets. Now that dog food manufacturers are aware of the problem, *the disease is less common*. The gross lesions are multiple, scaling, and crusted plaques, particularly affecting the muzzle, pressure points, distal extremities, and trunk. There is extreme thickening and fissuring of the footpads and, sometimes, the planum nasale. Secondary pyoderma may develop, and puppies often show a local lymphadenopathy.

The histologic lesions of both syndromes are usually typical of zinc deficiency, with papillary epidermal hyperplasia, marked spongiotic parakeratotic hyperkeratosis affecting the epidermis and follicular ostia, and multifocal neutrophilic crusts (Fig. 6-57B, C). Mild to moderate superficial perivascular mononuclear or eosinophil-rich dermatitis is present. Some reports indicate that the keratinization defect was sufficiently severe to induce dyskeratotic changes at all levels of the epidermis, whereas in others, orthokeratotic hyperkeratosis alone was found.

Differential diagnoses include superficial necrolytic dermatitis, lethal acrodermatitis, thallium toxicity, and chronic hypersensitivity dermatitis that may look very similar histologically. Dermatophytosis, pemphigus foliaceus, and pyoderma should be considered based upon gross lesions. *The signalment, history, lesion distribution, and pathologic changes should help to establish the diagnosis.* In some cases, response to dietary changes and/or zinc supplementation may be needed for confirmation of the suspected diagnosis. Serum and plasma zinc levels are not an accurate method of assessing zinc status. Values, even in a normal animal, are subject to marked variation according to sex, age, stress, concurrent disease, and collection methods. It is possible that dietary factors other than zinc are involved in some of these diseases, particularly those responding to dietary changes and not just to zinc supplementation.

Further reading

Campbell GA, Crow D. Severe zinc responsive dermatosis in a litter of Pharaoh Hounds. J Vet Diagn Invest 2010;22:663-666.

Romanucci M, et al. Oxidative stress in the pathogenesis of canine zinc-responsive dermatosis. Vet Dermatol 2011;22:31-38.

Superficial necrolytic dermatitis (hepatocutaneous syndrome)

A histologically distinct cutaneous reaction pattern characterized by the so called "red, white, and blue" *epidermal changes of parakeratosis, epidermal necrolysis or laminar intraepidermal edema, and basilar hyperplasia* has been recognized most often in the *dog*, and occasionally in the *cat*. The condition resembles necrolytic migratory erythema, a human paraneoplastic syndrome most often associated with α-cell neoplasms of the pancreas. *The pathogenesis of superficial necrolytic dermatitis (SND) is unknown*, but hepatic dysfunction and derangement of glucose and amino acid metabolism are clearly involved. Elevated glucagon levels alone are unlikely to be directly responsible for the skin lesions, as both dogs and humans may develop the disease in their absence, and dermatitis is not an inevitable result of the hyperglucagonemic state. Hypoaminoacidemia, the result of sustained gluconeogenesis and increased hepatic catabolism, is documented in both canine and human patients, and it has been postulated that it may deplete epidermal proteins and induce epidermal necrosis. Zinc and fatty acid metabolism may also be deranged. *The most likely pathogenesis of abnormal or impaired ability to properly use nutrients and the clinical and histologic similarities of this entity to zinc-responsive dermatoses* warrant discussion of SND in this section.

In dogs, SND has been reported to occur in association with a variety of systemic diseases, including *glucagon-secreting tumors of the pancreas, hyperglucagonemia, diabetes mellitus, and liver disease. Severe hepatopathy* is reported in >90% of the canine cases. The variety of concurrent diseases and the histologic appearance have led to terms for the characteristic cutaneous reaction pattern in dogs. These include superficial necrolytic dermatitis, hepatocutaneous syndrome, diabetic dermatopathy, metabolic epidermal necrosis, and necrolytic migratory erythema. Diabetes and hyperglucagonemia in some cases could be secondary to hepatic degeneration. Some dogs have a history of long-term phenobarbital administration. Rare reports in cats include a pancreatic carcinoma presumably of endocrine origin and a glucagon-producing primary hepatic neuroendocrine carcinoma.

Lesions have a roughly bilaterally symmetrical distribution. The muzzle, lips, periocular skin, edges of the pinnae, distal extremities, ventrum, and points of pressure or friction, such as the hocks, and the external genitalia are typically affected. Oral and mucocutaneous lesions are occasionally reported. Lesions are erythematous, erosive, ulcerative, and crusted. The footpads are markedly hyperkeratotic (Fig. 6-58A). Footpad lesions were not a feature of SND in the cat. *The histologic lesions of the "red, white, and blue" epidermis are virtually pathognomonic; the distinctive feature is a band of hydropic, pale-staining keratinocytes in the upper half of a usually acanthotic stratum spinosum* (Fig. 6-58B). Both intracellular and intercellular edema contribute to the epidermal pallor. As these cells degenerate, clefts and vesicles may form in the outer stratum spinosum. Neutrophils may accumulate to form subcorneal pustules. The stratum corneum is diffusely and markedly parakeratotic and appears hypereosinophilic in comparison to the subjacent pale-staining stratum spinosum of the epidermis. The epithelium of the follicular infundibulum can also be affected. The basal cell layer is basophilic and hyperplastic, forming small rete ridges. Individual necrotic keratinocytes may be located randomly in the epidermis and make distinction from erythema multiforme difficult in some cases. In SND, the necrotic keratinocytes lack satellitosis. Dermal inflammation is minimal, and predominantly mononuclear and perivascular. In eroded lesions, neutrophilic exocytosis is prominent, and inflammatory crust covers the surface.

In cases associated with liver disease, the most commonly associated gross lesion is a *nodular liver with intervening firm, collapsed parenchyma*. Histologically, there is loss of parenchyma and minimal inflammation. Hepatocytes are markedly vacuolated by a mix of lipid and glycogen. The nodules have been interpreted in some cases to represent regeneration and in others to be composed of nodular remnants of atrophic hepatic parenchyma.

The *diagnosis* is based on typical histologic findings. However, the pathognomonic epidermal edema may not be present in every biopsy. *Differential diagnoses* include other

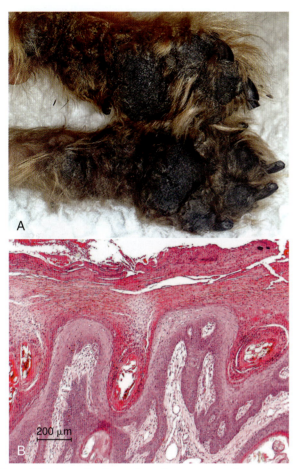

Figure 6-58 Superficial necrolytic dermatitis in a dog. **A.** Marked hyperkeratosis and crusting around the margins of the footpads and adjacent haired skin. **B.** The histologic changes of the epidermis make a characteristic "red (parakeratosis), white (intracellular edema in the spinous layer), and blue (basal layer hyperplasia)" pattern.

parakeratotic, hyperplastic dermatitides, such as the zinc-responsive dermatoses, lethal acrodermatitis of Bull Terriers, and thallium toxicity. The clinical differential is the same as listed for zinc-responsive dermatoses. The prognosis is generally considered poor because most cases have advanced liver disease. Cases associated with a pancreatic neoplasm may have resolution of skin lesions following tumor excision.

A similar syndrome has been described in horses with erosive, ulcerative, and exudative coronitis and concurrent liver pathology. The histopathologic changes in the skin are as described above, and may lead to necrosis and sloughing of the hoof wall.

Further reading

Asakawa MG, et al. Necrolytic migratory erythema associated with a glucagon-producing primary hepatic neuroendocrine carcinoma in a cat. Vet Dermatol 2013;24:466-469.

March PA, et al. Superficial necrolytic dermatitis in 11 dogs with a history of phenobarbital administration (1995-2002). J Vet Intern Med 2004;18:65-74.

Mizuno T, et al. Superficial necrolytic dermatitis associated with extrapancreatic glucagonoma in a dog. Vet Dermatol 2009;20:72-79.

ENDOCRINE DISEASES OF SKIN

Endocrine disorders frequently manifest clinically as skin disease, but these dermatoses are rarely specific for any one endocrinopathy. Although these dermatopathies are more common in dogs, they can occur in any species. **Clinical features** of many endocrine dermatoses include *a dry, coarse, brittle, dull, easily epilated haircoat that fails to regrow after clipping; hypotrichosis and hyperpigmentation; and alopecia that is frequently bilaterally symmetrical.* Secondary pyoderma and scaling are common. In addition, endocrine dermatoses share many **histologic features,** *including orthokeratotic hyperkeratosis, follicular dilation and keratosis, hair follicle atrophy, absence of hair shafts in follicles, increased numbers of telogen follicles, variably increased trichilemmal cornification (flame follicles) of follicles, and epidermal hyperpigmentation.* These histologic changes suggest an endocrine dermatosis but frequently are not pathognomonic for a specific endocrinopathy. *A combination of clinical and histologic features, together with clinical testing to demonstrate hormonal deficiency or excess, is required for confirmation.*

Hypothyroidism

Hypothyroidism, almost always primary hypothyroidism, is the most common endocrine dermatopathy in **dogs.** Histologically, the thyroid gland may have lymphoplasmacytic inflammation (lymphocytic thyroiditis) or atrophy without inflammation (idiopathic atrophy). *Lymphocytic thyroiditis* has been likened to Hashimoto's thyroiditis, a similar immune-mediated condition in humans. *Idiopathic thyroid atrophy* may represent the end stage of lymphocytic thyroiditis. In addition, hypothyroidism may be caused by developmental defects of the thyroid gland and rarely iodine deficiency. Congenital hypothyroidism with goiter has been reported in Tenterfield Terriers, as well as Toy Fox and Rat Terriers. The cause, so-called *dyshormonogenesis,* is caused by failure of the thyroid gland to produce sufficient hormone to inhibit pituitary release of thyroid-stimulating hormone (TSH). Pituitary neoplasia, or hypopituitarism, resulting in decreased secretion of TSH can lead to secondary hypothyroidism. It is a disease of middle-aged dogs, and there is no sex predilection, although the incidence is increased in neutered males and ovariohysterectomized females. Breeds that are predisposed include the Doberman Pinscher, Golden Retriever, Chow Chow, Great Dane, Irish Wolfhound, Boxer, English Bulldog, Dachshund, Afghan Hound, Newfoundland, Alaskan Malamute, Brittany Spaniel, Poodle, Irish Setter, and Miniature Schnauzer.

Clinical cutaneous changes include seborrhea, dry, coarse, brittle hair; hair that does not regrow after clipping; and hyperpigmentation and hypotrichosis with fine retained hairs that give the appearance of a "puppy coat." Alopecia typically develops on frictional areas, such as the elbows and hips, around the neck (from the collar), as well as the entire length of the tail (eFig. 6-12) ("rat tail"), and bridge of the nose. Pruritus is not a feature unless there is secondary pyoderma. Some cases may be presented with refractory pyoderma or chronic otitis externa. Hypothyroidism is thought to alter the skin barrier function; animal models suggest impaired lymphocyte and neutrophil function. Myxedema occurs in severe cases and may result in "tragic facial expression" see eFig. 6-12). Histologic changes can be nonspecific and simply suggest an endocrinopathy. The most common changes are orthokeratotic hyperkeratosis with follicular keratosis; normal

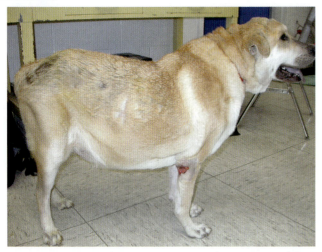

Figure 6-59 **Hyperadrenocorticism** in a dog. Note pendulous abdomen, truncal alopecia, and redistribution of adipose tissue. The dog has a decubital ulcer on the right elbow.

to mildly hyperplastic epidermis; sebaceous glands are atrophied, normal, or slightly hyperplastic; and most hair follicles in hairless telogen (kenogen). Myxedema is a more specific but less common finding. Occasionally, dysplastic follicles, flame follicles, vacuolated arrector pili muscles, and epidermal melanosis may occur.

Hypothyroidism occurs less frequently in other domestic animals, and usually in association with iodine deficiency and goiter. In **Merino sheep** and **Afrikander cattle,** a hereditary defect in the biosynthesis of thyroid hormone produces symmetrical hypotrichosis and thick, myxedematous, wrinkled skin. In **goats,** hypothyroidism occurs in a mixed strain of Saanen and dwarf goats in association with hereditary congenital thyroglobulin deficiency. Gross cutaneous changes include bilaterally symmetrical hypotrichosis and thick, myxedematous, scaly skin. Histologic findings include orthokeratotic hyperkeratosis, follicular keratosis, diffuse dermal mucinous degeneration (myxedema), and dermal thickening.

Hyperadrenocorticism

Hyperadrenocorticism is common in **dogs** and can be caused by bilateral adrenocortical hyperplasia resulting from a *pituitary tumor* (pituitary-dependent hyperadrenocorticism), a *neoplasm of the adrenal cortex* (usually unilateral), or exogenously administered glucocorticoids resulting in *iatrogenic hyperglucocorticism*. Of the naturally occurring forms, the pituitary-dependent form is considerably more common. The disease is seen most commonly in middle-aged or older dogs, and the Boxer, Boston Terrier, Dachshund, and Poodle are predisposed. Occasionally, skin lesions will be the only clinical sign of hyperadrenocorticism. Cutaneous changes can include *bilaterally symmetrical hypotrichosis or alopecia affecting primarily skin of the trunk, pendulous abdomen, thin skin that has decreased elasticity, slow wound healing, hyperpigmentation, telangiectasia, scaling, comedones, and calcinosis cutis* (Figs. 6-59, 6-60A). Lesions of calcinosis cutis occur most commonly in the dorsal neck region or axilla and groin. The lesions appear as firm erythematous papules or plaques that frequently ulcerate. Calcinosis cutis is most commonly the result of iatrogenic hyperadrenocorticism. Other causes of mineral deposits in the skin are discussed under Physical injury to skin.

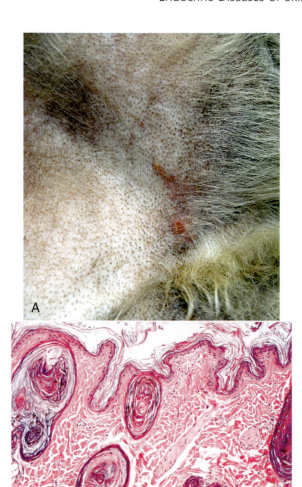

Figure 6-60 **Hyperadrenocorticism** in a dog. **A. Comedones** in a dog. Note gross appearance of distended follicles. **B.** Note thin epidermis and hair follicles distended with keratin.

Histologically, canine hyperadrenocorticism is characterized by thin epidermal and follicular epithelium, which can be 1-3 nucleated cell layers thick (Fig. 6-60B). If calcinosis cutis is present, the epidermis is frequently hyperplastic and can be ulcerated. Other changes can include orthokeratotic hyperkeratosis; marked follicular keratosis, sometimes with comedone formation; thin dermis; hair follicles that are frequently in telogen or kenogen; sebaceous gland atrophy; sebaceous melanosis; dysplastic follicles; and variable hyperpigmentation. *The presence of calcinosis cutis* (Fig. 6-61), *which can occasionally result in osseous metaplasia, is virtually pathognomonic for hyperadrenocorticism*, bearing in mind that mineralization of the external root sheath can be seen in normal old dogs and in Poodles. Cutaneous histologic lesions of hyperadrenocorticism can occur focally at the site of topical glucocorticoid application.

Hyperadrenocorticism is considerably less common in **cats.** As in dogs, the condition is more commonly pituitary dependent than adrenal dependent or iatrogenic. The clinical presentation in cats is similar to that in the dog; however, in addition, there is often concurrent diabetes mellitus, and marked skin fragility in which dermal collagen is reduced. This

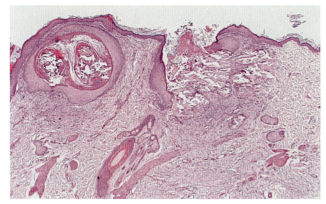

Figure 6-61 Calcinosis cutis in hyperadrenocorticism in a dog. The epidermis is hyperplastic. A large area of mineralized dermal collagen accompanied by granulomatous inflammation is undergoing transepidermal elimination.

can result in tearing and lacerations of the skin (*feline skin fragility syndrome*). Histologic lesions in the cat are similar to those in the dog; however, calcinosis cutis, and telangiectasia have not been reported.

Hyperadrenocorticism (referred to as pituitary dependent pars intermedia dysfunction) occurs in **horses** and is almost always seen in association with *hypertrophy, adenomatous hyperplasia, or functional neoplasms of the pars intermedia of the pituitary*. The disease affects primarily aged horses and has no breed or sex predilection. Gross cutaneous changes may include a coarse, brittle, long, shaggy haircoat (hirsutism), an abnormal shedding pattern, episodic hyperhidrosis, poor wound healing, decreased muscle tone, weight loss, and susceptibility to secondary skin infections.

Hyposomatotropism and hypersomatotropism

Hyposomatotropism, decreased production of growth hormone, occurs in young **dogs** with *congenital pituitary dwarfism*. The cause is a failure of the pharyngeal ectoderm to differentiate into hormone-secreting cell populations. Undifferentiated cells produce fluid, which causes *large cysts in the sella turcica*. The clinical signs are predominantly related to growth hormone deficiency, which may occur along with reduced levels of thyroid, adrenal, and sex hormones. In the German Shepherd dog and Karelian Bear dog, pituitary dwarfism is thought to be inherited as a simple autosomal recessive condition and is usually associated with a cystic Rathke's cleft. Clinically, the dogs are normal at birth, but show growth retardation and small stature. The most striking change is retention of the puppy haircoat.

Hypersomatotropism refers to the production of *excess growth hormone*, whereas *acromegaly* is the name of the syndrome that results from that state of excess growth hormone production. Acromegaly is very rare in dogs. Excessive somatotropin (growth hormone) production is associated with administration of progestins or with the metestrus (luteal) phase of the estrous cycle in intact female dogs. Cutaneous changes include thick, folded, myxedematous skin, especially on the head, neck, and distal extremities. The haircoat may be long and thick, and the nails may exhibit rapid overgrowth. Histologic findings in canine hypersomatotropism include thickened dermis resulting from increased production of glycosaminoglycans and collagen by dermal fibroblasts. Myxedema is present in about a third of cases. In cats, hypersomatotropism or acromegaly is caused by excess endogenous growth hormone secretion from a pituitary acidophil adenoma. Clinical signs include insulin-resistant diabetes mellitus, weight gain, broad facial features, inferior prognathia, heart murmur, organomegaly, and respiratory stridor.

Hyperestrogenism

Hyperestrogenism can occur in male or female **dogs.** In middle-aged to older intact male dogs, it is associated with *functional testicular neoplasms*, primarily Sertoli cell neoplasms, and occasionally functional interstitial cell tumors and seminomas. The Boxer, Shetland Sheepdog, Cairn Terrier, Pekingese, Collie, and Weimaraners are predisposed. Hyperestrogenism is also seen in middle-aged to older intact female dogs with *polycystic ovaries or functional ovarian neoplasms*. It can also occur in male or female dogs following estrogen administration. Rare cases can arise from physical contact with humans wearing topical estradiol compounds.

The clinical lesions of hyperestrogenism include *symmetrical hypotrichosis or alopecia*, which typically originates at the perineum and genital region and progresses cranially on the trunk. The hair is dry and dull, is easily epilated, can fail to regrow after clipping, and can be accompanied by hyperpigmentation, especially macular pigmentation. Male dogs may develop a pendulous prepuce, gynecomastia, or prostatomegaly with squamous metaplasia of the prostatic ducts. Females may develop an enlarged vulva. Histologic changes include hair follicles that are primarily in telogen, orthokeratotic hyperkeratosis, and follicular keratosis.

Alopecia X

Growth hormone/castration-responsive dermatosis has many synonyms, including hyposomatotropism of the adult dog, sex hormone alopecia, pseudo-Cushing's syndrome, testosterone-responsive dermatosis, estrogen-responsive dermatosis, congenital adrenal hyperplasia–like syndrome, and hair cycle arrest. This diversity in nomenclature reflects the differences in endocrine values and responses to various treatments and the fact that the pathogenesis of these conditions has not been fully characterized. *To simplify the nomenclature, the condition is now being referred to as* **alopecia X.** These dogs have normal thyroid function and adrenal function. Theories include genetics and hair follicle receptors, and most theories involve a deficiency or imbalance in sex hormones, such as a partial deficiency of 21-hydroxylase or other adrenocortical enzymes necessary for adrenal steroidogenesis and/or a growth hormone deficiency.

Alopecia X occurs most often in plush-coated Nordic breeds, such as the Pomeranian, Keeshond, Chow Chow, Samoyed, Siberian Husky, Alaskan Malamute, Norwegian Elkhound, American Eskimo Dog, and occasionally in other breeds. Affected dogs have a dull dry coat with loss of primary hairs. There is *symmetrical alopecia* of the trunk, perineum, caudal thighs, and neck, sparing the head and distal extremities (Fig. 6-62). Hyperpigmentation of exposed skin is common. Dark haircoats may fade. Coat changes can occur between 1 and 10 years of age, and either sex can be affected. These dogs tend to regrow tufts of hair at sites damaged by biopsy or surgery. Initial histologic changes are characterized by *follicular atrophy*; trichilemmal cornification in primary hairs can be quite prominent. Caution is warranted in making the diagnosis of alopecia X based exclusively on this feature because normal primary hair follicles of Nordic breeds can

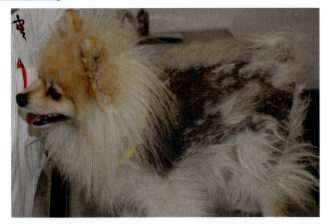

Figure 6-62 Alopecia X in a dog.

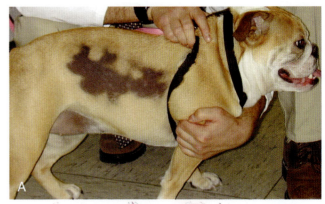
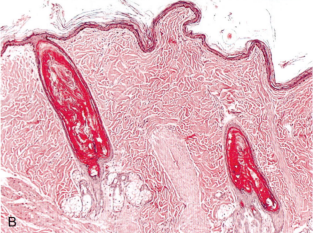

Figure 6-63 Recurrent flank alopecia. **A.** Large geographic area of hyperpigmentation and alopecia in the lateral thorax/flank area of an English Bulldog. **B.** Follicular infundibula are dilated and filled with keratin that extends into the openings of the primary and secondary atrophic follicles, giving the appearance of an inverted footprint.

have increased trichilemmal cornification. The histologic features must be interpreted in light of clinical findings.

Canine recurrent flank alopecia

Canine recurrent flank alopecia (seasonal flank alopecia, cyclical flank alopecia) is a condition seen most commonly in the Boxer, English Bulldog, Airedale Terrier, Schnauzer, and Griffon Korthal, but can occur in many, typically short-coated, breeds. It is characterized by alopecia of the skin of the flank that is usually bilaterally symmetrical, rarely unilateral, and occurs recurrently or seasonally. The first episode occurs at approximately 4 years of age but can be variable. In the Northern Hemisphere, the onset of alopecia is usually between November and March. There is spontaneous hair regrowth after 3-8 months; however, occasional dogs have progressively less hair regrowth after each episode. Rare dogs fail to regrow hair after the first episode; and some dogs have one episode of alopecia that never recurs.

Clinically, the bilaterally symmetrical lesions are usually confined to the thoracolumbar regions, have well-demarcated margins with abrupt transition from affected to unaffected skin, and are usually hyperpigmented (Fig. 6-63A). Histologic changes are those of *noninflammatory, nonscarring follicular atrophy*. Follicular infundibula are dilated and filled with keratin that can extend into the openings of the primary and secondary atrophic follicles, giving the appearance of an inverted footprint over the remnants of the follicular epithelium (Fig. 6-63B). Sebaceous melanosis may be seen. *Rarely, canine recurrent flank alopecia is associated with an interface dermatitis in Boxer dogs* (eFig. 6-13). The interface reaction is manifest by annular areas of scaling localized within the areas of alopecia.

Further reading

Frank LA. Comparative dermatology—canine endocrine dermatoses. Clin Dermatol 2006;24:317-325.

Frank LA. Endocrine and metabolic diseases. In: Miller WH, et al., editors. Muller & Kirk's Small Animal Dermatology. 7th ed. St Louis: Elsevier; 2013. p. 501-553.

Müntener T, et al. Canine noninflammatory alopecia: a comprehensive evaluation of common and distinguishing histological characteristics. Vet Dermatol 2012;23:206-e44.

Niessen SJ, et al. Hypersomatotropism, acromegaly, and hyperadrenocorticism and feline diabetes mellitus. Vet Clin North Am Small Anim Pract 2013;43:319-350.

Ris-Stalpers C, Bikker H. Genetics and phenomics of hypothyroidism and goiter due to TPO mutations. Mol Cell Endocrinol 2010;322: 38-43.

Scott-Moncrieff JC. Clinical signs and concurrent diseases of hypothyroidism in dogs and cats. Vet Clin North Am Small Anim Pract 2007;37:709-722.

Zur G, White SD. Hyperadrenocorticism in 10 dogs with skin lesions as the only presenting clinical signs. J Am Anim Hosp Assoc 2011;47:419-427.

IMMUNE-MEDIATED DERMATOSES

Hypersensitivity dermatoses

In the context of infection or vaccination, contact with exogenous antigens usually leads to induction of a protective response, but when the immune response causes damage to tissues, it is called *hypersensitivity or allergy*. Compounds such as pollens, food, drugs, insect components, various chemicals, and agents such as dust mites, *Staphylococcus*, and *Malassezia* spp. contain antigens that are normally innocuous but may induce allergic reactions in predisposed individuals. Most cutaneous hypersensitivity reactions are mediated by type I (immediate) hypersensitivity, type IV (cell-mediated or delayed) hypersensitivity, or by a combination of the 2 types. Hypersensitivity reactions cause a variety of dermatoses that

Immune-Mediated Dermatoses 591

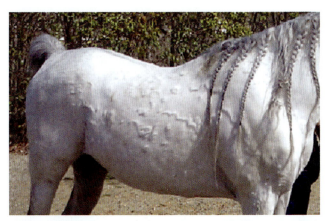

Figure 6-64 Urticaria in a horse. Discrete, well-circumscribed, serpiginous plaques with a flat top and steep sides. (Courtesy J. Greek.)

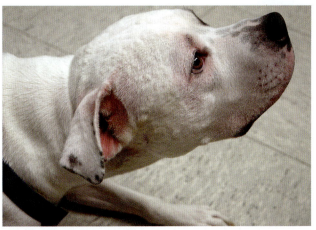

Figure 6-65 Acute atopic dermatitis in a dog. Note the perioral, periocular, and aural erythema.

range from annoying and uncomfortable (Fig. 6-64) to severely debilitating or life threatening. Allergic dermatoses are common and important in dogs, cats, and horses, but are rarely reported in food animals. Most of the research in allergy of domestic animals has focused on canine atopic dermatitis.

Atopic dermatitis

Atopy is a defined as an inherited tendency to produce IgE antibodies and develop clinical allergy to pollens and other environmental antigens. Atopy is a general term and when used as an adjective, "atopic," it describes a disease process in an organ system (e.g., atopic rhinitis, atopic asthma, atopic dermatitis [AD]).

A surge of investigations into pathogenesis atopic disorders has dramatically changed the understanding of AD. There are bodies of evidence that stress the "outside in" theory that begins with an abnormal skin barrier that results in a pathologic immune response, as opposed to the "inside out" theory that focuses on immunologic aberrations that result in skin disease. The strong link between an abnormal skin barrier and AD is corroborated by investigations into the genetics of ichthyosis vulgaris (IV). Individuals with IV are homozygous for mutations in the filaggrin gene. Heterozygous relatives are clinically normal but predisposed to AD and atopic asthma. Although filaggrin is not the only predisposing cause of atopic disease, loss of function mutations are present in about 10% of the population in Western Europe. During cornification, profilaggrin, located within keratohyaline granules of the stratum granulosum, is dephosphorylated to filaggrin. Filaggrin serves to anneal keratin intermediate filaments to form the strong central corneocyte core. Degradation products of filaggrin (e.g., urcanic acid) act as a natural moisturizing factor for the stratum corneum (SC). Even subtle defects in the organization or composition of the SC enable transepidermal allergen penetration and sensitization. Humans with AD have xerosis (dry skin), which is a result of increased transepidermal water loss (TEWL) and impairment of the water-holding capacity of the skin. In dogs, there is only limited evidence of an association between filaggrin and canine atopic dermatitis (CAD). Mutations in the filaggrin gene *FLG* do not appear to play a role in the development of CAD, although altered filaggrin expression may be present. There is reasonable evidence that dogs with CAD have an altered skin barrier: deranged lipid profiles in the SC (e.g., decreased free ceramides), ultrastructural changes in the SC of atopic dogs, and increased TEWL in both normal and abnormal skin.

Canine atopic dermatitis. Canine atopic dermatitis has been defined as a genetically predisposed inflammatory and pruritic allergic skin disease with characteristic clinical features most commonly associated with IgE antibodies to environmental allergens. It is a common condition that is estimated to affect 10% of the canine population, and runs second only to flea-bite hypersensitivity in geographic areas where fleas are endemic.

CAD is a multifactorial disease that involves immune dysregulation, allergen sensitization, skin barrier defects, environmental conditions, and altered microbial flora.

CAD has a strong genetic component, but the precise genetic basis remains unclear. Numerous studies (quantitative PCR, microarrays, single nucleotide polymorphism [SNP], genome-wide linkage, and genome-wide association) have implicated many genes that are differentially expressed in CAD; however, there is little concordance between studies both within and among breeds. In the United States, predisposed breeds include Labrador Retriever, Golden Retriever, West Highland White Terrier, Chinese Shar-Pei, Bull Terrier, Bichon Frise, and Tibetan Terrier; however, the predilection can vary geographically. In Britain, guide dogs (mainly Golden Retriever and Labrador Retriever guide dogs) are at high risk of developing CAD. Other breeds considered predisposed include the French Bulldog, Cairn Terrier, Basset Hound, Scottish Terrier, Lhasa Apso, Shih Tzu, Wirehaired Fox Terrier, Dalmatian, Pug, Irish Setter, Boston Terrier, Boxer, English Setter, Miniature Schnauzer, Belgian Tervuren, and Beauceron.

Caution is urged when attempting to differentiate causes of allergic skin disease based on histopathology. Although there may be histologic features that support CAD, *the diagnosis of CAD is based on a combination of historical findings, gross lesions, and exclusion of other allergic conditions (e.g., sarcoptic mange, flea-bite hypersensitivity, food hypersensitivity).* When interpreting skin biopsies, pathologists should be aware of the clinical presentation and characteristic clinical lesions. The *primary clinical sign is pruritus*, which frequently begins seasonally but eventually becomes perennial. Pruritus and erythema most commonly affect the face (Fig. 6-65), paws, distal extremities, and ventrum and is often manifested as face rubbing and foot chewing and licking. Skin lesions are usually due to self-trauma, secondary pyoderma, and *Malassezia* dermatitis. Secondary skin changes include alopecia and salivary staining of the hair, excoriations, scale, hyperpigmentation, lichenification, and pyotraumatic dermatitis (eFig. 6-14). Atopic dogs characteristically have an unpleasant odor that results from a combination of scaling, secondary bacterial or yeast infection, and hyperhidrosis. Atopic otitis externa is common. Noncutaneous clinical signs are rare and may include conjunctivitis, rhinitis, asthma, and gastrointestinal disorders.

The following criteria are significantly correlated with CAD: onset before 3 years of age, indoor living, pruritus prior to lesion onset, lesions on the forepaws, and concave pinnae. Lesions on the ear margins (sarcoptic mange) and dorsolumbosacral region (flea-bite hypersensitivity) do not support CAD. The presentation varies among different dog breeds. For example, West Highland White Terriers have lesions on the feet, flexural surfaces, dorsolumbosacral skin, and face, and often with generalized involvement. Boxers are more likely to have urticaria and otitis.

CAD was once considered a strictly Th2 cell–mediated disease; however, newer evidence shows that CAD reflects a slow progression from Th2 humoral inflammation (associated with high IgE) in the early phase to a Th1 cell–mediated response in the chronic phase. One hypothesis to explain the etiology of CAD begins with a defective skin barrier. For decades, **allergic inhalant dermatitis** was ingrained prominently in the veterinary literature as the consequence of an allergic reaction triggered by inhaled aeroallergens. There is strong evidence that transdermal exposure is more important, which predisposes to allergen penetration and sensitization. In dogs, transdermal exposure correlates with the distribution of lesions on sparsely haired areas (i.e., paws, ventrum, flexural folds). Allergens are captured by high-affinity receptors for IgE (FcεR1) receptors on Langerhans cells that process and present antigen to T lymphocytes. Atopic dogs and cats have increased and often aggregated Langerhans cells within the epidermis. Moreover, there are increased T cells in the epidermis, and the dermis contains clusters of perivascular dendritic cells. Functionally, these findings correlate with antigen capture by Langerhans cells (dendritic cells in the epidermis) and enhanced antigen presentation by dendritic cells to lymphocytes. The cytokine thymic stromal lymphopoietin (TSLP) is innately released by activated keratinocytes and serves as a potent activator of dermal dendritic cells. Dendritic cells activate allergen-specific T cells and drive the Th2 response.

Th2 cytokines (particularly interleukin-4 [IL-4], IL-5, IL-13) enhance eosinophilic inflammation and overproduction of allergen-specific IgE. IL-4 is a critical cytokine in the development of allergic diseases. It signals T cells to become Th2 cells, which are the major source of IL-4 production, thereby initiating a self-amplifying process. IL-4 induces expression of IgE receptors on Langerhans cells, resulting in enhanced antigen presentation capability. IL-4 and IL-13 induce the antibody isotype switch from IgM to IgE. They also upregulate expression of vascular cell adhesion molecule-1 (VCAM-1), an adhesion molecule expressed by cutaneous endothelial cells and involved in migration of eosinophils and mononuclear cells into sites of allergic inflammation. IL-5 promotes differentiation, vascular endothelial adhesion, and survival of eosinophils.

IgE appears to have a multifunctional role in the pathogenesis of atopic dermatitis (AD). An immediate type of hypersensitivity reaction develops within minutes of allergen exposure when mast cells bearing allergen-specific IgE bind allergen and release a variety of preformed mediators, most notably histamine. The skin histamine content has been found to be increased in humans and dogs with AD. Activated mast cells also release cytokines, such as IL-4, IL-5, IL-6, tumor necrosis factor-α, and platelet-activating factor (PAF), that further promote inflammation. An IgE-dependent late-phase reaction develops subsequently when expression of leukocyte adhesion molecules on postcapillary venule endothelium promotes influx of eosinophils, neutrophils, and mononuclear cells into the skin. Eosinophils release various mediators, including PAF, eosinophil major basic protein (MBP), eosinophil cationic protein (ECP), and cytokines that promote inflammation and cause tissue damage. Antigen-specific IgE antibodies also appear to be involved in a nonclassic role in antigen uptake and processing. IgE-bearing antigen-presenting cells (APCs), particularly Langerhans cells and dermal dendritic cells, bind, process, and present specific antigen locally to allergen-specific indeterminate T cells (Th0), thereby directing them to the Th2-cell phenotype. Moreover, IgE-mediated antigen presentation increases the presenting capacity of these APCs up to 100-fold, a mechanism known as "facilitated antigen presentation." Ultimately, B cells are stimulated to produce more allergen-specific IgE, which is bound to antigen-presenting cells, and a vicious cycle of facilitated antigen presentation is perpetuated.

In lesional skin of atopic dogs, superficial perivascular eosinophils, subcorneal eosinophilic micropustules, eosinophil degranulation, and increased CD4+ and CD8+ T cells are present. Tissue-selective homing of T cells is thought to be regulated at the level of T-cell recognition of vascular endothelial cells via interaction of differentially expressed T lymphocyte homing receptors, such as cutaneous lymphocyte antigen (CLA), and their endothelial cell ligands. Therefore it seems likely that the elevated expression of adhesion molecules by endothelial cells promotes migration of increased numbers of CLA+ T cells into the skin. The tendency to develop AD, as opposed to asthma or allergic rhinitis, may depend on differences in the memory/effector T cells that are specialized to home to the skin versus lung. Furthermore, cytokines released by Th2 cells (e.g., IL-31) appear to incite pruritus. IL-31 activates Janus kinase/signal transducer and activator of transcription (Jak/STAT) pathways in a broad range of immune cells, and receptors for IL-31 are also found on keratinocytes. As pruritus persists, self-trauma further compromises the skin barrier and facilitates additional allergen exposure.

With chronicity, the inflammation becomes Th1 polarized. Dendritic cells release IL-12, and a Th1 cytokine milieu (interferon-γ [IFN-γ], IL-2) ensues. In contrast to the Th2 response, Th1 cells produce IFN-γ, which inhibits IgE synthesis and differentiation of Th2 cells. The balance between Th1 and Th2 cells may be modulated by biochemical defects in monocytes. Peripheral blood mononuclear cells of individuals with AD have been shown to have increased activity of phosphodiesterase, which results in increased monocyte prostaglandin E_2 (PGE_2) production. PGE_2 tends to inhibit Th1 production of IFN-γ and accentuate secretion by Th2 cells. Histologically, the progression to a Th1-mediated immune response corresponds with a greater abundance of superficial perivascular lymphocytes and plasma cells, with eosinophils becoming a less prominent component of the inflammatory infiltrate.

Dogs and humans with AD are predisposed to superficial infections with *Malassezia* and *Staphylococcus*. Although *Staphylococcus pseudintermedius* is part of the normal canine flora, it is the most frequent cause of pyoderma in dogs with AD. Dogs with AD have higher levels of anti-staphylococcal IgE than non-atopic dogs. Multidrug resistance to *S. pseudintermedius* is not uncommon in dogs that have received multiple antibiotic courses. *Staphylococcus aureus* in humans is believed to augment allergen-induced skin inflammation in AD by secreting exotoxins that act as *superantigens*. Superantigens have the capacity to activate large numbers of T cells nonspecifically by virtue of their ability to bridge the linkage between the class II major histocompatibility complex molecule on the antigen-presenting cell (APC) and certain classes of the T-cell receptor without having to be processed and presented by the APC. IgE antibodies directed against these exotoxins have been identified in individuals with AD, and the severity of disease correlates with these IgE antibody titers, presumably because the locally produced exotoxins are absorbed through the skin surface and cause IgE-dependent mast cell degranulation within the dermis.

As in the dog, the diagnosis of AD in *cats* is made clinically by a *combination of historical findings, gross lesions, and specifically by exclusion of other allergic conditions* (e.g., flea-bite hypersensitivity; ectoparasites such as *Cheyletiella, Demodex gatoi, Notoedres*; and adverse food reaction). Devon Rex and Abyssinian breeds may be predisposed. Clinical signs usually develop at 6-24 months of age; however, AD can arise in older cats. The pruritus associated with AD in cats is often nonseasonal and severe. Clinical lesions of AD cannot distinguish causes of non–flea-induced hypersensitivity. Reaction patterns include self-induced alopecia, eosinophilic granuloma complex lesions, miliary dermatitis, recurrent swelling or ulceration of the lower lip, otitis externa, and pruritus of the face, pinnae, and neck, as well as the abdomen/axillae, dorsal trunk, and distal limbs and paws. In some cases, pruritus might not be obvious because of the secretive nature of cats. Instead, hair loss, secondary to covert licking and chewing, may be the only abnormality, and the skin may appear normal. *Miliary dermatitis is a clinical reaction pattern of cats* that consists of numerous small erythematous crust-covered papules. It is not specific for AD and may also occur in ectoparasite, food, and drug hypersensitivities. Noncutaneous signs associated with atopy in cats include sneezing, conjunctivitis, coughing, and asthma. Lymphadenopathy may be present in cats with miliary dermatitis or eosinophilic granulomas.

Pruritus is the primary clinical sign in **horses** with atopy. Some cases are manifested as recurrent pruritic urticaria. Onset is usually between 1.5 and 4 years of age. Skin lesions usually develop secondarily in response to self-trauma and include alopecia, excoriations, lichenification, and hyperpigmentation. The face, ears, ventrum, and legs are most commonly affected. Arabians and Thoroughbreds may be predisposed. A seasonal pruritic dermatosis typical of AD has been described in 2 **Suffolk ewes.**

Microscopic changes associated with AD have been considered nonspecific and usually consist of perivascular to interstitial dermatitis. In *dogs*, the epidermis is variably hyperplastic and may have mild, patchy intercellular edema; focal parakeratosis; and crusting. Erosion and ulceration may be present from self-trauma. Exocytosis of lymphocytes or eosinophils and small subcorneal accumulations of eosinophils may be seen. Dermal inflammation is superficial perivascular to interstitial, and consists of lymphocytes and macrophages primarily. Mast cells are in increased numbers and may be numerous. Eosinophils and neutrophils are usually in low numbers, but eosinophils may be missed because of degranulation. Sebaceous glands are hyperplastic, and apocrine sweat glands may be dilated in chronic lesions. Superficial dermal blood vessels may be congested, and the superficial dermis may be mildly edematous.

Histologic changes in the skin of *cats* with AD vary according to the lesions biopsied. The epidermis varies from normal to variably hyperplastic. Serocellular crusts, foci of intercellular edema and epidermal necrosis, and exocytosis of small numbers of eosinophils are usually present in lesions of miliary dermatitis. The dermis contains a superficial perivascular to interstitial infiltrate of mixed cells. Mast cells, eosinophils, lymphocytes, and neutrophils are typically present but vary in their proportions. Neutrophils are most numerous in areas of erosion or ulceration. In some cases, the lesions are those of an eosinophilic plaque. The microscopic lesion in *atopic horses and sheep* is hyperplastic perivascular dermatitis with a predominance of eosinophils.

Diagnosis of AD is based on compatible history and physical examination findings coupled with demonstration of allergen-specific IgE antibodies. In dogs, measurement of total serum IgE has not been found to be useful because there is no significant difference in IgE concentrations between atopic and clinically normal dogs. Intradermal skin testing (IDST) has been considered to be the most reliable method of identifying clinically relevant allergens. In vitro tests that measure concentrations of allergen-specific IgE are commercially available but generally have been found to correlate poorly with IDST results. However, newer procedures (radioallergosorbent test, ELISA, and liquid-phase immunoenzymatic assay) for measurement of allergen-specific IgE may be more accurate in identifying clinically relevant allergens in dogs and cats. Diagnosis may be complicated by the presence of concurrent hypersensitivity conditions; such as flea-bite allergy or food allergy, and solely histologic findings in these conditions are indistinguishable.

Further reading

Favrot C. Feline non-flea induced hypersensitivity dermatitis: clinical features, diagnosis and treatment. J Feline Med Surg 2013;15: 778-784.

Gonzales AJ, et al. Interleukin-31: its role in canine pruritus and naturally occurring canine atopic dermatitis. Vet Dermatol 2013;24: 48-53.

Kanda S, et al. Characterization of canine filaggrin: gene structure and protein expression in dog skin. Vet Dermatol 2013;24:25-31.

Klukowska-Rötzler J, et al. Expression of thymic stromal lymphopoietin in canine atopic dermatitis. Vet Dermatol 2013;24:54-59.

Marsella R, et al. Current understanding of the pathophysiologic mechanisms of canine atopic dermatitis. J Am Vet Med Assoc 2012; 241:194-207.

Nuttall T, et al. Canine atopic dermatitis what have we learned? Vet Rec 2013;172:201-207.

Olivry T. Is the skin barrier abnormal in dogs with atopic dermatitis? Vet Immunol Immunopathol 2011;144:11-16.

Ravens PA, et al. Feline atopic dermatitis: a retrospective study of 45 cases (2001-2012). Vet Dermatol 2014;25:95-102.

Voie KL, et al. Drug hypersensitivity reactions targeting the skin in dogs and cats. J Vet Intern Med 2012;26:863-874.

Urticaria and angioedema

Urticaria (hives, heat bumps) and **angioedema** (angioneurotic edema) *are variably pruritic, edematous skin lesions produced by mediators released by basophils and dermal mast cells.* Urticaria is most common in horses, uncommon in dogs, and rare in ruminants, pigs, and cats. Angioedema is rare. A wide variety of immunologic and nonimmunologic causes have been implicated, but frequently the specific causative agent cannot be determined for a particular individual. Immunologic causes of urticaria/angioedema are thought to involve type I hypersensitivity reactions primarily; type III hypersensitivity is involved occasionally. *Recognized initiators* in all species include foods and food additives, drugs, biological agents, stinging and biting arthropods, intestinal parasites, inhalant and contact allergens, and bacterial, fungal, and viral infections. *Nonimmunologic factors* associated with urticaria/angioedema include physical factors such as heat, cold, or pressure; mast cell degranulating agents such as radiocontrast media; and agents that result in perturbation of arachidonic acid metabolism. Deficiency of C1 esterase inhibitor is a genetic cause of chronic urticaria in humans. Aspirin and other nonsteroidal anti-inflammatory drugs, psychologic stress, and concurrent febrile illness may be *exacerbating factors,* if not causative ones, in humans with chronic urticaria. Another cause of chronic urticaria identified in humans is IgG autoantibody directed against the IgE receptor of cutaneous mast cells and circulating basophils. Binding of the autoantibody to this receptor induces release of histamine. T-helper 2 cytokines, eosinophils, mast cells, and macrophages have been suggested to play a role in the pathogenesis of equine recurrent urticaria. Regardless of cause, the *final common pathway is increased vascular permeability and resultant edema produced by histamine, the major mediator, and possibly also by kinins, eicosanoids, and neuropeptides.*

Drugs are probably the most frequent cause of urticaria in **horses.** A wide variety of systemic drugs and biological products have been implicated in initiating urticaria. *Wheals* frequently develop in minutes to hours after exposure to the offending drug and usually subside within several hours. *Cholinergic or heat-reflex urticaria,* induced by exercise or a hot bath, has been reported in a horse; pruritus in this horse appeared to be exacerbated by pelleted feed. An unusual form of urticaria called *dermatographism,* which is induced by blunt pressure to the skin, has also been described in the horse. In some instances, urticaria is thought to be caused by *overfeeding of grains,* especially those high in protein content ("protein bumps," "feed bumps"). Lesions occur anywhere on the body but are most common on the face, neck, and thorax. In **cattle,** a unique form of urticaria has been described in high-producing dairy cows, especially Jerseys and Guernseys, that become sensitized to casein in their own milk *(milk allergy).* Foods, drugs, biological agents, and venomous stings are reported most frequently as causes of urticaria and angioedema in **dogs** and **cats.**

Urticaria is characterized by *wheals (hives),* which are discrete, well-circumscribed, erythematous, edematous plaques with a flat-top and steep sides (see Fig. 6-64). They are cool and pit upon digital pressure. They vary in size and may coalesce to measure many centimeters in diameter. Wheals are usually round; but in some instances, they assume bizarre and irregular serpentine shapes. The overlying hair may stand erect, giving the impression of a follicular disease. The lesions may be localized to a single body region, for instance, lateral neck, head, or thorax, or they may involve the entire body. The individual lesions usually last <12-24 hours and disappear, leaving no residual skin changes unless pruritus results in self-mutilation. Although individual lesions are transient, new ones may erupt over a period of days or weeks. The occurrence in horses of one of the multiple hypersensitivities of recurrent airway obstruction, insect-bite hypersensitivity, and urticaria may predispose the horse to the other hypersensitivities.

Angioedema consists of larger, less well-demarcated swellings that originate subcutaneously. With time, the swellings may gravitate ventrally. Angioedema is a potentially serious condition because involvement of perilaryngeal tissues may cause asphyxiation. Approximately 50% of affected humans develop both lesions concurrently, but development of both wheals and angioedema does not seem to be as common in animals.

Microscopic lesions are variable and nonspecific. The epidermis is usually normal in nontraumatized lesions. Urticaria is characterized by *dermal edema,* which is visualized as widening of spaces between collagen fibers in the superficial and middle dermis. The change may be very subtle and can be missed. Edema is typically more severe and involves the deep dermis and subcutaneous tissue in angioedema. Small vessels are congested, and lymphatics are dilated. Inflammation is inconsistent. When present, it usually consists of perivascular granulocytes, mast cells, and fewer lymphocytes and macrophages. The reaction involves the upper and middle dermis in urticaria and the deep dermis and subcutis in angioedema. Vasculitis is not a typical feature of urticaria and angioedema.

Diagnosis is usually based on the history and appearance and transitory nature of the clinical lesions. Biopsy is performed to rule out other conditions when the lesions are recurrent or chronic, and the diagnosis is uncertain. Identification of a particular inciting cause relies on history and a combination of elimination trials, environmental alterations, intradermal skin testing, and insect control measures.

Further reading

Fadok VA. Update on equine allergies. Vet Clin North Am Equine Pract 2013;29:541-550.

Hinden S, et al. Characterization of the inflammatory infiltrate and cytokine expression in the skin of horses with recurrent urticaria. Vet Dermatol 2012;23:503-e99.

Kehrli D, et al. Multiple hypersensitivities including recurrent airway obstruction, insect bite hypersensitivity, and urticaria in 2 Warmblood horse populations. J Vet Intern Med 2015;29:320-326.

Cutaneous adverse food reaction

The term "adverse food reaction" is a broad term that has replaced "food allergy" and "food hypersensitivity" in veterinary medicine. It is often unclear if the pathologic mechanisms represent a specific immune-mediated response (e.g., type I hypersensitivity) to food antigens or if the mechanism is related to nonimmune-mediated intolerance to a component in the food. When an adverse food reaction is manifested by dermatologic signs, it is termed *cutaneous adverse reaction to food* (CARF); however, affected animals can have concurrent gastrointestinal signs. The skin may represent the second most frequent target organ, after the gastrointestinal tract, in adverse food reactions. The clinical distribution and histologic lesions are largely indistinguishable from atopic dermatitis (AD).

Food allergy in humans is thought to develop as a consequence of physiologic and immunologic immaturity, resulting in increased absorption of food antigens during early life in association with the inherited tendency for increased production of IgE antibody. Absorption of intact food proteins is limited by the intestinal mucosal barrier and by combination of the proteins with food allergen–specific IgA secreted into the gut. However, adult levels of IgA are not generally produced until puberty, and this relative IgA deficiency may contribute to increased permeability of the gastrointestinal barrier during childhood. Gastrointestinal infections and parasitism may also contribute to disruption of the mucosal barrier to increase absorption of food antigens. The majority of food allergens are *glycoproteins* molecular weight 10,000-80,000 Da, which tend to be resistant to proteolysis and are heat stable and water soluble. Even in the mature intestine, ~2% of ingested food antigens are absorbed into the circulation in an immunologic form. However, these immunologically recognizable proteins do not normally cause adverse reactions despite being transported throughout the body because tolerance develops in most individuals. Tolerance is thought to involve activation of CD8+ T suppressor cells in gut-associated lymphoid tissue (GALT) to suppress an immune response. The development of tolerance to food appears to have little effect on B cells, given that antibody production to food proteins is a universal phenomenon; although low concentrations of serum IgG, IgM, and IgA food-specific antibodies are found in normal individuals, they are of no clinical consequence. In genetically predisposed infants, however, ingested antigens result in excessive production of IgE antibodies. These food-specific antibodies bind high-affinity receptors on mast cells, dendritic cells, and macrophages in tissues and basophils in circulation. When food allergens penetrate mucosal barriers and reach the IgE bound to mast cells and basophils, mediators are released that induce the signs of immediate hypersensitivity. Activated mast cells also generate various mediators (such as IL-4, tumor necrosis factor-α (TNF-α), and platelet-activating factor) that may induce an IgE-mediated late-phase response in which eosinophils, lymphocytes, and monocytes are attracted to the site of reaction and release additional inflammatory mediators and cytokines that drive a Th2-mediated response. The development of dermatitis rather than respiratory signs in individuals with food allergy may be related to homing of allergen-specific T cells to the skin by way of cutaneous lymphocyte-associated antigen (CLA), a homing molecule that directs these cells to the skin.

In companion animal species, the pathogenesis of adverse food reactions is poorly understood and does not correlate with food hypersensitivity in humans. In humans, the disorder is seen most commonly in infants and young children; and in many cases, a loss of clinical sensitivity develops after 1-3 years of an appropriate food elimination diet. Although signs may initially develop in young animals, CARF is typically a disease of adult animals, and no loss of clinical sensitivity has been observed in affected animals. Because gastrointestinal parasitism and viral enteritides are relatively common in animals, disruption of the intestinal mucosal barrier may be an important factor in the development of CARF. Furthermore, laboratory tests that measure food-specific IgE or IgG antibodies in dogs are notoriously inaccurate.

In **dogs**, CAFR does not show breed or sex predilections. CARF may affect up to 8% of dogs and accounts for 7-25% of allergic skin disorders in dogs. A minor population of dogs with CARF shows gastrointestinal signs (10-15%). In dogs, cutaneous adverse food reactions arise before 1 year of age in 33-48% of cases, and 51-85% are manifested between 1-3 years. Fewer cases (16%) arise in dogs aged 4-11 years; 23-45% of dogs with CARF have concurrent hypersensitivity conditions, such as AD, flea-bite allergy, or both. Adverse food reactions may be provoked by more than one dog food ingredient. The most common allergens identified in dogs are beef, soy, chicken, milk, corn, wheat, and eggs.

The most consistent sign is nonseasonal pruritus affecting the ears, feet, face, ventrum, limbs, or perineal regions. CARF may mimic sarcoptic mange, flea allergy dermatitis, or AD. The pruritus may be unresponsive or poorly responsive to glucocorticoid therapy. Primary skin lesions may include erythema, papules, or pruritic urticaria-angioedema, but they are frequently obscured by self-trauma as a consequence of chronic pruritus. More commonly, only secondary lesions are seen, and these typically include excoriation, alopecia, hyperpigmentation, lichenification, scales, and crusts. In a small number of cases, pruritic otitis externa or recurrent superficial pyoderma may occur in the absence of any other clinical signs of food allergy. Bacterial pyoderma and *Malassezia* infection are common secondary complications. Some dogs also exhibit *concurrent gastrointestinal signs*, which include increased frequency of defecation most commonly, and mucus and/or blood in feces, tenesmus, flatulence, vomiting, and diarrhea. Neurologic signs, such as malaise and seizures, and respiratory signs have been reported rarely in conjunction with skin lesions in dogs with food allergy.

The prevalence of CARF in **cats** is estimated to be 1-6% of all feline dermatoses. Furthermore, CARF may affect 12-16% of cats with pruritus and 10% of cats with military dermatitis. No breed or sex predilection is apparent. Most cases are recognized in young adult cats. The major complaint is *severe pruritus* that is usually nonseasonal and frequently poorly responsive to glucocorticoid therapy. The face, ears, and neck are most commonly involved, but pruritus may be generalized (Fig. 6-66). Allergens identified include *fish, lamb, milk, whale meat, beef, chicken, rabbit, eggs, and pork*. Food-allergic cats may also have other hypersensitivity conditions, such as AD or flea-bite allergy. Skin lesions are extremely variable and include erythema, angioedema-urticaria, self-induced alopecia and excoriations, crusting, seborrhea, or

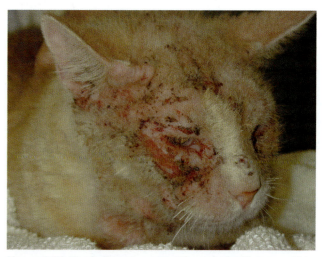

Figure 6-66 **Food allergy** in a cat with marked self-trauma. Note the preauricular and periocular crusting, and erythema.

miliary dermatitis. They may be localized to the face and head or generalized in distribution. Eosinophilic granuloma complex lesions may be a manifestation of food allergy. Concurrent gastrointestinal or respiratory signs are uncommon.

Cutaneous adverse food reaction has been reported rarely in **horses, cattle,** and **pigs.** Substances that have been incriminated include wheat, barley, bran, oats, concentrates, and tonics in horses; wheat, bran, corn, clover hay, rice bran, and soybeans in cattle; and clover pasture in pigs. Clinical signs in horses and cattle are pruritic papular eruptions, pruritic urticaria, and tail rubbing. A condition described as food allergy in white hogs on new clover pasture consisted of generalized erythema and skin pain, depression, and reluctance to move. However, the description of this condition is more suggestive of an adverse food reaction, such as photosensitization, than of food hypersensitivity.

The microscopic lesions associated with food allergy are variable and are not diagnostic. The epidermis is variably acanthotic and may be multifocally spongiotic. Crusting, erosion, and ulceration may be present. The superficial dermis is mildly to moderately edematous, and inflammation is variable. In dogs, inflammation may be perivascular, interstitial, or diffuse. The cells are mixed and include lymphocytes, macrophages, eosinophils, and mast cells. Neutrophils and plasma cells are present in numbers proportional to the degree of self-trauma. Sebaceous and epitrichial glands may be hyperplastic in chronic lesions. Rarely, eosinophilic vasculitis has been described in dogs with CARF. In cats, dermal inflammation may be a superficial perivascular mononuclear dermatitis but more commonly is characterized by eosinophilic inflammation that is perivascular to diffuse and extends into the subcutis. Mast cell numbers are commonly moderately to markedly increased throughout the dermis. Collagen flame figures may occur in areas of intense eosinophilic inflammation. Eosinophilic folliculitis and furunculosis and lesions of eosinophilic plaque are present in some cases of food allergy in cats. The microscopic lesion ascribed to food allergy in large animals is superficial perivascular dermatitis, with eosinophils comprising a significant proportion of the inflammatory cells.

The *diagnosis* of food allergy is made by a combination of appropriate clinical history, exclusion of other pruritic conditions, and resolution of pruritus with feeding of a novel protein diet. Intradermal skin testing and measurement of serum allergen-specific IgE levels have been found to be unreliable for diagnosis of food allergy in animals.

Further reading

Hardy JI, et al. Food-specific serum IgE and IgG reactivity in dogs with and without skin disease: lack of correlation between laboratories. Vet Dermatol 2014;25:447-e70.

Verlinden A, et al. Food allergy in dogs and cats: a review. Crit Rev Food Sci Nutr 2006;46:259-273.

Vogelnest LJ, Cheng KY. Cutaneous adverse food reactions in cats: retrospective evaluation of 17 cases in a dermatology referral population (2001-2011). Aust Vet J 2013;91:443-451.

Allergic contact dermatitis

Allergic contact dermatitis is an uncommon hypersensitivity condition in domestic animals. Although considered a typical delayed (type IV) hypersensitivity reaction, *there is considerable overlap in pathogenesis between allergic contact dermatitis and primary irritant dermatitis, and the rigid distinction between the 2 conditions is becoming blurred.* It has been estimated to account for 1-10% of dermatoses in dogs. The low incidence, as compared to that in humans, is thought to be due to the natural protection afforded by the haircoat of most animals and by the decreased exposure to potential allergens in cosmetics and industrial chemicals.

Allergic contact dermatitis is caused by contact with a nonirritating concentration of a substance to which an individual has previously become sensitized. The compounds involved are usually lipid-soluble haptens (low-molecular-weight substances) that become immunogenic only after penetrating the epidermis and binding covalently to an autologous structural or cell surface protein to form a complete antigen. This antigen is subsequently internalized and processed by Langerhans cells and presented to CD4+ T cells. Langerhans cells are crucial to development of allergic contact dermatitis, as depletion of these cells results in a decreased ability to induce contact sensitization. During the induction phase of the reaction, Langerhans cells present antigen to CD4+ cells in the paracortical region of regional lymph nodes, where the specifically sensitized T cells undergo clonal expansion and then circulate as memory cells in blood and home to skin by virtue of adhesion molecules that bind to addressins on endothelial cells. Development of allergic contact dermatitis depends on the nature of the allergen, frequency of contact, and state of the skin. *Factors that damage the integrity of the protective barrier of the skin predispose to development of allergic contact dermatitis.* The induction phase is typically a prolonged process, estimated to require 6-24 months to develop. Although strong immunogens can elicit sensitivity after as short a period of contact as 7-21 days, most contact allergens are weaker immunogens and require chronic repeated exposure for sensitization to develop. Upon subsequent exposure to the contact allergen, specifically sensitized T cells in skin and circulation are presented the antigen by Langerhans cells (elicitation phase), become activated, and elaborate various cytokines that attract and activate other inflammatory cells and stimulate proliferation of the epidermis. Only a very small fraction (<1%) of the infiltrating T cells are specific for a relevant antigen. Thus various amplification and recruitment mechanisms are involved in induction of the reactions. The activated T cells secrete a Th1 profile of cytokines, including interferon-γ (IFN-γ) and TNF-β, which recruit and activate a wide variety of inflammatory cells, affect keratinocyte function and differentiation, and induce expression of adhesion molecules on endothelial cells and keratinocytes. TNF-β and IFN-γ induce expression of intercellular adhesion molecule-1 (ICAM-1) on keratinocytes and endothelium, which promotes homing of T cells to the dermis and epidermis. Unlike the delayed-type hypersensitivity reaction that develops in response to antigen injected into the dermis, which primarily involves CD4+ cells, the response to hapten painted on the epidermis involves both CD4+ and CD8+ T cells. Local production of cytokines induces arrival of more T cells and further amplification of proinflammatory mechanisms. Irritated keratinocytes also release a variety of cytokines that induce or augment the inflammatory response.

Allergic contact dermatitis has been reported most frequently in *dogs and horses*, although most cases have not been confirmed by patch testing. Numerous *plants and chemicals* have been suspected or shown to cause allergic contact dermatitis in animals. In dogs, wandering Jew (*Tradescantia fluminensis*), spreading dayflower (*Cornelina diffusa*), doveweed (*Murdannia nudiflora*), leaves and bulbs of plants in the family *Amaryllidaceae*, dandelion leaves, cedar wood, and Asian jasmine have been implicated in cases of allergic contact dermatitis. Cobalt and nickel ions, pine oil resin found in cleaning products, topical medications such as neomycin, rubber, cement, and various fragrances such as those in shampoos and carpet deodorizers are a few of the chemical causes of allergic contact dermatitis in dogs and cats. Hairless dogs may have an increased frequency of allergic contact dermatitis. Contact hypersensitivity has been document in Mexican hairless dogs housed in stainless steel cages (chromium metal). In horses, pasture plants, insecticides, various dyes and preservatives of tack items, soaps, and bedding materials have been suggested as causes of allergic contact dermatitis.

The *clinical course* is typically prolonged, and lesions in dogs are usually confined to sparsely haired areas of the body, such as the lips, chin, ventral cervical and thoracic areas, abdomen, scrotum, perineum, and ventral interdigital skin. Footpads are usually protected by the thick stratum corneum; however, cracking of footpads of all 4 feet was a feature described in a cat with suspected allergic contact dermatitis to carpet deodorizer. Lesion distribution is also dependent on the contactant involved. *Primary lesions include erythema, papules, plaques, and vesicles*, but these are very transient and thus rarely seen. *Pruritus is variable*, ranging from mild to severe. Chronic secondary lesions are more commonly seen and include alopecia, lichenification, scaling, crusting, excoriations, and pigmentary changes. Secondary bacterial or fungal infection may complicate lesions.

Microscopic changes described in various reports of allergic contact dermatitis in animals have been conflicting. *Differences in histologic lesions no doubt reflect, at least in part, differences in stage of the reaction*. Whereas neutrophils have been the predominant cell type seen in some cases, lymphocytes or eosinophils predominated in others. The epidermis may be variably spongiotic and may develop vesicles in some areas. In allergic contact dermatitis produced experimentally in dogs by topical application of 1-chloro-2,4-dinitrochlorobenzene (DNCB), histologic changes at 48 and 72 hours postchallenge included mild acanthosis, mild dermal edema, and perivascular and perifollicular infiltrations of lymphocytes and macrophages. Mild and focal to widespread and marked epidermal necrosis may occur, both in patch test reaction sites as well as in spontaneous lesions. Exocytosis of inflammatory cells is a common feature, but the cells vary and may be neutrophils, lymphocytes, eosinophils, or a combination thereof. The superficial dermis may be edematous, and the predominant inflammatory cells may be lymphocytes, neutrophils, or eosinophils. Inflammation may be perivascular, diffuse interstitial, or lichenoid and frequently perifollicular. *The histologic changes of allergic contact dermatitis are frequently indistinguishable from those caused by irritant contact dermatitis.*

The list of *differential diagnoses* is extensive and includes a wide variety of allergic and parasitic conditions, bacterial and fungal infections, and irritant contact dermatitis. When a single animal of a group is affected, allergic contact dermatitis is considered more likely than irritant dermatitis. *Diagnosis is based on history, physical examination findings, exclusion of other dermatoses, and is confirmed by restriction followed by provocative exposure to the suspected allergen or patch testing.*

Further reading

Kimura T. Contact hypersensitivity to stainless steel cages (chromium metal) in hairless descendants of Mexican hairless dogs. Environ Toxicol 2007;22:176-184.

Walder EJ, Conroy JD. Contact dermatitis in dogs and cats: pathogenesis, histopathology, experimental induction and case reports. Vet Dermatol 1994;5:149-162.

Insect hypersensitivity

Insects are cosmopolitan in their distribution, and virtually all animals are exposed to them. Many insects are capable of inducing allergic reactions, including various dermatoses. *Antigens of insect origin that produce hypersensitivity are usually proteins, and sources include venom, saliva, whole bodies, shed skins, egg capsules, feces, and insect hemoglobin*. These antigens can be introduced via the bite or sting of insects or by inhalation, ingestion, or percutaneous absorption. In general, lesions associated with insect hypersensitivity are *seasonal* or seasonally more severe and *involve short- or sparsely haired regions*, such as the nose, muzzle, pinnae, inguinal area, and distal extremities. *Lesions typically consist of pruritic crusted papules and are characterized histologically by eosinophilic inflammation.*

The most well-known insect hypersensitivities of veterinary significance are those caused by an allergic reaction to salivary antigens, and these are *flea-bite hypersensitivity of dogs and cats* and *Culicoides hypersensitivity of horses*. *Hypersensitivity to mosquito bites has been recognized in cats*, and an *eosinophilic furunculosis of the face of dogs* is suspected to be a hypersensitivity response to the sting or bite of various insects. The first 3 of these conditions will be discussed in this section. Canine eosinophilic furunculosis of the face is discussed under Eosinophilic dermatitides.

Flea-bite hypersensitivity is a pruritic dermatitis caused by hypersensitivity to allergens in the saliva of fleas. *It is the most common allergic dermatosis of dogs and cats in flea-endemic regions*. The cat flea, *Ctenocephalides felis felis*, is the major initiator of the condition. Because many animals harbor large numbers of fleas without any apparent skin abnormalities, it is likely that animals develop skin disease as a result of flea infestation only if they are allergic to fleas.

Both type I and type IV hypersensitivity reactions are believed to be involved in the pathogenesis of flea-bite hypersensitivity. Participation of immediate hypersensitivity is supported by the fact that clinically allergic animals develop immediate skin reactions in response to intradermal injection of flea antigen and that IgE antibodies to flea antigen are demonstrable in sera from allergic animals. Histologic evidence also supports a role for immediate hypersensitivity and suggests that cell-mediated/delayed hypersensitivity is involved in the pathogenesis of flea allergy as well. Many flea-allergic animals also have delayed skin test reactions—further support for a type IV hypersensitivity component. Upregulation of mast cell proteases has been demonstrated during sensitization, with selective release of mast cell tryptase after exposure to flea antigen.

No breed or sex predilections have been reported in flea-bite hypersensitivity, and in cats, no age predilection has been recognized. In dogs, disease occurs most commonly between 3 and 5 years of age, unless naive dogs are moved to a flea-endemic area at a later age. Disease is rare prior to 6 months. Signs tend to be more severe in summer and fall in animals living in areas with cold winters but are year-round in those living in warm regions or where indoor infestation persists. Affected individuals may have other hypersensitivity conditions, such as atopic dermatitis (AD) or food allergy.

Flea-bite hypersensitivity in **dogs** is characterized by pruritus, erythema, wheals, and papules that may become crusted. *Primary lesions are usually obscured by secondary lesions that develop in response to chronic pruritus.* These may include hyperkeratosis, lichenification, hyperpigmentation, alopecia, excoriations, redundant skin folds on the rump and caudal thighs, and seborrhea. Lesions typically involve the dorsal lumbosacral area, flanks, caudal and medial aspect of the thighs, and ventral abdomen. In severely hypersensitive dogs, lesions may become generalized. Pyotraumatic dermatitis ("hot spots") and bacterial pyoderma are common secondary complications. Firm alopecic nodules ("fibropruritic nodules") may develop on the dorsal lumbosacral region secondary to self-trauma in chronically affected dogs. Differential diagnoses include other hypersensitivity conditions (AD, food allergy), sarcoptic mange, cheyletiellosis, and bacterial or yeast infection.

The lesions of flea-bite hypersensitivity in **cats** are extremely variable. The most common manifestation is multiple erythematous pruritic papules covered by brown crust *("miliary dermatitis")* on the dorsal lumbosacral area, flanks, caudal and medial aspect of the thighs, ventral abdomen, and neck. In some cats, the condition may be manifested as overzealous grooming rather than scratching, producing alopecia that may be ventral abdominal, bilaterally symmetrical along the lateral aspect of the trunk, or dorsal lumbosacral. The skin may appear completely normal grossly, or excoriations, crusts, scales, and hyperpigmented macules may be seen. Fleas or flea dirt may not be evident because of the fastidious grooming behavior typical of most cats. Eosinophilic granuloma complex lesions have also been associated with flea-bite hypersensitivity in cats. Secondary bacterial pyoderma is uncommon. Differential diagnosis is extensive because the manifestations of flea allergy are so varied in cats. *The most common differentials for miliary dermatitis include other hypersensitivity conditions (AD, food hypersensitivity), dermatophytosis, and cheyletiellosis.* Cases characterized by self-induced alopecia with normal-appearing skin may resemble an endocrinopathy.

Histopathology is useful in confirming the suspected diagnosis of a hypersensitivity condition, but the microscopic changes associated with flea-bite hypersensitivity are similar to those seen in other hypersensitivities, and the specific diagnosis cannot be made histologically. The epidermis is variably acanthotic, and foci of spongiosis and serocellular crusting are commonly seen. Mixed orthokeratotic and parakeratotic hyperkeratosis and self-induced erosion or ulceration may be present. Foci of epidermal necrosis and intraepidermal eosinophilic pustules may be evident. The superficial dermis is mildly to moderately edematous, and perivascular to interstitial infiltration of eosinophils, lymphocytes, fewer macrophages, and mast cells is present in the superficial to mid-dermis in dogs and may extend into the subcutis in cats. The proportion of eosinophils in relation to mononuclear cells varies, with eosinophils being most numerous in early lesions and mononuclear cells predominating in more chronic reactions. Melanophages are in variable numbers and may be numerous in chronic cases with prominent lichenification. Sebaceous and epitrichial glands may be hyperplastic in chronic lesions. Neutrophils are numerous in association with ulceration or bacterial infection. In cats, eosinophilic mural folliculitis and furunculosis have been seen in flea bites as have histologic lesions of eosinophilic granuloma complex.

***Culicoides* (insect) hypersensitivity** *is the most common allergic dermatosis of horses.* It occurs worldwide, and *Culicoides* spp. gnats are the most common cause. The condition is known by a variety of colloquial names worldwide, including Queensland itch, kasen, dhobie itch, sweet itch, muck itch, summer itch, and summer eczema. It is a major annoyance to horse and owner, and substantial economic losses can be incurred from treatment, prevention, and damage caused by scratching horses. *Culicoides* hypersensitivity is an *intensely pruritic dermatosis* that can render affected animals too restless and anxious to perform.

The insects are also called biting midges, punkies, and "no-see-ums." Hundreds of different species exist throughout the world, and they vary in their favored feeding sites and time of activity. They are most active when the ambient temperature is >10° C (50° F), when humidity is high, and when there is no breeze because they are weak fliers. The insects are in highest numbers in wetlands and swampy areas.

The hypersensitivity to salivary antigens of *Culicoides* gnats is thought to be mediated by *both type I and type IV hypersensitivity reactions.* Support for immediate hypersensitivity is provided by immediate skin test reactivity to *Culicoides* antigens, presence of specific IgE in affected horses, and peripheral eosinophilia and increased blood histamine concentrations during periods of insect activity. The presence of increased numbers of primarily CD4+ T lymphocytes and eosinophils in skin test reactions is also consistent with immediate hypersensitivity. Also, sulfidoleukotriene generation from peripheral blood leukocytes in response to *Culicoides* extract was increased in horses with insect hypersensitivity, indicating involvement of IgE-mediated hypersensitivity in the pathogenesis of *Culicoides* hypersensitivity. Delayed reactions (up to 48 hours) to intradermal skin tests suggest that type IV hypersensitivity may also be involved in the pathogenesis of the condition.

Culicoides hypersensitivity is typically a seasonal disease, but in warm climates it may be a problem virtually year-round. Horses of any breed and either sex are affected; pedigree studies suggest there may be a genetic basis. Lesions are uncommon in horses <2 years of age; however, in tropical and subtropical climates with a long insect season, sensitization and mild clinical disease may develop within the first year of exposure. The favored feeding sites vary with the species of *Culicoides* endemic to a particular environment, accounting for the varied distribution of skin lesions. Distribution may be dorsal and involve the head, ears, neck, withers, back, and tailhead, or it may be primarily ventral and involve the intermandibular space, legs, and ventral midline. In some areas, such as Florida in the United States, multiple species of *Culicoides* are active at different times and have different favored feeding sites, such that disease may be generalized. The *primary lesions are pruritic papules* that may be recognized initially by clusters of erect hairs and commonly become encrusted. Because of severe pruritus, however, self-mutilation obscures the primary lesions and results in *more commonly observed secondary lesions, such as excoriations, crusts, lichenification, pigmentary changes, broken hairs, alopecia, and a short stubbled tail ("rat tail")* (Fig. 6-67). The mane may be rubbed off, and the skin over the neck and withers may become thickened and rugose. Lesions typically heal during winter and recur in spring or summer and commonly worsen with age.

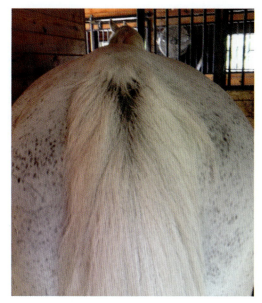

Figure 6-67 *Culicoides* hypersensitivity in a horse. Alopecia at the tail head caused by self-trauma ("rat tail"). (Courtesy N. Radwanski.)

Affected horses may scratch and bite themselves and rub objects in their environment, thereby causing damage to themselves, their riders, and environmental objects. Constant anxiety and restlessness may prevent severely affected animals from performing as riding or show animals. Also, because sweating exacerbates pruritus, affected horses cannot be worked vigorously. The differential diagnoses include ectoparasitism and other hypersensitivity dermatoses. The *diagnosis* is based on seasonality of the condition, location and appearance of lesions, sporadic occurrence of the condition in a group, eliminating other diseases, and response to therapy.

The *histologic lesions* of *Culicoides* hypersensitivity are typically *superficial or superficial and deep perivascular dermatitis consisting of eosinophils and lymphocytes primarily*. The epidermis is variably acanthotic, spongiotic, and hyperkeratotic with foci of parakeratosis, and may be focally necrotic. Increased numbers of T lymphocytes and Langerhans cells are present in the basal portion of the epidermis. Erosions and ulceration may be present as a result of self-trauma and are associated with neutrophilic inflammation. The dermis is variably edematous and increased numbers of mast cells, which may be degranulated, are present. In some cases, eosinophilic inflammation is diffuse, and collagen flame figures or eosinophilic folliculitis may also be seen.

A seasonal pruritic dermatosis attributed to *Culicoides* hypersensitivity has also been described in *cattle, sheep, and donkeys*. Affected sheep were 2-5 years of age and had an intensely pruritic, exudative dermatitis with loss of wool and marked skin thickening of the abdomen, udder, teats, and legs. Lesions in adult dairy cattle consisted of marked thickening and folding of the skin of the head, ears, and neck. Donkeys developed exudative dermatitis, alopecia, crusting, and skin thickening of the legs and head. Affected animals were restless and often bit at themselves, suggesting that they were intensely pruritic. Histologic examination of biopsies from affected sheep and cows showed primarily an eosinophilic dermal infiltrate.

Mosquito-bite hypersensitivity dermatitis is documented in the Mosquito-bite dermatitis section.

Further reading

Fadok VA. Update on equine allergies. Vet Clin North Am Equine Pract 2013;29:541-550.

Hobi S, et al. Clinical characteristics and causes of pruritus in cats: a multicentre study on feline hypersensitivity-associated dermatoses. Vet Dermatol 2011;22:406-413.

Kunkle GA, et al. Pilot study to assess the effects of early flea exposure on the development of flea hypersensitivity in cats. J Feline Med Surg 2003;5:287-294.

Lam A1, Yu A. Overview of flea allergy dermatitis. Compend Contin Educ Vet 2009;31:E1-E10.

von Ruedorffer U, et al. Flea bite hypersensitivity: new aspects on the involvement of mast cells. Vet J 2003;165:149-156.

Hormonal hypersensitivity

Pruritic dermatitis resulting from hypersensitivity to endogenous sex hormones is recognized in women ("autoimmune progesterone dermatitis") and is *very rare in dogs*. Results of intradermal skin tests with aqueous progesterone in women indicate that type I and/or type IV hypersensitivity are involved. *Most canine cases are in intact females, frequently with a history of irregular estrus or recurrent pseudopregnancy.* The condition is characterized by *intense pruritus* that develops or is exacerbated near the time of estrus or pseudopregnancy but tends to become more severe and protracted with each episode; pruritus is generally perennial in male dogs. Bilaterally symmetrical erythema and crusted papules typically begin in the dorsal lumbosacral, perineal, genital, and caudomedial thigh areas and progress cranially. In chronic cases, the condition is generalized, and the skin becomes alopecic and lichenified. Pruritus is usually unresponsive to glucocorticoid treatment. Differential diagnoses include other allergic conditions and sarcoptic mange. The microscopic lesion is a hyperplastic superficial perivascular dermatitis in which neutrophils, mononuclear cells, or eosinophils may predominate. *Diagnostic clues include poor response to glucocorticoid therapy and development or exacerbation of cutaneous signs coincident with estrus or pseudopregnancy.* Gonadectomy is curative.

Intestinal parasite hypersensitivity

Hypersensitivity to intestinal parasites has been suspected of causing pruritic dermatoses in *dogs, cats, horses, and humans*. The pathomechanism is unknown, but a type I hypersensitivity reaction has been proposed. *Ascarids, coccidia, hookworms, tapeworms, and whipworms have rarely been associated with pruritic dermatoses that resolve with elimination of the intestinal parasites*. Lesions that have been attributed to intestinal parasite hypersensitivity include multifocal or generalized papulocrustous eruptions, pruritic seborrheic disease, pruritic urticaria, and pruritus without skin lesions. The histologic changes described are superficial perivascular dermatitis with variable numbers of eosinophils, ranging from few to many. Diagnosis is based on fecal examination and resolution of the skin lesions following appropriate parasiticidal therapy.

Further reading

Cooper PJ. Intestinal worms and human allergy. Parasite Immunol 2004;26:455-467.

Marsella R, et al. Hypersensitivity disorders. In: Miller WH, et al., editors. Muller & Kirk's Small Animal Dermatology. 7th ed. St Louis: Elsevier; 2013. p. 417.

Autoimmune dermatoses

The autoimmune skin diseases are *uncommon to rare* but merit detailed consideration as many are debilitating to life threatening and require specific therapy. *Their characteristic microscopic lesions, combined with clinical information and careful interpretation of ancillary studies, often enable a specific diagnosis to be made.* In the vast majority of cases, the stimulus triggering the aberrant T- or B-cell responses against self-antigens is unknown. Drug therapy, underlying neoplasia (see Paraneoplastic pemphigus), tissue injury, infectious diseases, other autoimmune diseases, and genetic makeup are all factors known to be associated with the occurrence of autoimmune diseases. Penicillinamine, for example, may precipitate clinically, histologically, and immunologically classic cases of pemphigus in humans, which regress when the drug is withdrawn. Drug-induced forms of pemphigus are thought to be the result of haptenization of keratinocyte antigens, rendering them immunogenic. One theory suggests environmental agents, such as drugs, influence T cells by causing DNA methylation abnormalities that, in turn, alter gene expression. Exposure to ultraviolet light is known to exacerbate cutaneous autoimmune disease, perhaps by inducing keratinocyte intercellular adhesion molecule-1 (ICAM-1) expression and keratinocyte production of proinflammatory cytokines. Still another theory suggests that the structural similarities of peptide fragments of some infectious agents to host proteins may trigger postinfectious autosensitization.

The recognition that one autoimmune disease, tissue injury, inflammatory or neoplastic process in an individual may precede the onset of cutaneous autoimmune disease led to investigation of the phenomenon termed *epitope spreading.* Epitope spreading refers to the process by which the targets of the autoimmune response do not remain fixed but drift to include other epitopes on the same protein or nearby proteins of the same tissue. This may account for regional variations in pemphigus antigen expression and the clinical variation of cutaneous autoimmune diseases. Epitope spreading may also account for aberrant immune responses developing to tissue antigens after the tissue has been injured, possibly leading to the release or exposure of a previously sequestered antigen.

Selection of fully-developed lesions is crucial to diagnosis. Demonstration of tissue-bound or circulating autoantibody using appropriate immunologic tests may be helpful in confirming the diagnosis of an autoimmune skin disease. However, such tests (e.g., direct and indirect immunofluorescence testing, immunohistochemistry) are fraught with interpretation pitfalls (false-positive or false-negative test results) and should never be interpreted in the absence of histologic examination. Demonstration of autoantibodies does not necessarily confirm causative roles for these antibodies, just as negative results do not necessarily exclude the diagnosis of a cutaneous autoimmune disease. For example, the various entities of the pemphigus complex are characterized by the deposition of immunoglobulin, with or without complement, on the surface of keratinocytes or at the basement membrane zone using the techniques of direct immunofluorescence (IF) testing or immunohistochemistry (IHC). Unfortunately, false-negative (poor lesion selection, prior glucocorticoid therapy) and false-positive (any dermatosis in which spongiosis or numerous lymphocytes and plasma cells are present) reactions are frequent. In addition, normal epithelium of the canine nasal planum and footpad often label nonspecifically. Hence *these immunopathology tests can only be interpreted in the light of clinical and histopathologic findings.* Indirect immunofluorescence testing has variable usefulness in domestic animals with pemphigus as results may be falsely negative, or "pemphigus-like" antibodies can be occasionally found in nonpemphigus diseases. Indirect IF testing for canine PF can be useful provided the appropriate substrate (bovine esophagus) is used. In many of the putative cases of autoimmune skin disease in animals, the criteria for autoimmunity have not been met fully.

Further reading

Chan LS, et al. Epitope spreading: lessons from autoimmune skin diseases. J Invest Dermatol 1998;110:103-109.

White SD, et al. Putative drug-related pemphigus foliaceus in four dogs. Vet Dermatol 2002;13:195-202.

Autoimmune diseases characterized by vesicles, pustules, or bullae as the primary lesion

The pemphigus complex. Pemphigus refers to a group of autoimmune skin diseases characterized clinically by pustules, vesicles, bullae, erosions, and ulcers and histologically by loss of adhesion between cells *(acantholysis).* Autoantibodies directed against antigens within stratified squamous epithelia, including haired skin, mucocutaneous junctions, oral and genital mucosa, and esophagus, develop and can be detected via immunologic assays. Classic pemphigus in humans is divided into pemphigus vulgaris and pemphigus foliaceus. The clinical phenotypes correlate with the autoantibody profile in the skin. Autoantibodies are directed against components of keratinocyte transmembrane glycoproteins (i.e., extracellular domains of desmoglein 1 or desmoglein 3) that are responsible for keratinocyte cell-to-cell adherence. The autoantibodies cause loss of cohesion between keratinocytes (acantholysis) and blister formation. In pemphigus vulgaris, blisters occur in the lower layers of the epidermis (suprabasilar), where the antibody targets desmoglein-3, the predominant antigen at this location on mucous membranes. Pemphigus foliaceus lesions occur only on haired skin, and the antibody targets desmoglein-1, which resides in upper layers of the epidermis. Pemphigus vulgaris can have both mucous membrane and haired skin involvement if there is concurrent autoantibody formation to desmoglein-1. IgG autoantibodies can also occur in humans with paraneoplastic pemphigus.

The mechanisms leading to acantholysis are not completely understood. Antigen-antibody binding may result in a type II immune reaction or promote proinflammatory cytokine release from keratinocytes. The binding of pemphigus autoantibodies to keratinocyte antigens is associated with the synthesis and secretion of urokinase-type plasminogen activator (uPA), a serine protease that activates plasminogen. Activation of plasminogen may indirectly induce the cleaving of intercellular contacts. Anti-uPA antibodies or the specific inhibitor of uPA, plasminogen activator inhibitor type-2, inhibit lesion formation in vitro. Another hypothesis proposes that the binding of autoantibodies to keratinocyte antigens may disrupt the structural integrity of the adhesion molecule.

Immune-Mediated Dermatoses

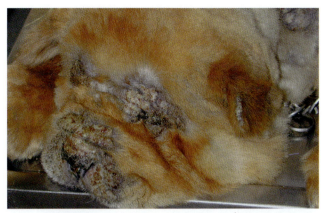

Figure 6-68 Pemphigus foliaceus in a Chow Chow. Note the thick pustules and crusts on the muzzle, nose, periocular area, and apical pinnae.

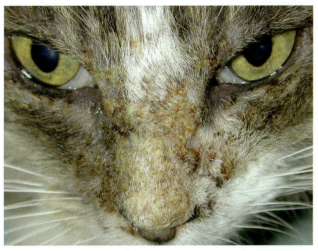

Figure 6-69 Pemphigus foliaceus in a cat. Note the thick crusts in the haired skin of the nasal area.

Experimental studies in mice have demonstrated that acantholysis in pemphigus foliaceus (PF) can occur with passive transfer of PF IgG autoantibody as well as with transfer of Fab fragments and F (ab')$_2$ fragments in both complement-sufficient and complement-deficient mice.

Pemphigus foliaceus is the *most common form of pemphigus in domestic animals and has been reported in the dog, cat, horse, goat, and a Barbary sheep. In humans, PF autoantibodies recognize the desmosomal protein, desmoglein 1. In contrast to humans, desmoglein 1 is only a minor autoantigen in dogs; the major autoantigen is desmocollin-1.* Desmocollin-1 is a transmembrane calcium-dependent desmosomal glycoprotein involved in intercellular adhesions. Desmocollin-1 is found primarily in the upper layers of the epidermis, where PF pustules typically arise. Pemphigus foliaceus often arises spontaneously; however, cases have been triggered by adverse drug reactions as well as topical flea and tick preventatives. PF has no sex predilection in **dogs,** but Akitas, Chow Chows, Bearded Collies, Collies, Chinese Shar-Peis, Dachshunds, Newfoundlands, Doberman Pinschers, Schipperkes, English Springer Spaniels, and Appaloosa horses appear predisposed. In dogs, most cases occur before 5 years of age. In all species, the clinical lesions are nonpruritic to mildly pruritic pustules that rupture and form thick crusts with scaling. On the face, the skin lesions are often bilaterally symmetrical (Fig. 6-68). Dogs and cats may have pawpad hyperkeratosis and crusting with involvement of the claw fold (paronychia). In **cats,** thick crusts are often bilaterally symmetrical on the face and ears (particularly pinnal margins) (Fig. 6-69). PF is the most common autoimmune skin disease in **horses;** lesions often begin on the face or distal extremities, or may be localized to coronets. In any species, the lesions may become generalized (Fig. 6-70A, B). Foals may also be affected with a benign form of PF that responds rapidly to treatment or may resolve spontaneously. Pain and pruritus may be present.

The histologic pattern of pemphigus foliaceus is a superficial intraepidermal pustular dermatitis that typically involves the corneal layer and granular cell layer (see Figs. 6-1 and 6-17). Either neutrophils or eosinophils may predominate. At the base of the pustule, acantholytic keratinocytes continue to detach and enter the pustule. Ruptured pustules form a thick inflammatory crust in which acantholytic cells are prominent. The external root sheath of the hair follicle undergoes a similar acantholytic process. Dermal infiltrates consist of mild

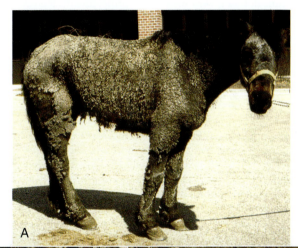

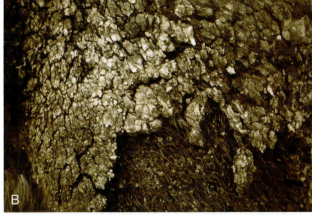

Figure 6-70 Pemphigus foliaceus in a horse. **A.** Generalized exfoliative dermatitis and alopecia. **B.** Detail of skin showing massive build-up of scales and crusts. (Courtesy K. Moriello.)

perivascular to interstitial neutrophils or eosinophils. There is dermal edema, vascular congestion, and occasionally hemorrhage. Rarely, a lichenoid inflammatory infiltrate is seen. Deposition of IgG at intercellular bridges in all layers of the suprabasilar epidermis or in the superficial epidermis demonstrated by IF or IHC is characteristic, but not specific, for PF. Secondary bacterial infection may complicate lesions. *The primary differential for PF is superficial bacterial folliculitis.*

Acantholytic cells are more numerous and can more often be found in rafts in PF than in superficial folliculitis. *The "cling-on" stratum granulosum cells are only present in PF.* In PF, pustules also span the interfollicular epidermis encompassing multiple follicles, whereas in superficial folliculitis pustules are more likely to be centered on single follicles. Evidence of recornification and reformation of pustules is often prominent in PF. Dermatophytosis and superficial pyoderma (impetigo) can also have similar gross and histologic lesions. Careful examination of skin sections with fungal and bacterial stains and possibly cultures may be needed for differentiation. Impetigo does not involve hair follicles, whereas PF may.

Pemphigus erythematosus (PE) and **pemphigus vegetans** are terms that have been loosely applied to veterinary diseases based on human comparisons. *Further studies suggest the conditions are not directly comparable.* Criteria for diagnosis and differentiation from PF were dependent upon the immunologic demonstration of both a diffuse cell surface IF or IHC pattern typical of the pemphigus group and a linear band of immunoglobulin, with or without complement, deposited at the basement membrane zone. For reasons stated previously, IF and IHC are not dependable. Pemphigus erythematosus is a poorly characterized facially oriented PF in dogs and cats. It is unclear if PE is indeed different from PF, a localized variant of PF, or if the disease is a crossover between discoid lupus and PF. Reported cases of pemphigus vegetans in veterinary patients are very limited and originally thought to be benign variants of pemphigus vulgaris. A documented case of pemphigus vegetans has been reported in a Greater Swiss Mountain dog. The dog had verrucous superficial PF pustules/crust and deep epidermal pemphigus vulgaris lesions. Panepidermal pustular pemphigus (PPP) is a term previously used to describe a deep epidermal form of pemphigus in the dog that encompassed some of the features of pemphigus foliaceus, pemphigus vegetans, and pemphigus erythematosus. PPP is now thought to be a histologic variant of PF.

Pemphigus vulgaris (PV) *is the most severe and rare form of pemphigus in animals.* This life-threatening disease has been reported in the *dog, cat, horse, goat, monkey, and llama.* There is no apparent breed or sex predilection. Middle-aged **dogs** are most commonly affected. In humans and dogs, PV autoantibodies recognize the desmosomal protein desmoglein 3. Desmoglein 3 also belongs to the cadherin family of cell-adhesion molecules and is most prominent in the area of the basal layer of keratinocytes of the epidermis and mucosal epithelium, hence lesions occur deeper in the epidermis and in the oral mucosa. The *fragile vesicles or bullae in the epidermis are extremely transient and readily rupture* to leave the more common presenting lesion of a roughly circular, shallow, flat-based erosion or ulcer. Firm sliding pressure to adjacent unaffected skin may induce fresh vesicle formation or dislodge the skin *(the Nikolsky sign)*. Lesions involve mucous membranes (Fig. 6-71A), mucocutaneous junctions and skin in the mechanically stressed areas, such as the inguinal and axillary regions. Oral involvement is present in 90% of cases, and in 50% of cases, the lesions commence in the mouth. Involvement of the nailbeds occurs also, and corneal ulceration may be present. Animals may be febrile, depressed, and anorectic and have leukocytosis. Drooling is often a presenting complaint.

Microscopically, *the earliest lesions consist of spongiosis and vacuolation of the suprabasilar epidermis progressing to suprabasilar acantholysis with intraepidermal clefts, vesicles, or bullae*

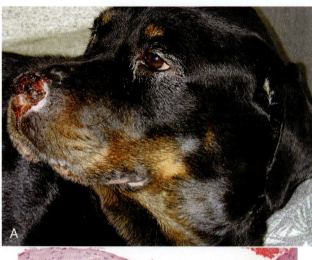

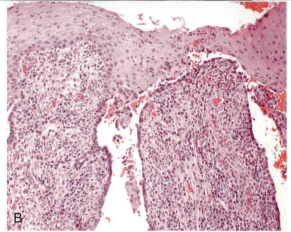

Figure 6-71 Pemphigus vulgaris in a Rottweiler. **A.** The nasal planum and lips are markedly ulcerated. **B.** Separation of the epidermis occurs between the stratum spinosum and stratum basale. Basal keratinocytes also lose intercellular contact, leaving the basal layer arranged to resemble a "row of tombstones."

between the stratum basale and the stratum spinosum (Fig. 6-71B). The basal keratinocytes, although separated from each other following disruption of intercellular contacts, are anchored to the basal lamina resembling a "row of tombstones." The outer layers of the epidermis form the roof of the vesicle that may contain a few acantholytic keratinocytes, singly or in clumps, but few or no inflammatory cells. The process may extend into the hair follicle epithelium. The dermal reaction in haired skin varies from a mild superficial perivascular to interstitial accumulation of mononuclear cells and eosinophils. A moderately intense lymphocytic-plasmacytic interface infiltrate may be present in mucosal lesions.

Clinical differentials include mucous membrane pemphigoid, erythema multiforme, bullous pemphigoid, toxic epidermal necrolysis, vesicular lupus erythematosus of Collies and Shetland Sheepdogs, mycosis fungoides, and other diseases resulting in oral ulcers. Histopathologic findings of primary lesions in PV are diagnostic.

Further reading

Bizikova P, et al. Cloning and establishment of canine desmocollin-1 as a major autoantigen in canine pemphigus foliaceus. Vet Immunol Immunopathol 2012;149:197-207.

Bizikova P, et al. Serum autoantibody profiles of IgA, IgE and IgM in canine pemphigus foliaceus. Vet Dermatol 2014;25:471-e75.

Brenner DJ, et al. Pemphigus foliaceus in a barbary sheep (Ammotragus lervia). Vet Rec 2009;165:509-510.

Oberkirchner U, et al. Metaflumizone-amitraz (Promeris)-associated pustular acantholytic dermatitis in 22 dogs: evidence suggests contact drug-triggered pemphigus foliaceus. Vet Dermatol 2011;22:436-448.

Olivry T, Linder KE. Dermatoses affecting desmosomes in animals: a mechanistic review of acantholytic blistering skin diseases. Vet Dermatol 2009;20:313-326.

Winfield LD, et al. Pemphigus vulgaris in a Welsh pony stallion: case report and demonstration of antidesmoglein autoantibodies. Vet Dermatol 2013;24:269-e60.

Paraneoplastic pemphigus. *Paraneoplastic pemphigus (PNP) is an aggressive form of pemphigus most often associated with solid or hematopoietic neoplasia.* PNP has been documented in *humans, 2 dogs, and a single putative case in a cat with thymic lymphoma and a horse with a sarcoma on the neck.* Of the 2 cases reported in dogs, one had thymic lymphoma and the other an undifferentiated sarcoma in the spleen. Cutaneous lesions may precede detection of the neoplastic process. The condition is resistant to treatment. Lesions consist of *severe mucosal and mucocutaneous blistering and erosions.* Histologically, lesions have a combined pattern of erythema multiforme and suprabasilar acantholysis characteristic of pemphigus vulgaris. Lymphohistiocytic, lichenoid interface dermatitis, and apoptosis of keratinocytes with lymphocytic satellitosis throughout the epidermis are characteristic. Immunologically, labeling of intercellular bridges and/or basement membrane is detected by IHC or IFA staining. Direct immunofluorescence studies implicate autoantibodies to a 190-kDa protein, the 210- and 250-kDa desmoplakin proteins, and to the 230-kDa BPAGI, one of the bullous pemphigoid antigens. Antidesmoglein IgG was recently documented in the serum of canine PNP. Not all cases with the above-described lesions and autoantibodies have underlying neoplasia. Histologic differentials include panepidermal pustular pemphigus and those listed for PV and mucous membrane pemphigoid.

Further reading

Elmore SA, et al. Paraneoplastic pemphigus in a dog with splenic sarcoma. Vet Pathol 2005;42:88-91.

Hill PB, et al. Putative paraneoplastic pemphigus and myasthenia gravis in a cat with a lymphocytic thymoma. Vet Dermatol 2013;24:646-649.

Nishifuji K, et al. IgG autoantibodies directed against desmoglein 3 cause dissociation of keratinocytes in canine pemphigus vulgaris and paraneoplastic pemphigus. Vet Immunol Immunopathol 2007;117:209-221.

Mucous membrane pemphigoid. Mucous membrane pemphigoid (MMP), also called cicatricial pemphigoid, is an autoimmune blistering disorder with a distinct clinical presentation of lesions localized to mucous membranes and mucocutaneous junctions. In dogs and cats, MMP is the diagnosis given to half of the patients with autoimmune subepidermal blistering diseases. The lesions typically appear as vesicles that ulcerate and then heal with scar tissue. In dogs, lesions typically arise on the nasal planum (Fig. 6-72A), medial canthus, oral cavity, ear canals, and genitalia. The lesions arise in adult

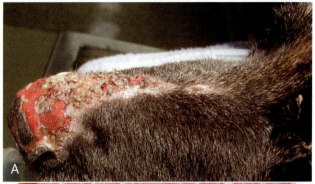

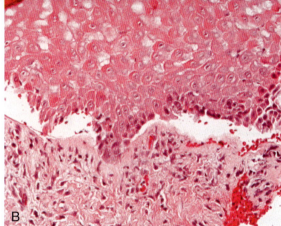

Figure 6-72 Mucous membrane pemphigoid in a dog. **A.** Ulcers on the nasal planum and dorsal muzzle. **B.** Subepidermal vesiculation. The basement membrane zone forms the floor of the vesicle. Note the lack of acantholysis.

dogs and cats. German Shepherd dogs account for about 30% of canine cases. Despite the unique clinical presentation, autoantibodies may be found toward various components of the basement membrane proteins, including BPAG2 and laminin V. Histologically, the cases have subepidermal clefting with various degrees of inflammation (Fig. 6-72B).

Further reading

Olivry T, et al. Laminin-5 is targeted by autoantibodies in feline mucous membrane (cicatricial) pemphigoid. Vet Immunol Immunopathol 2002;88:123-129.

Bullous pemphigoid. *Bullous pemphigoid (BP) is a chronic, autoimmune skin disease characterized clinically by vesicles, bullae, and ulcers, and histologically by subepidermal vesicles/bullae containing eosinophils or other leukocytes.* In humans, the autoantibodies are directed against BP antigen 1 (BPAG1, a 230-kDa intercellular antigen) and BP antigen 2 (BPAG2, also called type XVII collagen, a 180-kDa hemidesmosomal transmembrane molecule). In animals, only BPAG2 has been identified. The mechanism of dermoepidermal separation is thought to be the result of the release of proinflammatory cytokines IL-1, IL-5, IL-6, IL-8, and others by keratinocytes altered by antigen-antibody interactions. Cytokines recruit neutrophils and eosinophils, leading to the release of damaging proteases. Separation of basal cells from the underlying dermis may also be the direct result of disorganization or internalization of components of the hemidesmosomes. In almost all cases, the stimulus triggering the immune response is unknown, although drugs may precipitate clinically, histologically, and immunopathologically classic cases of pemphigoid that regress when the drug is withdrawn. Exposure to ultraviolet light is known to exacerbate BP.

The diagnosis of BP in dogs and cats has come under intense scrutiny in recent literature. *Many cases that have been reported as BP were cited before techniques were available to identify the target protein.* Although Collies are supposedly predisposed to BP, the disease process would currently be classified as cutaneous vesicular lupus erythematosus. Furthermore, additional cases in dogs and cats would now be classified as mucous membrane pemphigoid. One confirmed BP case was documented in 3-year-old dog with vesicles and erosions on the prepuce, trunk, face, and paws. The dogs was documented with IgG autoantibodies that targeted BPAG2 (XVII collagen). BP has been documented in horses and Yucatan minipigs. **In horses,** the lesions are often generalized with marked sloughing of the oral mucosa and signs of systemic illness. Lesions on the rump and back characterize the disease in **Yucatan minipigs.** Mucosal lesions have not been described in pigs.

Histologically, there is *a subepidermal bulla filled with fibrin and variable numbers of neutrophils, eosinophils, and mononuclear cells.* Eosinophils are not always present as they are in lesions of humans. *Acantholytic keratinocytes are not present.* The basal cells that line the roof of the bulla are not initially degenerate. The basement membrane zone lines the floor of the bulla as separation occurs within the lamina lucida. There is often marked subepidermal vacuolar alteration. The dermis is usually markedly edematous, capillaries are dilated and lined with swollen endothelial cells, and there is perivascular accumulation of neutrophils, eosinophils, and mononuclear cells. Mild to moderate lichenoid interface dermatitis may be present, particularly in mucocutaneous regions. *Histologic differential diagnoses* include pemphigus vulgaris, vesicular lupus erythematosus, mucous membrane pemphigoid, epidermolysis bullosa acquisita, toxic epidermal necrolysis (TEN), and thermal burns.

Classically, BP is characterized by the presence of *immunoglobulin (IgG, IgM, or IgA) and/or complement deposited at the basement membrane zone* within skin lesions. The BP180 antigen extends to the lateral and apical aspects of basal keratinocytes, and labeling may extend to these areas. Serum autoantibodies may be detected in some cases.

Further reading

Olivry T. An autoimmune subepidermal blistering skin disease in a dog? The odds are that it is not bullous pemphigoid. Vet Dermatol 2014;25:316-318.

Linear immunoglobulin A disease in dogs. Linear IgA disease (LAD) *is an acquired autoimmune subepidermal blistering disease occurring in humans and dogs.* IgG and/or IgA autoantibodies against LAD-1, defined as the processed extracellular domain of type XVII collagen, are demonstrable at the basement membrane zone of lesional skin and in the serum of affected dogs and humans. It is interesting to note the BP antigen is also type XVII collagen; however, in BP, antibodies recognize the transmembrane form of type XVII collagen. Clinically, LAD is characterized by erosions, ulcers, and crusts on the face, extremities, and in the oral cavity. Histologically, dermoepidermal clefting with little or no neutrophilic infiltration is present. *Differential diagnoses are similar to those listed for BP and TEN.* Differentiation of LAD from other subepidermal blistering diseases requires demonstration of linear IgA deposits at the basement membrane zone of skin lesions as well as identification of circulating autoantibodies against the target antigen, LAD-1. Too few cases have been documented in the dog to define the prognosis.

Epidermolysis bullosa acquisita in the dog. *Epidermolysis bullosa acquisita (EBA) is a subepidermal blistering disease characterized by vesicle formation in areas of concurrent neutrophilic superficial dermatitis.* The condition has been reported in dogs and humans. Circulating and tissue-bound autoantibodies targeting the distal end of anchoring fibrils in the sub-lamina densa of the lower basement membrane zone have been demonstrated using immunofluorescence and immunoelectron microscopy. The actual target antigen has been shown to be the amino-terminal globular noncollagenous domain of type VII collagen. Clinical lesions in the dog are characterized by erythematous and urticarial eruption with vesicles, bullae, or ulcerations arising in areas subject to friction, including oral ulcerations. Histologically, dermoepidermal separation is present in association with marked neutrophilic inflammation in the superficial dermis and within vesicles and bullae. Too few cases have been documented to provide information regarding triggering events or clinical outcome. Differentials include those listed for BP.

Further reading

Olivry T, Dunston SM. Usefulness of collagen IV immunostaining for diagnosis of canine epidermolysis bullosa acquisita. Vet Pathol 2010;47:565-568.

Lupus erythematosus

Lupus erythematosus (LE) represents a spectrum of inflammatory disorders that varies from mild skin-limited conditions to life-threatening systemic disease (*systemic lupus erythematosus,* SLE). *Cutaneous lupus erythematosus* (CLE) refers to the skin-specific effects of LE, regardless of whether or not there is systemic involvement (i.e., polyarthritis, glomerulonephritis, thrombocytopenia, etc.). In human medicine, CLE is subdivided into 3 major categories: chronic CLE (localized and generalized discoid lupus), subacute CLE, and acute CLE. The subsets serve as prognosticators and are based on the morphology of skin lesions, variations in the histologic reaction, and clinicopathologic findings. For example, chronic CLE is more likely to remain skin localized than acute or subacute CLE. However, patients with chronic CLE who have generalized skin involvement (i.e., disseminated discoid LE) have increased risk of developing systemic manifestations of LE. Acute CLE is the typical malar "butterfly" rash associated with flare-ups of SLE. Subacute CLE is characteristically provoked by solar exposure. The feature common to the lupus subsets is a distinct constellation of histopathologic changes affecting the basal layer and basement membrane zone: basal cell vacuolar degeneration, basement membrane thickening, mononuclear cell infiltration of the dermoepidermal junction and dermis and dermal edema/mucin deposition. It is important to note that lupus patients may develop a variety of skin lesions that are not histologically distinct for lupus (lupus nonspecific), and may be seen with another disease processes.

In veterinary and human medicine, the diagnosis of SLE is based on fulfillment of 4 of 11 criteria established by the American College of Rheumatology, with virtually all cases having a positive antinuclear antibody (ANA) titer. CLE and SLE are thought to have similar pathogenic mechanisms whether or not the disorder remains skin localized. The pathogenesis of CLE involves genetic predisposition (e.g., major histocompatibility complex [MHC] subtype) and generation of autoreactive antibodies that may be triggered by solar exposure, drugs, and tobacco smoke.

Veterinary medicine has historically classified LE into discoid lupus erythematosus (DLE) and SLE. Discoid lupus, the prototype in dogs, has a classic presentation on the nasal planum and/or lips and vulva or prepuce. Although having some features of DLE in humans, the overall disease is not comparable, and veterinarians/owners should be discouraged from applying generalizations from the human literature. The nosology of this disorder remains questionable. Furthermore, 2 diseases (lupoid dermatosis of German Shorthaired Pointers and idiopathic ulcerative dermatosis of Shetland Sheepdogs and Collies) have since been reclassified as variants of cutaneous lupus. Recently, case reports have documented disseminated forms of discoid lupus in dogs, which are more comparable to the disease in humans. It is likely that many unclassified "interface diseases" will fall into CLE as the dermatopathology expertise evolves in veterinary medicine.

Aside from a few exceptions in case reports, the following generalizations hold true for most cases of CLE in veterinary medicine.

- Cutaneous lupus in domestic animals generally does not precede the onset of systemic lupus.
- The frequency of SLE related skin disease is controversial. Although "skin disease" is considered a major sign of SLE, the precise lesions are often not defined, and inclusion may erroneously fulfill criteria for the diagnosis of SLE. "Dermatitis" associated with some cases of SLE may reflect "lupus nonspecific" skin lesions.
- Well-characterized CLE disorders in dogs are often breed specific and presumed hereditary.

Systemic lupus erythematosus. *Dogs, cats, and horses* have been documented with skin manifestations of SLE. Aside from one recent report in a dog, the cutaneous lesions do not herald the onset of SLE. SLE is reported to occur in middle-aged animals without age or sex predilections. German Shepherd dogs appear to be predisposed. SLE is a chronic condition that *may wax and wane.* Drug administration, pregnancy, extreme heat or cold, and ultraviolet (UV) radiation have been known to trigger onset of SLE. *Polyarthritis, thrombocytopenia, fever of unknown origin, anemia, stomatitis, and glomerulonephritis are common manifestations.* Although "dermatitis," is cited as a common manifestation, (i.e., occurring in ~⅓ of affected dogs) the type of skin lesion (i.e., "lupus specific" vs. lupus nonspecific) is generally not indicated. Contrary to citations in textbooks and reviews, *true cutaneous manifestations of SLE are probably rare.* The *gross lesions* that have been described are extremely variable, and range from a mucocutaneous, ulcerative dermatitis resembling pemphigus vulgaris and bullous pemphigoid to erythema, scaling, and alopecia. Lesions may occur in sun-exposed regions (i.e., face, ears, nose, lips) and sparsely haired, lightly pigmented, thin skin of other body regions.

The histopathology consists of a cell-poor to lichenoid interface dermatitis with hydropic degeneration of basal cells and a lymphohistiocytic infiltrate at the dermoepidermal junction. Lymphocytes predominate; however, plasma cells are intermixed at mucocutaneous sites. *Apoptosis of basal keratinocytes and pigmentary incontinence, a consequence of the basal cell degeneration, are key histologic lesions, as is subepidermal vacuolar change.* One well-documented case of SLE (bullous form) with IgG autoantibody against collagen VII has been reported in the dog and found to be similar to the condition in humans. Histologically, subepidermal bullae were associated with circulating IgG autoantibodies to type VII collagen as well as IgG deposits at the basement membrane zone. In the acute cutaneous lesions of SLE, there is dermal edema, capillary dilation, extravasation of leukocytes and erythrocytes, and variable lymphohistiocytic infiltrates around vessels of superficial and deep capillary plexuses. Mucinous degeneration may be prominent. With chronicity, a few cases may show thickening of the basement membrane caused by accumulation of antigen-antibody complexes. Fibrinoid deposits may also occur around superficial blood vessels. Leukocytoclastic vasculitis develops occasionally. Immunoglobulin and complement deposition at the basement membrane zone may be detectable by IF or IHC staining. An antinuclear antibody (ANA) titer of >256 is present in 97-100% of dogs with SLE but is not entirely specific for the disease. *Differential diagnoses* vary with the type of lesions present but may include other autoimmune skin diseases, drug eruption, vasculitis, ischemic dermatopathy, and dermatomyositis.

There are anecdotal cases of SLE with cutaneous manifestations in the **horse** and a documented case in a 2-year-old Standardbred filly. The horse developed weight loss, bilateral symmetrical alopecia with scaling oral ulcers, and lymphadenopathy. Abnormal findings included a Coombs test–positive hemolytic anemia and a positive ANA test result. An autopsy revealed membranous glomerulonephritis and fibrinous synovitis. Skin biopsies had an interface reaction with IgG deposition at the basement membrane zone.

SLE-like disease occurs in the **cat,** but with only a few case reports and case series, a cohesive dermatologic manifestation has not been revealed. Approximately 50% of SLE cases in cats are reported to have skin lesions (seborrhea, exfoliative erythroderma, symmetrical erythematous scaling and crusting); however, it is unclear how many cases with dermatitis had a lupus-specific reaction pattern. Glomerulonephritis, thrombocytopenia, and hemolytic anemia and neurologic disease have been cited. One case report documents a cat with LE-specific histologic lesions and criteria for the diagnosis of SLE (symmetrical facial dermatitis, thrombocytopenia, positive ANAs, oral ulceration).

Cutaneous lupus erythematosus. In dogs, localized forms of lupus include nasal planum discoid lupus, and disseminated discoid lupus, as well as breed-specific cutaneous vesicular lupus and exfoliative cutaneous lupus. **Nasal DLE,** a distinct entity in dogs and very rarely seen in cats, is currently under close scrutiny. The terminology for this clinicopathologic condition is likely to change, as the pathogenesis becomes understood. There does not appear to be a relationship between nasal planum DLE and SLE. The clinical findings are distinct on the nasal planum: loss of cobblestone architecture, depigmentation, erosions/ulcers, hyperkeratosis, and crusting. The condition affects the entire nasal planum, and may be exacerbated or triggered by solar exposure, which is the reason for a proposed name change *(photosensitive nasal dermatitis)*. Some dogs may have similar lesions around the eyes, lips, vulva, and prepuce. Biopsies are often complicated by surface bacterial infection. Histologic features consist of lichenoid lymphoplasmacytic interface dermatitis with pigmentary incontinence, mild vacuolar change in the basal cell layer, and a few individually necrotic basal keratinocytes. The epidermis may have elongated rete ridges, which are generally thin, as is the epidermis between the ridges. Many pathologists have been frustrated by these biopsies, as the features found in routine cases often represent a "blurred line" that cannot distinguish DLE from mucocutaneous pyoderma. This clinical distribution can be helpful because mucocutaneous pyoderma generally affects the junctions of the alar folds and haired skin rather than the entire nasal planum. Mucocutaneous pyoderma also lacks evidence of basal cell damage and is predominantly plasmacytic. Both conditions may be present simultaneously. Other differential diagnoses include parasympathetic nasal dermatitis, Labrador Retriever nasal parakeratosis, superficial dermatophytosis, adverse drug reaction, and uveodermatologic syndrome. The biopsy is most helpful to rule out other conditions (e.g., cutaneous lymphoma, pemphigus foliaceus, vitiligo). A final diagnosis is achieved with both histologic and clinical evaluation.

Cutaneous (discoid) lupus erythematosus is rarely described in horses. There are no age, breed, or sex predilections. Lesions commonly begin on the face, especially around mucocutaneous junctions, leading to annular and oval symmetrical areas of erythema, scaling, alopecia, and variable degrees of leukoderma and leukotrichia. Lesions may also occur on the pinna, neck, shoulders, perianal, perineal, and genital areas. As in other species, the disease is exacerbated by UV radiation.

Disseminated discoid lupus erythematosus has been documented in a 9-year-old Chinese Crested dog and a 3-year-old, female Spitz. Both dogs had generalized lesions affecting the haired skin without mucous membrane involvement. The Chinese Crested dog had annular and polycyclic hyperpigmented and scaly skin lesions with central erosions, hypopigmentation. Skin biopsies showed a lymphocyte-rich interface dermatitis with epidermal atrophy and dermoepidermal deposition of immunoglobulins and activated complement. The Spitz had diffuse erythema and scaling on the dorsal trunk with an interface dermatitis characterized by hydropic degeneration of the basal layer, plasmacytic perivascular dermatitis, and a plasma cell–rich interface mural folliculitis.

Exfoliative cutaneous lupus erythematosus (ECLE) in the German Shorthaired Pointer is a severe heritable variant form of CLE. Early in life, these dogs develop widespread skin lesions (scaling, erythema, erosions/ulcers, pigment loss) as well as variable lethargy and lameness. The inheritance is autosomal recessive and maps to canine chromosome 18. All dogs generally develop lesions by 6 months of age. The clinical and histologic features are diagnostic. The lesions are not solar associated. This first manifestation is adherent scale on the dorsal muzzle (Fig. 6-73). This is followed by erythema, with progression to hair loss, pigment alterations, erosions, and ulcers. As the lesions change, the distribution becomes truncal and involves the scrotum (often severe), limbs, and ears. The collar area is generally spared. The dogs are generally nonpruritic. Biopsies of peripheral lymph nodes reveal reactive lymphoid hyperplasia; nodes are often palpably enlarged before the onset of severe skin lesions. The dogs have consistent mild lymphopenia and hyperproteinemia, with some dogs having

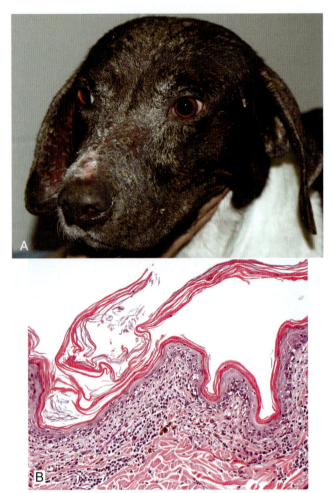

Figure 6-73 Exfoliative cutaneous lupus erythematosus in a German Shorthaired Pointer. **A.** Scaling, alopecia, and hypopigmentation on the muzzle and medial pinna. **B.** Lymphocytic interface dermatitis with basal layer vacuolar change, pigmentary incontinence, and marked orthokeratotic hyperkeratosis.

minimal to mild thrombocytopenia. ANA titers are negative. With time, the dogs develop progressive shifting leg lameness and a hunched "tucked up" stance. Joint aspirates, detailed radiographic studies, and postmortem examinations have failed to find a source for the apparent arthralgia. Both males and females are infertile. The males have oligospermia, and the females have delayed or absent estrus cycles.

The histologic changes are lupus specific and characteristic of ECLE. A subtle interface change can be detected as early as 6 weeks of age but typically is not fully developed until 4-6 months. The interface reaction is characterized by a sparse to mild lymphocytic superficial dermal inflammatory infiltrate, basal keratinocyte vacuolar change with individual basal keratinocyte necrosis, dermoepidermal clefting, and pigmentary incontinence. Some individually necrotic keratinocytes can be found in the spinous layer as in human CLE. The interface reaction affects outer root sheaths, and may be associated with patchy (not complete) sebaceous gland loss. With time, hair follicles undergo atrophy. The stratum corneum has marked orthokeratotic hyperkeratosis. Although the disease may wax and wane for several years, most dogs are eventually euthanized because of intractable skin disease. The main differential diagnosis is erythema multiforme.

Vesicular cutaneous lupus erythematosus is a disorder, formerly known as *idiopathic ulcerative dermatosis*, that is seen in Rough-coated Collies, Shetland Sheepdogs, and Border Collies. This condition was originally thought to be an adult-onset variant of dermatomyositis, but recent immunologic studies indicate the presence of autoantibodies that target nuclear antigens similar to that seen in CLE. Antinuclear antibody testing is negative. Lesions develop in middle-aged to older dogs. Clinical lesions consist of vesicles and bullae that evolve into erosions and ulcers. The inguinal and axillary regions are most commonly involved, but lesions may also occur on mucocutaneous junctions. Histologic changes consist of interface lymphocytic dermatitis with hydropic degeneration of basal cells, keratinocyte apoptosis, and extensive vesicles and bullae at the dermoepidermal junction.

Lupus panniculitis (lupus profundus) is *characterized by well-circumscribed subcutaneous nodules over the trunk and proximal extremities*. It is reported rarely in dogs, and because the features are identical to rabies vaccine–associated panniculitis, the "lupus" association is questionable. Histologically, it is initially a septal panniculitis with dense nodular infiltrates of lymphocytes and plasma cells and fewer macrophages. The fat lobules may undergo necrosis, often represented by hyalinization without mineralization. Usually *the dermis and epidermis show the typical microscopic features of lupus*, including hydropic degeneration of basal cells, pigmentary incontinence, thickened basement membrane zone, and sclerosis of the dermis. Abundant mucinous degeneration is usually prominent. Leukocytoclastic vasculitis may be present in the interlobular septa.

Further reading

Gibson I, Barnes J. Vesicular cutaneous lupus erythematosus in a border collie in New Zealand. N Z Vet J 2011;59:153.

Mauldin EA, et al. Exfoliative cutaneous lupus erythematosus in German shorthaired pointers: disease development, progression and evaluation of three immunomodulatory drugs (ciclosporin, hydroxychloroquine, and adalimumab) in a controlled environment. Vet Dermatol 2010;21:373-382.

Oberkirchner U, et al. Successful treatment of a novel generalized variant of canine discoid lupus erythematosus with oral hydroxychloroquine. Vet Dermatol 2012;23:65-70.

Olivry T, Linder KE. Bilaterally symmetrical alopecia with reticulated hyperpigmentation: a manifestation of cutaneous lupus erythematosus in a dog with systemic lupus erythematosus. Vet Pathol 2013;50:682-685.

Smee NM, et al. Measurement of serum antinuclear antibody titer in dogs with and without systemic lupus erythematosus: 120 cases (1997-2005). J Am Vet Med Assoc 2007;230:1180-1183.

Wilhelm S. Two cases of feline exfoliative dermatitis and folliculitis with histological features of cutaneous lupus erythematosus. Tierärztliche Praxis Ausgabe 2005;33:364.

Other immune-mediated dermatoses
Drug eruptions

Drug eruptions are occasionally reported in *dogs, cats, and horses* and rarely in other domestic animals. Drugs responsible for skin eruptions may be administered *orally, topically, or by injection or inhalation*. Any drug may cause an eruption, and any one drug consistently produces no specific type of reaction. Thus *drug eruption can mimic virtually any dermatosis*. Erythema multiforme, Stevens-Johnson syndrome, toxic epidermal necrolysis (TEN), and vasculitis are well-recognized dermatoses that can be manifestations of cutaneous drug eruptions and are described individually later in this section. Criteria for establishing a cutaneous reaction as a confirmed drug eruption include (1) elimination of other causes of the skin lesions, (2) timing of onset of reaction with administration of a suspect drug, (3) improvement upon drug withdrawal, (4) recognition that the suspect drug has been associated with similar reactions in other animals or species in the past, and (5) recurrence of lesions upon rechallenge of the patient with the drug. Understandably, all 5 of these criteria are not often met, particularly rechallenge as this can be associated with high morbidity or mortality. The time period between drug administration and onset of an adverse reaction varies widely from hours to months, and lesions can result from a single or repeated administration. *Drug-induced gross and histologic lesions are not pathognomonic* for an adverse cutaneous drug eruption, although histopathologic changes may often point to a limited list of differentials. *Histologic patterns that have been recognized as forms of adverse drug reactions include urticaria, perivascular dermatitis (allergy-like), hydropic and/or lichenoid interface dermatitis (erythema multiforme, TEN, lupus erythematosus-like), perforating folliculitis, vasculitis, intraepidermal vesiculopustular dermatitis (pemphigus-like), and subepidermal bullous reactions (pemphigoid-like)*. The pathogenesis of lesion formation in many types of drug eruptions is not known with certainty. Drug hypersensitivities are believed to involve all 4 types of hypersensitivity reactions, and in some cases are not thought to be immunologically mediated.

The most common drugs recognized to produce hypersensitivity reactions in domestic animals are the *sulfonamides (especially trimethoprim-potentiated) and penicillins*. Erythema multiforme, Stevens Johnson syndrome, and TEN (discussed later in this section) have been seen most commonly with *trimethoprim-potentiated sulfonamides, cephalosporins, and levamisole*. *Diethylcarbamazine* and *5-fluorocytosine* have been associated with fixed-drug eruption on the scrotum of dogs. The ulcerative lesions healed with hyperpigmentation when the drug was withdrawn but recrudescence at the same site, with vesiculation, occurred when the dog was rechallenged. *The mechanism underlying fixed-drug eruption is unknown*. In humans, the epidermal invasion of T cells in fixed-drug eruptions is associated with the expression of the intercellular adhesion molecule-1 (ICAM-1) on the surface of lesional keratinocytes. In dogs, *cyclosporine* has been reported to cause a lichenoid lymphoplasmacytic dermatitis as well as cutaneous papillomas and viral plaques. These changes are likely attributed to long-term immune suppression rather than an immune-mediated adverse drug reaction. *Urticaria and angioedema* have been associated with levamisole, barbiturates, and some antibiotics. Drug eruptions manifesting as *exfoliative erythroderma* have been seen in dogs treated with levamisole and lincomycin. Acute maculopapular eruptions with erythroderma are reported in dogs being treated for gastrointestinal illness, so-called Wells-like syndrome, but specific drugs have not been implicated.

Drug eruptions resembling bullous pemphigoid clinically, histologically, and immunohistochemically have been associated with *triamcinolone*. It is quite possible that some cases described as bullous pemphigoid actually represent drug eruptions. Pemphigus foliaccus–like drug cruptions have been described in cats treated with ampicillin or cimetidine and dogs receiving trimethoprim-sulfonamide. Lesions consisted of classic subcorneal pustules with acantholytic cells, with an additional feature of vasculitis in some cases. Systemic lupus–like drug reactions have been reported in dogs and in cats. Cutaneous vasculitis caused by immune complex deposition may be initiated by drug administration. Sulfadiazine administration in Doberman Pinschers causes a poorly defined skin rash as well as ocular, joint, kidney, and hematologic abnormalities suggestive of systemic vasculitis.

Further reading

Favrot C, et al. Evaluation of papillomaviruses associated with cyclosporine-induced hyperplastic verrucous lesions in dogs. Am J Vet Res 2005;66:1764-1769.

Mauldin EA, et al. Clinical associations with severe eosinophilic dermatitis in dogs: a retrospective study. Vet Dermatol 2006;17:338-347.

McKenna JK, Leiferman KM. Dermatologic drug reactions. Immunol Allergy Clin North Am 2004;24:399-423.

Werner AH. Psoriasiform-lichenoid-like dermatosis in three dogs treated with microemulsified cyclosporine A. J Am Vet Med Assoc 2003;223:1013-1016.

Cryopathies

Cryopathies are cold-related hypersensitivity syndromes that include **cold agglutinin disease,** *a condition in which erythrocyte autoantibodies react at lower temperatures to produce microvascular thrombosis in superficial dermal vessels.* Other cryopathies are small vessel vasculopathies associated with abnormal serum proteins (paraproteins) that precipitate out of the serum at cooler temperatures and redissolve upon warming. *Paraproteins include cryofibrinogens, cryoglobulins, macroglobulins, and γ heavy chains.* Cryoglobulins may be monoclonal IgG or IgM (type I cryoglobulinemia), or mixed monoclonal and polyclonal, with one antibody directed against the other, in which case, immune complexes are in the circulation (type II cryoglobulinemia). In type III cryoglobulinemia, the immunoglobulins are polyclonal. Type I cryoglobulinemia is often associated with underlying disease, such as multiple myeloma, leukemia, or lymphoma, whereas in type II or III, connective tissue disease, such as SLE, or a systemic infection is present. Type II and III may also be idiopathic. *Most cases reported in dogs and cats are the result of cold-reacting anti-erythrocyte antibodies.* Cold agglutinin disease has been reported rarely to cause skin disease in dogs and cats. Cold agglutinin disease as a postinfectious event has been reported in sheep, horses, and pigs. One report in Birman cats occurred in association with neonatal isoerythrolysis and suggested that group B blood group cats may be predisposed. A monoclonal cryoglobulinemia associated with multiple myeloma has been reported in a cat. Lead exposure and hemobartonellosis *(Mycoplasma haemofelis)* have also been implicated as predisposing factors in dogs and cats. Cryopathy caused by cryofibrinogens and cryoglobulins has also been reported in the dog.

Cutaneous signs associated with cryopathies result from vascular insufficiency (obstruction, stasis, spasm, and thrombosis). Lesions include erythema, purpura, cyanosis, necrosis, ulceration, and occasionally sloughing of extremities, and are precipitated or exacerbated by exposure to cold. The paws, pinnae, nose, and tip of the tail are typically involved. Skin biopsy usually reveals necrosis, ulceration, and often secondary suppurative changes. *Microvascular thrombosis* may be evident in cold agglutinin disease. In other types of cryopathies, paraproteins are precipitated and deposited throughout vessel walls and within vascular lumens. The proteins stain pink with H&E and bright red with PAS. *Hemorrhage* may be present. In type I cryopathies, inflammation is usually absent, whereas a leukocytoclastic vasculitis is often present in types II and III.

Diagnosis requires a test for cryoprecipitates and analysis of serum proteins. Erythrocyte agglutination on a cooled slide that reverses upon warming and a positive Coombs test at 4° C should be present in cases of cold agglutinating anti-erythrocyte antibodies. *Differential diagnoses* include frostbite, disseminated intravascular coagulation, SLE, dermatomyositis, and other causes of vasculitis.

Further reading

Hickford FH, et al. Monoclonal immunoglobulin G cryoglobulinemia and multiple myeloma in a domestic shorthair. J Am Vet Med Assoc 2000;217:1029-1033.

Nagata M, et al. Cryoglobulinaemia and cryfibrinogenaemia: a comparison of canine and human cases. Vet Dermatol 1998;9:277-281.

Graft-versus-host disease

Graft-versus-host disease (GVHD) occurs as a complication of bone marrow transplantation. It has been recorded in *humans, dogs, cats, and horses.* The disease results from donor T-lymphocyte responses to recipient histocompatibility antigens in the *acute phase,* and from immunocompetent recipient lymphocyte responses to transplantation antigens in the *chronic phase.* Principal target organs are the *skin, liver, and intestinal tract.* GVHD is considered the *classic example of cell-mediated attack upon the epidermis.* Proposed target cells in the skin include basal keratinocytes, follicular stem cells, and/or Langerhans cells. Studies indicate both CD8+ and CD4+ lymphocytes are active in the disease process, with CD8+ T cells found more often in the epidermis and CD4+ T cells in the dermal infiltrate. Natural killer (NK) cells may also play a role. T-cell production of interferon-γ (IFN-γ) results in keratinocyte expression of ICAM-1, the binding molecule for lymphocyte function-associated antigen 1 (LFA-1) found on infiltrating T cells. Tumor necrosis factor-α (TNF-α) production by activated keratinocytes and Langerhans cells and IFN-γ lead to keratinocyte production of IL-8 attracting more lymphocytes.

Skin lesions in the acute phase include generalized erythematous macules, multifocal alopecia, and ulcerative dermatitis. Oral lesions, epidermal detachment, and follicular papules may be present. In the chronic phase, erythema, irregular hyperpigmentation, dermal fibrosis, cutaneous atrophy, and cicatricial alopecia from chronic ulceration may occur. *Histologic findings* include various degrees of hydropic and/or lichenoid interface dermatitis with marked lymphocytic satellitosis of necrotic keratinocytes in all layers of the epidermis and the follicular epithelium. There are lymphocytic exocytosis and spongiosis. Dermal lymphocytic infiltrate is variable. Dermal-epidermal cleft or ulceration may also be present. Over time, epidermal atrophy and dermal sclerosis with loss of adnexa may occur. Basal layer vacuolation and inflammation persist. *Differential diagnoses* include erythema multiforme, toxic epidermal necrolysis (TEN) or other drug eruption, alopecia areata, and radiation dermatitis. *The history and the triad of cutaneous, hepatic, and intestinal signs should lead to the proper diagnosis of GVHD.*

Erythema multiforme/Stevens-Johnson syndrome/ toxic epidermal necrolysis

Historically, erythema multiforme (EM) has represented one end of the spectrum of diseases that includes Stevens-Johnson syndrome (also called erythema multiforme major) and TEN, based on comparison of veterinary diseases to the human literature. EM is considered the "mild" disease form (i.e., EM minor), with TEN being the most severe. In human medicine, it is now accepted that EM and Stevens-Johnson syndrome (SJS)/TEN are different entities and not a spectrum of disease. SJS and TEN are likely triggered by an adverse drug reaction. EM minor in human is associated with herpes simplex infection, and the name has now changed to "herpesvirus-associated EM." Only rare cases of EM minor are due to adverse drug reactions ("drug-associated EM").

In veterinary medicine, EM has been reported in dogs, cats, horses, cattle, swine, a ferret, and anecdotally in the goat. Adverse drug reaction has been firmly entrenched in the literature; however, this association has come under intense scrutiny. Two cases series have reported adverse drug reactions as the cause of EM at 19 and 59%, respectively. Many cases are idiopathic, and old dogs are more likely to have idiopathic EM rather than drug-induced EM. A number of drugs have been reported to trigger EM in animals (e.g., D-limonene–based dips, levamisole, cephalexin, trimethoprim-sulfa, gentamicin, penicillin). Many of cases in earlier literature would be putative, at best, if strict criteria or drug provocation testing was applied. A multicenter study reclassified cases of EM based on aspects of the human classification system. The study found that SJS/TEN in dogs was likely to be triggered by drugs, whereas EM was not. The study also showed that skilled pathologists were unable to distinguish EM from SJS or TEN on light microscopy.

To date, there is no consensus on the classification of these disorders in veterinary medicine. Although the diagnosis of EM/SJS/TEN requires histopathology, the diseases are separated by clinical features and not by microscopic differences. For example, SJS involves >50% of the skin with <10% epidermal detachment and involvement of more than one mucosal surface; whereas TEN has similar criteria, but there is >30% epidermal detachment. In humans, the specific type of clinical lesion is paramount to distinguishing the reactions: EM is raised and palpable, whereas SJS/TEN lesions are flat. A recent review of 3 dogs with TEN reports the clinical lesions as flat purpuric macules.

SJS in humans may also be associated with infectious disease, with the most common agent being *Mycoplasma pneumoniae*. Interestingly, TEN has been associated with *Mycoplasma bovis* infection in calves. There are also reports of parvovirus-associated EM in dogs. Unlike herpesvirus-associated EM in people, the lesions in dogs have parvoviral inclusions, indicating active virus replication and likely represent systemic viral infection with unusual skin involvement. *Equid herpesvirus-5*–associated dermatitis resembling herpes-associated erythema multiforme was described in a 9-year-old Holsteiner stallion. Skin lesions consisted of nonpruritic, multifocal, pustular dermatitis around the eyes, nostrils, and muzzle. Histopathologically, there was interface dermatitis with apoptotic keratinocytes and intranuclear inclusions within the stratum spinosum and stratum granulosum.

There are also anecdotal reports of EM in cats triggered by feline herpesvirus infections. The lesion of thymoma-associated dermatosis in cats has also been likened to erythema multiforme.

The pathogenesis of EM/SJS/TEN is poorly understood in animals. The histologic lesions, cellular infiltrates and types of lymphocytes present mirror that of GVHD, lending further support for a cell-mediated immune response. One study of GVHD and EM in dogs revealed similar populations of CD4 and CD8+ cells. In humans, the pathogenesis of herpesvirus-associated EM (HAEM) is thought to be markedly different from SJS/TEN. In HAEM, viral proteins on the surface of keratinocytes provoke a Th1 CD4+ αβ response. Activated T cells secrete IFN-γ profile, which leads to a cascade of cytokines. Effector CD8+ cytotoxic T cells and NK cells target keratinocytes expressing herpesvirus protein. Apoptosis is mediated by granzyme that enters keratinocytes via transient pores induced by perforin. In drug-induced SJS/TEN, it remains unclear how the drug causes sensitization and why only rare individuals are affected. The hapten model proposes that small drug moieties bind to host proteins and are recognized as immunogenic. Keratinocyte death is similarly mediated by CD8+ T cell and NK cells; however, the apoptosis in TEN/SJS is often confluent. Soluble mediators such as TNF-α, FAS-ligand, and granulysin may play a role. The reader is referred to the reference by Yager (2014) for a detailed review of EM.

A wide range of clinical lesions (maculopapular to vesiculobullous and ulcerative and hyperkeratotic) has been reported in animals. Many of the clinical lesions of EM are likely confused with SJS/TEN. EM is often manifest as erythematous macules, papules, and plaques with central clearing (Fig. 6-74A, B). Dogs may have very thick hyperkeratotic crusted plaques that ulcerate. For SJS/TEN, epidermal detachment with resultant ulcers is the hallmark lesion (Fig. 6-74C). Clinical lesions of SJS/TEN include urticarial plaques and vesiculobullous lesions. In SJS/TEN, the animals have widespread painful lesions with systemic signs (fever, lethargy, inappetance). Some cases may have a positive pseudo-Nikolsky sign (i.e., digital pressure causes separation of the inflamed skin). Dogs and cats often have ulcers involving mucocutaneous junctions; footpads may also be involved (Figs. 6-74D, 6-75). SJS/TEN cases are clinical emergencies, which require intense critical care. The mortality rate for TEN is high.

Histologically, the lesions of EM show the *characteristic cytotoxic (interface) dermatitis*. Necrotic keratinocytes, often with lymphocytic satellitosis, are scattered throughout the epidermis and the adnexal epithelia (see Fig. 6-11). A sparse lymphohistiocytic infiltrate occurs at the dermoepidermal junction and around superficial blood vessels. Vasculitis is not a feature. Although *full-thickness coagulative necrosis of the epidermis may be present, it is not always present and most likely represents a continuum of disease. It is very important to note that the dermis is not necrotic. This feature enables distinction of TEN/EM from a thermal burn or cutaneous infarct.*

Clinical differentials for SJS/TEN include thermal or caustic burns, vesicular cutaneous lupus erythematosus, urticaria, vasculitis, other immune-mediated dermatoses, epitheliotropic lymphoma, superficial necrolytic dermatitis, and necrotic arachnidism. Occasionally, lesions of EM may histologically resemble epitheliotropic T-cell lymphoma (CTCL). Important

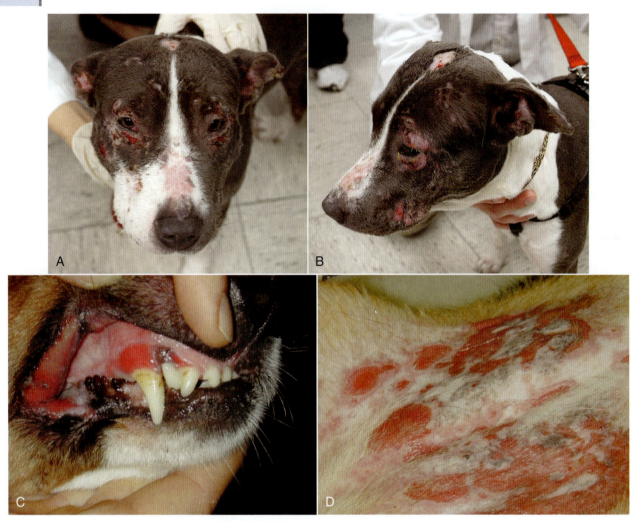

Figure 6-74 **Erythema multiforme and Stevens-Johnson syndrome. A, B.** Bilaterally symmetrical hyperkeratotic and ulcerative plaques in a dog with erythema multiforme. **C.** Bright red erythematous macules progressing to serpiginous erosions and ulcers in a dog with Stevens-Johnson syndrome. **D.** Ulcers and erosions on the lips and gums in a dog with Stevens-Johnson syndrome.

distinguishing features are atypical lymphocytes (CTCL), and apoptosis accompanied by lymphocytic satellitosis in all levels of the epidermis (EM). Chronic EM in old dogs is often idiopathic and is characterized by the additional changes of a proliferative epidermis with marked parakeratosis and extensive lymphocytic exocytosis.

Further reading

Herder V, et al. Equid herpesvirus 5-associated dermatitis in a horse resembling herpes-associated erythema multiforme. Vet Micro 2012;155:420-424.

Senturk S1, et al. Toxic epidermal necrolysis associated with *Mycoplasma bovis* in calves. Vet Rec 2012;170:566.

Woldemeskel M, et al. Canine parvovirus-2b associated erythema multiforme in a litter of English Setter dogs. J Vet Diagn Invest 2011;23:576-580.

Yager JA. Erythema multiforme, Stevens-Johnson syndrome and toxic epidermal necrolysis: a comparative review. Vet Dermatol 2014; 25:406-e64.

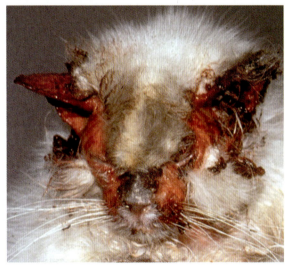

Figure 6-75 **Toxic epidermal necrolysis** in a cat. Severe epidermal sloughing and ulcers. (Courtesy T. Grieshaber.)

Vasculitis

Cutaneous vasculitis is characterized as an aberrant immune response directed toward dermal blood vessels. The pathophysiology is complex, often poorly understood, and involves a variety of mechanisms that lead to loss of vascular integrity, dermal edema, hemorrhage, and sometimes necrosis. The clinical presentation correlates with degree of vascular damage, type of vessels involved, and chronicity. Pathogenic mechanisms are diverse and may be associated with hypersensitivity reactions (type I, II, or III) infectious agents, malignancy, toxins, and many cases are idiopathic. Classic examples include infection with an endotheliotropic organism *(Rickettsia rickettsii)* and septicemia *(Erysipelothrix rhusiopathiae)*. In textbooks, systemic lupus erythematosus (SLE) is considered the classic example of immune complex (type III hypersensitivity)–induced cutaneous vasculitis; however, cases of true cutaneous involvement in domestic animals are exceedingly rare and poorly documented. Clinical signs of immune-complex cutaneous vasculitis have been documented in healthy and critically ill dogs given intravenous human albumin. Cutaneous vasculitis may be a secondary event associated with cutaneous diseases, such as staphylococcal infections. In veterinary medicine, drug-induced vasculitis is probably under-diagnosed. Dose-dependent vasculitis has been seen in dogs receiving itraconazole for cutaneous fungal disease. The mechanism is thought to be the result of haptenization of host proteins, direct drug toxicity against vessel walls, autoantibodies against endothelial cells, or possibly cell-mediated cytotoxic reactions against vessels.

Cutaneous vasculitis is seen most often in the *dog and horse* and is considered to be rare in cats, pigs, and cattle; ~50% of cases of vasculitis in dogs and horses are idiopathic. *Gross lesions suggestive of vasculitis include erythematous plaques or macules, palpable purpura, hemorrhagic bullae, edema, necrosis, and well-demarcated ulcers* (Fig. 6-76). Ischemic necrosis may occur leading to eschar formation and sloughing of the skin or distal extremities. Paws, pinnae, lips, tail, and oral mucosa are most commonly affected. Ischemic atrophy of folliculosebaceous units may lead to areas of alopecia and scaling in long-standing lesions of more subtle vasculitis.

Small arterioles, capillaries, and postcapillary venules are most often affected in cutaneous vasculitis. Histologic lesions in the classic case feature evidence of damage to the vessel wall, such as *necrotic cell debris and fibrinoid necrosis within the vessel wall, mural infiltrates of either neutrophils or lymphocytes, and intramural or perivascular edema, hemorrhage, or fibrin exudation* (see Fig. 6-15). Subtle cases of vasculitis may be characterized by edema, rare necrotic cells in the vicinity of vessels, and a mild interstitial mononuclear cell infiltrate. Microscopic evidence of vasculitis in the dog is often subtle and may lead to under-diagnosis of the condition. Some pathologists prefer to refer to very cell-poor cases of vasculitis as a *vasculopathy* rather than true vasculitis when degenerative lesions of vessel wall and evidence of ischemia are detected in the absence of inflammation of vessel walls. Edema, hemorrhage, and evidence of ischemia and homogenization of dermal collagen are helpful changes. *A preponderance of leukocytes in vessels walls rather than in the dermis suggests that vessels are the primary target of inflammation and not just serving to deliver leukocytes.* Vessels will stand out in the section because of the attraction of leukocytes to vessel walls.

Some generalizations regarding the pathogenesis of the vasculitis can be made from types of leukocytes present within vessel walls; however, the types of leukocytes present do not necessarily point to a particular etiology and may simply reflect the stage of the disease process.

- *Neutrophilic vasculitis* is most suggestive of a type III immune-complex hypersensitivity reaction and is often referred to as *leukocytoclastic vasculitis* if neutrophil degeneration and nuclear karyorrhexis are evident. Examples include the vasculitis associated with staphylococcal dermatitis in dogs, immune-mediated vasculitis as in SLE, some drug eruptions, and septicemia. In the case of septicemia, the vasculitis tends to be non-leukocytoclastic.
- *Lymphocytic vasculitis* may suggest a cell-mediated immune basis, such as rabies vaccine–induced cutaneous vasculitis and some drug eruptions.
- *Eosinophilic vascular infiltrates* are most suggestive of a type I hypersensitivity reaction. Eosinophils may be the predominant cells in some cases of equine vasculitis and in association with the markedly eosinophilic dermatitis seen in some arthropod bite lesions, mast cell tumors, or in lesions of the eosinophilic granuloma complex in the cat. Eosinophilic vasculitis has been documented in cases of drug reaction and in some dogs with food hypersensitivity.
- Involvement of deep dermal blood vessels in all cases may suggest systemic disease.
- In **dogs,** cutaneous vasculitis has been associated with drugs, systemic or localized infections (Rocky Mountain spotted fever, *Babesia,* staphylococcal pyoderma), malignancies, and connective tissue diseases. Three cases of cutaneous vasculitis have been reported in dogs seropositive for *Bartonella vinsonii;* all dogs responded to antimicrobial treatment.

Familial or inherited forms of vasculitis have also been recognized.

- A syndrome of cutaneous ulceration in conjunction with limb edema and/or acute renal failure, referred to as *cutaneous and renal glomerular vasculopathy (CRGV) of Greyhounds,* or in layman's terms "Alabama rot," has been reported sporadically in young Greyhounds throughout the United States. Multifocal cutaneous ulcers, renal afferent arteriolar and dermal arterial thrombosis, azotemia, microangiopathic hemolytic anemia, and thrombocytopenia

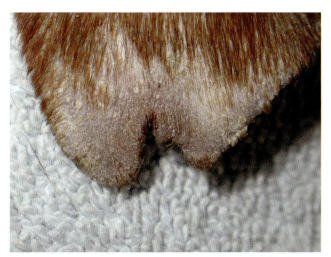

Figure 6-76 Typical punched-out ulcers on the margins of the ears caused by **vasculitis** in a dog. (Courtesy M.S. Canfield.)

with normal coagulation times characterize CRGV. Cutaneous lesions may occur in the absence of renal or other systemic disease. The syndrome has many features in common with the hemolytic-uremic syndrome in people caused by a Shiga-like toxin–induced endothelial cell necrosis. *Studies have failed to identify infectious agents, toxins, or evidence of an immune-mediated reaction in CRGV.* Exposure to Shiga-like toxin–producing *Escherichia coli* has not been completely ruled out. Affected dogs may be genetically predisposed to develop CRGV as outbreaks have occurred in related groups of dogs. Hemorrhage, fibrinoid arteritis, thrombosis with infarction, and ulceration characterize the skin lesions that are most often found on the limbs. Renal glomerular necrosis and tubular necrosis are present in the kidneys.

- An arteritis affecting the nasal philtrum has been documented in adult Saint Bernards, one Giant Schnauzer, and one Basset Hound. It has been reported anecdotally in several other breeds. The dogs develop deep deforming ulcers on the philtrum and may have episodes of arterial bleeding. Deep dermal arteries and arterioles have a subendothelial spindle cell proliferation with fibrosis and deposition of mucinous (Alcian blue–positive) matrix.
- A genodermatosis affecting *German Shepherd dog puppies* characterized by swelling, depigmentation; frequent ulceration of footpads, pinnae, and tail tips; and nasal planum depigmentation has been reported in Canada. A neutrophilic to mononuclear nodular dermatitis, dermal collagenolysis, and subtle vasculitis are present histologically. Nasal lesions correspond to a hydropic interface dermatitis. The cause is unknown but presumed to be immunologically mediated as lesions are temporally related to vaccination dates. Dogs recover by 5-6 months of age. The condition may also be related to an underlying collagen disorder, as musculoskeletal abnormalities are also present.
- Familial vasculitis has been reported in a litter of *Scottish Terriers*. Lesions were limited to the nasal epithelium and mucosa and were characterized by leukocytoclastic vasculitis and pyogranulomatous inflammation, leading to ulceration and destruction of the nasal planum.
- Cutaneous vasculitis has been reported in *Jack Russell Terriers*, leading to alopecia and ulcerative lesions of the extremities and bony prominences with histologic lesions virtually indistinguishable from dermatomyositis of Collies and Shetland Sheepdogs (see Congenital and hereditary diseases of skin).

In **horses**, cutaneous vasculitis has been seen with or following numerous infections, such as with *Streptococcus*, influenza A virus, equine arteritis virus, equine infectious anemia virus, *Ehrlichia*, *Rhodococcus equi*, and *Corynebacterium pseudotuberculosis*.

- Equine purpura hemorrhagica is an acute, usually streptococcal infection (strangles)-associated, leukocytoclastic vasculitis characterized clinically by urticaria and extensive edema of the distal limbs, ventrum, and head. These swellings may progress to exudation and sloughing.
- Pastern leukocytoclastic vasculitis is a syndrome unique to the horse that affects the unpigmented, sun-exposed skin of distal extremities and sometimes muzzle; hence ultraviolet radiation is thought to play a role in pathogenesis. Adult horses are most often affected. There is no evidence of liver disease or exposure to photosensitizing compounds. Interestingly, a single limb may be affected, although other limbs lack pigment as well. Lesions are crusty, eroded or ulcerated, sharply demarcated, and may be associated with extensive edema and pain. Histologically, leukocytoclastic vasculitis of the superficial dermal vessels is present. Chronic cases develop papillary hyperplasia of the epidermis, giving the lesion a verrucous appearance.
- Nodular eosinophilic vasculitis is seen as firm, painful, nodular to linear lesions on one or more legs. Lesions may ulcerate, bleed, and crust.

Cutaneous vasculitis in **pigs** is most commonly associated with *Erysipelothrix rhusiopathiae* infection. Systemic vasculitis affecting primarily the skin and kidneys occurs in pigs and has been called the *porcine dermatitis and nephropathy syndrome*. Skin lesions consist of irregularly enlarging hemorrhagic macules and papules on the ears, limbs, abdomen, thorax, and perineum. Leukocytoclastic vasculitis is present in the dermis, panniculus, synovium, and renal pelvis. Pigs have concurrent pneumonia and pathogenesis studies indicate that porcine circovirus 2 is associated with the condition.

Direct immunofluorescence testing or immunohistochemistry may demonstrate immunoglobulin and/or complement in vessel walls and occasionally at the basement membrane zone in suspected cases of vasculitis. Positive tests are most likely in lesions <24 hours old. False positives occur also. Adverse drug reactions, infection, familial vasculopathies, cryopathies, and systemic autoimmune diseases, such as SLE, should be ruled as possible causes. In many cases, a specific cause cannot be determined.

Further reading

Breitschwerdt EB, et al. Clinicopathological abnormalities and treatment response in 24 dogs seroreactive to *Bartonella vinsonii (berkhoffi)* antigens. J Am Anim Hosp Assoc 2004;40:92-101.

Innerå M. Cutaneous vasculitis in small animals. Vet Clin North Am Small Anim Pract 2013;43:113-134.

Jasani S, et al. Systemic vasculitis with severe cutaneous manifestation as a suspected idiosyncratic hypersensitivity reaction to fenbendazole in a cat. J Vet Intern Med 2008;22:666-670.

Niza MM, et al. Cutaneous and ocular adverse reactions in a dog following meloxicam administration. Vet Dermatol 2007;18:45-49.

Opriessnig T, Langohr I. Current state of knowledge on porcine circovirus type 2-associated lesions. Vet Pathol 2013;50:23-38.

Powell C, et al. Type III hypersensitivity reaction with immune complex deposition in 2 critically ill dogs administered human serum albumin. J Vet Emerg Crit Care (San Antonio) 2013;23:598-604.

Tasaki Y, et al. Generalized alopecia with vasculitis-like changes in a dog with babesiosis. J Vet Med Sci 2013;75:1367-1369.

Torres SM, et al. Dermal arteritis of the nasal philtrum in a Giant Schnauzer and three Saint Bernard dogs. Vet Dermatol 2002;13: 275-281.

Rabies vaccine–induced vasculitis and alopecia in dogs

This disease is characterized by a localized inflammatory and ischemic reaction to subcutaneously administered rabies vaccine in the dog. Although any breed can be affected, the disorder typically affects small-breed dogs such as Poodles, Yorkshire Terriers, and Silky Terriers. The pathogenesis remains unknown, but formation of antigen-antibody complexes that become lodged in vessel walls (a type III hypersensitivity response) has been proposed.

There are 2 clinical presentations: a localized form where the lesion arises at the site of vaccination and a generalized form that mimics canine familial dermatomyositis. The localized form is common and develops several months after vaccination. The gross lesion is a focal, typically depressed, alopecic, and hyperpigmented patch (Fig. 6-77A). The histologic features are characteristic and involve combination of changes in the subcutis, dermis, adnexa, and basement membrane zone/epidermis. Panniculitis is only present at the site of vaccination. The vascular lesions are subtle and not seen in all cases. Venules, arterioles, and small arteries develop a *very mild chronic lymphocytic vasculitis*, characterized by thickening of the vessel wall, a few intramural mononuclear inflammatory cells, scattered nuclear debris, and variable perivascular mononuclear infiltrates (Fig. 6-77B). Occasionally, a more florid leukocytoclastic vasculitis is seen. A cell-poor interface dermatitis with vacuolar change in the basal epithelial layer and pigmentary incontinence and mural folliculitis may be present in some cases. The dermis is atrophic and hyalinized, sometimes mucinous. Hair follicles are markedly atrophied and pale staining ("faded") (Fig. 6-77C). At the site of vaccination, the subcutis contains lymphocytic panniculitis, and some cases may have blue-grey material (vaccine product) extracellularly and within the cytoplasm of macrophages. The additional lesions of erosions and ulcers of the oral mucosa and skin of the extremities and bony prominences and ischemic myopathy in subjacent musculature have been reported in cases with multicentric involvement. Immunofluorescence staining has identified rabies antigen in the vessels and epithelium of the hair follicles. A low-grade immune-mediated vasculitis with resultant tissue anoxia, leading to the atrophic changes in the overlying skin has been suggested as the pathogenesis. Lesions may remain for months to years. Differential diagnoses include dermatomyositis, traction alopecia, idiopathic vasculopathy, and lupus profundus.

Further reading

Morris DO. Ischemic dermatopathies. Vet Clin North Am Small Anim Pract 2013;43:99-111.

Canine uveodermatologic syndrome (Vogt-Koyanagi-Harada [VKH] syndrome)

This syndrome, seen only in dogs and humans, is characterized by the concurrent *acute onset of bilateral uveitis and depigmentation of the nose, lips, eyelids, and occasionally the footpads and anus*. Although the cause of the disorder is unknown, a cell-mediated hypersensitivity to melanin has been hypothesized. VKH is discussed further under Disorders of pigmentation.

Plasma cell pododermatitis

This is a *rare disorder of cats* of all breeds, ages, and sex. A possible link to feline immunodeficiency virus (FIV) has been suggested, and one study demonstrated 50% of plasma cell pododermatitis cases tested positive for FIV. Although the pathogenesis is unknown, *an immune-mediated basis* is suggested by the tissue plasmacytosis, hypergammaglobulinemia, and beneficial response to immunosuppressive and immunomodulating drugs (e.g., doxycycline monohydrate). In addition, occasional cats have other abnormalities, such as renal amyloidosis, plasmacytic stomatitis, positive antinuclear

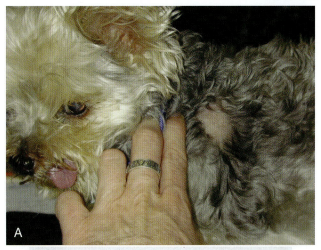
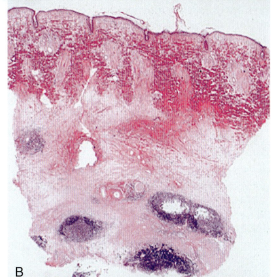
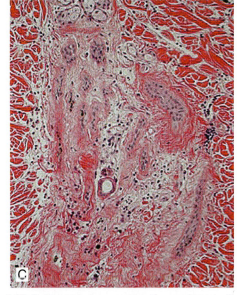

Figure 6-77 Rabies vaccine–associated vasculitis. **A.** Focal area of alopecia on the dorsum in a Yorkshire Terrier. **B.** Marked atrophy of follicles with smudged dermal collagen and lymphocytic panniculitis. **C.** Higher magnification showing marked follicular atrophy (faded follicles).

antibody tests, Coombs-positive anemia, polyclonal gammopathy, or glomerulonephritis with positive direct immunofluorescence testing (immunoglobulin deposited at the basement membrane zone). PCR testing of tissue digests has been performed to assess for infectious agents, and particularly those that may respond to the antimicrobial properties of doxycycline (e.g., *Bartonella* spp., *Ehrlichia* spp., *Anaplasma phagocytophilum*, *Chlamydophila*, *Mycoplasma* spp.). DNA of those pathogens was not amplified from tissue.

Clinically, plasma cell pododermatitis begins as soft, nonpainful swelling of multiple footpads on multiple paws. The central metacarpal or metatarsal pads are usually most severely affected. Affected pads feel soft resulting from collapse of the underlying fatpad. Footpad surfaces are crosshatched with white scaly striae but may become ulcerated or develop fleshy granulomatous proliferations that may hemorrhage. Lameness develops with progression of the lesions. Some cases spontaneously resolve or may recur seasonally.

Histologically, early lesions are characterized by *superficial and deep perivascular dermatitis with plasma cells predominating*. Later, there is a diffuse plasmacytic dermatitis. Russell bodies can be numerous. Leukocytoclastic vasculitis is rarely seen. Ulcerated or proliferative lesions show various degrees of superimposed suppurative-to-pyogranulomatous inflammation. The gross and histologic features are diagnostic.

Further reading

Bettenay SV, et al. An immunohistochemical and polymerase chain reaction evaluation of feline plasmacytic pododermatitis. Vet Pathol 2007;44:80-83.

Guaguere E, et al. Feline plasma cell pododermatitis: a retrospective study of 26 cases. Vet Dermatol 2004;15(Suppl. 1):27.

Cutaneous amyloidosis

The physical structure of amyloid gives it special properties, such as apple-green birefringence when Congo red–stained sections are polarized. *Primary cutaneous amyloidosis is thought to share a common pathway with other amyloid diseases*. The amyloid fibrils (AL amyloid) are derived from monoclonal immunoglobulin light chains. Cutaneous amyloidosis occurs rarely in *horses, dogs, and cats*. The cutaneous lesion in **dogs** has been associated with monoclonal gammopathy, dermatomyositis, and is seen occasionally in the stroma of plasmacytomas of skin and oral cavity (see Cutaneous plasmacytoma). In dogs with monoclonal gammopathy, purpuric lesions are seen, and cutaneous hemorrhage is easily induced by minor external trauma. The superficial dermis contains an amorphous, homogeneous, eosinophilic substance, and the walls of blood vessels in the involved area are thickened by deposits of the same substance. There may be a familial tendency in Abyssinian and Siamese **cats**. Cutaneous amyloidosis is usually associated with chronic inflammation, neoplasia, and accumulations of plasma cells.

The pathogenesis of amyloidosis in **horses** is unclear. The lesions are multiple, asymptomatic papules, nodules, and plaques that are seen most commonly on the head, neck, shoulders, and pectoral region. There is no established breed, age, or sex predisposition. The lesions are firm, well circumscribed, and 0.5-10 cm in diameter. The overlying skin and haircoat are normal. The initial lesions may be urticarial in type. The cutaneous lesions may be accompanied by similar nodules in the respiratory mucosa and regional lymph nodes but are seldom associated with systemic amyloidosis. Lesions may regress, become recurrent or progressively enlarge. Histologic findings include *nodular-to-diffuse granulomatous dermatitis and panniculitis*. Large extracellular deposits of amyloid appear as variably sized areas of homogeneous, amorphous, hyaline, eosinophilic material, which may contain clefts or fractures. Multinucleated histiocytic giant cells are usually numerous. *Clinical differentials* include infectious and noninfectious granulomas, cutaneous neoplasms, and eosinophilic granulomas.

Further reading

Borowicz J, et al. Nodular cutaneous amyloidosis. Skinmed 2011;9: 316-318.

Woldemeskel M. Primary localized nodular cutaneous amyloidosis in a male neutered Golden Retriever. Dtsch Tierarztl Wochenschr 2007;114:473-475.

Alopecia areata

Alopecia areata (AA) is a nonscarring, presumably autoimmune, alopecic inflammatory disorder directed against hair follicles in humans, nonhuman primates, dogs, cats, horses, and cattle. Alopecia areata may be focal, multifocal, or generalized *(alopecia universalis)*. Lesions occur most commonly on the face, neck, and trunk (Fig. 6-78A). Some horses may have hair loss on the mane and tail. Areas of alopecia are usually hyperpigmented and may exhibit sparse short and dystrophic hairs Leukotrichia may be seen in some animals initially. Lesions may be bilaterally symmetrical. There is no apparent age, breed, or sex predilection. Rodent models are available to study the condition—the C3H/HeJ mouse and the Dundee experimental bald rat.

Early, clinically active lesions are characterized histologically by an accumulation of lymphocytes ("swarm of bees") in and around the inferior segment of anagen hair follicles—the classic example of *peribulbar lymphocytic folliculitis* (Fig. 6-78B). Unfortunately, the classic lesion is not always evident, and more subtle bulbar inflammation is the rule. Bulbar keratinocytes are frequently vacuolated, apoptotic, or karyorrhectic. Pigmentary incontinence and melanophagia in the peribulbar region are also typical findings. Telogen follicles are unaffected, and dystrophic hair follicles may be present. Demonstration of the lymphocytic peribulbitis may be difficult and require examination of multiple sections from different levels of the paraffin-embedded biopsy specimen. Immunostaining to detect CD3+ lymphocytes may be helpful in some cases. Biopsies from the periphery of early, expanding lesions are most rewarding. *Histologic findings in chronic, clinically static lesions are nondiagnostic*, revealing a predominance of telogen hair follicles and follicular atrophy that may be misdiagnosed as an endocrine skin disorder. Immunologic studies in dogs and horses have indicated that the intrabulbar lymphocytes are primarily cytotoxic CD8+ lymphocytes. CD1+ dendritic antigen-presenting cells and both CD8+ and CD4+ lymphocytes are found in the peribulbar infiltrate. In addition, various autoantibodies targeting trichohyaline, hair keratins, and other components of the hair follicle have been demonstrated in various species, indicating a role for humoral immunity. In

VIRAL DISEASES OF SKIN

Cutaneous lesions occur in the course of a number of viral diseases in domestic animals. Viruses may induce skin lesions upon *local infection*, but the intact integument is resistant to viral penetration; injection via an arthropod bite or introduction through a cutaneous wound is a prerequisite for infection. Examples of local viral infection include papillomas induced by the papillomaviruses, bovine mammillitis induced by a herpesvirus, and the so-called milker's nodule in humans caused by a parapoxvirus. More often, viruses localize in the skin during the viremic phase of a *systemic infection*. Examples include some poxvirus infections, malignant catarrhal fever, and the vesicular diseases, such as vesicular stomatitis and foot-and-mouth disease. Pantropic viruses, such as canine distemper virus and classical swine fever virus, may cause cutaneous lesions; but *most viruses causing cutaneous lesions are epitheliotropic*. Some epitheliotropic viruses, in particular the poxviruses, have a predilection for the epithelium of the skin. Others, including the viruses associated with the mucosal diseases, cause primary lesions in the alimentary tract with lesser involvement of the skin.

A "rash," comprising erythematous macules caused by long-lasting dilation of dermal blood vessels, is often associated with systemic viral disease in humans. Such lesions are uncommon in animals, but may be hidden by the haircoat. Exceptions are the *cutaneous erythema* occurring in classical swine fever and African swine fever, and hemorrhagic diathesis of skin occurring with disseminated porcine adenovirus infection. In addition, a condition known as *dermatitis/nephropathy syndrome of pigs*, seen clinically as erythematous macules, papules, and plaques, caused by cutaneous and systemic necrotizing vasculitis, is associated with porcine circovirus 2 (PCV-2) infection.

Cutaneous viral diseases are *more common in food-producing animals than in pets*. Some of these diseases, notably sheeppox, cause significant mortality. Others have an economic impact because of their deleterious effect on production. Herpes mammillitis and pseudocowpox, for example, reduce milk yield in dairy cattle; contagious pustular dermatitis affects the growth rate of lambs by interfering with their ability to suckle. A few of the large animal viral dermatoses are extremely mild, for example, molluscum contagiosum in the horse.

Systemic viral diseases with cutaneous manifestations are rare in dogs and cats. Canine distemper virus is associated with nasodigital hyperkeratosis, so-called "hard pad" disease, and pustular dermatitis. In cats, rare occurrences of cutaneous disease occur with feline calicivirus infection. Cutaneous lesions caused by felid herpesvirus 1 can occur in the absence of respiratory disease, a presumed recrudescence of a latent herpesvirus infection.

Traditionally, viral diseases have been *diagnosed* by light and electron microscopy, serology, and viral culture. However, the development of monoclonal antibodies to specific viruses for use with immunofluorescence and immunoperoxidase techniques is increasingly being used for specific and rapid diagnosis. PCR testing can be used to detect virus-encoded DNA and RNA and identify many different viruses. In addition, viral genome DNA sequencing has led to the detection and understanding of the relationships among many different viruses.

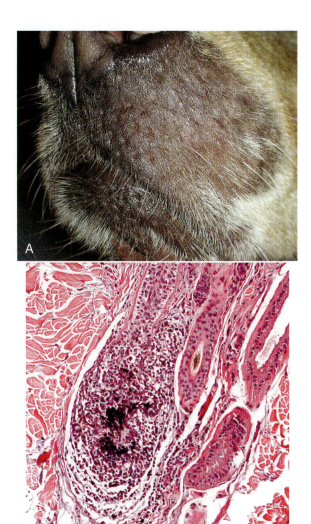

Figure 6-78 Alopecia areata in a dog. **A.** Note discrete area of non-inflamed, hyperpigmented alopecic skin. (Courtesy M.S. Canfield.) **B.** Peribulbar lymphocytic folliculitis. Lymphocytes are in and around the hair bulb.

dogs and horses, *AA frequently reverses spontaneously*; however, sometimes the hair regrowth is white.

Clinical differentials include telogen effluvium and many other causes of lymphocytic mural folliculitis, such as erythema multiforme (EM), systemic lupus erythematosus (SLE), graft-versus-host disease (GVHD), ischemia, and demodicosis, to name a few. *The distinguishing feature of AA is the fact that the hair bulb and inferior segment of anagen hairs are the primary targets of inflammation rather than the infundibulum or the isthmus*, although the isthmus has been reported to be affected in a horse.

Further reading

Rosychuk RA. Noninflammatory, nonpruritic alopecia of horses. Vet Clin North Am Equine Pract 2013;29:629-641.

Timm K, et al. Alopecia areata in Eringer cows. Vet Dermatol 2010;21:545-553.

Valentine BA, et al. Alopecia areata in two black Angus cows. J Vet Diagn Invest 2012;24:405-407.

Further reading

Koutinas AF, et al. Histopathology and immunohistochemistry of canine distemper virus-induced footpad hyperkeratosis (hard pad disease) in dogs with natural canine distemper. Vet Pathol 2004;41:2-9.

Segales J. Porcine circovirus type 2 (PCV2) infections: clinical signs, pathology and laboratory diagnosis. Vir Res 2012;164:10-19.

Poxviral infections

The *Poxviridae* is a large family of complex DNA viruses. *Highly epitheliotropic, they cause cutaneous and systemic disease in birds, wild and domestic mammals, and humans.* Some species of the *Poxviridae*, including *Sheeppox virus*, *Ectromelia virus*, *Monkeypox virus*, and the now eradicated *Variola virus* (human smallpox), cause severe systemic disease. Others cause mild, localized disease, for example, pseudocowpox, which chiefly affects the teats of milking cows. A few poxviruses are associated with hyperplastic or neoplastic conditions, such as molluscum contagiosum in horses and Shope fibroma of rabbits.

The *Poxviridae* share group-specific nucleoprotein antigens. Animal poxviruses are in the subfamily *Chordopoxvirinae*. The genera *(species names italicized)* include

- *Parapoxvirus: Orf virus* (contagious pustular dermatitis virus, contagious ecthyma virus), *Pseudocowpox virus* (milker's nodule virus), *Bovine papular stomatitis virus*, and *Parapox virus of red deer*. Unassigned members in the genus are Auzduk disease virus (camel contagious ecthyma virus), chamois contagious ecthyma virus, sealpox virus, and a virus that causes papillomatous dermatitis and pododermatitis in cattle.
- *Orthopoxvirus: Cowpox virus*, *Vaccinia virus* (buffalopox virus, rabbitpox virus), *Horsepox virus*, *Camelpox virus*, *Ectromelia virus* (mousepox virus), and *Monkeypox virus*; unassigned member of the genus is *Uasin Gishu disease virus*
- *Molluscipoxvirus: Molluscum contagiosum virus*
- *Capripoxvirus: Sheeppox virus, Goatpox virus, Lumpy skin disease virus*
- *Suipoxvirus: Swinepox virus*
- *Avipoxvirus: Fowlpox virus, Pigeonpox virus*, and many other avian poxviruses.
- *Leporipoxvirus: Myxoma virus; Rabbit fibroma virus* (Shope fibroma virus).
- *Yatapoxvirus: Tanapox virus*, Yaba monkey tumor virus

Many of the poxviruses are host specific; but the orthopoxviruses, such as *Cowpox virus* and *Vaccinia virus*, affect a wide range of species. Some poxviruses, for example *Pseudocowpox virus*, are zoonotic. *Infection is usually achieved by cutaneous or respiratory routes.* Poxviruses, whether acquired by the subcutaneous or respiratory routes, usually gain access to the systemic circulation via the lymphatic system, although multiplication at the site of injection in the skin may lead to direct entry into the blood and primary viremia. Secondary viremia disseminates the virus back to the skin and to other target organs.

Poxviruses induce lesions by a variety of mechanisms. Degenerative changes in the epithelium are caused by virus replication and induce *vesicular lesions* typical of many poxvirus infections. Degenerative lesions in the dermal or submucosal tissues sometimes result from ischemia secondary to vascular damage caused by viral multiplication in endothelial cells. Poxvirus infections also *induce proliferative lesions*. Poxviruses, such as *Orf virus*, replicating in the epidermis typically induce hyperplasia along with degenerative changes. Host cell DNA synthesis is stimulated before the onset of cytoplasmic virus-related DNA replication. Proliferative changes may be explained by a gene, present in several poxviruses, including *Molluscum contagiosum virus*, whose product has significant homology with epidermal growth factor. Poxviruses also encode for functions that may counteract host defenses. These include genes related to those encoding the serine protease inhibitors (SERPINs), a superfamily of related proteins important in regulating serine protease enzymes that mediate kinin, complement, fibrinolytic and coagulation pathways, and genes encoding anti-interferon activities.

Pox lesions have a typical developmental sequence. They commence as erythematous macules, become papular, and then vesicular. The vesicular stage is well developed in some pox infections, such as sheeppox, and is transient or non-existent in others, such as contagious pustular dermatitis. Vesicles develop into *umbilicated pustules with a depressed center and a raised, often erythematous border*. This lesion is the so-called "pock." The pustules rupture, and a crust forms on the surface. This crust may become very thick, as in lesions of contagious pustular dermatitis. Lesions heal and often leave a residual scar. The mucosal lesions are briefly vesicular and develop into ulcers rather than pustules.

Histologically, pox lesions begin as epidermal cytoplasmic swelling and vacuolation, usually first affecting the cells of the outer stratum spinosum. There is evidence, from experimental studies with the virus of contagious pustular dermatitis, that postinjury proliferating keratinocytes are the target for viral replication. Rupture of the damaged keratinocytes produces multiloculated vesicles, so-called *reticular degeneration*. The early dermal lesions include edema, vascular dilation, a perivascular mononuclear cell infiltrate, and a variable neutrophilic infiltrate. Neutrophils migrate into the epidermis and aggregate in vesicles to form microabscesses. Large intraepidermal pustules may form and sometimes extend into the superficial dermis. There is usually marked epithelial hyperplasia and sometimes pseudocarcinomatous hyperplasia of the adjacent epithelium. This contributes to the raised border of the umbilicated pustule. Rupture of the pustule produces an inflammatory crust, often colonized on its surface by bacteria.

Poxvirus lesions often contain *characteristic intracytoplasmic inclusion bodies*. These are single or multiple and of variable size and duration. The more prominent inclusions are designated *type A*. They are eosinophilic, reflecting their high protein content, and weakly Feulgen positive. *Smaller, basophilic, Feulgen-positive, type B* bodies also occur and represent the site of virus replication.

Diagnosis of poxvirus infections is usually based on *typical clinical appearance* and may be supported by *characteristic histologic lesions*. Parapoxviruses are ultrastructurally distinct from the other poxviruses that are morphologically similar to each other when viewed by electron microscopy.

Further reading

Mercer A, et al., editors. Poxviruses. Birkhauser Advances in Infectious Diseases. Basel: Birkhauser Biosciences; 2007.

Parapoxviral diseases

Contagious pustular dermatitis. Contagious pustular dermatitis is a highly contagious zoonotic poxviral disease of *sheep and goats*, with incidental infections occurring in humans, camelids, cattle, and many wild ruminants, and very rarely dogs. Dogs may acquire infection by eating infected lamb carcasses. The disease is caused by species **Orf virus** (ORFV), a *Parapoxvirus* closely related to *Pseudocowpox virus* and *Bovine papular stomatitis virus*. Synonyms for contagious pustular dermatitis include contagious ecthyma, orf, infectious labial dermatitis, soremouth, and scabby mouth.

The disease is geographically widespread and occurs wherever sheep or goats are raised. The virus can repeatedly infect sheep and goats, and although live-virus vaccines control the disease and decrease the severity of the disease, they also ensure its continuance by perpetuating infection in the environment. The economic significance of contagious pustular dermatitis results chiefly from loss of condition, because *affected animals neither suckle nor graze*. Morbidity in a susceptible population may reach 90%, but mortality rarely exceeds 1% unless secondary infection intervenes, or unless the animals are immunosuppressed or stressed, in which case mortality can be high. Mortality often results from the invasion of primary lesions by the larvae of the screwworm fly (*Cochliomyia hominivorax*) or by bacteria such as *Fusobacterium necrophorum* and occasionally *Dermatophilus congolensis*. Cellulitis may complicate pedal lesions, mastitis may complicate mammary lesions, and necrotizing stomatitis and aspiration pneumonia may complicate oral lesions.

Contagious pustular dermatitis affects sheep and goats of all breeds. *It is predominantly a disease of lambs and kids*. Infection is established through cutaneous abrasions, particularly those associated with dry and prickly pasture or forage. Clinically affected lambs may transmit the virus to the udder of the ewe. The virus is hardy and probably persists in a dry environment indefinitely in crust material shed from affected animals. Chronically infected, reinfected, or possibly, latently infected carrier animals may allow the virus to persist in a flock for several years.

Viral vascular endothelial growth factor (*VEGF*) is an important virulence gene in the pathogenesis of orf. Epidermal hyperplasia and capillary growth with increased vascular permeability allows increased virus replication and formation of crusts. Crusts rich in virus particles favor the chances of virus survivability in the environment for extended periods. Via the CD95 pathway, ORFV can induce apoptosis of antigen-presenting cells. By inhibiting Bcl-2 (B-cell lymphoma 2), the virus is also able to inhibit apoptosis of virally infected cells.

Gross lesions usually commence at the commissures of the lips and spread around the lip margins to the muzzle and sometimes on the face and around the eyes (Fig. 6-79A). In severe cases, lesions may develop on the gingiva, dental pad, palate, and tongue. Lesions mainly confined to the tongue must be differentiated from those of foot-and-mouth disease. The buccal lesions are raised, red, or gray foci with a surrounding zone of hyperemia. Very rarely, lesions extend to the esophagus, rumen, and omasum in the lower alimentary canal, causing ulcerative gastroenteritis, and in lungs and heart. Lesions on the limbs are less common than on the lips and tend to involve the coronet, interdigital cleft, and bulb of the heels. They may extend, in severe cases, to the knee or hock on the caudal aspect of the leg. Lesions of the mammary gland affect the teats and adjacent skin of the udder. Lesions may develop in other areas of sparsely wooled skin, such as the inner thigh, axilla, and the edge of wounds in recently earmarked lambs, or tail-dock sites. Proliferative lesions affecting predominantly the head, neck, and body have been described in Nubian goats.

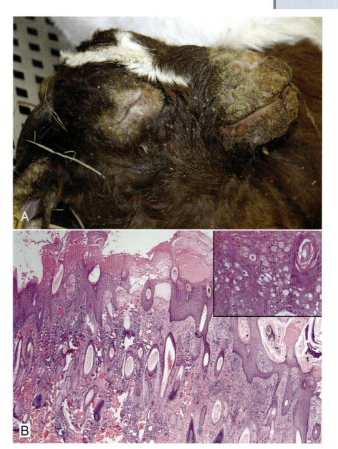

Figure 6-79 Contagious pustular dermatitis (orf). **A.** Crusted lesions around the eyes and at the margins of the lips in a goat. (Courtesy W.H. Miller). **B.** Epidermal hyperplasia with marked intracellular edema of keratinocytes, reticular degeneration, and intracytoplasmic eosinophilic inclusion bodies (see inset). Marked edema and perivascular dermatitis.

The lesions develop through the typical pox phases but are much more proliferative. The vesicular stage is transient and pustules are flat rather than umbilicated. The most significant feature of the gross lesion is the layer of thick brown-gray crust that may be elevated 2-4 mm above the skin surface. Depending on the degree of secondary infection, regression is usually complete by 4 weeks. Papillomatous growths, resulting from continued epidermal proliferation, sometimes occur.

A severe persistent and generalized form of the disease has been described in Boer goats and crosses. All affected animals have had multifocal severe proliferative dermatitis and peripheral lymphadenopathy that persisted for several months. A genetic defect or immune deficiency has been proposed. Premature thymic involution, suppurative arthritis, and pneumonia have been detected in many of these goats.

The microscopic lesions of contagious pustular dermatitis are characterized by vacuolation and swelling of keratinocytes in the stratum spinosum, reticular degeneration, marked epidermal proliferation, intraepidermal microabscesses, and accumulation of scale-crust (Fig. 6-79B). In experimentally abraded sheep skin, the active site of viral replication was found to be the newly proliferative keratinocyte population, growing up under the superficial necrotic layer. By ~30 hours postinfection, keratinocyte swelling and vacuolation commences in the outer stratum spinosum. It is accompanied by cytoplasmic basophilia, which corresponds ultrastructurally to an increased number of polyribosomes, presumably active in viral protein synthesis. Basophilic intracytoplasmic inclusion bodies are reported as early as 31 hours postinfection. By 72 hours postinfection, the keratinocytes show nuclear pyknosis and marked intracytoplasmic edema, leading to reticular degeneration. The term *ballooning degeneration* is often used, but the keratinocytes do not have the homogeneous eosinophilic cytoplasm typical of this condition. At this time, intracytoplasmic eosinophilic inclusion bodies appear (see Fig. 6-79B inset). The inclusion bodies persist for 3-4 days. The proliferative reaction in the epidermis is underway by 55 hours postinfection, with mitotic figures numerous in the stratum basale. By 3 days postinfection, the epithelium is 3-4 times normal thickness, and rete ridges are markedly elongated. Pseudocarcinomatous hyperplasia is common.

Dermal lesions include superficial edema, marked capillary dilation, and an early influx of neutrophils, followed by a marked accumulation of major histocompatibility complex class II dendritic cells, with CD4+ T cells, CD8+ T cells, and B cells. A thick layer of scale-crust is built up, composed of orthokeratotic and parakeratotic hyperkeratosis, proteinaceous fluid, degenerating neutrophils, cellular debris, and bacterial colonies. The subsequent microscopic appearance of the lesions depends on the degree of secondary bacterial infection.

Further reading

de la Concha-Bermejillo A, et al. Severe persistent orf in young goats. J Vet Diagn Invest 2003;15:423-431.

Hosamani M, et al. Orf: an update on current research and future perspectives. Expert Rev Anti Infect Ther 2009;7:879-893.

Ulcerative dermatosis of sheep. Ulcerative dermatosis is a disease of the epidermis of sheep that has been reported in the literature as being caused by an **unclassified poxvirus,** which is similar to *Orf virus*, but the viruses do not cross-protect. The disease has been reported in South Africa, where it is known as "pisgoed" or "pisgras"; in the United Kingdom as a contagious venereal infection; and in the United States, where it is known as "lip and leg ulceration," "anovulvitis," "infectious balanoposthitis," and "ulcerative vulvitis." The various names indicate the *essential features of the disease, which are ulcerative papules on the lips, face, legs, feet, vulva, prepuce, and occasionally, the glans penis*. The genital lesions are transmissible by coitus.

Presumably, infection results from viral contact with damaged skin. *The pathologic process is primarily ulcerative,* with ulcers of up to 4-5 cm in diameter and 3-5 mm deep. Pus covers the granulation tissue at the base of the ulcer and underlies a scab that is thin, brown and bloody, and unlike the thick parakeratotic crusts that develop in contagious pustular dermatitis. The underlying dermis is diffusely swollen, especially in distensible parts, such as the vulva and prepuce. The lesions on the hairy parts of the face tend to be fairly well circumscribed, but those of the feet tend to spread, especially on the interdigital skin. The vulval lesions usually begin on the tip and spread around the margins of the lips. An ulcerative ring tends to form around the preputial orifice, but the preputial mucosa is spared. Lesions on the glans penis remain moist. The urethral process may become necrotic. The labial and pedal lesions must be distinguished from those of contagious pustular dermatitis and foot-and-mouth disease, and the preputial lesions must be distinguished from noncontagious forms of balanoposthitis. *Detailed descriptions of the histopathology of ulcerative dermatitis are lacking;* the lesions are supposedly distinguishable from those of contagious pustular dermatitis by the *lack of epithelial hyperplasia*.

Pseudocowpox. Pseudocowpox is caused by species **Pseudocowpox virus**, genus *Parapoxvirus*. The virus is closely related to *Bovine papular stomatitis virus* and *Orf virus*. *It is a common endemic infection in cattle throughout most of the world.* Transmission occurs via contamination of skin abrasions. It affects chiefly milking herds and occasionally beef herds. Morbidity in a herd approaches 100%, but only 5-15% of cows are affected at any one time. The economic significance lies in the effect on milk production, either as a result of sore teats or because of secondary bacterial mastitis. Lesions typically affect the teats and udder and occasionally the perineum, medial thighs, and scrotum. Lesions usually start as erythematous macules and papules, and do not form the umbilicated pustules seen in cowpox and vaccinia infections. Instead, a *characteristic ring or horseshoe-shaped crust forms* that may become umbilicated as it expands, but infrequently ulcerates (Fig. 6-80). *The histologic appearance of lesions is typical of other poxviral infections*. The lesions usually heal within 6 weeks. Occasionally, lesions develop in the mouth and on the muzzle of suckling calves, and the infection can be spread by cross-suckling as well as poor hygiene in milking sheds. Transmission to people induces "milker's nodule." The lesion in humans starts as an erythematous papule that becomes a nodule with a target-like appearance, red center surrounded by a white ring and then red peripheral margin. There is a red oozing center that forms a crust.

Bovine papular stomatitis. Species ***Bovine papular stomatitis virus*** is distributed worldwide, and although it causes disease more commonly in *cattle <1 year of age*, it can occur

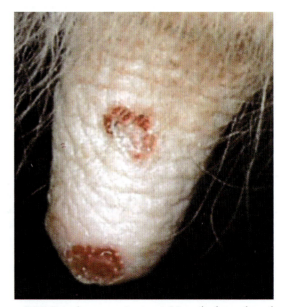

Figure 6-80 Pseudocowpox in a cow. Note the horseshoe-shaped red crust on the teat. (Courtesy E. Pichon.)

at any age and in any breed. Like pseudocowpox, transmission occurs via contamination of skin abrasions. Lesions occur on the *muzzle, nostrils, lips, and mouth*, although they can become more widespread (see Vol. 2, Alimentary system and peritoneum), and cows with suckling calves can develop *teat and udder lesions*. The appearance of initial lesions is similar to pseudocowpox; however, lesions may become papillomatous or undergo central necrosis and become crusted. Resolution of lesions occurs in days to weeks. A chronic and fatal form has been described in calves and is characterized by exudative necrotic dermatitis, proliferative and necrotizing stomatitis, and marked hyperkeratosis around the mouth, anus, and ventral tail. A necrotic dermatitis of the tail of feedlot cattle ("rat-tail syndrome") has been associated with bovine papular stomatitis. Affected cattle lose the tail switch, leaving an ulcerated area. *Transmission to humans induces lesions identical to "milker's nodule"* caused by *Pseudocowpox virus* infection. The histologic appearance of lesions is typical of other poxviral infections.

Further reading

Scott DW. Color Atlas of Farm Animal Dermatology. Ames, Iowa: Blackwell; 2007.

Parapox of red deer. A new addition to the genus *Parapoxvirus* is species **Parapox virus of red deer**, first noted in 1986 in farmed red deer in New Zealand. Morbidity is high, but mortality is low unless secondary infections are present. The virus causes crusty lesions on the lips, muzzle, face, ears, and neck, and on the antler velvet in stags. Removal of the crusts leaves a red raw ulcer. A more severe form of the disease was recently reported in red deer in Italy. These animals had proliferative lesions, erosion and ulcers on the lips and hard palate, and died as a result of starvation. Histologic lesions are characterized by *epithelial hyperplasia with marked intracellular edema, dyskeratosis, and eosinophilic cytoplasmic viral inclusions*. Like some of the other members of genus *Parapoxvirus*, viral VEGF is thought to contribute to the proliferative and highly vascular nature of the lesions.

Further reading

Scagliarini A, et al. Parapoxvirus infections of red deer, Italy. Emerg Infect Dis 2011;17:684-687.

Ueda N, et al. Parapoxvirus of red deer in New Zealand encodes a variant of viral vascular endothelial growth factor. Vir Res 2007; 124:50-58.

Orthopoxviral diseases

Cowpox. Species ***Cowpox virus*** is a zoonotic virus belonging to the genus *Orthopoxvirus*. Cowpox affects a range of species, including *wild and domestic felids, cattle, dogs*, rodents, humans, nonhuman primates, horses, and several zoo and circus animals, including elephants and rhinoceros. Cowpox is enzootic in Europe and in some western states of the former Soviet Union, and in adjacent areas of Northern and Central Asia. The natural reservoirs are wild rodents, with the highest seroprevalence in bank voles *(Clethrionomys glareolus)*. In cattle, poxvirus lesions most commonly develop on the *teats and udder*. A thick red crust, 1-2 cm in diameter is characteristic. In severe cases, lesions occur on the medial thighs, perineum, vulva, scrotum, and mouth of nursing calves. Human cowpox infection is rare, and most have been associated with infected cats.

Domestic **cats** develop cutaneous and, occasionally, respiratory lesions. Transmission is probably through rodent bites or feeding on rodents carrying the virus. Most cats have a single primary cutaneous lesion, usually on the head, neck, forelimbs, or paws (Fig. 6-81A). A secondary bacterial infection may develop, resulting in an abscess or cellulitis. A viremic period occurs 1-3 weeks following the initial infection, and affected cats may be febrile, inappetent, and depressed. Secondary skin lesions develop during this viremic phase and consist of multiple papules that enlarge to small nodules over 3-5 days and ulcerate, forming craters and crusts. Lesions are rarely vesicular except on the oral mucosa and inner aspect of the pinna. The ulcers heal with thick gray crusts over 2-3 weeks. Mucocutaneous junctions, oral mucosa, and the tongue may also be involved. Most cats recover within 4-5 weeks, and permanent scarring can occur. However, some cats develop more severe and sometimes fatal disease. Rarely, domestic cats can develop a fatal necrotizing pneumonia without typical skin lesions. Exotic felids, especially cheetahs, are at high risk of developing a rapidly fatal necrotizing pneumonia during the viremic period. More severe disease is rare in domestic cats and is often associated with severe secondary bacterial infection or immune suppression caused by concurrent infection with feline leukemia virus, feline immunodeficiency virus,

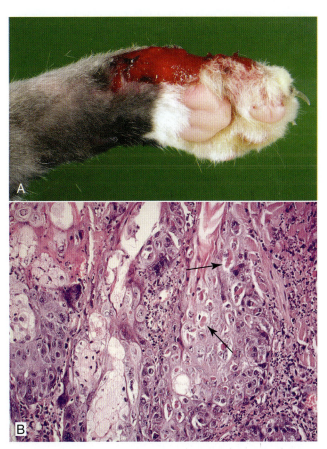

Figure 6-81 Cowpox in a cat. **A.** Ulcerative lesion on the paw. **B.** Necrotizing dermatitis with eosinophilic intracytoplasmic inclusions (arrows) within hair follicle epithelium and sebocytes at the edge of an ulcer. (Courtesy W. von Bomhard.)

feline panleukopenia virus, feline herpesvirus, or from glucocorticoid therapy.

A few cats exhibit clinical signs of upper respiratory tract disease. Lower respiratory tract lesions, which are rare in domestic cats, include pleural effusion and localized areas of cream-colored consolidation in the ventral lung lobes. They are thought to develop from systemic spread rather than from primary respiratory infection.

The *microscopic lesions* in naturally infected cats are *focal, sharply demarcated ulcers covered by fibrinonecrotic exudate*. The ulcers may extend to the deep dermis, subcutis, or even muscle. An intense dermal inflammatory cell infiltrate of neutrophils and mononuclear cells may be associated with the base of the ulcers. *Eosinophilic, homogeneous, intracytoplasmic inclusion bodies*, 3-7 μm in diameter, occur in keratinocytes in the hyperplastic epithelium at the margin of the ulcers and in the epithelium of the external root sheath and sebaceous gland (Fig. 6-81B). Epidermal lesions typical of poxvirus infections develop in cats experimentally infected intravenously or by skin scarification. These lesions include focal hyperplasia, with reticular degeneration and multilocular vesiculation. Epidermal cells bordering the vesicles contain eosinophilic intracytoplasmic inclusion bodies. Viral inclusions also occur in macrophages, fibroblasts, and endothelial cells. The extensive necrosis is probably ischemic in origin following viral damage to endothelial cells. The pulmonary lesion is necrotizing alveolitis in which eosinophilic inclusion bodies are present in the degenerating cells.

Electron microscopic examination of scabs reveals typical orthopox virions. *Cowpox virus* infection may be confirmed by immunohistochemical staining of lesions, PCR, or virus isolation. Serologic tests may be helpful in establishing retrospective diagnoses, as virus neutralizing antibodies persist for several years.

There have been outbreaks of severe orthopoxviral infections in several species of **nondomestic felids** in English and Russian zoos. Lions, cheetahs, pumas, jaguars, and ocelots have been affected. Rats were implicated as the source of infection in the Russian outbreaks. Two forms of the disease are recognized. The cutaneous form is rarely fatal. The lesions are ulcerative and crusted as described for domestic cats. The respiratory form is uniformly fatal and consists of severe fibrinous and necrotizing bronchopneumonia and pleuritis. A virus closely resembling *Cowpox virus* is responsible.

Cowpox has been described in 3 dogs, 2 of which were <1 year of age, and all had a solitary raised ulcerated nodule, clinically mimicking a canine cutaneous histiocytoma. None of the dogs showed signs of dissemination or systemic spread.

Raccoonpox virus, also belonging to the genus *Orthopoxvirus*, was reported to cause a localized ulcerative and exudative lesion on the forepaw of a 2-year-old cat in Canada.

Further reading

Godfrey DR, et al. Unusual presentations of cowpox infection in cats. J Small Anim Pract 2004;45:202-205.

Herder V, et al. Poxvirus infection in a cat with presumptive human transmission. Vet Dermatol 2011;22:220-224.

Miller WH, et al. Viral rickettsial and protozoal skin diseases. In: Miller WH, et al., editors. Muller & Kirk's Small Animal Dermatology. 7th ed. St Louis: Elsevier; 2013. p. 343-362.

Von Bomhard W, et al. Localized cowpox infection in a 5 month old Rottweiler. Vet Dermatol 2012;22:111-114.

Vaccinia. Species *Vaccinia virus* (VACV), and vaccinia-like viruses in genus *Orthopoxvirus*, infects horses, cattle, swine, and humans. This virus was used for the immunization of humans during the smallpox eradication campaign. *The origin of the virus is controversial*. One theory is that it represents the laboratory survival of horsepoxvirus, which is now considered extinct in nature, and that horse-derived material was the source of vaccine material used by Edward Jenner in 1817 to protect against variola or smallpox. It may have arisen from buffalopox virus, which is antigenically almost identical to VACV. Another theory is that VACV was derived from cowpox virus by repeated passage on the skin of cows, sheep, and other animals, and that "horsepox" was caused by the infection of horses with cowpox virus. Incidental infections in cattle, horses, and pigs were transferred from vaccinated people. The lesions in cattle are indistinguishable from those of cowpox, and in swine are indistinguishable from those of swinepox. When vaccinia is inoculated onto scarified skin of horses, papular lesions resembling a naturally occurring poxvirus infection described in horses in the United States results. Furthermore, inoculation of the skin of the flexor surface of the pastern produces lesions resembling the classic "grease heel" form of horsepox. Although most clinical descriptions of VACV are associated with vaccination, over the past decade, a number of outbreaks of VACV affecting dairy cattle and humans in Brazil have been reported. Coinfection by VACV and orf virus–like parapoxvirus has also been reported in dairy cattle in Brazil. An outbreak of orthopoxvirus involving 14 horses in Brazil had gross findings similar to those of the buccal form of horsepox, but molecular analysis showed a high nucleotide sequence homology (95-100%) with Brazilian VACV isolates.

Further reading

Brum MCV, et al. An outbreak of orthopoxvirus-associated disease in horses in southern Brazil. J Vet Diagn Invest 2010;22: 143-147.

Chapman JL, et al. Animal models of *Orthopoxvirus* infection. Vet Pathol 2010;47:852-870.

de Sant'Ana FJF, et al. Coinfection by *Vaccinia virus* and an *Orf virus*-like parapoxvirus in an outbreak of vesicular disease in dairy cows in midwestern Brazil. J Vet Diag Invest 2013;25:267-272.

Buffalopox. Buffalopox virus, an *Orthopoxvirus* closely related to *Vaccinia virus*, is the cause of buffalopox, an economically important disease of domestic buffaloes. It is thought that buffalopox virus is a subspecies of *Vaccinia virus* resident in the water buffalo population. First reported in India in 1967, it has subsequently been reported in Pakistan, Indonesia, Egypt, Italy, and Russia. In India, it is considered to be an emerging enzootic virus and can occur in epidemic form, with significant economic impact. Zebu cattle are apparently refractory to infection. Pox lesions predominantly affect the teats and udder and can lead to mastitis. Lesions can also occur on the medial aspects of the thighs, lips, and muzzle and may be generalized, especially in calves. *Buffalopox virus is zoonotic*, causing lesions primarily on the hands. Human-to-human transmission has been postulated following the occurrence of disease in children who had had no contact with infected animals. Experimentally, the virus can be transmitted to cattle, rabbits, guinea pigs, and mice.

Further reading

Essbauer S, et al. Zoonotic poxviruses. Vet Microbiol 2010;140: 229-236.

Camelpox. *Camelpox virus*, a distinct species of genus *Orthopoxvirus*, causes severe disease in Old World camelids (*Camelus dromedarius* and *Camelus bactrianus*). First reported in Russia and later India, the disease is known to occur throughout the camel breeding areas of Northern Africa, the Middle East, and Asia, but has not been reported in wild camels in Australia. It is characterized by *high morbidity and a relatively high mortality rate* in young animals. A major effect is a fall in milk production and loss of condition. The disease is characterized by fever, lymphadenopathy, and skin lesions. Lesions affect both *skin and mucous membranes* and follow the usual pattern of pox lesions. Lesions tend to be most concentrated around the face, including eyelids, nostrils, and margins of the pinnae. In severe cases, the whole head may be swollen. Intense pruritus may be seen in acute cases. Later, skin lesions may extend to the neck, limbs, genitalia, mammary glands, and perineum. Generalized skin lesions occur more typically in calves. Skin lesions may take 4-6 weeks to heal. Rarely, the infection can become systemic and involve the mucous membranes of the mouth, respiratory, and digestive tract. Fatalities are usually associated with *secondary bacterial infection leading to septicemia*, a phenomenon more prevalent in the rainy season. *The lesions can be identical to parapox* (camel contagious ecthyma), and laboratory tests such as ELISA, PCR, and immunohistochemistry, as well as electron microscopy, can be used to differentiate the infections. Histologic lesions are similar to those caused by other orthopoxviruses.

Further reading

Bhanuprakash V, et al. Camelpox: epidemiology, diagnosis and control measures. Expert Rev Anti Infect Ther 2010;8:1187-1201.

"Horsepox" and Uasin Gishu disease. Species **Horsepox virus** (HSPV), genus *Orthopoxvirus*, is the cause of horsepox. Horsepox was a common disease of horses in Europe before the 20th century. It is rare today, and some consider it extinct. It is thought that Jenner, in his "cowpox" vaccination experiments to protect humans from smallpox, was actually using horse-derived material as a source of the vaccine, and that *Vaccinia virus* may be the long-lost agent of horsepox. Experimental infection of horses with *Vaccinia virus* reproduces the "grease heel" lesions of Jenner's horsepox and the more generalized form known as *equine papular dermatitis*. Although there is a close genetic relationship between HSPV and known VACV-like viruses, HSPV is considered a unique virus.

Poxviral lesions in the horse take *several clinical forms*. Jenner originally described an exudative dermatitis of the flexor aspects of the hind pasterns. The condition is colloquially named *"grease heel"* because thick, yellow, grease-like exudate mats the hair. Unfortunately, poxvirus infection is only one manifestation of this clinical entity, sparking considerable controversy as to the true nature of equine pox.

A second form has a predilection for the *muzzle and buccal cavity* (contagious pustular stomatitis). The lesions, which develop in the typical sequence of a pock, affect the inner surface of the lips and cheeks, the gums, and the ventral surface of the tongue. Following the development of the buccal eruptions, crops of pocks may appear in the rostral nares, on the face, and on other parts of the body. It is a benign infection, sometimes seriously complicated by bacterial contamination.

Equine papular dermatitis or viral papular dermatitis, may be a variant of horsepox. It has been described as a highly contagious disease of horses in the United States, Australia, and New Zealand. The disease is characterized by a papular reaction and is reported to spread by direct contact and through infected harness, bedding, and grooming tools. The lesions are firm papules, up to 0.5 cm diameter, which tend to develop on the lateral neck and shoulder and thorax but become generalized. The papules become crusted, and the crusts slough to leave circular alopecic patches. Resolution may take 6 weeks.

There is one case report of a donkey from Kansas (United States) with horsepox-like lesions over the face, nares, lips, cheeks, and gingiva. Histologic lesions resembled those of other orthopoxviruses and pox virions were noted with electron microscopy, but the virus was not further characterized. The donkey was euthanized because of a femoral fracture.

Uasin Gishu disease in Kenya, caused by an *Orthopoxvirus*, is also characterized by generalized skin lesions, but the disease differs clinically from equine papular dermatitis. Lesions begin similarly as small papules but develop into crusted papillomatous proliferations, up to 2 cm diameter. Lesions eventually resolve, but the disease may continue for 2 years. The histologic lesions of Uasin Gishu disease are identical to molluscum contagiosum.

Further reading

Jayo MJ, et al. Poxvirus infection in a donkey. Vet Pathol 1986;23: 635-637.

Tulmas ER, et al. Genome of horsepox virus. J Virol 2006;80: 9244-9258.

Molluscipoxviral disease

Equine molluscum contagiosum. Species **Molluscum contagiosum virus** (MCV), genus *Molluscipoxvirus*, is most commonly reported in humans, with a few reports in the veterinary literature that include predominantly horses, with rare reports of macropods (kangaroos and quokkas), chimpanzees, donkeys, and anecdotal reports in dogs.

In situ hybridization experiments indicate there is very close homology between the equine and human MCV. It has been suggested that the disease may actually be transmitted from humans to horses. Attempts to grow both the human and equine MCV in culture have failed, and this can help differentiate the virus from the orthopoxvirus of Uasin Gishu, which produces histologically and clinically similar lesions, but which can be grown in culture. *Molluscipoxvirus* can also be identified with PCR.

Molluscum contagiosum virus can be found worldwide, with a higher distribution in tropical areas. In horses, it is a benign cutaneous infection characterized clinically by multiple, slightly raised, smooth to slightly roughened, white and shiny, 2-8 mm papules that may occur anywhere on the body but seem to occur more frequently on the neck, chest, shoulders, limbs, and inguinal region. Lesions may remain localized to one body region, such as the muzzle, prepuce, or scrotum,

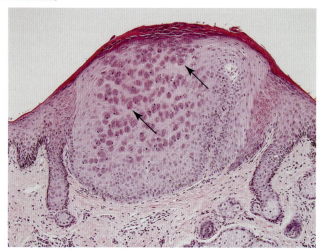

Figure 6-82 *Molluscum contagiosum* in a horse. Focal epidermal hyperplasia. Note large intracytoplasmic inclusion bodies referred to as "molluscum bodies" (arrows).

or they may become widespread with hundreds of lesions. As the lesions enlarge, papules become umbilicated and may bleed or have a central white to brown crust or horn projecting from the surface. Lesions may remain for months to years without regression.

The microscopic lesions of molluscum contagiosum are highly characteristic. *Well-demarcated foci of epidermal hyperplasia and hypertrophy form pear-shaped lobules.* The individual keratinocytes are markedly swollen and contain *large intracytoplasmic inclusions known as "molluscum bodies"* (Fig. 6-82). These occur initially as eosinophilic, floccular aggregates in the cells of the inner stratum spinosum. As the keratinocytes move toward the surface, the inclusions grow in size and density, compressing the nucleus against the cytoplasmic membrane until it is a thin crescent. The inclusion becomes increasingly basophilic so that cells of the stratum corneum contain deep-purple molluscum bodies. These exfoliate through a pore that forms in the stratum corneum and enlarges into a central crater. There is usually no dermal reaction. Molluscum bodies are easily identified in cytologic preparations.

Further reading

Fox R, et al. Molluscum contagiosum in two donkeys. Vet Rec 2012;170:649-651.

Scott DW, Miller WH. Viral and protozoal skin diseases. In: Scott DW, Miller WH, editors. Equine Dermatology. 2nd ed. St Louis: Elsevier Saunders; 2011. p. 251-262.

Thompson CH, Yager JA. Close relationship between equine and human molluscum contagiosum virus demonstrated by in situ hybridization. Res Vet Sci 1998;64:157-161.

Capripoxviral diseases

Sheeppox, goatpox, and lumpy skin disease of cattle are caused by viruses of the genus *Capripoxvirus* and cause significant economic losses in countries where they are endemic. The exact relationship between these viruses has been controversial. *It is believed that they represent strains of a single virus.* The evidence includes antigenic and biochemical similarity, a high degree of nucleotide sequence homology, lack of absolute host specificity in most strains, evidence of recombination in the field, and demonstration of cross-infection and cross-protection. The viruses are indistinguishable by conventional serology; nevertheless, the geographic distributions of the three are different, indicating the viruses are distinct. Most strains of *Capripoxvirus* show definite host preferences; however, some isolates can infect both species, and the disease caused by the same isolate can vary dramatically between sheep and goats. There is one report from China of an outbreak of sheeppox associated with goatpox virus in which 6 of 26 affected sheep died. PCR methods of identification of capripoxvirus have been developed so that classic virology methods based on live virus need not be used in areas of the world where the virus is exotic.

Further reading

Embury-Hyatt C, et al. Pathology and viral antigen distribution following experimental infection of sheep and goats with capripoxvirus. J Comp Pathol 2012;146:106-115.

Yan X, et al. An outbreak of sheep pox associated with goat poxvirus in Gansu province of China. Vet Microbiol 2012;156:425-428.

Sheeppox. *Sheeppox is the most serious of the pox diseases of domestic animals.* It exists in Africa, Asia, and the Middle East where, despite attempts at vaccination, it is responsible for cycles of epidemic disease, followed by periods of endemic maintenance with low morbidity. The disease is exotic to the Americas, Australia, and New Zealand. Eradication measures eliminated the disease from Britain in the mid-19th century but have only recently been successful in Eastern European countries. *Sheeppox causes extensive economic loss* through high mortality; reduced meat, milk, or wool yields; commercial inhibitions from quarantine requirements; and the cost of disease prevention programs.

Transmission of infection is by direct contact with diseased sheep or indirect contact via contaminated environment. Insect transmission has been demonstrated experimentally. Species **Sheeppox virus** is resistant to desiccation and remains viable for up to 2 months on wool or 6 months in dried crust. There are breed differences in disease susceptibility. Fine-wooled Merino sheep are particularly sensitive, whereas breeds native to endemic areas, such as Algerian sheep, are comparatively resistant. Sheeppox occurs in all ages of sheep with high morbidity, and mortality as high as 50%, but the disease is most severe in lambs, with mortality reaching 80-100%. A high level of background immunity, such as occurs in endemic areas of Kenya, is associated with low mortality, even in the young.

Sheeppox is a *systemic disease*. Infection is usually by the respiratory route but may occur through skin abrasions. The incubation period is 4-7 days and is followed by a leukocyte-associated viremia. The virus localizes in many organs, including the skin, where the virus concentration is highest 10-14 days postinfection. The initial clinical signs are fever, lacrimation, drooling, serous nasal discharge, and hyperesthesia. Skin lesions, which develop 1-2 days later, have a predilection for the sparsely wooled areas and typically involve eyelids, cheeks, nostrils, vulva, udder, scrotum, prepuce, ventral surface of the tail, and medial thigh.

The macroscopic lesions follow the typical pattern for pox infections. *Sheeppox lesions have a prominent vesicular stage* (Fig. 6-83A). The vesicles are umbilicated and, being

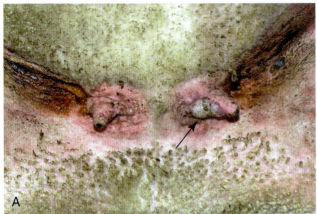

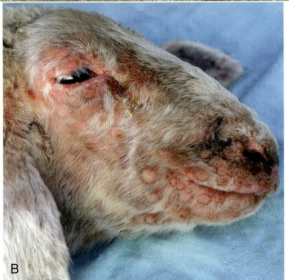

Figure 6-83 Sheeppox in a sheep. **A.** Vesicle (arrow) on teat. (Courtesy A. Alcaraz.) **B.** Erythematous papules, nodules, and plaques around the mouth, nose, and eyes. (Courtesy J.M. Gourreau.)

multilocular, yield only a small amount of fluid if punctured. Occasionally a large vesicle forms as a result of cleavage of necrotic epidermis from underlying dermis. The *pustule stage* is characterized by the formation of a thin crust. In severely affected animals, the lesions coalesce. There may be marked, gelatinous dermal edema. Highly susceptible animals often develop hemorrhagic papules early in the course of the disease and, later, ulcerative lesions in the gastrointestinal and respiratory tracts. Approximately ⅓ of animals develop multiple *foci of pulmonary consolidation*. There may be multiple fleshy nodules throughout the renal cortices.

Healing of the skin lesions is slow, taking up to 6 weeks, and a scar may remain. In the milder form of the disease, seen in endemic areas, the full range of pox lesions does not develop. Instead, epidermal proliferation produces papules covered by scale-crust, which heal with desquamation in a few days (Fig. 6-83B). Such lesions often occur on the ventral surface of the tail.

Sheeppox lesions have the epithelial changes typical for the group, including marked vacuolar degeneration of stratum spinosum keratinocytes, microvesiculation, eosinophilic intracytoplasmic inclusion bodies, and epidermal hyperplasia. The lesions affect both surface epithelium and that of the hair follicles.

There are, in addition, *marked dermal lesions* reflecting the systemic route of cutaneous involvement and possibly implicating immune-mediated lesions in addition to those caused by direct viral damage. The initial dermal lesions, corresponding to the macroscopic erythematous macule, are marked edema, hyperemia, and neutrophilic exocytosis. During the papular stage, large numbers of mononuclear cells accumulate in the increasingly edematous dermis. These cells are called "cellules claveleuses" or *"sheeppox cells"* and are characteristic of the disease. The nuclei of sheeppox cells are vacuolated and have marginated chromatin. The vacuolated cytoplasm contains single, occasionally multiple, *eosinophilic intracytoplasmic inclusion bodies*. Sheeppox cells are virus-infected monocytes, macrophages, and fibroblasts, but not endothelial cells. Sheep experimentally infected with capripoxvirus may develop large spindle-shaped syncytial cells with intracytoplasmic inclusions within the dermis. Approximately 10 days postinfection and corresponding with the most prominent epithelial lesions and peak of skin infectivity, severe necrotizing vasculitis develops in arterioles and postcapillary venules. Virus particles have not been identified in endothelial cells, and the vasculitis may be due to immune-complex deposition. Ischemic necrosis of the dermis and overlying epidermis follows.

The pulmonary lesions are proliferative alveolitis and bronchiolitis with focal areas of caseous necrosis. Alveolar septal cells contain intracytoplasmic inclusion bodies. Additional histologic lesions, characterized by the accumulation of sheeppox cells, may involve heart, kidney, liver, adrenals, thyroid, and pancreas.

The course and outcome of sheeppox depend not only on the usual host-virus relationship but also on the nature and location of secondary infections. The virus itself may cause death during the febrile, eruptive phase of the disease. Of great importance, however, are the secondary bacterial infections that rapidly develop in the necrotic tissue of the pocks. Death is often due to bacterial septicemia or pneumonia.

Goatpox. Goatpox, caused by species **Goatpox virus**, occurs in North Africa and the Middle East. A benign form of goatpox occurs in California and Sweden. The clinical signs of goatpox vary in different geographic areas. The disease has *many parallels with sheeppox, but is generally milder* with a low mortality rate (5%), although generalized eruption with mortality rates approaching 100% may occur. The cutaneous lesions have a predilection for the same areas as for sheeppox. In nursing kids, lesions may appear on the buccal mucosa or rostral nares. In animals with higher levels of resistance, the lesions may be confined to the udder, teats, inner aspects of thighs, or ventral surface of the tail. Occasionally, only nodular lesions are seen ("stone pox"), resembling lumpy skin disease of cattle.

Further reading

Embury-Hyatt C, et al. Pathology and viral antigen distribution following experimental infection of sheep and goats with capripoxvirus. J Comp Pathol 2012;146:106-115.

Scott DW. Color Atlas of Farm Animal Dermatology. Ames, Iowa: Blackwell; 2007.

Lumpy skin disease. Lumpy skin disease, caused by species **Lumpy skin disease virus** of the genus *Capripoxvirus*, is a disease of cattle, buffalo, and occasionally other wild species of hoofstock, characterized by the *eruption of multiple,* *well-circumscribed skin nodules, accompanied by fever, ventral edema, and generalized lymphadenopathy.* Lumpy-skin disease is found throughout the African continent and Madagascar, with sporadic reports from the Middle East and Israel.

Cattle of all ages, sex and breeds are affected, although the disease is more severe in Channel Island breeds. Both *Bos indicus* and *Bos taurus* cattle are susceptible; however, the disease can be less severe in Zebu breeds. The disease occurs in epidemics; a notable one in 1944 affected 8 million cattle. Transmission is believed to occur mainly by blood-feeding arthropods. Epidemics tend to follow periods of prolonged rainfall, which favor population increases in vector species. A forest maintenance cycle, probably involving Cape buffalo, is thought to be the reservoir of infection in the interepidemic periods. No reservoir host apart from cattle has been identified.

The morbidity is extremely variable, and inapparent infection is common. *Mortality is usually low;* around 1% but may be >50%. Economic losses are due to debilitation, loss of milk and meat production, damage to hides, and reproductive wastage resulting from fever-associated abortions and temporary sterility in bulls.

The natural incubation period of lumpy skin disease is 2-4 weeks, but this may be halved in experimental infection. In severely affected animals, the development of large numbers of cutaneous lesions over most of the body is preceded by fever, marked weight loss, profuse drooling, oculonasal discharge, ventral edema, and generalized lymphadenopathy. In the mild disease, there may be few isolated nodules and no prodromal fever. *The cutaneous lesions are firm, circumscribed, flat-topped papules and nodules, 0.5-5.0 cm in diameter.* They may coalesce. The nodules have a creamy gray color on cut section and involve the full width of the cutis, extending into the subcutis and occasionally adjacent muscles. Nodules affecting the scrotum, perineum, udder, vulva, glans penis, eyelids, and conjunctiva are usually flatter, and in nonpigmented tissue are surrounded by a zone of intense hyperemia. The fate of the nodules varies. *Typically, they undergo central necrosis and sequestration, but some may resolve rapidly and completely, and others may fail to separate but, instead, become indurated and persist as hard intradermal lumps for many months.* Sequestration is preceded by central necrosis in the nodule and occurs rapidly. Separation of the epidermis around the margin of the nodule exposes a rim of dermal granulation tissue. As the process of separation extends into the dermis, the nodule comes to contain a *core or sequestrum of necrotic material ("sit-fast")*, which is cone shaped and flat topped (Fig. 6-84). When the sequestrum is removed, a deep ulcer remains that is slowly filled with granulation tissue. *Secondary bacterial infections* develop in the necrotic cores of the nodules and contribute very significantly to the seriousness of the disease. Large craterous ulcers develop, which lead to lymphangitis and lymphadenitis. Local extension of lesions causes blindness, tenosynovitis, arthritis, or mastitis.

The mucous membranes of the upper respiratory and upper alimentary tracts often develop multiple, discrete ulcerative lesions, irrespective of the number of cutaneous nodules. Those in the respiratory tract may cause swelling sufficient to result in severe dyspnea and asphyxia. Aspiration may lead to pneumonia or, if the animal recovers, scarring may cause stenosis of the cranial portion of the trachea. Nodules occasionally occur in parenchymal organs, including kidneys, lungs, and testes.

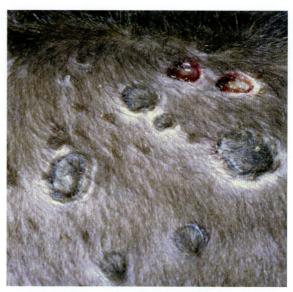

Figure 6-84 Lumpy skin disease in a calf. Circumscribed necrotic tissue ("sit-fasts") and deep ulcers. (Courtesy I. Yeruham.)

Although the virus is introduced percutaneously, *the infection is systemic.* A leukocyte-associated viremia disseminates the virus to various tissues, including the skin, where greatest virus concentration occurs 9-12 days postinfection. The virus infects a wide range of cells, including keratinocytes, mucous and serous glandular epithelium, fibrocytes, skeletal muscle, macrophages, pericytes, and endothelial cells. *Damage to endothelial cells causes vasculitis that is central to the pathogenesis of the lumpy skin disease lesions.*

Acute lesions consist of vasculitis, lymphangitis, thrombosis, marked dermal edema that sometimes induces dermoepidermal separation, and infarction. The epidermis shows the typical vacuolar changes associated with poxvirus infection. *Intracytoplasmic, eosinophilic, homogeneous, and occasionally granular inclusion bodies* occur in endothelial cells, pericytes, keratinocytes, macrophages, and fibroblasts. Virions in various stages of development are present in these inclusion-containing cells and in peripheral nerves. Neutrophils, macrophages and occasionally eosinophils migrate into the dermis in the acute lesions, to be replaced as the lesion ages by a predominantly mononuclear cell population. The infarcted tissue is sequestered and surrounded by granulation tissue. Inclusion bodies are absent from the resolving lesions but may be present in adjacent skin or sebaceous glands. Lymph nodes are edematous and hyperplastic.

The chief differential diagnosis is **pseudo–lumpy skin disease** *caused by a herpesvirus identical to the bovine herpes mammillitis virus but originally known as the Allerton virus.* Pseudo–lumpy skin disease is a milder condition clinically, and the nodules are superficial, resembling only the early stage of lumpy skin disease. Confirmation of the latter is best achieved by demonstration of poxvirus particles in fresh or formalin-fixed tissue.

Further reading

Tuppurainen ESM, Oura CAL. Review: lumpy skin disease: an emerging threat to Europe, the Middle East and Asia. Transbound Emerg Dis 2012;59:40-48.

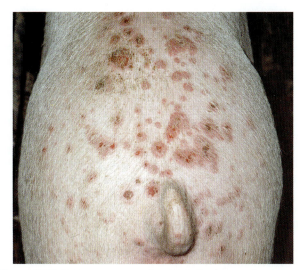

Figure 6-85 Swinepox in a piglet. Multifocal to coalescing erythematous macules and plaques, some with central necrosis. (Courtesy B. Sansot.)

Suipoxviral disease

Swinepox. The host-specific **Swinepox virus** (SWPV), the sole species in genus *Suipoxvirus*, is the chief cause of pox lesions in swine. In the past, *Vaccinia virus* was also responsible. The disease occurs worldwide and is endemic in areas of intensive swine production. The disease has received relatively little attention as it is *usually mild and mortality is negligible. It chiefly affects young, growing piglets* but occurs in neonates, promoting speculation that transplacental infection may be possible. Normally, SWPV is transmitted by contact. The virus is resistant and persists in dried crust from infected animals. The sucking louse *Haematopinus suis* often acts as a mechanical vector and also assists infection by causing skin trauma. *The gross lesions typically affect the ventral and lateral abdomen, lateral thorax, and medial foreleg and thigh.* Occasionally, lesions on the dorsum predominate (Fig. 6-85). In severe infection, lesions may be generalized and rarely involve the oral cavity, pharynx, esophagus, stomach, trachea, and bronchi. The morphology of the gross lesions follows the typical pattern of pox infection. The erythematous papules usually transform into umbilicated pustules without a significant vesicular stage. The inflammatory crust eventually sheds to leave a white macule.

The histologic lesions also follow the pattern for pox infections. The eosinophilic, intracytoplasmic inclusion bodies are quite transient and are not found in older lesions. Vacuoles develop in the nuclei of infected stratum spinosum keratinocytes early in the course of swinepox infection.

Further reading

Medaglia ML, et al. Swinepox virus outbreak, Brazil, 2011. Emerg Infect Dis 2011;17:1976-1978.

Thibault S, et al. Congenital swinepox: a sporadic skin disorder in nursing piglets. Swine Health Prod 1998;6:276-278.

Herpesviral infections

The *Herpesviridae* is a large family of *enveloped DNA viruses* responsible for important animal diseases, of which relatively few are primary skin diseases. ***Bovine herpesvirus 2*** (BoHV-2) causes primary cutaneous infections and is widespread in many parts of the world. It is responsible for 2 distinct clinical forms of skin disease: *bovine mammillitis of cattle*, which is the major cutaneous infection, and *pseudo—lumpy skin disease*. Skin lesions occur in systemic herpesvirus infections such as *malignant catarrhal fever*, and *infectious bovine rhinotracheitis* in cattle, and *pseudorabies* in pigs.

A unique form of alopecia and mural folliculitis has been described in sika deer with **Caprine herpesvirus 2** infection and in one goat with **Ovine herpesvirus 2** infection. Skin lesions consisted of nonpruritic scaling and crusting of the pinna, nares, and peribuccal skin in addition to papules, erythema, and scaling of the distal limbs. Microscopically, there was irregular epidermal hyperplasia with compact orthokeratotic and parakeratotic hyperkeratosis layered with inflammatory cells. The main feature was mural folliculitis with large numbers of macrophages, fewer lymphocytes, plasma cells, eosinophils, and occasional multinucleated giant cells.

Skin lesions associated with **Felid herpesvirus 1** infection are also recognized, usually in the absence of respiratory lesions. Vesicles, pustules, ulcers, and depigmentation are seen on the genital organs and occasionally the lips and nostrils of horses with **Equid herpesvirus 3** infection (equine coital exanthema), and in **Bovine herpesvirus 1** infection (infectious vulvovaginitis and balanoposthitis).

Further reading

Crawford TB, et al. Mural folliculitis and alopecia caused by infection with goat-associated malignant catarrhal fever virus in two sika deer. J Am Vet Med Assoc 2002;221:843-847.

Fenner F, et al. Veterinary Virology. 2nd ed. San Diego: Academic Press; 1993.

Foster AP, et al. Diagnostic exercise: generalized alopecia and mural folliculitis in a goat. Vet Pathol 2010;47:760-763.

Bovine herpesvirus 2 diseases

Pseudo—lumpy skin disease. Species *Bovine herpesvirus 2* (BoHV-2) is a member of the *Alphaherpesvirinae* subfamily and is antigenically related to human herpes simplex virus 1. First isolated in Africa in 1957 from lesions resembling lumpy skin disease, it was named the *Allerton virus*. The associated disease was subsequently named "pseudo—lumpy skin disease" to differentiate it from the more serious disease caused by *Lumpy skin disease virus*. Pseudo—lumpy skin disease is widespread in southern Africa, with sporadic reports from Australia, the United Kingdom, the United States, and Israel. It is characterized by a generalized eruption of superficial cutaneous nodules that develop a central depression but that heal without scar formation and do not produce the deep necrotic sequestra of true lumpy skin disease. The natural mode of transmission is not clear but is thought to be spread by inoculation into the dermis by biting flies.

Bovine herpes mammillitis. Bovine herpes mammillitis, or ulcerative mammillitis, is a localized form of BoHV-2 infection seen sporadically in the United States, Canada, Great Britain, Europe, Africa, and Australia. Serologic surveys indicate that *infection is much more common than disease*. In Africa, Asia, and Hungary, several species of wild animals have antibody titers or PCR detection of the virus, although clinical disease is not seen.

Herpes mammillitis is *chiefly a disease of lactating dairy cows* but occurs in heifers about to calve and in beef animals. The incidence is usually sporadic with occasional local epidemics in fully susceptible herds. In previously exposed herds, the disease affects only the recently introduced nonimmune, first-calf heifers. There is no mortality. The economic significance of teat lesions lies in the effect on milk production or secondary bacterial mastitis, which complicate ~20% of cases.

Intact teat skin is refractory to virus penetration, indicating that *some form of teat trauma precedes infection*. Transmission of the virus is presumed to involve mechanical vectors, particularly the milking machine, but biting flies, such as *Stomoxys calcitrans*, have also been implicated. In the latter instance, it is difficult to explain the localization of lesions to the teat and mammary gland. Local tissue temperature has, however, been shown to be critical in the pathogenesis, and environmental conditions have been associated with the occurrence of outbreaks. Experimental cutaneous inoculation of BoHV-2 results in higher virus titers and larger and more persistent lesions when the site is kept cold. The increased prevalence of disease in the autumn months may also be related to the temperature sensitivity of the virus. The source of infection within a herd is not known, but latency, a characteristic of herpesviruses, is likely important. Latency has been demonstrated in experimental BoHV-2 infections.

The macroscopic lesions affect the teats, less frequently the udder, and occasionally the perineum of lactating cows. Transmission of infection to nursing calves may result in ulcerative lesions of the muzzle, chin, lips, and occasionally the oral cavity. Teat lesions develop after a 3- to 7-day incubation period. *The teat becomes very swollen and painful and develops 1- to 2-cm diameter plaques*. Vesicles are rare. The epidermis in the center of the plaque becomes necrotic and sloughs to expose an erythematous, irregularly shaped ulcer. Exuded serum mixed with blood forms a thin brown crust, which is easily displaced by the teat cups. The lesions heal beneath the crust, and there is no residual scar. Lesions on the udder are often diffuse, giving rise to the term "gangrene of the udder." Regional lymph nodes are swollen in the early stages.

The microscopic lesions are characterized by the formation of epithelial syncytia containing prominent intranuclear eosinophilic inclusion bodies. The inclusion bodies are typical Cowdry type A. The nuclear chromatin is marginated, and the eosinophilic inclusions are surrounded by a clear halo. The inclusions are numerous from the time of the first macroscopic lesion until the fifth day. Thereafter, they are very difficult to find. Syncytial cell formation commences early in groups of cells in the stratum basale and inner stratum spinosum. The process extends to involve the full thickness of the epidermis, the outer root sheath of the hair follicle infundibulum, and the sebaceous gland. By day 5, after macroscopic lesions develop, the epidermis is necrotic, although the outlines of syncytial cells are apparent. The inclusion bodies lose their sharp outline and fill the entire nucleus. Some are free in the necrotic epidermis, released from fragmenting nuclei. The necrotic epidermis and adnexa are infiltrated with large numbers of neutrophils. Loss of the necrotic epithelium leaves an ulcer, which is covered by hemorrhagic and fibrinous exudate and a band of degenerating neutrophils. Deeper, there is dermal edema and a predominantly mononuclear cell infiltrate. In the healed lesion, the epithelium is re-established; there is superficial dermal fibrosis and a perivascular infiltrate of predominantly mononuclear cells.

The diagnosis of herpes mammillitis is confirmed by isolation of the virus. A rapid provisional diagnosis may be made by examining clinical material by electron microscopy. Biopsy is diagnostic if lesions are collected before the fifth day. Cytology smears prepared from an early lesion are diagnostic if syncytial cells containing eosinophilic intranuclear inclusion bodies are found. Serologic tests allow a retrospective diagnosis, provided paired samples are collected and a rising titer identified.

Experimental intravenous inoculation of **sheep** with BoHV-2 results in lesions resembling those of similarly inoculated cattle. Naturally occurring outbreaks of dermatitis of the pasterns caused by BoHV-2 have been described in captive Dahl sheep. Goats will only develop skin lesions following intravenous inoculation.

Further reading

Brenner J, et al. Herpesvirus type 2 in biopsy of a cow with possible pseudo-lumpy skin disease. Vet Rec 2009;165:539-540.

d'Offay JM, et al. Use of a polymerase chain reaction assay to detect bovine herpesvirus type 2 DNA in skin lesions from cattle suspected to have pseudo-lumpy skin disease. J Am Vet Med Assoc 2003; 222:1404-1407.

Janett F, et al. Bovine herpes mammillitis: clinical symptoms and serologic course. Schweiz Arch Tierheilkd 2000;142:375-380.

Torres FD, et al. Distribution of latent bovine herpesvirus 2 DNA in tissues of experimentally infected sheep. Res Vet Sci 2009;87: 161-166.

Bovine herpesvirus 4 diseases

A strain of species *Bovine herpesvirus 4* (BoHV-4) can cause udder lesions on dairy cows **(mammary pustular dermatitis)**; the teats are not involved. The macroscopic lesions are *vesicles, pustules, ulcers, and crusts*, originally 2-4 mm in diameter, becoming larger with coalescence. The microscopic lesion is *intraepidermal pustular dermatitis*. The etiologic association between BoHV-4 and the cutaneous disease is controversial, however, because the virus is a ubiquitous herpesvirus of cattle that can produce no disease when experimentally inoculated into susceptible cattle and can be isolated from cell cultures prepared from clinically normal cattle. Although not a primary mastitis pathogen, BoHV-4 may prolong cases of bacterial mastitis. BoHV-4 infection is considered a risk factor for abortion in cows, and is reported as a cause of endometritis in postparturient dairy cows.

Further reading

Frazier K, et al. Endometritis in postparturient cattle associated with bovine herpesvirus-4 infection: 15 cases. J Vet Diagn Invest 2001;13:502-508.

Kalman D, et al. Role of bovine herpesvirus 4 in bacterial bovine mastitis. Microb Pathog 2004;37:125-129.

Equine herpesvirus

Equine herpes coital exanthema is caused by species **Equid herpesvirus 3** (EHV-3) and is found in most parts of the world. Lesions include papules, vesicles, or pustules that may enlarge to plaques and bullae on the penis, prepuce, and scrotum of stallions, and on the vagina, vulva, and perineum of mares. Lesions may also occur on the muzzles of foals in contact with infected mares. Lesions heal over 2-5 weeks, and depigmentation may occur where lesions have healed. Microscopically, there is ballooning degeneration of keratinocytes with eosinophilic intranuclear inclusion bodies. Species *Equid herpesvirus* 2 (EHV-2) occurs worldwide and is isolated from normal horses and foals with respiratory disease. One horse was reported to have multiple plaques over the neck and chest. Microscopically, the lesions were composed of deep dermal infiltrates of neutrophils, lymphocytes, plasma cells, macrophages, and multinucleated giant cells, and thrombosed blood vessels with necrosis. Eosinophilic intranuclear inclusions were present within the macrophages and multinucleated giant cells. Species *Equid herpesvirus* 5 (EHV-5)–associated dermatitis resembling herpes-associated erythema multiforme was described in a 9-year-old Holsteiner stallion. Skin lesions consisted of nonpruritic, multifocal, pustular dermatitis around the eyes, nostrils, and muzzle. Histologically, there was interface dermatitis with apoptotic keratinocytes and intranuclear inclusions within the stratum spinosum and stratum granulosum.

Further reading

Herder V, et al. Equid herpesvirus 5-associated dermatitis in a horse resembling herpes-associated erythema multiforme. Vet Microbiol 2012;155:420-424.

Scott DW, Miller WH. Viral and protozoal skin diseases. In: Scott DW, Miller WH, editors. Equine Dermatology. 2nd ed. St Louis: Elsevier Saunders; 2011. p. 251-262.

Felid herpesvirus 1

Species *Felid herpesvirus 1* (FeHV-1, Feline viral rhinotracheitis virus), a well-recognized pathogen of the upper respiratory tract, is commonly associated with oral ulceration. It can also be associated with *focal ulcerative lesions, primarily on the haired skin of the face or on the nasal planum*, with rare reports of lesions on the feet and trunk. The lesions generally occur in the absence of clinical respiratory signs. In common with other herpesviruses, FeHV-1 can establish latency in the trigeminal ganglion. As affected cats often have a history of previous respiratory disease or recent stress, recrudescence of a latent herpesvirus infection is likely. *The macroscopic lesions consist of crusts, ulcers, and vesicles, frequently on the face or nasal planum, which can be persistent or recurrent* (Fig. 6-86A). Microscopically, the lesions are *ulcerative and necrotizing*, and the mixed dermal inflammation frequently includes numerous eosinophils. There may be foci of degranulating eosinophils around collagen fibers (flame figures). *Large amphophilic or glassy intranuclear inclusions* are present in the surface and adnexal epithelium (Fig. 6-86B). They are variable in number and sometimes hard to find in small rafts of epithelial cells surrounded by necrotic debris. The similarity of the inflammatory component in this condition with that of the feline hypersensitivity conditions, such as mosquito-bite hypersensitivity or feline eosinophilic granuloma complex, warrants close scrutiny of eosinophilic necrotizing cutaneous lesions for intranuclear inclusions or examination by molecular techniques.

A similar FeHV-1 associated eosinophilic dermatitis, although reportedly more severe and widespread, occurs in captive cheetahs.

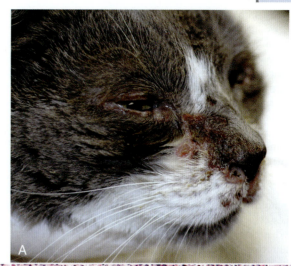

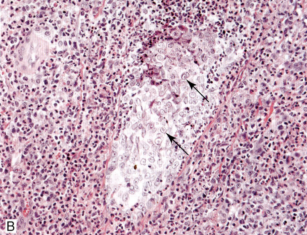

Figure 6-86 Feline herpesviral dermatitis. **A.** Ulceration and crusting around eyes and nose. (Courtesy W.H. Miller.) **B.** Eosinophilic intranuclear inclusion bodies (arrows) within hair follicle epithelium surrounded by eosinophilic dermatitis.

Further reading

Hargis AM, et al. Ulcerative facial and nasal dermatitis and stomatitis in cats associated with feline herpesvirus 1. Vet Dermatol 1999;10:267-274.

Munson L, et al. Chronic eosinophilic dermatitis associated with persistent feline herpes virus infection in cheetahs (*Acinonyx jubatus*). Vet Pathol 2004;41:170-176.

Persico P, et al. Detection of feline herpes virus 1 via polymerase chain reaction and immunohistochemistry in cats with ulcerative facial dermatitis, eosinophilic granuloma complex reaction patterns and mosquito-bite hypersensitivity. Vet Dermatol 2011;22: 521-527.

Retroviral infections

Several skin disorders have been associated with retroviral infections caused by species *Feline leukemia virus* (FeLV) and *Feline immunodeficiency virus* (FIV) in **cats**. Because both viruses are immunosuppressive, *most dermatologic conditions are considered secondary*. However, primary viral infection of keratinocytes has been reported. Scaling, crusting, and alopecic lesions affecting primarily the head and face, with occasional involvement of trunk and extremities is seen rarely in FeLV-infected cats. Histologically, syncytial keratinocytes are seen in the epidermis and superficial follicular epithelium, accompanied by individual cell necrosis (apoptosis), pustules, and ulcers. Immunohistochemical staining demonstrates FeLV antigen in epithelial cells and giant cells. In addition, cutaneous keratin horns seen in FeLV-infected cats have been reported as a primary effect of viral infection of keratinocytes. Recurrent pyoderma and paronychia have been attributed to the immunosuppressive effects of FeLV. Dermatologic diseases associated with naturally occurring chronic FIV infection include generalized demodectic mange, notoedric mange, dermatophytosis, *Malassezia* dermatitis, cowpoxvirus infections, bowenoid in situ lesions, atypical mycobacteriosis, and abscesses. Cats that are FIV positive are more frequently diagnosed as having subcutaneous abscesses and cellulitis than are noninfected cats. Because the virus is shed in high titer in the saliva, and bite wounds are thought to be an important mode of transmission, this finding may simply reflect a greater tendency for cats that fight to become FIV positive. Many of the associations made between retroviral infection and specific diseases are anecdotal. A nonpruritic generalized skin disorder characterized by a papulocrustous eruption with alopecia and scaling most severe on the head and limbs has been described in 3 FIV-positive cats. Microscopically, there was hydropic interface dermatitis with occasional giant cells and pale basal epidermal cells. Degenerative mucinotic mural folliculitis is described rarely in cats infected with FIV (see Miscellaneous skin conditions).

Further reading

Gross TL, et al. Degenerative mucinotic mural folliculitis in cats. Vet Dermatol 2001;12:279-283.

Merchant SR, Taboada J. Systemic diseases with cutaneous manifestations. Vet Clin North Am Small Anim Pract 1995;25:945-959.

Miller WH, et al. Viral, rickettsial and protozoal skin diseases. In: Miller WH, et al., editors. Muller & Kirk's Small Animal Dermatology. 7th ed. St Louis: Elsevier; 2013. p. 343-362.

Parvoviral infections

More typically associated with reproductive problems, species **Porcine parvovirus** (PPV) has been implicated in outbreaks of vesicular and ulcerative dermatitis and glossitis in 1-4 week-old piglets in the midwestern United States. Various clinical signs, including diarrhea and sneezing, accompanied the skin lesions. *Small slit-like erosions, ruptured vesicles, and extensive ulceration were seen on the tongue, lips, snout, coronary band, and interdigital spaces.* Severe lesions sometimes led to separation and sloughing of the hoof wall. Intact vesicles were seen rarely. Sporadic cases have been reported in which the lesions were exudative rather than ulcerative. They were grossly indistinguishable from those of exudative epidermitis. PPV has been cultured from skin and internal organs of affected piglets, and PPV antigen has been detected in hair follicles of lesional skin. Skin lesions were reproduced with tissue culture–origin PPV, but were not as severe as those induced with crude suspensions prepared from the skin lesions. In the sporadic cases, *Staphylococcus* spp. and swinepox virus were also recovered. It is likely that the severe clinical disease results from dual bacterial and viral infection.

Caliciviral infection

Species *Feline calicivirus* belongs to the genus *Vesivirus*. Many different strains exist. The most common clinical signs associated with infection are oral vesicles, ulcers, depression, pyrexia, sneezing, and conjunctivitis with ocular and nasal discharge. An unusual pustular dermatitis of the shaved ventral abdomen was described in 2 cats following routine ovariectomy. The histopathology showed panepidermal pustulosis and necrotizing dermatitis. Virulent systemic calicivirus has been associated with facial and paw edema and with ulcers and crusting of the skin of the nose, lips, pinnae, periocular region, and distal limbs. Cutaneous vasculitis is seen in some of these cats.

Further reading

Declercq J. Pustular calicivirus dermatitis on the abdomen of two cats following routine ovariectomy. Vet Dermatol 2005;16:395-400.

Pesavento PA, et al. Pathologic, immunohistochemical, and electron microscopic findings in naturally occurring virulent systemic feline calicivirus infection in cats. Vet Pathol 2004;41:257-263.

Papillomaviral infections

Papillomaviruses are associated with a variety of proliferative skin lesions, typically benign epithelial neoplasms, although they have also been shown to be associated with proliferative cutaneous plaques and papules. Although these lesions are almost always benign and often self-limiting, there is evidence that, in some cases, both in humans and animals, the virus can be a factor in the development of malignant tumors. Papillomaviruses tend to be species-specific viruses that affect stratified squamous epithelium in all domestic and numerous wildlife species. Papillomavirus-associated lesions are discussed under Tumors of the epidermis.

Miscellaneous viral infections of the skin

Foot-and-mouth disease, vesicular stomatitis, vesicular exanthema of swine, swine vesicular disease, bovine viral diarrhea, and bluetongue are discussed in Vol. 2, Alimentary system and peritoneum.

Feline infectious peritonitis (FIP), caused by a mutated feline coronavirus, is a systemic viral disease with rare cutaneous manifestations. Multiple papular to nodular, nonpruritic lesions over the head, neck, trunk, and limbs have been described. Histologically, these lesions have been characterized by pyogranulomatous perivascular to nodular dermatitis, pyogranulomatous vasculitis, and folliculitis. Immunohistochemistry for the detection of intracellular feline coronavirus (FCoV) antigen in macrophages is required to confirm the diagnosis. Ulcerative lesions around the head and neck associated with superficial dermal vasculitis have been described in experimentally infected cats.

Further reading

Bauer BS, et al. Positive immunostaining for feline infectious peritonitis (FIP) in a Sphinx cat with cutaneous lesions and bilateral panuveitis. Vet Ophthalmol 2013;16(Suppl. 1):160-163.

Declercq J, et al. Papular cutaneous lesions in a cat associated with feline infectious peritonitis. Vet Dermatol 2008;19:255-258.

Miller WH, et al. Viral rickettsial and protozoal skin diseases. In: Miller WH, et al., editors. Muller & Kirk's Small Animal Dermatology. 7th ed. St Louis: Elsevier; 2013. p. 343-362.

BACTERIAL DISEASES OF SKIN

Normal skin of healthy individuals is highly resistant to invasion by bacteria because of natural defense mechanisms, consisting of physical, chemical, immunologic, and microbial components. The stratum corneum is composed of tightly packed keratinized cells and intercellular substance derived from lamellar granules that form an impermeable physical barrier. Furthermore, this layer continually desquamates, and any adherent bacteria are lost as the outer cells are shed. The sebum-sweat emulsion, which spreads along the skin surface, contains a variety of antibacterial substances, including fatty acids, inorganic salts, and proteins such as complement components, transferrin, and immunoglobulins. Finally, the normal skin microflora prevents pathogenic bacteria from multiplying and becoming established on the skin. These normal resident bacteria are a mixture of organisms that live in symbiosis and maintain static, consistent populations restricted to the superficial layers of the stratum corneum and hair follicle infundibula. They inhibit colonization of invading organisms by competition for limited nutrients and production of antibacterial substances. The protective effect of bacterial interference is well documented. For example, the development of exudative epidermitis has been prevented by exposing piglets to avirulent strains of *Staphylococcus hyicus*.

The normal skin flora is established shortly after birth, and it is difficult subsequently to introduce other bacteria. The normal resident flora of skin has been investigated most extensively in dogs. Coagulase-negative staphylococci, *Micrococcus* spp., some aerobic gram-negative species, and *Clostridium* spp. are most numerous and are probably residents of canine skin. Although *Staphylococcus pseudintermedius* is the most frequent bacterial pathogen isolated from canine clinical specimens, it is also a part of the normal cutaneous microflora and colonizes the skin, hair follicles/coat, and in particular, mucocutaneous sites, such as the nose, mouth, and anus. It is thought to be part of the resident biota of these regions, and these sites can be spread to other regions of the body. *S. pseudintermedius* constitutes about 90% of staphylococci isolated from canine healthy carriers and from dogs with underlying skin disease. In all species, skin surface humidity and temperature are important factors in determining the composition and density of skin microflora, with hot humid conditions being associated with increased numbers of skin bacteria. Regional variation in numbers and types of bacteria occurs, and moist intertriginous areas and oily skin have the highest numbers of bacteria.

Cutaneous bacterial infections are typically pyogenic and are thus commonly called **pyodermas**. They can be categorized as *primary and secondary* or *superficial and deep*. Primary pyodermas are those for which no underlying cause can be found. However, *it is now thought that the vast majority of pyodermas are secondary to underlying cutaneous, endocrine, or immunologic abnormalities*. Localized disruption of normal host defenses may be produced by maceration, biting ectoparasites, scratching, abrasions and other skin wounds, or introduction of foreign bodies, such as plant thorns or awns; such disruption promotes development of clinical infection. Allergic, seborrheic, and follicular disorders are the most common predisposing causes of bacterial skin infection in dogs. Hypothyroidism and spontaneous and iatrogenic hyperadrenocorticism are common metabolic conditions associated with pyoderma. Primary immunologic abnormalities are uncommon to rare predisposing factors.

Bacterial skin disease is seen much more frequently in dogs than in any other mammalian species, and pyoderma is one of the most common skin diseases in dogs. This apparent increased susceptibility of dogs to pyoderma has been attributed to the relatively thin compact stratum corneum, the small amount of intercellular lipids in the stratum corneum, lack of a protective lipid seal at the entrance of canine hair follicles, and the relatively high pH of canine skin. *S. pseudintermedius* is the predominant bacterial isolate from canine pyodermas. It is also frequently isolated from canine ear and wound infections and can be a complicating factor in immunomodulatory-responsive lymphocytic-plasmacytic pododermatitis. The pathogenesis of *S. pseudintermedius* infection is poorly understood. It is an opportunistic pathogen and does not cause disease unless the resistance of the host is lowered or the skin barrier is altered by atopic dermatitis, medical and surgical procedures, and/or immunosuppressive disorders. Similar to *Staphylococcus aureus*, *S. pseudintermedius* produces a variety of virulence factors, including enzymes such as coagulase, thermonuclease, and proteases; surface proteins such as clumping factor and protein A; and toxins such as cytotoxins, exfoliative toxin, and enterotoxin. It has also been shown to form biofilms. A major rapidly emerging problem with this organism has been multidrug resistance generally characterized by methicillin resistance and the presence of the *mecA* gene. The *mecA* gene encodes an altered, surplus cell wall penicillin-binding protein 2a (PBP2a), which has a low affinity to virtually the entire class of β lactam antibiotics.

Coagulase-positive staphylococci are also the most common bacteria isolated from pyoderma in horses (*S. aureus*, *S. delphini*) and in cattle, goats, and sheep (*S. aureus*). *S. hyicus* causes exudative epidermitis in piglets and has been associated with superficial pyoderma in several other species. Many other bacteria cause skin infections. *Dermatophilus congolensis* is responsible for superficial pyoderma in many species. Many gram-negative bacteria are opportunistic pathogens that can invade already diseased or compromised skin. Organisms that are typically associated with infections of other organ systems occasionally cause skin disease. *Listeria monocytogenes* has been found to be the cause of pyoderma in a small number of humans and a dog with multiple nodules over the back. Although bacterial infections are typically associated with neutrophilic inflammation, certain bacteria, such as mycobacteria, *Actinomyces*, and *Nocardia*, typically produce *pyogranulomatous dermatitis or panniculitis*.

Further reading

Bannoehr J, Guardabassi L. *Staphylococcus pseudintermedius* in the dog: taxonomy, diagnostics, ecology, epidemiology and pathogenicity. Vet Dermatol 2012;23:253-266.

Foster AP. Staphylococcal skin disease in livestock. Vet Dermatol 2012;23:342-351.

Lloyd D. Bacterial skin disease. In: Miller WH, et al., editors. Muller & Kirk's Small Animal Dermatology. 7th ed. St Louis: Elsevier; 2013. p. 184-222.

Superficial bacterial pyoderma

Superficial pyodermas involve the epidermis and/or superficial portion of hair follicles. They occur more commonly than deep pyodermas. Superficial pyodermas usually are of short duration, heal without scarring, and are not usually associated

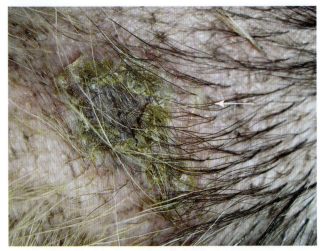

Figure 6-87 Pustule (arrow) and annular erythematous lesion with central hyperpigmentation and **epidermal collarette**. (Courtesy M.S. Canfield).

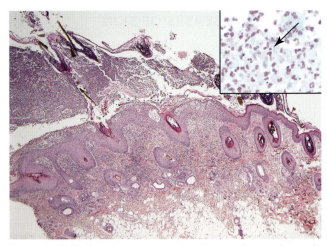

Figure 6-88 **Bullous impetigo** in a dog. Large subcorneal pustule spans multiple follicles and contains degenerate neutrophils and gram-positive bacterial cocci (arrow, see inset).

with systemic illness. *Gross lesions are extremely variable* and include papules, pustules, crusts, circular scaling areas of alopecia with epidermal collarettes (Fig. 6-87), hyperpigmented or erythematous macules, a moth-eaten appearance to the haircoat, diffuse erythroderma, and hyperpigmented lichenified plaques. *Microscopic lesions* consist of subcorneal or loosely organized, spongiotic superficial epidermal pustules, superficial folliculitis, and crusts. Neutrophils are the predominant inflammatory cell. Bacteria are not always visible histologically, and culture may be necessary to confirm the etiology.

Impetigo

Impetigo is a superficial pustular dermatitis that does not involve hair follicles. It is most common in dogs but also occurs in kittens, piglets, cows, sheep, and goats. Impetigo is usually caused by *coagulase-positive staphylococci. In puppies, it tends to occur before or at the time of puberty for no apparent reason.* In other animals, it is usually seen in association with predisposing causes, such as moist and dirty environments, cutaneous abrasions, parasitism, stress, and poor nutrition. Lesions develop in young kittens as a result of excessive wetting of the skin by the queen as she transports the kittens. Bullous impetigo is more often seen in adult dogs and is usually associated with diabetes mellitus, hypothyroidism, and natural or iatrogenic hyperglucocorticism. In these cases, other bacteria such as *Escherichia coli* and *Pseudomonas* spp. may be present.

The lesions begin as small erythematous papules that develop into superficial pustules. They are fragile and rupture easily, leaving a honey-colored crust adherent to a shallow erosion. A *bullous form of impetigo* consists of large flaccid pustules. In *puppies*, the lesions are most common on the glabrous skin of the inguinal and axillary areas. In *kittens*, the lesions are usually confined to sites that are most commonly in contact with the queen's mouth; these include the back of the neck, head, and shoulder areas. Lesions in *cows and does* are usually on the udder, especially at the base of the teats and the intermammary sulcus. Occasionally, the infection extends to involve the teats, ventral abdomen, medial thighs, perineum, and ventral surface of the tail. In general, these lesions are nonpruritic, nonpainful, and heal spontaneously. Spread of infection by the milker to other cows or does and to the hands of milkers has been suggested. One outbreak of contagious impetigo in a herd of dairy cattle was associated with crowding and intensive showering of the cows to decrease heat stress during the heat of summer.

The microscopic lesion of impetigo is a subcorneal pustule composed primarily of neutrophils. The pustules usually extend above the skin surface and are located between hair follicles. Bullous impetigo consists of larger pustules that span several hair follicles (Fig. 6-88). Acantholysis may be mild. Gram-positive cocci are present within intact pustules (see Fig. 6-88 inset). The epidermis is mildly to moderately acanthotic, and variable intercellular edema is common beneath pustules. The superficial dermis is edematous, and superficial perivascular to interstitial inflammation is composed predominantly of neutrophils. *The principal differential diagnosis is pemphigus foliaceus.* However, in contrast to pemphigus, acantholysis is absent or minimal in impetigo, and bacteria are present in intact pustules of impetigo.

Mucocutaneous pyoderma primarily affects the lips and perioral skin of dogs and rarely horses. German Shepherd dogs and their crosses are at increased risk. Lesions are symmetrical and include erythema, swelling, crusting, erosions, and depigmentation of the lips. *Histologically*, this condition has features similar to discoid lupus erythematosus. There is epidermal hyperplasia with a *lichenoid infiltrate of lymphocytes and plasma cells and pigmentary incontinence*. In addition, there are moderate to large numbers of *neutrophils in the epidermis and superficial dermis*, and the basement membrane is not obscured. Hydropic degeneration and apoptosis of the stratum basale are usually not present. The etiology is unknown; however, the condition responds to antibiotic therapy.

Exudative epidermitis of pigs

Exudative epidermitis is an acute, exudative, superficial pyoderma of young pigs most commonly caused by *Staphylococcus hyicus* subsp. *hyicus*. There may be other staphylococcal bacteria involved, such as *S. chromogenes* and *S. sciuri*. The disease has also been called **greasy-pig disease,** impetigo contagiosa suis, and seborrhea oleosa. The infection is common and occurs worldwide. It is most common in *piglets 5-35 days of age,* but mild cases occur in older pigs also. The morbidity ranges from 10-90% and mortality from 5-90%. Mortality is higher in young pigs with lower resistance. Usually, when a litter is affected, all piglets develop the disease. *The infection may cause significant economic loss.* Autogenous vaccines prepared from toxigenic strains of bacteria have been used to prevent infection in some situations.

The *pathogenesis* of exudative epidermitis is incompletely understood. Both virulent and nonvirulent strains of *S. hyicus* are part of the normal skin flora of healthy pigs; it is carried on the conjunctiva, snout, ear skin, and vagina. The highest rates of carriage of the organism are found in the youngest piglets, suggesting that the organisms are acquired at birth. It is thought that infection develops as a result of *trauma* that breaches the skin barrier. Other factors that may predispose piglets to developing clinical disease include *agalactia of the sow, concurrent infections, and nutritional deficiencies.* The presence of porcine circovirus 2 and porcine parvovirus have been suggested as predisposing factors. The most important factor in the pathogenesis of this skin disease is considered to be the presence of bacterial strains that express *exfoliative toxins* known as *ExhA, ExhB, ExhC, ExhD, SHETA, and SHETB*. The *Exh toxins have been shown to digest desmoglein-1 in the epidermis of porcine skin*. This disease process is considered to involve the same mechanisms as staphylococcal scalded skin syndrome and bullous impetigo in humans.

The disease can be divided into acute, subacute, and chronic forms:
- In the **acute form,** most common in piglets only a few days old, there is abrupt onset of lesions around the eyes, snout, chin, and on the ears, with extension to the medial aspect of the legs. Lesions then rapidly spread to the thorax, abdomen, entire legs, and coronets. Lesions begin as peeling of small areas of the stratum corneum, leaving red, glistening, moist areas. These areas are quickly covered by *greasy, dark brown exudate*. Lesions become generalized in 24-48 hours, and the entire body is erythematous and covered with brown, greasy, malodorous exudate. Erosions of the coronary bands and heels commonly develop. Conjunctivitis also occurs frequently and typically causes matting together of the eyelids and results in an inability to see. Death occurs within 3-5 days as a result of dehydration, electrolyte imbalance, negative energy balance, and septicemia.
- In the **subacute form,** the course is more protracted. The skin becomes thick and wrinkled, and the exudate covering the entire body becomes dry, hard, and cracked, producing a generalized furrowed appearance. The underlying skin visible in the furrows is red (Fig 6-89).
- The **chronic form** occurs in older piglets, and skin lesions are milder and usually confined to the head and ears and consist of erythema and waxy brown crusts. Older piglets with less severe forms of disease frequently survive; however, recovery is slow, and the piglets are severely stunted. Lesions that may also occur in affected piglets are subcutaneous abscesses, necrosis of the ears and tail, and polyarthritis.

The earliest *microscopic lesion is subcorneal vesicular to pustular dermatitis*. Extension of infection to hair follicles results in a superficial purulent luminal folliculitis. In fully developed lesions, the skin is covered with a thick crust composed of orthokeratotic and parakeratotic keratin, lakes of serum, accumulations of neutrophils, necrotic debris, and microcolonies of gram-positive cocci. The epidermis is variably acanthotic and rete ridges are elongated. Cells in the outer stratum spinosum exhibit variable intracellular edema. Neutrophilic exocytosis, intercellular edema, and spongiotic pustules may be seen in the epidermis and infundibular portion of hair follicles. The dermis is edematous, dermal vessels are congested, and there is a perivascular to interstitial neutrophilic infiltrate. Dermal inflammation is more intense and diffuse in areas of ulceration. In chronic cases, exudation is less severe, and there is more marked epidermal hyperplasia and hyperkeratosis. Inflammation in the dermis becomes primarily mononuclear.

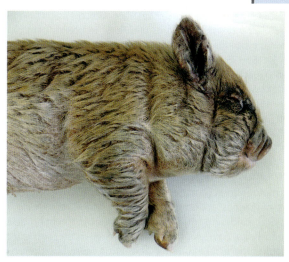

Figure 6-89 Exudative epidermitis in a piglet. Parallel rows of matted hair ("furrows") separated by erythematous waxy skin.

Microscopic lesions may also be seen in *other tissues*. Lymph nodes draining severely affected areas of skin contain foci of hemorrhage, purulent inflammation, and occasional microcolonies of bacterial cocci. Renal lesions are common, and bacteremia is not required for them to be present. The lesions are distinctive, with early vacuolation of the epithelium of collecting ducts and renal pelvis progressing to epithelial degeneration and exfoliation. Intratubular casts of desquamated epithelium may be sufficiently severe to be evident macroscopically, leading to linear striations of the renal pelvis, and accumulation of cellular sediment in the pelvis and ureters. The process may be sufficiently severe to occlude the ureters. In cases in which bacteremia is present, purulent pyelonephritis is common. Animals with greasy pig disease may also have lesions in the oral cavity and conjunctiva, and the causative organism has been associated with abortion in sows.

S. hyicus has been associated with skin lesions in *other species*. The organism is common in cattle and has been associated with concurrent psoroptic mange. The organism was isolated from skin lesions of a young pygmy goat with chronic generalized seborrheic dermatitis and alopecia. The microscopic lesion was a purulent exudative epidermitis similar to that in pigs. *S. hyicus* has been cultured from a number of horses with exudative crusty alopecic skin lesions on the distal limbs that resembled "grease heel" clinically.

Further reading

Foster AP. Staphylococcal skin disease in livestock. Vet Dermatol 2012;23:342-351.

Fudaba Y, et al. *Staphylococcus hyicus* exfoliative toxins selectively digest porcine desmoglein 1. Micro Pathogen 2005;39:171-176.

Iyori K, et al. Identification of a novel *Staphylococcus pseudintermedius* exfoliative toxin gene and its prevalence in isolates from canines with pyoderma and healthy dogs. FEMS Microbiol Lett 2010; 312:169-175.

Lloyd D. Bacterial skin disease. In: Miller WH, et al., editors. Muller & Kirk's Small Animal Dermatology. 7th ed. St Louis: Elsevier; 2013. p. 184-222.

Scott DW. Color Atlas of Farm Animal Dermatology. Ames, Iowa: Blackwell; 2007.

Dermatophilosis

Dermatophilosis (cutaneous streptothricosis, mycotic dermatitis, cutaneous actinomycosis, lumpy wool, strawberry foot rot, rain scald, rain rot, Kirchi, Gasin-Gishu, Senkobo disease, Drodo-Boka, Savi, Ambarr-Madow) is an acute, subacute, or chronic superficial exudative dermatitis caused by the actinomycete **Dermatophilus congolensis.** The disease occurs worldwide and has a wide host range, but it is *most common in the hot humid tropics and subtropics and in areas with heavy prolonged rains*. In hot monsoon climates, cattle are the primary animals affected, and the disease is endemic in some portions of Africa. In more temperate climates, sheep and goats are involved primarily. The disease is occasional in horses and camels; it is rare in dogs, cats, pigs, and humans. Anecdotal reports exist for alpacas. Cases of dermatophilosis have also been reported in a wide variety of wild and captive mammals and reptiles. There is no apparent sex or age predilection, and congenital infections have been reported in calves and lambs.

In cattle and sheep, dermatophilosis causes important economic losses by virtue of decreased meat and milk production, damaged hides, wool loss, infertility, and early culling. Severe udder and teat lesions may interfere with suckling by calves and result in decreased growth rate. Affected animals are predisposed to secondary infections and cutaneous myiasis. Severely affected animals of any species may become emaciated and die.

Dermatophilus congolensis is a gram-positive facultative anaerobic bacterium whose natural habitat is unknown. Attempts to culture it from soil have been unsuccessful. Studies have shown that the organism's survival in soil is dependent on the type of soil and the water content but not the pH. Clinically normal carrier animals and crusts from infected animals probably serve as sources of infection. Zoospores can remain viable in crusts at a temperature of 28-31° C for up to 42 months. *D. congolensis* has a distinctive life cycle in which coccoid bodies germinate to produce branching filaments. These filaments undergo transverse and longitudinal septation to form parallel rows of coccoid bodies. The cocci are resistant to unfavorable conditions and are reproductively dormant until the appropriate wet conditions occur and they are activated to become motile zoospores.

Dermatophilosis cannot be reproduced experimentally to resemble natural disease, even with large doses of the organism. Multiple factors appear to be involved in pathogenesis of the natural disease. Two factors that appear to be most important are *trauma to the skin and prolonged wetting*. Zoospores are unable to overcome the protective barriers of the hair, surface lipid film, and stratum corneum, and their entry is facilitated by breaks in the skin surface. Trauma from ectoparasites, shearing, dipping, barbed wire injuries, sharp stones, and scratches from sharp vegetation can act as portals of entry for the zoospores. Besides producing skin trauma, external parasites such as flies, mites, lice, ticks, and mosquitoes also act as mechanical vectors. In addition to skin trauma, prolonged moisture is needed for the activation, proliferation, and spread of the zoospores. Wetting may also act to breach skin barriers by dissolving the surface lipid film and softening the stratum corneum. Outbreaks of dermatophilosis are frequently associated with periods of unusually heavy rainfall, housing in pastures or paddocks with standing water or mud, or after intensive high-pressure washing of animals.

Other factors involved in development of disease are less well understood. Genetic factors may be involved, because some breeds of cattle appear to be more resistant to disease than are others. Skin color appears to have an effect because some light-skinned breeds or light-skinned areas may be more susceptible to infection. A definite association between infestation with the tick *Amblyomma variegatum* and occurrence of dermatophilosis in cattle has been found. In herds with effective tick prevention, there is a much lower incidence or diminished severity of the disease. Because the lesions of dermatophilosis do not correspond to sites of tick attachment, a systemic effect on the animal's immune system has been suspected. In addition, concurrent diseases or stresses, including intestinal parasitism, nutritional deficiencies, stress of pregnancy or migration, and viral infections may contribute to the development of dermatophilosis by compromising the host's immune system.

Once the normal skin surface has been disrupted and activated zoospores gain access to the epidermis, infection can develop. The zoospores are apparently attracted to the low carbon dioxide concentration of the normal epidermis, and there they germinate to form filaments that invade the viable epidermis and outer root sheaths of hair follicles. Only rarely do the bacteria proliferate in the dermis or deeper tissues. The means by which *D. congolensis* invades the epidermis is unknown, but it is thought that the bacteria produces exoenzymes. As the filaments invade the epidermis, keratinocytes at sites of penetration begin to cornify, and numerous neutrophils accumulate beneath and migrate into the epidermis, which subsequently separates from the underlying dermis. The neutrophils inhibit further invasion by the organism, and the epidermis re-forms from cells in adjacent external hair follicle sheaths. This new epidermis is again invaded by organisms arising from the hair follicles to initiate another cycle of epidermal penetration, neutrophilic exocytosis, and epidermal detachment. These repeated sequences of bacterial invasion, inflammation, and epidermal regeneration produce the *thick laminar and parakeratotic crusts characteristic of dermatophilosis*.

The earliest lesions of dermatophilosis consist of patches of slight erythema that are visible only in unpigmented areas. Very small papules and pustules develop next and are more evident by palpation than by visual inspection. As the lesions become covered by exudate and hairs become entrapped within the developing crust, they form small tufts that resemble paintbrushes (Fig. 6-90A). As these small lesions coalesce, they form the typical large oval to circular domed yellow-brown adherent scabs that when removed leave a moist hyperemic base that may bleed. The lesions are painful and nonpruritic. In chronic cases, lesions progress to form thick layers of dry spongy material involving extensive areas of long hair or hard wart-like crusts that protrude above the hair surface, usually in areas with a short haircoat.

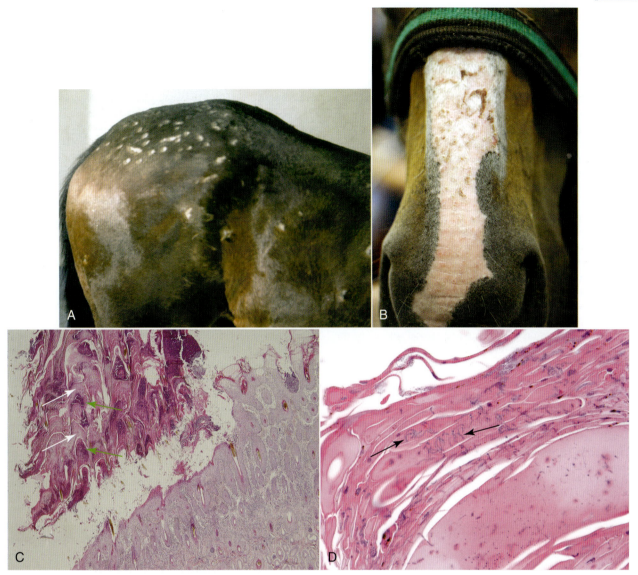

Figure 6-90 **Dermatophilosis**. **A.** Tufted papules and annular areas of alopecia over the rump and sides of a horse. (Courtesy D.W. Scott.) **B.** Crusted papules and erythema on the muzzle of a horse. **C.** Skin biopsy from a calf shows large surface crust composed of thick alternating layers of hyperkeratosis (white arrows) and degenerate neutrophils (green arrows) parallel to the skin surface. **D.** Coccoid organisms forming branching filaments ("railroad tracks") (arrows) within the surface keratin.

The distribution of lesions in **cattle** is variable. Lesions confined to the face and ears are most often seen in young suckling calves. In other forms of the disease, lesions occur on the brisket, axillae, and inguinal areas, or on the udder and teats of cows, and scrotum and prepuce of bulls. Cattle standing in deep water or mud develop lesions on the legs. Lesions located in the perineum and tail are assumed to result from trauma caused by mounting by other animals. In many cases, lesions are diffusely distributed over the head, topline of the neck and body to the tail, and dorsal sides. Animals with >50% of body involvement often show weight loss, dehydration, and death. Rare instances of subcutaneous abscesses, lymphadenitis, and oral lesions have been reported.

In **sheep,** infection of the wooled areas is frequently missed in early stages, and some animals recover spontaneously during the acute stage of infection. If the disease continues to progress, the wool of the neck, back, and flank becomes matted with exudate to form dense pyramidal masses (lumpy wool, mycotic dermatitis) that may last for months to years in some individuals. "Strawberry foot rot" is an infection that begins at the coronet regions and may progress to involve the skin to the carpi and/or tarsi. In some cases, crusts may be confined to the ears, nose, and face, a clinical form common in lambs. Concurrent infection with contagious ecthyma and pox has been reported.

Dermatophilosis in **goats** frequently consists of 2-3 mm crusty lesions on the pinnae and tail of kids and large pyramidal crusts on the dorsal midline, sides, caudal thighs, and scrotum of adults. Lesions involving the distal limbs resemble strawberry footrot of sheep. Concurrent infection with contagious ecthyma and pox may occur, and secondary infections with staphylococci, streptococci, or corynebacteria may develop. In addition, as with cattle, tick infestations (*Amblyomma variegatum* and *Boophilus decoloratus*) are a risk factor for clinical dermatophilosis.

In **horses,** lesions of dermatophilosis are frequently located on the dorsal aspect of the body and look as if large drops of liquid have scalded the skin ("rain scald"). Horses kept in wet, marshy, or muddy enclosures, and undergoing trauma to the legs, develop lesions of the distal extremities primarily (grease heel, scratches, mud fever). Lesions on the legs may be associated with swelling, pain, and lameness. In some instances, only the head is affected. Unpigmented skin may be more susceptible to infection, and lesions on these areas are typically very erythematous (Fig. 6-90B). These lesions may represent a type of photodermatitis caused by *D. congolensis* ("dew poisoning"). Outbreaks in show horses have been associated with frequent high-pressure washing.

Dermatophilosis cases reported in **cats** are notable in that they have all been subcutaneous or extracutaneous infections. The lesions consisted of draining nodules involving, or in the area of, the popliteal lymph nodes or the subcutaneous tissue of a paw and masses on the tongue and serosal surface of the urinary bladder. In at least one of the cats with subcutaneous infection, superficial wounds suggestive of a recent cat fight were seen, prompting speculation that the infection was traumatically introduced.

Dermatophilosis lesions in **camels** are present, especially on the rump, neck, flanks, and lower abdomen. The legs are generally spared. In one study, infected camels were often infested with *Hyalomma* spp. ticks, suggesting that ticks may have an important role in the pathogenesis of dermatophilosis in camels.

The earliest *histologic lesions* of dermatophilosis are superficial dermal congestion, edema, and neutrophil infiltration of the superficial dermis. Exocytosis of neutrophils becomes more pronounced as lesions progress, and intraepidermal or subcorneal pustules may develop. Eventually, repeated cycles of bacterial invasion and inflammation result in thick crusts composed of *alternating layers of parakeratotic and orthokeratotic keratin, serous fluid, degenerate inflammatory cells, and bacterial filaments composed of multiple parallel rows of cocci* "palisading crust" (Fig. 6-90C, D). The epidermis is acanthotic, with orthokeratotic and parakeratotic hyperkeratosis. Purulent luminal folliculitis with intralesional bacterial filaments is also usually present. Dermal inflammation is usually mild and superficial perivascular. In cases of dermatophilosis in cats and rare instances of subcutaneous and lymph node infection in cattle, the lesions consist of granulomas or pyogranulomas with scattered necrotic foci that contain typical *D. congolensis* filaments. In one 3-year-old pony, the infection was seen as only granulomatous lymphadenitis.

Ovine fleece rot

So-called "fleece rot" in sheep is caused by excessive moisture (6 days of continual wet wool and skin) and subsequent proliferation of *Pseudomonas* spp. The bacterial proliferation causes acute inflammation with serum exudation and matting of the wool. The *wool becomes discolored by chromogenes* produced by the bacteria and has a rotten odor. *Histologically,* there are epidermal pustules and superficial suppurative luminal folliculitis. Affected sheep are predisposed to myiasis.

Further reading

Byrne BA, et al. Atypical *Dermatophilus congolensis* infection in a three-year-old pony. J Vet Diagn Invest 2012;22:141-143.

Chatikobo P, et al. Bovine dermatophilosis, a re-emerging pandemic disease in Zimbabwe. Trop Anim Health Prod 2009;41:1289-1297.

Hargis AM, Ginn PE. The integument. In: Zachary JF, McGavin MD, editors. Pathologic Basis of Veterinary Disease. 5th ed. St Louis: Elsevier Mosby; 2012. p. 972-1084.

Norris BJ, et al. Fleece rot and dermatophilosis in sheep. Vet Micro 2008;128:217-230.

Scott DW. Color Atlas of Farm Animal Dermatology. Ames, Iowa: Blackwell; 2007.

Scott DW, Miller WH. Bacterial skin disease. In: Scott DW, Miller WH, editors. Equine Dermatology. 2nd ed. St Louis: Elsevier Saunders; 2011. p. 130-170.

Deep bacterial pyoderma

Deep pyodermas are serious bacterial infections that involve the hair follicle, dermis, and/or subcutis. They are often chronic or recurrent, heal with scarring, and are commonly associated with regional or generalized lymphadenopathy and systemic signs. The clinical appearance of deep pyoderma is tremendously diverse. Lesions commonly seen in deep pyodermas include dark red or violaceous raised nodules, poorly demarcated areas of tissue swelling, hemorrhagic bullae, draining tracts, abscesses, purulent or serosanguineous exudate that dries to form crusts, and necrotic or ulcerated skin covered by crusts. Pain may be severe. Microscopic changes associated with deep pyodermas include folliculitis, furunculosis, nodular-to-diffuse dermatitis or panniculitis, and variable fibrosis. Bacteria may not be seen microscopically even with special stains.

Staphylococcal folliculitis and furunculosis

Staphylococcus spp. are the most common cause of folliculitis in domestic animals. Other organisms less frequently or rarely associated with folliculitis include *Streptococcus* spp., *Corynebacterium* spp., *Pseudomonas* spp., *Bacillus* spp., and *Pasteurella multocida*. Inflammation of the deep portion of hair follicles frequently results in rupture of the follicular wall (furunculosis) and extension of infection to the surrounding dermis and panniculus. *Staphylococcal folliculitis and furunculosis are very common in the dog; common in horses, goats, and sheep; and uncommon in cats, cattle, and pigs.* Skin lesions associated with folliculitis and furunculosis are extremely variable. The earliest skin lesion is a follicular papule with one or several hairs protruding from the center. The papule develops into a pustule, but these are very fragile, break easily, and are thus very transient. Consequently, crusted papules are seen more commonly than are pustules. In shorthaired dogs, horses, and cattle, the earliest clinical sign is a dishevelment of the haircoat produced by small groups of hairs tufting together above the skin surface, an appearance that can be confused with urticaria. As the hairs fall out of infected follicles, multiple small foci of alopecia and scaling develop. The haircoat develops a moth-eaten appearance as the areas of alopecia become progressively larger. Lesions often enlarge and develop a central ulcer that discharges purulent or serosanguineous exudate that dries to form a crust. When furunculosis occurs, dark red to violaceous nodules, draining fistulae, ulcers, and extensive tissue swelling develop (Fig. 6-91A). Hemorrhagic bullae may be prominent in some cases (Fig. 6-91B). Scarring,

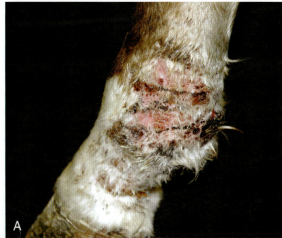

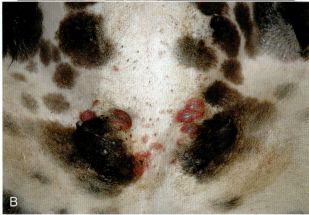

Figure 6-91 Deep bacterial folliculitis and furunculosis. **A.** Draining tracts in the distal limb of a horse. **B.** Hemorrhagic bullae on the ventrum of a dog. (Courtesy W.H. Miller.)

alterations in pigmentation of the hair and skin, and lichenification may result. Regional and generalized lymphadenopathy are common. Constitutional signs, such as fever and anorexia, may occur when infection is severe or extensive.

The *microscopic changes* of staphylococcal folliculitis and furunculosis are as varied as the gross lesions. The epidermis is variably acanthotic and may be ulcerated. Serocellular crusting is common. Staphylococcal folliculitis is characterized by *neutrophilic inflammation*, but the relative number of neutrophils is extremely variable, depending on the duration of the infection and presence of furunculosis. Pustules composed of neutrophils may be seen within the infundibulum or ostium of hair follicles. Small numbers of eosinophils may be seen and in some cases may indicate a concurrent allergy or ectoparasite. Neutrophils accumulate within the lumen of hair follicles, distending the lumen and frequently causing rupture of the hair follicle wall (see Fig. 6-5B). Neutrophils, eosinophils, macrophages, and plasma cells form dense sheets in the dermis and may extend to the panniculus. Hemorrhagic bullae consist of large pustules with hemorrhage in the interfollicular dermis. Large dermal pustules may form cavitary lesions. Release of hair and keratin into the dermis or panniculus induces an *intense foreign-body reaction* that may completely efface the follicle (see Fig. 6-6). Fragments of hair or keratin may be surrounded by discrete granulomas *(trichogranuloma)* composed of multinucleated giant cells, epithelioid macrophages, and neutrophils. Eosinophils may be numerous around the fragments of hair and keratin. Inflammation may become diffuse as adjacent furuncles coalesce and completely replace normal dermal structures. Hemorrhage and fibroplasia are variable. Bacteria may not be evident even with special stains, such as tissue Gram stain or Giemsa stain.

Deep pyoderma is not as common as superficial pyoderma but is still a relatively common disease in **dogs**. *Staphylococcus pseudintermedius* is usually the primary pathogen in bacterial folliculitis and furunculosis in dogs. However, gram-negative bacteria, such as *Proteus, Pseudomonas,* and *Escherichia coli* are common secondary invaders. Rarely, acute deep pyoderma presenting with dorsal truncal pain has been associated with a pure culture of *Pseudomonas aeruginosa* in dogs. In some cases, this condition may be associated with self-service dog-grooming facilities or aggressive grooming, such as back-clipping and back-combing. Deep pyoderma may be localized or widespread. *Localized forms* of staphylococcal deep pyoderma commonly involve the bridge of the nose, the chin ("canine acne"), paws (interdigital "pedal" folliculitis-furunculosis), and pressure points. A particularly refractory form of staphylococcal pyoderma has been recognized in German Shepherd dogs. **German Shepherd pyoderma** is a genetically inherited characteristic clinical syndrome that can be triggered by a variety of other diseases in susceptible individuals. This condition affects middle-aged German Shepherd dogs and their crosses. Rump, back, ventral abdomen, and thighs are the typical distribution. In some cases, lesions are more generalized. These dogs have a disproportionately severe form of pyoderma. Typical lesions include papules, pustules, erosions, and crusts, followed by ulcers, draining tracts, furunculosis, alopecia, and hyperpigmentation. Lesions are pruritic and may be painful. An immunologic abnormality is suspected because most affected dogs have a relative increase in the CD8+ T lymphocytes and relative decrease in the CD4+ and CD21+ lymphocytes in peripheral blood. Whether these changes are a cause or effect of the disease is unknown, and in addition, some believe that in general normal German Shepherd dogs have lower lymphocyte subpopulations with a relative increase of CD8+ T lymphocytes. Examination of T and B lymphocytes in histologic sections found a marked paucity of T lymphocytes in lesions of deep pyoderma of German Shepherd dogs as compared to similar lesions from dogs of other breeds. Although not always apparent, there is generally thought to be another factor that triggers the condition (e.g., flea-bite hypersensitivity, atopic dermatitis, adverse food reactions, ehrlichiosis, or hypothyroidism).

Staphylococcal folliculitis and furunculosis in **horses** are usually secondary to trauma and various physiologic stresses. Lesions most often involve the harness, saddle (saddle scab, saddle boils), neck, and dorsal lumbosacral regions. *Friction from tack* is considered an important initiating factor. It is most common in the summer, coincident with excessive sweating, higher environmental temperature and humidity, and increased numbers of biting insects. Lesions are usually painful rather than pruritic. *Staphylococcal pyoderma may be one of many causes of pastern dermatitis (grease heel, scratches)* in which lesions involve the caudal aspect of the pastern and fetlock areas of one or more legs. In *tail pyoderma,* the dorsal surface of the tail is particularly affected, and infection is usually secondary to skin abrasions caused by tail rubbing associated with insect bites, mange, biting lice, pinworms, yeast dermatitis, herpes coital exanthema, or vice. Although much less common, *Corynebacterium pseudotuberculosis* can cause folliculitis and clinical lesions ("contagious acne") similar to those with staphylococcal folliculitis.

Staphylococcal folliculitis and furunculosis are common in **goats and sheep,** frequently are secondary to trauma or moisture, and *Staphylococcus aureus* is most commonly isolated. Lesions include papules, pustules, crusting, and alopecia. Common locations in goats are periocular areas, pinnae, distal limbs, dorsal trunk, neck, ventral abdomen, and medial thighs. Severe infections, particularly those with secondary mastitis, may produce pyrexia, anorexia, depression, and septicemia. In sheep, lesion distribution is muzzle, tail, and perineum of otherwise healthy 3-4 week-old lambs that usually regresses spontaneously within 3 weeks. A generalized skin infection with septicemia similar to *porcine exudative epidermitis* has been described in neonatal lambs. *Staphylococcus xylosus*, a coagulase-negative staphylococcus, was isolated from the skin and various tissues. In adult sheep, lesions of bacterial folliculitis and furunculosis usually occur on the poorly wooled areas of the face (periocular, pinna, base of the horn, nasal bones, maxillary ridge) and include pustules, crusts, erosions, and ulcerations. These lesions are commonly associated with crowded feeding in troughs, with head rubbing and fighting (facial eczema, eye scab), particularly of adult ewes just prior to lambing. In both goats and sheep, lesions are generally nonpruritic, but furunculosis can be painful.

Staphylococcal folliculitis and furunculosis occur occasionally in cattle, pigs, cats, and alpacas. Infection in **cattle** is seen most commonly in young bulls on the tail, perineum, scrotum, and face, and *S. aureus* is most commonly isolated. Trauma and poor hygiene may be initiating factors. Staphylococcal folliculitis in **pigs** usually occurs on the hindquarters, abdomen, and chest of piglets <8 weeks of age and spontaneously regresses. Pustules covering much of the body rupture, forming brown crusts that are neither painful nor pruritic. Bacterial folliculitis and furunculosis is uncommon in **cats** and is usually secondary to other underlying conditions, such as feline acne and hypersensitivity conditions. Lesions may consist of a crusted papular eruption on the face, head, or over the dorsum that clinically resembles miliary dermatitis. Bacterial folliculitis in **alpacas** may be associated with insect-bite hypersensitivity, contact dermatitis, or idiopathic. Lesions consist of erythematous papules, pustules, brown-to-yellow crusts, epidermal collarettes and annular areas of alopecia and scaling, and are most common over the muzzle, back, ventrum, and distal hindlegs. Pruritus is more likely with an underlying hypersensitivity.

Further reading

Bannoehr J, Guardabassi L. *Staphylococcus pseudintermedius* in the dog: taxonomy, diagnostics, ecology, epidemiology and pathogenicity. Vet Dermatol 2012;23:253-266.

Foster AP. Staphylococcal skin disease in livestock. Vet Dermatol 2012;23:342-351.

Hillier A, et al. Pyoderma caused by *Pseudomonas aeruginosa* infection in dogs: 20 cases. Vet Dermatol 2006;17:432-439.

Lloyd D. Bacterial skin disease. In: Miller WH, et al., editors. Muller & Kirk's Small Animal Dermatology. 7th ed. St Louis: Elsevier; 2013. p. 184-222.

Rosser EJ. German shepherd dog pyoderma. Vet Clin North Am Small Anim Pract 2006;36:203-211.

Scott DW. Color Atlas of Farm Animal Dermatology. Ames, Iowa: Blackwell; 2007.

Abscesses and cellulitis

Abscesses *are well-circumscribed accumulations of pus.* **Cellulitis** *is a severe, deep, suppurative infection that is poorly defined and tends to dissect through tissue planes. The lesions are usually painful, often warm, and overlying skin is often friable, dark, devitalized, and may be sloughed.* The wounds frequently have a putrid smell and may be emphysematous if the organism is a gas producer (*Clostridium* spp., *Bacteroides* spp.). Pyrexia and regional lymphadenopathy may be present. Abscesses and cellulitis are fairly common in large animals and are *one of the most common disorders in cats*, where they are a frequent sequel to fight wounds. Other predisposing causes include traumatic puncture wounds, foreign bodies, injections, and shearing and clipping wounds. *Microscopically*, abscesses consist of central accumulations of neutrophils and/or necrotic debris, frequently surrounded by a wall of granulation tissue or dense collagenous connective tissue, depending on duration. In contrast, cellulitis is poorly circumscribed and consists of extensive purulent to pyogranulomatous dermal and subcutaneous inflammation that may be accompanied by hemorrhage, necrosis, and thrombosis. Bacteria may or may not be visible histologically.

A wide variety of aerobic and anaerobic bacteria have been associated with abscesses and cellulitis. The most common organisms include *Staphylococcus* spp. (dogs, horses, cattle, goats, pigs), *Clostridium* spp. (malignant edema, gas gangrene, and big head in horses, cattle, sheep, goats, pigs, and dogs), *Pasteurella multocida* (cats), and *Corynebacterium pseudotuberculosis* (abscesses in horses, goats, cattle, alpacas, and sheep; ulcerative lymphangitis in horses, cattle, sheep, and goats; caseous lymphadenitis in sheep and goats; pyogranulomas in cats), and *Trueperella pyogenes* (abscesses in cattle, goats, sheep, pigs, horses; ulcerative lymphangitis in cattle and goats). *Rhodococcus equi*, most commonly associated with pneumonia in young horses, has been isolated from cutaneous abscesses and cellulitis in young horses and rarely in cats. *Pasteurella granulomatis* has been associated with a disease in southern Brazil called lechiguana, which is characterized by large subcutaneous fibrosing eosinophilic abscesses. Lesions are most commonly located in the scapular region, and the condition is frequently fatal if untreated. Various mycoplasmas and mycoplasma-like organisms have been recovered from abscesses in cats and from decubital abscesses in calves.

Streptococcus canis, Lancefield group G, has been isolated in most cases of **necrotizing fasciitis.** This is a rare condition that has been described most commonly in dogs, very rarely in cats, and one 2-year-old bull. *Staphylococcus pseudintermedius* and *E. coli* have been isolated from a few affected dogs. *Arcanobacterium haemolyticum* was isolated from the bull. Necrotizing fasciitis is a severe life-threatening disease that usually starts as a localized infection but spreads rapidly and aggressively within hours. The condition is characterized grossly by *extensive exudation along fascial planes and necrosis of subcutaneous fat and fascia*, resulting in extensive sloughing of necrotic skin. The *microscopic lesions* of necrotizing fasciitis include *severe necrosis, suppuration, fibrinous exudation, and hemorrhage of the dermis and subcutaneous fat, fascia, and muscle*. In some instances, the epidermis and superficial dermis are infarcted as a result of *thrombosis of dermal and subcutaneous blood vessels*. Colonies of bacterial cocci may be evident in the inflamed subcutaneous tissue.

A condition histologically identical to **toxic shock syndrome (TSS)** in humans has been described in dogs. TSS in humans is associated with *S. aureus* and group C streptococci infections. Bacterial toxins, including toxic shock syndrome toxin-1 (TSST-1), are thought to induce massive cytokine release (including tumor necrosis factor-α and interleukin-1), increased sensitivity to cytokines, and endothelial damage. In dogs, TSS has been associated with *S. pseudintermedius* infection. *Lesions* include macular erythema and edema of the trunk and limbs initially with vesicles, ulcers, and variable crusting seen later. Fever, depression, anorexia and hypoalbuminemia are common. Disseminated intravascular coagulation is a consistent finding in dogs that succumb to infection. *Histologically*, there is epidermal and follicular epithelial spongiosis, with individual keratinocyte necrosis (apoptosis) associated with neutrophils and occasionally eosinophils surrounding the necrotic cells. There may also be suppurative epidermitis, crusts, and confluent epidermal necrosis. In the dermis, there is edema, extravasation of erythrocytes, and variable perivascular neutrophils and fewer eosinophils.

In dogs, *Streptococcus canis* and *S. pseudintermedius* have also been associated with a toxic shock–like syndrome where infected dogs rapidly develop sepsis. *Acinetobacter baumannii* was isolated from a cat with necrotizing fasciitis and toxic shock. Toxic shock–like syndrome was reported in a 3-year-old Thoroughbred gelding with *S. aureus* pneumonia.

L-form infections are described in dogs and cats. L-forms are bacterial variants that lack a cell wall and divide by a variety of processes. Lesions occur as one or more draining abscesses, usually over joints. Some animals may be febrile or depressed. L-forms cannot be cultured by routine techniques.

Melioidosis, caused by the gram-negative, intracellular bacterium *Burkholderia pseudomallei*, produces abscesses in multiple organs. This organism is a soil saprophyte, and infection may occur through inhalation, arthropod-bite and wound contamination. Skin lesions include multiple small nodules that tend to rupture and drain. In addition, horses may develop papulocrustous dermatitis and lymphangitis of the limbs. *Glanders*, like melioidosis, can have systemic involvement, and both infections are commonly fatal. Glanders is caused by *Burkholderia mallei*. The cutaneous form of this disease is called *farcy*. Horses are highly susceptible and are considered the natural reservoir. In the acute form, clinical signs include fever, respiratory signs, painful and enlarged submaxillary lymph nodes, skin nodules on the legs and abdomen, and death caused by septicemia. The chronic form is more common, and skin lesions include nodules forming chains along lymphatics, ulceration, and exudation. Both of these organisms have been eradicated from many parts of the world.

Further reading

Brachelente C, et al. A case of necrotizing fasciitis with septic shock in a cat caused by *Acinobacter baumanni*. Vet Dermatol 2007;18:432-438.

Gross TL, et al. Necrotizing diseases of the epidermis. In: Gross TL, et al., editors. Skin Diseases of the Dog and Cat: Clinical and Histopathological Diagnosis. 2nd ed. Oxford, UK: Blackwell; 2005. p. 75-104.

Holbrook TC, et al. Toxic shock syndrome in a horse with *Staphylococcus aureus* pneumonia. J Am Vet Med Assoc 2003;222:620-623.

Scott DW, Miller WH. Bacterial skin diseases. In: Scott DW, Miller WH, editors. Equine Dermatology. 2nd ed. St Louis: Elsevier Saunders; 2011. p. 130-170.

Slovak JE, et al. Toxic shock syndrome in two dogs. J Am Anim Hosp Assoc 2012;48:434-438.

Cutaneous bacterial granulomas

A wide variety of bacteria are capable of producing granulomatous inflammation of the skin. The organisms are frequently of *low virulence* and are introduced by *traumatic implantation*. These infections are typically *slowly progressive* and produce *cutaneous or subcutaneous nodules*. Inflammation is nodular or diffuse, granulomatous, or pyogranulomatous, and involves the dermis, panniculus, or both. *Diagnosis commonly requires special stains, such as tissue Gram stain and routine acid-fast (Ziehl-Neelsen) or modified acid-fast (Fite-Faraco) stains*. Staining frozen sections of formalin-fixed tissue may be necessary to demonstrate the bacteria in some atypical mycobacterial infections. Organisms are so infrequent in some cases that confirmation of the bacterial etiology cannot be made histologically and depends instead on cultural isolation of the agent or PCR testing.

Actinomycosis and nocardiosis

Actinomycosis and nocardiosis are uncommon subacute-to-chronic opportunistic cutaneous, pulmonary, and disseminated infections that develop secondary to wound contamination, inhalation, or ingestion. The diseases are discussed together because of their clinical and histologic similarities. *Actinomyces* and *Nocardia* are the most common actinomycetes, so-called higher bacteria, which cause disease, but occasional reports of infections in animals by other actinomycetes include *Streptomyces* and *Actinomadura*. The infections occur sporadically and are worldwide in distribution. They are not considered of public health significance.

Actinomyces spp. are gram-positive, non–acid-fast, filamentous anaerobic or microaerophilic rods that are *commensal inhabitants of the oral cavity, intestine, and upper respiratory tract*. Infection is usually secondary to penetrating wounds of the oral mucosa and skin. Cutaneous actinomycosis occurs in cattle, dogs, horses, camelids, goats, pigs, and cats. In cattle, lesions are most commonly on the mandible and maxilla *(lumpy jaw)* and are most commonly caused by *A. bovis*. These are firm, variably painful, swellings due to osteomyelitis, with extension into the skin resulting in nodules, abscesses, and draining tracts (Fig. 6-92A). Osteomyelitis caused by actinomycosis has also been described in dogs, camelids, goats, and a horse. Actinomycosis is rare in horses but has been associated with mandibular lymphadenitis and abscesses, fistulous withers, and poll evil. Hunting or field dogs in warm climates are most commonly affected. It can take months to years for signs to develop after injury. Lesions in dogs and cats are usually tender, subcutaneous, may or may not have draining tracts, and are most common on the head or neck, thoracic, paralumbar, or abdominal regions. In pigs, nodules are most common in the udder and ventral abdomen. In goats, they have been described in the leg and shoulder.

Nocardia spp. are *ubiquitous saprophytes* occurring in *soil, straw, grasses, decaying vegetable matter, and water*. Unlike *Actinomyces* spp., they are not part of the normal flora of mammals. They are opportunistic pathogens that cause infection by wound contamination, inhalation, or ingestion, particularly in immunocompromised animals. Several cases have been reported in dogs receiving immunomodulatory therapy for atopic dermatitis. *Nocardia* spp. are aerobic, gram-positive,

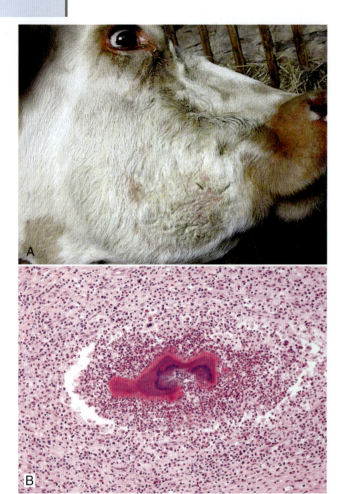

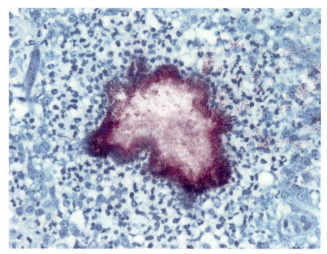

Figure 6-92 *Actinomyces bovis.* **A.** Firm swelling with alopecia and crusting over the mandible in a cow *(lumpy jaw).* (Courtesy J.M. Nicol.) **B.** Clusters of filamentous organisms surrounded by eosinophilic Splendore-Hoeppli material forming a "sulfur granule."

Figure 6-93 Nocardiosis in a cat. Filamentous organisms are acid fast with Fite-Faraco stain.

branching filamentous organisms that are variably acid fast. Pathogenic *Nocardia* spp. are facultative intracellular bacteria. Major virulence factors are the complex cell wall lipids and resistance to phagocytosis. *Nocardia* spp. also have the ability to invade blood vessels, leading to vascular necrosis and ischemia. Cutaneous nocardiosis is reported most frequently in cats, dogs, horses, and cattle, with very rare occurrence in goats. In cattle, *Nocardia* spp. are more commonly associated with mastitis. There are >30 named *Nocardia* spp., and different species are correlated with differences in disease features and pathogenicity. The most commonly isolated organisms are *Nocardia asteroides* complex types I-VI, which include *N. nova, N. farcinica, N. brasiliensis,* and *N. otitidis-caviarum.*

The *gross lesions* of actinomycosis and nocardiosis are usually indistinguishable. In **cats,** nocardia panniculitis is clinically indistinguishable from panniculitis caused by rapidly growing mycobacteria. Lesions consist of abscesses, cellulitis, ulcerated nodules, draining tracts, and dense fibrous masses. *When the triad of clinical signs consisting of tumefaction, draining tracts, and tissue grains is present, the lesion can be termed an* **actinomycotic mycetoma.** Lesions progress slowly by local extension. They occur most commonly on the head, neck, and extremities. Pleural and retroperitoneal infections may extend to involve the subcutaneous tissues of the lateral thoracic wall and flank area, respectively. The exudate is variable and ranges from thin serosanguineous to thick purulohemorrhagic. It may be odorless or foul smelling and contain white, yellow, tan, or gray **"sulfur granules."** Sulfur granules are more common in actinomycosis than in nocardiosis. Regional lymphadenopathy frequently accompanies skin lesions. Mandibular and maxillary osteomyelitis may occur in dogs and cats.

Microscopically, actinomycosis and nocardiosis are characterized by *pyogranulomatous dermatitis and panniculitis.* The epidermis is variably acanthotic and may be ulcerated. The dermis and subcutis contain central accumulations of neutrophils surrounded by a wall of epithelioid macrophages and variable numbers of multinucleated giant cells. Necrosis may be prominent within the central abscess. The pyogranulomas are separated by granulation tissue or dense fibrous connective tissue containing lymphocytes and plasma cells. Fibrosis tends to be more common and severe in actinomycosis than in nocardiosis. Organized masses, measuring 30-3,000 μm or more in diameter, of basophilic- or amphophilic-staining organisms, may be seen in the centers of the abscesses (Fig. 6-92B). They are commonly bordered by a clubbed corona of brightly eosinophilic *Splendore-Hoeppli material. These structures correspond to the sulfur granules seen grossly in the exudate.* Although granule formation is a more common feature of actinomycosis, *Nocardia* spp. may form granules in cutaneous lesions that are morphologically indistinguishable from those of *Actinomyces.* In nocardiosis, the bacteria tend to be distributed singly and are more difficult to identify in H&E-stained sections. With Gram stain, the bacteria are evident as delicate, branched, and beaded filaments, from 10-30 μm or more long and 0.5-1.0 μm wide. The beaded appearance is due to alternating gram-positive and gram-negative regions within the filament and is less prominent with *Actinomyces* than with *Nocardia* spp. Most *Nocardia* spp. are at least partially acid fast when using a modified acid-fast stain such as Fite-Faraco stain in tissue sections (Fig. 6-93), whereas *Actinomyces* spp. and other anaerobic actinomycetes are not acid fast. Definitive diagnosis can be made with anaerobic culture for *Actinomyces* and aerobic culture for *Nocardia* spp. Diagnosis of specific *Nocardia* spp. can be made by molecular sequencing of 16S rRNA.

Further reading

Fielding CL, et al. *Actinomyces* species as a cause of abscesses in nine horses. Vet Rec 2008;162:18-20.

Lloyd D. Bacterial skin disease. In: Miller WH, et al., editors. Muller & Kirk's Small Animal Dermatology. 7th ed. St Louis: Elsevier; 2013. p. 184-222.

Malik R. *Nocardia* infections in cats: a retrospective multi-institutional study of 17 cases. Aust Vet J 2006;84:235-245.

Scott DW. Color Atlas of Farm Animal Dermatology. Ames, Iowa: Blackwell; 2007.

Scott DW, Miller WH. Bacterial skin disease. In: Scott DW, Miller WH, editors. Equine Dermatology. 2nd ed. St Louis: Elsevier Saunders; 2011. p. 130-170.

Mycobacterial infections

Mycobacterial infections are caused by bacteria that belong to the family *Mycobacteriaceae*, order Actinomycetales. *Mycobacterium* is a genus comprising morphologically similar, aerobic, gram-positive, acid-fast, non–spore-forming, nonmotile, pleomorphic bacilli with wide variations in host affinity and pathogenic potential. Cutaneous mycobacterial infections are caused by obligate pathogens, such as the tuberculosis groups *(Mycobacterium tuberculosis, M. bovis, M. microti,)* the leprosy group *(M. lepraemurium, M. visibilis)*, and the opportunistic group considered to be saprophytes or facultative pathogens (subdivided based on growth rate and pigment production). Rapid-growing opportunistic organisms *(M. fortuitum, M. smegmatis, M. chelonae, M. abscessus, M. thermoresistible)* and slow-growing opportunistic organisms *(M. avium-intracellulare complex, M. kansasii, M. ulcerans)* are inhabitants of soil, water, and decomposing vegetation, and cutaneous infections are usually acquired via wound contamination or traumatic implantation. Most mycobacteria are intracellular pathogens that are able to persist in tissue by entering macrophages. They survive and replicate in macrophages by inhibiting fusion with lysosomes. Tissue destruction results from persistence of antigen in the tissue and a cell-mediated inflammatory response. Mycobacterial organisms produce *granulomatous to pyogranulomatous dermatitis and panniculitis with variable necrosis* in many domestic animal species, particularly **cats,** less frequently dogs and cattle, and rarely in horses and other species. The number of organisms within lesions may be rare to numerous and are best visualized with acid-fast (Ziehl-Neelsen) or modified acid-fast (Fite-Faraco) stains. Because many of these organisms are fastidious and difficult to culture, diagnosis is often made by molecular techniques such as PCR.

Cutaneous infections caused by slow-growing mycobacteria

Tuberculosis. Cutaneous infections caused by *M. tuberculosis* and *M. bovis* (the "bovine bacillus") are rare but can occur in cattle, dogs, cats, and possibly horses. *M. tuberculosis* causes tuberculosis in humans. *M. bovis*, which infects many animals, historically spread to humans when they began drinking milk following cattle domestication. These facultative or obligate intracellular parasites grow best in tissue with high oxygen concentrations, such as lungs. Pulmonary and alimentary infections are more common in cattle, horses, and dogs, but skin infections can develop alone or in combination with disseminated infection. Most cases of tuberculosis in cats are cutaneous, with alimentary and respiratory forms less frequent. *M. microti* (the "vole bacillus") causes cutaneous tuberculosis in cats, llamas, and rarely dogs. *M. microti* infection is believed to be transmitted via direct contact with wild rodents and other small mammals. In **cats,** most cases of *M. microti* involve *submandibular lymphadenopathy* and/or cutaneous lesions that typically affect the "fight and bite" sites: face, legs, and tail base. In some cases, the infection can become disseminated with spread to the lungs. Tuberculous mycobacteria possess mycolate-containing molecules in their cell walls, including the original cord factor *trehalose 6,6'-dimycolate*. These substances are associated with *virulence and the production of characteristic tubercles*. To be maintained in nature, they require infection of reservoir mammalian hosts because environmental survival is limited to a maximum of a few weeks on infected fomites.

Cutaneous lesions are single or multiple ulcers, plaques, nodules, or abscesses that exude thick yellow to green fluid. Lesions are most common on the head, neck, and limbs. Patients usually have systemic signs, such as anorexia, weight loss, fever, and localized or generalized lymphadenopathy. *Histology* of skin lesions shows a *nodular-to-diffuse granulomatous to pyogranulomatous dermatitis and panniculitis* with *central caseous necrosis*. There may be small numbers of multinucleated giant cells and mineralization with *few to many acid-fast bacteria*.

Nontuberculous mycobacteria. The *Mycobacterium avium-intracellulare* complex (MAC) includes *M. avium* subspp. *avium, hominissus,* and *paratuberculosis*. These are slow-growing opportunistic organisms that are associated with 2 forms of disease: *localized infections of the skin and subcutis in immunocompetent hosts and disseminated disease in immunocompromised animals*. Clustering of cases within breeds (Bassett Hounds, Siamese cats, Somali cats, and Abyssinian cats) suggests a genetic predisposition. Affected animals have signs of respiratory and/or gastrointestinal disease, generalized lymphadenopathy, or nodular skin disease with regional lymphadenopathy. Failure to regrow hair after clipping is a unique feature of disseminated MAC infection in Abyssinian cats. Although mycobacteriosis is rare in horses, the most common isolate is *M. avium* subsp. *avium*. Lesions in horses range from fairly localized granulomatous dermatitis and panniculitis to exfoliative dermatitis with ulcers, to swollen painful limbs with areas of necrosis, to severe systemic disease. Histologically, there is granulomatous dermatitis and panniculitis without formation of tubercles. Lesions tend to have numerous organisms, and therefore they may be visible in aspirates of masses and various tissues.

Opportunistic cutaneous mycobacterial infections occur in **cattle** *(bovine cutaneous opportunistic mycobacteriosis)*. *Mycobacterium kansasii* has been isolated from some of these lesions. Lesions occur as single or multiple nodules 1-8 cm in diameter in the dermis and subcutis. Lesions in cattle are usually unilateral and affect the distal leg. They may spread to the thigh, shoulder, or abdomen. *Papules and nodules may be single or multiple, hard or fluctuant, and often occur in chains with intralesional large and palpable ("corded") lymphatics.* Lesions may rupture and discharge thick, yellow to gray pus. Regional lymph nodes are normal, animals are otherwise healthy, and pruritus and pain are absent. *Histologically*, there is nodular-to-diffuse granulomatous dermatitis and panniculitis with intracellular acid-fast bacilli and variable fibrosis and mineralization. Small lesions may spontaneously resolve, but larger lesions persist.

Mycobacterium ulcerans is the causative agent of Buruli ulcer, a chronic localized infection of the skin and subcutis of humans typically associated with necrotizing skin ulcers with undermined edges. The extensive tissue destruction is associated with *mycolactone, a necrotizing cytotoxin and immunosuppressant*. The disease is most prevalent in West Africa but also occurs in coastal Victoria and Queensland, Australia. The infection is most commonly reported in marsupial species of Australia but has also been diagnosed in dogs, horses, alpacas, and a cat.

Cutaneous infections caused by rapidly growing mycobacteria (atypical mycobacteriosis). Rapidly growing mycobacteria (RGM) (formerly Runyon Group IV or atypical mycobacteria) are by definition characterized by the ability to form colonies on solid media within 7 days of incubation. These bacteria are ubiquitous free-living organisms that are usually harmless and commonly found in *water, soil, and decaying vegetation*. RGM cause opportunistic disease in both healthy and immunocompromised individuals. These organisms are opportunistic environmental saprophytes. Infections are most common in **cats,** less frequent in dogs and rare in cattle, horses, and other species. Infection has been reported in Australia, the United States, Canada, New Zealand, France, Finland, the Netherlands, Italy, and Switzerland. Three syndromes are recognized: *mycobacterial panniculitis involving chronic infection of the subcutis and skin, pyogranulomatous lobar pneumonia, and disseminated systemic disease in immunocompromised individuals*. Panniculitis is the most common clinical presentation, especially in Australian cats. Rapidly growing mycobacteria reported to cause cutaneous granulomas in dogs and cats are the *Mycobacterium fortuitum* group (including *M. fortuitum, M. perigrinum*, and the third biovariant complex), the *Mycobacterium chelonae/abscessus* group (including *M. chelonae* and *M. abscessus*), the *M. smegmatis* group (including *M. smegmatis sensu stricto, M. goodii, M. wolinskyi*), and a variety of other species, including *M. phlei* and *M. thermoresistibile*. *M. smegmatis* is the most commonly isolated organism in Australia; *M. fortuitum* is most common in the United States. *M. smegmatis* was isolated from a firm, painful, subcutaneous abscess in the stifle region of a horse.

Lesions can occur anywhere but are *most common in the cat in the caudal abdomen, inguinal region, or lumbar region*. The causative organisms *thrive in fatty tissues*. The bacterial cell wall contains *glycolipids*. It is thought that the lipid may provide nutrients for the organisms to grow and protect them from the immune response. A lipid-rich environment activates virulent mycolic acids in the bacterial cell walls, resulting in granulomatous inflammation. Lesions may or may not be painful, and the regional lymph nodes may not be enlarged. With solitary lesions, systemic illness is rarely observed. In immunocompromised animals, lesions may be widespread, and anorexia, fever, and inappetence may be observed. Lesions generally develop slowly over a period of weeks to months after a history of a penetrating wound or cat fight. *Lesions include single or multiple cutaneous and subcutaneous nodules, plaques, purpuric macules, or diffuse swellings*. Multiple punctate ulcers or large draining tracts frequently develop and discharge serous, serosanguineous, or purulent exudate that is not usually malodorous (Fig. 6-94).

The *microscopic lesions* of atypical cutaneous mycobacteriosis are usually *multinodular-to-diffuse pyogranulomatous dermatitis and panniculitis*, often with circular clear vacuoles surrounded by a rim of neutrophils and a wider outer zone of

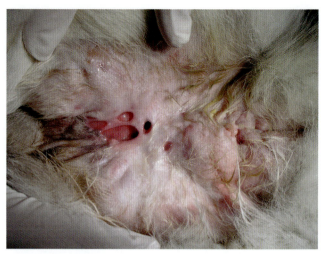

Figure 6-94 Multiple draining tracts on the ventral abdomen of a cat caused by **atypical mycobacteriosis.** (Courtesy M.S. Canfield.)

epithelioid macrophages and variable numbers of neutrophils among more diffuse inflammation composed of macrophages, neutrophils, and lymphoid cells. Multinucleated giant cells are infrequent. *Organisms are characteristically rare and difficult to find but are usually located in small clumps within the clear vacuoles*. Small numbers of organisms may also be found within macrophages. The bacilli may stain more intensely with modified acid-fast stain than with routine acid-fast stain. In some instances, staining frozen sections of formalin-fixed tissue may result in enhanced acid-fast staining. The organisms are long rods to short filamentous bacilli. Intracellular bacteria tend to be shorter rods. The organisms stain unevenly positive with tissue Gram stains, resulting in a beaded appearance to the bacilli. *Because of the scarcity of organisms, any single section may lack organisms, and the diagnosis will be missed*. In rare instances, fibroplasia may be marked, and the lesion may be confused for a spindle cell tumor. *The specific diagnosis of opportunistic mycobacterial infection requires identification by culture or molecular-based techniques*. Because of the scarcity of organisms in some lesions, diagnosis may require multiple attempts at biopsy, culture, and PCR.

Feline leprosy. *Feline leprosy is a rare localized cutaneous infection caused by mycobacteria that are not culturable by standard mycobacteriologic methods*. Cases occur worldwide, although certain mycobacterial species have strong geographic predilections. *Mycobacterium* spp. associated with feline leprosy include *M. lepraemurium, M. visibile, M.* spp. strain Tarwin, and a novel species found in New Zealand and the East Coast of Australia. *M. lepraemurium* infections have been reported from the United Kingdom, the Netherlands, France, Greece, Australia, New Zealand, Canada, and the United States. Feline leprosy has no zoonotic potential; however, lesions can be clinically and microscopically indistinguishable from lesions caused by tuberculosis bacteria *(M. bovis* and *M. microti)* and members of *M. avium* complex (MAC).

Young male cats with access to the outdoors are overrepresented, and lesions are most common over the head, neck, and limbs. **Cats** may present with *single or multiple cutaneous papules and nodules 2-40 mm in diameter often accompanied by lymphadenopathy*. The nodules are generally *firm, well circumscribed, alopecic, and some may ulcerate*. The location of lesions on cats suggests inoculation of organisms through insect bites, rodent bites, or fight wounds. The development of the disease is due to a complex and incompletely understood interaction between the organism and the immune response of the host. Some organisms (*M.* spp. strain Tarwin) are associated with localized disease in an immunocompetent host, whereas others (*M. visible* and the novel Australian East Coast species) are associated with hematogenously disseminated (usually limited to the skin) in the immunodeficient host. **Feline leprosy syndrome** has a progressive and occasionally aggressive clinical course, depending on the causal species, the size of the infective inoculum, and the immunologic response of the host. In some cases, widespread lesions can develop, and large tuberculoid lesions may ulcerate.

Histologically there are 2 distinct morphologic patterns of inflammation. In **lepromatous leprosy,** there is nodular-to-diffuse dermal to subcutaneous granulomatous inflammation without necrosis and with large numbers of intracellular acid-fast bacilli. These large granulomas are composed of solid sheets of *large, pale, foamy epithelioid macrophages* with smaller numbers of multinucleated histiocytic giant cells often containing bacilli. Variable numbers of lymphocytes and plasma cells surround vessels. In some cases, there are scattered neutrophils resembling pyogranulomas. *This lepromatous reaction pattern is generally indicative of a poor host immune response.* Differential diagnoses for the lepromatous form includes cutaneous xanthoma/xanthogranuloma. Xanthomas are sterile granulomatous lesions composed of foamy macrophages. In **tuberculoid leprosy,** there are dermal to subcutaneous granulomas with central caseous necrosis surrounded by a zone of lymphocytes. Few to moderate numbers of acid-fast bacilli are generally limited to the areas of necrosis. Variable numbers of lymphocytes surround blood vessels.

In most mycobacterial infections, bacilli are not visible in routine H&E-stained sections. However, *M. visible* and the novel Australian East Coast species can be seen in H&E-stained sections because they weakly take up the hematoxylin. Regional lymph nodes are characterized by variable architectural disruption by infiltrates of macrophages. Acid-fast bacteria are rare within lymph nodes.

Canine leproid granuloma. Canine leproid granuloma is a cutaneous to subcutaneous localized nodular granulomatous skin disease that is usually confined to the *head, especially pinna,* but can occur anywhere. This condition is thought to be caused by a single novel mycobacterium that has not been fully characterized. The condition can be seen worldwide but is most common in Australia and Brazil. Affected dogs are otherwise healthy and *generally short-coated breeds,* particularly Boxers and their crosses, Doberman Pinschers, and Bullmastiffs. Lesions consist of one or more asymptomatic nodules, 2-5 cm in diameter, confined to the skin and subcutis. Larger lesions may ulcerate (Fig. 6-95). Regional lymph nodes are generally not enlarged. The route of infection is unknown, but it is speculated, based on the propensity for pinnal lesions in short-coated breeds, that biting insects or arthropods may introduce the mycobacteria directly into the skin. Lesions within the dermis and subcutis are characterized by nodular-to-diffuse pyogranulomatous inflammation composed of epithelioid macrophages, Langerhans-type giant cells with scattered neutrophils, plasma cells, and small numbers of lymphocytes. The number and morphology of the acid-fast bacilli is highly variable. Bacteria range from long slender filaments in parallel sheaves to short variably beaded bacilli or highly

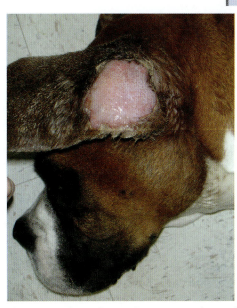

Figure 6-95 **Canine leproid granuloma.** Large ulcerated nodule on the pinna of a dog. (Courtesy M.S. Canfield.)

beaded to coccoid forms. Lesions can be disfiguring and cause irritation, especially when they are secondarily infected with bacteria. Lesions may spontaneously resolve over the course of several months, but some persist.

Miscellaneous mycobacterial infections. **Farcy** is a common pyogranulomatous disease of the skin and lymphatics that occurs in **cattle** in tropical and subtropical climates of Africa, Asia, Latin America, and the Caribbean. Historically it was thought to be caused by *Nocardia farcinica*, but is now known to be caused by *Mycobacterium senegalense* and *M. farcinogenes*. The mycobacterial organisms gain entry via skin wounds, particularly those caused by tick bites. Skin lesions are most common on the head, neck, shoulder, and legs. Firm, painless, *slow-growing subcutaneous nodules may ulcerate and discharge thick, stringy, odorless, gray or yellow material.* Enlarged "corded" lymphatics and regional lymphadenopathy are present. *Histopathology* shows nodular-to-diffuse pyogranulomatous dermatitis and panniculitis with intracellular gram-positive acid-fast bacilli. Farcy has a prolonged course and may have widespread organ involvement, emaciation, and death. Economic losses are high in endemic areas.

Further reading

Couto SS, Artacho CA. *Mycobacterium fortuitum* pneumonia in a cat and the role of lipid in the pathogenesis of atypical mycobacterial infections. Vet Pathol 2007;44:543-546.

Davies JL, et al. Histological and genotypical characterization of feline cutaneous mycobacteriosis: a retrospective study of formalin-fixed paraffin-embedded tissue. Vet Dermatol 2006;17: 155-162.

Greene CE, Gunn-Moore DA. Mycobacterial infections. In: Greene CE, editor. Infectious Diseases of the Dog and Cat. 4th ed. St Louis: Elsevier Saunders; 2012. p. 495-521.

Hamid ME. Epidemiology, pathology, immunology and diagnosis of bovine farcy: a review. Prev Vet Med 2012;105:1-9.

Lloyd D. Bacterial skin disease. In: Miller WH, et al., editors. Muller & Kirk's Small Animal Dermatology. 7th ed. St Louis: Elsevier; 2013. p. 184-222.

Malik R, et al. Ulcerated and nonulcerated nontuberculous cutaneous mycobacterial granulomas in cats and dogs. Vet Dermatol 2013;24:146-e33.

Bacterial pseudomycetoma

Bacterial pseudomycetoma (botryomycosis, bacterial pseudomycosis, bacterial granuloma) is *a chronic infection caused by nonfilamentous bacteria that form colonies visible as tissue grains or granules within lesions*. Clinically and histologically, the condition resembles actinomycotic and eumycotic mycetomas. The disease occurs in humans and all domestic animals, including alpacas. Although reported rarely, the condition is probably not uncommon. Lesions are usually localized in the skin and subcutis but may extend deep to involve underlying bone and muscle. Disseminated infection with visceral involvement is rare. Coagulase-positive staphylococci are involved most commonly, but *Streptococcus, Pseudomonas, Actinobacillus, Pasteurella, Proteus, Escherichia, Trueperella,* and *Bibersteinia* have also been isolated from lesions. Infection is thought to develop as a result of wound contamination or trauma, such as bites, lacerations, or puncture wounds with foreign bodies.

Lesions typically consist of *firm, nonpruritic single or multiple nodules that ulcerate and develop draining tracts*. They discharge purulent material that frequently contains *white to yellow sand-like grains*. The most common lesion sites in **horses** are limbs, lips, chin, and scrotum. The microscopic lesion is characterized by the presence of *basophilic granules within the center of neutrophilic abscesses or pyogranulomas in the dermis or subcutis*. These granules correspond to the grains seen grossly in the discharge. They are surrounded and separated by fibrous tissue that may be quite extensive. Plant debris or other foreign material may also be seen in the lesions and indicate the means of infection. The granules consist of compact bacterial colonies that are usually surrounded by amorphous, deeply eosinophilic, radially arranged Splendore-Hoeppli material (Fig. 6-96A). This material is thought to be antigen-antibody complexes. The bacteria are not well delineated in H&E-stained sections; thus *special stains are usually necessary to distinguish the organisms from actinomycotic bacteria and fungi*. Individual cocci or bacilli within the granules are seen most clearly in sections stained with tissue Gram or Brown-Brenn stains (Fig. 6-96B). The granulomatous reaction is thought to develop as a result of a delicate balance between the virulence of the organism and the response of the host. The host is able to isolate the infection but is unable to eradicate it. It is speculated that this may be associated with a polysaccharide slime coating produced by the bacteria.

Further reading

Lloyd D. Bacterial skin disease. In: Miller WH, et al., editors. Muller & Kirk's Small Animal Dermatology. 7th ed. St Louis: Elsevier; 2013. p. 184-222.

Scott DW, et al. Skin diseases in the alpaca *(Vicugna pacos)*: a literature review and retrospective analysis of 68 cases (Cornell University 1997-2006). Vet Dermatol 2010;22:2-16.

Scott DW, Miller WH. Bacterial skin disease. In: Scott DW, Miller WH, editors. Equine Dermatology. 2nd ed. St Louis: Elsevier Saunders; 2011. p. 130-170.

Spagnoli S, et al. Subcutaneous botryomycosis due to *Bibersteinia trehalosi* in a Texas Longhorn steer. Vet Pathol 2012;49:775-778.

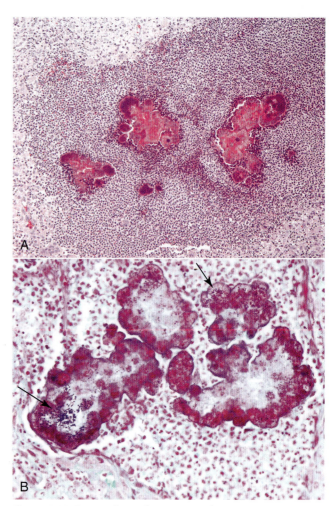

Figure 6-96 Bacterial pseudomycetoma (botryomycosis). **A.** Pyogranulomatous dermatitis surrounding multiple angular eosinophilic tissue grains. **B.** Gram stain reveals gram-positive cocci (arrows).

Bacterial pododermatitis of horses and ruminants

Proliferative pododermatitis (equine canker)

Equine hoof canker is a destructive painful chronic hypertrophic pododermatitis of the frog, sole, and hoof wall in equids. The condition can affect one or more feet and occur in all breeds, although it is more common in draft breeds. A moist and softer hoof horn may account for the higher occurrence of the disease in these breeds. The cause is unknown; however, the condition has been associated with the presence of a variety of gram-positive and gram-negative bacteria, including *Bacteroides* spp. and *Fusobacterium necrophorum*. Spirochetes identified as *Treponema* spp. have been isolated in some cases. Recent research suggests that bovine papillomavirus 1 and 2 may be involved in the pathogenesis of this condition. Humid environment and poor sanitation and hoof care may be contributing factors; however, the condition also occurs in well-cared-for horses.

Grossly, early lesions consist of focal pink raised tissue on the frog, resembling granulation tissue. This is surrounded by a gray to brown zone that will progress to excessive soft white filiform papillomatous proliferations associated with foul-smelling caseous white exudate. Histologically, the lesions are characterized by marked papillary epidermal hyperplasia with hyperkeratosis and radiating bands of neutrophilic inflammation in the epidermis. There may be marked intracellular edema of the stratum spinosum. There often is superficial interstitial neutrophilic and lymphoplasmacytic dermatitis.

Necrotizing pododermatitis (equine thrush)
Necrotizing pododermatitis is a *painful necrotizing condition of the frog and central and lateral sulci of the hoof* caused by *Fusobacterium necrophorum*. The condition can affect all hooves but is most common in the hindfeet. Wet humid conditions allow for softening of the frog and bacterial colonization. *F. necrophorum* produces leukotoxin as the major virulence factor. Grossly, lesions consist of softening of the frog with black discoloration and a very foul odor. Over time deeper tissues become involved, and there is foul-smelling black exudate with loss of frog tissue. Histologically, the lesions are characterized by necrosis and suppurative inflammation of the frog epithelium and sometimes deeper tissues.

Necrobacillosis of cattle
Necrobacillosis of cattle has a similar etiology and pathogenesis as equine thrush. Trauma to the interdigital skin leads to invasion and colonization by *F. necrophorum* and *Prevotella melaninogenica*, and subsequent lameness. Grossly, lesions are characterized by interdigital dermatitis and cellulitis with fissures and necrosis. In severe cases, necrosis and inflammation can extend to deeper structures, such as tendons, bones, and joints. Cutaneous infection with *F. necrophorum* can occur in other body sites of cattle (especially axillae, groin, and udder). Infection is associated with necrosis, ulceration, crusting, foul odor, and variable systemic signs.

Necrobacillosis of pigs
In pigs, cutaneous infections with *F. necrophorum* occur especially on the lips, cheeks, legs, and teats.

Necrobacillosis of sheep
In sheep, necrobacillosis includes both interdigital dermatitis and foot abscesses. *F. necrophorum* and *Trueperella pyogenes* may be isolated. Foot abscesses occur more in heavy adult sheep during the wet season and include heel and toe abscesses.

Contagious footrot
Footrot is a highly contagious bacterial infection of the digits of *sheep, cattle, and goats* with worldwide distribution. It has also been reported in *pigs*. The multistrain, gram-negative, slow-growing obligate anaerobe **Dichelobacter nodosus** is the essential causal pathogen, with *F. necrophorum* playing an important synergistic role in infection.

The pathogenesis of footrot is complex and has been studied most extensively in sheep. The disease is initiated by *maceration of the interdigital skin* brought about by wet conditions along with minor wounds and abrasions. The damaged epidermis then becomes colonized by *F. necrophorum*, aerobic diphtheroids, coliforms, and other common bacteria originating from the soil, skin, and feces. *Footrot develops if the dermatitis is subsequently complicated by infection with D. nodosus.* The bacterium is an obligate parasite of the ruminant hoof, and carrier animals serve as the source for uninfected stock. Transmission of infection requires adequate moisture and a mean ambient temperature >10° C. Direct contact between susceptible and infected sheep is not required for transmission of infection. Contact with contaminated substrate for <1 hour has been shown to be adequate for transmission, and outbreaks have been associated with contact with environment contaminated by affected animals as long as 4 days previously. *D. nodosus* produces a variety of *extracellular proteases* (the major one is AprV5) that are thought to digest the horn and allow bacterial invasion of the epidermal matrix of the horn. It also produces a *heat-stable soluble factor (AprV2)* that enhances the growth and invasiveness of *F. necrophorum*. Type IV fimbriae promote close contact between *D. nodosus* and host cells and allow the bacteria to translocate to a more anaerobic environment that is necessary for bacterial growth and protease production. *F. necrophorum* produces a *leukocidal exotoxin* that reduces phagocytosis. The separation of horn is caused by lysis of the epidermal matrix as a result of the local inflammatory response rather than from direct bacterial attack. *T. pyogenes* and other aerobic bacteria are usually located superficially in the lesion, where they remove oxygen, destroy hydrogen peroxide, and create the anaerobic environment necessary for the growth of the 2 anaerobic pathogens.

The severity of **ovine footrot** can vary from benign to a virulent form. *Benign footrot*, also called *foot-scald*, is a milder, less persistent form of the condition. It is typically characterized by moderate interdigital dermatitis that causes mild lameness and minimal production loss. The benign form has a greater propensity for self-cure. Virulence of *D. nodosus* varies widely from strain to strain. Virulent strains of the bacterium produce more extracellular proteases, including elastase, and proteases from virulent strains tend to be more thermostable than those from benign strains. The *virulent form of footrot in sheep* is the serious, persistent form of the disease characterized by severe necrotic damage to the hoof and extensive separation of hoof horn in more than one foot in a high percentage of the sheep. The infection may persist for more than 1 year if not treated, and chronically infected sheep may die of emaciation as a result of severe pain and lameness. Affected animals are also predisposed to fly strike.

Footrot in sheep develops ~10-20 days after exposure and *begins as interdigital dermatitis in the axial bulbar notch*. At this early stage, the interdigital skin is pale, swollen, and moist. Inflammation progressively extends forward and caudad around the bulb of the heel. Separation of the horn usually occurs 7 days later, beginning at the skin-horn junction and spreading to the bulb and sole. The animal is severely lame at this stage. From the sole, the process spreads to the hoof wall to involve the axial and abaxial surfaces of the digits. Exudation is minimal and consists of a small amount of gray, greasy malodorous material in the cleft beneath the horn. Because the infection does not destroy the germinative layers of the horn, new horn is continually being regenerated but is rapidly destroyed as long as the infection continues. Chronically infected hooves become long and misshapen.

Benign footrot is indistinguishable from the early stages of virulent footrot. However, *in benign footrot, the erosions usually remain confined to the caudal aspect of the interdigital cleft*. Occasionally, there is separation of the soft horn of the heel and caudal portion of the sole, but there is no separation of the hard horn. Affected sheep may appear normal or exhibit mild, temporary lameness. The effect of benign footrot on production is minimal.

Diagnosis of footrot in sheep is based on clinical signs, demonstration of *D. nodosus* in smears from lesional material, and culture and biochemical characterization of isolates to identify antigenic and virulence variants. Because the organism is slow to grow, culture and biochemical testing is time consuming and may require 10-14 days.

Footrot of **cattle and goats** is typically a *less severe disease* and resembles the benign form of footrot of sheep. Infection with *D. nodosus* is more common than is clinical disease. Direct transmission can occur between sheep and goats in the same environment, but this is less common in goats. The lesions in goats tend to stay confined to the interdigital skin. Under-running lesions are not common in goats and are usually restricted to a portion of the soft horn. *D. nodosus* isolates from *cattle* with footrot tend to be relatively benign strains. Footrot in cattle usually begins at the caudal aspect of the interdigital space, spreads laterally on the bulbs of the heels, and eventually involves the entire interdigital space. *Lesions usually remain confined to the interdigital skin*, which may be eroded, ulcerated, or become deeply fissured. The fissures are covered with necrotic material with a characteristic fetid odor. Lesions may extend to the heels, and mild separation of the soft horn may develop. Extensive undermining of the horn, as occurs in sheep, does not typically occur in cattle. Affected animals stand on their toes. In rare severe cases, fever, anorexia, recumbency, and decreased milk production may develop.

Contagious ovine digital dermatitis

Contagious ovine digital dermatitis (CODD) is a condition of the ovine hoof reported in the United Kingdom and Ireland. Initially, this condition was thought to be a severe form of virulent footrot (VFR). Features that distinguish this condition from VFR are the acute severe nature, lesion distribution, and poor response to conventional therapy and vaccination. The cause of this condition is unknown; however, several studies have implicated *Treponema* as likely playing a role in the pathogenesis. Affected sheep have acute severe lameness. Grossly, lesions are characterized by coronary band ulceration with progression to the abaxial wall lining the hoof, with hoof wall loss in severe cases. Interdigital lesions are not reported, whereas lesions of VFR affect the heel and interdigital region.

Papillomatous digital dermatitis

Papillomatous digital dermatitis (PDD) is a painful, contagious dermatitis of the feet of *cattle* that occurs worldwide. The condition is also called *footwarts* and *hairy heelwarts*, and clinically and histologically, it appears to be the same disease as *digital dermatitis, interdigital papillomatosis, verrucose dermatitis, and digital papillomatosis*. Papillomatous digital dermatitis is economically important because it frequently causes moderate to severe lameness that results in weight loss, decreased milk production, and poor reproductive performance.

The *vast majority of cases are in dairy cows*, but it has also been reported in beef cattle. Although the disease occurs in all ages, the highest incidence appears to be in *replacement heifers*. The pathogenesis of papillomatous digital dermatitis is unknown; however, it is speculated that noninfectious skin lesions lead to a keratinization defect allowing for a suitable growth medium for bacteria. Because *Dichelobacter nodosus* has been isolated in many cases, some believe that this bacterium may be a first invader, and proteolytic enzymes of *D. nodosus* allow secondary invasion by various phylotypes of *Treponema* spp. Proliferation of various treponemes then leads to the proliferative lesions of PDD. It is generally thought that more than one treponemal species is involved in this

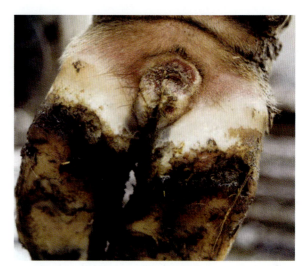

Figure 6-97 Papillomatous digital dermatitis. Interdigital wart-like growth in a cow. (Courtesy V. Serre.)

multifactorial disease. The condition has been compared to chronic periodontitis in humans because both are tissue-destructive diseases with multibacterial etiology in which spirochetes appear to be predominant. The condition is also usually associated with management conditions in which the feet of cattle remain wet for prolonged periods. Some research has indicated that there is upregulation of interleukin-8 (IL-8) by keratinocytes. This may explain the epidermal hyperplasia in these lesions because IL-8 is known to have a stimulatory effect on the migration and proliferation of keratinocytes. IL-8 also plays a key role in the recruitment of neutrophils, which are common in the epidermis of these lesions.

Papillomatous digital dermatitis most commonly affects the skin proximal and adjacent to the interdigital space at the back of the hindfeet (Fig. 6-97). The front feet are less frequently involved, and usually only one foot is affected. The cranial aspect of the foot and the interdigital skin are rarely involved. Lesions are painful, forcing the animal to shift its weight to the toe of the foot and resulting in clubbing of the affected foot and atrophy of the bulbs of the heels. Early lesions are well circumscribed, round to oval, red plaques up to 6 cm in diameter with a moist granular surface prone to bleeding and with a very strong, pungent odor. They are partially to completely alopecic and may be bordered by hypertrophied hairs 2-3 times longer than normal. The lesions become progressively more proliferative and less painful with time. Mature lesions are irregular wart-like growths or filamentous papillae that measure 0.5-1.0 mm in diameter, 1 mm to 3 cm in length, and are pale yellow, gray, or brown.

The early *microscopic changes* of papillomatous digital dermatitis consist of mild epidermal hyperplasia with *foci of erosion, necrosis, marked intracellular edema*, and microabscesses. The basal layer exhibits an increased mitotic index. The dermis contains minimal perivascular inflammation. Mixed bacteria may be present in the outer necrotic debris, but only spirochetes are present in the deeper viable epidermis. Two morphologically distinct spirochetes have been demonstrated to be in large numbers in early lesions. One is a long thin type with few twists, and the other is a short, thick spirochete with many twists. The spirochetes are oriented perpendicular to the epidermis and appear to invade the keratinocytes. The older lesions are composed of frond-like projections or plaques of markedly hyperplastic epidermis with parakeratotic hyperkeratosis. *Foci of necrosis and hemorrhage, marked intracellular edema, and aggregates of neutrophils are scattered throughout the hyperplastic epidermis.* At this later stage, inflammation is more intense in the dermis, and plasma cells may be numerous.

Further reading

Bennett G, et al. *Dichelobacter nodosus, Fusobacterium necrophorum* and the epidemiology of footrot. Anaerobe 2009;15:173-176.

Kennan RM, et al. The pathogenesis of ovine footrot. Vet Microbiol 2011;153:59-66.

Moe KK, et al. Detection of treponemes in canker lesions of horses by 16S rRNA clonal sequencing analysis. J Vet Med Sci 2010;72:235-239.

Rasmussen M, et al. Bovine digital dermatitis: possible pathogenic consortium consisting of *Dichelobacter nodosus* and multiple *Treponema* species. Vet Microbiol 2012;160:151-161.

Scott DW. Color Atlas of Farm Animal Dermatology. Ames, Iowa: Blackwell; 2007.

Porcine ear necrosis syndrome

Porcine ear necrosis syndrome (PENS, ulcerative spirochetosis of the ear) is a condition of 8-9 week-old pigs (weaners). The pathogenesis is uncertain, but **spirochetes** are often isolated from these lesions. In one study, some isolates were identified as *Treponema* spp. *Staphylococcus hyicus*, β-hemolytic streptococci, and *Trueperella pyogenes* have also been isolated from these lesions but are thought to be secondary invaders. In another study, in addition to many cases with *Staphylococcus* and *Streptococcus* isolated, 7 piglets were positive for porcine reproductive and respiratory syndrome virus, one was positive for *Mycoplasma*, one had antibodies to *Sarcoptes scabiei* var. *suis*, and in 15 samples, no infectious agents were detected. Mycotoxins were detected in some of the feed samples. *These results suggest that PENS is multifactorial with no one triggering factor.*

Grossly, lesions begin as bilateral small erythematous areas at the base of the pinnae that progress to *necrosis* and can involve the *entire length of the margin of the pinna.* The pinnae are bilaterally thickened and may be discolored gray, red, or black. The lesions are covered by thick flat crusts. *Histologically,* there is *vasculitis* of the arterioles and venules characterized by hyaline degeneration, medial hypertrophy, and thrombosis, with suppurative dermatitis, epidermal hyperplasia, hyperkeratosis, ulcerations, and crusts. Some lesions may be granulomatous. Spirochetes can be seen with silver stains (modified Steiner) at the junction of granulation tissue and necrosis in some cases. Coccoid or coccobacilli bacteria are frequently seen on the surface in early lesions and in the dermis in chronic lesions. Differential diagnoses for pinnal necrosis in pigs are ear biting, erysipelas, and septicemia.

Further reading

Pringle M, et al. Isolation of spirochetes of genus *Treponema* from pigs with ear necrosis. Vet Microbiol 2009;139:279-283.

Weissenbacher-Lang C, et al. Porcine ear necrosis syndrome: a preliminary investigation of putative infectious agents in piglets and mycotoxins in feed. Vet J 2012;194:392-397.

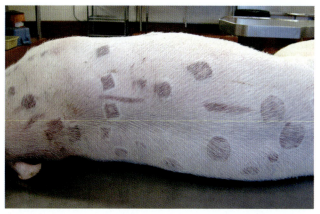

Figure 6-98 Linear, round, and diamond skin lesions in ***Erysipelothrix rhusiopathiae*** infection in a pig. (Courtesy L.L. Pittman.)

Skin lesions in systemic bacterial disease

Skin lesions may develop during the course of systemic bacterial infection. They frequently arise *as a result of vasculitis and/or thrombosis*. This occurs most commonly in **pigs.** Swine erysipelas is caused by *Erysipelothrix rhusiopathiae*, a facultative, non–spore-forming, small, gram-positive bacillus. Pigs 3 months to 3 years of age are most commonly affected. Swine erysipelas is seen in 3 forms: *acute, subacute, and chronic.*

- Acute erysipelas is characterized by general signs of septicemia and sudden death. There is depression, anorexia, lameness, and blue-to-purple discoloration of the skin, especially the abdomen, pinnae, and legs. Pink to red macules and papules may be seen.
- In the subacute form, animals do not appear sick and have erythematous papules and wheals that enlarge to form square, rectangular, or rhomboid plaques ("diamond skin disease") (Fig. 6-98).
- In the chronic form, there is necrosis and sloughing of the plaques, resulting in black, dry, firm areas of skin that peel away to reveal ulcers. Distal extremities may slough.

Microscopic findings include marked dermal congestion, *neutrophilic vasculitis, cutaneous necrosis, and suppurative hydradenitis.* Erysipelas is a zoonosis and is of great economic importance in the swine industry because multiple animals are usually affected. Various gram-negative septicemias, in particular septicemic salmonellosis caused by *S. choleraesuis*, may produce blue-purple discoloration of the skin of the ears, ventral abdomen, snout, and tail, primarily as a result of *endotoxin-induced venous thrombosis. Pasteurella multocida* may cause similar skin lesions in pigs. *Edema disease*, caused by a hemolytic *Escherichia coli*, may be associated with subcutaneous edema secondary to vascular hyaline degeneration, fibrinoid necrosis, and mural edema. *Shiga toxin 2e* (verotoxin 2e) damages the endothelium and tunica media of vessels.

Skin lesions occur less commonly in other domestic species with systemic bacterial infection. *Salmonella enterica* ser. Dublin infections in **cattle** may produce gangrene of distal extremities, tail, and pinnae as a consequence of vascular thrombosis. Cutaneous salmonellosis secondary to septicemia has also been described in horses.

Cutaneous lesions are uncommon in **dogs** with systemic infections. Rocky Mountain spotted fever, caused by *Rickettsia rickettsii*, is most often associated with skin lesions. This organism is transmitted by ticks, *Dermacentor andersoni* and *Dermacentor variabilis*. Cutaneous lesions consist of *petechiae, edema,* necrosis, and ulceration as a result of direct endothelial cell damage and vasculitis. Acral dermal necrosis occurs rarely. Dogs may also have ocular, genital, and oral lesions.

Bartonella

Bartonella spp. are highly fastidious gram-negative intracellular bacterial pathogens that infect erythrocytes, endothelial cells, and macrophages. There are at least 22 species and subspecies, and each is highly adapted to preferential mammalian reservoir hosts in which they cause a long-lasting intraerythrocytic bacteremia. Infection is transmitted via various blood-sucking arthropods. *Bartonella* infection has been described in humans, dogs, and cattle, and *endocarditis* is most common. Various cutaneous manifestations have been rarely reported in dogs. Three dogs were reported to have pyogranulomatous meningoradiculoneuritis and multiple *pyogranulomatous nodular dermatitis or panniculitis* in association with **Bartonella vinsonii subsp. berkhoffi** infection. All 3 dogs responded to surgical decompression and appropriate antibiotic therapy. Another dog with α1-proteinase inhibitor deficiency developed multiple subcutaneous nodules consistent with granulomatous panniculitis, polyarthritis, and meningitis in association with *Bartonella* spp. bacteremia. In these cases, DNA of the organism was found by PCR within the blood but not in the skin lesions.

Several species of *Bartonella*, including *B. vinsonii* subsp. *berkhoffii* and *B. henselae*, have been shown to cause proliferative vascular diseases in animals. *B. vinsonii* subsp. *berkhoffii* induces activation of hypoxia-inducible factor-1 and production of vascular endothelial growth factor. A dog undergoing immunosuppressive therapy for pancytopenia was diagnosed with **bacillary angiomatosis** caused by *B. vinsonii* subsp. *berkhoffii*. This dog developed multiple erythematous, raised round, variably alopecic, papular to nodular lesions, 5-13 mm in diameter, in the skin of the trunk, limbs, face, and footpads. *Histologically*, the lesions were located in the subcutis and composed of *multifocal proliferations of capillaries* lined by plump endothelium with areas of *fibrinoid degeneration*. Capillary clusters were separated by edematous connective tissue and lightly infiltrated by degenerate inflammatory cells, including neutrophils and macrophages. Warthin-Starry silver stain showed large numbers of bacilli consistent with *Bartonella*. Bacillary angiomatosis has also been described in immunocompromised humans, and in those cases, like this one, bacteria can be seen with silver stains.

Borreliosis

Borreliosis (Lyme disease) is caused by **Borrelia burgdorferi**, a gram-negative spirochete that is transmitted from small rodents to mammals by *Ixodes* spp. ticks. The predominant clinical sign in all species is polyarthritis. **Borrelia-associated cutaneous pseudolymphoma** has been reported in humans and a horse. Cutaneous pseudolymphoma is a benign self-limiting lymphoproliferative condition in the skin causing papular to nodular asymptomatic lesions. The reported horse was a 10-year-old Belgian-Warmblood mare with multiple, 2-7 mm, dermal papules over the right masseter. The lesions were not alopecic, ulcerated, or painful. The lymphatics around the lesions and the right mandibular lymph node were enlarged. *Microscopically*, there was a dermal infiltrate composed of small mature CD3+ T cells, CD79a+ B cells, and small numbers of eosinophils with aggregates of CD79a+ B cells and clusters of larger blastic CD3+ T cells around capillaries with hyperplastic endothelial cells (postcapillary high-endothelial venule). *B. burgdorferi* was detected in the horse's serum by ELISA and Western blot and in the skin biopsy by PCR.

In humans, a characteristic expanding ring-like macule or papule (erythema chronicum migrans) is the most common cutaneous lesion associated with Lyme borreliosis and develops 1-2 weeks post–tick bite. This lesion has been reported in dogs, although no histologic studies were performed, and this lesion has not been experimentally reproduced in dogs. Rarely, seropositive dogs are described to have urticaria, rash, or moist dermatitis. Tetracycline-responsive pyotraumatic dermatitis has been described in seropositive dogs.

Further reading

Beerlage C, et al. *Bartonella vinsonii* subsp. *berkhoffii* and *Bartonella henselae* as potential causes of proliferative vascular diseases in animals. Med Microbiol Immunol 2012;201:319-326.

Lloyd D. Bacterial skin disease. In: Miller WH, et al., editors. Muller & Kirk's Small Animal Dermatology. 7th ed. St Louis: Elsevier; 2013. p. 184-222.

Scott DW, Miller WH. Bacterial skin disease. In: Scott DW, Miller WH, editors. Equine Dermatology. 2nd ed. St Louis: Elsevier Saunders; 2011. p. 130-170.

Sears KP, et al. A case of *Borrelia*-associated cutaneous pseudolymphoma in a horse. Vet Dermatol 2011;23:153-156.

Wang Q, et al. *Erysipelothrix rhusiopathiae*. Vet Microbiol 2010;140: 405-417.

FUNGAL DISEASES OF SKIN

Fungi are ubiquitous in the environment, but of the thousands present, only a few are capable of causing infection in animals. The vast majority of fungi in nature are incapable of causing infection because they are unable to breach 2 major physiologic barriers to fungal growth in tissue: temperature and oxidation-reduction potential. Many fungi have an optimal growth range considerably below the temperature of the body and cannot survive the relatively high temperature of the body. Other fungi are thermotolerant. The propensity of fungi to cause infection is dependent not only on their ability to adapt to the tissue environment and temperature, but also to withstand the lytic activity of the host's cellular defenses. Some fungi are *true pathogens* with the ability to cause disease in normal individuals, whereas many more organisms are *opportunistic pathogens* that infect individuals who have become immunologically or otherwise compromised and are unable to resist and suppress the fungal invasion. Immunocompromise by various infectious agents, as well as pharmacologic immunosuppression, are important predisposing factors in development of some fungal infections. However, many mycotic infections occur in individuals without any clinically overt immune impairment. These infections are likely a consequence of an overwhelming exposure to the infectious propagules or mild immunologic defects that are not readily apparent. Mycotic infections are commonly divided into 3 categories: cutaneous, subcutaneous, and systemic.

- **Cutaneous mycoses** are the most common fungal diseases in veterinary medicine. The infections are generally confined to the nonliving cornified layers of the skin, hair, and claws.

- **Subcutaneous mycoses** are fungal infections that involve the skin and subcutaneous tissues. They are caused by a wide variety of saprophytic fungi that gain entry by traumatic implantation. Infection is a very indolent process and usually remains localized to the site of entry with slow spread to surrounding tissue.
- **Systemic mycoses** are infections of the internal organs. Cutaneous involvement usually occurs as a result of hematogenous dissemination. Skin lesions from direct cutaneous inoculation in systemic mycoses are rare. These infections include blastomycosis, cryptococcosis, coccidioidomycosis, and histoplasmosis. Occasionally, the diagnosis of a systemic fungal infection/mycosis, particularly blastomycosis in dogs and cryptococcosis in cats, is made by biopsy of skin lesions.

Histopathology is an important diagnostic tool for fungal infections. It is a relatively rapid and inexpensive means to make a definitive or presumptive diagnosis of mycotic infection. In many cases, fungal infections are mistaken for neoplasms, and the entire lesion is fixed and submitted for histologic examination. Consequently, only fixed tissue is available, and the pathologist has the responsibility for the final diagnosis because the organism cannot be cultured. Some fungal organisms have distinctive enough morphologic features that, if present in sufficient numbers, they can be identified with a high degree of certainty, for instance, *Blastomyces*, *Cryptococcus*, and *Coccidioides*. Other mycotic infections are caused by a variety of fungi that are similar in appearance in tissues and cannot be specifically identified, although the disease can be named, for instance, dermatophytosis, phaeohyphomycosis, and eumycotic mycetoma. In some cases, fungi may be detectable in tissues but may be impossible to identify, and only the conclusion that mycotic infection exists can be made. Although immunofluorescence and immunohistochemical methods for identification of fungi in formalin-fixed, paraffin-embedded tissue sections have been developed, the specific antisera are not readily available, and *culture remains the mainstay for identification of fungal pathogens*. Some fungi stain with H&E, but many fungi do not stain or stain very poorly with H&E. However, even in these cases, fungal infection can be suspected because of the presence of clear circular or linear structures, representing unstained fungal hyphae, within the lesion. *Special fungal stains*, such as Gomori methenamine silver (GMS), which stains fungi black, PAS, which stains fungi pink-red, delineate the fungi so that their morphology can be examined. In general, GMS is better for screening tissue because some fungal-like organisms (e.g., *Pythium*) stain poorly with PAS. Fungal stains may mask the natural color of fungi, however. To determine whether a fungus is pigmented, it can be examined in unstained cleared and mounted sections, or a melanin stain, such as Fontana-Masson, can be applied to the tissue.

Further reading

Guarner J, Brandt ME. Histopathologic diagnosis of fungal infections in the 21st century. Clin Microbiol Rev 2011;24:247-280.

Cutaneous fungal infections

Cutaneous mycoses are infections in which the fungal organisms are generally confined to the nonliving keratinized tissues, that is, *stratum corneum, hair, claw, and horn*. Pathologic changes, which occur in response to the infectious agent and its metabolic products, involve the epidermis and dermis and may vary from minimal to severe and extensive. These infections include candidiasis, *Malassezia* dermatitis, and dermatophytosis.

Candidiasis

Candidiasis (candidosis, moniliasis, thrush) is a rare opportunistic infection of skin, mucocutaneous junctions, external ear canal, and the claw bed. Candida spp. yeasts are normal inhabitants of the upper respiratory, alimentary, and genital tracts but are not normally present on the skin except at mucocutaneous junctions of body orifices. Factors that alter the superficial keratin barrier (such as maceration, chronic trauma, or burns), upset normal flora (such as prolonged broad spectrum antibiotic therapy), or produce immunosuppression (such as diabetes mellitus, hyperadrenocorticism, neoplasia, viral infections, cytotoxic chemotherapy, or prolonged glucocorticoid treatment) predispose to infection with the organism. Because neutrophils are a major defense mechanism against *Candida*, prolonged neutropenia renders an individual more susceptible to candidiasis. The other major mechanism for eliminating *Candida* from the skin surface is T-cell–mediated immunity.

Cutaneous infections have been described in *dogs, cats, pigs, horses, goats, and a llama*. Lesions are variable and may begin as erythematous papules, pustules, and vesicles, which evolve into crusts and characteristic *sharply delineated ulcers with erythematous borders and a malodorous surface with moist gray-white exudate*. Chronic lesions consist of thickened alopecic hyperkeratotic skin with prominent folds. Histologic changes include hyperkeratosis, parakeratosis, serocellular crusts, subcorneal or superficial epidermal neutrophilic pustules, and spongiosis. The dermis is edematous and contains a superficial perivascular to interstitial mixed infiltrate. *Yeasts, pseudohyphae, and hyphae may be numerous but are best visualized with PAS or GMS stains.* Generally, yeasts are most numerous on the surface of the lesions, whereas hyphae and pseudohyphae extend into the epidermis.

Infection with *Candida guilliermondii* is reported in a horse with multiple firm painful cutaneous nodules. *Histologically, there was nodular granulomatous dermatitis with numerous budding 2-6 μm blastoconidia within macrophages and multinucleated histiocytic giant cells.*

Further reading

Lamm CG, et al. Pathology in practice. J Am Vet Med Assoc 2009;234:1013-1015.

Mueller RS, et al. Cutaneous candidiasis in a dog caused by *Candida guilliermondii*. Vet Rec 2002;150:728-730.

Scott DW, Miller WH. Fungal skin diseases. In: Scott DW, Miller WH, editors. Equine Dermatology. 2nd ed. St Louis: Elsevier Saunders; 2011. p. 171-211.

Malassezia dermatitis

The genus *Malassezia* consists of at least 13 species of lipophilic yeasts, which are components of the cutaneous microflora of many mammals, including humans. ***Malassezia pachydermatis*** is the only species that does not require lipid supplementation during culture in vitro and is thus characterized as lipophilic, non–lipid dependent. All other species are lipid dependent. Of all the species, *M. pachydermatis* is most commonly associated with skin disease in dogs and cats. It is also the species most commonly isolated from the skin, mucosa, and ear canals of healthy dogs and cats. When associated with skin disease, it is currently believed that *Malassezia* infection is due to *overgrowth of normal flora resulting from disturbances of the normal physical, chemical, or immunologic mechanisms controlling the skin surface microenvironment and host defenses*. *Virulence factors* associated with *M. pachydermatis* include the production of various *hydrolases*, including lipases, phospholipases, aspartyl proteases, and acid sphingomyelinases. Isolates of *M. pachydermatis* have also been shown to form biofilms on surfaces of various materials.

Malassezia dermatitis is most common in **dogs**. Greater than 70% of dogs have concurrent dermatoses, including allergies, keratinization defects, endocrinopathies, and bacterial pyoderma. Predisposed breeds include West Highland White Terrier, Bassett Hound, American Cocker Spaniel, Shih Tzu, English Setter, Toy and Miniature Poodle, Boxer, Cavalier King Charles Spaniel, Australian and Silky Terriers, German Shepherd dog, and Dachshund. Excessive surface lipid or cerumen, high humidity, or failure of host defense mechanisms to control overgrowth of the yeast may predispose an animal to develop clinical disease. Dogs with *Malassezia* dermatitis develop high serum titers of specific IgG antibody and exhibit significantly greater skin test reactions in response to intradermal injection of *M. pachydermatis* extracts than dogs without evidence of *Malassezia* dermatitis, suggesting that *hypersensitivity may be involved in the pathogenesis of clinical disease*. Lesions associated with *Malassezia* dermatitis include erythema, alopecia, greasiness, yellow-gray scaly plaques, lichenification, and hyperpigmentation (Fig. 6-99A). A rancid offensive odor is typical, and moderate to severe pruritus is a common feature. Lesions may be localized or generalized, and the most common sites include lips, ear canals, axillae, groin, ventral neck, inguinal area, interdigital skin, perianal area, and intertriginous regions. *Malassezia* paronychia and/or claw infections produce red-brown discoloration of paronychial hairs or claws (Fig. 6-99B). Involvement of one or several of these areas is more common than generalized disease.

Malassezia dermatitis in **cats** is less common and is generally associated with black ceruminous otitis externa, chronic chin acne, facial dermatitis with large dark brown to black scales and follicular casts, with refractory paronychia, or generalized erythematous scaly to waxy dermatitis. Devon Rex and Sphynx cats have been shown to have a higher *Malassezia* spp. colonization compared to other breeds of cats. Devon Rex cats may be predisposed to greasy seborrheic dermatitis associated with increased *Malassezia* colonization and paronychia. In cats, *Malassezia* dermatitis is an opportunistic infection, and it has been associated with localized exfoliative dermatitis, chin acne, idiopathic facial dermatitis of Persian cats, allergic dermatitis, thymoma-associated dermatitis, paraneoplastic alopecia, and in cats with feline leukemia virus and feline immunodeficiency virus infections.

Malassezia dermatitis is uncommon in **goats**. Poor nutrition and debilitating underlying disease appear to be predisposing factors. Lesions are nonpruritic to mildly pruritic and nonpainful, and are characterized by erythema, hyperpigmentation, scale, greasiness, yellow waxy crusts, and lichenification. Lesions are multifocal, often over the back and trunk, and typically become generalized but tend to spare the head and legs.

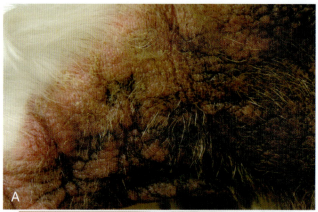
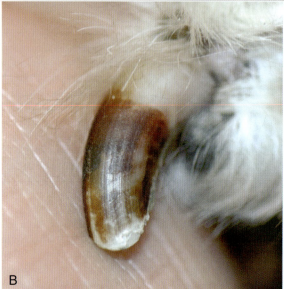
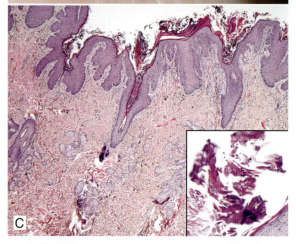

Figure 6-99 *Malassezia* dermatitis in a dog. **A.** The skin is erythematous, alopecic, lichenified, hyperpigmented, and covered with some scale. (Courtesy W.H. Miller.) **B.** Red-brown discoloration of claw. (Courtesy W.H. Miller.) **C.** Skin biopsy shows irregular epidermal hyperplasia with parakeratotic hyperkeratosis, superficial interstitial dermatitis, and hyperplastic sebaceous glands in disarray. *Malassezia* spp. yeast can be seen within the surface keratin (see inset).

Malassezia dermatitis is rarely reported in **horses.** As in dogs and cats, it is associated with pruritic, greasy to waxy, occasionally foul-smelling dermatitis in intertriginous areas, including axillae, groin, udder, and prepuce. Predisposing conditions include humidity, hormonal alterations, keratinization defects, hypersensitivity disorders, immunosuppressive disease, and immunosuppressive therapy. One horse diagnosed with *Malassezia* dermatitis had concurrent alopecia areata.

Malassezia otitis externa is common in **cattle** in South America. There is a ceruminous to suppurative otitis externa caused by predominantly thermotolerant *M. sympodialis* in the summer and a predominantly less thermotolerant species, *M. globosa* in the winter.

Histologic features of *Malassezia* dermatitis of dogs consist of multifocal parakeratotic hyperkeratosis, irregular epidermal hyperplasia, intercellular edema (spongiosis), and lymphocytic and eosinophilic exocytosis (Fig. 6-99C). In dogs, intraepidermal eosinophilic microabscesses, pigmentary incontinence, and subepidermal linear accumulation of mast cells may be seen. There is variable edema and perivascular to interstitial infiltration of mixed cells (lymphocytes, plasma cells, histiocytes, eosinophils) in the superficial dermis. *Malassezia* organisms are *oval to footprint- or peanut-shaped 2 × 4–µm yeasts located in the stratum corneum or in crusts* (see Fig. 6-99C inset). They are usually seen in focal aggregates rather than diffusely distributed, and they can best be visualized with PAS or GMS stains. The organism will be missed if the skin surface was scrubbed prior to obtaining the biopsy or if the surface debris is lost during processing. Histologic findings in **cats** and **horses** are probably similar, but reports are few. In **goats,** there tends to be marked surface and follicular orthokeratotic hyperkeratosis and mild lymphocytic perivascular dermatitis. Numerous budding yeasts are seen, which is in contrast to few or none seen in biopsy samples from other species.

Further reading

Eguchi-Coe Y, et al. Putative *Malassezia* dermatitis in six goats. Vet Dermatol 2011;22:497-501.

Miller WH, et al. Fungal and algal skin diseases. In: Miller WH, et al., editors. Muller & Kirk's Small Animal Dermatology. 7th ed. St Louis: Elsevier; 2013. p. 184-222.

Nardoni S, et al. Occurrence, distribution and population size of *Malassezia pachydermatis* on skin and mucosae of atopic dogs. Vet Microbiol 2007;122:172-177.

Ordeix L, et al. *Malassezia* spp. overgrowth in allergic cats. Vet Dermatol 2007;18:316-323.

Scott DW, Miller WH. Fungal skin diseases. In: Scott DW, Miller WH, editors. Equine Dermatology. 2nd ed. St Louis: Elsevier Saunders; 2011. p. 171-211.

Dermatophytosis

Dermatophytosis ("ringworm") is a highly contagious, zoonotic, superficial fungal infection generally confined to the keratin layers of the skin, hair, and claws, affecting cats, cattle, horses, dogs, goats, pigs, sheep, and rarely alpacas. In rare instances, deeper tissues are involved. The infection is caused by fungi of the genera *Microsporum, Trichophyton,* and *Epidermophyton,* which are cosmopolitan in distribution. They are commonly divided according to the host preference and natural habitat of the fungus.

- **Geophilic** dermatophytes are normal soil inhabitants. The most common species to infect dogs and cats is *Microsporum gypseum.*
- **Zoophilic** dermatophytes (e.g., *M. canis, M. equinum, T. equinum*) are adapted to living on animals and are rarely found in the soil. They occasionally infect humans.
- **Sylvatic** dermatophytes (e.g., *T. mentagrophytes, M. persicolor*) are zoophilic dermatophytes adapted to living on rodents or hedgehogs.
- **Anthropophilic** dermatophytes (e.g., *T. tonsurans, T. rubrum*) are primarily adapted to humans and do not survive in the soil. Animals occasionally develop infections with these organisms as a reverse zoonosis from infected humans.

Incidence and prevalence of dermatophytosis vary with individual host factors, health status, climate, season, natural reservoirs, and local environment. Predisposing host factors for dermatophyte infection include young age, stress, poor nutrition, debilitating disease, compromised immune status, and areas of chronically warm moist skin. Environmental factors include hot, humid weather, with wet, poorly ventilated unsanitary conditions, and decreased exposure to sunlight. Transmission of dermatophytes occurs by direct contact with infected animals or indirectly by exposure to infective hair and scales in the environment (contaminated grooming equipment, bedding, saddles, cages, etc.). *Hair fragments containing infectious arthrospores are the most effective means of transmission.* They can remain infectious for more than 18 months if protected from the deleterious effects of ultraviolet light. This material is the major source of persistent environmental contamination. Certain dermatophytes are associated with specific sources. *M. canis,* despite its name, is most commonly associated with cats, and the cat is considered the reservoir for this dermatophyte. *T. mentagrophytes* dermatophytosis is typically acquired from small rodents; infection with *M. gypseum* is assumed to be acquired from digging or rooting in contaminated soil.

Normal skin is relatively inhospitable to fungal growth because of low moisture conditions, antifungal substances in the surface film, and normal resident flora. Sebum contains fatty acids that are fungistatic and play an important role in resistance to infection. The process by which the stratum corneum (SC) is continually renewed may also present a form of defense against organisms because the process results in continuous shedding of the SC and thus removes infecting organisms with the sloughed keratin. Disruption of the SC, either by microabrasions or maceration, appears to be important in facilitating invasion by the fungus. Fungal cells adhere to keratinocytes and migrate to the follicular orifice. Dermatophytes produce keratinolytic enzymes, endoproteases, and exoproteases, which hydrolyze keratin and enable them to penetrate and invade the hair shaft. They grow downward within the hair shaft toward the hair bulb until they reach the keratogenous zone (Adamson's fringe), where they stop because they cannot grow in viable tissue. Infection continues as long as the downward growth of the fungus is in equilibrium with keratin production; if not, the fungus is sloughed and the hair is cleared of infection. When the hair enters telogen phase, keratin production stops and fungal growth ceases. Hair shafts are weakened as a result of penetration by the fungi, and they become brittle and easily broken.

Dermatophytosis in healthy individuals is *usually self-limiting,* with lesions resolving in several weeks to 2-3 months.

Chronic dermatophyte infections have been reported in dogs. *Trichophyton* spp. and *M. persicolor* dermatophyte infections, lasting up to 5 years in some cases, have been described in dogs without any other evidence of immunodeficiency, suggesting that these organisms may produce inhibitory substances that prevent development of an effective immune response and elimination of the organism.

The *clinical signs* of dermatophytosis are highly variable and depend on the host-fungus interaction. Pruritus varies from absent to severe. Well-adapted species, such as *M. canis* infection in cats, produce minimal inflammation, whereas less-adapted species, such as the zoophilic dermatophyte *M. gypseum*, produce more significant inflammation and more prominent lesions. *Expanding circular patches of scaling and alopecia or stubbled hairs are considered the classic lesion of dermatophytosis.* Follicular papules and pustules, more extensive inflammation caused by furunculosis, and crusting are prominent in some cases. Lesions are typically nonpruritic, but occasionally pruritus is intense. *Infection of claws is called* **onychomycosis** and is characterized by misshapen, crumbly or easily broken, and split claws that may be sloughed. **Kerions** are rapidly developing tender erythematous alopecic nodules that may ulcerate and develop draining tracts. They are usually solitary and most common on the face and forelimbs of dogs that dig in the dirt (Fig. 6-100A). These lesions result from *severe furunculosis* producing locally extensive inflammation that may be confused for a tumor. A rare form, the **dermatophytic pseudomycetoma** seen almost exclusively in Persian cats, occurs as *subcutaneous nodules*.

The microscopic lesions of dermatophytosis are as variable as the clinical lesions. *Histopathology is not considered as sensitive as culture for diagnosis*, but it can be used to confirm infection when the significance of a cultured organism is in question. It is most useful in the nodular forms, such as kerion and pseudomycetoma, which are frequently negative when superficial material is cultured. Biopsies should be taken within the outer border of expanding alopecia as this is the most active site of infection, and organisms are most likely to be present. In most cases, fungal organisms are evident in H&E-stained sections, but *in some instances, fungal stains (PAS, GMS) are necessary to demonstrate infection*. Dermatophytes occur as septate hyphae that break up into chains of round to oval arthrospores in the surface and follicular keratin. *Hyphae are also usually present in the hair shafts, and arthrospores are formed on the outside of the hairs (ectothrix) or within the hairs (endothrix).* In some cases, fungal organisms are present only in the surface keratin (*T. mentagrophytes* and *M. persicolor* in dogs); if this material was removed in preparing the skin for obtaining the biopsy or is lost during tissue processing, the diagnosis will be missed. *Orthokeratotic and parakeratotic hyperkeratosis* is a typical feature of dermatophytosis, and acanthosis is variable, ranging from mild to marked (Fig. 6-101A). Inflammation may be very mild and consist of low numbers of perivascular and perifollicular lymphocytes and macrophages (Fig. 6-101B). This is the case when infection is caused by a species of dermatophyte that is well adapted to its host. *Neutrophilic luminal folliculitis* is a common lesion in dermatophytosis and may result in *follicular rupture and development of discrete granulomas* surrounding fragments of hair at the base of the follicles (Fig. 6-101C). *Eosinophils* may be numerous in these trichogranulomas. Kerions consist of diffuse pyogranulomatous inflammation in the deep dermis produced by extensive furunculosis (see Fig. 6-100B). This form of

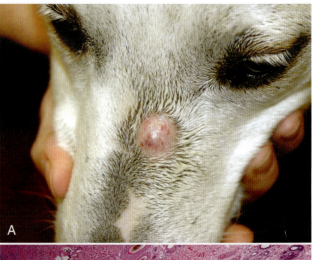

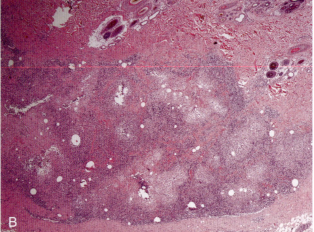

Figure 6-100 Dermatophytosis. A. Kerion on the muzzle of a dog. (Courtesy W.H. Miller.) **B.** Multifocal furunculosis grouped together forming a pyogranulomatous nodular dermatitis.

inflammation is most commonly caused by poorly adapted organisms, such as the geophilic dermatophyte *M. gypseum*. Hair fragments containing hyphae and arthrospores are frequently present among the inflammatory cells but may be destroyed by the intense inflammatory reaction. *In some cases, the pattern of inflammation may be confused with autoimmune diseases.* Lymphocytic lichenoid interface dermatitis, lymphocytic mural folliculitis, and subcorneal pustules containing neutrophils and acantholytic cells have been reported in several cases of dermatophytosis in dogs and horses; however, organisms were evident with fungal stains. The *dermatophytic pseudomycetoma* is characterized by masses of fungal elements surrounded by granulomatous or pyogranulomatous inflammation in the deep dermis and subcutis.

Cattle. Dermatophytosis is *common* in cattle and is most prevalent in calves. *T. verrucosum* is the most frequent isolate; others include *T. mentagrophytes, T. equinum, M. gypseum, M. nanum,* and *M. canis*. Outbreaks are associated with *crowding and confinement indoors during fall and winter*. Lesions occur on the *neck, head, pinnae, and pelvic area* most commonly. The intermandibular space and dewlap are common sites for lesions in bulls. Lesions vary from tufted papules to *circular areas of alopecia with variable crusting or scaling* (Fig. 6-102). In calves, the entire neck may become alopecic, crusty,

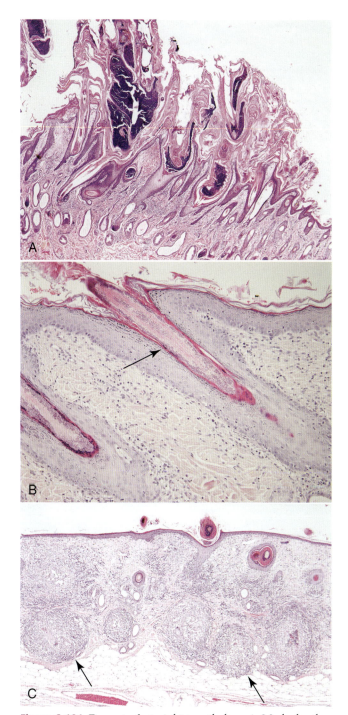

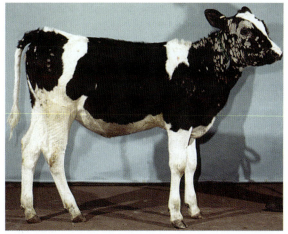

Figure 6-102 **Dermatophytosis** in a calf. Annular, thick, gray crusts predominantly on the face and neck. (Courtesy D.W. Scott.)

Figure 6-101 **Dermatophytosis** histopathology. **A.** Marked orthokeratotic and parakeratotic hyperkeratosis with suppurative luminal folliculitis in a calf. **B.** Mild lymphocytic mural folliculitis with intraluminal dermatophytes (arrow) in a dog. **C.** Multiple trichogranulomas (arrows) in a dog.

thickened, and corrugated. Pruritus is rare. The disease may be of some economic significance because of damage to hides or restrictions on showing or marketing of infected animals. In very severe cases, loss of condition and weight loss or decreased milk production may result.

Sheep and goats. Dermatophytosis is *common* in goats but *uncommon* in sheep and is most commonly caused by *T. verrucosum*. Lesions of annular areas of alopecia, scaling, erythema, and yellow crusts are usually on the *head, face, pinnae, neck, and limbs* in goats. In sheep, *T. verrucosum* typically affects the *haired areas of the head, face, and pinnae*, whereas *M. canis* and *M. gypseum* are more likely to affect the *wooled areas*, with lesions characterized by *matted wool with brown crusts and exudates*. Infection in show lambs in the United States has been most commonly associated with *M. gypseum*. Pruritus and pain are uncommon.

Pigs. Dermatophytosis is uncommon in pigs and most commonly caused by *M. nanum. T. verrucosum* occurs in pigs housed in premises previously occupied by cattle. Infections also are also caused by *T. mentagrophytes, M. canis*, and *M. gypseum*. The lesions of *M. nanum* are especially common on the face, behind the pinnae, and on the trunk, and consist of irregular dark patches with fine brown scales or crusts. Alopecia and pruritus are rare. Lesions may resolve spontaneously or spread slowly to involve extensive areas.

Horses. Dermatophytosis is common in the horse *(girth itch, tinea)* and is caused by a variety of organisms but most frequently by *T. equinum*. Infections with *T. mentagrophytes* and *M. gypseum* are also common; *T. verrucosum* and *M. canis* infections are less frequent. Outbreaks of dermatophytosis caused by *M. gypseum* have been associated with periods of humid weather and a high prevalence of mosquitoes and stable flies. In some training establishments, >30% of the horses have ringworm, and the causative agent is *M. gypseum*. Lesions occur most often in *areas in contact with the saddle and tack: face, neck, dorsolateral thorax, and girth*. In some cases, the caudal aspect of the pastern may be the only site affected and resembles "grease heel" or "scratches." The mane and tail areas are not usually affected. Initial lesions may be tufted papules and resemble fly bites or urticaria, but within several days, they become the more typical scaly or crusty circular alopecic foci. Pruritus varies from severe to absent. Lesions may continue to expand for 1-2 months and then regress as an immune response develops. Several horses with *T. equinum* dermatophytosis that resembled pemphigus foliaceus have been described. Two adult horses developed rapidly progressive painful widespread dermatitis consisting of papules, pustules, crusting, scaling, and erosions. Microscopically, lesions were characterized by prominent acantholysis. However, fungal arthrospores and hyphae were also evident and lesions resolved with antifungal therapy.

Dogs. *M. canis* is considered the most common cause of dermatophytosis in dogs, but in some areas, infections caused by *M. gypseum* predominate. *T. mentagrophytes* infection is less frequent. Infections with anthropophilic species *Epidermophyton floccosum* and *T. rubrum* have been reported and suspected to have been acquired from infected humans. Dermatophyte infections are most often localized, with lesions occurring most commonly on the face, pinnae, paws, and tail. Most cases are seen in dogs <1 year of age. However, sylvatic ringworm is more common in adults. Most cases of dermatophytosis in dogs are follicular, and thus lesions are most commonly one or more peripherally expanding circular patches of alopecia with variable papules, pustules, scaling, and crust.

The lesions of dermatophytosis are grossly indistinguishable from demodicosis or bacterial folliculitis. *Trichophyton* infection may result in folliculitis or furunculosis affecting one leg or paw. Infection by *M. persicolor* may produce lesions characterized by prominent scaling but minimal alopecia. This dermatophyte does not invade hair, and thus fungal organisms are seen only in the surface keratin. In some cases, dermatophytosis can occur as generalized greasy scaling resembling seborrhea. Pruritus is usually absent but may be severe in some cases. Cases of dermatophytosis caused by *T. mentagrophytes*, *T. terrestre*, and *M. persicolor* with a very long duration (1-5 years) have been reported. These infections suggest that there is *little tendency for spontaneous resolution in some infections*, a situation analogous to chronic dermatophytosis in humans. Kerions are often associated with *M. gypseum* or *T. mentagrophytes* infections. *Onychomycosis is rare* and may consist of chronic inflammation of the ungual fold or infection of the claw alone, producing deformity or fragility of the claw.

Several cases of *Trichophyton* dermatophytosis with clinical and histologic features resembling pemphigus erythematosus or foliaceus have been reported. These dogs had symmetrical nasal or facial to periocular folliculitis and furunculosis with alopecia and crusting. Rarely lesions are generalized. Microscopically, lesions included *lymphoplasmacytic lichenoid to interface dermatitis with mural folliculitis*, with or without *intraepidermal pustules with acantholytic keratinocytes*, suggestive of an immune-mediated disease. However, fungal elements were demonstrable with fungal stains. *T. mentagrophytes* has been isolated in most cases, and *M. persicolor*, less frequently. These organisms tend to colonize the stratum corneum preferentially over the hair, and thus the lesions are not follicularly oriented. Acantholysis may be due to complement-mediated transepidermal neutrophilic chemotaxis as well as dermatophyte-produced proteolytic enzymes. Some cases lack intraepidermal pustules and acantholysis but have striking interface dermatitis with spreading facial scaling and hair loss (Fig. 6-103A-C).

Certain breeds of dogs may be predisposed to dermatophytosis. In Europe, dermatophyte infections are more common in the Parson Russell Terrier (especially *T. mentagrophytes*), Yorkshire Terrier (especially *M. canis*), and Pekingese (especially *M. canis*). Severe dermatophytosis and dermatophytic pseudomycetoma with lymph node involvement has been reported in Yorkshire Terriers with *M. canis* and *T. mentagrophytes* infections.

Cats. Dermatophytosis is a *common* disease in cats. It is more common in cats than dogs, and longhaired and pedigree cats are at particular risk. Persian and Himalayan cats are

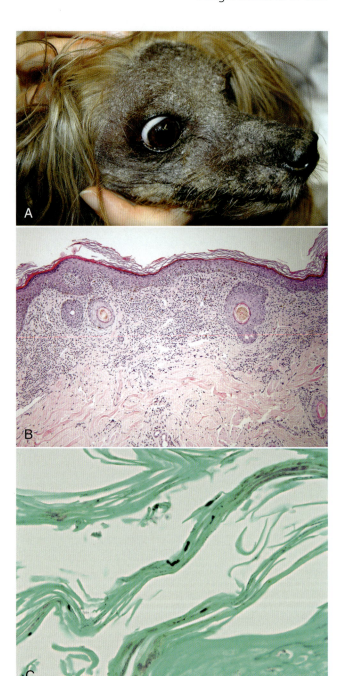

Figure 6-103 *Trichophyton mentagrophytes* in a dog. **A.** Spreading facial alopecia and scaling. **B.** Skin biopsy shows a lichenoid infiltrate with pigmentary incontinence. **C.** Small numbers of fungal hyphae are seen in the surface keratin with a silver stain.

predisposed to *M. canis* dermatophytosis. Infection may be endemic in large catteries, with up to 35% of cats culture positive. The vast majority of cases (>90%) are caused by *M. canis*, which is of considerable public health significance because of its zoonotic potential. Despite the name, this dermatophyte is well adapted to the cat and induces minimal host response. Geographic differences may influence the prevalence of various dermatophytes. A survey of dermatophytes isolated from cats in shelters in the United States found *M. canis* to predominate in the southeastern United States; whereas in cats from the northern United States, anthropophilic organisms were cultured, and *M. canis* was not isolated from any cat.

Lesions are extremely variable. They are most common on the face, pinnae, and paws, and may become generalized. As with dogs, dermatophytosis is more common in cats <1 year of age, but sylvatic ringworm is more common in adults. Pruritus is uncommon but may be moderate. Classic circular foci of alopecia and crusting or scaling are more common in kittens. In adult cats, lesions may be extremely subtle and consist of patchy mild alopecia or broken hairs with little skin change. This is especially true of longhaired cats that may have a poor haircoat and excessive shedding. Scaling and crusting may be absent or severe. Lesions may be hyperpigmented. Recurring chin folliculitis resembling feline acne or dermatitis of the dorsal tail resembling "stud tail" may occur. Focal pruritic lesions that resemble eosinophilic plaques can occur. Kerions are uncommon in cats, but longhaired cats, especially Persian cats, can develop dermatophytic pseudomycetomas, usually over the dorsal trunk or tail base, and tissue grains may be seen.

Widespread, pruritic papulocrustous miliary dermatitis is an uncommon manifestation of *M. canis* infection. Other uncommon clinical presentations associated with *M. canis* are widespread pruritic exfoliative erythroderma, recurrent otitis externa, asymmetrical paronychia or onychodysplasia, generalized seborrhea-like eruptions, and clinical signs suggestive of pemphigus foliaceus with crusting over the bridge of the nose, pinnae, and paronychia.

Microscopic findings are variable. In some cases, organisms are infrequent, and only a single infected hair may be found in a biopsy, whereas in other cases, organisms may be numerous. *Pseudomycetomas* are subcutaneous nodules. They are an atypical form of dermatophytosis caused by *M. canis* in which the deep dermis and subcutis are involved. There is frequently also a history of previous or concurrent superficial dermatophyte infection. Lesions are usually focal and measure 2-3 cm in diameter; but in some instances, they are multiple and may even have systemic lesions. They consist of discrete masses of bizarre, distorted, septate fungal hyphae; larger thick-walled fungal cells resembling *chlamydospores*; and chains of round structures surrounded by a hyaline eosinophilic Splendore-Hoeppli reaction. These granules are surrounded by granulomatous or pyogranulomatous inflammation. Fungal organisms are not necessarily present in the hair and keratin of the overlying skin. In contrast to pseudomycetoma, true mycetomas contain more abundant organisms and have a less pronounced Splendore-Hoeppli reaction.

Further reading

Baldo A, et al. Mechanisms of skin adherence and invasion by dermatophytes. Mycoses 2012;55:218-223.

Bond R. Superficial veterinary mycoses. Clin Dermatol 2010;28:226-236.

García-Sánchez A, et al. Outbreak of ringworm in a traditional Iberian pig farm in Spain. Mycoses 2011;54:179-181.

Miller WH, et al. Fungal and algal skin diseases. In: Miller WH, et al., editors. Muller & Kirk's Small Animal Dermatology. 7th ed. St Louis: Elsevier; 2013. p. 184-222.

Pittman JS, Roberts JD. Ringworm in lactating sows. J Swine Health Prod 2005;13:86-90.

Scott DW. Color Atlas of Farm Animal Dermatology. Ames, Iowa: Blackwell; 2007.

Scott DW, Miller WH. Fungal skin diseases. In: Scott DW, Miller WH, editors. Equine Dermatology. 2nd ed. St Louis: Elsevier Saunders; 2011. p. 171-211.

Subcutaneous fungal infections

Subcutaneous mycoses are fungal infections that have invaded beyond the skin and hair follicles. These infections produce granulomatous to pyogranulomatous inflammation and can be destructive. These are a heterogeneous group of infections caused by a wide variety of *saprophytic fungi* that normally exist in soil or vegetation. Infection generally requires mechanical introduction into tissue. The ability of the organism to adapt to the tissue environment and elicit disease is variable. The clinical course is usually insidiously progressive over a period of months to years. Infection usually remains localized to the site of entry and surrounding tissues. Slow extension by way of lymphatics occurs in some diseases, but widespread dissemination is rare.

- **Mycetoma**: The organism has mycelial morphology in tissue and is surrounded by eosinophilic hyaline material (Splendore-Hoeppli reaction: antigen-antibody complexes) resulting in a macroscopic granule or grain.
  - **Eumycotic**: The cause is fungal.
  - **Actinomycotic**: The cause is a member of the order Actinomycetales, such as *Actinomyces* and *Nocardia*.
  - **Chromomycosis**: A subcutaneous and systemic disease caused by pigmented (dematiaceous) fungi.
    - **Chromoblastomycosis**: The fungus is present in tissue as large (4-15 μm diameter) rounded, dark-walled cells (sclerotic bodies, chromo bodies, Medlar bodies).
    - **Phaeohyphomycosis**: Organisms are pigmented and have mycelial and yeast morphology in tissue.
- **Hyalohyphomycosis**: It is a subcutaneous and systemic disease caused by nondematiaceous (nonpigmented, hyaline) fungi. Organisms have septate branching or nonbranching hyphal (mycelial) tissue morphology.
- **Pseudomycetoma**: The organism is present in tissue as granules or grains, but the formation of the granule is different from that of true mycetomas. Pseudomycetomas are formed by dermatophytes (dermatophytic pseudomycetoma) or bacteria (bacterial pseudomycetoma).

Eumycotic mycetoma

Mycetomas are characterized clinically by the triad of tumefaction (swelling), draining tracts, and grains in the discharge. Eumycotic mycetomas have been reported worldwide but are most frequent near the Tropic of Cancer. They occur in humans, occasionally in dogs and horses, and rarely in cattle and cats. A wide variety of fungi that exist as saprophytes in the soil or on plants have been associated with mycetomas. The organisms involved may also cause other clinical diseases, for instance, phaeohyphomycosis and mycotic granulomas, when all 3 criteria are not present for a diagnosis of a mycetoma. Mycetomas usually involve skin and subcutaneous tissues and sometimes extend to involve underlying bone. *Curvularia* spp. and the *Scedosporium/Pseudallescheria* complex are most commonly involved in mycetomas in animals.

Lesions in animals most frequently occur on the extremities and face. Lesions are usually solitary, but rarely, disseminated infections occur. Lesions begin as small dermal or subcutaneous papules that gradually enlarge to form nodules

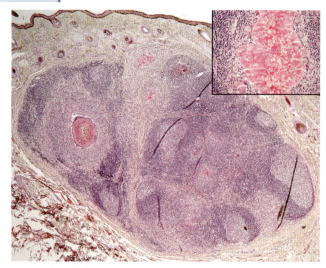

Figure 6-104 **Eumycotic mycetoma** in a horse. Nodular pyogranulomatous dermatitis with multifocal intralesional tangles of fungal hyphae embedded in amorphous eosinophilic material forming white tissue grains (see inset).

over a period of months to years. As the lesion slowly enlarges, they can become alopecic, hyperpigmented, firm, ulcerated, and develop draining tracks. The discharge is serous, purulent, or hemorrhagic and contains tissue grains. *The grains or granules are composed of aggregates of fungal organisms* and vary in size from 0.1 mm to several millimeters in size and may be white, yellow, pink-red, brown, or black. The color, size, shape, and texture of the grains may be sufficiently characteristic to suggest the etiologic agent, but *definitive identification of the fungus requires culture. Curvularia* spp. and *Madurella* spp. have been associated with black-grained mycetomas, whereas the *Scedosporium/Pseudallescheria complex* is usually associated with white grains.

The salient histologic feature is the presence of granules in a tumor-like mass of chronically inflamed tissue. Microscopically, the lesions are characterized by nodular infiltrates of pyogranulomatous to granulomatous inflammation in the subcutis and/or dermis surrounding tissue grains (Fig. 6-104). The grains (0.2-6 mm) are irregularly shaped (spherical, lobular, or scroll-shaped) masses and consist of densely tangled hyphae in the center with an outer rim of chlamydoconidia (terminal cystic dilations, 5-20 μm in diameter). The fungal hyphae may be embedded in an amorphous eosinophilic "cement-like" substance (see Fig. 6-104 inset). The granules of some mycetomas are surrounded by an amorphous eosinophilic radially arranged or smoothly contoured Splendore-Hoeppli reaction. *Fragments of plant material* may be seen within the lesion adjacent to the granules and are suspected to be the vehicle of infection. Nodules are surrounded by a chronic inflammatory reaction consisting of epithelioid macrophages, multinucleated histiocytic giant cells, and fewer plasma cells and lymphocytes. Fibrous connective tissue of variable maturity separates the inflammatory foci. In some cases, *special stains may be needed to determine if the grains are composed of bacteria or fungi.* Culture is the usual means of identification for definitive diagnosis.

Further reading

Elad D, et al. Disseminated pseudallescheriosis in a dog. Med Mycol 2010;48:635-638.

Elad D, et al. Eumycetoma caused by *Madurella mycetomatis* in a mare. Med Mycol 2010;48:639-642.

Elad D. Infections caused by fungi of the *Scedosporium/Pseudallescheria* complex in veterinary species. Vet J 2011;187:33-41.

Miller WH, et al. Fungal and algal skin diseases. In: Miller WH, et al., editors. Muller & Kirk's Small Animal Dermatology. 7th ed. St Louis: Elsevier; 2013. p. 184-222.

Chromomycosis (phaeohyphomycosis and chromoblastomycosis)

Phaeohyphomycosis (chromomycosis) is an uncommon opportunistic subcutaneous, cerebral, or systemic infection caused by a wide variety of fungi that are all characterized by formation of dematiaceous, or pigmented, hyphae and/or yeast in tissue. The pigmentation is due to the presence of melanin, which may act as a virulence factor in the development of infection. The organisms responsible for these infections are numerous and include *Alternaria* spp., *Bipolaris* spp., *Cladosporium* spp., *Curvularia* spp., *Exophiala* spp., *Phialophora* spp., and *Wangiella* spp. These organisms are worldwide in distribution and are widespread in the soil, on wood, and in vegetation. Some of the organisms can also be cultured from the skin of healthy people and animals. Subcutaneous infection is thought to result from wound contamination or traumatic implantation of wood slivers, thorns, sticks, and the like.

Phaeohyphomycosis has been reported most frequently in *cats* and occasionally in *horses, dogs, cattle, and goats*. The disease also occurs in humans. No underlying immune deficiency is apparent in most cases of subcutaneous phaeohyphomycosis, whereas disseminated infections have been associated with immunologic compromise or debilitating disease. German Shepherd dogs may be predisposed. Subcutaneous infection with *Staphylotrichum coccosporum*, a fungus previously thought to be nonpathogenic, was described in a cat positive for feline leukemia virus. Subcutaneous infection is insidiously progressive and evolves over months to years.

Lesions of phaeohyphomycosis consist of *single or multiple subcutaneous nodules*. The *fungal pigmentation may be grossly visible in the tissue* and, in some cases, the nodule is so dark it may be mistaken for a melanoma. In *cats*, lesions are usually single and occur most commonly on the *face (nose and pinnae) and paws.* Firm to fluctuant subcutaneous nodules grow slowly and may be ulcerated or have draining tracts. Multiple recurrences following surgical excision are common. The clinical course in some reported cases has been several years. Lesions in *horses* are frequently multiple and located on several different parts of the body. Occasionally, nodules may be generalized. Multiple ulcerated cutaneous nodules are the usual form of the infection described in *cattle*, and lesions may also be present in the nasal mucosa. Lesions in *dogs* are also frequently multiple and may be extensive. They consist of poorly circumscribed ulcerated or draining nodules or plaques on the paws and legs. In one affected dog, lesions consisted of multiple nodules in the area of ascending lymphatics of a leg and an enlarged regional lymph node, a clinical appearance similar to the cutaneous-lymphatic form of sporotrichosis.

The histologic diagnosis of phaeohyphomycosis is made by demonstrating pigmented hyphae within the tissue. The lesions consist of nodular-to-diffuse pyogranulomatous dermatitis and panniculitis (Fig. 6-105A). The overlying epidermis is acanthotic or multifocally to diffusely ulcerated. Microabscesses with foci of necrosis are frequently prominent. Necrosis may

Fungal Diseases of Skin

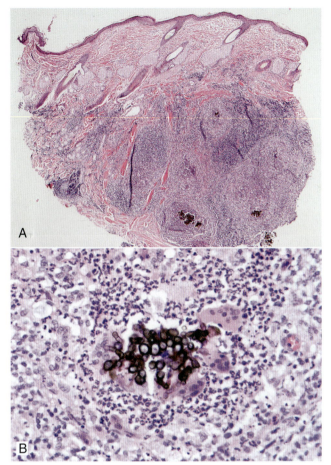

Figure 6-105 Phaeohyphomycosis in a horse. **A.** Nodular pyogranulomatous dermatitis with intralesional dematiaceous fungi. **B.** Dematiaceous fungal hyphae surrounded by multinucleated giant cells, neutrophils, and macrophages.

be extensive. Fungi are distributed throughout the lesion as scattered small aggregates and individual hyphae. *The hyphae are septate, 2-6 μm wide, and branched or unbranched.* They are often constricted at their prominent thick septations and may contain single or chains of thick-walled vesicular swellings, 25 μm or more in diameter, that resemble chlamydospores (Fig. 6-105B). *The innate brown pigment may not be readily apparent in tissue sections, especially in cases of Alternaria* spp. Melanin stains, such as Fontana-Masson, can be used to confirm the presence of melanin in the hyphae. Fungal stains demonstrate the organisms well but can mask the natural color. The etiologic agents are so similar in appearance within tissues that they cannot be identified on the basis of their morphology. Culture is always needed for specific identification of the fungi. Phaeohyphomycosis has been confused with eumycotic mycetomas caused by dematiaceous fungi. *The fungi in mycetomas form discrete organized granules, whereas those of phaeohyphomycosis appear as individual hyphae and small aggregates scattered throughout the lesion.* The aggregates of hyphae in phaeohyphomycosis may be surrounded by Splendore-Hoeppli material, but this does not constitute a granule. The fungal elements of phaeohyphomycosis are frequently intracellular within epithelioid macrophages and multinucleated histiocytic giant cells; granules of mycetomas are nearly always extracellular.

Hyalohyphomycosis

Hyalohyphomycosis (adiaspiromycosis) are opportunistic infections by nonpigmented saprophytic fungi normally found in soil and water. Numerous fungi have been implicated as a cause of hyalohyphomycosis, including *Acremonium* spp., *Fusarium* spp., *Geotrichium* spp., *Paecilomyces* spp., and the *Scedosporium/Pseudallescheria* complex. *Aspergillus* spp. are not included. Some organisms such as *Geotrichium* may be part of the normal flora of the host, oral cavity, gastrointestinal tract, and integument. Infections occur via wound contamination or invasion through mucosal surfaces. Common cutaneous sites of infection in dogs and cats are *clawbeds, face, head, eyes, and joints*. As with phaeohyphomycosis, German Shepherd dogs may be predisposed, and disseminated infection may occur in immunocompromised individuals. Gross lesions vary from well-circumscribed ulcers covered by exudate to nonulcerated nodular masses with variable alopecia and desquamation. Infection may be pruritic in horses. *Microscopic findings* are similar to phaeohyphomycosis with the important exception that the fungal elements are nonpigmented.

Further reading

Dye C, et al. *Alternaria* species infection in nine domestic cats. J Fel Med Surg 2009;11:332-336.

Miller RI. Nodular granulomatous fungal skin diseases of cats in the United Kingdom: a retrospective review. Vet Dermatol 2009;21:130-135.

Miller WH, et al. Fungal and algal skin diseases. In: Miller WH, et al., editors. Muller & Kirk's Small Animal Dermatology. 7th ed. St Louis: Elsevier; 2013. p. 184-222.

Seyedmousavi E, et al. Phaeohyphomycosis, emerging opportunistic diseases in animals. Clin Microbiol Rev 2013;26:19-35.

Sporotrichosis

Sporotrichosis is an uncommon chronic infection usually limited to skin and subcutaneous tissue caused by the opportunist fungal pathogen **Sporothrix schenckii**. The organism is a dimorphic fungus, growing as hyphae at environmental temperatures and in yeast form in tissue. *S. schenckii* exists as a saprophyte distributed worldwide in the soil, on plants, and on various plant materials. It is more common in tropical, subtropical, and temperate zones and is endemic in Central and South America and Africa. Since 1998, there has been an ongoing epidemic affecting cats, dogs, and humans in Rio de Janeiro and Southern Brazil. Sporotrichosis has been reported in cats, dogs, horses, mules, donkeys, cattle, goats, swine, camels, humans, and a variety of other animal species. The infection has been *reported most often in cats, horses, and dogs.* Infection is usually acquired by wound contamination or inoculation of the organism into tissue by puncture wounds caused by thorns, wood splinters, or contaminated claws. Pulmonary infection is occasionally acquired by inhalation of spores. In humans, the disease is considered an occupational hazard for those who work with the soil, plants, or plant materials.

Sporotrichosis is considered a zoonotic disease. Transmission of the infection from cats to humans has been reported many times, and *infected cats pose a significant public health danger.* Veterinarians, other veterinary professionals and students, and owners exposed to ulcerated wounds or exudates from infected cats have developed infections. The organism may be able to penetrate intact skin because not all patients who develop lesions can recall having wounds or being bitten or scratched by infected cats. The large number of organisms typically present in lesions from cats is thought to be the reason for the transmission of disease from cats to humans. However, even when the lesions in cats had few organisms, transmission to humans has occurred. In contrast, infection was not transmitted from a dog with multiple cutaneous lesions containing relatively numerous organisms to several adults and children with whom the dog had had frequent contact for the 2-year duration of infection. These cases suggest that factors in addition to absolute numbers of yeasts are involved in the apparent ease of cat-to-human transmission.

Sporotrichosis is subdivided into 3 *clinical forms*.
- The **primary cutaneous form** consists of multiple scattered raised alopecic, ulcerated, crusted nodules or plaques that remain confined to the point(s) of entry of the organism. It is thought that this form results from a *high degree of host immunity*, preventing spread of infection. Nodules may become ulcerated and associated with seropurulent exudate and crust formation. The normal grooming behavior of cats may result in autoinoculation and spread of lesions to distant sites. The cutaneous form may have a very chronic course. An unusual case of sporotrichosis in a dog consisted of otitis externa characterized by multiple cutaneous nodules that persisted for >5 years. A donkey with sporotrichosis had multiple slowly progressive facial lesions for 2 years before the disease was diagnosed.
- The **cutaneous-lymphatic form** involves the skin, subcutaneous tissue, and associated lymphatics. Lesions begin as firm round nodules at the site of entry, usually on an extremity, and spread proximally along lymphatics. Lymphatic vessels become thick and corded, and a series of secondary nodules forms as the infection progresses. The nodules may break open and discharge seropurulent material. Lesions may cavitate and expose extensive areas of underlying muscle and bone. Regional lymphadenopathy is common. This is the most common form in *horses and humans*. Lesions generally involve the proximal forelimbs, chest, and thigh, but usually no regional lymph node involvement is evident. *Dogs* usually have the cutaneous or cutaneous-lymphatic form. The head, pinnae, and trunk are involved most frequently. In *cats*, lesions are usually located on the head, distal limbs, and base of the tail (Fig. 6-106A). The initial draining puncture wounds may be indistinguishable from cat-inflicted fight wound infections.
- The **extracutaneous/disseminated form** may involve a single extracutaneous tissue, such as osteoarticular sporotrichosis, or multiple internal organs. It develops as a sequela to cutaneous-lymphatic infection or following inhalation of the fungus. The disseminated form of sporotrichosis *occurs most frequently in cats*, and no immunosuppressive factors are usually identified. In experimentally induced sporotrichosis in cats, organisms were shown by culture to have disseminated to viscera in 50% of the cases. Cats with disseminated sporotrichosis are often febrile, depressed, and anorexic. This is a rare presentation in dogs.

Microscopically, sporotrichosis is usually a *nodular-to-diffuse pyogranulomatous or granulomatous inflammatory reaction involving the dermis and subcutaneous fat*. The epidermis is acanthotic or ulcerated. Neutrophils, epithelioid macrophages,

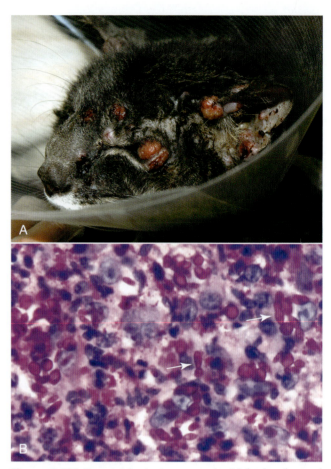

Figure 6-106 Sporotrichosis in a cat. **A.** Multiple ulcerated nodules over the face and pinnae. **B.** Diffuse pyogranulomatous dermatitis with numerous periodic acid–Schiff–positive intralesional round and "cigar-shaped" yeast (arrows).

multinucleated histiocytic giant cells, and fewer lymphocytes and plasma cells form discrete granulomas or extensive sheets of inflammation replacing dermal and subcutaneous tissues. Fibrosis is variable; and necrosis may be extensive. *Yeast(s) surrounded by a stellate radial corona of brightly eosinophilic material (asteroid body/Splendore-Hoeppli reaction) are seen in some* cases. The yeasts appear as round, oval, or elongated ("cigar"-shaped) single or budding cells that measure 2-6 μm or more in diameter for the round and oval forms and 2×3 to 3μ 10 μm for the cigar form (Fig. 6-106B). The cigar forms are considered characteristic of *Sporothrix*, but they may not be regularly found. *In general, organisms are numerous in lesions from cats and rare in tissues from dogs and horses*. However, some reports indicate that visible organisms may be few or absent in some cats. In immunosuppressed dogs, yeasts may be numerous. The yeasts may be extracellular or within neutrophils and macrophages. The yeasts have a refractile cell wall from which the cytoplasm may shrink during processing and give the appearance of a capsule. In such instances and when no cigar forms are evident, the organism may be mistaken for *Cryptococcus neoformans* or *Histoplasma capsulatum*. Yeasts stand out clearly with fungal stains, but serial sections may be needed to demonstrate even a single organism. Without a significant number of cigar-shaped forms, identification may not be possible. Tissue culture, immunohistochemistry, or *fluorescent antibody staining* may be necessary for definitive identification of the organism. The yeast can usually be cultured from tissue obtained from areas of active inflammation even in dogs and horses, which typically have very few organisms in tissue. In cats, cytologic examination of exudates and material obtained by fine-needle aspiration of nodules is frequently diagnostic because sufficient numbers of yeasts are usually present to identify the organism.

In certain geographic regions, for instance, southern Brazil, a main differential diagnosis for canine sporotrichosis is American tegumentary leishmaniosis. These 2 diseases are clinically similar, are both endemic to this region, and present cross-reactivity in serologic tests. Organisms can be difficult to identify microscopically in both conditions. Although these 2 infections are histopathologically similar, in one study, well-formed granulomas with marked neutrophilic infiltration were more commonly associated with sporotrichosis.

Further reading

Crothers SL, et al. Sporotrichosis: a retrospective evaluation of 23 cases seen in northern California (1987-2007). Vet Dermatol 2009;20:249-259.

Madrid IM, et al. Feline sporotrichosis in the Southern region of Rio Grande do Sul, Brazil: clinical, zoonotic and therapeutic aspects. Zoonoses Public Health 2010;57:151-154.

Miranda LHM, et al. Comparative histopathological study of sporotrichosis and American tegumentary leishmaniosis in dogs from Rio de Janeiro. J Comp Path 2010;143:1-7.

Miranda LHM, et al. Evaluation of immunohistochemistry for the diagnosis of sporotrichosis in dogs. Vet J 2011;190:408-411.

Schubach TMP, et al. Canine sporotrichosis in Rio de Janeiro, Brazil: clinical presentation, laboratory diagnosis and therapeutic response in 44 cases (1998-2003). Med Mycol 2006;44:87-92.

Cutaneous oomycosis (pythiosis and lagenidiosis)

Oomycosis refers to infection by **Pythium insidiosum** and **Lagenidium** spp. organisms, both of which are aquatic dimorphic water *molds* and members of the Oomycetes in the kingdom Stramenopila (Chromista). These opportunistic pathogens live in warm stagnant water and are most often reported in regions with tropical to subtropical environments. The organisms are thought to enter the skin through cutaneous wounds, and infection may involve the dermis, subcutis, or distant tissue. These organisms are often associated with devastating and often fatal infections.

Pythiosis (leeches, kunkers, swamp cancer, bursattee) is a chronic cutaneous-subcutaneous, gastrointestinal, or multisystemic infection of horses, dogs, humans, cattle, cats, and sheep, with rare reports in camels and other species. The infection is most common in tropical, subtropical, and temperate regions throughout the world, especially Thailand, Australia, India, Indonesia, and Costa Rica. In North America, infections are most common in the Gulf Coast region but have been reported as far north as New Jersey and as far west as Arizona and California. *Pythium* spp. are aquatic organisms. *Pythium insidiosum* is the etiologic agent of pythiosis in mammals. Microscopically, *P. insidiosum* develops mycelium-like fungi, but it is not a true fungus because its cell walls do not contain chitin but are composed of cellulose and β-glucan, its cytoplasmic membrane lacks ergosterol, the sexual process is oogamy, and the organism develops biflagellate zoospores in wet environments. The infective stage of the organism is a biflagellate aquatic zoospore that is released seasonally in association with warm weather and moisture. Most infections occur in late summer and fall. Infection is thought to be acquired from prolonged contact with stagnant fresh water containing the newly emerged zoospores that are motile and are attracted chemotactically to animal hair, damaged skin, and intestinal mucosa. Once the zoospores are in contact, they encyst on the surface of injured tissue. The encysted zoospores secrete a sticky amorphous glycoprotein that mediates the adhesion of zoospores to tissue. The body temperature of the host stimulates the encysted zoospores to develop a germ tube (hypha) that extends into the infected tissue and can later infiltrate blood vessels. These organisms also produce proteases that weaken host tissue, enhancing the ability of the hyphae to invade tissue. The zoospore stage is not known to form in tissue, and the infection is thus *not considered to have zoonotic potential*. Not all animals with pythiosis have a history of contact with permanent bodies of water, suggesting that the organism may proliferate in temporary stands of water or even on wet grasses.

Cutaneous pythiosis has been reported most frequently in **horses**. No age, breed, or sex predilection is recognized. Lesions occur most commonly on the *limbs, distal to the carpus and hock*, and on the ventral aspect of the thorax and abdomen, sites that are most likely to be in contact with stagnant water and would be traumatized by aquatic plants or vegetation. Affected horses frequently have a history of prolonged contact with water in lakes, ponds, swamps, or flooded areas. Lesions are usually single, but occasional horses develop lesions in several separate sites. Lesions begin as nodules that enlarge very rapidly to become circular masses of granulation tissue. The masses ulcerate or develop multiple draining tracts that discharge thick purulohemorrhagic material. The tracts also contain characteristic gray-white to pale yellow coral-like concretions (called *leeches* or *kunkers*) that may be extruded at the skin surface (Fig. 6-107A). The colloquial name leeches is based on the initial misidentification of the masses. *These structures are unique to the horse* and are not seen in other animals with pythiosis. Lesions are frequently extremely pruritic, and biting or rubbing the lesion contributes to tissue damage. The largest lesions usually develop on the thorax and abdomen and may attain a size of 45 cm or more in diameter. In chronic cases, underlying bone may be invaded. Regional lymph nodes may be involved, but visceral spread is rare. *The clinical appearance of the lesions may resemble basidiobolomycosis, cutaneous habronemiasis, excessive granulation tissue, and neoplasia (particularly sarcoid and squamous cell carcinoma).*

In **dogs**, cutaneous pythiosis has been reported less frequently than the gastrointestinal form. The disease occurs most often in young adult, large-breed dogs, and German Shepherd dogs and Labrador Retrievers may be predisposed. Most lesions are on the extremities, face, and tailhead. In most cases, a single body region is involved. *The initial lesion is a poorly circumscribed dermal nodule that rapidly expands peripherally and extends into the subcutis to form multiple secondary nodules* (Fig. 6-107B). The nodules develop into spongy masses that ulcerate, become necrotic, and develop multiple draining tracts that discharge purulohemorrhagic exudate. Early lesions on the legs may resemble acral lick dermatitis. Pruritus is not as constant a feature in dogs as it is in horses with

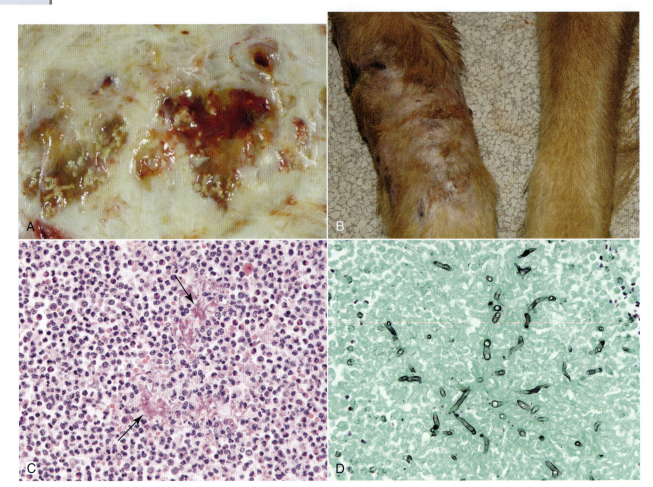

Figure 6-107 Pythiosis. A. Cut surface reveals multiple foci of necrosis with pale yellow linear concretions ("kunkers") in a horse. (Courtesy R. Miller.) **B.** Alopecic nodular lesion with draining tracts on the limb of a dog. (Courtesy M.S. Canfield.) **C.** Negatively staining hyphae (arrows) surrounded by a small amount of eosinophilic Splendore-Hoeppli material and large numbers of eosinophils, neutrophils, and macrophages. **D.** Fungal hyphae are Gomori methenamine silver positive.

pythiosis. A common clinicopathologic abnormality is absolute eosinophilia.

Pythiosis has been reported infrequently in **cattle** and **sheep**. There are a few reports of epizootic outbreaks in these species. Most reported cases of pythiosis in cattle have been in beef calves <12 months of age. In sheep, the condition appears to have no age, breed, or sex predisposition. In cattle, most lesions are located on the distal extremities, and in sheep lesions are most common on the limbs, ventral abdomen, and prescapular region. Lesions consist of irregular swellings that may or may not be ulcerated with multiple draining tracts. Although no concretions have been present, the tissue contains numerous yellow punctate foci. Secondary bacterial contamination with anaerobes and other bacteria is common in cattle. The lesions may be very painful and lead to recumbency, starvation, and death in calves. However, there have also been reports of spontaneous resolution. Internal spread, especially to lungs, may be more common in sheep than other species. Spontaneous resolution has not been reported in sheep.

Reports of pythiosis in **cats** are rare. As in other species, lesions usually are located on the extremities. In at least 2 cats, the lesions progressed very slowly, and the clinical course was much more protracted than is typical of the disease in dogs and horses. Ulceration is uncommon. Nodules usually remained confined to the subcutaneous tissues.

Microscopically, the lesions vary depending on the infected host species. In horses, skin lesions are usually extensively ulcerated with surface fibrin, neutrophils, and bacterial colonies. There is abundant fibrous connective tissue extending from the dermis to the subcutis. There are coalescing foci of granulation tissue with scattered macrophages surrounding eosinophilic material ("kunkers"). The kunkers are composed of necrotic tissue containing dense collections of eosinophils. A moderate to large number of negatively stained hyphae are present at the periphery of the kunkers and may be surrounded by many eosinophils and smaller numbers of lymphocytes, plasma cells, and mast cells. The hyphae are broad, sparsely septate, and have smooth, almost parallel walls with inconspicuous dilations. Deeply eosinophilic granular material (Splendore-Hoeppli material) is present around many hyphae. Degenerate or thrombosed arteries may be seen.

Two inflammatory patterns are seen in canine cutaneous pythiosis. The first pattern *(necro-eosinophilic)* is characterized by broad zones of eosinophilic necrosis, cell debris, and variable numbers of eosinophils. Some areas of necrosis are similar to equine kunkers. The second pattern *(granulomatous)* consists of epithelioid macrophages and Langerhans giant cells and may be surrounded by connective tissue. Both patterns may be seen in a single lesion. Negatively stained hyphae are more commonly seen in the necroeosinophilic lesions (Fig. 6-107C). Fibrinoid necrosis of arterial walls and small arterial thrombi may be seen. Angioinvasion is noted rarely. Angioinvasion has also been reported in one cat with gastrointestinal pythiosis but did not result in distant spread.

In **cattle** and **sheep,** there are multifocal necrotic areas within the dermis and subcutis, with numerous multinucleated histiocytic giant cells, eosinophils, neutrophils, macrophages, and plasma cells. Short poorly stained hyphal elements are observed within giant cells and necrotic areas. There is prominent eosinophilic material around hyphae (Splendore-Hoeppli phenomenon).

Because *Pythium* does not produce chitin, it stains poorly or not at all with PAS. It is readily stained with Gomori methenamine silver (GMS) and appears as *thick-walled, sparsely septate hyphae, 2-7 µm in diameter, with occasional branching* (Fig. 6-107D). Organisms are usually most numerous in necrotic foci and may also be seen in walls of small arterioles in some species. They are rare in areas of granulomatous inflammation, and they are not usually present in intervening connective tissue. The hyphae are similar to those of the zygomycetes *Basidiobolus* and *Conidiobolus*. The hyphae of these organisms tend to be broader, ranging from 5-20 µm in diameter; however, the differentiation of *Pythium* spp. from the zygomycetes in tissue is frequently impossible.

Diagnosis of pythiosis is based on the appearance of the gross lesions, microscopic lesions, and culture of the organism. Pythium is readily cultured in most instances, but it cannot be grown in some cases. PCR assays, immunohistochemistry, and immunoblot analyses have been developed for identification and differentiation of *Pythium insidiosum, Lagenidium,* and the zygomycetes. Not all assays are available for each organism, but a combination of assays and evaluation of the clinical information and laboratory results can lead to a definitive diagnosis.

Cutaneous lagenidiosis is remarkably similar to cutaneous pythiosis in geographic occurrence and clinical and histologic lesions. Lagenidiosis has been reported only in dogs, and most have been young to middle-aged living in the southeastern United States. Gross lesions consist of firm dermal or subcutaneous nodules of the limbs, mammary and inguinal regions, perineum, or trunk. Lesions may be ulcerated with areas of necrosis and draining tracts. Regional lymphadenopathy consisting of granulomatous to pyogranulomatous lymphadenitis is common and may precede skin lesions. The disease can be very aggressive, and affected dogs frequently develop lesions of the great vessels, mediastinum, lungs, and esophagus. Sudden death caused by great vessel rupture has been reported. Gastrointestinal lesions have not been observed. In some dogs, lesions may be slowly progressive, chronic, and limited to cutaneous and subcutaneous tissues. *Microscopically, there is severe eosinophilic and granulomatous inflammation with numerous multinucleated histiocytic giant cells centered around broad 7-25 µm infrequently septate hyphae.* Pyogranulomatous vasculitis may occur. Again, clinical presentation, PCR assays, immunohistochemistry and immunoblot analyses are needed to differentiate these infections.

Further reading

Gaastra W, et al. *Pythium insidiosum:* an overview. Vet Microbiol 2010;146:1-16.

Grooters AM. Pythiosis, lagenidiosis, and zygomycosis in small animals. Vet Clin North Am Small Anim Pract 2003;33:695-720.

Martins TB, et al. A comparative study of the histopathology and immunohistochemistry of pythiosis in horses, dogs, and cattle. J Comp Pathol 2012;146:122-131.

Miller WH, et al. Fungal and algal skin diseases. In: Miller WH, et al., editors. Muller & Kirk's Small Animal Dermatology. 7th ed. St Louis: Elsevier; 2013. p. 184-222.

Moriello KA, DeBoer DJ. Cutaneous fungal infections. In: Greene CE, editor. Infectious Diseases of the Dog and Cat. 4th ed. St Louis: Elsevier Saunders; 2012. p. 588-709.

Zygomycosis

Zygomycosis refers to subcutaneous, systemic, or rhinocerebral infections caused by a wide variety of zygomycete fungi. The class Zygomycetes is composed of 2 orders that cause disease in animals. The order Mucorales includes *Rhizopus, Mucor, Lichtheimia (Absidia), Saksenaea,* among other genera, and diseases caused by these organisms have been called **mucormycosis.** The order Entomophthorales contains the genera *Basidiobolus (B. ranarum)* and *Conidiobolus (C. coronatus, C. incongruous, and C. lamprauges),* and disease caused by these fungi is called **entomophthoromycosis.** In humans and animals, Mucorales organisms tend to cause acute, rapidly progressive disease in immunocompromised individuals, whereas Entomophthorales organisms typically cause localized infections in the subcutaneous tissues or nasal submucosa of immunocompetent individuals. Reports of mucormycosis are very uncommon in veterinary species, especially small animals. Zygomycetes are widespread in nature and occur as soil saprophytes, agents of decay, insect pathogens, or as components of normal skin and hair flora. They are common laboratory contaminants and are thus sometimes ignored when cultured from clinical specimens. The portal of entry may be cutaneous (via traumatic implantation or biting insects), gastrointestinal, or respiratory. Zygomycosis is not a contagious disease; the environment is the source of all infections. Infections are typically nonseasonal.

Zygomycosis is a rare disease of humans and animals, including dogs, cats, horses, llamas, sheep, and pigs. It occurs most commonly in tropical and subtropical areas, including the southeastern United States, South America, Australia, and India.

In humans, horses, sheep, and other mammalian species, **conidiobolomycosis** occurs most often in the nasopharyngeal region with or without extension into the tissues of the face, retropharyngeal region, and retrobulbar space. In horses, most lesions are found on the external nares or nasal passages. Lesions may be unilateral or bilateral, single or multifocal. Within the nasal passages, there are usually multifocal to coalescing firm nodules (1-5 cm) with either a cobblestone appearance or ulceration. Small (0.5 mm) foci of yellow friable material (leeches) may be present. Rhinopharyngeal conidiobolomycosis is an important disease of sheep in Brazil. Unlike the protracted clinical course typical of most cases of zygomycosis, nasal zygomycosis in sheep caused by *C. incongruus* results in loss of condition and death within a period of 7-10 days after initial clinical signs. This infection produces prominent asymmetrical swelling of the face, extending from the nostrils to the eyes, and marked thickening of the skin and subcutaneous tissue. In advanced cases, the nasal skin is alopecic and necrotic.

Lesions may be associated with exophthalmos and appear as white to yellow firm masses. Nasal conidiobolomycosis has been reported in several dogs and one llama. The llama and one dog had ulcerative dermatitis of the nasal planum. Two dogs also had ulcerative lesions of the hard palate. Subcutaneous zygomycosis caused by *Conidiobolus* of unknown species has been reported in a young adult dog. Lesions involved the skin of a hind leg and the thoracic wall but not the nasal mucosa or skin surrounding the nose. The lesions on the leg began as an ulcerated mass that progressed to circumferential swelling and induration with numerous coalescing ulcers draining serosanguineous fluid. The condition exhibited some waxing and waning, but new lesions continued to develop. No immunologic compromise or predisposing factors were apparent.

In horses, **basidiobolomycosis** is usually caused by *B. ranarum*. Most lesions are found on the trunk, head, and neck. They are characterized by large (up to 50 cm) circular, ulcerative granulomas with serosanguineous discharge. Small irregular gritty masses of yellow-white material (kunkers, leeches) may discharge to the surface. Lesions are usually solitary with moderate to severe pruritus. A discontinuous undulating band of yellow-white material that sharply demarcates the superficial hemorrhagic, edematous tissue from the underlying fibrogranulation tissue characterizes the cut surface of granulomas. The clinical lesions are similar to those of pythiosis but may sometimes be differentiated in the horse by differences in anatomic location, number and appearance of kunkers, and epidemiology. Basidiobolomycosis is a rare cause of pulmonary disease and ulcerative draining skin lesions in dogs. Disseminated infection involving the gastrointestinal tract and other abdominal organs has been described in 2 dogs.

Microscopically, zygomycosis is characterized by *multifocal-to-diffuse eosinophilic and granulomatous dermatitis and panniculitis with multifocal necrosis.* Necrotic foci consist of eosinophilic coagulated material corresponding to the kunkers seen grossly. Eosinophils, neutrophils, epithelioid macrophages, and multinucleated histiocytic giant cells surround the eosinophilic coagula and are separated by fibrovascular connective tissue. Fungi are usually located in necrotic foci and may be seen as clear linear or circular hyphal "ghosts" often surrounded by a thick (2.5-25 µm) eosinophilic sleeve (Splendore-Hoeppli phenomenon). This finding helps differentiate zygomycosis from pythiosis and lagenidiosis, in which eosinophilic sleeves tend to be thin or absent. In addition, the hyphal diameter (as measured in tissue) tends to be significantly larger for *Basidiobolus* spp. (5-20 µm). *Conidiobolus* spp. are 5-13 µm wide, and *P. insidiosum* are 2-7 µm wide. Basophilic granular protoplasm may be visible with H&E stain, but the organisms are usually better visualized with GMS stain. They frequently stain poorly with PAS. Hyphae are thin walled and have occasional septations and uncommon branching. Folded, twisted, or compressed hyphae may be seen. The lesions of nasal zygomycosis caused by *C. incongruus* in sheep are characterized by segmental necrosis and thrombosis of subcutaneous blood vessels. Many fungal hyphae are visible in necrotic foci, in thrombi, and within vessel walls. This *propensity to invade blood vessels* is common with *Mucorales* but is an unusual feature for the Entomophthorales.

The microscopic lesions of basidiobolomycosis and conidiobolomycosis are similar to those of pythiosis, and the diseases may be histologically indistinguishable, especially when the width of hyphae is at the narrow end of the range. All members of the zygomycetes are morphologically similar in tissue, and consequently culture, PCR, or immunohistochemistry are necessary for specific identification.

Further reading

de Paula DAJ, et al. Molecular characterization of ovine zygomycosis in central western Brazil. J Vet Diagn Invest 2010;22:274-277.

Grooters AM. Pythiosis, lagenidiosis, and zygomycosis in small animals. Vet Clin North Am Small Anim Pract 2003;33:695-720.

Tan RM, et al. Severe chronic diffuse pyogranulomatous, necrohemorrhagic and eosinophilic rhinitis caused by *Conidiobolus*. J Am Vet Med Assoc 2010;236:831-833.

Ubiali DG, et al. Pathology of nasal infection caused by *Conidiobolus lamprauges* and *Pythium insidiosum* in sheep. J Comp Pathol 2013;149:137-145.

Miscellaneous fungal infections of skin

Infections with various opportunist fungi are reported sporadically in animals. These organisms are ubiquitous in the environment, common contaminants of laboratory cultures, and frequently also a component of skin and hair flora of normal animals. Thus *diagnosis of infection is difficult to make by culture alone and requires histologic demonstration of tissue invasion by morphologically compatible organisms.* In humans, these infections are usually associated with immunosuppression and neutropenia, but predisposing factors are only occasionally identified in animals.

Aspergillus spp. are distributed widely in nature and are found in soil, dust, and decaying vegetation. *Aspergillus* spp. are not commonly associated with skin infections. Subcutaneous infection with *Aspergillus versicolor* producing a nodular mass on the upper lip was reported in an adult Saddlebred mare. The lesion recurred once following surgical excision but had not recurred 1 year after the second surgical excision. *A. terreus* has been associated with subcutaneous granulomas in an adult Holstein cow without any lesions elsewhere. Dogs with disseminated aspergillosis may rarely develop cutaneous lesions secondarily. Nasal and cutaneous aspergillosis caused by *A. niger* was reported in a goat from Brazil. Lesions included a large mass in the nasal cavity and several raised nodules over the nares (2-3 cm) and pinnae (0.3-1 cm). *Microscopically*, there was pyogranulomatous rhinitis and dermatitis with central necrosis and intralesional fungal hyphae. Hyphae are *septate, branching, 5-7 µm in diameter, have thick walls, and occasionally have bulbous apical dilations.*

Piedra is a fungal infection of the extrafollicular portion of the hair shaft caused by *Piedraia hortae* ("black piedra") and *Trichosporon beigelii* ("white piedra"). These organisms are ubiquitous saprophytic yeast-like fungi. Piedra is an opportunistic infection and has been associated with cutaneous infections, urinary tract infections, systemic infections, pneumonitis, valvular endocarditis, fatal mastitis, and abortions. In humans, disseminated systemic infections usually occur in immunocompromised patients with granulocytopenia. *Cutaneous white piedra* has been described in humans, monkeys, horses, dogs, and cats. The infection is more common in temperate climates of South America, Europe, Asia, Japan, and the southern United States. The infection is characterized by *firm, irregular white or pale brown nodules on hair shafts*. In horses, the long hairs of the mane, tail, and forelock are affected. *The nodules consist of tightly packed septate hyphae that are held together by a cement-like substance.* Trichosporon spp. has rarely been reported to cause nasal granulomas in cats and in one cat was reported to cause an ulcerated mass on the distal leg at the site of a previous cat-bite wound. *Microscopically*, the organisms consist of spherical to oval, 3-8 μm, narrow-based, budding yeast cells and septate, nonpigmented, branching hyphae with nonparallel sides.

Rhodotorula spp. are normal inhabitants of the skin, ear canal, and alimentary tract. These yeast-like fungi are opportunistic pathogens in immunosuppressed patients. Cutaneous infection has been reported in one cat with feline immunodeficiency virus and feline leukemia virus infections. This cat had adherent brown-red crusts over the nasal planum, nostrils, bridge of nose, periocular region, and one digit.

Further reading

do Carmo PM, et al. Nasal and cutaneous aspergillosis in a goat. J Comp Pathol 2014;150:4-7.

Fleming RV, et al. Emerging and less common fungal pathogens. Infect Dis Clin North Am 2002;16:915-933.

Miller WH, et al. Fungal and algal skin diseases. In: Miller WH, et al., editors. Muller & Kirk's Small Animal Dermatology. 7th ed. St Louis: Elsevier; 2013. p. 184-222.

Sharman MJ, et al. Clinical resolution of a nasal granuloma caused by *Trichosporon loubieri*. J Fel Med Surg 2010;12:345-350.

PROTOZOAL DISEASES OF SKIN

Cutaneous lesions occur in several **systemic or localized protozoal** infections. Differentials for protozoal dermatitis should include *Besnoitia* spp., *Leishmania* spp., *Caryospora* spp., *Neospora* spp., *Toxoplasma* spp., *Sarcocystis* spp., and *Babesia* spp. Cutaneous lesions have also been associated with *Theileria* infection (see Vol. 3, Hematopoietic system). *Trypanosoma equiperdum* and dourine are discussed in Vol. 3, Female genital system.

Besnoitiosis

Besnoitia is an apicomplexan protozoal parasite in the family Sarcocystidae. It is closely related to *Toxoplasma* and *Neospora*. Besnoitiosis has a worldwide distribution and affects both wild and domestic animals. Infections are reported in cattle, donkeys, horses, goats, sheep, and a number of wild animals, including reindeer, caribou, zebras, rodents, rabbits, the Virginia opossum, and lizards. Currently, there are 10 known species of *Besnoitia*, but the life cycle of only 4 of those is understood. A feline definitive host has been identified for *B. oryctofelis, B. darling, B. neotomofelis*, and *B. wallacei*, which affects rabbits, opossums, southern plains woodrat, and rodents, respectively. The pathogenesis, life cycle, and route of infection are poorly understood for the 4 *Besnoitia* spp. that affect ungulates: *B. besnoiti* (cattle), *B. bennetti* (equids), *B. caprae* (goats, sheep), and *B. tarandi* (reindeer, caribou).

In the 4 species in which the definitive host is known to be a felid, sexual reproduction is thought to occur in the intestinal tract of the definitive host, and the sporulated oocysts are passed in the feces. *The exact mode of infection of the intermediate hosts is not known*, but mechanical transmission by blood-sucking insects is regarded as an important natural mode of transmission. Some studies suggest that direct transmission from intermediate host to intermediate host is possible, such as through mating. Tachyzoites in the intermediate host proliferate in endothelial cells, monocytes, and neutrophils. In the later phases of infection, tissue cysts occur. Infection, however, may be generalized and is typically so in some infections in rodents and wild animals. *The tissue cysts represent parasitized host cells, for instance, fibroblasts, myofibroblasts, endothelial cells, or smooth muscle cells*. The bradyzoites multiply in cellular vacuoles and induce hyperplastic and hypertrophic changes in the host cells. These often divide to form multinucleated cells. The enlarging mass of crescent-shaped bradyzoites compresses the cell cytoplasm and nuclei into a thin rim forming an inner coat to the cyst. A hyalinized collagenous cyst wall is laid down around the parasitized cell. The cysts, which measure up to 500 μm with a 10- to 50-μm thick wall, are visible to the naked eye. Ingesting parasitized tissue from the intermediate host infects the definitive host.

Besnoitiosis is an emerging disease of cattle in Europe and donkeys in the United States. **Bovine besnoitiosis** caused by *B. besnoiti* is enzootic in Africa and Asia, and both enzootic and epizootic in parts of Europe. It has been reported in France, Spain, Portugal, Italy, and Germany. The disease also occurs in Israel, Russia, South Korea, and Venezuela. The disease is of *high economic importance in Africa*, causing mortality in up to 10% and morbidity in >80%. In Europe, mortality is <1%, and although many animals in an endemic area may be seropositive, most are subclinically infected. Predilections for age, breed, and sex appear to vary between geographic regions. In the enzootic regions of France, bovine besnoitiosis occurs preferentially from spring to autumn. Two- to 4-year-old males are more susceptible than females and have more acute signs with higher mortality rates. In the French Alps, where the disease is epizootic, females are more susceptible. Infection appear to be rare in calves <6 months of age. In clinically affected animals, there is an acute and a chronic stage. The acute stage can be confused with bluetongue or malignant catarrhal fever and is characterized by fever, generalized edema, weakness, anorexia, and lymphadenopathy. During this stage, tachyzoites proliferate in macrophages, fibroblasts, and endothelial cells, resulting in vasculitis and thrombosis, especially in small vessels of the dermis, subcutis, fascia, testes, and upper respiratory mucosa. Pregnant cows may abort, and bulls may develop orchitis and sterility. *Besnoitiosis is usually recognized as a chronic disease* characterized by alopecia; marked thickening and folding of the skin, especially around the neck, shoulders, and rump; scaling; exudation; and fissuring. Animals lose condition, have decreased milk production, have permanent sterility in some bulls, have significant hide damage, and up to 10% mortality may occur during the chronic stage. Lesions may be painful. During the chronic stage of besnoitiosis, only tissue cysts are found. Tissue cysts are most concentrated around mucous membranes (nares, conjunctiva, vulva, perineum) and sclera ("scleral pearls") but also occur commonly in the dermis; subcutis; fascia; muscle; epididymis; testes; in the mucosa of the pharynx, larynx, and trachea; and less commonly in the spleen, liver, lung, lymph nodes, periosteum, endosteum, and heart muscle. It is not certain if new tissue cysts are formed during the chronic stage and how long the cysts persist in cattle.

Although some tissue cysts do degenerate and cause inflammation, there is no evidence that besnoitiosis can be reactivated from the chronic to acute stage. This is unlike the biology of rodent *Besnoitia* spp., where it has been shown that chronic *B. jellisoni* infection in rodents can be reactivated by experimentally induced immunosuppression.

Equid besnoitiosis is caused by *B. bennetti* and was first described in isolated cases of horses and donkeys in Africa. Besnoitiosis has become an emerging disease of donkeys in the United States, with outbreaks occurring in Michigan, Pennsylvania, and Oregon. No cases have been reported in horses outside of Africa. The disease is also reported in mules and a zebra in Africa. Clinical disease is characterized by tens to hundreds of nonpruritic, white, pinpoint papular lesions in the skin and mucous membranes, especially over the nares, conjunctiva, sclera, pinnae, limbs, and perineum (Fig. 6-108A). As with bovine besnoitiosis, the presence of *scleral pearls* is a valuable diagnostic feature. Tissue cysts also occur in the dermis, subcutis, fascia, muscle, epididymis, testes, and in the mucosa of the pharynx, larynx, and trachea. There is variable hair loss and lichenification. For unknown reasons, some infected donkeys remain healthy, whereas others become cachectic and debilitated. Internal dissemination of tissue cysts has not been reported in equid besnoitiosis. Risk factors for infection in donkeys have been suggested to be young age (most affected donkeys have been <3 years of age) and stressful, crowded, or unhygienic conditions.

Caprine besnoitiosis caused by *B. caprae* is clinically and pathologically similar to bovine besnoitiosis but has only been reported in Iran and Kenya. The prevalence of disease is higher in older goats and rare in goats <1 year of age. In an outbreak affecting >500 domestic goats in Kenya, ocular cysts were the most common finding, but cysts were found in many body systems. Dorper **sheep** were also affected in that outbreak. A disease resembling besnoitiosis was reported in New Zealand lambs.

Histologically, protozoal cysts are 150-500 μm in diameter with 10-50 μm thick 3-layered walls (Fig. 6-108B, C). The mature cyst wall has *4 distinct layers*. Outermost is a condensed, hyalinized, laminated, eosinophilic to amphophilic birefringent layer of collagen fibers. Next is a very thin homogeneous intermediate zone. The third layer is the cytoplasm of the host cell, and in this layer lie several giant, vesicular but compressed host cell nuclei. A thin inner membrane forms the parasitophorous vacuole containing a myriad of tightly packed 7 × 2 μm basophilic crescentic bradyzoites. These may be separated from the wall by an artifactual shrinkage space. Some cysts have no tissue reaction, and some are surrounded by small to moderate numbers of lymphocytes, plasma cells, eosinophils, and histiocytes. Ruptured or degenerate cysts are often surrounded by inflammation (as noted previously) and multinucleated giant cells. Other histopathologic features in donkeys include epidermal hyperplasia, mild orthokeratotic to parakeratotic hyperkeratosis with occasional cellular crusts, intercellular edema in the epidermis, lymphocytic exocytosis, mild lymphocytic mural folliculitis, and mild to moderate diffuse superficial to mid-dermal perivascular infiltrates composed of mixed mononuclear cells, and variable numbers of eosinophils. In cattle in the acute phases, there is epidermal hyperplasia with dermal edema and perivascular accumulations of lymphocytes, plasma cells, and large histiocytes. *Crescent-shaped trophozoites occur in arterioles and lymphatics and free in tissue spaces*. Occasionally, they may be detected in

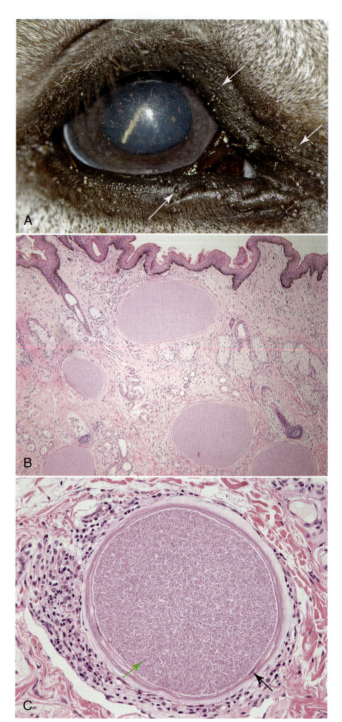

Figure 6-108 Besnoitiosis in a donkey. **A.** Multiple periocular pinpoint pale tan to white papules representing encysted protozoa (arrows). **B.** Five protozoal cysts in the dermis. **C.** Note the compressed host cell nucleus (black arrow) in the cyst wall and the intraluminal bradyzoites (green arrow).

macrophages. In some cases, there is vasculitis, thrombosis, and extensive dermal and epidermal necrosis. As the parasites become encysted, inflammation and edema diminish (chronic stage). In cattle and goats, cysts are sometimes present within blood vessels.

Diagnosis of besnoitiosis is based on clinical findings and skin biopsies. Serologic tests can be used to detect subclinical infections; however, these tests have a low level of specificity, it takes several weeks for antibodies to be formed in the animal after infection, and some infected animals have low antibody titers. PCR testing has superior sensitivity compared with serology in acutely affected animals.

Further reading

Alvarez-Garcia G, et al. A century of bovine besnoitiosis: an unknown disease re-emerging in Europe. Trends Parasitol 2013;29:407-415.

Elsheikha HM, et al. An outbreak of besnoitiosis in miniature donkeys. J Parasitol 2005;91:877-881.

Jacquiet P, et al. Bovine besnoitiosis: epidemiological and clinical aspects. Vet Parasitol 2010;174:30-36.

Ness SL, et al. Investigation of an outbreak of besnoitiosis in donkeys in northeastern Pennsylvania. J Am Vet Med Assoc 2012;240:1329-1337.

Oryan A, et al. Histopathologic and ultrastructural studies on experimental caprine besnoitiosis. Vet Pathol 2011;48:1094-1100.

Leishmaniasis

Leishmaniasis is a zoonotic infection caused by an intracellular, diphasic protozoan of the genus *Leishmania*. More than 30 *Leishmania* spp. have been identified. Species vary by geographic region, but *Leishmania infantum* is the most commonly reported cause of visceral disease in the endemic regions of Europe. The disease is most commonly reported in humans and dogs but occurs in a wide variety of domestic mammals and wildlife. Three forms of clinical leishmaniasis are recognized: *cutaneous, mucocutaneous, and visceral*. Cutaneous leishmaniasis occurs worldwide in dogs, cats, horses, and cattle. It is endemic in Mediterranean countries, Portugal, and in parts of Africa, India, and Central and South America. Endemic foci have also been reported in the United States and include regions of Texas, Oklahoma, Ohio, Michigan, and Alabama. Leishmaniasis is also endemic in Foxhound populations in the United States.

The most common mode of transmission is through the bite of a female *blood-sucking sandfly* of the genera *Phlebotomus* and *Lutzomyia*. The biting sandfly injects promastigotes and saliva into the skin of the host. *The sandfly saliva has potent vasodilating, anticoagulant, anesthetic, and immunomodulatory properties.* Other modes of transmission have been suggested, such as blood transfusions and vertical transmission. Domestic and wild dogs, cats, rodents, and other wild mammals act as reservoirs. The parasite's life cycle and manifestations of visceral disease are discussed in Vol. 3, Hematopoietic system.

Leishmaniasis can manifest as a subclinical infection, self-limiting disease, or severe systemic illness. A variety of host and parasite factors are likely important in determining whether the host is resistant or susceptible. Leishmaniasis is a chronic disease with an incubation period that varies from weeks to years. The disease can occur at any age but is more common in young adults. Studies in mice and dogs indicate that resistance to infection is dependent upon a Th1-type of immune response, whereas susceptibility is associated with a Th2-type of immune response. The alopecic form of the cutaneous disease in the dog has been shown to be associated with fewer organisms and a more appropriate cellular immune response in terms of number of antigen-presenting Langerhans cells, major histocompatibility complex II–positive keratinocytes, and infiltrating T cells. In contrast, dogs with the nodular form lacked antigen-presenting cells and had more numerous macrophages containing large numbers of organisms. It has been suggested that the clinical and histologic lesions may be useful in establishing a prognosis for remission in that the character of the lesions that develops reflects epidermal immunocompetence. For example, papular dermatitis caused by *Leishmania* spp. in dogs has been associated with good response to treatment and reduced antibody titers, which are suggestive of immunocompetence and a favorable prognosis.

Skin lesions occur in >80% of dogs with visceral involvement. The most common presentation is exfoliative dermatitis with silvery white scales. Lesions are most pronounced on the head, pinnae, and extremities but may be generalized. Involved skin may be hypotrichotic to alopecic, and nasodigital hyperkeratosis may also occur. Periocular alopecia *"lunettes"* is common. Ulcerative dermatitis is the next most common presentation. Other gross lesions include onychogryphosis, paronychia, sterile pustular dermatitis, nasal depigmentation with ulceration, and papular to nodular dermatitis. Papular and nodular lesions are generally nonpainful and nonpruritic and are most common on the ventral abdomen, inner aspect of the pinnae, eyelids, and face but can be anywhere on the body. *Nodular mucosal leishmaniasis* affecting the oral cavity, tongue, nose, and penis has been reported in the dog.

Histologically, 9 inflammatory patterns have been recognized. The 3 most common patterns are granulomatous perifolliculitis, superficial and deep perivascular dermatitis, and interstitial dermatitis. Other patterns reported include lichenoid interface dermatitis, nodular dermatitis, lobular panniculitis, suppurative folliculitis, and intraepidermal pustular epidermitis. Dogs commonly have more than one pattern. Orthokeratotic and parakeratotic hyperkeratosis are usually prominent, and the inflammatory infiltrate typically is composed of macrophages with fewer lymphocytes and plasma cells. Multinucleated histiocytic giant cells may be present. The infiltrate in areas of ulceration includes neutrophils. Sebaceous adenitis with total obliteration of the sebaceous glands occurs in ~45% of cases. *Leishmania* amastigotes are found intracellularly (macrophages, leukocytes, endothelial cells, or fibroblasts) or extracellularly in 50% of the cases. Organisms are often contained within round, clear, intracellular parasitophorous vacuoles, many of which contain more than a dozen amastigotes at their periphery. Amastigotes are round to oval, 2-4 μm in diameter, and contain a round basophilic nucleus and a small rod-like kinetoplast. *Leishmania* organisms can often be seen with routine H&E stains; however, they are best visualized with Giemsa stain. Some animals have infiltrates consisting primarily of large, foamy macrophages with numerous organisms and fewer plasma cells and lymphocytes, whereas other animals have larger numbers of lymphocytes and plasma cells, indicating a more effective cellular immune response. Histologically, the perifollicular pattern with granulomatous inflammation and sebaceous gland destruction may need to be differentiated from sebaceous adenitis and sterile granuloma syndrome.

Feline leishmaniasis is rare and generally occurs as a cutaneous disease without visceral involvement, although visceral involvement can occur. It has been reported in the Mediterranean region and South America, where the disease is endemic, as well as Switzerland, Iran, and the United States. *Leishmania mexicana* is endemic in Texas, where it is the confirmed cause of cutaneous leishmaniasis in cats. Clinically, cats most commonly have *one to multiple variably smooth,*

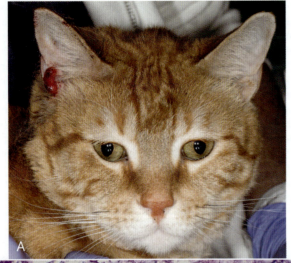

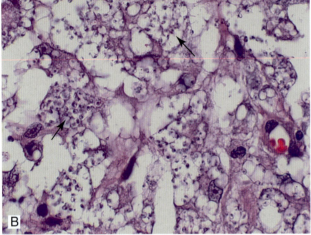

Figure 6-109 Leishmaniasis in a cat. **A.** Ulcerated nodule at the base of the pinna. **B.** Numerous intrahistiocytic amastigotes (arrows) in the dermis. (Courtesy B.F. Porter.)

ulcerated or scaly papules and nodules on the pinnae and muzzle (Fig. 6-109A). Histologically, a nodular-to-diffuse pattern of granulomatous dermatitis with numerous intrahistiocytic amastigotes and a variable number of lymphocytes and plasma cells is the most common inflammatory reaction pattern seen in cats (Fig. 6-109B).

Cutaneous leishmaniasis has been reported in **horses, mules, and donkeys** in Europe, South America, North America, and Puerto Rico. Reports in **cattle** are rare: one cow from Switzerland with *L. siamensis* and one suspected case from Zimbabwe. Lesions in equids consist of *single to multiple crusted or ulcerated papules and nodules* on the pinnae, head, and neck, or less commonly, the legs, scrotum, and penis. In cattle, lesions have been described on the muzzle, pinnae, udder, and legs. Histologically, the dermis contains nodular-to-diffuse infiltrates of macrophages and lymphocytes or distinct granulomas with organisms identified in macrophages or free within the interstitium. Numerous eosinophils and foamy macrophages were described in a case of a 7-year-old Brown Swiss cow from Switzerland. Cutaneous lesions may not be associated with systemic infection.

Diagnosis can be made through finding the organism on cytologic or histologic evaluation of tissues, PCR, immunohistochemistry, in situ hybridization, serology demonstrating anti-*Leishmania* antibodies, or a positive skin test reaction.

Further reading

Miller WH, et al. Fungal and algal skin diseases. In: Miller WH, et al., editors. Muller & Kirk's Small Animal Dermatology. 7th ed. St Louis: Elsevier; 2013. p. 184-222.

Muller N, et al. Occurrence of *Leishmania* sp. in cutaneous lesions of horses in Central Europe. Vet Parasitol 2009;166:346-351.

Navarro JA, et al. Histopathological lesions in 15 cats with leishmaniosis. J Comp Pathol 2010;143:297-302.

Petersen CA. Leishmaniasis, an emerging disease found in companion animals in the United States. Top Companion Anim Med 2009;24:182-188.

Saridomichelakis MN. Advances in the pathogenesis of canine leishmaniosis: epidemiologic and diagnostic implications. Vet Dermatol 2009;20:471-489.

Trainor KE, et al. Eight cases of feline cutaneous leishmaniasis in Texas. Vet Pathol 2010;47:1076-1081.

Miscellaneous coccidian parasites

Toxoplasma gondii, an apicomplexan intracellular coccidian parasite, has been reported rarely as a cause of cutaneous lesions in humans, cats, and dogs. This parasite has worldwide distribution and is most commonly associated with disseminated and often fatal infections in immunocompromised hosts. Necrotizing hepatitis and pneumonia are most common and are discussed elsewhere in this book. The cat is the definitive host, and most mammals can serve as an intermediate host. Most reports of cutaneous toxoplasmosis have been associated with systemic fatal infections. All 3 dogs described in the literature were on immunosuppressive therapy. Skin lesions are described as single to multiple ulcerated and non-ulcerated nodules. One dog was described to have generalized cutaneous pruritic pustules. Histologically, there is severe pyogranulomatous dermatitis and panniculitis with vasculitis, vascular thrombosis, edema, and necrosis. The tachyzoites are 2 × 6 μm and have a crescent shape with pale basophilic cytoplasm and a dark nucleus. They can be single or arranged in clusters, some of which are extracellular or within the cytoplasm of follicular, epidermal, and glandular epithelial cells, and within macrophages, fibroblasts, and endothelial cells.

Caryospora spp., apicomplexan parasites whose primary hosts are reptiles and raptors, rarely cause *pyogranulomatous dermatitis in puppies*. Immunosuppression and concurrent disease, such as canine distemper, likely play a facilitatory role. Lesions involve skin and draining lymph nodes and comprise diffuse pyogranulomatous dermatitis. Macrophages contain large numbers of intracellular organisms, including schizonts, gamonts, oocysts, and caryocysts. Caryocysts have a thin cyst wall enclosing the host cell nucleus and contain up to 3 sporozoites. Not all stages of the life cycle may be present in tissue sections, precluding a microscopic diagnosis in some cases. Immunohistochemical studies identified the agent in one case as *Caryospora bigenetica*. Experimental oral infection of immunosuppressed puppies infected with *C. bigenetica* induced typical skin lesions affecting the muzzle, periocular skin, footpads, ears, and abdomen within 10 days of inoculation.

Neospora caninum is a cyst-forming apicomplexan protozoal parasite. The definitive hosts are *domestic and wild dogs,* and intermediate hosts include *dogs, cattle, sheep, goats, horses, and deer*. It is best known as a cause of bovine abortion capable of transplacental transmission. This parasite is a primary pathogen in dogs and has been associated with progressive ascending paralysis, polymyositis, multifocal central nervous system disease, myocarditis, pneumonia, and hepatitis. Cutaneous lesions occur rarely in adult dogs, often with underlying immunosuppression from drug therapy or concurrent disease. It is not known whether the disease in adult dogs results from a reactivated congenital infection or from a recently acquired infection. Lesions have been described as *multifocal-to-generalized, ulcerative papulonodular dermatitis*. Histologically, there is pyogranulomatous and sometimes eosinophilic, to necrotizing and hemorrhagic, dermatitis. Numerous tachyzoites, 4-7 µm × 1.5-5 µm, may be seen in macrophages, keratinocytes, and neutrophils, and rarely in endothelial cells and fibroblasts. Tissue cysts are not present in the cutaneous lesions. Cutaneous infection with both *N. caninum* and *L. infantum* was reported in one dog from Italy. To differentiate neosporosis from toxoplasmosis, immunohistochemistry, electron microscopy, or PCR is necessary.

An unidentified **Sarcocystis-like protozoan** was associated with *multiple cutaneous abscesses and disseminated visceral lesions in a dog*. The skin lesions were diffuse, necrotizing, hemorrhagic, and suppurative. Large numbers of protozoa were present, primarily in macrophages and neutrophils, and occasionally in fibroblasts and endothelial cells. Some vessels contained thrombi, and there was associated dermal and epidermal infarction. The organism did not stain with antisera to the other apicomplexan parasites, so far identified as causing dermatitis in dogs, namely, *N. caninum*, *T. gondii*, and *Caryospora* spp.

Infection with **Babesia canis** and **B. gibsoni** have been reported to rarely cause cutaneous lesions in dogs. *Babesia* is a hemoprotozoal parasite that is transmitted through the bite of a tick or through saliva in fighting dogs. Skin lesions include petechiae, ecchymoses, edema, ulceration, and necrosis of extremities, pressure points, and frictional areas—most commonly pinnae, axillae, groin, limbs, and scrotum. In one dog, generalized alopecia was reported. Histologically, there is *leukocytoclastic vasculitis* with or without vascular necrosis.

Further reading

Hoffmann AR, et al. Cutaneous toxoplasmosis in two dogs. J Vet Diagn Invest 2012;24:636-640.

Kul O, et al. Clinicopathologic diagnosis of cutaneous toxoplasmosis in an Angora cat. Berl Munch Tierarztl Wochenschr 2011;124:386-389.

Miller WH, et al. Fungal and algal skin diseases. In: Miller WH, et al., editors. Muller & Kirk's Small Animal Dermatology. 7th ed. St Louis: Elsevier; 2013. p. 184-222.

Tarantino C, et al. *Leishmania infantum* and *Neospora caninum* simultaneous skin infection in a young dog in Italy. Vet Parasitol 2001;102:77-83.

Tasaki Y, et al. Generalized alopecia with vasculitis-like changes in a dog with babesiosis. J Vet Med Sci 2013;75:1367-1369.

ALGAL DISEASES OF SKIN

Protothecosis is an uncommon disease caused by *Prototheca* spp. organisms, achlorophyllic algae-like unicellular organisms belonging to the family *Chlorellaceae*. The organism is ubiquitous in organic matter and in fresh and marine waters. Reports of infection in humans and domestic and wild animals are worldwide, but the majority of cases are from the southeastern United States. The 2 most common species associated with infection are **Prototheca wickerhamii** and **P. zopfii**. Mastitis in cows and disseminated disease in dogs are more common than cutaneous-subcutaneous infection. In humans, the cutaneous form is the most common and is thought to be initiated by traumatic implantation, resulting in a protracted and indolent clinical course. *Cutaneous protothecosis has been reported in dogs and cats* in the United States, Australia, England, and Spain, and a goat in Brazil. In those cases in which the organism was speciated, *P. zopfii* is most often associated with disseminated disease, whereas the cutaneous form has been caused by *P. wickerhamii*.

Despite widespread distribution of *Prototheca* spp., *the prevalence of infection is very low*, and attempts to reproduce infection experimentally have met with mixed success. This has led to speculation that the organism is an *opportunist with low pathogenicity* that requires an underlying immunologic dysfunction for the development of disease. Most humans with cutaneous protothecosis have a concurrent disease condition that may alter the immune response to the organism; however, immunocompromise has not been documented in most affected animals.

Dermatologic lesions include *single to multiple papules and nodules, often over pressure points or nodules and ulcerations involving mucocutaneous junctions (especially nostrils), scrotum, and pawpads* (Fig. 6-110A). *Nasal planum depigmentation may be striking*. Histologically, there is pyogranulomatous to granulomatous dermatitis and panniculitis with epithelioid macrophages, multinucleated histiocytic giant cells, neutrophils, and lymphoid cells are in variable numbers, and foci of necrosis may be present. *Organisms are typically numerous, but they are only lightly stained with H&E and therefore are poorly visualized*. The cell wall and internal contents are readily stained with fungal stains, for instance, Gridley (GF), Gomori methenamine silver (GMS), and periodic acid–Schiff (PAS). The organisms vary from 3–30 µm in diameter and consist of cells called sporangia that divide by internal cleavage to form multiple *endospores* (Fig. 6-110B). Identification of *Prototheca* can be made reliably by examination of tissue sections, but species identification usually requires culture or immunofluorescence methods because differences in the 2 species are subtle. *P. wickerhamii* sporangia are smaller (3-15 µm) and round in comparison to the larger (7-30 µm) and oval or cylindrical shape of most *P. zopfii*. Prototheca must be *differentiated from Chlorella algae*, whose natural green pigmentation is removed in fixation and routine tissue processing. In contrast to *Prototheca* cells, *Chlorella* sporangia contain many large starch granules that are stained by GF, GMS, and PAS.

Further reading

Hollingsworth SR. Canine protothecosis. Vet Clin North Am Small Anim Pract 2000;30:1091-1101.

Macedo JTSA, et al. Cutaneous and nasal protothecosis in a goat. Vet Pathol 2008;45:352-354.

Miller WH, et al. Fungal and algal skin diseases. In: Miller WH, et al., editors. Muller & Kirk's Small Animal Dermatology. 7th ed. St Louis: Elsevier; 2013. p. 184-222.

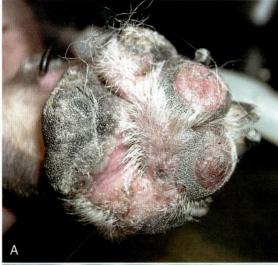

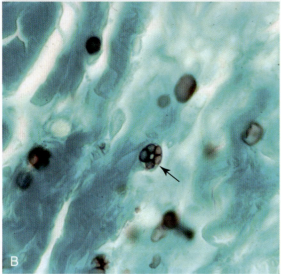

Figure 6-110 *Prototheca* **spp. infection** in a dog. **A.** Multiple ulcerations of the pawpad. (Courtesy R. Last, D. Miller.) **B.** *Prototheca* spp. sporangium (arrow) stained with Gomori methenamine silver. (Courtesy D.W. Scott.)

ARTHROPOD ECTOPARASITES

Of the parasitic arthropods, very few are parasites of domestic animals, but the harmfulness of these is quite out of proportion to their number. Some, such as the mites, are pathogens in their own right, but *most owe their immense importance to their ability to act as mechanical or biological transmitters for many pathogenic viruses, bacteria, protozoa, and helminths*. Their role as vectors is discussed in relation to the specific diseases throughout these volumes.

The parasites of concern to us here belong to the 2 large classes, Insecta and Arachnida. The class Insecta contains 4 important orders: Diptera *(flies)*, Siphonaptera *(fleas)*, Mallophaga *(chewing lice)*, and Siphunculata *(sucking lice)*. The class Arachnida contains the order Acarina, in which *ticks and mites* are classified. For information on biological characters and classification, reference should be made to texts on entomology.

Many **arthropod bites or stings** go unreported and are of minimal consequence. The type and number of arthropods inflicting the bite or sting and the individual host response determine the severity of the injury. In general, most arthropod bites initially appear as circular, erythematous lesions, 0.5-2.0 cm in diameter. Lesions may progress to focal areas of necrosis with ulceration, alopecia, and crust formation. Histologically, the area of necrosis and inflammation may have a triangular outline with one point of the triangle in the deep dermis or panniculus. In early lesions, the inflammation is perivascular to diffuse and includes variable numbers of eosinophils, neutrophils, lymphocytes, and macrophages. Edema and hemorrhage may be present. As the lesion ages, the area may become nodular to form *"arthropod-bite granuloma"* composed of macrophages, lymphocytes, mast cells, eosinophils, and plasma cells. Lymphoid nodules with follicle formation may develop. More specific details concerning injury inflicted by various arthropods, if known, are discussed in the following sections.

Further reading

Gross TL, et al. Nodular and diffuse diseases of the dermis with prominent eosinophils, neutrophils or plasma cells. In: Gross TL, et al., editors. Skin Diseases of the Dog and Cat: Clinical and Histopathological Diagnosis. 2nd ed. Oxford, UK: Blackwell; 2005. p. 342-372.

Steen CJ, et al. Arthropods in dermatology. J Am Acad Dermatol 2004;50:819-842.

Flies

Flies belong to the insect order Diptera. Different species have various degrees of adaptation to a parasitic existence. Adult flies feed on blood, sweat, tears, saliva, feces, urine, and other body secretions. Nonbiting, nuisance flies accomplish this by feeding only at the body surface on wounds or natural body orifices, whereas biting flies puncture the skin to feed. *Musca* are facultative feeders. Some, such as the *Simuliidae* and parasitic species of *Culicidae* and *Ceratopogonidae*, are obligate blood-suckers, although usually only the females draw blood. At the other end of the spectrum are the *Oestridae*, whose larvae are obligate parasites, and some members of the *Hippoboscidae* that are obligate parasites in the adult stage.

Because of the variety of parasitic modes, it is not possible to generalize on the effects of flies on domestic animals, nor, with the exception of a few obligate parasites, is it possible to be specific because there is little information available on primary pathogenicity. Flies adversely affect domestic animals by *causing annoyance*, by *direct toxicity* that may be fatal following massive insect attack, by *indirect toxicity* resulting from the deposition of larva into damaged skin (myiasis), by *local irritant effects* causing dermatitis that may predispose to secondary bacterial infection or to myiasis, by *injection of antigens* that induce hypersensitivity reactions, by *blood-feeding activities* that cause anemia, and by the biological or mechanical *transmission of other pathogens*. It has been estimated that tabanid flies could transmit 35 pathogens, including equine infectious anemia virus and trypanosomes. *Musca* spp. have been implicated in the mechanical transmission of anthrax, mastitis, *Habronema* spp., and conjunctivitis in animals. *Stomoxys calcitrans*, the stable fly, is thought to be the primary transmitter of habronemiasis in horses.

Animal annoyance, so-called *fly-worry*, is an important source of economic loss to the cattle, sheep and, to a lesser extent, swine industries. Fly worry refers to the behavioral disturbances in animals brought about by the attempted feeding of flies. Biting flies inflict pain, whereas nonbiting flies cause annoyance by clustering around the eyes and nostrils, where they feed on lacrimal or nasal secretions *(Musca autumnalis* and *Hydrotaea irritans)* or by other means, such as simulating the sound of a bumble bee *(Hypoderma* spp.). Fly-worry occasionally induces such apprehension that the animals run aimlessly ("gadding"), and severe injury or death may result from misadventure. Deaths are usually sporadic, but high levels of mortality have been reported. Of much greater economic importance is the *loss of production* associated with fly-worry. When the insects are numerous, they cause considerable annoyance to livestock, interfere with feeding and resting, and cause reduced milk production and reduced weight gain. Fly-worry has been attributed to biting flies such as the horn fly *(Haematobia [Lyperosia] irritans)*, the stable fly *(Stomoxys calcitrans)*, and horse flies (several genera in the family Tabanidae), and to nonbiting species such as house flies *(Musca* spp.), *Hypoderma* spp., and the sheep-head fly *(Hydrotaea irritans)*. *Culicoides* spp. biting midges can cause pruritus and restlessness in horses. Horses that develop a hypersensitivity response to *Culicoides* spp. bites may suffer weight loss as a result of severe pruritus and irritation (see Immune-mediated dermatoses). Louse flies *(Hippobosca* spp.) parasitize large animals in many parts of the world. They suck blood and tend to cluster in the perineal and inguinal region. Once the fly lands on its host, it sheds its wings and burrows into the skin to feed. They remain on their host for long periods and are a source of irritation and fly-worry.

Mortality may arise from direct toxic effect as well as from misadventure. Death may be the result of urticarial swelling of the head and neck or shock. Many flies are attracted to exhaled carbon dioxide and can occasionally cause *death by suffocation* of cattle, horses, or other animals when large numbers of flies are inhaled. Mosquitoes, especially aggressive species, such as *Aedes vigilex*, may cause significant mortality among piglets and puppies. The Simuliidae (black flies or buffalo gnats) are responsible for massive animal mortalities, particularly in temperate latitudes and river valleys following extensive flooding, when the insect population expands. They feed on cattle, horses, sheep, goats, poultry, wild mammals, and birds. *Simuliid flies exert systemic effects through inoculation of a heat-stable toxin*, which causes increased vascular permeability and abnormalities in cardiorespiratory function, which may cause death.

The hematophagous flies seldom cause serious loss of blood; however, anemia may result from heavy infestations by *Haematobia irritans*, mosquitoes, the sheep ked *Melophagus ovinus*, and *Stomoxys calcitrans*, which may ingest as much as 16 mg of blood per feeding.

In **dogs**, 3 forms of fly-bite dermatitis have been described. The first form is characterized by annular, macular targetoid lesions with a central puncture surrounded by an edematous zone with a peripheral erythematous rim on the abdomen, axillae, and lateral surfaces of the pinnae (Fig. 6-111). These lesions are associated with black fly *(Simulium* spp.) bites. The second form occurs as erythematous crusted papules that are dark red to black and hemorrhagic on the abdomen and lateral surfaces of the pinnae. The third form has ulcers covered with red to black crusts on the tips and folds of the pinnae. Only the third type is associated with clinical signs of variable pruritus. Both the second and third forms are thought to be associated with bites of stable flies *(Stomoxys calcitrans)* or deer flies *(Chrysops* spp.).

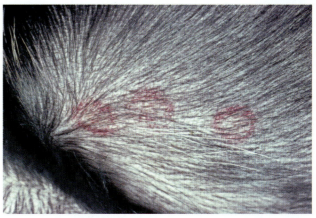

Figure 6-111 **Fly-bite dermatitis** caused by black flies in a dog. (Courtesy W.H. Miller.)

In **horses,** simulids tend to bite thinly haired, areas such as the face, pinnae, neck, ventrum, and legs. Lesions may be localized to the intermandibular region. Lesions are painful papules, wheals, ulcers, or circumscribed areas of necrosis. Simulid bites may be involved in the pathogenesis of ear papillomas and insect-bite hypersensitivity in horses.

Local irritant effect results from *injection of salivary fluids into the host*. Very little is known of the nature of the cutaneous lesions produced in animals by these insects. The character and severity of the local lesions vary. Pruritus is often intense, resulting in secondary traumatic lesions. The primary lesions are usually erythematous papules or wheals often surrounding a central bleeding point (mosquitoes) or small puncture wounds (biting flies). The wheals are usually transient but may persist for several weeks. The puncture wounds often develop an exudative crust. Some flies *(Simuliidae)* feed by lacerating the skin until a pool of blood forms on the surface from which they feed.

Histologically, there may be *intraepithelial eosinophilic spongiform pustules* or focal areas of epidermal necrosis indicating the penetration point. The dermal reaction is superficial perivascular to interstitial in pattern and contains predominantly eosinophils, lymphocytes, and plasma cells. Occasionally, there is acute necrosis of the surface of the papules, including both dermis and epidermis.

The injected salivary substances are irritant, and many are allergenic; hypersensitivity reactions probably contribute to the severity of the local lesions caused by a variety of biting flies. Hypersensitivity reactions to *S. calcitrans* are recognized in cattle; affected animals develop coalescing blisters on the forelimbs. An important allergic dermatitis of horses is caused by hypersensitivity to *Culicoides* spp. Black flies have also been associated with insect-bite hypersensitivity in horses.

Rather more important than the blood-sucking or biting flies are those species whose larvae are highly destructive facultative or obligate parasites. Infestations with such larvae cause *myiasis*, which is discussed later.

Further reading

Miller WH, et al. Parasitic skin disease. In: Miller WH, et al., editors. Muller & Kirk's Small Animal Dermatology. 7th ed. St Louis: Elsevier; 2013. p. 284-342.

Scott DW, Miller WH. Parasitic diseases. In: Scott DW, Miller WH, editors. Equine Dermatology. 2nd ed. St Louis: Elsevier Saunders; 2011. p. 212-250.

Scott DW, Miller WH. Fly-bite dermatitis in dogs: a retrospective study of 35 cases (1988-1998). Jpn J Vet Dermatol 2012;18:239-243.

Myiasis

Myiasis is the infestation of the tissue of living animals with the larvae of dipterous flies. The larvae are referred to as *maggots* or *grubs* and may be facultative or obligate parasites. The important families are *Cuterebridae, Sarcophagidae* (*Wohlfahrtia* spp.), *Gasterophilidae* (stomach bots of horses), *Oestridae* (nasal bots, warbles), and *Calliphoridae* (blowflies). Calliphorids feed only on dead tissue. Only those flies whose larvae cause cutaneous or subcutaneous lesions are discussed here. Nasal and stomach bots are described elsewhere. Agents of facultative myiasis affecting the skin live in decaying organic matter, and the females oviposit in wounded, infected, or heavily soiled skin of warm-blooded vertebrate hosts. The larvae feed on host tissues and eventually drop to the ground to pupate. *Cochliomyia hominivorax*, the screwworm fly, has a widespread geographic distribution, feed only on living tissue and has been eliminated from North America. They produce larvae that are obligatory parasites and are discussed separately.

Cuterebra. The larvae of ***Cuterebra*** spp. (order Diptera; family *Oestridae*; subfamily *Cuterebrinae*) are obligate parasites of rodents and rabbits, but occasionally aberrant infestations occur in cats and rarely in dogs, pigs, and humans. Larvae attach to the host's fur and either enter via ingestion through grooming, direct skin penetration, or through natural orifices to migrate to the subcutaneous tissues to produce an initially firm, then fluctuant, cyst-like subcutaneous abscess in which the larvae mature. The larvae breathe through a draining tract in the skin through which they are visible, and feed off tissue debris. Wounds heal slowly after larvae are removed or released, and secondary bacterial infection may occur. The majority of infections occur in late summer or fall. *In cats, the larvae have a predilection for the neck area* (Fig. 6-112), often over the submandibular salivary gland, but swellings also occur in the scrotal region. Larvae may locate in aberrant locations, such as the pharynx, nasal cavity, eye, and brain.

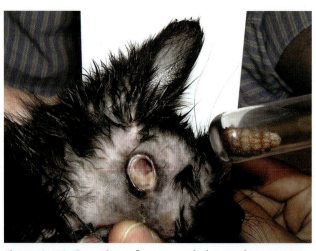

Figure 6-112 *Cuterebra* infestation with draining lesion in a cat. (Courtesy W.H. Miller.)

In South and Central America, ***Dermatobia hominis*** *(furuncular myiasis)* (order Diptera; family *Oestridae*; subfamily *Cuterebrinae*) affects horses, cattle, sheep, goats, pigs, rabbits, and people, and rarely dogs and cats. It is also known as the *human bot fly*. The adult fly captures another carrier insect to which it attaches its eggs. The eggs hatch when the carrier insect visits a host. The larvae then attach to the host and penetrate the skin to form local subcutaneous nodules that can be pruritic. The mature larvae exit the nodule through holes that leave the host susceptible to fly strike. A case report of an infected dog from the Netherlands described lesions as painful, erythematous, exudative nodules with a central pore.

Wohlfahrtia magnifica (order Diptera; superfamily *Oestoidea*; family *Sarcophagidae*) is an *obligate larval parasite of warm-blooded vertebrates* in the Mediterranean basin, Eastern and Central Europe, and Asia Minor. The female fly deposits larvae on the host near body orifices or in wounds. Larvae mature and drop to the ground to pupate in 5-7 days. *W. magnifica* causes myiasis in sheep, camels, poultry, and to a lesser extent in cattle, horses, pigs, and dogs. Fecal soiling in sheep is a predisposing condition. *W. vigil* is a parasite of mink, foxes, rabbits, and occasionally dogs and cats in North America. The larvae can penetrate the tender skin of young animals, hence the young are most often affected. *W. nubia* is a secondary facultative invader of wounds in camels in North Africa and the Middle East.

Further reading

Glass EN, et al. Clinical and clinicopathologic features in 11 cats with *Cuterebra* larvae myiasis of the central nervous system. J Vet Intern Med 1998;12:365-368.

Orfanou DC, et al. Myiasis in a dog shelter in Greece: epidemiological and clinical features and therapeutic considerations. Vet Parasitol 2011;181:374-378.

Verocai GG, et al. Furuncular myiasis caused by the human bot-fly *Dermatobia hominis* in a domestic cat from Brazil. J Fel Med Surg 2010;12:491-493.

Warbles. Warbles (hypodermiasis, grubs) is caused by the larval stages of ***Hypoderma*** **spp.** (***H. bovis*** **and** ***H. lineatum***) (order Diptera; family *Oestridae*; subfamily *Hypodermatinae*). It is common in cattle and seen occasionally in horses, sheep, and goats in the Northern Hemisphere. *H. bovis, H. lineatum,* and *H. sinense* are present in Europe and Asia. Intensive eradication programs have eliminated *Hypoderma* spp. from some northern European countries and have greatly reduced their populations in much of the United States and Canada. *Przhevalskiana silenus* affects sheep and goats in Asia and Eastern Europe. *H. diana*, a parasite of roe deer in Europe, has been identified in horses and sheep.

Warble flies are also called heel flies because the eggs are deposited predominantly on the hair of the legs. Larvae emerge 4-6 days later and burrow directly into the skin or into hair follicles, causing minimal irritation. Larvae migrate along fascial planes leaving tracks of green gelatinous material known as "butcher's jelly." The first instar larvae of *H. bovis* overwinter in the epidural fat, whereas those of *H. lineatum* develop in the esophageal submucosa. In the esophageal lesions, collagen bundles around the first instar larvae of *H. lineatum* appear fragmented, as if undergoing enzymatic digestion. A collagenase has been isolated from *H. lineatum*. In the epidural lesions of *H. bovis*, it is the fat tissue that appears necrotic. In the spring, the larvae migrate dorsally to the subcutaneous tissue of the back to form subcutaneous nodules ~3 cm in diameter with a central pore for respiration. The lesions, known as "warbles," may be painful and last for 4-6 weeks, during which the larvae undergo 2 molts. The mature third-instar larvae emerge from the breathing hole and pupate in the soil. In horses, the lesions are commonly seen over the withers and are often "blind" in that the larvae do not complete their development. Fatalities resulting from aberrant migration into the central nervous system are reported in horses.

Histologically, the cellular reaction is composed of neutrophils and eosinophils, but may be pyogranulomatous to granulomatous. It is the eosinophilic infiltrate that gives "butcher's jelly" its green coloration. However, the most intense inflammatory reactions occur at sites of previous migration rather than around the viable larvae, suggesting that in naive hosts the parasites depress any effective host responses. Proteinases with the capacity to cleave bovine complement C_3 have been isolated from the first-instar larvae of *H. lineatum*. Such enzymes could well ablate the host's inflammatory responses. The actual "warble" is lined by a wall of granulation tissue that matures to form a connective tissue capsule in which lie islands of eosinophils. The cystic cavity between the cuticle of the parasite and the granulation tissue fills with fibrin and a few inflammatory cells, chiefly eosinophils. Cuticle sloughed during ecdysis, or remnants of dead larva, incite a marked foreign-body giant cell reaction. Once the larvae emerge, the cavity is repaired by fibrosis, but small foreign-body granulomas may persist for months.

Warbles are economically important. The buzzing of the adult *H. bovis* (*H. lineatum* is silent) disturbs cattle, causing considerable loss in milk and meat production. Larval tracks in the tissues decrease carcass value, and the larval-induced holes markedly depreciate the value of the hide. Larval rupture, either accidental or deliberate, may induce a fatal anaphylactic reaction. This may result from systemic effects of the warble toxin, from type I hypersensitivity reactions or a combination of both.

Further reading

Oryan A, Bahrami S. Pathology of natural *Przhevalskiana silenus* infection in goats. Trop Biomed 2012;29:524-531.

Scott DW, Miller WH. Parasitic diseases. In: Scott DW, Miller WH, editors. Equine Dermatology. 2nd ed. St Louis: Elsevier Saunders; 2011. p. 212-250.

Calliphorine myiasis. Calliphorine myiasis (blowfly strike) is a common disorder of large animals in most areas of the world. It is *most common in sheep* and can be of major economic importance. The flies involved are members of the subfamily *Calliphoridae* (**blowflies**). Important blowfly genera are *Lucilia, Calliphora, Condylobia, Protophormia, Phormia,* and *Chrysomia*. The larvae (maggots) adopt a *facultative parasitic mode*, which is an adaptation of their beneficial and important role in the breakdown of carrion. Adult flies lay eggs on moist, warm skin of weakened or debilitated animals, in wounds or areas of heavy soiling with feces, urine, or other body fluids. Hence any species of animal can be susceptible.

Moisture, whether provided by rain, dew, urine, sweat, or inflammatory exudate, predisposes to bacterial proliferation. The odor induced by the bacterial proliferation and resultant inflammatory exudate attracts the primary flies, which deposit batches of 50-200 ova. The larvae of primary flies emerge within 12-24 hours and grow rapidly, feeding on inflammatory exudates. *The primary larvae secrete proteolytic enzymes*, including collagenases, which liquefy the host tissues and provide predigested nutrients. The *cutaneous necrosis* that results attracts the secondary flies to oviposit. The resulting larvae *tunnel into the adjacent viable tissue* and markedly expand the lesion. The putrefactive odor attracts more flies, and the process is further exacerbated. The lesions of fly strike are often extensive and *leave large areas of undermined skin with punched-out holes*. The subcutaneous tissues may become cavitated. Muscle may be destroyed and body cavities invaded. Lesions may result in death from *shock, debilitation, toxemia, or bacterial septicemia*.

The species of fly involved in fly strike differs with geographic location: *Lucilia cuprina* is the most important primary fly in Australia, *Phormia regina* in the United States and Canada, and *Lucilia sericata* in Great Britain. Several different species of flies are involved in the development of the lesion of cutaneous myiasis. Primary flies, such as *L. cuprina*, are capable of initiating a strike on living animals. Secondary flies, such as *Chrysomia rufifaces*, are not able to initiate a strike, but greatly exacerbate the lesions initiated by the primary fly. They may also displace the maggots developing from the eggs laid by the primary fly. Tertiary flies, such as the housefly *Musca domestica*, attack at a later stage and do not contribute significantly to the skin damage.

The development of fly strike depends upon abundance of primary flies, susceptible animals, and moisture. The prevalence of the disease tends to follow the rise and fall in the population of primary flies. In general, the flies require warm and moist but not hot conditions. Thus there is usually a double wave of primary flies, peaking in the spring and autumn. In sheep, the lesions are most common in the perineum *(breech strike)*, particularly in sheep with a narrow conformation and/or marked skin wrinkling, which favor urine or fecal soiling. Lesions may affect the preputial orifice *(pizzle strike)*, particularly in animals with narrow urethral orifices, which predispose to urine soiling. Rams with deep head folds may develop *poll strike*, possibly predisposed to by fight wounds. *Wound strike* occasionally follows castration or tail docking, and *body strike* follows prolonged wetting, which in turn predisposes to *fleece rot* or dermatophilosis.

Gross lesions consist of "honeycombed" foul-smelling ulcers with scalloped margins that are filled with larvae (maggots). The lesions are irritating and pruritic. Occasionally, the maggots migrate deeper into the muscle.

Further reading

Hall MJ. Traumatic myiasis of sheep in Europe: a review. Parasitologia 1997;39:409-413.

Scott DW, Miller WH. Parasitic diseases. In: Scott DW, Miller WH, editors. Equine Dermatology. 2nd ed. St Louis: Elsevier Saunders; 2011. p. 212-250.

Screwworm myiasis. Screwworm flies differ from blowflies in that *screwworm fly larvae are obligate parasites, invading edges of fresh, uncontaminated wounds on live animals*. **Cochliomyia hominivorax** and **C. macellaria** occur in North, Central, and South America. The African and Asian screwworm fly is

Chrysomyia bezziana. Eradication programs have led to a significant reduction in this condition in North and Central America.

Screwworm myiasis affects all domestic animals and humans and is an important cause of mortality in wildlife. The flies oviposit in cutaneous wounds, such as those caused by castration, dehorning, branding, or accidental injuries. The navel of neonatal calves, the perineum of recently calved cows, and tick bites are also favorable sites for oviposition. The larvae feed in groups, to penetrate and liquefy fresh, live host tissue with the aid of proteolytic enzymes. Blood-stained fluid, often containing incompletely digested shreds of tissue, oozes from the wound, which contains clusters of voraciously feeding larvae. A distinctive and particularly foul odor emanates from the lesion. The lesions are extremely painful and pruritic and may expand rapidly, leading to death from toxemia and septicemia in untreated animals. Screwworm infestation is a reportable condition in many countries.

Further reading

Scott DW, Miller WH. Parasitic diseases. In: Scott DW, Miller WH, editors. Equine Dermatology. 2nd ed. St Louis: Elsevier Saunders; 2011. p. 212-250.

Sheep ked infestation

Melophagus ovinus (Diptera: *Hippoboscidae*) *is a wingless fly that causes chronic, pruritic dermatitis of sheep.* Goats are also affected. Of worldwide distribution, the disease's chief economic importance is the associated *loss of wool production.*

Melophagus ovinus is an obligate ectoparasite. The eggs develop into larvae within the female until they are ready to pupate. The female attaches its larva to wool fibers with the aid of a sticky substance. The immotile larva transforms into a chestnut-brown pupa ~3-4 mm long. The pupal stage lasts 3-5 weeks, and the adult keds live 4-5 months. The adults are 4-7 mm and red-brown. They prefer the sides of the neck and body and are difficult to detect in fully fleeced animals. Severe pruritus leads to broken wool, alopecia, and excoriations. Heavy infestations can lead to anemia and stained wool from fly excrement. Wool loss and vertical ridging of the skin leads to a condition referred to as "cockle." The irritation induced by the bites also affects weight gain. Sheep keds can transmit several important infectious agents such as bluetongue virus.

Histologic lesions reported are superficial and deep perivascular dermatitis, with eosinophils and lymphocytes predominating. Fibrinoid necrosis of small arterioles is also described.

Further reading

Scott DW. Color Atlas of Farm Animal Dermatology. Ames, Iowa: Blackwell; 2007.

Horn fly dermatitis

Although mainly an obligate parasite of cattle, the **horn fly (*Haematobia irritans*)** is one cause of *seasonal ventral midline dermatitis in the horse.* In **cattle,** the flies feed in groups primarily on the back, withers, and head. They leave the animal only briefly to mate and lay eggs. Horn flies require fresh bovine feces to lay eggs. Large numbers of horn flies in cattle can result in significant loss of blood, wounds that attract other flies, and in loss of production. *H. irritans* is also thought to transmit the skin parasitic nematode of cattle, *Stephanofilaria stilesi.*

Haematobia irritans was associated with teat atresia in a herd of Limousin cattle in Texas. Only first-calf heifers were affected. A cord of firm tissue was palpated in the area of the teat canal in the majority of teats of the affected calves. Histologically, the papillary duct was replaced by mature fibrous connective tissue. The teat and mammary skin of all glands had fibrosis and superficial and deep, perivascular and interstitial dermatitis with perivascular mast cells and fewer eosinophils. Institution of a horn fly control program eliminated the problem in this herd.

In **horses,** horn flies cluster on the ventral abdomen (and occasionally on the neck or periocular region), producing bites marked by tiny drops of dried blood. A few days later pruritic, scaling, alopecic patches develop. These become lichenified and heal with either leukoderma or melanosis. The lesions are often single, usually well circumscribed, and occur near the umbilicus. Pruritus is variable. Histologically, lesions are perivascular and eosinophilic, typical of many insect-bite–induced dermatopathies. If ulcerated, lesions predispose to infection by *Habronema* spp. nematodes. Lesions of *Culicoides* hypersensitivity (see Immune-mediated dermatoses) and onchocerciasis may also occur on the ventrum, but these are diffuse, often extending from the axillae to the groin. Both *Culicoides* hypersensitivity and onchocerciasis are sporadic diseases, whereas up to 80% of horses in a group may be affected with horn fly–bite dermatitis.

Further reading

Edwards JF, et al. Bovine teat atresia associated with horn fly (*Haematobia irritans irritans* [L.])–induced dermatitis. Vet Pathol 2000;37:360-364.

Perris EE. Parasitic dermatoses that cause pruritus in horses. Vet Clin N Am Equine Pract 1995;11:14-15.

Mosquito-bite dermatitis

Mosquito bites in animals are common, and the bite itself is of little consequence most of the time. Mosquitoes serve as *vectors* for a number of important diseases, including malaria in humans, canine and feline heartworm disease, equine viral encephalitis and equine infectious anemia, and rabbit myxomatosis. In **cats,** mosquito bites can induce a severe papular, crusting dermatitis characterized by dense eosinophilic infiltrates. Experimental studies in cats, by using intradermal skin tests and Prausnitz-Kustner tests, indicate that these lesions develop only in cats hypersensitive to mosquito-bite antigens and are initiated by a type I hypersensitivity reaction. The disease is seasonal and often pruritic. Clinically, cats initially develop wheals progressing to erythematous papules and plaques that eventuate into crusted, ulcerated, and sometimes hypopigmented lesions (Fig. 6-113A, B). Sparsely haired regions of the body are most often affected, such as the bridge of the nose, the pinnae, and pawpad margins. The pinnae may develop symmetrical lesions of miliary dermatitis. The severity of lesions varies by individual, leading to scar formation in the more severe cases.

Histologic lesions include intraepidermal eosinophilic microabscessation and perivascular to diffuse interstitial

Arthropod Ectoparasites 671

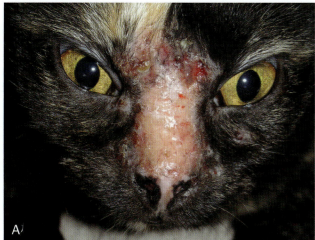

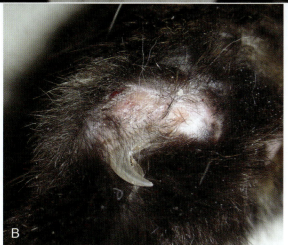

Figure 6-113 Mosquito-bite dermatitis in a cat. **A.** Ulcerative and depigmented lesions on the bridge of the nose and nasal planum. **B.** Similar lesions on the pawpad margin. (Courtesy M.S. Canfield.)

infiltrates of eosinophils, mast cells, macrophages, and lymphocytes. The epidermis is often spongiotic and hyperplastic. Nodular eosinophilic granulomas with collagen flame figures may be present. Infiltrative and necrotizing eosinophilic and mural folliculitis with mucinosis are common findings. Cats may have regional lymphadenopathy and peripheral eosinophilia.

Miscellaneous insects

Fire ants have a venomous bite. The venom is composed of *solenopsin A*, which is cytotoxic and hemolytic. Skin lesions include erythematous variably pruritic swellings to a pustular rash, with each pustule surrounded by an erythematous halo. Lesions usually resolve within 48 hours. Histopathologic findings vary. The pustular lesions are neutrophilic intraepidermal pustules with interstitial neutrophilic dermatitis. The swellings tend to be vertically oriented bands of full thickness dermal necrosis surrounded by edema and eosinophils.

Certain **caterpillar larvae** can cause cutaneous reactions most commonly in dogs. Pine and oak caterpillars (*Thaumetopoea* spp.) have bristles that contain *thaumetopoein*, which causes mast cell degranulation and histamine release. Skin lesions are most common on the lips and muzzle and include urticaria, facial pruritus, angioedema, or necrosis. The tongue may also be involved.

Further reading

Miller WH, et al. Parasitic skin disease. In: Miller WH, et al., editors. Muller & Kirk's Small Animal Dermatology. 7th ed. St Louis: Elsevier; 2013. p. 284-342.

Nagata M, Ishida T. Cutaneous reactivity to mosquito bites and its antigens in cats. Vet Dermatol 1997;8:19-26.

Power HT, Ihrke PJ. Selected feline eosinophilic skin diseases. Vet Clin N Am: Small Anim Pract 1995;25:838-840.

Lice

Lice are host-specific obligate parasites of the class Insecta. They are dorsoventrally flattened wingless insects that are common ectoparasites in most parts of the world. Two orders of lice are recognized. The *Mallophaga* are *chewing lice* that have mouth parts specially adapted for feeding on the epithelial scales, feathers, and sebaceous secretions of birds and mammals. The *Anoplura* have piercing mouth parts and are the *sucking lice* of mammals. Lice spend their complete life cycle on the host and cannot live away from their hosts for more than a few days. Nits (1-2 mm–long operculated eggs) are attached to hairs by a clear adhesive secretion by female lice (3-6 mm). Spread of infection occurs most commonly via direct contact, but transmission via indirect contact also occurs. Because various species of lice have adapted to different microenvironments within the host pelage, it is possible for an animal to carry several species at once.

Infestation with lice is called **pediculosis**. It tends to be a seasonal problem, being worse in winter. Lice do not breed at temperatures above 30° C and die at temperatures around 50° C. The signs associated with pediculosis are extremely variable. In most instances, lice do not pose a significant threat to the host. *Heavy infestations signal an underlying contributing condition, such as poor sanitation, overcrowding, ill thrift, or poor nutrition.* In some cases, animals are asymptomatic carriers or only have scaling with variable pruritus. *Most lesions result from skin irritation and pruritus, which ranges from mild to severe. Lesions include scaling, crusting, erythema, papules, excoriations, hair loss,* and damage to wool or hide caused by rubbing or biting. *Sucking lice may induce anemia, especially in young animals,* that is occasionally fatal in heavy infestations. Weight loss and decreased milk production are associated with the constant irritation seen in some lice infestations.

Lice are usually host specific, but *Heterodoxus longitarsus*, normally parasitic on kangaroos, has become an important ectoparasite of Australian dogs. *Phthirus pubis*, the human crab louse, has been reported to infest dogs living with infested humans. The dog louse, *Heterodoxus spiniger* has been detected on cats in several countries. Poultry lice feed on horses, dogs, and cats.

Louse infestation occurs in **cattle** more often than in other domestic species. *Haematopinus eurysternus*, the short-nosed louse; *H. quadripertusus*, the tail-switch louse; *H. tuberculatis*, the buffalo louse; *Linognathus vituli*, the long-nosed louse; and *Solenoptes capillatus*, the little blue cattle louse are sucking lice of cattle. *Damalinia (Bovicola) bovis* is the one chewing species. The various species have preferred habitats. *Damalinia bovis* tend to cluster about the neck, withers, and tail head. Sucking lice are commonly found on the poll, pinnae, muzzle, periocular region, neck, brisket, withers, tail, axillae, and groin. Heavy periorbital infestation of heifers by *H. quadripertusus* has caused keratoconjunctivitis and periorbital papillomatosis. Bovine pediculosis usually has little deleterious effect on weight gain and other production parameters. Economic consequences are due to deterioration of hide quality, damage to fences, and costs of treatment. One exception is *H. eurysternus* infestation, which may cause anemia and death in some uniquely susceptible cattle. *L. vituli* has been associated with severe anemia and mortality in young buffaloes. Sucking lice can serve as vectors of severe diseases, including anaplasmosis, theileriosis, and dermatomycosis.

The species of sucking lice affecting **sheep** include *Linognathus ovillus* (the face or blue louse), *L. africanus* (also called the blue louse), and *L. pedalis* (the foot louse). *Damalinia ovis* is a chewing louse and is most common over the dorsum. *L. ovillus* affects the face, and *L. pedalis* the legs and scrotum. Although goat and sheep lice are considered host specific, there are reports of naturally occurring transmission of the goat louse *Damalinia caprae* to sheep and experimental transmission of *D. ovis* to goats.

In **goats,** the sucking lice are *Linognathus stenopsis* and *L. africanus*. The chewing lice are *Damalinia caprae, D. limbata,* and *D. crassipes*. Lice are most commonly seen on the head, neck, dorsum, and groin. The haircoat of Angora goats may be seriously damaged by the irritation induced by pediculosis.

Two species of lice occur on **horses.** *Haematopinus asini*, a sucking louse, prefers the head, neck, back, thighs, and fetlocks. *Werneckiella (Damalinia) equi*, a chewing louse, favors the head, mane, and base of the tail. The populations of lice fluctuate considerably, being highest when the hair is long as in winter or in debilitated animals that have not shed their hair. In warm weather, the populations decline but some lice persist in the long hair of the mane and tail.

One species, *Haematopinus suis*, a sucking louse is parasitic on **pigs.** Preferential sites include the ears and skin folds of the neck, axillae, flanks, and inguinal areas. The lice are vectors for swinepox virus, African swine fever virus, and *Eperythrozoon suis.*

Pediculosis in **alpacas** is caused by 2 species of lice: *Bovicola (Lepikentron) breviceps*, a chewing louse and *Microthoracius mazzi (praelongiceps)*, a sucking louse. *B. breviceps* is also known to affect llamas. Chewing lice may be more numerous on the rump, dorsal trunk, and neck, and sucking lice on the head, neck, and shoulder.

Linognathus setosus is a sucking louse, and *Trichodectes canis* and *Heterodoxus spiniger* are chewing lice of **dogs.** *Trichodectes canis* may serve as an intermediate host for the tapeworm, *Dipylidium caninum*. Pediculosis is a rare disease in pet dogs. Breeds with moderately long, fine hair may provide a more favorable environment for lice, and the disease is more prevalent in the cooler winter months. Lice accumulate under mats of hair and around the ears and body openings. Pediculosis may resemble flea-bite hypersensitivity in dogs. Infestation in the absence of pruritus may be an incidental finding.

Only one species, the chewing louse, *Felicola subrostratus*, occurs on **cats.** Infestation may be an incidental finding, or it may be associated with severe pruritus with dermatitis and hair loss over the back. Pediculosis may resemble miliary dermatitis in cats.

Further reading

Arther RG. Mites and lice: biology and control. Vet Clin North Am Small Anim Pract 2009;39:1159-1171.

Cortinas R, Jones CJ. Ectoparasites of cattle and small ruminants. Vet Clin North Am Food Anim Pract 2006;22:673-693.

Norhidayu S, et al. The dog louse *Heterodoxus spiniger* from stray cats in Penang, Malaysia. Trop Biomed 2012;29:301-303.

Scott DW. Color Atlas of Farm Animal Dermatology. Ames, Iowa: Blackwell; 2007.

Scott DW, et al. Skin diseases in the alpaca *(Vicugna pacos):* a literature review and retrospective analysis of 68 cases (Cornell University 1997-2006). Vet Dermatol 2010;22:2-16.

Fleas

Fleas are ubiquitous and obligate parasites, and their survival depends upon temporary episodes of feeding and a habitat where the host is periodically available. Fleas are wingless and have a laterally compressed body. They primarily parasitize hosts that return on a regular basis to a nest, burrow, bedding, or lair. Hence animals such as ungulates rarely have fleas, and carnivores, rabbits, rodents, and bats often do. Most fleas can parasitize a range of hosts. An exception to this general rule is the more recent finding that cat fleas spend more of their lifetime on the cat than fleas infesting other species. Fleas are chiefly a problem in cats, dogs, pigs, and humans. Flea bites damage the host by irritation, pruritus, blood loss, and possible transmission of infectious agents. *Ctenocephalides felis felis*, the cat flea; *Ctenocephalides canis*, the dog flea; and *Pulex irritans*, the human flea are intermediate hosts for the dog tapeworm *Dipylidium caninum* and the filarid nematode *Acanthocheilonema (Dipetalonema) reconditum*. Fleas are also vectors for *Rickettsia* spp., *Bartonella* spp., *Haemoplasma (Mycoplasma)* spp., the promastigotes of *Leishmania* spp., *Francisella tularensis, Yersinia pestis,* and rabbit myxomatosis. Flea saliva is injected into the host as the flea feeds, leading to hypersensitivity reactions in some animals.

Fleas are the most common ectoparasites of **cats** and **dogs.** The most important species are *Ctenocephalides felis felis*, the cat flea, and *C. canis*, the dog flea. However, infestations also occur with *P. irritans* (human flea), *Leptopsylla segnis* (rat flea), *Echidnophaga gallinacea* (chicken stick-tight flea), *Spilopsyllus cuniculi* (European rabbit flea), and *Ceratophyllus* spp. (bird and hedgehog fleas). *C. felis felis* is the most common flea found on both dogs and cats in North America and northern Europe.

The clinical manifestations of flea infestation are highly variable. Most species of fleas move freely around their host's body and can be found virtually anywhere. In general, *C. felis felis* prefers the rump and inguinal areas. *E. gallinacea* has a preference for the face. *S. cuniculi*, the rabbit flea, has a preference for the pinnae and periauricular region. Typically, hunting cats, primarily in parts of Europe and Australia, acquire the infestation from their prey. Macroscopic lesions are crusted, alopecic papules on both aspects of the pinnae and periauricular areas. Histologically, there are perivascular to interstitial eosinophils. *Tunga penetrans*, most common in South America and Africa, burrows into the skin and produces significant damage at the site of attachment. Some animals, despite heavy infestations, remain asymptomatic carriers. Some animals may develop **flea-bite dermatitis,** which is a reaction to the many irritant substances in the flea's saliva, but the vast majority of animals that develop lesions do so because of hypersensitivity reactions to allergenic components of the flea saliva. **Flea-allergy dermatitis** is an extremely common and very important disease of the dog and cat; it is discussed in detail under Immune-mediated dermatoses. Finally, the blood-sucking activities of fleas may induce blood loss, iron deficiency anemia in heavily infested animals, particularly in kittens, puppies, or debilitated adults.

The 2 fleas most commonly associated with **swine** are the human flea *(P. irritans)* and the chicken stick-tight flea *(E. gallinacea)*. Infestation with *C. felis felis* and *C. canis* have also been reported. In Africa, *Tunga penetrans*, the chigoe flea or jigger, has been associated with swine infestations, although it is chiefly a human parasite. The female flea burrows into the skin, causing ulcerative lesions. Favored sites are the skin around the coronary band, on the scrotum, and on the snout. Infestations of the teat canal have been associated with agalactia in sows. Fleas may act as vectors for swinepox virus. Heavy infestations with *Ctenocephalides* spp. in Africa lead to anemia, reduced weight gain, and even death in **sheep and goats,** particularly in the young. Fleas may also trigger allergic dermatitis in sheep. *C. felis felis* has been rarely reported in **cattle.** Heavy infestation with *C. felis felis* was reported to cause mortality in calves, lambs, and kids in Israel. Rarely, **horses** may become infested with *C. felis felis*, *E. gallinacea*, or *T. penetrans*. Dermatologic signs include various degrees of rubbing, scratching, chewing, alopecia, excoriations, nonfollicular papules, and crusts. The face, distal limbs, and trunk are typical sites. Heavily infested animals can become anemic.

Further reading

Dobler G, Pfeffer M. Fleas as parasites of the family Canidae. Parasit Vectors 2011;4:139-151.

Miller WH, et al. Parasitic skin disease. In: Miller WH, et al., editors. Muller & Kirk's Small Animal Dermatology. 7th ed. St Louis: Elsevier; 2013. p. 284-342.

Scott DW. Color Atlas of Farm Animal Dermatology. Ames, Iowa: Blackwell; 2007.

Scott DW, Miller WH. Parasitic diseases. In: Scott DW, Miller WH, editors. Equine Dermatology. 2nd ed. St Louis: Elsevier Saunders; 2011. p. 212-250.

Traversa D. Fleas infesting pets in the era of emerging extra-intestinal nematodes. Parasit Vectors 2013;6:59-74.

Mites
Sarcoptic mange

Sarcoptes scabiei (Acarina: *Sarcoptidae*) is responsible for scabies (sarcoptic mange) in humans and many species of mammals worldwide. It is known to cause severe disease in a number of wildlife species. This species of mite has been divided into morphologically indistinguishable host-adapted varieties that rarely cross-infect between species of animals. Most can parasitize people but will not complete their life cycle on a human. People in contact with infected animals often develop lesions, most commonly pruritic erythematous papules. Sarcoptic mange is common in pigs, dogs, and goats and is uncommon to rare in cattle, sheep, horses, and cats. It is the most important ectoparasite of swine. In regions where ivermectin is used regularly in large animal species, this condition is much less common. It is a reportable disease in some countries.

In the normal host, the parasite completes its life cycle in tunnels burrowed into and under the stratum corneum. After mating in a "molting pocket" close to the surface, the female burrows through the stratum corneum to feed on cells of the stratum granulosum and stratum spinosum and lays ~1-4 eggs per day for ~6 weeks before dying. The eggs develop through the larval and nymphal stages in the same tunnel or in new ones, to reach maturity in 10-15 days, depending on the host species. The entire cycle takes 2-3 weeks. In general, both parasites and ova have poor viability in the external environment; however, low temperature and high humidity may allow some mites and nymphs to persist in the environment up to 21 days. The disease, which is *highly contagious*, is transmitted largely by direct contact, but may occur following indirect contact with contaminated objects such as bedding. The adult female mite is 200-400 µm in diameter, oval and white with 2 pairs of short legs anteriorly that bear long unjointed stalks with suckers. Two pairs of posterior legs are rudimentary but carry long bristles, and there is a terminal anus.

The *pathogenesis* of lesions in *S. scabiei* infestation is due to *direct damage* inflicted by the parasite mechanically, by the *irritant effects* of its secretions and excreta, and by an *allergic reaction* developed against mite antigens, including proteins in the cuticle, saliva, and feces. Scabies is a complex hypersensitivity reaction involving both humoral and cell-mediated components and circulating immune complexes. In an otherwise normal infected individual, a cell-mediated immune response is mounted against mite antigens, and this acquired immunity limits the spread of mites, preventing overwhelming infestation. In undernourished or immuno-compromised individuals, there may be widespread lesions and large numbers of mites.

In most animal hosts, sarcoptic mange is an *intensely pruritic disease*, and typically multiple animals are affected. In a herd situation, there may be decreased feed intake, weight loss, decreased milk production, hide and fiber damage, difficulty in breeding, and secondary bacterial infections and myiasis. In some wildlife species, sarcoptic mange is very severe and can lead to death. The cause for this is not completely understood but may be related to scarcity of food and animals spending much less time feeding because of intense pruritus. In addition, severe skin lesions can lead to ulceration, myiasis, secondary bacterial infections, toxemia, and sepsis.

The primary parasite-related lesions of sarcoptic mange are erythematous, crusted, nonfollicular papules that progress to scaling, oozing, larger crusts, and alopecia. Peripheral lymphadenopathy may be marked. In animals with heavy mite infestations, the lesions are characterized by alopecia, marked lichenification, accumulation of thick gray scale-crust, and fissuring. Chronic hypersensitivity lesions include excoriations, marked alopecia, scaling, and lichenification.

The distribution of the lesions is characteristic in the various species. In **pigs**, sarcoptic mange is caused by *S. scabiei* var. *suis*, and 2 clinical syndromes exist. *The most common (hypersensitivity) form* is seen mostly in young growing pigs, with intense pruritus. Lesions include papules, crusts, and excoriations on and in the ears. Aural hematomas sometimes develop. Subsequently, a widespread maculopapular eruption appears over the rump, flanks, and abdomen. In chronic cases, there is lichenification with crusts. The *second (hyperkeratotic, chronic) form* is seen in multiparous sows or debilitated animals. Lesions include thick asbestos-like crusts on the pinnae, head, neck, and legs. Pruritus is moderate to severe.

In **dogs**, the condition is caused by *S. scabiei* var. *canis*, and the preferred sites are the lateral elbows, hocks, ventral thorax and abdomen, and lateral margin of the pinna. The vast majority of dogs have widespread lesions, but some dogs have localized lesions limited to one area of their body. Localization to the face or pinnae is most common. In most cases, the dorsum is spared. Asymptomatic carriers exist, and some dogs are minimally pruritic. Dogs with compromised immune systems, resulting from coexistent immunosuppressive disease or therapy with corticosteroids or cytotoxic drugs, may be infested by much larger populations of mites.

Infestation with *S. scabiei* can occur rarely in **cats**. The primary lesions are crusting on the pinnae, bridge of the nose, paws, and tail. In contrast to most other animal hosts, affected cats are often nonpruritic and mites are easily found with deep skin scrapings. In some cases, the condition in cats has been likened to "crusted scabies" or "Norwegian scabies" in humans. Crusted scabies tends to occur in patients with impaired cell-mediated immunity, and mites multiply unchecked and reach extremely large numbers in skin and scale. The skin reacts to the infestation by increasing keratinocyte turnover, which leads to thick adherent crusts. In humans with Norwegian scabies, pruritus is absent in up to 50% of cases.

In **cattle**, scabies is caused by *S. scabiei* var. *bovis* ("head mange"), the lesions chiefly affect the face, pinnae, neck, shoulders, and rump but may become generalized. The disease in **goats**, caused by *S. scabiei* var. *caprae*, causes lesions most commonly on the face, pinnae, neck, and legs but may become generalized (Fig. 6-114A). Scabies in **sheep** is caused by *Sarcoptes scabiei* var. *ovis*. Lesions are most common on the non-wooled regions, such as the face, in particular the lips, nostrils, external surface of the pinna, and occasionally the legs. Generalized lesions occur in the more hairy desert sheep of the Sudan. Sarcoptic mange, caused by *S. scabiei* var. *equi*, is rare in **horses**. Lesions begin on the head, pinnae, and neck and may spread caudally.

In **alpacas**, sarcoptic mange, caused by *S. scabiei* var. *auchinae*, is a significant cause of weight loss and decreased fiber production in alpacas. The disease often begins on the ventral abdomen and chest, axillae, and groin, with gradual extension to the medial thighs, prepuce, perineum, legs, interdigital spaces, face, and pinnae.

Histologically, lesions vary with the balance between allergic reaction and parasitic infestation and chronicity. *Definitive diagnosis requires demonstration of the parasite.* Rarely, sections of mites or ova may be present within the epidermis or surface crusts (Fig. 6-114B). Lesions consist of a mild to severely hyperplastic epidermis with variable orthokeratotic to patchy parakeratotic hyperkeratosis. In fully developed lesions, there is marked spongiosis, mixed leukocytic exocytosis, serocellular crusts, and possibly intraepidermal eosinophilic pustules. Vasodilation, endothelial swelling, and edema may also be present. Immunosuppressed animals with large numbers of adult mites in epidermal burrows often have a markedly parakeratotic stratum corneum. Dermal lesions consist of a mild to moderate superficial to mid-level perivascular to interstitial infiltrate with a variable ratio of lymphohistiocytic cells and eosinophils. The chronic allergic lesions reflect continued trauma, with dermal fibrosis, epidermal hyperplasia with prominent rete ridge formation, hyperpigmentation, and a predominantly mononuclear cell perivascular infiltrate.

Diagnosis of the typical allergic form of the disease depends chiefly on the clinical signs of extreme pruritus and the nature

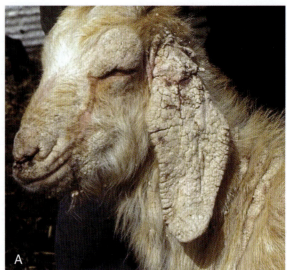
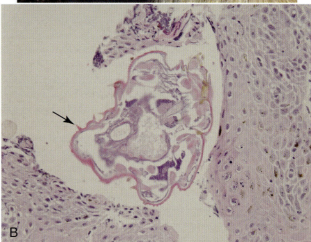

Figure 6-114 Sarcoptic mange. A. Alopecia and thick crusts over the pinna, face, and neck of a goat. (Courtesy I. Yeruham.) **B.** Note the dorsal spines (arrow) on the mite burrowing into the epidermis of a dog.

and distribution of the cutaneous lesions. Mites are characteristically difficult to demonstrate, either in skin scrapings or in microscopic section. Approximately 50-80% of affected dogs fail to yield parasites even when multiple scrapings are performed. Mites are more commonly recovered from puppies than adult dogs. *The microscopic lesions are not diagnostic, being indistinguishable from other allergic and parasitic dermatoses that feature eosinophils. Fifty to 100% of dogs with scabies that have pinnal lesions will have a positive pinnal-pedal reflex.* The most useful diagnostic procedure is response to appropriate therapy. In the chronic form of sarcoptic mange associated with poorly developed hypersensitivity reactions, mites are plentiful in scrapings and in tissue section.

Further reading

Huang H, Lien Y. Feline sarcoptic mange in Taiwan: a case series of five cats. Vet Dermatol 2013;24:457-459.

Malik R, et al. Crusted scabies (sarcoptic mange) in four cats due to *Sarcoptes scabiei* infestation. J Fel Med Surg 2006;8: 327-339.

Miller WH, et al. Parasitic skin disease. In: Miller WH, et al., editors. Muller & Kirk's Small Animal Dermatology. 7th ed. St Louis: Elsevier; 2013. p. 284-342.

Pin D, et al. Localised sarcoptic mange in dogs: a retrospective study of 10 cases. J Small Anim Pract 2006;47:611-614.

Scott DW. Color Atlas of Farm Animal Dermatology. Ames, Iowa: Blackwell; 2007.

Scott DW, et al. Skin diseases in the alpaca (Vicugna pacos): a literature review and retrospective analysis of 68 cases (Cornell University 1997-2006). Vet Dermatol 2010;22:2-16.

Notoedric mange

Notoedres cati (Acarina: *Sarcoptidae*) is the cause of *feline scabies* and is also a parasite of the rabbit, and occasionally foxes, dogs, and humans. *The disease in cats is uncommon to rare*, although there are some endemic areas of higher prevalence. The mite has a life cycle similar to that of *S. scabiei*. *The infestation is highly contagious*, with transmission chiefly by direct contact. The major clinical sign is *pruritus*. The lesions in cats commence on the head and ears, particularly on the margin of the pinna but may extend to the neck, paw, or become generalized (Fig. 6-115A, B). Female mites burrow into the horny layer of the epidermis between hair follicles. These burrows appear on the skin surface in the center of minute papules. Lesions include partial alopecia, thickening and wrinkling of the skin, and in chronic cases, the formation of tightly adherent yellow-gray crusts. There may be accompanying regional lymphadenopathy. Lesions in dogs are indistinguishable from sarcoptic mange. Histologically, the epidermis is hyperplastic to spongiotic, and there is eosinophil-rich, superficial perivascular to interstitial dermatitis with marked focal parakeratosis. Mite segments may be found within the superficial epidermis. *The diagnosis is based on history, clinical signs, and demonstration of typical mites in section or skin scrapings. Notoedres* spp. mites are readily found in skin scrapings from infected cats. These mites are smaller than *S. canis* and have medium-length unjointed sucker-bearing stalks on their legs, more body striations, and a dorsal anus, whereas *Sarcoptes* has a terminal anus.

Further reading

Leone F. Canine notoedric mange: a case report. Vet Dermatol 2007;18:127-129.

Miller WH, et al. Parasitic skin disease. In: Miller WH, et al., editors. Muller & Kirk's Small Animal Dermatology. 7th ed. St Louis: Elsevier; 2013. p. 284-342.

Psoroptic mange

Psoroptic mange caused by **Psoroptes** mites (Acarina: *Psoroptidae*) is highly contagious and infests *sheep, cattle, horses, rabbits, and goats* as well as other nondomestic species. Humans are not susceptible. There are actually fewer species of psoroptic mites than originally thought, as mites from one host can often infect another host, and morphologic distinctions overlap. Based on critical literature review and molecular genetic analyses, the *Psoroptes* mites are conspecific, and, by rule of priority, belong to the **one genus *P. equi*** (Hering, 1838). Valid species include *P. cervinus*, *P. cuniculi*, *P. natalensis*, and *P. ovis*, and they are synonyms of *P. equi*. *P. ovis* infests sheep, cattle, goats, rabbits, and horses. *P. cuniculi* is an ear mite of several species, including rabbit, horse, donkey, mule, goat, and sheep, and is a body mite in horses. *P. natalensis* infests cattle, zebu, water buffaloes, and horses in South Africa, South America, and Europe. *P. cervinus* occurs as an ear mite in bighorn sheep and as a body mite in wapitis in the western part of the United States. Transmission occurs via direct and indirect contact.

Psoroptic mange is a serious disease in cattle and sheep and is a reportable disease in several countries. Bovine psoroptic mange showed a recrudescence in North America during the 1970s and early 1980s but has been brought under control by the effective use of ivermectin. Ovine psoroptic mange has been eradicated from many countries, including New Zealand, the United States, and Canada. *The economic importance* in sheep and cattle results from a marked decrease in weight gain, reduced milk production, reduced fleece weight and quality, occasional mortality, and costs related to prevention and eradication campaigns.

Psoroptic mites do not burrow into the outer epidermis, as do the sarcoptic mites, but instead complete their life cycle on the skin surface. Lipids from the stratum corneum provide a major source of nutrients in the early stages of infestation, probably supplemented by serous and hemorrhagic inflammatory exudates in the later stages.

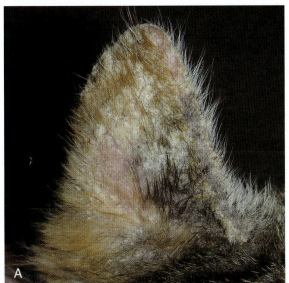

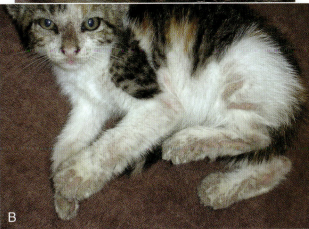

Figure 6-115 **Notoedric mange** in a kitten. **A.** Alopecia and thick adherent crust on the pinna. **B.** Alopecia, erythema and crusting on all paws and distal limbs. (Courtesy M.S. Canfield.)

Psoroptic mange is characterized by *intensely pruritic dermatitis*. The pathogenicity of the mite has been attributed to its local irritant effect on the epidermis, but this does not readily explain the marked loss of condition induced by *Psoroptes* infestation in some species, particularly cattle. The detrimental systemic effects may derive directly or indirectly from a *chronic hypersensitivity reaction* rather than from local dermatitis. The histologic lesions, in which the predominant inflammatory cells in the superficial dermis are eosinophils, mast cells, and lymphocytes, are consistent with an *allergic pathogenesis*. Constant pruritus resulting from allergy markedly reduces feed intake, and secondary bacterial infection or myiasis may further contribute to loss of condition. There is little evidence to support the hypothesis that the mites inoculate a toxic compound along with their saliva.

Histologically, lesions are similar in all species. The pattern of inflammation is superficial perivascular to interstitial dermatitis with predominantly spongiotic, exudative, or hyperplastic reactions, depending on chronicity. The eosinophil is the most numerous of the infiltrating leukocytes, followed by lymphocytes, other mononuclear cells, and mast cells. Eosinophilic microabscesses and focal areas of epidermal edema, leukocytic exocytosis, and necrosis may be found. Dermal edema may be marked. Mites are rarely seen but if present are both on top of and under the surface scale-crust. Sebaceous gland hyperplasia has been described in lesions in sheep and cattle.

Psoroptic mange in **sheep,** also called *sheep scab,* is common to uncommon in most parts of the world and is caused by *Psoroptes ovis.* Psoroptic mange may occur as a latent infection in which mites persist in the ears, infraorbital fossae, inguinal and perineal folds, and at the base of the horns. In rams, mites may be found on the scrotum or prepuce in small, dry lesions. Latency occurs in the summer months, when the fleece microclimate is less favorable to parasite proliferation. In autumn and winter or with debilitation of the host, the parasitic population explodes and lesions are induced. The withers and sides are particularly affected. The initial lesions are vesicles and yellow-green pustules that rupture, ooze, and develop into yellow crusts. The individual lesions expand at the periphery and may coalesce to become diffuse over most of the body surface. Fleece overlying the skin lesions becomes stained, moist, soiled, and matted. Tufts and clumps of matted wool may be shed or pulled out by self-trauma because of the intense pruritus. Affected sheep scratch, kick, rub, and tear out the fleece with their teeth.

Excoriations, ulcerations, and secondary myiasis and bacterial infections occur. In addition, *P. cuniculi* is an occasional cause of "ear mites" in sheep, and in some cases, clinical signs are limited to the ears and may be due to *P. cuniculi* or *P. ovis.* Aural hematomas may result from head shaking, rubbing, and scratching at the pinnae.

In **cattle,** psoroptic mange is sometimes referred to as *body mange.* It is uncommon to common in most parts of the world. Mite populations are usually higher during cold weather, and thus clinical signs are more severe in the winter. Lesions in naturally affected cattle usually commence about the poll, withers, or at the base of the tail, and chiefly result from persistent licking, rubbing, and scratching induced by intense pruritus. Early lesions include papules, pustules, exudation, and excoriations. Infested areas are fairly well defined as areas of alopecia. Alopecic areas become lichenified and covered by dry gray crusts and scales. Severely affected calves may develop mild anemia, lymphopenia, and marked neutropenia.

Psoroptic mange is uncommon in **goats** and is caused by *P. cuniculi (the ear canker mite)* and *P. ovis* (previously *P. caprae*). *P. cuniculi* is found in the ear canal, and clinically, signs range from absent to head shaking, ear scratching, and variable degree of excessive cerumen, crusted lesions on the inner surface, and alopecia on the outer surface of the pinna. Otitis media and otitis interna are possible if the tympanic membrane ruptures. In debilitated or stressed animals, thick brown-yellow, dry scale-crust accumulates on the inner aspect of the pinna and, rarely, spreads to involve the poll, body, and the legs. Concurrent *Mycoplasma* and *P. cuniculi* infections have been described in the ears of goats; however, *Mycoplasma* may be cultured from the ears of clinically normal animals, placing some doubt on the significance of the finding. *P. ovis* has been reported to cause otitis externa, crusts, scales, and alopecia of the pinnae, head, face, pasterns, and interdigital areas. Pruritus is variable.

In **horses,** *P. cuniculi* is found quite frequently in the ear. Clinical signs are variable, but when present, the main distribution is the topline affecting the ears, mane, and tail and, less commonly, the dorsal trunk. Infested horses may be asymptomatic. Signs of ear disease include head shaking, ear scratching, head shyness, or a lop-eared appearance. Pruritus is variable but can be intense. In mildly pruritic horses, there may be mane and tail seborrhea. In the more pruritic horses, there are commonly nonfollicular papules, crusts, excoriations, and alopecia. *P. ovis (P. equi)* infestations are rare; lesions are crusted papules with alopecia, and the preferred sites are at the base of the mane, forelock, and tail.

The mite responsible for psoroptic mange in **alpacas** has been referred to as *P. communis* var. *auchinae.* The varieties *P. auchinae, P. cuniculi,* and *P. ovis,* however, have not been officially named. The condition is usually pruritic, and lesions are most commonly present on the head, neck, and pinnae but can become more widespread, involving the shoulders, back, rump, sides, and perineum. In some cases, clinical signs are limited to the ears and include head shaking, ear twitching, scaling in the ear canals, and occasionally purulent exudate caused by secondary bacterial infections. Skin lesions include papules, crusts, exudation, and alopecia.

Further reading

Losson BJ. Sheep psoroptic mange: an update. Vet Parasitol 2012;189:39-43.

Lusat J, et al. Mange in alpacas, llamas and goats in the UK: incidence and risk. Vet Parasitol 2009;163:179-184.

Scott DW. Color Atlas of Farm Animal Dermatology. Ames, Iowa: Blackwell; 2007.

Scott DW, et al. Skin diseases in the alpaca *(Vicugna pacos):* a literature review and retrospective analysis of 68 cases (Cornell University 1997-2006). Vet Dermatol 2010;22:2-16.

Scott DW, Miller WH. Parasitic diseases. In: Scott DW, Miller WH, editors. Equine Dermatology. 2nd ed. St Louis: Elsevier Saunders; 2011. p. 212-250.

Chorioptic mange

Chorioptic mange, most commonly caused by ***Chorioptes bovis*** (Acarina: *Psoroptidae*), affects horses, cattle, sheep, and goats. *C. texanus* has also been reported to affect cattle, goats, elk, and reindeer. Not host specific, C. bovis is an obligate parasite that lives on the surface of the skin. The mite populations tend to fluctuate considerably as a result of host and environmental factors. As with *Sarcoptes* spp. and *Psoroptes* spp. infestations, mite numbers and thus severity of clinical signs are more prominent in the winter. Mites do not survive, and numbers decline when the environment is hot and dry. Inapparent infections allow persistence in the population. Pruritus is variable. It is absent to intense in the horse, goat, and cattle; tends to be intense in sheep; and tends to be absent to mild in alpacas. Lesions usually occur as erythema and papules progressing to scaling, oozing, crusts, and alopecia. In some cases, lesions may become lichenified, depending upon the duration of the disease and the degree of self-trauma inflicted. The condition is contagious and transmission occurs via direct and indirect contact.

Chorioptic mange (foot mange, tail mange) is uncommon in **cattle** in most parts of the world. It predominantly affects *housed dairy cows* and is most prevalent in winter. Subclinical infections are probably quite common. The major clinical sign is *pruritus*, but this is not as severe as in sarcoptic or psoroptic mange. Chorioptic mange is, in general, a less serious condition than psoroptic mange in cattle, although a syndrome of highly pruritic coronitis was associated with falling milk production. The typical distribution of lesions is perineum, tail, scrotum, udder, and caudal areas of thigh, hindlimbs, and rump. Lesions are predominantly alopecia, erythema, lichenification, and wrinkling of the skin.

The disease in **horses** is common. As indicated by the colloquial name "leg mange," lesions occur preferentially on the lower limb around the fetlock but may extend proximally to the thigh and ventral abdomen and rarely become widespread. Draft horses, with thick-feathered fetlocks, are affected more often.

Chorioptic mange is common in **goats**. Lesions are most common on the feet and hindlegs, although lesions can also be on the forelegs, perineum, tail, udder, teats, scrotum, ventrum, and may spread to the lateral trunk, neck, and face.

In **sheep**, chorioptic mange (foot mange, scrotal mange) is uncommon in most parts of the world. Lesions are more common in the nonwooled regions, particularly lower hindlimbs (including pastern and interdigital skin) and scrotum. The scrotum may be affected, and the resultant scrotal dermatitis may lead to infertility in rams. Lesions may also be present on the forelegs, udder, teats, and rump. Severe infestations can reduce growth rates and milk and meat yields. Chorioptic mange has been eradicated from the sheep population in the United States. It is a reportable disease in some countries.

Chorioptes bovis is the most common mite infestation of **alpacas**. Lesions include scale, crust, and alopecia on the ventral tail, perineal region, ventral abdomen, and medial thighs (Fig. 6-116A). Lesions can spread to the axillae, tips and lateral surface of the pinnae, face, neck, dorsum, and feet. In severe cases, erosions, ulcers and lichenification can be seen. Interestingly, heavily infested alpacas can be clinically normal, and alpacas with extensive lesions can have low numbers of mites.

Definitive diagnosis is based on history, physical examination, and demonstration of mites by scraping, brushing, or combing affected areas and examining those samples microscopically. Mites are active, fast moving, and usually easy to demonstrate during cool weather. Histopathology reveals

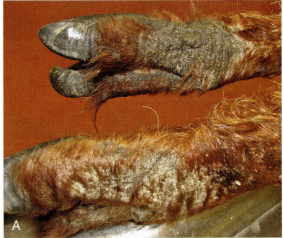

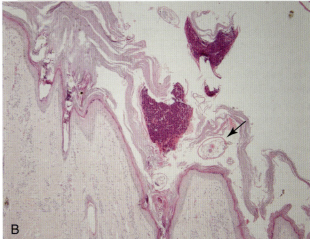

Figure 6-116 Chorioptic mange in an alpaca. **A.** Alopecia, crusting, and lichenification of the distal hindlimbs. **B.** Mild perivascular dermatitis with marked hyperkeratosis. Note the cross-sections of mites (arrow) within the surface keratin.

variable degrees of superficial perivascular to interstitial dermatitis with numerous eosinophils. Eosinophilic epidermal microabscesses and focal epidermal edema, exocytosis, and necrosis ("epidermal nibbles") may be seen. Mites are not usually seen in skin biopsy specimens (Fig. 6-116B).

Further reading

Scott DW, Miller WH. Parasitic diseases. In: Scott DW, Miller WH, editors. Equine Dermatology. 2nd ed. St Louis: Elsevier Saunders; 2011. p. 212-250.

Suh G, et al. The first outbreak of *Chorioptes texanus* (Acari: *Psoroptidae*) infestation in a cattle farm in Korea. Korean J Parasitol 2008;46:273-278.

Otodectic mange

Otodectes cynotis (Acarina: *Psoroptidae*) is an obligate parasite of the external skin surface of *dogs, cats, and ferrets*. Although the mite may be found at several body sites, its preferred habitat is the *external ear canal*. The major lesion is thus *otitis externa* (see Vol. 1, Special senses). Focal, erythematous, alopecic, or excoriated lesions occur occasionally on the face, paws, neck, or tailhead. Self-trauma and head shaking can lead to aural hematomas. The mites are contagious, particularly in young animals, and can live off the host for extended periods of time. *Diagnosis is by direct visualization;* however, mites may be difficult to demonstrate in some cases. Mites can cause a transient papular dermatitis in humans or rarely otitis externa.

Cheyletiellosis

Members of the genus **Cheyletiella** (Acarina: *Cheyletidae*) affect *dogs, cats, rabbits, wild animal species, and, incidentally, humans*. Three species are involved: *C. parasitivorax* is chiefly a parasite of rabbits, although formerly considered as a canine pathogen; *C. yasguri* is the major canine cheyletid; and, the species most commonly associated with feline infestation is *C. blakei*. Host specificity is weak, and cross-infestations are common. The mites are large, ovoid, 400 μm, obligate parasites with curved palpal claws. The mites live in the keratin layer of the epidermis; they do not burrow, but they pierce the skin with stylet-like chelicerae to feed on lymph. Ova are non-operculated, smaller than louse nits, and are attached to hairs by fine fibrillar strands. Fully developed nymphs emerge from eggs. The entire life cycle is completed on one host and is about 21 days. Adult female mites can live up to 10 and possibly 30 days off their host without feeding, and thus transmission can be both indirect and direct. The mites are highly contagious.

Pruritus is variable, ranging from absent to intense, and some animals have nonlesional pruritus. The gross lesions in both the dog and cat reflect the mite's *predilection for the dorsal midline*. Lesions often commence over the caudal back and progress cranially but may become generalized. The typical lesion is a moderate to marked exfoliation of small, dry, white scales (seborrhea sicca). The mites crawl in "pseudotunnels" in the loose keratin debris, and their movement has produced the colloquial name *walking dandruff* for cheyletiellosis. Hair loss may occur because of scratching and overgrooming, and pruritus tends to increase. The intensity of the pruritus may outweigh the number of mites, suggesting a hypersensitivity reaction. Some animals may develop exfoliative erythroderma or a scabies-like condition with similar distribution of lesions and intensity of pruritus. Cats may develop, in addition, focal, multifocal, or generalized erythematous papules or crusted lesions (miliary dermatitis). Other cats may develop self-induced dorsal hypotrichosis with few or no skin lesions. Free-living cheyletids *(Cheyletus eruditus)* can also infest dogs and cats. These mites do not induce clinical signs.

Diagnosis depends upon demonstration of the mites via direct examination of the animal, skin scraping, acetate tape, vacuum cleaning, or flea-combing techniques. *Cheyletiella* eggs and occasionally mites can often be found in feces, especially in grooming cats. Histopathology shows a spongiotic hyperplastic superficial perivascular dermatitis with variable numbers of eosinophils. In some cases, an interface lichenoid lymphoplasmacytic dermatitis is seen. Mite segments are occasionally found within the stratum corneum. Humans in contact with affected animals often develop a pruritic maculopapular rash on the arms and trunk. Individual human cases of a bullous eruption with systemic lupus erythematosus, bullous pemphigoid, and peripheral eosinophilia with elevated immune complexes and joint pain with decreased mobility and numbing of fingertips associated with *C. blakei* have been reported. As the mites do not complete their life cycle on humans, skin lesions usually regress once the animal is treated.

Further reading

Dobrosavljevic DD, et al. Systemic manifestations of *Cheyletiella* infestation in man. Int J Dermatol 2007;46:397-399.

Miller WH, et al. Parasitic skin disease. In: Miller WH, et al., editors. Muller & Kirk's Small Animal Dermatology. 7th ed. St Louis: Elsevier; 2013. p. 284-342.

Saevik BK, et al. *Cheyletiella* infestation in the dog: observations on diagnostic methods and clinical signs. J Small Anim Pract 2004; 45:495-500.

Sotiraki ST. Factors affecting the frequency of ear canal and face infestation by *Otodectes cynotis* in the cat. Vet Parasitol 2001;96: 309-315.

Psorergatic mange

Psorergates (Psorobia) ovis (Acarina: *Cheyletidae*) is a parasite of the integument of *sheep. The* disease is uncommon and occurs in Australia, New Zealand, South Africa, and South America. It is thought to have been eradicated from the United States and has not been reported in Europe. The mite (100-200 μm), which is much smaller than sarcoptid mites, is an *obligate parasite and goes through its life cycle on the skin surface in the loose keratin debris.* The mite does not penetrate deeper than the stratum corneum. Infestations occur predominantly in the winter and spring. Sheep experience intense pruritus with rubbing, chewing, and kicking at fleece. There may be scaling and matted, chewed, broken, and absent wool over the lateral thorax, flanks, and thighs. In affected areas, the wool resembles bleached, twisted tufts that give the fleece a ragged, tasseled appearance. Fleece damage is more severe in the fine-wooled Merino.

Psorergates (Psorobia) bos is the cause of psorergatic mange in cattle. The disease is uncommon and has been reported in North America, Africa, Australia, and Europe. Clinical signs vary from absent to severe alopecia, scaling, and pruritus over the dorsal head, neck, shoulders, rump, and back.

Further reading

Cortinas R, Jones CJ. Ectoparasites of cattle and small ruminants. Vet Clin North Am Food Anim Pract 2006;22:673-693.

Scott DW. Color Atlas of Farm Animal Dermatology. Ames, Iowa: Blackwell; 2007.

Demodectic mange

More than 140 **Demodex** (Acarina: *Demodicidae*) species or subspecies have been identified in hair follicles, sebaceous glands, Meibomian glands, and ceruminous glands of numerous mammals, including dogs, cats, cattle, goats, horses, sheep, pigs, deer, and hamsters. *Demodex gatoi* in cats lives in the superficial stratum corneum rather than in the follicles. In small numbers, *Demodex* spp. are normal inhabitants of the hair follicles and sebaceous glands in dogs, humans, and probably most mammals, and their position is invariably head-down. Transmission of follicular mites usually occurs from mother to young during the first 3 days of life through close physical contact while nursing. *Demodex* spp. *are obligate parasites completing their life cycle on the host.* Mites feed on cells, sebum, and epidermal debris. They are rapidly killed by desiccation on the surface of the skin, but mites move from follicle to follicle, and it is probably at this time that transmission to another host takes place. Two or more *Demodex* spp. can simultaneously parasitize the same mammalian host. Demodicosis or demodectic mange refers to a proliferation of mites associated with clinical signs and is often, but not always, associated with immunocompromise in the host.

Canine demodicosis. Canine demodicosis (demodectic mange, follicular mange, red mange) is one of the most common skin disorders of **dogs** in North America. Two species of *Demodex* have been identified: ***D. canis*** (300 µm) and ***D. injai*** (the long-bodied mite, 334-368 µm). Recent genetic studies have demonstrated that *D. cornei* (the short-tailed mite, 90-148 µm) should be considered a morphologic variant of *D. canis* rather than a separate species. Two types of demodicosis are generally recognized in dogs with *D. canis* infestations: localized and generalized. **Localized demodicosis** occurs as one to several, small, well-circumscribed, erythematous, scaly, nonpruritic to occasionally pruritic areas of alopecia, most commonly on the face (periocular and around lips) and forelegs (Fig. 6-117A). Most cases resolve spontaneously. In some cases, the condition is limited to the external ear canal, and these dogs have pruritic ceruminous otitis externa. **Generalized demodecosis** is defined as involvement of an entire body region, multiple localized regions or complete involvement of 2 paws or more. Generalized demodecosis usually starts between 3 and 18 months of age. Over time, lesions, as described above, enlarge and may coalesce to form patches. Follicular casts may be pronounced. Peripheral lymphadenopathy may be marked. Lesions that become secondarily infected with bacteria display edema, exudation, and crusting (Fig. 6-117B). In some cases, lesions are nodular, especially in English Bulldogs. Spontaneous resolution occurs in >50% of cases; however, if lesions do not spontaneously resolve and if the dog does not receive adequate treatment, lesions will likely continue into adulthood. This condition can be very severe and even fatal. Dogs that first develop the disease at 4 years of age or older are considered to have *adult-onset generalized demodicosis*. Disorders associated with adult-onset demodicosis include hypothyroidism, hyperglucocorticism, leishmaniasis, malignant neoplasia, and immunosuppressive therapy. In >50% of cases, no underlying disease can be documented at the time of demodicosis diagnosis but may become evident weeks to months into therapy.

The pathogenesis of juvenile-onset generalized demodecosis appears to be multifactorial and not completely understood. The disease is thought to be a genetically mediated specific immunodeficiency that allows the proliferation of *Demodex* mites. The condition is more common in purebred dogs, and breeds at risk include American Staffordshire Terrier, Staffordshire Bull Terrier, and Shar Pei. Although some studies have suggested a decrease in T lymphocytes or premature apoptosis of peripheral blood leukocytes, most dogs are not lymphopenic, and rather, the problem is depressed T-cell function, not decreased numbers. It also appears that immune suppression is worse in those with secondary bacterial pyoderma. One study concluded that dogs with reoccurring demodicosis have higher interleukin-10 (IL-10) levels than healthy dogs and those suffering the disease for the first time. IL-10 can inhibit cytokine secretion by Th1 cells, including IL-1, interferon-γ (IFN-γ) and tumor necrosis factor-β. IL-10 has anti-inflammatory and suppressive effects on most hematopoietic cells, and it indirectly suppresses cytokine production and proliferation of antigen-specific CD4+ T effector cells

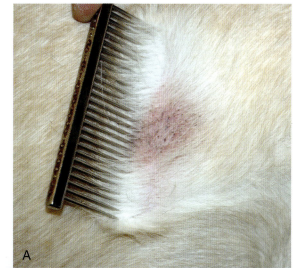
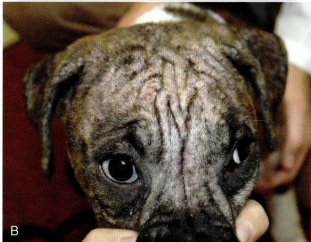
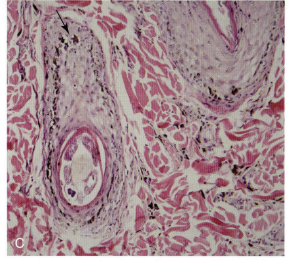

Figure 6-117 *Demodex canis* in a dog. **A.** Localized demodecosis. (Courtesy E. Smith.) **B.** Generalized demodecosis. **C.** Mural interface folliculitis with vacuolar degeneration and apoptosis (arrow) of the outer root sheath, intraluminal mites, and perifollicular pigmentary incontinence.

by inhibiting the antigen-presenting capacity of antigen-presenting cells.

Dogs with infestations with *D. injai* generally have a different clinical presentation than those with *D. canis*. Terriers,

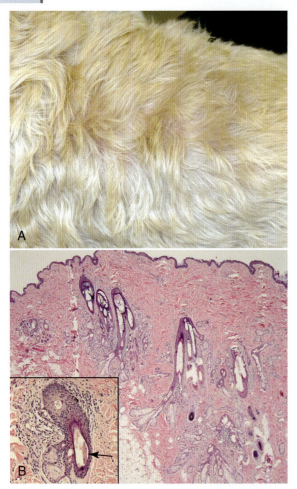

Figure 6-118 *Demodex injai* in a dog. **A.** Erythema and greasy haircoat over the dorsal trunk. (Courtesy W.H. Miller.) **B.** Sebaceous gland hyperplasia with perifollicular inflammation and lymphocytic mural folliculitis. Rare intraluminal mites (arrow) are detected (see inset).

CD8+ cytotoxic T cells, whereas the perifollicular infiltrates were found to be composed of approximately equal numbers of CD4+ and CD8+ lymphocytes. The external root sheath may be hyperplastic. Current research suggests lymphocyte-mediated follicular wall injury may be directed against keratinocytes expressing either altered self-antigens or *Demodex* antigens. It is not known whether or not the presence of cytotoxic T lymphocytes indicates an appropriate host reaction to eliminate the parasite or if it represents an inappropriate and self-damaging host response.

Perifolliculitis is also a consistent feature with infiltrates of plasma cells, macrophages, and lymphocytes in periadnexal regions. Mast cells and eosinophils may be present in smaller numbers. Marked follicular hyperkeratosis is associated with variable numbers of mites in the upper third of the follicle. Mural folliculitis is also consistently present at later stages and in cases with secondary bacterial infection, but may not be the predominant pattern. In some cases, follicles may contain numerous mites but have no evidence of folliculitis, possibly indicating a poor immune response. Typically, large numbers of mites occupy the hair follicles at all levels and also occlude the opening of the sebaceous gland into the pilar canal. Marked follicular hyperkeratosis and build-up of mite products causes follicular plugging. Bacterial proliferation, chiefly *Staphylococcus* spp., within the plugged follicle often induces suppurative luminal folliculitis. The combined effects of *follicular keratosis*, mite proliferation, and folliculitis lead to *follicular rupture* and release of mites, bacteria, keratin, sebum, and other irritant products into the dermis. The keratin and other irritant substances stimulate a pyogranulomatous reaction, chiefly of neutrophils; epithelioid macrophages; and fewer multinucleated histiocytic giant cells. Epidermal lesions include hyperplasia, orthokeratotic and parakeratotic hyperkeratosis, and variable spongiosis, neutrophilic exocytosis, ulceration, and inflammatory crusting. Longer-standing lesions consist of perifollicular mid to deep dermal or occasionally subcuticular granulomas, sometimes containing remnants of mites. Chronic lesions also have marked dermal fibrosis, often with obliteration of adnexa. Mites or fragments of mites are found in the subcapsular zone of regional lymph nodes associated with a local granulomatous inflammatory response. These do not indicate active invasion but rather passive transport to the node, via lymphatic channels. Through blood and lymph drainage, dead and degenerate mites in all stages can also be found in the spleen, lung, intestinal wall, liver, kidney, urinary bladder, thyroid gland, blood, urine, and feces.

Histopathologic changes in the skin of dogs with *D. injai* are somewhat different. Usually, there is marked sebaceous gland hyperplasia, especially in the skin of the dorsal trunk (Fig. 6-118B). In general, very few, if any, mites are detected within the hair follicles of biopsy specimens (see Fig. 6-118B inset). In one study, pyogranulomatous sebaceous adenitis was observed in 2 of 5 cases biopsied. Lymphoplasmacytic periadnexal dermatitis is a typical feature.

Three species of *Demodex* mites are associated with **feline demodecosis**. *D. gatoi* appears to be the most common, and it is the shortest, measuring 91-108 μm. It is a broad mite that inhabits the stratum corneum. *D. cati* is a long (182-291 μm) slender mite with similar morphology to *D. canis*. Like *D. canis*, this mite resides within hair follicles, sebaceous glands, and their ducts. The third unnamed species has rounded edges and measures 139 ± 4.5 μm. It has been found along hair shafts of plucked hairs and therefore is thought to reside

especially the West Highland White Terrier, Shih Tzu, and Wirehaired Fox Terrier are predisposed. Most dogs are middle-aged to older dogs with generalized disease that is characterized by mild to intense pruritus and greasy seborrhea, especially of the face and topline (Fig. 6-118A). Erythema, hyperpigmentation, and comedones have been described, but hypotrichosis, alopecia, and secondary bacterial skin infections are rare. Many affected dogs have had prior histories of allergic dermatitis, immunosuppression, or immunomodulatory drug use. One 12-year-old spayed female Beagle undergoing immunomodulatory therapy for immune-mediated polyarthritis was reported to have bilateral ceruminous otitis externa associated with *D. injai*.

Histologically, demodicosis has a variable appearance, depending on the stage of the disease and presence of secondary bacterial infection. Early, uncomplicated lesions are characterized by a predominantly *lymphocytic mural interface folliculitis*. Lymphocytic infiltration of the isthmus and infundibulum, accompanied by various degrees of vacuolar degeneration and apoptosis of keratinocytes of the outer root sheath; follicular melanosis or pigment clumping in the outer root sheath; and perifollicular pigmentary incontinence, are present (Fig. 6-117C). Immunophenotyping has identified infiltrating lymphocytes as within hair follicles; however, this mite has not been demonstrated in biopsy samples.

Demodex gatoi is a contagious mite that is most commonly associated with pruritus and overgrooming; however, some cats are asymptomatic carriers. Affected cats generally have self-induced alopecia over the ventral abdomen, thorax, and medial aspects of the limbs. The skin may be erythematous, scaly, or hyperpigmented, depending on the chronicity and severity of the pruritus. The mite may be difficult to find in cats that groom excessively. Histologically, minimal inflammation is observed. The epidermis may be irregularly hyperplastic, and hyperkeratotic and mites can sometimes be observed within the stratum corneum. In severely pruritic cases, there may be erosions, ulcerations, and crusts with mild to moderate perivascular to diffuse infiltrates of lymphocytes, histiocytes, eosinophils, and mast cells. Neutrophils are prominent in ulcerated areas.

Demodex cati infestation results in a localized or generalized dermatitis as with *D. canis* in dogs. Localized disease is rare and can involve the eyelids, periocular area, head, or neck. It can occur as ceruminous otitis externa. Skin lesions are variably pruritic with patchy alopecia, papules, comedones, erythema, scaling, and crusting. Generalized feline demodicosis is rare and not usually as severe as the canine form. Lesions are primarily on the face and head, but may be on the neck, trunk, and limbs. Generalized demodicosis caused by *D. cati* is usually associated with underlying disease, such as diabetes mellitus, hyperglucocorticism, feline immunodeficiency virus, or feline leukemia virus, which presumably suppresses normal cell-mediated immune responses.

Histologic lesions include mild to moderate epidermal hyperplasia with follicular keratosis and mild crusting. There tends to be mild perifollicular inflammation with lymphocytes, macrophages, and neutrophils. There is variable mural follicular inflammation, spongiosis, and mucinosis. In feline viral plaques and bowenoid in situ carcinoma, mites have been found within lesional follicles; adjacent skin is normal.

Cats infested with the third unnamed species generally have concurrent illness or have recently recovered from a systemic illness. Pruritus is variable. Hair is generally easily epilated, and mites have been found on skin scrapings or hair trichograms. Histopathologic findings are described as moderate nonsuppurative and mastocytic dermatitis with moderate superficial orthokeratotic hyperkeratosis. Mites have not been noted on biopsy specimens.

Demodectic mange is uncommon in **cattle** but occurs worldwide. Three species exist in cattle: *D. bovis*, *D. ghanensis*, and *D. tauri*. Only *D. bovis* is known to cause clinical disease. It is assumed that all animals experiencing disease resulting from the excessive replication of this normal mite resident are in some way immunocompromised because of concurrent disease, poor nutrition, stress, or genetic predisposition. Economic significance lies largely in the damage that mite infestation produces in hides. In some parts of Africa and Madagascar, demodectic mange in cattle may become generalized and fatal, with this outcome contributed to by other debilitating conditions, such as malnutrition, tick-worry, and tropical heat. There is one report of a 2-year-old heifer from Africa with severe granulomatous nodular dermatitis with marked hyperkeratosis and thick nodular folds over the head, neck, and shoulder caused by concurrent infection with *D. bovis* and *Sarcoptes scabiei*. This animal died despite antiparasitic treatment.

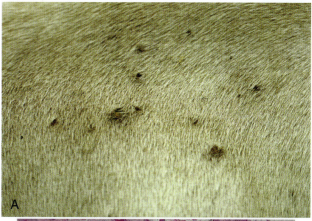

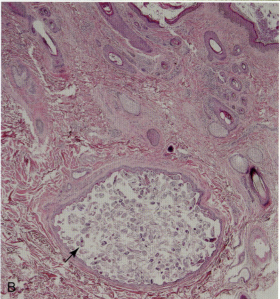

Figure 6-119 Demodecosis. A. Multiple crusted papular to nodular lesions in a cow. (Courtesy D.W. Scott.) **B.** Dilated hair follicle in a goat filled with numerous mites (arrow).

Typical gross lesions are *multiple cutaneous papules or nodules* varying in number from a few to several hundred (Fig. 6-119A). The nodules are visible in smooth-coated cattle, often indicated by overlying tufts of erect hairs. In rough-coated cattle, such as Herefords, detection usually requires palpation. The preferred sites are the shoulders, neck, dewlap, and muzzle, but in heavy infestations, nodules may be present over most of the body. The content of the nodules is thick, waxy, or caseous material, sometimes stained with blood. The contents may liquefy and discharge to the surface, forming a thick crust, or rupture of the nodule into the dermis may generate a pyogranulomatous reaction. Lesions are neither painful nor pruritic, and there may be a seasonal increase in the number of lesions in the spring and summer.

Histologically, the nodules are follicular cysts lined by flattened squamous epithelium and filled with keratin squames and large numbers of demodicid mites (Fig. 6-119B). Adult parasites occur occasionally in sebaceous glands and rarely in epitrichial sweat glands. A mild mononuclear cell infiltrate may occur around the epithelial lining. Rupture of a follicular cyst induces a marked nodular granulomatous reaction in which degenerating and occasionally mineralized segments of parasites and keratin debris are surrounded by epithelioid macrophages, multinucleated histiocytic giant cells, lymphocytes, plasma cells, and eosinophils.

Demodectic mange is common in **goats.** The lesions in goats, caused by *D. caprae*, are similar to those described for cattle in both distribution and morphology. Some affected goats are mildly depressed, inappetent, and have decreased milk production. Generally, the chief economic significance of caprine demodicosis lies in damage to the hides.

Demodectic mange, caused by *D. ovis* and *D. aries*, is rare in **sheep.** Lesions occur as asymptomatic papules and nodules on especially the face, chin, and pinnae. Widespread lesions and secondary bacterial infections may be seen in debilitated sheep. *D. ovis* infestation occurs in the medium to coarse-wooled sheep, affecting the Meibomian glands of the eyelid and the sebaceous glands of the primary follicles on the body, particularly the neck, flank, and shoulders. *D. aries* infests the large sebaceous glands of the vulva, prepuce, and nostrils. *D. ovis* infestation has been associated with matted fleece ("stringy wool"). Histologically, the mites are present in sebaceous glands or the pilar canal, occasionally inciting folliculitis or furunculosis.

Although *Demodex* spp. are found commonly in the Meibomian glands of the **horse,** demodectic mange is a very rare disease. As in other species, follicular demodecosis probably only occurs in horses that are immunocompromised. In horses, demodecosis has been reported in association with chronic treatment with systemic glucocorticoids and in horses with pituitary pars intermedia dysfunction. *D. caballi* (264-453 μm) parasitizes the pilosebaceous units of the eyelids and muzzle, whereas *D. equi* (179-236 μm) infestation occurs over the body. Lesions occur on the head, neck, and shoulder but may become generalized. They include asymptomatic hypotrichosis, alopecia, scaling, and crusting. Histologically, hair follicles are distended to various degrees with keratin and demodectic mites. Inflammation may be minimal up to various degrees of perifolliculitis, folliculitis, furunculosis, and foreign-body granuloma formation.

Demodex phylloides of **pigs** is uncommon and is relatively unimportant in comparison to sarcoptic mange. The principal economic loss results from damage to the hide. The mites reside in the pilosebaceous units. Proliferation of mites is thought to be due to concurrent immunocompromise. The lesions typically involve the ventral abdomen, ventral neck, eyelids, and snout and they are neither painful nor pruritic. They commence as small red macules, developing into cutaneous nodules covered by surface scale. Follicular hyperkeratosis with comedo formation may develop. Incision of the nodules releases thick, white, caseous debris that is full of mites. The histologic lesions are as described in cattle.

Rarely, demodicosis has been described in **alpacas** and one **llama.** In the reported llama, lesions were described as multiple pruritic papules with erythema, alopecia, hyperkeratosis, lichenification, and hyperpigmentation on the medial thigh, axilla, inguinal region, and dorsal skin of the lower limb. *Demodex* spp. (200-280 μm) were identified via skin scraping and microscopy but were not seen in biopsy specimens. Histologically, there was folliculitis, hyperkeratosis of the epidermis, and infiltration of mainly eosinophils and mononuclear cells in the dermis. A nodular pyogranulomatous reaction was occasionally observed in the dermis.

Definitive *diagnosis* can be made by history, physical examination, and identification of the *Demodex* mite. In dogs, cats, horses, and llamas with follicular demodecosis, manually squeezing the skin lesions with deep skin scrapings may be necessary to recover the mite. In dogs with *D. injai*, multiple deep scrapes may need to be performed because mite numbers are generally low. In cats with *D. gatoi*, multiple surface scrapings should be performed. Mites may also be recovered on fecal flotation. In highly pruritic cats, mites may be difficult to recover, and therefore a treatment trial may help make the diagnosis. In those species with nodular demodicosis (cattle, goats, sheep, pigs), nodules can be incised or manually expressed to reveal multiple mites. Skin scrapings may reveal cigar-shaped larvae, nymphs, and adult mites or elongated ovoid eggs. Adults and nymphs have 4 pairs of legs, whereas larvae have 3 pairs. In dogs, PCR techniques can be used to make a definitive diagnosis regarding mite species.

Further reading

Beale K, et al. Feline demodecosis a consideration in the itchy or over-grooming cat. J Fel Med Surg 2012;14:209-213.

Eo K, et al. Skin lesions associated with *Demodex* sp. in a llama (*Lama peruana*). J Zoo Wildl Med 2010;41:178-180.

Felix AOC, et al. Comparison of systemic interleukin 10 concentrations in healthy dogs and those suffering from recurring and first time *Demodex canis* infestations. Vet Parasitol 2013;193: 312-315.

Hill FI, et al. *Demodex* spp. infestation and suspected demodicosis of alpacas (*Vicugna pacos*) in New Zealand. NZ Vet J 2008;56:148-149.

Moriello KA, et al. Five observations of a third morphologically distinct feline *Demodex* mite. Vet Dermatol 2013;24:460-462, e106.

Ordeix L, et al. *Demodex injai* infestation and dorsal greasy skin and hair in eight wirehaired fox terrier dogs. Vet Dermatol 2009;20: 267-272.

Sadtre N, et al. Phylogenetic relationships in three species of canine *Demodex* mite based on partial sequences of mitochondrial 16S rDNA. Vet Dermatol 2012;23:509-e101.

Trombiculiasis

The nymphs and adults of trombiculid mites are free living or parasitize plants or other arthropods; the larvae are parasitic and are known as "harvest mites," "chiggers," or "red bugs." The parasitic larvae are 6-legged, red to orange to yellow, and 0.2-0.4 mm in length, just visible to the naked eye. The mites attach themselves to the skin and make a channel into the epidermis, called a *stylostome*, through which salivary enzymes are injected and digested tissue fluids are withdrawn. The mites engorge to twice their original size over a period of 3-5 days, after which they drop off and complete their life cycle in the soil. *Intensely pruritic dermatitis* develops at the sites of attachment, probably as a result of an allergic reaction to the salivary secretions delivered through the stylostome; the allergic reaction caused by larval trombiculid mites is known as *trombidiosis*.

Wild vertebrates are the usual hosts for the trombiculid mite larvae, but food-producing domestic animals, pets, and humans may be accidentally infested. The disease tends to have a seasonal incidence, occurring in the *late summer and autumn* when climatic conditions favor an expansion of the mite population. Factors such as soil type also influence the prevalence of trombiculiasis in different geographic regions. Animals exposed to fields and woodlands are more often infested.

Trombicula (Neotrombicula) autumnalis, the European harvest mite, attacks most domestic species. *T. sarcina,* an Australian species known as the leg-itch mite, is an important parasite of sheep, although its principal host is the gray kangaroo. *T. (Eutrombicula) alfreddugesi* (North American chigger) and *T. splendens* are some of the species implicated in trombiculiasis in cats, dogs, and horses. *Straelensia cynotis,* normally residing on foxes, has been reported to infest dogs and cats in France, Spain, and Portugal. *S. cynotis* has a different clinical presentation, histopathologic features, and response to treatment compared to the other trombiculids.

Lesions caused by most trombiculids tend to occur in areas close to ground contact in animals exposed to wild or semi-wild areas. Pruritus is variable but can be intense. Different responses to the infestations may be due to individual hypersensitivity reactions to the mites. In **cattle** and **sheep**, the legs, face, pinnae, axillae, and groin are the most commonly affected sites. In **goats**, legs, face, and ventrum are most commonly affected. The mite in **horses** is known as the "heel-bug" because of its tendency to parasitize the feathered area of the pastern. Lesions may also occur on the muzzle, nares, face, ears, and neck. Horses may sneeze or head-shake. In **cats**, lesions affect the paws, head, ears, and ventrum, but an atypical generalized form of the disease may occur in association with *Walchia americana* infestation. The interdigital web, concave surface of the pinnae, face, and ventral abdomen are the predilection sites in the **dog** infested with species other than *S. cynotis.* In a massive infestation reported in 2 dogs, temporary hindlimb paresis developed.

The gross lesions caused by all species, with the exception of *S. cynotis,* are erythematous crusted papules on which are clustered tiny (0.2-0.4 mm) bright red, orange, or yellow mites. The mites leave a small, shallow ulceration that oozes a serous discharge and becomes crusted. Pruritus induces marked self-trauma, which may incite secondary bacterial infection. Histologically, *the mite may be present in tunnels within the stratum spinosum or in the stratum corneum.* The presence of the mites induces both hyperplastic and degenerative changes in the epidermis. The stylostome appears as a pale staining, hyalinized tube with undulating margins oriented vertical to the skin's surface and extending into the dermis. A large zone of necrotic cellular debris usually surrounds the stylostome. The surrounding dermis has a superficial perivascular infiltrate, with eosinophils and mast cells predominating.

Dogs infested with *S. cynotis* (straelensiosis) have multiple alopecic erythematous papules and nodules over the head, neck, dorsum, extremities, and lumbar regions. The ventral thorax and abdomen are rarely involved. Pustules, purulent exudate, crusts, and ulcerations are sometimes very extensive. Uncomplicated lesions are generally nonpruritic. Histologically, hair follicles are dilated, and most contain an intrafollicular larval mite. Marked *pseudoepitheliomatous hyperplasia and perifollicular mucinosis are considered pathognomonic.* Eosinophilic, sometimes mineralized, dense and amorphous material often surrounds larvae. Dermal inflammation is generally mild, consisting of lymphocytes, plasma cells, and a few mast cells. Eosinophils are rare. There is a striking proliferation of vascular channels surrounding some lesions and occasionally replacing hyperplastic follicular epithelium. The epidermis is hyperplastic with hyperkeratosis, focal spongiosis, and serocellular crusts.

Diagnosis of trombiculosis is confirmed by isolation and identification of mites through visual inspection of the infested animal in most species and histopathology in the case of straelensiosis.

Further reading

Ramirez GA, et al. Clinical, histopathological and epidemiological study of canine straelensiosis in the Iberian Peninsula (2003-2007). Vet Dermatol 2008;20:35-41.

Scott DW. Color Atlas of Farm Animal Dermatology. Ames, Iowa: Blackwell; 2007.

Scott DW, Miller WH. Parasitic diseases. In: Scott DW, Miller WH, editors. Equine Dermatology. 2nd ed. St Louis: Elsevier Saunders; 2011. p. 212-250.

Seixas F, et al. Dermatitis in a dog induced by *Straelensia cynotis*: a case report and review of the literature. Vet Dermatol 2006;17:81-84.

Other mite-induced dermatoses

The **cat fur mite**, *Lynxacarus radovsky,* infests cats and is widely distributed worldwide. The mite attaches to the hair shafts rather than to the skin surface. Mites are usually located along the topline, including the tail tip, tail head, and perineum. The mite infestation mimics seborrhea sicca, giving the coat a characteristic "salt and pepper" appearance. The infestation is not usually associated with lesions, although crusted, exudative, and pruritic lesions and alopecia have been described.

The **straw-itch mite** *(Pyemotes tritici)* is normally found in straw or grain, where it parasitizes the larvae of soft-bodied grain insects. The parasite may occasionally infest mammals, causing pruritic dermatitis. Mildly pruritic lesions may develop in horses fed infested hay. Multiple papules and wheals may occur on the muzzle, neck, withers, legs, and ventral thorax and abdomen. *Acarus (Tyroglyphus) farinae* and *A. (Tyroglyphus) longior* may cause a pruritic, exudative, crusting, and alopecic dermatosis in horses exposed to contaminated grain or hay.

Horses, cattle, goats, cats, and dogs may be infested on rare occasions with the **poultry mite,** *Dermanyssus gallinae.* Adult mites are 0.6 to 1 mm and suck blood. They live and lay eggs in cracks and crevices in the walls of poultry houses or in bird nests. Lesions consist of pruritic papules and crusts. In **dogs** and **cats,** the lesions are usually over the back and extremities and in **horses** lesions tend to be on muzzle, limbs and ventrum, and sometimes the topline, especially if birds are nesting above the horse's stall. Predilection sites in **cattle** and **goats** include legs and ventrum.

Ornithonyssus syviarum, the **northern fowl mite,** is another blood-sucking parasite that can parasitize horses. Adult mites can live off the host for 1-3 weeks. Lesions tend to begin as topline dermatitis because infestations are most commonly due to birds nesting above the horse's stall. Pruritus is variable.

House-dust mites, *Dermatophagoides farinae* and *D. pteronyssinus,* are associated with allergic dermatitis in dogs and cats.

Sheep may, on rare occasions, become infested with the **stored-product mite,** *Sancassania berlesei.* These mites cannot infest dry skin; infestations are secondary to other conditions such as myiasis.

Further reading

Miller WH, et al. Parasitic skin disease. In: Miller WH, et al., editors. Muller & Kirk's Small Animal Dermatology. 7th ed. St Louis: Elsevier; 2013. p. 284-342.

Norhidayu JJ, et al. The cat fur mite, *Lynxacarus radovskyi* Tenorio, 1974 (Acarina: Astigmata: *Listrophoridae*) from cat, *Felis catus* in peninsular Malaysia. Trop Biomed 2012;29: 308-310.

Scott DW. Color Atlas of Farm Animal Dermatology. Ames, Iowa: Blackwell; 2007.

Scott DW, Miller WH. Parasitic diseases. In: Scott DW, Miller WH, editors. Equine Dermatology. 2nd ed. St Louis: Elsevier Saunders; 2011. p. 212-250.

Ticks

Ticks belong to the class Arachnida, subclass Acari. Ticks are divided into 2 families, the *Argasidae* (soft ticks) and the *Ixodidae* (hard ticks). Ticks harm their host most importantly by transmitting various bacterial, viral, protozoal, and rickettsial infections. Ticks are small, attach firmly to their hosts, use multiple hosts, live for prolonged periods of time, and can often survive without feeding for long periods of time. These factors make ticks important in the possible transport and transmission of diseases from one host to another and between countries or continents. Importation of animals harboring ticks can pose a threat to animals in areas free of certain diseases. Babesiosis, Rocky Mountain spotted fever, ehrlichiosis, tularemia, Lyme borreliosis, heartwater disease, Q fever, louping ill, and anaplasmosis are a few examples of tick-transmitted diseases.

If infestation is heavy, fatalities may result. The local injury may predispose to myiasis and secondary bacterial infection, particularly to staphylococcal cutaneous abscesses or septicemia in lambs. Heavy infestations are also capable of causing anemia as a result of the blood-sucking activities of the ticks, but ixodid ticks, which engorge only once at each instar, are much less important in this respect than are argasid ticks, which as adults engorge repeatedly. Tick bites may also induce hypersensitivity reactions. Severe hypersensitivity reactions to the larvae of *Boophilus microplus* have been described in horses in Australia. Within 30 minutes of reinfestation, sensitized horses develop intensely pruritic papules and wheals, chiefly on the lower legs and muzzle. As tick-bite lesions progress, they are often typified by the "arthropod-bite granuloma" described earlier in this section. Twelve ixodid species have been associated with tick paralysis, and they include *Ixodes rubicundus* and *Rhipicephalus evertsi* of South Africa, *I. holocyclus* of Australia, and *R. sanguineus*, *Dermacentor andersoni* and *D. variabilis* in North America. These ticks have neurotoxins in salivary secretions that can cause paralysis of the host. It may be secreted by the ovaries because it is associated with egg production.

The *Argasidae* are the so-called soft ticks, lacking the scutum that characterizes the *Ixodidae*. This group of ticks is more common in warm climates. Adults lay eggs in sheltered spots in the environment, and larvae and nymphs suck blood and lymph and drop off the host to become adults. Included in this group is *Otobius megnini* and *Ornithodoros* spp. *Otobius megnini*, known as the "spinose ear-tick," is parasitic to all domestic animals causing severe blood and lymph loss, parasitic otitis externa, vigorous head-shaking and scratching, and secondary bacterial infections or myiasis. In some cases, the ear canal becomes packed with immature ticks. *Ornithodoros coriaceus*, occurring along the Pacific coast of the United States, has a painful bite, and is a vector of epizootic bovine abortion.

Most of the pathogenic species of tick are found in the **Ixodidae.** Ixodid ticks, such as *Dermacentor* spp., *Rhipicephalus* spp., and *Amblyomma* spp., lay their eggs in sheltered areas. Larvae climb onto grass and shrubbery and wait for a suitable host to come by. Infestations of larval and nymphal *Ixodes* spp. have been described in dogs and cats. Most cases occur in late summer and autumn. Clinical signs include asymptomatic clusters of tick larvae on the neck, back, and scrotum to multiple variably pruritic erythematous papules on the trunk and thighs. In North America, "seed tick infestation" has been associated with *Amblyomma americanum* larvae, and in Australia "scrub itch" has been associated with *I. holocyclus* and *Haemaphysalis longicornis* larvae. Histologic features of "seed and scrub itch" are as follows: Ticks are attached in well-demarcated deep invaginations ("tick craters") of the epidermis, variable epidermal hyperplasia and necrosis, and mild to marked diffuse perivascular to interstitial eosinophilic and neutrophilic dermal inflammation.

The *local reaction to adult ticks is variable*, depending on properties of the tick, for example, its ability to secrete prostaglandins, and on host factors such as the level of tick resistance. Primary tick bite lesions are papules, wheals, and nodules. Crusts, erosions, ulcerations, and alopecia may develop. Pain and pruritus are variable. In **horses,** tick bites are most common on the face, ears, neck, mane, axillae, groin, distal limbs, and tail. In **cattle, goats, sheep, and pigs,** tick bites are most common on the ears, face, neck, axillae, groin, and legs.

Histologically, the primary lesions are characterized by focal epidermal edema and necrosis with adjacent dermal edema and infiltration of neutrophils, eosinophils, and mononuclear cells. Reactions in previously infested hosts are characterized by marked spongiosis with eosinophilic and basophilic microabscesses, subepidermal edema, and marked dermal infiltration with basophils, eosinophils, and mononuclear cells. In some cases, especially horses, there may be persistent nodular lesions. These are characterized by diffuse dermatitis composed of lymphocytes, histiocytes, and fewer eosinophils and plasma cells. Lymphoid nodules with developing follicles, resembling pseudolymphoma, may occur.

Further reading

Baxter CG, et al. Dermatoses caused by infestations of immature *Ixodes* spp. on dogs and cats in Sydney, Australia. Aust Vet J 2009; 87:182-187.

Cortinas R, Jones CJ. Ectoparasites of cattle and small ruminants. Vet Clin North Am Food Anim Pract 2006;22:673-693.

Scott DW. Color Atlas of Farm Animal Dermatology. Ames, Iowa: Blackwell; 2007.

Scott DW, Miller WH. Parasitic diseases. In: Scott DW, Miller WH, editors. Equine Dermatology. 2nd ed. St Louis: Elsevier Saunders; 2011. p. 212-250.

HELMINTH DISEASES OF SKIN

The skin is the natural portal of entry of a number of metazoal parasites that have their final habitat in the gastrointestinal tract or elsewhere. As a rule, those infective larvae that can invade percutaneously are not host specific, thus infection of aberrant hosts occurs. Such parasites are quite varied in their nature and include infective larvae of trematodes, such as *Schistosoma*, and of the nematodes of various genera, including *Strongyloides, Gnathostoma, Ancylostoma, Bunostomum, Uncinaria*, and others. Infective larvae of the filariids, such as *Dirofilaria* and *Setaria*, are deposited in the skin by the biting insects that are their vectors. The first percutaneous invasion of one of these parasites in its natural hosts takes place very quickly (for example, the larvae of *Strongyloides* and *Bunostomum* reach the dermis in 15 minutes) and provokes little reaction. Repeated invasions in a natural host or single invasion in an unnatural host are met with some resistance that is manifested as acute dermatitis limited to the invaded area. The cutaneous lesions are, except under experimental circumstances, seldom observed in animals. It is on the glabrous nonpigmented skin of people that they are easily observed and well recognized as the so-called "creeping eruption." There the larvae produce acutely inflamed, serpiginous, vesicular to papular tracts that may advance several centimeters a day. Usually, aberrant larvae die in the skin, but some enter the vessels and become lodged in the lungs or other tissues. Nematode larvae most often incriminated are *Ancylostoma braziliense, A. caninum*, and *Uncinaria stenocephala*, the canine hookworm larvae. *Bunostomum phlebotomum, Gnathostoma spinigerum, Dirofilaria* sp., *Strongyloides procyonis*, and *S. westeri* are nematode parasites of other domestic and wild animals that have also been reported to cause cutaneous larval migration in humans.

Hookworm dermatitis, caused by aberrant migration of *Ancylostoma* spp. and *U. stenocephala*, occurs in dogs kept on grass or dirt and subjected to poor sanitation. *A. caninum* can complete its life cycle via skin penetration. Although *U. stenocephala* rarely completes its life cycle via this route, it can produce marked dermatitis as a result of skin penetration. Third-stage larvae enter the dog's skin on areas of the body that frequently contact the ground. Larvae enter the skin via pressure, leaving no visible penetrating point. Other species of hookworm larvae cause loss of epidermal integrity. Lesions consist of pruritic red papules on parts of the body exposed to the ground. Lesions become erythematous, thickened, and alopecic. Distal limbs and feet are especially affected. The footpads and interdigital regions of the feet may be edematous and painful. Claw deformities may occur. Pruritus varies from mild to severe. Histologically, hyperplastic spongiotic perivascular dermatitis with eosinophils and neutrophils is present. Larval tracts may be present in the epidermis or dermis lined by degenerating leukocytes. Inflammation is thought to be due to a hypersensitivity reaction to migrating larvae. *B. phlebotomum* cases pruritic dermatitis of feet, legs, and ventrum in cattle. *B. trigonocephalum* can cause a similar syndrome in sheep.

The cutaneous lesions produced by the blood flukes, and those nematodes that pass through the skin on the way to the gut are discussed elsewhere with the mature parasites (see Vol. 2, Alimentary system and peritoneum). The dermatitis produced by the larvae of *Elaeophora* is discussed in Vol. 3, Cardiovascular system. To be discussed in more detail here are those helminthic infestations that remain more or less localized to the dermis.

Cutaneous habronemiasis

The aberrant deposition of the larvae of the spirurid nematodes *Habronema majus (microstoma), H. muscae*, and *Draschia megastoma* by transmitting flies at cutaneous or mucocutaneous sites causes this *common disease of equids* (horses, donkeys, mules). The adult worms normally develop in the stomach of horses following the ingestion of infective larva (see Vol. 2, Alimentary system and peritoneum). The cutaneous disease occurs sporadically in horse populations in temperate or tropical climates during the summer when the transmitting flies, *Musca* spp. and *Stomoxys calcitrans*, are active. Horses with a hypersensitivity response to the larvae are affected, and the condition is recurrent each summer, hence the term *"summer sores."* Lesions are consistently pruritic.

The location of the lesions is in the moist exposed areas of the body that attract flies. The most common sites are the *medial canthus of the eye (Fig. 6-120A), the glans penis and*

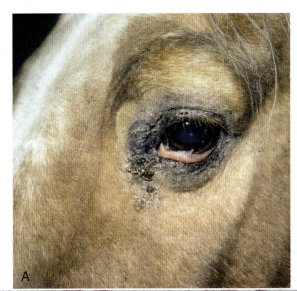

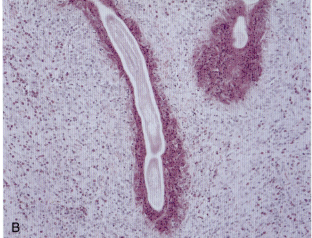

Figure 6-120 Cutaneous habronemiasis in a horse. **A.** Crusted papular lesion below medial canthus. (Courtesy D.W. Scott.) **B.** Longitudinal section of *Habronema* spp. larva surrounded by a palisading eosinophilic granuloma.

prepuce, and any cutaneous wound. Because lacerations are more common on the distal extremities, these too are predilection sites for habronemiasis. Fly bites alone are sufficient to initiate an infestation. Ulcerative diseases initiated by other causes can be complicated by habronemiasis.

The gross lesions are rapidly progressive and proliferative in nature, comprising *ulcerated, tumorous masses of red-brown granulation tissue.* The surface is friable and bleeds readily. Lesions may be single or multiple and range in size from 5-15 cm in diameter and from 0.5-1.5 cm in depth. They are often irregular in shape in the early stages but become circular as they enlarge. On cut section, multiple small (1-5 mm) yellow-white, caseous, and occasionally gritty foci are scattered through the granulation tissue. These are often confused with the "kunkers" of pythiosis, but lack the characteristic branching pattern of the true kunker. In the deeper parts of the lesion, the more mature connective tissue has a dense, white appearance. The lesions on the conjunctiva and eyelids do not usually exceed 2 cm. Commencing with a serous conjunctivitis, small ulcerated, proliferative nodular lesions develop on the mucous membrane of the third eyelid and at the medial canthus. Lacrimal duct involvement characteristically produces a lesion 2-3 cm below the medial canthus. The entire conjunctiva may be affected, resulting in profuse lacrimation, photophobia, chemosis, and inflammation of the eyelid. On cut section, *the nodular lesions of brown-red granulation tissue contain the typical caseous or mineralized foci.* Involvement of the penis and prepuce may cause prolapse of the urethral process and dysuria. On rare occasions, *Habronema* granulomas are found in the lung. Gross lesions of cutaneous habronemiasis may resemble those of exuberant granulation tissue, bacterial pseudomycetoma, pythiosis, equine sarcoid, and squamous cell carcinoma. Habronemiasis may complicate a pre-existing lesion; secondary *Habronema* infestations occur with pythiosis, *Corynebacterium pseudotuberculosis* infection, and in skin tumors, particularly squamous cell carcinoma of the penis.

Histologically, there is nodular-to-diffuse dermatitis with numerous eosinophils and mast cells. Multifocal coagulative necrosis with dense aggregates of degranulating eosinophils is a characteristic feature. In 50% of cases, nematode larvae are found within the necrotic foci. Palisading granulomas containing epithelioid macrophages and multinucleated histiocytic giant cells may develop around these foci. (Fig. 6-120B). Larvae are usually degenerate and sometimes mineralized. The fibrous connective tissue is heavily and diffusely infiltrated with eosinophils and with fewer numbers of mast cells, lymphocytes, and plasma cells. The surface of the lesion is usually covered with fibrinonecrotic exudate overlying highly vascular granulation tissue infiltrated with neutrophils.

In addition to equids, cutaneous habronemiasis has been reported in a **dog** and a **dromedary camel.** Lesions in the dog developed on the face but, unlike the equine disease, were not characterized by rapid proliferation of granulation tissue. The dog was housed under unsanitary conditions in the company of several heavily parasitized ponies. The camel had a nonhealing, severely pruritic, ulcerative fibrotic plaque at the medial canthus. Histologic findings were similar to those for equids.

Definitive *diagnosis* is based on history, physical examination, direct smears, and biopsy. PCR may help confirm the diagnosis if larvae are not visible within cytology or biopsy specimens.

Further reading

Myers DA, et al. Cutaneous periocular *Habronema* infection in a dromedary camel (*Camelus dromedarius*). Vet Dermatol 2010;21: 527-530.

Pusterla N, et al. Cutaneous and ocular habronemiasis in horses: 63 cases (1988-2002). J Am Vet Med Assoc 2003;222:978-982.

Sanderson TP, Niyo Y. Cutaneous habronemiasis in a dog. Vet Pathol 1990;27:208-209.

Stephanofilariasis

Members of the genus **Stephanofilaria** (Spirurida: Setariidae) are parasites of **cattle.** Stephanofilariasis is uncommon. All stephanofilarid parasites cause similar cutaneous lesions, but the species are geographically separated, and the lesions occur on different parts of the host's body. *Stephanofilaria stilesi* occurs in North America (especially the west and southwest), affecting the abdominal skin near the midline (including udder, teats, scrotum, and flanks); in Australian cattle, initial lesions develop at the medial canthus of the eye; *S. dedoesi* in Indonesia causes dermatitis, known locally as "cascado," on the sides of the neck, dewlap, withers, and around the eyes; *S. assamensis* causes "hump-sore" of Zebu cattle in India and the Soviet Union; *S. kaeli* causes dermatitis of the legs of cattle from the Malay Peninsula; *S. dinniki* affects the shoulder of black rhinoceros; *S. boomkeri* causes severe dermatitis in pigs in Zaire; *S. zaheeri* causes dermatitis of the ears of buffalo, and *S. okinawaensis* causes lesions on the teats and muzzle of cattle in Japan. There is one report of scrotal dermatitis caused by *S. stilesi* in France. *Stephanofilaria kaeli, S. assamensis,* and *S. dedoesi* cause crusting dermatitis of the face, neck, shoulders, and feet in **goats.**

Flies transmit stephanofilariasis. The horn fly, *Haematobia irritans,* is the vector of *S. stilesi* in North America, and the buffalo fly, *Haematobia irritans exigua,* is the major vector for stephanofilariasis in Australia. *Musca conducens* transmits *S. assamensis* and *S. kaeli.* The flies ingest microfilariae when feeding on cutaneous lesions. After a period of development in the fly, the infective larva is deposited on the skin by the biting species of fly or onto cutaneous wounds in the case of the nonbiting vectors such as *M. conducens*. The adults of *S. stilesi* live in cystic diverticula off the base of the hair follicles. The parasites are very small, with males reaching 3 mm and females 8 mm in length.

The *initial macroscopic lesions* in *S. stilesi* infections are circular patches 1 cm or less in diameter in the skin of the ventral midline, in which the hairs are moist and erect, and the underlying epidermis is spotted with small hemorrhages and droplets of serum. These initial foci enlarge and coalesce, sometimes to produce a lesion 25 cm or more in diameter. As the foci enlarge, new spots of hemorrhage and exudation develop at the periphery, whereas, in the central areas, the hair is shed and the exudate builds up into scabs or rough dry crusts through which the few remaining hairs penetrate. The lesions are mildly pruritic, and rubbing may aggravate them. In the healing stage, the affected areas remain as alopecic, lichenified plaques (Fig. 6-121A).

Histologically, sections of adult parasites may be seen in the cystic diverticula from hair follicles or lying free in the adjacent dermis (Fig. 6-121B). They may be identified as *Stephanofilaria* spp. with some confidence if microfilariae are seen in the uteri of females because this parasite is viviparous;

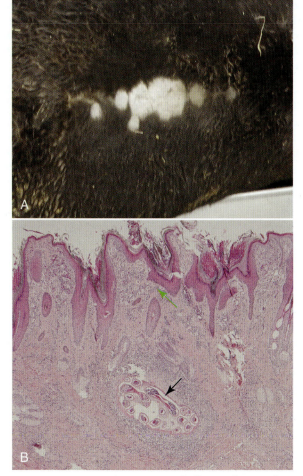

Figure 6-121 Stephanofilariasis in a bull. **A.** Chronic alopecic lichenified plaque on the ventrum. (Courtesy R.J. Ossiboff.) **B.** Multiple cross sections of nematodes (black arrow) within a dilated hair follicle and numerous microfilariae (green arrow), each surrounded by a vitelline membrane in the superficial dermis.

if ova rather than larvae are found, it is more likely for the parasite to be of the genus *Rhabditis*. Microfilariae occur free in the dermis or in dermal lymphatics, enclosed within their own vitelline membranes *(S. stilesi)*, or may be found free or unhatched in surface exudate *(S. kaeli)*. In general, there is little dermal reaction to the microfilariae or to the adults enclosed in cystic hair follicles, but the presence of adults in the dermis stimulates a mononuclear inflammatory reaction. There is accompanying superficial and deep perivascular dermatitis characterized by accumulations of eosinophils and mononuclear cells, chiefly lymphocytes. The epidermis is hyperplastic, spongiotic, and often covered by orthokeratotic and parakeratotic hyperkeratosis and inflammatory crust. Spongiform microabscesses containing eosinophils and mononuclear cells are also described; such lesions are more typically associated with the bites of arthropod ectoparasites. It is difficult to assess the relative contributions made to the lesion by the stephanofilarial parasite and by the bites of the fly that acts as the vector.

Diagnosis is usually made on the basis of the typical gross lesions, by histologic examination of biopsy specimens, or by demonstration of microfilariae by deep scrapings.

Further reading

Scott DW. Color Atlas of Farm Animal Dermatology. Ames, Iowa: Blackwell; 2007.
Watrelot-Virieux D, et al. Chronic eosinophilic dermatitis in the scrotal area associated with stephanofilariasis infestation of Charolais bull in France. J Vet Med 2006;53:150-152.

Onchocerciasis

Cutaneous onchocerciasis caused by *Onchocerca* spp. (Spirurida: *Onchocercidae*) affects horses, cattle, people, and some wild mammals, including deer and moose. Historically, the prevalence of infection was very high in cattle and horses, ranging up to 100% in some studies. However, the widespread use of avermectins has dramatically reduced the incidence, and in some areas, cutaneous onchocerciasis is quite rare. *Onchocerca* microfilariae cause cutaneous lesions in some horses; in cattle, the adults cause the cutaneous lesions.

In dogs, onchocerciasis has been associated with nodular lesions of the palpebral conjunctiva, third eyelid, sclera, cornea, and retrobulbar space. Degenerating or mineralized adult *Onchocerca* spp. parasites were found in the center of pyogranulomas comprising the masses.

Equine cutaneous onchocerciasis

Onchocerca cervicalis, *O. reticulata*, and *O. gutturosa* microfilariae are associated with cutaneous lesions in horses in different parts of the world. *Culicoides* spp. serve as intermediate hosts for all three, *Simulium* spp. may also be an intermediate host for *O. gutturosa*, and mosquitoes may serve as intermediate hosts for *O. cervicalis*. *O. gutturosa* infests horses in North America, Africa, Australia, and Europe. Adult worms can measure up to 60 cm long and *inhabit the lamellar part of the ligamentum nuchae*. Microfilariae (200-230 μm) can be found in the dermis of the face, neck, back, and ventral midline. *O. reticulata* infests horses in Europe and Asia. Adults live in the connective tissue of the *flexor tendons and suspensory ligament of the fetlock*. Microfilariae (310-395 μm) are found in the dermis of the ventral midline and legs. *O. cervicalis* infests horses worldwide, and adult worms, measuring up to 30 cm, live in the *funicular portion of the ligamentum nuchae*. Microfilariae (200-240 μm) are found in the dermis of the ventral midline, face, and neck.

Cutaneous onchocerciasis is thought to represent a hypersensitivity reaction to microfilarial antigens, and most cases are associated with *O. cervicalis*. Dead and dying microfilariae provoke the most intense inflammation. *O. cervicalis* can invade ocular tissues, and these lesions are discussed in Vol. 1, Special senses. Affected horses are usually 4 years of age or older. Clinical signs are rare in horses <2 years of age. Lesions are most common on the face and neck, especially around the mane, and ventral chest and abdomen. The ventral lesions are indistinguishable grossly from those of *Culicoides* hypersensitivity, but onchocerciasis does not cause lesions at the base of the tail. It is likely that onchocerciasis and *Culicoides* hypersensitivity can exist simultaneously.

Lesion morphology ranges from focal annular areas of alopecia, scaling, crusting, and inflammatory plaques to widespread areas of alopecia, erythema, ulceration, oozing, crusting, and lichenification. *An annular lesion in the center of the forehead is very characteristic of onchocerciasis.* Pruritus is variable. Cutaneous lesions include partial or complete alopecia,

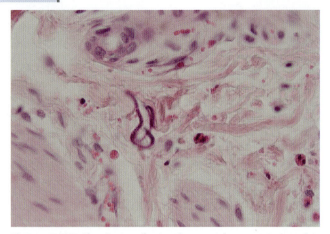

Figure 6-122 Skin biopsy from a horse with **cutaneous onchocerciasis** reveals microfilariae in the dermis, accompanied by small numbers of perivascular to interstitial eosinophils.

scaling, crusting, and leukoderma. Secondary excoriations or ulcerative dermatitis are induced by self-trauma in pruritic animals. Horses infested with adult worms of O. *reticulata* may have extensive swelling and lameness.

The microscopic lesions reveal various degrees of superficial and deep perivascular to interstitial to diffuse dermatitis with numerous eosinophils. Microfilariae may be present in large numbers or may be very sparse (Fig. 6-122). Other reported histopathologic findings are eosinophilic mural and necrotizing folliculitis, palisaded eosinophilic granulomas, and deep dermal to subcutaneous lymphoid nodules. It is important to note that microfilariae can be seen in skin of normal horses, and thus histopathologic findings should be correlated with historical and physical examination findings. Microfilariae are best recovered from unfixed biopsies that are minced and incubated in saline at 37° C.

Viable adult parasites in the nuchal ligament are not associated with significant lesions. In older horses, there is an increased frequency of caseated, mineralized, and granulomatous lesions associated with death of the parasite. Histologic examination shows that this parasite does not penetrate the elastic tissue of the ligament, and the inflammatory reaction is localized around the worm. They are usually encased in a chronic, fibrosing, and pyogranulomatous to granulomatous mass that may also have dystrophic mineralization. Adult O. *gutturosa* may also be associated with a similar inflammatory response. Mineralization is the fate of degenerate *Onchocerca gutturosa* worms, in contrast to caseation with O. *cervicalis*.

Bovine cutaneous onchocerciasis
Cattle can be infected by 3 species of *Onchocerca*. Cattle infested with O. *gibsoni* (Africa, Asia, Australia) develop multiple asymptomatic subcutaneous nodules, 2-9 cm in diameter. Lesions may be hard or soft, depending on the degree of mineralization and fibrosis or the degree of caseation and suppuration. Lesions predominantly affect the brisket but also the stifle and hip. Histologic assessment of O. *gibsoni* nodules revealed dead worms and associated degenerative changes, such as mineralization in 30% of nodules. Eosinophilic infiltration is more marked around viable worms, with eosinophils apparently adherent to the cuticle. In O. *gutturosa* infestations (North America, Europe, Africa, Australia), the worm is found in the nuchal ligament and connective tissue around tendons and ligaments of the shoulder, hip, and stifle. It may not form nodules and thus is sometimes overlooked. In O. *ochengi* (Africa) infestations, asymptomatic firm dermal and subcutaneous papules and nodules form on the scrotum, udder, flanks, lateral thorax, and head. *Onchocerca* spp. microfilariae may be associated with papules, plaques, and ulcers over the teats.

Further reading
Abraham D, et al. Immunity to *Onchocerca* spp. in animal hosts. Trends Parasitol 2002;18:164-171.
Achukwi MD, et al. *Onchocerca ochengi* transmission dynamics and the correlation of O. *ochengi* microfilaria density in cattle with the transmission potential. Vet Res 2000;31:611-621.
Eberhard ML, et al. Ocular *Onchocerca* infections in two dogs in western United States. Vet Parasitol 2000;90:333-338.
Scott DW. Color Atlas of Farm Animal Dermatology. Ames, Iowa: Blackwell; 2007.
Scott DW, Miller WH. Parasitic diseases. In: Scott DW, Miller WH, editors. Equine Dermatology. 2nd ed. St Louis: Elsevier Saunders; 2011. p. 212-250.

Pinworms
Oxyuris equi infection of the equine cecum and colon can be associated with *pruritic dermatitis of the perineal region*, leading to self-induced excoriations and alopecia of the tail known as "rat tail." The adult female parasite crawls out of the anus to deposit eggs on the hair and skin using a gelatinous material that can induce pruritus. *Diagnosis* is made by using the tape method in the perianal region for identification of characteristic operculated eggs. Oxyuriasis affects horses in most parts of the world.

Further reading
Perris EE. Parasitic dermatoses that cause pruritus in horses. Vet Clin North Am Equine Pract 1995;11:11-28.

Parafilariasis
Parafilaria multipapillosa occurs in horses in Eastern Europe and Great Britain. *Parafilaria bovicola* is endemic in cattle in Africa, India, and parts of Europe. *Parafilaria bassoni* has been reported in African buffalo and springbok in Namibia. The parasites are thin, thread-like worms, 2-7 cm long. The adults inhabit subcutaneous and intermuscular connective tissues producing nodules 1-2 cm in diameter. Lesions are most common over the neck, shoulders, and trunk, and pain and pruritus are variable. In the spring and summer, the nodules rapidly enlarge, burst open, hemorrhage, and heal. This coincides with the migration of the fully gravid female into the more superficial dermis to oviposit and to release infective microfilariae. The vectors, flies such as *Haematobia atripalpis* in Russia and *Musca* spp., are infected when they feed from these bleeding points, known as "blood nodules." Secondary subcutaneous abscesses may occur.

Further reading
Gibbons LM, et al. Redescription of *Parafilaria bovicola* Tubangui, 1934 (Nematoda: *Filarioidea*) from Swedish cattle. Acta Vet Scand 2000;41:85-91.

Van Wuijckhuise L, et al. Parafilariasis: a new parasitic disease of cattle in The Netherlands. Tijdschr Diergeneeskd 2007;132: 820-824.

Pelodera dermatitis

Some of the biological characteristics of the *Rhabditidae* have been discussed with the principal parasitic genus, *Strongyloides*, in Vol. 2, Alimentary system and peritoneum. Here it is necessary only to describe the cutaneous lesions produced occasionally by the small free-living worms of this family. Those worms that are found in the lesions are usually classified as ***Pelodera (Rhabditis) strongyloides.***

Pelodera dermatitis occurs most commonly in **dogs**, occasionally in **cattle**, and rarely in **horses, sheep,** and **humans**. Although most reported cases are sporadic, outbreaks involving multiple animals have been described in cattle and sheep. These worms live as saprophytes in warm moist soil that is rich in organic matter, and significant infestations probably require that the host's skin should be continually moist and filthy. Affected dogs often have a history of being bedded on straw. *Pruritus is moderate to marked in most species, but is variable and can be absent in cattle*. The lesions develop on contact areas (feet, legs, perineum, ventral trunk, tail), particularly at the margins of areas caked with dirt. The gross lesions include erythema, papules, excoriations, scaling, exudation, and crusting, with partial to complete alopecia (Fig. 6-123A). Pustules may occur, particularly in dogs. In sheep and cattle, lesions become lichenified. Affected sheep may have complete loss of wool.

Histologically, the worms (0.6 mm long) are in the lumina of the hair follicles (Fig. 6-123B) or in the dermis surrounded by eosinophilic and pyogranulomatous inflammation. There is perivascular and perifollicular eosinophilic and lymphoplasmacytic dermatitis and perifolliculitis. Definitive *diagnosis* is based upon environmental history and deep skin scrapings or biopsy. The infestation is self-limiting once the animal is removed from the source of contamination.

Nematodes of the genus *Rhabditis* are associated with otitis externa in cattle living in tropical environments. Lesions are painful with brown to yellow purulent foul-smelling discharge.

Further reading

Rashmir-Raven AM, et al. Papillomatous pastern dermatitis with spirochetes and *Pelodera strongyloides* in a Tennessee Walking Horse. J Vet Diagn Invest 2000;12:287-291.

Saari SAM, Nikander SE. *Pelodera* (syn. *Rhabditis*) *strongyloides* as a cause of dermatitis—a report of 11 dogs from Finland. Acta Vet Scand 2006;48:18-24.

Yeruham I, et al. Dermatitis in a dairy herd caused by *Peloderma strongyloides* (Nematoda: *Rhabditidae*). J Vet Med 2005;52:197-198.

Miscellaneous helminths

Dracunculus medinensis (Spirurida: *Dracunculidae*) is the "guinea worm" of humans in Asia and Africa. It has been introduced into America, the West Indies, and Fiji. The parasite has been reported in *dogs, cats, horses, and cattle* as well as other species in endemic areas. *Dracunculus insignis* is the species of the nematode that occurs in dogs, cats, and wild carnivores in North America. Infection is particularly prevalent in *raccoons and mink* that appear to be the natural definitive species. The intermediate host is a crustacean copepod, but frogs may act as paratenic hosts. The definitive host ingests the intermediate host, and the larvae are released during digestion and proceed to migrate through the body. The adult worms mature in the connective tissue of the host in ~1 year. The parasite occurs typically in the subcutaneous tissues of the limbs. The mature female may measure up to 70 cm in length, resulting in the formation of a 2-4 cm nodule. Lesions are usually solitary occurring on the limbs and abdomen. The gravid female produces an intraepidermal bulla with her anterior end by means of toxin secretion. Rupture of the bulla forms a shallow ulcer from which a milky exudate drains. When these lesions contact water, the worm is stimulated to release very large numbers of larvae that are ingested by copepods in the water. Fine-needle aspiration of the cutaneous nodules reveals rhabditiform *Dracunculus* larvae, ~500 μm long and covered by a striated cuticle. The adults lie in a pseudocyst lined by fibrous connective tissue and infiltrated with eosinophils, lymphocytes, and multinucleated giant cells. Ulcerated lesions are seen as draining tracts that may be painful or pruritic. The parasite can be identified by morphologic features.

Parelaphostrongylus tenuis, a common parasite of white-tailed deer, is an occasional cause of neurologic disease in several domestic species, including goats, sheep, llamas, and alpacas. Some affected goats also develop an unusual dermatitis, often restricted to one side of the body. Lesions are vertically oriented, alopecic, ulcerated, crusted, or scarred linear tracks on the shoulder, thorax, or flanks. The lesions have been

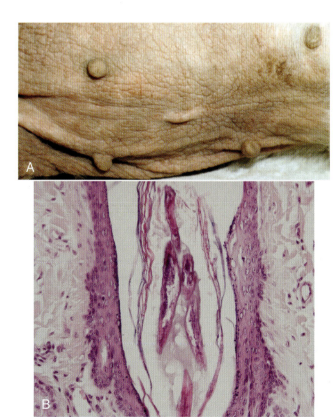

Figure 6-123 *Pelodera strongyloides* in a dog. **A.** Alopecia and lichenification along the ventral abdomen. (Courtesy D.W. Scott.) **B.** Adult rhabditiform parasites within hair follicle.

explained tentatively on the basis of ganglioneuritis, leading to irritation of dermatomes. Histologically, the lesion is a fibrosing dermatitis with focal areas of basal keratinocyte hydropic degeneration.

Strongyloides papillosus can cause pruritic dermatitis of the feet, legs, and ventrum of cattle, goats, and sheep. *Strongyloides* spp. have been reported to cause a rough, dull, dry haircoat, hemorrhagic pododermatitis, and crusted lesions on the tail, limbs, and ventrum in puppies.

Larval migrans caused by ***Anatrichosoma*** spp. has been reported in 2 cats. Clinical signs included lameness with necrosis, ulceration, and sloughing of multiple pawpads on all paws. This same parasite was reported to produce an erythematous scaling nodular lesion on a dog.

Dirofilaria immitis microfilariae can occasionally lead to cutaneous lesions in dogs harboring the adult parasite. A series of 5 cases document a scabies-like, papular to nodular, variably ulcerated, pruritic dermatitis of the skin of the head, trunk, and extremities in dogs infected with *D. immitis*. Histologic examination of affected skin revealed angiocentric and pyogranulomatous dermatitis with intralesional microfilariae. The numbers of eosinophils is variable. A type II hypersensitivity response was proposed as a pathogenic mechanism based on positive immunoreaction of microfilariae with anti-IgG serum. Lesions resolved with antiparasitic treatment. Ectopic adult *D. immitis* have been recovered from cutaneous abscesses and interdigital cysts in parasitized dogs and cats. In addition, a generalized cutaneous syndrome characterized by a pruritic papular and crusting dermatitis without intralesional microfilariae has been apparently associated with infection with *D. immitis* and was thought to be a manifestation of an unusual hypersensitivity reaction. Parasites are not present in the cutaneous tissues. Lesions also resolved with antiparasitic treatment. *Dirofilaria repens* can cause subcutaneous dirofilariasis in dogs, cats, and wild carnivores in Europe and parts of Africa and Asia. Like *D. immitis*, mosquitoes are the intermediate host. During a mosquito's blood meal, L3 larvae penetrate into the subcutaneous tissues of a dog, where they molt to L4 and remain for 6-7 months before developing into adults. Adults are 5-17 cm in length. Adult nematodes are rarely found but are occasionally recovered from skin nodules. Other clinical signs include various degrees of erythema, papules, alopecia, scaling, and crusting. *Acanthocheilonema* (*Dipetalonema*) *reconditum* affects dogs in Europe, America, and Asia. Generally, it is not associated with clinical signs; however, there is one report of 10 dogs with an *Acanthocheilonema*-like parasite showing single to multiple pruritic papules and plaques with alopecia, scarring, erythema, ulceration, and crusting over the head, neck, and shoulders. Histologic changes included ulceration and perivascular, periglandular, or interstitial mixed inflammatory cell infiltrates with variable eosinophils and plasma cells. Microfilariae were free within the dermis or subcutis and within microgranulomas. No microfilariae were present within vessels. One adult nematode was also present in the cutaneous tissues and was determined to be a *Acanthocheilonema* sp. Microfilariae are much thinner (4-5 µm wide) than *D. immitis* (5-7.5 µm wide) and *D. repens* (7-8 µm wide) and have a hook-shaped tail.

Various ***Cercopithifilaria*** spp. are transmitted by ticks to dogs and cats. This organism has been reported in southern and eastern Europe, Australia, Brazil, Malaysia, and South Africa. The lesion described in the dermis of dogs is erythematous papular and pruritic dermatitis with perivascular to interstitial inflammatory infiltrates of neutrophils, eosinophils, and lymphocytes surrounding microfilaria. Adult nematodes occur subcutaneously.

Suifilaria suis occurs in pigs in South Africa. The worms are 2-4 cm long and live in the subcutaneous and intermuscular connective tissues, sometimes producing small white nodules. The female is oviparous, and the eggs are released to the surface via small vesicular eruptions in the epidermis. The remainder of the life cycle is unknown.

Subcutaneous abscesses have been reported in dogs with a number of trematodes, cestodes, and nematodes, including *Paragonimus kellicotti*, *Habronema* spp., *Gnathostoma spinigerum*, *Lagochilascaris major*, and in cats with *L. major* and *Gordius robustus*. The larval cestode of *Sparganum proliferum* was reported to cause painful erythematous to violaceous nodules in the axillary region of a dog with spread to internal organs. *Schistosoma cercariae* can penetrate the skin of many warm-blooded abnormal hosts and produce dermatitis. Skin lesions are intensely pruritic and include macules and wheals that develop into papules and vesicles.

Further reading

Cortes HC, et al. Diversity of *Cercopithifilaria* species in dogs from Portugal. Parasit Vectors 2014;7:261.

Gabrielli S, et al. Chronic polyarthritis associated to *Cercopthifilaria bainae* infection in a dog. Vet Parasitol 2014;205:401-404.

Langlais L. Dracunculosis in a German shepherd dog. Can Vet J 2003;44:682.

Lucio-Forster A, et al. First report of *Dracunculus insignis* in two naturally infected cats from the northeastern USA. J Fel Med Surg 2013;16:194-197.

Miller WH, et al. Parasitic skin disease. In: Miller WH, et al., editors. Muller & Kirk's Small Animal Dermatology. 7th ed. St Louis: Elsevier; 2013. p. 284-342.

Tarello W. Clinical aspects of dermatitis associated with *Dirofilaria repens* in pets: a review of 100 canine and 31 feline cases (1990-2010) and a report of a new clinic case imported from Italy to Dubai. J Parasitol Res 2011;2011:578385.

MISCELLANEOUS SKIN CONDITIONS
Canine juvenile cellulitis

Canine juvenile cellulitis (juvenile sterile granulomatous dermatitis, puppy strangles, juvenile pyoderma) is an idiopathic disease typically affecting puppies <4 months of age. The cause and pathogenesis are unknown; however, heritability is supported by the fact that the condition is seen more commonly in certain breeds, such as the Golden Retriever, Dachshund, Gordon Setter, Labrador Retriever, and Lhasa Apso, and the condition is sometimes seen in more than one puppy from a litter. An underlying immune dysfunction is strongly suspected because the lesions are sterile when cultured, nontransmissible, and respond to corticosteroids and cyclosporine. Special stains and electron microscopy have also failed to identify intralesional infectious agents. Given the young age of onset, some have suggested vaccine reaction as a possible cause; however, reproduction of the disease with subsequent vaccinations does not occur. Depressed in vitro lymphocyte blastogenesis responses have been reported but likely represent the result not the cause of the disease. A condition clinically and histopathologically identical to juvenile cellulitis

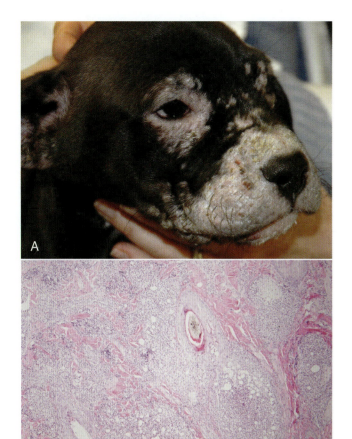

Figure 6-124 Canine juvenile cellulitis in a puppy. **A.** Facial edema with alopecia, papules, and crusts around the eyes and muzzle. **B.** Nodular pyogranulomatous perifollicular dermatitis.

Further reading

Miller WH, et al. Miscellaneous skin diseases. In: Miller WH, et al., editors. Muller & Kirk's Small Animal Dermatology. 7th ed. St Louis: Elsevier; 2013. p. 695-723.

Neuber AE, et al. Dermatitis and lymphadenitis resembling juvenile cellulitis in a four-year-old dog. J Small Anim Pract 2004;45:254-258.

Park C, et al. Combination of cyclosporin A and prednisolone for juvenile cellulitis concurrent with hindlimb paresis in 3 English cocker spaniel puppies. Can Vet J 2010;51:1265-1268.

Cutaneous paraneoplastic syndromes

Cutaneous paraneoplastic syndromes are dermatoses associated with internal neoplasms. The neoplasms may be malignant or benign but are most often malignant. In keeping with the definition of a paraneoplastic syndrome, *these conditions cannot be directly attributed to the anatomic location of the neoplasm.* The skin or mucosal lesions may precede, concur with, or follow the diagnosis of the underlying neoplasm. Removal or elimination of the tumor should alleviate the cutaneous lesions; relapse of the dermatosis signals recurrence of the underlying neoplasm. The majority of cutaneous paraneoplastic syndromes in animals do not have a defined pathogenesis and often have only been reported a limited number of times. These syndromes are better documented in humans, but the increased recognition and clinical significance in domestic animals warrants mention in this chapter. The well-recognized cutaneous lesions seen with functional pituitary, adrenal, or testicular tumors are discussed elsewhere (see Endocrine diseases of skin). Cutaneous lesions associated with the cryoglobulinemia associated with multiple myelomas have been discussed elsewhere (see Other immune-mediated dermatoses).

A unique dermatosis reported in aged cats is characterized by symmetrical ventrally distributed alopecia affecting the trunk and limbs (Fig. 6-125A) and has been reported to be associated with a concurrent **pancreatic carcinoma** or **bile duct carcinoma.** Crusting and brown-black waxy debris tends to be associated with a secondary *Malassezia* dermatitis. Pawpads may have concentric circular scales and fissures. The alopecia is due to *marked follicular atrophy* (Fig. 6-125B). Hair follicles are diffusely in telogen and appear miniaturized. Surrounding sebaceous glands are usually normal but may be atrophic in some cases. The epidermis is mildly hyperplastic and often lacks a stratum corneum, giving the regions of affected skin the characteristic "glistening" or moist appearance. The lack of the stratum corneum may be due to licking by the cat. In some areas, there may be parakeratotic hyperkeratosis. Inflammation is not a feature unless complicated by secondary infection. Pawpads may be softened and hyperkeratotic. The pancreatic carcinoma is usually in an advanced stage, often with hepatic metastasis at the time of diagnosis, and the prognosis is grave. The condition must be differentiated from hyperadrenocorticism and feline psychogenic alopecia.

Thymoma and concurrent **exfoliative dermatitis** has been reported in cats. Cats are usually aged and may have signs such as dyspnea and coughing referable to an intrathoracic mass. Cutaneous lesions may be well developed prior to onset of respiratory signs. The cutaneous lesions consist of dry exfoliative dermatitis with large scales over the head, neck, and pinnae that may become generalized. Brown, waxy material

has also been reported in adult dogs; however, this is controversial.

Cutaneous lesions comprise papules, pustules, crusts, alopecia, and very marked edema (Fig. 6-124A). Skin of the muzzle, face, ears, and occasionally the feet, abdomen, vulva, prepuce, and anus are affected. Otitis externa is common, and the pinnae are frequently thickened and edematous. Lymphadenopathy of the mandibular nodes is common and may precede the onset of the skin lesions. Lymphadenitis may also occur in nodes distant to the skin lesions and may occur in the absence of skin lesions. The cutaneous lesions are bilaterally symmetrical, painful, but not pruritic. Some puppies develop concurrent sterile pyogranulomatous panniculitis with firm to fluctuant subcutaneous nodules that may develop draining tracts. Anorexia, fever, malaise, and arthritis affecting multiple joints are common. Lameness and paresis can be seen. One dog was reported to develop juvenile cellulitis 2 weeks after hypertrophic osteodystrophy was diagnosed.

Histologically, the lesions are pyogranulomatous nodular-to-diffuse dermatitis with furunculosis and pyogranulomatous lymphadenitis (Fig 6-124B). Sebaceous glands and epitrichial sweat glands may be obliterated. Inflammation often extends into the panniculus. In some dogs, the condition is self-limiting, resolving in 1-3 months and rarely recurs.

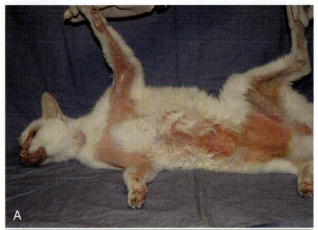

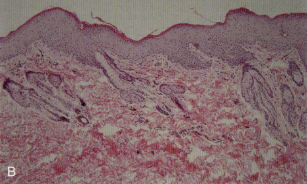

Figure 6-125 Feline paraneoplastic alopecia. **A.** Extensive alopecia of the entire ventrum, medial limbs, paws, periocular, and muzzle region in a bilaterally symmetrical distribution. Note the glistening appearance to the skin that is a striking feature of this disease (Courtesy M.S. Canfield.) **B.** Epidermal hyperplasia and marked follicular atrophy.

often accumulates at mucocutaneous junctions and in interdigital spaces and clawbeds. Some lesions may have erythema, thickened skin, and marked crusting with alopecia. The condition is generally nonpruritic unless there is a secondary pyoderma or *Malassezia* dermatitis. Histologically, there is a cell-poor to cell-rich predominantly lymphocytic interface dermatitis with mild transepidermal and follicular apoptosis and marked orthokeratotic hyperkeratosis, with patchy parakeratotic hyperkeratosis. The interface changes include Civatte bodies, hydropic degeneration, and pigmentary incontinence with a band-like lymphocytic infiltrate with fewer plasma cells and mast cells. Lymphocytic interface to infiltrative mural folliculitis is a consistent feature, and sebaceous glands are frequently reduced to absent. Some cases have been reported to also have an overgrowth of *Malassezia pachydermatis* and bacteria. It has been speculated that the presence of a thymoma initiates abnormal immunologic responses responsible for the dermatitis, which at times can resemble erythema multiforme or graft-versus-host dermatitis histologically. This condition has been reported in a rabbit and anecdotally in dogs.

Necrolytic migratory erythema (hepatocutaneous syndrome, superficial necrolytic dermatitis) has been reported in dogs and occasionally the cat. The condition is sometimes associated with *endocrine tumors of the pancreas* (see Nutritional diseases of skin).

Multiple collagenous hamartomas (**nodular dermatofibrosis**) of the distal limbs, head, and pinnae have been reported in middle-aged German Shepherd dogs and occasionally other breeds (Golden Retriever, Boxer, Belgian Shepherd, mixed breed) in association with *renal cysts, renal cystadenocarcinomas, and/or uterine leiomyomas.* Both kidneys are often affected. The cutaneous lesions range from 2-40 mm. The overlying skin may be normal, thickened, hyperpigmented, alopecic, or ulcerated. Histologically, the skin lesions are nodules composed of increased numbers of slightly thickened collagen bundles within the subcutis or occasionally the dermis. Animals are usually presented for examination of the cutaneous lesions prior to signs referable to the internal neoplasms. Death occurs most often because of complications of the renal lesions. Multiple collagenous hamartomas are suspected to be *inherited* in an autosomal dominant manner in German Shepherd dogs.

Severe **generalized pruritus** without primary gross or histologic cutaneous lesions or other identifiable cause for pruritus has been reported in the dog and horse in association with underlying *malignant lymphoma*. Self-trauma can lead to extensive excoriations and secondary infection. This condition is also reported in humans with lymphoma and a variety of other internal malignancies. The mechanism of the development of pruritus is not understood but is speculated to be related to tumor-induced release of chemical mediators. Pruritus can only be relieved by successful treatment of the malignancy.

Paroxysmal **cutaneous flushing** of extensive areas of the skin without pruritus has been reported in a German Shepherd dog with an intrathoracic mast cell tumor and pulmonary adenocarcinoma. Functional pheochromocytomas upon rare occasion can lead to cutaneous flushing in the dog. Flushing is due to vasodilation and is usually caused by vasoactive mediators.

Occasionally, **vesicular, pustular, or bullous dermatoses** virtually identical to idiopathic autoimmune skin diseases may be associated with an underlying malignancy. The tumor is suspected to trigger the production of autoantibodies. These types of paraneoplastic dermatoses must be differentiated from true autoimmune skin diseases as the prognosis may vary. Differentiation is based on ruling out the presence of an underlying neoplasm and resolution of the skin lesions with tumor removal. A *subepidermal bullous stomatitis* microscopically identical to bullous pemphigoid has been reported in a horse in association with a hemangiosarcoma. Immunoprecipitation studies indicated the horse had antibodies to desmoplakin I and II, the bullous pemphigoid 230 antigen, and a 190-kDa antigen. This immunoprecipitation profile was consistent with that reported for **paraneoplastic pemphigus** as reported in humans and the dog. Paraneoplastic pemphigus is a form of pemphigus that is sometimes associated with an underlying malignancy and has been previously discussed (see Immune-mediated dermatoses).

Further reading

Castellano MC, et al. Generalized nodular dermatofibrosis and cystic renal disease in five German Shepherd dogs. Canine Pract 2000;25:18-21.

Miller WH, et al. Pigmentary abnormalities. In: Miller WH, et al., editors. Muller & Kirk's Small Animal Dermatology. 7th ed. St Louis: Elsevier; 2013. p. 618-629.

Pascal-Tenoria A, et al. Paraneoplastic alopecia associated with internal malignancies in the cat. Vet Dermatol 1997;7:221-226.

Rottenberg S, et al. Thymoma-associated exfoliative dermatitis in cats. Vet Pathol 2004;41:429-433.

Turek MM. Cutaneous paraneoplastic syndromes in dogs and cats: a review of the literature. Vet Dermatol 2003;14:279-296.

Eosinophilic dermatitides

Eosinophilic dermatitis is not a disease but rather a cutaneous reaction pattern to a variety of stimuli, including environmental allergens, food, insects, parasites, drugs, endogenous (e.g., free keratin in the dermis) and exogenous (embedded insect parts) foreign material, and even some viral infections, such as feline herpesvirus 1 in cats. Eosinophils are one of the major sources of inflammatory mediators associated with type I hypersensitivity reactions. Eosinophils can phagocytize small antigens, and they can kill large parasites by releasing toxic substances via degranulation. Eosinophils have 4 major granules containing a wide variety of proteins and enzymes: primary granules, secondary granules, small granules, and lipid bodies. Secondary granules contain major basic protein, eosinophilic cationic protein, eosinophilic peroxidase, and eosinophil-derived neurotoxin. Small granules contain arylsulfatase and acid phosphatase. Lipid bodies are responsible for eicosanoid formation. Eosinophils also produce transforming growth factor-β that is associated with chronic inflammation and fibrosis. Taken as a whole, the contents within eosinophil granules are responsible for inflammation and tissue destruction. They have profound vasoactive and neurogenic properties that manifest clinically as erythema, wheals, and pruritus. Eosinophilic inflammation in the horse and cat is a common tissue reaction, and it seems that the chemotactic stimuli that attract neutrophils in most species attract both eosinophils and neutrophils in these 2 species.

Feline eosinophilic granuloma complex

The **eosinophilic granuloma complex** (EGC) includes a group of lesions *(feline eosinophilic granuloma, eosinophilic plaque, indolent ulcer)* that affect the skin, mucocutaneous junctions, and oral cavity of cats. These lesions can occur separately or together and, rather than a specific disease, are considered a *mucocutaneous reaction pattern*. In most cases, an underlying allergic etiology, particularly to environmental allergens, food, and insect bites (fleas and mosquitoes), are suspected. In human patients with severe atopic dermatitis (AD), there is some evidence to suggest that although the disease is initiated by environmental allergens, some patients may form IgE antibodies directed against human proteins (self-antigens) generated through self-trauma from scratching. *Felis domesticus* allergen I (Feld I) could be an autoallergen responsible for chronic inflammatory reaction in cats with EGC. And in other cases, the lesions spontaneously resolve and do not recur, making allergy an unlikely trigger in those cases. Bacterial involvement may be a significant factor, especially with indolent ulcers and eosinophilic plaques, and in some cases, lesions resolve with antibiotic therapy alone. In some cases, the oral and lip lesions are thought to be due to embedded foreign material such as insects or plants. Because this condition has been reported in several groups of related cats, there is some evidence to suggest heritable eosinophil dysregulation. Clinically and histologically, these 3 conditions have distinct features, although histologically the features can overlap.

Feline eosinophilic plaque is a common cutaneous lesion in cats. Lesions are pruritic, and affected cats lick them constantly,

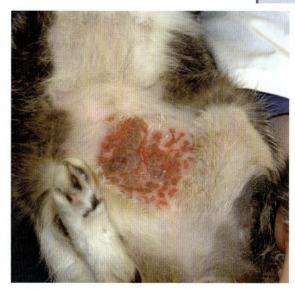

Figure 6-126 Eosinophilic plaque on the ventral abdomen of a cat. (Courtesy W.H. Miller.)

resulting in well-demarcated, singular to multiple, raised, erythematous, alopecic, eroded to ulcerated to oozing plaques that can develop peracutely (Fig. 6-126). Lesions occur most commonly on the ventral abdomen, perineum, and medial thigh. Secondary bacterial infection is common. Peripheral lymphadenopathy may be present. *Histologically, the lesions are characterized by epidermal hyperplasia and moderate to marked spongiosis with exocytosis of eosinophils.* In some cases, there is epidermal and follicular epithelial mucinosis characterized by pale basophilic or gray mucin between keratinocytes. Inflammation in the dermis is perivascular to interstitial and sometimes diffuse, containing numerous eosinophils, and may extend into the subcutis. Mast cells, lymphocytes, and macrophages are present in smaller numbers.

Feline eosinophilic granuloma (linear granuloma) is a common cutaneous, mucocutaneous, and oral lesion in cats. This lesion is the most variable in its clinical presentation and, of the 3 lesions in the EGC, is the most likely to be considered idiopathic. It is often nonpruritic. It can occur at any age; however, it is *more common in young cats*. Spontaneous regression can occur, especially in cats <1 year of age. A genetic predisposition has been documented in some cases. The lesions can be papular, nodular, or linear, and occur on the skin, pawpads, mucocutaneous junctions, and in the oral cavity. Linear lesions are more common on the caudal or medial thigh, and nodular lesions are more common on the lips, chin, oral cavity, and face (Fig. 6-127). The lesions are raised, pink to orange-yellow, and frequently alopecic. Some, especially oral lesions, may be ulcerated with multifocal pinpoint yellow to white foci over the surface. Histologically, the lesions are characterized by *diffuse dermal inflammation composed primarily of eosinophils*, with fewer mast cells, macrophages, and occasional lymphocytes. *Within the inflammation are large irregular foci of collagen fibers and degranulated and degenerating eosinophils (flame figures).* These foci may be surrounded by macrophages and multinucleated histiocytic giant cells. Older lesions tend to have palisading granulomas around flame figures with fewer eosinophils. Mucinosis of the epidermis and hair follicle outer root sheath, focal infiltrative to necrotizing mural eosinophilic folliculitis or furunculosis, and

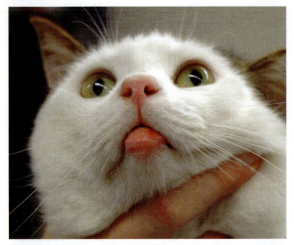

Figure 6-127 *Eosinophilic granuloma* on the chin of a cat. (Courtesy of W.H. Miller.)

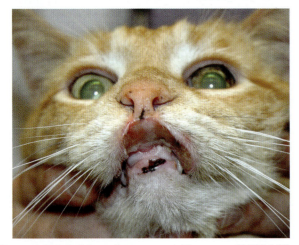

Figure 6-128 *Indolent ulcer* in a cat. (Courtesy of W.H. Miller.)

focal eosinophilic panniculitis may be present. The epidermis may be acanthotic or ulcerated.

Indolent ulcer (rodent ulcer) is a common and clinically distinct condition in cats. *Clinically, the condition is characterized by an ulcerated lesion on the upper lip adjacent to the philtrum, which can be unilateral or bilateral* (Fig. 6-128). The ulcers are not pruritic or painful. Peripheral lymphadenopathy may be present. Histologically, the acute lesions are characterized by diffuse infiltrates of neutrophils with variable numbers of eosinophils, mast cells, and macrophages; however, the lesions are more often biopsied in the chronic phase when the inflammation is composed almost entirely of lymphocytes, plasma cells, macrophages, and neutrophils, together with fibrosis. The numbers of neutrophils vary according to the degree of ulceration. Concurrent bacterial infection is common, and some lesions resolve with antibiotic therapy alone.

Further reading

Bloom PB. Canine and feline eosinophilic skin diseases. Vet Clin North Am Small Anim Pract 2006;36:141-160.

Buckley L, Nuttall T. Feline eosinophilic granuloma complex(ities) some clinical clarification. J Fel Med Surg 2012;14:471-481.

Miller WH, et al. Miscellaneous skin diseases. In: Miller WH, et al., editors. Muller & Kirk's Small Animal Dermatology. 7th ed. St Louis: Elsevier; 2013. p. 695-723.

Scott DW, Miller WH. Idiopathic eosinophilic granuloma in cats: a retrospective study of 55 cases (1988-2003). Jpn J Vet Dermatol 2012;18:13-18.

Canine eosinophilic granuloma

This is a *rare condition in dogs* that has many histologic similarities to feline eosinophilic granuloma. Any breed and age can be affected; however, the condition appears to be more common in Siberian Huskies, in dogs <3 years of age, and males. There may be a genetic basis for the disease in Siberian Huskies and Cavalier King Charles Spaniels. The etiology is unknown, although a hypersensitivity has been proposed, because of the fact that the lesions are corticosteroid responsive, the eosinophilic nature of the lesions, and that there is occasionally circulating eosinophilia. *The lesions can be nodules or plaques, and occur most commonly in the mouth and on the tongue.* Skin lesions are less frequent, although singular to multiple papules, nodules, or plaques have been described on the ventral abdomen, prepuce, digits, flanks, muzzle, external ear canal, nasal planum, and eyelid. *Histologically, the lesions are composed of diffuse dermal eosinophilic inflammation within which are foci of degranulating eosinophils sometimes surrounded by epithelioid macrophages.* The overlying epithelium or epidermis may be acanthotic or ulcerated.

Further reading

Bredal WP, et al. Oral eosinophilic granuloma in three Cavalier King Charles spaniels. J Small Anim Pract 1996;37:499-504.

Vercelli A, et al. Eyelid eosinophilic granuloma in a Siberian husky. J Small Anim Pract 2005;46:31-33.

Equine eosinophilic nodular diseases

Eosinophilic inflammation is a common reaction pattern in the horse, and cutaneous nodules, either single or multiple, are common skin lesions in the horse. Nodular conditions of unknown etiology and pathogenesis include eosinophilic granuloma, axillary nodular necrosis, and unilateral papular dermatosis. Other eosinophilic nodular conditions with known etiologies, such as cutaneous habronemiasis, can look histologically similar (see Helminth diseases of skin). Cutaneous mast cell tumors in the horse can also be seen clinically as cutaneous nodular lesions, and, as histologically, they may contain significant numbers of eosinophils and areas of necrosis, care should be taken to differentiate this tumor from an inflammatory eosinophilic lesion.

Eosinophilic granuloma is the *most common* of the equine cutaneous eosinophilic nodular diseases and is the most common inflammatory nodular skin disease of the horse. The condition is seen most often in the spring and summer, but can occur at any time of year. The etiology is unknown but probably multifactorial. Proposed causes include insect-bite hypersensitivity, atopic dermatitis, food allergy, localized trauma, injections from silicone-coated needles, and close-clipping with free hair shafts embedded in the dermis provoking the inflammatory response. The lesions occur as single or multiple, firm, raised, well-circumscribed, round papules or nodules measuring 0.5-10 cm in diameter, most commonly on

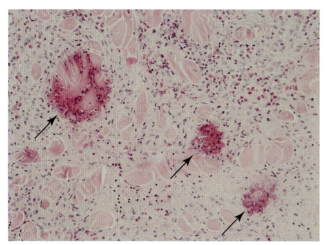

Figure 6-129 Multiple "flame figures" (arrows) in an **equine eosinophilic granuloma**.

the withers, neck, and back, but can occur anywhere on the body and can be generalized. The lesions are neither painful nor pruritic, and the overlying skin and haircoat are typically normal. *Histologically, there are nodular-to-diffuse infiltrates of eosinophils and granulomatous inflammation in the dermis and panniculus. There may be multiple collagen flame figures surrounded by palisading granulomas* (Fig. 6-129). Other histologic features include eosinophilic folliculitis and furunculosis, lymphoid nodules, and dystrophic mineralization. The granulomatous process is fairly linear in silicone-needle injection reactions. Free hair shafts within the lesion suggest previous close-clipping.

Axillary nodular necrosis (girth galls) is a rare dermatosis of the horse. The cause and pathogenesis are unknown. The cutaneous and subcutaneous nodules are firm, round, well circumscribed, 1-10 cm in diameter, and can be single or multiple, usually not more than 10. They are usually unilateral and occur on the trunk behind the axilla. Lesions may also be seen caudal to the shoulder and on the proximal medial aspect of the forelimb. The overlying skin and haircoat are usually normal, and lesions are neither pruritic nor painful. Lesions are sometimes arranged in a linear pattern. Histologically, the lesions are characterized by interstitial to nodular-to-diffuse eosinophilic granulomatous dermatitis and panniculitis with foci of coagulative necrosis, collagen flame figures, dystrophic mineralization, palisaded granulomas, and lymphoid nodules. *Eosinophilic arteritis is characterized by intimal mucinosis and karyorrhectic nuclear debris in the tunica media.* Necrotizing arteritis may be seen.

Unilateral papular dermatosis is an uncommon condition in horses, seen worldwide but reported primarily in the United States, and is more common in spring and summer. It has been seen in many breeds, although Quarter Horses appear to be over-represented. The etiology is unknown; however, the seasonality of the lesions together with the eosinophilic nature of the histologic findings *suggests ectoparasite hypersensitivity*. It has further been suggested that the unilateral distribution may indicate direct contact hypersensitivity to an ectoparasite inhabiting bedding. *Clinically, the lesions are multiple cutaneous papules and nodules measuring 2-10 mm, which occur in a unilateral distribution, usually on the trunk* but sometimes on the neck, shoulders, or abdomen. There is neither pruritus nor pain; however, some lesions become crusted and alopecic. The histologic lesions are characterized by *eosinophilic folliculitis and furunculosis*. Eosinophilic granulomas and collagen flame figures may be present in the surrounding dermis.

Further reading

Scott DW, Miller WH. Miscellaneous skin diseases. In: Scott DW, Miller WH, editors. Equine Dermatology. 2nd ed. St Louis: Elsevier Saunders; 2011. p. 436-467.

Slovis NM, et al. Injection site eosinophilic granulomas and collagenolysis in 3 horses. J Vet Intern Med 1999;13:606-612.

Multisystemic, eosinophilic, epitheliotropic disease in the horse

This rare disease typically occurs in young horses (mean 3-4 years of age) and is characterized by eosinophilic infiltration of many organs, including skin. The cause of multisystemic, eosinophilic, epitheliotropic disease is unknown. A genetic basis has been proposed; Standardbreds and Thoroughbreds are over-represented. Recurrent episodes of type I hypersensitivity caused by dietary, inhaled, or parasitic antigens has been suggested in several reports. There is one report of this condition occurring concurrently with intestinal lymphoma, and several other unpublished cases that appear identical to the case described; the authors suggest that the clonal proliferation of T lymphocytes triggers proliferation of eosinophils by secretion of cytokines such as interleukin-5. This mechanism has also been proposed in humans who have concurrent abnormal T-lymphocyte proliferations and hypereosinophilic syndrome.

Affected horses often display severe weight loss, pitting edema, and exudative, exfoliative dermatitis that usually originates at the coronary bands or head and becomes generalized. Chronically, there is scaling, crusting, and alopecia. Early findings include well-demarcated ulcers on the coronary bands, muzzle, mucocutaneous junctions, and mouth. Vesicles, bullae, and wheals are rarely noted. Pruritus is variable, and peripheral lymph nodes may be enlarged. Approximately 50% of horses have diarrhea and fever. Peripheral eosinophilia is only present in ~14% of cases. Histologically, the condition is characterized by *eosinophilic and lymphoplasmacytic infiltration of multiple organs, sometimes with eosinophilic granuloma formation*. Organs most commonly affected include *skin, pancreas, liver, common bile duct, gastrointestinal tract, and lungs*. In the skin, the inflammatory pattern is variable, including perivascular, lichenoid interface, interstitial, diffuse, and granulomatous. Eosinophils, lymphocytes, and plasma cells predominate. There is marked epidermal hyperplasia with hyperkeratosis that is orthokeratotic and parakeratotic. An epitheliotropic infiltrate of eosinophils and lymphocytes is common, and apoptotic keratinocytes may be prominent. Eosinophilic folliculitis, furunculosis, and eosinophilic microabscesses may be seen. Collagen flame figures and lymphoid nodules are seen occasionally. Most horses suffer a chronic course of progressive weight loss and dermatitis and die or are euthanized within 8 months of diagnosis.

Further reading

Bosseler L, et al. Equine multisystemic eosinophilic epitheliotropic disease: a case report and review of literature. N Z Vet J 2013;61: 177-182.

La Perle KMD, et al. Multisystemic, eosinophilic, epitheliotropic disease with intestinal lymphosarcoma in a horse. Vet Pathol 1998; 35:144-146.

Sterile eosinophilic folliculitis and furunculosis

In **dogs,** eosinophilic folliculitis and furunculosis is a condition that typically affects the face. The etiology of this condition has not been fully characterized, but *a hypersensitivity reaction to insect stings and arthropod bites is strongly suspected*. The condition is most common in young, large-breed dogs, and lesions are seen primarily on the dorsal muzzle, around the eyes, ears, and less commonly in the axillae, inguinal areas, and ventrum. Lesions are characterized by sudden onset of vesicles, papules, nodules, crusts, erosions, and ulcers. Pruritus is variable but can be intense. Lesions are painful in some dogs.

In **horses,** sterile eosinophilic folliculitis and furunculosis can be seen in horses with atopic dermatitis, insect-bite hypersensitivity, food allergy, unilateral papular dermatosis, and onchocerciasis. Lesions are characterized by tufted papules that become alopecic and crusted in a generally symmetrical and multifocal distribution anywhere on the body; however, the neck, shoulders, chest, and dorsolateral thorax are most commonly affected. Pruritus is variable but is commonly moderate to marked.

Sterile eosinophilic folliculitis has been reported in **cattle** and is characterized by nonpainful, nonpruritic, symmetrically distributed, multiple crusting, or alopecic papules and plaques primarily on the head, neck, and trunk. The condition in nonseasonal, and the cause is unknown. In **cats,** sterile eosinophilic folliculitis and furunculosis may be seen as a bystander lesion in any allergic dermatitis; however, it is more commonly seen in mosquito-bite hypersensitivity and feline herpesvirus dermatitis, both of which are most commonly located on the face and head.

Histologically, sterile eosinophilic folliculitis and furunculosis are characterized by infiltrative eosinophilic mural folliculitis, luminal eosinophilic folliculitis, and eosinophilic furunculosis. Within the dermis, there is marked edema and mucin accumulation along with variable numbers of eosinophils, neutrophils, and mononuclear cells. Dermal hemorrhage may be prominent in dogs. Collagen flame figures may be present. There is moderate to severe epidermal hyperplasia, spongiosis, and serocellular crusts. There may also be erosions and ulcerations.

Canine sterile eosinophilic pinnal folliculitis is an uncommon, nonseasonal, bilaterally symmetrical dermatosis with variable pruritus and an unknown cause and pathogenesis. Erythematous papules and crusts are present on the concave surface of the pinnae. Eosinophilic folliculitis and furunculosis are seen with histopathology.

Sterile eosinophilic pustulosis

This is a rare idiopathic dermatosis of dogs characterized by peripheral eosinophilia, sterile tissue eosinophilia, and responsiveness to systemic glucocorticoids. Skin lesions include multifocal to generalized pruritic, erythematous, follicular, and nonfollicular papules and pustules that evolve into annular targetoid lesions with erosions, epidermal collarettes, and hyperpigmentation. Histopathology is characterized by subcorneal pustules containing eosinophils and fewer neutrophils. There may be various degrees of flame figures and eosinophilic folliculitis and furunculosis.

Further reading

Gross TL, et al. Pustular and nodular diseases with adnexal destruction. In: Gross TL, et al., editors. Skin Diseases of the Dog and Cat: Clinical and Histopathological Diagnosis. 2nd ed. Oxford, UK: Blackwell; 2005. p. 406-459.

Hargis AM, et al. Ulcerative facial and nasal dermatitis and stomatitis in cats associated with feline herpesvirus 1. Vet Dermatol 1999;10:267-274.

Miller WH, et al. Miscellaneous skin diseases. In: Miller WH, et al., editors. Muller & Kirk's Small Animal Dermatology. 7th ed. St Louis: Elsevier; 2013. p. 695-723.

Scott DW, Miller WH. Miscellaneous skin diseases. In: Scott DW, Miller WH, editors. Equine Dermatology. 2nd ed. St Louis: Elsevier Saunders; 2011. p. 436-467.

Eosinophilic dermatitis with edema

This is a unique condition in dogs characterized by severe erythema and erythematous to hemorrhagic macules or plaques most pronounced on the ventral abdomen and limbs. Some dogs have lesions with central clearing (targetoid macules), wheals, facial swelling, or generalized edema. The cause is unknown; however, about ¾ of the reported cases have been dogs treated for vomiting and diarrhea; thus drug association has been suspected in many cases. The histologic lesions are marked perivascular to diffuse eosinophilic dermatitis with edema. Collagen flame figures are seen in some cases. Eosinophilic intraepidermal pustules may be present.

Further reading

Mauldin EA, et al. Comparison of clinical history and dermatologic findings in 29 dogs with severe eosinophilic dermatitis: a retrospective analysis. Vet Dermatol 2006;17:338-347.

Sterile neutrophilic dermatoses

Sterile neutrophilic dermatosis is a very rare condition, described in dogs, with marked similarities to the human disease known as acute febrile neutrophilic dermatosis (Sweet's syndrome). Reported lesions include painful red papules, nodules, and plaques with variable degrees of edema and ulceration. Other clinical signs include fever, arthritis, pneumonia, and circulating neutrophilia. The pathogenesis is unknown; however, it is believed to be an antigen-induced T-cell–mediated immune reaction. Possible triggers include drugs, respiratory and gastrointestinal infections, and neoplasia. Three cases have been associated with carprofen. Histologically, there is moderate to severe interstitial neutrophilic dermatitis with variable eosinophils and neutrophilic infiltration into the epidermis forming small pustules.

Subcorneal pustular dermatosis is a very rare, sterile, superficial, pustular condition of dogs with an unknown cause and pathogenesis. Miniature Schnauzers are over-represented. Lesions are multifocal to generalized, symmetrical, and commonly affect the head and trunk. They include intact nonfollicular transient green to yellow pustules that evolve into areas of alopecia, epidermal collarettes, and hyperpigmentation. Lesions may spread peripherally into annular and serpiginous formations. Pruritus is variable and may be extreme. Pawpads are rarely affected.

Auricular chondritis

Auricular chondritis (relapsing polychondritis) is a rare condition in the cat and dog characterized by inflammation and destruction of the auricular cartilage. The condition was named after a similar human condition thought to be an immune-mediated attack directed against type II collagen and known to affect other cartilaginous sites, such as the nose, trachea, and cardiac valves. The cause is unknown in cats and dogs, in most cases only affects the pinnae, is generally not reported to relapse, and an autoimmune or immune-mediated pathogenesis has not been supported. In one case, cartilaginous lesions were also noted in the costae, larynx, trachea, and limbs, and the cat had multicentric lymphoma. Trauma or damage to the pinnal cartilage has been proposed as a possible initiator. In a few cases, chronic otitis externa has preceded the development of the disease. Clinically, the condition occurs in young to middle-aged cats and dogs; one or both pinnae are swollen, erythematous, deformed, and often painful. Histologically, the auricular cartilage may be thinned, curled, or wrinkled, with loss of basophilic staining. Lymphoplasmacytic infiltrates and variable numbers of neutrophils surround areas of necrosis of the auricular cartilage. Variable amounts of granulation tissue and fibrosis may be seen.

Nodular auricular chondropathy has been described rarely in horses. The condition occurs as nonprogressive, single to multiple, unilateral to bilateral, firm, raised, nonmoveable, nonpainful papules and nodules along the pinnal margins and tips. Affected cartilage is disorganized, necrotic, or mineralized.

Further reading

Baba T, et al. Auricular chondritis associated with systemic joint and cartilage inflammation in a cat. J Vet Med Sci 2009;71:79-82.

Gerber B, et al. Feline relapsing polychondritis: two cases and a review of the literature. J Feline Med Surg 2002;4:189-194.

Follicular lipidosis

Follicular lipidosis is characterized by regional alopecia of areas of mahogany colored points of the hair of the paws and face of Rottweiler puppies. Histologically, the lesions are characterized by marked swelling, caused by lipid accumulation, of the hair matrix cells of primary anagen hair follicles. Matrix cells of the bulb are most severely affected, whereas cells of the internal and external root sheath are affected to a lesser degree. Scattered hair shafts may contain vacuoles and have irregular, thickened, or frayed cuticles. *This condition may represent yet another type of color-associated follicular dysplasia.* Too few cases have been recognized to clearly predict the clinical course of the alopecia, or to identify associated abnormalities or the mode of inheritance, if any.

Further reading

Gross TL, et al. Follicular lipidosis in three Rottweilers. Vet Dermatol 2001;8:33-40.

Follicular mucinosis (alopecia mucinosa)

Follicular mucinosis is characterized by collections of mucin in the outer root sheath of the follicular epithelium and of sebaceous glands. Intraepithelial cysts filled with mucin may form. Grossly, the lesions consist of progressive alopecia and scaling that may become generalized. A disease resembling follicular mucinosis in humans has been described in the **cat** and **dog**. The condition described in 2 cats chiefly affected the head, neck, and shoulders. Histologically, there was mucinous degeneration of the outer root sheath of the follicular infundibulum. Both cats had swollen facial skin and developed epitheliotropic lymphoma within several months of the initial biopsy. Follicular mucinosis has been reported in 2 older dogs. The skin of the head, limbs, and some areas of the trunk was affected. In addition to the histologic lesions described above, there was a perivascular and perifollicular lymphocytic to plasmacytic infiltrate. The epidermis was mildly acanthotic with compact orthokeratotic hyperkeratosis and multifocal spongiosis with lymphocytic exocytosis. The basal cell layer demonstrated hydropic degeneration, mild apoptosis, and prominent pigmentary incontinence. No follow-up information was available. In humans, follicular mucinosis can resolve spontaneously or become a chronic relapsing condition. Many cases are thought to progress to epitheliotropic lymphoma. It should be noted that *epidermal and epithelial mucinosis can be seen in various allergic dermatitides of the cat.*

A condition in cats described as **degenerative mucinotic mural folliculitis** has many similarities to follicular mucinosis. Seven cats have been described, and they all had a several-month to 2-year history of progressive hair loss that started on the face or neck and led to generalized alopecia. The skin of the face, particularly the muzzle, of all the cats was thickened and swollen. There was variable scaling, crusting, and hyperpigmentation. Most of the cats were lethargic, 4 were pruritic, 3 had concurrent feline immunodeficiency virus, and 2 had weight loss. Six of the cats were euthanized because of progressive disease. Histologically, there was moderate to severe mucin accumulation in the superficial outer root sheath. Most cases had follicular atrophy with infiltrative mural folliculitis consisting of lymphocytes, plasma cells, macrophages, and neutrophils focused primarily on the isthmus with extension to the perifollicular dermis. In some cases, pyogranulomas effaced the isthmus of some follicles. In addition, there was moderate epidermal hyperplasia, compact hyperkeratosis, and neutrophilic crusts. In contrast to alopecia mucinosa, interface changes were not described, and none of these cats developed epitheliotropic lymphoma.

Feline scleromyxedema

Scleromyxedema is the generalized form of lichen myxedematosus, *a primary dermal mucinosis.* This condition is *very rare* and is characterized by dermal mucin deposits on the head and legs, increased numbers of fibroblasts, variable fibrosis, absence of thyroid disease, and a monoclonal gammopathy. Mucin deposits are also detected on thoracic and abdominal organs.

Further reading

Bell A, Oliver F. Alopecia mucinosa (follicular mucinosis) in a dog. Vet Dermatol 1995;6:221-226.

Ishida M, et al. Adult T-cell leukemia/lymphoma accompanying follicular mucinosis: a case report with review of the literature. Int J Clin Exp Pathol 2013;6:3014-3018.

Müntener T, et al. Scleromyxedema-like syndrome with systemic involvement in a cat. Vet Pathol 2010;47:346-350.

Localized scleroderma (morphea) and cicatricial alopecia

Localized scleroderma (morphea) is a rare disease described in humans, dogs, cats, and a horse. The cause is unknown; but in humans, vascular injury, abnormal collagen metabolism, and an immune-mediated pathogenesis, such as drug reaction, have all been proposed. *Asymptomatic, well-demarcated, sclerotic plaques that are alopecic, smooth, and shiny characterize the condition. Hypopigmentation may occur.* Lesions tend to be oval to linear and occur on the trunk, limbs, and head. Histologically, the epidermis is normal, and the dermis is replaced by collagenous connective tissue. Pilosebaceous units are essentially absent. A very mild superficial and deep perivascular accumulation of lymphohistiocytic cells is present. Spontaneous resolution has been reported.

Cicatricial alopecia is grossly and microscopically very similar; however, in this condition, lesions are permanent. Causes include a variety of insults that result in fibrous tissue deposition: injection-site reactions, furunculosis, vasculitis, dermatomyositis, post-traumatic scarring, and so on. Histologically, there is *laminar arrangement of collagen replacing the dermis, and the epidermis is hyperplastic.* Scattered orphaned sweat glands may be seen.

Generalized scleroderma is a rare multisystemic disorder that results in progressive fibrosis of the skin, lungs, gastrointestinal tract, kidneys, and heart. It has been described in humans and a horse.

Further reading

Frank LA, et al. Diffuse systemic sclerosis in a Paso Fino mare. Comp Cont Educ Pract Vet 2000;22:274.

Miller WH, et al. Miscellaneous skin diseases. In: Miller WH, et al., editors. Muller & Kirk's Small Animal Dermatology. 7th ed. St Louis: Elsevier; 2013. p. 695-723.

Psoriasiform dermatitis of goats

This is a rare condition described in pygmy goats and alpine goats most commonly. Affected animals range from 3 months to young adults. Lesions are nonpruritic and begin on the face and pinnae and may also affect the neck, ventrum, and distal limbs. There is erythema, scaling, and variable degrees of crusting, thickened skin, and alopecia. Lesions wax and wane. Psoriasiform epidermal hyperplasia, neutrophilic intraepidermal microabscesses with neutrophilic perivascular dermatitis, and marked orthokeratotic and parakeratotic hyperkeratosis are described histologically.

Porcine juvenile pustular psoriasiform dermatitis

This disease of weanling pigs was originally named **pityriasis rosea**. Because the clinical signs and gross lesions bear little relationship to those of the human disease for which it was originally named, the new designation, porcine juvenile pustular psoriasiform dermatitis, has been suggested. *The disease is of no significance, except esthetic. The cause is not known.* A hereditary predisposition has been suggested but not proved, particularly in Landrace pigs. Lesions develop most often in weaned pigs 3-14 weeks of age. Entire litters or just a few piglets may be affected.

The disease begins with symmetrical, nonpruritic, scaly, erythematous papules on the skin of the abdomen and inner thighs. The papules expand centrifugally to produce, at first, scaly plaques and later, when the central areas return to normal, ring-shaped, erythematous lesions (Fig. 6-130). As the rings expand, they coalesce to produce mosaic patterns and may extend to the sides and perineum. The acute histologic lesion is superficial and comprises deep perivascular dermatitis with eosinophils, neutrophils, and mononuclear cells. There may be epidermal spongiosis with intraepidermal eosinophilic and neutrophilic pustules. Superficial epidermal necrosis may extend into the ostia of the hair follicles. As the lesions heal, marked psoriasiform hyperplasia and parakeratotic scale-crusts predominate. The condition spontaneously resolves within about 4 weeks.

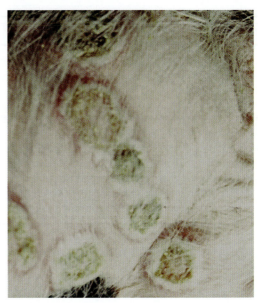

Figure 6-130 Porcine juvenile pustular psoriasiform dermatitis. Multifocal to coalescing crusted annular lesions with central depressions. (Courtesy D.W. Scott.)

Miscellaneous porcine dermatoses

Idiopathic hyperkeratosis is commonly described in intensively housed sows and boars. Brown, waxy material accumulates on the dorsal neck and shoulders, dorsum, or flanks. The underlying skin is normal, and the condition is nonpruritic.

Porcine ulcerative dermatitis syndrome is uncommon and mostly described in adult sows. Annular to polycyclic chronic ulcers with thickened margins and crusts are present on the perineum, lateral thorax, abdomen and thighs, mammae, and convex surface of the pinnae. Lesions may resolve during lactation but recur with weaning. Variable features and patterns have been reported histologically. They include epidermal necrosis, hyperkeratosis, dermal perivascular eosinophils with fewer neutrophils and plasma cells, as well as cell-poor lymphoplasmacytic and histiocytic interface dermatitis and folliculitis with hydropic degeneration, apoptotic keratinocytes, and vesicle formation at the dermal-epidermal junction. The latter pattern suggests that this condition may be a form of vesicular cutaneous lupus erythematosus.

Recurrent dermatosis of sows is a rare idiopathic condition characterized by nonpruritic, erythematous macules and patches that enlarge and become scaly, especially on the trunk and only in white skin. Hairs within the lesion become discolored brown. Lesions tend to occur while farrowing and resolve when out of the farrowing house.

Further reading

Kimura T, Doi K. Clinical and histopathological findings in pustular psoriasiform dermatitis (pityriasis rosea) in pigs. J Vet Med Sci 2004;66:1147-1150.

Lopez A, et al. Porcine ulcerative dermatitis syndrome in sows: a form of vesicular cutaneous lupus erythematosus? Vet Rec 2009;165: 501-506.

Straw BE, et al. eds Skin. In: Straw BE, et al., editors. Diseases of Swine. 8th ed. Ames, Iowa: Iowa State University Press; 1999. p. 955.

Spiculosis

Spiculosis is a dysplastic and dyskeratotic condition of the hair follicle that results in 1-2 mm diameter and 0.5-2.0 cm long brittle spicules (hair shafts) protruding from hair follicles. The condition has been reported in humans and intact male **Kerry Blue Terriers.** Clinically, the condition is characterized by multiple hard, brittle, follicular spicules on various areas of the body but are most common on the lateral hocks. Affected dogs may chew or lick at the spicules. Histologically, hair follicles have enlarged hair bulbs that may have 2 dermal papillae. Enlargement of the hair bulb results from collections of heavily pigmented matrix cells that keratinize prematurely to form hyperpigmented keratinized amorphous masses or columns of unpigmented keratin in place of normal hairs.

Further reading

McKeever PJ, et al. Spiculosis. J Am Anim Hosp Assoc 1992;28: 257-261.

Sebaceous gland dysplasia

Abnormal sebaceous gland differentiation (sebaceous gland dysplasia) is a rare dermatosis in **cats** and **dogs.** The lesion develops at a young age, usually <1 year, as variable degrees of scaling, poor-quality haircoat, follicular casting, and hair loss. In kittens, it is characterized by hypotrichosis with scaling that is apparent as early as 4 weeks of age (eFig. 6-15). Lesions tend to start on the face and, whereas hair loss is the main clinical sign in kittens, scaling and follicular cast formation is the most common lesion in dogs. The cause is unknown; however, the juvenile onset suggests a genetic defect leading to abnormal sebaceous gland development.

Histologically, sebaceous glands are markedly reduced in size with irregular profiles and composed of haphazardly arranged basaloid epithelial cells and sebocytes. Scattered shrunken sebocytes with hypereosinophilic cytoplasm and pyknotic nuclei are often observed. Sebaceous glands lack the normal differentiation from reserve (basal) cells to mature sebocytes. The lobules have irregularly sized sebocytes intermixed with vacuolated immature basaloid cells (eFig. 6-16).

Further reading

Peters-Kennedy J, et al. Scaling dermatosis in three dogs associated with abnormal sebaceous gland differentiation. Vet Dermatol 2014;25:23-e8.

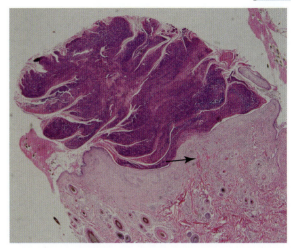

Figure 6-131 Perforating dermatitis in a cat. Vertically oriented collagen fibers (arrow) extending down from a conical shaped crust.

Yager JA, et al. Abnormal sebaceous gland differentiation in 10 kittens ("sebaceous gland dysplasia") associated with generalized hypotrichosis and scaling. Vet Dermatol 2012;23:136-144.

Perforating dermatitis

Perforating dermatitis is a rare, distinctive reaction pattern in **cats** and humans. Clinically, there are multiple, conical, brown, firm horn-like papules and plaques. Lesions have been reported on the shoulder, neck, axilla, flank, hip, trunk, legs, and nose. The lesions may be arranged in a linear configuration. Histologically, this is a *very distinctive lesion* with a *large conical crust containing a large number of degenerate inflammatory cells and numerous vertically oriented degenerate collagen fibers protruding into it* (Fig. 6-131). The superficial to deep dermis contains moderate to marked infiltrates of eosinophils, mast cells, neutrophils, and fewer mononuclear cells. There may be subepidermal fibrosis. Pruritus is variable, ranging from absent to severe. The cause is unknown, although some cases may occur secondary to self-trauma from allergic skin disease. It has been proposed that this condition is the result of abnormal wound healing possibly caused by abnormal collagenesis. There is no age, sex, or breed predisposition. Masson trichrome staining of affected collagen fibers demonstrates segmental red cores; however, this finding is not specific for this condition.

Further reading

Albanese F, et al. Feline perforating dermatitis resembling human reactive perforating collagenosis: clinicopathological findings and outcome in four cases. Vet Dermatol 2009;20:273-280.

Olivry T. Is feline acquired reactive perforating collagenosis a wound healing defect? Treatment with topical betamethasone and halofuginone appears beneficial. Vet Dermatol 2010;21:434-436.

Sterile granulomas and pyogranulomas

Sterile granulomatous or pyogranulomatous dermatoses have been reported in dogs and less commonly in cats and horses.

Sterile pyogranuloma syndrome

The sterile granuloma/pyogranuloma syndrome (SPGS) is uncommon in **dogs** and rare in **cats** and **horses.** The cause is unknown; however, negative tissue cultures, negative special stains for microbial agents, absence of foreign material with polarization, and good response to immunomodulatory therapy have suggested an *immune-mediated pathogenesis*. It has been hypothesized by some that SPGS may be caused by an immune response against persistent endogenous or exogenous antigens, such as *Leishmania* spp. and/or *Mycobacterium* spp. These agents have been identified by PCR in some cases. Lesions are solitary or multiple, and localized or generalized firm, hair-covered to partially alopecic, erythematous papules, nodules, and plaques (Fig. 6-132A). Lesions may become ulcerated and secondarily infected. Affected animals are otherwise healthy. Histologic findings include *large perifollicular granulomas or pyogranulomas* that are elongated and vertically oriented and that track hair follicles but do not invade them (Fig. 6-132B). Older lesions may become diffuse, obliterating adnexal structures and extending into the subcutis. Histiocytes, lymphocytes, and neutrophils predominate, with occasional plasma cells or multinucleated histiocytic giant cells. In horses and some cats, multinucleated histiocytic giant cells may be numerous. There are no age or sex predispositions.

In **dogs,** Collies, Boxers, Great Danes, Weimaraners, English Bulldogs, Doberman Pinschers, Dachshunds, and Golden Retrievers appear to be predisposed. In most dogs, the lesions are multiple, nonpainful, nonpruritic, and can occur anywhere on the body; however, the face and distal extremities are the most common sites. Lymphadenopathy occurs in some cases, and rarely, there can be pyogranulomatous lymphadenitis. The condition may spontaneously resolve or wax and wane. In **horses,** as in dogs, lesions are generally asymptomatic. They are usually single on the lip, eyelid, or pastern, or multiple and scattered over the body.

In **cats,** lesions tend to be symmetrical and pruritic. Common sites are periauricular, pinna, and head, less commonly on the paws and trunk. Lesions are violaceus or orange-yellow and may become red to purple when palpated.

Cutaneous xanthoma

Xanthomas *(xanthogranulomas)* are single to multiple nodular lesions occurring rarely in the **cat** and very rarely in the **dog** and **horse.** Disorders of metabolism, such as hyperlipidemia in cats, diabetes mellitus, or high-fat diets, lead to the formation of xanthogranulomas in most cases; other cases, particularly solitary xanthomas, are idiopathic. In horses, xanthomas have been described in conjunction with equine pituitary pars intermedia dysfunction. Clinically, the lesions are *yellow to white papules, plaques, or nodules with erythematous margins. They can be painful or pruritic*. The head, distal extremities, paws, and bony prominences are typical sites. *Histologically*, there are nodular-to-diffuse infiltrates of foamy macrophages in the dermis, with variable numbers of multinucleated histiocytic giant cells and lipid lakes.

Sarcoidosis

Sarcoidosis in humans is a systemic granulomatous disease of undetermined etiology. The granulomas are characteristic, being composed predominantly of epithelioid macrophages with few lymphocytes ("naked" granulomas).

A *sterile "sarcoidal" granulomatous dermatitis* has been described in dogs and horses. **Dogs** develop multiple erythematous papules, nodules, and plaques that were neither pruritic nor painful. The lesions most commonly affected the neck, trunk, face, and pinnae. Nodular-to-diffuse sarcoidal granulomatous inflammation was present histologically. This condition is suspected to be part of SPGS.

Equine sarcoidosis (idiopathic generalized or systemic granulomatous disease) is rare and may be seen as a generalized or localized exfoliative dermatitis and/or as granulomatous inflammation in multiple organs. The cause is unknown; however, an immune-mediated pathogenesis, *Mycobacterium* spp., and hairy vetch toxicosis have been implicated. Sarcoidosis has been categorized into 3 clinical presentations: *generalized, partially generalized, and localized*. Peripheral lymphadenopathy may occur in the former two. The *localized form* is defined as localized areas of nonpruritic exfoliative dermatitis on 1 or 2 lower limbs with variable pain, edema, and lameness. The *partially generalized form* is characterized by exfoliative dermatitis on 1 or 2 limb(s) and/or (sub)cutaneous nodular lesions on a limited body region. The *generalized form* shows nonpruritic cutaneous signs and or (sub)cutaneous nodules all over the body with one or more of the following signs: low-grade fever, exercise intolerance, pain when touched,

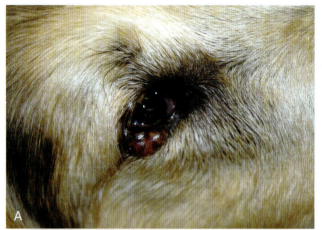

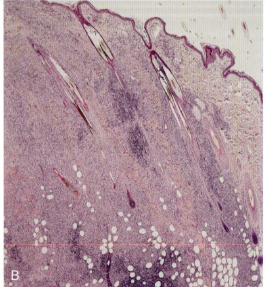

Figure 6-132 Sterile granuloma syndrome in a dog. **A.** Alopecic nodule under the lower eyelid. (Courtesy Cornell University Hospital for Animals, Clinical Dermatology Service.) **B.** Note the vertically oriented perifollicular lymphohistiocytic infiltrates.

respiratory distress, weight loss, and/or peripheral lymphadenopathy. The onset may be insidious or rapid. There are no age, breed, or sex predilections, although most horses are >3 years of age. The skin lesions are characterized by well-demarcated, focal, multifocal, or generalized scaling and crusting, with various degrees of alopecia and increased local skin temperature. Lesions are most common on the lower limbs. Internal nodules may be found in the lung, lymph nodes, liver, gastrointestinal tract, spleen, kidneys, bones, and central nervous system. In some generalized cases, skin lesions may not be present. *Histopathology* shows multifocal nodular-to-diffuse, lymphogranulomatous dermatitis with *multinucleated histiocytic giant cells*. *Vasculitis* may be present, particularly in the localized form. The prognosis is poor for the generalized and partially generalized forms, with most horses being euthanized within months of diagnosis. Prognosis for survival is good for the localized form but guarded for the localized skin disease. Spontaneous resolution has been reported in the generalized and localized form.

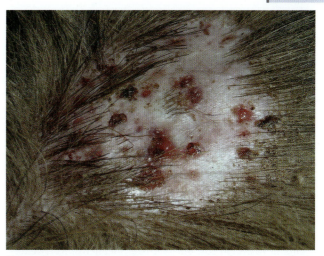

Figure 6-133 Sterile nodular panniculitis in a dog. Note multiple grouped ulcerative draining lesions on the trunk. (Courtesy M.S. Canfield.)

Further reading

Oliveira-Filho JP, et al. *Mycobacterium* DNA detection in liver and skin of a horse with generalized sarcoidosis. J Vet Diagn Invest 2012;24:596-600.

Panich R, et al. Canine cutaneous sterile pyogranuloma/granuloma syndrome: a retrospective analysis of 29 cases (1976 to 1988). J Am Anim Hosp Assoc 1991;27:519-528.

Santoro D, et al. Cutaneous sterile granuloma/pyogranulomas, leishmaniasis and mycobacterial infections. J Small Anim Pract 2008;49:552-561.

Sloet van Oldruitenborgh-Oosterbaan MM, Grinwis GCM. Equine sarcoidosis: clinical signs, diagnosis, treatment and outcome of 22 cases. Vet Dermatol 2013;24:218-e48.

Sterile nodular panniculitis

Panniculitis refers to inflammation of the subcutaneous adipose tissue. Panniculitis has many causes, most of which have been discussed in previous sections (bacteria, fungi, immune-mediated disease, trauma, injection of irritant substances, foreign bodies, nutritional disorders, adverse reactions to vaccines or other injections, pancreatic disease). *The syndrome of sterile nodular panniculitis (SNP) currently is considered to be idiopathic and either primary in origin or associated with a variety of other illnesses, including pancreatic nodular hyperplasia, pancreatic neoplasia, pancreatitis, or immune-mediated disease, such as rheumatoid arthritis and systemic lupus erythematosus.* Concurrent inflammation of the fat in the abdomen, epidural space, and bone (steatitis) can occur in dogs with SNP.

It is a rare condition affecting **dogs, cats, horses,** and **cattle.**

The *gross lesions* are single to multiple, firm or soft, well-delineated or ill-defined, subcutaneous papules to nodules that may become cystic, ulcerate, or develop draining tracts. The exudate may be oily, serosanguineous, or hemorrhagic. Lesions may be grouped or distributed widely (Fig. 6-133). Affected animals with single lesions may be asymptomatic; animals with multiple lesions often have pyrexia, lethargy, and anorexia. Pain is variable. A normochromic, normocytic non-regenerative anemia is seen in chronically affected animals with multiple extensive lesions. Some cases spontaneously regress. Most lesions in dogs and cats respond to immunosuppressive doses of glucocorticoids. The condition can be recurrent. There is a tendency for the canine lesions to affect the trunk, and Dachshunds and Poodles are over-represented. Lesions in the horse are most often found on the neck, thorax, abdomen, and proximal limbs, and may elicit pain upon palpation. Shetland ponies may be predisposed. In cats, most lesions are solitary and occur most commonly over the ventral abdomen and ventral thorax. Lesions in cattle have been described over the neck, trunk, and proximal limbs.

The microscopic lesion is a lobular to diffuse infiltrate in the subcutis and deep dermis composed predominantly of neutrophils and macrophages and lesser numbers of lymphocytes and plasma cells. Discrete granulomas and pyogranulomas may be present. Adipocytes may appear necrotic or infiltrated with foamy macrophages. Lipid released from damaged lipocytes hydrolyzes to glycerol and fatty acids. Fatty acids incite further inflammation that perpetuates the lesions. *Sterile panniculitis may be indistinguishable histologically from the panniculitides of infectious cause, and thus tissue culture and special stains for microbial agents are necessary for a definitive diagnosis.*

The presence of saponification of fat and fat necrosis, along with diffuse infiltrates of pyogranulomatous inflammation, is associated with pancreatic disease and vitamin E deficiency in cats. The latter is also associated with ceroid deposits. Septal panniculitis is often associated with vasculitis. Sterile panniculitis resulting from trauma often occurs as a single lesion of lobular fat necrosis surrounded by fibrosis. Panniculitis resulting from repositol injection is usually characterized by fat necrosis and large numbers of degenerate neutrophils. Postinjection panniculitis also occurs with focal necrosis in the subcutis, but this area is surrounded by predominantly foamy macrophages and multinucleated histiocytic giant cells. Rabies vaccine-induced panniculitis is discussed under Immune-mediated dermatoses.

Further reading

German AJ, et al. Sterile nodular panniculitis and pansteatitis in three weimaraners. J Small Anim Pract 2003;44:449-455.

Gross TL, et al. Diseases of the panniculus. In: Gross TL, et al., editors. Skin Diseases of the Dog and Cat: Clinical and Histopathological Diagnosis. 2nd ed. Oxford, UK: Blackwell; 2005. p. 538-558.

Menzies-Gow NJ, et al. Chronic nodular panniculitis in a three-year-old mare. Vet Rec 2002;151:416-419.

O'Kell AL, et al. Canine sterile nodular panniculitis: a retrospective study of 14 cases. J Vet Intern Med 2010;24:278-284.

Waitt LH, et al. Panniculitis in a horse with peripancreatic and pancreatic fibrosis. J Vet Diagn Invest 2006;18:405-408.

Symmetrical lupoid onychitis

Symmetrical lupoid onychitis or onychodystrophy (SLO) is a disease of young to middle-aged **dogs** *characterized by onychalgia, onycholysis, and onychomadesis of multiple claws on multiple paws.* The cause is unknown, but studies showing that dog leukocyte antigen class II is significantly associated with SLO support an immune-mediated pathogenesis. A genetic predisposition has been established in certain breeds. The condition occurs in many breeds, but German Shepherds, Rottweilers, and Gordon Setters are predisposed. The condition is painful and often leads to lameness. Amputation of the third phalanx of affected digits to include clawbed epithelium is often needed to establish the diagnosis. Histologic lesions are most pronounced on the dorsal aspect of the claw. *The most common changes are a lichenoid interface onychitis with lymphocytic exocytosis and spongiosis and multifocal hydropic degeneration of the basal epidermis.* Pigmentary incontinence may be severe, and there may be dermal hemorrhage or fibrosis and mucinosis of the deep dermis. Claws regrow but are misshapen, dry, soft or brittle, and discolored. Secondary bacterial infection may occur. *The pathogenesis of SLO is not known* and, in fact, the possibility that SLO is not a specific disease entity but merely an inflammatory reaction typical for the clawbed is possible. Similar clinical and histopathologic changes have been described in cases of leishmaniasis, systemic lupus erythematosus, food allergy, drug reaction, and idiopathic and antibiotic-responsive disease.

Further reading

Ovrebo Bohnhorst J, et al. Antinuclear antibodies (ANA) in Gordon setters with symmetrical lupoid onychodystrophy and black hair follicular dysplasia. Acta Vet Scand 2001;42:323-329.

Wilbe M, et al. DLA class II alleles are associated with risk for canine symmetrical lupoid onychodystrophy (SLO). PLoS ONE 2010;5:1-6.

Laminitis

The hoof wall is a complex structure composed of an epidermis and dermis that attaches to the underlying distal phalanx. The distal phalanx is held in place by interdigitation of the epidermal lamina of the inner hoof wall and the dermal lamina of the corium that is attached to the third phalanx. When these laminae fail, the forces of body weight, motion, and tendons lead to sinking and rotation of P3, shearing of vessels that supply these tissues, and damage to the corium of the sole and coronet. *The separation of the distal phalanx (coffin bone, P3) from the inner hoof wall is responsible for the severe clinical signs in laminitis*, rather than a primary inflammatory process. Laminitis occurs in all hoofed species, but particularly affects **horses** and **cattle**. *Laminitis is one of the most devastating of equine diseases, often leading to chronic debilitation or euthanasia.*

Traditionally, it has been thought that laminitis is caused by one common pathophysiologic pathway. Currently, it is thought that there are *3 phases* and *3 distinct forms* of laminitis. The 3 phases are *developmental, acute, and chronic*. Laminitis is a cutaneous manifestation of a systemic problem, and thus there are many risk factors and potential causes that can be categorized into 3 forms.

- The first form is *inflammatory laminitis*, which includes starch/grain overload; black walnut–induced laminitis, sepsis, and systemic inflammation caused by gastrointestinal disease, pneumonia, and septic metritis. Following release of inflammatory toxins, there is degradation of the lamellar basement membrane and dyshesion of the epithelial cells from the basement membrane. There is matrix metalloproteinase activation and leukocyte infiltration as well as profound hemodynamic changes.
- *Endocrinopathic laminitis/laminopathy* is the second form and includes horses with insulin resistance, obesity, pituitary pars intermedia dysfunction, and possibly corticosteroid-induced laminitis. This form is characterized by little if any inflammation and stretching of the secondary epidermal lamellae as opposed to early separation from the basement membrane. This will still lead to eventual basement membrane separation at the tips of the secondary epidermal lamellae.
- The third form, *contralateral limb laminitis/laminopathy*, is thought to be initiated by poor blood flow and ischemia and likely involves subsequent enzyme activation and degradation of the lamellar basement membrane in conjunction with the effects of tension and stretch on the lamellar tissues.

These different forms of laminitis are not entirely exclusive. Laminitis is a syndrome with many contributing factors, and although there may be different pathways, *the common lesion in all forms of the disease is dermal-epidermal separation at the interface of the lamellar basal epithelial cells and the underlying basement membrane and dermis.*

The earliest changes evident in the laminar tissue anatomy during acute laminitis are elongation and disorganization of basal and parabasal keratinocytes and attenuation of the tips of the secondary epidermal laminae. The basement membrane of the secondary laminae detaches first in the region of parabasal cell attachment and subsequently in the region of the basal cells, leaving aggregates of degenerating basement membrane components within the connective tissue space between the laminae. *Loss of the basement membrane leads to separation of the dermal and epidermal laminae of the hoof wall and is crucial in loss of structural integrity of the P3/hoof wall attachment.* Collapse of secondary laminae leads to loss of capillaries normally present within the connective tissue between the epidermal laminae. The loss of capillaries leads to increased resistance to blood flow, arteriovenous shunting, and eventual ischemic damage. This early stage is characterized clinically by a bounding digital pulse.

Acute laminitis is seen as sudden lameness and severe pain affecting most commonly the forefeet but may affect all feet, or just the hind feet. An increase in the hoof wall temperature and a bounding digital pulse indicate marked vascular engorgement in the hoof tissues. In horses, pain is often severe enough to provoke systemic disturbances. A section through an acutely affected hoof reveals little gross alteration beyond congestion of the laminar dermis and occasionally hemorrhage. There is no hoof deformity, although the skin above the coronary band may be swollen. Horses with diffuse swelling and depression along the coronary band are often found to have acute separation and displacement of P3 and are referred to as "sinkers," a manifestation of acute laminitis. Microscopic changes are as described above. In addition, the dermis may be congested, edematous, and have mild hemorrhage and mild infiltrates of mononuclear cells. In time, coagulative necrosis of the secondary laminae may be evident.

Chronic laminitis (founder) refers to the stage of laminitis associated with *radiographic or physical evidence of rotational or vertical displacement of the third phalanx relative to the hoof wall*. The rotation has been attributed to loss of the interlocking force normally supplied by the epidermal laminae. In chronic cases, the ventral deviation is caused also by irregular hyperplasia of epidermal laminae placing a wedge of epidermis between the phalanx and the immovable hoof wall. The weight of the animal, the leverage forces placed on the toe, and the pulling forces of the deep digital flexor tendon contribute mechanically to the rotation. *In severely affected animals, the third phalanx may penetrate the sole*, which becomes convex. A mid-sagittal section through the hoof wall at this point will show obvious separation of P3 from the dorsal hoof wall, sinking, and various degrees of rotation of P3. The corium at the coronary band and sole may be edematous or hemorrhagic. In long-standing cases, the space between the dorsal hoof wall and P3 is filled with firm white tissue (proliferative epidermis). The toe usually turns up, and the cranial aspect of the hoof becomes concave and wrinkled by encircling horizontal ridges.

Laminitis occurs sporadically in *dairy cows, heifers, fattening cattle, and young bulls*. In cattle, carbohydrate overload is also an important predisposing cause of laminitis. Others include metritis, mastitis, and ketosis. A heritable form has been reported in Jersey cattle in South Africa, the United States, and the United Kingdom. *Laminitis, not related to traumatic and metabolic episodes, occurs in all species but is important only in ungulates*. Erysipelas in lambs; the various causative types of footrot in pigs, sheep, and cattle; and bluetongue in sheep are examples of diseases in which degenerative and inflammatory changes occur in the laminae of the hoof.

The chief microscopic lesion in chronic equine laminitis is marked irregular hyperplasia of the epidermal laminae. The regenerating secondary laminae may not regain their orderly arrangement and instead form irregular and anastomosing epidermal cords. The epidermal laminae, both primary and secondary, become markedly hyperkeratotic. The reason for the hyperkeratosis is not known. Both physical and physiologic influences on keratogenesis are likely altered in chronic laminitis. There is also osteoclastic resorption, boney remodeling, and medullary fibromyxoid proliferation in P3. Similar epidermal lesions occur in chronic bovine laminitis, although parakeratotic hyperkeratosis develops in addition to the orthokeratotic hyperkeratosis. Alterations in the dermal vasculature are most prominent in cattle. Moderate to marked arteriolosclerosis occurs in chronic bovine laminitis, especially in the solar dermis. Other changes in laminitis in cattle include chronic dermal granulation tissue, organized and recanalized vascular thrombi, perineural fibrosis, and perivascular accumulations of macrophages, often containing hemosiderin.

Further reading

Eades SC. Overview of current laminitis research. Vet Clin Equine 2010;26:51-63.

Engiles JB. Pathology of the distal phalynx in equine laminitis: more than just skin deep. Vet Clin North Am Equine Pract 2010;26: 155-165.

Katz LM, Bailey SR. A review of recent advances and current hypotheses on the pathogenesis of acute laminitis. Equine Vet J 2012; 44:752-761.

NEOPLASTIC AND REACTIVE DISEASES OF THE SKIN

Epithelial tumors of the skin

Epithelial tumors of the skin are classified according to the predominant pattern of differentiation and the biological behavior. Most of the following tumors are named according to the World Health Organization International Histological Classification of Tumors of Domestic Animals, second series (1998), and Skin Disease of the Dog and Cat: Clinical and Histopathological Diagnosis, 2nd ed. (2005). The decision to classify a given tumor as one or another of the epidermal or adnexal tumors is often quite arbitrary. A neoplasm of the multipotential germinal cells of the epidermis may differentiate into a number of types of epithelial cells characteristic of mature cells of the various components of the epidermis or adnexa. Sometimes the differentiation results in a distinctive group of tumor cells, making precise identification unequivocal. At other times, the tumor cells may differentiate toward several skin structures forming squamous cells, sebaceous cells, or components of the hair follicle. The tumor can then be named according to the most aggressive or dominant cell type within the tumor. *Other than squamous cell carcinomas, the majority of tumors derived from the epidermis or adnexa exhibit benign behavior.*

- *Tumors of the epidermis* include squamous papilloma, squamous cell carcinoma, and basal cell tumors.
- *Adnexal tumors of follicular origin* include infundibular keratinizing acanthoma (intracutaneous cornifying epithelioma, keratoacanthoma), tricholemmoma, trichofolliculoma, trichoblastoma, trichoepithelioma, and pilomatricoma.
- *Adnexal tumors arising from glandular structures* include sebaceous gland tumors, epitrichial (apocrine) gland tumors, and atrichial (eccrine) gland tumors.

Also included in this section are varieties of tumor-like or keratin-filled cystic lesions that can be confused with true neoplasms. Mention will be made also of tumors that metastasize to the skin.

Cysts, hamartomas, and tumor-like lesions
Cysts

A cyst is a non-neoplastic, simple sac-like structure with an epithelial lining. Classification of cysts depends on identification of the lining epithelium or structure from which the cyst arose. *Follicular cysts* are classified according to the level of the hair follicle from which they develop. *Infundibular, isthmus, matrical, and hybrid* are named based on their epithelial lining and type of keratinization. Epithelial and follicular cysts occur in multiple species of animals, including cats, horses, cattle, sheep, alpacas, and camels. They are most common in dogs. In long-standing lesions, the epithelial wall may become very thin, and rupture may release entrapped keratin to stimulate pyogranulomatous dermal inflammation.

Infundibular cysts (epidermoid cyst, epidermal cyst, epidermal inclusion cyst) arise from the infundibular portion of the hair follicle, are lined by squamous epithelium with an obvious granular layer, and filled with laminated concentrically arranged keratin. They may be single or multiple, smooth, most often unilocular, spherical dermal papules or nodules seldom larger than 1 cm in diameter. The keratin may appear as loose flakes. Infundibular cysts may arise from dilation of the infundibulum of occluded hair follicles, and indeed, occasionally one can detect superficial dermal scarring that may support this hypothesis. As well, such cysts may contain fragments of mature hair shafts. One report in the dog documents multiple squamous cell carcinomas arising from multiple infundibular cysts. Some cysts are thought to arise from traumatic, developmental, or surgical implantation of epidermal fragments into dermis or subcutis. Penetrating grass seeds cause implantation of epidermal fragments in sheep. One dog was reported to have >100 infundibular cysts in the perianal area, possibly resulting from chronic external trauma to the perianal area as a response to anal sacculitis. Occasionally, an infundibular cyst can be found within the bone of the third phalanx of the dog *(subungual epidermal inclusion cyst)*.

Isthmus cyst (trichilemmal cyst) is lined by keratinizing epithelium that lacks a granular layer. The inner layers of the epidermis lining the cyst have large amounts of pale eosinophilic cytoplasm and inconspicuous intercellular bridges resembling the outer root sheath of the middle segment of an anagen follicle and the mid to lower portion of a catagen follicle. There is trichilemmal cornification and the cyst contents are paler and more homogeneous than in the infundibular cyst.

Matrical cyst (pilar cyst) is derived from the inferior segment of the anagen hair follicles and is lined by small basaloid epithelial cells with scant cytoplasm and hyperchromatic nuclei. The epithelium keratinizes abruptly forming "ghost" cells.

Hybrid cyst (trichoepitheliomatous cyst, panfollicular cyst) is lined by 2 or all 3 types of follicular epithelium. The presence of 2 or 3 types of keratin may help support this diagnosis (Fig. 6-134).

Dilated pore of Winer is a flask-shaped epidermal cyst on the head or neck of middle-aged or old cats and rarely dogs and horses. It is connected to the skin surface by a pore. *It is a variant of the infundibular cyst.* The stratified keratinizing epithelium of the cyst wall near its base is hyperplastic with very regular rete ridges in parallel columns (Fig. 6-135). Keratin may protrude through the pore, forming a cutaneous horn.

Keratoma (horn cyst, horn tumor, keratin cyst) is a keratin-filled cyst that develops between the hoof wall and the distal phalanx. They are thought to originate from the epidermal horn-producing cells of either the coronary or solar corium. They are rare but do occur in both simple- and cloven-hoofed animals. Most are reported in **horses.** The cysts are usually solitary, 1-5 cm in diameter, and often exert pressure on P3, leaving an area of bone resorption that can be seen radiographically. There are rare reports of horses with multiple keratomas. Keratomas are painful, causing lameness and bulging of the affected area of the hoof wall. Histologically, the cyst is lined by squamous epithelium of the primary epidermal lamellae and filled with laminated keratin that in some cases may mineralize. Trauma to the hoof wall and

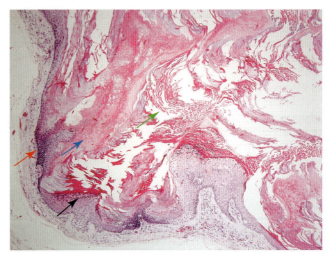

Figure 6-134 Hybrid follicular cyst in a dog. The cyst wall is lined by stratified squamous epithelium with a prominent granular cell layer (black arrow) and lamellar flaky keratin (green arrow) resembling an infundibular cyst. The cyst wall is also lined by small basaloid epithelium (red arrow) resembling a matrical cyst with abrupt keratinization into ghost cells (blue arrow).

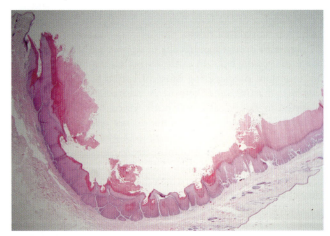

Figure 6-135 Dilated pore of Winer in a cat. Cystically dilated follicular infundibulum communicates with the skin surface, produces trichilemmal cornification and is lined by thickened squamous epithelium with psoriasiform hyperplasia.

infection have been suggested, although not proven, causes of keratomas.

Dermoid cysts (dermoid sinus) are congenital lesions found in young animals, often along the dorsal midline. They arise by developmental failure of epidermal closure along embryonic fissures that maroons an island of multipotential ectoderm within the dermis or subcutis. Some dermoid cysts may extend deep into the tissue and be connected to the dura mater of the spinal cord. Some, such as those occurring in Rhodesian Ridgeback **dogs,** actually retain a sinus pore to the skin surface (see Congenital and hereditary diseases of skin). Dermoid cysts are common in some families of Boxer dogs, and affected animals have multiple cysts along the midline of the skin over the forehead. In the **horse,** dermoid cysts occur most often on the midline between the withers and the rump. Dermoid cysts contain keratin and hair fragments and sometimes sebaceous secretions. The dermis abutting the cyst wall has numerous hair follicles, sebaceous glands, and occasionally epitrichial sweat glands. Hair follicles are attached to and radiate from the cyst wall. Specimens with only hair follicle differentiation may be confused with unilocular trichoepitheliomas, but the dermoid cyst has gradual keratinization rather than abrupt trichilemmal cornification.

Epitrichial (apocrine) cysts may be single or multiple and are filled with clear secretions and lined by a single layer of cuboidal to columnar epithelial cells. Multiple cysts at multiple sites are referred to as epitrichial (apocrine) cystomatosis. This is an uncommon lesion that occurs in middle-aged to older dogs for unknown reasons.

Sebaceous duct cysts are extremely rare. They are usually solitary and may occur in Meibomian glands. They are lined by a thin layer of stratified squamous epithelium that has a sparse granular cell layer. Atrophic sebaceous gland lobules surround the cyst.

Hamartomas

Hamartomas are benign tumor-like nodules composed of *disorganized and excessive amounts, or enlarged components, of mature tissue elements indigenous to the site in which they arise*. **Nevus** refers to any congenital malformation of the skin. *Thus the term hamartoma is more inclusive than nevus* and is the preferred nomenclature for most lesions that are regarded as malformations, either congenital or acquired.

- **Epidermal hamartomas** (pigmented epidermal nevus, linear epidermal hamartoma, verrucous epidermal nevus) grossly appear as focal hyperkeratotic plaques or papules forming one or more linear arrays on the trunk or legs. Some lesions are hyperpigmented. Histologically, there is abrupt irregular epidermal papillary hyperplasia with marked laminated hyperkeratosis. The stratum granulosum may have enlarged keratohyaline granules. In the dog, an association with papilloma virus infection has been documented in some cases. Linear epidermal hamartomas are thought to be a genetically inherited lesion in Belgian horses. Lesions develop at <1 year of age and are seen as bilateral linear vertically oriented bands of hyperkeratosis and alopecia on the caudal aspect of the rear cannon bones.
- **Follicular hamartomas** have been reported in the dog and consist of one or more clusters of very large anagen hair follicles that extend more deeply than adjacent normal follicles. Associated glands surround the follicles and sebaceous glands may be enlarged. There is normal orientation of follicles and adnexal glands. Clinically, there are single to multiple grouped plaques or small nodules ranging from 0.3 to several centimeters in diameter, and the skin is irregularly thickened. In some cases, locally extensive areas are affected.
- **Fibroadnexal hamartoma** (adnexal nevus, focal adnexal dysplasia, folliculosebaceous hamartoma) is a common lesion in dogs and consists of aggregates of markedly distorted and variably inflamed folliculosebaceous units surrounded by dense collagen and lacking a connection to the skin surface. Hair bulbs are not present. These lesions are typically solitary, raised, well circumscribed, and 1-4 cm in diameter. They are most common on the distal limbs, pressure points, and interdigital areas. Some pathologists believe this type of lesion is a result of trauma and is not a true hamartoma.
- **Sebaceous hamartoma** is an uncommon variant of fibroadnexal hamartoma and thus is clinically similar. Histologically, it is composed predominantly of large sebaceous lobules with random distribution. Hair follicles are small and malformed.
- **Sweat gland hamartomas** are rare in domestic animals but have been described in cats and dogs. Histologically, there are proliferating sweat glands in the superficial dermis. The ductal and secretory epithelia are cytokeratin 8 positive.
- **Trichofolliculoma** is also thought to be a hamartoma. It is uncommon in dogs and rare in cats. It is a well-circumscribed, nonencapsulated dermal mass composed of one or more large dilated primary follicles that open to the surface, forming a pore seen clinically. Secondary follicles radiate out from the primary follicles, and associated adnexal glands are present. Tumors with large sebaceous glands are called **sebaceous trichofolliculomas.**

Tumor-like lesions

Idiopathic squamous papillomas *(warts) are 1-5 mm papillary masses composed of hyperplastic stratified squamous epithelium supported by dermal projections*. The maturation of the epidermis is orderly and does not show viral-induced cytopathic effects as seen in viral papillomas. These lesions are most often seen on the eyelids, face, conjunctiva, or pawpads of older dogs and occasionally cats, and they may be traumatic in origin. One report describes 11 dogs with idiopathic squamous papillomas of the penile mucosa. Congenital papillomas, which may actually represent epidermal hamartomas, have been reported in newborn foals and fetuses. Two cases of nonviral congenital fibropapilloma have been reported in piglets.

Cutaneous horns *are rare exophytic cylindrical formations of compact keratin* a few millimeters in diameter and 1-2 cm in length, formed by an underlying markedly hyperplastic epithelium. Orthokeratotic hyperkeratosis predominates. Cutaneous horns may arise from viral papillomas, actinic keratosis, squamous cell carcinoma (bowenoid in situ or invasive), infundibular keratinizing acanthomas, or dilated pores of Winer. Cutaneous horns of the pawpad of cats have been associated with feline leukemia virus infection.

Warty dyskeratoma is a rare a cystic cup-shaped dermal mass lined by stratified squamous epithelium resembling the follicular infundibulum. The base of the structure has many filiform projections. There is extensive acantholysis, individual dyskeratosis, and apoptosis of keratinocytes. The lumen is filled with orthokeratotic and parakeratotic debris.

Further reading

Callan MB, et al. Multiple papillomavirus-associated epidermal hamartomas and squamous cell carcinomas in situ in a dog following chronic treatment with prednisone and cyclosporine. Vet Dermatol 2005;16:338-345.

Nishiyama S, et al. Congenital cutaneous fibropapillomatosis with no evidence of papillomavirus infection in a piglet. J Vet Med Sci 2011;73:283-285.

Park J, et al. Multiple perianal infundibular follicular cysts in a dog. Vet Dermatol 2010;21:303-306.

Redding WR, O'Grady SE. Nonseptic diseases associated with the hoof complex: keratoma, white line disease, canker and neoplasia. Vet Clin North Am Equine Pract 2012;28:407-421.

Scott DW, Miller WH. Neoplasms, cysts, hamartomas, and keratoses. In: Scott DW, Miller WH, editors. Equine Dermatology. 2nd ed. St Louis: Elsevier Saunders; 2011. p. 468-516.

Tumors of the epidermis
Papillomas and papillomavirus-induced lesions

Cutaneous papillomas are benign proliferative epithelial neoplasms that have a complex etiology and pathogenesis. The differences in site preference, clinical course, and histology of such lesions have been made more understandable by the discovery that *most papillomas are caused by infection with a host- and often site-specific papillomavirus* of the family *Papillomaviridae*. Not all papillomas are caused by or contain viruses. The nonviral lesion is considered to be an idiopathic squamous papilloma and is described under Tumor-like lesions.

Many papillomaviruses (PVs) have been identified using in situ hybridization, PCR, and DNA sequencing, and they exist in most domestic and nondomestic mammals. *Papillomaviruses are double-stranded DNA viruses that reproduce in keratinocyte nuclei*. They gain access through defects in the epithelium and infect cells of the stratum basale. However, for viral replication to occur, infected cells must become terminally differentiated, and therefore PVs attempt to increase both proliferation of basal cells and terminal keratinocyte differentiation. PV types are grouped into genera. Most of the >100 human PVs (HPVs) are classified as alpha or beta PVs. *Alpha-PV genus* includes the oncogenic mucosal types. The *beta-PV genus* contains cutaneous PVs that are usually associated with immunosuppression. The *delta-PV type* is important in nonhuman mammals because it is associated with benign fibropapillomas in both ungulates and cats. Although most *papillomaviruses* are species specific, delta-PVs have the unique ability to infect multiple species.

Immunocompromised animals have increased susceptibility to papillomavirus infection. Papillomaviruses induce and/or are associated with several types of cutaneous lesions, including **squamous papilloma, inverted papilloma, feline viral plaques, canine pigmented viral plaques, bowenoid in situ carcinoma (BISC), invasive squamous cell carcinoma (ISCC),** and **fibropapillomas, including equine and feline sarcoids.**

Viral papillomas may regress as a result of cell-mediated immune attack, may persist, or may progress to squamous cell carcinomas. Although some viral and host factors are known to influence the behavior of viral-induced papillomas and fibropapillomas, many other factors are not yet defined.

The typical papilloma is a 1-2 cm wart-like, filiform, exophytic, and hyperkeratotic mass composed of hyperplastic epidermis supported by thin, inconspicuous dermal stalks with dilated capillaries (Fig. 6-136A). Lesions can be anatomically extensive and multiple. The stratum corneum exhibits variable degrees of orthokeratotic to parakeratotic hyperkeratosis. Most of the hyperplasia is due to marked expansion of stratum spinosum cells, which have pale basophilic cytoplasm. Cells of the spinous and/or granular layer have swollen eosinophilic to lightly basophilic cytoplasm (ballooning degeneration) and enlarged, condensed, or multiple nuclei (koilocytes) (Fig. 6-136B). Degenerating keratinocytes may have condensed *eosinophilic cytoplasmic inclusions that represent aggregates of keratin*, a result of the viral cytopathic effect. These inclusions should not be confused with the cytoplasmic inclusions associated with poxvirus infections. The stratum granulosum has large, variably sized and shaped basophilic keratohyaline granules. Cells of the stratum spinosum and granulosum may have vesicular nuclei with intranuclear pale basophilic viral inclusions that contain virus particles visible with electron

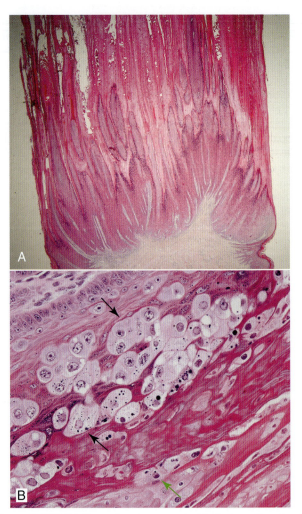

Figure 6-136 Papillomavirus in a cow. **A.** Marked papillated epidermal hyperplasia, hypergranulosis, and hyperkeratosis. **B.** Multiple koilocytes (black arrows) in the stratum granulosum and a few intranuclear inclusion bodies in the stratum corneum (green arrow).

microscopy and viral antigen detectable by immunohistochemistry, but these may not be numerous.

Fibropapillomas *appear as nodules or plaques covered by a variably hyperplastic and hyperkeratotic epidermis*. Classic examples of fibropapillomas are bovine fibropapilloma, equine sarcoid, and feline sarcoid *(feline fibropapilloma)*. Microscopic lesions typical of fibropapillomas include the features of acanthosis, hyperkeratosis, and downgrowth of rete ridges, but *dermal proliferation predominates* (Fig. 6-137A). The proliferating cell is a large, plump fibroblast. The cells are arranged in haphazard whorls and fascicles rather than in perpendicular sheets, as in granulation tissue. In some, the epidermal proliferation is minimal and is seen only as slight acanthosis and accentuation of rete pegs, whereas, in others, the hyperplasia resembles full-fledged papillomas.

Cattle. Thirteen bovine papillomaviruses (BPVs) have been described (BPV 1-13) (Table 6-1). Bovine papillomatosis may be a herd problem in that the virus is easily transmitted by animal-to-animal contact and by fomites. Depending on the anatomic site and papillomavirus type, both morphologic and biological features of lesions may differ. BPV-1 causes typical fibropapillomas on the teats and penis. BPV-2 causes

Table • 6-1

Bovine papillomaviruses

Virus	PV genus	Lesion
BPV-1	Delta	Cutaneous, teat, rumen, and genital fibropapilloma; rumen papilloma; urinary bladder neoplasia; equine sarcoid
BPV-2	Delta	Cutaneous, teat, rumen, and genital fibropapilloma; rumen papilloma; urinary bladder neoplasia; equine sarcoid
BPV-3	Xi	Cutaneous papilloma
BPV-4	Xi	Oral/esophageal/rumen papilloma, urinary bladder neoplasia
BPV-5	Epsilon	Teat and rumen fibropapilloma, cutaneous and rumen papilloma
BPV-6	Xi	Teat papilloma
BPV-7	Dyoxi	Teat papilloma, healthy skin
BPV-8	Epsilon	Cutaneous papilloma, fibropapilloma
BPV-9	Xi	Teat papilloma
BPV-10	Xi	Teat papilloma, tongue papilloma
BPV-11	Xi	Cutaneous papilloma
BPV-12	Xi	Tongue papilloma
BPV-13	Delta	Ear papilloma, equine sarcoid

BPV, bovine papillomavirus.

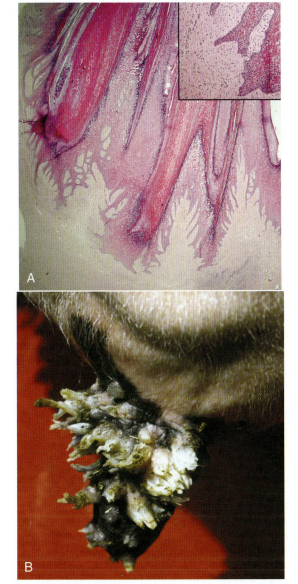

Figure 6-137 Fibropapilloma in a cow. A. Marked papillated epidermal hyperplasia, koilocytes with rete pegs, and dermal fibroblast proliferation (see inset). **B.** "Teat fronds" caused by infection with bovine papilloma virus-1 (BPV-1), BPV-2, and BPV-5. (Courtesy J.M. Gourreau.)

typical fibropapillomas on the head, neck, dewlap, shoulder, and occasionally the legs and teats. Both of these viruses tend to produce multiple lesions in animals <2 years of age, and the lesions often spontaneously regress within 1 year. BPV-3 causes "atypical warts" in cattle of all ages. The lesions are low, flat, circular, and nonpedunculated and have delicate to thick frond-like projections on their surfaces. These rarely spontaneously regress and can occur anywhere on the body, including the teats. "Teat frond" warts caused by BPV-5 (Fig. 6-137B) are small, white, elongated hyperkeratotic, and do not spontaneous regress. BPV-6 causes nonpedunculated, conical to branch-like, hyperkeratotic, frond-like papillomas on the teats in cattle of all ages. These lesions sometimes break off, leaving ulcers that commonly become secondarily infected with bacteria.

Some BPVs are associated with neoplastic transformation in the skin, alimentary tract, and urinary bladder. An angiokeratomatous papilloma has been described in association with PV in an 8-month-old Simmental calf. Many factors are involved, including viral proteins that promote cell dysregulation and immune evasion. BPVs are composed of early (E) and late (L) genes. E5, E6, and E7 are the transforming proteins. E5 is the major BPV transforming oncoprotein. It is believed to be critical in driving cell transformation, especially by activating platelet-derived growth factor receptor β (PDGFRβ). The binding of BPV-1 E5 to PDGFRβ results in activation of the phosphatidylinositol-3-kinase (PI3K)-AKT-cyclin D pathway, leading to cell cycle deregulation. BPV-1 can also down-regulate the expression of toll-like receptor 4 (TLR-4) through the E2 and E7 oncoproteins. TLR-4 down-regulation is expected to contribute to immune evasion and viral persistence. In conjunction with several BPVs (BPV-1, BPV-2, and BPV-4), the ingestion of bracken fern *(Pteridium aquilinum)* has been associated with various epithelial and mesenchymal urinary bladder neoplasms. This plant is known to promote genomic instability, resistance to apoptosis, and cell cycle deregulation by inactivating p53 and activating ras and preventing the immune system from clearing viral papillomas.

Congenital papillomatosis was described in a Holstein heifer, and although BPV-3 was suspected, a viral etiology was not proved, and thus these lesions may be hamartomas.

Horses. Currently, there are 3 distinct clinical syndromes in the horse caused by *Equus caballus papillomaviruses* (EcPV 1-7) (Table 6-2). **Classic equine viral papillomatosis** caused by *Equus caballus papillomavirus-1* (EcPV-1) is a contagious disease and most commonly causes exophytic viral papillomas on the muzzle and lips of horses <3 years of age (Fig. 6-138).

Table • 6-2

Equine papillomaviruses

Virus	PV genus	Lesion
EcPV1	Zeta	Equine viral papillomatosis
EcPV2	Dyoiota	Genital papilloma, in situ and invasive SCC
EcPV3	Dyorho	Ear papilloma
EcPV4	Dyoiota	Ear papilloma, vulvar and inguinal plaques
EcPV5	Dyoiota	Ear papilloma
EcPV6	Dyorho	Ear papilloma
EcPV7	Dyorho	Undiagnosed penile mass

EcPV, Equus cabalus papillomavirus; *SCC*, squamous cell carcinoma.

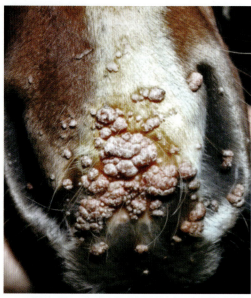

Figure 6-138 **Viral papillomatosis** on the muzzle of a young horse. (Courtesy D.W. Scott.)

Lesions begin as 1-mm diameter raised, round, white to gray smooth papules and develop into broad-based to pedunculated gray to white plaques and nodules with a hyperkeratotic frond-like surface. Spontaneous remission occurs in ~2-3 months. **Equine genital papillomas** caused by EcPV-2 usually occur on older horses and are not known to spontaneously resolve. This virus has been associated with malignant transformation of penile and vulvar lesions to squamous cell carcinoma (SCC) in situ and invasive squamous cell carcinoma (ISCC). **Equine ear papillomas** (aural plaques) occur in horses of all ages, rarely spontaneously resolve, and are associated with EcPV 3-6. Early lesions are grossly similar to viral papillomatosis, with the exception of generally being confined to the pinnae. Fully developed lesions are usually bilaterally symmetrical and appear as 1-3 cm white hyperkeratotic plaques. Blackfly bites may be important in the transmission. Aural plaques are similar histologically to exophytic papillomas; however, the epidermis is less papillated, and hypomelanosis may be striking. EcPV-4 has also been isolated from vulvar and inguinal plaques, and EcPV-7 was isolated from an undiagnosed penile mass in a horse. *Congenital papillomas* have been reported in foals (see the section Hamartomas).

The most important papillomavirus-induced lesion in the horse is the **sarcoid**, known to be associated with BPV-1, BPV-2, and most recently BPV-13. *Sarcoids are locally aggressive, nonmetastatic fibroblastic skin tumors of horses, mules, donkeys, and zebras.* They are the *most common skin tumor of horses*, accounting for up to 90% of tumors. A combination of factors appears to be involved in development of the tumors, including *exposure to a viral agent, cutaneous trauma, and a genetic predilection*. Viral etiology has been deduced based on reports of epizootics of cases, transmission studies, detection of viral particles in cultured tumor cells, and demonstration of DNA sequences very similar or identical to that of BPV-1 or BPV-2 genome in tumor cells of horses and donkeys. BPV DNA has been demonstrated in normal skin of healthy horses and horses with inflammatory conditions, suggesting that there are more factors involved in sarcoid development than simply viral infection. Sarcoids frequently develop in areas subjected to trauma or at sites of wounds 6-8 months after wound healing. In horses, there is a breed predilection for Appaloosas, Quarter Horses, Arabians, and Thoroughbreds and a lower incidence in Standardbreds and Lipizzaners. In Thoroughbreds and Warmbloods, the increased risk has been associated with major histocompatibility complex (MHC)-1 A3 and W13 alleles, whereas, in Standardbreds and Lipizzaners, a decreased risk is associated with decreased W13 allele and a lack of W13, respectively.

Sarcoids develop anywhere but are most common on the *head, legs, and ventral trunk*. They may be single or multiple. Young horses 1-7 years of age are at increased risk, with rare reports in older horses. The tumors are classified according to their gross appearance as *occult, verrucous, nodular, fibroblastic, mixed*, and *malignant (malevolent)*. Many horses have multiple tumors, and all types of sarcoids can be present in the same horse. **Occult sarcoids** are focal areas with alopecia, scaling, hyperkeratosis, and hyperpigmentation (Fig. 6-139A). Common locations are neck, face, sheath, medial thigh, and shoulder. The **verrucous sarcoid** is a small wart-like growth, usually measuring <6 cm in diameter, with a dry, rough surface and variable alopecia (Fig. 6-139B). This type is usually found in the head, neck, axilla, and groin. **Nodular sarcoids** are spherical dermal to subcutaneous masses. The overlying skin may be normal but can become alopecic and ulcerated. This type is common on the eyelid, groin, and prepuce. The **fibroblastic sarcoid** is more variable in appearance and may range from a well-circumscribed firm nodule with intact surface to large masses, >25 cm in diameter, with an ulcerated surface prone to hemorrhage and resembling exuberant granulation tissue. Common locations are axilla, groin, legs, and periocular. **Malignant/malevolent sarcoids** are aggressive and locally invasive. These tumors extend widely into the adjacent skin and subcutis and infiltrate lymphatic vessels. The occult and verrucous and, to a lesser extent, the nodular sarcoid can remain static for years if not traumatized. Any type of sarcoid lesion can develop into an aggressive fibroblastic or malignant/malevolent tumor if traumatized. *Spontaneous remission is rare*. The tumors are characterized by a high rate of recurrence, up to 50%, following surgical excision.

Histopathology is necessary for definitive diagnosis of a sarcoid. Sarcoids are typically *biphasic tumors composed of both epidermal and dermal components.* The epidermal component

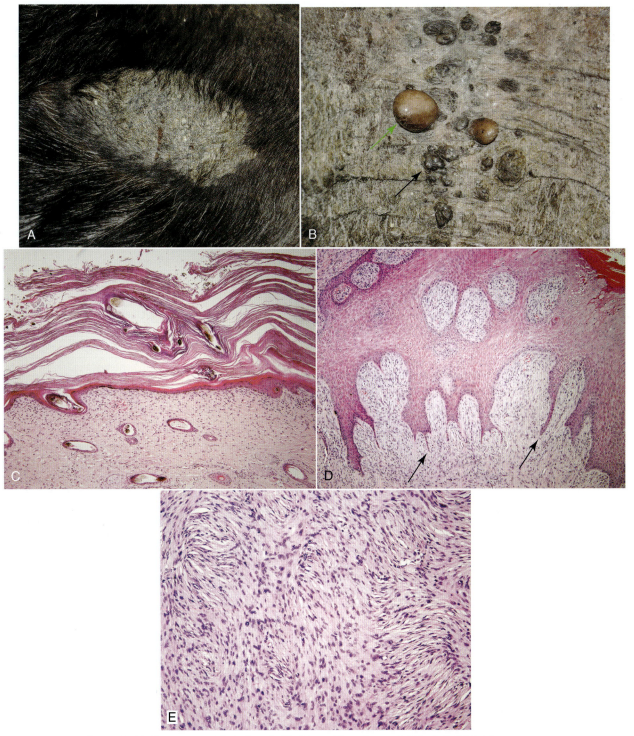

Figure 6-139 Equine sarcoid. **A.** Occult (flat) sarcoid on the medial thigh. **B.** Multiple **verrucous** (black arrow) and **nodular** (green arrow) **sarcoids** on the groin of the same horse. (Courtesy D.W. Scott.) **C.** Note the subtle fibroblast proliferation in the superficial dermis, marked orthokeratotic hyperkeratosis, and lack of an epidermal response in this early **occult sarcoid**. **D.** Prominent fibroblast proliferation and multiple thin rete pegs (arrows). **E.** The neoplastic fibroblasts of this **nodular sarcoid** are arranged in whorls and interlacing bundles resembling a peripheral nerve sheath tumor.

may be minimal or absent in some tumors, especially nodular and early occult sarcoids (Fig. 6-139C). When the epidermis is intact, hyperkeratosis and irregular epidermal hyperplasia with thin rete pegs extending deep into the dermis are common features (Fig. 6-139D). The dermal component consists of fibroblasts and collagen in various proportions. The fibroblasts have plump nuclei, and nucleoli may be prominent. The mitotic index is usually low. *Fibroblasts at the dermal-epidermal junction are frequently oriented perpendicular to the basement membrane in a "picket fence" pattern, which is a distinctive histologic feature seen in most sarcoids.* The cells are arranged in whorls, interlacing bundles, or haphazard arrays of variable density (Fig. 6-139E). Tumor margins are typically indistinct, and adequacy of excision is frequently difficult to determine. When the tumor is ulcerated, it may not be possible to differentiate a sarcoid from granulation tissue, fibroma, well-differentiated fibrosarcoma, and peripheral nerve sheath tumor. Immunohistochemical staining for S-100 protein may be useful in confirming a peripheral nerve sheath tumor. Additional biopsies to include intact epidermis may be required to make a diagnosis. BPV infection of equine fibroblasts appears to be mainly nonproductive with respect to producing complete viruses, and therefore there is no histologic or immunohistochemical evidence of PV infection.

Sheep and goats. Papillomas are uncommon in sheep and goats. Three papillomaviruses have been described in sheep. *Ovis aries papillomavirus 1 and 2 (OaPV-1, OaPV-2) are delta-PVs and are associated with fibropapillomas.* OaPV-3 (dyolambda-PV) has been associated with SCC. SCC is the most common skin neoplasm of sheep. Filiform squamous papillomas occur in young sheep, especially on the fetlock area of the lower legs. Lesions are 1-3 cm in diameter, raised, and frond-like. Similar lesions may occur on the scrotum of rams. Fibropapillomas occur on the face, pinnae, legs, and teats of adult sheep. Lesions are 0.5-1 cm, raised, hyperkeratotic, and pedunculated. Two clinical entities involving cutaneous papillomas have been described in goats. In one, papillomas occur on the face, pinnae, neck, shoulder, and forelegs, and spontaneous regression occurs in 1-12 months. In the second form, papillomas occur on the udder and teats of white goats especially; cutaneous horns may develop. There is no spontaneous regression, and malignant transformation to SCC can occur. In both forms, lesions are multiple, hyperkeratotic, and verrucous. PV DNA sequenes have only been detected in some goats with mammary lesions. *Capra hircus papillomavirus 1*, a phi-PV, has been isolated from healthy goat skin.

Dogs. Cutaneous papillomas are common in the dog, and at least 5 different clinical syndromes are recognized. Fifteen *Canis familiaris papillomaviruses* (CfPVs) or *Canine papillomaviruses* (CPVs) have been described (Table 6-3). Canine oral papillomatosis has been associated with CPV-1 (*Canine oral papillomavirus*, COPV) and CPV-13. This is usually a self-limiting disease confined to the mucosa of the oral cavity or lips of young dogs (Fig. 6-140). It occasionally affects the conjunctiva and external nares. Lesions are commonly multiple and are characterized by white to gray pedunculated or cauliflower-like hyperkeratotic masses up to 3 cm in diameter. Oral papillomatosis is occasionally associated with immunosuppression. It has been described in Beagles with IgA deficiency, in dogs undergoing immunosuppressive therapy with cyclosporine, and in a Chinese Shar-Pei in association with glucocorticoid therapy.

Cutaneous (exophytic) papillomas occur in dogs of any age, but they are usually young or elderly. They are associated with CPV-1, CPV-2, and CPV-7. They may be single to multiple, occurring mainly on the head, eyelids, and paws. These lesions are usually smaller than 0.5 cm, pedunculated to cauliflower-like, soft to firm, well circumscribed, alopecic, and smooth to hyperkeratotic. These lesions usually spontaneously regress.

Cutaneous inverted papillomas are usually seen in young adult dogs <3 years of age and have been associated with CPV-1, CPV-2, and CPV-6. Lesions are single to multiple, 1-2 cm in diameter, raised, firm, and contain a central pore

Table • 6-3

Canine papillomaviruses

Virus	PV genus	Lesion
CPV-1	Lambda	Oral/cutaneous papilloma, inverted papilloma, invasive SCC
CPV-2	Tau	Cutaneous papilloma, inverted papilloma, invasive SCC
CPV-3	Chi	Pigmented plaque, in situ SCC, invasive SCC
CPV-4	Chi	Pigmented plaque
CPV-5	Chi	Pigmented plaque
CPV-6	Lambda	Cutaneous inverted papilloma
CPV-7	Tau	Cutaneous papilloma, in situ SCC
CPV-8	Chi	Pigmented plaque
CPV-9	Chi	Pigmented plaque
CPV-10	Chi	Pigmented plaque
CPV-11	Chi	Pigmented plaque
CPV-12	Chi	NR
CPV-13	Tau	Oral papilloma
CPV-14	Chi	Pigmented plaque
CPV-15	Chi	NR

CPV, canine papilloma virus; *NR*, not reported; *SCC*, squamous cell carcinoma.

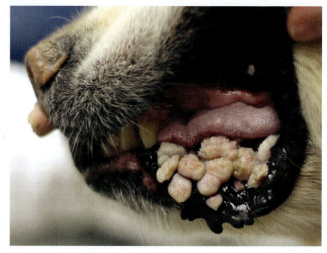

Figure 6-140 Canine oral papillomatosis. Multiple white to gray pedunculated frond-like masses in the mouth and nasal philtrum of a dog.

filled with keratin (Fig. 6-141A). They occur most commonly on the ventral abdomen and groin, can occur on limbs and digits and most do not regress spontaneously. *Histologically, these lesions are cup shaped with a central core of keratin that may be parakeratotic* (Fig. 6-141B). The cup is lined by hyperplastic squamous epithelium with centripetal papillary projections. The cells may exhibit koilocytes or blue-gray cytoplasm. Large keratohyaline granules and intranuclear inclusions may be present. Malignant transformation has been associated with CPV-2 infection in immunosuppressed dogs.

Canine pigmented plaques may be heritable because they are most commonly reported in certain breeds: Miniature

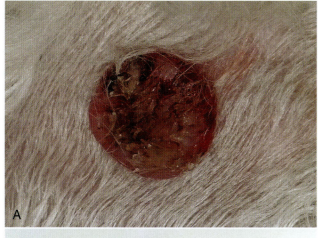
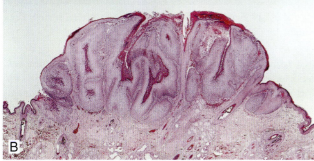

Figure 6-141 **Inverted papilloma** in a dog. **A.** Cup-shaped inverted papilloma. (Courtesy A. Alcaraz, M. Heil.) **B.** Papillated epidermal hyperplasia with hypergranulosis and koilocytes projects from a cup-shaped wall, and the center is filled with keratin. (Courtesy J. Tran.)

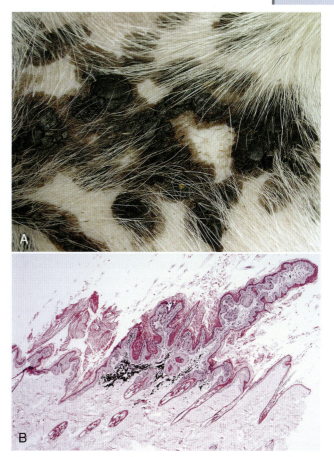

Figure 6-142 **Pigmented viral plaques** in a pug. **A.** Melanotic macules, papules, and plaques on the ventral abdomen. (Courtesy M.S. Canfield.) **B.** Well-demarcated epidermal hyperplasia, hyperpigmentation, hyperkeratosis, scalloped configuration, and pigmentary incontinence.

Schnauzers and Pugs. Affected dogs are usually young adults. Plaques in other breeds tend to be restricted to immunocompromised dogs. Lesions are most common on the ventral abdomen and groin and are characterized by melanotic macules, papules, and plaques that often have a scaly surface (Fig. 6-142A). *Histologically, there is well-demarcated, moderate epidermal hyperplasia with a scalloped configuration, hyperpigmentation of the lower layers of the epidermis, and clumped keratohyaline granules in the stratum spinosum* (Fig. 6-142B). Koilocytes and viral inclusions are rare to absent. The potential for transformation to bowenoid in situ carcinoma (BISC), and ISCC has been reported in lesions infected with CPV-3.

Canine pigmented papules have been rarely associated with long-term glucocorticoid therapy. Lesions are single to multiple, black papules up to 2 mm in diameter. *Histologically, there are well-demarcated, cup-shaped foci of epidermal hyperplasia with marked parakeratotic hyperkeratosis.* These lesions may resolve after cessation of glucocorticoid therapy.

Like other PVs, some CPVs have been associated with ISCC and some with BISC. Anecdotally, the author has seen 2 young dogs with generalized demodecosis associated with CPV. One dog had multiple oral and cutaneous papillomas, oral SCC associated with CPV-1, and was thought to have T-cell dysfunction. The other dog had numerous viral plaques that were positive by IHC for canine papillomavirus.

Cats. Papillomavirus infection has been associated with *cutaneous papillomas, feline viral plaques, feline sarcoid (feline fibropapilloma), BISC, and ISCC* in cats. PV-induced exophytic cutaneous papillomas are rare in domestic cats, with only 2 cases reported. One developed on the eyelid of a previous surgical site, and the other developed on the nasal planum of an older cat with actinic keratosis. Interestingly, human papillomavirus 9 was isolated from the latter. Feline viral plaques are uncommon and occur as multiple scaly, flat, variably pigmented lesions that can develop anywhere on the body. *Felis catus papillomavirus 1* (FcaPV-1), also called *Felis domesticus* PV-1 (FdPV-1), a lambda-PV, and FcaPV-2, a dyotheta-PV, have been isolated from these lesions; however, FcaPV-2 has also been isolated from many cats with no skin lesions. Viral plaques may spontaneously resolve; however, some have been known to progress to BISC. In fact, FcaPV-2 DNA has been detected in many feline BISC lesions and up to 50% of ISCC lesions and is thought to play a role in the pathogenesis of these lesions. Feline viral plaques have been associated with immunosuppression in some cats but have also been noted in healthy cats. *Histologically, they are well-demarcated foci of epidermal hyperplasia and hyperkeratosis.* The granular layer is thickened and irregular, and keratohyaline granules are frequently enlarged. Small numbers of koilocytes may be present in the stratum granulosum.

Feline BISC (a **multicentric squamous cell carcinoma in situ**) usually appears as multiple crusting, hyperpigmented, roughly circular plaques in middle-aged to older cats. Solitary lesions may occur. The face, neck, and limbs may be predisposed. It is uncommon to rare. Lesions may be more severe

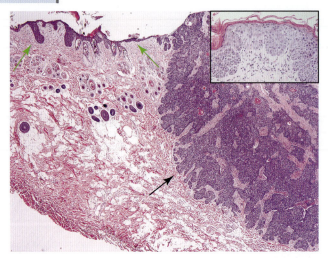

Figure 6-143 Feline bowenoid in situ carcinoma and invasive squamous cell carcinoma. In situ carcinoma is characterized by abrupt hyperplasia and dysplasia of the epidermis and outer root sheath (green arrows; also see inset). Squamous cell carcinoma is characterized by invasive anastomosing islands and trabeculae of neoplastic epithelial cells (black arrow) with multiple keratin pearls.

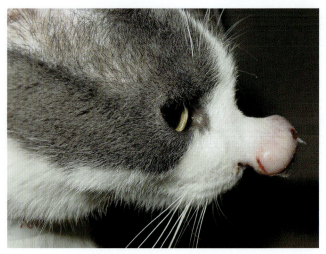

Figure 6-144 Feline sarcoid on the nose of a cat. (Courtesy C.G. Knight.)

in hairless breeds. FcaPV-2 and FcaPV-3 (tau-PV) have been detected from many of these lesions. Rarely, intrafollicular *Demodex cati* can be found in these lesions, sometimes in association with feline immunodeficiency virus infection. *Microscopically, there is abrupt hyperplasia and dysplasia of the epidermis and follicular outer root sheath that remain confined to the basement membrane* (Fig. 6-143). The basal and spinous layers are most affected. Mitotic activity is present in all layers of the epidermis, and keratin pearl formation may be present. Tumor cells often have large hyperchromatic nuclei and may have vacuolated cytoplasm, cytoplasmic pallor, or occasionally are multinucleated. Groups of dysplastic cells have elongated nuclei that tend to orient in one direction ("wind-blown") appearance. The tumors are often pigmented and may have papillomatous epidermal projections with marked hyperkeratosis, occasionally forming a cutaneous horn. These lesions may progress to ISCC. Distant metastasis is very rare but was reported in a 7-year-old Devon Rex cat.

Invasive squamous cell carcinomas are the most common malignant cutaneous neoplasms of cats. They are discussed later under Squamous cell carcinoma.

Papillomaviruses have also been associated with **feline sarcoids**. These are rare cutaneous neoplasms that tend to occur on the nose, lips, or digits of young to middle-aged cats from rural areas (Fig. 6-144). Feline sarcoids are firm, smooth, exophytic, and can become ulcerated. Recurrence is common, but metastasis has not been documented. Histologic features virtually identical to the equine sarcoid have been described and found to be associated with papillomavirus DNA via PCR. The implicated virus feline sarcoid-associated PV (FeSarPV) is thought to be a novel bovine papillomavirus (BPV), given the similarity in its DNA sequences to BPV-1, BPV-2, and ovis aries papillomavirus 2 (OaPV-2).

Camelids. Fibropapillomas associated with papillomaviruses have been described in both llamas and alpacas. Lesions were located on the nose, lips, and cheeks and histologically resembled equine sarcoids. Of 6 reported cases, all lesions were cured by surgical excision, with the exception of one that recurred and spread. One viral squamous papilloma was reported on the cornea of a dromedary camel. The specific PV was not identified in that case. *Camelus dromedarius papillomavirus 1* (delta-PV) has been associated with fibropapillomas in Arabian camels.

Rabbits. Domestic **rabbits** develop oral papillomatosis caused by infection with *Rabbit oral papillomavirus*. Papillomas, which are multiple and found most often under the tongue, are grossly and histologically typical of viral-induced squamous papillomas.

Further reading

Bergvall KE. Sarcoids. Vet Clin North Am Equine Pract 2013;29:657-671.

Gil da Costa RM, Medeiros R. Bovine papillomavirus: opening new trends for comparative pathology. Arch Virol 2014;159:191-198.

Gorino AC, et al. Use of PCR to estimate the prevalence of *Equus caballus papillomavirus* in aural plaques in horses. Vet J 2013;197:903-904.

Knight CG, et al. Equine penile squamous cell carcinomas are associated with the presence of equine papillomavirus type 2 DNA sequences. Vet Pathol 2011;48:1190-1194.

Lange CE, Favrot C. Canine papillomaviruses. Vet Clin Small Anim 2011;41:1183-1195.

Munday JS. Bovine and human papillomaviruses: a comparative review. Vet Pathol 2014;51:1063-1075.

Munday JS. Papillomaviruses in felids. Vet J 2014;199:340-347.

Nasir L, Campo MS. Bovine papillomaviruses: their role in the aetiology of cutaneous tumours of bovids and equids. Vet Dermatol 2008;19:243-254.

Rector A, Van Ranst M. Animal papillomaviruses. Virol 2013;445:213-223.

Schulman FY, et al. Camelid mucocutaneous fibropapillomas: clinicopathologic findings and association with papillomavirus. Vet Pathol 2003;40:103-107.

Torres SMF, Koch SN. Papillomavirus-associated diseases. Vet Clin North Am Equine Pract 2013;29:643-655.

Squamous cell carcinoma

Squamous cell carcinoma (SCC) *is a relatively common, locally invasive, and occasionally metastatic neoplasm of most domestic* *species*. The behavior of squamous cell carcinoma (SCC) of the skin is usually that of locally destructive spread. Its metastatic potential is low, with certain qualifications depending on location. Those initiated by sunlight are slow to metastasize, and usually only to local lymph nodes. In contrast, those originating on the canine digit may be more prone to metastasize, but even these are cured by amputation in virtually all but the most neglected cases.

Development of SCC has been associated with papillomaviruses in multiple species, including dogs, cats, horses, and sheep (see cutaneous papillomas). *Sunlight is probably the most important carcinogenic stimulus for these tumors.* The action of sunlight may be related to overexpression of p53 protein as a result of ultraviolet (UV)-induced mutations of the p53 tumor suppressor gene. Chronic sun exposure, lack of pigment, and thin haircoat in the area of tumor development are predisposing factors. In these cases, SCC is usually preceded by *actinic keratosis* and is seen more frequently in geographic regions exposed to long periods of intense sunlight (see Actinic diseases of skin). Affected animals are usually middle aged to older. In **cats**, predilection sites for UV-induced SCC are eyelids, pinnae, and nasal planum (Fig. 6-145). In **dogs**, the ventral trunk, digits, limbs, scrotum, and lips are the most common sites. The nasal planum is rarely affected, and when it is affected, it is usually secondary to depigmentation from a chronic inflammatory condition, such as discoid lupus erythematosus. **Subungual squamous cell carcinomas** in **dogs** may be multiple and are seen most often in black dogs, particularly large breeds such as Labrador Retrievers and Standard Poodles. Although papillomaviruses have been a suspected etiology, one study did not support a viral pathogenesis. In **horses**, the periocular region, penis, and perianal regions are predilection sites, and Appaloosas, American Paint horses, Quarter Horses, and males are predisposed. In **cattle**, Herefords and Ayrshires are at increased risk, and lesions are most common on the face, eyelids, pinnae, back, vulva, and distal legs. In **goats**, Angoras and Boers may be at increased risk, and lesions are most common in sparsely haired skin of the udder, perianal region, horn base, pinnae, vulva, and eyelid. In **sheep**, cutaneous SCC is most common on the muzzle, lips, eyelids, pinnae, perineum, and vulva, and Merinos may be at risk. SCC in **llamas** and **alpacas** has been reported in ocular tissue, perineum, and haired skin. SCCs are rare in **pigs** but usually occur in white skin.

Rarely, SCC has been reported to arise from burn scars, nonhealing wounds, and chronic inflammation. Brand keratomas in cattle have been reported to undergo malignant transformation to SCC. SCC with regional metastasis was reported in a 12-year-old llama with an 18-month history of a nonhealing wound. SCC have been reported to arise from follicular cysts in both dogs and sheep. Equine smegma has been implicated in the development of preputial SCC.

Squamous cell carcinoma in situ refers to a malignant tumor of cells with squamous differentiation that is *confined by the basement membrane*. Multicentric SCC in situ in cats (bowenoid in situ carcinoma) is discussed under Papillomas and papillomavirus-induced lesions.

Invasive squamous cell carcinomas (ISCC) are plaque-like, crateriform, or papillary masses that vary from a few millimeters to several centimeters in diameter. Alopecia, erythema, ulceration, and crusting are usually present. Lesions may be single to multiple. On cut section, they are firm and white. In some locations (eye, penis), they are raised and papillary, even though the surface is ulcerated.

Histologically, several subtypes have been described and they include *well-differentiated, poorly differentiated, acantholytic, spindle cell,* and *verrucous* variants. The **well-differentiated SCC** is a plaque-like lesion composed of islands, cords, and trabeculae of squamous cells that originate from the epidermis or rarely hair follicles or follicular cysts, breach the basement membrane, and extend into the dermis. Intercellular bridges between keratinocytes may be prominent, and there is often formation of central accumulations of compact laminated keratin *(keratin pearls)* within islands of invasive neoplastic epithelial cells. There is a fairly orderly progression from polyhedral, nonkeratinized basal cells at the periphery of the neoplastic epithelial structures to large polygonal keratinized cells at the centers. Neoplastic cells have vesicular nuclei with one or multiple very prominent nucleoli. Cytoplasm is usually abundant and eosinophilic. There is often a desmoplastic reaction in the surrounding dermis. There may be marked crusting and hyperkeratosis. **Poorly differentiated SCCs** tend to be composed of mostly cords and nests of neoplastic epithelial cells. Neoplastic cells have amphophilic cytoplasm with hyperchromatic nuclei and prominent nucleoli. There is moderate to high mitotic activity and frequent mitotic atypia. Keratin pearls are not observed, and instead, there are individual dyskeratotic cells or clusters of partially keratinized cells.

Acantholytic squamous cell carcinoma is an uncommon variant. Pseudoglandular to pseudocystic structures are formed by drop-out of partially keratinized cells from the centers of epithelial islands and trabeculae resulting from loss of intercellular junctions. This type of tumor must be carefully distinguished from an adenocarcinoma by identifying tumor cell keratinization. **Spindle cell squamous cell carcinoma** is a rare variant of poorly differentiated SCC and is composed of large pleomorphic spindle and polygonal cells that have abundant pale or amphophilic cytoplasm. Nuclei are large and vesicular with prominent nucleoli. The mitotic index is high. Rare foci of individual cell keratinization will help distinguish this neoplasm from a sarcoma. **Verrucous squamous cell carcinoma** is a rare variant of SCC only described in dogs. It is a low-grade malignancy. It is both exophytic and endophytic, and the broad trabeculae have smooth rounded margins. There may

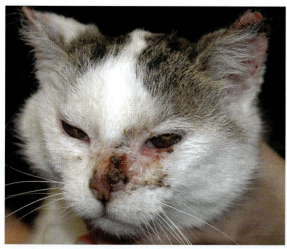

Figure 6-145 Ultraviolet light–induced **squamous cell carcinoma** in a white cat. Erythematous, ulcerative, crusted lesions on the tips of the pinna, nasal planum, and eyelids.

be large tubular invaginations with sloughed keratinocytes. Keratin pearls are absent. There is mild cellular pleomorphism and low mitotic activity.

Carcinoma of the horn of cattle is almost exclusive to castrated male adult cattle in India and neighboring countries. The tumor gradually infiltrates and destroys the horn core and may invade adjacent sinuses and cranial bone. The histology is of well-differentiated squamous cell carcinoma, but neither the site of origin nor the reason for its peculiar site and sex preference is understood.

Basal cell carcinoma

Basal cell carcinomas (BCCs) are uncommon in cats and dogs and rare in other domestic species. These tumors are thought to arise from epithelial cells of the basal layer of the epidermis and adnexa. They are the most common malignant neoplasms in humans, and chronic exposure to UV radiation is a key factor in the development of these tumors. In cats, chronic UV exposure may also play a role. However, in some cats, BCC arises from BISC, and therefore papillomaviruses may also play a role in pathogenesis. The pathogenesis is unknown in dogs. BCC usually occur as single to occasionally multiple, alopecic and crusted, ulcerated plaques or umbilicated nodules measuring a few millimeters to several centimeters in diameter. The skin may have a black or blue tint because of melanin pigment in the neoplasm. BCC in cats occurs most commonly on the face, nose, and pinnae. BCC in dogs are usually on the trunk. They generally occur in middle-aged to older animals. They are generally considered a low-grade malignancy. Rates of recurrence and metastasis are very low.

There are 3 histopathologic variants: *solid, keratinizing, and clear cell*. BCC have a horizontal plaque-like configuration extending multifocally from the epidermis. The neoplastic cells of **solid basal cell carcinoma** resemble basal cells of the epidermis or hair follicles. Each has an oval, deeply basophilic nucleus, a single nucleolus, and scant eosinophilic cytoplasm with indistinct cell boundaries. In contrast to normal stratum basale, there are no intercellular bridges. The cells extend into the dermis as islands, trabeculae, or grow expansively as solid sheets embedded in a moderately cellular stroma of fibrous or fibromyxoid tissue. Caseation necrosis, sometimes with cystic degeneration, is often present in the centers of large epithelial islands. Solid BCCs may have small foci of squamous differentiation. Mitotic figures and nuclear pleomorphism are variable. Tumor cells may contain melanin, and melanophages may be present in the intervening stroma. **Keratinizing basal cell carcinomas** have similar features to the solid type; however, melanin and cystic degeneration are uncommon. Angular islands and trabeculae of neoplastic epithelium predominate. Mitotic activity is moderate to high, and mitotic atypia can usually be detected. Many of the epithelial islands contain central or peripheral foci of abrupt squamous differentiation that is cytologically benign and may or may not have keratinization. **Clear cell basal cell carcinomas** are rare. The epithelial cells are larger and have clear to finely granular cytoplasm. Nuclei lack pleomorphism, nucleoli are small, and mitotic activity is variable. Necrosis is common.

Basosquamous carcinoma

This rare tumor has features of both SCC and BCC and has been described in the cat and dog. It is clinically indistinguishable, and histologically it has a similar silhouette. **Basosquamous carcinomas** are composed primarily of dermal lobules of basaloid cells with centralized foci of atypical abruptly keratinized cells. The squamous component has histologic features of malignancy and lacks differentiation of the follicular isthmus or bulb. These 2 features help differentiate it from a keratinizing BCC. The basaloid population may have foci of dyskeratosis or melanization. Tumor lobules may or may not be connected with the epidermis.

Further reading

De Lorimier L, Garrett LD. Neoplastic and non-neoplastic tumors. In: Miller WH, et al., editors. Muller & Kirk's Small Animal Dermatology. 7th ed. St Louis: Elsevier; 2013. p. 774-843.

Gross TL, et al. Epithelial tumors. In: Gross TL, et al., editors. Skin Diseases of the Dog and Cat: Clinical and Histopathological Diagnosis. 2nd ed. Oxford, UK: Blackwell; 2005. p. 562-603.

Schaffer PA, et al. Cutaneous neoplastic lesions of equids in the central United States and Canada: 3,351 biopsy specimens from 3,272 equids (2000-2010). J Am Vet Med Assoc 2013;242:99-104.

Valentine BA. Survey of equine cutaneous neoplasia in the Pacific Northwest. J Vet Diagn Invest 2006;18:123-126.

Valentine BA, Martin JM. Prevalence of neoplasia in llamas and alpacas (Oregon State University, 2001-2006). J Vet Diagn Invest 2007;19:202-204.

Tumors with adnexal differentiation
Tumors arising from hair follicles

Hair follicle (pilar) neoplasms occur in most domestic species but are most commonly encountered in the dog and cat. Their classification is rather complex; however, *the majority of tumors arising in animals share a benign biological behavior*. Exceptions exist as follows:

Infundibular keratinizing acanthoma (intracutaneous cornifying epithelioma) is a benign cystic tumor of the skin of dogs. Tumors are 0.5-4 cm in diameter and classically have a central pore with a hard keratinized plug. Common sites are the dorsum of the neck and back. Subungual lesions also occur. Usually, there is only a single tumor, but Norwegian Elkhounds and Keeshonds are predisposed to developing a generalized form affecting the entire body.

The histologic lesion is a well-demarcated cup-shaped dermal mass oriented around a central cyst filled with concentric laminated to amorphous keratin (Fig. 6-146). With fortuitous sectioning, a central pore opening to the surface will be seen. The epithelium surrounding the cyst consists of large polygonal cells with abundant pale-pink glassy cytoplasm. There is a sparse granular layer. The periphery of the cyst wall consists of orderly basal cells. Extending into the deeper dermis from the cyst wall are small secondary horn cysts resembling keratin pearls interconnected by narrow cords of basal epithelium. The stroma is poorly cellular and often mucinous. Cartilaginous and osseous metaplasia are occasionally seen. Focal rupture is common, inciting a granulomatous or pyogranulomatous reaction in surrounding dermis.

Trichoepitheliomas are common in dogs, uncommon in cats, and reported in horses, cattle, and an alpaca. However, in this author's opinion, the report in the alpaca was probably a hybrid follicular cyst. Trichoepithelioma is *a tumor of primitive hair germ that exhibits rudimentary differentiation toward all 3 segments of the follicle: the infundibulum, isthmus, and the inferior segment*. Trichoepitheliomas are single or multiple alopecic skin tumors occurring anywhere on the body, with a slight

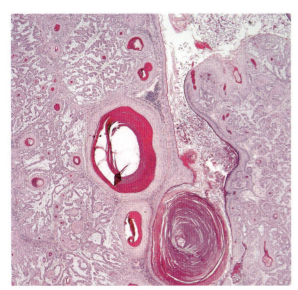

Figure 6-146 Infundibular keratinizing acanthoma. Cup-shaped mass oriented around a central cyst. Cords of epithelium and secondary horn cysts in mucinous stroma extend out from the cyst wall.

preference for the back in dogs and tail in cats. Persian cats are predisposed. Tumors are usually <2 cm in diameter but on occasion can be very large and ulcerated. Multiple tumors occur most frequently in Basset Hounds. Histologically, the tumor is well circumscribed, unencapsulated, and composed of multiple variably sized epithelial islands and cystic structures. These structures are partially or fully lined by squamous epithelium with or without a granular layer or basaloid epithelial cells resembling matrical epithelium surrounded by a thickened basement membrane. The cystic structures are filled with infundibular, trichilemmal, or keratinized "ghost cells," depending upon the lining epithelium (Fig. 6-147A, B).

The outer layer of basal cells usually shows peripheral palisading and may abut the fibrous stroma or send out basal cell ribbons into a mucinous stroma. Some trichoepitheliomas have several large primary cystic areas surrounded by many smaller cysts. Rupture of some of the keratinaceous cysts stimulates pyogranulomatous inflammation within the stroma and even within the cyst, sometimes accompanied by mineralization and foreign body giant cells. Mineralization and inflammation are more typical of the closely related pilomatricoma.

Malignant trichoepitheliomas have only been described in dogs. They are generally larger, asymmetrical, and poorly circumscribed compared to their benign counterpart. Other features include atypical mitotic figures, central caseous necrosis within the islands of matrical cells, minimal squamous component, and invasion of subcutis sometimes accompanied by desmoplasia. Lymphatic invasion is considered an essential finding to confirm malignancy by some pathologists. Regional and pulmonary metastasis is possible. *Trichoepitheliomas are distinguished from all other epidermal or appendage tumors by the abrupt (matrical) keratinization and the follicle-like basal cell nests that surround it.* Other tumors or cysts simulating trichoepithelioma lack one or both of these features.

Tricholemmoma is a rare, *benign, and nonrecurring* pilar tumor of the outer root sheath recognized in dogs and cats. There are 2 types: one in which the tumor cells differentiate

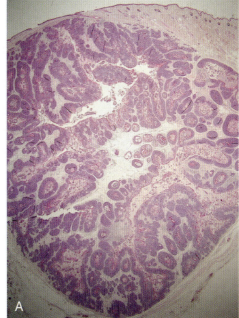

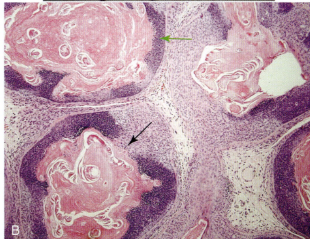

Figure 6-147 Trichoepithelioma. **A.** Well-demarcated dermal mass composed of numerous small cystic epithelial structures with a fibromyxoid stroma. **B.** Note the abrupt keratinization and differentiation toward the isthmus (black arrow) and inferior segment (green arrow) of the follicle.

into cells characteristic of the inferior segment of the hair follicle (**inferior tricholemmoma**) external root sheath or the second type, the isthmus (**isthmic tricholemmoma**) section of the external root sheath. *Inferior tricholemmomas* are very rare, only recognized in dogs, 1-7 cm diameter firm nodules on the head and neck. Tumor cells form nests separated by a fine collagenous stroma. The tumor cells have abundant eosinophilic cytoplasm that is pale (clear cells) peripherally and more intensely eosinophilic toward the center of the nests. Pallor of the outermost layer of cells is due to marked cytoplasmic glycogen storage, seen in histologic section as cytoplasmic clearing. These are thought to represent differentiation toward outer root sheath cells. Each tumor follicle is surrounded by a thick, homogeneous basal lamina resembling the vitreous sheath of the normal follicle. *Isthmic tricholemmomas* are very rare, raised, alopecic papules and nodules <2 cm in diameter, recognized in cats and dogs. The epithelial cells are

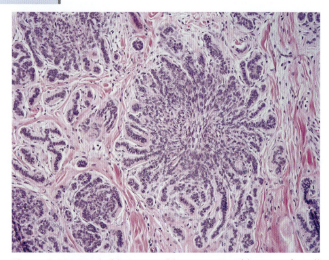

Figure 6-148 Trichoblastoma, ribbon type. Double rows of small basaloid epithelial cells arranged in branching and winding patterns.

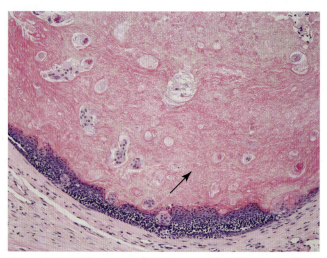

Figure 6-149 Pilomatricoma. Cystic mass lined by matrical epithelium with abrupt keratinization into the lumen. Note the numerous evenly spaced vacuoles (arrow) within the keratin (keratin ghost cells).

arranged as islands, and radiating cords that may intersect or be associated with the epidermis. The tumor cells show central trichilemmal cornification. The granular layer is absent.

Trichoblastoma (basal cell tumor) is *a benign tumor derived from the primitive hair germ of embryonic follicular development.* There are ribbon, trabecular, granular, spindle cell (with outer root sheath differentiation) variants. These are common in dogs and cats, seen occasionally in horses, and rare in cattle and sheep. Lesions are generally solitary, firm, raised alopecic nodules 1-2 cm in diameter, although they can sometimes be much larger and ulcerated. The head, neck, and base of the ear are common locations, especially in dogs and cats.

- The **ribbon (garland, medusa-head) trichoblastoma** is a well-demarcated dermal to subcutaneous tumor formed by long, narrow (2-cells thick), branching or winding cords of small basaloid epithelial cells (Fig. 6-148) that may join or radiate from a large central aggregate (medusoid pattern). A mucinous stroma is frequently associated with the medusoid pattern. Nuclei in tumors arranged in cords often palisade perpendicular to the long axis of the cord. Mitotic figures may be numerous. Abundant collagen that may appear hyalinized is more common in dog tumors. This pattern is common in dogs and rare in cats and other species.
- **Trabecular trichoblastomas** are well-demarcated dermal masses composed of islands and broad trabeculae of basal keratinocytes with prominent peripheral palisading. The cells that are centrally located have more abundant cytoplasm. Connection to the overlying epidermis is minimal. Stroma is sparse and may be collagenous to mucinous and is of low cellularity. Keratin microcysts may be present. This is the most common variant of cats.
- **Granular trichoblastoma** is a rare variant with the same architecture as a ribbon trichoblastoma, but the neoplastic epithelial cells are larger and contain abundant, finely granular or vacuolated cytoplasm. Nuclei are small, angular, and eccentric.
- **Spindle cell trichoblastomas** are most often seen in cats. They are well-demarcated dermal masses composed of trabeculae and lobules of elongated, streaming, basaloid epithelial cells within a poorly cellular collagenous stroma.

Peripheral palisading in not a prominent feature. There is often a broad zone of connection to the epidermis. Tumor cells have scant cytoplasm, oval nuclei with inconspicuous nucleoli, and rare mitoses. Melanin may be present in the tumor cells and accompanying melanophages. Keratinization is rare.

- **Trichoblastomas with outer root sheath differentiation** are recognized by some pathologists. These are rare, well-demarcated masses in the dermis to subcutis composed of multiple lobules and trabeculae and areas of cystic degeneration. Small epithelial cells form anastomosing cords similar to the ribbon type, and these merge into islands of cells with markedly vacuolated cytoplasm resembling anagen suprabulbar outer root sheath or pale pink isthmus-type keratinocytes that line the cystic zones.

Pilomatricoma (pilomatrixoma, epithelioma of Malherbe, necrotizing and calcifying epithelioma) is an uncommon benign tumor of dogs and is believed to be derived from primitive hair matrix and thus shows incomplete differentiation towards hair cortex. This tumor macroscopically resembles trichoepithelioma but is often more heavily mineralized and consists of fewer, larger cysts than does trichoepithelioma. They usually occur as single, firm to hard, raised, 1-10 cm diameter nodules most commonly on the proximal legs and dorsal trunk over the rump and shoulders. Poodles, Kerry Blue Terriers, and Old English Sheepdogs and other breeds with continuously growing coats, and thus a higher proportion of anagen follicles, are predisposed. *The typical microscopic morphology is of one or more large, thick-walled cysts partially filled with so-called shadow or ghost cells* (Fig. 6-149) *typical of matrical differentiation*. These cells are flattened eosinophilic epithelial cells with a central empty halo in place of the lysed nucleus. The cyst wall is composed of multiple layers of basal cells, resembling matrical epithelium of the hair bulb, and showing a sudden zonal degeneration to form the central laminations of shadow cells. Small zones of squamous epithelium may be seen. Small foci resembling rounded dermal papilla-like structures may be present in the cyst wall. These tumors are not connected to the overlying epidermis. There is sparse collagenous to mucinous stroma. Mitotic activity may be high. Mineralization of shadow cells is very common, and cyst rupture results in the pyogranulomatous inflammation that is very typical of these tumors. Foci of necrosis within the tumor are frequently seen, and mineralization or even ossification within the stroma occurs occasionally. **Melanocytic matricoma,** reported in one dog, is similar to pilomatricoma with the additional feature of neoplastic melanocyte proliferation.

Malignant pilomatricomas (matrical carcinoma, pilomatrix carcinoma) are rare in dogs and not reported in other domestic species. They are locally aggressive and may invade bone, and have been reported to metastasize to multiple distant sites, including lung, central nervous system, and bone. This malignant variant is poorly circumscribed and may extend into the subcutis. Compared to its benign counterpart, there is usually an increased ratio of basaloid cells to keratinized ghost cells, infiltrative borders, increased mitotic activity, and mitotic atypia. Ulcerations and necrosis are common, and some neoplasms are connected to the epidermis. Additional features include desmoplastic stroma, and mineralization or ossification of keratin. Lymphatic invasion is the most important feature to support malignancy.

Tumors arising from sebaceous or modified sebaceous glands

Tumors of sebaceous glands include *nodular sebaceous hyperplasia, sebaceous adenoma, sebaceous epithelioma, and sebaceous carcinoma.* **Modified sebaceous glands** include the Meibomian glands of the eyelid and perianal (hepatoid, circumanal) glands. Tumors of the Meibomian gland include *Meibomian gland adenomas, epitheliomas, and carcinomas* that are histologically identical to the corresponding sebaceous gland lesion and will not be described separately. Perianal glands are only present in canids and are located in the perianal skin as well as around the proximal third of the tail, dorsal lumbosacral area, lateral to the prepuce, and along the ventral midline as far cranial as the neck. Tumors of perianal glands include perianal gland hyperplasia, perianal gland adenomas, epitheliomas, and carcinomas. *Epitheliomas are considered to be low-grade malignancies.* Sebaceous gland tumors are common in dogs, uncommon in cats and rare in other species.

Nodular sebaceous hyperplasia is common and accounts for 50% of the sebaceous gland tumors in dogs. Lesions are single or multiple, raised, yellow-orange, multilobulated, wart-like, waxy to hyperkeratotic masses. They are most common in Cocker Spaniels and Poodles on the head, eyelids, limbs, and trunk. Size varies but most are <1 cm in diameter. Many are ulcerated by continued tumor growth or by trauma. Histologically, there are multiple, enlarged sebaceous lobules clustered around one or more dilated sebaceous duct(s) and hair follicle(s). Secondary erosion and inflammation are common. The sebaceous cells (sebocytes) are fully mature, and the peripheral rim of basal (reserve) cell population is inconspicuous. There is no increase in basal reserve cells. Occasionally, some sebaceous lobules exhibit a metaplastic transformation to perianal gland cells.

Sebaceous adenomas are grossly similar to nodular sebaceous hyperplasia. *Sebaceous adenomas differ from hyperplasia in that there are more basal (reserve) cells than in hyperplasia, and the lobular proliferation is greater and less symmetrical.* Lesions are uncommon in cats, with the exception of Persian cats. Histologically, they are divided into *simple* and *compound.* Compound adenomas are more common. In the *simple variant, ducts are not a prominent feature.* Lesions are composed of multiple large lobules of sebocytes that show normal maturation. The *compound variant (ductal adenoma) contains glandular lobules and ducts in various proportions.* The sebaceous lobules are grouped in radiating clusters around ductal structures. As in nodular hyperplasia, perianal gland metaplasia is rarely observed. There may be compression of adjacent structures. Melanization in reserve cells is common in eyelid tumors.

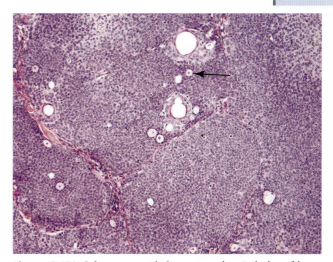

Figure 6-150 Sebaceous epithelioma in a dog. Lobules of basaloid epithelium with a few scattered mature sebocytes (arrow).

Sebaceous epitheliomas are grossly similar to sebaceous adenomas. They are common in dogs, occurring most commonly in Shih Tzus and Lhasa Apsos. Histologically, these masses are composed of multiple large irregular lobules of epithelial reserve cells with multiple small foci of distinct sebaceous differentiation (Fig. 6-150). Mitotic activity may be high in the basal reserve cells, but mature sebocytes are not mitotically active. Small ducts lined by mature squamous epithelium are usually present. These lesions, especially Meibomian epitheliomas, are variably pigmented. This tumor is considered to be a low-grade malignancy. Sebaceous and Meibomian epitheliomas may recur if incompletely excised; rarely, sebaceous epitheliomas have been reported to invade lymphatics and metastasize to regional lymph nodes and, in one case, lung and central nervous system.

Sebaceous carcinomas are rare malignant neoplasms in dogs and cats. Cocker Spaniels may be predisposed. These lesions are usually solitary, firm nodules, up to 7 cm in diameter and most common on the head. Ulceration and alopecia are common. Histologically, some pathologists divide these tumors into 2 variants: *sebocytic* and *epitheliomatous.* **Sebocytic carcinomas** are multilobular dermal masses that are irregular in shape but well circumscribed and may extend into the subcutis. Neoplastic cells are polygonal and larger than basal reserve cells. Orderly progression from basaloid reserve cells to mature sebocytes is markedly distorted or absent. Neoplastic cells are pleomorphic with eosinophilic cytoplasm that is variably vacuolated. Nuclei are large with prominent nucleoli, and mitotic activity is moderate to high. There may be atypical mitotic figures. Other possible features include ulceration, necrosis, cystic degeneration, squamous differentiation, keratinization, or occasional glandular structures. **Epitheliomatous sebaceous carcinomas** are composed predominantly of slightly larger and more pleomorphic than normal basaloid reserve cells in islands, cords, and trabeculae. There are scattered foci of mature sebocytes. There may be multifocal connections to the epidermis. They are commonly ulcerated, and margins may be infiltrative and can extend into the subcutis. Distinction between **epitheliomatous carcinoma** and **sebaceous epithelioma** includes the following proposed criteria: Carcinomas have an increased nuclear size, a higher mitotic rate, atypical mitotic figures, and mitotic figures in the mature sebocytes. They may be locally aggressive but reports of distant metastasis are rare.

The cause of perianal gland tumors is unknown; however, they are known to be modulated by sex hormones and contain both androgen and estrogen receptors. **Nodular perianal gland hyperplasia** may occur as either discrete nodules of variable size or as a diffuse bulging ring around the anus. Histologically, there are multiple enlarged lobules of *well-differentiated perianal gland cells with a single peripheral layer of basaloid reserve cells. Lobules are organized around small ducts*. Mitotic activity is low.

Perianal (hepatoid) gland adenomas are common and occur only in dogs. Males are predisposed. The *gross appearance* of perianal gland adenomas is of one or more raised rubbery masses that may grow to 10 cm or more in diameter, most commonly around the anus but can occur anywhere perianal glands exist. Adenomas are well-circumscribed nodular or multinodular masses composed of *broad, anastomosing trabeculae or islands of well-differentiated perianal gland cells surrounded by a single layer of basal reserve cells* (Fig. 6-151). There is low mitotic activity, delicate fibrovascular to collagenous stroma, and compression of adjacent glands and structures. Ulceration is common in large tumors. Distinguishing adenomas from hyperplasia can be difficult, but the main difference is that the lobular architecture is maintained in hyperplastic lesions, and adenomas may be highly vascular. Local excision and castration is usually curative and prevents the development of new benign perianal gland tumors.

Perianal (hepatoid) gland epitheliomas are rare tumors and may be benign or of low-grade malignancy. They are composed of predominantly (>90%) basal reserve cells with small scattered foci of mature perianal gland cells. Neoplastic cells are arranged in sheets, islands, and anastomosing trabeculae. The tumor margin is irregular and mildly infiltrative. Small ducts may be present. Mitotic activity is increased in comparison to the adenomas, but nuclear atypia is not present, and mitotic figures are not observed within mature perianal gland cells.

Perianal (hepatoid) gland carcinomas are uncommon, and when they occur, they are usually perianal in location. They are grossly similar to adenomas, and most are 2 cm or greater diameter. Histologically, they vary from *well differentiated* to *poorly differentiated*. Well-differentiated tumors have similar architecture to adenomas but have variable infiltrative growth at the margins. Mature and basal reserve cells are disorganized and scattered haphazardly within neoplastic islands and trabeculae. Nuclei are larger than those in benign lesions, slightly pleomorphic, and may have multiple prominent nucleoli. Mitotic activity is low to moderate with mitotic atypia and mitoses of mature cells. There may be small scattered foci of squamous metaplasia. Ulceration, hemorrhage, and necrosis are common. Poorly differentiated tumors are rare. They are poorly circumscribed and infiltrative, composed of cords and trabeculae of pleomorphic polygonal cells. Neoplastic cells have eosinophilic to amphophilic cytoplasm that is variably vacuolated. Nuclei are large and vesicular with prominent nucleoli. Mitotic activity is high, and atypia is common. Lymphatic invasion must be diagnosed with caution because compression of reserve cells by lobular expansion may simulate a tumor embolus surrounded by lymphatic endothelium. Carcinomas tend to grow more rapidly and ulcerate more than adenomas. Metastasis to regional lymph nodes occurs in 30% of cases. Direct extension into the pelvic canal can occur. Castration is generally not effective treatment for carcinomas.

Tumors arising from sweat glands

Epitrichial (apocrine) gland tumors can be benign or malignant. Adenomas are more common and occur in cats, dogs, and rarely in horses, cattle, and pigs. They are usually solitary, 0.5-10 cm in diameter, and ulcerated. Cystic tumors may be blue to purple. In dogs, adenomas are more common on the head, neck, dorsal trunk, and limbs. Similar sites are affected in cats, with the addition of pinnae and tail. Pinnae and vulva are common sites in horses. Carcinomas more commonly occur on the legs and may be poorly circumscribed and infiltrative. Adenoma variants include *cystadenoma, simple and complex secretory adenoma, and ductular adenomas, which are divided into canine, feline, and solid-cystic ductular adenomas*. **Epitrichial cystadenomas** (apocrine hidrocystoma) are well-circumscribed, dermal masses composed of one or more cystic structures generally lined by a single layer of cuboidal to columnar epithelium. Some cysts contain simple or branching papillary aggregates, and if this is a dominant feature, then the term *papillary cystadenoma* is appropriate. Small glandular structures may be present. In cats, the majority of these tumors are on the head, including ear canal and eyelid (glands of Moll), and lesions may be multiple in Himalayan and Persian cats. **Simple secretory epitrichial adenomas** are well-circumscribed dermal neoplasms with acinar, tubular, or papillary patterns. Cystic cavities and glandular lumens may contain pale eosinophilic homogeneous secretory material.

Complex (mixed) secretory epitrichial adenomas are analogous to complex and benign mixed mammary adenomas.

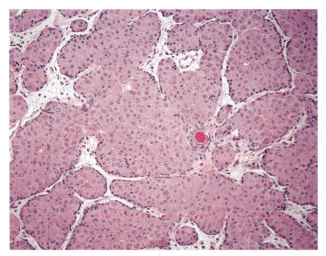

Figure 6-151 Perianal (hepatoid) gland adenoma in a dog. Anastomosing islands and trabeculae of well-differentiated perianal (hepatoid) gland cells surrounded by a single layer of basaloid reserve cells embedded in a delicate fibrovascular stroma. There is a small focus of squamous metaplasia.

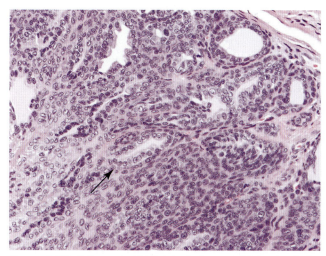

Figure 6-152 Feline epitrichial ductal adenoma. Multiple tubular structures are lined by a double layer of cuboidal epithelium (arrow).

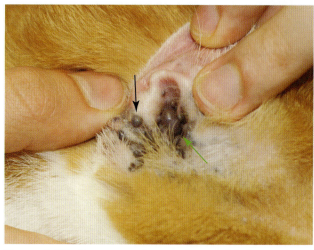

Figure 6-153 Ceruminous (apocrine) cysts (black arrow) and cystadenoma (green arrow) on the pinna and ear canal of a cat.

Stroma may be myxoid or have chondroid differentiation. Osseous metaplasia is uncommon. **Canine epitrichial ductular adenomas** are circumscribed, multinodular, and located in the deep dermis to subcutis. Lobules are composed of tightly packed tubular structures lined by a double layer of cuboidal epithelium that resemble basal cells. There are multiple small foci of squamous metaplasia. There is moderate collagenous stroma, moderate mitotic activity, and no secretory activity. **Feline epitrichial ductular adenomas** are similar to those of dogs (Fig. 6-152). The centers of the lobules may be irregularly cystic and partially lined by cuboidal epithelium. Mitotic activity is low and stroma is sparse. **Solid-cystic epitrichial adenomas** are multinodular, circumscribed, and often vertically oriented in the dermis. There is cystic degeneration of larger lobules. These neoplasms are formed of 2 distinct cell types: a small basaloid cuboidal cell and slightly larger polygonal cells. The smaller cells form occasional short, double rows with or without an obvious, often sharp, angular lumen (ductal structures). Melanization is common in this variant.

Epitrichial (apocrine) carcinomas have similar histologic variants to the adenomas: *cystadenocarcinoma; simple and complex (mixed) adenocarcinoma; and ductal, solid-cystic ductal, and clear cell ductal carcinoma.* Lesions are generally solitary, frequently alopecic, and may be ulcerated. They occur most commonly on the legs in dogs, and on head, legs, and abdomen in cats. In general, these lesions are histologically similar to their benign counterparts, although they tend to be larger and less well circumscribed and have cytologic features of malignancy. Nuclei are larger and more pleomorphic; there may be loss of nuclear polarity, and nucleoli may be prominent. Mitotic activity varies. Atypical mitotic figures may be seen. Well-differentiated lesions do not produce a desmoplastic response, and lymphatic invasion is rare. Poorly differentiated variants are infiltrative, have ill-defined borders, more desmoplasia, and are often ulcerated. The myoepithelial component of the complex adenocarcinoma usually has a benign histologic appearance. However, in some cases, it predominates over the epithelial component. On rare occasions, both glandular and myoepithelial components demonstrate features of malignancy, and the tumor is referred to as an **epitrichial gland carcinosarcoma** or **mixed malignant epitrichial gland tumor**.

Ductal epitrichial carcinomas tend to have more desmoplasia, lymphatic invasion, and higher mitotic activity with mitotic atypia than secretory adenocarcinomas. In contrast to ductal adenomas, ductal carcinomas have more irregular infiltrative borders, larger nuclei, prominent nucleoli, larger areas of squamous metaplasia, and zones of necrosis. **Solid-cystic epitrichial carcinomas** only occur in cats and have a horizontal rather than vertical orientation. **Clear cell epitrichial carcinomas** (follicular stem cell carcinoma, clear cell hidradenocarcinoma, clear cell adnexal carcinoma) are composed of large polygonal cells in lobules and nests with zones of cystic degeneration. The neoplastic cells have moderate to abundant pale eosinophilic to finely vacuolated cytoplasm. Multinucleated cells are usually seen. Subtle tubules lined by 1-3 layers of cells are present. There is sparse to moderate stroma, and chondroid metaplasia may occur. Occasional nests of small mesenchymal cells consistent with follicular papillary bodies are identified in the stroma. Immunohistochemistry using specific cytokeratin such as CAM5.2, CK7/8, and CK13 may be necessary to support this diagnosis. Lymphatic invasion, regional lymph node, and pulmonary metastasis are reported.

Tumors of **atrichial (eccrine) glands** are extremely rare and occur only on the footpads of dogs and cats. These tumors are usually malignant, although a few adenomas are described. Lesions are usually poorly circumscribed, ulcerated, and may be seen as swollen pawpad(s) or digit(s). These are aggressive neoplasms that often recur locally and may metastasize rapidly to local lymph nodes. Pulmonary metastasis has been reported. Histologically, they are infiltrative, have desmoplastic stroma, and may invade bone and cause bone lysis. Neoplastic cells form tubular, acinar, cribriform, or papillary structures. Tumor cells are polygonal, have pale amphophilic or eosinophilic cytoplasm, large hyperchromatic nuclei, prominent nucleoli, high mitotic activity, and atypical mitotic figures.

Ceruminous glands *can give rise to cysts, cystomatosis, adenomas, complex and mixed adenomas, and the malignant versions of these tumors* (Fig. 6-153). Morphologic features are very similar to those described for the epitrichial (apocrine) gland counterpart, with the additional distinguishing feature of *brown luminal secretions* on H&E-stained sections. In addition, foci of tumor cells may be found within the overlying epithelium, and secondary inflammation is more common.

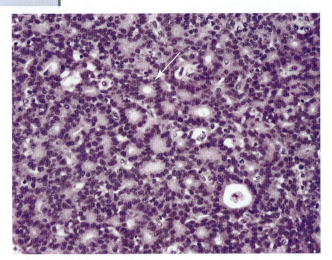

Figure 6-154 Carcinoma of the apocrine glands of the anal sac. Multifocally, neoplastic cells palisade around a central point or clear central lumen (rosettes) (arrow).

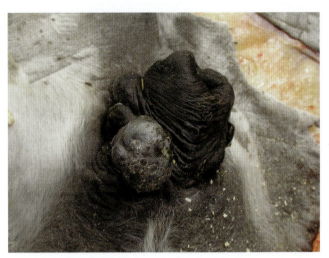

Figure 6-155 Melanoma on the prepuce of a horse. (Courtesy P. Habecker.)

Carcinoma of the apocrine glands of the anal sac is a rare neoplasm of dogs. These tumors occur as unilateral or bilateral masses ventrolateral to the anus. *Paraneoplastic hypercalcemia occurs in 25-90% of cases and is associated with a shorter survival. Metastasis is primarily to regional lymph nodes but is also reported to occur in the lung, spleen, liver, and bone in 50-80% of cases.* The tumor varies histologically from solid, rosette, to tubular types. The solid form consists of sheets of relatively monomorphic polygonal cells with scant eosinophilic cytoplasm and round to oval hyperchromatic nuclei. In the rosette form, tumor cells with peripheral nuclei are arranged radially, sometimes surrounding small amounts of eosinophilic secretory material (Fig. 6-154). The tubular arrangement has larger cells with abundant eosinophilic cytoplasm and hyperchromatic nuclei. Tubules are filled with eosinophilic secretions. These tumors are invasive and induce a desmoplastic response. Tumor growth is often directed inward through the pelvic canal so that a grossly visible perianal mass is seen in only ~50% of cases.

Further reading

Bettini G, et al. Central nervous system and lung metastasis of sebaceous epithelioma in a dog. Vet Dermatol 2009;20:289-294.

Carroll EE, et al. Malignant pilomatricoma in 3 dogs. Vet Pathol 2010;47:937-943.

Gross TL, et al. Gross TL, et al., editors. Skin Diseases of the Dog and Cat: Clinical and Histopathological Diagnosis. 2nd ed. Oxford, UK: Blackwell; 2005. p. 562-603.

Saito S, et al. Melanocytic matricoma in a dog. Vet Pathol 2005;42:499-502.

Schulman FY, et al. Canine cutaneous clear cell adnexal carcinoma: histopathology, immunohistochemistry, and biologic behavior of 26 cases. J Vet Diagn Invest 2005;17:403-411.

Melanocytic tumors

Tumors derived from melanocytes or melanoblasts are of *neuroectodermal origin*. They have been reported in most species of domestic animals and many wildlife species, although they are most common in dogs, horses, and some breeds of swine.

There are some species differences in melanocytic tumors. In **dogs**, *melanomas in the oral cavity and nonhaired skin of the lip have been historically cited as "almost invariably malignant";* however, newer studies have shown a subpopulation of oral and lip melanocytic neoplasms with a favorable prognosis. Tumors of the nailbeds also are frequently malignant, whereas cutaneous tumors are more commonly benign. In **horses**, melanomas occasionally occur as congenital tumors; however, they are most common in *older gray horses, with a site predilection for the perineum, genital area, and distal limbs* (Fig. 6-155). The behavior of melanomas in horses is difficult to predict based on histologic features. They can be clinically malignant and aggressive from the outset, or they may demonstrate slow growth for years with a sudden onset of malignant behavior, or growth can be slow for many years without evidence of metastasis. In some breeds of **swine**, such as Sinclair miniature swine and Hormel crosses (MeLiM strain, melanoma-bearing Libechov minipigs), melanomas can occur as *congenital tumors*, and these breeds have been extensively used in biomedical research. Melanomas are uncommon in **cats** and are often *amelanotic*. Melanomas in **cattle** may occur as a congenital lesion, or they may occur at any age. Most are benign in cattle, although occasional tumors are malignant. Melanocytic tumors are uncommon in **goats** and **sheep** and are generally pigmented.

The *histologic diagnosis* of melanocytic tumors is complicated by the fact that they can display various degrees of pigmentation, from heavily pigmented to amelanotic. In addition, neoplastic melanocytes can be pleomorphic, and melanocytic tumors can display a variety of cell shapes, including *spindle cell, balloon cell (clear cell), epithelioid cell, and signet-ring cell*, thus making them difficult to distinguish from poorly differentiated sarcomas and carcinomas. *Junctional activity can be helpful in identification* (Fig. 6-156), because the only other tumors to display this activity are epitheliotropic lymphoma, and rarely, cutaneous histiocytomas and mast cell tumors. The advances in development of immunohistochemical detection of melanocytic markers has aided greatly in diagnosis of these tumors, particularly in the diagnosis of amelanotic melanomas. Although antibodies against vimentin, S-100, and neuron-specific enolase are sensitive for tumors of melanocytic origin, they are not specific for these tumors and react with many other tumors. For tumor cell specificity and sensitivity, the

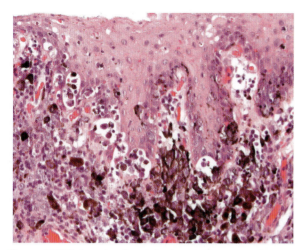

Figure 6-156 Junctional activity in a **malignant melanoma**.

current recommendation is to perform immunohistochemical labeling with Melan-A, PNL2, TRP-1, and TRP-2 as single antibodies, or as a cocktail.

The **mitotic index** (MI) is a key prognostic indicator for clinical behavior of canine melanocytic neoplasms, and it should be determined on all melanocytic tumors. The MI is determined by counting the number of mitotic figures in 10 consecutive high-power (400×) fields (HPFs), commencing in the area of highest mitotic activity for oral and lip neoplasms and in random fields for cutaneous neoplasms. Ulcerated regions should be avoided. *Oral and lip tumors that are heavily pigmented and composed of well-differentiated melanocytes with a low mitotic index (<4/10 HPFs) have a favorable prognosis.* Currently, Melan A is the most specific immunohistochemical marker for melanomas, albeit not 100% sensitive, and has been shown to be useful in many species, including the dog, cat, and horse. Dogs with cutaneous melanocytic neoplasms that have an MI of >3/10 HPFs are expected to have shorter survival times. Nuclear atypia, presence of ulceration, and deep infiltration beyond the dermis are also associated with a poor outcome, and readers are referred to the publication by Smedley (2011) for more detailed information and a thorough review of prognostic features.

Benign melanocytic tumors

Lentigo (lentigo simplex). *A lentigo is a proliferation of melanocytes that is usually confined to the epidermis, resulting clinically in a pigmented circumscribed macule.* This lesion is considered to be a hyperplastic melanocytic lesion rather than neoplastic (see Disorders of pigmentation).

Melanocytoma (benign melanoma, melanocytic nevus). Cutaneous melanocytomas are usually solitary, black, brown, or gray cutaneous nodules. Histologically, melanocytomas can be *junctional* (confined to the epidermis and dermoepidermal junction), *compound* (involving both epidermis and dermis), or *dermal*. Of these, the most common in domestic animals are compound and dermal melanocytomas. They are moderately circumscribed but not encapsulated and may be composed of any melanocytic cell type, that is, spindle, epithelioid, balloon cell (clear cell), or signet ring. Most commonly, they are composed of spindle cells, epithelioid cells, or a mixture of these cell types. The epithelioid cells often occur in nests in the dermis or in the epidermis and along the dermoepidermal junction, or in follicular epithelium. The spindle cell component may form whorls and fingerprint patterns in the dermis. The degree of pigmentation can vary, with the epithelioid cells commonly being darkly pigmented, and the spindle cells lightly pigmented or amelanotic. Mitotic figures are rare, and in the dog, a mitotic index of <3 is reported to predict benign behavior.

Balloon cell melanocytoma is a well-recognized variant in which the circumscribed dermal mass is composed of large epithelioid to polygonal cells with plentiful pale amphophilic to eosinophilic cytoplasm that has a faintly granular appearance. Fine melanin granules can sometimes be detected in low numbers of tumor cells. The nuclei are small, hyperchromatic, and uniform.

Melanocytoma-acanthoma (melanoacanthoma). This tumor is composed of both melanocytic and epithelial cells. It is well described in humans but is rare in domestic animals and has been reported only in dogs. The tumors are seen as solitary pigmented nodules, generally ≤1 cm in diameter. Histologically, the tumor is a *combination of a junctional melanocytoma with a benign epithelial tumor*. The epithelial population forms a mass in the dermis composed of cords and nests with occasional small cystic structures containing keratin. Melanocytic cells form nests in the epidermis and sometimes in the cords of epithelial cells within the dermal mass; melanocytic spindle cells can form whorls and bundles between the epithelial cords and nests.

Malignant melanoma

Malignant melanomas are generally tumors of older animals; however, they have been reported in juvenile animals of many species. Criteria for malignancy and prognosis are described in the introduction to this section; *in the dog, a mitotic index of 3 or greater appears to be the most accurate predictor of a poor prognosis*. In addition, several studies have indicated that *the degree of pigmentation and the histologic pattern are not correlated with prognosis*. Malignant melanomas can be composed of a variety of cell morphologies, including spindle cells, epithelioid cells, a mixture of spindle cells and epithelioid cells, signet-ring cells, or balloon cells (clear cells). In addition, the cells can be heavily pigmented or amelanotic and form bundles, sheets, nests, and whorled patterns. Focal areas of chondroid or osseous metaplasia within the tumor may be seen on rare occasion. The most common types of malignant melanoma are composed of epithelioid cells, a mixture of epithelioid and spindle cells, or spindle cells alone, forming an unencapsulated mass in the dermis or subcutis. Various degrees of junctional activity may be present in the epithelioid cell form and in the mixed epithelioid-spindle cell form. The epithelioid cells tend to form clusters and nests, and the spindle cells tend to form sheets, bundles, or whorls. The neoplastic cells have variable nuclear pleomorphism, usually single prominent basophilic nucleoli, 3 or more mitotic figures per 10 HPFs (400×), and mitotic atypia (Fig. 6-157). Cytoplasm is generally moderate to abundant, and the degree of pigmentation is highly variable, from darkly pigmented to amelanotic. An infrequent form of spindle cell melanoma, composed entirely of amelanotic spindle cells, can be impossible to distinguish from fibrosarcoma or neurofibrosarcoma without the aid of immunohistochemistry. Although the epithelioid and spindle cell forms of melanoma are usually pigmented to some degree, the uncommon balloon cell form and signet-ring cell form are usually unpigmented or poorly pigmented.

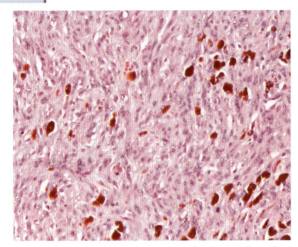

Figure 6-157 Malignant melanoma on the haired skin of a dog with prominent nuclei and mitotic figures.

Balloon cell malignant melanomas are dermal masses that are sometimes multilobulated, and exhibit no junctional activity. The cells are large, with large vesicular nuclei, prominent nucleoli, a relatively low mitotic index, and plentiful clear cytoplasm without visible melanin. Rare cells may have fine pale cytoplasmic dust-like granules. Occasional multinucleated cells can be present.

Signet-ring malignant melanomas are composed of round to polygonal cells that have eccentric nuclei compressed by abundant faintly eosinophilic or amphophilic cytoplasm that is not visibly pigmented. Occasional cells have fine pale brown granules. Nucleoli are prominent. Occasional multinucleated cells can be present.

Further reading

Campagne C, et al. Canine melanoma diagnosis: RACK1 as a potential biological marker. Vet Pathol 2013;50:1083-1090.

Espinosa de Los Monteros A, et al. Immunohistopathologic characterization of a dermal melanocytoma-acanthoma in a German Shepherd dog. Vet Pathol 2000;37:268-271.

Jiang L, et al. Constitutive activation of the ERK pathway in melanoma and skin melanocytes in Grey horses. BMC Cancer 2014;14:857.

Löhr CV. One hundred two tumors in 100 goats (1987-2011). Vet Pathol 2013, 50:668-675.

Munday JS, et al. Cutaneous malignant melanoma in an 11-month-old Russian blue cat. N Z Vet J 2011;59:143-146.

Okomo-Adhiambo M, et al. Gene expression in Sinclair swine with malignant melanoma. Animal 2012;6:179-192.

Phillips JC, Lembcke LM. Equine melanocytic tumors. Vet Clin North Am Equine Pract 2013;29:673-687.

Ramos-Vara JA, et al. Retrospective study of 338 canine oral melanomas with clinical, histologic, and immunohistochemical review of 129 cases. Vet Pathol 2000;37:597-608.

Smedley RC, et al. Prognostic markers for canine melanocytic neoplasms: a comparative review of the literature and goals for future investigation. Vet Pathol 2011;48:54-72.

Trappler MC, et al. Scrotal tumors in dogs: a retrospective study of 676 cases (1986-2010). Can Vet J 2014;55:1229-1233.

Tuohy JL, et al. Outcome following curative-intent surgery for oral melanoma in dogs: 70 cases (1998-2011). J Am Vet Med Assoc 2014;245:1266-1273.

Spindle cell tumors

Tumors arising from spindle-shaped cells of the skin are common in dogs and cats, sporadic in horses, and uncommon to rare in other domestic species. *Classification of these tumors may be difficult, and the nomenclature is inconsistent and controversial.* The tumors are classified according to the mature tissue they resemble, but histologic differences are frequently subtle, and morphologic appearance may not be specific enough to reflect histogenesis, particularly for malignant spindle cell tumors. Consequently, *accurate diagnosis by morphologic features alone may not be possible for many tumors.* An immunohistochemical study of canine cutaneous fibrosarcoma, hemangiopericytoma, and schwannoma found poor correlation between morphologic diagnosis and tumor cell differentiation. Although electron microscopy and immunohistochemistry may be helpful in determining the line of differentiation exhibited by tumor cells, some tumors defy identification because of conflicting results because of loss or alteration in antigens normally present or acquisition of novel antigens. Classification of spindle cell neoplasms is considered important because of the expectation that it will provide a prediction of the biological behavior of the tumor. Exact identification of spindle cell sarcomas of the skin may not be essential, however, because *most soft tissue spindle cell tumors exhibit similar behavior and prognosis. The tumors are typically locally invasive, recur frequently after surgical excision, but metastasize infrequently.* On gross examination, soft tissue sarcomas can appear well circumscribed or even encapsulated; however, *finger-like microextensions of tumor may commonly infiltrate into the surrounding tissue to give rise to satellite lesions that are not visible grossly.* The apparent tumor circumscription commonly results in incomplete excision, leaving microscopic foci of tumor tissue that result in recurrence. Wide surgical excision may be curative, however. Because determination of adequacy of excision is prognostic, *surgical margins should be marked.*

The *proposed grading system* for soft tissue sarcomas is based on the combination of 3 morphologic features: differentiation score (i.e., how well the sarcoma resembles normal tissue (1-3 with the higher number being poorly differentiated), mitotic index (scores 1-3), and tumor necrosis (0-2). A grade of I, II, or III is assigned by the total score of each category (i.e., ≤3 for grade 1; 4-5 for grade II; ≥6 for grade III). The grading system is useful for predicting which neoplasms are likely to recur and metastasize. For any grade, tumors with complete margins are unlikely to recur. Grade III tumors with close surgical margins are likely to recur, whereas grade I tumors infrequently recur, and grade II have an intermediate risk of recurrence. Metastasis is very rare for grade 1 tumors, rare to infrequent for grade II, and grade III tumors have an increased risk. The reader is referred to the Dennis, et al., 2011 reference for more information.

The *mitotic index* is more important than the tumor type in predicting the biologic behavior of most soft tissue sarcomas in dogs.

Benign spindle cell tumors

Skin tags (fibrovascular papilloma, acrochordon, skin polyp) are benign, fibrovascular lesions of middle-aged and older dogs that may be a *proliferative response to trauma or inflammation rather than actual neoplasms.* They are solitary or multiple; soft, polypoid, or filiform; hairless masses up to 1 cm in diameter and 2-3 cm long that occur most commonly on the *trunk,* sternum, *and bony prominences* of the limbs. Microscopically, skin tags are composed of mature collagenous tissue that is more highly vascular than normal dermis and covered by an irregularly hyperplastic, hyperkeratotic, and hyperpigmented epidermis. Adnexal structures are absent, and mononuclear inflammatory cells may be present in low numbers. Ulceration and neutrophilic inflammation are common sequelae to trauma.

Collagenous hamartomas (collagen nevi) *are focal nodular accumulations of excessive dermal collagen that are relatively common in middle-aged and older dogs.* They are typically solitary, alopecic, firm, dome-shaped nodules up to 1 cm in diameter. Microscopically, they are composed of haphazardly arranged bundles of collagen and low numbers of mature fibroblasts that entrap adnexal structures and result in their distortion or atrophy. Collagenous hamartomas are usually located in the dermis, but large masses may extend into the subcutis. The primary differential is fibroma, which tends to be larger and located deeper in the dermis, displaces and compresses adjacent structures, and is more cellular than a collagenous hamartoma. Some veterinary pathologists believe that collagen hamartomas are actually fibromas of low cellularity.

A syndrome called **nodular dermatofibrosis**, characterized by *multiple cutaneous collagenous hamartomas*, has been reported as *a marker of renal epithelial neoplasia in German Shepherd dogs* (see also the previous section Cutaneous paraneoplastic syndromes). The condition is thought to be inherited in an autosomal dominant manner. Affected dogs are adults, and most have bilateral renal cystadenocarcinomas. Nodules may number in the hundreds and are located anywhere on the body. Individual cases in several other breeds have also been reported. Histologically, the lesions are similar to collagen hamartomas and are differentiated primarily on the basis of the large number of lesions present and the breed affected.

Fibromas *are uncommon benign tumors of fibroblasts and collagen that occur in adult and aged animals of all species.* Fibromas are usually solitary, soft to firm, well-circumscribed, round, dome-shaped, or pedunculated masses that vary from 1-50 cm in diameter. They are usually alopecic and may be hyperpigmented. Large tumors may be ulcerated secondary to trauma. Microscopically, fibromas are well-circumscribed, nonencapsulated, dermal or subcutaneous nodules composed of fibroblasts and abundant collagen. The fibroblasts have uniform, oval to elongate, bland nuclei that may be slightly larger than fibroblasts in the normal dermis and have fine chromatin, inconspicuous nucleoli, and rare mitotic figures. The cytoplasm merges imperceptibly with collagen that is arranged in whorls and interwoven bundles that are thicker and more dense than those in the normal dermis. Adnexal structures are usually displaced and compressed peripherally. Some tumors contain substantial amounts of *mucinous or myxomatous matrix material in addition to the collagen*, in which case the term **fibromyxoma** may be used. In contrast to collagenous hamartomas, fibromas are typically larger, more highly cellular, and displace rather than incorporate adnexal structures.

Myxomas (myxofibromas) are *rare cutaneous neoplasms arising from fibroblasts or multipotential mesenchymal cells and containing abundant glycosaminoglycan stroma.* They usually occur in adult or aged animals as solitary, infiltrative, soft masses that are poorly circumscribed and may extend along fascial planes. The tissue is pale and exudes clear viscous fluid on cut surface. A report of a myxoma developing at the site of a subcutaneously implanted pacemaker in a dog raised the question of whether the implant may have induced the tumor. Microscopically, myxomas are nonencapsulated dermal or subcutaneous masses composed of small stellate to spindle cells randomly distributed within abundant basophilic mucinous stroma with scant, fine collagen fibers. Cellularity is typically low, and the cells have small hyperchromatic nuclei and rare mitotic figures. *Recurrence is common because of the infiltrative growth pattern.* Myxomas are difficult to differentiate from myxosarcomas because both are poorly circumscribed, locally infiltrative, and have low mitotic activity. However, nuclear and cellular pleomorphism is more apparent, and atypical mitotic figures may be seen in myxosarcomas.

Locally infiltrative and malignant spindle cell tumors

Canine perivascular wall tumors (PWTs) are mesenchymal neoplasms that were previously referred to as *hemangiopericytomas*. The tumors *are relatively common, histologically distinctive spindle cell tumors of dogs.* The nomenclature was changed to reflect the origin of the tumor (i.e., derived from components of the vascular wall but not the endothelium). The category of PWT includes the following: **glomus tumor, true hemangiopericytoma, angioleiomyoma/sarcoma, angiomyofibroblastoma, and angiofibroma.** A large battery of immunohistochemical stains is necessary to differentiate the subtypes, but is generally not needed. *All PWTs have similar biological behaviors, and are infiltrative, often invading along fascial planes, and are commonly recurrent;* metastasis is uncommon. Increased cellular pleomorphism is seen with each subsequent recurrence. Occasional tumors with similar microscopic features are seen in horses and cats The tumors usually occur on the *limbs of older dogs* of either sex and any breed but are most common in large-breed (>30 kg) dogs. They are usually solitary, slow-growing, multinodular masses that appear grossly well circumscribed and measure up to 25 cm in diameter. The tissue is usually pale, and the consistency varies from soft to very firm. The tumors *frequently recur following excision* because of the difficulty in identifying tumor margins and inability to perform wide surgical excision because of anatomic constraints. *Metastasis is uncommon*, however.

Perivascular wall tumors are usually located in the dermis and subcutis and are primarily composed of uniform plump spindle cells with oval nuclei, fine chromatin, and small central nucleoli. The characteristic microscopic feature of PWTs is *plump spindle cells arranged in concentric layers to form whorls, sometimes with small vessels within the centers* (Fig. 6-158). Sheets and interlacing bundles of similar spindle cells, occasional polygonal cells and multinucleated cells, and variable amounts of collagen also comprise most tumors. Densely cellular areas alternate with loose, myxomatous-appearing areas. Aggregates of lymphocytes may be scattered within some tumors and are usually most prominent along the periphery. At the margins of the tumor, *finger-like microextensions* of tumor cells commonly infiltrate along fascial planes and are the reason many tumors are incompletely excised despite the clinical impression that they are well circumscribed.

Recent investigations in the prognosis of perivascular wall tumors has aided the ability to predict behavior. The tumors fall into 1 of 3 prognostic profiles. **Profile 1** are tumors on the limbs that exhibit expansile growth in the subcutis. Limb

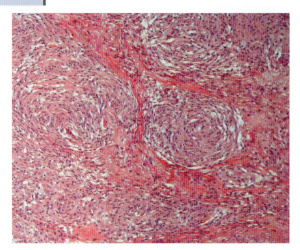

Figure 6-158 **Perivascular wall tumor** ("hemangiopericytoma") in a dog. Note the plump spindle cells arranged in concentric layers to form whorls, sometimes with small vessels within the centers.

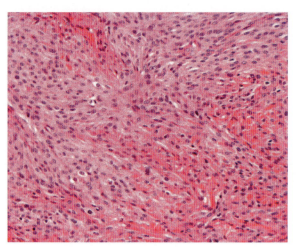

Figure 6-159 **Peripheral nerve sheath tumor** taken from the ear of a cat.

tumors with incomplete or close surgical margins have an intermediate risk of recurrence. **Profile 2** includes tumors that not located on extremities that exhibit infiltrative growth or satellite nodules that extend to skeletal muscle. Profile 2 tumors with incomplete or close margins have a high risk of recurrence. **Profile 3** tumors are similar to profile 2, except that the tumor depth reaches only to the subcutis and not to the depth of skeletal muscle. Profile 3 tumors have a low risk of recurrence with any margins (complete, incomplete, close). The *size of the tumors* has been associated with increased relapse probability. Dogs with tumors >5 cm were about 6 times greater to relapse than dogs with tumors <5 cm. Fortunately, *cases in any profile with complete surgical margins typically do not recur.* For more information, see Avallone et al., 2014. PWTs should be differentiated from fibrosarcomas, rhabdomyosarcomas, and hemangiosarcomas.

Cutaneous tumors of neural origin are uncommon in domestic animals but are likely under-diagnosed because of their histologic similarity to other more common tumors of the skin. They can be composed of one or more elements of a nerve, that is, axon, Schwann cell, and perineurial fibroblast. Consequently, these tumors are histologically heterogeneous, and the histogenesis is frequently uncertain, resulting in various and confusing classifications and terminologies in the literature. They have been called neurofibromas/neurofibrosarcomas, neurilemmomas, neurinomas, and schwannomas/malignant schwannomas. The name **peripheral nerve sheath tumor** is a broad term proposed to include all tumors arising from peripheral nerves; however, because most tumors are composed of Schwann cells, the term **schwannoma** is appropriate for the majority of the tumors. Both benign and malignant forms occur; however, tumors that appear histologically benign commonly recur. Schwannomas are common in **cattle** but occur primarily in the heart and rarely involve the skin. A condition termed **neurofibromatosis** has been observed in cattle of all ages and may occur congenitally. It is characterized by multiple neural tumors that usually involve deep nerves and viscera but sometimes also the skin.

Cutaneous peripheral nerve sheath tumors are usually solitary, well-circumscribed, slow-growing, soft to firm nodules in middle-aged to aged animals. In cats, the head and distal limbs may be involved most frequently. Schwannomas are usually subcutaneous in dogs; in cats, they may be confined to the dermis. Microscopically, *schwannomas are most commonly composed of small spindle cells characterized by oval, spindle-shaped, or wavy nuclei; fine chromatin; small inconspicuous nucleoli; and pale indistinct cytoplasm. The spindle cells form whorls, interlacing fascicles, and palisades reminiscent of nerve* (Fig. 6-159). A delicate collagenous stroma is moderately abundant, and a mucinous matrix may be prominent in some tumors. Delicate finger-like projections of tumor cells commonly extend into adjacent tissues and between fascial planes, accounting for frequent recurrences. Cellularity is increased, cellular pleomorphism is more prominent, and there is a decreased tendency to form whorls and palisades in malignant tumors. Mitotic figures are uncommon in benign tumors but may be moderately numerous in malignant peripheral nerve sheath tumors. Histologically and behaviorally, peripheral nerve sheath tumors may be difficult to differentiate from fibromas, well-differentiated fibrosarcomas, and PWTs. However, *neural tumors express S-100 protein, myelin basic protein, neuron-specific enolase, and glial fibrillary acidic protein, whereas the other more common cutaneous tumors do not.* In dogs, malignant peripheral nerve sheath tumors may arise within the peripheral nervous system (PNS) or within non-PNS soft tissue. It is important to distinguish those tumors arising within peripheral nerves from non-PNS nerve sheath tumors, as the former have a poor prognosis. Tumors arising within peripheral nerves have been shown to have higher S-100 and Olig 2 expression than peripheral nerve sheaths tumors arising in soft tissue. Immunohistochemical staining of **granular cell tumors** (granular cell myoblastomas) has demonstrated S-100 protein, myelin basic protein, and neuron-specific enolase within tumor cells, suggesting that they also represent a form of peripheral nerve sheath tumor.

Traumatic neuroma (tail dock neuroma, amputation neuroma) is considered an exuberant but non-neoplastic proliferation of the proximal nerve stump occurring in response to injury or surgery. In veterinary medicine, this lesion is rare and occurs most frequently as a result of tail docking in **dogs.** The tumors develop in young dogs, usually within 1 year after caudectomy. They are typically painful, self-traumatized, alopecic, hyperpigmented, lichenified lesions adherent to the underlying deep tissues at the tip of the tail. Microscopically, traumatic neuromas are well-circumscribed nodules composed of *haphazardly arranged myelinated nerve bundles of variable size randomly distributed within a relatively abundant connective tissue stroma.*

Fibrosarcomas are malignant tumors of fibroblasts that show no other evidence of cell differentiation. They commonly recur and may metastasize. *Fibrosarcomas are undoubtedly over-diagnosed*, as virtually any anaplastic highly cellular spindle cell sarcoma containing collagen is diagnosed as a fibrosarcoma when more specific histogenesis is not apparent. However, as *immunohistochemistry* has become a routine technique in most diagnostic laboratories, fibrosarcoma can be separated from other spindle cell tumors, such as peripheral nerve sheath tumor, leiomyosarcoma, rhabdomyosarcoma, amelanotic malignant melanoma, spindle cell carcinoma, and others.

Fibrosarcomas are common in dogs and cats and uncommon in other domestic species. In **dogs**, they usually occur in older animals and are most common on the trunk and limbs. They usually arise in the subcutis and are poorly circumscribed masses of variable size that may be soft to firm in consistency. Large tumors are often ulcerated and alopecic. Most canine fibrosarcomas are low-grade malignancies that commonly recur locally and metastasize infrequently. Similarities have been noted between canine fibrosarcomas from presumed injection sites and feline postvaccinal fibrosarcomas, suggesting that postinjection sarcomas may also occur in dogs.

Fibrosarcoma is the most common malignant mesenchymal tumor of **cats**, and 3 forms of fibrosarcoma have been recognized: virus-induced, solitary in older cats, and postvaccinal.

Virus-induced fibrosarcoma is rare. *Feline sarcoma virus* (FeSV) is the cause of multicentric fibrosarcoma in cats usually <5 years of age. FeSV is a replication-defective retrovirus that requires *Feline leukemia virus* (FeLV) as a helper virus. The genetic recombination of the 2 viruses produces an acutely transforming virus that induces multiple simultaneous rapidly growing fibrosarcomas after a short incubation period. FeSV-induced fibrosarcomas are typically locally invasive and metastasize to lung and other sites.

Solitary fibrosarcomas in older cats are much more common than virus-induced multicentric tumors. These may arise in the dermis or subcutis. Subcutaneous tumors are usually on the trunk and limbs; dermal tumors primarily involve the digits and pinnae. The clinical appearance and behavior of this type of fibrosarcoma are similar to those in dogs.

Epidemiologic evidence supports a relationship between vaccine administration in cats and the development of **postvaccinal fibrosarcomas** and, to a lesser extent, other sarcomas in injection sites. Vaccination site fibrosarcomas have also been reported in ferrets and putatively in dogs. The interval between vaccination and tumor development is 3 months to 3.5 years. The mechanism of tumor development is unknown, but persistent injection-site–induced inflammation leading to deranged fibrous connective tissue repair response and eventual neoplastic transformation in genetically predisposed cats has been postulated. Alterations in oncogene and growth factor expression may be involved in the pathogenesis. Postvaccinal fibrosarcomas typically develop in the subcutis of the dorsal cervical and interscapular area, dorsal and lateral thorax, flank, and musculature of the thigh, locations that are all *common vaccination sites*. These tumors arise in cats that are younger (median age 8 years) than those with fibrosarcomas at nonvaccination sites (median age 10.5 years) and are larger than nonvaccination site fibrosarcomas. The masses frequently have cystic centers, firm attachments to dorsal spinous processes or other deep structures, and ill-defined margins. *They are biologically aggressive and commonly recur multiple times within a period of weeks to months when removed*. The metastatic rate is not well characterized, but was found to be as high as 24% in one study. The lungs and regional lymph nodes are the most common sites of metastasis. Wide surgical excision prolongs the interval to recurrence but often fails to remove the tumor completely. Radiation therapy and chemotherapy are under evaluation as adjunctive treatment to prevent local recurrence and systemic spread, respectively.

Microscopically, *fibrosarcomas consist of interlacing and intersecting bundles of immature fibroblastic cells.* The tumors show a great deal of variation with respect to cellular pleomorphism and density, mitotic activity, and amount and maturity of collagen. Multinucleated giant cells are seen in many fibrosarcomas but are not numerous. The tumors are dermal, subcutaneous, or both. They are usually nonencapsulated, and local invasion is evident as finger-like projections of tumor cells extending along fascial planes and into surrounding tissues. These microscopic extensions of the tumor account for the difficulty in excising the tumor completely and resultant recurrences. Although collagen is the primary stromal element, mucin may also be produced in small amounts. Immunohistochemical staining is *positive for vimentin* only. *Retrospective studies have found only the mitotic index* (total number of mitotic figures in 10 [400×] HPFs) *to be significant in predicting tumor behavior*. In dogs, a mitotic index <9 was associated with greater survival than a mitotic index of 9 or greater. Likewise, cats with solitary fibrosarcomas with a mitotic index of 5 or less had significantly greater survival time than cats with tumors with mitotic index of 6 or greater. Poorly differentiated fibrosarcomas may be difficult to differentiate from a number of other mesenchymal and nonmesenchymal tumors, including malignant schwannoma, malignant fibrous histiocytoma, leiomyosarcoma, and spindle cell forms of amelanotic melanoma and squamous cell carcinoma. In such cases, immunohistochemical staining is necessary to exclude other tumors by showing lack of immunoreactivity to antigens typical of other cell types. In small biopsies with a limited amount of tissue to evaluate, it may be difficult to differentiate fibrosarcoma from reactive granulation tissue.

Postvaccinal fibrosarcomas are typically subcutaneous and have large cavitated centers as a result of extensive necrosis. An inflammatory reaction, consisting of lymphocytes and macrophages that sometimes contain gray-brown or blue globular material typical of a vaccine reaction, is commonly present at the periphery of the tumor. Mitotic activity and cellular pleomorphism tend to be high. Tumor cells of vaccination-site fibrosarcomas have been reported to be consistently strongly immunoreactive for platelet-derived growth factor and its receptor, epidermal growth factor and its receptor, and transforming growth factor-β, whereas non–vaccine-associated fibrosarcomas are negative or only slightly positive.

Undifferentiated pleomorphic sarcoma *(malignant fibrous histiocytoma, giant cell tumor of soft parts, extraskeletal giant cell tumor) is an uncommon tumor of controversial histogenesis.* It was originally believed to be derived from malignant cells of monocyte-macrophage origin capable of acting as "facultative" fibroblasts. Ultrastructural and immunohistochemical findings, however, indicate that malignant fibrous histiocytoma may not be a distinct entity but rather a *collection of anaplastic mesenchymal and nonmesenchymal tumors*. Historically, the diagnosis of malignant fibrous histiocytoma was made for those neoplasms characterized histologically by the *combination of fibroblast-like spindle cells, vacuolated histiocyte-like cells, and variable numbers of pleomorphic multinucleated giant cells, along with a collagenous stroma*. The tumors may now be classified into specific soft tissue tumors (e.g., histiocytic sarcoma) or pleomorphic undifferentiated sarcoma.

Other mesenchymal tumors

Tumors arising from subcutaneous lipocytes occur in all species. **Lipomas** are most common in dogs and may be multiple. In all species, they usually occur in adult and aged animals and are most commonly located on the trunk and proximal limbs. *Lipomas are masses of well-differentiated lipocytes indistinguishable from normal fat*, except for a compressed boundary of delicate stroma that normally serves to delineate the margin between tumor and adjacent normal adipose tissue. Some lipomas contain cartilage, bone, collagen, or blood vessels. In addition, some mesenchymal tumors contain roughly equal proportions of adipose tissue mixed with other mesenchymal components. These form distinctive variants, such as *angiolipomas, fibrolipomas,* and *leiomyolipomas*. Occasionally, hemangiosarcomas and mast cell tumors may be found arising within lipomatous masses, suggesting that lipomas may sometimes provide a local environment suitable for the emergence of these more sinister neoplasms. Necrosis, hemorrhage, fibrosis, and mild macrophage inflammation may occur as a result of trauma to lipomas.

Infiltrative lipomas are uncommon tumors of dogs. They are usually large, poorly delineated, deep subcutaneous masses composed of well-differentiated lipocytes that infiltrate subcutaneous muscle and fascia. They may cause pain or interfere with limb function and may invade through the body wall.

Liposarcomas are malignant tumors of lipocytes and are uncommon in all species. Liposarcomas in cats have been associated with retrovirus infection and with vaccination sites; a liposarcoma in a dog was associated with a glass foreign body. *Liposarcomas may recur but rarely metastasize. They are usually well-circumscribed, nonencapsulated, highly cellular masses of round to polyhedral cells primarily and fewer stellate, spindle, and multinucleated cells*. Lipocyte origin is recognized by the presence of *cytoplasmic vacuolation* that may be numerous fine vacuoles or a single large clear vacuole that displaces the nucleus peripherally. Mitotic figures are generally infrequent. *Myxoid liposarcomas* have prominent mucinous ground substance. Liposarcomas may be difficult to differentiate from anaplastic sebaceous carcinomas and balloon cell or clear cell melanomas. The tumor cells of liposarcoma are usually arranged in solid sheets of vacuolated cells, whereas in sebaceous carcinoma, the cells tend to be subdivided into nests and lobules. The presence of rare cells with cytoplasmic dusting of very fine brown granules can differentiate melanoma from the other 2 tumors; however, immunohistochemical staining for cytokeratin, vimentin, and a melanocytic marker (such as Melan A) may be needed to differentiate the tumors.

Tumors originating from muscle are rare in the skin of animals. Smooth muscle tumors, **leiomyomas** and **leiomyosarcomas**, can arise from arrector pili muscles (*piloleiomyomas*), cutaneous blood vessels (*angioleiomyomas*), and specialized muscles of genital skin. These tumors are usually solitary, firm, and well-circumscribed in animals. In humans, piloleiomyomas are commonly multiple; and multiple piloleiomyomas have been reported in an old cat. Microscopically, leiomyomas are small, well-circumscribed dermal masses adjacent to and surrounding hair follicles. They are composed of uniform long spindle cells in whorling and interlacing bundles. The cells have bland elongate nuclei with blunt ends ("cigar-shaped") and moderately abundant pale eosinophilic cytoplasm. Mitotic figures are rare. Leiomyosarcomas exhibit nuclear pleomorphism and low to moderate mitotic activity. Angioleiomyomas consist of interlacing bundles of smooth muscle cells between numerous vascular channels. Smooth muscle tumors may be confused with fibromas, fibrosarcomas, or malignant schwannomas. In such cases, *immunohistochemical staining for actin and desmin can confirm muscle origin*.

Cutaneous tumors of skeletal muscle, **rhabdomyomas** and **rhabdomyosarcomas,** are extremely rare. Rhabdomyomas of the ear pinna have been reported in 4 white-eared cats. The tumors were thinly haired, red-purple, nonulcerated discoid nodules 1-2 cm in diameter on the convex surface of the pinna. Histologically, they were well-circumscribed masses composed of whorls and bundles of long spindle cells with cross-striations evident in a few tumor cells. Mitotic figures were rare. Surgical excision was curative.

Further reading

Avallone G, et al. Canine perivascular wall tumors: high prognostic impact of site, depth, and completeness of margins. Vet Pathol 2014;51:713-721.

Avallone G, et al. The spectrum of canine cutaneous perivascular wall tumors: morphologic, phenotypic and clinical characterization. Vet Pathol 2007;44:607-620.

Choi H, et al. Undifferentiated pleomorphic sarcoma (malignant fibrous histiocytoma) of the head in a dog. J Vet Med Sci 2011;73:235-239.

Dennis MM, et al. Prognostic factors for cutaneous and subcutaneous soft tissue sarcomas in dogs. Vet Pathol 2011;48:73-84.

Munday JS, et al. Histology and immunohistochemistry of seven ferret vaccination-site fibrosarcomas. Vet Pathol 2003;40:288-293.

Vascellari M, et al. Fibrosarcomas at presumed sites of injection in dogs: characteristics and comparison with non-vaccination site fibrosarcomas and feline post-vaccinal fibrosarcomas. J Vet Med A Physiol Pathol Clin Med 2003;50:286-291.

Vascular tumors

Cutaneous vasoformative tumors are common in dogs, occasional in cats and horses, and uncommon in other species. The majority are benign in dogs and horses, whereas malignant tumors are more common in cats. Vascular tumors may be associated with thrombocytopenia, disseminated intravascular coagulation, and other hemostatic abnormalities.

Hemangioma *is a benign neoplasm of blood vessel endothelium that can originate in the dermis or subcutis*. The tumor is usually a solitary, well-circumscribed, fluctuant to firm, blue to red-black, slow-growing mass. Cutaneous hemangioma in **dogs** usually occurs in older animals (mean, 9-10 years) without apparent sex predilection. The tumor can occur anywhere, but lightly pigmented, sparsely haired, ventral abdominal, and inguinal skin may be predisposed. Chronic solar damage has been suggested as a cause of dermal hemangiomas in this location, and they may be multiple. Surgical excision is curative.

Benign cutaneous vascular lesions in **horses** frequently occur in animals <1 year of age, and some are congenital, raising the question of whether the lesions are true neoplasms or vascular malformations (hamartoma or nevus). The confusion in categorizing these vascular lesions in young horses has resulted in *inconsistent nomenclature,* and they have been referred to as **lobular capillary hemangioma** and **vascular nevus** in the literature. The lesions are most commonly located on the limbs and occur as a cauliflower or nodular mass or diffuse skin thickening that may become alopecic and ulcerated. The lesions may recur following excision. In some instances, they are too extensive to be excised, necessitating euthanasia of the affected animal. Cutaneous hemangiomas usually occur in adult and aged **cattle;** congenital hemangiomas have been reported also, and these are frequently multiple.

Microscopically, hemangiomas consist of nonencapsulated dermal or subcutaneous masses composed of blood-filled channels lined by a single layer of flattened, mature endothelium (Fig. 6-160). Mitotic figures are rare. Subcutaneous tumors are usually well circumscribed, whereas those in the dermis may not be as well defined and may incorporate adnexal structures within the mass. The tumors are classified as *capillary* or *cavernous,* depending on the size of the vascular spaces. The cavernous type is more common in dogs. The vascular channels are usually separated by collagenous septa that contain variable numbers of mast cells, lymphoid cells, and hemosiderin-laden macrophages. Occasional vascular channels contain fibrin thrombi. *Solar-induced dermal hemangiomas* of glabrous skin are located in the superficial dermis and may be associated with solar elastosis.

A variant of hemangioma, called **angiokeratoma,** is a raised superficial dermal hemangioma with prominent, irregular hyperplasia of the epidermis that extends down to separate and partially surround the vascular channels. The *lobular capillary hemangioma/vascular nevus of young horses* consists of multiple discrete dermal lobules of closely packed, haphazardly arranged vascular structures of small caliber. The vessels are lined by endothelial cells with plump oval nuclei and low-mitotic activity.

Cutaneous angiomatosis is a vascular endothelial proliferative disorder, characterized by irregular blood-filled capillaries in the dermis and subcutis. Lesions can appear as red to purple macules, papules, nodules, or plaques. It occurs in cattle and horses most commonly and also is reported in dogs, cats, llamas, and goats. *Bacillary angiomatosis* caused by infection with *Bartonella* spp. has been described in an immunocompromised dog. *Multisystem progressive angiomatosis* affecting the skin, gastrointestinal tract, and visceral surface of the abdominal organs, a syndrome resembling blue rubber bleb nevus syndrome, has been described in one dog. Further, there is a report of cutaneous angiomatosis causing sepsis in one dog.

Hemangiosarcoma, the malignant form of a tumor of blood vessel endothelium, can occur in the skin as a primary site or as a result of metastatic disease from a primary visceral tumor. These tumors usually occur in adult and aged animals. In one study of cutaneous vascular tumors of cats, hemangiosarcomas occurred most frequently in white-haired sites and most commonly involved the pinnae and head. Cutaneous hemangiosarcoma commonly recurs following excision and has the potential for widespread local invasion and metastasis; but in general, it appears to be less aggressive, has a longer clinical course, and prolonged survival when compared to visceral hemangiosarcomas. In contrast to the subcutaneous form, dermal hemangiosarcoma may be cured by wide surgical excision alone.

The degree of differentiation is extremely variable, ranging from well-differentiated tumors with well-defined vascular channels to poorly differentiated tumors with minimal lumen formation. *Usually hemangiosarcomas consist of plump pleomorphic endothelial cells arranged in single or multiple layers along trabeculae of collagen or pre-existing dermal collagen fibers to form a poorly circumscribed meshwork of blood-filled spaces.* Collagenous trabeculae lined by endothelial cells commonly protrude blindly into the vascular spaces. Mitotic activity may be high. Frequently, portions or entire tumors are composed entirely of sheets or intersecting and anastomosing bundles of pleomorphic spindle cells, and they may be indistinguishable from fibrosarcoma or other poorly differentiated spindle cell sarcomas. The presence of slit-like spaces containing erythrocytes between tumor cells may be the only clue to the diagnosis. Immunohistochemical staining may be required to identify the cells in anaplastic tumors. Endothelial cells express vimentin, factor VIII–related antigen (von Willebrand factor), and CD31 (platelet-endothelial cell adhesion molecule/PECAM). However, *immunostaining must be interpreted with knowledge of limitations of the procedure;* in poorly differentiated tumors, very anaplastic cells may not express typical antigens, and immature reactive stromal endothelial cells may be mistaken for tumor cells.

Tumors arising from endothelium of lymphatic vessels are rare in domestic animals. Both the benign, **lymphangioma,** and malignant, **lymphangiosarcoma,** forms occur in young animals, and it has been suggested that they represent lymphatic malformations resulting from a failure of connection between lymph vessels and the venous system rather than being true neoplasms. *The skin and subcutis appear to be the most common site of tumors of lymphatic endothelium, and the caudal ventral abdomen and inguinal areas appear to be predisposed.* They typically occur as poorly defined fluctuant or edematous masses that are present for many months and drain clear serous to milky fluid. Rarely, they occur as multiple clear turgid vesicles or bullae. It may be difficult to distinguish between lymphangioma and lymphangiosarcoma

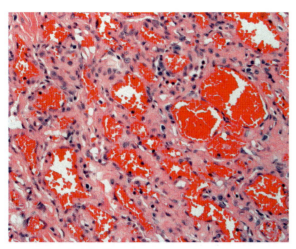

Figure 6-160 Cutaneous **hemangioma** in a dog.

histologically because the histologic appearance may not correlate well with the biologic behavior of the tumor. Tumors that appear histologically benign commonly recur and may be locally invasive. Lymphangiosarcomas commonly invade local tissues extensively and metastasize to distant sites. They are poorly defined and difficult to remove completely, resulting in poor wound healing and recurrence. In contrast to tumors of vascular endothelium, *lymphangiomas/lymphangiosarcomas are composed of spaces largely devoid of material*. They may contain only small amounts of proteinaceous fluid and low numbers of erythrocytes and/or lymphoid cells. The connective tissue stroma separating the vascular spaces is loose or edematous and may contain aggregates of lymphoid cells. These tumors have been reported to be immunoreactive for factor VIII–related antigen (von Willebrand factor); CD31 reactivity is variable. Ulceration, hemorrhage, granulation tissue proliferation, and inflammation are frequently present because of the chronic clinical course and may result in misdiagnosis when a small biopsy is taken. It may not be possible to differentiate a poorly differentiated lymphangiosarcoma from hemangiosarcoma. Further complicating diagnosis is a condition called **lymphangiomatosis**, which is considered a developmental disorder composed of bland dilated lymph channels involving skin, soft tissue, bone, and parenchymal organs.

Feline ventral abdominal lymphangiosarcoma is a tumor that causes marked swelling on the abdominal skin, with erythema and ulcers that ooze serous fluid. The abdomen often has a bruised appearance. These neoplasms were previously termed "angiosarcomas," but a detailed case series confirmed a lymphatic origin via a positive-staining marker for lymphatic vessels ((LYVE-1, lymphatic vessel endothelial receptor 1), and ultrastructural findings. The tumors are markedly infiltrative, difficult to completely excise, and commonly recur. Metastasis is rare.

Further reading

Asa SA, et al. Expression of platelet-derived growth factor and its receptors in spontaneous canine hemangiosarcoma and cutaneous hemangioma. Histol Histopathol 2012;27:601-607.

Curran KM, et al. Lymphangiosarcoma in 12 dogs: a case series (1998-2013). Vet Comp Oncol 2014;doi:10.1111/vco.12087; [Epub ahead of print].

Galeotti F, et al. Feline lymphangiosarcoma—definitive identification using a lymphatic vascular marker. Vet Dermatol 2004;15:13-18.

Sluiter KL, et al. Bacterial sepsis resulting in severe systemic illness and euthanasia in a dog with cutaneous angiomatosis. Can Vet J 2013;54:397-402.

Woldemeskel M, Rajeev S. Mast cells in canine cutaneous hemangioma, hemangiosarcoma and mammary tumors. Vet Res Commun 2010;34:153-160.

Histiocytic proliferative disorders

Histiocytic proliferative disorders are commonly observed in dogs, less often in cats, and rarely in piglets. There is a case report of malignant histiocytosis in an Arabian filly and a case report of a histiocytic sarcoma in the nasal cavity of a Dutch Warmblood horse. Histiocytic proliferative diseases recognized in dogs include **histiocytoma, cutaneous Langerhans cell (LC) histiocytosis, cutaneous histiocytosis, systemic histiocytosis,** and **histiocytic sarcoma (localized** and **disseminated)**. In cats, **feline progressive histiocytosis, feline pulmonary LC histiocytosis,** and **histiocytic sarcoma** have been described. **Congenital cutaneous histiocytosis** has been described in piglets.

Histiocytes differentiate from CD34+ stem cell precursors found in the bone marrow into macrophages and several dendritic cell (DC) lineages, such as LCs and interstitial DCs. DCs and macrophages have overlapping functions in that both can function as antigen-presenting cells and can act as effector cells. *Macrophages* are primarily effector cells and act as elements of the innate immune system, whereas *dendritic cells* function primarily in antigen presentation and hence provide a strong influence on the adaptive immune system. The morphologic features of neoplastic or abnormally reactive histiocytes are similar and can mimic tumor cells of different histogenic origin or be confused with granulomatous inflammation. Differentiation often requires immunophenotyping and sometimes ultrastructural characterization.

Canine cutaneous histiocytoma

Canine cutaneous histiocytomas (CCH) are tumors arising from proliferations of the intraepidermal dendritic cell, the Langerhans cell. Canine cutaneous histiocytomas are most often solitary, benign tumors that usually undergo spontaneous regression in 1-2 months. More than 70% of CCH occur in *dogs <4 years of age* and are most often found on the *head (pinna)*, but can occur anywhere on the body at any age. There is no sex predilection. Boxers and Dachshunds are predisposed. Grossly, the tumors are raised, red, frequently ulcerated and alopecic, 0.5-4 cm, papular to nodular lesions that grow rapidly. Metastasis of a solitary histiocytoma to a local lymph node has been reported, and in all reported cases with follow-up, there was spontaneous regression. The tumors are well demarcated but unencapsulated and located primarily in the dermis, with the base of the tumor smaller in configuration than the more superficial aspect ("top heavy"). Microscopically, *tumor cells form diffuse sheets that displace adnexal structures and dermal collagen, and extend from the epidermis and superficial dermis into the dermis.* Care must be taken to differentiate the lesion from epitheliotropic lymphoma. The epidermis is often attenuated or ulcerated, and associated edema may lead to *vertical rowing of tumor cells* near the surface. Ulceration is associated with infiltrates of neutrophils. The intact epidermis may be hyperplastic. Individual tumor cells are round to oval with moderate to abundant eosinophilic, slightly foamy cytoplasm. Nuclei are centrally located, round to oval, indented or convoluted with vesicular chromatin, and most often have a single nucleolus that may be inconspicuous. *Mitotic figures are variable but most often numerous*, with up to 10-15/HPF. The base of the tumor may have infiltrates of CD8+ cytotoxic T lymphocytes, a sign of *host-mediated spontaneous tumor regression*. Infiltrates of lymphocytes may also be found in perivascular or periadnexal regions. In older lesions, the lymphocytic infiltrates may be more extensive than the remaining tumor cell infiltrates, leading to a misinterpretation of primary inflammatory process or inflamed nonepitheliotropic T-cell lymphoma. *Tumor cell apoptosis and zones of necrosis are common findings*, particularly in regressing lesions but are not present in all CCH. As the function of LCs is to capture antigen and migrate to regional lymph nodes, regional lymph nodes may be enlarged but are not painful and should regress to normal size after tumor removal.

Tumor histiocytes in CCH consistently express vimentin, CD1a, CD11a/CD18, CD11c/CD18, CD44, CD45, and MHC II. They do not express CD90 (Thy-1) or CD45RA. They may also express E-cadherin, lysozyme, CD11d/CD18, and CD54.

Canine cutaneous Langerhans cell histiocytosis
Affected dogs may have hundreds of raised, red, alopecic, and ulcerated cutaneous papules and nodules that are *histologically similar to CCH*. Lesions may involve mucocutaneous junctions and the oral cavity. Lesions are generally limited to skin and draining lymph nodes initially, but spread to internal organs can also occur rarely. The condition occurs in many breeds, although Shar Peis are over-represented. Delayed regression of lesions is common, with some lesions persisting for 10 months. About 50% of affected dogs are euthanized because of complications such as ulceration and secondary bacterial infections. Those with *metastasis* to lymph nodes or widespread metastasis have a worse prognosis. Metastasis to lungs and other viscera has been observed. Histologically, lesions are similar to those of CCH; however, individual lesions may be larger *extending into the subcutis and muscle*. Also there may be a high degree of *cellular atypia* with more anisocytosis and multinucleated cells and a lack of T-cell infiltration. Lymphatic invasion may occur.

Cutaneous and systemic reactive histiocytosis
Cutaneous reactive histiocytosis (CRH) *is an inflammatory lymphohistiocytic proliferative disorder involving the skin, subcutis, and sometimes the local lymph nodes*. Lesions are often multiple and occur as cutaneous to subcutaneous nodules up to 4 cm in diameter, often with overlying ulceration (eFig. 6-17). Common sites are face, nose, neck, trunk, extremities, including pawpads, perineum, and scrotum. Lesions may wax and wane, disappear and reappear in other locations, or spontaneously regress.

Systemic reactive histiocytosis (SRH) is *the term used to designate a similar condition that affects not only the skin, but also lymph nodes and other body organs*. Cutaneous reactive histiocytosis does not necessarily lead to systemic reactive histiocytosis, and not all cases of systemic histiocytosis have cutaneous lesions. SRH has a tendency to involve the skin, ocular and nasal mucosae, and peripheral lymph nodes. It generally affects young to middle-aged dogs, and although it was first described in Bernese Mountain dogs, it has been described in many breeds. Lesions are often multiple, and common sites are nasal planum, eyelids, and scrotum. Clinical signs may include anorexia, weight loss, conjunctivitis, chemosis, and stertorous respiration. Lesions and signs may wax and wane. *Widespread metastasis* to lung, liver, bone marrow, spleen, peripheral and visceral lymph nodes, kidneys, testes, orbital tissues, and nasal mucosa have been described.

Histologically cutaneous lesions are "bottom-heavy," extending from the mid-dermis into the subcutis. *Dermal interstitial DC and T cells infiltrate blood vessel walls in the mid-dermis, leading to lymphohistiocytic vasculitis, which may cause vascular compromise and infarction* (eFig. 6-18). Lymphocytes may comprise 50% of the infiltrate. Smaller numbers of neutrophils, plasma cells, and eosinophils may also be present. Discrete perivascular lesions in the mid-dermis, seen initially, coalesce and form nodular infiltrates extending into the deep dermis and subcutis. Older lesions extend into the more superficial dermis and may have a periadnexal distribution. Epitheliotropism is not a feature. Infiltrates of other tissues and organs in SRH are morphologically similar to the cutaneous infiltrates. Histiocytes express CD1a, C11c/CD18, MHC II, CD4, and Thy-1 (CD90). Histiocytes lack expression of E-cadherin.

The *histologic differential diagnoses* include a response to infectious agents; other causes of periadnexal granulomas, such as idiopathic sterile pyogranulomas; drug reactions; cutaneous histiocytoma; and lymphomatoid granulomatosis.

The prognosis for CRH is good for survival but guarded for cure without long-term therapy. The prognosis for SRH is guarded. Lesions may wax and wane, and the minority of cases of CRH spontaneously regress. Many times, the lesions are slowly progressive and require long-term management with immunomodulatory therapy and often lead to death, particularly if there is systemic involvement.

Histiocytic sarcoma complex
Histiocytic sarcoma (HS) complex includes a number of distinct syndromes: hemophagocytic HS, articular/periarticular HS, central nervous system HS, dendritic cell leukemia, and feline progressive histiocytosis. Here we will focus only on those conditions with cutaneous involvement: localized HS and feline progressive histiocytosis.

Histiocytic sarcomas can be localized, affecting one site, or disseminated (malignant histiocytosis). Once the lesion spreads beyond the draining lymph node, it is considered disseminated. HSs are usually derived from interstitial dendritic cells. The condition occurs in dogs and is rare in cats. Animals are generally middle-aged to older. Bernese Mountain dogs, Rottweilers, Golden Retrievers, and Flat-coated Retrievers are predisposed. Bernese Mountain dogs and Flat-coated Retrievers have abnormalities in tumor suppressor gene loci (*CDKN2A/B*, *RB1*, and *PTEN*). Clinical signs depend on the organ involved and often include anorexia, weight loss, and lethargy. Mild nonregenerative anemia and hypercalcemia may be seen. In the hemophagocytic form, there are no skin lesions, but there is marked, regenerative, hemolytic anemia and thrombocytopenia.

Localized histiocytic sarcomas (LHS) *are rapidly growing malignant neoplasms occurring most often in the skin, subcutis, and associated soft tissues of the extremities.* The tumors are often found in periarticular regions and invade the joint capsule, tendons, and muscles of the region. Other reported primary sites for LHS include the spleen, lymph node, lung, bone marrow, and central nervous system. Grossly, masses are infiltrative and destructive and have a uniform smooth cut surface and are pale tan. Articular HS has a distinctive tan multinodular appearance under the synovial lining.

Disseminated histiocytic sarcoma *is the term now used to refer to the previously described condition of malignant histiocytosis*. Histologically and immunophenotypically, the lesions are identical. It is unclear whether the disseminated histiocytic sarcoma represents metastasis of a primary lesion or multicentric malignant transformation of histiocytes. Secondary sites can be widespread but consistently include liver and lung with primary lung disease and hilar lymph nodes with primary lung disease. Cutaneous involvement is rare with this form. The prognosis is extremely poor, and the condition is rapidly progressive.

Histologically, histiocytic sarcomas consist of a mixture of pleomorphic, anaplastic, plump, round histiocytic cells, and multinucleated histiocytic giant cells. There is marked cytologic atypia with numerous bizarre mitotic figures. Tumor cells have abundant eosinophilic cytoplasm and large oval to indented or twisted vesicular nuclei. Some lesions contain pleomorphic spindle-shaped cells. Mitotic activity is high, and phagocytosis may be evident, although it is much more profound in hemophagocytic HS.

Immunophenotypically, the histiocytic cells comprising these lesions are variable but most consistent with a *dendritic cell origin or occasionally macrophage origin*. Tumors of interstitial dendritic cell origin express CD1a, MDCII, and CD11c/CD18. Expression of CD4 in not observed. In contrast, expression of CD4 in canine reactive histiocytosis indicates an activation phenotype. In hemophagocytic HS, histiocytes express markers most consistent with macrophage differentiation (CD11d/CD18).

Feline progressive histiocytosis

Feline progressive histiocytosis (FPH) originates in the skin from interstitial DCs in middle-aged to older cats. Cutaneous lesions occur as solitary or more commonly multiple firm, nonpruritic, nonpainful, alopecic and ulcerated papules, nodules, and plaques. Head, trunk, and lower extremities are common sites. Lesions may wax and wane, but there is a poor long-term prognosis. Some cats develop invasive, expansile masses in the lymph nodes, lungs, kidneys, spleen, and/or liver. *Histologically, lesions consist of a diffuse dermal infiltrate of morphologically normal histiocytes* that may extend into the subcutis. The epidermis may be ulcerated. About 40% of lesions have epitheliotropism characterized by intraepidermal accumulations of one to multiple clusters of histiocytes. Mitotic activity varies. Late-stage lesions resemble HS. Neoplastic cells express CD1a, CD18, and MHC-II. They lack expression of E-cadherin and about half express CD5.

Congenital histiocytosis is a very rare condition of neonatal *piglets*. Multiple cutaneous macules, papules, and plaques may be widely distributed. On cut surface, they are mottled gray to tan. Histologically, there is a dense infiltrate of spindle cells in short bundles and storiform arrangement in the dermis, extending into the subcutis with variable numbers of histiocytoid cells. A few lymphocytes, plasma cells, and eosinophils may be scattered. There is no epidermotropism, and mitotic activity is low. In one case, expression of lysozyme, CD204, and CD163 within the neoplastic cells supported a histiocytic origin.

Further reading

Affolter VK, Moore PF. Feline progressive histiocytosis. Vet Pathol 2006;43:646-655.

Helie P, et al. Congenital cutaneous histiocytosis in a piglet. Vet Pathol 2013;51:812-815.

Lester GD, et al. Malignant histiocytosis in an Arabian filly. Equine Vet J 1993;25:471-473.

Moore PF. A review of histiocytic disease of dogs and cats. Vet Pathol 2014;51:167-184.

Paciello O, et al. Histiocytic sarcoma of the nasal cavity in a horse. Res Vet Sci 2013;94:648-650.

Mast cell tumors

Single or multiple nodular dermal proliferations of mast cells occur in all domestic species but are *most common in dogs* (Fig. 6-161). When the mast cells are present in large numbers and as an essentially pure population, a diagnosis of mast cell tumor is usually made. Some, more cautiously, consider such growths as *cutaneous mastocytosis* until invasive growth or morphologic evidence of anaplasia confirms their neoplastic nature. As heavy accumulations of mast cells may occur in a variety of parasitic, mycotic, allergic, and idiopathic inflammatory syndromes, caution is warranted; however, sheets of mast cells are not present in these other conditions. Multiple spontaneously regressing mast cell tumors have been reported in young dogs, cats, pigs, calves, foals, and humans, suggesting the underlying process may have been mast cell hyperplasia rather than true neoplasia. Diffuse dermal and subcutaneous infiltrates of well-differentiated mast cells occurring over large areas of the body have been reported in cats, dogs, and a foal. The condition has been compared to *urticaria pigmentosa* in humans.

The histologic lesion is seldom a diagnostic challenge, except in the very poorly differentiated tumors. *The mast cells form diffuse loose sheets or densely packed cords of round cells with a central round nucleus, abundant granular basophilic cytoplasm, and distinct cell membrane* (see Fig. 6-161B). Scattered diffusely among the tumor cells are mature eosinophils. Even solid tumors tend to have some areas composed of cords of tumor cells alternating with collagen bundles, particularly at the infiltrative border of the tumor. They are never encapsulated or even well demarcated, except at their superficial edge. A Grenz zone typically separates them from an intact epidermis. Ulceration in large or traumatized tumors may bring the skin surface in contact with the tumor. Eosinophils are few to numerous. Edema may be very severe, giving the tumor an appearance that macroscopically and microscopically resembles acute inflammation. Foci of tumor necrosis, eosinophilic or mononuclear leukocytic vasculitis, vascular necrosis, mineralization, mucinous extracellular matrix, collagen degeneration, or tumor cells with giant or multiple nuclei are all occasionally encountered. Degenerating collagen may incite granulomatous inflammation. Collagen flame figures may be found in some tumors.

In **dogs**, *mast cell tumors (MCTs) account for 15-20% of skin tumors and are the most frequent malignant or potentially malignant tumor of the skin*. The mean age of affected dogs is ~9 years, with a range of 3 weeks to 19 years. Boxers, Terriers, Boston Terriers, Labrador Retrievers, Beagles, and Schnauzers are reportedly predisposed. Shar-Peis are also predisposed and, in this breed, mast cell tumors often occur at an earlier age than in other breeds. The *macroscopic appearance* of canine mast cell tumors varies widely with their stage of progression and degree of histologic differentiation. Well-differentiated tumors most often appear as a rubbery, nodular nonencapsulated variably alopecic dermal mass 1-4 cm in diameter that clinically resembles a lipoma. Poorly differentiated tumors tend to achieve a large size more quickly, are less circumscribed, and often associated with inflammation and edema of the surrounding dermis and possible satellite lesions. Tumors of intermediate grade have a gross appearance that varies between those described previously.

Other clinical signs may occasionally result from the release of histamine or other vasoactive products from the mast cells. *Gastroduodenal ulceration* is relatively frequent in dogs with disseminated disease, occurring in 35-83% of cases. Histamine release stimulates the specific H2 gastric parietal cell receptors, resulting in increased acid secretion and perhaps local mucosal ischemia. Ulceration follows and may lead to fatal

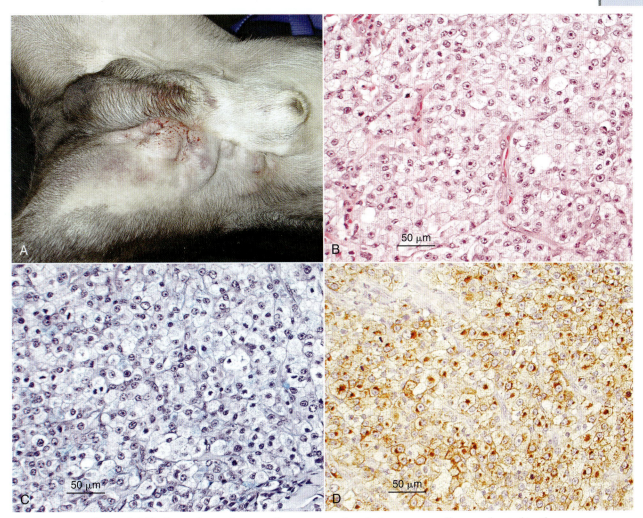

Figure 6-161 Gross photo of **mast cell tumor** in a dog. **A.** Large mast cell tumor located in the inguinal region of a dog, with numerous satellite nodules. **B.** High-grade mast cell tumor. Note the mitoses and karyomegaly. **C.** Toluidine blue stain from the tumor in B showing faint metachromatic granules in the cytoplasm of neoplastic cells. **D.** Cytoplasmic staining with c-Kit in a high-grade mast cell tumor.

exsanguination. *Hypotensive shock* from massive synchronous degranulation, as may occur with cryosurgery, is a rarely reported complication.

Several grading systems have been used for MCTs; until recently the **Patnaik system** was the most widely used. This system designated grade 1 MCTs as well-differentiated tumors with good prognosis, whereas grade 3 MCTs were poorly differentiated tumors with poor prognosis. Grade 2 MCTs were of intermediate differentiation with intermediate prognosis. The histologic features of each grade are as follows: grade 1 (well-differentiated cells, confined to the dermis, no mitoses or necrosis), grade 2 (moderately to highly cellular, extends into the lower dermis/subcutis, 0-2 mitoses/HPF, necrosis/edema/hyalinized collagen), and grade 3 (densely cellular, pleomorphic cells with vesicular nuclei and prominent nucleoli, 3-6/HPF, subcutis involvement, hemorrhage/necrosis/hyalinized collagen). This system left a large gray zone for the prognostication of grade 2 tumors and discordance among pathologists who were grading the tumors.

A newer and more reliable approach is a **2-tiered grading system** that divides MCTs into *high grade* (see Fig. 6-161B) and *low grade. The mitotic index (MI) appears to be a distinct indicator of clinical behavior.* The MI is defined as the number of mitotic figures/10 consecutive HPFs (400×), and within the region of the tumor with the highest overall mitotic activity. In the 2-tier system, the designation of high grade is based on any one of the following criteria: 7 or greater mitotic index, 3 or more multinucleated (3 or more nuclei) cells in 10 HPFs; 3 or more bizarre nuclei in 10 HPFs; karyomegaly (i.e., nuclear diameters of at least 10% of neoplastic cells vary by at least 2-fold). The designation of low-grade MCT is based on the lack of any high-grade criteria. In this system, high-grade tumors had a shorter time to metastasis or new tumor development and shorter survival time. The median survival time was <4 months for high-grade MCTs but >2 years for low-grade MCTs. Additional studies have corroborated the importance of a MI in grading MCTs.

For many MCTs, additional tests are needed to better define the prognosis, and are often requested by veterinary oncologists. High proliferation indices (Ki-67, AgNOR) have been associated with a worse prognosis and poor survival times. The mast/stem cell growth factor receptor (proto-oncogene *c-kit*, CD117) appears to be involved in MCT tumorigenesis. The *KIT* gene encodes the receptor tyrosine kinase that has an extracellular ligand-binding domain (exons 8 and 9), a transmembrane domain (exon 10), a negative regulatory juxtamembrane domain (exons 11 and 12), and a split cytoplasmic kinase. The ligand for *KIT* is stem cell factor (*KIT* ligand, mast cell growth factor). Activating mutations in *KIT* as well as aberrant *c-kit* expression has been demonstrated in canine MCTs. Approximately 15-40% of MCTs show *c-kit* mutations, including internal tandem duplications (ITDs) in the juxtamembrane domain, resulting in constitutive activation of *KIT* in the absence of ligand binding and activating point mutations in *c-kit* extracellular domains. Canine mast cell tumors that are positive for the activating duplication mutation in exon 11 have a shorter disease-free interval and shorter survival times than tumors without the *c-kit* mutation. Tumors with mutations in exon 8 or 11 have an increased likelihood of therapeutic success with tyrosine kinase inhibitors. The Kit staining pattern and protein location also has prognostic significance. The staining is defined as follows: pattern I (perimembrane), pattern II (focal or stippled cytoplasmic staining), and pattern III (diffuse cytoplasmic staining). Increased cytoplasmic staining is associated with increased rate of local recurrence and decreased survival time (see Fig. 6-161D).

Mast cell tumor margin evaluation is routinely performed on all tumors submitted for histopathology. The surgical guidelines for MCTs suggest that these tumors be resected with surgical margins of 2-3 cm laterally and one tissue plane in depth to minimize recurrence. Wide margins are probably not needed for low-grade MCTs, In one study, 29% (15/51) of low-grade tumors had a histologic margin of 3 mm or less, and only 4% (2/51) recurred locally; 36% of high-grade tumors with complete surgical margins recurred locally.

Mast cell tumors in **cats** occur as *primary cutaneous mast cell tumors* and as *visceral mastocytosis*; these are separate diseases. MCTs are the second most common cutaneous neoplasm in the cat, and account for 20% of skin tumors of cats in the United States. The metastatic potential of feline cutaneous MCTs is very low (~5%), and those destined for behavioral malignancy are easily detected by anisocytosis, hyperchromasia, and *mitotic activity*. An MI of >5 has been shown to negatively affect survival time. Apparent recurrence at the surgical site or elsewhere in the skin is seen in 25-50% of cases, but most of these probably represent multicentric origin. Cats with multiple MCTs are often feline immunodeficiency virus–positive. Cats with >5 cutaneous MCTs have a more guarded prognosis. There is *no widely accepted grading system* for feline MCTs.

Mast cell tumors in cats appear as one or several firm, raised pink, alopecic papules ranging in size from millimeters to several centimeters. Less commonly, the tumor appears as a poorly defined area of swelling resulting from an infiltrative rather than nodular lesion. The head and neck are preferred sites. There are 2 histologic subtypes: the *mastocytic type* and the *histiocytic (atypical) type*. Histologically, the cells are usually extraordinarily uniform, polygonal to round, and grow in a diffuse sheet interrupted only by small clusters of lymphocytes and rare eosinophils. The cytoplasm is clear, eosinophilic, or only faintly basophilic. Obvious granularity is infrequent. The nucleus is round, central, and relatively hyperchromatic compared with that of canine mast cells. Even with metachromatic stains, such as Giemsa or toluidine blue, cytoplasmic granules may stain poorly, yet ultrastructurally they are abundant. Occasionally, binucleated, multinucleated, or cells with giant nuclei measuring up to 25 μm may be seen. Eosinophils are seen in only a small number of feline MCTs. The tumor is not encapsulated and is most often confined to the dermis. Collagen degeneration and stromal proliferation are rare. Much less frequent is the *histologic type (atypical, histiocytic)*, seen most often in young cats as multiple, simultaneous, or sequential tumors located at the junction of the dermis and subcutis. Siamese cats are predisposed. The tumor mast cells resemble histiocytes, and the lesion may be mistaken for granulomatous inflammation. Toluidine blue or Giemsa staining may be equivocal. The cells are confirmed as mast cells on electron microscopic examination. Eosinophils, lymphoid aggregates, well-circumscribed growth habit, and benign behavior are similar to the more usual MCT of cats described previously.

Mast cell tumors in **horses** have been cautiously termed *cutaneous mastocytosis*, but the growths are comparable to the cutaneous tumors of other species. They most commonly occur as solitary nodules on the head, trunk, neck, and limbs. The tumors may be hyperpigmented, alopecic, or ulcerated. Collagen degeneration, large aggregates of eosinophils, necrosis, and focal mineralization are more prominent. Although in some respects resembling such lesions as cutaneous onchocerciasis, habronemiasis, or eosinophilic granulomas, none of these 3 is characterized by sheets of mast cells. Multiple congenital MCTs that spontaneously regress have been reported. There are no reports of metastasis of MCTs in the horse.

Mast cell tumors in **ferrets** resemble the well-differentiated feline MCT grossly, histologically, and in terms of biological behavior.

In **pigs,** mast cell nodules have been described as tumors and as multifocal inflammatory aggregates, perhaps in response to *Eperythrozoon*. Their morphology resembles that of well-differentiated feline tumors. In pigs with multiple skin lesions, visceral aggregates were also found.

In **cattle,** scant data suggest that the cutaneous tumors are usually multiple and are associated with visceral mast cell aggregates, although purely cutaneous tumors have been reported. Congenital cutaneous MCTs consisting of well-circumscribed 1-7 cm nodules randomly distributed all over the body have also been reported. Histologically, the tumors had features of well-differentiated MCTs. There are more reports of cutaneous metastases of multicentric visceral tumors than there are of primary skin disease. Cattle of any age, including calves, may be affected. There is one report of a calf with congenital diffuse cutaneous mastocytosis. The skin was described as diffusely thickened and wrinkled, with particularly prominent folds on the head, ventrum, and legs. Histologically, there was diffuse dermal infiltration by neoplastic mast cells.

Further reading

Donnelly L, et al. Evaluation of histological grade and histologically tumour-free margins as predictors of local recurrence in completely excised canine mast cell tumours. Vet Comp Oncol 2015;13:70-76.

Kiupel M, et al. Proposal of a 2-tier histologic grading system for canine cutaneous mast cell tumors to more accurately predict biological behavior. Vet Pathol 2011;48:147-155.

Romansik EM, et al. Mitotic index is predictive for survival for canine cutaneous mast cell tumors. Vet Pathol 2007;44:335-341.

Thompson JJ, et al. Canine subcutaneous mast cell tumor: characterization and prognostic indices. Vet Pathol 2011;48:156-168.

Vascellari M, et al. Expression of Ki67, BCL-2, and COX-2 in canine cutaneous mast cell tumors: Association with grading and prognosis. Vet Pathol 2012;50:110-121.

Webster JD, et al. Cellular proliferation in canine cutaneous mast cell tumors: associations with c-KIT and its role in prognostication. Vet Pathol 2007;44:298-308.

Webster JD, et al. The role of c-KIT in tumorigenesis: evaluation in canine cutaneous mast cell tumors. Neoplasia 2006;8:104-111.

Cutaneous lymphoma

Lymphomas in the skin can be a primary cutaneous neoplasm or can be part of a multicentric lymphocytic neoplasm. Cutaneous lymphomas have been reported in most domestic animals and in many wildlife species; however, the tumor has been most closely studied in the dog, cat, horse, and in cattle. The body of information about cutaneous lymphomas in veterinary dermatopathology has expanded rapidly in recent years, and is still a subject under close study.

Cutaneous lymphomas in domestic animals are usually divided into 2 groups: *epitheliotropic cutaneous lymphomas*, in which the neoplastic lymphocytes invade the epidermis and/or adnexal epithelium, and *nonepitheliotropic lymphomas*, which involve the dermis and subcutis.

Cutaneous epitheliotropic T-cell lymphoma (CTCL) has been reported in the *dog, cat, horse, rabbit, and cattle*. The misnomer "mycosis fungoides" is an accepted synonym in the human and veterinary literature. CTCL must be differentiated from non-epitheliotropic lymphoma (NEL) or dermal lymphoma. CTCL is classically divided into a localized form **pagetoid reticulosis** (Woringer-Kolopp disease), **classic mycosis fungoides,** and **Sézary syndrome;** however, it is unclear if this classification has any clinical relevance in veterinary medicine. CTCL is a disease of *older animals*. The clinical presentation varies from an erythematous, exfoliative dermatitis, to multiple plaques and nodules, and mucous membrane/mucocutaneous junction depigmentation (Fig. 6-162). Histologically, the neoplastic lymphoid infiltrate involves epidermis and the epithelium of adnexal structures (Fig. 6-163). The lymphoid infiltrate in the epithelium can be diffuse, scattered, or form aggregates *(Pautrier's microabscesses)* (see Fig. 6-163A). Dermal involvement varies from a mixed perivascular cellular component that contains low numbers of neoplastic lymphocytes to a more fulminating diffuse monomorphic neoplastic infiltrate. CTCL frequently causes ulcers, and verification of the epitheliotropic nature of the neoplasm can be difficult; however, a neoplastic lymphocytic component that abuts the ulcerated epidermis suggests epidermotropism. The neoplastic lymphocytes can vary from a small cell type, with a low mitotic index, hyperchromatic nucleus, and scant cytoplasm, to a large cell type, with moderate mitotic index together with moderate amounts of pale basophilic to clear cytoplasm. Although less well characterized than the human form of mycosis fungoides, epitheliotropic lymphomas in domestic animals also express T-cell surface antigens such as CD3. In contrast to human epitheliotropic lymphomas, which are reported to express CD4 in ~90% of cases as well as αβ T-cell receptor, 80% of epitheliotropic lymphomas in domestic animals express CD8 and the γδ T-cell receptor. CTCL with a leukemic blood component (Sézary syndrome) has been reported in the dog, cat, horse, and cow. Canine pagetoid reticulosis (Woringer-Kolopp disease) is a localized solitary plaque form of epitheliotropic lymphoma that is well

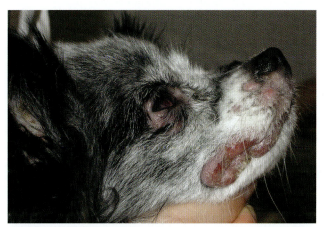

Figure 6-162 Dog with cutaneous **epitheliotropic T-cell lymphoma**. Note the swelling and depigmentation of the lips, nasal planum, rostral muzzle, and periocular skin.

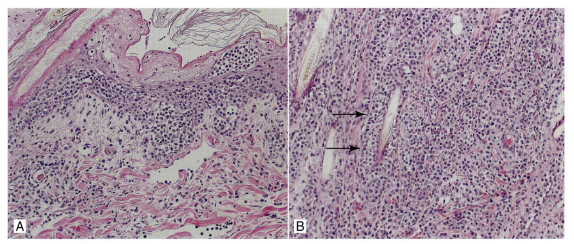

Figure 6-163 Cutaneous **T-cell epitheliotropic lymphoma** in a dog. **A.** Large aggregates of neoplastic cells (Pautrier's microabscesses) infiltrate the epidermis. **B.** Neoplastic cells infiltrate and efface outer root sheaths of hair follicles (arrows).

recognized in humans and has been reported rarely in the dog. In this form, the neoplastic lymphocytes are confined primarily to the epidermis and the dermal component is a mixture of mature lymphocytes and macrophages. This may represent an early form of CTCL, as it is unclear if there is a true difference in clinical behavior in the dog.

In **cats,** cutaneous epitheliotropic lymphoma is very rare and tends to be a more challenging clinical diagnosis. Affected cast have erythematous to scaly plaques and patches or ulcerated nodules and plaques. Adnexal involvement may be less common than in the dog.

An indolent form of **cutaneous nonepitheliotropic T-cell lymphoma** that resembles or arises from **cutaneous lymphocytosis** has been reported in dogs and cats. In cats, the disease occurs at a mean age of 12 years, with no breed predilection. The majority of the lesions appear as solitary areas of alopecia with scaling, erythema, and ulcers. Skin lesions are frequently located on the lateral thorax but may also be found on any region of haired skin or the nasal planum. Pruritus is a common clinical feature. The dermis contains sheets of small lymphocytes (CD3+) with fewer aggregates of C79a+ B cells. PCR for the feline T-cell receptor γ has demonstrated clonality of T cells in lesions from 14 of 20 cats with cutaneous lymphocytosis. Although the disease tends to be very slowly progressive, infiltration of internal organs by lymphocytes may occur along with clinical signs of systemic disease, such as lethargy, inappetence, and weight loss. The histologic features do not predict clinical outcome.

In dogs, **indolent cutaneous T-cell lymphoma** was characterized by erythematous and scaly macules patches or plaques in 8 dogs. The superficial to mid-dermis contained a band of monomorphic lymphocytes (CD3) without epitheliotropism; 7 of the 8 dogs showed T-cell receptor clonality. The lesions remained stable for years. A few dogs were euthanized because of lesion progression or development of high-grade lymphoma (one dog).

Inflamed nonepitheliotropic T-cell lymphoma is form of cutaneous lymphoma in dogs that can be difficult to differentiate morphologically from cutaneous reactive histiocytosis. The lesions are nonpruritic and range from nodules and plaques to masses, which often ulcerate. Lesions may be found on the mucocutaneous junctions of the face, extremities, neck, and trunk. Histologically, the neoplastic cells form *"bottom-heavy" nodules in the dermis and subcutis*, often with a Grenz zone. Atypical lymphocytes (intermediate to large) are intermixed with small lymphocytes, plasma cells, histiocytes, neutrophils, and variable numbers of eosinophils. Immunophenotyping is necessary to distinguish inflamed T-cell lymphoma from histiocytic proliferative diseases. The neoplastic cells can efface adnexal structures, but invasion into the epidermis or adnexal epithelium is very unusual. Although the clinical course is variable, the median survival time is only 9 months.

Other nonepitheliotropic cutaneous lymphomas are often of B-cell origin. An interesting form of nonepitheliotropic lymphoma is the **T-cell-rich B-cell lymphoma,** which is well recognized in humans and has been reported in the *cat, pig, dog, and horse*. In the horse, it appears to be the most common form of cutaneous lymphoma. In this form, the nodular masses are composed of large neoplastic B lymphocytes accompanied by a background population of smaller reactive T lymphocytes that usually comprise the majority of the cell population. The large neoplastic B cells exhibit cellular atypia, with large vesicular nuclei and numerous mitotic figures that are often atypical. Because the neoplastic population is often the minority population, the mitotic index should be evaluated carefully, taking into account the fact that the majority population is non-neoplastic small T lymphocytes with normal morphology and low mitotic index. These tumors also usually contain macrophages, epithelioid macrophages, and occasionally multinucleated giant cells. The mixed nature of the population can lead to this tumor being mistaken for inflammation, or a neoplasm of T lymphocytes. T-cell–rich B-cell lymphomas in the horse appear to be histologically the same as the neoplasm referred to in the older literature as *equine cutaneous histiolymphocytic lymphosarcoma.*

Angiocentric lymphoma (lymphomatoid granulomatosis) in the skin is usually a cutaneous manifestation of pulmonary lymphoma; however, it is thought to occur rarely as a primary cutaneous disease. Although well described in humans, this form of lymphoma has been reported infrequently in domestic animals. It is characterized by *angiocentric, angioinvasive, and angiodestructive neoplastic lymphocytes in the dermis and subcutis, resulting in intramural and extravascular neoplastic infiltrates*, in contrast to the luminal accumulations of lymphocytes in malignant angioendotheliomatosis. The neoplastic cells are medium- to large-sized lymphoid cells that can have a histiocytic appearance, with a cleaved or reniform nucleus. Inflammatory cells such as eosinophils, plasma cells, and small lymphocytes may accompany the neoplastic cells. In the small number of cases reported, the neoplastic lymphocytes have been identified as T lymphocytes by immunophenotyping. Clinically, the presentation is one of multiple alopecic and frequently ulcerated dermal or subcutaneous nodules. The angiodestructive nature of the neoplasm can result in multifocal necrotic or infarctive lesions.

Intravascular lymphoma (malignant angioendotheliomatosis, intravascular lymphomatosis, angiotropic large-cell lymphoma) is characterized by *intravascular neoplastic lymphocytes in the vessels of the skin and other organs in the absence of a primary mass or circulating neoplastic cells*. This condition is rare in humans and was originally thought to be a proliferation of endothelial cells, which lead to the original name of malignant angioendotheliomatosis. At present, it has been reported rarely in the dog and cat. Clinically, the skin lesions appear as plaques and nodules, and histologically vessels in the dermis and subcutis are partially or completely filled with *large atypical lymphoid cells.* In humans, the intravascular neoplastic cells are of B-lymphocyte origin; however, in dogs, the majority of cases so far have been of T-lymphocyte origin.

Cutaneous pseudolymphomas are *benign reactive proliferations of lymphocytes that mimic cutaneous lymphomas histologically and sometimes clinically*. These proliferations are poorly characterized in the veterinary literature, but are well recognized in humans as forming both a band-like infiltrate in the superficial dermis *(T-cell pattern)* and nodular-to-diffuse infiltrates in the dermis and subcutis *(B-cell pattern)*. Pseudolymphomas in humans can be due to many antigenic stimuli, such as drug eruptions, arthropod or tick-bite reactions, and contact dermatitis. *Borrelia burgdorferi*–associated cutaneous pseudolymphoma has been reported in one horse; the organism was identified by PCR in the biopsy tissue taken at the site of a tick bite. *Differentiation between benign inflammatory lesions and early cutaneous lymphoma can be extremely difficult.* Although immunophenotyping can distinguish between T-cell and B-cell lymphomas, methods to distinguish between inflammatory and malignant lymphocyte proliferations may require PCR for analysis for clonality.

Further reading

Affolter VK, et al. Indolent cutaneous T-cell lymphoma presenting as cutaneous lymphocytosis in dogs. Vet Dermatol 2009;20:577-585.
Fontaine J, et al. Cutaneous epitheliotropic T-cell lymphoma in the cat: a review of the literature and five new cases. Vet Dermatol 2011;22:454-461.
Gilbert S, et al. Clinical, morphological and immunohistochemical characterization of cutaneous lymphocytosis in 23 cats. Vet Dermatol 2004;15:3-12.
Moore PF, et al. Canine epitheliotropic cutaneous T-cell lymphoma: an investigation of T-cell receptor immunophenotype, lesion topography and molecular clonality. Vet Dermatol 2009;20:569-576.
Willemze R, et al. EORTC classification for primary cutaneous lymphomas: a proposal from the cutaneous lymphoma study group of the European Organization for Research and Treatment of Cancer. Blood 1997;90:354-371.

Cutaneous plasmacytoma

Cutaneous plasmacytomas are common in dogs and rare in cats. Most cases are benign; however, malignant cutaneous plasmacytomas demonstrating local invasion and tissue destruction do occur. It has not been described in other species. It occurs most often in *middle-aged or old dogs*, with a marked predilection for the *feet, ear canal, and mouth.* The typical tumor is a small spherical mass grossly similar to benign cutaneous histiocytoma, but its histology is distinctive. *Sheets of pleomorphic round cells are divided into solid lobules by a fine fibrous stroma.* The cells often have marked variation in nuclear size and degree of basophilia, with binucleation or multinucleation, and numerous mitotic figures. *At least some of the cells retain a perinuclear halo (suggesting a Golgi zone), "clockface" nucleus, and basophilic cytoplasm considered typical of plasma cells.* Russell bodies are sometimes seen even in very atypical cells, and the cytoplasm of most cells is pyroninophilic. Cells recognizable as plasma cells are most easily found near the periphery (Fig. 6-164). A grenz zone is usually present, and there is no epithelial invasion. Electron microscopy or immunohistochemistry for canine immunoglobulin confirms the diagnosis, but seldom are these tests necessary. Occasionally, a particularly anaplastic example must be distinguished from amelanotic epithelioid melanoma or lymphoma. The distinction is critical, because even bizarre plasmacytomas are cured by excision. Immunophenotyping may be helpful. The antibody Mum-1p is reasonably specific for plasma cell tumors and appears to be superior to CD79a and CD20. Rare B-cell lymphomas can stain positively for Mum-1p. Extracellular amyloid (AL) is found in a small percentage (perhaps up to 10% of plasmacytomas). They bear no apparent relationship to multiple myeloma. Multiple tumors, rarely >2-3, have been reported, as has a very low prevalence (~5%) of local recurrence.

Further reading

Ramos-Vara JA, et al. Immunohistochemical detection of multiple myeloma 1/interferon regulatory factor 4 (MUM1/IRF-4) in canine plasmacytoma: comparison with CD79a and CD20. Vet Pathol 2007;44:875-888.
Smithson CW, et al. Multicentric oral plasmacytoma in 3 dogs. J Vet Dent 2012;29:96-110.

Merkel cell tumor

Merkel cell tumors (Merkel cell carcinoma) have rarely been reported in the **dog and cat.** Clinically, the tumors appear as nodular lesions that may resemble a histiocytoma. Too few cases have been reported to establish age, site, or sex predilections. Microscopically, the tumors are comprised of *dermal infiltrates of round cells arranged as solid nests or clusters separated by collagenous stroma.* Individual tumor cells are reported to have indistinct margins and moderate amounts of pale to vacuolated cytoplasm. The nuclei are oval or spherical with dispersed chromatin. The nucleolus may or may not be conspicuous. Anisocytosis is mild to moderate. Mitotic activity varies. *Differential diagnoses* include round cell tumors, such as cutaneous plasmacytoma, balloon cell melanocytoma, and metastatic neuroendocrine carcinoma.

Definitive diagnosis requires ultrastructural examination or immunohistochemistry. Merkel cell tumors label for cytokeratin (CK), CK20, chromogranin A, neuron-specific enolase, and synaptophysin. Cytokeratin 20 is specific for Merkel cells and has been shown to be useful in the diagnosis of Merkel cell carcinoma in the cat. CK 20 is a low-molecular-weight cytokeratin whose expression is restricted to the gastrointestinal epithelium, urothelium, and Merkel cell. Electron microscopic evaluation demonstrates *electron-dense–core granules typical of neuroendocrine cells.* Merkel cell tumors in the dog are most often benign, with only one report documenting metastasis. Multicentric cutaneous tumors have also been reported in a dog. Recurrence and metastasis has been reported in cats.

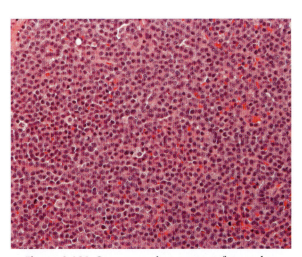

Figure 6-164 Cutaneous **plasmacytoma** from a dog.

Further reading

Dohata A, et al. Clinical and pathologic study of feline merkel cell carcinoma with immunohistochemical characterization of normal and neoplastic Merkel cells. Vet Pathol 2015;pii:0300985815570484. [Epub ahead of print].
Joiner KS, et al. Multicentric cutaneous neuroendocrine (Merkel cell) carcinoma in a dog. Vet Pathol 2010;47:1090-1094.
Ozaki K1, Narama I. Merkel cell carcinoma in a cat. J Vet Med Sci 2009;71:1093-1096.

Tumors metastatic to the skin

A variety of tumors can metastasize to the skin, but *the process is uncommon*. Cutaneous metastasis may be the first sign of an undiagnosed visceral malignancy. The usual routes of lymphatic, hematogenous, or implantation from a surgical procedure apply. A thorough search for a primary tumor, knowledge of prior history of a tumor, and an awareness of a few unique tumor patterns of metastasis are necessary to help establish the condition as a metastatic process. Clinically, a wide array of cutaneous lesions have been reported, including erythema, papules, pustules, vesicles, dermal to subcutaneous nodules, and ulcers. Cutaneous metastases in dogs have been reported to occur with the following neoplasms: transitional cell carcinoma (TCC), mammary carcinoma, mast cell tumors, lymphoma, hemangiosarcoma, duodenal and colonic adenocarcinoma, gastric mucinous adenocarcinoma, inflammatory mammary carcinosarcoma, seminoma, osteosarcoma, nasal neuroendocrine carcinoma, and rhabdomyosarcoma.

Cutaneous metastasis of **transitional cell carcinoma** is uncommon in dogs; however, it has been reported to occur after previous abdominal surgery for TCC and to occur through lymphatics and blood vessels. Transepidermal metastasis has been suggested, because in most cases, cutaneous lesions are in close proximity to the vulva and prepuce. Some believe neoplastic cells from the urine may seed eroded urine scalded skin. Cutaneous lesions appear as plaques, papules, and nodules and most often occur in the perineal, inguinal, or ventral abdominal dermis or subcutis in dogs with or without history of surgery. Many affected dogs also have lymph node and distant metastasis.

Visceral **hemangiosarcomas** may metastasize to the subcutis in the dog. Subcutaneous hemangiosarcomas, particularly if multiple, should prompt the clinician to search for a primary visceral tumor. Metastatic tumors may be fairly well differentiated or anaplastic.

Mammary gland carcinomas in the dog may metastasize to the dermis of the inner thigh. Spread of tumor cells occurs via direct invasion of dermal lymphatics or from retrograde metastasis of tumor cells from the external inguinal lymph node. Mammary gland carcinomas in the cat may also metastasize to the ventral abdominal tissues by using similar pathways. Primary epitrichial gland carcinoma of the skin may be difficult to distinguish. Cutaneous metastasis of mammary adenocarcinoma has also been reported in a llama. The llama was 8 years old and had nonhealing ulcerative cutaneous lesions distant from the mammary gland region.

Cutaneous metastasis of internal tumors is rare in **cats** and have been reported in association with mammary adenocarcinoma and digestive and respiratory carcinoma. **Pulmonary carcinoma** is the most common cause of tumor metastasis to the skin in cats. Pulmonary carcinomas in the cat have a propensity to metastasize to the digits, often prior to onset of clinical signs referable to the primary tumor. Clinically, the lesions are suggestive of paronychia. Histologically, nests, solid sheets, and glandular structures formed by malignant epithelial cells are found in the dermis and subcutis. Bony lysis of the third phalanx may be evident radiographically and histologically. Tumor cells have abundant eosinophilic cytoplasm, basally oriented nuclei, and frequently, apical cilia. Squamous differentiation is also common. Desmoplasia is usually present.

Abdominal surgeries to remove **transitional cell, colonic, or prostatic carcinomas** have the potential for implantation of tumor cells in the skin at the surgical site. Tumor cells may also reach the skin via retrograde lymphatic metastasis.

Further reading

Favrot C, Degeorge-Rubiales F. Cutaneous metastases of a bronchial adenocarcinoma in a cat. Vet Dermatol 2005;16:183-186.

Reed LT, et al. Cutaneous metastasis of transitional cell carcinoma in 12 dogs. Vet Pathol 2012;50:676-681.

 For more information, please visit the companion site: PathologyofDomesticAnimals.com.

INDEX

Entries followed by "f," "b," and "t" refer to figures and tables, respectively. The volume number of the entry is indicated in *italics* at the beginning of the page number.

A

Abdominal distention, 2:44
Abdominal fat necrosis, 2:76-77, 2:249, 2:249f
Abdominal trauma, 2:246-247, 2:246f
Abdominal wall, ventral hernia, 2:80
Abdominally retained testis, 3:470f
Aberdeen Angus cattle
   bovine familial convulsions and ataxia, 1:319
   brachygnathia inferior, 2:3
   hip dysplasia, 1:135-136
Abiotrophy, 1:265
   cerebellar, 1:276, 1:276f, 1:318-326
Abomasal fistulae, 2:49
Abomasal helminthosis, 2:205-211, 2:205f
Abomasitis, 2:52
   associated with viral infection, 2:54
   chemical, 2:52
   mycotic, 2:54, 2:54f
Abomasum. *See* Stomach and abomasum
Abortion, 3:395, 3:398-440. *See also* Female genital system; Gestation
   bacterial causes of, 3:402-417
   diagnosing infectious causes of, 3:399-402
   epizootic bovine, 3:419-420
   infectious causes of, 3:399b
   in mares, 3:417-418
   mycotic, 3:418-419, 3:418f-419f
   protozoal causes of, 3:420-424
Abscess(es), 1:636-637
   Brodie's, 1:98, 1:98f
   cerebral, 1:358-362, 1:358f, 1:360f
   epidural/subdural, 1:353-354, 1:354f
   jowl, 3:208-209, 3:208f-209f
   liver, 2:315-316, 2:315f
   lung, 2:520
   lymph node, 3:203f, 3:203.e1f
   meningitis, 1:359f
   ovarian, 3:371
   pancreatic, 2:361
   pulmonary hemorrhage and, 2:490
   splenic, 3:183-184, 3:184f
   subdural/intradural, 1:354f
   uterine, 3:390
Abyssinian cats
   atopic dermatitis, 1:593
   feline ceruminous cystomatosis, 1:507
   retinal degeneration, 1:469-470
Acacia cambadgei, 3:34
Acacia georginae, 3:34
Acanthamoeba, 2:574
Acanthocephalan infections, 2:227
Acantholysis, 1:518, 1:518f
Acantholytic cells, 1:518
Acantholytic dermatoses
   cattle, 1:537-538
   dogs, 1:537-538, 1:537.e1f
Acanthomatous ameloblastomas, 2:22-23, 2:23f-24f
Acanthosis, 1:518
Accessory adrenal cortical tissue, 3:338, 3:338f

Accessory cortical nodules, 3:343
Accessory lung, 2:484-485
Accessory pancreatic tissue, 2:356
Accessory spleens, 3:162-163, 3:163f
Accessory thyroid tissue, 3:310
Accreditation, laboratory, 1:14
Acetaminophen, 2:327
Acetylcholine, 2:45
Acetylcholinesterase, 1:170
Achalasia, esophageal, 2:33
Achlorhydria, 2:47
Achondroplasia, 1:37t
Acid-base imbalance, 2:384
Acidophil adenomas, 3:286, 3:286f
Acidosis, carbohydrate overload, 2:40-43
Acid treatment, of hemoglobin, 2:55-56
Acid urine, antibacterial effect of, 2:459
Acinar cells, 2:355
   necrosis, 2:356
Acinic cell carcinomas, 2:30
   nasal, 2:478-479
Acne, 1:549
Acorn poisoning, acute, 2:85
Acoustic trauma, 1:493
Acquired cysts, 2:396
Acquired deafness, 1:493
Acquired diaphragmatic hernia, 2:246-247, 2:246f
Acquired Fanconi syndrome, 2:428
Acquired hyperpigmentation, 1:554
Acquired hypopigmentation, 1:557, 1:557f
Acquired melanosis, 2:270
Acquired platelet disorders, 3:260
Acquired porphyria, 1:59-60
Acquired portosystemic shunts
   liver, 2:290, 2:298-299, 2:299f
   vascular, 2:266f
Acquired thrombocytopenia, 3:258
Acral lick dermatitis, 1:561-562, 1:561f-562f
Acrocyanosis, 3:65
Acrodermatitis, lethal, 1:533, 1:533.e1f
Acromegaly, 3:286, 3:286f
Acromelanism, 1:555
Actinic diseases of skin, 1:575-580
Actinobacillosis, 2:18-19, 2:18f
Actinobacillus equuli, 2:113-114, 2:433, 2:433f, 2:452, 2:543, 3:417-418, 2:433.e1f
   endocarditis and, 3:30-31
   liver and, 2:314-315
   myocarditis and, 3:42
Actinobacillus pleuropneumoniae (APP), 2:531-532, 2:531f, 2:543, 3:69
Actinobacillus seminis, 3:490
Actinobacillus suis, 2:543
Actinobaculum, 2:459
Actinobaculum suis, 2:459
Actinomyces spp.
   cutaneous, 1:637-639, 1:638f
   inflammation in buccal cavity due to, 2:13-14
   tonsillitis, 2:20
   tooth decay and, 2:9

Actinomyces weissii, 2:19
Activated clotting time (ACT), 3:263
Activated partial thromboplastin time (APTT)
   prolonged, 3:263
Active hyperemia, 3:169
Acute arthritis in cats, 1:154
Acute bacterial endocarditis, 3:32
Acute bovine liver disease, 2:343-344, 2:343.e1f
Acute eosinophilic (or acidophilic) degeneration, 1:253-254, 1:253f
Acute hepatitis, 2:301
Acute intermittent porphyria, 1:59
Acute interstitial lung disease in feedlot cattle, 2:513f, 2:513.e1
Acute kidney injury (AKI), 2:398
Acute local peritonitis, 2:39
Acute lymphadenitis, 3:202-203
Acute lymphocytic-plasmacytic chorioretinitis, 1:474
Acute lymphoid leukemia (ALL), 3:132-133, 3:133f
Acute myeloid leukemia (AML), 3:129-134, 3:130f-132f
Acute osteomyelitis, 1:95, 1:95f
Acute pancreatic necrosis, 2:357-360, 2:359f-360f
Acute pancreatitis, 2:360
Acute polyradiculoneuritis, 1:394
Acute renal failure (ARF), 2:383-384, 2:398, 2:418
Acute rupture of chordae tendineae, 3:27
Acute selenium toxicosis, 3:36
Acute serous uveitis, 1:448-449
Acute toxic hepatic injury, 2:327, 2:328f
Acute tubular injury (ATI), 2:383, 2:386, 2:398, 2:421-422
   epithelial injury, 2:422f
Acute tubular necrosis (ATN), 2:382, 2:398, 2:422
Addison's disease, 1:225
Adenocarcinomas. *See* Carcinomas/adenocarcinomas
Adenohypophysis, 3:276
   bacterial septicemia, 3:289
   functional cytology, 3:276-277
   hypothalamic control of, 3:277, 3:278f
   inflammation, 3:289-290
Adenoid cystic carcinomas, 2:478-479
Adenomas, 2:462. *See also* Carcinomas/adenocarcinomas
   acidophil, 3:286, 3:286f
   adrenal cortex, 3:344-345, 3:345f
   aortic body, 3:354-355, 3:354f
   carotid body, 3:355-356
   corticotroph (ACTH-secreting), 3:281-282, 3:281f, 3:283f-284f
   endocrine gland, 3:271
   exocrine pancreatic, 2:366
   hepatocellular, 2:346, 2:346f
   lactotroph, 3:286-287

Adenomas *(Continued)*
  mammary, 3:460, 3:461f
  papillary
    ears, 1:500
    pulmonary, 2:495
    thyroid, 3:327
  parathyroid glands, 3:302
  pars distalis, 3:287-288
  pars intermedia, 3:282-285, 3:283f-284f
  somatotroph, 3:285-286, 3:285f-286f
  testicular, 3:496
  thyroid, 3:322, 3:323f, 3:326-327, 3:327f-328f
    C-cell, 3:333, 3:334f
  thyrotroph, 3:286
Adenomatous hyperplasia
  focal papillary/papillotubular proliferation, 2:104
  Lawsonia intracellularis, 2:105
  rectal papillary adenoma, 2:104
Adenomatous polyposis coli (APC), 2:102-103
Adenomyosis, 3:385, 3:385f, 3:497
Adenosine triphosphate (ATP) in rigor mortis, 1:186
Adenosquamous (mucoepidermoid) carcinomas, 2:478-479
  pulmonary, 2:497, 2:498f
Adenovirus, 2:116, 2:432
  cattle, 2:143, 2:143f-144f, 2:542
  deer, 2:145, 2:145f
  dogs, 2:577
  horses, 2:145, 2:569
  pigs, 2:144-145, 2:144f
  sheep and goats, 2:557
Adhesion(s)
  peritoneal, 2:76-77
  platelet, 3:256
Adiaspiromycosis, 2:584-585, 2:585f
Adipocytes, 1:187, 1:188f
Adrenal glands, 3:336-348, 3:336f
  biosynthesis and hormone action, 3:337-338
  development, structure, and function, 3:336-338
  diseases, 3:338-343, 3:338f
  neoplasms, 3:343-348
  pituitary adenomas and, 3:288, 3:288f
Adrenal medulla, 3:348-354
  development, structure, and function, 3:348-354
  neoplasms, 3:349-352
Adrenal sex hormones, 3:337
Adrenal tissue, accessory or ectopic, 3:479, 3:480f
Adrenocorticotropic hormone (ACTH), 3:270-272
  biosynthesis, 3:337-338
  corticotroph (ACTH-secreting) adenoma, 3:281-282, 3:281f, 3:283f-284f
  functional cytology of adenohypophysis and, 3:276-277
Adult polycystic disease, liver 2:265
Adventitia, vascular system, 3:54
Adventitial placentation, 3:396-397
Adventitious bursae, 1:155
Adynamic ileus, 2:74-75, 2:77
Aelurostongylus abstrusus, 2:590-591, 2:590.e5f
Afghan dogs
  hypothyroidism, 1:587
  myelopathy, 1:340f
  necrotizing myelopathy, 1:340, 1:340f

Afibrinogenemia, 3:265
Aflatoxins, 2:333-334, 2:334f, 2:333.e1f
African horse sickness (AHS), 3:72-74, 3:74f, 3:72.e2f
African swine fever (ASF), 3:74-76, 3:75f-76f, 3:181-182, 3:181f-182f, 3:75.e1f, 3:181.e1f
Afrikander cattle, hypothyroidism in, 1:588
Agammaglobulinemia, 3:139
Agenesis, 2:392
  adrenal gland, 3:338
  cerebellar, 1:275-276, 1:275f
  corpus callosum, 1:269, 1:269f
  ovary, 3:366
  pancreas, 2:355
Aggrecan (ACAN) gene, 1:38
Aggregation, platelet, 3:257-258
Aging changes
  canine nasodigital hyperkeratosis, 1:549-550
  choroid plexus, 1:304, 1:304f
  gross examination of, 1:7
  hearing, 1:493
  meninges, 1:304
  "old dog" encephalitis and, 1:384-385
  ovaries, 3:371, 3:371f
  pancreas, 2:358
  spermatogenesis, 3:467
  tendon, 1:247
  vascular system, 3:56
Agnathia, 2:4
Aino virus (AINOV), 1:280, 1:381, 3:438
Airedale Terrier dogs
  dilated cardiomyopathy, 3:48
  recurrent flank alopecia, 1:590
Airway, upper, 2:466-467, 2:466f
  disease, 2:500-504, 2:500.e1f
Akabane virus (AKAV), 1:280, 1:381, 3:437-438
Akita dogs
  canine uveodermatologic syndrome, 1:557
  peripheral vestibular disease, 1:494
  polyarthritis, 1:158
  sebaceous adenitis, 1:551
Alaria spp., 2:225-227
Alaskan Husky dogs
  gangliosidosis, 1:58-59
  spongy encephalomyelopathies, 1:346-347
Alaskan Malamute dogs
  alopecia X, 1:589-590
  canine uveodermatologic syndrome, 1:557
  chondrodysplasia, 1:43f
  cone dysplasia, 1:469
  Factor VII deficiency, 3:264
  hypothyroidism, 1:587
  motor neuropathy, 1:335
  vitiligo, 1:555-556
  zinc-responsive dermatoses, 1:585-586
Alaskan sled dogs, 3:51
Albumin, 2:401
Alcelaphine herpesvirus 1 (AlHV-1), 2:132
Alcelaphine herpesvirus 2 (AlHV-2), 2:132
Aleutian mink cattle, Chediak-Higashi syndrome in, 3:259
Alexander disease, 1:262, 1:341
Algal diseases of skin, 1:665
Alimentary system, 1:250-406. *See also* Entries beginning gastrointestinal; specific components; specific infections/organisms
  bacterial diseases, 2:158-201
  buccal cavity and mucosa, 2:12-19

Alimentary system *(Continued)*
  diagnosis of gastrointestinal disease, 2:111-117
  diarrhea
    bovine coronavirus, 2:112
    bovine herpesvirus 1, 2:112
    bovine torovirus, 2:112
    in calves, 2:112-113
    Chlamydophila infection, 2:113
    Cryptosporidium parvum, 2:112
    enterotoxigenic *E. coli*, 2:112
    rotavirus, 2:112
    salmonellosis, 2:112
  enteritis
    cats, 2:117
    dogs, 2:116-117
    horses, 2:116
  esophagus, 2:30-35
  forestomachs, 2:35-44
  gastroenteritis
    cattle, 2:114-115
    sheep, 2:115
    swine, 2:115-116
  infectious/parasitic diseases, 2:117-244
    bovine viral diarrhea virus (BVDV), 2:122-128, 2:125f
      fetal infections, 2:122
      mucosal disease, 2:123
      PI calves, 2:122
    vesicular stomatitis (VS), 2:119-120
    viral diseases, foot-and-mouth disease (FMD), 2:117-119
  mycotic diseases, 2:201-203
  neonatal animals, undifferentiated diarrhea of, 2:111
  oral cavity, 2:2-28
  protistan infections, 2:227-244
  salivary glands, 2:28-30
  stomach and abomasum, 2:44-60
Alkali disease, 1:571
Alkaline phosphatase, 1:27
Alkaline urine pH, 2:456
Alkaloids, pyrrolizidine, 2:336-338, 2:337f, 2:337.e1f
Allantoic sac, 3:397
Allergic reactions, 1:590-600
  contact dermatitis, 1:596-597
  to food, 1:594-596, 1:595f
  inhalant dermatitis, 1:592
  rhinitis, 2:476, 2:476.e1f
All-*trans*-retinoic acid (ATRA), 1:82
Alopecia
  areata, 1:614-615, 1:615f
  canine recurrent flank, 1:590, 1:590f, 1:590.e1f
  cicatricial, 1:698
  color-dilution, 1:557
  congenital hypotrichosis, 1:538-539
    associated with pigmentary alteration, 1:539-541
    cats, 1:539
    cattle, 1:538-539
    dogs, 1:539, 1:539.e1f
  equine linear, 1:550, 1:550f
  feline paraneoplastic, 1:691, 1:692f
  mucinosa, 1:697
  psychogenic, 1:561
  rabies vaccine-induced vasculitis and, 1:612-613
  traction, 1:560
  X, 1:589-590, 1:590f
A1-Antitrypsin deficiency, 2:304-305
α-cells, endocrine pancreas, 2:368

INDEX

α-dystroglycan deficiency, 1:196
α-1,4-glucosidase deficiency, 1:290
α-granules, 3:257
α-L-fucosidosis, 1:289
α-L-iduronidase, 1:289
α-Mannosidosis, 1:288, 1:288f
α-naphthylthiourea (ANTU), 2:519-520
Alphaherpesviruses
    cattle, 2:537
    horses, 2:568, 2:568.e2f
Alphaviruses, 1:376-377, 1:377f
Alport syndrome, 2:415-416, 2:417f, 2:415.e3f. See also Hereditary nephritis
Alsike clover, 1:579, 2:341-342, 2:341f
Altered gut flora, 2:71-72
Aluminum, 3:298
    phthalocyanine tetrasulfonate, 2:329
Alveld, 2:340
Alveolar atrophy, 2:7-8
Alveolar ducts, 2:467
Alveolar emphysema, 2:486
Alveolar filling disorders, 2:516-518
Alveolar histiocytosis, 2:517
Alveolar macrophages, 2:470-472
Alveolar microlithiasis, 2:517, 2:517f
Alveolar overinflation, 2:486, 2:487.e1f
Alveolar parenchyma, 2:469
Alveolar phospholipidosis, 2:517, 2:517.e1f
Alveolar proteinosis, 2:517
Alveolar rhabdomyosarcoma, 1:241-243
Alveolar stage of lung growth, 2:484, 2:484.e1f
Alzheimer type II cells, 1:262, 1:262f, 2:88
Amanitins, 2:330-331
Amaranthus retroflexus, 2:386, 2:427
    toxicity, 2:427f
Amblyomma maculatum, 1:506
Amebiasis, 2:242
Amebic encephalitis, 1:386, 1:386f
Amelanotic malignant melanoma, glomerular micrometastasis of, 2:444.e1f
Ameloblastic fibroma, 2:24
Ameloblastic fibro-odontomas, 2:24
Ameloblastomas, 2:22-23, 2:23f
Ameloblasts, 2:5
Amelogenesis imperfecta, 2:7
American Brown Swiss cattle, bovine hypomyelinogenesis in, 1:338-339
American Bulldogs, ichthyosis in, 1:531, 1:531.e1f
American Cocker Spaniel dogs
    chronic hepatitis, 2:304, 2:305f
    phosphofructokinase (PFK) deficiency, 1:204-205
American Eskimo dogs, alopecia X in, 1:589-590
American Hairless Terrier dogs, congenital hypotrichosis in, 1:538
American Staffordshire Terrier dogs, demodectic mange in, 1:679
Amikacin, 1:494, 2:424
Amine precursor uptake decarboxylation (APUD), 2:105-106
Aminoglycosides
    nephrotoxicity, 2:424
    tubulotoxic effects of, 2:424
Amiodarone, 2:329
Ammonia toxicity, 2:291
Amniotic plaques, 3:397
Amniotic sac, 3:397

Amphotericin B, 1:562
Amycolatopsis, 3:417
Amylo-1,6-glucosidase deficiency, 1:290
Amyloid
    definitive characterization, 2:415
    degeneration, 1:297-298
    deposition in adrenal glands, 3:339
    eosinophilic in H&E sections, 2:415
    fibrils, 2:413-414
    histologically, 2:414-415
    localization of, 2:414
    medullary interstitial amyloidosis, 2:415f
    pale amorphous, 2:91f
    -producing odontogenic tumors, 2:23
Amyloidosis, 2:91, 3:298f
    cutaneous, 1:614
    liver, 2:278-279, 2:279f, 2:278.e1f
    nasal, 2:473, 2:474f
    parathyroid gland, 3:297-298
    spleen, 3:163-164, 3:165f, 3:164.e1f
    thyroid, 3:315, 3:315f
Amylopectinosis, 1:290
Anaerobiospirillum sp., 2:99, 2:199
Anagen phase, hair, 1:516
Angioleiomyomas, 3:52
Anagyrine, 1:90
Anal glands, 1:517
Anal sac, aprocrine adenocarcinoma of, 3:307f-308f, 3:308
Anaphylaxis, 2:512-513
Anaplasma centrale, 3:117
Anaplasma marginale, 3:116, 3:116f
Anaplasma phagocytophilum, 3:111, 3:178
Anaplasma platys, 3:128-129
Anaplasmosis, 3:116-117
Anaplastic diffuse large B-cell lymphomas (DLBCLs), 3:221
Anaplastic large T-cell lymphoma (ALTCL), 3:230
Anatrichosoma spp., 1:690
Anchoring filaments, 1:513-514
Ancylostoma spp., 2:214
Andersen disease, 1:290
Andersonstrongylus milksi, 2:587
Androgen in bone, 1:25t
Anemia, 1:539, 2:73, 3:112
    aplastic, 3:127-128, 3:128f
    blood loss, 3:112-114
    classification by mechanism, 3:113t
    of decreased production, 3:126-128
    hemolytic, 3:114-126
    immunohemolytic, 3:114, 3:115f
    of inflammatory disease (AID), 3:127
    iron deficiency, 3:112-114, 3:114f
    in uremic animals, 2:385
Anencephaly, cerebral, 1:266-267, 1:266f
Anesthesia
    deaths, 1:2-3
    postanesthethic myopathy in horses, 1:213
Aneurysmal bone cysts, 1:126
    cats, 1:126f
Aneurysms, 3:62-63, 3:62f
    congenital, 3:23
    portal vein, 2:266
Angiocentric lymphoma, 1:734
Angioedema, 1:594
Angiofibroma, nasopharyngeal, 2:480
Angioimmunoblastic T-cell lymphoma, 3:230
Angioinvasive lymphoma, 2:499, 2:499f
Angiokeratoma, 1:727, 3:99

Angioma, 3:99
Angiopathy, cerebrospinal, 1:298, 1:298f
Angiosarcomas, 3:99-101
Angiostrongylus vasorum, 1:390-391, 1:451-452, 2:586-587
Angiotensin converting enzyme (ACE), into angiotensin II, 2:379
Angora goats
    aural melanoma, 1:504-505
    spongy encephalomyelopathies, 1:347
Angular limb deformities, 1:31-33, 1:32f
    horses, 1:31-32
    sheep, 1:32, 1:33f
Angus cattle
    bovine hypomyelinogenesis, 1:338-339
    brachygnathia superior, 2:3
    genetic acantholytic dermatoses, 1:537-538
    hip dysplasia, 1:135-136
    osteopetrosis, 1:51
Anichkov cells, 3:37, 3:38f
Aniline derivatives, 3:325
Ankyloglossia, 2:4
Ankylosing spondylosis
    dogs, 1:145-146, 1:145f
    pigs, 1:146
Annual ryegrass toxicosis, 1:298, 1:298f
Annular pancreas, 2:355
Annulus fibrosus, 1:128-129
Anodontia, 2:6
    cattle, 1:538
Anoikis, 2:280
Anomalous pulmonary venous drainage, 2:485
Anophthalmos, 1:410, 1:410f
Anorexia, 2:69, 2:72
Anovulatory cystic ovarian disease, 3:372
Anovulatory luteinized cysts, 3:373, 3:373f
Anoxia, 1:305-307
Anterior segment dysgenesis, 1:416, 1:416f
Anterior staphyloma, 1:437
Anterior synechiae, 1:432, 1:432f
Anterior uveitis, 1:446
Anterograde degeneration, 1:256
Anthracosis, 2:518, 3:200, 3:200.e1f
Anthrax, 3:171-174, 3:172.e1f
    cattle, 3:172, 3:173f
    dogs, 3:174
    horses, 3:173
    pigs, 3:173-174
    sheep, 3:173
Anthropophilic dermatophytes, 1:649
Antibiotic-responsive diarrhea (ARD), 2:86
Antibody defense proteins, lung, 2:471
Antibody-dependent cytotoxicity (ADCC), 3:143-144
Antibody-mediated rejection, acute, 2:387
Anticoagulants, endogenous, 3:265-266
Anticonvulsant drugs and osteoporosis, 1:67
Antidiuretic hormone (ADH), 2:377, 2:401, 2:430, 3:10, 3:290
Anti-GBM glomerulonephritis, 2:408
Antimicrobial factors in lungs, 2:472
Antithrombin (AT), 3:265
Antithrombosis, 3:55
    balance between thrombosis and, 3:53.e1f
Aorta
    coarctation, 3:23, 3:23f
    complete transposition of pulmonary artery and, 3:22.e1f
    double arch, 3:23

Aorta *(Continued)*
  rupture, 3:62-63, 3:62f
  vascular anomalies, 3:23-24, 3:23f
Aortic-iliac thrombosis, 3:64, 3:64.e1f
Aorticopulmonary septal defect, 3:23
Aortic valve
  aortic and subaortic stenosis, 3:20-21, 3:21f
  semilunar, 3:2-3
  subendocardial fibrosis, 3:30
Aphakia, 1:422
Aplasia
  cerebral, 1:266-267, 1:266f
  enamel, 2:5
  pancreas, 2:355
  paramesonephric duct, 3:368, 3:369f
  pure red cell, 3:127-128, 3:128f
  segmental, 1:277-279
Aplastic anemia, 3:127-128, 3:128f
Apocrine glands, 1:517
  carcinoma, 1:720, 1:720f
Aponeuroses, 1:247-249
Apophyses, 1:30
Apoptosis, 1:186, 1:518
  liver, 2:279-280, 2:279f
Appaloosa horses, osteopetrosis in, 1:52
Aprocrine adenocarcinoma of anal sac, 3:307f-308f, 3:308
Aptyalism, 2:28
Aqueous flare, 1:448-449
Arabian horses
  atlantoaxial subluxations, 1:137
  cerebellar abiotrophy, 1:319
  equine adenovirus, 2:569
  severe combined immunodeficiency (SCID), 3:139-141
Arachnoid cysts, 1:279, 1:280f
Arachnomelia, 1:48-49
Argasidae, 1:684
"Armadillo Westie syndrome", 1:553
Arnold-Chiari malformation, 1:276-277, 1:277f
Arrector pili muscles, 1:515
Arrhythmogenic right ventricular cardiomyopathy (ARVC)
  dogs, 3:49, 3:49f
  -like syndrome in cats, 3:47
Arsenic poisoning, 1:327-328, 1:570
Arterial embolism, 3:63-66, 3:63f-64f
Arterial hypertrophy, 3:66-67
Arterial thrombosis, 3:63-66, 3:63f, 3:63.e1f
Arteries, 3:54, 3:56-88
  bronchial, 2:467-468, 2:468f
  congenital anomalies, 3:56
  degeneration, 3:56-61
  hepatic, 2:260
  mineralization, 3:60-61, 3:61f
  obstructions, 1:299-300, 1:299f
  pulmonary, 2:467-468, 2:468f
  rupture, 3:62-63, 3:62f
  transposition, 3:22.e1f
Arteriopathy, plexiform, 2:492, 2:492f
Arteriosclerosis, 3:36, 3:56-57, 3:59-60
Arteriovenous fistula, 3:56
Arteritis
  MCF microscopic, 2:135
  severe, 2:398.e1f
Arthritis
  coliform, 1:151
  erysipelas, 1:149-150
  fibrinous, 1:146-147, 1:147f
  fungal, 1:154-155
  infectious, 1:148-155

Arthritis *(Continued)*
  myocplasmal, 1:153-154
  protozoal, 1:155
  purulent (suppurative), 1:147-148, 1:148f
  rheumatoid, 1:157, 1:157f
  staphylococcal, 1:151
  streptococcal, 1:150-151
  viral, 1:154
Arthrogryposis, 1:137, 1:187-189, 1:188f, 1:281f
Arthropod ectoparasites, 1:666-684
Arthropod infections and central nervous system, 1:389-391
Articular capsule, 1:130
  fibrinous arthritis, 1:147
Articular cartilage, 1:129
  response to injury, 1:131-132
Articular disks, 1:130
Artiodactyla. See Malignant catarrhal fever (MCF)
Arylsulfatase-B deficiency, 1:290
Asbestosis, 2:518
Ascarid nematodes, 2:76, 2:255
Ascaris suum, 2:116, 2:218, 2:218f, 2:319, 2:319f, 2:536-537
  respiratory system and, 2:536-537, 2:556-557, 2:557f, 2:537.e1f
Ascarops spp., 2:54
Ascending pyelonephritis, acute, 2:441.e1f
Ascites, 2:248-249, 2:294-295
Asian cat breeds, peripheral vestibular disease in, 1:494
Aspartate aminotransferase (AST)
  canine dermatomyositis, 1:198
  canine X-linked muscular dystrophy, 1:192-193
  centronuclear myopathy of Labrador Retrievers, 1:197
  congenital myotonia in cats, 1:201
  diaphragmatic dystrophy in cattle, 1:199
  masticatory myositis, 1:226
  polymyositis, 1:227
  purpura hemorrhagica, 1:229
Aspergillus clavatus, 1:327
Aspergillus flavus, 2:426
Aspergillus fumigatus, 3:417-418
  bronchitis and, 2:502, 2:502.e1f
  mycotic rhinitis, 2:579, 2:580f
Aspergillus niger, 2:426
Aspergillus spp., 1:156, 1:156f, 1:660, 2:201
  abortion and, 3:399-400
  liver toxicity, 2:333
  pulmonary, 2:573, 2:573f
  pulmonary vasculitis and, 2:494
Aspergillus terreus, 3:183, 3:184f, 3:183.e1f
Aspiration pneumonia, 2:508-509, 2:508f-509f, 2:508.e1f
  meconium, 2:516, 2:516.e1f
Assimilation, epithelial phase of, 2:69-70
Asthma, feline, 2:502-503, 2:503.e1f
Astrocytes, 1:260-262, 1:261f
Astrocytoma, 1:398-399, 1:399f
Astrovirus, 2:117
Asynchrony, esophageal, 2:33
Atadenovirus, 2:145
Ataxia, 2:425
  bovine familial convulsions and, 1:319
  enzootic, 1:328-329, 1:328f
  progressive, 1:341f
Atelectasis, 2:486, 2:486.e2f
  fetal, 2:486.e2f

Atherosclerosis, 3:57-59, 3:58f-59f, 3:57.e2f
  with hypothyroidism, 3:318-319, 3:319f
Atlantoaxial subluxations, 1:137
  horses, 1:137
Atopic dermatitis, 1:591-593, 1:591f, 1:592.e1f
Atresia ani, 2:74
Atresia coli, 2:74
Atresia ilei, 2:74
Atresia intestinalis, 2:74
Atria, heart, 3:2
  restricted filling, 3:6
Atrial natriuretic factor (ANF), 3:3, 3:10
Atrial septal defect (ASD), 3:16, 3:16f
Atrichial sweat glands, 1:518
  tumors, 1:719
Atrioventricular (AV) valves, 3:3
  dysplasia of right, 3:21-22
  malformation of, 3:19-22, 3:19f
  septal defect, 3:17, 3:17f
Atrioventricular (AV) waves, 3:2
Atrophic dermatosis, 1:529-530, 1:529f
Atrophic rhinitis, 2:533
  nonprogressive (NPAR), 2:533
  pigs, 1:102
  progressive (PAR), 2:533
Atrophy, 1:174f
  alveolar, 2:7-8
  brain and spinal cord, 1:304-305
  cerebellar, 1:276, 1:276f, 1:318-326
  cerebrocortical, 1:7f
  denervation, 1:173-178, 1:175f-177f
  disuse, 1:175-177, 1:177f
  dog, 1:176f
  endocrine disease, 1:178, 1:178f
  endometrium, 3:382
  epidermis, 1:518-519
  exocrine pancreas, 2:362-363, 2:362f
  follicular, 1:520, 3:316f
  heart, 3:34
  hepatocellular, 2:269, 2:269f, 2:269.e1f
  horse, 1:176f
  hypertrophy, 1:178-180, 1:178f-179f
  hypothyroidism and, 1:224
  idiopathic follicular, 3:315-316, 3:315f, 3:317f
  lymphoid, 3:198, 3:199f
  male genital glands, 3:504
  myopathic, 1:178, 1:178f
  neuronal, 1:253
  parathyroid gland, 3:308, 3:309f
  pericardial fat, 3:25, 3:25f
  resulting from malnutrition or cachexia, 1:177, 1:177f
  testicular, 3:481-485, 3:482f-483f
  thymic, 1:6f, 3:123, 3:144-147, 3:145f
Attaching-effacing *E. coli* (AEEC), 2:161-163, 2:162f
Atypical adenomatous hyperplasia, 2:495
Atypical mycobacteriosis, 1:640, 1:640f
Atypical pneumonia, 2:509
Auditory tube, 1:495-496
Aujeszky's disease, 2:20
Aural hematoma, 1:504
Aural melanoma, 1:504-505
Aural plaques, 1:504
Auricular chondritis, 1:504, 1:697
Australian Cattle dogs
  cochleosaccular degeneration, 1:492
  spongy encephalomyelopathies, 1:346
  spongy myelinopathy, 1:343

INDEX

Australian Kelpie dogs, globoid cell leukodystrophy in, 1:339
Australian Shepherd dogs
 choroidal hypoplasia, 1:413
 cobalamin deficiency, 3:127
 cochleosaccular degeneration, 1:492
 spindle cell tumor, 1:486
Autoimmune dermatoses, 1:600-607
 pemphigus complex, 1:518, 1:600-603
Autolytic changes in retina after death, 1:467
Autopsy. *See* Gross and histologic examinations
Autopsy-in-a-jar pathology, 1:2
Autosomal recessive congenital ichthyoses (ARCI), 1:530, 1:531f
Autosomal recessive PKD (ARPKD), 2:396
Autosomal recessive severe combined immunodeficiency, 3:140-141
Avascular chorion, 3:397
Avipoxvirus, 1:616
AV node, 3:2
 heart examination and, 3:13-14
 impulse formation disturbances, 3:5
Avocado poisoning, 3:38
Axillary nodular necrosis, 1:695
Axonal dystrophy, 1:257-258, 1:258f, 1:324-325
Axonopathy, 1:256, 1:318-334
 distal, 1:257
 peripheral, 1:334-336
 proximal, 1:257, 1:257f
Axons, 1:255-258, 1:256f
 growth disorders, 1:268-269
Ayrshire cattle, cropped and notched pinnae in, 1:502

B

Babesia bigemina, 3:119
Babesia bovis, 3:118
Babesia caballi, 3:119-120
Babesia canis, 1:665, 3:119, 3:119.e1f
Babesia divergens, 3:119
Babesia felis, 3:120
Babesia gibsoni, 1:665, 2:412
Babesia major, 3:119
Babesia rossi, 3:119
Babesia spp., 1:611, 3:117-120, 3:117f
 differential diagnosis, 3:119
 splenic babesiosis, 3:161, 3:161f
Baccharis cordifolia, 2:89
Baccharis megapotamica, 2:89
Baccharis pteronioides, 2:89
Bacillary angiomatosis, 1:646
Bacillary hemoglobinuria, 2:317, 2:317f
Bacillus anthracis, 3:171-174
Bacillus fragilis, 2:113
Bacillus piliformis, 3:42
Bacterial arthritis, 1:148-154
Bacterial diseases, tooth surface, 2:9
Bacterial endophthalmitis, 1:449
Bacterial enterotoxin, 2:71
Bacterial granulomas, 1:637-642
Bacterial hemolysins, 3:126
Bacterial infections
 abortion and stillbirth due to, 3:398, 3:399b, 3:402-417
 alimentary tract, 2:158-201
 central nervous system, 1:353-365
 endocarditis, 3:30-33, 3:31f

Bacterial infections *(Continued)*
 liver, 2:314-318
 lungs and, 2:472-473
 myocarditis, 3:42
 pneumonia, 2:562-563, 2:562f
 respiratory system, 2:531-532, 2:531f
  cats, 2:589
  cattle, 2:542-551
  dogs, 2:577-579
  horses, 2:569-573
  pigs, 2:531-533
  sheep and goats, 2:562-563
 skin, 1:629-646
  lesions in, 1:645-646
 teeth, 2:9
Bacterial osteomyelitis, 1:98-103, 1:98f-99f
 cats, 1:99-100
 cattle, 1:99
 dogs, 1:99-100
 horses, 1:99, 1:99f, 1:101f
Bacterial overgrowth, small intestine, 2:364
Bacterial pododermatitis of horses and ruminants, 1:642-645
Bacterial pseudomycetoma, 1:642, 1:642f
Bacterial septicemia, 3:289, 3:290f
Bacteriology, 1:10-11
Bacteroides fragilis, 2:113, 2:199
Bacteroides spp., 2:9
Balanoposthitis, 3:507
Balantidium, 2:243-244, 2:244f
Baldy calf syndrome, 1:538
Bali cattle, Jembrana disease in, 3:195-196, 3:195f
Balloon cell malignant melanomas, 1:722
Ballooning degeneration of epidermis, 1:519, 1:519f
Bandera's neonatal ataxia, 1:318-319
Banzi virus, 1:281
Barbados Blackbelly sheep, osteogenesis imperfecta in, 1:50
Bartholin's glands, 3:442
Bartonella, 1:646
 endocarditis and, 3:30-31
 liver and, 2:318
Bartonella berkhoffi, 1:646
Bartonella henselae, 3:42
Bartonella vinsonii, 1:99-100, 1:646
Basal cell carcinomas, 1:714
Basement membrane zone (BMZ), 1:513-514
Basic multicellular unit (BMU), 1:26
Basidiobolomycosis, 1:660
 granulomatous rhinitis and, 2:476
Basilar membrane, 1:489-490
Basophilia, 3:111
Basophilic intranuclear viral inclusions, 2:22
Basosquamous carcinomas, 1:714
Basset Hound dogs
 canine atopic dermatitis, 1:591
 degenerative diseases of cartilaginous joints, 1:143-144
 globoid cell leukodystrophy, 1:339
 granulomatous hepatitis, 2:318
 platelet dysfunction, 3:259
 seborrhea, 1:548
 severe combined immunodeficiency (SCID), 3:139
Baylisascaris procyonis, 1:390-391
B-cells
 chronic lymphocytic leukemia/small lymphocytic lymphoma (B-CLL/SLL), 3:219-220

B-cells *(Continued)*
 diffuse large B-cell lymphomas, 3:220-222, 3:221f
 follicular-derived B-cell lymphomas, 3:222-226, 3:223f
 lymphoid hyperplasia, 3:201
 in masticatory myositis, 1:226-227
 Reed-Sternberg cell, 3:219
 T-cell-rich B-cell lymphoma, 3:221-222, 3:222f
Beagle dogs
 chondrodysplasia, 1:44, 1:45f
 cobalamin deficiency, 3:127
 Factor VII deficiency, 3:264
 globoid cell leukodystrophy, 1:339
 hypertrophy type 1 and 2, 1:225
 iatrogenic acromegaly, 3:286f
 lymphomas, 3:238
 osteogenesis imperfecta, 1:50
 osteoporosis, 1:67
 pain syndrome, 1:158, 3:70
 peripheral vestibular disease, 1:494
 selective deficiencies of immunoglobulins, 3:139
Beagle pain syndrome. *See* Steroid-responsive meningitis-arteritis
Beauceron dogs, canine atopic dermatitis in, 1:591
Bedlington Terriers, 2:303, 2:303.e1f
Belgian Blue cattle
 dermatosparaxis, 1:48
 osteopetrosis, 1:51-52
Belgian Gorenendael Shepherd dogs, canine X-linked muscular dystrophy in, 1:192
Belgian Malinois dogs, vitiligo in, 1:556.e1f
Belgian Tervuren dogs
 canine atopic dermatitis, 1:591
 vitiligo, 1:555-556
Benign bone cysts, 1:126
Benign cortical fibromas, 2:447
Benign epithelial neoplasms, 2:478-479, 2:479f
Benign mammary neoplasms, 3:460
Benign melanocytic tumors, 1:721
Benign spindle cell tumors, 1:722-723
Benign tumors of joints, 1:160-162
Bergmann's glia, 1:261
Bergmeister's papilla, 1:417-419, 1:418f
Bernese Mountain dogs
 afibrinogenemia, 3:265
 Alexander disease, 1:341
 canine hypomyelinogenesis, 1:338
 degenerative radiculomyelopathy, 1:330
 vasculitis, 3:70
Besnoitiosis, 1:661-663, 1:662f
 granulomatous rhinitis and, 2:476
Besnoitia spp., 2:239
B-cells, endocrine pancreas, 2:368
β-glucuronidase-deficient MPS, 1:290
β-Mannosidosis, 1:289, 1:492
B_2-microglobulin, 2:385
Betaherpesviruses, 2:537
Bibersteinia trehalosi, 2:543, 2:562-563
Bichon Frise dogs, canine atopic dermatitis, 1:591
Bilateral extraocular muscle myositis of dogs, 1:228
Bilateral hypoplasia, 2:392
Bile cast nephropathy, 2:430
Bile peritonitis, 2:250

Bilharziasis, 3:91-94
Biliary tract
  ducts, 2:261
    hyperplasia, 2:287-288, 2:289f
    necrosis, 2:285, 2:286f
  hyperplastic and neoplastic lesions, 2:344-352
  infarcts, 2:292-293
  inflammatory diseases, 2:300-309
  obstruction, 2:308-309
  pigmentation, 2:270-271
  plugs, 2:271f
Biomarkers of glomerular disease, 2:401
Biopsy
  bone marrow, 3:105f
  endometrial, 3:393
  formats, 1:2
  interpretation, 2:62
  specimen trimming, 1:8-9
  techniques, 2:383
Biosafety/biocontainment, 1:14
Biotin deficiency, 1:582
Birbeck granules, 1:513
Bird tongue, 2:4
Birman cats
  congenital hypotrichosis, 1:539
  peripheral and central distal axonopathy, 1:333
Birnavirus, 2:113
Biventricular failure, 3:6
Black disease, 2:316
Black hair follicular dysplasia, 1:540, 1:540f, 1:557
Black Labrador dogs, diffuse uveal melanocytosis in, 1:484-485
Blackleg, 1:230-233, 1:231f, 3:34
Bladder
  cells, 1:442
  neoplasia, 2:462
  wall
    hypertrophy, 2:452
    rupture, 2:452
Blastomas
  hepato-, 2:347-348, 2:348f
  pulmonary, 2:498
Blastomyces dermatitidis, 1:104, 1:449, 2:580, 3:491
  lymph nodes and, 3:206f
Blastomycosis, 1:449-450, 1:450f, 2:580-582, 2:582f, 2:580.e1f
Blebs, 2:487, 2:487f, 2:487.e1f
Blepharitis, 1:423
Blind staggers, 1:571
Blister beetle, 2:52
  myocardial necrosis and, 3:36
Bloat line in esophagus, 2:37f
Block vertebrae, 1:57
Blood-brain barrier (BBB), 1:263, 1:350
Blood cells
  erythrocyte disorders, 3:112
  hemostasis disorders, 3:255-268
  leukocyte disorders, 3:109-112
  platelet disorders, 3:128-129
Blood-cerebrospinal fluid barrier (BCSFB), 1:350
Blood clots, 2:37
Bloodhound dogs, gastric volvulus in, 2:49
Blood left shift, 3:109
Blood loss. *See also* Hemorrhage
  anemia, 3:112-114
  chronic, 2:73

Blood supply
  bone, 1:27-28, 1:28f
  brain, 1:296-301, 1:296f
  heart, 3:2, 3:5
    abnormal pattern of flow, 3:6
    regurgitant flow, 3:5
  hepatic, 2:260, 2:288
  pituitary gland, 3:278
  spleen, 3:158-162, 3:160f
"Blue-eye disease", 2:530
Blue-green algae, 2:330
Bluetick Hound dogs, globoid cell leukodystrophy in, 1:339
Bluetongue virus (BTV), 1:281, 2:136-139, 2:137f, 3:430-431
  cattle, 2:138
  sheep, 2:138-139
B-lymphocytic acute myeloid leukeumia, 3:132-133, 3:133f
Body mange, 1:676
Bone-forming tumors, 1:109-116, 1:109f
Bone-lining cells, 1:18
Bone marrow, 3:103-138, 3:103f
  in anemia, 3:116
  biopsy, 3:105f
  chronic inflammation and leukocytosis, 3:104-106, 3:106f
  erythroid hyperplasia, 3:106f
  histologic examination, 3:107, 3:107t
  sample procurement and processing, 3:107-109, 3:108f
Bone(s). *See also* Joint(s)
  ash, 1:30
  blood supply, 1:27-28, 1:28f
  cellular elements, 1:17-19, 1:17f
  development and anatomy, 1:21-24, 1:22f
  diseases, 1:17-127
    general considerations, 1:17
    genetic and congenital, 1:36-60, 1:37t
    hyperostotic, 1:91-94
    inflammatory and infectious, 1:97-107
    nutritional and hormonal, 1:60-84
    osteonecrosis, 1:94-97
    toxic, 1:84-91
    tumors and tumor-like lesions, 1:107-127
    viral infections, 1:104-105
  fracture repair, 1:33-36, 1:34f-35f
  growth plate damage, 1:30-31
  hypercalcemia with tumors metastatic to, 3:309
  matrix, 1:19-20
    mineralization, 1:20
  modeling, 1:24-25
  periosteal damage, 1:33
  postmortem examination of, 1:28-30
  remodeling, 1:26-27
  response to mechanical forces and injury, 1:30-36
  sialoprotein, 1:19
  skull, 1:21
    congenital abnormalities, 1:56, 1:56f
    craniomandibular osteopathy, 1:91-92, 1:92f
    fractures, 1:302-303
    sutures, 1:128
  stress-related lesions in horse, 1:36
  structure and function, 1:17-28
  tissue, 1:20-21
Bony labyrinth of ear, 1:488, 1:489f

Border Collie dogs
  cobalamin deficiency, 3:127
  cochleosaccular degeneration, 1:492
  myopathy, 1:198
  sensory and autonomic neuropathy, 1:334
Border disease virus (BDV), 1:104, 1:282-283, 2:128
  goats, 3:426-427
  pigs, 1:104
  sheep, 1:104, 3:426-427
Border Leicester sheep, congenital myopathy in, 1:200
Border-Leicester-Southdown sheep, collagen dysplasia in, 1:544
Bordetella bronchiseptica
  cats, 2:589
  dogs, 2:578, 2:578f
Borna disease virus (BDV), 1:377-378, 1:378f
Borrelia burgdorferi, 1:147, 1:152
Borreliosis, 1:152, 1:646
  dogs, 1:152
Borzoi dogs, gastric volvulus in, 2:49
Boston Terrier dogs
  canine atopic dermatitis, 1:591
  color dilution alopecia, 1:539-540
  corneal edema, 1:429
  corneal endothelial dystrophy, 1:433
  hyperadrenocorticism, 1:588
  malignant melanoma, 2:26
  myxomatous valvular degeneration, 3:27
  vascular ring anomalies, 2:33
Botryoid rhabdomyosarcoma, 1:244f, 2:463f, 2:464
Botryomycosis, 1:233-234
Botulism, 1:317
Bouvier des Flandres dogs
  motor neuropathy, 1:335
  myopathy, 1:198
Bovine adenovirus (BAdV), 2:143, 2:143f-144f, 2:542
Bovine alimentary papillomatosis, 2:43-44
Bovine anthrax, 3:172, 3:173f, 3:172.e1f
Bovine besnoitiosis, 1:661-662
Bovine cardiomyopathies, 3:50-51, 3:50f
Bovine chondrodysplasia, 1:38, 1:38f
Bovine congenital hematopoietic porphyria, 1:579
Bovine coronavirus (BCoV), 2:112, 2:148-150, 2:149f, 2:541-542, 2:542.e1f
Bovine cutaneous angiomatosis, 3:99
Bovine cutaneous onchocerciasis, 1:688
Bovine ephermeral fever virus (BEFV), 3:79
Bovine erythropoietic protoporphyria, 1:579
Bovine familial convulsions and ataxia, 1:319
Bovine farcy, 3:96
Bovine generalized glycogenesis type II, 3:46, 3:50
Bovine herpesviral encephalitis, 1:381-382, 1:381f
Bovine herpesvirus 1, 1:625-627
Bovine herpesvirus 2, 1:625-627
Bovine herpesvirus 4, 1:626, 3:435
Bovine herpesvirus in pregnant uterus, 3:433-435
Bovine hypomyelinogenesis, 1:338-339
Bovine kidney, 2:395
Bovine leukemia virus (BLV), 3:235
Bovine lymphoma, 3:235-237
Bovine malignant catarrhal fever-associated uveitis, 1:453
Bovine mastitis, 3:452-457, 3:452f
Bovine metabolic myopathy, 1:208

Bovine necrotizing meningoencephalitis, 1:381-382, 1:381f-382f
Bovine ovarian lymphosarcoma, 3:378, 3:379f
Bovine papillomaviruses, 1:706-707, 1:707f, 2:22
Bovine papular stomatitis virus (BPSV), 1:616, 1:618-619, 2:39-40, 2:139-140, 2:140f
Bovine parainfluenza virus 3 (BPIV-3), 2:541
Bovine paramyxoviral meningoencephalomyelitis, 1:382
Bovine parvovirus (BPV), 2:157-158, 3:429-430
–induced papilloma, 2:44
Bovine respiratory syncytial virus (BRSV), 2:539-541, 2:540f, 2:540.e2f, 2:540.e1f
Bovine rhinitis virus (BRAV), 2:542
Bovine rotaviral infection, 2:151-152, 2:152f
Bovine spongiform encephalopathy (BSE), 1:349
Bovine torovirus, 2:112
Bovine trypanosomiasis, 3:122-124
Bovine tuberculosis, 2:547-551, 2:549f
Bovine viral diarrhea virus (BVDV), 1:104, 1:105f, 1:281-283, 2:112, 2:114, 2:122-128, 2:123f-125f, 2:542, 2:542.e3f
  esophageal lesions, 2:124, 2:124f
  fetal infections, 2:122
  mucosal disease, 2:123
  -negative cattle, 2:413
  noncytopathic (NCP), 2:122-128
  PI calves, 2:122
  pregnant uterus, 3:425-426
  secondary infections, 2:127
  severe acute, 2:122-123
  thymic atrophy and, 3:145
Bowie, 1:90-91
Bowman's capsules, 2:406-407, 2:437-438, 2:407.e1f
  thickening and lamination, 2:407.e1f
Bowman's space, 2:406-407
Boxer dogs
  acne, 1:549
  canine atopic dermatitis, 1:591
  canine leproid granuloma, 1:503, 1:641
  canine persistent (recurrent) ulcer syndrome, 1:434, 1:435f
  chondrosarcoma, 1:118
  congenital myotonia, 1:201
  degenerative radiculomyelopathy, 1:330
  diffuse fibrous hyperplasia, 2:21-22
  dilated cardiomyopathy, 3:48
  factor VII deficiency, 3:264
  hyperadrenocorticism, 1:588
  hyperestrogenism, 1:589
  hypothyroidism, 1:587, 3:315
  immune-mediated myositis, 1:228
  intestinal lymphomas, 3:239
  lymphomas, 3:238
  malignant lymphoma, 1:123-124
  malignant oral tumors, 2:21
  myotonic dystrophy-like disorder, 1:202-203
  progressive axonopathy, 1:329-330
  recurrent flank alopecia, 1:590
  spongy encephalomyelopathies, 1:346
  typhlocolitis, 2:97-98, 2:98f
Brachycephalic airway syndrome, 2:482, 2:482f

Brachycephalic type dwarfism, 1:39, 1:39f
Brachydont teeth, 2:5
Brachygnathia inferior, 1:56, 1:56f, 2:3
Brachygnathia superior, 1:56, 2:3
Brachyspina, 1:57
Brachyspira pilosicoli, 2:182
Brachyspira hyodysenteriae, 2:182
Brachyspira spp., 2:98
Bracken fern, 1:471, 2:461
Brain. *See also* Spinal cord
  age changes in, 1:304
  atrophy, 1:304-305
  cerebellar hypoplasia, 1:275f
  cerebellum
    agenesis, hypoplasia, and dysplasia, 1:275-276, 1:275f
    Arnold-Chiari malformation, 1:276-277, 1:277f
    atrophy, 1:276, 1:276f
    Dandy-Walker syndrome, 1:277
    development, 1:274-277
    hypoplasia, 1:275f
    intracranial arachnoid cyst, 1:280f
    vascular leakage, 1:298f
  cerebrum, 1:266-274
    cerebral aplasia, anencephaly, 1:266-267, 1:266f
    defects in cerebral corticogenesis, 1:268
    disorders of axonal growth, 1:268-269
    encephalocele, meningocele, 1:267, 1:267f
    holoprosencephaly, 1:269-270, 1:269f
    hydranencephaly, porencephaly, 1:272-274, 1:272f
    hydrocephalus, 1:270-272, 1:271f
    periventricular leukomalacia of neonates, 1:274
  edema, 1:293-295, 1:295f
  embolism, 2:490
  increased intracranial pressure, 1:293-295
  lesions of blood vessels and circulatory disturbances, 1:296-301, 1:296f
    hemorrhagic, 1:300-301
    ischemic, 1:297-300, 1:297f
  microcirculation of, 1:263-264, 1:264f, 1:263.e1f
  traumatic injuries, 1:301-303
  tumors, 1:296f
Branched-chain α-ketoacid decarboxylase deficiency, 1:344, 1:345f
Brangus cattle, Chediak-Higashi syndrome in, 3:259
Brassica rapa, 2:342
Braunvieh x Brown Swiss cattle, congenital myopathy in, 1:199-200
Braxy, 2:53, 2:53f
Braxy-like clostridial abomasitis, 2:53f
Brazilian Terrier dogs, Sly syndrome in, 1:58
Breda virus, 2:112
Breed-related nephropathies, 2:388t-390t
  in domestic species, 2:388t-390t
Brick inclusions, 2:430
Brittany Spaniel dogs
  canine X-linked muscular dystrophy, 1:192
  hypothyroidism, 1:587
  late-onset progressive spinocerebellar degeneration, 1:319
Brodie's abscess, 1:98, 1:98f
Bronchi, 2:468-469

Bronchial arteries, 2:467-468, 2:468f
Bronchial atresia, 2:485
Bronchial gland carcinoma, 2:497
Bronchiectasis, 2:503-504, 2:503f, 2:503.e3f, 2:501.e1f
Bronchiolar necrosis and inflammation, 2:504-506, 2:504f
Bronchioles, 2:469
Bronchiolitis obliterans, 2:504, 2:504f, 2:504.e2f
Bronchioloalveolar hyperplasia, 2:505, 2:504.e2f
Bronchitis, 2:500-504
  cats, 2:502-503
  chronic, 2:501-503, 2:502.e1f
Bronchogenic cysts, 2:484-485
Bronchointerstitial pneumonia, 2:511-512, 2:514.e2f
  foals, 2:514
Bronchopneumonia, 2:506-509, 2:506f, 2:507t
  bacterial, in cattle, 2:542-546, 2:545f
  caseonecrotic, 2:553f
  chronic suppurative, 2:508, 2:508.e1f
  death from, 2:507-508
  morphology, 2:507
  opportunistic bacterial pathogens and, 2:532-533
  reduced lung function, 2:508
  resolution and sequelae, 2:507-508
  sequestrum, 2:508
Bronchopneumopathy, eosinophilic, 2:501-502, 2:502f, 2:501.e1f
Bronchopulmonary dysplasia, 2:516
Bronchopulmonary segment, 2:467
Bronchus-associated lymphoid tissue (BALT), 2:472
Brown recluse spider, 1:568
Brown Swiss cattle, progressive myeloencephalopathy of, 1:325
Brucella abortus, 3:402-406, 3:485-487, 3:490
Brucella canis, 1:449, 3:490
  abortion and, 3:403-404, 3:404f, 3:406
Brucella melitensis, 3:406
Brucella ovis, 3:405-406, 3:405f
  abortion and, 3:473-474, 3:490
Brucella suis, 3:490
  abortion and, 3:404-405
Bruch's membrane, 1:445
Brugia, 3:98
Brunn nests, 2:449
Brush cells, 2:469
Bubalus arnee, 2:117-118
Buccal cavity, 2:12-19
  circulatory disturbances, 2:12-13
  foreign bodies in, 2:13
  inflammation of, 2:13-19
  parasitic diseases, 2:19
  pigmentation, 2:12
  salivary glands, 2:28-30
  tonsil diseases, 2:19-20
Buccal mucosal bleeding time (BMBT), 3:257
Bucked shins, 1:36
Budd-Chiari syndrome, 2:298
Budgerigars, 3:286
Bufadienolide cardiac glycoside-containing plants, 3:35
Buffalopox virus, 1:620-621

Bulbourethral gland, 3:500-504, 3:500f
  disorders of sexual development, 3:500-501, 3:500f
  hyperplasia and metaplasia, 3:502-503, 3:502f
  inflammation, 3:501-502, 3:501f
  neoplasms, 3:503-504, 3:504f
Bullae, 1:524
  pneumothorax and, 2:487, 2:487f
Bullmastiff dogs
  acne, 1:549
  calvarial hyperostosis of, 1:92
  canine leproid granuloma, 1:503, 1:641
  spongy encephalomyelopathies, 1:346-347
Bullous immune skin diseases, 2:14
Bullous pemphigoid (BP), 1:603-604, 2:15
Bull Terrier dogs, 2:416-417
  autosomal recessive acrodermatitis, 3:141
  canine atopic dermatitis, 1:591
  cochleosaccular degeneration, 1:492
  lethal acrodermatitis, 1:533, 1:533.e1f
  melanocytopenic hypomelanosis, 1:555
  subvalvular aortic stenosis, 3:20
Bully Whippets, 1:191, 1:191f
Büngner's bands, 1:256
Bunina bodies, 1:255
Burkholderia mallei, 2:573
Burkholderia pseudomallei, 1:637, 3:491
  respiratory system and, 2:563
  splenic abscesses, 3:183-184
  splenic lesions, 3:188-189, 3:188f
Burkitt-like lymphoma (BKL), 3:226
Burmese cats, primary endocardial fibroelastosis in, 3:22
Burns, 1:564-566, 1:565f
Bursitis, 1:155-156
  sheep, 1:155f
Butterfly vertebrae, 1:57

C

Cabugi breed sheep, 1:42
Cachectic atrophy, lymph node, 3:198-199
Cache valley virus (CVV), 1:280, 3:438-439
Cachexia, atrophy resulting from, 1:177, 1:177f
Cadmium, 1:67
Caffey's disease, 1:53
Cairn Terrier dogs
  canine atopic dermatitis, 1:591
  diabetes mellitus, 2:373
  globoid cell leukodystrophy, 1:339
  hyperestrogenism, 1:589
  polycystic kidney and liver disease, 2:265
  primary portal vein hypoplasia, 2:267-268
  progressive neuronopathy, 1:332-333
Calcinosis circumscripta, 1:563, 1:563f
Calcinosis cutis, 1:562, 1:588, 1:589f
Calcinosis universalis, 1:562-563
Calcitonin, 1:62, 3:296-297
  biological actions, 3:297
  biosynthesis and secretion, 3:297
  in physis, 1:25t
Calcitriol
  biological action, 3:295-296
  biosynthesis, 3:295
Calcium
  carbonate, 1:562, 2:458
  chelation, 2:426
  chloride, 1:562

Calcium (Continued)
  crystal-associated arthropathy (pseudogout), 1:156-157
    dogs, 1:156-157
  deficiency, 2:8. See also Hypocalcemia
    odontodystrophy, 2:8
    osteoporosis, 1:61, 1:65-66
    rickets, 1:61, 1:66, 1:69
    vitamin D, 1:61
  functions, 3:291-292
  hypercalcemia, 3:305-310, 3:305f
  hypocalcemia, 3:299
  malabsorption, 2:70
  muscle necrosis and, 1:181-182, 1:181f
  oxalate, 2:457
  phosphate, 2:458
  phosphorus homeostasis and, 1:61-63
  -regulating hormones, 3:291-310, 3:291f
  salts, deposition of, 1:443, 1:519
Calculi, 2:452
  salivary, 2:29
  urinary, 2:453t
Calf diphtheria, 2:17
Calcium pyrophosphate dihydrate, 1:156-157
Calicivirus, 1:154, 1:628, 2:117
California encephalitis virus meningoencephalomyelitis, 1:383
Call-Exner body, 3:376
Calliphorine myiasis, 1:669
Callipyge phenotype in sheep, 1:191
Calluses, 1:524, 1:559-560
Calodium hepaticum, 2:320
Calvarial hyperostosis of Bullmastiffs, 1:92
Camelostrongylus, 2:54-55
Camelpox virus, 1:616, 1:621
Campylobacter fetus, 3:406-408, 3:408f, 3:424, 3:507
  liver and, 2:314-315
Campylobacter spp., 2:98, 2:117
  enteritis associated with, 2:180-181
Canalicular domain, liver, 2:262
Canalicular stage of lung growth, 2:484
Canal of Hering, 2:262
Cancrum oris, 2:18
Candida albicans, 1:647, 2:32, 2:202, 2:459
Candida parapsilosis, 3:30-31
  granulomatous rhinitis and, 2:476
Candida tropicalis, 2:202
Candidiasis, 2:202
Canid herpesvirus 1, 3:507
Canine acanthosis nigricans, 1:555
Canine adenovirus 1 (CAV-1), 1:105, 1:452-453, 2:410
  hepatitis, 2:310-312, 2:311.e1f
Canine adenovirus 2 (CAV-2), 2:577
Canine atopic dermatitis, 1:591-593
Canine blastomycosis, 2:459
Canine bocavirus, 2:577
Canine cardiomyopathies, 3:48-49, 3:48f
Canine colitis, 2:94
Canine congenital myasthenia, 1:209
Canine coronavirus (CCoV), 2:116, 2:150
Canine cutaneous histiocytoma (CCH), 1:728-729, 3:243-245, 3:244f-245f, 3:244.e1f, 3:243.e1f
Canine cutaneous Langerhans cell histiocytosis, 1:729, 3:245-246, 3:246f
Canine cyclic hematopoiesis, 3:110
Canine demodicosis, 1:679-682, 1:679f
Canine dermatomyositis, 1:198, 1:541-542, 1:542f-543f

Canine dietary factors, 2:457
Canine distemper virus (CDV), 1:104-105, 1:384-385, 1:474, 2:116-117, 2:574-576, 2:575.e1f
  acquired deafness and, 1:493
  lymph nodes and, 3:207f
  thymic atrophy and, 3:145
Canine dynamin 1 (DNM1) gene, 1:198
Canine ehrlichiosis, 1:474-475
Canine eosinophilic granuloma, 1:694
Canine epitrichical ductular adenomas, 1:718-719
Canine exertional rhabdomyolysis, 1:223
Canine familial glomerulonephritides, 2:412
Canine familial nephropathies, 2:391
Canine hepacivirus, 2:577
Canine hepatozoonosis, 1:94, 1:94f
Canine herpesvirus-1 (CaHV-1), 2:577, 3:431-432, 3:432f, 3:434f
  encephalitis, 1:383
Canine hypomeylinogenesis, 1:337-338
Canine immune-mediated hemolytic anemia, 3:265
Canine infectious respiratory disease (CIRD) complex, 2:574
Canine influenza, 2:577
Canine juvenile cellulitis, 1:690-691, 1:691f
Canine juvenile pancreatic atrophy, 2:363, 2:363f
Canine kidneys, 2:378
Canine leproid granuloma, 1:503, 1:641, 1:641f
Canine lymphomas, 3:238-239, 3:239f, 3:239.e1f, 3:239.e2f, 3:238.e2f
Canine minute virus (CnMV), 2:157, 3:430
Canine monocytotropic ehrlichiosis, 3:111
Canine multifocal retinopathy, 1:469
Canine nasodigital hyperkeratosis, 1:549-550
Canine necrotizing meningoencephalitis (NME), 1:392-393, 1:392f
Canine panosteitis, 1:106-107, 1:107f
Canine papillomavirus 1 (CPV1), 2:22, 2:22f
Canine parainfluenza (CPIV), 2:576
Canine parvovirus, 2:116-117
  thymic atrophy, 3:145
Canine parvovirus 2 infection (CPV-2), 2:156-157, 2:156f-157f
Canine perivascular wall tumors (PWTs), 1:723, 1:724f
Canine persistent (recurrent) ulcer syndrome, 1:434, 1:435f
Canine pigmented plaques, 1:710-711, 1:711f
Canine pneumovirus, 2:577
Canine pseudoplacentational endometrial hyperplasia, 3:383, 3:384f
Canine pulmonary veno-occlusive disease (PVOD), 2:493, 2:493f, 2:493.e1f
Canine reactive histiocytosis, 3:247-250, 3:248f, 3:247.e1f
  cutaneous, 3:247-249, 3:248f, 3:249.e1f, 3:247.e1f
  systemic, 1:729, 3:249-250, 3:249f
Canine recurrent flank alopecia, 1:590, 1:590f, 1:590.e1f
Canine respiratory coronavirus (CRCoV), 2:576
Canine transmissible veneral tumor (CTVT), 3:448-449, 3:449f, 3:509, 3:510f
Canine tubulointerstitium, 2:382f
Canine urothelial cell carcinomas, 2:462-463
Canine uveodermatologic syndrome, 1:557, 1:557f-558f, 1:613

INDEX

Canine X-linked muscular dystrophy, 1:192-194, 1:193f-195f, 3:49
Capillaries, 3:54
Capillarization, liver, 2:288
Capped elbow, 1:155
Capped hocks, 1:155
  pigs, 1:156
Capillarization of sinusoids, 2:260
Caprine arthritis-encephalitis virus (CAEV), 1:154, 1:154f, 1:378-380, 1:379f, 2:558-560, 2:559.e1f
  mastitis with, 3:458
Caprine besnoitiosis, 1:662
Caprine herpesvirus 2, 1:625-627
Caprine herpesvirus 3, 2:132
Caprine lymphomas, 3:237
Capripoxvirus, 1:616, 1:622-624
Capsular pseudocysts, 2:396f
Capsular sclerosis, 3:339
Capture myopathy, 1:223
Cara inchada, 2:12
Carbadox, 3:343
Carbohydrate overload, 2:40-43
Carbolic dips, 2:519
Carbon dioxide excretion, 2:381
Carbon monoxide poisoning, 1:306
Carboxyterminal telopeptide of type I collagen (ICTP), 1:27
Carcinoids, 2:497-498
  hepatic, 2:349, 2:350f
Carcinomas/adenocarcinomas, 2:30, 2:463. See also Neoplasia; Tumors
  adrenal gland, 3:345-346, 3:346f
  aortic body, 3:354-355, 3:354f
  carotid body, 3:355-356
  derived from apocrine glands of the anal sac, 3:307f-308f, 3:308
  endometrium and cervix, 3:449-450, 3:450f
  exocrine pancreatic, 2:366-367, 2:367f
  feline pulmonary, 2:497.e1f
  gastrointestinal, 2:101-104
  of gland of the third eyelid, 1:482
  hepatocellular, 2:346, 2:346.e1f
  lower urinary tract, 2:462
  mammary, 3:460-463, 3:462f, 3:463t
  nasal, 2:478, 2:478f-479f
  ovine pulmonary, 2:560-562, 2:561f, 2:561.e1f
  pulmonary, 1:736, 2:495-500, 2:496t, 2:497f-498f, 2:495.e2f
  rectal, 2:103f
  splenic, 3:194, 3:194f
  testicular, 3:496
  thymic, 3:156-157, 3:157f
  thyroid, 3:329-332, 3:330f
  tracheal, 2:483
Carcinosarcoma, 2:497
Cardenolide cardiac glycoside, 3:35
Cardiac dilation, 3:7-9, 3:7f
Cardiac fibrosis, 2:298
Cardiac gland mucosa, 2:44, 2:46
Cardiac hypertrophy, 3:7-9
Cardiac myocytes, 3:3
Cardiac output no-reflow phenomenon, 2:398
Cardiac rhabdomyomas, 1:241
Cardiac rhabdomyosarcomas, 1:243
Cardiac skeleton, 3:2
Cardiac syncope, 3:10

Cardigan Welsh Corgi dogs, severe combined immunodeficiency (SCID) in, 3:139
Cardiomyopathies, 3:44-51, 3:45.e1f
  cats, 3:46-48, 3:46.e2f
  cattle, 3:50-51, 3:50f
  dogs, 3:48-49, 3:48f, 3:48.e2f
Cardiovascular system, 3:1-101. See also Circulatory disturbances
  conduction system diseases, 3:51
  endocardial disease, 3:27-33
  heart
    congenital abnormalities, 3:14-24
    diseases, 3:2-54
    examination, 3:12-14
    failure, 3:6-12
    neoplasms, 3:52-54, 3:52f
  lymphatics, 3:94-98
  myocardial disease, 3:33-51
  pericardial disease, 3:24-27
  vascular system diseases, 3:54-101
  veins, 3:88-94
Cardiovirus, 3:43
Caries, dental, 2:9-11, 2:10f
Caroli disease, 2:265
Carotid body adenoma and carcinoma, 3:355-356
Carpal hygromas, 1:154
Carprofen, 2:329
Cartilage, articular, 1:129
  response to injury, 1:131-132
Cartilage-forming tumors, 1:116-121
Cartilaginous emboli, 1:299f
Cartilaginous end plates, 1:128-129
Cartilaginous joints, 1:128-129
  degenerative diseases of, 1:143-145
  dogs, 1:143-144
Caruncles, 3:400
Caryospora spp., 1:664
Case coordination, 1:12
Case interpretation and client service in postmortem examinations, 1:12-14, 1:13f
Casein clot formation, 2:38
Caseonecrotic bronchopneumonia, 2:553f
Caseous lymphadenitis (CLA), 2:562, 3:204-208, 3:207f-208f, 2:562.e1f, 3:205.e1f
Caseous tuberculosis, 3:389
Cassia occidentalis, 1:220, 1:220f
  myocardial necrosis and, 3:36
Castor beans, 2:117
Catagen phase, hair, 1:516
Cataract, 1:442-444, 1:442f
  congenital, 1:422
  deposition of calcium salts in, 1:443
  diabetic, 1:443
  galactose-induced, 1:443
  megavoltage X-radiation, 1:444
  Soemmering ring, 1:444, 1:444f
  sunlight-induced, 1:443-444
  uveitis and, 1:447-448
Catarrhal bronchitis, 2:501
Catarrhal stomatitis, 2:14
Catecholamine, 3:271
  hormone biosynthesis, 3:348-349, 3:350f
Caterpillar cells, 3:37
Cat fur mite, 1:683
Cattle, epidermolysis bullosa in, 1:534-535
Cauda equina, neuritis of, 1:394-395
Caudal fossa, 1:274-277

Caudal regression syndrome, 1:56-57
Cauliflower-like growths, 2:103-104
Cavalier King Charles Spaniel dogs, 2:457
  caudal fossa, 1:277
  ichthyosis, 1:531-532
  inherited thrombocytopenia, 3:258
  muscle hypertonicity, 1:203
  myxomatous valvular degeneration, 3:27
  oral eosinophilic granuloma, 2:16
  otitis media with effusion, 1:498
Cavitating leukodystrophy, 1:339-340
CCNU (1-(2-chloroethyl)-3-cyclohexyl-1-nitrosourea), 2:329
CD8+ T-cells
  in masticatory myositis, 1:226-227
  in polymyositis, 1:228-229
CD4+ T-cells in masticatory myositis, 1:226-227
Cebocephaly, 1:270
Cecal dilation, 2:78
Cecocolic intussusception, 2:84f
  in horse, 2:84
Cell-mediated immunity, 2:548-549
Cellular crescent, 2:406.e1f
Cellular elements of bone, 1:17-19, 1:17f
Cellularity, of glomerular tuft, 2:405
Cellular swelling, acute, 2:421-422
Cellulitis, 1:636-637
  canine juvenile, 1:690-691, 1:691f
Celomic epithelium tumors, 3:377, 3:377f
Cementing lines, 1:27, 1:27f
Cementum, 2:5-6
  hyperplasia, 2:6
  hypertrophy, 2:6-8
Central and peripheral neuronopathies, 1:326-334
Central chromatolysis, 1:252f-253f, 1:314, 1:333f
Central nervous system (CNS). See also Nervous system
  anoxia and, 1:305-307
  degeneration, 1:303-350
  fixed macrophage system, 1:262
  inflammation, 1:350-396, 1:351t-352t
    bacterial and pyogenic infections, 1:353-365
    chlamydia disease, 1:391-392
    helminth and arthropod infections, 1:389-391
    idiopathic inflammatory diseases, 1:392-396, 1:392f
    microsporidian infections, 1:385-386
    parasitic infections, 1:386-391
    viral infections, 1:365-385
  injury and myocardial necrosis, 3:39
  malformations, 1:264-284
    with BVDV, 3:426-427
    viral causes, 1:280-284
  microcirculation, 1:263-264, 1:264f, 1:263.e1f
  muscular defects, 1:187-189
  neoplastic diseases, 1:396-406
  oligodendrocytes in, 1:258
  spinal cord, 1:277-279
    arachnoid cysts, 1:279
    diplomyelia, 1:278f
    dysraphism, 1:278f
    embolism, 2:490
    lymphoma, 3:240f
    myelodysplasia, 1:277-279, 1:278f
    segmental hypoplasia of, 1:277f

INDEX

Central nervous system (CNS) *(Continued)*
    spina bifida, *1*:57, *1*:279
        subdural hemorrhage of, *1*:303*f*
        subdural/intradural abscess, *1*:354*f*
        syringomyelia, *1*:278*f*
    storage diseases, *1*:284-293
    traumatic injuries, *1*:301-303
    Wallerian-like degeneration, *1*:256-257
Central osteosarcomas, *1*:110
Centrilobular liver
    fibrosis, *2*:289, *2*:289*f*
    necrosis, *2*:282
Centronuclear myopathy of Labrador Retrievers, *1*:197, *1*:197*f*
Cercopithifilaria spp., *1*:690
Cerebellar atrophy, *1*:276, *1*:276*f*
Cerebellar cortical degeneration, *1*:318-320
Cerebellum
    agenesis, hypoplasia, and dysplasia, *1*:275-276, *1*:275*f*
    Arnold-Chiari malformation, *1*:276-277, *1*:277*f*
    atrophy, *1*:276, *1*:276*f*
    Dandy-Walker syndrome, *1*:277
    development, *1*:274-277
    hypoplasia, *1*:275*f*
    intracranial arachnoid cyst, *1*:280*f*
    vascular leakage, *1*:298*f*
Cerebral abscess, *1*:360*f*
Cerebral aplasia, *1*:266-267, *1*:266*f*
Cerebral corticogenesis defects, *1*:268
Cerebral edema, *1*:295*f*
Cerebral swelling, *1*:293-295
Cerebrocortical necrosis, *1*:5*f*
Cerebrocortical atrophy, *1*:7*f*
Cerebrospinal angiopathy, *1*:298, *1*:298*f*, *3*:60
Cerebrospinal fluid (CSF), *1*:270-272
Cerebrospinal vasculitis, *1*:298-299, *1*:298*f*
Cerebrum, *1*:266-274
    cerebral aplasia, anencephaly, *1*:266-267, *1*:266*f*
    defects in cerebral corticogenesis, *1*:268
    disorders of axonal growth, *1*:268-269
    encephalocele, meningocele, *1*:267, *1*:267*f*
    holoprosencephaly, *1*:269-270, *1*:269*f*
    hydranencephaly, porencephaly, *1*:272-274, *1*:272*f*
    hydrocephalus, *1*:270-272, *1*:271*f*
    periventricular leukomalacia of neonates, *1*:274
Ceroid/lipofuscin, *1*:254
Ceroid-lipofuscinoses, *1*:290-292, *1*:291*f*
Ceroid lipofuscinosis, *1*:291*f*
Certification of pathologists, *1*:14
Ceruminous glands
    cysts and tumors, *1*:719
    neoplasms, *1*:507-508
Cervical vertebral malformation-malarticulation, *1*:136, *1*:136*f*
    dogs, *1*:136, *1*:136*f*
    horses, *1*:136, *1*:136*f*
Cervicitis, *3*:441-442
Cervicovaginitis, bovine, *3*:443
Cervix
    carcinoma, *3*:449-450, *3*:450*f*
    dilations and diverticula, *3*:369
    hypoplasia, *3*:368-369
    pathology, *3*:441-442
Cestodes, *2*:221-223, *2*:319-320
    central nervous system and, *1*:389
Cestrum spp., *2*:331
Chabertia ovina, *2*:215-216

Chabertia spp., *2*:215-216
Chagas disease, *3*:44, *3*:44*f*
Chain-of-custody, *1*:2
Chalazion, *1*:423, *1*:423*f*
Channel Island cattle, spontaneous rupture of gastrocnemius muscle, *1*:211
Channelopathies, *1*:200
Characteristic granular pattern, *2*:407-408
Charolais cattle
    hip dysplasia in, *1*:135-136
    progressive ataxia, *1*:341, *1*:341*f*
Chediak-Higashi syndrome (CHS), *1*:556, *3*:110, *3*:259
Chemical abomasitis, *2*:52
Chemical gastritis, *2*:52
Chemical injury
    lungs, *2*:518-520
    parathyroid glands, *3*:298
    rodenticide intoxication, *3*:264
    to skin, *1*:566-575
Chemical peritonitis, *2*:250
Chemodectomas, *3*:354-356
    aortic body adenoma and carcinoma, *3*:354-355, *3*:354*f*
    carotid body adenoma and carcinoma, *3*:355-356
    development, structure, and function, *3*:354
    extra-adrenal paragangliomas, *3*:356
    heart-base tumors derived from ectopic thyroid, *3*:356
Chemokines, *2*:408
Chemosensory cells, *2*:469
Chemotactic cytokines, *2*:408
Chesapeake Bay Retriever dogs
    degenerative radiculomyelopathy, *1*:330
    follicular dysplasia, *1*:540-541, *1*:540.e1f*
Cheyletiellosis, *1*:678
Chief cell adenoma, *3*:302, *3*:303*f*
Chief cells, *2*:45
Chihuahua dogs
    axonal dystrophy, *1*:325
    color dilution alopecia, *1*:539-540
    corneal edema in, *1*:429
    corneal endothelial dystrophy, *1*:433
    myxomatous valvular degeneration, *3*:27
Chimerism, *3*:363
Chinaberry tree, *2*:89
Chinese Crested dogs
    congenital hypotrichosis, *1*:538-539
    hereditary striatonigral and cerebello-olivary degeneration, *1*:319
Chinese Shar Pei dogs
    canine atopic dermatitis, *1*:591
    cobalamin deficiency, *3*:127
    cutaneous mucinosis, *1*:546
    demodectic mange, *1*:679
    familial AA amyloidosis, *2*:278-279
    familial Chinese Shar Pei fever, *1*:158
    intestinal lymphomas, *3*:239
    seborrhea, *1*:548
    selective deficiencies of immunoglobulins, *3*:139
    vasculitis, *3*:70
Chlamydia, *2*:53
    abortion and, *3*:414, *3*:415*f*
    arthritis, *1*:152-153
    central nervous system and, *1*:391-392
    respiratory system and, *2*:551, *2*:563, *2*:590
Chlamydia abortus, *3*:414, *3*:415*f*
Chlamydophila felis, *1*:425, *2*:590

Chlamydophila psittaci, *2*:551, *2*:590
Chlamydophila spp., *2*:53, *2*:113
Chlorella algae, *1*:665
Choanal atresia, *2*:473
Cholangiocarcinomas, *2*:348, *2*:349*f*
Cholangiocellular tumors, *2*:348-349, *2*:348*f*
    mixed hepatocellular and, *2*:349, *2*:349.e1f*
Cholangiocytes, *2*:262
Cholangiohepatitis, *2*:301, *2*:307-308, *2*:307.e1f*
Cholangitis, *2*:301, *2*:307-308, *2*:308*f*
Cholecalciferol, *3*:295-296
    -25-hydroxylase, *3*:295
Cholestasis, *3*:265
Cholecystitis, *2*:301, *2*:306-307
Choledochal cysts, *2*:265-266
Choledochitis, *2*:301
Cholelithiasis, *2*:308-309, *2*:309*f*
Cholestasis, *2*:292-294, *2*:292*f*
Cholestatis injury, *2*:327
Cholesteatoma, *1*:499, *1*:499*f*
Cholesteatosis of choroid plexus, *1*:304, *1*:304*f*
Cholesterol granuloma, *1*:304*f*
    middle ear and, *1*:497
Chondritis, laryngeal, *2*:481-482, *2*:481.e2f*
Chondroblastic osteosarcomas, *1*:113-114, *1*:113*f*
Chondrocytes, *1*:22-24
Chondrodysplasias, *1*:37-46, *1*:37*t*
    cats, *1*:45-46, *1*:46*f*
    cattle, *1*:38-39, *1*:38*f*
    dogs, *1*:37-46, *1*:43*f*-44*f*
    horses, *1*:42, *1*:43*f*
    pigs, *1*:42
    sheep, *1*:40-42, *1*:40*f*-42*f*
Chondrodystrophy, *1*:37
    dogs, *1*:143-144
    manganese deficiency in, *1*:80
Chondroid bone, *1*:21
Chondromas, *1*:116
    laryngeal, *2*:482, *2*:482.e1f*
Chondromatosis, synovial, *1*:162, *1*:162*f*
Chondrosarcomas, *1*:118-121, *3*:52
    dogs, *1*:118, *1*:119*f*
    nasal, *2*:480, *2*:480.e1f*
Chordoma, *1*:404, *1*:404*f*
Chorioallantoic membranes, *3*:400
Chorioptic mange, *1*:676-677, *1*:677*f*
Chorioretinitis, *1*:446
Choristoma, *1*:520
Choroidal hypoplasia, *1*:413, *1*:414*f*
Choroidal melanocytomas, *1*:483
Choroiditis, *1*:357*f*
Choroid of uvea, *1*:445
Choroid plexus, *1*:262
    age changes, *1*:304, *1*:304*f*
    carcinoma, *1*:401*f*
    papilloma, *1*:401, *1*:401*f*
Chow Chow dogs
    alopecia X, *1*:589-590
    canine hypomyelinogenesis, *1*:337
    color dilution alopecia, *1*:539-540
    congenital myotonia, *1*:200*f*, *1*:201
    early onset diabetes mellitus, *2*:373
    hypothyroidism, *1*:587
    malignant melanoma, *2*:26
Chromatolysis, *1*:252*f*, *1*:314
    central, *1*:252*f*-253*f*, *1*:314, *1*:333-334, *1*:333*f*
    peripheral, *1*:253
Chromoblastomycosis, *1*:654-655
Chromogranin A, *3*:294

Chromomycosis, 1:654-655, 1:655f
Chromosomes
  disorders of sexual development and, 3:469
  sex
    disorders, 3:363-365, 3:363f-365f, 3:469
    genotype, 3:360
Chronic bronchitis, 2:501-502, 2:502.e1f
  cats, 2:503
Chronic cardiac glycoside poisoning, 3:35
Chronic degenerative joint disease, 1:138-140, 1:140f
Chronic endometritis, 3:389-390
Chronic eosinophilic enteritis in horses, 2:96
Chronic erosive colitis, 2:93f
Chronic erysipelas, 1:149-150
Chronic gingivostomatitis, 2:15-16
Chronic hepatitis, 2:301-306
  cats, 2:305
  dogs, 2:302-305, 2:305f
  horses, 2:305, 2:305.e1f
Chronic hepatotoxic injury, 2:328
Chronic hypertrophic pyloric gastropathy, 2:48
Chronic inflammatory bowel disease, 2:2, 2:92
Chronic interstitial pancreatitis, 2:360, 2:361f
Chronic lymphadenitis, 3:203-204, 3:203f, 3:204.e1f
Chronic lymphocytic leukemia (CLL), 3:136
Chronic lymphocytic leukemia/small lymphocytic lymphoma (B-CLL/SLL), 3:219-220
Chronic metabolic acidosis, 1:67
Chronic polypoid cystitis, 2:460-461
Chronic pressure overload, 3:7
Chronic renal disease, 2:16-17
  anemia and, 3:127
  hyperparathyroidism secondary to, 3:300-301, 3:300f
  hypertension and, 3:59
Chronic renal failure (CRF), 2:377-378, 2:384, 2:413-414
Chronic rhinitis, 2:475
Chronic suppurative bronchopneumonia, 2:508, 2:508.e1f
Chronic suppurative sinusitis, 2:477-478, 2:477.e1f
Chronic ulcerative paradental syndrome, 2:16
Chronic ulcerative stomatitis, 2:16
Chronic volume overload, 3:7
Chronic wasting disease (CWD), 1:349
Chrysomyia bezziana, 1:669-670
Chuzan virus (CHUV), 1:281, 3:431
Chylothorax, 2:521, 3:95-96, 2:521.e3f
Chylous ascites, 3:96
Cicatricial alopecia, 1:698
Cicuta douglasii, 3:36
Cilia-associated respiratory bacillus (CAR), 2:547, 2:547f
Ciliary body of uvea, 1:445
Ciliary dyskinesis, 1:496
Ciliated cells, 2:469
Circoviruses, 2:116
  circoviral antigen stains, 2:116
Circovirus postweaning multisystemic wasting syndrome (PMWS), 2:527-529, 3:210-212, 3:210f-212f, 3:440, 3:440f
Circulating nonhematopoietic neoplastic cells, 3:137-138

Circulation, micro-, 1:263-264
Circulatory disturbances, 2:51-52
  brain, 1:296-301, 1:296f
  buccal cavity and mucosa, 2:12-13
  circulatory failure, 3:6, 3:10-12
  edema, 2:51
  gastric venous infarction, 2:51
  hyperemia, 2:51
  lung, 2:487-494
  muscle, 1:210-213, 1:211f
    compartment syndrome, 1:211
    downer syndrome, 1:212
    muscle crush syndrome, 1:212
    postanesthethic myopathy in horses, 1:213
    vascular occlusive syndrome, 1:212, 1:212f
  nasal cavity, 2:473-474
  ovary, 3:381-382
  spleen, 3:169-171
  stomach, 2:51-52
  testes, 3:491-492
  uremic gastritis, 2:51
Circumventricular organs (CVOs), 1:263, 1:263.e1f
Cirrhosis, 2:289-290
  hepatic fatty, 2:276, 2:276.e1f
  hypertrophic hepatic, 2:306
Cisplatin, 1:494
Citrobacter koseri, 3:42
Classical swine fever virus (CSFV), 1:283, 3:77-79, 3:78f, 3:178-181, 3:179f-180f, 3:77.e1f, 3:78.e1f, 3:79.e1f
  pigs, 1:104
  pregnant uterus, 3:79, 3:424-425
  sheep, 1:104
  thymic atrophy and, 3:145
Classic equine viral papillomatosis, 1:707-710, 1:708f, 1:708t
Classic hepatic lobule, 2:261
Classification of lymphomas, 3:215-243, 3:217t
Clear cell basal cell carcinomas, 1:714
Clear cell epitrichial carcinomas, 1:719
Cleft palates, 2:3, 2:3f
  primary, 2:3
  secondary, 2:3f
Clefts, epidermal, 1:519, 1:519f
Clonality, 3:215
Clonorchis sinensis, 2:323-324
Clostridial myositis, 1:230-233, 1:231f
Clostridium botulinum, 2:77, 2:183-194
Clostridium chauvoei, 2:183-194, 3:42
Clostridium difficile, 2:100, 2:183-194, 2:192f-194f
  acute necro-hemorrhagic colitis, 2:99f
Clostridium haemolyticum, 3:126
  liver and, 2:317
Clostridium novyi, 3:126
  liver and, 2:316
Clostridium perfringens, 2:53-54, 2:183-194, 2:187f, 2:452, 3:126
  gastritis, 2:57
  type A, 2:113
  type C, 2:84, 2:100, 2:113, 2:187, 2:187f-188f
  type D enterotoxemia, 2:115, 2:188-191, 2:189f-190f
Clostridium piliforme, 2:98-99, 2:113-114, 2:183-194, 3:42
  liver and, 2:314-315, 2:317, 2:317f-318f

Clostridium septicum, 2:53, 2:183-194
Clotting times, 3:263
Club cells, 2:469, 2:469.e1f
Coagulase-positive staphylococci, 2:456
Coagulation
  liver disease and, 3:264-265
  regulation of, 3:265-266
Coagulative myocytolysis, 3:37
Coagulative necrosis, 3:37
  gastric wall, 2:56
  liver, 2:281
Coarctation of the aorta, 3:23, 3:23f
Coat color
  dilution and black hair follicular dysplasia, 1:557
  -linked hair follicle dysplasia, 1:540
Cobalamin
  deficiency, 3:127
  malabsorption, 2:69-70
Coccidioides immitis, 1:449-450, 2:583-584, 2:584f
  adrenal cortex and, 3:340
Coccidioides posadasii, 2:583-584
Coccidioides spp., 1:103-104, 1:104f, 2:115-116
  respiratory system and, 2:583-584
Coccidiosis, 2:227-235
  cattle, 2:229-231, 2:230f
  dogs and cats, 2:235-239
  horses, 2:233-234
  pigs, 2:234-235, 2:234f
  sheep and goats, 2:231-233, 2:232f
Cochlear duct, 1:489, 1:489f
Cochleosaccular degeneration, 1:492
Cochliomyia hominivorax, 1:669-670, 2:43
Cochliomyia macellaria, 1:669-670
Cocker Spaniel dogs
  axonal dystrophy, 1:325
  dilated cardiomyopathy, 3:48
  lymphomas, 3:238
  malignant melanoma, 2:26
  malignant oral tumors, 2:21
  multisystem neuronal degeneration, 1:320
  myxomatous valvular degeneration, 3:27
  peripheral vestibular disease, 1:494
  seborrhea, 1:548
Codman's triangle, 1:33
Coenurus cerebralis, 1:389
Coffee senna plant, 1:219-220
COL4A3 gene, 2:416
COL4A4 gene, 2:416
COL4A5 gene, 2:415-416
Cold agglutinin disease, 1:608
Cold injury, 1:564
Coliform arthritis, 1:151
Coliform mastitis, 3:454-455, 3:454f-455f
Colitis. See also Clostridium difficile
  cats, 2:98-99
  cystica profunda, 2:97
  idiopathic mucosal, 2:92-93
    canine, 2:94
  necrotic, 2:99, 2:99f
  spirochetal, in pigs, 2:181-183
  weaner colitis of sheep, 2:180-181
Collagen dysplasia, 1:543-544
  cats, 1:545, 1:545f
  cattle, 1:544
  dogs, 1:544-545, 1:545f
  horses, 1:544, 1:544.e1f
  sheep, 1:544

Collagen fibers, 1:129
  degeneration, 1:519
  dermal, 1:514
Collagenofibrotic glomerulonephropathy, 2:419f, 2:418.e1f
Collagenous hamartomas, 1:723
Collagenous metaplasia, 1:304
Collapse, tracheal, 2:483f, 1:192.e1
Collie dogs
  afibrinogenemia, 3:265
  axonal dystrophy, 1:324
  canine dermatomyositis, 1:198
  choroidal hypoplasia, 1:413
  Collie eye anomaly, 1:413-414, 1:414f
  hereditary deafness, 1:492
  hyperestrogenism, 1:589
  melanocytopenic hypomelanosis, 1:555
  motor neuron disease, 1:331
  retinal folding, 1:419
Collie eye anomaly (CEA), 1:413-414, 1:414f
Colliquative myocytolysis, 3:37
Colloid goiter, 3:322, 3:322f
Colloid mineralization, 3:314, 3:315f
Coloboma, 1:412, 1:412f
Colon
  adenocarcinoma
    cats, 2:103f
      metastasis, 2:102-103
  bacteria, 2:65
  colonic glands, 2:61-62
  epithelial cell proliferation, 2:68
  impaction, 2:76
  invasive carcinoma, 2:105f
  lamina propria, 2:62
  left dorsal displacement, 2:78-79, 2:79f
  mesenteric attachments anomaly, 2:74
  neoplasms, 2:117
  osmotic overload, 2:71-72
  right dorsal displacement, 2:78
  tympany, 2:78
  volvulus, 2:79
Color dilution alopecia, 1:539-540, 1:540f, 1:557
Combined ocular and skeletal dysplasia, 1:45
Comedo, 1:524
Committed myoblasts, 1:167
Compact cell carcinoma of thyroid, 3:330, 3:331f
Compartment syndrome, 1:211
Complement-leukocyte-dependent mechanism, 2:408
Complete blood count (CBC), 3:257
Complex partial cluster seizures with orofacial involvement, 1:307-308
Complex secretory epitrichial adenomas, 1:718-719
Complex vertebral malformation (CVM), 1:57
Compositae/asteracae, 2:331
Compound granular corpuscles, 1:263
Compressive atelectasis, 2:486
Compressive optic neuropathy, 1:320
Computed tomography (CT), 1:30
Concentric cardiac hypertrophy, 3:8, 3:8f
Concussion, 1:302
Conduction, heart impulse, 3:5
Conduction hearing loss, 1:496
Condylar fractures, 1:36
Cone dysplasia, 1:469
Congenital absence of the pericardium, 3:22
Congenital aneurysm, 3:23

Congenital atelectasis, 2:486
Congenital chondrodystrophy of unknown origin (CCUO), 1:80
Congenital colonic aganglionosis, 2:74
Congenital corneal opacities, 1:421-422
Congenital cystic adenomatoid malformation, 2:485, 2:485.e1f
Congenital diaphragmatic clefts, 1:191-192
Congenital dilation of large and segmental bile ducts, 2:265
Congenital duplication cysts, 2:31
Congenital enzyme defects of adrenal cortex, 3:339
Congenital erythropoietic porphyria, 1:59-60, 1:59f
  cats, 1:59
  cattle, 1:59-60
  pigmentation of teeth in, 2:7
Congenital flexures, 1:189
Congenital follicular parakeratosis, 1:532
Congenital hearing impairment, 1:491-492
Congenital heart abnormalities, 3:14-24, 3:15t, 3:66-67
Congenital hematomas, 3:22-23
  endocardium, 3:30
Congenital hepatic fibrocystic diseases, 2:265
Congenital hepatic fibrosis, 2:265, 2:265f-266f
Congenital histiocytosis, 1:730
Congenital hyperostosis (diaphyseal dysplasia), 1:53, 1:53f
Congenital hypothyroidism with dyshormonogenic goiter, 3:314, 3:323f
Congenital hypotrichosis, 1:538-539
  associated with pigmentary alteration, 1:539-541
  cats, 1:539
  cattle, 1:538-539
  dogs, 1:539, 1:539.e1f
Congenital idiopathic megaesophagus (CIM), 2:33-34
Congenital inguinal hernia, 2:80
Congenital intrahepatic arterioportal fistulae, 2:266f
Congenital melanosis, 2:270
Congenital myasthenia gravis, 1:209
Congenital spinal stenosis, 1:81
Congenital status spongiosus of Gelbvieh-cross calves, 1:347
Congenital stenosis of pancreatic duct, 2:355-356
Congenital tremor (CT), 1:338
Congenital trigeminal nerve hypoplasia, 1:187, 1:188f
Congenitally ectopic lenses, 1:422
Congestion, pulmonary, 2:487
Congestive brain swelling, 1:294
Congestive heart failure, 2:115, 3:6, 3:10-12, 3:11f, 3:9.e1f
Congo red (CR) stain, 2:415
Conidiobolomycosis, 1:659-660
  granulomatous rhinitis and, 2:476
Conium maculatum, 1:90, 2:3
Conjunctiva, 1:424-427
  neoplasms, 1:479-480, 1:479f-480f
  tumors, 1:481-482
Conjunctivitis, 1:424-427
  eosinophilic, 1:426
  feline lipogranulomatous, 1:427, 1:427f
  immune-mediated, 1:426-427
  ligneous, 1:426-427
Connective tissue disorders, 1:542-546

Constrictive pericarditis, 3:26, 3:27f
Contact activation pathway, 3:261
Contact dermatitis
  allergic, 1:596-597
  irritant, 1:566-568, 1:567f
  phytophoto, 1:578-579
Contagious agalactia, 3:458
Contagious bovine pleuropneumonia (CBPP), 2:551-552
Contagious caprine pleuropneumonia (CCPP), 2:563-564
Contagious equine metritis (CEM), 3:445, 3:445f
Contagious footrot, 1:643-644
Contagious ovine digital dermatitis (CODD), 1:644
Contagious pustular dermatitis, 1:617-618, 1:617f
Continuing education for pathologists, 1:14-15
Contractility disturbances, 3:4-5
Contractures, muscle, 1:213-214
Contusions, head, 1:302
Convulsions, bovine familial, 1:319
Coonhound paralysis, 1:394
Cooperia spp., 2:213
Coopworth sheep, 1:324
Copper
  deficiency, 1:559f, 2:115
    myocardial necrosis and, 3:34
    neonatal, 1:328-329, 1:328f
    osteochondrosis and, 1:81
    osteoporosis and, 1:66
    pigmentation and, 1:558, 1:558f
  liver toxicity, 2:342-343
  staining in liver, 2:303, 2:303f
Corgi dogs
  canine dermatomyositis, 1:198
  degenerative diseases of cartilaginous joints in, 1:143-144
  degenerative radiculomyelopathy, 1:330
  severe combined immunodeficiency (SCID), 3:139
  tongue atrophy, 1:228
Cornea, 1:427-441
  anomalies, 1:421-422
  cutaneous metaplasia, 1:429, 1:429f
  degeneration, 1:434-436
  dermoid, 1:421, 1:422f
  dystrophies and deposits, 1:433-434
    endothelial dystrophy, 1:433
    keratitis, 1:436-441
    lipid and crystalline, 1:433
    normal, 1:428f
    secondary to injury, 1:434, 1:434f
    secondary to metabolic disease, 1:433-434, 1:433f
    wound healing, 1:429-432, 1:430f, 1:431t, 1:432f
  edema, 1:428-429, 1:428f, 2:136f
  perforation, 1:437, 1:437f
  sequestrum in horses, 1:435
Corneodesmosomes, 1:513
Cornified envelope (CE), 1:513
Coronary embolism, 3:36
Coronavirus, 2:146-151
  cats, 2:117, 2:150-151, 2:587-588
  cattle, 2:112, 2:148-150, 2:149f, 2:541-542, 2:542.e1f
  dogs, 2:150, 2:576
  horses, 2:150
  pigs, 2:113, 2:115, 2:147-148, 2:529

Corpora amylacea, 3:504-505
 -like bodies, 3:314
Cor pulmonale, 3:6
Corpus callosum, agenesis of, 1:269, 1:269f
Cortical adenomas, 3:344-345, 3:345f
Cortical dysplasia, 1:268
Cortical granuloma, 2:442.e3f
Cortical nephrons, 2:377
Corticogenesis, cerebral, 1:268
Corticosteroid-induced osteoporosis, 1:67
Corticosteroids, hypokalemia, 2:394
Corticotroph (ACTH-secreting) adenoma, 3:281-282, 3:281f, 3:283f-284f
Corticotropin-releasing hormone (CRH), 3:338
Cortisol levels and hyperadrenocorticism, 1:224-225, 3:346-347, 3:347f
Cor triatriatum, 3:22
 dexter, 3:22
Corynebacterium pseudotuberculosis, 1:230, 2:433, 3:69, 3:97
 caseous lymphadenitis and, 3:204-208, 3:207f-208f, 3:205.e1f
 splenic abscesses, 3:183-184
Corynebacterium renale, 2:459
Corynetoxin poisoning, 1:309
Coughing, 2:471-472
Countercurrent exchange system, 2:379, 2:381
Cowdriosis, 3:80-82
Cowpox virus, 1:616, 1:619-620, 1:619f
 cats, 2:587-588
Coxiella burnetti, 3:416-417, 3:416f
Coyotillo, 1:219-220
 poisoning, 1:326
Cranial bones, 1:21
Cranial nerves
 internal ear neoplasia and, 1:494
 nuclei, 2:77
 peripheral vestibular disease and, 1:494
Craniomandibular osteopathy, 1:91-92
 dogs, 1:91, 1:92f
Craniopharyngioma, 1:404, 3:287, 3:287f
Creatine kinase (CK)
 canine dermatomyositis, 1:198
 canine X-linked muscular dystrophy, 1:192-193
 centronuclear myopathy of Labrador Retrievers, 1:197
 congenital myotonia in cats, 1:201
 diaphragmatic dystrophy in cattle, 1:199
 glycogenosis type II, 1:208
 ischemic damage, 1:211
 masticatory myositis, 1:226
 nemaline myopathy of cats, 1:198
 polymyositis, 1:227-229
 purpura hemorrhagica, 1:229
Crenosoma vulpis, 2:586
Crescentic proliferative glomerulonephritis, 2:412f
Cretan Hounds, canine hypomyelinogenesis in, 1:338
Cricopharyngeal dysphagia, 2:33
Crofton weed, 2:519
Cropped pinnae, 1:502
Crossiella equi, 3:417
Crossed renal ectopia, 2:392
Crotalaria retusa, 2:3
Crooked-calf disease, 1:90
Crusts, 1:519, 2:123-124

Cryopathies, 1:608
Cryptococcus gatti, 2:582
Cryptococcus neoformans, 1:449
 adrenal cortex and, 3:340
 granulomatous rhinitis and, 2:476
 lymph nodes and, 3:207f
 respiratory system and, 2:582, 2:583f
Cryptococcus osteomyelitis, 1:104, 1:104f
Cryptococcus spp., 1:104, 1:104f, 1:450, 1:450f, 2:582-583
Cryptocotyle, 2:225-227
Cryptorchidism, 3:476-478, 3:476f-477f
Cryptosporidiosis, 2:239-241, 2:240f-241f
Cryptosporidium andersoni, 2:54-55, 2:241
Cryptosporidium parvum, 2:111, 2:241, 3:140
Crystal-associated cholangiohepatopathy, 2:340, 2:340f
Crystalline dystrophies, corneal, 1:433
Cytauxzoon felis, 3:120-121
Culicoides hypersensitivity, 1:598-599, 1:599f
Culicoides oxystoma, 3:431
Cushing's disease, 1:224-225, 3:346-347, 3:347f
Cutaneous adverse food reaction, 1:594-596, 1:595f
Cutaneous amyloidosis, 1:614
Cutaneous anaplastic large T-cell lymphoma, 3:234-235, 3:234f
Cutaneous and systemic reactive histiocytosis (CRH), 1:729, 1:729.e1f
Cutaneous angiomatosis, 1:727
Cutaneous asthenia, 1:545, 1:545f
Cutaneous bacterial granulomas, 1:637-642
Cutaneous epitheliotropic T-cell lymphoma (CTCL), 1:733-734
Cutaneous habronemiasis, 1:685-686, 1:685f
Cutaneous histiocytoma, canine, 3:243-245, 3:244f-245f, 3:244.e1f, 3:243.e1f
Cutaneous horns, 1:551, 1:705
Cutaneous iodism, 1:570
Cutaneous Langerhans cell histiocytosis, 1:729, 3:245-246, 3:246f
Cutaneous leishmaniasis, 3:174-175
Cutaneous lupus erythematosus, 1:605-607
Cutaneous lymphomas, 1:733-735, 1:733f, 3:237.e1f
Cutaneous mucinosis, 1:546
Cutaneous oomycosis, 1:657-659
Cutaneous paraneoplastic syndromes, 1:691-693
Cutaneous plasmacytoma, 1:735, 1:735f, 3:228f, 3:226.e1f
Cutaneous pseudolymphomas, 1:734-735
Cutaneous reactive histiocytosis, 3:247-249, 3:248f-249f, 3:249.e1f
Cutaneous T-cell lymphoma (CTCL), 3:232-235
Cutaneous tumors of neural origin, 1:724
Cutaneous xanthoma, 1:700
Cuterebra spp., 1:391, 1:426, 1:668, 1:668f
Cutting cones, 1:64
Cyanide poisoning, 1:305-306
Cyanobacteria, 2:330
Cycadales, 2:331
Cycad poisoning, 1:322, 1:323f
Cyclic adenosine monophosphate (cAMP), 2:71
 toxin-stimulated, 2:71
Cyclic hematopoiesis, 1:556-557

Cyclitic membrane, 1:447
Cyclooxygenase-2 expression, neoplastic urinary bladder epithelium, 2:462-463
Cyclopamine, 1:90
Cyclophosphamide-induced lesions, 2:460
Cyclopia, 1:269, 1:269f, 1:410-411, 1:411f
Cyclosporin and osteoporosis, 1:67
Cylicospirura felineus, 2:211
CYP isozymes, 2:519
Cystadenomas
 epitrichial, 1:718
 thyroid, 3:326
Cystic adenomas, 3:326-327
Cystic dental inclusions, 2:7
Cystic dilation of pancreatic duct, 2:355-356
Cystic diseases, of kidney, 2:394
Cystic endometrial hyperplasia, 3:382-385, 3:382f-383f, 3:391, 3:391f-392f
Cystic epoophoron, 3:371
Cysticerci, 2:255
Cysticercosis, 1:239-240, 1:239f
Cysticercus bovis, 1:239, 1:389
Cysticercus cellulosae, 1:239, 1:239f, 1:389
Cysticercus ovis, 1:239-240, 1:239f
Cysticercus tarandi, 1:240
Cysticercus tenuicollis, 3:473-474
 liver and, 2:318-319, 2:319f
Cystic eye, 1:411-412, 1:411f
Cystic follicular disease, 3:372
Cystic mucinous hyperplasia, 2:345
Cystic nasal conchae, 2:478
Cystic ovarian disease in cows, 3:372-374, 3:373f
Cystic paroophoron, 3:371
Cystic placental mole, 3:396
Cystic rete, 3:371, 3:372f
Cystic septum pellucidum, 1:269
Cystic subsurface epithelial structures of the bitch, 3:371-372
Cystic uterus masculinus, 3:501, 3:501f
Cystine stones, 2:458
Cystitis, 2:439, 2:459-461
 chronic, 2:460-462
 emphysematous, 2:459, 2:460f
 eosinophilic, 2:460
 feline interstitial, 2:460
 follicular, 2:460-461, 2:460f
 sterile hemorrhagic, 2:460
Cystocaulus ocreatus, 2:565, 2:565t, 2:567
Cystoisospora spp., 2:235-239
Cystoisospora suis, 2:113, 2:234-235, 2:234f
Cysts, 1:703-705
 adrenal cortex, 3:339, 3:339f
 arachnoid, 1:279, 1:280f
 bone
  benign, 1:126
  subchondral (juxtacortical), 1:126, 1:134, 1:134f
 bronchogenic, 2:484-485
 cerebral cortex, 1:299f
 cervical, 3:441
 congenital duplication, of esophagus, 2:31
 dentigerous, 2:6-7, 2:7f
 epidermal inclusion, 2:478
 epidermoid, 1:404
 epithrichial, 1:705
 hepatic, 2:264
 liver fatty, 2:274-275, 2:274f
 Neospora caninum, 1:388f
 odontogenic, 2:6-7

INDEX

Cysts *(Continued)*
  orbital, *1*:478
  ovarian, *3*:371-372, *3*:372f
    germinal inclusion, *3*:372, *3*:372f
    and uterine remnants, *3*:366-367, *3*:367f-368f
  paranasal sinus, *2*:478
  parathyroid, *3*:297-302
  peritoneum, *2*:256
  pharyngeal, *2*:29
  pituitary, *3*:279-281, *3*:280f
  prostatic, *3*:500-501
  retrobulbar, *1*:412, *1*:412f
  Sarcocystis, *1*:234-236
  serosal inclusion, *3*:386-387, *3*:387f
  skin
    dermoid, *1*:547, *1*:704-705
    epithelial, *1*:500
    epitrichial, *1*:705
    ganglion, *1*:162-163
    hybrid, *1*:704
    infundibular, *1*:704
    isthmus, *1*:704
    lacrimal duct, *1*:424
    matrical, *1*:704
    sebaceous duct, *1*:705
  splenic, *3*:189
  subepiglottic, *2*:481
  synovial, *1*:162-163
  thymic, *3*:151, *3*:152f, *3*:151.e1f
  thyroglossal duct, *2*:29, *3*:310, *3*:314
  uveal, *1*:446, *1*:446f
  vaginal, *3*:442
  valvular, *3*:30
Cytauxzoonosis, *3*:120-121, *3*:120f
  splenic histiocytosis, *3*:184f
Cytoarchitectural changes in muscle fibers, *1*:185, *1*:185f
Cytochrome P450 (CYP) isozymes, *2*:519
Cytokeratin-7 expression, *2*:462.e1
Cytokines in degenerative joint diseases, *1*:140-141
Cytopathic (CP) biotype, *2*:122
Cytoplasmic basophilia, *2*:67
Cytoplasmic plaque, *1*:513-514
Cytotoxic edema, *1*:294
Cytotoxic hepatocellular injury, *2*:327

D

Dachshund dogs
  canine acanthosis nigricans, *1*:555
  canine congenital myasthenia, *1*:209
  cochleosaccular degeneration, *1*:492
  color dilution alopecia, *1*:539-540
  corneal edema, *1*:429
  degenerative diseases of cartilaginous joints, *1*:143-144
  familial myoclonic epilepsy, *1*:205
  hyperadrenocorticism, *1*:588
  hypothyroidism, *1*:587, *3*:315
  malignant melanoma, *2*:26
  motor neuron disease, *1*:331
  myxomatous valvular degeneration, *3*:27
  osteogenesis imperfecta, *1*:50
  osteopetrosis, *1*:52
  seborrhea, *1*:548
  sensory and autonomic neuropathy, *1*:334
  sick sinus syndrome, *3*:51
  vitiligo, *1*:555-556
Dacryoadenitis, *1*:423-424
Dactylomegaly, *1*:54-55
Daft lambs, *1*:319

Dalmatian dogs
  canine atopic dermatitis, *1*:591
  canine hypomyelinogenesis, *1*:337
  canine X-linked muscular dystrophy in, *1*:192
  cavitating leukodystrophy, *1*:339-340
  chronic hepatitis, *2*:304
  deafness, *3*:51
  hereditary deafness, *1*:492
  interstitial lung disease, *2*:515
  melanocytopenic hypomelanosis, *1*:555
  motor neuropathy, *1*:335
  nephritis, *2*:416-417
  solar radiation and, *1*:566
Dandy-Walker syndrome, *1*:277
Darier disease (DD), *1*:537
Deafness
  acquired, *1*:493
  hereditary, *1*:492-493, *1*:492f
  traumatic causes of, *1*:493-494
Death
  adenosine triphosphate (ATP) in rigor mortis, *1*:186
  bronchopneumonia, *2*:507-508
  causes of unexpected, *1*:4t
  diapedesis of red cells, *1*:301
  embryonic, *3*:395-396
  fetal, *3*:395
  gastric rupture and, *2*:48
  liver, *2*:295-296
    cell, *2*:279-285
  muscle changes after, *1*:186
  Phalaris poisoning and sudden, *1*:293
  retina after, *1*:467
  ruminal mucosa after, *2*:36
Decision analysis, *1*:12, *1*:13f
Decreased protein intake, *2*:72
Decubitus ulcers, *1*:559
Deep bacterial pyoderma, *1*:634-637, *1*:635f
Deep plexus, dermal, *1*:514
Deep stomatitides, *2*:17-19
Deer fly fever, *3*:184-186, *3*:185f
Defective mineralization, *1*:68
Deforming cervical spondylosis, *1*:88
Degeneration
  adrenal cortex, *3*:339-340, *3*:339f
  amyloid, *1*:297-298
  arteries, *3*:56-61
  arteriosclerosis, *3*:59-60
  atherosclerosis, *3*:57-59, *3*:57.e2f
  central nervous system, *3*:317-336
  cerebellar cortical, *1*:276, *1*:276f
  corneal, *1*:434-436
  endocardium, *3*:27-30
  exocrine pancreas, *2*:356-364
  fibrinoid, *1*:520
  hydropic, *1*:522, *1*:522f
  myocardial, *3*:34, *3*:34f
  nervous system, *1*:303-350
  optic nerve, *1*:476
  ovarian, *3*:371, *3*:371f
  parathyroid gland, *3*:297-298
  pleura, *2*:520
  reticular, *1*:523
  retinal, *1*:468-469
  spleen, *3*:163-165
  teeth and dental tissue, *2*:7-9
  testicular, *3*:481-485, *3*:482b, *3*:483f
  thyroid gland, *3*:314-315
  uvea, *1*:445-446
  vacuolar, *1*:185, *1*:185f, *1*:254, *1*:254f, *1*:522

Degenerative joint diseases, *1*:137-146
  cats, *1*:143
  cattle, *1*:143, *1*:143f
  chronic, *1*:138-140, *1*:140f
  dogs, *1*:138, *1*:138f-139f, *1*:142-145, *1*:143f-144f
  gross lesions, *1*:138, *1*:138f
  horses, *1*:141-142, *1*:141f-142f
  synovial joints, *1*:137-143
Degenerative mucinotic mural folliculitis, *1*:697
Degenerative myopathies, *1*:221-224
Degenerative radiculomyelopathy of adult dogs, *1*:330
Degenerative suspensory desmitis, *1*:247
Degradation of hormone, *3*:275
Dehydration, *2*:384, *2*:399
Dells, *1*:524
β-cells, endocrine pancreas, *2*:368
Demodecosis, *1*:681, *1*:681f
Demodectic mange, *1*:678-682, *1*:680f
Demodex cati, *1*:681
Demodex gatoi, *1*:681
Demodex injai, *1*:679-680, *1*:680f
Demodex phylloides, *1*:682
Demodex spp., *1*:506, *1*:678-682
Demyelinating diseases, *1*:259
Demyelinating neuropathy, *1*:341-342
Dendritic cells
  lung, *2*:470
  trafficking, *2*:64
Dendritic reticular cells, lymph node, *3*:197-198
Denervation atrophy, *1*:173-175, *1*:174f-177f
Dental attrition, *2*:7-8
Dental calculus, *2*:9
Dental caries, *2*:9-11, *2*:10f
Dental follicle, *2*:4
Dental lamina, *2*:4
Dental lesions with canine distemper virus, *2*:576
Dentigerous cysts, *2*:6-7, *2*:7f
Dentin, *2*:5
  pigmentation of, *2*:7
Deoxypyrolidine (DPD), *1*:27
Deoxyribonucleic acid (DNA) extraction, *1*:30
Deposits
  calcium salts, on lens, *1*:443
  corneal, *1*:433-434
  cutaneous tissue, *1*:562-564
Depression, *2*:425
Dermal edema, *1*:519
Dermal fibers, *1*:514
Dermal perivascular unit, *1*:515
Dermanyssus gallinae, *1*:683
Dermatitis
  acral lick, *1*:561-562, *1*:561f
  atopic, *1*:591-593, *1*:591f, *1*:592.e1f
  contact
    allergic, *1*:596-597
    phytophoto-, *1*:578-579
    primary irritant, *1*:566-568, *1*:567f
  with edema, eosinophilic, *1*:696
  eosinophilic, *1*:693-696
  fibrosing, *1*:528
  fly-bite, *1*:552, *1*:666-671
  hookworm, *1*:685
  horn fly, *1*:670
  interface, *1*:525, *1*:526f
  intraepidermal vesicular and pustular, *1*:527, *1*:528f

Dermatitis *(Continued)*
   Malassezia, 1:548-549, 1:553, 1:593, 1:647-649, 1:648f
   nodular and diffuse, 1:526-527
   papillomatous digital, 1:644-645, 1:644f
   Pelodera, 1:689, 1:689f
   perforating, 1:699, 1:699f
   perivascular, 1:525, 1:525f
   photosensitization, 1:577-580, 1:578f
   porcine juvenile pustular psoriasiform, 1:698, 1:698f
   psoriasiform, 1:698
   pyotraumatic, 1:560
   pyrexia with, 1:574
   radiant heat, 1:566
   solar, 1:576, 1:576f
   subepidermal vesicular and pustular, 1:527-528, 1:528f
   superficial necrolytic, 1:586-587, 1:587f
   thymoma and exfoliative, 1:691-692
Dermatobia hominis, 1:668
Dermatohistopathology, 1:518-530
   gross terminology, 1:524
   histologic terms, 1:518-524
   pattern analysis, 1:524-530
Dermatologic diseases of external ear, 1:503-504
Dermatomyositis, canine, 1:198, 1:541-542, 1:542f-543f
Dermatophagoides farinae, 1:683
Dermatophagoides pteronyssinus, 1:683
Dermatophilosis, 1:503, 1:632-634, 1:633f
Dermatophilus congolensis, 2:19
Dermatophytosis, 1:649-653, 1:650f-651f
   cats, 1:652-653
   cattle, 1:650-651, 1:651f
   dogs, 1:652, 1:652f
   horses, 1:651-652
   pigs, 1:651
   sheep and goats, 1:651
Dermatoses
   acantholytic, 1:537-538
   atrophic, 1:529-530, 1:529f
   autoimmune, 1:600-607
   hypersensitivity, 1:590-600, 1:670-671
   immune-mediated, 1:590-615
   mineral-responsive, 1:583-586, 1:584f
   photoaggravated, 1:580
   porcine, 1:698-699
   vitamin-responsive, 1:581-583, 1:582f
Dermatosis vegetans, 1:546-547, 1:546f
Dermatosparaxis, 1:544
Dermis, 1:514-515
   muscles, 1:515
Dermoid cysts, 1:547, 1:704-705
Dermoid sinus, 1:279
Descemet's membrane, 1:427, 1:432, 1:439-440
Desmoglein, 2:14
Desmoplasia, 1:519
Destructive cholangitis, 2:308
Developmental anomalies/diseases
   central nervous system, 1:264-284, 3:426-427
      viral causes, 1:280-284
   ear
      external, 1:501-502
      middle, 1:496

Developmental anomalies/diseases *(Continued)*
   eye, 1:409-427
   joints, 1:132-137
      cervical vertebral malformation-malarticulation, 1:136
      hip dysplasia, 1:135-136
      luxations and subluxations, 1:137
      osteochondrosis, 1:132-135
   liver, 2:264-268
   lungs, 2:484-485, 2:485.e1f
   muscle, 1:186-210
      malignant hyperthermia, 1:209-210
      metabolic myopathies, 1:204-209
      muscular defects, 1:189-192
      muscular dystrophy, 1:192-197
      myasthenia gravis, 1:209
      myopathies, 1:197-200
      myotonic and spastic syndromes, 1:200-204
      primary central nervous system conditions, 1:187-189
   pancreas, exocrine, 2:355-356
   peritoneum, 2:245
   pleura, 2:520
   ureters, 2:449-450
Devon Rex cats
   atopic dermatitis, 1:593
   α-dystroglycan deficiency, 1:196
   vitamin-K-dependent γ-glutamyl carboxylase deficiency, 3:264
Dexter chondrodysplasia, 1:38
Dextrocardia, 3:23
Diabetes, fatty liver of, 2:275
Diabetes insipidus, 3:290
Diabetes mellitus, 2:370-373, 2:371f
   cats, 2:372, 2:373f
   cattle, 2:372
   diabetic cataract, 1:443
   dogs, 2:373
   horses, 2:372
   metabolic neuropathies, 1:335
   retinopathies, 1:472
Diagnosis. *See also* Gross and histologic examinations
   defined, 1:1
   genetics, 1:12
   imaging, 1:11-12
   introduction to, 1:1
   purpose of gross and histologic examinations in, 1:2-15
Diapedesis of red cells, 1:301
Diaphragm
   congenital clefts of, 1:191-192
   diaphragmatic hernias, 2:80
   myopathy in cattle, 1:199
Diaphyseal dysplasia, 1:53, 1:53f
Diaphysis, 1:22
Diaporthe toxica, 2:334
Diarrhea, 2:111-112, 2:542, 2:542.e3f. *See also* Bovine viral diarrhea virus (BVDV)
   Bacteroides fragilis associated, 2:199
   bovine coronavirus, 2:112
   bovine herpesvirus 1, 2:112
   bovine torovirus, 2:112
   calves, 2:112-113
   in calves, 2:112-113
   Chlamydophila infection, 2:113
   chronic erosive colitis in cat, 2:93f

Diarrhea *(Continued)*
   Cryptosporidium parvum, 2:112
   enterotoxigenic *E. coli*, 2:112
   foals, 2:113-115
   neonatal ruminants, 2:113
   neonatal swine, 2:113
   rotavirus, 2:112, 2:151-153
   salmonellosis, 2:112, 2:169
Diarthrodial joints, 1:129-131
Diazepam, 2:329
Dichelobacter nodosus, 1:643-644
Dicrocoelid flukes, 2:322, 2:322f
Dicrocoelium dendriticum, 2:323, 2:323f, 2:323.e1f
Dicrocoelium hospes, 2:322-323
Dictyocaulus filaria, 2:565-567, 2:565t, 2:574, 2:566.e2f
Dictyocaulus viviparus, 2:554-556, 2:556f, 2:555.e1f
Dieffenbachia, 2:13-14
Diffuse alveolar damage (DAD), 2:509-511, 2:510f, 2:514.e2f
Diffuse cortical hyperplasia, 3:343
Diffuse fibrinous pleuritis, 2:522, 2:521.e1f
Diffuse fibrous hyperplasia, 2:21-22
Diffuse gastric mucosal hypertrophy, 2:53
Diffuse hyperplasia, 3:300, 3:300f
Diffuse idiopathic skeletal hyperostosis (DISH), 1:146
Diffuse large B-cell lymphomas (DLBCLs), 3:220-222, 3:221f
   anaplastic, 3:221
Diffuse sclerosing actinobacillosis, 2:18-19
Diffuse tissue mineralization, pathogenesis of, 2:387
Diffuse transmural inflammation, 2:38
Diffuse uveal melanocytosis, 1:484-485
DiGeorge syndrome, 3:144
Digits, defects of, 1:37t
Diiodotyrosine (DIT), 3:311
Dilated cardiomyopathy (DCM), 3:45, 3:47f
   cats, 3:46-47
   cows, 3:50, 3:50f
   dogs, 3:48, 3:48f
Dilated lymphatics, 2:87
Dilated pore of Winer, 1:704, 1:704f
Dilation
   abomasal, 2:51
   bladder, 2:451
   gastric, 2:48-50, 2:49f
   of rumen, forestomach, 2:36, 2:37f
   salivary ducts, 2:29
Dimethylnitrosamine, 2:340
Dioctophyma renale, 2:255, 2:443f, 2:443.e1f
Dipetalonema reconditum, 3:83-84
Diphtheria, 2:17
Diphyllobothrium spp., 2:223
Diplodiosis, 1:345-346
Diplomyelia, 1:278f
Diplostomum spathaceum, 1:451-452
Direct inguinal hernia, 2:80
Direct salt poisoning, 1:314
Dirofilaria immitis, 1:451-452, 1:690, 2:418, 3:83-85, 3:84f, 3:85.e1f
   microfilaria, 2:411f
   pulmonary vasculitis and, 2:494
Dirofilariasis, chronic, 2:410-411

Diskospondylitis, *1*:156, *1*:156f
  dogs, *1*:156, *1*:156f
  horses, *1*:156
  pigs, *1*:156
  sheep, *1*:156f
Dislocation of the lens, *1*:441-442
Disproportionate dwarfism, *1*:41
  dogs, *1*:45
  sheep, *1*:41-42
Disseminated cavernous hemangiomas, 3:99
Disseminated discoid lupus erythematosus, *1*:606, 3:65b
Disseminated histiocytic sarcoma, *1*:729
Disseminated intravascular coagulation (DIC), 2:84, 2:398-399, 3:64-66, 3:266-268, 3:68.e1f
Distal axonopathy, *1*:257
Distichiasis, *1*:421
Distribution of edema, 3:11
Disturbance of retrograde axonal transport, *1*:257-258
Disuse atrophy, *1*:175-177, *1*:177f
Disuse osteoporosis, *1*:67
Diverticula, 2:450
  bladder, 2:450
  esophageal, 2:31
DNA damage, 3:341
Doberman Pinscher dogs
  acne, *1*:549
  canine leproid granuloma, *1*:641
  cervical vertebral malformation-malarticulation, *1*:136
  chronic hepatitis, 2:303
  color dilution alopecia, *1*:539-540
  dilated cardiomyopathy, 3:48
  follicular dysplasia, *1*:540-541
  hepatitis, 2:318
  hypothyroidism, *1*:587, 3:315
  maxillary or mandibular fibrosarcoma, *1*:121
  motor neuron disease, *1*:331
  myxomatous valvular degeneration, 3:27
  nephritis, 2:417
  neuroepithelial degeneration, *1*:492
  peripheral vestibular disease, *1*:494
  seborrhea, *1*:548
  spastic syndromes, *1*:203
  sudden unexpected death, 3:51
  vitiligo, *1*:555-556
Dogues de Bordeaux
  dysplasia of right atrioventricular valve, 3:21-22
  ichthyosis, *1*:532
  subvalvular aortic stenosis, 3:20
Dolichocephalic dwarfs, *1*:39
Donkey pulmonary fibrosis (DPF), 2:514, 2:514.e2f
Dorsal and ventral longitudinal ligaments, *1*:129
Dorsal displacement of soft palate, 2:481
Dorset Down sheep, wattles in, *1*:532
Double aortic arch, 3:23
Double-chambered right ventricle, 3:22
Double muscling, *1*:190-191
Dourine, 3:445-447
Downer syndrome, *1*:212
Doxorubicin cardiotoxicosis, 3:39
Doxycycline, 2:424
Dracunulus medinensis, *1*:689
Draschia megastoma, 2:54, 2:210f

Drug
  eruptions, *1*:607-615
  -induced disorders
    liver injury, 2:326, 2:329
    platelet dysfunction, 3:260
    polyarthritis, *1*:158
    thrombocytopenia, 3:258
  reactions and lung injury, 2:520
Dryland distemper, *1*:230
Dual energy X-ray absorptiometry (DEXA), *1*:30
Ductal cells, pancreas, 2:355
Ductal epitrichial carcinomas, *1*:719
Ductal plate malformations, 2:265, 2:265f
Ductular reaction, 2:262
Duodenal lesions, 2:116
Duodenal sigmoid flexure volvulus, 2:83
Duodenal stenosis, 2:59
Duodenitis-proximal jejunitis, 2:116
Duodenum, 2:354
Duplication
  of ovaries, 3:366, 3:366f
  of spleen, 3:163
Dwarfism
  dogs, *1*:45
  horses, *1*:42
  pigs, *1*:42
  sheep, *1*:41-42
Dynamin 1 gene, *1*:198
Dysautonomia, *1*:333-334, 2:77
  distinctive ultrastructural appearance, 2:77
Dysentery
  swine, 2:100, 2:181-182, 2:182f
  winter, 2:149, 2:150f
Dysgerminoma, 3:377
Dyshormonogenesis, *1*:587
Dyskeratosis, *1*:518-519
  cattle, *1*:539
Dysmyelinating diseases, *1*:260
Dysontogenic (cartilaginous or osseous) metaplasia, 2:393
Dysphagia, 2:33-34, 2:34f
Dysplasia
  adrenal gland, 3:338, 3:338f
  black hair follicular, *1*:540, *1*:540f
  cerebellar, *1*:275-276, *1*:275f
  coat-color-linked hair follicle, *1*:540
  collagen, *1*:543-544
    cats, *1*:545, *1*:545f
    cattle, *1*:544
    dogs, *1*:544-545, *1*:545f
    horses, *1*:544, *1*:544.e1f
    sheep, *1*:544
  cortical, *1*:268
  epidermal, *1*:519
  inherited epidermal, *1*:538
  pectinate ligament, *1*:462-463
  right atrioventricular valve, 3:21-22
  sebaceous gland, *1*:699, *1*:699.e2f
Dysraphism, *1*:278f
Dysrhythmias, 3:4-5
Dystrophic epidermolysis bullosa, *1*:534
  dogs, *1*:536
  goats, *1*:535
Dystrophic mineralization, *1*:519
Dystrophies
  axonal, *1*:257-258, *1*:258f, *1*:324-325
  corneal, *1*:433-434
  equine coronary band, *1*:553-554
  follicular, *1*:520
Dystrophin in muscular dystrophy, *1*:194, *1*:195f

E
Ear(s), *1*:488-508. See also Hearing
  external, *1*:500-508
    dermatologic diseases of, *1*:503-505
    developmental disease, *1*:501-502
    hearing and, *1*:501
    histologic preparation and examination, *1*:508
    otitis externa, *1*:497, *1*:502-503, *1*:502f, *1*:497.e2f
    parasitism, *1*:505-507
    pinnal tumor-like growths and neoplasia, *1*:504-505
  general considerations, *1*:488
  internal, *1*:488-495
    hearing and, *1*:491
      impairment, *1*:491-494
    Horner and Pourfour du Petit syndromes, *1*:494-495
    neoplasia, *1*:494
    peripheral vestibular disease, *1*:494
  margin dermatosis, *1*:553
  middle, *1*:495-500
    developmental disease, *1*:496
    epithelial neoplasia, *1*:500
    hearing and, *1*:496
    jugulotympanic paragangliomas, *1*:500
    non-neoplastic and neoplastic disease, *1*:498-499
    otitis media, *1*:496-498, *1*:497.e1f
    parasites, *1*:498
    temporohyoid osteoarthropathy, *1*:500
  porcine ear necrosis syndrome (PENS), *1*:503, *1*:645, *1*:503.e1f
East Coast fever, 3:176-178, 3:177f, 3:177.e1f
Ebstein's anomaly, 3:21-22
Eccentric cardiac hypertrophy, 3:8, 3:8f-9f
Ecchondromas, *1*:116
Echinochasmus, 2:225-227
Echinococcus equinus, 2:574, 2:574.e2f
Echinococcus granulosus, 2:319, 2:320f, 2:556-557, 2:567
Echinococcus multilocularis, 2:319-320, 2:320f
Economic considerations in postmortem examinations, *1*:13
Ectopia cordis, 3:22, 3:23f
Ectopic adrenal tissue, 3:498
  ovaries, 3:366, 3:367f
Ectopia lentis, *1*:441-442
Ectopic ossification, *1*:127
Ectopic pancreatic tissue, 2:356
Ectopic ureter, 2:449-450, 2:449f
Ectromelia virus, *1*:616
Edema, 2:401
  ascites and, 2:294-295
  cerebral, *1*:293-295, *1*:295f
    cytotoxic, *1*:294
    vasogenic, *1*:294, *1*:295f
  corneal, *1*:428-429, *1*:428f, 2:136f
  dermal, *1*:519
  disease, *1*:298, *1*:298f, 2:163-166, 2:164f
  distribution of, 3:11
  eosinophilic dermatitis with, *1*:696
  fluid, 3:6
  of gastric rugae, 2:51
  intracellular, *1*:522
  laryngeal, 2:481
  pulmonary, 2:487-489, 2:488b, 2:489.e1f
  serosal, 2:195-196, 2:196f
  tracheal, *1*:192, 2:483f
Egyptian Mau cats, spongy myelinopathy in, *1*:343-344

Ehlers-Danlos syndrome (EDS), 1:543-544
Ehrlichia canis, 2:414, 2:418, 3:111
  platelet dysfunction, 3:260
Ehrlichia platys, 3:260
Ehrlichia ruminantium, 3:80-82
Ehrlichiosis, 1:449
Eimeria alabamensis, 2:230-231
Eimeria apsheronica, 2:233
Eimeria arloingi, 2:232, 2:232f
Eimeria auburnensis, 2:230
Eimeria bareillyi, 2:231
Eimeria bovis, 2:229
Eimeria bukidnonensis, 2:230-231
Eimeria caprina, 2:231
Eimeria christenseni, 2:231-232
Eimeria crandallis, 2:233
Eimeria gilruthi, 2:54-55
Eimeria leuckarti, 2:233-234, 2:233f
Eimeria ninakohlyakimovae, 2:231
Eimeria ovinoidalis, 2:231
Eimeria zuernii, 2:229
Elaeophora bohmi, 3:88
Elaeophora poeli, 3:88, 3:88.e1f
Elaeophora schneideri, 1:390, 1:451-452, 3:88
Elaeophoriasis, 3:88
Elaphostrongylus cervi, 1:390
Elaphostrongylus panticola, 1:390
Elaphostrongylus rangifera, 1:390
Elastic fibers, dermal, 1:514
  abnormalities of, 1:545
Elbow hygroma, 1:155, 1:155f
Electrical burns, 2:13
Electrolytes
  abnormalities and myopathies, 1:225
  balance, 2:384
Ellipsoids, 1:256
Ellis van Creveld syndrome 2, 1:39, 1:39f
Elokomin fluke fever, 3:149
Embolic pneumonia, 2:520, 2:520.e2f
Embolic suppurative myocarditis, 3:42.e1f
Embolism
  arterial, 3:63-66, 3:63f-64f
  coronary, 3:36
  pulmonary, 2:489, 2:490f
    fat, 2:490
    septic, 2:490
  septic, 1:358-362, 1:358f
Embryonal carcinoma, 3:496
Embryonal rhabdomyosarcoma, 1:241-243, 1:243f
Embryonal tumors, 1:401-403
Embryonic death, 3:395
  with persistence of membranes, 3:396
Embryonic stage of lung growth, 2:484
Emmonsia crescens, 2:584
Emmonsia parva, 2:584
Emphysema
  fetal, 3:396
  lymph node, 3:199
  pulmonary, 2:486-487, 2:487f
Emphysematous cystitis, 2:459, 2:460f
Emphysematous pyelonephritis, 2:440
Empyema, 1:353-354
  of sinus, 2:477, 2:477f
Enamel, 2:5
  hypoplasia, 2:7f
  loss, 2:10
Encephalitozoon, 1:451

Encephalitozoon cuniculi, 1:385-386, 2:431, 3:418
Encephalocele, 1:267, 1:267f
Encephalomalacia, 1:307
  focal symmetrical, 1:300-301, 1:301f
    pigs, 1:308-309
  nigropallidal, 1:314, 1:314f
Encephalomyelopathies, spongy, 1:342f, 1:345f, 1:346-347
Encephalomyocarditis virus (EMCV), 3:43
Enchondromatosis, 1:116
Endoarteritis, 2:84
Endocardiosis, 3:27, 3:28f-29f
Endocarditis, 3:30-33, 3:31f, 3:31.e1f
Endocardium, 3:3
  disease, 3:27-33
    degenerative lesions, 3:27-30
  mural and valvular, 3:4
Endochondral ossification, 1:22, 1:22f
  rickets and, 1:71-72
Endocrine cells, 2:45
Endocrine pancreas, 2:368-375
  diabetes mellitus, 2:370-373, 2:371f
    cats, 2:372, 2:373f
    cattle, 2:372
    diabetic cataract, 1:443
    dogs, 2:373
    horses, 2:372
    retinopathies, 1:472
  hyperplastic and neoplastic diseases, 2:373-375, 2:374f
Endocrine system, 3:269-357
  adrenal cortex, 3:336-348
  adrenal medulla, 3:348-354
  diseases/disorders, 2:384-385
    atrophy of, 1:178, 1:178f
    mechanisms, 3:272-276
    myopathies associated with, 1:224-225
    of skin, 1:587-590
  general considerations, 3:270-276
  hormones
    calcium-regulating, 3:291-310, 3:291f
    catecholamine and iodothyronine, 3:271
    steroid, 3:271
    thyroid, 3:311-312
    types, 3:270-271
  multiple endocrine neoplasia (MEN), 3:356-357
  paragangliomas, 3:354-356
  parathyroid gland, 3:292-295, 3:292f
  pituitary gland, 3:276-291
  proliferative lesions, 3:271-272
  thyroid gland, 3:310-336
  tumors, 3:272
Endogenous anticoagulants, 3:265-266
Endogenous lipid pneumonia, 2:517
Endogenous protein, 2:72-73
Endolymph, 1:489
Endometrial biopsy, 3:393
Endometrial cups, 3:394, 3:394f
Endometrial polyps, 3:385, 3:386f
Endometritis, 3:388-389, 3:388f
  chronic, 3:389-390
Endometrium, 3:382-387, 3:382f
  carcinoma, 3:449-450
  cysts, postpartum, 3:440
  endometritis, 3:388-389, 3:388f
Endophthalmitis, 1:446
  bacterial, 1:449
  mycotic, 1:449-451

Endophthalmitis *(Continued)*
  parasitic, 1:451-452
  protozoal, 1:451
  viral, 1:452
Endothelial cells
  hepatic, 2:262-263
  sinusoidal, 2:260
  vascular, 3:55
    disorders, 3:255-268
Endothelial protein C receptor (EPCR), 3:265-266
Endothelium-mediated fibrinolysis, 3:266
End-stage kidneys, 2:377-378
English Bulldogs
  acne, 1:549
  brachycephalic airway syndrome, 2:482, 2:482f
  demodectic mange, 1:679
  factor VII deficiency, 3:264
  hypothyroidism, 1:587, 3:315
  keratoconjunctivitis sicca, 1:436
  recurrent flank alopecia, 1:590
English Cocker Spaniel hereditary nephritis, 2:416
English Pointer dogs
  chondrodysplasia, 1:44
  motor neuron disease, 1:331
  sensory and autonomic neuropathies, 1:334
English Setter dogs, atopic dermatitis in, 1:591
English Springer Spaniel dogs
  canine congenital myasthenia, 1:209
  canine hypomyelinogenesis, 1:337
  chronic hepatitis, 2:304
  gangliosidosis, 1:58-59
  lichenoid-psoriasiform dermatosis, 1:552-553
  malignant hyperthermia, 1:210
  persistent atrial standstill, 3:51
  phosphofructokinase (PFK) deficiency, 1:204-205
  polymyopathy, 1:198
  prolonged APTT, 3:263
  retinal folding, 1:419
  seborrhea, 1:548
  sensory and autonomic neuropathy, 1:334
Enrofloxacin, 1:472
Entamoeba histolytica, 2:98-99, 2:242
Enteric clostridial infections, 2:183-194
Enteric coronaviral infections, 2:146-151
Enteric disease, pathophysiology of, 2:69-73, 2:107
  anemia, 2:73
  diarrhea, 2:70-72
    increased intestinal motility, 2:72
    increased permeability, 2:71
    large-bowel, 2:71
    malabsorptive, 2:71
    secretory, 2:71
    small-bowel, 2:71
  inappetence/anorexia, 2:69
  malassimilation, 2:69-70
    assimilation of fat, 2:70
    lipids, malabsorption of, 2:70
    polysaccharides, maldigestion of, 2:70
    protein maldigestion, 2:70
  protein-energy malnutrition, 2:69

Enteric disease, pathophysiology of *(Continued)*
  protein metabolism, 2:72-73
    albumin, elevated hepatic synthesis of, 2:73
    anorexia, 2:72
    decreased protein intake, 2:72
    peptides/amino acids, malabsorption of, 2:72
    protein-losing gastroenteropathy, 2:72
Enteric nervous system, 2:62
Enteritis
  adenoviral, 2:143, 2:143f-144f, 2:542, 2:568
  Campylobacter spp., 2:180-181
  Enterococcus spp., 2:198-199
  eosinophilic, 2:96
  granulomatous, 2:97
  necrotizing, 2:187, 2:187f-188f
  parvoviral, 2:153-158
Enteroaggregative *E. coli* heat stabile toxin (EAST1), 2:160, 2:160f-161f
Enterococcus durans, 2:113-114
Enterococcus spp. enteritis, 2:198-199
Enterocolitis, protothecal, 2:203-204
Enterocytes, 2:60-61
  invasion and salmonellosis, 2:168
Enteroendocrine cells, 2:60
Enterohemorrhagic colibacillosis, 2:112, 2:162f
Enterohemorrhagic *E. coli* (EHEC), 2:162
Enteroinvasive *E. coli*, 2:166
Enteroliths, 2:75
Enteropathogenic colibacillosis, 2:161-163
Enteropathy-associated T-cell lymphoma (EATL), 3:230-232, 3:231f, 3:232.e1f
Enterotoxemia, 2:115, 2:188-191, 2:189f-190f
Enteroviral encephalomyelitis, 1:373f
Enterovirus/teschovirus polioencephalomyelitis of pigs, 1:372-373, 1:373f
Entheses, 1:130
Entomophthoromycosis, 1:659-660, 2:201, 2:573-574
Envenomation, 1:568
Environmental contaminants
  liver and, 2:330-333
  thymic atrophy and, 3:144
Enzootic ataxia, 1:328-329, 1:328f
Enzootic bovine leukosis, 3:235-236, 3:236f, 3:236.e1f, 3:236.e2f
Enzootic hematuria, 2:461-462
  hemorrhagic urinary bladder mucosa, 2:461f
Enzootic nasal tumor, 2:560, 2:560f
Enzootic pneumonia, 2:539
Enzyme(s)
  defects of adrenal cortex, 3:339
  lysosomal, 1:284
Eosinophilia, 3:111
Eosinophilic bronchopneumopathy, 2:501-502, 2:502f, 2:501.e1f
Eosinophilic conjunctivitis, 1:426
Eosinophilic cystitis, 2:460
Eosinophilic dermatitis, 1:693-696
  with edema, 1:696
Eosinophilic enteritis
  cats, 2:96, 2:96f
  dogs, 2:92f
  horses, 2:96

Eosinophilic epitheliotropic disease, 2:16
Eosinophilic folliculitis and furunculosis, 1:696
Eosinophilic gastroenteritis, 2:96
Eosinophilic granuloma
  complex (EGC), feline, 1:693-694, 1:693f-694f
  dogs, 1:694
  horses, 1:694-695, 1:695f
Eosinophilic interstitial pneumonia, 2:513.e1
Eosinophilic meningoencephalitis, 1:396
Eosinophilic myocarditis, 3:43
Eosinophilic myositis, 1:236-237, 1:236f-237f, 2:34
Eosinophilic pulmonary granulomatosis, 2:513.e1
Eosinophilic pustulosis, 1:696
Eosinophilic rhinitis, 2:476, 2:476.e1f
Eosinophilic sialoadenitis, 2:29-30
Eosinophilic ulcers, 2:16
Eosinophilic vascular infiltrates, 1:611
Eosinophilic vasculitis, 1:526
Eosinophils, 1:527
Ependymal cells, 1:262
Ependymoma, 1:400-401, 1:401f
Epicardium, 3:3
Epicauta spp., 2:52
Epidermal collarette, 1:524
Epidermal growth factor (EGF), 2:46, 3:257, 3:257f
Epidermal hamartomas, 1:705
Epidermal inclusion cysts, 2:478
Epidermal mast cells, 1:519
Epidermal vesicles, 2:118
Epidermis, 1:512-513, 1:520
  basement membrane zone, 1:513-514
  dermatohistopathology, 1:518-530
  disorders of differentiation, 1:547-554
    acne, 1:549
    canine nasodigital hyperkeratosis, 1:549-550
    ear margin dermatosis, 1:553
    equine coronary band dystrophy, 1:553-554
    exfoliative dermatoses, 1:553
    hyperplastic dermatosis of West Highland White Terriers, 1:553
    ichthyosis, 1:554
    keratoses, 1:550-551
    Labrador Retriever nasal parakeratosis, 1:550
    lichenoid-psoriasiform dermatosis, 1:552-553
    Schnauzer comedo syndrome, 1:549
    sebaceous adenitis, 1:551-552, 1:552f
    seborrhea, 1:548-549, 1:549f
    tail gland hyperplasia, 1:549
    vitamin A-responsive dermatosis, 1:552
  tumors, 1:706-714, 1:706f
Epidermoid cysts, 1:404
Epidermolysis bullosa, 1:533-537, 1:534f, 2:15
  cats, 1:536-537
  cattle, 1:534-535
  dogs, 1:536, 1:536f
  dystrophic, 1:534
  goats, 1:535
  horses, 1:535-536
  junctional, 1:534
  sheep, 1:535
  simplex, 1:534-535
Epidermolysis bullosa acquisita (EBA), 1:604

Epidermolytic ichthyosis, 1:531, 1:531.e1f
Epididymis. *See* Testes and epididymis
Epididymitis, 3:473-474, 3:474f, 3:487-491, 3:488f-489f
  boars, 3:490
  bulls, 3:489-490
  dogs and cats, 3:490-491
  infectious bovine, 3:443
  small ruminants, 3:490
  stallions, 3:490
Epidural/subdural abscess, 1:353-354, 1:354f
Epilepsy, familial myoclonic, 1:205
Epinephrine, 3:348, 3:350f
Epiphyseal arteries, 1:27
Epiphysiolysis, 1:31
Epiphysis, slipped, 1:31
Epiploic foramen, herniation through, 2:79
Episclerokeratitis, 1:476
Epistaxis, 2:473-474
Epithelial cells, 2:61-62
  of neonate, 2:63
Epithelial cysts, 1:500
Epithelial hyperplasia, 1:442-443, 3:151, 3:151f
Epithelial inclusions, 3:22
Epithelial integrity, restoration of, 2:67
Epithelial neoplasia, middle ear, 1:500
Epithelial regeneration, 2:422-423
Epithelial renewal
  large intestine, 2:68-69
  small intestine, 2:66-67
  villus atrophy, 2:67-68
Epithelial rests of Malassez, 2:6
Epithelial tumors
  pulmonary, 2:495
  skin, 1:703
  thymic, 3:152-153
Epitheliogenesis imperfecta, 2:4, 2:4f
Epithelioid macrophages, 1:527
Epitheliomas, sebaceous, 1:717
Epitheliomatous sebaceous carcinomas, 1:717-718
Epitheliotropic T-cell tumors, 2:107-108
Epitheliotropism, 3:232
Epithelium
  exfoliation in coronavirus, 2:146
  nasal, 2:466, 2:466f
Epithrichial cysts, 1:705
Epitrichial sweat glands, 1:517-518
  carcinomas, 1:719
  tumors, 1:718
Epizootic bovine abortion (EBA), 3:148, 3:149f, 3:419-420
Epizootic catarrhal enteritis of ferrets (ECE), 2:150-151
Epizootic hemorrhagic disease virus (EHDV), 2:39-40, 2:137, 2:137f, 3:431
Epizootic lymphangitis, 3:97-98
ε-cells, endocrine pancreas, 2:368
Epulis, 2:20, 2:24, 2:24f
Equid alphaherpesviruses (EHV), 2:568
Equid besnoitiosis, 1:662
Equid gammaherpesviruses, 2:568-569
Equid herpesvirus 1, 3:435-437, 3:436f, 2:568.e2f
  spleen and, 3:183f
  thymic atrophy and, 3:145-146
Equid herpesvirus 2, 1:626-627, 2:514
Equid herpesvirus 3, 1:625-627
Equid herpesvirus 5, 1:626-627
Equine anterior uveal melanocytomas, 1:483

Equine arteritis virus (EVA), 3:71-72, 3:72f, 3:427-428
Equine aural plaques, 1:504
Equine bacterial pneumonia, 2:571-572
Equine bone fragility syndrome, 1:91, 1:91f
Equine canker, 1:642-643
Equine cannon keratosis, 1:550
Equine coital exanthema, 3:507
Equine coronary band dystrophy, 1:553-554
Equine coronavirus (EqCoV), 2:150
Equine cutaneous onchocerciasis, 1:687-688
Equine degenerative myeloencephalopathy (EDM), 1:322-324
Equine ear papillomas, 1:707-708
Equine encephalitides, 1:376-377, 1:377f
Equine encephalitis, 1:377f
Equine eosinophilic nodular diseases, 1:694-695, 1:695f
Equine exercise-induced fatal pulmonary hemorrhage (EAFPH), 2:491-492, 2:491.e1f
Equine exercise-induced pulmonary hemorrhage (EIPH), 2:490-491, 2:491f, 2:490.e1f
Equine genital papillomas, 1:707-708
Equine grass sickness, 3:51
Equine herpesviral myeloencephalopathy, 1:383-384, 1:384f
Equine hyperlipemia, 2:276-277
Equine infectious anemia virus (EIAV), 3:114-116
Equine influenza, 2:567-568, 2:567.e3f
Equine intestinal clostridial diseases, 2:99
Equine laryngeal hemiplegia, 1:334-335
Equine linear alopecia, 1:550, 1:550f
Equine lymphomas, 3:237-238, 3:238f, 3:238.e1f
Equine multinodular pulmonary fibrosis (EMPF), 2:568, 2:569f
Equine onchocerciasis, 1:452
Equine polysaccharide storage myopathy, 1:205-207, 1:206f-207f
Equine postanesthetic degenerative myopathy, 1:224
Equine protozoal myeloencephalitis, 1:386-387, 1:387f
Equine purpura hemorrhagica, 1:612
Equine recurrent ophthalmitis, 1:455-456
Equine sarcoidosis, 1:700-701
Equine self-mutilation syndrome, 1:562
Equine serum hepatitis, 2:313-314, 2:314f
Equine stringhalt, 1:335
Equine strongylosis, 2:216
Equine suprascapular neuropathy, 1:335
Equine systemic calcinosis, 1:223-224, 1:224f
Equine thrush, 1:643
Equine viral arteritis, 3:71.e2f
Ergotism, 1:572-573, 1:573f
Erosions
  BVDV, 2:123-124, 2:124f
  erosive and ulcerative stomatitides, 2:15-17
  erosive esophagitis, 2:31-32
  erosive polyarthritis, 1:157-158
  laryngeal, 2:481, 2:481.e2f
  teeth, 2:9-11
Eructation, 2:36-37, 2:40
Eryptosis, 3:114
Erysipelas
  pigs, 1:149-150, 1:150f
  sheep, 1:150

Erysipelothrix rhusiopathiae, 1:150, 2:20, 2:433, 3:30-31
Erysipelothrix tonsillarum, 3:30-31
Erythema multiforme (EM), 1:607, 1:609-610, 1:610f
Erythrocyte disorders, 3:112, 3:255-268. See also Anemia
  hereditary, 3:126
Erythrocytosis, 3:128
Erythroid hyperplasia, 2:73, 3:106f
Erythrosine, 3:325
Eschar, 1:524
Escherichia coli, 2:51, 2:111, 2:115, 2:158-167, 2:159f, 2:452, 2:589
  abortion and, 3:417
  bovine, 2:112
  in Boxer dogs, 2:95
  coliform arthritis due to, 1:151
  edema disease and, 2:163-166, 2:164f
  endocarditits and, 3:30-31
  enteroinvasive, 2:166
  enterotoxigenic, 2:112
  epididymitis due to, 3:491
  gastric venous infarction due to, 2:51
  mastitis, 3:454-455, 3:454f
  penis and prepuce injury, 3:507
E-selectin, 1:515
Eskimo Spitz dogs, platelet dysfunction in, 3:259
Esophageal diverticula, 2:31
Esophageal sarcocysts, 2:34
Esophagitis, 2:31-32, 2:32f
Esophagorespiratory fistulae, 2:31
Esophagus, 2:30-35
  anomalies, epithelial metaplasia, and similar lesions, 2:31
  anomalies/epithelial metaplasia/similar lesions, 2:31
  congenital duplication cysts, 2:31
  dysphagia, 2:33-34, 2:34f
    congenital idiopathic megaesophagus (CIM), 2:33-34
    cricopharyngeal dysphagia, 2:33
    megaesophagus, 2:33
    pharyngeal dysphagia, 2:33
  esophageal diverticula, 2:31
  esophageal obstruction/stenosis/ perforation, 2:32-33
  esophagitis, 2:31-32
    erosive/ulcerative esophagitis, 2:30
    hiatus hernia, 2:32
    reflux esophagitis, 2:32
    thrush, 2:32
  esophagorespiratory fistulae, 2:31
  lesions, 2:124, 2:124f
  neoplasia, 2:43-44
  obstruction, stenosis, and perforation, 2:32-33, 2:33f
  papillomas, 2:43-44
  parasitic diseases, 2:34-35, 2:35f
    Spirocerca lupi, 2:34-35
Estrela Mountain dogs, dilated cardiomyopathy in, 3:48
Estrogen in physis, 1:25t
Ethylene glycol, 2:425
  intoxication, 2:425f
Eucoleus aerophilus, 2:585, 2:591
Eucoleus boehmi, 2:585
Eumycotic mycetoma, 1:653-654, 1:654f
Eupatorium rugosum, 3:36

Eurytrema, 2:365
Eventration, 2:78
Eversion, of the bladder, 2:451
Excess free cytosolic calcium, 2:399
Excessive moderator bands, 3:47
Excess renal tissue, 2:392
Excitotoxicity, 1:254
Excrete metabolic wastes, 2:384
Exertional myopathies, 1:221-223
  dogs, 1:223
  horses, 1:221-223, 1:222f
  other species, 1:223
Exfoliative cutaneous lupus erythematosus (ECLE), 1:606, 1:606f
Exfoliative dermatitis, 1:691-692
Exfoliative dermatoses, 1:553
Exocrine pancreas, 2:353-368
  atrophy, 2:362-363, 2:362f
  developmental anomalies, 2:355-356
  hyperplastic and neoplastic lesions, 2:365-368, 2:365f-366f
  insufficiency, 2:69, 2:363-364
  necrosis, 2:357-360, 2:359f-360f
  pancreatitis, 2:360-362
  parasitic diseases, 2:365
  regressive changes, 2:356-364
Exocytosis, 1:519-520
Exogenous porcine growth hormone, 1:225
Exogenous steroids, 3:341
Exostoses, 1:33
  osteitis and, 1:97-98
  vitamin A toxicity and, 1:87
Expansile nodules, symptomatic tumors of, 2:110
ExPEC, 2:578
Experimental disease, 1:3
External acoustic meatal stenosis, 1:502
External ear, 1:500-508
  dermatologic diseases of, 1:503-505
  developmental disease, 1:501-502
  hearing and, 1:501
  histologic preparation and examination, 1:508
  otitis externa, 1:497, 1:502-503, 1:502f, 1:497.e2f
  parasitism, 1:505-507
  pinnal tumor-like growths and neoplasia, 1:504-505
External hernias, 2:79-81, 2:245
External hordeolum, 1:423
Extra-adrenal paragangliomas, 3:356
Extrahepatic biliary anomalies, 2:265-266, 2:266.e1f
Extramedullary hematopoiesis (EMH), 2:300-301, 2:441, 3:191
Extramedullary plasmacytomas (EMP), 2:27-28, 2:109, 3:226-228, 3:226.e1f
Extranodal T-cell lymphoma, 3:232
Extraskeletal osteosarcomas, 1:115
Extrathyroidal lesions in hypothyroidism, 3:318-319
Extrinsic compression, 2:74
Exuberant fracture callus, 1:127
Exuberant granulomas, 2:13
Exudative epidermitis, 2:17
  of pigs, 1:630-632, 1:631f
Eyelid(s)
  abortion and, 3:401
  canine cutaneous histiocytoma, 3:244f
  developmental anomalies and acquired diseases, 1:423

Eyelid(s) *(Continued)*
  neoplasms
    Meibomian adenoma, *1*:480-481, *1*:481*f*
    squamous cell, *1*:479-480, *1*:479*f*-480*f*
Eye(s), *1*:408-488
  developmental anomalies, *1*:409-427
    anomalies of mesenchyme, *1*:413-414
    anomalies of neuroectoderm, *1*:419-421
    anomalies of surface ectoderm, *1*:421-423
    defective differentiation, *1*:413-423
    defective organogenesis and, *1*:410-412, *1*:410*f*
    defects primarily in anterior chamber mesenchyme, *1*:415-417
    early ocular organogenesis and, *1*:409-410
    incomplete atrophy of posterior segment mesenchyme, *1*:417-419
  general considerations, *1*:408-409
  histologic section, *1*:408-409, *1*:409*f*
  lesions with canine distemper virus, *2*:576
  lymphomas, *3*:239*f*, *3*:239.e1*f*
  neoplasia, *1*:478-488
    melanocytic tumors, *1*:482-485
    ocular neuroectoderm, *1*:485-486, *1*:485*f*
  ocular adnexa, *1*:423-427
  ocular fixation, *1*:408-409

F

Facial clefts, *2*:2-3, *2*:3*f*
Facial eczema, *2*:335
Factor IX deficiency, *3*:263
Factor VII deficiency, *3*:264
Factor VIII deficiency, *3*:263-264
Factor XII deficiency, *3*:263-264
Fading follicular hyperplasia (FFH), *3*:222-223
Failure of omasal transport, *2*:39
Falciform ligament, *2*:245
Fallopian tubes pathology, *3*:379-380
False tendons, *3*:22
Familial AA amyloidosis, *2*:278-279
Familial Chinese Shar Pei fever, *1*:158
Familial hyperlipoproteinemia, *2*:277-278
Familial myoclonic epilepsy, *1*:205
Fanconi anemia, *1*:57
Fanconi syndrome, *2*:428, *2*:428*f*
Farcy, *1*:641-642, *3*:96
Fasciola gigantica, *2*:322, *2*:556-557
Fasciola hepatica, *2*:255, *2*:320, *2*:321*f*, *2*:556-557, *2*:322.e1*f*, *2*:321.e1*f*
Fascioloides magna, *2*:322, *2*:322.e1*f*
Fat, muscle steatosis and, *1*:191, *1*:191*f*
Fatal gastric hemorrhage, *2*:58
Fat embolism, *2*:490
Fat-granule cells, *1*:263
Fatty acid deficiency, *1*:581
Fatty cysts, liver, *2*:274-275, *2*:274*f*
Fatty liver, *2*:275-276
Feeding rations deficient, *2*:40
Feedlot cattle
  acute interstitial lung disease, *2*:513*f*, *2*:513.e1
  bloat, *2*:37
  peracute fibrinous bronchopneumonia, *2*:545*f*
  pleuritis, *2*:522*f*
Felid herpesvirus 1, *1*:425, *1*:625-627, *1*:627*f*, *2*:588-589, *2*:588.e2*f*
Feline buccal bone expansion, *1*:99-100
Feline calicivirus (FCV), *2*:15, *2*:589

Feline cardiomyopathies, *3*:46-48, *3*:46.e2*f*
Feline ceruminous cystomatosis, *1*:507
Feline chronic gingivostomatitis, *2*:16
Feline chronic progressive polyarthritis, *1*:158
Feline congenital myasthenia, *1*:209
Feline corneal sequestrum, *1*:434, *1*:434*f*
Feline coronavirus (FCoV), *2*:117, *2*:150-151, *2*:587-588
Feline enteric coronavirus (FECV), *2*:117, *2*:150-151, *2*:587-588
Feline demodecosis, *1*:680-681
Feline diffuse iris melanomas, *1*:483-484, *1*:484*f*
Feline eosinophilic granuloma complex (EGC), *1*:693-694, *1*:693*f*-694*f*
Feline eosinophilic keratitis, *1*:438-439, *1*:439*f*
Feline epitrichial ductular adenomas, *1*:718-719, *1*:719*f*
Feline hepatic steatosis, *2*:277, *2*:277*f*
Feline hereditary cerebellar cortical atrophy, *1*:319
Feline herpesvirus, *1*:105
Feline hippocampal necrosis, *1*:307-308
Feline hyperesthesia, *1*:199
Feline idiopathic pulmonary fibrosis (IPF), *2*:497
Feline immunodeficiency virus (FIV), *1*:627-628, *3*:240
Feline inductive odontogenic tumor, *2*:24
Feline infectious peritonitis virus (FIPV), *2*:253-255, *2*:254*f*, *3*:90, *3*:90*f*
  -associated uveitis, *1*:453, *1*:453*f*
  lymph nodes and, *3*:206*f*
  spleen and, *3*:184*f*
Feline interstitial cystitis, *2*:460
Feline ischemic encephalopathy, *1*:297, *1*:297*f*
Feline leishmaniasis, *1*:663-664, *1*:664*f*
Feline leprosy, *1*:640-641
Feline leukemia virus (FeLV), *1*:105, *1*:627-628
  anemia and, *3*:127, *3*:127*f*
  lymphomas, *3*:235, *3*:239-240
  thymic atrophy and, *3*:145
Feline lipogranulomatous conjunctivitis, *1*:427, *1*:427*f*
Feline lower urinary tract disease (FLUTD), *2*:456, *2*:460
Feline lymphomas, *3*:239-241
Feline mannosidosis, *1*:288*f*
Feline multifocal uveal melanocytoma, *1*:483
Feline Niemann-Pick disease type C, *1*:325
Feline panleukopenia virus (FPLV), *1*:283-284, *2*:98-99, *2*:153-156, *2*:155*f*
Feline paraneoplastic alopecia, *1*:691, *1*:692*f*
Feline parvoviral infection, *3*:145
Feline plasma cell gingivitis-pharyngitis, *2*:16
Feline post-traumatic sarcoma, *1*:486, *1*:487*f*
Feline progressive histiocytosis (FPH), *1*:730, *3*:252*f*-253*f*, *3*:253-254, *3*:253.e1*f*
Feline proliferative necrotizing otitis externa, *1*:503-504
Feline pulmonary adenocarcinoma, *2*:497.e1*f*
Feline pulmonary Langerhans cell histiocytosis, *2*:499, *3*:246-247, *3*:246.e1*f*
Feline scleromyxedema, *1*:697
Feline spinal myelinopathy, *1*:341
Feline spongiform encephalopathy (FSE), *1*:349
Feline ulcerative stomatitis, *2*:16
Feline ventral abdominal lymphangiosarcomas, *1*:728

Feline viral rhinotracheitis, *2*:16, *2*:588-589
Feline X-linked muscular dystrophy, *1*:194-195, *1*:195*f*
Felty's syndrome, *1*:157
Female genital system, *3*:358-464. *See also* Abortion; Gestation
  endometrium, *3*:382-387, *3*:382*f*
  mammae, *3*:451-459
  neoplastic conditions of tubular genitalia, *3*:447-450
  normal sexual differentiation, *3*:360-361
  ovaries, *3*:366, *3*:366*f*
    pathology, *3*:370-375
  pathology
    of cervix, vagina, and vulva, *3*:441-442
    of gravid, *3*:393-398
    of nongravid, *3*:359-441
  sexual development disorders, *3*:360-370, *3*:361*f*-362*f*
  uterine (fallopian) tube pathology, *3*:379-380
  uterus
    cysts arising from, *3*:366-367
    mucometra, *3*:374, *3*:374*f*
    pathology, *3*:380-382, *3*:380*f*
  vaginal anomalies, *3*:369-370
Femoral hernias, *2*:80
Ferrets, *2*:52
  adrenal tumors in, *3*:347-348, *3*:349*f*
  epizootic catarrhal enteritis of, *2*:150-151
  fibrous osteodystrophy in, *1*:78*f*
  gastritis, *2*:52
Fescue toxicosis, *1*:573
Festoons, *1*:520
Fetlock joint, synovial pad proliferation of, *1*:163
Fetus
  atelectasis, *2*:486.e2*f*
  bovine viral diarrhea and, *2*:122
  death, *3*:395
  endocrine function, *3*:274-275, *3*:275*f*
  infections, *2*:122
  lobulations, kidney, *2*:392-393
  lung development, *2*:484
  maceration and emphysema, *3*:396, *3*:396*f*
  mummification of, *3*:395-396, *3*:395*f*
  pneumonia, *3*:404, *3*:404*f*
Fiber balls, *2*:75-76
Fibrin exudation, in urinary space, *2*:405-406
Fibrin formation, *3*:262-263
  disorders, *3*:265
  laboratory evaluation, *3*:262-263
Fibrinocellular crescent, *2*:406*f*, *2*:405.e1*f*
Fibrinogen, *3*:256
  concentration, *3*:262-263
Fibrinoid
  degeneration, *1*:520
  necrosis, *1*:520, *2*:492.e1*f*
Fibrinoid leukodystrophy, *1*:341
Fibrinolysis, *3*:266-267
  endothelium-mediated, *3*:266
  plasma-mediated, *3*:266-267
Fibrinonecrotic bronchitis, *2*:501
Fibrinonecrotic (diphtheritic) membranes, *2*:474-475
Fibrinopurulent arthritis, *1*:147-148
Fibrinopurulent exudate, *1*:356*f*
Fibrinosuppurative exudate with mastitis, *3*:453-454, *3*:453*f*
Fibrinous arthritis, *1*:146-147
  cattle, *1*:147*f*
Fibrinous exudate, *1*:6*f*

Fibrinous inflammation, 1:353
Fibrinous pericarditis, 3:25-26, 3:26f
Fibroadenomatous hyperplasia, 3:460, 3:460f
Fibroadnexal hamartomas, 1:705
Fibroblast growth factor 23 (FGF23), 1:18, 3:296
Fibroblastic metaplasia, 1:442-443
Fibroblastic osteosarcomas, 1:114, 1:114f
Fibroblastic sarcoids, 1:708
Fibroblasts
  alveolar wall, 2:470
  dermal, 1:514
Fibrodysplasia ossificans progressiva (FOP), 1:127, 1:128f, 1:248-249, 1:249f
Fibrohistiocytic nodules of spleen, 3:190-191, 3:190f-191f, 3:191.e1f
Fibromas, 1:723, 2:463-464
  ear, 1:505
  ossifying, 1:109, 1:109f
Fibromatous disorders of tendons and aponeuroses, 1:248-249
  fibrodysplasia ossificans progressiva, 1:127, 1:128f, 1:248-249, 1:249f
  musculoaponeurotic fibromatosis, 1:248, 1:248f
Fibromatous epulis, 2:25f
  of periodontal ligament origin, 2:24, 2:24f-25f
Fibronectins, 1:514
Fibropapillomas, 2:44
  epidermis, 1:706
  esophagus, 2:44
  penis and prepuce, 3:508
  vulva, 3:449
Fibroplasia, 1:520
Fibrosarcomas, 1:121, 1:121f, 1:725, 2:27
  dogs, 2:21
  ear, 1:505
  liver, 2:350
  nasal, 2:480
  solitary, 1:725
  Spirocerca granuloma and, 2:35f
  vaccinal, 1:725
  virus-induced, 1:725
Fibrosis, 1:528
  donkey pulmonary (DPF), 2:514, 2:514.e2f
  equine multinodular pulmonary fibrosis (EMPF), 2:568, 2:569f
  idiopathic pulmonary fibrosis in cats, 2:515, 2:515f, 2:515.e2f
  interstitial, 2:510
    cats, 2:515, 2:515f
    dogs, 2:514-515, 2:515f
  liver, 2:288-289, 2:289f
  muscle, 1:184-185
  subendocardial, 3:30
  thymic, 3:147f
Fibrotic myopathies, 1:213-214
Fibrous astrocytes, 1:260-261
Fibrous capsule, 1:130
Fibrous dysplasia, 1:109-110
Fibrous epulis (fibrous hyperplasia), 2:21, 2:21f
Fibrous hyperplasia, 2:21, 2:21f
Fibrous joints, 1:128
Fibrous osteodystrophy, 1:61, 1:74-80
  cats, 1:77, 1:77f-78f, 1:80f
  dogs, 1:77, 1:78f-79f

Fibrous osteodystrophy *(Continued)*
  goats, 1:76, 1:77f
  gross lesions, 1:75
  horse, 1:75, 1:76f
  horses, 1:76, 1:76f
  pigs, 1:76, 1:76f
  premature osteoclastic resorption of trabeculae in, 1:79-80, 1:80f
Fibrous tumors of bone, 1:121-122, 1:121f-122f
Filaggrin, 1:513
Filaroides hirthi, 2:587
Filtration secretion, 2:71-72
Fimbriae, 2:168
Final reports in postmortem examinations, 1:14
Fire ants, 1:671
First-degree burns, 1:564-566
Fissures
  caries, 2:10
  splenic, 3:163, 3:163f
Fistulae, esophagorespiratory, 2:31
Fistulous tract, 3:472, 3:472f
Fistulous withers, 1:155-156
5′-deiodinase, 3:325
Fixed macrophage system of CNS, 1:262
Flagellates, 2:242-243
Flame figure, 1:519
Flame follicles, 1:520, 1:520f
Flaviviral encephalitides, 1:373-376
Flea, 1:672-673
  -bite hypersensitivity, 1:597-598
  collar dermatitis, 1:566-567
Fleece rot, 1:634
Flexispira rappini, 3:408
Flies, 1:552, 1:666-671
  myiasis, 1:668-670
  warbles, 1:668-669
Fluid accumulation in heart failure, 3:9
Fluid volume regulation, 2:384
Fluorescent markers, 1:29-30
Fluorine poisoning, 2:8
Fluoroacetate poisoning, 1:306, 3:37-38
Fluorosis, 1:84-86
  cattle, 1:85f-86f
  dogs, 1:86
  pigs, 1:86
Foam cells, 1:527, 2:418
Foamy (synctium-forming) virus, 1:154
Focal atrophy of brain and spinal cord, 1:305
Focal contused injuries, 1:302
Focal hepatitis, 2:282, 2:282f
Focal hyperplasia
  C cells, 3:332-333, 3:333f
  thymus, 3:151
Focal macular melanosis, 1:554
Focal myocardial necrosis, 3:36, 3:38f
Focal necrosis, 2:281-282, 2:282f
Focal scarring/fibrosis of ventricular wall, 3:5
Focal segmental glomerulosclerosis (FSGS), 2:405f, 2:417, 2:401.e5f
Focal symmetrical encephalomalacia, 1:300-301, 1:301f
  pigs, 1:308-309
Focal symmetrical poliomyelomalacia, 1:308, 1:308f
Foci of hematopoietic cells, 3:339
Follicle-stimulating hormone (FSH), 3:276-277

Follicular atrophy, 1:520
Follicular cell adenomas, 3:326-327, 3:327f-328f
Follicular cell carcinomas, 3:329-332, 3:330f
Follicular cystitis, 2:460-461, 2:460f
Follicular-derived B-cell lymphomas, 3:222-226, 3:223f
Follicular dystrophy, 1:520
Follicular hamartomas, 1:705
Follicular hyperplasia, 3:222-223, 3:223f
  thymus, 3:150-151, 3:150f
Follicular keratosis, 1:520
Follicular lipidosis, 1:697
Follicular lymphoma (FL), 3:223-224, 3:224f
Follicular mucinosis, 1:697
Folliculitis, 1:520, 1:521f
  Staphylococcal, 1:634-636, 1:635f
  sterile eosinophilic, 1:696
Food reaction, cutaneous, 1:594-596, 1:595f
Foot-and-mouth disease (FMD), 1:233, 1:233f, 2:117, 2:118f-119f
Foothills abortion, 3:419
Footrot, 1:643-644
  virulent, 1:644
Foreign bodies, 2:75
  forestomachs, 2:38
  oral cavity, 2:13, 2:13f
  in peritoneal cavity, 2:247-249
  salivary glands, 2:29
  stomach and abdomen, 2:50-51
Foreign-body glossitis, 2:13f
Foreign-body stomatitis, 2:13
Forelimb-girdle muscular anomaly, 1:189
Forensic autopsy, 1:2
Forestomachs, 2:35-44
  dilation of rumen, 2:36-38
  dystrophic and hyperplastic changes in ruminal mucosa of, 2:36, 2:36f
  foreign bodies in, 2:38
  inflammatory lesions, 2:39-40
  mild inflammation of, 2:40
  neoplasia, 2:43-44
  neoplasia of esophagus, 2:43-44
    fibropapillomas, 2:44
    mesenchymal tumors, 2:44
  parasitic diseases, 2:43, 2:43f
  postmortem change, 2:36
  rumen dilation, 2:36-38
    primary tympany, 2:36
    secondary tympany, 2:37-38
  rumenitis, 2:39-40
    and acidosis caused by carbohydrate overload, 2:40-43
  rumenitis/acidosis caused by carbohydrate overload, 2:40-43
    Fusobacterium necrophorum, 2:41
    mycotic rumenitis, 2:42
  ruminal mucosa, dystrophic/hyperplastic changes, 2:36
  traumatic reticuloperitonitis, 2:38-39
    pericarditis, 2:39
  tympanitic distention of, 2:36
Formalin, 1:8, 1:408
4-Ipomeanol, 2:519
Fourth-degree burns, 1:565
Foveolar mucous cells, 2:45
Fowlpox virus, 1:616

Fox Terrier dogs
  motor neuron disease, 1:331
  myxomatous valvular degeneration, 3:27
Fractional catabolic rate, 2:72
Fractures, 1:33-36
  micro-, 1:34, 1:34f
  repair
    complications of, 1:35-36
    process, 1:34-35, 1:35f
  skull, 1:302-303
  stress-related, in horses, 1:36
  types of, 1:34
Fragile histidine triad (Fhit) protein, 2:462.e1
Francisella tularensis, 3:184-186
Frank-Starling relationship, 3:7
Freemartinism, 3:470f
Free-radical–mediated damage, 2:81
Free radicals, 1:215
Freeze branding, 1:564
French Bulldogs
  canine atopic dermatitis, 1:591
  typhlocolitis, 2:97-98
Friesian cattle, 2:38
  bovine hypomyelinogenesis, 1:338-339
  congenital axonopathy, 1:325
  congenital myopathy, 1:200
  hypertrichosis, 1:541
  lethal trait A46, 3:141
  spastic syndromes, 1:203
  vitiligo, 1:555-556
Frostbite, 1:564
  scrotal, 3:472, 3:472f
Froth, tracheal, 2:483, 2:483f, 2:483.e1f
Frothy bloat, 2:36, 2:37f
Frozen tail, 1:214
Full-thickness intestinal biopsy, 2:89
Fumonisin, 2:334, 2:519-520
Functional obstruction, 2:74-75
Fundic/oxyntic gland acid-secretory mucosa, 2:44
Fungal arthritis, 1:154-155
Fungal infections
  fungal osteomyelitis, 1:103-104
    dogs, 1:104f
  gastrointestinal tract, 2:201
  liver and, 2:324-325, 2:324f, 2:330-331
  lymph nodes and, 3:206f
  respiratory system, 2:535-536, 2:554, 2:573-574, 2:579-585
  skin
    cutaneous, 1:646-661
    subcutaneous, 1:653-661
Furocoumarins, 1:578-579
Furunculosis, 1:520, 1:521f, 1:528
  staphylococcal, 1:634-636, 1:635f
  sterile eosinophilic, 1:696
Fusarium spp., 3:442-443
Fusobacterium equinum, 2:18
Fusobacterium necrophorum, 2:17, 2:39, 2:41, 2:41f-42f
  laryngitis and, 2:481
  liver and, 2:316, 2:316.e1f
  rhinitis and, 2:474-475
  splenic abscesses, 3:183-184, 3:183.e1f
Fusobacterium spp., 2:13-14

G

Galactocerebrosidosis, 1:288
Galactose-induced cataract, 1:443
Galactosialidosis, 1:288
Galenia africana, 3:35

Gallbladder
  agenesis, 2:266.e1f
  anomalies, 2:265-266
  duplication of, 2:355-356
  infarction, 2:307, 2:307f
  mucocele, 2:307, 2:345, 2:345f
Gallotannins, 2:427-428
Galloway cattle, hip dysplasia in, 1:135-136
Gallstones, 2:308-309, 2:309f
Gammaherpesviruses, equid, 2:568
Gammel Dansk Høneshund, canine congenital myasthenia in, 1:209
Gangioneuroma, 3:353
Gangliocytomas, 1:401
Ganglion cysts, 1:162-163
Ganglioneuritis, 1:373f
Gangliosidoses, 1:286f-287f, 1:287-288
  cats, 1:58-59
  cattle, 1:58-59
  dogs, 1:58-59
  sheep, 1:58-59
Gangrene, 3:65
Gangrenous ergotism, 1:572-573, 1:573f
Gangrenous stomatitis, 2:18
Gartner's ducts, 3:442, 3:442f
Gas gangrene, 1:232
Gasterophilus spp., 2:19, 2:34
  esophagus and, 2:34
Gastric adenocarcinoma, 2:102f
Gastric biopsies, 2:47
Gastric carcinomas, 2:102
Gastric changes, 2:94
Gastric dilation
  abomasal volvulus, 2:49-50
  displacement, 2:48-50, 2:49f
  gastric rupture, 2:48
  gastroduodenal intussusception, 2:50
  gastroesophageal intussusception, 2:50
  pylorogastric intussusception, 2:50
  volvulus, 2:49
Gastric distention, 2:31
Gastric foreign bodies
  impaction, 2:50-51
    by inspissated content in horses, 2:50
    primary abomasal impaction in cattle, 2:50
Gastric lymphomas, 2:107-109, 3:241f, 3:241.e1f
Gastric motility, 2:45-46
Gastric mucosa, 2:46
  atrophy, 2:94
  barrier, 2:46
  hypertrophy, 2:53
  mineralization, 2:386f
  mucous metaplasia and hyperplasia, 2:47
  parietal cell mass, atrophy of, 2:47
  response, 2:46-48
  restitution, 2:46
Gastric parasitism, 2:209-210, 2:209f
Gastric rupture, 2:48
Gastric secretion, 2:44
Gastric squamous cell carcinomas, 2:106-107, 2:106f
Gastric ulcers, 2:59
Gastric venous infarction, 2:51
Gastric volvulus, 2:49, 2:49f
  dogs, 2:49f
Gastrin, 2:45

Gastrinomas, 2:375
Gastritis, 2:52-55
  abomasitis associated with viral infection, 2:54
  braxy, 2:53f
  chemical, 2:52
  chemical gastritis/abomasitis, 2:52
  Chlamydophila, 2:53
  diffuse gastric mucosal hypertrophy, 2:53
  due to hypertrophic antritis, 2:53
  due to infection, 2:52, 2:55
  Gasterophilus, 2:54
  gastric mucosal hypertrophy, 2:53
  Helicobacter pylori, 2:52
  hypertrophic antritis, 2:53
  infectious agents, in small animals, 2:52
  mechanical, 2:52
  mycotic, 2:54
  mycotic gastritis/abomasitis, 2:54
  parasitic, 2:54
  parasitic gastritis, 2:54
Gastroduodenal intussusception, 2:50
Gastroduodenal ulceration, 2:55-60
  abomasal ulcers in cattle, 2:57
  acid hypersecretion, factors implicated, 2:55
  duodenal ulcers, 2:56
  gastric ulcers in swine, 2:57
  horses, ulcers, 2:59
  mucosal protective mechanisms, 2:55
  peptic ulcers in dogs, 2:56
  Zollinger-Ellison syndrome, 2:56
Gastroesophageal intussusception, 2:32, 2:50
Gastrointestinal adenocarcinomas, 2:101-104
  adenocarcinoma of stomach, 2:102
  intestinal adenocarcinomas, 2:102-103
  intestinal carcinomas, 2:104
Gastrointestinal carcinomas, histologic lesion of, 2:101
Gastrointestinal disease, diagnosis of, 2:111-117
  diarrhea
    in calves, 2:112-113
    in foals, 2:113-115
    in neonatal ruminants, 2:113
    in neonatal ruminants, swine, and horses, 2:111-112
    in neonatal swine, 2:113
  diarrhea, in calves
    bovine coronavirus, 2:112
    bovine herpesvirus 1, 2:112
    bovine torovirus, 2:112
    Chlamydophila infection, 2:113
    Cryptosporidium parvum, 2:112
    enterotoxigenic *E. coli*, 2:112
    rotavirus, 2:112
    salmonellosis, 2:112
  enteritis
    cats, 2:117
    dogs, 2:116-117
      ascarid infection, 2:117
      canine parvovirus 2, 2:116-117
      Salmonella infection, 2:117
    horses, 2:116
    horses, duodenitis-proximal jejunitis, 2:116
  gastroenteritis
    cattle, 2:114-115
    sheep, 2:115
    swine, 2:115-116

Gastrointestinal disease, diagnosis of *(Continued)*
   gastroenteritis, cattle, gastrointestinal parasitism, 2:114
   neonatal animals, undifferentiated diarrhea of, 2:111
Gastrointestinal helminthosis, 2:204-227
Gastrointestinal malabsorption in humans, 1:69
Gastrointestinal mast cell tumors, 2:109
Gastrointestinal microbiota, 2:65
Gastrointestinal mucosal defense, 2:63
Gastrointestinal mucosal mast cell tumors, 2:109
Gastrointestinal neuroendocrine carcinomas, 2:105-106
   goblet-cell carcinoids, 2:106
Gastrointestinal parasitism, 2:114
Gastrointestinal tract, 2:62-63
   bacterial diseases, 2:158-201
   carcinoid tumors, 2:106
   mycotic diseases, 2:201-203
   neoplasms metastatic, 2:101
Gastrointestinal ulceration, 2:109
Gedoelstia spp., 1:426
Geeldikkop, 2:338-339
Gelbvieh cattle
   congenital status spongiosus, 1:347
   motor neuron disease, 1:332
   necrotizing vasculopathy, 1:200, 1:200f
Geminous teeth, 2:6
Gemistocytes, 1:261-262, 1:261f
Generalized cerebral edema, 1:294
Generalized Shwartzman-like reaction (GSR), 3:65
Generalized skeletal dysplasias, 1:37
Genetic disease/disorders
   of bone, 1:36-60, 1:37t
   connective tissue, 1:542-546
   indirectly affecting the skeleton, 1:57-60
   of muscles, 1:186-210
   osteochondrosis, 1:132
   rickets, 1:69-70
   vasculitis, 3:70
Genetics, diagnostic, 1:12
Genital tritrichomoniasis, 3:423-424
Gentamicin, 1:494, 2:424
Geophilic dermatophytes, 1:649
German Boxer dogs, cleft palate in, 2:3
German Pinscher dogs, vascular ring anomalies in, 2:33
German Shepherd dogs
   acquired protoporphyria, 2:271
   bronchitis, 2:502
   canine panosteitis, 1:107f
   chondrosarcoma, 1:118
   congenital idiopathic megaesophagus, 2:33-34
   corneal edema, 1:429
   corneal endothelial dystrophy, 1:433
   degenerative radiculomyelopathy, 1:330
   diskospondylitis, 1:156, 1:156f
   fibrotic myopathy, 1:213-214
   giant axonal neuropathy, 1:330
   hyposomatotropism, 1:589
   malignant lymphoma, 1:123-124
   masticatory myositis, 1:226
   maxillary or mandibular fibrosarcoma, 1:121
   motor neuron disease, 1:331

German Shepherd dogs *(Continued)*
   motor neuropathy, 1:335
   mucous membrane pemphigoid, 2:15
   myxomatous valvular degeneration, 3:27
   panhypopituitarism, 3:280, 3:280f
   pannus keratitis, 1:438
   peripheral vestibular disease, 1:494
   platelet dysfunction, 3:259-260
   primary parathyroid hyperplasia, 3:301
   pyoderma, 1:635
   pyotraumatic dermatitis, 1:560
   seborrhea, 1:548
   selective deficiencies of immunoglobulins, 3:139
   Sly syndrome, 1:58
   subvalvular aortic stenosis, 3:20
   sudden unexpected death, 3:51
   vascular ring anomalies, 2:33
   vasculitis, 1:612, 3:70
   vitiligo, 1:555-556
German Shorthaired Pointer dogs
   acne, 1:549
   canine X-linked muscular dystrophy, 1:192
   epidermolysis bullosa, 1:536
   malignant oral tumors, 2:21
   sensory and autonomic neuropathy, 1:334
   subvalvular aortic stenosis, 3:20
   vitiligo, 1:555-556
Germ cell tumors
   ovary, 3:377-378
   suprasellar, 1:403-404, 3:287, 3:287f
   testes, 3:495-496, 3:495f
   thymic, 3:158
Gestation, 3:393-398. *See also* Female genital system
   abortion and stillbirth, 3:395, 3:398-440
      diagnosing infectious causes of, 3:399-402
      in mares, 3:417-418
      protozoan infections causing, 3:420-424
   adventitial placentation, 3:396-397
   amniotic plaques, placental mineralization, and avascular chorion, 3:397
   embryonic death, 3:395
      with persistence of membranes, 3:396
   fatty liver in, 2:275
   fetal death, 3:395
   fetal maceration and emphysema, 3:396
   general considerations, 3:393-394
   hydramnios and hydrallantois, 3:397
   mummification of fetus, 3:395-396, 3:395f
   mycotic abortion in cattle, 3:418-419
   postpartum uterus, 3:440-441
   prolonged, 3:397-398
   toxemia, 2:275
   viral infections during, 3:424-440
Ghrelin, 2:368
Giant axonal neuropathy of German Shepherds, 1:330
Giant cell
   granuloma, peripheral, 2:21
   hepatitis, 2:306, 2:306f, 2:438
   multinucleated syncytial, 3:297-298, 3:298f
   -rich osteosarcomas, 1:114
   sarcomas, 1:244
   thyroid carcinoma, 3:331, 3:331f
   tumor
      of bone, 1:122
      of tendon sheath, 1:161-162

Giant Schnauzer dogs, cobalamin deficiency in, 3:127
Giardia, 2:113, 2:242-243
Gingivitis, 2:11-12
   foreign-body stomatitis and, 2:13, 2:13f
Gitter cells, 1:263, 1:263f
Gla-containing proteins, 1:19
Gland acid–secretory mucosa, 2:44
Glanders, 2:573
Glandular structures, 2:452
Glanzmann thrombasthenia, 3:259
Glasser's disease, 1:151-152
Glaucoma, 1:459-465
   histologic lesions of, 1:460-462, 1:460f
   lesions causing, 1:462-465
   retinal changes in, 1:460, 1:461f
Glial fibrillary acidic protein (GFAP), 1:10f, 1:261-262
Glia limitans, 1:261
Glial reactions, 1:366
Gliomatosis cerebri, 1:400f
Gliosis, focal and diffuse, 1:262-263, 1:263f
Glipizide, 2:329
Glisson's capsule, 2:260
Global assays of hemostasis, 3:263
Global glomerulosclerosis, 2:401.e6f
Globe and orbit tumors, 1:488
Globoid cell leukodystrophy, 1:339-342, 1:339f
Glomangiomas, 3:99
Glomerular amyloidosis, 2:414, 2:416f, 2:415.e2f
Glomerular basement membrane (GBM), 2:377, 2:380f
   anti-GBM glomerulonephritis, 2:408
   familial abnormalities of, 2:415-417
   size-dependent barrier, 2:380
   thickening/remodeling, 2:406
   type IV collagen, 2:415-416
Glomerular capillary walls, 2:406
Glomerular cellular crescent, 2:406f
Glomerular cystic atrophy, 2:407
Glomerular damage, monocytes, 2:409
Glomerular disease, 2:377-378, 2:401-421
   amyloidosis, 2:413-414
   in dog, 2:416f, 2:415.e2f
   eosinophilic in H&E sections, 2:415
   histologically, 2:414-415
   familial glomerulopathies, in dog breeds, 2:416f
   immune-complex, 2:413-415
   renal amyloidosis, in cat, 2:414f
   global glomerulosclerosis, 2:401.e6f
   glomerular blood flow, 2:401
   glomerulonephritis (GN), 2:401
      classification, 2:401
   glomerulosclerosis, focal segmental, 2:401.e5f
   membranoproliferative glomerulonephritis (MPGN), 2:404f, 2:401.e4f
   membranous glomerulonephropathy (MGN), 2:402f, 2:401.e2f
   mesangioproliferative glomerulonephropathy, 2:403f, 2:401.e3f
   proliferative glomerulonephropathy, 2:403f, 2:401.e3f

Glomerular filtration, 2:400
  membrane, 2:379-380
Glomerular filtration rate (GFR), 2:377, 3:10
  intrarenal blood flow, 2:379
Glomerular hyperperfusion, 2:387
Glomerular injury
  mechanisms of, 2:408-409
  nonimmunologic causes of, 2:409
Glomerular lipid emboli, 2:420f, 2:418.e4f
Glomerular lipidosis, 2:418-421, 2:420f, 3:319, 3:319f, 2:418.e3f
Glomerular sites immune complexes
  localization of, 2:408
  modification of, 2:408
Glomerular tuft, cellularity of, 2:405
Glomeruli, 2:401
  in neonatal kidneys, 2:382
  reactions, 2:383
Glomerulitis, 2:401
Glomerulocystic atrophy, 2:407f, 2:407.e2f
Glomerulocystic disease, 2:396, 2:396f
Glomerulonephritis (GN), 2:381-382, 2:401
  acute fatal, 2:412-413
  acute phase of proliferative, 2:409
  anti-GBM, 2:408
  capillary walls, hyalinosis of, 2:407f, 2:406.e2f
  cellular crescent, 2:406.e1f
  cellularity, 2:405
  chronic, 2:409f
  classification of, 2:401
  factor H deficiency, 2:412-413
  glomerulocystic atrophy, 2:407f, 2:407.e2f
  histologic changes, 2:405-407
  immunologic evidence, 2:413
  membranoproliferative, 3:123-124
  morphology of, 2:409-410
    acute glomerulonephritis, 2:409
    chronic glomerulonephritis, 2:409f
    intratubular red blood cell cast, 2:409.e1f
  nonglomerular histologic changes, 2:407
  pathogenesis of, 2:407-408
  prevalence of, 2:410-413
    cat glomerulonephritides, 2:412
    crescentic proliferative, 2:412f
    dogs, 2:410-412
    horses, 2:412
    ruminants, 2:413
    swine, 2:412-413
  subacute, 2:409
  swelling of foot processes, 2:406
  thickening
    and lamination, 2:407.e1f
    remodeling, 2:406
  tubulointerstitium, 2:407f
Glomerulopathy, 2:401
Glomerulosclerosis, 2:417-418
  global, 2:405f
  segmental, 2:418
Glomerulus, 2:377
Glomus jugulare tumors, 3:99
Glomus pulmonale tumors, 3:99
Glossitis, 2:16-17
  necrotic, 2:17f
  stomatitis and, 2:17f
Glucagon and hypoglycemic effects of insulin, 2:368
Glucagonomas, 2:374-375
Glucocerebrosidosis, 1:287

Glucocorticoids, 2:55
  biosynthesis, 3:337
  in physis, 1:25t
Glucose-6-phosphatase deficiency, 1:290
Gluten-sensitive enteropathy, 2:69-70, 2:95
Glycogen brancher enzyme deficiency, 1:207, 1:208f
Glycogenoses, 1:290
Glycogenosis type II (Pompe's disease), 1:208
Glycogen storage disease type Ia, 2:273
Glycogen storage disease type II, 1:204
Glycogen storage disease type III, 2:273
Glycogen storage disease type IV, 1:205, 1:205f, 2:273
Glycoproteinoses, 1:288-289, 1:492
Glycoproteins, 1:514
Gnathostoma, 2:54
Gnathostoma spinigerum, 2:210-211
Goatpox virus, 1:616, 1:622-624, 2:557
Goblet-cells, 2:60
  carcinoids, 2:106
  hyperplasia, 2:60
Goiter, 1:6f, 3:273
  colloid, 3:322, 3:322f
  congenital, 3:321, 3:321f
  congenital hypothyroidism with dyshormonogenic, 3:314, 3:323f
  goitrogenesis, 3:320-323, 3:320f, 3:324f
  inherited dyshormonogenic, 3:322-323
  nodular, 3:322, 3:322f
Golden Retriever dogs
  bilateral extraocular muscle myositis, 1:228
  canine atopic dermatitis, 1:591
  canine X-linked muscular dystrophy, 1:192, 3:49
  chondrosarcoma, 1:118
  cobalamin deficiency, 3:127
  demyelinating neuropathy, 1:341-342
  epidermolysis bullosa, 1:536
  hypothyroidism, 1:587, 3:315
  ichthyosis, 1:531, 1:531.e1f
  iris cysts, 1:446
  lymphomas, 3:238
  malignant oral tumors, 2:21
  maxillary or mandibular fibrosarcoma, 1:121
  motor neuron disease, 1:331
  osteogenesis imperfecta, 1:50
  peliosis hepatis, 2:318
  peripheral hypomyelination, 1:338
  pyotraumatic dermatitis, 1:560
  subvalvular aortic stenosis, 3:20
  vitiligo, 1:555-556
Gomen disease, 1:319-320
Gomphoses, 1:128
Gonad phenotype, 3:360
Gongylonema pulchrum, 2:34, 2:35f, 2:43
Gongylonema spp., 2:19, 2:35f
  esophagus and, 2:34
Goniodysgenesis, 1:417, 1:417f
Gordon Setter dogs, canine hypomyelinogenesis in, 1:338
Gossypol, 1:220
"Gotch ear", 1:506, 1:506f
Gousiekte, 3:38
Graft-versus-host disease (GVHD), 1:608-609
Granular cell tumors, 1:245, 2:27
  heart, 3:52-53
  laryngeal, 2:482, 2:482.e1f
  pulmonary, 2:498

Granular trichoblastomas, 1:716
Granular vulvitis, 3:443, 3:443f
Granulation tissue, 1:520
Granulomas, 1:527
  exuberant, 2:13
  nasal, 2:476
  oral eosinophilic, 2:16
  pigment, 2:274-275, 2:275f
  spermatic, 3:480-481, 3:480f-481f, 3:497
  sterile, 1:699-702
  testicular degeneration, 3:484
Granulomatous and pyogranulomatous meningoencephalomyelitis, 1:362, 1:362f
Granulomatous encephalitis, 1:393f-394f
Granulomatous enteritis, 2:97
Granulomatous infections, pancreatic, 2:361
Granulomatous inflammation, 1:353, 2:38
Granulomatous interstitial pneumonia, 2:513
Granulomatous lesions, 1:233-234
Granulomatous lympadenitis, 3:203-204, 3:203f
Granulomatous lymphangitis, 2:196, 2:196f
Granulomatous meningoencephalomyelitis (GME), 1:362f, 1:393-394, 1:393f-394f
Granulomatous pneumonia, 1:6f
Granulomatous radiculitis, 1:396
Granulomatous typhlocolitis, 2:100
Granulomatous uveitis, 1:449
Granulosa-theca cell tumors, 3:375, 3:376f-377f
Grass sickness, in horses, 2:77
Greasy-pig disease, 1:630-632, 1:631f
Great Dane dogs
  acne, 1:549
  calcium crystal-associated arthropathy (pseudogout), 1:157
  cervical vertebral malformation-malarticulation, 1:136
  cochleosaccular degeneration, 1:492
  congenital idiopathic megaesophagus, 2:33-34
  gastric volvulus, 2:49
  hypothyroidism, 1:587, 3:315
  inherited myopathy, 1:197-198
  melanocytopenic hypomelanosis, 1:555
  motor neuropathy, 1:335
Greater Swiss Mountain dogs, Chediak-Higashi syndrome in, 3:259
Great Pyrenees dogs
  canine multifocal retinopathy, 1:469
  chondrodysplasia, 1:44
  cochleosaccular degeneration, 1:492
  prolonged APTT, 3:263
Grenz zone, 1:520
Greyhound dogs
  canine exertional rhabdomyolysis, 1:223
  erosive polyarthritis, 1:157-158
  hip dysplasia, 1:135
  malignant hyperthermia, 1:210
  periodontal osteomyelitis, 1:101f
  vasculitis, 3:70
Griffon Briquet Vendéen dogs, motor neuron disease in, 1:331
Griffon Korthal dogs, recurrent flank alopecia in, 1:590
Griseofulvin, 2:329
Gross and histologic examinations, 1:2-15
  acute pancreatic necrosis, 2:359
  aging changes and other incidental lesions, 1:7
  bone marrow, 3:107-109, 3:108f
  case interpretations and client service, 1:12-14, 1:13f

Gross and histologic examinations *(Continued)*
  classification of tumors, *1*:107, *1*:108*b*
  diagnostic imaging, *1*:11-12
  external ear, *1*:508
  eye, *1*:408-409, *1*:409*f*
  feline panleukopenia, *2*:155
  genetics, *1*:12
  heart, *3*:6, *3*:12-14, *3*:12*f*, *3*:13*t*
  hematoxylin and eosin (H&E) stains, *1*:9, *1*:29
  immunohistochemistry, *1*:9, *1*:10*f*
  immunology, *1*:11
  initial and ongoing competence of pathologists in, *1*:14-15
  liver, *2*:277
  lungs, *2*:489
  male genital tract, *3*:465-466
  methodologies, *1*:2
  microbiology, *1*:10-11
  molecular biology, *1*:11
  morphologic diagnosis in, *1*:5
  osteosarcoma, *1*:112-114, *1*:113*f*
  parasitology, *1*:11
  photography, *1*:12
  problem-oriented, *1*:7
  quality assurance of pathology services and, *1*:14
  sample selection and preservation, records, *1*:8
  of severely osteoporotic bones, *1*:64
  skeleton, *1*:28
  special stains, *1*:9
  systematic, *1*:4-6
  techniques and stains in postmortem examination of skeleton, *1*:28-29, *1*:29*f*
    preparation artifacts in, *1*:29, *1*:29*f*
  toxicology, *1*:11
  trimming of fixed autopsy and biopsy specimens, *1*:8-9
  types of investigations, *1*:2-3, *1*:3*f*
Ground substance, congenital abnormalities of, *1*:545-546
Ground (interstitial) substance, dermis, *1*:514
Growing axonal sprouts, *1*:256
Growth arrest line, *1*:60, *1*:60*f*, *1*:64
Growth factors in bone matrix, *1*:20
Growth hormone (GH), *1*:25*t*, *3*:276-277
  adenomas, *3*:285-286, *3*:285*f*-286*f*
  castration-responsive dermatosis, *1*:589
Growth plate, *1*:22, *1*:22*f*, *1*:24
  bulldog type chondrodysplasia, *1*:38, *1*:38*f*
  copper deficiency and, *1*:81
  damage, *1*:30-31
  fibrous osteodystrophy and, *1*:79-80
  hormonal regulation of, *1*:24, *1*:25*t*
  mucopolysaccharidoses, *1*:58
  thickness, *1*:23-24
Growth rate
  growth retardation lattices, *1*:104, *1*:105*f*
  osteochondrosis, *1*:132
Guernsey cattle, cyclopia in, *1*:269-270
Guinea pigs
  ptyalism, *2*:29
  scurvy, *1*:83, *1*:83*f*-84*f*
Gurltia paralysans, *1*:390-391
Gut
  external muscle, *2*:62
  flora, *2*:65
  immune reactions, *2*:67-68

Guttural pouch, *1*:495-496, *2*:480-481
  disease, *1*:498
  myocosis, *2*:480-481, *2*:480*f*
  squamous cell carcinoma of, *1*:500
Gynecomastia, *3*:471
Gyr cattle, *Rhabditis bovis* in, *1*:507

H

Habronema spp., *2*:567, *3*:508
  splenic abscesses, *3*:183-184
Haematobia irritans, *1*:670
Haemonchus, *2*:54-55
Haemonchus contortus, *3*:112-114
Haemophilus, *1*:151-152
Haemophilus parasuis, *2*:543
Haflinger horses, axonal dystrophy in, *1*:324
Hailey-Hailey disease (HHD), *1*:537
Hair
  congenital and hereditary diseases of
    congenital hypotrichosis, *1*:538-541
    hypertrichosis, *1*:539-541
  follicles, *1*:515-517
    tumors arising from, *1*:714-717
Hairy vetch, *1*:574, *2*:306, *3*:43
Halicephalobus gingivalis, *1*:98, *1*:390, *1*:390*f*, *2*:19, *2*:444*f*
Halogenated hydrocarbons, *2*:332
Halogenated salicylanilide toxicosis, *1*:345
Halogeton glomeratus, *2*:425-426
Halothane, *2*:329
Hamartomas, *1*:404, *1*:520, *1*:705, *3*:98
  collagenous, *1*:723
  liver, *2*:264, *2*:264*f*
  ovarian, *3*:366, *3*:378-379
  pulmonary, *2*:485
Hammondia, *2*:239
Hampshire sheep, abomasal dilation and emptying defect in, *2*:51
Hansen type II intervertebral disk herniations, *1*:144*f*, *1*:145
Hansen type I intervertebral disk herniations, *1*:144, *1*:144*f*
Hard callus, *1*:35
Harlequin ichthyosis, *1*:530, *1*:531*f*
Hassall's corpuscles, *3*:142
Havanese dogs, sebaceous adenitis in, *1*:551
Haversian systems, *1*:20, *1*:21*f*
Head. *See also* Brain
  defects, *1*:37*t*
  traumatic injuries, *1*:301-303
Hearing. *See also* Ear(s)
  external ear and, *1*:501
  impairment, *1*:491-494
    acquired deafness, *1*:493
    congenital, *1*:491-493
    traumatic causes of deafness and, *1*:493-494
  internal ear and, *1*:491
  middle ear and, *1*:496
Heart
  -base tumors dervied from ectopic thyroid, *3*:356
  blood supply, *3*:2
  cardiac rhabdomyomas of, *1*:241
  cholesterol granuloma, *1*:304*f*
  congenital abnormalities, *3*:14-24, *3*:15*t*, *3*:66-67
  diseases, *3*:2-54
    cardiomyopathies, *3*:44-51, *3*:48.*e2f*, *3*:45.*e1f*, *3*:46.*e2f*
    conduction system, *3*:51

Heart *(Continued)*
    endocardial, *3*:27-33
    heart failure and, *3*:2.*e1f*
    morphologic patterns, *3*:4-5
    pathophysiologic patterns, *3*:5-6
  examination, *3*:12-14, *3*:12*f*, *3*:13*t*
  failure, *2*:493, *2*:493*f*, *3*:6-12, *2*:493.*e1f*
    congestive, *3*:6, *3*:10-12, *3*:11*f*, *3*:9.*e1f*
    heart disease and, *3*:2.*e1f*
    systemic responses in, *3*:9-10
  hemorrhages, *3*:33
  neoplasms, *3*:52-54, *3*:52*f*
  valves, *3*:4
  weight, *3*:2
Heartwater, *3*:80-82, *3*:81*f*-82*f*
Heartworm disease, *3*:83-85, *3*:84*f*, *3*:85.*e1f*
Heat-stable toxin, *2*:160
Heinz bodies, *3*:126*f*, *3*:238.*e1f*
Helcococcus ovis, *2*:562
Helianthrones, *1*:578
Helichrysum blandowskianum, *2*:331
Helicobacter acinonychis, *2*:52
Helicobacter heilmannii, *2*:58
Helicobacter pylori, *2*:52
  gastritis and, *2*:52, *2*:55
  liver and, *2*:318
Helicobacter spp., *2*:55
  chronic, *2*:52
  colonization, *2*:52
Helminthic infections
  central nervous system and, *1*:389-391
  gastrointestinal, *2*:204-227
  liver, *2*:318-324
  skin, *1*:685-690
Hemal nodes, *3*:162, *3*:162*f*, *3*:162.*e1f*
Hemangioendothelioma (HE), *3*:98
Hemangiomas, *1*:122, *1*:726-727, *1*:727*f*, *2*:28, *2*:447, *3*:98-99
  conjunctival, *1*:481-482, *1*:482*f*
  liver, *2*:349-350
  ovarian, *3*:378
  scrotal, *3*:472
Hemangiosarcomas, *1*:122, *1*:244-245, *1*:245*f*, *1*:727, *3*:99-101, *3*:100*f*-101*f*
  ear, *1*:505
  metastasis, *1*:736
  splenic, *3*:192-194, *3*:193*f*, *3*:192.*e1f*
Hematin, *2*:271
Hematocele, *3*:473
Hematogenous osteomyelitis, *1*:98
Hematomas
  aural, *1*:504
  congenital, *3*:22-23
  endocardium, *3*:30
  progressive ethmoid, *2*:477
  splenic, *3*:166*f*
  thymic, *3*:147-148, *3*:147*f*-148*f*, *3*:146.*e2f*
Hematopoiesis, *2*:264, *2*:264*f*
Hematopoietic neoplasia, *3*:129-136, *3*:129*t*
Hematopoietic stem cells (HSC), *3*:103
Hematopoietic system, *3*:102-268. *See also* Lymphomas
  bone marrow, *3*:103-138, *3*:103*f*
  histiocytic proliferative diseases, *3*:243-255
  leukocyte disorders, *3*:109-112
  lymph nodes, *3*:196-243
  lymphoid organs, *3*:139-141

Hematopoietic system *(Continued)*
  sample procurement and processing, 3:107-109, 3:108f
  spleen and hemolymph nodes, 3:158-196
  thymus, 3:141-158
Hematopoietic tumors, 1:403
Hematoxylin and eosin (H&E) stains, 1:9, 1:29
Hemerocallin, 1:345
Hemidesmosomes, 1:513-514
Hemimelia, 1:55-56
Hemivertebrae, 1:57
Hemochromatosis, 2:272
Hemoconcentration, 3:343
Hemocysts, 3:30
Hemodynamic effects of valvular abnormalities, 3:4.e1f
Hemoglobinuria, 2:436
  -associated ATI, 2:422-423
Hemolysis, intravascular, 3:114, 3:115f
Hemolytic anemia, 3:114-126
Hemolytic-uremic syndrome (HUS), 3:65
Hemomelasma ilei, 2:216-217, 2:217f
Hemonchosis, 2:207-208, 2:207f-208f
Hemopericardium, 3:25, 3:25f
Hemoperitoneum, 2:247
Hemophagocytic histiocytic sarcoma, 3:254-255, 3:254f-255f, 3:254.e1f
Hemophilia A, 3:263-264
Hemophilia B, 3:263
Hemorrhage, 2:57
  adrenal gland, 3:339-340, 3:340f
  central nervous system, 1:300-301
  heart, 3:33, 3:78.e1f
  intrafollicular (ovary), 3:370
  liver, 2:294
  lymph node, 3:200f
  pulmonary, 2:490-492, 2:490.e1f
  retinal, 1:473
  septicemia of cattle, 2:546-547
  subendocardial, 3:4
  testicular, 3:492, 3:492f
  thymic, 3:147-148, 3:146.e2f
  tracheal, 1:192, 2:483f
Hemorrhagic adrenal necrosis, 3:65
Hemorrhagic bowel syndrome, 2:114. *See also* Jejunal hematoma
Hemorrhagic glomeruli turkey egg pattern, 2:399
Hemorrhagic infarcts, 1:299f-300f
Hemorrhagic inflammation, 1:353
Hemorrhagic shock, 2:84
Hemosiderin, 1:434, 2:271, 3:165, 3:165f
Hemosiderosis, chronic hemolytic anemia, 2:429
Hemostasis disorders, 3:255-268
  dysregulation of hemostasis, 3:267-268
  fibrin formation, 3:265
  fibrinolysis, 3:266-267
  platelet plug formation, 3:255-257
  regulation of coagulation, 3:265-266
  thrombin formation, 3:260-261, 3:263-265
Hemothorax, 2:521, 2:521.e3f
Hemotropic mycoplasmas, 3:124-125
Hendra virus, 2:569
Henle loop, 2:377
Hepatic acinus of Rappaport, 2:261
Hepatic arterial buffer effect, 2:260
Hepatic arteriovenous malformations, 2:266, 2:266f
Hepatic artery, 2:260
  injury, 2:296-300

Hepatic carcinoids, 2:349, 2:350f
Hepatic coccidiosis, 2:324, 2:324f
Hepatic cysts, 2:264
Hepatic dendritic cells, 2:263
Hepatic dysfunction, 2:290-295
Hepatic encephalopathy (HE), 1:262, 1:262f, 1:344, 1:344f, 2:291-292
Hepatic endothelial cells, 2:262-263
Hepatic fatty cirrhosis, 2:276, 2:276.e1f
Hepatic iron overload, 2:272
Hepatic lipodystrophy, 2:278
Hepatic progenitor cells (HPCs), 2:262
Hepatic regeneration, 2:286-287
Hepatic sinusoids, 2:260
Hepatic stellate cells (HSC), 2:263
Hepatic susceptibility, 2:325-326, 2:260
Hepatic veins, 2:260
  injury, 2:296-297
  thrombosis, 2:298
Hepatitis
  acute, 2:301
  B antigen, 3:71
  chronic, 2:301-306, 2:305.e1f
    cats, 2:305
    dogs, 2:302-305, 2:305f
    horses, 2:305
    lobular dissecting, 2:305, 2:305f, 2:305.e1f
  equine serum, 2:313-314, 2:314f
  focal, 2:282, 2:282f
  giant cell, 2:306, 2:306f
  infectious canine, 2:310-312, 2:310f-311f, 2:311.e1f
  necrotic, 2:316, 2:316.e1f
  nonspecific reactive, 2:306
  periportal interface, 2:301-302, 2:302f, 2:304f
Hepatoblastomas, 2:347-348, 2:348f
Hepatocellular atrophy, 2:269, 2:269f, 2:269.e1f
Hepatocellular carcinoma, 2:346, 2:346.e1f
  mixed cholangiocellular and, 2:349, 2:349.e1f
Hepatocellular cholestasis, 2:293
Hepatocellular hypertrophy, 2:269-270, 2:269f
Hepatocellular steatosis, 2:273-278, 2:274f-276f, 2:274.e1f, 2:276.e1f
Hepatocutaneous syndrome, 1:586-587, 2:295, 2:329, 2:295.e1f
Hepatocytes, 2:261-264
Hepatocytotropic T-cell lymphoma (HC-TCL), 3:232
Hepatogenous photosensitization, 1:579-580, 2:294, 2:294f
Hepatoid glands, 1:517
Hepatopancreatic ampullary carcinoma (HC-TCL), 2:367
Hepatorenal syndrome, 2:294, 2:430
Hepatosis dietetica, 2:284, 2:285f
Hepatosplenic T-cell lymphoma (HS-TCL), 3:232
Hepatozoon americanum, 1:98, 1:240, 2:414, 3:110-111
Hepatozoon canis, 3:110
Hepatozoonosis, 1:240
Hereditary deafness, 1:492-493, 1:492f
  cryptorchidism, 3:476-478, 3:476f
Hereditary equine regional dermal asthenia (HERDA), 1:544
Hereditary footpad hyperkeratosis, 1:532
Hereditary hypopigmentation, 1:555-557

Hereditary nephritis, 2:417f, 2:415.e3f
Hereditary nephropathy, 2:388-391
Hereditary renal diseases, 2:391
Hereditary striatonigral and cerebello-olivary degeneration, 1:319
Hereditary zinc deficiency, 1:532-533
Heredity. *See* Genetic disease/disorders
Hereford cattle
  bovine familial convulsions and ataxia, 1:319
  bovine hypomyelinogenesis, 1:338-339
  Chediak-Higashi syndrome, 3:259
  congenital hypotrichosis, 1:538-539
  hip dysplasia, 1:135-136
  idiopathic spongy myelinopathies, 1:342-343
  motor neuron disease, 1:332, 1:332f
  osteopetrosis, 1:51
Hernias
  acquired diaphragmatic, 2:246-247, 2:246f
  diaphragmatic, 2:80
  direct inguinal, 2:80
  external, 2:79-81, 2:245
  femoral, 2:80
  hernial contents, 2:79-80
  hiatal, 2:32
  indirect inguinal, 2:80
  inguinal, 2:80, 3:498
  internal, 2:79
  mesenteric, 2:79
  omental, 2:79
  pelvic, 2:79
  perineal, 2:80
  prepubic, 2:80
  scrotal, 3:498
  sequelae of, 2:80
  through natural foramen, 2:79
  umbilical, 2:80
  ventral hernia of abdominal wall, 2:80
Herniation, natural foramen, 2:79
Herpesviral infections, 1:625-627
  adrenal cortex and, 3:340
  alphaherpesviruses
    cattle, 2:537
    horses, 2:568, 2:568.e2f
  Canid herpesvirus-1 (CaHV-1), 2:577, 3:431-432, 3:432f, 3:434f
  cats, 1:425, 1:625-627, 1:627f, 2:588-589, 2:588.e2f
  general features, 2:537
  male goats, 3:507
  myocardial necrosis and, 3:34
  pigs
    causing abortion in, 3:432-433
    pregnant uterus, 3:433
    pups and pregnant bitches, 3:431-432, 3:432f
Herpetic keratitis of cats, 1:438
Hertwig's epithelial root sheath (HERS), 2:4-5
Heterobilharzia americana, 2:323, 3:93-94, 3:94f
Heterophilic otitis media, 1:493, 1:493.e2f
Heterotopic polyodontia, 2:6
Hexachlorophene poisoning, 1:344-345, 1:345f
Hiatal hernia, 2:32
Hidradenitis, 1:520
"High-altitude disease" of cattle, 3:66
High-endothelial venules (HEV), 3:196
Highland cattle, cropped or notched pinnae in, 1:502

Highly chlorinated naphthalene toxicosis, 1:571
Himalayan cats, feline corneal sequestrum in, 1:434, 1:434f
Hip dysplasia
　cats, 1:135
　cattle, 1:135-136
　dogs, 1:135-136, 1:135f
Hirano-like bodies, 1:255
Histamine, 2:45
Histiocytes in nodular and diffuse dermatitis, 1:526
Histiocytic proliferative disorders, 1:728-730, 3:243-255
　canine cutaneous histiocytoma, 3:243-245, 3:244f-245f, 3:244.e1f, 3:243.e1f
　canine cutaneous Langerhans cell histiocytosis, 1:729, 3:245-246, 3:246f
　canine reactive histiocytosis, 3:247-250, 3:248f-249f, 3:247.e1f, 3:249.e1f
　feline progressive histiocytosis (FPH), 1:730, 3:252f-253f, 3:253-254, 3:253.e1f
　feline pulmonary Langerhans cell histiocytosis, 2:499, 3:246-247, 3:247f, 3:246.e1f
　hemophagocytic histiocytic sarcoma, 3:254-255, 3:254f-255f, 3:254.e1f
　histiocytic sarcoma (HS), 1:159-160, 1:160f, 1:729-730, 3:250-253, 3:250f-252f, 3:250.e2f, 3:250.e1f
Histiocytic sarcoma (HS), 1:159-160, 1:160f, 1:403, 1:729-730, 3:250-253, 3:250f-252f, 3:250.e2f, 3:250.e1f
　multifocal, 2:448f
　pulmonary, 2:498-499, 2:499f
Histiocytic ulcerative colitis, 2:97-98, 2:98f
Histochemical fiber types, 1:169-170, 1:169f-170f
Histologic examinations. See Gross and histologic examinations
Histophilus somni, 1:151-152, 1:364f-365f
　abortion and, 3:414
　cattle, 2:543-544, 2:546, 2:546.e1f
　central nervous system and, 1:364-365, 1:364f-365f
　liver and, 2:314-315
　pleuritis, 2:522f
　pulmonary vasculitis and, 2:494
　sheep, 2:562
Histoplasma capsulatum, 1:104, 1:449-450, 1:450f, 2:98, 2:202, 2:203f, 3:97, 3:340, 2:324.e1f
　spleen and, 3:186-187, 3:186f-187f, 3:186.e2f
Histoplasmosis, 1:450, 1:450f
　intestinal, 2:202-203, 2:203f
H3N8 influenza A virus, 2:577
HoBi-like BVDV, 2:122
Hodgkin-like lymphomas (HLL), 3:219
Holoprosencephaly, 1:269-270, 1:269f
Holstein cattle, 2:38
　bovine hypomyelinogenesis, 1:338-339
　cardiomyopathies, 3:50
　congenital axonopathy, 1:325
　congenital hypotrichosis, 1:538-539
　degenerative joint disease, 1:143
　diaphragmatic dystrophy, 1:199
　prolonged APTT, 3:263
　vitiligo, 1:556

Hookworms
　dermatitis, 1:685
　of ruminants, 2:214-215
Hormonal hypersensitivity, 1:599
Hormones
　abnormal degradation of, 3:275
　adrenal, 3:337-338
　calcium-regulating, 3:291-310, 3:291f
　catecholamine and iodothyronine, 3:271, 3:348-349, 3:350f
　excess, syndromes of iatrogenic, 3:275-276
　hypersecretion by non-endocrine tumors, 3:274
　pancreatic, 2:368, 2:369f
　polypeptide, 3:270-271, 3:270f
　steroid, 3:271
　thyroid, 3:311-312
　types, 3:270-271
Horn cysts, 1:520
Horner syndrome, 1:494-495
Horn fly dermatitis, 1:670
"Horsepox", 1:621
Horsepox virus, 1:616, 1:621
Horseshoe kidney, 2:392, 2:393f
"Hot spots", 1:560, 1:598
House-dust mites, 1:683
Howship's lacunae, 1:18, 1:19f, 1:78-79
Humans
　arrhythmogenic right ventricular cardiomyopathy, 3:49
　atherosclerosis, 3:57
　benign bone cysts, 1:126
　carcinoids, 2:497-498
　Fanconi anemia, 1:57
　Hashimoto's disease, 3:316
　ichthyosis, 1:530
　infantile cortical hyperostosis, 1:53
　inflammatory bowel disease, 1:66-67
　light-induced retinal degeneration, 1:470
　metabolic myopathies, 1:204
　muscular dystrophy, 1:192
　necrotizing sialometaplasia, 2:30
　ocular onchocerciasis, 1:452
　osteochondromatosis, 1:54
　osteoporosis, 1:63-64, 1:67
　renal failure, 1:80
　rickets and osteomalacia, 1:69
　steroid-induced bone necrosis, 1:95
　tuberculosis in, 2:548
　Werdnig-Hoffman disease, 1:331
Humoral hypercalcemia of malignancy (HHM), 3:274, 3:305-310, 3:306f
Hunter syndrome, 1:58
Hurler's syndrome, 1:58
Hyaline arteriosclerosis, 3:60
Hyaline droplets, 2:421-422
Hyaline necrosis, 1:297-298
Hyaline scars, 2:504, 2:504.e2f
Hyalinization of dural collagen, 1:304
Hyalinosis, 2:406, 3:60, 3:60f
　of capillary walls, 2:407f, 2:406.e2f
　pulmonary, 2:517
Hyalohyphomycosis, 1:653, 1:655
Hyaluronan, 1:131
Hybrid cysts, 1:704
Hybrid sorghum, 1:91
Hydatid disease, 2:537
Hydrallantois, 3:397

Hydramnios, 3:397
Hydranencephaly, 1:272-274, 1:272f
　orbiviruses and, 1:281
Hydrocarbons, halogenated, 2:332
Hydrocele, 3:473
Hydrocephalus, 1:270-272, 1:271f
Hydrogen ion excretion, 2:381
Hydrometra, 3:386, 3:386f
Hydromyelia, 1:278
Hydronephrosis, 2:400-401
　development of, 2:400
　glomerular filtration, 2:400
　gross changes, 2:400-401
　microscopically, 2:401
　in sheep, 2:400f
Hydropericardium, 3:24-25, 3:24f
Hydropic degeneration, 1:522, 1:522f
Hydrosalpinx, 3:379-380, 3:379f
Hydrothorax, 2:521.e3f
Hydroureter, 2:451
　in goat, 2:451.e1f
Hydroxyapatite, 1:20
Hydroxyl radical, 2:81
Hyena disease, 1:88
Hygroma, 1:155, 1:155f, 1:559
Hygromycin B, 1:444
Hymen, 3:368-369, 3:370f
Hymenopteran insects, 1:568
Hymenoxon odorata, 2:52
Hyostrongylus rubidus, 2:210
Hyostrongylus spp., 2:47
Hyperacute infection, 2:437
Hyperadrenocorticism, 1:224-225, 1:588-589, 1:588f, 3:346-347, 3:347f
　muscle myopathies and, 1:224-225
　spontaneous and iatrogenic, 1:67
Hypercalcemia, 2:441, 3:305-310, 3:305f, 3:343
　with tumors metastatic to bone, 3:309
Hypercalcemic nephropathy, 2:383, 2:441, 2:441f, 2:456
　cause, 2:441
　mineralization, 2:441
　renal failure, 2:441
Hypercellularity, 2:405
Hypercementosis, 2:6
Hypercholesterolemia, 3:318-319
Hyperemia, 2:51
　lungs and, 2:487
　mastitis, 3:453-454, 3:453f
Hyperestrogenism, 1:589
Hyperfibrinogenemia, 3:265
Hypergammaglobulinemia, 2:95
Hyperglobulinemia, 2:72-73
Hypergranulosis, 1:520
Hyperimmune states, 3:163
Hyperkalemic periodic paralysis (HYPP), 1:186-187, 1:202
Hyperkeratosis
　canine nasodigital, 1:549-550
　esophageal epithelium, 2:31
　hereditary footpad, 1:532
　hypothyroidism with, 3:318
　perivascular dermatitis with, 1:525
　stratum corneum, 1:520, 1:522f
Hyperkinetic equilibrium, 2:72-73
Hyperlipemia, equine, 2:276-277
Hypermotility, 2:72
Hypernatremia, 1:225

Hyperostotic diseases, 1:91-94
    calvarial hyperostosis of Bullmastiffs, 1:92
    canine hepatozoonosis, 1:94, 1:94f
    craniomandibular osteopathy, 1:91-92, 1:92f
    hypertrophic osteopathy, 1:92-94, 1:93f
Hyperoxaluria, primary, 2:426
Hyperparathyroidism, 3:273-274
    nutritional, 3:274
        secondary, 1:75
    primary, 1:74, 3:304-305
    renal secondary, 1:74-75, 1:77-78
    secondary, 1:74
        to renal disease, 3:300-301, 3:300f
        secondary to nutritional imbalances, 3:301
Hyperpigmentation, 1:520-521, 1:554-555
    acquired, 1:554
    focal macular melanosis, 1:554
    hypothyroidism with, 3:318
Hyperplasia, 2:387. See also Neoplasia
    adrenal cortex, 3:343, 3:344f
    adrenal medullary, 3:352
    atypical adenomatous, 2:495
    bile duct, 2:287-288, 2:289f
    bronchiolar epithelial, 2:505, 2:504.e2f
    cementum, 2:6
    dermatosis of West Highland White Terriers, 1:553
    diffuse, 3:300, 3:300f
    ductular epithelium, 2:365-366
    endocrine gland nodular, 3:271
    endometrial, 3:382-385, 3:382f-384f, 3:391, 3:391f-392f
    epidermal, 1:521, 1:522f
        perivascular dermatitis with, 1:525
    epithelial, 1:442-443, 3:151, 3:151f
    erythroid, 3:106f
    esophageal epithelium, 2:31
    fibroadenomatous, 3:460, 3:460f
    follicular, 3:222-223, 3:223f
    liver, 2:344-352
    lymph node, 3:200-202
    male genital system
        prostate and bulbourethral gland, 3:502-503, 3:503f
        testicular, 3:470f, 3:493
    mucous, 2:47
    muscular, 1:190-191
    nodular
        adrenal cortex, 3:343
        liver, 2:344, 2:344f
        spleen, 3:189-190, 3:190f, 3:189.e2f
        thyroid, 3:322, 3:322f
    pancreas
        endocrine, 2:373-375
        exocrine, 2:365, 2:365f-366f
    parathyroid, 3:299-300, 3:299f-300f
        primary, 3:301
    pharyngeal lymphoid, 2:480.e3f
    plasma cell, 3:201
    pseudoepitheliomatous, 3:151
    sebaceous gland, 1:523
    Sertoli cell, 3:477f
    splenic, 3:169f, 3:189-191, 3:189f
    tail gland, 1:549
    thymic, 3:150-151, 3:150f
    thyroid, 1:6f, 3:320-323, 3:320f
Hyperplastic dermatosis of West Highland White Terriers, 1:553
Hypersensitivity dermatoses, 1:590-600
    hormonal, 1:599
    insect, 1:597-599, 1:670-671

Hypersensitivity pneumonitis, 2:512-513
Hypersensitivity-related idiosyncrasies, 2:327
Hypersomatotropism, 1:589
Hypertension, 2:398, 3:59-60
    portal, 2:297
    pulmonary, 2:492-494, 3:60
        canine pulmonary veno-occlusive disease (PVOD), 2:493, 2:493f, 2:493.e1f
        causes, 2:492b
        pulmonary arterial hypertension (PAH), 2:492-494, 2:492f, 3:66-67
Hypertensive retinopathy, 1:472, 1:473f
Hyperthyroidism
    associated with thyroid tumors, 3:327-329, 3:328f
    concentric cardiac hypertrophy and, 3:9
    muscle myopathies and, 1:224
    osteoporosis and, 1:67
Hypertrichosis, 1:541, 3:284, 3:284f
Hypertrophic antritis, 2:53
Hypertrophic cardiomyopathy (HCM), 3:45
    cats, 3:46, 3:47f
    cattle, 3:50
    dogs, 3:49
Hypertrophic osteodystrophy (HOD), 1:105-106, 1:105f
Hypertrophic osteopathy, 2:444
    dogs, 1:92-94, 1:93f
    horses, 1:93f
Hypertrophic pulmonary osteopathy, 2:35
Hypertrophic reaction, 1:262-263
Hypertrophic zone, 1:23
Hypertrophy, 1:178-180, 1:178f-179f, 3:2
    arterial, 3:66-67
    cardiac, 3:7-9
    cementum, 2:6-8
    gastric mucosal, 2:53
    hepatocellular, 2:269-270, 2:269f
    of pulmonary arteries of cats, 3:67, 3:67f
    smooth muscle of esophagus, 2:31
    testicular, 3:485
    of the tongue, 2:4
Hypoadrenocorticism, 1:225
    lesions, 3:341-343, 3:342f
Hypoalbuminemia, syndromes of, 2:95
Hypoalbuminemic animal, 2:73
Hypocalcemia, 3:299
Hypoderma bovis, 1:668-669
Hypoderma lineatum, 1:668-669, 2:34
Hypoderma spp., 1:668-669
Hypoglycemia, 3:343
    nervous system and, 1:306-307
Hypoglycin A., 1:220
Hypokalemia, 2:430
    cats, 1:225
    cattle, 1:225
Hypomyelinating diseases, 1:259-260, 1:260f
Hypomyelination, 1:336-337
Hypoparathyroidism, 3:298-299
Hypophosphatemia, 1:225
Hypophosphatemic rickets, 1:70, 1:70f
Hypophyseal form of diabetes insipidus, 3:290
Hypopigmentation
    disorders, 1:555-558
        acquired, 1:557, 1:557f
        hereditary, 1:555-557
        leukoderma and leukotrichia, 1:555
    epidermis, 1:521-522
    iris, 1:415
Hypoplasia
    adrenal cortex, 3:338-339
    cerebellar, 1:275-276, 1:275f

Hypoplasia (Continued)
    cervical, 3:368-369
    corpus callosum, 1:269, 1:269f
    enamel, 2:5
    iris, 1:415
    optic nerve, 1:420-421, 1:421f
    ovaries, 3:366
    pancreas, 2:355
    penile and preputial, 3:505
    pulmonary, 2:484, 2:484.e3f
    renal, 2:392
    segmental, 1:277-279, 1:277f
    splenic, 3:163
    testicular, 3:478-479, 3:478f
    thymic, 3:144
    thyroid, 3:314, 3:314f
    tracheal, 2:482, 2:482f
Hypoproteinemia, 2:73, 2:248
Hypopyon, 1:356f, 1:449
Hyposomatotropism, 1:589
Hypospadias, 3:470, 3:470f
Hypotension, 2:398
Hypothalamic neurons, 3:277
Hypothalamus, 2:377
    control of adenohypophysis, 3:277, 3:278f
Hypothyroidism, 1:31-32, 1:224, 1:587-588, 3:273, 3:315-319, 3:315f, 3:318f, 1:587.e2f
    acquired myasthenia gravis and, 1:229
Hypotrichosis, congenital, 1:538-539
    associated with pigmentary alterations, 1:539-541
    cats, 1:539
    cattle, 1:538-539
    dogs, 1:539, 1:539.e1f
Hypotrophy, muscle, 1:187, 1:188f
Hypovitaminosis A, 1:470-471, 1:581-583
Hypoxia, 2:37, 2:275
Hypsodont teeth, 2:5

I

Iatrogenic acromegaly, 3:286f
Ibaraki disease, 2:138-139
Ibex MCF virus, 2:132
Ibizan hounds, multisystem axonal degeneration in, 1:325
I-cell disease, 1:58
Ichthyosis, 1:530-532, 1:530f, 1:554, 1:531.e1f
    harlequin, 1:530, 1:531f
    nonepidermolytic, 1:531-532
    vulgaris, 1:530
IC-mediated glomerulonephritis (ICGN), 2:401-404
Idiopathic follicular atrophy, 3:315-316, 3:315f-317f
Idiopathic generalized or systemic granulomatous disease, 1:700-701
Idiopathic granulomatous marginal blepharitis, 1:423
Idiopathic immune-mediated uveitis, 1:453-455, 1:454f
Idiopathic inflammatory bowel disease, 2:91-96
Idiopathic lymphocytic uveitis in dogs, 1:456
Idiopathic lymphonodular uveitis in cats, 1:456
Idiopathic lymphoplasmacytic rhinitis, 2:476
Idiopathic mucosal colitis, 2:92-93
    cats, 2:98-99
Idiopathic multifocal osteopathy
    cattle, 1:54
    dogs, 1:54

Idiopathic polyarthritis, 1:158
Idiopathic pulmonary fibrosis in cats, 2:515, 2:515f, 2:515.e2f
Idiopathic spongy myelinopathies, 1:342-344
Idiopathic squamous papillomas, 1:705
Idiopathic thyroid atrophy, 1:587
Idiosyncratic hepatotoxins, 2:327
IgA-producing lymphocytes, 2:64
IgE autoantibodies, 2:15
IGF-1, 1:25t
IgG autoantibodies, 2:15
IgG-producing plasma cells, 2:64
Iliac thromboembolism, 3:46
Imaging, diagnostic, 1:11-12
Immune-mediated disorders, 1:225-230, 1:226f
  acquired myasthenia gravis, 1:229-230
  conjunctivitis, 1:426-427
  dermatoses, 1:590-615
  glomerulonephritis, 2:410b
  horses, 1:229
  immune-mediated thrombocytopenia (IMT), 3:129
  masticatory myositis of dogs, 1:226-227, 1:226f
  other myositides of dogs, 1:228
  polyarthritis, 1:157-159
  polymyositis
    cats, 1:228-229
    dogs, 1:227-228, 1:228f
  pulmonary immune responses and, 2:472
  rabies vaccine-induced vasculitis and alopecia, 1:612-613
  thrombocytopenia (ITP), 3:258
Immune privilege, 1:454
Immune system
  male genital system, 3:468
    testes and, 3:467-468
  skin and, 1:515
  upper respiratory tract, 2:474
Immunocompromise, 2:44
Immunodeficiency syndromes, lymphoid systems, 3:139-141
Immunofluorescence (IF), 2:384
  evaluation, 2:383
Immunoglobulin A (IgA), 2:13-14
Immunoglobulin deficiencies, 3:139
Immunoglobulin-derived amyloidosis, 2:414
Immunoglobulin G (IgG), 2:401
Immunohemolytic anemia, 3:114, 3:115f
Immunohistochemical reactivity, 2:110
Immunohistochemistry, 1:9, 1:10f, 2:445
Immunoinflammatory, 2:65
Immunologically mediated tubulointerstitial disease, 2:431
Immunology, 1:11
Immunoperoxidase techniques, 2:384
Immunophenotyping, 3:214-215
Immunoreactive peptides, 3:285, 3:285f
Immunosuppressive therapy, complications of, 2:387
Immunosuppressive agents and osteoporosis, 1:67
Impaction, gastric, 2:50-51
Impairment of steroidogenesis, 3:340
Imperforate hymen, 3:368-369, 3:370f
Imperforate pectinate ligament, 1:462-463
Impetigo, 1:630, 1:630f
Imported fire ants, 1:568
Impulse formation disturbances, 3:5

Inappetence, 2:69
Incidental lesions, gross examination of, 1:7
Incisor anodontia, 1:538
Inclusion bodies
  neuronal diseases, 1:320
  in neurons, neuroglia, and microglia, 1:367
  rhinitis, 2:529-530, 2:530f
Inclusion cysts
  ovarian, 3:372, 3:372f
  serosal, 3:386-387, 3:387f
Incomplete atrophy of anterior chamber mesenchyme, 1:415, 1:415f
Incomplete atrophy of posterior segment mesenchyme, 1:417-419, 1:418f
Incomplete cortical fractures, 1:36
Increased intestinal motility, 2:72
Indirect inguinal hernia, 2:80
Indirect salt poisoning, 1:315
Indolent cutaneous T-cell lymphoma, 1:734
Indolent ulcer, 1:694, 1:694f
Indospicine, 2:340-341, 2:341.e1f
Indubrasil cattle, *Rhabditis bovis* in, 1:507
Induced storage diseases, 1:292-293
Infantile cortical hyperostosis, 1:53
Infarction
  adrenal cortex, 3:340, 3:340f
  cerebral, 1:299-300, 1:299f-300f
  gallbladder, 2:307, 2:307f
  laryngeal, 2:481
  lymph node, 3:199
  pulmonary, 2:490.e1f
  retinal, 1:473
  splenic, 3:170f-171f, 3:170.e1f
Infection(s)
  abortion due to, 3:399-402, 3:399b
  acquired platelet disorders and, 3:260
  arthritis, 1:148-155
    fibrinous, 1:147
  bacterial. *See* Bacterial infections
  BVDV secondary, 2:127
  canine hepatitis, 2:310-312, 2:310f
  fungal. *See* Fungal infections
  gastritis due to, 2:52, 2:55
  granulomatous rhinitis and, 2:476
  liver
    bacterial, 2:314-318
    helminthic, 2:318-324
    viral, 2:309-325, 2:309f-310f
  lymphoid tissues, 3:171-182
  microsporidian, 1:385-386
  mycoplasmal. *See* Mycoplasmal infections
  myositis due to, 1:230-234
    clostridial, 1:230-233, 1:231f
    granulomatous lesions, 1:233-234
    malignant edema and gas gangrene, 1:232
    muscle changes secondary to systemic infections, 1:234, 1:234f
    specific diseases with muscle alterations, 1:233
    suppurative, 1:230, 1:230f
    Toxoplasma and *Neospora* myositis, 1:237
  nervous system changes with, 1:351t-352t
  parasitic. *See* Parasitic infections
  parvoviral, 1:628
  respiratory tract, 2:149
  retroviral, 1:627-628
  small intestinal bacterial overgrowth, 2:364
  viral. *See* Viral infections

Infectious bovine cervicovaginitis and epididymitis, 3:443
Infectious bovine keratoconjunctivitis, 1:440
Infectious bovine rhinotracheitis (IBR), 1:425, 2:140-142, 2:525f, 2:537-539, 2:538f
Infectious canine hepatitis, 2:310-312, 2:310f-311f, 2:311.e1f
Infectious keratoconjunctivitis of sheep and goats, 1:440-441
Infectious pustular vulvovaginitis of cattle, 3:443-445, 3:444f
Infertility, 2:438
Infiltrative variant of lipoma, 1:245, 1:246f, 1:726
Inflamed nonepitheliotropic T-cell lymphoma, 1:734
Inflammation/inflammatory response
  adenohypophysis, 3:289-290
  adrenal cortex, 3:340, 3:340f
  anemia of inflammatory disease, 3:127
  bronchiolar, 2:504-506, 2:504f
  central nervous system, 1:350-396, 1:351t-352t
    bacterial and pyogenic infections, 1:353-365
    helminth and arthropod infections, 1:389-391
    idiopathic inflammatory diseases, 1:392-396, 1:392f
    viral infections, 1:365-385
  corneal, 1:436-441
  diseases of bone, 1:97-107
    bacterial osteomyelitis, 1:98-103, 1:98f-99f
    canine panosteitis, 1:106-107
    fungal osteomyelitis, 1:103-104
    metaphyseal osteopathy, 1:105-106, 1:105f
    viral infections of bones, 1:104-105
  dysregulation of hemostasis and, 3:267-268
  endothelial cells and, 3:55
  epidermal
    fibrosis, 1:528
    interface dermatitis, 1:525
    intraepidermal vesicular and pustular dermatitis, 1:527, 1:528f
    nodular and diffuse dermatitis, 1:526-527, 1:527f
    panniculitis, 1:528-529, 1:529f
    perifolliculitis, folliculitis, and furunculosis, 1:528
    perivascular dermatitis, 1:525, 2:363f
    subepidermal vesicular and pustular dermatitis, 1:527-528, 1:528f
    vasculitis, 1:525-526, 1:526f
  epididymitis, 3:473-474, 3:474f, 3:487-491, 3:489f
  exocytosis, 1:519-520
  forestomachs, 2:42
  gross diagnosis, 1:5
  joints
    degenerative joint diseases, 1:141
    diseases, 1:146-159
  large intestine, 2:97-100
    colitis cystica profunda, 2:97
    colitis in cats, 2:98-99
      feline panleukopenia virus (FPLV), 2:98-99
      necrotic colitis, 2:99

Inflammation/inflammatory response (Continued)
  typhlocolitis in dogs, 2:97-98
  typhlocolitis in horses, 2:99-100
    ciliate protozoa, 2:99
    equine intestinal clostridial diseases, 2:99
    Potomac horse fever, 2:99
    subacute/chronic diarrhea in horses, 2:99
  typhlocolitis in ruminants, 2:100
  typhlocolitis in swine, 2:100
    dysentery, 2:100
    postweaning colibacillosis, 2:100
  lesions of joint structures, 1:155-159
  liver and biliary tract, 2:300-309, 2:326
  lupus erythematosus (LE), 1:604-607
  lymph nodes, 3:202-212
  male genital system
    penis and prepuce, 3:506-508
    prostate and bulbourethral gland, 3:501-502, 3:502f
    spermatic cord, 3:498-499
    testis and epididymis, 3:485-491
    vesicular glands, 3:499-500, 3:499f
  mammae, 3:451-452
  mucosa, 2:47
  muscle necrosis and, 1:182, 1:182f
  myocarditis, 3:41-44, 3:42f, 3:42t
  nervous system and, 1:351t-352t
  oral cavity, 2:13-19
    salivary glands, 2:29
  spleen, 3:182-189, 3:182.e1f
  teeth, 2:9-12
  thymus, 3:148-150
  uterine (fallopian) tubes, 3:380
  uterus, 3:387-393
  vaginal and vulval, 3:443
  vasculitis, 3:67-88, 3:68b
Inflammatory airway diseases, 2:506
Inflammatory aural polyps, 1:498-499, 1:498.e2f
Inflammatory bowel disease (IBD), 1:66-67, 2:91, 2:93f
  idiopathic, 2:91-96
Inflammatory ceruminous otitis externa, 1:548
Influenza
  cats, 2:587-588
  dogs, 2:577
  horses, 2:567-568, 2:567.e3f
  pigs, 2:526-527, 2:526f, 2:526.e1f, 2:527.e1f
Infractions, 1:34, 1:34f
Infundibular cysts, 1:704
Infundibular keratinizing acanthoma, 1:714, 1:715f
Infundibular necrosis, 2:10, 2:10f
  horses, 2:10, 2:10f
Infundibular stalk, 3:277
Infundibulum, 1:516
Ingesta, 2:247
Inguinal hernias, 2:80, 3:498
Inhalation
  oxygen, 2:518
  smoke
    lung injury, 2:518
    trachea and, 2:483, 2:483f
  toxic gases, 2:518
Inherited dyshormonogenic goiter, 3:322-323
Inherited erythrocyte enzyme deficiencies, 3:126
Inherited myopathy of Great Dane dogs, 1:197-198
Inherited photoreceptor dysplasias, 1:469
Inherited storage diseases, 1:286-292, 1:287f
Inherited thrombocytopenia, 3:258
Injections
  interstitial lung disease reactions to, 2:512
  site reactions, 1:560
Injury. See Trauma; specific injuries
Inorganic (mineral) component of bone matrix, 1:20
Insects
  caterpillar larvae, 1:671
  fire ants, 1:671
  fleas, 1:672-673
  flies, 1:666-671
  horn fly, 1:670
  hypersensitivity, 1:597-599, 1:670-671
  lice, 1:671-672
  mites, 1:673-684
  mosquito, 1:599, 1:670-671, 1:671f
Insulin, 2:368
Insulinomas, 2:374
Intact nephron hypothesis, 2:377-378
Integumentary system. See Skin
Intercellular adhesion molecules (ICAMs), 3:198
Interface dermatitis, 1:525, 1:526f
Interferons, 2:548-549
Interfollicular smooth muscles, 1:515
Interglobular dentin, 2:5
Interleukins, 2:263, 2:548-549
Internal ear, 1:488-495
  hearing, 1:491
    impairment, 1:491-494
  Horner and Pourfour du Petit syndromes, 1:494-495
  neoplasia, 1:494
  peripheral vestibular disease, 1:494
Internal hernias, 2:79
Internal hordeolum, 1:423
Interphalangeal joints, 1:142
Interstitial cells
  of Cajal, 2:62
  tumors of testes, 3:493, 3:493f
Interstitial edema, 1:294
Interstitial emphysema, 2:486
Interstitial fibrosis, 2:510
  cats, 2:515, 2:515f
  dogs, 2:514-515, 2:515f
Interstitial lesions, miscellaneous, 2:441-442
  acute ascending pyelonephritis, 2:441.e1f
  bone, 2:442
  extramedullary hematopoiesis, 2:441
  renal telangiectasia, 2:442
Interstitial lung disease, 2:509, 2:510f, 2:511b
  dogs, 2:514-515, 2:515f
  eosinophilic, 2:513
  feedlot cattle, 2:513f, 2:513.e1
  foals, 2:514
  granulomatous, 2:513
  noninfectious, 2:512-520
Interstitial macrophages, 2:471
Interstitial myocarditis, 3:42
Interstitial nephritis, 2:431-432
  acute, 2:431
  chronic, 2:431
Interstitial orchitis, 3:486
Interstitial pneumonia, 2:509
Interstitium, 3:3
Intertrigo, 1:559

Intervertebral disk diseases, 1:128-129
  degenerative, 1:143, 1:144f
  Hansen type I intervertebral disk herniations, 1:144, 1:144f
  Hansen type II intervertebral disk herniations, 1:144f, 1:145
Intestinal adenocarcinomas, 2:102
Intestinal carcinomas, 2:104, 2:104f
  microscopic appearance, 2:103
Intestinal/colonic biopsies, interpretation of, 2:62
Intestinal diverticula, 2:74
Intestinal emphysema, 2:87f
Intestinal encephalopathy, 2:88
Intestinal eosinophils, 2:64
Intestinal fluke infection, 2:225-227
Intestinal histoplasmosis, 2:202-203, 2:203f
Intestinal ischemia
  arterial thromboembolism, 2:84
  colon, 2:81
  infarction, 2:81-86
  reduced perfusion, 2:84-86
    acute acorn poisoning in horse, 2:85
    nonsteroidal anti-inflammatory drugs (NSAIDs), 2:85
    shock gut, 2:85
    transient/noninfarctive slow flow, 2:85
  reperfusion injury, 2:81
  sequelae of, 2:81-82
  small intestine, 2:81
  venous infarction, 2:82-84
    cecal inversion, 2:84
    cecocolic intussusception in horse, 2:84
    displacements of, 2:83
    duodenal sigmoid flexure volvulus, 2:83
    intussusception, 2:83
    mesenteric volvulus, 2:83
    segmental ischemic necrosis of small colon, 2:84
    volvulus, large colon, 2:83
Intestinal lipofuscinosis, 2:86-87, 2:86f
Intestinal lymphangiectasis, 3:95
Intestinal lymphomas, 3:239-241, 3:240f, 3:240.e1f
Intestinal mucosa
  mast cells, 2:64
  microscopic lesion, 2:125-126
Intestinal mucus, 2:60
Intestinal obstruction, 2:74-78
  extrinsic obstruction, 2:76-77
    neoplasms, 2:76-77
  functional obstruction, 2:77-78
    adynamic (paralytic) ileus, 2:77
    feline dysautonomia, 2:77
    grass sickness in horses, 2:77
    intestinal smooth muscle, intrinsic disease of, 2:77-78
    megacolon in Clydesdale foals, 2:77
    pseudo-obstruction, 2:77
  proximal to obstruction, 2:75
  stenosis/obturation, 2:75-76
    cecal rupture, 2:76
    cecum/colon in horses, 2:76
    enteroliths, 2:75
    fiber balls, 2:75-76
    foreign bodies, 2:75
    impaction of colon, 2:76
    small intestinal obstruction, 2:76
Intestinal parasite hypersensitivity, 1:599-600
Intestinal phycomycosis, 2:201
Intestinal sclerosis, 2:77-78

INDEX

Intestinal smooth muscle, intrinsic disease of, 2:77-78
Intestinal spirochetosis, 2:100
Intestinal stromal tumors, 2:110-111
  gastrointestinal, 2:110
  leiomyoma, 2:110
  leiomyosarcoma, 2:110
Intestinal T-cell lymphomas, 2:107-108
Intestinal tract, miscellaneous conditions, 2:86-89
  chinaberry tree, 2:89
  idiopathic muscular hypertrophy, 2:87
  intestinal emphysema, 2:87
  intestinal encephalopathy, 2:88
  intestinal lipofuscinosis, 2:86-87
  jejunal hematoma, 2:88
  muscular hypertrophy of, 2:87
  oleander toxicosis, 2:89
  rectal prolapse, 2:88
  small intestinal bacterial overgrowth (SIBO), 2:86
  small intestine, pseudodiverticulosis of, 2:87
Intestinal trichostrongylosis, 2:212-213
Intestine
  large, 2:97-100
    colitis cystica profunda, 2:97
    colitis in cats, 2:98-99
      feline panleukopenia virus (FPLV), 2:98-99
      necrotic colitis, 2:99
    typhlocolitis in dogs, 2:97-98
    typhlocolitis in horses, 2:99-100
      ciliate protozoa, 2:99
      equine intestinal clostridial diseases, 2:99
      Potomac horse fever, 2:99
      subacute/chronic diarrhea in horses, 2:99
    typhlocolitis in ruminants, 2:100
    typhlocolitis in swine, 2:100
      dysentery, 2:100
      postweaning colibacillosis, 2:100
  small, 2:81, 2:82f, 2:92
    amyloid deposition, 2:91
    cardinal finding, 2:92
    eosinophilic enteritis, 2:96
      chronic, 2:96
    gastric changes, 2:94
    granulomatous enteritis, 2:97
      transmural granulomatous enteritis, 2:97
    idiopathic inflammatory bowel disease, 2:91-96
    idiopathic mucosal colitis, 2:92-93
    lymphangiectasia, 2:90-91, 2:90f
    lymphocytic-plasmacytic, 2:94
    mucosa, 2:124
      hypoplasia, 2:74
      vascular supply, 2:61
    obstruction, 2:76
      dogs, 2:75f
    pseudodiverticulosis of, 2:87
    small intestinal bacterial overgrowth (SIBO), 2:86, 2:364
Intestines
  B/T lymphoblasts, 2:64
  cecum and colon, 2:61
  congenital anomalies of, 2:73-74
    atresia ani, 2:74
    atresia coli, 2:74

Intestines (Continued)
  congenital colonic aganglionosis, 2:74
  intestinal diverticula, 2:74
  persistent Meckel's diverticulum, 2:74
  segmental anomalies, 2:73
  short colon, 2:74
  small intestinal mucosa, hypoplasia of, 2:74
displacements, 2:78-81, 2:83
  cecal/colonic dilation, 2:78
  colonic volvulus, 2:79
  eventration, 2:78
  external hernia, 2:79-81
    abdominal wall, ventral hernia of, 2:80
    diaphragmatic hernias, 2:80
    direct inguinal hernia, 2:80
    femoral hernias, 2:80
    indirect inguinal hernias, 2:80
    inguinal hernia, 2:80
    perineal hernias, 2:80
    prepubic hernias, 2:80
    sequelae of hernias, 2:80
    umbilical hernia, 2:80
  internal hernia, 2:79
  torsion, 2:78
  tympany, 2:78
electrolyte and water transport, 2:65-66
enteroendocrine cells, 2:60
gastrointestinal mucosal barrier, 2:62-65
gastrointestinal mucosal defense, elements of, 2:63
globule leukocytes, 2:63
IgA-producing lymphocytes, 2:64
IgG-producing plasma cells, 2:64
immune elements, 2:62-65
immunoinflammatory events, 2:66
interpretation and colonic biopsies, 2:62
intestinal intraepithelial T lymphocytes, 2:63
intestinal mucosal mast cells, 2:64
intussusception, 2:83f
lamina propria, 2:61-62
muscular hypertrophy, 2:87
normal form/function, 2:60-62
oligomucous cells, 2:60
Paneth cells, 2:60
segmental anomalies of, 2:73
stem cells, 2:60
submucosa, 2:62
Intima, vascular system, 3:54
Intimal bodies, 3:61, 3:61f
Intimal sclerosis of testicular veins, 3:498
Intoxication
  hepatic steatosis by, 2:276
  steroidal sapogenins, 2:338-340
  vitamin D, 3:301-302, 3:301f
Intracelluar edema, 1:522
Intracranial pressure, 1:293-295
Intracranial thrombophlebitis, 1:300
Intracytoplasmic inclusion bodies, 2:448f
Intradural abscess, 1:354f
Intraepidermal vesicular and pustular dermatitis, 1:527, 1:528f
Intrafollicular hemorrhage of ovaries, 3:370
Intranuclear inclusions, 2:270
Intraosseous epidermoid cysts, 1:126-127
Intrapancreatic hepatocytes, 2:356
Intratubular orchitis, 3:486, 3:486f
Intratubular red blood cell cast, 2:409.e1f
Intravascular hemolysis, 3:114, 3:115f

Intravascular lymphoma, 1:734, 3:99
Intrinsic cardiac responses, 3:6-9, 3:7f
Intrinsic disorders of platelet function, 3:259-260
Intrinsic hepatotoxins, 2:327
Intrinsic lesion, 2:74
Intrinsic obstruction, 2:32
Intrinsic pathway, 3:261
Intussusception, 2:82-83
Invasive tumors of bones, 1:125
Involucrum, 1:96, 1:96f, 1:98
Involution
  B-dependent tonsillar lymphoid follicles, 2:20
  thymic, 3:144-147, 3:146f
Iodine, 1:570
  deficiency and goiter, 3:320-322, 3:320f
  excess, 3:325
  ion and thyroid function, 3:273, 3:311
  uptake blockage, 3:325
Iodism, 1:570
Iodothyronine, 3:271
Ionophore toxicosis, 1:219
Iridociliary epithelial tumor, 1:485, 1:485f
Iridovirus, 2:430
Iriki virus, 1:280
Iris
  atrophy of, 1:447
  hypopigmentation, 1:415
  hypoplasia, 1:413-415, 1:415f
  melanomas, feline diffuse, 1:483-484, 1:484f
  normal, 1:445, 1:445f
Irish Dexter cattle, cropped or notched pinnae in, 1:502
Irish Setter dogs
  canine atopic dermatitis, 1:591
  color dilution alopecia, 1:539-540
  congenital idiopathic megaesophagus, 2:33-34
  gastric volvulus, 2:49
  globoid cell leukodystrophy, 1:339
  hypothyroidism, 1:587
  seborrhea, 1:548
  selective deficiencies of immunoglobulins, 3:139
  vascular ring anomalies, 2:33
Irish Terrier dogs
  canine X-linked muscular dystrophy, 1:192
  ichthyosis, 1:532
Irish Wolfhound dogs
  dilated cardiomyopathy, 3:48
  hypothyroidism, 1:587
  iris cysts, 1:446
Iron
  deficiency anemia, 3:112-114, 3:114f, 3:127
  in hemoglobin synthesis, 3:107
  hepatotoxicity, 2:272, 2:333
Irradiation, cataract due to, 1:443-444
Ischemic damage, 1:211, 1:211f
  brain, 1:297-300, 1:297f
  heart failure and, 3:9
Ischemic tubular necrosis, 2:423f
Ischemic ulcers, 2:82
Islands of Calleja, 1:262
Islet amyloid polypeptide (IAPP)-derived amyloidosis, 2:414
Islet cells, 2:355, 2:370f
  hyperplasia and nesidioblastosis, 2:373

Isthmus, hair follicle, 1:516
Isthmus cysts, 1:704
Italian Greyhound dogs, color dilution alopecia in, 1:539-540
Italian Spinones dogs, motor neuropathy in, 1:335
Ixodidae, 1:506, 1:684

J

Jaagsiekte, 2:560-562
Jack Russell Terrier dogs
  canine congenital myasthenia in, 1:209
  ichthyosis, 1:531
  multisystem axonal degeneration, 1:325
  sensory and autonomic neuropathy, 1:334
  severe combined immunodeficiency (SCID), 3:139-141
  severe factor X deficiency, 3:264
Japanese cattle
  Chediak-Higashi syndrome, 3:259
  congenital hypotrichosis, 1:538-539
  forelimb-girdle muscular anomaly, 1:189
  neuronal inclusion-body diseases, 1:320
  prolonged APTT, 3:263
  vitiligo, 1:556
Japanese encephalitis virus (JEV), 1:376
Japanese quail, metabolic myopathy in, 1:208-209
Jaundice, 2:292-294, 2:292f
Jejunal hematoma, 2:88, 2:88f
Jembrana disease virus (JDV), 2:136, 3:195-196, 3:195f-196f, 3:195.e1f
Jersey cattle
  bovine hypomyelinogenesis, 1:338-339
  brachygnathia superior, 2:3
  cyclopia, 1:269-270
  degenerative joint disease, 1:143
Jimsonweed, 1:90
Johne's disease, 2:100, 2:115, 2:194-197, 2:195f-197f, 3:205f, 3:204.e1f
Joint(s). *See also* Bone(s)
  cartilaginous, 1:128-129, 1:143-145
  degenerative diseases of, 1:137-146
  developmental diseases of, 1:132-137
  diseases, 1:128-163
  fibrous, 1:128
  inflammatory diseases of, 1:146-159
  synovial, 1:129-131, 1:137-143
    fibrinous arthritis, 1:146-147
  tumors and tumor-like lesions of, 1:159-163
    benign, 1:160-162
    malignant, 1:159-160
Jones' methenamine silver (JMS) stain, 2:383
Jowl abscess, 3:208-209, 3:208f-209f
Jugulotympanic paragangliomas, 1:500
Junctional epidermolysis bullosa, 1:534
Juvenile nephropathy, 2:388-391
Juvenile-onset distal myopathy, 1:198
Juvenile-onset polyarthritis, 1:158
Juvenile panhypopituitarism, 3:280, 3:280f
Juvenile polycystic disease, 2:265
Juxtaglomerular apparatus (JGA), 2:379
Juxtamedullary nephrons, 2:377, 2:378f, 2:381

K

Kallikrein, 3:261
Kanamycin, 2:424
"Kangaroo gait" of lactating ewes, 1:336
K antigen, 2:459
Karakul sheep, wattles in, 1:532

Karelian Bear dogs
  chondrodysplasia, 1:43-44
  hyposomatotropism, 1:589
Karwinskia humboldtiana, 3:36
Keeshond dogs
  alopecia X, 1:589-590
  early onset diabetes mellitus, 2:373
Keratic precipitates, 1:449
Keratinizing basal cell carcinomas, 1:714
Keratinocytes, 1:515
Keratin pearls, 1:520
Keratitis, 1:436-441
  feline eosinophilic, 1:438-439, 1:439f
  herpetic, of cats, 1:438
  infectious bovine keratoconjunctivitis, 1:440
  infectious keratoconjunctivitis of sheep and goats, 1:440-441
  mycotic, 1:439-440, 1:439f
  pannus, 1:438
Keratoconjunctivitis sicca, 1:436
Keratomalacia, 1:436-437, 1:437f
Keratomas, 1:704
Keratoses, 1:550-551
  cutaneous horns, 1:551
  equine cannon, 1:550
  equine linear alopecia, 1:550, 1:550f
  follicular, 1:520
  lichenoid, 1:551
  lichenoid reaction patterns, 1:551
  linear epidermal nevi, 1:551
  seborrheic, 1:550-551, 1:551.e1f
  solar, 1:577
Kerry Blue Terrier dogs
  diffuse uveal melanocytosis, 1:484-485
  hereditary striatonigral and cerebello-olivary degeneration, 1:319
  prolonged APTT, 3:263
  spiculosis, 1:699
Ketoconazole, 2:329
Ketosis, acute, 2:275
Kidney(s)
  Actinobacillus equuli embolic nephritis, 2:433f, 2:433.e1f
  acute tubular injury, 2:433f
  anatomy of, 2:378-381
  anomalies of development, 2:391-397
  β-mannosidosis in a newborn term Salers calf, 2:429.e1f
  Cloisonné kidney, 2:429
  cortex. *See* Renal cortex
  cortical and juxtamedullary nephrons, diagram, 2:378f
  defined, 2:377
  diffuse diseases, 2:382
  Dioctophyma renale, 2:443.e1f
  disease. *See* Renal disease
  duplication of, 2:392
  embolic nephritis, 2:432-433
  endogenous factors, 2:387
  endogenous oxalates, 2:426
  failure. *See* Renal failure
  giant kidney worm, 2:442
  glomerulus, 2:379-381
  gross appearance, 2:399
  gross examination, 2:381-382
  heart failure and, 3:10
  hematoxylin and eosin (H&E), 2:383-384
  histologic appearance, 2:399
  histologic examination, 2:382-383
  horses, 2:433

Kidney(s) (*Continued*)
  horseshoe, 2:393f
  hypoplastic, 2:392
  IgA deposition, 2:412
  interstitium, 2:381
  leptospiral serovars, 2:434t
    maintenance and incidental, 2:435t
  leptospirosis, 2:433-439
  lipofuscinosis, 2:429
  lymphoma, 3:240f-241f
  malformation, 2:391
  malposition, 2:392
  miscellaneous tubular conditions, 2:430-431
    glycogen accumulation, 2:430
    hepatorenal syndrome, 2:430
    hypokalemic nephropathy, 2:430
    miscellaneous histologic changes, 2:430-431
    nephrogenic diabetes insipidus, 2:430
  multifocal renal cortical hemorrhages, 2:432f
  parasitic lesions, 2:442-443
    Dioctophyma renale, 2:442-443
    Halicephalobus gingivalis, 2:443
    Klossiella equi, 2:443
    Pearsonema plica, 2:443
    Stephanurus dentatus, 2:442
    Toxocara canis, 2:442
  perivascular pyogranulomatous nephritis, 2:432f
  pigmentary changes, 2:429-430
    brown pigmentation, 2:429
    cloisonné kidney, 2:429
    dark brown to black, 2:429f
    green-yellow discoloration, 2:429-430
  primary mesenchymal tumors, 2:447
  pulpy, 2:381-382
  renal biopsy, 2:383-384
  renal blood flow, 2:377
  sagittal section, 2:437.e1f
  suppurative interstitial nephritis, 2:432
  swelling of, 2:409
  toxic and hypoxic insults, 2:399
  tubules, 2:381
  tubulointerstitial nephritis, chronic, 2:433.e1f
  urate calculi in renal medulla, 2:385f
  vascular supply, 2:379
  vitamin D, metabolism of, 2:377
  white-spotted kidney, 2:431f, 2:431.e1f
Kiel classification, 3:215, 3:217
Kinesin, 1:251-252
KIRREL2 gene, 2:418
Klebsiella pneumoniae, 2:113-114, 3:388, 3:417
Klossiella equi, 2:443f
Kupffer cells, 2:260, 2:263, 2:263f, 2:271
  in acute hepatitis, 2:301
Kürsteiner's cysts, 3:297, 3:297f
Kuvasz dogs, spongy encephalomyelopathies in, 1:346-347
Kwashiorkor, 2:362
Kyphosis, 1:37t

L

Laboratory accreditation, 1:14
Labrador Retriever dogs
  Alexander disease, 1:341
  axonopathy, 1:325
  canine atopic dermatitis, 1:591
  canine X-linked muscular dystrophy, 1:192
  cavitating leukodystrophy, 1:339-340

Labrador Retriever dogs *(Continued)*
  centronuclear myopathy, *1*:197, *1*:197f
  chondrodysplasia, *1*:45
  chronic hepatitis, *2*:304
  dysplasia of right atrioventricular valve, *3*:21-22
  exercise-induced collapse, *1*:198
  hip dysplasia, *1*:135
  Hunter syndrome, *1*:58
  hypothyroidism, *3*:315
  ichthyosis, *1*:532
  laryngeal paralysis, *2*:481
  lymphomas, *3*:238
  malignant hyperthermia, *1*:210
  myxomatous valvular degeneration, *3*:27
  nasal parakeratosis, *1*:550
  pyotraumatic dermatitis, *1*:560
  seborrhea, *1*:548
  spongy myelinopathy, *1*:343
  true retinal dysplasia, *1*:420
  vitiligo, *1*:555-556
  X-linked myotubular myopathy, *1*:197
Labyrinthitis, *1*:493, *1*:493.e2f
Laceration, *1*:302
Lacrimal system, *1*:423-424
La Crosse virus, *1*:280, *1*:383
Lactate dehydrogenase (LDH)
  diaphragmatic dystrophy in cattle, *1*:199
  nemaline myopathy of cats, *1*:198
Lactation, "kangaroo gait" and, *1*:336
Lactational osteoporosis, *1*:65-66
  cattle, *1*:66, *1*:66f
Lactotroph adenomas, *3*:286-287
Lafora bodies, *1*:255, *1*:255f
Lafora disease (LD), *1*:292
Lagenidiosis, *1*:657-659
Lamellar bodies, *1*:512-513
Lamellar bone, *1*:20-21
Lamina cribosa, *1*:476
Lamina densa, *1*:513-514
Lamina fibrous zone, *1*:513-514
Lamina lucida, *1*:513-514
Lamina propria, *2*:51, *2*:61
Laminitis, *1*:702-703
Landrace pigs, *1*:42
Landseer-European Continental Type (ECT) dogs, platelet dysfunction in, *3*:259
Langerhans cells
  canine cutaneous histiocytosis, *1*:729, *3*:245-246, *3*:246f
  feline pulmonary Langerhans cell histiocytosis, *3*:246-247, *3*:247f, *3*:246.e1f
  histiocytosis, *3*:243
  immune function, *1*:515
  skin, *1*:513
Lantana camara, *3*:36
  toxicity, *2*:293, *2*:338
Lapland dogs, glycogen storage disease type II in, *1*:204
Large-bowel diarrhea, *2*:70-71
Large cell carcinoma, *2*:497
Large-cell/lymphoblastic lymphoma, *2*:108
Large dark fibers in muscular dystrophy, *1*:193
Large granular lymphocytic leukemia, *3*:235
Large granular lymphocytic lymphoma (LGL), *3*:231, *3*:231f
Large granular lymphoma, *2*:108

Large intestine, inflammation of, *2*:97-100
  colitis cystica profunda, *2*:97
  colitis in cats, *2*:98-99
    feline panleukopenia virus (FPLV), *2*:98-99
    necrotic colitis, *2*:99
  typhlocolitis in dogs, *2*:97-98
  typhlocolitis in horses, *2*:99-100
    ciliate protozoa, *2*:99
    equine intestinal clostridial diseases, *2*:99
    Potomac horse fever, *2*:99
    subacute/chronic diarrhea in horses, *2*:99
  typhlocolitis in ruminants, *2*:100
  typhlocolitis in swine, *2*:100
    dysentery, *2*:100
    postweaning colibacillosis, *2*:100
Large White X Essex pigs, *1*:545
Larval paramphistomes, *2*:43
Larval strongyles, *2*:319, *2*:319f
Larynx, *2*:467, *2*:481-482, *2*:481f
  equine laryngeal hemiplegia, *1*:334-335
  laryngitis, *2*:481
  paralysis, *2*:481, *2*:481f
  rhabdomyomas, *1*:177f, *1*:241, *1*:242f
L-asparaginase, *3*:298
Late-onset progressive spinocerebellar degeneration, *1*:319
Lateral domain, liver, *2*:262
Lathyrus odoratus, *1*:91
Lawsonia intracelluaris, *2*:177-180, *2*:178f, *3*:202, *3*:202f
Lead poisoning, *1*:86, *1*:87f, *1*:316-317
Lectin staining, *2*:445
Left atrioventricular valvular insufficiency or stenosis, *3*:22
Left atrium, heart, *3*:2
  failure, *3*:6
Left-sided heart failure, *3*:10-11
Left ventricle, heart, *3*:2
Legg-Calvé-Perthes disease, *1*:31, *1*:96, *1*:96f
  dogs, *1*:97, *1*:97f
Leiomyomas, *1*:726, *2*:110, *2*:463-464, *3*:378, *3*:447-448, *3*:447f-448f
  gastrointestinal, *2*:110
  liver, *2*:350
Leiomyometaplasts, *2*:87
Leiomyosarcomas, *1*:726, *2*:110, *2*:110f
  female genital system, *3*:447-448, *3*:448f
  gastrointestinal, *2*:110, *2*:110f
  liver, *2*:350
  urinary system, *2*:463-464
Leishmania infantum, *1*:240, *2*:19
Leishmania spp., *1*:98, *1*:240, *1*:503, *1*:663-664, *2*:412
  feline, *1*:663-664, *1*:664f
  penis and prepuce lesions, *3*:508
  spleen, *3*:174-175, *3*:175f-176f, *3*:175.e1f
Lens, *1*:441-444
  anomalies, *1*:422-423
  aphakia, *1*:422
  cataract, *1*:442-444, *1*:442f
  congenital cataract, *1*:422
  congenitally ectopic, *1*:422
  ectopia lentis, *1*:441-442
  -induced uveitis, *1*:453-454, *1*:457-459
  lenticonus and lentiglobus, *1*:422
  microphakia, *1*:422
Lenticonus, *1*:422
Lentiglobus, *1*:422
Lentigo simplex, *1*:554, *1*:721

Lentiviral encephalomyelitis of sheep and goats, *1*:378-380
Lentiviruses, *2*:558-560, *2*:559f, *2*:558.e1f
Leonberger dogs
  leukoencephalomyelopathy, *1*:340-341
  motor neuropathy, *1*:335
Leporipoxvirus, *1*:616
Lepromatous leprosy, *1*:641
Leprosy, feline, *1*:640-641
Leptomeningitis, *1*:354-358, *1*:355f-357f
Leptospira borgpetersenii, *2*:435-436
Leptospira fainei, *2*:438
Leptospira interrogans, *2*:431, *2*:433-434
Leptospiral serovars, *2*:434t
Leptospira spp., *2*:435t
  abortion and stillbirth in horses and, *3*:411
  abortion in cattle and, *3*:409-410
  abortion in sheep and, *3*:411
  abortion in swine and, *3*:410-411
  hemolytic anemia and, *3*:126
  liver and, *2*:317-318, *2*:317.e1f
Leptospires, *2*:435, *2*:437-438
Leptospirosis, *2*:433-439
  abortion, *2*:435
  cattle, *2*:435-437
  dogs, *2*:437-438
  in domestic animals, *2*:434t
  horses, *2*:438-439
  maintenance and incidental hosts, *2*:435t
  renal failure, *2*:435
  sheep, goats, and deer, *2*:437
  swine, *2*:438
Lesions. *See also* Non-neoplastic lesions
  adrenal, *3*:341-343
  brain
    ischemic, *1*:297-300, *1*:297f
  bronchopneumonia, *2*:506f
  canine distemper virus, *2*:576
  degenerative joint diseases, *1*:138, *1*:138f
  dental, *2*:576
  diffuse alveolar damage, *2*:509
  endocardial, *3*:27-30
  endocrine gland, *3*:271-272
  esophageal, *2*:124, *2*:124f
  exocrine pancreas, *2*:365-368
  glaucoma-causing, *1*:462-465
  granulomatous, *1*:233-234
  hypothyroidism, *3*:318-319
  incidental, *1*:7
  laryngeal, *2*:481-482, *2*:481.e2f
  liver and bile ducts, *2*:344-352
  microcirculatory, *1*:301
  middle ear, *1*:498-499
  muscle, *1*:171
  oral cavity, *2*:20-28
  osteomalacia, *1*:73
  osteoporosis, gross, *1*:63-64
  ovarian, *3*:370-371
  pericardium, *3*:24-25, *3*:24f
  photographs of, *1*:8
  photosensitization dermatitis, *1*:578
  postpartum uterus, *3*:440-441
  pulmonary idiopathic hypertension, *2*:492
  pyelonephritis, *2*:383
  retinitis, *1*:474-475
  rickets, microscopic, *1*:72, *1*:72f
  rinderpest, *2*:129, *2*:129f
  sepsis, *1*:358-362, *1*:358f, *2*:512f

Lesions (Continued)
  skin, in systemic bacterial disease, 1:645-646
  splenic, 3:188-189, 3:188f
  stomach and intestine, 2:100-111, 2:101t
Lethal acrodermatitis, 1:533, 1:533.e1f
Lethal trait A46, 3:141
Leukocyte disorders, 3:109-112
Leukoderma, 1:555
Leukodystrophic and myelinolytic diseases, 1:339-342, 1:339f
Leukoencephalitis, necrotizing, 1:392-393
Leukoencephalomalacia, mycotoxic, 1:315-316, 1:315f-316f
Leukoencephalomyelopathy, 1:340-341, 1:340f
Leukomalacia, 1:307-308
  periventricular, 1:274
Leukotrichia, 1:555
  reticulated, 1:557-558
Lewy bodies, 1:255
L-form infections, 1:637
Lhasa Apso dogs
  afibrinogenemia, 3:265
  keratoconjunctivitis sicca, 1:436
  sebaceous adenitis, 1:551
  sebaceous epitheliomas, 1:717
Lice, 1:671-672
Lichenification, 1:524
Lichenoid keratoses, 1:551
Lichenoid-psoriasiform dermatosis, 1:552-553
Lichenoid reaction patterns, 1:551
Lichtheimia corymbifera, 3:417
Lieberkühn, epithelial lining, 2:125-126
Ligaments, 1:130
Light-induced retinal degeneration, 1:470
Lightning strikes, 1:564f
Ligneous conjunctivitis, 1:426-427
Liliaceae family, 2:428
Limbal (epibulbar) melanocytoma, 1:482-483
Limb defects, 1:37t
  congenital flexures, 1:189
  dysplasias, 1:54-56, 1:54f
Limb dysplasias
  cats, 1:54-56
  dogs, 1:54-56
Limber tail, 1:214
Limbus, 1:424
Limiting plate, liver, 2:261-262
Limnatis africana, 2:557
Limnatis nilotica, 2:19, 2:557
Linear epidermal nevi, 1:551
Linear foreign bodies, 2:75, 2:76f
Linear immunoglobulin A disease, 1:604
Linguatula serrata, 2:19, 2:585
Lining cells, bone, 1:17
Lion jaw, 1:91-92
Lipidosis, 3:319, 3:319f
Lipid(s)
  dystrophies, corneal, 1:433
  epidermal, 1:512-513
  keratopathy, 1:433-434, 1:433f
  malabsorption of, 2:90
  pneumonia, 2:516-518, 2:516.e1f
  storage myopathy, 1:205
  vacuoles, 1:185, 1:185f
Lipofuscin, 2:262, 2:271, 3:200, 3:314
  ceroid-lipofuscinoses, 1:290-292, 1:291f
Lipofuscinosis, 2:86-87
Lipolysis, 2:70

Lipomas, 1:726
  infiltrative, 1:245, 1:246f, 1:726
  peritoneal, 2:256, 2:257f
Lipomatosis, 2:356
Lipomeningocele, 1:279
Lipopolysaccharide (LPS) moiety of *Salmonella*, 2:168-169
Lipoprotein lipase activity, 1:336
Liposarcomas, 1:123, 1:726
Liquefactive necrosis, 1:254
Lissencephaly, 1:268
Listeria monocytogenes, 1:363f, 1:449
  abortion and, 3:408-409, 3:409f
  central nervous system and, 1:362-364, 1:363f
  liver and, 2:314-318, 2:314f
  myocarditis and, 3:42
Liver, 2:258-352
  abscesses, 2:315-316, 2:315f
  acquired portosystemic shunting, 2:290
  cell death, 2:279-285
    apoptosis, 2:279-280, 2:279f
    lobular necrosis, 2:282-284
    necrosis, 2:280-281, 2:280f-281f, 2:283f, 2:285.e1f
    tissue patterns, 2:281-285
  cells, 2:261-264
  cholestasis and jaundice, 2:292-294, 2:292f
  cirrhosis, 2:276, 2:289-290, 2:276.e1f
  developmental disorders, 2:264-268
    congenital vascular anomalies, 2:266-268
    cysts, 2:264
    ductal plate malformations, 2:265, 2:265f
    extrahepatic biliary anomalies, 2:265-266
    hamartomas, 2:264, 2:264f
  disease, 3:264-265
    acute bovine, 2:343-344, 2:343.e1f
  displacement, torsion, and rupture, 2:268
  dysfunction, 2:290-295
    edema and ascites, 2:294-295
    enlargement and heart failure, 3:11
    failure, 2:290-295
    hemorrhage and, 2:294
  fatty, 2:275-276
  fibrosis, 2:288-289, 2:289f
  general considerations, 2:259-264
    cells, 2:261-264
    origin, structure, and function, 2:259-261, 2:259f
  hepatic encephalopathy (HE), 1:262, 1:262f, 1:344f, 2:291-292
  hepatitis, 2:301
    acute, 2:301
    B antigen, 3:71
    cats, 2:305
    chronic, 2:301-306, 2:305.e1f
    dogs, 2:302-305, 2:305f, 2:310-312, 2:310f, 2:311.e1f
    focal, 2:282, 2:282f
    giant cell, 2:306, 2:306f
    horses, 2:305
    lobular dissecting, 2:305, 2:305f, 2:305.e1f
    nonspecific reactive, 2:306
    periportal interface, 2:301-302, 2:302f, 2:304f
  hepatocellular adaptations and intracellular accumulation, 2:269-279, 2:269f, 2:269.e1f
    amyloidosis, 2:278-279, 2:279f, 2:278.e1f
    atrophy, 2:269, 2:269f, 2:269.e1f

Liver (Continued)
  hypertrophy, 2:269-270, 2:269f
  intranuclear inclusions, 2:270
  lysosomal storage diseases, 2:278, 2:278f, 2:278.e1f
  pigmentation, 2:270-272, 2:271f, 2:270.e1f
  polyploidy and multinucleation, 2:270
  steatosis, 2:273-278, 2:274f-276f, 2:274.e1f, 2:276.e1f
  vacuolation, 2:272-273, 2:272f
hepatocutaneous syndrome, 1:586-587, 2:295, 2:295.e1f
hyperplastic and neoplastic lesions, 2:344-352
infectious diseases
  bacterial, 2:314-318
  fungal, 2:324-325, 2:324f
  helminthic, 2:318-324
  protozoal, 2:324
  viral, 2:309-325, 2:310f
inflammatory diseases, 2:300-309
  nonspecific reactive hepatitis, 2:306
injury
  mechanisms, 2:326
  responses, 2:285-290, 2:287f
necrobacillosis, 2:42f
nephropathy, 2:294
photosensitization, 2:294, 2:294f
postmortem and agonal changes, 2:295-296
regeneration, 2:286-287, 2:290f
toxic hepatic disease, 2:325-344
  adverse drug reactions, 2:329
  agents, 2:328
tumor metastasis to, 2:351f-352f, 2:351.e1f
vascular factors in injury and circulatory disorders of, 2:296-300
  acquired portosystemic shunts, 2:298-299, 2:299f
  efferent hepatic vessels, 2:297-298
  hepatic artery, 2:296
  peliosis hepatis/telangiectasis, 2:299-300, 2:299f-300f, 2:299.e1f
Lobar bronchus, 2:467
Lobar pneumonia, 2:507
Lobular bronchopneumonia, 2:507
Lobular capillary hemangioma, 1:727
Lobular dissecting hepatitis, 2:305, 2:305f, 2:305.e1f
Lobulated kidney, 2:392.e3f
Localized bacterial periostitis, 1:102
Localized histiocytic sarcomas (LHS), 1:729
Localized scleroderma, 1:698
Localized skeletal dysplasias, 1:54-57, 1:54f
Locoweed, 1:91
Long-headed dwarfs, 1:39
Lordosis, 1:37t
Louisiana Catahoula Cattle dogs, cochleosaccular degeneration in, 1:492
Louping-ill, 1:367f
Lubricin, 1:131
Lukes-Collins classification, 3:215
Luminal folliculitis, 1:528
Lumpy jaw, 1:102-103
Lumpy skin disease virus, 1:616, 1:622-624, 1:624f
Lungs, 2:484-520
  abortion and, 3:401-402
  abscesses, 2:520
  atelectasis, 2:486, 2:486.e2f

Lungs *(Continued)*
    cellular architecture and cell biology, 2:468-471
    circulatory disturbances, 2:487-494
    congenital anomalies, 2:484-485, 2:485.e1f
    defenses, 2:471-473
    development and growth, 2:484, 2:484.e1f
    heart failure and, 3:11
    hemorrhage, 2:490-492, 2:490.e1f
    injury, 2:500-520, 2:500f
        airway disease, 2:500-504, 2:500.e1f
    interstitial lung disease, 2:509, 2:510f, 2:511b
    lobes, 2:467
        torsion, 2:485-486, 2:485f
    mineralization, 2:494-495, 2:494f
    neoplasia, 2:495-500, 2:495b
    organization of, 2:467
    pulmonary emphysema, 2:486-487
    pulmonary hypertension, 2:492-494
    thrombosis, embolism, and infarction, 2:489-490, 2:489b
    toxic injury, 2:518-520
    vascular supply to, 2:467-468, 2:468f
Lungworms, 2:564-567, 2:565t, 2:566f, 2:565.e2f
Lupins, 1:90
Lupinus arbustus, 2:3
Lupinus formosus, 2:3
Lupus erythematosus (LE), 1:604-607
    cutaneous, 1:605-607
    disseminated discoid, 1:606
    exfoliative cutaneous, 1:606, 1:606f
    systemic, 1:158-159, 1:605
    vesicular cutaneous, 1:607
Lupus panniculitis, 1:607
Luteinized cysts, 3:373, 3:373f
Luxations and subluxations, 1:137, 1:137f
Lycoperdon spp., 2:584-585
Lyme disease. *See* Borreliosis
Lyme nephritis, definitive diagnosis, 2:411-412
Lymph, overproduction of, 2:248
Lymphadenitis
    acute, 3:202-203
    caseous, 3:204-208, 3:207f-208f, 3:205.e1f
    chronic, 3:203-204, 3:203f, 3:204.e1f
    suppurative, 3:203-204, 3:204f
Lymphadenopathy, 3:200-201
Lymphangiectasia, 2:89-90, 2:90f
Lymphangiomas, 1:727-728, 3:99
Lymphangiomatosis, 1:727-728
Lymphangiosarcomas, 1:727-728, 3:101
Lymphangitis, 2:195-196, 2:196f, 3:96-98, 3:96f
    epizootic, 3:97-98
    granulomatous, 2:196, 2:196f
    parasitic, 3:98
    ulcerative, 3:97
Lymphatic capillaries, 3:54-55
Lymphatics, 3:94-98. *See also* Lymphomas
    congenital anomalies, 3:94-95
    developmental diseases, 3:139-141
    dilation and rupture, 3:95-96, 3:95f
    liver and, 2:260-261
    lung, 2:468
    lymphangitis, 3:96-98, 3:96f
        epizootic, 3:97-98
        parasitic, 3:98
        ulcerative, 3:97

Lymphatics *(Continued)*
    lymphoid organs, 3:138-141
    spleen, 3:158-162
    vessels, dermal, 1:514
Lymphatic sinus ectasia, 3:199, 3:199f
Lymphedema, 3:94, 3:95f
Lymph nodes, 3:196-243
    developmental diseases, 3:198
    hyperplasia, 3:200-202
    inflammatory diseases, 3:202-212
    neoplastic metastatic diseases, 3:212-213, 3:212f-213f
    parasitic diseases, 3:212
    scrotal, 3:498
    structure and function of normal, 3:196-198, 3:196f
Lymphocytes
    dermal, 1:514
    liver, 2:263
    in masticatory myositis, 1:226-227
    thymic cortical, 3:143
    thymic medullary, 3:143
Lymphocytic cholangitis, 2:308, 2:308f
Lymphocytic parathyroiditis, 3:298-299
Lymphocytic-plasmacytic enteritis, 2:95
    in cat, 2:92f
Lymphocytic-plasmacytic stomatitis, 2:16
Lymphocytic-plasmacytic synovitis, 1:147-148
Lymphocytic-plasmacytic uveitis, 1:449
Lymphocytic thyroiditis, 3:316, 3:317f-318f
Lymphocytic vasculitis, 1:526, 1:611
Lymphocytosis, 1:147, 3:111, 3:241.e2f
Lymphoglandular complexes, 2:64
Lymphoid atrophy, 3:198, 3:199f
Lymphoid hyperplasia, 3:201
    adrenal cortex, 3:343
    pharyngeal, 2:480.e3f
    spleen, 3:189, 3:189f
Lymphoid nodules, 1:522
Lymphoid tissue, 2:62-63
Lymphomas, 1:403, 2:107, 3:213-243, 3:309, 3:309f
    angiocentric, 2:499, 2:499f
    cats, 3:239-241, 3:241.e1f
    cattle, 3:235-237, 3:236f-237f, 3:236.e2f, 3:236.e1f
    classification, 3:215-243, 3:217t
    clinical features, 3:214
    cutaneous, 1:733-735, 1:733f
    diagnosis, 3:214-215, 3:218f
    dogs, 3:238-239, 3:239f, 3:238.e2f, 3:239.e2f, 3:239.e1f
    gastric, 2:107-109, 3:241f, 3:241.e1f
    heart, 3:53, 3:53f
    Hodgkin-like, 3:219
    horses, 3:237-238, 3:238f, 3:238.e1f
    intestinal, 3:239-241, 3:240f, 3:240.e1f
    intravascular, 1:734, 3:99
    malignant, 1:123-124, 1:245, 1:245f, 3:241.e1f
    cats, 3:241.e1f
    cattle, 1:124
    pigs, 3:242f, 3:241.e2f
    multicentric, 3:241, 3:241f
    nasal and nasopharyngeal, 2:479-480, 3:239f, 3:241, 3:241f, 3:239.e1f
    ocular, 1:482
    pigs, 3:241-243, 3:242f, 3:241.e2f
    renal, 2:447, 3:240f-241f

Lymphomas *(Continued)*
    sheep and goats, 3:237, 3:237f
    skin, 3:237, 3:237f, 3:239f, 3:237.e1f, 3:239.e1f
    spinal cord, 3:240f
    thymic, 3:157-158, 3:157f-158f, 3:237, 3:240f, 3:157.e1f
    viral etiology and, 3:235
Lymphomatoid granulomatosis (LYG), 3:99, 3:222
Lymphopenia, 3:111
Lymphoplasmacytic, 2:107
Lymphoplasmacytic cystitis, chronic, 2:460.e1f
Lymphoplasmacytic myocarditis, 3:44, 3:44f
Lymphoplasmacytic stomatitis, 2:15
Lymphosarcomas, 1:403
    bovine ovarian, 3:378, 3:379f
    uterus, 3:450, 3:450f
Lynxacarus radovsky, 1:683
Lysosomal enzymes, 1:284
Lysosomal phospholipidosis, 2:424
Lysosomal storage diseases, 1:284-293, 1:285f-286f, 2:429
    liver, 2:278, 2:278f, 2:278.e1f
    skeleton, 1:57-59
    spinal cord, 1:285f-286f
Lyssavirus infections, 1:367-370

M
Maceration, fetal, 3:396, 3:396f
Macracanthorhynchus hirudinaceus, 2:227
Macrocyclic trichothecene toxins, 1:573
Macrophages, 2:64
    hyperplasia, 3:201-202
    multinucleated, 2:540.e2f
    in muscle regeneration, 1:182-183
    pulmonary, 2:470
        alveolar, 2:470-472
        interstitial, 2:471
        intravascular, 2:471, 2:471.e1f
Macroscopic hematuria, 2:461
Macroscopic lesions in horses, 2:108
Macrovesicles, 2:274
Macula densa, 2:380f
Macules, 1:524
Maduramicin, 1:219, 3:34-35
Maedi-visna, 2:413, 2:558-560, 2:559f, 2:558.e1f
Magnesium ammonium phosphate hexahydrate, 2:455
Main Drain virus, 1:280
Malabsorptive, 2:95
Malacia, 1:299f, 1:307-317
    cerebral, 1:299-300, 1:299f
Malassez, epithelial rests of, 2:4-6
Malassezia dermatitis, 1:548-549, 1:553, 1:593, 1:647-649, 1:648f
Malassimilation, 2:89-97
Maldevelopment of filtration angle, 1:417, 1:417f
Male genital system, 3:465-510
    accessory genital glands, 3:499-505, 3:499f
    genital considerations, 3:465-468
    oxidative stress and testicular function, 3:467
    penis and prepuce, 3:505-510
        inflammation, 3:506-508
        neoplasms, 3:508-510
    prostate and bulbourethral glands, 3:500-504, 3:500f

Male genital system (Continued)
  sampling of male genital tract, 3:465-466
  scrotum, 3:471-473
  sexual development disorders, 3:468-471, 3:476f, 3:499-501, 3:505
  spermatic cord, 3:497-499
  spermatogenesis, 3:466-467
  testis and epididymis, 3:474-497
    circulatory disturbances, 3:491-492
    disorders of sexual development, 3:476-481, 3:476f
    hypoplasia, 3:478-479, 3:478f
    neoplasms, 3:492-497
    testicular immune function, 3:467-468
    vaginal tunics, 3:473-474, 3:473f-474f
Malignant angioendotheliomatosis, 3:99
Malignant catarrhal fever (MCF), 2:131-136, 2:133f-136f, 2:459-460
Malignant edema and gas gangrene, 1:232
Malignant hyperthermia, 1:209-210
  dogs, 1:210
  horses, 1:210
  pigs, 1:209-210
Malignant lymphomas, 1:123-124, 1:245, 1:245f, 2:107-109
  cats, 3:241.e1f
  cattle, 1:124
  large-cell/lymphoblastic lymphoma, 2:108
  large granular lymphoma, 2:108
  pigs, 3:242f, 3:241.e2f
  small-cell lymphocytic villus lymphoma, 2:107-108
Malignant/malevolent sarcoids, 1:708
Malignant melanomas, 1:721-722, 2:26-27, 2:26f, 2:240f
  cats, 2:26-27
  iris, 1:483-484, 1:484f
  dogs, 2:21, 2:26, 2:26f
Malignant mixed thyroid tumors, 3:331, 3:331f
Malignant neoplasms, 2:100-101
Malignant pheochromocytoma, 3:349-351
Malignant pilomatricomas, 1:717
Malignant transformation, 2:22
Malignant trichoepitheliomas, 1:715
Malignant tumors of joints, 1:159-160
  histiocytic sarcoma, 1:159-160
  synovial cell sarcoma, 1:159
Malleus, 1:495
Malnutrition. See Nutritional deficiency/disease
Maltese dogs
  cochleosaccular degeneration, 1:492
  myelinolytic leukodystrophy, 1:341
Mammae, 3:451-459
  benign neoplasms, 3:460
  bovine mastitis, 3:452-457, 3:452f
  carcinomas, 3:451t, 3:460-463, 3:461f-462f, 3:463t
    cats, 3:463-464, 3:464f
  coliform mastitis, 3:454-455, 3:454f
  developmental biology, 3:451, 3:451t
  inflammatory disease, 3:451-452
  innate and acquired resistance of, 3:451-452
  masses including neoplasia, 3:459-464, 3:459f
  mycoplasma mastitis, 3:456, 3:456f
  sarcomas, 3:463, 3:463f
  streptococcal mastitis, 3:455
  summer mastitis, 3:455-456
Mammomonogamus auris, 1:498

Mammary gland carcinomas, 1:736
Mammomonogamus ierei, 2:557
Mammomonogamus laryngeus, 2:557
Mammomonogamus nasicola, 2:557, 2:567
Mandibular osteomyelitis, 1:103f
  cattle, 1:102-103
Mandibular osteopathy, 2:9
Manganese chloride, 2:329
Manganese deficiency, 1:80
  cattle, 1:80, 1:81f
Mange
  chorioptic, 1:676-677, 1:677f
  demodectic, 1:678-682, 1:680f
  notoedric, 1:675, 1:675f
  otodectic, 1:677-678
  psorergatic, 1:678
  psoroptic, 1:675-676
  sarcoptic, 1:673-675, 1:674f
Mannheimia haemolytica, 2:557, 3:69
  liver and, 2:314-315
  respiratory system and, 2:543-544, 2:545f, 2:562-563, 2:540.e2f
Mantle cell lymphoma (MCL), 3:226, 3:227f
Manx cats, corneal endothelial dystrophy in, 1:433
Maple syrup urine disease, 1:344, 1:345f
Mare reproductive loss syndrome, 3:417
Marginal zone lymphoma (MZL), 3:224, 3:225f, 3:226.e1f
Marked acute tubular necrosis, 2:428.e1f
Markers of remodeling, 1:27
Maroteaux-Lamy syndrome, 1:58
Marshallagia, 2:54-55
Massive fat necrosis in cattle, 2:249
Massive liver necrosis, 2:284-285, 2:284f
Masson trichrome
  method, 1:29
  stain, 2:383
Mastadenovirus, 2:145
Mast cells, 1:514-515
  epidermal, 1:519
  liver, 2:264
  tumors, 1:730-733, 1:731f, 2:27, 2:109
    conjunctival, 1:482
    gastrointestinal, 2:109
    mastocytosis, 3:137
    metastasis to lymph nodes, 3:212-213, 3:213f
    metastasis to spleen, 3:194
Masticatory myositis of dogs, 1:226-227, 1:226f-227f
Mastitis
  bovine, 3:452-457, 3:452f
  camelids, 3:458-459
  coliform, 3:454-455, 3:454f-455f
  dogs and cats, 3:458, 3:458f
  fibrinosuppurative exudate with, 3:453-454, 3:453f
  horses, 3:457
  mycoplasma, 3:456, 3:456f
  nocardia, 3:457, 3:457f
  staphylococcal, 3:452-454
  streptococcal, 3:453-455, 3:454f
  summer, 3:455-456
  swine, 3:457
  tuberculosis, 3:456-457
Mastocytosis, 3:137
Materia alba, 2:9
Maternal leptospiremia, 2:435
Matrical cysts, 1:704
Matrix vesicles, 1:20

Mature (peripheral) B-cell neoplasms, 3:219-228
Mature (peripheral) T-cell neoplasms, 3:228-229
Maxillary or mandibular fibrosarcoma, 1:121, 1:121f-122f
M cells, 2:63-64
Mean platelet volume (MPV), 3:258
Mebendazole, 2:329
Mechanical forces and injury effects on bones, 1:30-36
Mechanical gastritis, 2:52
Mecistocirrus, 2:54-55
Meconium aspiration syndrome, 2:516, 2:516.e1f
Media, vascular system, 3:54
Medial hypertrophy of pulmonary arteries, 3:67, 3:67f
Medullary necrosis, gross lesions of, 2:399-400
Medullary rays, 2:378
Medullary solute washout, 2:381
Medulloblastoma, 1:402, 1:402f
Medulloepitheliomas, 1:485-486, 1:486f
Megacolon, in Clydesdale foals, 2:77
Megaesophagus, 2:33-34, 2:34f
  congenital, 2:34
Megakaryocytes, 3:106-107
  hypoplasia, 3:258
  pulmonary embolism and, 2:490
Megalencephaly, 1:268
Megalocornea, 1:421
Megalocytosis, 2:270, 2:337f
Megavoltage X-radiation and cataract, 1:444
Megestrol acetate, 2:329
Meibomian adenoma, 1:480-481, 1:481f
Melanin, 1:513
  disorders of pigmentation, 1:554-558
  lymph node, 3:200
Melanocortin receptor (MR2), 3:270-271
Melanocytes, 1:513
  dermal, 1:514
  tumors, 1:720-722, 1:720f-721f
Melanocyte-stimulating hormone (MSH), 3:276-277
Melanocytic tumors of eye, 1:482-485
Melanocytoma-acanthoma, 1:721
Melanocytomas, 1:481, 1:721
Melanocytopenic hypomelanosis, 1:555-556
Melanomas, 1:720-722, 1:720f-721f
  malignant, 1:721-722, 2:26-27, 2:240f
  cats, 2:26-27
    iris, 1:483-484, 1:484f
  dogs, 2:21, 2:26, 2:26f
  lymph node, 3:213.e1f
Melanopenic hypomelanosis, 1:556-557
Melanosis, congenital and acquired, 2:270, 2:270.e1f
Melanotic tumors, cytologic evaluation of, 2:26
Melia azedarach, 2:89
Melioidosis, 1:637, 2:563, 3:188-189, 3:188f
Melophagus ovinus, 1:670
Membrane permeability transition (MPT) pore, 2:281
Membrane receptor (RANK), 3:294-295
Membranoproliferative glomerulonephritis (MPGN), 2:404f, 2:411f, 2:411.e1f, 2:401.e4f, 3:123-124
  proteinuria and azotemia, 2:412
Membranous glomerulonephropathy (MGN), 2:402f, 2:401.e2f

Membranous labyrinth of ear, 1:488-489
Meningeal hemorrhages, 1:301
Meningeal sarcomatosis, 1:398
Meninges
  age changes in, 1:304
  tumors, 1:396-398
Meningioangiomatosis, 1:404, 3:99
Meningiomas, 1:396-398, 1:397f
  intracranial, 1:494
  nasal, 2:480
  optic nerve, 1:487, 1:487f
Meningitis, 1:355f-357f, 1:359f
Meningocele, 1:267, 1:267f, 1:279
Meningoencephalitis, necrotizing, 1:392-393, 1:392f
Meningoencephalocele, 1:267f
Meningoencephalomyelitis, granulomatous and pyogranulomatous, 1:362, 1:362f
Meningomyelocele, 1:279
Menisci, 1:130
Mercury toxicosis, 1:570
Merino sheep
  Alexander disease, 1:341
  axonal dystrophy, 1:324
  brachygnathia inferior, 2:3
  congenital myopathy, 1:200
  focal macular melanosis, 1:554
  hypothyroidism, 1:588
  wattles, 1:532
Merkel cells, 1:513
  tumor, 1:735
Mesangial cells, 2:409
Mesangial hyaline droplets, 2:421
Mesangial matrix, 2:380-381
Mesangioproliferative glomerulonephropathy, 2:403f, 2:401.e3f
Mesangium, 2:380-381
Mesenchymal liver hamartomas, 2:264
Mesenchymal progenitor cells, 1:21-22
Mesenchymal tumors, 2:44, 2:463-464
  of ear, 1:504
  lipomas, 1:245, 1:246f, 1:726
Mesenchyme, anomalies of, 1:413-414
  anterior chamber, 1:415-417
Mesenteric hernia, 2:79
Mesenteric lymph nodes, 2:107-108
Mesenteric volvulus, 2:83
Mesocestoides spp., 2:223
Mesodermal somites, 1:167
Mesodermal tumor(s), 2:349-351, 2:350f
Mesodiverticular band, 2:245
Mesonephric and paramesonephric structures disorders, 3:480-481, 3:480f
Mesonephric (Wolffian) ducts, 3:360-361
  cysts, 3:368f, 3:371
Mesothelial cells, 2:81, 2:244
Mesotheliomas
  peritoneal, 2:256-257, 2:256f
  pleura, 2:523, 2:523.e2f
  vaginal tunic, 3:474f
Mesquite toxicosis, 1:326
Metabolic acidosis, 2:75, 2:381
Metabolic alkalosis, 2:50
Metabolic bone diseases, 1:61
Metabolic disease, 2:41
  corneal deposits secondary to, 1:433-434, 1:433f
Metabolic myopathies, 1:204-209
  cats, 1:205
  cattle and sheep, 1:207-208
  dogs, 1:204-205

Metabolic myopathies (Continued)
  horses, 1:205-207, 1:206f-207f
Metanephric blastema, 2:391
Metanephros formation, 2:391
Metaphyseal arteries, 1:27
Metaphyseal osteopathy, 1:106f
  dogs, 1:105-106, 1:105f-106f
Metaphysis, 1:22, 1:24, 1:26f
Metaplasia, 2:393
  fibroblastic, 1:442-443
  mucous, 2:47
  myeloid, 3:107, 3:191
  osseous, 1:304, 2:517, 2:517.e1f
  osteocartilaginous, 3:34, 3:34f
  peribronchiolar, 2:495, 2:495.e2f
  prostate and bulbourethral gland, 3:502-503, 3:502f
Metastases, tumor, 1:245-246, 2:102-103, 2:447
  to adrenal medulla, 3:353-354, 3:353f
  to central nervous system, 1:404
  within the globe and orbit, 1:488
  hypercalcemia with, 3:309
  to liver, 2:351-352, 2:351f-352f, 2:351.e1f
  to lung, 2:499-500
  to lymph nodes, 3:212-213, 3:212f-213f, 3:213.e1f
  metastatic bone disease, 1:124, 1:124f
    dogs, 1:124, 1:124f
  to ovaries, 3:378
  to pancreas, 2:367
  to peritoneum, 2:257
  to pituitary gland, 3:288-289
  to pleura, 2:523
  to skin, 1:736
  to spleen, 3:194, 3:194f
Metastrongylus spp., 2:536, 2:536.e2f
  respiratory system and, 2:536, 2:536.e2f
Metazoan parasites and pancreas, 2:365
Methimazole, 2:329
Methotrexate, 2:329
Methoxyflurane anesthesia, 2:426
Methoxyflurane, 2:329
Metorchis conjunctus, 2:323
Metritis, 3:389-393
  contagious equine, 3:445, 3:445f
Meuse-Rhine-Issel cattle, 2:38
  diaphragmatic dystrophy, 1:199
Mexican Hairless dogs, congenital hypotrichosis in, 1:538-539
Mexican Hairless pigs, congenital hypotrichosis in, 1:538
Mibolerone, 2:329
Microabscess, 2:440.e1f
Microangiopathic hemolytic anemia (MHA), 3:65
Microbiology, diagnostic, 1:10-11
Microcirculation, 1:263-264, 1:264f, 3:54, 1:263.e1f
  lesions, 1:301
Microcornea, 1:421
Microcystiis aeruginosa, 2:330
Microcystin-LR, 2:330
Microencephaly, 1:268
Microfractures, 1:34, 1:34f
Microglia, 1:262-263, 2:392.e3f
Microglial nodules, 1:262-263
Microgliomatosis, 1:403
Microhematuria, 2:461
Microlithiasis, alveolar, 2:517, 2:517f
Micronodular thymomas, 3:154, 3:155f

Microphakia, 1:422
Microphthalmos, 1:410, 1:410f
Microradiography, 1:30
Microscopic agglutination test (MAT), 2:434-435
Microscopic lesions, 2:399-400
  intestinal mucosa, 2:125-126
Microscopic polyangiitis, 3:71
Microscopic structure of muscle fibers, 1:165-167, 1:166f
Microsporidian infections, 1:385-386
Microthrombi, 2:85
Microvascular injury, 2:85-86
Microvascular maturation, 2:484
Microvascular steatosis, 2:273-274, 2:274f
Microvilli, 2:61
Microwave burns, 1:565
Middle ear, 1:495-500
  developmental disease, 1:496
  epithelial neoplasia, 1:500
  jugulotympanic paragangliomas, 1:500
  non-neoplastic and neoplastic disease, 1:498-499, 1:498.e2f
  otitis media, 1:496-498, 1:497.e1f
  parasites, 1:498
  temporohyoid osteoarthropathy, 1:500
Middle plexus, dermal, 1:514
Midstromal corneal vascular ingrowth from limbus, 1:437-438
Midzonal liver necrosis, 2:283, 2:283f
Mild morphologic damage, 2:81
Mimosine toxicosis, 1:572
Mineralocorticoids, 3:337
Mineral deficiency, 1:583-586
Mineral deposition
  corneal, 1:434
  cutaneous tissue, 1:562-564
Mineralization, 2:386f
  adrenal glands, 3:339
  arterial, 3:60-61, 3:61f
  cartilage matrix, 1:23
  colloid, 3:314, 3:315f
  defective, 1:68
  dystrophic, 1:519
  enamel, 2:5
  fibrous osteodystrophy and, 1:78-79, 1:79f
  front, bone, 1:20
  heart, 3:34
  matrix, 1:20
  parathyroid suppression associated with vitamin D intoxication, 3:302, 3:302f
  placenta, 3:397
  pulmonary, 2:494-495, 2:494f
  subendocardial, 3:4, 3:30, 3:30f
  testicular degeneration, 3:484
Miniature Poodle dogs
  Alexander disease, 1:341
  chondrodysplasia, 1:44, 1:44f
  diabetes mellitus, 2:373
  epidermolysis bullosa, 1:536
  globoid cell leukodystrophy, 1:339
  malignant melanoma, 2:26
  pancreatic necrosis, 2:358
Miniature Schnauzer dogs
  canine atopic dermatitis, 1:591
  congenital idiopathic megaesophagus, 2:33-34
  congenital myotonia, 1:201

Miniature Schnauzer dogs *(Continued)*
  demyelinating neuropathy, *1*:341-342
  factor VII deficiency, *3*:264
  hypothyroidism, *1*:587
  pancreatic necrosis, *2*:358
  pigmented plaques, *1*:710-711
  Schnauzer comedo syndrome, *1*:549
  sick sinus syndrome, *3*:51
  XY disorder of sexual development, *3*:471, *3*:471f
Minimal change disease, *2*:418, *2*:420f, *2*:418.e2f
Minimata disease, *1*:321
Miscellaneous glomerular lesions, *2*:418-421
Misshapen teeth, *2*:6
Mites, *1*:673-684
  Demodex, *1*:678-682
  trombiculiasis, *1*:682-683
Mitochondria, *1*:251-252
Mitochondrial cytochrome P450 enzymes, *3*:341
Mitochondrial myopathy
  dogs, *1*:205
  horses, *1*:207
Mitochondrial outer membrane permeabilization (MOMP), *2*:280
Mitotic index (MI), *1*:721
Mittendorf's dot, *1*:417-418
Mixed-breed dogs, *2*:415-416
  factor VII deficiency, *3*:264
  severe factor X deficiency, *3*:264
Mixed germ cell-sex cord stromal tumor, *3*:496
Mixed liver hamartomas, *2*:264
Mixed neuronal-glial tumors, *1*:401
Mixed toxic insults, liver, *2*:327
Modeling, *1*:24-25, *1*:26f
Molecular biology, *1*:11
Molluscipoxvirus, *1*:616, *1*:621-622, *1*:622f
Molybdenosis, *1*:84
Molybdenum, *1*:81-82
Monensin, *1*:219, *3*:34-35
Monkeypox virus, *1*:616
Monocytes, dermal, *1*:514
Monoiodotyrosine (MIT), *3*:311
Monomyelocytic leukemia, *2*:352f
Monorchia, *3*:479
Moraxella bovis, *1*:425
  infectious bovine keratoconjunctivitis and, *1*:440
Morgagnian globules, *1*:442
Morgan horse, axonal dystrophy in, *1*:324
Morphea, *1*:698
Morphologic diagnosis, *1*:5
Mortierella wolfii, *2*:554
Mortierellosis, *2*:554
Mosaicism, *3*:383
Mosquito-bites
  dermatitis, *1*:670-671, *1*:671f
  flaviviruses, *1*:374-376
  hypersensitivity, *1*:599
Motility and salmonellosis, *2*:168
Motor neuron disease, *1*:255, *1*:255f, *1*:330-332, *1*:331f-332f
  "shaker calf", *1*:332, *1*:332f
Motor units, muscular, *1*:165
Mouth. *See* Buccal cavity; Oral cavity
Mucinosis, *1*:522-523
Mucocele
  gallbladder, *2*:307, *2*:345, *2*:345f
  paranasal, *2*:477, *2*:477.e4f
  salivary, *2*:29

Mucociliary clearance, *2*:471-472
Mucocutaneous leishmaniasis, *3*:174
Mucocutaneous pyoderma, *1*:630
Mucocyte bodies, *1*:255
Mucoepidermoid carcinomas, *2*:30
Mucolipidoses, *1*:290
Mucometra, *3*:374, *3*:374f, *3*:382-383, *3*:383f, *3*:386
Mucoperiosteal exostoses, *1*:499, *1*:499f
Mucopolysaccharidoses (MPS), *1*:58, *1*:58f, *1*:289-290
  hearing and, *1*:491-492
Mucosa. *See also* Buccal cavity
  -associated lymphoid tissue (MALT), *2*:20
  -associated lymphoid tissue (MALT)oma, *3*:225f
  buccal cavity and, *2*:12-19
  disease, *2*:114, *2*:123
  hypertrophy, *2*:48
  infarction, *2*:385-386
  microscopic appearance, *2*:67
  nasal cavity, *2*:466
  polyps, *2*:104f
  ulcers, *2*:82
Mucous cells, *2*:469
Mucous glands, *2*:378
Mucous membrane pemphigoid, *1*:603, *1*:603f, *2*:15
Mucous metaplasia and hyperplasia, *2*:47
Mucous neck cells, *2*:45
Mucus, *2*:471
Mucus-producing carcinomas, *2*:101-102
Muellerius capillaris, *2*:565, *2*:565t, *2*:566f, *2*:565.e2f
Mulberry heart disease, *1*:217, *3*:39-41, *3*:39f-41f, *3*:39.e1f
Multicentric lymphoma, *3*:241, *3*:241f
Multidrug-resistance-associated protein-2 (MRP-2), *2*:293
Multifocal intramural myocardial infarction, *3*:36
Multifocal necrotizing panniculitis, *2*:360
Multifocal osseous metaplasia, *2*:517, *2*:517.e1f
Multifocal polyphasic necrosis, *1*:218
Multifocal renal cortical hemorrhages, *2*:432f
Multifocal symmetrical myelinolytic encephalopathy, *1*:341
Multilobular tumor of bone, *1*:117-118, *1*:117f-118f
Multinucleated giant cells, *1*:527, *2*:27
Multinucleated keratinocytes, *1*:523
Multinucleated macrophages, *2*:540.e2f
Multinucleated syncytial giant cells, *3*:297-298, *3*:298f
Multinucleation, liver, *2*:270
Multiple acquired cortical cysts, *2*:396f
Multiple cartilaginous exostosis, *1*:54
Multiple endocrine neoplasia (MEN), *3*:356-357
Multiple epiphyseal dysplasia, *1*:44, *1*:45f
Multiple hepatic peribiliary cysts, *2*:264
Multiple myeloma (MM), *3*:137, *3*:138f, *3*:228, *3*:228f
Multiple persistent vitelline duct cysts, *2*:74
Multisystemic, eosinophilic, epitheliotropic disease in the horse, *1*:695-696
Multisystemic epitheliotropic syndrome, *2*:96
Multisystem neuronal degeneration of Cocker Spaniel dogs, *1*:320
Mummification of fetus, *3*:395-396, *3*:395f
Munro's microabscess, *1*:523

Mural endocarditis, *3*:32
Mural folliculitis, *1*:528
Murray Grey cattle, inherited progressive spinal myelopathy of, *1*:325
Muscle crush syndrome, *1*:212
Muscle(s), *1*:165-246. *See also* Tendons
  basic reactions of, *1*:173-186
    atrophy, *1*:173-178
    fibrosis, *1*:184-185
    hypertrophy, *1*:178-180
    injury and necrosis, *1*:180-182
    other myofiber alterations, *1*:185-186
    postmortem changes, *1*:186
    regeneration, *1*:182-183
  circulatory disturbances of, *1*:210-213
    compartment syndrome, *1*:211
    downer syndrome, *1*:212
    muscle crush syndrome, *1*:212
    postanesthetic myopathy in horses, *1*:213
    vascular occlusive syndrome, *1*:212
  congenital and inherited diseases, *1*:186-210
    malignant hyperthermia, *1*:209-210
    metabolic myopathies, *1*:204-209
    muscular defects, *1*:189-192
    muscular dystrophy, *1*:192-197
    myasthenia gravis, *1*:209
    myopathies, *1*:197-200
    myotonic and spastic syndromes, *1*:200-204
    primary central nervous system conditions, *1*:187-189
  degenerative myopathies, *1*:221-224
    equine systemic calcinosis, *1*:223-224
  dermal, *1*:515
  histochemical fiber types, *1*:169-170, *1*:169f-170f
  immune-mediated conditions, *1*:225-230
    masticatory myositis of dogs, *1*:226-227
  microscopic structure, *1*:165-167, *1*:166f
  myogenesis, *1*:167-169
  myopathies
    associated with endocrine disorders, *1*:224-225
    associated with serum electrolyte abnormalities, *1*:225
  myositis resulting from infection, *1*:230-234
    clostridial, *1*:230-233
    malignant edema and gas gangrene, *1*:232
    suppurative myositis, *1*:230
  neoplastic diseases of, *1*:240-246
    muscle pseudotumors, *1*:246, *1*:246f
    nonmuscle primary tumors of muscle, *1*:244-245
    rhabdomyoma, *1*:241, *1*:242f
    rhabdomyosarcoma, *1*:241-243, *1*:243f-244f
    secondary tumors of skeletal muscle, *1*:244-246, *1*:245f-246f
  nutritional myopathy, *1*:214-218
    cattle, *1*:215-216
    etiology and pathogenesis, *1*:214-215
    horses, *1*:218
    other species, *1*:218
    pigs, *1*:217
    sheep and goats, *1*:216-217

Muscle(s) (Continued)
  parasitic diseases and, 1:234-240
    cysticercosis, 1:239-240, 1:239f
    eosinophilic myositis, 1:236-237, 1:236f-237f
    hepatozoonosis, 1:240
    leishmaniasis, 1:240
    sarcocystosis, 1:234-236, 1:235f
    Toxoplasma and *Neospora* myositis, 1:237-238
    trichinellosis, 1:237-238
  physical injuries of, 1:213-214
    ossifying fibrodysplasia, 1:213
    strains/tears/ruptures/fibrotic myopathies/contractures, 1:213-214
  repair, 1:166-167
  specialized structures, 1:170-171, 1:170f
  spindles, 1:171, 1:171f
  steatosis, 1:191, 1:191f
  structure and development, 1:165-173
  techniques for study of, 1:171-173
  toxic myopathies, 1:218-220
    ionophore toxicosis, 1:219
    toxic plants and plant-origin toxins, 1:90-91, 1:219-220
  ultrastructure, 1:167
Muscular dystrophy, 1:185, 1:185f, 1:192-197
  canine X-linked, 1:192-194, 1:193f-195f
  α-dystroglycan deficiency and, 1:196
  feline X-linked, 1:194-195, 1:195f
  ovine, 1:196-197, 1:196f
Musculoaponeurotic fibromatosis, 1:248, 1:248f
Myasthenia gravis, 1:209, 3:157
  acquired, 1:229-230
  cats, 1:209
  dogs, 1:209
Mycetoma, 1:653
Mycobacterial infections, 1:639
  canine leproid granuloma, 1:503, 1:641, 1:641f
  feline leprosy, 1:640-641
  liver and, 2:314-315, 2:315f
  nontuberculous, 1:639-640
  spleen and, 3:183f
  tuberculosis, 1:639
Mycobacterium avium, 2:194, 2:548
Mycobacterium bovis, 2:547-551
Mycobacterium tuberculosis, 2:548
Mycobacterium ulcerans, 1:640
Mycology, 1:10-11
Mycoplasma agalactiae, 2:564
Mycoplasma alkalescens, 2:554
Mycoplasma arginini, 2:554
Mycoplasma bovigenitalium, 2:554
Mycoplasma bovirhinis, 2:459, 2:554
Mycoplasma bovis, 1:153-154, 1:498, 2:552-554, 2:553f, 2:552.e2f
Mycoplasma canis, 2:554, 3:491
  epididymitis due to, 3:491
Mycoplasma capricolum, 2:563-564
Mycoplasma cynos, 2:579
Mycoplasma dispar, 2:554
Mycoplasma haemofelis, 3:124, 3:125f
Mycoplasma haemosuis, 3:168t, 3:170
Mycoplasma hyopneumoniae, 2:534-535, 2:535f, 3:25-26
Mycoplasma hyorhinis, 1:153
Mycoplasmal arthritis, 1:153-154
  cats, 1:154

Mycoplasmal arthritis (Continued)
  dogs, 1:154
  goats, 1:153, 1:153f
  pigs, 1:153
  sheep, 1:153
Mycoplasmal infections, 1:646-661, 2:459
  abortion and, 3:399b
  guttural pouch, 2:480-481, 2:480f
  respiratory system, 2:533-535, 2:551-554, 2:563-564, 2:573, 2:579, 2:590
Mycoplasma mastitis, 3:456, 3:456f
Mycoplasma mycoides, 1:153f, 1:154, 2:551, 2:564
Mycoplasma ovipneumoniae, 2:564
Mycoplasma putrifaciens, 2:564
Mycoplasmas, hemotropic, 3:124-125
Mycoplasmology, 1:10-11
Mycosis fungoides (MF), 3:232, 3:233f
Mycotic abomasitis, 2:54, 2:54f
Mycotic abortion in cattle, 3:418-419, 3:418f-419f
Mycotic diseases of gastrointestinal tract, 2:201-203
Mycotic endophthalmitis, 1:449-451
Mycotic epididymitis, 3:491
Mycotic gastritis, 2:54
Mycotic keratitis, 1:439-440, 1:439f
Mycotic omasitis, 2:42
Mycotic rhinitis, 2:579, 2:580f
Mycotic rumenitis, 2:42, 2:42f
Mycotoxic leukoencephalomalacia, 1:315-316, 1:315f-316f
Mycotoxicosis, 1:472
  ergotism, 1:572-573, 1:573f
Myelination, 1:259
Myelinic edema, 1:260
Myelin in Wallerian degeneration, 1:256-257, 1:257f
Myelinolytic leukodystrophy, 1:341
Myelinopathies, 1:336-347
  spongy, 1:342-346, 1:342f-343f
Myelin sheath, 1:258-260
Myeloblasts, 3:104-106
Myelodysplasia, 1:188f, 1:277-279
Myelodysplastic syndrome (MDS), 3:129-136, 3:135f-136f
Myelofibrosis (MF), 3:136-138, 3:137f
Myeloid metaplasia, 3:107
  spleen, 3:191
Myelolipomas, 2:351f, 3:343-344
  liver, 2:350-351
Myelomalacia, 1:307
Myelomas
  multiple, 3:137, 3:138f, 3:228, 3:228f
  plasma cell, 1:123, 1:123f, 2:27-28, 3:226-228, 3:226.e1f
Myelopathy, necrotizing, 1:340, 1:340f
Myeloproliferative neoplasm (MPN), 3:129-134, 3:134f-135f
Myiasis, 1:668-670
  calliphorine, 1:669
  of rumen, 2:43
  screwworm, 1:669-670
Myocardial bridges, 3:22
Myocardial conduction system, 3:2, 3:3f
  diseases, 3:51
Myocarditis, 3:41-44, 3:42f, 3:42t
  embolic suppurative, 3:42.e1f

  parasitic, 3:43-44, 3:44.e1f
Myocardium, 3:3-5
  contractile strength, 3:5
  disease, 3:33-51
    causes, 3:33t
    degeneration, 1:217
    myocarditis, 3:41-44, 3:42f, 3:42t
    necrosis, 3:34-41, 3:36f-37f
Myofibers, 1:165, 1:166f, 1:167
  congenital trigeminal nerve hypoplasia, 1:187, 1:188f
  vacuolar degeneration, 1:185, 1:185f
Myofibrillar hypoplasia, 1:190, 1:190f
Myofibrils, 1:167
Myofibroblasts, 2:60-61
Myofilaments, 1:167
Myogenesis, 1:167-169
Myoglobin-induced acute tubular injury, 2:423f
Myopathic atrophy, 1:178, 1:178f
Myopathies
  degenerative, 1:221-224
  endocrine disorder-associated, 1:224-225
  exertional, 1:221-223
  inherited and congenital, 1:197-200
    breed-associated, in dogs, 1:197-198, 1:197f
    cats, 1:198-199
    cattle, 1:199-200
    horses, 1:200
    sheep, 1:200
  metabolic, 1:204-209
  nutritional, 1:214-218
    cattle, 1:215-216, 1:216f
    horses, 1:218
    pigs, 1:217
    sheep and goats, 1:216-217
  serum electrolyte abnormalities and, 1:225
  toxic, 1:218-220
    ionophore toxicosis, 1:219
Myophosphorylase deficiency, 1:186-187, 1:208, 1:290
Myoporaceae, 2:331-332, 2:332f
Myosin heavy chains (myHC), 1:167-168
Myositis
  clostridial, 1:230-233, 1:231f
  eosinophilic, 1:236-237, 1:236f-237f
  granulomatous lesions, 1:233-234
  infectious, 1:230-234
  malignant edema and gas gangrene, 1:232
  muscle changes secondary to systemic infections, 1:234, 1:234f
  specific diseases with muscle alterations, 1:233
  suppurative, 1:230f
  Toxoplasma and *Neospora*, 1:237
Myospherulosis, 1:560
Myostatin defects leading to muscular hyperplasia, 1:190-191
Myotonia, 1:200-204
  cats, 1:201
  dogs, 1:200f, 1:201
  goats, 1:201-202
  myotonic dystrophy-like disorders in dogs and horses, 1:202-203, 1:203f
  periodic paralyses, 1:202
  spastic syndromes, 1:203f
Myotonic dystrophy-like disorders in dogs and horses, 1:202-203, 1:203f
Myotonic syndromes, 1:318
Myotubes, 1:167

Myriad tubular functions, 2:377
Myringitis, 1:497, 1:497f, 1:497.e2f
Myxedema with hypothyroidism, 3:318, 3:318f
Myxobdella, 2:19
Myxomas, 1:723, 3:52
Myxomatous valvular degeneration, 3:27-29, 3:28f-29f
Myxoma virus, 1:616

N

N-acetylglucosamine-6-sulfatase deficiency, 1:289-290
NADPH oxidase mechanisms, 2:81
Nanophyetus salmincola, 2:225-226, 3:148-149
Nasal-associated lymphoid tissue (NALT), 2:474
Nasal cavity, 2:466, 2:473-480
　circulatory disturbances, 2:473-474
　congenital anomalies, 2:473
　general considerations, 2:473
　nasal amyloidosis, 2:473, 2:474f
　neoplasms, 2:478-480, 2:478f
　non-neoplastic proliferative disorders, 2:477-478
　paranasal sinus diseases, 2:477, 2:477f
　polyps, 2:477-478, 2:477f, 2:579
　rhinitis, 2:474-477, 2:475b
　tumors, 2:560, 2:560f
Nasal chondrosarcoma, 1:119f-120f, 2:480.e1f
Nasal granulomas, 2:476
Nasal lymphomas, 3:239f, 3:241, 3:241f, 3:239.e1f
Nasal/nasopharyngeal stenosis, 2:475
Nasal papillomas, 2:479, 2:479.e1f
Nasomaxillary tumors of young horses, 2:480
Nasopharyngeal angiofibroma, 2:480
Nasopharyngeal polyps of cats, 2:477-478, 2:477f
Nasopharynx, 2:467
Natural killer (NK) cells, 2:260, 2:263, 3:219
Naturally occurring disease, 1:2
Navicular syndrome, 1:142, 1:142f
NCP biotype and BVDV, 2:122
Nebovirus, 2:113
Necrobacillary rumenitis, 2:41-42
Necrobacillosis, 2:17
　　cattle, 1:643
　　hepatic, 2:316
　　pigs, 1:643
　　rumen, 2:41f
Necrohemorrhagic vasculitis, 1:299f
Necrolytic migratory erythema, 1:692
Necrosis, 2:386f
　abdominal fat, 2:76-77, 2:249, 2:249f
　bronchial, 2:501, 2:504-506, 2:504f
　epidermal, 1:523
　fibrinoid, 1:520
　hyaline, 1:297-298
　infundibular, 2:10, 2:10f
　liquefactive, 1:254
　liver cell, 2:280-284, 2:280f-283f, 2:286f, 2:285.e1f
　　massive, 2:284-285, 2:284f
　　piecemeal, 2:285
　muscle, 1:180-182, 1:180f-181f
　　muscular dystrophy, 1:193, 1:194f
　myocardial, 3:34-41
　with neuronophagia, 1:254
　pancreatic, 2:356-360, 2:359f-360f

Necrosis (Continued)
　retinal, 1:419
　tail tip, 1:560
　thymic, 3:145-146, 3:146f, 3:145.e1f
Necrosuppurative epididymitis, 3:489f
Necrotic bone. *See* Osteonecrosis
Necrotic colitis, 2:99, 2:99f
Necrotic hepatitis, 2:316, 2:316.e1f
Necrotic laryngitis, 2:17
Necrotic orchitis, 3:486
Necrotic stomatitis, 2:17, 2:17f
Necrotic vaginitis and vulvitis, 3:445, 3:445f-446f
Necrotizing enteritis, 2:187, 2:187f-188f
Necrotizing fasciitis, 1:636
Necrotizing leukoencephalitis, 1:392-393
Necrotizing meningoencephalitis, 1:392-393, 1:392f
Necrotizing myelopathy, 1:340, 1:340f
Necrotizing pododermatitis, 1:643
Necrotizing scleritis, 1:477, 1:478f
Necrotizing sialometaplasia, 2:30
Necrotizing vasculitis, 1:200, 1:200f, 3:69, 3:69f
Negative nitrogen balance, 2:73
Nemaline rods
　cats, 1:198-199, 1:199f
　dogs, 1:185, 1:198
Nematodes
　central nervous system and, 1:389-391
　external ear, 1:507
　liver, 2:320
　spirurid, 2:210
Nematodirus spp., 2:213
Neomycin, 2:424
Neonatal alloimmune thrombocytopenia, 3:258
Neonatal copper deficiency, 1:328-329, 1:328f
Neonatal maladjustment syndrome of foals, 1:297
Neonatal periventricular leukomalacia, 1:274
Neonatal respiratory distress syndrome, 2:515-516, 2:516.e1f
　familial forms, 2:516
Neoplasia, 2:76-77, 2:89-90, 2:462. *See also* Carcinomas/adenocarcinomas; Metastasis, tumor
　adrenal cortex, 3:343-348
　adrenal medullary secretory cells, 3:349-352
　classification of, 2:101
　ear
　　external acoustic meatal, 1:507-508
　　internal, 1:494
　　middle, 1:498-499
　endocrine system, 3:356-357
　esophagus and forestomachs, 2:43-44
　female genital system, 3:447-450
　　cervix, 3:449-450, 3:450f
　　ovaries, 3:375-379
　　uterus, 3:449-450, 3:450f
　heart, 3:52-54, 3:52f
　hematopoietic, 3:129-136, 3:129t
　hypercalcemia associated with nonparathyroid, 3:305-310, 3:305f
　invasion of veins, 3:89, 3:89f
　liver, 2:344-352
　lymphoid. *See* Lymphomas
　male genital system
　　penis and prepuce, 3:508-510
　　prostate and bulbourethral gland, 3:503-504, 3:504f

Neoplasia (Continued)
　　spermatic cord, 3:498-499
　　testis and epididymis, 3:492-497
　　vaginal tunic, 3:474
　mammary masses including, 3:459-464, 3:459f, 3:463f
　muscle, 1:240-246
　　muscle pseudotumors, 1:246, 1:246f
　　nonmuscle primary tumors of muscle, 1:244-245
　　rhabdomyoma, 1:241, 1:242f
　　rhabdomyosarcoma, 1:241-243, 1:243f-244f
　　secondary tumors of skeletal muscle, 1:245-246, 1:245f-246f
　nasal cavity and sinuses, 2:478-480, 2:478f
　nervous system, 1:396-406
　ocular, 1:478-488
　oral cavity, 2:20-28
　ovary, 3:375-379
　pancreas
　　endocrine, 2:373-375, 2:374f
　　exocrine, 2:365-368
　parathyroid glands, 3:302-305
　peritoneum, 2:256-257, 2:256f
　pinnal tumor-like growths and, 1:504-505
　pituitary gland, 3:281-289, 3:281f
　pleura, 2:523
　pulmonary, 2:495-500, 2:495b
　salivary glands, 2:30
　skin, 1:703-736
　splenic, 3:169f, 3:191-196
　stomach and intestine, 2:100-111, 2:101t
　systemic inflammation, 3:267-268
　thymic, 3:151-158, 3:152t
　thyroid gland, 3:326-336
　vascular, 3:98-101
Neorickettsia helminthoeca, 2:225-226, 3:148-149, 3:150f, 3:149.e1f
Neorickettsia risticii, 2:200-201
Neospora caninum, 1:387-389, 1:388f, 1:664-665
　abortion and, 3:421-423, 3:422f-423f
　cysts, 1:388f
　myocarditis and, 3:44
Neospora myositis, 1:237
Neosporosis, 1:387-389, 1:388f, 2:238-239
Neostrongylus linearis, 2:565t, 2:567
Nephroblastomas, 2:446-447, 2:446f
　grossly, 2:446
　renal and perirenal lymphosarcoma, 2:447f
　renal cystadenocarcinoma, 2:446.e1f
　true embryonal tumors, 2:446
　urothelial cell carcinoma, 2:447f
Nephrogenic form of diabetes insipidus, 3:291
Nephroliths, 2:453
Nephrons, 2:379, 2:382, 2:391
　atrophy, 2:400
Nephropathy, 2:294, 2:388
　familial, 2:388-391
Nephrosis, 2:422
Nephrotic syndrome, 2:401, 2:414
Nephrotoxicity, 2:426
　ATI, 2:423
　in domestic animals, 2:424b
　nephritis, 2:408
Nerium oleander, 2:89
Nerve sheath neoplasms, 1:245
Nervous system
　astrocytes, 1:260-262, 1:261f
　axon, 1:255-258, 1:256f

Nervous system *(Continued)*
  cytopathology, 1:251-264
  degeneration, 1:303-350
  ependymal cells, 1:262
  infectious agents/diseases inducing inflammatory changes in, 1:351t-352t
  microcirculation, 1:263-264, 1:264f, 1:263.e1f
  microglia, 1:262-263
  neuron, 1:251-258, 1:252f
  oligodendrocytes, Schwann cells, and the myelin sheath, 1:258-260
Nesidioblastosis, 2:373
Nestin, 1:261
Nests, 1:523
  of residual glia, 1:262
Netherlands cattle, diaphragmatic dystrophy in, 1:199
Neural plate, 1:265
Neural tube, 1:265
  defects, 1:265
Neuritis of cauda equina, 1:394-395
Neuroaxonal dystrophies, 1:257-258
Neuroblastomas, 1:402, 3:352-353, 3:353f
  olfatory, 2:479, 2:479f
Neuroblasts, 1:252
Neurodegenerative diseases, 1:317-336
  central neuronopathies and axonopathies, 1:318-326
Neuroectoderm
  anomalies of, 1:419-421
  tumors of ocular, 1:485-486, 1:485f
Neuroendocrine carcinomas, 2:27, 2:478-479
Neuroendocrine cells, 2:27
Neuroendocrine tumors, 2:497-498
Neuroepithelial tissue
  degeneration, 1:492
  tumors, 1:398-403
Neurofibromas, 1:405, 3:53, 3:53f, 3:53.e1f
Neurofibromatosis, 1:724
Neurogenic diabetes insipidus, 2:430
Neurogenic disorders of micturition, 2:451
Neurohypophysis, 3:277-278
  diseases, 3:290-291
Neuromelanins, 1:254-255
Neuromuscular junction, 1:170, 1:170f
Neuromycotoxicoses, tremorgenic, 1:322
Neuronal atrophy, 1:253
Neuronal inclusion-body diseases, 1:320
Neuronal storage diseases, 1:285, 1:473
Neuronal tumors, 1:401
Neuronal vacuolar degeneration of Angora goats, 1:347
Neuronopathies, 1:318-326
Neuronophagia, 1:263, 2:77
Neuronophagic nodules, 1:253f, 1:254
Neurons, 1:251-258
  axons, 1:255-258, 1:256f
  concussion and, 1:302
  degenerative changes, 1:252-255, 1:252f
Neutropenia, 3:109-110
  congenital, 3:110
Neutrophilic cholangitis, 2:307-308, 2:308f
Neutrophilic dermatoses, sterile, 1:696
Neutrophilic vasculitis, 1:526, 1:611
Neutrophils
  in immune-mediated polyarthritis, 1:157-159

Neutrophils *(Continued)*
  in nodular and diffuse dermatitis, 1:526
  production, 3:109
Nevi, linear epidermal, 1:551
Newfoundland dogs
  dilated cardiomyopathy, 3:48
  focal bone dysplasia, 1:56
  hypothyroidism, 1:587
  subvalvular aortic stenosis, 3:20
  vitiligo, 1:555-556
New Zealand Huntaway dogs, 1:334
Niacin, 1:582
Nicotiana tabacum, 1:90
Nictitans gland, protrusion of, 1:424
Nigropallidal encephalomalacia, 1:314, 1:314f
Nipah virus, 1:380-381, 2:501, 2:501f, 2:530
Nitrate toxicity, 1:91
  nervous system and, 1:306
Nitrite poisoning, 1:306
Nitrogen dioxide, 2:518
Nitrosamines, 2:340
Nocardia asteroides, 2:314-315
Nocardia mastitis, 3:457, 3:457f
Nocardioform placentitis, 3:417
Nocardiosis, 1:637-639, 1:638f
Nodal lymphomas, 3:238.e2f
Nodal T-cell lymphomas, 3:229-230
Nodular and diffuse dermatitis, 1:526-527, 1:527f
Nodular auricular chondropathy, 1:697
Nodular dermatofibrosis, 1:692, 1:723
Nodular eosinophilic vasculitis, 1:612
Nodular goiter, 3:322, 3:322f
Nodular granulomatous episcleritis (NGE), 1:476, 1:477f
Nodular hyperplasia
  adrenal cortex, 3:343
  liver, 2:344, 2:344f
  spleen, 3:189-190, 3:190f, 3:189.e2f
Nodular pancreatic hyperplasia, 2:365, 2:365f-366f
Nodular perianal gland hyperplasia, 1:718
Nodular sarcoids, 1:708, 1:709f
Nodules
  accessory cortical, 3:343
  hamartoma, 1:520, 1:705
  lymphoid, 1:522
  neuronophagic, 1:253f, 1:254
  splenic, 3:167-169, 3:167f-168f, 3:169.e1f, 3:191.e1f
Noma, 2:18
Non-angiogenic, nonhematogenic splenic sarcomas, 3:192-194, 3:192f
Non-B, non-T leukocytic neoplasm, 1:403
Noncystic endometrial hyperplasia, 3:383
Nonepidermolytic ichthyosis, 1:531-532
Nonepithelial neoplasms, 2:367
Non-erosive polyarthritis, 1:158-159
Noninfarctive "slow flow", 2:85
Noninflammatory thrombosis of cranial dural sinuses, 1:300
Nonkeratinocytes, epidermal, 1:513
Nonmuscle primary tumors of muscle, 1:244-245
Non-neoplastic lesions, 1:162-163
  mammary enlargement and masses, 3:459-460, 3:459f
  middle ear, 1:498-499
  nasal cavity and sinuses, 2:477-478

Non-neoplastic lesions *(Continued)*
  synovial chondromatosis, 1:162, 1:162f
  synovial cysts, 1:162-163
  synovial pad proliferation, 1:163
Nonparenchymal cells, 2:261-264
Nonprogressive atrophic rhinitis (NPAR), 2:533
Nonspecific reactive hepatitis, 2:306
Nonsteroidal anti-inflammatory drugs (NSAIDs), 2:55-57, 2:85
  cyclooxygenase (COX), 2:55
  gastroduodenal ulceration, 2:55
  toxicity, 2:399, 2:400f
Nonsuppurative meningoencephalomyelitis, 2:121
Nonsuppurative vasculitis and perivasculitis, 1:298f
Nontuberculous mycobacteria, 1:639-640
Nonviral eosinophilic cytoplasmic inclusion bodies, 1:255
Norepinephrine, 3:348, 3:350f
Norfolk Terrier dogs, inherited thrombocytopenia in, 3:258
Normal canine glomerular filtration barrier, transmission electron micrograph of, 2:380f
Normal canine glomerulus, 2:380f
Northern fowl mite, 1:683
Norwegian Dala sheep, collagen dysplasia in, 1:544
Norwegian Dunker dogs, cochleosaccular degeneration in, 1:492
Norwegian Elkhound dogs
  alopecia X, 1:589-590
  chondrodysplasia, 1:43-44
  nephritis, 2:417
Norwegian Forest cats, glycogen storage disease type IV in, 1:205, 1:205f
Notched pinnae, 1:502
Notoedres cati, 1:675
Notoedric mange, 1:675, 1:675f
NPHS1 gene, 2:418
Nuclear glycogenosis, 2:430
Nuclear margination, 1:252-255, 1:252f
Nucleus pulposus, 1:128-129
Nutmeg liver, 2:298
Nutrient arteries, 1:27
Nutrients, assimilation of, 2:69
Nutritional deficiency/disease, 1:60
  atrophy resulting from, 1:177
  of bone, 1:60-84
  exocrine pancreas and, 2:355, 2:362, 2:364
  fatty liver, 2:276
  hyperparathyroidism secondary to, 3:301
  mineral imbalances, 1:80-82
  myocardial necrosis and, 3:34, 3:35f
  myopathy, 1:214-218
    cattle, 1:215-216, 1:216f
    horses, 1:218
    pigs, 1:217
    sheep and goats, 1:216-217
  nutritional secondary hyperparathyroidism, 1:75
  odontodystrophies and, 2:9
  osteochondrosis, 1:132
  retinopathy, 1:470-471
  of skin, 1:580-587
  tooth development and, 1:65
  vitamin imbalances, 1:82-84, 1:581-583

INDEX

O

Oak poisoning, acute, 2:428
Oak shrubs, 2:427-428
Obstructions
  cerebrospinal artery, 1:299-300, 1:299f
  cerebrospinal veins, 1:300
  esophageal, 2:32-33, 2:33f
  obstructive atelectasis, 2:486
  obstructive cholestasis, 2:293
  obstructive urolithiasis, 2:455f
  obstructive uropathy, 2:461.e1
  pancreatic ductal drainage, 2:362
Obturation, 2:74
Occlusion of testicular artery, 3:491
Occult dirofilariasis, 3:84
Occult sarcoids, 1:708, 1:709f
Occupational health and safety, 1:14
Ochratoxin A (OTA), 2:427
Ocular adnexa, 1:423-427
  conjunctiva, 1:424-427
  eyelids, 1:423
  lacrimal system, 1:423-424
  tumors, 1:481-482
Ocular fundus, 1:466
Ocular habronemiasis, 1:425, 1:426f
Ocular neoplasia, 1:478-488
  feline post-traumatic sarcoma, 1:486, 1:487f
  melanocytic tumors, 1:482-485
  ocular neuroectoderm, 1:485-486, 1:485f
  optic nerve tumors, 1:487, 1:487f
  orbital, 1:487-488
  spindle cell tumor of blue-eyed dogs, 1:486
Ocular onchocerciasis, 1:425-426, 1:452
Ocular tuberculosis, 1:449
Odocoileus adenovirus 1, 2:145, 2:145f
Odontoameloblastoma, 2:24
Odontoblasts, 2:4-5, 2:8
Odontoclastic resorptive lesions, 2:10-11
Odontodysplasia cystica congenita, 2:7
Odontodystrophies, 2:8-9
  effects of, 2:9
Odontogenic cysts, 2:6-7
Odontogenic epithelium, 2:23
Odontomas, 2:24
Oesophagostomum radiatum, 2:114-115
Oesophagostomum spp., 2:116, 2:215-216
Oestrus ovis, 2:564-565, 2:564.e3f
Oil of pennyroyal, 2:329
Old dog encephalitis, 1:384-385, 2:576
Old English Sheepdogs
  cochleosaccular degeneration, 1:492
  mitochondrial myopathy, 1:205
  vitiligo, 1:555-556
Oleander poisoning, 2:89, 3:35, 3:35f
  intoxication in llama, 2:89f
Olfactory neuroblastomas, 1:401, 2:479, 2:479f
Oligoastrocytoma, 1:400
Oligodendrocytes, 1:258-260
Oligodendroglioma, 1:400, 1:400f
Oligodontia, 2:6
Oliguria, 2:423
Olivopontocerebellar atrophy, 1:319
Ollulanus tricuspis, 2:211
Omasal transport, failure of, 2:39
Omasitis, 2:42
Omental hernia, 2:79
Omphalomesenteric duct, 2:245
Onchocerca armillata, 3:87-88

Onchocerca cervicalis, 1:248, 1:451-452, 1:687-688
Onchocerca gibsoni, 1:247-248, 1:688
Onchocerca gutturosa, 1:248, 1:687-688
Onchocerca lienalis, 1:248
Onchocerca reticulata, 1:248, 1:687-688
Onchocerciasis, 1:687-688, 1:688f, 3:87-88
Onchocercidae, 1:247
Oncicola canis, 2:227
Oncocytic metaplasia, 2:28
Oncocytomas, 2:478-479
$1,25(OH)_2D_3$, 1:25t
Oophoritis, 3:370-371, 3:371f
Ophthalmitis, equine recurrent, 1:455-456
Ophthalmomyiasis, 1:426
Opisthorchid flukes, 2:323
Opisthorchis felineus, 2:323-324
Opportunisitc bacterial pathogens in foals, 2:571
Optic disc cupping, 1:460, 1:462f
Optic nerve, 1:475-476
  degeneration, 1:476
  hypoplasia, 1:420-421, 1:421f
  tumors, 1:487, 1:487f
Optic neuritis, 1:474-475
  chronic, 1:476
Optic neuropathy, compressive, 1:320
Optimal cutting temperature compound (OCT), 2:383
Oral actinobacillosis, 2:19
Oral candidiasis, 2:14
  neoplastic and like lesions, 2:20-28
Oral cavity, 2:2-28. See also specific components
  buccal cavity/mucosa diseases
    actinobacillosis, 2:18
    bullous pemphigoid, 2:15
    catarrhal stomatitis, 2:14
    circulatory disturbances, 2:12-13
    deep stomatitides, 2:17-19
    eosinophilic ulcer, 2:16
    erosive/ulcerative stomatitides, 2:15-17
    feline calicivirus, 2:15
    feline chronic gingivostomatitis, 2:16
    feline plasma cell gingivitis-pharyngitis, 2:16
    feline ulcerative stomatitis, 2:16
    feline viral rhinotracheitis, 2:16
    foreign bodies, 2:13
    gingivostomatitis, chronic, 2:15
    glossitis, 2:16
    horses, with eosinophilic epitheliotropic disease, 2:16
    inflammation, 2:13-19
    lymphocytic-plasmacytic stomatitis, 2:16
    mucous membrane pemphigoid, 2:15
    oral dermatophilosis, 2:19
    oral eosinophilic granuloma, 2:16
    pemphigus vulgaris, 2:14
    pigmentation, 2:12
    superficial stomatitis, 2:13-14
    thrush/oral candidiasis, 2:14
    uremia, 2:16-17
    vesicular stomatitides, 2:11
  buccal/mucosal disease, 2:12-19
  congenital anomalies, 2:2-4
    brachygnathia inferior/micrognathia, 2:3
    epitheliogenesis imperfecta, 2:4
    facial clefts, 2:2-3
    primary cleft palate, 2:3
    prognathism, 2:3

Oral cavity (Continued)
  dental tissue tumors, 2:22-25
  foot-and-mouth disease lesions, 1:233, 1:233f
  foreign bodies, 2:13, 2:13f
  inflammation, 2:13-19
  neoplastic and like lesions, 2:20-28
  neoplastic/lesions of, 2:20-28
    dental tissues, tumors of, 2:22-25
      acanthomatous ameloblastoma, 2:23
      amyloid-producing odontogenic tumors, 2:23
      feline inductive odontogenic tumor, 2:24
      periodontal ligament origin, fibromatous epulis of, 2:24
    epulis, 2:20
    fibrosarcomas, 2:27
    granular cell tumors, 2:27
    mast cell tumors, 2:27
    melanomas, malignant melanomas, 2:26
    miscellaneous tumors, 2:28
    neuroendocrine carcinomas, 2:27
    oral papillomatosis, 2:22
    pharynx, 2:27
    plasmacytomas, 2:27-28
      extramedullary plasmacytomas, 2:27
    reactive/hyperplastic lesions, 2:21-22
      fibrous hyperplasia, 2:21
      peripheral giant cell granuloma, 2:21
      pyogenic granuloma, 2:21
    squamous cell carcinoma (SCC), 2:25-26
    vascular tumors, 2:28
  papillomatosis, 2:22
  parasitic diseases, 2:19
  reactive and hyperplastic lesions, 2:21-22
  teeth and tooth development
    fluorosis and, 1:84-86
    mandibular osteomyelitis and, 1:103, 1:103f
    undernutrition and, 1:65
    vitamin A deficiency and, 1:82-83
  teeth/dental tissue disease, 1:20-21
  teeth/dental tissues diseases, 2:4-12
    cementum, 2:5-6
    degenerative conditions of, 2:7-9
      abnormal wear, 2:8
      calcium deficiency, 2:8
      dental attrition, 2:7-8
      odontodystrophies, 2:8-9
      phosphorus deficiency, 2:8
      pigmentation, 2:7
      subnormal wear, 2:8
    developmental anomalies of, 2:6-7
      anodontia, 2:6
      cystic dental inclusions, 2:7
      heterotopic polyodontia, 2:6
      odontogenic cysts, 2:6-7
      polyodontia, 2:6
    enamel, 2:5
    hypercementosis, 2:6
    malassez, epithelial rests of, 2:6
    periodontal ligament, 2:6
  teeth/periodontium, infectious/inflammatory diseases of, 2:9-12
    bacterial diseases, involving tooth surfaces, 2:9
    cara inchada, 2:12
    cats, 2:10-11
    cattle, 2:10
    dental calculus, 2:9

Oral cavity *(Continued)*
  dental caries, 2:9-11
    pit/fissure caries, 2:10
    smooth-surface caries, 2:10
  gingivitis, 2:11
  infundibular necrosis, 2:10
  materia alba, 2:9
  periodontal disease, 2:11-12
  pulpitis, 2:11
  sheep, 2:10
  tonsils, diseases, 2:19-20
Oral dermatophilosis, 2:19
Oral dysphagia, 2:33
Oral eosinophilic granuloma, 2:16
Oral lesions, 2:121
Oral papillomatosis, 2:22, 2:22f
Orbit, 1:477-478
  neoplasms, 1:487-488
Orbital celluitis, 1:478
Orbital myositis, 1:478
Orbital (extra-adrenal) paragangliomas, 3:356
Orbivirus, 1:281, 3:430-431
Orchitis, 3:485-487
  boars, 3:486-487
  bulls, 3:486
  camelids, 3:487
  dogs and cats, 3:487, 3:488f
  interstitial, 3:486
  intratubular, 3:486, 3:486f
  necrotic, 3:486
  small ruminants, 3:487
  stallions, 3:487
Orf virus, 1:616-617
Organic anion-transporting polypeptide (OATP), 2:293, 2:325
Organobromine, 1:571-572
Organochlorine, 1:571-572
Organogenesis
  eye, 1:410-412, 1:410f
  pancreas, 2:353-354, 2:354f
Organomercurial poisoning, 1:320-321, 1:321f
Organophosphate poisoning, 1:326
Ornithonyssus syviarum, 1:683
Orthobunyaviruses, 1:280
Orthopoxvirus, 1:616, 1:619-621
Oslerus osleri, 2:586, 2:586f
Oslerus rostratus, 2:591
Osmotic diuresis, 2:425
Osseous drift, 1:24-25
Osseous metaplasia, 1:304, 2:517, 2:517.e1f
Osseous sequestration, 1:97
Ossification, endochondral, 1:22, 1:22f
  rickets and, 1:71-72
Ossification centers, 1:22
Ossification groove of Ranvier, 1:23
Ossifying fibrodysplasia, 1:213
Ossifying fibroma, 1:109, 1:109f
Ossifying pachymeningitis, 1:304
Osteitis, 1:97
Osteoarthritis, 1:137
Osteoblastic osteosarcomas, 1:113, 1:113f
Osteoblasts, 1:17-19, 1:17f
  modeling, 1:24, 1:26f
  necrotic bone and, 1:96
  osteosarcoma, 1:111-112
  remodeling, 1:26
  in vitamin D toxicity, 1:89

Osteocalcin, 1:19, 1:27
Osteocartilaginous metaplasia, 3:34, 3:34f
Osteochondrodysplasia, 1:44-45
  cats, 1:45-46
Osteochondromas, 1:116-117, 1:117f
  cats, 1:117, 1:117f
  horses, 1:116
Osteochondromatosis, 1:54
  dogs, 1:54, 1:117f
  horses, 1:54
Osteochondrosis, 1:81, 1:132-135
  dissecans, 1:132-134, 1:133f-134f
  horses, 1:134, 1:134f
  latens, 1:132, 1:132f
  manifesta, 1:132, 1:133f
  pigs, 1:133-134
  sheep, 1:135
Osteoclastic bone resorption, 1:18-19
Osteoclasts, 1:17-19
  remodeling, 1:26
Osteocytes, 1:17-18
Osteofluorosis, 1:85
Osteogenesis imperfecta
  cats, 1:50
  cattle, 1:37t, 1:46-50, 1:47f-49f
  dogs, 1:50
  sheep, 1:49, 1:49f-50f
Osteoid, 1:17-19
  seam, 1:20
    rickets and, 1:73, 1:73f
Osteoliposarcoma, 1:123
Osteolysis, 1:109
Osteoma, 1:109
Osteomalacia, 1:61, 1:66, 1:68-74
  calcium deficiency in, 1:69
  lesions of, 1:73
  phosphorus deficiency in, 1:68-69
  vitamin D deficiency, 1:68
Osteomyelitis, 1:97, 2:12
  acute, 1:95, 1:95f
  bacterial, 1:98-103, 1:98f-99f
  cats, 1:99-100
  cattle, 1:99
  dogs, 1:99-100
  fungal, 1:103-104, 1:104f
  horses, 1:99, 1:99f, 1:101f
  mandibular, 1:102-103, 1:103f, 2:11
  periodontal, 1:101f
  suppurative, 1:100-101, 1:102f
  vertebral, 1:101-102, 1:102f
Osteonecrosis, 1:94-97
  morphology and fate of necrotic bone in, 1:95-97
Osteonectin, 1:19
Osteons, 1:20, 1:21f
Osteopathy, metaphyseal, 1:105-106, 1:105f-106f
Osteopenia, 1:61
Osteopetrosis, 1:37t, 1:50-53
  cattle, 1:51-52, 1:51f
  deer, 1:52
  dogs, 1:52
  horses, 1:52, 1:52f
  sheep, 1:52, 1:52f
Osteopontin, 1:19
Osteoporosis, 1:61, 1:63-68
  copper deficiency in, 1:81
  corticosteroid-induced, 1:67
  definition, 1:63
  disuse, 1:67
  gross lesions of, 1:63-64

Osteoporosis *(Continued)*
  growth arrest lines and, 1:64
  histologic examination, 1:64
  lactational, 1:65-66, 1:66f
  nutritional, 1:61, 1:64-66
  parasite-induced, 1:67f
  pigs, 1:64f
  postmenopausal, 1:64
  senile, 1:64
  starvation, 1:64-65, 1:65f
  vitamin A toxicity and, 1:67, 1:87
Osteoprotegerin (OPG), 1:26, 3:295
Osteosarcomas, 1:95, 1:110-116, 1:110f
  cats, 1:110
  cytology, 1:111, 1:111f
  dogs, 1:95, 1:110, 1:110f
  extraskeletal, 1:115
  grading systems, 1:115
  nasal, 2:480
  parosteal, 1:115, 1:115f
  radiography, 1:111
  subtypes, 1:113-114
Ostertagia spp., 2:54-55
Ostertagiosis, 2:205-207, 2:206f
Otitis externa, 1:497, 1:502-503, 1:502f, 1:497.e2f
  feline proliferative, necrotizing, 1:503-504
Otitis interna, 1:493, 1:493.e2f
Otitis media, 1:496-498, 1:497.e1f
  with effusion, 1:498
Otoacariasis, 1:505-506
Otobius megnini, 1:507
Otodectes cynotis mite, 1:505, 1:506f
Otodectic mange, 1:677-678
Otognathia, 1:496
Otosclerosis, 1:493, 1:496
Ototoxicity, 1:494, 1:494.e1f
Outer hair cells of ear, 1:491
Ovarian hemangiomas, 3:378
Ovarian remnants, 3:366
  cysts arising from, 3:366-367, 3:367f-368f
Ovarian suspensory ligaments, 2:76-77
Ovaries, 3:366, 3:366f-367f
  age-related degenerative changes, 3:371, 3:371f
  circulatory disturbances, 3:381-382
  cysts, 3:371-372, 3:372f
  neoplastic conditions, 3:375-379
  pathology, 3:370-375
Overinflation of alveoli, 2:486, 2:487.e1f
Ovine fleece rot, 1:634
Ovine herpesvirus 2, 1:625-627, 2:132
Ovine lymphomas, 3:237, 3:237f
Ovine muscular dystrophy, 1:196-197, 1:196f
Ovine parainfluenza virus, 2:557
Ovine progressive pneumonia, 2:558-560, 2:559f, 2:558.e1f
Ovine pulmonary adenocarcinoma (OPA), 2:560-562, 2:561f, 2:561.e1f
Ovine respiratory syncytial virus, 2:557
Ovine white-liver disease, 2:276
Ovotestes, 3:361-362, 3:362f, 3:365f
Oxalate calculi, 2:456-457
Oxalate uroliths, 2:457
  prevalence of, 2:457
Oxalic acid, 2:456
Oxibendazole-diethylcarbamazine, 2:329
Oxidative stress and testicular function, 3:467
Oxygen exposure and lung injury, 2:518

Oxyphilic adenomas, 3:327
Oxyuris equi, 1:688
Ozone, 3:298

P

Pachygyria, 1:268
Pagetoid reticulosis (PR), 3:232-234, 3:233f
Paint horses
    deafness in, 1:493
    equine systemic calcinosis in, 1:223-224
    melanocytopenic hypomelanosis, 1:555
Palyam virus, 3:431
Panarteritis, 3:71
Pancreas, 2:353-375
    abscesses, 2:361
    diabetes mellitus and, 2:370-373, 2:371f
    endocrine, 2:368-375
        diabetes mellitus, 2:370-373, 2:371f
            cats, 2:372, 2:373f
            cattle, 2:372
            diabetic cataract, 1:443
            dogs, 2:373
            horses, 2:372
            retinopathies, 1:472
        hyperplastic and neoplastic diseases, 2:373-375, 2:374f
    exocrine, 2:353-368
        atrophy, 2:362-363, 2:362f
        hyperplastic and neoplastic lesions, 2:365-368
        insufficiency, 2:363-364
        necrosis, 2:357-360, 2:359f-360f
        organogenesis, 2:353-354, 2:354f
        pancreatitis, 2:360-362
        parasitic diseases, 2:365
    general considerations, 2:353
    necrosis, 2:249
Pancreatic bladder, 2:355-356
Pancreatic endocrine neoplasia, 2:373-375
Pancreatic hypoplasia, 2:355
Pancreatic lipofuscinosis, 2:356
Pancreatic phlegmon, 2:361
Pancreatic polypeptide, 2:368
Pancreatic polypeptide-secreting islet neoplasia (PPoma), 2:375
Pancreatitis, 2:360-362, 2:361f
Pancreatolithiasis, 2:361-362
Paneth cells, 2:61-63
Panhypopituitarism, 3:280, 3:280f
Panicum spp., 2:339, 2:339f
Panniculitis, 1:523, 1:528-529, 1:529f
    sterile nodular, 1:701-702, 1:701f
Pannus keratitis, 1:438
Panophthalmitis, 1:446
Panthothenic acid, 1:582
Pantropic canine coronavirus, 2:577
Pan-vasculitis, 3:72
Papillary adenomas
    ears, 1:500
    pulmonary, 2:495
    thyroid, 3:327
Papillary carcinomas of thyroid, 3:330
Papillary hyperplasia, 2:462
Papilledema, 1:475
Papillomas, 2:462
    cats, 1:711-712, 1:712f
    cattle, 1:706-707
    choroid plexus, 1:401, 1:401f
    conjunctival, 1:481
    cutaneous, 1:706-712, 1:706f
    dogs, 1:710-711, 1:710f, 1:711f
    epidermal, 1:706-712

Papillomas *(Continued)*
    horses, 1:707-710
    idiopathic squamous, 1:705
    laryngeal, 2:482
    nasal, 2:479, 2:479.e1f
    pigs, 3:449
    sheep and goats, 1:710
Papillomatosis, 1:523
Papillomatous digital dermatitis (PDD), 1:644-645, 1:644f
Papillomaviruses, 1:628
    aural plaques and, 1:504
    camelids, 1:712
    cats, 1:711-712, 1:712f
    cattle, 1:530, 1:706-707, 1:707f
    dogs, 1:710-711, 1:710f, 1:710t
    horses, 1:707-710, 1:708f, 1:708t
    lesions of epidermis, 1:706-712, 1:706f
    rabbits, 1:712
    sheep and goats, 1:710
Papillon dogs, axonal dystrophy in, 1:325
Papules, 1:524
Paracentral liver necrosis, 2:283-284, 2:284f
Paracortical tissue, lymph node, 3:197
Parafilaria multipapillosa, 1:688-689
Parafilariasis, 1:688-689
Paragangliomas, 1:406, 3:354-356
    aortic body adenoma and carcinoma, 3:354-355, 3:354f
    carotid body adenoma and carcinoma, 3:355-356
    development, structure, and function, 3:354
    extra-adrenal, 3:356
    heart-base tumors derived from ectopic thyroid, 3:356
Paragonimus spp., 2:537, 2:591, 2:591f, 2:591.e2f
Parahyperthyroidism, 1:75
Parainfluenza virus, 2:557
    canine, 2:576
Parakeratosis
    Labrador Retriever nasal, 1:550
    swine, 1:584
Paralysis, laryngeal, 2:481, 2:481f
Paramesonephric (Müllerian) ducts, 3:360-361, 3:361f
    arrested development of, 3:367-369, 3:368f
    cysts, 3:371
Parametritis, 3:390, 3:390f
Paramphistomatidae, 2:43, 2:43f
Paramphistome, 2:226
Paramphistomum spp., 2:43, 2:43f
Paramyxoviral encephalomyelitis of pigs, 1:380-381
Paramyxovirus, 2:116
Paranasal meningioma, 1:396, 1:397f
Paranasal sinus diseases, 2:477, 2:477f, 2:477.e4f
    cysts, 2:478
    paranasal meningioma, 1:397f
Paraneoplastic hypoglycemia, 2:111
Paraneoplastic necrotizing myopathy, 1:224
Paraneoplastic syndromes, cutaneous, 1:691-693
Paranesoplastic pemphigus, 1:603
Parapoxviral infections, 2:139-142
    bovine papular stomatitis virus (BPSV), 1:616, 1:618-619, 2:39-40, 2:139-140, 2:140f

Parapoxviral infections *(Continued)*
    infectious bovine rhinotracheitis (IBR), 1:425, 2:140-142, 2:525f, 2:537-539, 2:538f
    parapox virus of red deer, 1:616, 1:619
Paraquat, 2:519
Parasagittal fractures, 1:36
Parascaris equorum, 2:219, 2:574
Parasite hypersensitivity, 1:599-600
Parasite-induced osteoporosis, 1:67f
Parasitic arthropods, 1:666-684
Parasitic endocarditis, 3:32
Parasitic gastritis, 2:54
Parasitic infections, 1:234-240
    abortion and, 3:421-423
    central nervous system and, 1:386-391
    conjunctivitis, 1:425-426
    cysticercosis, 1:239-240, 1:239f
    ear
        external, 1:505-507
        middle, 1:498
    endophthalmitis, 1:451-452
    eosinophilic myositis, 1:236-237, 1:236f-237f
    erythrocyte, 3:114
    esophagus, 2:34-35, 2:35f
    forestomachs, 2:43, 2:43f
    gastric, 2:209-210, 2:209f
    gastritis, 2:54
    hepatozoonosis, 1:240
    leishmaniasis, 1:240
    liver pigments and, 2:272
    lymphangitis, 3:98
    lymph nodes, 3:212
    myocarditis and, 3:43-44, 3:44.e1f
    oral cavity, 2:19
    pancreas, 2:365
    peritoneum, 2:255
    respiratory system and, 2:536-537, 2:554-557, 2:564-567, 2:574, 2:585-587, 2:590, 2:590f, 2:536.e2f
    sarcocystosis, 1:234-236, 1:235f
    tendons, 1:247-248
    thrombophlebitis, 3:91-94
    Toxoplasma and *Neospora* myositis, 1:237
    trachea, 2:483
    trichinellosis, 1:237-238
Parasitic lymphangitis, 3:98
Parasitic thrombophlebitis, 3:91-94
Parasitology, 1:11
Parastrongylus cantonensis, 1:389, 1:390f
Parathyroid glands, 3:292-295, 3:292f
    carcinomas, 3:304, 3:304f
    diseases, 3:297-302
Parathyroid hormone (PTH), 1:18, 1:25t, 1:61-62, 2:385, 3:272, 3:292-295, 3:292f
    biological action, 3:294-295
    biosynthesis and secretion, 3:292-294
    -related protein, 3:274, 3:305-306
Paratuberculosis. See Johne's disease
Parbendazole, 1:91
Parelaphostrongylus tenuis, 1:390, 1:689-690
Parenchymal cells, 2:261-262
Parietal cells, 2:45, 2:51
    atrophy, 2:47
    atrophy of parietal cell mass, 2:47
    mass, atrophy of, 2:47
    presumably loss of, 2:47
Parietal pericardium, 3:3
Parosteal osteosarcoma
    cats, 1:115, 1:115f
    dogs, 1:115

Pars distalis, 3:276, 3:277f
  adenoma, 3:287-288, 3:288f
Pars intermedia, 3:276
  adenomas, 3:282-285, 3:283f-284f
Pars nervosa, 3:277
Parson Russell Terrier dogs, 1:325
Pars tuberalis, 3:276
Particle deposition in lungs, 2:471
Parturient paresis, 3:299
Parvoviral enteritis, 2:153-158
  cats, 2:153, 2:155f
  cattle, 2:44, 2:157-158, 3:429-430
  dogs, 2:156-157, 2:156f-157f
Parvoviral infections, 1:628
  myocardial necrosis and, 3:34
  myocarditis and, 3:42, 3:43f
  in pregnant uterus, 3:429-430
  thymic atrophy and, 3:145
Passive congestion
  of liver, 2:297-298, 2:298f, 2:298.e1f
  of spleen, 3:169
Pastern leukocytoclastic vasculitis, 1:612
Pasteurellacae, 2:543, 2:562
Pasteurella multocida, 1:230, 2:543-544, 2:562
Patellar luxations, 1:137, 1:137f
  dogs, 1:137, 1:137f
  horses, 1:137
Patent ductus arteriosus (PDA), 3:17-18, 3:18f-19f
Pathologic fracture, 1:33-36
Pathologists, competence of, 1:14-15
Patnaik system, 1:731
Pattern recognition, 1:3-4, 1:3f
  molecules, 2:63
Pautrier's microabscess, 1:523, 1:523f
Pax genes, 1:21-22
PCR-based diagnosis, 2:435
PCR for antigen receptor rearrangements (PARR) assay, 3:215, 3:216f
Pearsonema mucronata, 2:443
Pediculosis, 1:671
Peer review, 1:14
Pekingese dogs
  degenerative diseases of cartilaginous joints, 1:143-144
  hyperestrogenism, 1:589
Pelger-Huët anomaly (PHA), 3:110
Peliosis hepatis/telangiectasis, 2:299-300, 2:299f-300f, 2:299.e1f
Pelodera dermatitis, 1:689, 1:689f
Pelvic flexure, infarction of, 2:85f
Pelvic hernia, 2:79
Pelvis deformities, 1:56-57
Pembroke Welsh Corgi dogs. *See* Corgi dogs
Pemphigus complex, 1:518, 1:600-603
Pemphigus erythematosus (PE), 1:602
Pemphigus foliaceus, 1:601, 1:601f
Pemphigus vegetans, 1:602
Pemphigus vulgaris (PV), 1:602, 1:602f, 2:14
Pendrin, 3:311-312
Penis and prepuce, 3:505-510, 3:506f
  inflammation, 3:506-508
  neoplasms, 3:508-510
Pentachlorophenol (PCP), 1:572
Pentastomiasis, 2:585
Pepsin, 2:45
Peptic ulcers, 2:55
  chronic, 2:56
Peptides, immunoreactive, 3:285, 3:285f

Perendale sheep, 1:324
Perforating dermatitis, 1:699, 1:699f
Perforation, 2:48
  corneal, 1:437, 1:437f
  esophageal, 2:32-33
  rectal, 2:247
Perianal glands, 1:517
  adenomas, 1:718, 1:718f
  carcinomas, 1:718
  epitheliomas, 1:718
Periapical abscess, 2:11
Periarteriolar lymphoid sheaths (PALS), 3:159-160
Periarteriolar macrophage sheath (PAMS), 3:160-161
Periarteritis nodosa, 3:71
Periarticular fibroma, 1:161
Periarticular histiocytic sarcoma, 3:252f, 3:250.e1f
Peribronchiolar metaplasia, 2:495, 2:495.e2f
Pericardial sac, 3:2-3
Pericarditis, 3:25-27
  constrictive, 3:26, 3:27f
  fibrinous, 3:25-26, 3:26f
  purulent, 3:26
  traumatic, 3:39
Pericardium, 3:5
  congenital absence of, 3:22
  disease, 3:24-27
    noninflammatory lesions, 3:24-25, 3:24f
  hemo-, 3:25, 3:25f
  hydro-, 3:24-25, 3:24f
  serous atrophy of fat of, 3:25, 3:25f
Perichondrial ring of LaCroix, 1:23
Periciliary liquid layer, 2:471-472
Perifolliculitis, 1:528
  demodectic mange and, 1:680
Perilla ketone, 2:519
Perimetritis, 3:390
Perineal hernias, 2:80
Perinephric abscess, 2:439
Perinephric pseudocyst, 2:396.e2f
Perineurioma, 1:405
Periodic acid-Schiff (PAS) positive, amylase-resistant inclusions, 1:204
Periodic acid-Schiff stain, 2:383
Periodic paralyses, 1:202
Periodontal bone expansion, 1:101f
Periodontal disease, 2:11-12, 2:12f
Periodontal ligament, 2:5-6
Periodontal ligament origin
  fibromatous epulides of, 2:24-25
  fibromatous epulis of, 2:24
Periodontal osteomyelitis, 1:101f
Periodontium, 2:6
  infectious and inflammatory diseases of, 2:9-12
Perioophoritis, 3:371
Periorchitis, 3:473-474, 3:474f
Periosteal damage, 1:33
Periosteal fibrosarcomas, 1:121
Periosteum, 1:24, 1:24f
Periostitis, 1:97
Peripheral axonopathies, 1:334-336
Peripheral chromatolysis, 1:253
Peripheral circulatory failure, 3:10
Peripheral giant cell granuloma, 2:21
Peripheral nerve sheath tumors, 1:404-405, 1:406f

Peripheral nervous system tumors, 1:404-406
Peripheral neuroblastic tumors, 1:405-406
Peripheral T-cell lymphomas, 3:229, 3:229f
Peripheral vestibular disease, 1:494
Peripheral vestibular function, 1:490
Periportal interface hepatitis, 2:301-302, 2:302f, 2:304f
Periportal liver necrosis, 2:283
Perirenal edema, 2:427f
Peritoneal milky spots, 2:244
Peritoneopericardial diaphragmatic hernia, 2:245, 3:22
Peritoneum and retroperitoneum, 2:244-257
  abnormal contents in, 2:247-249
  anomalies, 2:245
  ascites, 2:248-249
  cysts, 2:256
  general considerations, 2:244-245
  neoplasia, 2:256-257, 2:256f
  parasitic diseases, 2:255
  peritonitis, 2:249-255
  reactions to injury, 2:245-246
Peritonitis, 2:249-255
  cats, 2:253-255, 2:254f, 3:90, 3:90f
    -associated uveitis, 1:453, 1:453f
    lymph nodes and, 3:206f
    spleen and, 3:184f
  cattle, 2:251-252, 2:251f
  consequences of, 2:250-251
  dogs, 2:252-253
  horses, 2:251
  pigs, 2:252, 2:252f
  sheep and goats, 2:252
Peritubular capillaries, 2:398
Perivascular cuffing, 1:263, 1:264f, 1:366
Perivascular dermatitis, 1:525, 1:525f
Perivascular pyogranulomatous nephritis, 2:432f
Perivascular Virchow-Robin space, 1:263
Perivascular wall tumor (PWTs), 1:723, 1:724f
Perivasculitis, cerebrospinal, 1:298-299, 1:298f
Periventricular leukomalacia of neonates, 1:274
Peromelia, 1:56
Perosomus elumbus, 1:57, 1:277-278
Persian cats
  Chediak-Higashi syndrome, 3:259
  epidermolysis bullosa, 1:536
  feline ceruminous cystomatosis, 1:507
  feline corneal sequestrum, 1:434, 1:434f
Persistence of the right aortic arch, 3:23-24, 3:23f
Persistent atrial standstill, 3:51
Persistent hyaloid artery, 1:417
Persistent hyperplastic primary vitreous, 1:417-418, 1:418f
Persistently infected (PI) calf, 2:122
Persistent Meckel's diverticulum, 2:74
Persistent posterior perilenticular vascular tunic, 1:417
Persistent pupillary membrane, 1:415, 1:416f
Persistent vitelline artery, 2:245
Persistent vitelline duct, 2:245
Peruvian Paso horses, osteopetrosis in, 1:52
Peste des petits ruminants virus (PPRV), 2:115, 2:130-131, 2:131f, 2:557
Pestiviruses, 1:281-283, 2:122-128
Petechiae, 2:397

Peundculated lipoma, 2:256, 2:257f
Peyer's patches, 2:63, 2:124-126
PFK. See Phosphofructokinase (PFK) deficiency
Phacoclastic uveitis, 1:457-459, 1:458f-459f
Phacolytic uveitis, 1:457
Phaeohyphomycosis, 1:654-655, 1:655f
Phalaris poisoning, 1:292-293, 1:293f
  myocardial necrosis and, 3:36
Pharyngeal (branchial) cysts, 2:29
Pharyngeal dysphagia, 2:33
Pharynx, 2:480-481
  cysts, 2:29
  dysphagia, 2:33
  lymphoid hyperplasia, 2:480.e3f
  neuroendocrine carcinoma of, 2:27
Phenobarbital, 2:329
Phenothiazine photosensitization, 1:579
Phenotype, gonad, 3:360
Phenotypic sexual development, 3:360
Phenytoin, 2:329
Pheochromocytoma, 3:89, 3:89f, 3:349-351, 3:350f-352f
Phlebectasia, 3:89
Phlebitis, 3:90, 3:90f
Phlebothrombosis, 3:89-91
Phomopsin, 2:334-335, 2:335f
Phosphate-buffered 10% formalin, 1:8
Phosphatonins, 1:63
Phosphofructokinase (PFK) deficiency, 1:186-187, 1:290, 3:126
  English Springer Spaniels and American Cocker Spaniels, 1:204-205
Phospholipidosis, 2:278
  alveolar, 2:517, 2:517.e1f
Phosphorus
  calcium homeostasis and, 1:61-63
  deficiency, 1:61, 2:8
    odontodystrophy and, 2:8
    osteoporosis and, 1:66
    rickets and osteomalacia and, 1:68-69
  liver toxicity, 2:332-333
Phosphotungstic acid hematoxylin (PTAH), 1:241
Photoaggravated dermatoses, 1:580
Photoallergy, 1:575
Photography, 1:12
Photomicroscopy, 1:12
Photosensitization, 1:575, 2:294, 2:294f
  dermatitis, 1:577-580, 1:578f
  hepatogenous, 1:579-580
  phenothiazine, 1:579
  primary, 1:578-579
  resulting from defective pigment synthesis, 1:579
Phthisis bulbi, 1:448
Phycomycosis, intestinal, 2:201
Phylloerythrin, 1:579-580
Physaloptera spp., 2:54, 2:211
Physeal dysplasia in cats, 1:46, 1:46f
Physicochemical diseases of skin, 1:558-575
  chemical injury, 1:566-575
  physical injury, 1:559-566
Physiologic steatosis, 2:275
Physis, 1:22, 1:22f
  bacterial osteomyelitis, 1:98-99, 1:99f
  hormonal regulation of, 1:24, 1:25t
  osteoporosis, 1:64, 1:65f
  rickets, 1:70-71, 1:71f
Physocephalus spp., 2:54
Phytobezoars, 2:38, 2:50, 2:75-76
Phytophoto-contact dermatitis, 1:578-579

Pick bodies, 1:255
Picornaviridae, 2:117, 3:43
Piebaldism, 1:555
Piecemeal liver necrosis, 2:285
Piedra, 1:660-661
Pigeon fever, 1:230
Pigeonpox virus, 1:616
Pigmentary incontinence, 1:523
Pigmentation
  buccal cavity, 2:12
  disorders, 1:554-558
    acquired hyperpigmentation, 1:554
    acquired hypopigmentation, 1:557
    acromelanism, 1:555
    canine acanthosis nigricans, 1:555
    copper deficiency, 1:558, 1:558f-559f
    focal macular melanosis, 1:554
    hyper-, 1:554-555
    hypo-, 1:555-558
    leukotrichia, 1:557-558
  drug-induced thyroid, 3:325
  liver, 2:270-272, 2:271f
  tooth, 2:7
Pigment granuloma, 2:274-275, 2:275f
Pigments storage, 1:254
Pilar cysts, 1:704
Pilomatricomas, 1:716-717, 1:716f
Pilus adhesins, 2:168
Pimelea spp., 2:519-520
Pineal tumors, 1:403
Pinnae, 1:501
  cropped or notched, 1:502
  dermatologic diseases, 1:503-504
  tumor-like growths and neoplasia, 1:504-505
Pinnal necrosis in pigs, 1:503, 1:503.e1f
Pinworms, 1:688
Pit caries, 2:10
Pithomyces chartarum, 2:335
Pituicytoma, 3:291, 3:291f
Pituitary gland, 3:276-291
  blood supply to, 3:278
  chromophobe carcinoma, 3:288
  cysts, 3:279-281, 3:280f
  development, structure, and function, 3:276-278, 3:276f
  diseases, 3:278-281, 3:279f
  neoplasia, 3:281-289, 3:281f
  tumors
    granular cell, 3:289
    metastatic to, 3:288-289, 3:289f
PKD1 gene defect, 2:395-396
Placenta
  adventitial, 3:396-397
  mineralization, 3:397
  subinvolution of placental sites, 3:441, 3:441f
Placentitis, 3:415, 3:415f, 3:418f
  mycotic, 3:419, 3:419f
  nocardioform, 3:417
Plant toxicities, 1:90-91, 1:219-220
  avocado, 3:38
  coyotillo, 1:326
  cyanide poisoning, 1:305-306
  cycad, 1:322, 1:323f
  fluoracetate, 3:38
  gousiekte, 3:38
  hepatogenous photosensitization and, 1:580
  horses, 1:91
  liver and, 2:329-344
  mesquite, 1:326

Plant toxicities *(Continued)*
  myocardial necrosis and, 3:34-41, 3:35f
  parathyroid suppression associated with, 3:301-302, 3:301f
  Romulea, 1:322
  sheep, 1:90-91
Plaque, 2:9
Plaques, 1:524
  amniotic, 3:397
  canine pigmented, 1:710-711, 1:711f
Plasma cells
  gingivitis-pharyngitis, 2:16
  hemostasis disorders, 3:255-268
  hyperplasia, 3:201
  myeloma
    cats, 1:123
    dogs, 1:123, 1:123f
    horses, 1:123
  in nodular and diffuse dermatitis, 1:527
  pododermatitis, 1:613-614
  tumor, 1:403
Plasmacytic/lymphocytic synovitis, 1:159
Plasmacytomas, 2:27-28, 3:226-228, 3:228f, 3:226.e1f
  laryngeal, 2:482
Plasma-mediated fibrinolysis, 3:266-267
Plasma membrane, BMZ, 1:513-514
Plasmacytomas, 1:735, 1:735f
Platelet-activating factor (PAF), 3:256
Platelet-derived growth factor (PDGF), 3:257, 3:257f
Platelet Function Analyzer (PFA), 3:257-258
Platelet integrin, $\alpha IIb\beta III$ (or GPIIb/IIIa), 3:256
Platelets
  adhesion, 3:256
  aggregation, 3:256-257
    test, 3:257-258
  disorders, 3:257-260
    acquired, 3:260
    intrinsic, 3:259-260
    thrombocytopenia, 3:258
    von Willebrand disease, 3:258-259
  function evaluation, 3:257-258
  hyperreactivity, 3:260
  plug formation, 3:255-257
Platynosomum fastosum, 2:322
Pleomorphic adenomas, 2:30
Pleomorphic rhabdomyosarcoma, 1:241-243, 1:244f
Pleura, 2:520-523
  neoplasms, 2:523
    mesothelioma, 2:523, 2:523.e2f
  noninflammatory pleural effusions, 2:521
  pleural effusions, 2:520
    noninflammatory, 2:521
  pleuritis, 2:521-523, 2:522f, 2:521.e3f, 2:521.e1f
  pneumothorax, 2:487, 2:487f, 2:521, 2:521.e3f
Pleuritis, 2:521-523, 2:522f, 2:521.e3f
  suppurative, 2:522, 2:521.e1f
Pleuropneumonia, 2:571-572
Plexiform arteriopathy, 2:492, 2:492f
Pneumatosis cystoides intestinalis, 2:87
Pneumoconiosis, 2:518
Pneumocystis carinii, 2:536f, 3:140
  respiratory system and, 2:535-536, 2:536f
Pneumonia
  aspiration, 2:508-509, 2:508f-509f, 2:508.e1f
  meconium, 2:516, 2:516.e1f

Pneumonia *(Continued)*
  atypical, 2:509
  bacterial, 2:542-546, 2:545f, 2:562-563, 2:562f
    equine, 2:571-572
  bronchointerstitial, 2:511-512, 2:514.e2f
  caseonecrotic broncho-, 2:553f
  dogs, 2:577
  embolic, 2:520, 2:520.e2f
  eosinophilic interstitial, 2:513.e1
  granulomatous interstitial, 2:513
  hypersensitivity, 2:512-513
  interstitial, 2:509
  lipid, 2:516-518, 2:516.e1f
  ovine progressive, 2:558-560, 2:559f, 2:558.e1f
  proliferative and necrotizing, 2:529, 2:529.e1f
Pneumonyssoides caninum, 2:585
Pneumoperitoneum, 2:247
Pneumothorax, 2:487, 2:487f, 2:521, 2:521.e3f
Poisoning
  arsenic, 1:327-328, 1:570
  carbon monoxide, 1:306
  copper, 2:343
  corynetoxin, 1:309
  coyotillo, 1:326
  cyanide, 1:305-306
  cycad, 1:322, 1:323f
  fluoracetate, 1:306
  gangrenous ergotism and fescue toxicosis, 1:572-573, 1:573f
  hexachlorophene, 1:344-345, 1:345f
  lead, 1:86, 1:87f, 1:316-317
  mercury, 1:570
  mimosine, 1:572
  myocardial necrosis and, 3:35, 3:37-38
  nitrate/nitrite, 1:306
  organochlorine/organobromine, 1:571-572
  organomercurial, 1:320-321, 1:321f
  organophosphate, 1:326
  Phalaris, 1:292-293, 1:293f
  quassinoid, 1:574-575
  salt, 1:314-315
  selenium, 1:570 571, 1:571f
  solanum, 1:321-322
  thallium, 1:568-569, 1:569f
  trachyandra, 1:292
  trichothecene toxicoses, 1:573-574
  vetch, 1:574
  vitamin D, 3:61
  yellow-wood tree, 2:428
Polioencephalomalacia, 1:297, 1:297f, 1:310f-311f, 2:43
  ruminants, 1:309-312, 1:310f-311f
Poliomalacia, 1:307-308
Poll evil, 1:155-156
Polypay sheep, osteopetrosis in, 1:52, 1:52f
Polyalveolar lobe, 2:485
Polyarteritis nodosa, 3:71
Polyarthritis, 1:148
  erosive, 1:157-158
  feline chronic progressive, 1:158
  idiopathic, 1:158
  immune-mediated, 1:157-159
  non-erosive, 1:158-159
  -polymyositis syndrome, 1:158

Polycystic kidney disease (PKD), 2:395-396, 2:395f
  congenital, 2:396
  mutation of, 2:394
Polycystic liver disease, 2:265
Polycystic ovarian disease, 3:374-375, 3:375f
Polydactyly, 1:55, 1:55f
Polymelia, 1:55, 1:55f
Polymerase chain reaction (PCR), 1:11
Polymicrogyria, 1:268
Polymyositis
  cats, 1:228-229
  dogs, 1:227-228, 1:228f
Polyodontia, 2:6
Polypeptide hormones, 3:270-271, 3:270f
Polyploidy, liver, 2:270
Polypoid intestinal adenocarcinomas, 2:102
Polyps
  endometrial, 3:385, 3:386f
  inflammatory aural, 1:498-499
  nasal, 2:477-478, 2:477f, 2:579
Pomeranian dogs
  alopecia X, 1:589-590
  myxomatous valvular degeneration, 3:27
Pompe's disease, 1:208, 3:50
Poodle dogs
  amelogenesis imperfecta, 2:7
  color dilution alopecia, 1:539-540
  dilated cardiomyopathy, 3:48
  hyperadrenocorticism, 1:588
  hypothyroidism, 1:587
  myxomatous valvular degeneration, 3:27
  osteogenesis imperfecta in, 1:50
  rabies vaccine-induced vasculitis and alopecia, 1:612
  sebaceous adenitis, 1:551
Poorly differentiated chondrosarcoma, 1:119-120, 1:120f
Poorly differentiated osteosarcoma, 1:113, 1:113f
Poorly differentiated sarcomas, 1:244
Porcine adenovirus, 2:144-145, 2:144f
Porcine circovirus 2 (PCV-2), 2:116, 2:412-413, 2:527-529, 3:210-212, 3:210f-211f, 3:440, 3:440f
  encephalopathies, 1:382-383
Porcine deltacoronavirus (PDCoV), 2:147-148
Porcine dermatitis and nephropathy syndrome (PDNS), 2:412f, 3:210-212, 3:210f
Porcine dermatoses, 1:698-699
Porcine ear necrosis syndrome (PENS), 1:503, 1:645, 1:503.e1f
Porcine encephalitis associated with PRRSV infection, 1:383
Porcine epidemic diarrhea virus (PEDV), 2:113, 2:147
Porcine erysipelas, 1:149
Porcine hemagglutinating encephalomyelitis virus (HEV), 1:372
Porcine hypomyelinogenesis, 1:338
Porcine intestinal spirochetosis, 2:182
Porcine juvenile pustular psoriasiform dermatitis, 1:698, 1:698f
Porcine lymphomas, 3:241-243
Porcine parvovirus (PPV), 3:429
Porcine proliferative enteropathy, 2:179, 2:179f

Porcine reproductive and respiratory syndrome (PRRS), 2:523-526, 2:525f, 3:424
Porcine reproductive and respiratory syndrome virus (PRRSV), 1:383
Porcine respiratory coronavirus (PRCoV), 2:147, 2:529
Porcine salmonellosis, 2:170-172, 2:170f-172f
Porcine stress syndrome (PSS), 1:209-210, 3:39
Porcine ulcerative dermatitis syndrome, 1:698
Porencephaly, 1:272-274, 1:272f, 1:285f
  orbiviruses and, 1:281
Porphyromonas gingivalis, 2:11
Porphyromonas spp., 2:9, 2:11
Portal hypertension, 2:297
Portal tract, liver, 2:261, 2:261f
Portal veins
  aneurysms, 2:266
  hypoplasia, 2:267-268
  injury, 2:296-297
  thrombosis, 2:297f
Portosystemic shunting, 2:298-299, 3:127
Portosystemic vascular anomalies, 2:267, 2:267f
Portuguese Water dogs
  dilated cardiomyopathy, 3:48
  follicular dysplasia, 1:540-541
Portulacca oleracea, 2:425-426
Postanesthetic myopathy in horses, 1:213
Posterior staphyloma, 1:413
Posterior tunica vasculosa lentis, 1:418
Posterior uveitis, 1:446
Postinfectious encephalomyelitis, 1:395-396
Postmortem examination. *See* Gross and histologic examinations
Postmortem rupture of viscus, 2:247
Postnecrotic scarring, 2:284, 2:289, 2:289f
Postoperative conjunctival inclusion cysts, 1:478
Postpartum uterus, lesions of, 3:440-441
Postparturient vascular lesions, 3:370
Postrenal azotemia, 2:384-385
Postvaccinal canine distemper encephalitis, 1:384
Postweaning colibacillosis, 2:100, 2:165, 2:165f
Postweaning diarrhea, 2:115
Postweaning multisystemic wasting syndrome (PMWS), 2:527-529, 2:528f, 3:210-212, 3:210f-212f, 3:440, 3:440f
Potassium depletion, chronic, 2:430
Potomac horse fever, 2:99, 2:200-201
Poultry mite, 1:683
Pourfour du Petit syndrome, 1:494-495
Poxviral infections, 1:616-625
  sheep and goats, 2:557
  trachea and, 2:483
PP cells, endocrine pancreas, 2:368
Precipitation of pentobarbital salts, 1:8f
Precursor lymphoblastic leukemia/lymphoma, 3:219, 3:220f
Pregnancy. *See* Abortion; Gestation
Pregnancy toxemia in sheep, 2:419-421
Pre-iridal fibrovascular membrane, 1:447, 1:448f
Prekallikrein deficiency, 3:263
Preparation artifacts in histologic sections, 1:29, 1:29f

Prepubic hernias, 2:80
Preputial diverticulitis, 3:507-508, 3:507f
Prerenal azotemia, 2:384
Presa Canario dogs, dilated cardiomyopathy in, 3:48
Presbycusis, 1:493
Preservation, sample, 1:8
Primary abomasal impaction in cattle, 2:50
Primary ciliary dyskinesia, 2:504
Primary cleft palate, 2:3
Primary endocardial fibroelastosis, 3:22
Primary epithelial neoplasms of liver, 2:345-346
Primary gastric dilation, 2:48
Primary glaucoma, 1:462-463, 1:463f
Primary hairs, 1:515-516
Primary hyperaldosteronism, 1:225
Primary hyperfunction of endocrine gland, 3:272
Primary hyperparathyroidism, 1:74, 3:304-305
Primary hypofunction of endocrine gland, 3:272-273
Primary idiopathic hyperlipidemia, 2:277-278
Primary irritant contact dermatitis, 1:566-568, 1:567f
Primary ossification center, 1:22
Primary parathyroid hyperplasia, 3:301
Primary photosensitization, 1:578-579
Primary portal vein hypoplasia (PVH), 2:267-268
Primary spongiosa, 1:23, 1:23f
Primary synovial chondromatosis, 1:162, 1:162f
Primary thyroid hypoplasia, 3:314
Primary tympany of forestomachs, 2:36, 2:37f
Primary vascular disease, 2:398
Primidone, 2:329
Primordial germ cells (PGC), 3:469
Principal bronchus, 2:467
Prion diseases, 1:347-350
Prion proteins, 2:20
Probiotics, 2:65
Procoagulant activities, 3:55
Proficiency testing of pathologists, 1:14
Profilaggrin, 1:513
Progesterone, 3:383
Prognathism, 2:3
Progressive ataxia, 1:341f
  of Charolais cattle, 1:341, 1:341f
Progressive atrophic rhinitis (PAR), 2:533
Progressive axonopathy of Boxer dogs, 1:329-330
Progressive ethmoid hematomas (PEH), 2:477
Progressive motor neuron disease, 1:255, 1:255f, 1:330-332, 1:331f-332f
Progressive neuronopathy of Cairn Terrier, 1:332-333
Progressive renal mineralization, 2:441
Proinflammatory cytokines, 2:72
Prolactin, 3:276-277
Prolapse, female genital organ, 3:381
Proliferative and necrotizing pneumonia, 2:529, 2:529.e1f
Proliferative arthritis, 1:147-148
Proliferative glomerulonephropathy, 2:403f, 2:401.e3f
Proliferative hemorrhagic enteropathy, 2:179-180, 2:180f
Proliferative optic neuropathy, 1:476
Proliferative pododermatitis, 1:642-643
Proliferative zone, growth plate, 1:22-23
Prolonged gestation, 3:397-398
Prolonged renal ischemia, 2:422-423
Pro-opiomelanocortin (POMC), 3:285, 3:285f
Prosencephalic hypoplasia, 1:266-267, 1:266f
Prostaglandins, 2:46
Prostate gland, 3:500-504, 3:500f
  disorders of sexual development, 3:500-501, 3:500f
  hyperplasia and metaplasia, 3:502-503, 3:503f
  inflammation, 3:501-502, 3:501f
  neoplasms, 3:503-504, 3:504f
Prostatitis, 3:501, 3:502f
Protein-calorie deficiency, 1:581
Protein core, epidermal, 1:513
Protein C pathway, 3:265-266
Protein-energy malnutrition, 2:69
Protein hydrolysis, 2:45
Protein-losing gastroenteropathy, 2:72
Protein-losing nephropathy (PLN), 2:418
Protein-losing syndromes, 2:89-97
Protein maldigestion, 2:70
Proteinuria, 2:401
Proteoglycans, 1:19-20, 1:514
  deficiency, 1:545-546
Protistant infections, 2:227-244
Protoplasmic astrocytes, 1:260-261
Protostrongylus rufescens, 2:565-566, 2:565t
Prototheca, 1:451, 1:665, 1:666f
  enterocolitis, 2:203-204
Prototheca wickerhamii, 2:476
Prototheca zopfii, 2:433, 2:476
Protozoal infections
  abortion and, 3:399b, 3:420-424, 3:420f
  arthritis, 1:155
  diseases of skin, 1:661-665
  endophthalmitis, 1:451
  liver and, 2:324
Protrusion of nictitans gland, 1:424
Proud flesh, 1:560-561
Proximal axonopathy, 1:257, 1:257f
Proximal esophagus, segmental aplasia of, 2:31
Psammoma bodies, 1:304
Psammomatous meningioma, 1:397, 1:397f
Pseudallescheria boydii, 2:476
Pseudamphistomum truncatum, 2:324
Pseudoachondroplastic dysplasia, 1:44
Pseudoaneurysms, 2:398
Pseudoanodontia, 2:6
Pseudoarthrosis, 1:36
Pseudo-blackleg, 1:233
Pseudocowpox virus, 1:616, 1:618
Pseudocysts, pancreatic, 2:361
Pseudoepitheliomatous hyperplasia, 3:151
Pseudoglandular stage of lung growth, 2:484
Pseudohepatorenal syndromes, 2:430
Pseudomembranous stomatitis, 2:18
Pseudomembranous rhinitis, 2:474-475
Pseudomonas aeruginosa, 3:30-31
Pseudomonas spp., 2:459
Pseudomycetoma, 1:653
Pseudo-obstruction, 2:77
Pseudo-oligodontia, 2:6
Pseudoplacentational endometrial hyperplasia, 3:383, 3:384f
Pseudopolyodontia, 2:6
Pseudorabies, 1:370-372, 1:371f, 2:530
Pseudotuberculosis, 3:209-210, 3:209f
Pseudotumors, muscle, 1:246, 1:246f
Psorergatic mange, 1:678
Psoriasiform dermatitis of goats, 1:698
Psoroptes spp., 1:505-506
Psoroptic mange, 1:675-676
Psychogenic alopecia, 1:561
Psychogenic injury, 1:561-562, 1:561f
Pteridium spp., 2:173-180
Ptyalism, 2:28-29
Puerperal tetany, 3:299
Pug dogs
  canine atopic dermatitis, 1:591
  canine necrotizing meningoencephalitis, 1:392-393
  hereditary stenosis of common bundle, 3:51
  motor neuron disease, 1:331
  pigmented plaques, 1:710-711, 1:711f
Pulmonary adenocarcinoma, 2:447
Pulmonary arterial hypertension (PAH), 2:492-494, 2:492f, 3:66-67, 2:492.e1f
Pulmonary artery, 2:467-468, 2:468f
  transposition with aorta, 3:22.e1f
Pulmonary aspergillosis, 2:573, 2:573f
Pulmonary blastomas, 2:498
Pulmonary carcinomas/adenocarcinomas, 1:736, 2:495-500, 2:497f, 2:495.e2f, 2:497.e1f
  classification, 2:496t
Pulmonary edema, 2:487-489, 2:488b, 2:489.e1f
Pulmonary emphysema, 2:486-487, 2:487f
Pulmonary hamartoma, 2:485
Pulmonary hemorrhage, 2:490-492, 2:490.e1f
Pulmonary hyalinosis, 2:517
Pulmonary hypertension, 2:492-494, 3:60
  canine pulmonary veno-occlusive disease (PVOD), 2:493, 2:493f, 2:493.e1f
  causes, 2:492b
  pulmonary arterial hypertension (PAH), 2:492-494, 2:492f, 3:66-67
Pulmonary hypoplasia, 2:484, 2:484.e3f
Pulmonary immune responses, 2:472
Pulmonary infarcts, 2:490.e1f
Pulmonary intravascular macrophages (PIMs), 2:471, 2:471.e1f
Pulmonary Langerhans cell histiocytosis, 2:499, 3:246-247, 3:247f, 3:246.e1f
Pulmonary macrophages, 2:470
Pulmonary mineralization, 2:494-495, 2:494f
Pulmonary neoplasia, 2:495-500, 2:495b
Pulmonary surfactant, 2:470
Pulmonary thromboembolism, 2:489, 2:489b, 2:489.e1f
Pulmonary vasculitis, 2:494, 2:494.e2f
Pulmonary veins, 2:467-468, 2:468f
Pulmonary venous hypertension, 2:492-493
Pulmonic stenosis, 3:19, 3:19f
Pulmonic valves, 3:2-3
Pulpitis, 2:11
Pure red cell aplasia, 3:127-128, 3:128f
Pure silica stones, 2:455
Purified protein derivatives (PPD), 2:548
Purkinje fibers, 3:2
Purpura hemorrhagica, 1:229, 1:229f
Purulent (suppurative) arthritis, 1:147-148, 1:148f
Purulent bronchitis, 2:501
Purulent pericarditis, 3:26
Purulent splenitis, 3:183-184
Purulent streptococcal meningitis, 1:357f

Pustules, 1:524
  infectious pustular vulvovaginitis of cattle, 3:443-445
  sterile eosinophilic pustulosis, 1:696
Pyelonephritis, 2:382, 2:431, 2:439-441
  acute, 2:440-441, 2:440f
  cattle, 2:441
  chronic, 2:439, 2:440f
  dogs and cats, 2:440
  microabscess, 2:440.e1f
  swine, 2:440-441
  thyroidization, 2:440f
  urinary tract defenses, 2:439
  vesicoureteral reflux, 2:439
  virulence of bacteria, 2:439
Pyemotes tritici, 1:683
Pyencephaly, 1:361, 1:361f
Pyloric mucosa, 2:45
Pyloric smooth muscle, hypertrophy of, 2:48
Pyloric stenosis, 2:48
  chronic hypertrophic pyloric gastropathy, 2:48
Pylorogastric intussusception, 2:50
Pyodermas, 1:629
  deep bacterial, 1:634-637, 1:635f
  mucocutaneous, 1:630
  superficial bacterial, 1:629-634, 1:630f
Pyogenic granuloma, 2:21
Pyogenic infections and central nervous system, 1:353-365
Pyogranulomas, 2:18
  sterile, 1:699-702
Pyogranulomatous meningoencephalomyelitis, 1:362, 1:362f
Pyometra, 3:390-393, 3:390f-391f
  cows, 3:392-393
  mare, 3:393
Pyonephrosis, 2:439
Pyosalpinx, 3:380
Pyothorax, 2:521.e1f
Pyotraumatic dermatitis, 1:560
Pyrenean Mountain dogs, motor neuropathy in, 1:335
Pyrexia with dermatitis, 1:574
Pyridoxine, 1:582
Pyridoxine (vitamin B_6) deficiency, 2:426
Pyrrolizidine alkaloids, 2:336-338, 2:337f, 2:519-520, 2:337.e1f
Pyruvate kinase (PK) deficiency, 3:126
Pythiosis, 1:657-659, 1:658f, 2:203
Pythium insidiosum, 2:476, 2:573f

Q

Quality assurance of pathology services, 1:14
Quarter Horses
  agammaglobulinemia, 3:139
  degenerative myopathy and rapid muscle atrophy, 1:229
  equine polysaccharide storage myopathy, 1:205-207
  equine systemic calcinosis, 1:223-224
  fiber hypertrophy, 1:179
  glycogen branching enzyme deficiency, 1:208f
  hereditary equine regional dermal asthenia, 1:544
  hyperkalemic periodic paralysis, 1:202
  lymphomas, 3:238
  malignant hyperthermia, 1:210

Quarter Horses (Continued)
  myotonic dystrophy-like disease, 1:202-203
Quassinoid toxicosis, 1:574-575
Quercus spp., 2:427-428

R

Rabbit fibroma virus, 1:616
Rabbit oral papillomavirus, 1:712
Rabies, 1:367-370, 1:369f
  vaccine, 1:560
    -induced vasculitis and alopecia, 1:612-613, 1:613f
Racing sled dogs, exertional myopathies in, 1:223
Radiant heat dermatitis, 1:566
Radiation
  deafness and, 1:493
  injury, 1:566
  thyroid carcinogenesis and, 3:332
Radiculomyelopathy, degenerative, 1:330
Radiography
  aneurysmal bone cysts, 1:126
  bone tumors, 1:108
  osteosarcoma, 1:111
Ragged fibers, 1:185
Raillietia spp., 1:505-506
Rangelia vitalii, 3:125, 3:125f
RANKL, 1:18, 1:26
Ranula, 2:29
Rapeseed oil, 3:36
Rapidly growing mycobacteria (RGM), 1:640, 1:640f
Rappaport classification, 3:215
Rathke's pouch, 3:280-281
Rats, plant toxicitiies in, 1:91
"Rat-tail syndrome", 1:539
Rat Terrier dogs
  canine hypomyelinogenesis, 1:338
  canine X-linked muscular dystrophy, 1:192
Reactive astrocytes, 1:261-262, 1:261f
Reactive astrogliosis, 1:262
Reactive histiocytosis, 3:247-250, 3:248f, 3:247.e1f
  cutaneous, 3:247-249, 3:248f-249f, 3:247.e1f, 3:249.e1f
  systemic, 1:729, 3:249-250, 3:249f
Reactive systemic amyloidosis, 2:414
Receptor ligand (receptor activator of nuclear factor κB [NFκB] ligand [RANKL], 3:294
Rectal papillary adenoma, 2:104, 2:105f
Rectal perforation, 2:247
Rectal prolapse, in sheep, 2:88
Rectal stricture, 2:100
Rectovaginal fistula, 2:450
Recurrent airway obstruction in horses (RAO), 2:505-506, 2:505f
Recurrent dermatosis of sows, 1:698-699
Recurrent uveitis, 2:438-439
Recurrent vomiting, 2:48
Red and wapiti-red crossbred (elk) deer, 1:32-33, 1:33f
Red blood cells (RBC), 3:112
  diapedesis of, 1:301
Red pulp, spleen, 3:161
Reduced enamel epithelium, 2:5
Reduced water intake, 2:452-453
Reed-Sternberg cell, 3:219
Reflux esophagitis, 2:32, 2:32f, 2:56

Regeneration
  liver, 2:286-287, 2:290f
  muscle, 1:182-183, 1:183f-184f
  pancreatic cells, 2:355
Reinfection syndrome, Dictyocaulus viviparus, 2:554-556
Remodeling, 1:26-27
  markers of, 1:27
Renal adenoma, 2:444f
Renal agenesis, 2:392
Renal amyloidosis, 2:414f
Renal and perirenal lymphosarcoma, 2:447f
Renal arterioles, lipid embolization of, 2:418
Renal biopsies, 2:383, 2:412
Renal blood flow, 2:377
Renal cell carcinomas (RCC), 2:444-446, 2:444f-445f, 2:445.e1f
  oncocytic form, 2:445-446
Renal collecting system, 2:378
Renal cortex
  hemorrhages, 2:397
  olive-green coloration, 2:429
Renal cortical necrosis, 2:398-399
Renal cortical petechiae, 2:397f
Renal crest, 2:378
  necrosis, 2:400f, 2:399.e2f
Renal cystadenocarcinomas, 2:446, 2:446f
  histopathology of, 2:446.e1f
Renal cysts, 2:394-397
  acquired cysts, 2:396
  autosomal dominant, 2:395-396
  autosomal recessive PKD (ARPKD), 2:396
  glomerulocystic disease, 2:396
  mechanisms, 2:394
  simple renal cysts, 2:394-395
Renal disease, 2:384-388. See also Renal failure; specific conditions
  anemia, 2:385
  chronic, 2:16-17
    anemia and, 3:127
    hyperparathyroidism secondary to, 3:300-301, 3:300f
    hypertension and, 3:59
  CRF tends to be progressive, 2:387
  electrolyte balance, 2:384
  endocrine function, disturbances, 2:384-385
  end-stage, 2:384
  fluid volume regulation, 2:384
  nonrenal lesions of uremia, 2:385
  systemic arterial lesions, 2:386
  transplantation, 2:387
  uremia, renal lesions of, 2:387
  uremic encephalopathy, 2:387
  uremic toxins, 2:385
Renal dysplasia, 2:388-391, 2:393, 2:394f, 2:449.e2f
  microscopic criteria, 2:393
Renal ectopia, 2:392
Renal encephalopathy, 1:344
Renal enlargement, 2:381-382
  acute inflammation, 2:381-382
Renal failure, 2:384-388, 2:435. See also Kidney(s); Renal disease
  hypercalcemic nephropathy, 2:441
  volume of urine of low specific gravity, 2:410
Renal glomerular vasculopathy, 2:418-419
Renal glucosuria, primary, 2:429

Renal hemorrhages, 2:397
Renal hyperemia, 2:397
Renal hypoplasia, 2:392
Renal infarcts, 2:397-398, 2:397f
Renal insufficiency, 2:384
Renal interstitial cell tumors, 2:447
Renal lesions, 2:393
Renal lobule, 2:378
Renal lymphomas, 3:240f-241f
Renal lymphosarcoma, 2:447.e1f
Renal medulla, 2:383
Renal medullary necrosis, 2:399-400
　amyloidosis, 2:399
　analgesic nephropathy, 2:399
　dehydration, 2:399
　gross lesions, 2:399-400
　pyelonephritis, 2:399
　urinary obstruction, 2:399
Renal neoplasia, 2:444-448
　adenoma, 2:444
　nephroblastoma, 2:446f
　renal carcinoma, 2:444-446
　renal cell carcinoma, 2:445f, 2:445.e1f
　renal cystadenocarcinoma, 2:446f
Renal oncocytomas, 2:447
Renal pelvis
　urothelium of, 2:449
　worms, 2:443
Renal position anomalies, 2:392-393
Renal secondary hyperparathyroidism, 1:74-75, 1:77-78
Renal telangiectasia, 2:398, 2:442, 2:442.e1f
Renal tissue
　abnormalities, 2:392
　agenesis, 2:392
　hypoplasia, 2:392
Renal transplantation, 2:387
Renal tubular acidosis, 2:384, 2:428-429
Renal tubules degeneration, 1:5f
Renal vasoconstriction, 2:424-425
Ren arcuatus, 2:392
Renin-angiotensin-aldosterone system (RAAS), 2:377, 2:401, 3:10, 3:337
Reoviridae, 3:430-431
Reparative dentin, 2:5
Repeat breeder, 2:438
Reperfusion injury, 2:81
Reports, final, 1:14
Reproductive system
　abnormalities with hypothyroidism, 3:318
　female, 3:358-464
　male, 3:465-510
Respiratory bronchioles, 2:467
Respiratory distress syndrome, 2:515-516, 2:516.e1f
　familial, 2:516
Respiratory system, 2:465-591
　general considerations, 2:465-473
　　organization of lung, 2:467
　　upper airway, 2:466-467, 2:466f
　infectious diseases, 2:523-591
　　bacterial, 2:531-533, 2:542-551, 2:562-563, 2:569-573, 2:577-579, 2:589
　　cats, 2:587-591
　　cattle, 2:537-557
　　dogs, 2:574-587
　　fungal, 2:535-536, 2:554, 2:579-585
　　horses, 2:567-574
　　mycoplasmal, 2:533-535, 2:563-564, 2:573-574, 2:579

Respiratory system (Continued)
　　parasitic, 2:536-537, 2:554-557, 2:564-567, 2:574, 2:585-587, 2:590, 2:590f
　　sheep and goats, 2:557-567
　　viral, 2:523-531, 2:537-542, 2:557-562, 2:567-569, 2:574-577, 2:587-589
　larynx, 2:467, 2:481-482, 2:481f
　　laryngitis, 2:481
　　paralysis, 2:481, 2:481f
　　rhabdomyomas, 1:241, 1:242f
　lungs, 2:484-520
　　abortion and, 3:401-402
　　abscesses, 2:520
　　atelectasis, 2:486, 2:486.e2f
　　cellular architecture and cell biology, 2:468-471
　　circulatory disturbances, 2:487-494
　　congenital anomalies, 2:484-485, 2:485.e1f
　　defenses, 2:471-473
　　development and growth, 2:484, 2:484.e1f
　　heart failure and, 3:11
　　hemorrhage, 2:490-492, 2:490.e1f
　　injury, 2:500-520, 2:500f
　　　airway disease, 2:500-504, 2:500.e1f
　　　interstitial lung disease, 2:509, 2:510f, 2:511b
　　lobes, 2:467
　　　torsion, 2:485-486, 2:485f
　　mineralization, 2:494-495, 2:494f
　　neoplasia, 2:495-500, 2:495b
　　organization of, 2:467
　　pulmonary emphysema, 2:486-487
　　pulmonary hypertension, 2:492-494
　　thrombosis, embolism, and infarction, 2:489-490, 2:489b
　　toxic injury, 2:518-520
　　vascular supply to, 2:467-468, 2:468f
　nasal cavity, 2:466, 2:473-480
　　circulatory disturbances, 2:473-474
　　congenital anomalies, 2:473
　　general considerations, 2:473
　　nasal amyloidosis, 2:473, 2:474f
　　neoplasms, 2:478-480, 2:478f
　　non-neoplastic proliferative disorders, 2:477-478
　　paranasal sinus diseases, 2:477, 2:477f
　　rhinitis, 2:474-477, 2:475b
　pharynx, 2:480-481
　　cysts, 2:29
　　dysphagia, 2:33
　　lymphoid hyperplasia, 2:480.e3f
　　neuroendocrine carcinoma of, 2:27
　pleura, 2:520-523
　　neoplasms, 2:523
　　noninflammatory pleural effusions, 2:521
　　pleural effusions, 2:520
　　pneumothorax, 2:487, 2:487f, 2:521, 2:521.e3f
　　pleuritis, 2:521-523, 2:522f, 2:521.e3f
　　suppurative, 2:522, 2:521.e1f
　pneumonia
　　aspiration, 2:508-509, 2:508f-509f, 2:516, 2:516.e1f, 2:508.e1f
　　atypical, 2:509
　　bacterial, 2:562-563, 2:562f
　　bronchointerstitial, 2:511-512, 2:514.e2f
　　embolic, 2:520, 2:520.e2f
　　eosinophilic interstitial, 2:513.e1

Respiratory system (Continued)
　　granulomatous interstitial, 2:513
　　hypersensitivity, 2:512-513
　　interstitial, 2:509
　　lipid, 2:516-518, 2:516.e1f
　　proliferative and necrotizing, 2:529, 2:529.e1f
　　pulmonary carcinomas/adenocarcinomas, 1:736, 2:495-500, 2:497f, 2:495.e2f, 2:497.e1f
　　classification, 2:496t
　sinuses
　　diseases, 2:477, 2:477f
　　neoplasms, 2:478-480, 2:478f
　　non-neoplastic proliferative disorders, 2:477-478
　trachea, 1:201, 2:467-469, 2:482-483
　　bronchus, 2:467
　　collapse, 2:483f, 1:192.e1
　　smoke inhalation and, 2:483, 2:483f
　　transitional metaplasia, 2:501, 2:501.e1f
Respiratory tract infection, 2:149
Resting lines, 1:27
Resting zone, growth plate, 1:22-23
Restrictive cardiomyopathy (RCM), 3:45
　cats, 3:46
Retained cartilage core, 1:32, 1:32f
Retarded endochondral ossification, 1:32
Rete testis, 3:497
Reticular degeneration, 1:523
Reticulin fibers, 2:260
Retina, 1:465-475
　degeneration, 1:468-469
　　inherited, in cats, 1:469-470
　　light-induced, 1:470
　　miscellaneous retinopathies, 1:472-474
　　non-inherited, 1:470
　　nutritional, 1:470-471
　　taurine-deficiency, 1:471
　　toxic retinopathies, 1:471-472
　dysplasia, 1:419-420, 1:420f
　　in cats, 1:469-470
　　inherited photoreceptor, 1:469
　　true, 1:420
　folding, 1:419, 1:419f
　general pathology, 1:466-467
　histopathology, 1:467
　necrosis, 1:419
　nonattachment, 1:411-412, 1:414f
　normal, 1:465-466, 1:465f
　retinitis, 1:474-475, 1:474f
　separation, 1:467-468, 1:467f-468f
　vasculature, 1:466
Retinal pigment epithelial dystrophy, 1:469
Retinitis, 1:474-475, 1:474f
Retinoblastomas, 1:485
Retinol, 1:82
Retrobulbar cyst, 1:412, 1:412f
Retrocaval ureter, 2:449, 2:449f
Retroflexion, of the bladder, 2:451
Retroperitoneal pelvic fat bulges, 2:80
Retroperitoneum, 2:245. *See also* Peritoneum and retroperitoneum
　diseases, 2:257
Retroviral infections, 1:627-628
Reversal lines, 1:27
Revised European-American Classification of Lymphoid Neoplasms (REAL), 3:217
Rhabditis bovis, 1:507
Rhabdomyolysis, 1:221-224
　exertional, in horses, 1:221-223, 1:222f

Rhabdomyomas, 1:241, 1:242f, 1:726, 3:52, 3:52f
  ear, 1:505
  laryngeal, 2:482, 2:482f, 2:482.e1f
Rhabdomyosarcomas, 1:241-243, 1:243f-244f, 1:726, 2:464
Rheumatoid arthritis, 1:157, 1:157f
Rheum rhaponticum, 2:425-426
Rhinitis, 2:474-477
  allergic, 2:476, 2:476.e1f
  atrophic, 2:533
    nonprogressive (NPAR), 2:533
      pigs, 1:102
    progressive, 2:533
  bovine rhinitis virus, 2:542
  causes, 2:475b
  chronic, 2:475
  idiopathic lymphoplasmacytic, 2:476
  inclusion body, 2:529-530, 2:530f
  mycotic, 2:579, 2:580f
Rhinosporidium seeberi, 2:476, 2:579-580, 2:581f
Rhipicephalus sanguineus, 1:240, 1:506
Rhizoctonia leguminicola, 2:29
Rhodesian Ridgeback dogs
  congenital myotonia in, 1:201
  degenerative radiculomyelopathy, 1:330
  dermoid cysts, 1:547, 1:704-705
  myotonic dystrophy-like disorder, 1:202-203
Rhodococcus equi, 2:113-114, 2:197-198, 2:198f, 2:514, 3:418
  lymph nodes and, 3:206f, 3:204.e1f
  respiratory system and, 2:569-571, 2:571f
  splenic abscesses, 3:183-184
Rhodotorula glutinis, 3:491
Rhodotorula spp., 1:661
Rib and sternum congenital abnormalities, 1:56
Ribbon trichoblastoma, 1:716, 1:716f
Riboflavin deficiency, 1:582
Ribonucleic acid (RNA) extraction, 1:30
Rickets, 1:61, 1:66, 1:68-74, 3:82-83, 3:274, 3:296
  calcium deficiency in, 1:61, 1:66, 1:69
  hereditary, 1:69
    vitamin D-resistant, 1:70
  hypophosphatemic, 1:70, 1:70f
  microscopic lesions of, 1:72, 1:72f
  phosphorus deficiency in, 1:68-69
  rickettsial vasculitides, 3:80-83
  sheep, 1:70, 1:70f
  vitamin D deficiency in, 1:68
  vitamin D-dependent type I, 1:69-70
Rift Valley fever virus (RVFV), 1:281, 2:312-313, 3:439-440, 2:312.e1f
Right atrioventricular valve dysplasia, 3:21-22
Right atrium, heart, 3:2
  failure, 3:6
Right-sided heart failulre, 3:11
Right ventricle, heart, 3:2
  double-chambered, 3:22
Rigor mortis, 1:186
Rinderpest, 2:128-130, 2:129f-130f, 3:182-183, 3:183f, 3:182.e1f
Ringbinden, 1:185, 1:185f
Ringbone, 1:142
Ringworm, 1:649-653

Rocky Mountain spotted fever, 1:449, 1:474-475, 3:82-83
Rod cells, 1:262-263
Rodenticides, 3:301-302, 3:301f
  hemothorax, 2:521.e3f
  intoxication, 3:264
Roeckl's granuloma of cattle, 1:234
Romney sheep
  axonal dystrophy, 1:324
  osteogenesis imperfecta, 1:49, 1:49f
Romulea poisoning, 1:322
Rosenthal fibers, 1:262
Rotavirus, 2:112, 2:115-117, 2:151-153, 2:152f
Rottweiler dogs
  axonal dystrophy, 1:324
  canine X-linked muscular dystrophy in, 1:192, 1:193f
  diabetes mellitus, 2:373
  ichthyosis, 1:532
  juvenile-onset distal myopathy, 1:198
  leukoencephalomyelopathy, 1:340-341, 1:340f
  motor neuropathy, 1:335
  nephritis, 2:417
  neuroepithelial degeneration, 1:492
  severe combined immunodeficiency (SCID), 3:140-141
  spongy encephalomyelopathies, 1:346
  static spinal stenosis in, 1:136, 1:136f
  vitiligo, 1:555-556
Rouge-des-prés calves, central and peripheral axonopathy of, 1:332
Roughage, 2:36
Row of tombstones, 2:14-15
Rubriblasts, 3:104
Rumen
  fluid, 2:455
  flukes, 2:43, 2:43f, 2:226
  mycotic inflammatory lesions of, 2:39-40
  papillae, adhesion of, 2:36f
Rumenitis, 2:39-40, 2:41f-42f
  and acidosis caused by carbohydrate overload, 2:40-43
  mycotic, 2:42
Rumenitis-liver abscess complex, 2:41-42
Ruminal acidosis, 2:40
  diagnosis of, 2:41
Ruminal carcinomas, 2:44
Ruminal drinkers, 2:38
Ruminal mucosa, 2:36, 2:36f
  microscopic examination of, 2:41
Ruminal papillae, 2:36
Ruminant forestomachs, 2:44
Ruptures
  abomasal, 2:50-51
  arterial, 3:62-63, 3:62f
  biliary tract, 2:309
  gastric, 2:48
  liver, 2:268
  muscle, 1:213-214
  spleen, 3:165-166, 3:166f, 3:166.e1f
  vaginal and vulval, 3:442
  vein, 3:89

S

Sabulous cystitis, in horse, 2:451f
Sabulous (matrix-crystalline) urethral plugs, in male cats, 2:456
Saccharated iron, 3:34-35

Saccular stage of lung growth, 2:484
Saint Bernard dogs
  dilated cardiomyopathy, 3:48
  gastric volvulus, 2:49
  pyotraumatic dermatitis, 1:560
  subvalvular aortic stenosis, 3:20
Salinomycin, 3:34-35
Salivary calculi (sialoliths), 2:29
Salivary glands, 2:28-30
  acute reactions to injury, 2:28
  dilations of duct, 2:29
  foreign bodies, 2:29
  necrotizing sialometaplasia, 2:30
  neoplasms, 2:30
  ptyalism, 2:29
  salivary mucocele/sialocele, 2:29
  sialoadenitis, 2:29
Salmonella Arizonae, 2:115
Salmonella choleraesuis, 2:170
Salmonella enterica, 2:99
Salmonella Typhimurium, 2:100, 2:171, 2:173f, 2:175f
Salmonella typhisuis, 2:172
Salmonellosis, 2:117, 2:167-176
  abortion and, 3:401, 3:412-413
  asymptomatic carriage of, 2:167-168
  bacterial osteomyelitis and, 1:99, 1:99f, 1:101f
  canivores, 2:176
  cattle, 2:174-175, 2:174f
  gastric venous infarction due to, 2:51
  horses, 1:99f, 2:172-174, 2:173f
  infectious arthritis and, 1:148
  liver and, 2:314-315
  pathogenesis of salmonellosis, 2:168
  pigs, 2:170-172, 2:170f-172f
  salmonellosis, 2:99, 2:112
  sheep, 2:175-176
  suppurative rhinitis and, 2:476
  in tonsils of swine, 2:20
Salmon poisoning disease, 2:117, 2:226, 3:148-149, 3:150f, 3:149.e1f
Salpingitis, 3:380
Salt poisoning, 1:314-315
Saluki dogs
  color dilution alopecia, 1:539-540
  motor neuron disease, 1:331
Samoyed dogs
  alopecia X, 1:589-590
  canine hypomeylinogenesis, 1:337
  canine uveodermatologic syndrome, 1:557
  canine X-linked muscular dystrophy in, 1:192
  chondrodysplasia in, 1:45
  early onset diabetes mellitus, 2:373
  sebaceous adenitis, 1:551
  spongy myelinopathy, 1:343
  true retinal dysplasia, 1:420
Samoyed hereditary glomerulopathy, 2:415-416
Samoyed hereditary nephropathy, 2:415-416
Sample selection and preservation, 1:8
  for study of muscle, 1:171-172, 1:172f-173f
San Angelo virus, 1:280
Sancassania berlesei, 1:683-684
San Miguel sea lion virus (SMSV), 2:121
Sarcina-like bacteria, 2:50
Sarcobatus vermiculatus, 2:425-426

Sarcocystis canis, 1:389
Sarcocystis gigantea, 2:34
Sarcocystis-like protozoans, 1:665
Sarcocystis spp., 1:234-236, 1:235f, 2:239
    abortion and, 3:423, 3:423f
    myocarditis and, 3:43-44
Sarcoidosis, 1:700-701
Sarcoids, 1:708, 1:709f
Sarcomas, 1:245
    feline post-traumatic, 1:486, 1:487f
    hemophagocytic histiocytic, 3:254-255, 3:254f-255f, 3:254.e1f
    histiocytic, 1:159-160, 1:160f, 1:729-730, 3:250-253, 3:250f-252f, 3:250.e2f, 3:250.e1f
        pulmonary, 2:498-499, 2:499f
    mammary, 3:463, 3:463f
    splenic, 3:192-194, 3:192f-193f, 3:192.e1f, 3:192.e2f
    undifferentiated pleomorphic, 1:725-726
    vaccine-associated, 1:560
Sarcomeres, 1:167, 1:168f, 3:3
Sarcoplasm, 1:167
Sarcoptic mange, 1:673-675, 1:674f
Sarcosporidiosis, 2:34
Satellite cells, 1:166-167
Satellitosis, 1:523, 1:523f
"Sawdust", 1:29
Sawfly larvae, 2:332
Scales, 1:524, 1:554
Scars, splenic, 3:166f
Scheibe-type deafness, 1:492
Schipperke dogs, myopathy in, 1:198
Schistosoma mattheei, 2:459-460
Schistosoma nasalis, 2:556-557, 2:567
Schistosomiasis, 2:227, 3:91-94, 3:92f, 3:93.e1f
Schmallenberg virus (SBV), 1:280, 1:281f, 3:438
Schnauzer dogs
    canine X-linked muscular dystrophy, 1:192
    myxomatous valvular degeneration, 3:27
    recurrent flank alopecia, 1:590
Schwann cells, 1:256, 1:258-260
Schwannomas, 1:405, 1:405f, 1:494, 1:724
Sclera, 1:476-477
Scleral ectasia, 1:413
Scleroderma, 2:77-78
    localized, 1:698
Scleromyxedema, feline, 1:697
Sclerosis, 1:523
Sclerotic masses, 2:104
Scoliosis, 1:37t
Scottish Blackface sheep, epidermolysis bullosa in, 1:535
Scottish Deerhound dogs, chondrodysplasia in, 1:44-45
Scottish Fold cats, osteochondrodysplasia in, 1:45-46
Scottish Terrier dogs
    Alexander disease, 1:341
    axonal dystrophy, 1:325
    canine atopic dermatitis, 1:591
    diffuse uveal melanocytosis, 1:484-485
    idiopathic multifocal osteopathy, 1:54
    malignant melanoma, 2:26
    spastic syndromes, 1:203, 1:318
Scrapie-associated prion protein, 1:348, 2:20
Screwworm fly, 2:43
Screwworm myiasis, 1:669-670

Scrotum, 3:471-473
    frostbite, 3:472, 3:472f
    hernia, 3:498
    varicose tumor of, 3:99
Scurvy, 1:83, 1:83f-84f
Sealyham Terrier dogs, melanocytopenic hypomelanosis in, 1:555
Sebaceous adenitis, 1:551-552, 1:552f
Sebaceous carcinomas, 1:717-718
Sebaceous duct cysts, 1:705
Sebaceous epitheliomas, 1:717
Sebaceous glands, 1:517
    dysplasia, 1:699, 1:699.e2f
    hyperplasia, 1:523
    tumors, 1:717-718, 1:717f
Sebaceous hamartomas, 1:705
Seborrhea, 1:548-549, 1:549f
Seborrheic keratoses, 1:550-551, 1:551.e1f
Secondary cleft palate, 2:3, 2:3f
Secondary demyelination, 1:257
Secondary glaucoma, 1:463-464, 1:464f
Secondary hair follicles, 1:515-516
Secondary hyperfunction of endocrine gland, 3:272
Secondary hyperparathyroidism, 1:74
    nutritional, 1:75
    renal, 1:74-75, 1:77-78
Secondary hypertension, 3:59-60
Secondary hypofunction of endocrine gland, 3:273
Secondary immune-mediated thrombocytopenia, 3:258
Secondary spongiosa, 1:23
Secondary synovial chondromatosis, 1:162, 1:162f
Secondary thyroid hypoplasia, 3:314, 3:314f
Secondary tumors of skeletal muscle, 1:244-245, 1:246f
Secondary tympany of forestomachs, 2:37-38
Second-degree burns, 1:564-566
Second opinions, 1:14
Secretory granules, 3:271
Segmental aplasia, 1:277-279
    of esophagus, 2:31
    of the mesonephric duct (SAMD), 3:480, 3:480f, 3:499
    paramesonephric duct, 3:368, 3:369f
Segmental cerebellar atrophy, 1:305
Segmental glomerulosclerosis (GS), 2:401
Segmental hypoplasia of spinal cord, 1:277-279, 1:277f
Segmental ischemic necrosis, of small colon, 2:84
Seizures, 3:51
Selenium
    -accumulator plants, 2:519-520
    deficiency, 1:214-215, 1:217
    toxicosis, 1:570-571, 1:571f
Sellar region tumors, 1:403-404
Semicircular canals, 1:490
Semihairlessness, 1:538
Seminomas, 3:496, 3:496f
Semiplacenta diffusa, 3:396-397
Senile atrophy
    of brain, 1:304-305
    of lymph nodes, 3:198-199
Senile osteoporosis, 1:64
Senile retinopathy, 1:473-474
Senna plant, 1:219-220, 2:341
Sensory ganglioneuritis, 1:395
Sensory hair cells, 1:489-490, 1:490f
Sepsis, 2:511, 2:512f
Septic arthritis, 1:147-148

Septic embolism, 2:490
Septicemia
    hemorrhagic, 2:546-547
    salmonellosis, 2:173
Septicemic colibacillosis, 2:166-167
Septicemic pasteurellosis, 2:562-563
Septic infection, 1:31-32
Sequestrum, 1:35-36, 1:94-96, 1:96f
    bronchopneumonia, 2:508
Serology, 1:11
Serosal edema, 2:195-196, 2:196f
Serosal inclusion cysts, 3:386-387, 3:387f
Serous atrophy of pericardial fat, 3:25, 3:25f
Serous retinal separation, 1:448-449
Sertoli cells, 3:466
    development, 3:469
    hyperplasia, 3:477f
    toxicants and testicular degeneration, 3:484
    tumor, 3:494-495, 3:494f
Serum albumin, 2:108
Serum calcium "set-point", 3:294
Serum electrolyte abnormalities and myopathies, 1:225
Serum protein levels, 2:40
Serum total and bone-specific alkaline phosphatase (ALP), 1:115
Setaria digitata, 1:390, 2:255
Setaria labiatopapillosa, 3:473-474
Severe acute respiratory syndrome (SARS), 2:587-588
Severe combined immunodeficiency (SCID), 3:139-141, 3:141f
Severe factor X deficiency, 3:264
Severe gastrointestinal parasitism, 1:66
Sex chromosome
    disorders of sexual development, 3:363-365, 3:363f-364f
    genotype, 3:360
Sex cord-gonadal stromal tumors
    in females, 3:375-377
    in males, 3:492-495
Sexual development disorders (DSD)
    female, 3:360-370, 3:364f-365f
    male, 3:468-471, 3:476-481, 3:476f, 3:499
Sézary syndrome, 3:232-234
"Shaker calf", 1:332, 1:332f
Shaker dog disease, 1:395
Sharpey's fibers, 1:130
Shear mouth, 2:8
Sheep-associated MCF, 2:132
Sheep grazing estrogenic pastures, 2:458
Sheep ked infestation, 1:670
Sheeppox virus, 1:616, 1:622-624, 1:623f, 2:557
Sheep scab, 1:676
Shetland Sheepdogs
    canine dermatomyositis, 1:198
    canine X-linked muscular dystrophy, 1:192
    choroidal hypoplsia, 1:413
    hyperestrogenism, 1:589
    spongy myelinopathy, 1:343
Shiga toxin, 2:112
Shiga toxin-producing *E. coli* (STEC), 2:162
Shih Tzu dogs
    keratoconjunctivitis sicca in, 1:436
    lymphomas, 3:238
    myelinolytic leukodystrophy, 1:341
    sebaceous epitheliomas, 1:717
Shipping-fever pneumonia, 2:542-543
Shock, 3:6
Shock gut, 2:85

Shorter-acting sulfonamides, crystalline nephropathy, 2:424
Shorthorn cattle
  bovine hypomyelinogenesis, 1:338-339
  lethal trait A46, 3:141
Shoulder joint, degenerative joint disease of, 1:143
Shunted blood flow to heart, 3:6
  malformation causing, 3:16-18, 3:16f
Shunts, hepatic, 2:267, 2:267f, 2:267.e1f
  acquired portosystemic, 2:290, 2:298-299, 2:299f
Shwartzman reaction, 2:398-399
Sialoadenitis, 2:29
Sialocele
  nasopharyngeal, 2:477.e4f
  salivary, 2:29
Siamese cats
  congenital hypotrichosis, 1:539
  congenital idiopathic megaesophagus, 2:34
  Maroteaux-Lamy syndrome, 1:58
  photosensitization, 1:579
  vitiligo, 1:556
Siberian Husky dogs
  alopecia X, 1:589-590
  canine uveodermatologic syndrome, 1:557
  degenerative radiculomyelopathy, 1:330
  motor neuropathy, 1:335
  oral eosinophilic granuloma, 2:16
  vitiligo, 1:555-556
  zinc-responsive dermatoses, 1:585-586
Sick sinus syndrome, 3:51
Siderocalcinosis, 3:61
Siderosis, 1:297, 1:298f
Sideritic pigmentation, 1:255
Siderotic plaques, splenic, 3:163, 3:164f, 3:163.e2f
Signet ring cells, 2:101-102
Signet-ring malignant melanomas, 1:722
Silica calculi, 2:455
Silicate pneumoconiosis, 2:518
Silicates, 2:518
Silky Terrier dogs
  rabies vaccine-induced vasculitis and alopecia, 1:612
  spongy myelinopathy, 1:343-344
Silo gas, 2:518
Silver fox
  spongiform myelinopathy, 1:343f, 1:344
  status spongiosus, 1:342f
Simmental cattle
  epidermolysis bullosa simplex, 1:535
  inherited progressive spinal myelopathy, 1:325
  osteopetrosis, 1:51
Simondsia spp., 2:54
Simple follicles, 1:515-516
Simple renal cysts, 2:394-395
Simple secretory epitrichial adenomas, 1:718
Sinus erythrocytosis, 3:199-200, 3:200f, 3:200.e1f
Sinuses
  diseases, 2:477, 2:477f
  neoplasms, 2:478-480, 2:478f
  nonflammatory thrombosis of cranial dural, 1:300
  non-neoplastic proliferative disorders, 2:477-478
Sinus hairs, 1:517
Sinusitis, chronic suppurative, 2:477-478, 2:477.e1f

Sinus node, 3:2
Sinusoidal domain, liver, 2:262
Sinusoidal endothelial cells, 2:260
Sinusoidal leukocytosis, 2:300-301
Sinusoidal lining cells necrosis, 2:285
Size-dependent barrier, 2:380
Skeletal dysplasias, 1:37t
  localized, 1:54-57, 1:54f
  osteochondromatosis, 1:54
Skeletal muscles, dermal, 1:515
Skeleton. *See also* Bone(s)
  genetic and congenital diseases of, 1:36-60, 1:37t
  genetic diseases indirectly affecting, 1:57-60
  manganese deficiency and, 1:80
  postmortem examination of, 1:28-30, 1:29f
Skin, 1:509-736
  actinic diseases of, 1:575-580
  algal diseases of, 1:665
  bacterial diseases of, 1:629-646
  basement membrane zone (BMZ), 1:513-514
  canine cutaneous histiocytoma, 3:243-245, 3:244f-245f, 3:244.e1f, 3:243.e1f
  canine juvenile cellulitis, 1:690-691, 1:691f
  canine reactive histiocytosis, 3:247-250, 3:248f, 3:247.e1f
  congenital and hereditary diseases of, 1:530-547
  dermal muscles, 1:515
  dermatohistopathology, 1:518-530
    gross terminology, 1:524
    histologic terms, 1:518-524
    pattern analysis, 1:524-530
  dermis, 1:514-515
  endocrine diseases of, 1:587-590
  epidermal differentiation disorders, 1:547-554
  epidermis, 1:512-513
  fungal diseases of, 1:646-661
  general considerations, 1:511-518
  hair follicles, 1:515-517
  helminth diseases of, 1:685-690
  immune-mediated dermatoses, 1:590-615
    autoimmune dermatoses, 1:600-607
    drug eruptions, 1:607-608
    hypersensitivity, 1:590-600
  immunologic function, 1:515
  lesions with canine distemper virus, 2:576
  lymphomas, 3:237, 3:237f, 3:239f, 3:239.e1f
  neoplastic and reactive diseases, 1:703-736
  nutritional diseases of, 1:580-587
  paraneoplastic syndromes, 1:691-693
  perianal glands, 1:517
  physiochemical diseases of, 1:558-575
    chemical injury, 1:566-575
    physical injury, 1:559-566
  pigmentation disorders, 1:554-558
  protozoal diseases of, 1:661-665
  sebaceous glands, 1:517
  subcutis, 1:518
  sweat glands, 1:517-518
  tags, 1:722-723
  tumor-like lesions, 1:705
  viral diseases of, 1:615-628
Skin-associated lymphoid tissue (SALT), 1:515
Skin-homing memory T-cells, 1:515

Skin immune system (SIS), 1:515
Skull bones, 1:21
  congenital abnormalities, 1:56, 1:56f
  craniomandibular osteopathy, 1:91-92, 1:92f
  fractures, 1:302-303
  sutures, 1:128
Skye Terrier dogs, chronic hepatitis in, 2:304
Slaframine, 2:29
SLC2A9 gene, 2:457
SLC3A1 genes, 2:458
SLC7A9 genes, 2:458
Slipped epiphysis, 1:31
Sly syndrome, 1:58
Small-bowel diarrhea, 2:70-71
Small-cell carcinoma
  neuroendocrine, 2:497-498
  thyroid, 3:330-331
Small-cell lymphocytic villus lymphoma, 2:107-108
Small intestinal bacterial overgrowth (SIBO), 2:86, 2:364
Small intestine, 2:81, 2:82f
  cardinal finding, 2:92
  idiopathic inflammatory bowel disease, 2:92
  lymphangiectasia, 2:90f
  mucosa, 2:124
    hypoplasia, 2:74
    vascular supply, 2:61
  obstruction, 2:76
    dogs, 2:75f
  pseudodiverticulosis of, 2:87
Small ruminant lentiviruses, 2:558-560, 2:559f, 2:558.e1f
Smoke inhalation
  lung injury, 2:518
  trachea and, 2:483, 2:483f
Smooth Fox Terrier dogs
  canine congenital myasthenia, 1:209
  multisystem axonal degeneration, 1:325
Smooth muscle cells, lungs, 2:469
Smooth-surface caries, 2:10
Snakebite envenomation, 1:568
Snowshoe hare virus, 1:383
Snorter dwarfism, 1:39, 1:39f
Sodium absorption, 2:65-66
Sodium fluoroacetate, 3:37-38
Sodium iodide symporter (NIS), 3:311
Soemmering ring cataract, 1:444, 1:444f
Soft callus, 1:34-35
Soft tissue sarcomas, 1:245
Solanaceae, 2:331
Solanum glaucophyllum, 3:301-302, 3:301f-302f
Solanum poisoning, 1:321-322
Solar dermatitis, 1:576, 1:576f
Solar elastosis, 1:577, 1:577f
Solar keratoses, 1:577
Solar radiation
  burns and, 1:566
  direct effect of, 1:575-577
Solid basal cell carcinoma, 1:714
Solid-cystic epitrichial adenomas, 1:718-719
Solid-cystic epitrichial carcinomas, 1:719
Solitary biliary cysts, 2:264
Solitary mucosal lymphoid nodules, 2:64
Somatostatin, 2:368
Somatostatinoma, 2:375
Somatotroph adenomas, 3:285-286, 3:285f-286f

South Dorset Down sheep, epidermolysis bullosa in, 1:535
Space of Disse, 2:260, 2:263
Spargana, 2:255
Spastic syndromes, 1:203-204, 1:318
Spavin, 1:142
Special stains, 1:9
Spermatic cord, 3:497-499
Spermatic granulomas, 3:497
   of the epididymal head, 3:480-481, 3:480f-481f
Spermatogenesis, 3:466-467
Spherocytes, 3:114
Spheroids, 1:257
Sphincter mechanism incompetence, 2:451-452
Sphingolipidoses, 1:287-288, 1:287f
Sphynx cats
   congenital hypotrichosis, 1:538
   α-dystroglycan deficiency in, 1:196
Spiculosis, 1:699
Spider bites, 1:568
Spider lamb syndrome, 1:40, 1:40f-41f
   sheep, 1:40, 1:40f-41f
Spina bifida, 1:57, 1:279
   occulta, 1:279
Spinal cord, 1:277-279. *See also* Brain
   arachnoid cysts, 1:279
   atrophy, 1:304-305
   diplomyelia, 1:278f
   dysraphism, 1:278f
   embolism, 2:490
   lymphoma, 3:240f
   myelodysplasia, 1:277-279, 1:278f
   nephroblastoma, 1:402-403, 1:403f
   segmental hypoplasia of, 1:277f
   spina bifida, 1:57, 1:279
   subdural hemorrhage of, 1:303f
   subdural/intradural abscess, 1:354f
   syringomyelia, 1:278f
   traumatic injuries, 1:303, 1:303f
Spinal defects, 1:37t
Spinal nephroblastoma, 1:403f
Spindle cells
   trichoblastomas, 1:716
   tumors, 1:722-726
     benign, 1:722-723
     of blue-eyed dogs, 1:486
     locally infiltrative and malignant, 1:723-726
Spindles, muscle, 1:171, 1:171f
Spiral colon, of ruminants, 2:66
Spiral ganglion cells, 1:490
Spiral mucosal folds, 2:60
Spiral osseous lamina, 1:489
Spirocerca-associated sarcoma, 2:35
Spirocerca lupi, 2:34-35, 2:35f
Spirochetal colitis, 2:181-183
Spirochetes, 1:645
Spirurid nematodes, 2:210
Splayleg, 1:189-190, 1:189f-190f
Spleen
   abscesses, 3:183-184, 3:184f
   circulatory diseases, 3:169-171
   cysts, 3:189
   degenerative diseases, 3:163-165
   developmental diseases, 3:162-163, 3:163f
   fibrohistiocytic nodules, 3:190-191, 3:190f-191f
   hematopoietic alterations, 3:191
   hyperplastic diseases, 3:189-191, 3:189f
   infarct, 3:170f-171f, 3:170.e1f

Spleen *(Continued)*
   inflammatory diseases, 3:182-189, 3:182.e1f
   lymphomas, 3:239f
   neoplastic diseases, 3:191-196
   rupture, 3:165-166, 3:166f, 3:166.e1f
   specific infections and, 3:171-182
   splenomegaly and splenic nodules, 3:167-169, 3:167f-168f, 3:169.e1f
   structure and normal function, 3:158-162, 3:160f
   thrombosis, 3:171f
   vascular neoplasms, 3:169f
   volvulus, 3:167, 3:167f
Splenic artery, 3:159
Splenic follicles, 3:116
Splenic infarct, 3:170f
Splenomegaly, 3:167-169, 3:167f-168f
Splenosis, 3:166, 3:166f
Spondylosis
   cattle, 1:145-146
   dogs, 1:146
   horses, 1:146
   pigs, 1:146
   sheep, 1:146
Spongiform myelinopathy, 1:343f
Spongiform pustule of Kogoj, 1:523
Spongiosis, 1:523, 1:524f
   perivascular dermatitis with, 1:525
Spongy encephalomyopathies, 1:342f, 1:345f, 1:346-347
Spongy myelinopathies, 1:342-346, 1:342f-343f
Spontaneous and iatrogenic hyperadrenocorticism, 1:67
Spontaneous chronic corneal epithelial defects (SCCED), 1:434
Spontaneous hemorrhages in brain, 1:300-301
Sporadic lymphangitis, 3:96
Sporidesmin, 2:335-336, 2:336f, 2:336.e1f
Sporotrichosis, 1:655-657, 1:656f
Spotted leukotrichia, 1:557-558
Squamous cell carcinoma (SCC), 1:125, 1:125f, 2:25-26, 2:25f, 2:44, 2:106, 2:106f, 2:447, 2:463
   acantholytic, 1:713-714
   cats, 2:21, 2:25, 2:44
   cattle, 2:26, 2:44
   dogs, 2:21, 2:25, 2:25f, 2:44
   esophagus and forestomachs, 2:44
   eyelid and conjunctival, 1:479-480, 1:479f-480f
   gastric, 2:106-107, 2:106f
   guttural pouch, 1:500
   horses, 2:25-26
   invasive, 1:713
   laryngeal, 2:482
   nasal, 2:478-479
   papillomaviruses and, 1:713, 1:713f
   penis and prepuce, 3:509, 3:509f
   pinnae, 1:504
   poorly differentiated, 1:713
   pulmonary, 2:497
   sheep and goats, 2:44
   well-differentiated, 1:713
Squamous eddies, 1:523
Squamous epithelium, 2:58
Squamous metaplasia of tracheal epithelium, 2:483
Squamous papilloma, 3:509
Srichinella spiralis, 2:19

Stachybotryotoxicosis, 1:573
Stachybotrys alternans, 2:14
Staffordshire Terrier dogs
   congenital myotonia, 1:201
   demodectic mange, 1:679
   spongy enceephalomyelopathies, 1:346
Staghorn calculus, 2:454f
Standardbred horses, agammaglobulinemia in, 3:139
Stanozolol, 2:329
Stapes, 1:495
Staphylococcal granuloma, 1:233-234
Staphylococcus aureus, 1:593
   abortion and, 3:417
   bacterial osteomyelitis and, 1:98, 1:100
   mastitis, 3:452-454
   polyarthritis, 1:151
Staphylococcus capitis, 3:473-474
Staphylococcus hyicus, 1:151
Staphylococcus pseudintermedius, 1:156
Staphylococcus spp., 2:455
   folliculitis and furunculosis, 1:634-636, 1:635f
Starvation, 1:60, 1:581
   osteoporosis and, 1:64-65, 1:65f
Status spongiosus, 1:342f, 1:345f, 1:346-347
Steatitis, 1:218, 2:249
Steatosis, hepatocellular, 2:273-278, 2:274f-276f, 2:274.e1f, 2:276.e1f
Stellate cells, 2:355
Stenosis, 2:73-74
   aortic and subaortic, 3:20-21, 3:21f
   cervical, 3:441
   esophageal, 2:32-33
   left atrioventricular valvular, 3:22
   nasal/nasopharyngeal, 2:475
   pulmonic, 3:19, 3:19f
   vaginal, 3:369, 3:370f
Stephanofilariasis, 1:686-687, 1:687f
Stephanofilaria zaheeri, 1:507
Stephanurus dentatus, 1:391, 2:255, 2:319
   encysted, 2:442f
Step mouth, 2:8
Sterile eosinophilic folliculitis and furunculosis, 1:696
Sterile eosinophilic pustulosis, 1:696
Sterile granulomas and pyrogranulomas, 1:699-702
Sterile hemorrhagic cystitis, 2:460
Sterile neutrophilic dermatoses, 1:696
Sterile nodular panniculitis, 1:701-702, 1:701f
Sterile pyogranuloma syndrome (SPGS), 1:700, 1:700f
Sternum and rib congenital abnormalities, 1:56
Steroidal sapogenins, 2:338-340
Steroid hormones, 3:271
   impairment, 3:340, 3:341f
Steroid-induced bone necrosis, 1:95
Steroid-responsive meningitis-arteritis, 1:158, 1:298-299, 1:298f, 1:395
Stevens-Johnson syndrome, 1:607, 1:609-610, 1:610f
Stilesia hepatica, 2:319-320
Stillbirth, 3:395, 3:398-440
Stomach and abomasum, 2:44-60
   adenocarcinoma of, 2:102
   circulatory disturbances, 2:51-52
   displacement, 2:49, 2:50f
   foreign bodies and impaction, 2:50-51

Stomach and abomasum *(Continued)*
  gastric dilation and displacement, 2:48-50
  gastric mucosal barrier, 2:46
  gastritis, 2:52-55
  gastroduodenal ulceration, 2:55-60
  heart failure and, 3:11-12
  neoplastic/proliferative lesions, 2:100-111, 2:101t
    tumors of lower gastrointestinal tract, 2:100-101
  normal form/function, 2:44-46
    mucous neck cells, 2:45
  pyloric stenosis, 2:48
  response of gastric mucosa to injury, 2:46-48
  rupture, 2:50-51
  volvulus, 2:49-50, 2:50f
Stomatitis
  catarrhal, 2:14
  chronic gingivostomatitis, 2:15-16
  chronic ulcerative, 2:16
  deep stomatitides, 2:17-19
  feline ulcerative, 2:16
  foreign-body, 2:13, 2:13f
  lymphocytic/plasmacytic, 2:16
  necrotic, 2:17, 2:17f
  superficial, 2:13-14
  vesicular, 2:14-15, 2:117-158, 2:120f
Storage diseases, 1:284-293
  ceroid-lipofuscinoses, 1:290-292
  glycogenoses, 1:290
  glycoproteinoses, 1:288-289
  induced, 1:292-293
  inherited, 1:286-292, 1:287f
  Lafora disease, 1:292
  lysosomal, 1:284-293, 1:285f-286f, 2:429
    liver, 2:278, 2:278f, 2:278.e1f
    skeleton, 1:57-59
    spinal cord, 1:285f-286f
  mucolipidoses, 1:290
  mucopolysaccharidoses (MPS), 1:58, 1:58f, 1:289-290
    hearing and, 1:491-492
  neuronal, 1:285, 1:473
Stored-product mite, 1:683-684
Strains, muscle, 1:213-214
Strangles, 2:572, 3:208-209, 3:208f, 3:208.e2f
Strangulation obstruction, 2:74-75
Stratum basale, 1:512
Stratum corneum (SC), 1:511-512
  seborrhea, 1:548-549
Stratum granulosum, 1:512
Stratum spinosum, 1:512
Straw-itch mite, 1:683
Streptococcal adenitis, 3:208-209, 3:208f
  dogs, 3:209
  pigs, 3:208-209
Streptococcal arthritis, 1:150-151, 1:151f
Streptococcal mastitis, 3:453-455, 3:454f
Streptococcal polyarthritis, 1:148
Streptococcus canis, 1:636
Streptococcus dysgalactiae, 1:151
Streptococcus equi, 2:412
  associated purpura hemorrhagica, 1:229, 1:229f
  cats, 2:589
  endocarditis and, 3:30-31
  splenic abscesses, 3:183-184
  strangles, 2:572, 3:208-209, 3:208f, 3:208.e2f

Streptococcus equi (Continued)
  suppurative myositis and, 1:230
Streptococcus equi
  Streptococcus porcinus, 3:208-209, 3:208f
Streptococcus spp. in sheep, 1:151, 2:562
Streptococcus suis, 1:150-151
  tonsils, 2:20
Streptococcus zooepidemicus, 2:578
Streptomyces, 3:417
Streptomycin, 2:424
Stress-related lesions, horses, 1:36
Striated myofibrils, 1:167
Stromal tumors, intestinal, 2:110-111
  gastrointestinal, 2:110
  leiomyoma, 2:110
  leiomyosarcoma, 2:110
Strongyloides felis, 2:212
Strongyloides papillosus, 1:690, 2:212, 3:507
Strongyloides ransomi, 2:212
Strongyloides spp., 2:211-227, 2:211f
Strongyloides stercoralis, 2:212
Strongyloides tumefaciens, 2:212
Strongyloides westeri, 2:212
Strongylus edentatus, 2:216, 2:255
Strongylus equinus, 2:216, 2:255
Strongylus vulgaris, 2:84, 2:216-217, 3:85-87, 3:86f, 3:87.e1f
Struvite calculi, 2:455-456
Strychnine poisoning, 1:317
Stypandra toxicosis, 1:345
Subcapsular nephrogenic zone, 2:382.e1f
Subchondral (juxtacortical) bone, 1:129
  cysts, 1:126, 1:134, 1:134f
Subcorneal pustular dermatosis, 1:696
Subcutaneous fungal infections, 1:653-661
Subcutaneous mast cell tumors, 1:245
Subcutaneous "panniculitis-like" T-cell lymphoma, 3:234, 3:234f
Subcutis, 1:518
Subdural abscess, 1:353-354, 1:354f
Subdural hemorrhage of spinal cord, 1:303f
Subendocardial fibrosis, 3:30
Subendocardial hemorrhage, 3:4
Subendocardial mineralization, 3:4, 3:30, 3:30f
Subendothelial connective tissues, 3:55
Subepidermal vesicular and pustular dermatitis, 1:527-528, 1:528f
Subepiglottic cysts, 2:481
Subintima, 1:130-131
Subinvolution of placental sites, 3:441, 3:441f
Subluxations, vertebral, 1:303
Submucosa, 2:62
Subnormal wear, 2:8
Substituted phenols, 3:325
Subungual squamous cell carcinomas, 1:713
Subvalvular aortic stenosis, 3:20-21
Sudan grass, 1:91
Suffolk sheep
  abomasal dilation and emptying defect, 2:51
  axonal dystrophies, 1:324
  epidermolysis bullosa, 1:535
Suid herpesvirus 1 (SuHV-1), 2:530, 3:432-433
  pseudorabies and, 1:370, 1:371f
Suid herpesvirus 2 (SuHV-2), 2:529-530, 3:433

Suifilaria suis, 1:690
Suipoxvirus, 1:616, 1:625, 1:625f
Sulfides, absorption of, 2:40
Sulfonamides, 3:324
Sulfur compounds and PEM, 1:312
Summer mastitis, 3:455-456
Sunlight-induced cataract, 1:443-444
Superficial bacterial pyoderma, 1:629-634, 1:630f
Superficial necrolytic dermatitis, 1:586-587, 1:587f
Superficial plexus, dermal, 1:514
Superficial stomatitis, 2:13-14
Suppurative arthritis, 1:148f
Suppurative hypophysitis, 3:289, 3:290f
Suppurative lymphadenitis, 3:203-204, 3:204f
Suppurative meningitis, 1:355f
Suppurative myocarditis, 3:42
Suppurative myositis, 1:230, 1:230f
Suppurative osteomyelitis, 1:100-101
  cattle, 1:102f
Suppurative pleuritis, 2:522, 2:521.e1f
Suppurative rhinitis, 2:476
Suppurative streptococcal encephalitis, 1:360f
Suppurative thymitis, 3:148, 3:149f
Suppurative uveitis, 1:449
Suprabasilar acantholysis, 2:14-15
Supragingival plaque, 2:9
Suprasellar germ cell tumor, 1:403-404, 3:287, 3:287f
Surface ectoderm, anomalies of, 1:421-423
Surgical pathology, 1:2
Surveillance, 1:1-2
Sutures, 1:21-22, 1:128
Swainsonine, 1:292, 2:29
Swayback, 1:328-329, 1:328f
Sweat glands, 1:517-518
  hamartomas, 1:705
  tumors, 1:718-720
Swedish Golden Retrievers, 1:334
Swedish Lapland dogs, motor neuron disease in, 1:331
Swelled head, 1:232
Swelling
  brain, 1:293-295, 1:295f
  of foot processes, 2:406
  vulval, 3:442-443
Swine dysentery, 2:100, 2:181-182, 2:182f
Swine influenza, 2:526-527, 2:526f, 2:526.e1f, 2:527.e1f
Swinepox virus, 1:616, 1:625, 1:625f
Swine rotaviral infection, 2:152, 2:152f
Swine vesicular disease (SVD), 2:121
Sylvatic dermatophytes, 1:649
Symmetrical lupoid onychitis (SLO), 1:702
Sympathetic nervous system neoplasms, 3:352-353
Symphyses, 1:128
Syncerus caffer, 2:117-118
Synchondroses, 1:128
Syndactyly, 1:54
Syndesmoses, 1:128
Synophthalmos, 1:411f
Synovial bursae, 1:155-156
Synovial cell sarcoma, 1:159
Synovial chondromatosis, 1:162, 1:162f
Synovial cysts, 1:162-163

Synovial fluid, 1:131
  purulent arthritis, 1:147-148
  synovial cysts, 1:162-163
Synovial fossae, 1:130, 1:130f
  goats, 1:130, 1:130f
  horses, 1:130, 1:130f
Synovial joints, 1:129-131
  degenerative diseases of, 1:137-143
  fibrinous arthritis, 1:146-147
Synovial membrane, 1:130
Synovial myxoma, 1:160-162, 1:161f
Synovial pad proliferation, 1:163
Synoviocytes, 1:131
Syringomyelia, 1:278, 1:278f
Systemic arterial lesions, 2:386
Systemic cardiac responses, 3:6
Systemic granulomatous disease, 2:306
Systemic hypertension, 3:59
Systemic inflammation and neoplasia, 3:267-268
Systemic lupus erythematosus (SLE), 1:158-159, 1:605
  polymyositis and, 1:227
Systemic reactive histiocytosis (SRH), 1:729, 3:249-250, 3:249f

T

Taenia krabbei, 1:240
Taenia multiceps, 1:389
Taenia ovis, 1:239-240
Taenia saginata, 1:239, 1:389
Taenia solium, 1:239, 1:389
Taeniid tapeworms, 2:223-225
Tail gland hyperplasia, 1:549
Tail tip necrosis, 1:560
Tamm-Horsfall mucoproteins, 2:421-423, 2:456, 2:458-459
Tanapox virus, 1:616
Tannerella forsythia, 2:9
Tapeworms, 2:222-225, 2:222f
Target cell response failure, 3:274
Targetoid fibers, 1:185
Tarsal joint, spavin of, 1:142
Tartar, tooth, 2:9
Tartrate resistant acid phosphatase (TRAP), 1:18, 1:27
Taurine-deficiency retinopathy, 1:471
Taylorella equigenitalis, 3:445
T-cell receptor (TCR), 2:107-108
T-cells
  anaplastic large T-cell lymphoma (ALTCL), 3:230
  angioimmunoblastic T-cell lymphoma, 3:230
  cutaneous epitheliotropic lymphoma, 1:733-734
  cutaneous T-cell lymphoma (CTCL), 3:232-235
  enteropathy-associated T-cell lymphoma (EATL), 3:230-232, 3:231f, 3:232.e1f
  epitheliotropic T-cell tumors, 2:107-108
  extranodal T-cell lymphoma, 3:232
  graft-versus-host disease and, 1:608-609
  hepatocytotropic T-cell lymphoma (HC-TCL), 3:232
  hepatosplenic T-cell lymphoma (HS-TCL), 3:232
  immunodeficiency, 3:141
  Langerhans cells and, 1:513
  large granular lymphocytic leukemia, 3:235
  large granular lymphocytic lymphoma, 3:231, 3:231f

T-cells (Continued)
  in masticatory myositis, 1:226-227
  mature (peripheral) T-cell neoplasms, 3:228-229
  mycosis fungoides (MF), 3:232, 3:233f
  nodal T-cell lymphoma, 3:229-230
  pagetoid reticulosis (PR), 3:232-234, 3:233f
  PCR for antigen receptor rearrangements (PARR) assay, 3:215, 3:216f
  -rich B-cell lymphoma, 1:734, 3:221-222, 3:222f
  skin-homing memory, 1:515
  subcutaneous "panniculitis-like" T-cell lymphoma, 3:234, 3:234f
  t-zone lymphomas (TZL), 3:229-230, 3:230f
  unspecified, peripheral T-cell lymphomas, 3:229, 3:229f
Tears, muscle, 1:213-214
Technetium labeling, 1:30
Teeth
  abnormal wear, 2:8
  buds, 2:4
  degenerative conditions, 2:7-9
    dental attrition, 2:7-8
    infectious and inflammatory diseases, 2:9-12
    odontodystrophies, 2:8-9
    pigmentation, 2:7
  development, 2:4-12
    anomalies of, 2:6-7
    fluorosis and, 1:84-86
    mandibular osteomyelitis and, 1:103, 1:103f
    undernutrition and, 1:65
    vitamin A deficiency and, 1:82-83
  pituitary dwarfism and, 3:281
  structure of, 2:4-12
  subnormal wear, 2:8
Teladorsagia, 2:54-55
Teladorsagia circumcincta, 1:66, 2:205
Telangiectasis, 3:99
  adrenal cortex, 3:340
  liver, 2:299-300, 2:299f-300f, 2:299.e1f
Telangiectatic osteosarcoma, 1:111, 1:111f, 1:114, 1:114f
Telemark lethal bovine chondrodysplasia, 1:38-39
Telepathology, 1:3-4, 1:3f
Telogen phase, hair, 1:516
Temporal odontomas, 1:502
Temporohyoid osteoarthropathy, 1:500
Tendons, 1:130, 1:246-249. *See also* Muscle(s)
  aging and injury, 1:247
  aponeuroses and, 1:247-249
  fibromatous disorders of tendons and aponeuroses, 1:248-249
    fibrodysplasia ossificans progressiva, 1:248-249, 1:249f
    musculoaponeurotic fibromatosis, 1:248, 1:248f
  general considerations, 1:246-247
  parasitic diseases of, 1:247-248
Tension lipidosis, 2:275-276, 2:276f
Tephrosia cinerea, 2:342
Teratomas
  ovaries, 3:377, 3:378f
  testes, 3:496
Terminal acinus, 2:467

Terminal deoxynucleotide transferase-mediated dUTP nick-end labeling (TUNEL) technique, 2:280
Terminal hepatic venules, 2:260-261
Terminalia oblongata, 2:428
Terminal ileitis of lambs, 2:115
Terminal pulmonary edema, 2:386
Testes and epididymis
  abdominally retained, 3:470f
  atrophy and degeneration, 3:481-485, 3:482b, 3:482f-483f
  circulatory disturbances, 3:491-492
  epididymitis, 3:473-474, 3:474f, 3:487-491, 3:488f-489f
  equine fetal, 3:475, 3:475f
  hemorrhage, 3:492, 3:492f
  hypertrophy, 3:485
  hypoplasia, 3:478-479, 3:478f
  immune function, 3:467-468
  inflammation, 3:485-491
  mesonephric and paramesonephric structure disorders, 3:480-481, 3:480f
  neoplasms, 3:492-497
  oxidative stress and, 3:467
  size variations, 3:481-485
Test validation, 1:14
Tetanic/paretic syndromes, 1:318
Tetanus, 1:317
Tetrathyridia, 2:255
Tetrology of Fallot, 3:20, 3:20f-21f
Texas Brangus cattle, epidermolysis bullosa in, 1:535
Texel sheep, 1:41, 1:41f-42f
Thallium, 3:34-35
Thallotoxicosis, 1:568-569, 1:569f
Thebesian veins, 3:56
Theileria equi, 3:119-120
Theileria spp., 3:176-178, 3:177f
Theiler's disease, 2:313-314, 2:314f
Thelazia, 1:425
Thermal injury, 1:564-566, 1:564f-565f
Thiacetarsemide, 2:329
Thiamine deficiency, 3:34
  nervous system and, 1:312-314, 1:313f
Thin filaments, 1:167, 1:168f
Thioamides, 3:324-325
Thiocyanate, 1:306
Third-degree burns, 1:564-566
Thoracic empyema, 2:521.e1f
Thoracolumbar spinal tumor of young dogs, 1:402-403, 1:403f
Thoroughbred horses, agammaglobulinemia in, 3:139
3-methylindole (3-MI) toxicity, 2:519
Threlkeldia proceriflora, 2:425-426
Thrombi, 3:27, 3:90, 3:90f, 3:64.e1f
Thrombin, 3:55
  formation, 3:260-261
    amplification of thrombin generation, 3:261, 3:261f
    fibrin formation, 3:262-263
    inherited disorders, 3:263-264
    laboratory evaluation, 3:262-263
  functions of, 3:255, 3:256f
  receptors, 3:256
Thrombin-activatable fibrinolysis inhibitor (TAFI), 3:262, 3:262f
Thrombocytopenia, 3:258
Thrombocytopenic syndrome, 2:122
Thrombocytosis, 3:129
Thromboelastography (TEG), 3:258

Thromboembolism (TE), 3:63-66, 3:63f, 3:265
  pulmonary, 2:489, 2:489b, 2:489.e1f
Thrombophlebitis, 3:89-91
  caudal vena cava, 3:90.e1f
  intracranial, 1:300
  parasitic, 3:91-94
Thrombosis
  aortic, 1:6f
  aortic-iliac, 3:64, 3:64.e1f
  arterial, 3:63-66, 3:63f, 3:63.e1f
  balance between antithrombosis and, 3:53.e1f
  caudal vena cava, 2:298, 2:299f
  cerebrospinal arterioles, 1:299, 1:299f
  portal vein, 2:297f
  pulmonary, 2:489.e1f
  splenic, 3:171f
  testicular arteries, 3:491
Thrombotic microangiopathy, 2:421f, 2:419.e1f
Thromboxane A2 (TxA2), 3:256
Thrush, 2:14, 2:32
Thymitis, 3:148, 3:149f
Thymomas, 1:691-692, 3:153-157, 3:153f-154f, 3:153.e1f
Thymus, 3:141-158
  atrophy, 1:6f, 3:123, 3:144-147, 3:145f
  carcinomas, 3:156-157, 3:157f
  cortical lymphocytes, 3:143
  cysts, 3:151, 3:152f, 3:151.e1f
  developmental diseases, 3:144
  fibrosis, 3:147f
  germ cell tumors, 3:158
  hematomas, 3:147-148, 3:147f-148f, 3:146.e2f
  hemorrhage, 3:147-148, 3:146.e2f
  hyperplasia, 3:150-151, 3:150f
  hyperplastic and neoplastic diseases, 3:150-158
  inflammatory diseases, 3:148-150
  involution and atrophy, 1:6f, 3:123, 3:144-147, 3:145f-146f
  lymphomas, 3:157-158, 3:157f-158f, 3:237, 3:240f, 3:157.e1f
  medullary lymphocytes, 3:143
  necrosis, 3:145-146, 3:146f, 3:145.e1f
  neoplasms, 3:151-158, 3:152t
  remnants, 3:147f, 3:153f
  structure and function of normal, 3:141-144, 3:142f, 3:142.e1f
  thymomas, 1:691-692, 3:153-157, 3:153f-154f, 3:153.e1f
  with anaplasia, 3:157
Thyroglossal duct
  cysts, 2:29, 3:310, 3:314
  neoplasms, 3:332, 3:332f
Thyroid gland, 3:310-336
  biosynthesis of thyroid hormones, 3:311-312
  C cells, 3:296-297
    tumors, 3:332-336, 3:333f, 3:335f
  development, structure, and function, 3:310-314, 3:310f
  diseases, 3:314-326, 3:314f
  effects of drugs and chemicals on, 3:323-326
  function evaluation, 3:319
  hormones, 1:25t

Thyroid gland *(Continued)*
  action, 3:313-314
  release blockage, 3:325
  secretion, 3:312-313, 3:313f
  -stimulating hormone (TSH), 3:276-277
  thyroxine, 3:272
  hyperplasia, 3:320-323, 3:320f
  hypofunction, 3:315-319, 3:315f
  location, 3:293f
  neoplasms, 3:326-336
Thyroidization, 2:440f
Thyrotroph adenomas, 3:286
Thyrotropin-releasing hormone (TRH), 3:312-313
Thyroxine, 3:311
  -binding globulin, 3:312
Thysanosoma actinoides, 2:319-320, 2:319.e1f
Tibetan Mastiffs, hypertrophic neuropathy in, 1:341-342
Tibetan Terrier dogs
  canine atopic dermatitis, 1:591
  diabetes mellitus, 2:373
Ticks, 1:152, 1:684
  Babesia transmission by, 1:611, 3:117-120, 3:117f
  -borne fever, 3:178
  external ear, 1:506-507
  flaviviral encephalitides, 1:373-376
  Hepatozoon transmission by, 3:110
Tiger-stripe pattern, 2:125
Tissue-activatable fibrinolysis inhibitor (TAFI), 3:266
Tissue factor pathway, 3:260-261
  inhibitor (TFPI), 3:261, 3:266
Tissue samples. *See* Gross and histologic examinations
T lymphoblasts, 2:64
Tobramycin, 2:424
Toluidine blue stains, 1:29
Tongue abnormalities, 2:4, 2:4f
Tonsillar crypts, 2:20
Tonsillar diseases, 2:19-20
Tonsillitis, 2:13-19, 2:13f
  pigs, 2:13f
Tonsillophilus, 2:20
Tonsils, 2:20
Torsion, 2:78
  bladder, 2:451
  liver lobe, 2:268
  lung lobe, 2:485-486, 2:485f
  testis, 3:491-492
Total myeloschisis, 1:279
Toxascaris canis, 2:219
Toxascaris leonina, 2:219-220
Toxemia, pregnancy, 2:275
Toxic bone diseases, 1:84-91
  fluorosis, 1:84-86
  lead toxicity, 1:86, 1:87f
  molybdenosis, 1:84
  plant toxicities, 1:90-91
  vitamin A toxicity, 1:67, 1:86-89
  vitamin D toxicity, 1:89-90
Toxic epidermal necrolysis (TEN), 1:607-615, 1:610f
Toxic hepatic disease, 2:325-344
  agents, 2:328
Toxic insult, acute, 2:425
Toxicities, plant, 1:90-91, 1:219-220
  avocado, 3:38
  fluoroacetate, 3:38

Toxicities, plant *(Continued)*
  gousiekte, 3:38
  hepatogenous photosensitization and, 1:580
  horses, 1:91
  liver and, 2:329-344
  myocardial necrosis and, 3:34-41, 3:35f
  parathyroid suppression associated with, 3:301-302, 3:301f
  sheep, 1:90-91
Toxic lung injury, 2:518-520
Toxic metabolite-dependent idiosyncrasies, 2:327
Toxic myocardial degeneration, 3:34-35
Toxic myopathies, 1:218-220
  ionophore toxicosis, 1:219
Toxicology, 1:11
Toxicopathology, 1:3
  anoxia and nervous system, 1:305-307
  thyroid gland, 3:323-326
Toxicosis. *See* Poisoning
Toxic retinopathies, 1:471-472
Toxic shock syndrome (TSS), 1:636-637
Toxocara canis, 2:219, 2:220f, 2:442
Toxocara vitulorum, 2:220
Toxoplasma gondii, 1:451, 1:664, 2:236-238
  abortion and, 3:420-424, 3:420f-421f
  adrenal cortex and, 3:340
  central nervous system and, 1:389
  myositis, 1:237
  respiratory system and, 2:590, 2:590f, 2:590.e3f
Toy Manchester Terrier dogs, dilated cardiomyopathy in, 3:48
Trabecular adenomas, 3:326-327
Trabecular meshwork, 1:461-462, 1:462f
Trabecular trichoblastomas, 1:716
Trachea, 2:467-469, 2:482-483
  bronchus, 2:467
  collapse, 2:483f, 1:192.e1
  smoke inhalation and, 2:483, 2:483f
  transitional metaplasia, 2:501, 2:501.e1f
Tracheal puddle, 2:571-572
Trachyandra poisoning, 1:292
Traction alopecia, 1:560
Traction diverticulum, 2:31
Transepidermal elimination, 1:524
Transglutaminases, 1:513
Transitional cell carcinoma, 1:736
  nasal, 2:478-479, 2:479f
Transitional metaplasia of trachea, 2:501, 2:501.e1f
Transmissible gastroenteritis virus (TGEV), 2:113, 2:147, 2:148f
Transmissible genital papilloma, 3:508-509, 3:509f
  pig, 3:449
Transmissible mink encephalopathy (TME), 1:349
Transmissible spongiform encephalopathies (TSEs), 1:347
Transmural granulomatous enteritis, 2:97
Transphyseal blood vessels, 1:27-28, 1:28f
Transposition complexes, 3:22
Trans-synaptic degeneration, 1:254
Transverse ridge arthrosis, 1:142
Trapped neutrophil syndrome, 3:110
Trauma
  abdominal, 2:246-247, 2:246f
  acute conjunctival, 1:424

Trauma (Continued)
  articular cartilage response to, 1:131-132
  blood loss anemia and, 3:112-114
  central nervous system, 1:301-303
  chronic conjunctival, 1:424
  corneal, 1:429-432, 1:430f, 1:431t, 1:432f
    deposits secondary to, 1:434, 1:434f
  deafness caused by, 1:493-494
  head, 1:301-303
  hemolytic anemia due to, 3:125-126
  infectious arthritis and, 1:149
  ischemic damage to muscle fibers, 1:211, 1:211f
  liver, 2:285-290, 2:287f, 2:326
    hepatic artery, 2:296
    portal vein, 2:296-297
  lung, 2:500-520, 2:500f, 2:500.e1f
    toxic, 2:518-520
    ventilator-induced, 2:511
  mammae, 3:451
  muscle, 1:180-182, 1:180f, 1:213-214
  myocardial necrosis secondary to neural, 3:39
  neurons response to, 1:252-256, 1:252f
  osteochondrosis, 1:132
  peritoneal, 2:245-246
  response of gastric mucosa to, 2:46-48
  retinal, 1:473
  skin, 1:559-561
    mechanical, frictional, and traumatic, 1:559-566
    psychogenic, 1:561-562, 1:561f
  spinal cord, 1:128
  tendon, 1:247
  tracheal, 2:483
Traumatic lens rupture, 1:444
Traumatic neuroma, 1:724-725
Traumatic pericarditis, 2:39
Traumatic reticuloperitonitis of forestomachs, 2:38-39
Traumatic synovitis, 1:141
Trematodes, 1:391, 2:320-324
Trema tomentosa, 2:331
Tremor, congenital, 1:338
Tremorgenic mycotoxicoses, 1:318, 1:322
Trianthema portulacastrum, 2:425-426
Tribulosis, 2:338-340
Trichiasis, 1:421
Trichinella spiralis, 2:19
  myocarditis and, 3:44
Trichinellosis, 1:237-238
Trichobezoars, 2:38, 2:50, 2:76f
Trichobezoars, 2:50
Trichoblastomas, 1:716, 1:716f
Trichoepitheliomas, 1:714-715, 1:715f
Trichofolliculomas, 1:705
Tricholemmoma, 1:715-716
Trichomegaly, 1:421
Trichophytobezoars, 2:50
Trichophyton, 1:652, 1:652f
Trichostrongylus axei, 2:54-55, 2:208-209
Trichostrongylus colubriformis, 1:66, 2:212
Trichostrongylus rugatus, 2:212
Trichostrongylus spp., 3:112-114
Trichostrongylus vitrinus, 2:212
Trichothecene toxicoses, 1:573-574
Trichuriasis, 2:115-116
Trichuris spp., 2:220-221, 2:221f
Trichuris vulpis, 2:98
Trifolium hybridum, 2:341-342, 2:341f
Trifolium subterraneum, 2:458

Triiodothyronine, 3:272, 3:311
Trimethoprim-sulfonamides, 2:329
Trimming of fixed autopsy and biopsy specimens, 1:8-9
Tritrichomonas foetus, 2:98, 2:243, 3:423-424
Troglostrongylus acutum, 1:391
Troglostrongylus brevior, 2:591
Troglostrongylus subcrenatus, 2:591
Trombiculiasis, 1:682-683
Trueperella pyogenes, 2:19
Trueperella (Arcanobacterium) pyogenes, 1:102, 1:230, 3:507
  abortion in cattle and sheep and, 3:412
  endocarditis and, 3:30-31, 3:31f
  infectious arthritis and, 1:148
  oral cavity lesions, 2:19
  splenic abscesses, 3:183-184
True retinal dysplasia, 1:420
Trypanosoma brucei brucei, 3:124, 3:473-474
Trypanosoma cruzi, 3:44, 3:121, 3:124
Trypanosoma equinum, 3:124
Trypanosoma equiperdum, 3:121, 3:445-447, 3:508
Trypanosoma evansi, 3:124
Trypanosoma simiae, 3:124
Trypanosomatidae, 3:174
Trypanosoma vivax, 3:121f, 3:491
Trypanosomiasis, 3:121-124, 3:121f
Trypanosom suis, 3:124
T-2 toxin, 1:573
Tuberculoid granuloma, 2:549
Tuberculoid leprosy, 1:641
Tuberculoproteins, 2:548
Tuberculosis, 1:639. See also Mycobacterial infections
  bovine, 2:547-551, 2:549f
  caseous, 3:389
  dogs and cats, 2:550
  horses, 2:550
  liver and, 2:315f
  lymph nodes and, 3:204f-205f, 3:203.e1f
  mastitis, 3:456-457
  pigs, 2:550
Tubular backleak, 2:423
Tubular basement membranes, 2:422-423
Tubular cells, degeneration and swelling of, 2:421-422
Tubular diseases, 2:421-431
  acute tubular injury (ATI), 2:421-428
    ischemic tubular necrosis, 2:423f
    with karyomegaly, 2:428f
      epithelial injury, 2:428.e3f
    myoglobin-induced acute tubular injury, 2:423f
    nephrotoxic, 2:423
    amaranthus, 2:427
    aminoglycosides, 2:424
    amphotericin B, 2:424-425
    chelation of calcium, 2:426
    cyanuric acid, 2:426-427
    degeneration and swelling, 2:421-422
    ethylene glycol, 2:425
    grapes and raisins, 2:428
    marked acute tubular necrosis, 2:428.e1f
    melamine acid, 2:426-427
    mycotoxins, 2:427
    nephrotoxic in domestic animals, 2:424b
    oxalate poisoning, 2:425-426
    plant toxicoses, 2:427-428
    primary renal glucosuria, 2:429
    specific tubular dysfunctions, 2:428-429
    sulfonamides, 2:424
    tetracyclines, 2:424

Tubular epithelial injury, acute, 2:428.e3f, 2:421.e2f
Tubular genitalia development, 3:360-361, 3:361f
Tubular injury, acute, 2:427f-428f, 2:433f
Tubular necrosis, acute, 2:398-399
  caused by ethylene glycol intoxication, 2:426f, 2:425.e2f
Tubular protein casts, 2:407
Tubules, 2:383
Tubule segment, structure, 2:381
Tubuloglomerular feedback, 2:379
Tubulointerstitial diseases, 2:431-443
  chronic interstitial nephritis, 2:431
  Encephalitozoon cuniculi, 2:431
  histologic features, 2:431
  Leptospira interrogans, 2:431
  nonsuppurative interstitial nephritis, 2:431-432
Tubulointerstitial nephritis, chronic, 2:433.e1f
Tubulointerstitium, from proteinuric dog, 2:407f
Tubulorrhectic ATI, 2:422-423
Tularemia, 3:184-186, 3:185f
Tumoral calcinosis, 1:127, 1:127f
Tumor-like proliferative lesions, 2:101t
Tumor necrosis factor-α, 2:548-549
Tumors, 2:447-448. See also Lymphomas; Metastases, tumor; Non-neoplastic lesions
  adrenal medullary, 3:349-352
  benign cortical fibromas, 2:447
  bone, 1:107-127
    cartilage-forming, 1:116-121
    fibrous, 1:121-122, 1:121f
    forming, 1:109-116, 1:109f
    giant cell, 1:122
    secondary, 1:124-125
    vascular, 1:122
  brain, 1:296f
  carcinoma, 2:447
  cholangiocellular, 2:348-349, 2:348f
  dental tissue, 2:22-25
  endocrine gland, 3:271-272
  epithelial
    pulmonary, 2:495
    skin, 1:703
    thymic, 3:152-153
  granular cell, 1:245, 2:27
    heart, 3:52-53
    laryngeal, 2:482
    pulmonary, 2:498
  hemangioma, 2:447
  hepatocellular, 2:345-348, 2:346f
  hypersecretion of hormones by, 3:274
  interstitial cell, 2:447
  intestinal stromal tumors, 2:110-111
    gastrointestinal, 2:110
    leiomyoma, 2:110
    leiomyosarcoma, 2:110
  -like lesions
    of bones, 1:125-127
    of joints, 1:159-163
  liver mesodermal, 2:349-351, 2:350f
  lymphoma, 2:447
  male genital system
    germ cell, 3:495-496, 3:495f
    interstitial testicular, 3:493, 3:493f
    Sertoli cell, 3:494-495, 3:494f
    sex cord-gonadal stromal, 3:492-495

INDEX

Tumors *(Continued)*
  mast cell, 2:27
  mesenchymal, 2:44
  metastatic, 2:447
  nasomaxillary, 2:480, 2:560, 2:560f
  neuroendocrine, 2:497-498
  pedicles of, 2:76-77
  pituitary gland, 3:281-289, 3:289f
  plasmacytomas, 2:27-28
  primary mesenchymal, 2:447
  pulmonary adenocarcinoma, 2:447
  renal oncocytomas, 2:447
  skin, 1:703, 1:705
    adnexal differentiation, 1:714-720
    epidermis, 1:706-714
    mast cell, 1:730-733
    melanocytic, 1:720-722, 1:720f
    metastasis to, 1:736
    sebaceous gland, 1:717-718, 1:717f
    spindle cell, 1:722-726
    sweat gland, 1:718-720
    vascular, 1:726-728
  stomach and intestine, 2:100-111, 2:101t
  thymic epithelial, 3:152-153
  thyroid, 3:327-329
  urothelial papilloma, 2:447
Tumor(s)
  embryonal, 1:401-403
  mengingeal, 1:396-398
  neuroepithelial tissue, 1:398-403
  sellar region, 1:403-404
Tumor(s), peritoneal, 2:256-257
Tunica vaginalis, indirect inguinal hernia, 2:80
Turning sickness, 3:178, 3:178f
25- hydroxycholecalciferol-1-α-hydroxylase, 3:295
2,8-DHA urolithiasis, 2:430.e1
2,8-dihydroxyadenine, 2:272
Tylecodon toxicosis, 1:345
Tympanic cavities, 1:495
  otitis media, 1:496-498
Tympanic cavity inflammation. *See* Otitis media
Tympanic membrane, 1:491, 1:495
Tympanic ring, 1:495, 1:495.e2f
Tympanokeratoma, 1:499, 1:499f
Type AB thymomas, 3:156, 3:156f
Type 2A histochemical fiber type, 1:169
Type A thymomas, 3:154, 3:154f
Type 2B histochemical fiber type, 1:169
Type B2 thymomas, 3:155-156, 3:155f-156f
Type B3 thymomas, 3:156, 3:156f
Type 1 histochemical fiber type, 1:169, 1:170f
Type I collagen, 1:19
Type II pneumocytes, 2:470
Type I pneumocytes, 2:469-470
Type 2X histochemical fiber type, 1:169
Typhlitis, 2:97
Typhlocolitis, 2:97-98, 2:98f
  horses, 2:99-100
  pigs, 2:100
Tyrosine, 3:311
Tyzzer's disease, 2:317, 2:317f-318f
T-zone lymphomas (TZL), 3:229-230, 3:230f

U

Uasin Gishu disease, 1:621
Ulcerating fibrosarcoma, 2:35f

Ulceration, 2:385f
  BVDV, 2:123-124, 2:124f
  corneal, 1:429-432, 1:430f, 1:431t, 1:432f
  decubitus, 1:559
  gastroduodenal, 2:55-60
  indolent, 1:694, 1:694f
  laryngeal, 2:481
  mucosal protective mechanisms, 2:55
  of squamous mucosa, 2:59f
Ulcerative balanitis, 3:508
Ulcerative colitis, 2:86f
Ulcerative dermatosis of sheep, 1:618
Ulcerative duodenitis, 2:59
Ulcerative esophagitis, 2:31-32
Ulcerative keratitis, 1:436
Ulcerative lymphangitis, 3:97
Ulcerative mural endocarditis, 3:32, 3:33f
Ulcerative posthitis
  bulls, 3:507
  of wethers, 3:508
Ulcerative stomatitis, chronic, 2:16
Ulegyria, 1:268
Ulex europaeus agglutinin I, 2:445
Ulmaceae, 2:331
Ultimobranchial body, 3:296
Ultimobranchial gland, 3:296
Ultimobranchial tumors of thyroid, 3:334-336
Ultrastructure, muscle, 1:167
Umbilical hernia, 2:80
Uncinaria stenocephala, 2:214
Undifferentiated carcinomas, 2:463
  nasal, 2:478-479
Undifferentiated diarrhea of neonatal animals, 2:111, 2:112f
Undifferentiated neonatal diarrhea, 2:112f
Undifferentiated pleomorphic sarcomas, 1:725-726
Undifferentiated thyroid carcinomas, 3:330-331
Unexpected death, causes of, 1:4t
Unfolded protein response (UPR), 2:280
Unilateral agenesis of adrenal gland, 3:338
Unilateral papular dermatosis, 1:695
Unilateral renal hypoplasia, 2:392f
Unipyramidal, 2:378
Unspecified, peripheral T-cell lymphomas (PTCL), 3:229, 3:229f
Upper airway, 2:466-467, 2:466f
  disease, 2:500-504, 2:500.e1f
Upper respiratory tract, 2:473
  immunology, 2:474
Urate calculi, 2:385f
Ureaplasma diversum, 1:154, 2:554
  abortion and, 3:411-412, 3:412f
Ureaplasma spp., 3:401
Urea-splitting organisms, 2:457
Urea toxicity, 2:35-36
Uremia, 2:16-17, 2:384-388, 3:60, 3:260
  diffuse tissue mineralization, pathogenesis of, 2:387
  nonrenal lesions of, 2:385
  renal lesions of, 2:387
Uremic acidosis, 2:384
Uremic encephalopathy, 2:387
Uremic gastritis, 2:51
Uremic pneumonitis, 2:386, 2:387.e1f
Uremic pneumonopathy, 2:494-495, 2:494f
Uremic toxins, 2:385
Ureteral duplication, 2:449.e2f
Ureterocele, 2:450

Ureters
  anomalies, 2:449-450
  displacements, 2:451
  duplication of, 2:392
Urethra, 2:448
Urethral atresia, 2:450
Urethral caruncles, 2:452
Urethral hypoplasia, 2:450
Urethral plugs, 2:452
Urethrorectal, 2:450
Urinary bladder, 2:448
  duplication, 2:450
Urinary hydroxyproline, pyridinoline (PYD), 1:27
Urinary system
  calculi, 2:453t
  defenses, 2:439
  infections. *See* Urinary tract infection (UTI)
  kidneys. *See* Kidney(s)
  neoplasms, 2:462
  obstruction, 2:399
  pH, 2:452-453
  urea excretion, 2:73
Urinary tract, lower, 2:448-464
  anomalies of, 2:449-452
    acquired anatomic variations, 2:451-452
    ectopic ureter, 2:450
    renal dysplasia in pig, 2:449.e2f
    ureteral duplication in pig, 2:449.e2f
    ureters, 2:449-450
    urethra, 2:450-451
    urinary bladder, 2:450
  circulatory disturbances, 2:452
  clover stones, 2:458
  cystine calculi, 2:458
  cystitis, 2:459-461
  enzootic hematuria, 2:461-462
  inflammation of, 2:458-462
    mycoplasmas, 2:459
  neoplasms of, 2:462-464
    epithelial tumors, 2:462-463
    mesenchymal tumors, 2:463-464
  obstructive urolithiasis, 2:455f
  oxalate calculi, 2:456-457
  oxalate uroliths, in cats, 2:457
  ruminants, 2:456
  silica calculi, 2:455
  staghorn calculus in renal pelvis of dog, 2:454f
  struvite calculi, 2:455-456
  types of calculi, 2:458
  urate calculi, 2:457
  ureters, urinary bladder, and urethra, 2:448
  uric acid, 2:457
  urinary calculi, composition and importance, 2:453t
  urinary pH and reduced water intake, 2:452-453
  urolithiasis, 2:452-458
    dog, 2:454f
  urothelium, 2:448-449
  xanthine calculi, 2:457-458
Urinary tract infection (UTI), 2:458-459
  predisposition, 2:458-459
  risk factors, 2:458-459
Urine
  osmolality, 2:459
  in peritoneal cavity, 2:452
  protein to urine creatinine (UPC), 2:401
  supersaturation, 2:452-453

Uriniferous pseudocyst, 2:451
Urolithiasis, 2:454f
Urolith initiation
   crystallization-inhibition theory, 2:453
   matrix-nucleation theory, 2:453
Uroperitoneum, 2:247
Uroplakins, 2:462.e1
Urothelial cell carcinomas, 2:447f, 2:462-463, 2:462f, 2:447.e1f
   metastasize, 2:462-463
Urothelial papilloma, 2:447
Urothelium, 2:448
Urticaria, 1:594
Uterine (fallopian) tubes pathology, 3:379-380
Uterus
   abscess, 3:390
   accumulation of secretory or inflammatory exudates, 3:386-387
   carcinoma, 3:449-450, 3:450f
   cysts arising from, 3:366-367
   inflammatory diseases of, 3:387-393
   mucometra, 3:374, 3:374f
   neoplasia, 3:449-450, 3:450f
   pathology, 3:380-382, 3:380f, 3:393-398
   postpartum, 3:440-441
   rupture, 3:381, 3:381f
UVA/UVB radiation. *See* Solar radiation
Uvea, 1:445-465
   degenerations, 1:445-446
   glaucoma, 1:459-465
   melanocytoma, 1:482-483, 1:483f
   uveitis, 1:446-459
      bacterial endophthalmitis, 1:449
      significance of, 1:447-448, 1:447f-448f
Uveitis, 1:446-459
   bacterial endophthalmitis, 1:449
   bovine malignant catarrhal fever-associated, 1:453
   canine adenovirus I, 1:452-453
   equine recurrent ophthalmitis, 1:455-456
   feline infectious peritonitis-associated, 1:453, 1:453f
   histologic classification, 1:448-449
   idiopathic immune-mediated, 1:453-455, 1:454f
   idiopathic lymphocytic, in dogs, 1:456
   idiopathic lymphonodular, of cats, 1:456
   lens-induced, 1:453-454, 1:457-459
   mycotic endophthalmitis, 1:449-451
   protozoal endophthalmitis, 1:451
   significance of, 1:447-448, 1:447f-448f
   uveodermatologic syndrome, 1:453-454, 1:456-457, 1:457f
   viral endophthalmitis, 1:452
Uveodermatologic syndrome, 1:453-454, 1:456-457, 1:457f

V

Vaccinal fibrosarcomas, 1:725
Vaccine administration and injection-site reactions, 1:560
Vaccine-induced polyarthritis, 1:158
Vaccinia virus, 1:616, 1:620
Vacuolar degeneration, 1:185, 1:185f, 1:254, 1:254f, 1:522
Vacuolation, 2:272-273, 2:272f
Vagal indigestion, diagnosis of, 2:39
Vagal lesions, 2:39
Vagina
   anomalies, 3:369-370, 3:370f
   inflammatory diseases, 3:443
   pathology of, 3:442-447, 3:442f

Vaginal eventration, 2:78
Vaginal stenosis, 3:369, 3:370f
Vaginal tunics, 3:473-474, 3:473f-474f
Vaginitis, necrotic, 3:445, 3:445f-446f
Vagus indigestion, 2:39
Valgus deformity, 1:31
Valvular cysts, 3:30
Valvular endocarditis, 3:30-31, 3:31.e1f
Vanishing bone disease, 1:54
Varicocele, 3:497-498, 3:498f
Varicose tumor of the scrotum, 3:99
Variola virus, 1:616
Varus deformity, 1:31
Vascular anomalies
   heart, 3:23-24, 3:23f
   liver, 2:266-268
Vascular endothelial growth factor (VEGF) receptors, 2:421
Vascular-epithelial structure, 2:379-380
Vascular hamartomas of ovary, 3:366, 3:378-379
Vascular malformation, 3:99
Vascular neoplasia, 3:98-101
Vascular nevus, 1:727
Vascular occlusive syndrome, 1:212, 1:212f
Vascular ring anomalies, 2:33
Vascular smooth muscle cells, 3:55-56
Vascular system
   arteries, 3:56-88
   congenital abnormalities, 3:14-24
   dermal, 1:514-515
   diseases, 3:54-101
   hemodynamic effects of valvular abnormalities, 3:4.e1f
   leakage, 1:298f
   liver, 2:266-268, 2:296-300
   lungs, 2:467-468, 2:468f
   neoplasms, 3:98-101
   retina, 1:466
   spleen, 3:161, 3:161f
   tumors
      bone, 1:122
      dogs, 1:122
      oral cavity, 2:28
      skin, 1:726-728
   veins, 3:88-94
Vasculitis, 1:525-526, 1:526f, 1:607, 3:67-88, 3:68b, 3:68.e1f
   cerebrospinal, 1:298-299, 1:298f-299f
   chronic fibrosing, 3:71, 3:71f
   cutaneous, 1:611-612, 1:611f
   lymphocytic, 1:526, 1:611
   male genital system, 3:498
   necrotizing, 1:200, 1:200f, 3:69, 3:69f
   neutrophilic, 1:526, 1:611
   nodular eosinophilic, 1:612
   pastern leukocytoclastic, 1:612
   photoactivated, 1:580
   pulmonary, 2:494, 2:494.e2f
   rabies vaccine-induced, 1:612-613, 1:613f
Vasoactive intestinal polypeptide, 2:368
Vasogenic edema, 1:294, 1:295f
Vasopressin. *See* Antidiuretic hormone (ADH)
Veins, 3:54, 3:88-94
   drainage, 2:18
   hepatic, 2:260
   infarction, 2:82f
   inflammation. *See* Phlebitis
   invasion by neoplasms, 3:89, 3:89f
   obstruction of cerebrospinal, 1:300
   pulmonary, 2:467-468, 2:468f

Vena caval syndrome, 3:85
Venom, 1:568
Venous drainage, 2:18
Venous infarction, 2:82f
Ventilator-induced lung injury, 2:511
Ventral hernia of abdominal wall, 2:80
Ventricles, heart, 3:2
   restricted filling, 3:6
   wall thickness, 3:5
Ventricular pre-excitation, 3:51
Ventricular septal defect (VSD), 3:17, 3:17f-18f
Veratrum californicum, 1:90, 1:269-270, 2:3
   cleft palate and, 2:3
Verminous arteritis, 3:83-88
Verminous endoarteritis, 2:84
Verminous granulomas, 3:498
Vernonia rubricaulis, 2:331
Verotoxin-producing *E. coli* (VTEC), 2:162
Verrucous sarcoids, 1:708, 1:709f
Vertebrae
   congenital abnormalities, 1:57
   diskospondylitis, 1:156, 1:156f
   osteomyelitis, 1:101-102, 1:102f
   subluxations, 1:303
Very low-density lipoproteins (VLDLs), 2:273, 2:276-277
Vesicle, 1:524
Vesicoureteral reflux, 2:439
Vesicular adenitis, 3:499-500, 3:499f
Vesicular cutaneous lupus erythematosus, 1:607
Vesicular exanthema (VE), of swine, 2:120-121
Vesicular exanthema of swine virus (VESV), 2:121
Vesicular stomatitis (VS), 2:14-15, 2:117-158, 2:120f
Vestibular membrane, 1:489
Vestibular window, 1:489
Vestibulocochlear nerve, 1:489-491
Vetch toxicosis, 1:574
Vicia villosa, 3:36
Villaneuva's bone stain, 1:29
Villus, 1:524
Villus atrophy, 2:67-68, 2:96
Villus fusion, 2:146
Vimentin, 1:261
Viral agents, 2:57
Viral antigen, 2:22
Viral arthritis, 1:154
Viral endophthalmitis, 1:452
Viral inclusion bodies, 1:255
Viral infections
   abortion and stillbirth due to, 3:398, 3:399b
   alimentary tract, 2:117-158
   bone, 1:104-105
   central nervous system and, 1:365-385
   developmental defects of central nervous system and, 1:280-284
   liver, 2:309-325
      lobular necrosis and, 2:282
   lymphomagenesis and, 3:235
   myocarditis and, 3:42, 3:43f
   parvo-, 1:628
   pregnant uterus, 3:424-440
   respiratory system, 2:523-531
      cats, 2:587-589
      cattle, 2:537-542

Viral infections *(Continued)*
　　dogs, 2:574-577
　　horses, 2:567-569
　　sheep and goats, 2:557-562
　skin, 1:615-628
　thymic atrophy and, 3:145
Viral vasculitides, 3:71-80
Virology, 1:10-11
Virtual microscopy, 1:3-4, 1:3f
Virulent footrot (VFR), 1:644
Virus-induced fibrosarcomas, 1:725
Virus titers, 2:121
Visceral larva migrans, 1:452
Visceral leishmaniasis, 3:174-175
Visna-maedi virus (VISNA), 1:378-380
Vitamin A
　deficiency, 1:82, 1:581-582, 1:582f, 2:8, 2:29-30
　　hydrocephalus, 1:271, 1:271f
　　odontodystrophies and, 2:8
　　pigs, 1:82-83
　　salivary gland inflammation, 2:29-30
　excess, 1:89
　function, 1:82
　-responsive dermatosis, 1:552
　toxicity, 1:86-89
　　cats, 1:88, 1:88f
　　cattle, 1:88
　　horses, 1:89
　　osteoporosis and, 1:67, 1:87
　　pigs, 1:88
Vitamin B deficiency, 1:582
Vitamin C
　deficiency, 1:83, 1:582-583
　　cataract and, 1:443
　　scurvy and, 1:83, 1:83f
　function, 1:83
Vitamin D
　cholecalciferol, 3:295-296
　deficiency, 1:61
　　cats, 1:68
　　cattle, 1:68
　　dogs, 1:68
　　pigs, 1:68
　　rickets and, 1:68
　-dependent rickets type I, 1:69-70
　metabolism disorders. *See* Rickets
　parathyroid hormone and, 1:62
　parathyroid suppression associated with intoxication of, 3:301-302, 3:301f
　poisoning, 3:61
　-resistant rickets, 1:70
　toxicity, 1:89-90
　　cats, 1:89
　transport, 1:62
Vitamin E
　deficiency, 1:583, 2:86-87
　nutritional myopathy, 1:214-215, 1:217
Vitamin K, 1:19
　antagonism, 3:264
　-dependent γ-glutamyl carboxylase deficiency, 3:264
Vitamins. *See also* specific vitamins
　imbalances, 1:82-84
　lipid malabsorption, 2:90
Vitiligo, 1:555, 1:556f, 1:556.e1f
Vizsla dogs
　afibrinogenemia, 3:265
　sebaceous adenitis, 1:551

Vogt-Koyanagi-Harada syndrome, 1:453-454, 1:456-457, 1:457f, 1:613
Volvulus, 2:83
　abomasal, 2:49-50, 2:50f
　gastric, 2:49, 2:49f
　splenic, 3:167, 3:167f
Von Hippel-Lindau *(VHL)* gene, 2:444-445
Von Kossa stains, 1:29
Von Meyenburg complex, 2:264, 2:265f
Von Willebrand disease (vWD), 3:258-259
Von Willebrand factor (vWF), 3:256
Vulva, 3:442-447
　fibropapilloma, 3:449
　inflammatory diseases, 3:443
　swelling, 3:442-443
Vulvitis
　granular, 3:443, 3:443f
　necrotic, 3:445, 3:445f-446f
Vulvovaginitis, infectious pustular, 3:443-445, 3:444f

W

Waardenburg syndrome, 1:555-556
Wallerian degeneration, 1:256-257, 1:257f
Warbles, 1:668-669
Warts. *See* Papillomas
Warty dyskeratomas, 1:705
Water
　diuresis, 2:381
　salinity, 1:314
　urolithiasis and, 2:454f
Waterhouse-Friderichsen syndrome, 3:65
"Watery mouth", 2:167
Wattles, 1:532
Wave mouth, 2:8
Weaner colitis of sheep, 2:180-181
Wedelia glauca, 2:331
Weighting of competing etiologies, cut-offs, explanation, 1:12-13
Weimaraner dogs
　canine hypomyelinogenesis, 1:337-338
　follicular dysplasia, 1:540-541
　hydromyelia, 1:278
　hyperestrogenism, 1:589
　malignant oral tumors, 2:21
　subvalvular aortic stenosis, 3:20
　syringomyelia, 1:278, 1:278f
　T-cell immunodeficiency, 3:141
Weisses Alpenschaf sheep, epidermolysis bullosa in, 1:535
Werdnig-Hoffman disease, 1:331
Wesselsbron virus (WESSV), 1:281, 2:312, 2:313f, 3:428-429
West Highland White Terrier dogs
　canine atopic dermatitis, 1:591
　chronic hepatitis, 2:304
　cochleosaccular degeneration, 1:492
　globoid cell leukodystrophy, 1:339
　hyperplastic dermatosis, 1:553
　interstitial fibrosis, 2:514-515, 2:515f
　keratoconjunctivitis sicca in, 1:436
　polycystic kidney and liver disease, 2:265
　seborrhea, 1:548
　sick sinus syndrome, 3:51
　spongy enceophalomyelopathies, 1:346
West Nile virus, 1:281
　encephalomyelitis, 1:374-375, 1:375f
Wheal, 1:524

Whippet dogs
　color dilution alopecia, 1:539-540
　muscle hypertrophy, 1:191, 1:191f
　myxomatous valvular degeneration, 3:27
Whipworms, 2:220-221, 2:221f
White pulp, spleen, 3:161-162
White-spotted kidneys, 2:431f, 2:436, 2:431.e1f
White-tailed deer, osteopetrosis in, 1:52
Whorled muscle fibers, 1:185, 1:185f
WHO system of classification of hematopoietic neoplasms, 3:217, 3:217t
Wild black cherry, 1:90
Wildebeest-associated MCF, 2:132
Wild lupins, 1:90
Winchester syndrome, 1:54
Winter dysentery, 2:149, 2:150f
Wohlfahrtia magnifica, 1:668
Wolff's law, 1:30
Wolfhound dogs, gastric volvulus in, 2:49
Wooly haircoat and cardiomyopathy, 3:50
Worms. *See* Helminthic infections; Nematodes
Woven bone, 1:21, 1:21f, 1:78-79, 1:79f, 1:108f

X

Xanthine calculi, 2:457
Xanthium pungens, 2:331
Xanthomas, 1:641
　cutaneous, 1:700
Xanthosis, 3:34
Xenobiotics, 3:324-326, 3:326f
　liver and, 2:325
Xipapillomavirus, 2:22
Xiphoid, 2:39
X-linked hypohidrotic ectodermal dysplasia (XHED), 1:539, 1:539.e1f
X-linked ichthyosis, 1:530
X-linked myotubular myopathy in Labrador Retrievers, 1:197
X-linked severe combined immunodeficiency, 3:140
Xnathium pungens, 2:329-330
XXY chromosomes, 3:469
XY disorders of sexual development, 3:365, 3:365f
Xylitol, 2:329

Y

Yaba monkey tumor virus, 1:616
Yatapoxvirus, 1:616
Y chromosome, 3:365, 3:469
Yeast bodies
　Blastomyces dermatitidis, 1:104, 1:449, 2:580, 3:491
　Coccidioides immitis, 1:449-450, 2:583-584, 2:584f
Yellow fat disease. *See* Steatitis
Yersinia enterocolitica, 2:176, 3:210
Yersinia pestis, 3:210, 3:210f
Yersinia pseudotuberculosis, 2:176, 2:177f, 3:209-210, 3:209f
　liver and, 2:314-315
Yersinia spp. and abortion, 3:401, 3:413-414, 3:413f
Yersiniosis, 2:176-177
Yorkshire Terrier dogs
　color dilution alopecia, 1:539-540
　pancreatic necrosis, 2:358

Yorkshire Terrier dogs *(Continued)*
   primary portal vein hypoplasia, 2:267-268
   rabies vaccine-induced vasculitis and alopecia, *1*:612, *1*:613f
   spongy encephalomyelopathies, *1*:346-347
Yucatan minipigs, *1*:604

Z

Zalophus californianus, 2:121
Z bands, *1*:167
   in muscular dystrophy, *1*:193-194, *1*:194f
Zenker's degeneration, *1*:181-182
Zenker's fixative, *1*:408, *1*:449, 3:474-475
Zinc
   chemical abomasitis and, 2:52
   deficiency, *1*:583-585, *1*:584f
      dogs, *1*:585-586, *1*:585f
      hereditary, *1*:532-533
   toxicity and pancreas, 2:356, 2:357f
Z-line streaming, *1*:190, *1*:193-194, *1*:194f
Zollinger-Ellison syndrome, 2:55-56, 2:375
Zona fasciculata, 3:336
Zona glomerulosa, 3:336
   hyperplasia, 3:343, 3:344f
Zona reticularis, 3:336-337
Zone of degeneration, growth plate, *1*:23
Zonisamide, 2:329
Zoophilic dermatophytes, *1*:649
Zoospores, *1*:632, 2:203
Zoo ungulates, *1*:214-215
Zygomycetes, *1*:659, 2:42, 2:324, 2:324f, 2:573
Zygomycosis, *1*:659-660